Drug Information Handbook  Physician Assistants

2nd Edition **2000-2001**

Michael J. Rudzinski, RPA-C, RPh
J. Fred Bennes, RPA, RPh

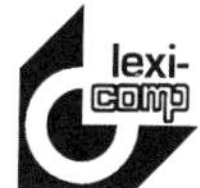

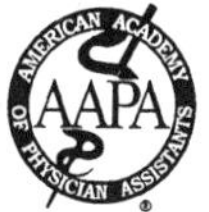

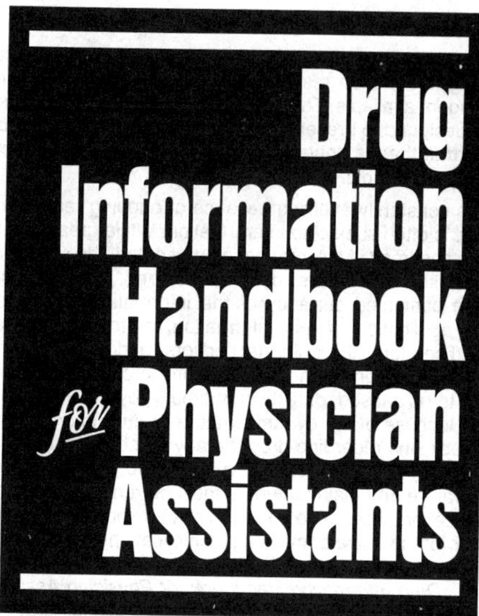

2nd Edition 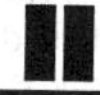 **2000-2001**

Edited by:

Michael J. Rudzinski, RPA-C, RPh
Physician Assistant
Promedicus Health Group
Buffalo, New York

J. Fred Bennes, RPA, RPh
Clinical Professor of Pharmacy
University of Buffalo School of Pharmacy
Director of Quality and Resource Management
Promedicus Health Group
Buffalo, New York

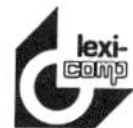

LEXI-COMP, INC
Hudson (Cleveland)

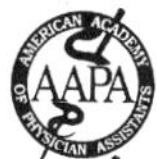

NOTICE

This handbook is intended to serve the user as a handy quick reference and not as a complete drug information resource. It does not include information on every therapeutic agent available. The publication covers commonly used drugs and is specifically designed to present certain important aspects of drug data in a more concise format than is generally found in medical literature or product material supplied by manufacturers.

Drug information is constantly evolving because of ongoing research and clinical experience and is often subject to interpretation. While great care has been taken to ensure the accuracy of the information presented, the reader is advised that the authors, editors, reviewers, contributors, and publishers cannot be responsible for the continued currency of the information or for any errors, omissions, or the application of this information, or for any consequences arising therefrom. Therefore, the author(s), editors, and/or the publisher shall have no liability to any person or entity with regard to claims, loss, or damage caused, or alleged to be caused, directly or indirectly, by the use of information contained herein. Because of the dynamic nature of drug information, readers are advised that decisions regarding drug therapy must be based on the independent judgment of the clinician, changing information about a drug (eg, as reflected in the literature and manufacturer's most current product information), and changing medical practices. The editors are not responsible for any inaccuracy of quotation or for any false or misleading implication that may arise due to the text or formulas as used or due to the quotation of revisions no longer official. Further, the *Drug Information Handbook for Physician Assistants* is not offered as a guide to dosing. The reader, herewith, is advised that information shown under the heading **Usual Dosage** is provided only as an indication of the amount of the drug typically given or taken during therapy. Actual dosing amount for any specific drug should be based on an in-depth evaluation of the individual patient's therapy requirement and strong consideration given to such issues as contraindications, warnings, precautions, adverse reactions, along with the interaction of other drugs. The manufacturers most current product information or other standard recognized references should always be consulted for such detailed information prior to drug use.

The editors and contributors have written this book in their private capacities. No official support or endorsement by any federal agency or pharmaceutical company is intended or inferred.

If you have any suggestions or questions regarding any information presented in this handbook, please contact our drug information pharmacist at

1-877-837-LEXI (5394)

This manual was produced using the FormuLex™ Program – a complete publishing service of Lexi-Comp Inc.

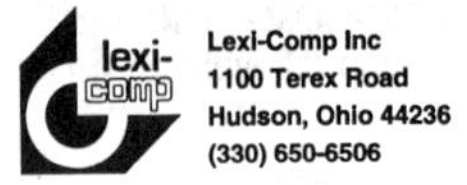

ISBN 1-930598-31-9

TABLE OF CONTENTS

ABOUT THE EDITORS

Michael J. Rudzinski, RPA-C, RPh

Michael (Mike) Rudzinski received his Bachelor's of Science degree in Pharmacy from the State University of New York at Buffalo in 1975 and his Bachelor's of Science degree as a Physician Assistant from the University of Oklahoma in 1979.

Mike started working in his local neighborhood pharmacy in 1967, and has been active in pharmacy ever since. He has practiced as a clinical pharmacist in hospital and retail settings for 25 years, and is currently practicing in a community pharmacy. In addition to his pharmacy work, Mike has been practicing as a physician assistant in a staff model HMO for 19 years, in primary care, and orthopedic medicine. He is currently employed with Promedicus Health Group.

Mike gives presentations yearly at the national American Academy of Physician Assistants Annual PA Conference and serves on the editorial board for the *Clinician Reviews Journal.* He is a clinical preceptor for D'Youville College's physician assistant program, Daemen College's physician assistant program, and the State University of New York at Buffalo Schools of Pharmacy, Nurse Practitioners, and Medicine. He also serves as adjunct faculty for the D'Youville College PA program. He is a member of the American Academy of Physician Assistant (AAPA), the New York State Society of Physician Assistants (NYSSPA), and the Pharmacist Society of the State of New York (PSSNY). Mike would also like to acknowledge all the help and guidance he has received throughout his career from family, friends, and colleagues.

J. Fred Bennes, RPA, RPh

Fred Bennes received a Bachelor of Science in Pharmacy (1973) from the University of North Carolina, Chapel Hill and a Physician Associate Certificate (1974) from Duke University. Since then he has practiced as a primary care physician assistant in rural, inner city, and suburban settings both in North Carolina and New York. Additionally, Fred has been on the faculty of the State University of New York at Buffalo for the Schools of Pharmacy, Graduate Nursing, and Medicine. Besides clinical practice and didactic teaching, he has developed and directed a seven pharmacy practice at a staff model HMO and served as the Practice Administrator for a 85-physician medical group.

Currently, Fred is Clinical Professor of Pharmacy at the University of Buffalo School and Pharmacy and the Director of Quality and Resource Management at Promedicus Health Group, a large multispecialty group practice with designs on the innovative practice of healthcare. Fred was an early supporter of certification for Physician Assistants, being so certified from 1976-1998 when he retired from active practice to pursue teaching and administrative challenges.

ABOUT THE AUTHORS

Charles F. Lacy, PharmD, FCSHP

Dr Lacy received his doctorate from the University of Southern California School of Pharmacy. With over 18 years of clinical experience at one of the nation's largest teaching hospitals, he has developed a reputation as an acknowledged expert in drug information and critical care drug therapy.

In his current capacity as Coordinator of Clinical Services for the Department of Pharmacy at Cedar-Sinai Health System in Los Angeles, Dr Lacy plays an active role in the education and training of the medical, pharmacy, and nursing staff. He manages the Drug Information Center, the development of medical center clinical pathways, the pharmacists' clinical certification and staff development program, the department's continuing education program, and the pharmacy residency clinical assessment, training, and longitudinal experience program. He also supervises the activities of clinical specialists in medication use evaluation, antibiotic use review, infection control, investigational drug protocols, transplant pharmacy services, the Adverse Drug Reaction Monitoring Program, the Medical Center's Medication Error Detection and Remedy Program, and directs the maintenance of the Medical Center Formulary Program, is editor of the Medical Center's *Drug Formulary Handbook*, and associate editor of the drug information newsletter *Prescription*.

Presently, Dr Lacy holds teaching affiliations with the University of Southern California School of Pharmacy, the University of California at San Francisco School of Pharmacy, the University of the Pacific School of Pharmacy, Western University of Health Sciences School of Pharmacy, the Nevada School of Pharmacy in Las Vegas, and the University of Alberta at Edmonton, School of Pharmacy and Health Sciences.

Dr Lacy is an active member of numerous professional associations including the American Society of Health-System Pharmacists (ASHP), the California Society of Hospital Pharmacists (CSHP), the American Society of Consultant Pharmacists (ASCP), American Pharmaceutical Association (APhA), and the American College of Clinical Pharmacy (ACCP).

Lora L. Armstrong, RPh, PharmD, BCPS

Dr Armstrong received her bachelor's degree in pharmacy from Ferris State University and her Doctor of Pharmacy degree from Midwestern University. Dr Armstrong is a Board Certified Pharmacotherapy Specialist (BCPS).

In her current position, Dr Armstrong serves as a clinical pharmacist in Clinical Services at Caremark RX, Inc, Prescription Services Division. Caremark is a prescription benefit management company (PBM). She is responsible for the development and enhancement of clinical management programs, physician and staff education, and formulary management. She participates in the development and evaluation of clinical programs which include Formulary Management, Concurrent Interventions, Retrospective Case Management, Physician Profiling, and Utilization Review Pharmacy Management. Dr Armstrong also provides support for Caremark's National Pharmacy and Therapeutics Committee activities.

Prior to joining Caremark RX, Dr Armstrong served as the Director of Drug Information Services at the University of Chicago Hospitals. She obtained 17 years of experience in a variety of clinical settings including critical care, hematology, oncology, infectious diseases, and clinical pharmacokinetics. Dr Armstrong played an active role in the education and training of medical, pharmacy, and nursing staff. She coordinated the Drug Information Center, the medical center's Adverse Drug Reaction Monitoring Program, and the continuing Education Program for pharmacists. She also maintained the hospital's strict formulary program and was the editor of the University of Chicago Hospitals' *Formulary of Accepted Drugs* and the drug information center's monthly newsletter *Topics in Drug Therapy*.

Dr Armstrong is an active member of the Academy of Managed Care Pharmacy (AMCP), the American Society of Health-Systems Pharmacists (ASHP), the American Pharmaceutical Association (APhA), and the American College of Clinical Pharmacy (ACCP). She also serves on the Editorial Advisory Board of the *Journal of the American Pharmaceutical Association* and the *Drug INFO Line* Newsletter.

ABOUT THE AUTHORS *(Continued)*

Morton P. Goldman, PharmD, BCPS

Dr Goldman received his bachelor's degree in pharmacy from the University of Pittsburgh, College of Pharmacy and his Doctor of Pharmacy degree from the University of Cincinnati, Division of Graduate Studies and Research. He completed his concurrent 2-year hospital pharmacy residency at the VA Medical Center in Cincinnati. Dr Goldman is presently the Assistant Director of Pharmacotherapy Services for the Department of Pharmacy at the Cleveland Clinic Foundation (CCF) after having spent over 3 years at CCF as an Infectious Disease pharmacist and 4 years as Clinical Manager. He holds faculty appointments from Case Western Reserve University, College of Medicine; The University of Toledo, College of Pharmacy; and The University of Cincinnati, College of Pharmacy. Dr Goldman is a board-certified Pharmacotherapy Specialist.

In his capacity as Assistant Director of Pharmacotherapy Services at CCF, Dr Goldman remains actively involved in patient care and clinical research with the Department of Infectious Disease, as well as the continuing education of the medical and pharmacy staff. He is an editor of CCF's *Guidelines for Antibiotic Use* and coordinates their annual Antimicrobial Review retreat. He is a member of the Pharmacy and Therapeutics Committee and many of its subcommittees. Dr Goldman has authored numerous journal articles and lectures locally and nationally on infectious diseases topics and current drug therapies. He is currently a reviewer for the *Annals of Pharmacotherapy* and the *Journal of the American Medical Association*, an editorial board member of the *Journal of Infectious Disease Pharmacotherapy*, and coauthor of the *Drug Information Handbook* and the *Drug Information Handbook for the Allied Health Professional* produced by Lexi-Comp, Inc. He also provides technical support to Lexi-Comp's Clinical Reference Library™ publications.

Dr Goldman is an active member of Cleveland's local clinical pharmacy society, the Ohio College of Clinical Pharmacy, the Society of Infectious Disease Pharmacists, the American College of Clinical Pharmacy, and the American Society of Health-Systems Pharmacy.

Leonard L. Lance, RPh, BSPharm

Leonard L. (Bud) Lance has been directly involved in the pharmaceutical industry since receiving his bachelor's degree in pharmacy from Ohio Northern University in 1970. Upon graduation from ONU, Mr Lance spent four years as a navy pharmacist in various military assignments and was instrumental in the development and operation of the first whole hospital I.V. admixture program in a military (Portsmouth Naval Hospital) facility.

After completing his military service, he entered the retail pharmacy field and has managed both an independent and a home I.V. franchise pharmacy operation. Since the late 1970s Mr Lance has focused much of his interest on using computers to improve pharmacy service and to advance the dissemination of drug information to practitioners and other health care professionals.

As a result of his strong publishing interest, he serves in the capacity of pharmacy editor and technical advisor as well as pharmacy (information) database coordinator for Lexi-Comp. Along with the *Drug Information Handbook for the Allied Health Professional* edition, he provides technical support to Lexi-Comp's *Pediatric Dosage Handbook, Laboratory Test Handbook, Diagnostic Procedure Handbook, Infectious Diseases Handbook, Poisoning & Toxicology Handbook*, and *Geriatric Dosage Handbook* publications. Mr Lance has also assisted approximately 120 major hospitals in producing their own formulary (pharmacy) publications through Lexi-Comp's custom publishing service.

Mr Lance is a member and past president (1984) of the Summit Pharmaceutical Association (SPA). He is also a member of the Ohio Pharmacists Association (OPA), the American Pharmaceutical Association (APhA), and the American Society of Health-System Pharmacists (ASHP).

EDITORIAL ADVISORY PANEL

EDITORIAL ADVISORY PANEL *(Continued)*

Eugene S. Olsowka, MD, PhD
Pathologist
Institute of Pathology PC
Saginaw, Michigan

Thomas E. Page, MA
Drug Recognition Expert and Instructor
Pasadena, CA

Frank P. Paloucek, PharmD
Clinical Associate Professor
University of Illinois
Chicago, Illinois

Christopher J. Papasian, PhD
Director of Diagnostic Microbiology and Immunology Laboratories
Truman Medical Center
Kansas City, Missouri

Bradley G. Phillips, PharmD, BCPS
Assistant Professor
University of Iowa College of Pharmacy
Iowa City, Iowa
Clinical Pharmacist
Veterans Affairs Medical Center
Iowa City, Iowa

Martha Sajatovic, MD
Assistant Professor of Psychiatry
Case Western Reserve University
Cleveland, Ohio

Todd P. Semla, PharmD
Associate Director of the Psychopharmacology Clinical and Research Center
Department of Psychiatry and Behavioral Sciences
Evanston Northwestern Healthcare
Evanston, Illinois
Clinical Assistant Professor of Pharmacy Practice in Medicine, Section of Geriatric Medicine
University of Illinois at Chicago
Chicago, Illinois

Dominic A. Solimando, Jr, MA
Oncology Pharmacist
Director of Oncology Drug Information
cancer**education**.com
Arlington, VA

Virend K. Somers, MD, DPhil
Consultant in Hypertension and Cardiovascular Disease
Mayo Clinic
Professor
Mayo Medical School
Rochester, Minnesota

Carol K. Taketomo, PharmD
Pharmacy Manager
Children's Hospital of Los Angeles
Los Angeles, California

Lowell L. Tilzer MD
Associate Medical Director
Community Blood Center of Greater Kansas City
Kansas City, Missouri

Beatrice B. Turkoski, RN, PhD
Professor, Advanced Pharmacology and Applied Therapeutics
Kent State University School of Nursing
Kent, Ohio

Richard L. Wynn, PhD
Professor and Chairman of Pharmacology
Baltimore College of Dental Surgery
Dental School
University of Maryland at Baltimore
Baltimore, Maryland

PREFACE

Physician assistants, other nonphysician primary care providers, pharmacists, and physicians are increasingly confronted with information that is becoming more intense. The need to access relevant drug information in an efficient manner is a challenge that is equally as intense.

When we created the first edition of this book, we tried hard to keep it small enough so that it could be employed as a handbook (that is, keep it portable without compromising content and extensiveness). This edition actually increases the number of agents; however, due to the fact that portability is an important focus, we have condensed many monographs. HIV medications are one of the groups of monographs that we have shortened into 11 important fields of information; most compound drugs include only 3 fields of information as the individual components have complete monographs; and other selected monographs, at the editor's discretion, have been condensed to include 7 fields of information (ie, Pharmacologic Class, Use, Usual Dosage, U.S. Brand Names, Contraindications, Pregnancy Risk Factor, and Pronunciation). Also, we have eliminated the alphabetical index, since the book works nicely by simply looking through the text listings which have the index "embedded" within them. We did not appreciate this feature until we began to use it, but now we think it is the more efficient way to look up an agent. Another new feature to the monograph section is the running header at the top of the pages. Very similar to a dictionary, you will now see the name of the drug that begins or ends on the page. We hope that you find this new format useful and convenient.

In continuing to survey the needs of practitioners, we have tried to develop a reference that is useful at the point of the patient encounter. The annotated organization of the material is hopefully pertinent and logical. Features include more herbal drug monographs, dosing information for adults/pediatrics/geriatrics for each monograph, and appendices with updated guidelines, unique categorical listings, and clinical calculation tools.

A portable text cannot allow for information on every therapeutic agent available. We believe, though, that you will find the consistent and comprehensive format to be useful in your therapeutic decision making. We would welcome any comments to improve future editions.

ACKNOWLEDGMENTS

The *Drug Information Handbook for Physician Assistants* has been extracted from the *Drug Information Handbook*, 7th ed, by Lacy, Armstrong, Goldman, and Lance (also published by Lexi-Comp, Inc) and adapted to the specific information needs of physician assistants. Special acknowledgment is also extended to the *Drug Information Handbook for Nursing,* Turkoski B and Lance B (Lexi-Comp, Inc), for information related to Patient Education.

The *Drug Information Handbook for Physician Assistants* exists in its present form as the result of the concerted efforts of the following individuals: Robert D. Kerscher, publisher and president of Lexi-Comp Inc; Lynn D. Coppinger, managing editor; Barbara F. Kerscher, production manager; David C. Marcus, director of information systems; Elizabeth Tomsik, PharmD, pharmacotherapy specialist; Ginger Conner, project manager; Kristin M. Thompson, product manager; and Tracey J. Reinecke, graphic designer.

Special acknowledgment to all Lexi-Comp staff for their contributions to this handbook.

Much of the material contained in this book was a result of pharmacy contributors throughout the United States and Canada. Lexi-Comp has assisted many medical institutions to develop hospital-specific formulary manuals that contain clinical drug information as well as dosing. Working with clinical pharmacists, hospital pharmacy and therapeutics committees, and hospital drug information centers, Lexi-Comp has developed an evolutionary drug database that reflects the practice of pharmacy in these major institutions.

In addition, the authors and editors wish to thank their families, friends, and colleagues who supported them in their efforts to complete this handbook.

DESCRIPTION OF SECTIONS AND FIELDS USED IN THIS HANDBOOK

The *Drug Information Handbook for Physician Assistants* is divided into four sections.

The first section is a compilation of introductory text pertinent to the use of this book.

The drug information section of the handbook, in which all drugs are listed alphabetically, details information pertinent to each drug. Extensive cross-referencing is provided by U.S. brand names, Canadian brand names, and synonyms. Commonly-used natural products have also been included. The fields of information in each monograph have been carefully chosen by the editors to reflect the professional responsibilities and decisions of physician assistants. Many combination-product monographs have been condensed with only brand names and forms available; for more information, see the individual components.

The third section is an invaluable appendix which offers a compilation of tables, guidelines, nomograms, algorithms, and conversion information which can be helpful when considering patient care.

The last section of this handbook contains a Pharmacologic Index.

The **Alphabetical Listing of Drugs** is presented in a consistent format and provides the following fields of information:

Generic Name	U.S. adopted name
Pronunciation	Phonetic pronunciation guide
Pharmacologic Class	Unique systematic classification of medications
U.S. Brand Names	U.S. trade names (manufacturer-specific)
Generic Available	Indicates if drugs are available in generic form
Mechanism of Action	How the drug works in the body to elicit a response
Use	Information pertaining to appropriate indications of the drug. Includes both FDA approved and non-FDA approved indications.
Usual Dosage	The amount of the drug to be typically given or taken during therapy for children and adults; also includes any dosing adjustment/comments for renal impairment or hepatic impairment and other suggested dosing adjustments (eg, hematological toxicity)
Dosage Forms	Information with regard to form, strength, and availability of the drug. The field is strung with the forms bolded and uses the following abbreviations: Aero = aerosol; Cap = capsule; Crm = cream; Inf = infusion; Inh = inhalation; Inj = inject; Liq = liquid; Oint = ointment, Soln = solution; Supp = suppository; Susp = suspension; Syr = syrup; Tab = tablet; Top = topical.
Contraindications	Information pertaining to inappropriate use of the drug
Warnings/ Precautions	Precautionary considerations, hazardous conditions related to use of the drug, and disease states or patient populations in which the drug should be cautiously used

Pregnancy Risk Factor	Five categories established by the FDA to indicate the potential of a systemically absorbed drug for causing birth defects
Pregnancy Implications	Information pertinent to or associated with the use of the drug as it relates to clinical effects on the fetus, breast-feeding/lactation, and clinical effects on the infant
Adverse Reactions	Side effects are grouped by percentage of incidence (if known) and/or body system; in the interest of saving space, <1% effects are grouped only by percentage
Drug Interactions	If a drug has demonstrated involvement with cytochrome P-450 enzymes, the initial line of this field will identify the drug as an inhibitor, inducer, or substrate of specific isoenzymes (ie, CYP1A2). A summary of this information can also be found in a tabular format within the appendix section of this handbook. The remainder of the field presents a description of the interaction between the drug listed in the monograph and other drugs or drug classes. May include possible mechanisms and effect of combined therapy. May also include a strategy to manage the patient on combined therapy (ie, quinidine).
Alcohol Interactions	Information supplied if there is an interaction
Onset	The time after drug administration when therapeutic effect is observed. May also include time for peak therapeutic effect.
Duration	Length of therapeutic effect
Half-life	The reported half-life of elimination for the parent of metabolites of the drug.

Education and Monitoring Issues

Patient Education	Specific information pertinent for the patient
Dietary Considerations	Information is offered, when appropriate, regarding food and/or nutrition
Monitoring Parameters	Laboratory tests and patient physical parameters that should be monitored for safety and efficacy of drug therapy
Reference Range	Therapeutic and toxic serum concentrations listed including peak and trough levels

Manufacturer	Name of manufacturer is supplied if there is only one manufacturer of that specific drug. Phone number, address, and web site information can be found in the Pharmaceutical Manufacturers Directory located in the Appendix
Related Information	Cross-reference to other pertinent drug information found elsewhere in this handbook

SAFE WRITING PRACTICES

Health professionals and their support personnel frequently produce handwritten copies of information they see in print; therefore, such information is subjected to even greater possibilities for error or misinterpretation on the part of others. Thus, particular care must be given to how drug names and strengths are expressed when creating written healthcare documents.

The following are a few examples of safe writing rules suggested by the Institute for Safe Medication Practices, Inc.*

1. There should be a space between a number and its units as it is easier to read. There should be no periods after the abbreviations mg or mL.

Correct	Incorrect
10 mg	10mg
100 mg	100mg

2. Never place a decimal and a zero after a whole number (2 mg is correct and 2.0 mg is **incorrect**). If the decimal point is not seen because it falls on a line or because individuals are working from copies where the decimal point is not seen, this causes a tenfold overdose.
3. Just the opposite is true for numbers less than one. Always place a zero before a naked decimal (0.5 mL is correct, .5 mL is **incorrect**).
4. Never abbreviate the word unit. The handwritten U or u, looks like a 0 (zero), and may cause a tenfold overdose error to be made.
5. IU is not a safe abbreviation for international units. The handwritten IU looks like IV. Write out international units or use int. units.
6. Q.D. is not a safe abbreviation for once daily, as when the Q is followed by a sloppy dot, it looks like QID which means four times daily.
7. O.D. is not a safe abbreviation for once daily, as it is properly interpreted as meaning "right eye" and has caused liquid medications such as saturated solution of potassium iodide and Lugol's solution to be administered incorrectly. There is no safe abbreviation for once daily. It must be written out in full.
8. Do not use chemical names such as 6-mercaptopurine or 6-thioguanine, as sixfold overdoses have been given when these were not recognized as chemical names. The proper names of these drugs are mercaptopurine or thioguanine.
9. Do not abbreviate drug names (5FC, 6MP, 5-ASA, MTX, HCTZ, CPZ, PBZ, etc) as they are misinterpreted and cause error.
10. Do not use the apothecary system or symbols.
11. Do not abbreviate microgram as µg; instead use mcg as there is less likelihood of misinterpretation.
12. When writing an outpatient prescription, write a complete prescription. A complete prescription can prevent the prescriber, the pharmacist, and/or the patient from making a mistake and can eliminate the need for further clarification. The legible prescriptions should contain:
    a. patient's full name
    b. for pediatric or geriatric patients: their age (or weight where applicable)
    c. drug name, dosage form and strength; if a drug is new or rarely prescribed, print this information
    d. number or amount to be dispensed
    e. complete instructions for the patient, including the purpose of the medication
    f. when there are recognized contraindications for a prescribed drug, indicate to the pharmacist that you are aware of this fact (ie, when prescribing a potassium salt for a patient receiving an ACE inhibitor, write "K serum leveling being monitored")

*From "Safe Writing" by Davis NM, PharmD and Cohen MR, MS, Lecturers and Consultants for Safe Medication Practices, 1143 Wright Drive, Huntington Valley, PA 19006. Phone: (215) 947-7566.

ALPHABETICAL LISTING OF DRUGS

- **A-200™ Shampoo [OTC]** *see* Pyrethrins *on page 795*

Abacavir (a BAK a veer)

Pharmacologic Class Antiretroviral Agent, Reverse Transcriptase Inhibitor (Nucleoside)

U.S. Brand Names Ziagen™

Use Treatment of HIV infections in combination with other antiretroviral agents

USUAL DOSAGE Oral:

Children 3 months to 16 years: 8 mg/kg body weight twice daily (maximum: 300 mg twice daily) in combination with other antiretroviral agents

Adults: 300 mg twice daily in combination with other antiretroviral agents

Contraindications Prior hypersensitivity to abacavir (or carbovir) or any component of the formulation; do not rechallenge patients who have experienced hypersensitivity to abacavir

Warnings/Precautions Should always be used as a component of a multidrug regimen. Fatal hypersensitivity reactions have occurred. **Patients exhibiting symptoms of fever, skin rash, fatigue, and GI symptoms (eg, abdominal pain, nausea, vomiting) or respiratory symptoms such as pharyngitis, dyspnea, or cough, should discontinue therapy immediately and call for medical attention. Ziagen™ SHOULD NOT be restarted because more severe symptoms may occur within hours, including LIFE-THREATENING HYPOTENSION AND DEATH. To report these events on abacavir hypersensitivity, a registry has been established (1-800-270-0425).** Use with caution in patients with hepatic dysfunction; prior liver disease, prolonged use, and obesity may be risk factors for development of lactic acidosis and severe hepatomegaly with steatosis.

Pregnancy Risk Factor C

Adverse Reactions Note: Hypersensitivity reactions, which may be fatal, occur in ~5% of patients (see Warnings). Symptoms may include anaphylaxis, fever, rash, fatigue, diarrhea, abdominal pain, nausea and vomiting. Less common symptoms may include edema, lethargy, malaise, myalgia, shortness of breath, mouth ulcerations, conjunctivitis, lymphadenopathy, hepatic failure and renal failure.

Rates of adverse reactions were defined during combination therapy with lamivudine. Adverse reaction rates attributable to abacavir alone are not available.

Adults:

Central nervous system: Insomnia (7%)

Gastrointestinal: Nausea (47%), vomiting (16%), diarrhea (12%), anorexia (11%), pancreatitis

Neuromuscular & skeletal: Weakness

Endocrine & metabolic: Hyperglycemia, hypertriglyceridemia (25%)

Miscellaneous: Elevated transaminases

Children:

Central nervous system: Fever (19%), headache (16%)

Dermatologic: Rash (11%)

Gastrointestinal: Nausea (38%), vomiting (38%), diarrhea (16%), anorexia (9%)

Drug Interactions

Ethanol may increase the risk of toxicity

Abacavir increases the AUC of amprenavir

Manufacturer GlaxoWellcome

Related Information

Pharmaceutical Manufacturers Directory *on page 1020*

- **Abbokinase** *see* Urokinase *on page 963*
- **Abbokinase® Injection** *see* Urokinase *on page 963*
- **Abenol®** *see* Acetaminophen *on page 17*
- **Abitrate®** *see* Clofibrate *on page 211*
- **Absorbine® Antifungal [OTC]** *see* Tolnaftate *on page 931*
- **Absorbine® Antifungal Foot Powder [OTC]** *see* Miconazole *on page 600*
- **Absorbine® Jock Itch [OTC]** *see* Tolnaftate *on page 931*
- **Absorbine Jr.® Antifungal [OTC]** *see* Tolnaftate *on page 931*

Acarbose (AY car bose)

Pharmacologic Class Antidiabetic Agent (Miscellaneous)

U.S. Brand Names Precose®

Mechanism of Action Competitive inhibitor of pancreatic α-amylase and intestinal brush border α-glucosidases, resulting in delayed hydrolysis of ingested complex carbohydrates and disaccharides and absorption of glucose; dose-dependent reduction in postprandial serum insulin and glucose peaks; inhibits the metabolism of sucrose to glucose and fructose

Use

Monotherapy, as indicated as an adjunct to diet to lower blood glucose in patients with noninsulin-dependent diabetes mellitus (NIDDM) whose hyperglycemia cannot be managed on diet alone

Combination with a sulfonylurea, metformin, or insulin in patients with NIDDM when diet plus acarbose do not result in adequate glycemic control

USUAL DOSAGE Oral:

Adults: Dosage must be individualized on the basis of effectiveness and tolerance while not exceeding the maximum recommended dose

Initial dose: 25 mg 3 times/day with the first bite of each main meal

Maintenance dose: Should be adjusted at 4- to 8-week intervals based on 1-hour postprandial glucose levels and tolerance. Dosage may be increased from 25 mg 3 times/day to 50 mg 3 times/day. Some patients may benefit from increasing the dose to 100 mg 3 times/day.

Maintenance dose ranges: 50-100 mg 3 times/day.

Maximum dose:

≤60 kg: 50 mg 3 times/day

>60 kg: 100 mg 3 times/day

Patients receiving sulfonylureas: Acarbose given in combination with a sulfonylurea will cause a further lowering of blood glucose and may increase the hypoglycemic potential of the sulfonylurea. If hypoglycemia occurs, appropriate adjustments in the dosage of these agents should be made.

Dosing adjustment in renal impairment: Cl_{cr} <25 mL/minute: Peak plasma concentrations were 5 times higher and AUCs were 6 times larger than in volunteers with normal renal function; however, long term clinical trials in diabetic patients with significant renal dysfunction have not been conducted and treatment of these patients with acarbose is not recommended

Dosage Forms TAB: 50 mg, 100 mg

Contraindications Known hypersensitivity to the drug and in patients with diabetic ketoacidosis or cirrhosis; patients with inflammatory bowel disease, colonic ulceration, partial intestinal obstruction or in patients predisposed to intestinal obstruction; patients who have chronic intestinal diseases associated with marked disorders of digestion or absorption and in patients who have conditions that may deteriorate as a result of increased gas formation in the intestine

Warnings/Precautions Hypoglycemia: Acarbose may increase the hypoglycemic potential of sulfonylureas. Oral glucose (dextrose) should be used in the treatment of mild to moderate hypoglycemia. Severe hypoglycemia may require the use of either intravenous glucose infusion or glucagon injection.

Elevated serum transaminase levels: Treatment-emergent elevations of serum transaminases (AST and/or ALT) occurred in 15% of acarbose-treated patients in long-term studies. These serum transaminase elevations appear to be dose related. At doses >100 mg 3 times/day, the incidence of serum transaminase elevations greater than 3 times the upper limit of normal was 2-3 times higher in the acarbose group than in the placebo group. These elevations were asymptomatic, reversible, more common in females, and, in general, were not associated with other evidence of liver dysfunction.

When diabetic patients are exposed to stress such as fever, trauma, infection, or surgery, a temporary loss of control of blood glucose may occur. At such times, temporary insulin therapy may be necessary.

Pregnancy Risk Factor B

Pregnancy Implications Breast-feeding/lactation: It is not known whether acarbose is excreted in human milk

Adverse Reactions

>10%:

Gastrointestinal: Abdominal pain (21%) and diarrhea (33%) tend to return to pretreatment levels over time, and the frequency and intensity of flatulence (77%) tend to abate with time

Hepatic: Elevated liver transaminases

<1%: Erythema, gastrointestinal distress (severe), headache, sleepiness, urticaria, vertigo, weakness

Drug Interactions Decreased effect: Thiazides and other diuretics, corticosteroids, phenothiazines, thyroid products, estrogens, oral contraceptives, phenytoin, nicotinic acid, sympathomimetics, calcium channel-blocking drugs, isoniazid, intestinal adsorbents (eg, charcoal), digestive enzyme preparations (eg, amylase, pancreatin)

Alcohol Interactions Limit use especially with other diabetic agents (may cause hypoglycemia)

Education and Monitoring Issues

Patient Education: Take this medication exactly as directed, with the first bite of each main meal. Do not change dosage or discontinue without first consulting prescriber. Do not take other medications with or within 2 hours of this medication unless so advised by prescriber. It is important to follow dietary and lifestyle recommendations of prescriber. If combining acarbose with other diabetic medication (eg, sulfonylureas, insulin), keep source of glucose (sugar) on hand in case hypoglycemia occurs. You may experience mild side effects during first weeks of acarbose therapy (eg, bloating, flatulence, diarrhea, abdominal discomfort); these should diminish over time. Report severe or persistent side effects, fever, extended vomiting or flu, or change in color of urine or stool.

Monitoring Parameters: Postprandial glucose, glycosylated hemoglobin levels, serum transaminase levels should be checked every 3 months during the first year of treatment and periodically thereafter

(Continued)

Acarbose *(Continued)*

Manufacturer Bayer Corp (Biological and Pharmaceutical Division)

Related Information

Hypoglycemic Drugs and Thiazolidinedione Information *on page 1240*
Pharmaceutical Manufacturers Directory *on page 1020*

- **Accolate®** *see* Zafirlukast *on page 986*
- **Accupril®** *see* Quinapril *on page 800*
- **Accuretic®** *see* Quinapril and Hydrochlorothiazide *on page 801*
- **Accutane®** *see* Isotretinoin *on page 492*

Acebutolol (a se BYOO toe lole)

Pharmacologic Class Antiarrhythmic Agent, Class II; Beta Blocker (with Intrinsic Sympathomimetic Activity)

U.S. Brand Names Sectral®

Generic Available No

Mechanism of Action Competitively blocks $beta_1$-adrenergic receptors with little or no effect on $beta_2$-receptors except at high doses; exhibits membrane stabilizing and intrinsic sympathomimetic activity

Use Treatment of hypertension, ventricular arrhythmias, angina

USUAL DOSAGE Oral:

Adults:

Hypertension: 400-800 mg/day (larger doses may be divided); maximum: 1200 mg/day

Ventricular arrhythmias: Initial: 400 mg/day; maintenance: 600-1200 mg/day in divided doses

Elderly: Initial: 200-400 mg/day; dose reduction due to age related decrease in Cl_{cr} will be necessary; do not exceed 800 mg/day

Dosing adjustment in renal impairment:

Cl_{cr} 25-49 mL/minute/1.73 m^2: Reduce dose by 50%

Cl_{cr} <25 mL/minute/1.73 m^2: Reduce dose by 75%

Dosing adjustment in hepatic impairment: Use with caution

Dosage Forms CAP: 200 mg, 400 mg

Contraindications Hypersensitivity to beta-blocking agents, avoid use in uncompensated congestive heart failure; cardiogenic shock; bradycardia or heart block; sinus node dysfunction; A-V conduction abnormalities. Although acebutolol primarily blocks $beta_1$-receptors, high doses can result in $beta_2$-receptor blockage. Use with caution in bronchospastic lung disease and renal dysfunction (especially the elderly).

Warnings/Precautions Abrupt withdrawal of beta-blockers may result in an exaggerated cardiac beta-adrenergic responsiveness. Symptomatology has included reports of tachycardia, hypertension, ischemia, angina, myocardial infarction, and sudden death. It is recommended that patients be tapered gradually off of beta-blockers over a 2-week period rather than via abrupt discontinuation.

Pregnancy Risk Factor B (per manufacturer); D (2nd and 3rd trimester, based on expert analysis)

Adverse Reactions

>10%: Central nervous system: Fatigue (11%)

1% to 10%:

Cardiovascular: Chest pain (2%), edema (2%), bradycardia, hypotension, congestive heart failure

Central nervous system: Headache (6%), dizziness (6%), insomnia (3%), depression (2%), abnormal dreams (2%), anxiety, hyperesthesia, hypoesthesia, impotence

Dermatologic: Rash (2%), pruritus

Gastrointestinal: Constipation (4%), diarrhea (4%), dyspepsia (4%), nausea (4%), flatulence (3%), vomiting, abdominal pain

Genitourinary: Micturition frequency (3%), dysuria, nocturia, impotence (2%)

Neuromuscular & skeletal: Arthralgia (2%), myalgia (2%), back pain, joint pain

Ocular: Abnormal vision (2%), conjunctivitis, dry eyes, eye pain

Respiratory: Dyspnea (4%), rhinitis (2%), cough (1%), pharyngitis, wheezing

<1% (limited to important or life-threatening symptoms): Increased transaminases, increased bilirubin, increased alkaline phosphatase, hepatotoxic reaction, ventricular arrhythmias, A-V block, facial edema, xerostomia, anorexia, impotence, urinary retention, cold extremities, systemic lupus erythematosus, palpitations, exacerbate pre-existing renal insufficiency

Case reports: Pleurisy, pulmonary granulomas, pneumonitis, lichen planus, lupus erythematosus, drug-induced lupus-like syndrome

Potential adverse effects (based on experience with other beta-blocking agents) include reversible mental depression, disorientation, catatonia, short-term memory loss, emotional lability, slightly clouded sensorium, laryngospasm, respiratory distress, allergic reactions, erythematous rash, agranulocytosis, purpura, thrombocytopenia, mesenteric artery thrombosis, ischemic colitis, alopecia, Peyronie's disease, claudication

Drug Interactions

Alpha-blockers (prazosin, terazosin): Concurrent use of beta-blockers may increase risk of orthostasis

Clonidine: Hypertensive crisis after or during withdrawal of either agent

Drugs which slow A-V conduction (digoxin): Effects may be additive with beta-blockers

Glucagon: Acebutolol may blunt the hyperglycemic action of glucagon

Insulin and oral hypoglycemics: Acebutolol masks the tachycardia from hypoglycemia

NSAIDs (ibuprofen, indomethacin, naproxen, piroxicam) may reduce the antihypertensive effects of beta-blockers

Salicylates may reduce the antihypertensive effects of beta-blockers

Sulfonylureas: Beta-blockers may alter response to hypoglycemic agents

Verapamil or diltiazem may have synergistic or additive pharmacological effects when taken concurrently with beta-blockers

Alcohol Interactions Limit use (may increase risk of hypotension or dizziness)

Onset 1-2 hours

Duration 12-24 hours

Half-Life 6-7 hours average

Education and Monitoring Issues

Patient Education: Take exactly as directed; do not increase, decrease, or adjust dosage without consulting prescriber. Take pulse daily, prior to medication, and follow prescriber's instruction about holding medication. Do not take with antacids. Do not use alcohol or OTC medications (eg, cold remedies) without consulting prescriber. If diabetic, monitor serum sugars closely (may alter glucose tolerance or mask signs of hypoglycemia). May cause fatigue, dizziness (use caution when driving or engaging in tasks that require alertness until response to drug is known); postural hypotension (use caution when changing position from lying or sitting to standing or when climbing stairs); or alteration in sexual performance (reversible). Report chest pain or palpitations, unresolved swelling of extremities or unusual weight gain, difficulty breathing or new cough, skin rash, unresolved fatigue, unresolved constipation or diarrhea, unusual muscle weakness, or CNS disturbances.

Monitoring Parameters: Blood pressure, orthostatic hypotension, heart rate, CNS effects, EKG

Related Information

Beta-Blockers Comparison *on page 1233*

♦ **Aceon®** *see* Perindopril Erbumine *on page 717*

♦ **Acephen® [OTC]** *see* Acetaminophen *on page 17*

♦ **Aceta® [OTC]** *see* Acetaminophen *on page 17*

♦ **Acet-Am Expectorant** *see* Theophylline and Guaifenesin *on page 906*

Acetaminophen (a seet a MIN oh fen)

Pharmacologic Class Analgesic, Miscellaneous

U.S. Brand Names Acephen® [OTC]; Aceta® [OTC]; Apacet® [OTC]; Arthritis Foundation® Pain Reliever, Aspirin Free [OTC]; Aspirin Free Anacin® Maximum Strength [OTC]; Children's Silapap® [OTC]; Feverall™ [OTC]; Feverall™ Sprinkle Caps [OTC]; Genapap® [OTC]; Halenol® Childrens [OTC]; Infants Feverall™ [OTC]; Infants' Silapap® [OTC]; Junior Strength Panadol® [OTC]; Liquiprin® [OTC]; Mapap® [OTC]; Maranox® [OTC]; Neopap® [OTC]; Panadol® [OTC]; Redutemp® [OTC]; Ridenol® [OTC]; Tempra® [OTC]; Tylenol® [OTC]; Tylenol® Extended Relief [OTC]; Uni-Ace® [OTC]

Generic Available Yes

Mechanism of Action Inhibits the synthesis of prostaglandins in the central nervous system and peripherally blocks pain impulse generation; produces antipyresis from inhibition of hypothalamic heat-regulating center

Use Treatment of mild to moderate pain and fever; does not have antirheumatic effects (analgesic)

USUAL DOSAGE Oral, rectal (if fever not controlled with acetaminophen alone, administer with full doses of aspirin on an every 4- to 6-hour schedule, if aspirin is not otherwise contraindicated):

Children <12 years: 10-15 mg/kg/dose every 4-6 hours as needed; do **not** exceed 5 doses (2.6 g) in 24 hours; alternatively, the following doses may be used. See table.

Acetaminophen Dosing

Age	Dosage (mg)	Age	Dosage (mg)
0-3 mo	40	4-5 y	240
4-11 mo	80	6-8 y	320
1-2 y	120	9-10 y	400
2-3 y	160	11 y	480

Adults: 325-650 mg every 4-6 hours or 1000 mg 3-4 times/day; do **not** exceed 4 g/day

Dosing interval in renal impairment:

Cl_{cr} 10-50 mL/minute: Administer every 6 hours

(Continued)

Acetaminophen *(Continued)*

Cl_{cr} <10 mL/minute: Administer every 8 hours (metabolites accumulate)

Hemodialysis: Moderately dialyzable (20% to 50%)

Dosing adjustment/comments in hepatic impairment: Appears to be well tolerated in cirrhosis; serum levels may need monitoring with long-term use

Dosage Forms CAPLET: 160 mg, 325 mg, 500 mg; Extended: 650 mg. **CAP:** 80 mg. **DROPS:** 48 mg/mL (15 mL); 60 mg/0.6 mL (15 mL); 80 mg/0.8 mL (15 mL); 100 mg/mL (15 mL, 30 mL). **ELIX:** 80 mg/5 mL, 120 mg/5 mL, 160 mg/5 mL, 167 mg/5 mL, 325 mg/5 mL. **LIQ, oral:** 160 mg/5 mL, 500 mg/15 mL. **SOLN:** 100 mg/mL (15 mL); 120 mg/2.5 mL. **SUPP, rectal:** 80 mg, 120 mg, 125 mg, 300 mg, 325 mg, 650 mg. **SUSP:** Oral: 160 mg/5 mL; Oral drops: 80 mg/0.8 mL. **TAB:** 325 mg, 500 mg, 650 mg; Chewable: 80 mg, 160 mg

Contraindications Patients with known G-6-PD deficiency; hypersensitivity to acetaminophen

Warnings/Precautions May cause severe hepatic toxicity on overdose; use with caution in patients with alcoholic liver disease; chronic daily dosing in adults of 5-8 g of acetaminophen over several weeks or 3-4 g/day of acetaminophen for 1 year have resulted in liver damage

Pregnancy Risk Factor B

Adverse Reactions Percentage unknown: May increase chloride, bilirubin, uric acid, glucose, ammonia, alkaline phosphatase; may decrease sodium, bicarbonate, calcium

<1%: Analgesic nephropathy, anemia, blood dyscrasias (neutropenia, pancytopenia, leukopenia), hypersensitivity reactions (rare), nausea, nephrotoxicity with chronic overdose, rash, vomiting

Drug Interactions CYP1A2 enzyme substrate (minor), CYP2E1 and 3A3/4 enzyme substrate

Decreased effect: Rifampin can interact to reduce the analgesic effectiveness of acetaminophen

Increased toxicity: Barbiturates, carbamazepine, hydantoins, sulfinpyrazone can increase the hepatotoxic potential of acetaminophen; chronic ethanol abuse increases risk for acetaminophen toxicity; effect of warfarin may be enhanced

Alcohol Interactions Avoid use or limit to <3 drinks/day

Onset <1 hour

Duration 4-6 hours

Half-Life Adults: Normal renal function: 1-3 hours; End-stage renal disease: 1-3 hours

Education and Monitoring Issues

Patient Education: Take exactly as directed (do not increase dose or frequency); most adverse effects are related to excessive use. Take with food or milk. While using this medication, avoid alcohol and other prescription or OTC medications that contain acetaminophen. Maintain adequate hydration (2-3 L/day of fluids unless instructed to restrict fluid intake). This medication will not reduce inflammation; consult prescriber for anti-inflammatory, if needed. Report unusual bleeding (stool, mouth, urine) or bruising; unusual fatigue and weakness; change in elimination patterns; or change in color of urine or stool.

Dietary Considerations: Food: May slightly delay absorption of extended-release preparations; rate of absorption may be decreased when given with food high in carbohydrates

Monitoring Parameters: Relief of pain or fever

Reference Range:

Therapeutic concentration (analgesic/antipyretic): 10-30 µg/mL

Toxic concentration (acute ingestion) with probable hepatotoxicity: >200 µg/mL at 4 hours or 50 µg/mL at 12 hours after ingestion

Related Information

Acetaminophen, Isometheptene, and Dichloralphenazone *on page 19*

Hydrocodone, Chlorpheniramine, Phenylephrine, Acetaminophen, and Caffeine *on page 446*

Phenyltoloxamine, Phenylpropanolamine, and Acetaminophen *on page 730*

Propoxyphene and Acetaminophen *on page 786*

Acetaminophen and Codeine (a seet a MIN oh fen & KOE deen)

Pharmacologic Class Analgesic, Combination (Narcotic)

U.S. Brand Names Capital® and Codeine; Phenaphen® With Codeine; Tylenol® With Codeine

Dosage Forms CAP: #2: Acetaminophen 325 mg and codeine phosphate 15 mg (C-III); #3: Acetaminophen 325 mg and codeine phosphate 30 mg (C-III); #4: Acetaminophen 325 mg and codeine phosphate 60 mg (C-III). **ELIX:** Acetaminophen 120 mg and codeine phosphate 12 mg per 5 mL with alcohol 7% (C-V). **SUSP, oral,** (alcohol free): Acetaminophen 120 mg and codeine phosphate 12 mg per 5 mL (C-V). **TAB:** Acetaminophen 500 mg and codeine phosphate 30 mg (C-III); acetaminophen 650 mg and codeine phosphate 30 mg (C-III); **TAB:** #1: Acetaminophen 300 mg and codeine phosphate 7.5 mg (C-III); #2: Acetaminophen 300 mg and codeine phosphate 15 mg (C-III); #3: Acetaminophen 300 mg and codeine phosphate 30 mg (C-III); #4: Acetaminophen 300 mg and codeine phosphate 60 mg (C-III)

Alcohol Interactions Avoid use (may increase central nervous system depression)

Acetaminophen, Isometheptene, and Dichloralphenazone

(a seet a MIN oh fen, eye soe me THEP teen, & dye KLOR al FEN a zone)

Pharmacologic Class Analgesic, Non-narcotic

U.S. Brand Names Isocom®; Isopap®; Midchlor®; Midrin®; Migratine®

Dosage Forms CAP: Acetaminophen 325 mg, isometheptene mucate 65 mg, dichloralphenazone 100 mg

Pregnancy Risk Factor B

Alcohol Interactions Avoid use or limit to <3 drinks/day

- **Acetasol® HC Otic** *see* Acetic Acid, Propylene Glycol Diacetate, and Hydrocortisone *on page 20*
- **Acetazolam®** *see* Acetazolamide *on page 19*

Acetazolamide (a set a ZOLE a mide)

Pharmacologic Class Anticonvulsant, Miscellaneous; Carbonic Anhydrase Inhibitor; Diuretic, Carbonic Anhydrase Inhibitor; Ophthalmic Agent, Antiglaucoma

U.S. Brand Names Diamox®; Diamox Sequels®

Use Lowers intraocular pressure to treat glaucoma, also as a diuretic, adjunct treatment of refractory seizures and acute altitude sickness; centrencephalic epilepsies (sustained release not recommended for anticonvulsant)

USUAL DOSAGE Note: I.M. administration is not recommended because of pain secondary to the alkaline pH

Neonates and Infants: Hydrocephalus: To slow the progression of hydrocephalus in neonates and infants who may not be good candidates for surgery, acetazolamide I.V. or oral doses of 5 mg/kg/dose every 6 hours increased by 25 mg/kg/day to a maximum of 100 mg/kg/day, if tolerated, have been used. Furosemide was used in combination with acetazolamide.

Children:

- Glaucoma:
  - Oral: 8-30 mg/kg/day or 300-900 mg/m²/day divided every 8 hours
  - I.M., I.V.: 20-40 mg/kg/24 hours divided every 6 hours, not to exceed 1 g/day
- Edema: Oral, I.M., I.V.: 5 mg/kg or 150 mg/m² once every day
- Epilepsy: Oral: 8-30 mg/kg/day in 1-4 divided doses, not to exceed 1 g/day; sustained release capsule is not recommended for treatment of epilepsy

Adults:

- Glaucoma:
  - Chronic simple (open-angle): Oral: 250 mg 1-4 times/day or 500 mg sustained release capsule twice daily
  - Secondary, acute (closed-angle): I.M., I.V.: 250-500 mg, may repeat in 2-4 hours to a maximum of 1 g/day
- Edema: Oral, I.M., I.V.: 250-375 mg once daily
- Epilepsy: Oral: 8-30 mg/kg/day in 1-4 divided doses; **sustained release capsule is not recommended for treatment of epilepsy**
- Altitude sickness: Oral: 250 mg every 8-12 hours (or 500 mg extended release capsules every 12-24 hours)
  - Therapy should begin 24-48 hours before and continue during ascent and for at least 48 hours after arrival at the high altitude
- Urine alkalinization: Oral: 5 mg/kg/dose repeated 2-3 times over 24 hours

Elderly: Oral: Initial: 250 mg twice daily; use lowest effective dose

Dosing adjustment in renal impairment:

- Cl_{cr} 10-50 mL/minute: Administer every 12 hours
- Cl_{cr} <10 mL/minute: Avoid use → ineffective

Hemodialysis: Moderately dialyzable (20% to 50%)

Peritoneal dialysis: Supplemental dose is not necessary

Contraindications Hypersensitivity to sulfonamides or acetazolamide, patients with hepatic disease or insufficiency; patients with decreased sodium and/or potassium levels; patients with adrenocortical insufficiency, hyperchloremic acidosis, severe renal disease or dysfunction, or severe pulmonary obstruction; long-term use in noncongestive angle-closure glaucoma

Pregnancy Risk Factor C

Related Information

Epilepsy Guidelines *on page 1091*

Acetic Acid (a SEE tik AS id)

Pharmacologic Class Antibacterial, Otic; Antibacterial, Topical

U.S. Brand Names Aci-jel®; VōSol®

Generic Available Yes

Use Irrigation of the bladder; treatment of superficial bacterial infections of the external auditory canal and vagina

(Continued)

Acetic Acid *(Continued)*

USUAL DOSAGE

Irrigation (note dosage of an irrigating solution depends on the capacity or surface area of the structure being irrigated):

For continuous irrigation of the urinary bladder with 0.25% acetic acid irrigation, the rate of administration will approximate the rate of urine flow; usually 500-1500 mL/24 hours

For periodic irrigation of an indwelling urinary catheter to maintain patency, about 50 mL of 0.25% acetic acid irrigation is required

Otic: Insert saturated wick; keep moist 24 hours; remove wick and instill 5 drops 3-4 times/day

Vaginal: One applicatorful every morning and evening

Dosage Forms JELLY, vag: 0.921% with oxyquinolone sulfate 0.025%, ricinoleic acid 0.7%, and glycerin 5% (85 g). **SOLN:** Irrigation: 0.25% (1000 mL); Otic (VōSol®): Acetic acid 2% in propylene glycol (15 mL, 30 mL, 60 mL)

Contraindications During transurethral procedures; hypersensitivity to drug or components

Warnings/Precautions Not for internal intake or I.V. infusion; topical use or irrigation use only; use of irrigation in patients with mucosal lesions of urinary bladder may cause irritation; systemic acidosis may result from absorption

Pregnancy Risk Factor C

Adverse Reactions <1%: Hematuria, systemic acidosis, urologic pain

Related Information

Acetic Acid, Propylene Glycol Diacetate, and Hydrocortisone *on page 20*
Aluminum Acetate and Acetic Acid *on page 41*

Acetic Acid, Propylene Glycol Diacetate, and Hydrocortisone

(a SEE tik AS id, PRO pa leen GLY kole dye AS e tate, & hye droe KOR ti sone)

Pharmacologic Class Antibiotic/Corticosteroid, Otic

U.S. Brand Names Acetasol® HC Otic; VōSol® HC Otic

Dosage Forms SOLN, otic: Acetic acid 2%, propylene glycol diacetate 3%, and hydrocortisone 1% (10 mL)

Acetylcholine (a se teel KOE leen)

Pharmacologic Class Cholinergic Agonist

U.S. Brand Names Miochol-E®

Use Produces complete miosis in cataract surgery, keratoplasty, iridectomy and other anterior segment surgery where rapid miosis is required

USUAL DOSAGE Adults: Intraocular: 0.5-2 mL of 1% injection (5-20 mg) instilled into anterior chamber before or after securing one or more sutures

Contraindications Hypersensitivity to acetylcholine chloride and any components; acute iritis and acute inflammatory disease of the anterior chamber

Pregnancy Risk Factor C

Acetylcysteine (a se teel SIS teen)

Pharmacologic Class Antidote; Mucolytic Agent

U.S. Brand Names Mucomyst®; Mucosil™

Generic Available No

Mechanism of Action Exerts mucolytic action through its free sulfhydryl group which opens up the disulfide bonds in the mucoproteins thus lowering mucous viscosity. The exact mechanism of action in acetaminophen toxicity is unknown; thought to act by providing substrate for conjugation with the toxic metabolite.

Use Adjunctive mucolytic therapy in patients with abnormal or viscid mucous secretions in acute and chronic bronchopulmonary diseases; pulmonary complications of surgery and cystic fibrosis; diagnostic bronchial studies; antidote for acute acetaminophen toxicity

USUAL DOSAGE

Acetaminophen poisoning: Children and Adults: Oral: 140 mg/kg; followed by 17 doses of 70 mg/kg every 4 hours; repeat dose if emesis occurs within 1 hour of administration; therapy should continue until all doses are administered even though the acetaminophen plasma level has dropped below the toxic range

Inhalation: Acetylcysteine 10% and 20% solution (Mucomyst®) (dilute 20% solution with sodium chloride or sterile water for inhalation); 10% solution may be used undiluted

Infants: 1-2 mL of 20% solution or 2-4 mL 10% solution until nebulized given 3-4 times/day

Children: 3-5 mL of 20% solution or 6-10 mL of 10% solution until nebulized given 3-4 times/day

Adolescents: 5-10 mL of 10% to 20% solution until nebulized given 3-4 times/day

Note: Patients should receive an aerosolized bronchodilator 10-15 minutes prior to acetylcysteine

Meconium ileus equivalent: Children and Adults: 100-300 mL of 4% to 10% solution by irrigation or orally

Dosage Forms SOLN: 10% [100 mg/mL] (4 mL, 10 mL, 30 mL); 20% [200 mg/mL] (4 mL, 10 mL, 30 mL, 100 mL)

Contraindications Known hypersensitivity to acetylcysteine

Warnings/Precautions Since increased bronchial secretions may develop after inhalation, percussion, postural drainage and suctioning should follow; if bronchospasm occurs, administer a bronchodilator; discontinue acetylcysteine if bronchospasm progresses

Pregnancy Risk Factor B

Pregnancy Implications Clinical effects on the fetus: There are no adequate and well controlled studies in pregnant women; use if only clearly needed

Adverse Reactions

>10%:

Gastrointestinal: Vomiting

Miscellaneous: Unpleasant odor during administration

1% to 10%:

Central nervous system: Drowsiness, chills

Gastrointestinal: Stomatitis, nausea

Local: Irritation

Respiratory: Bronchospasm, rhinorrhea, hemoptysis

Miscellaneous: Clamminess

<1%: Skin rash

Onset Oral: Peak plasma levels 1-2 hours; Inhalation: Mucus liquefaction occurs maximally within 5-10 minutes

Duration Oral: Can persist for >1 hour

Half-Life Oral: Reduced acetylcysteine: 2 hours; Total acetylcysteine: 5.5 hours

Education and Monitoring Issues

Patient Education: Pulmonary treatment: Prepare solution (may dilute with sterile water to reduce concentrate from impeding nebulizer) and use as directed. Clear airway by coughing deeply before using aerosol. Wash face and face-mask after treatment to remove any residual. You may experience drowsiness (use caution when driving) or nausea or vomiting (small frequent meals may help). Report persistent chills or fever, adverse change in respiratory status, palpitations, or extreme anxiety or nervousness.

Reference Range: Determine acetaminophen level as soon as possible, but no sooner than 4 hours after ingestion (to ensure peak levels have been obtained); administer for acetaminophen level >150 μg/mL; toxic concentration with probable hepatotoxicity: >200 μg/mL at 4 hours or 50 μg at 12 hours

- **Aches-N-Pain® [OTC]** *see* Ibuprofen *on page 458*
- **Achromycin® Ophthalmic** *see* Tetracycline *on page 903*
- **Achromycin® Topical** *see* Tetracycline *on page 903*
- **Aci-jel®** *see* Acetic Acid *on page 19*
- **Acilac** *see* Lactulose *on page 506*
- **Aciphex™** *see* Rabeprazole *on page 805*
- **Aclovate® Topical** *see* Alclometasone *on page 29*

Acrivastine and Pseudoephedrine (AK ri vas teen & soo doe e FED rin)

Pharmacologic Class Antihistamine

U.S. Brand Names Semprex®-D

Use Temporary relief of nasal congestion, decongest sinus openings, running nose, itching of nose or throat, and itchy, watery eyes due to hay fever or other upper respiratory allergies

USUAL DOSAGE Adults: 1 capsule 3-4 times/day

Dosing comments in renal impairment: Do not use

Dosage Forms CAP: Acrivastine 8 mg and pseudoephedrine hydrochloride 60 mg

Duration 12 hours

Half-Life 1.5 hours

Education and Monitoring Issues

Patient Education: Take as directed; do not exceed recommended dose. Avoid use of other depressants, alcohol, or sleep-inducing medications unless approved by prescriber. You may experience drowsiness or dizziness (use caution when driving or engaging in hazardous activity until response to drug is known); or dry mouth, nausea or vomiting (frequent small meals, frequent mouth care, chewing gum, or sucking lozenges may help). Report persistent dizziness, sedation, or agitation; chest pain, rapid heartbeat, or palpitations; difficulty breathing or increased cough; changes in urinary pattern; muscle weakness; or lack of improvement or worsening of condition.

- **ACT® [OTC]** *see* Fluoride *on page 376*
- **Actagen-C®** *see* Triprolidine, Pseudoephedrine, and Codeine *on page 958*
- **ActHIB®** *see Haemophilus* b Conjugate Vaccine *on page 427*
- **Acti-B_{12}®** *see* Hydroxocobalamin *on page 451*
- **Acticin® Cream** *see* Permethrin *on page 719*
- **Acticort 100®** *see* Hydrocortisone *on page 447*
- **Actidose-Aqua® [OTC]** *see* Charcoal *on page 175*

- **Actidose® With Sorbitol [OTC]** *see* Charcoal *on page 175*
- **Actifed® Allergy Tablet (Day) [OTC]** *see* Pseudoephedrine *on page 792*
- **Actigall™** *see* Ursodiol *on page 965*
- **Actinex® Topical** *see* Masoprocol *on page 555*
- **Actiprofen®** *see* Ibuprofen *on page 458*
- **Actiq®** *see* Fentanyl *on page 355*
- **Activase®** *see* Alteplase *on page 39*
- **Actonel™** *see* Risedronate *on page 825*
- **Actos™** *see* Pioglitazone *on page 738*
- **Actron® [OTC]** *see* Ketoprofen *on page 500*
- **ACU-dyne® [OTC]** *see* Povidone-Iodine *on page 756*
- **Acular** *see* Ketorolac Tromethamine *on page 501*
- **Acular® Ophthalmic** *see* Ketorolac Tromethamine *on page 501*
- **Acutrim® 16 Hours [OTC]** *see* Phenylpropanolamine *on page 729*
- **Acutrim® II, Maximum Strength [OTC]** *see* Phenylpropanolamine *on page 729*
- **Acutrim® Late Day [OTC]** *see* Phenylpropanolamine *on page 729*

Acyclovir (ay SYE kloe veer)

Pharmacologic Class Antiviral Agent

U.S. Brand Names Zovirax®

Generic Available Yes

Mechanism of Action Acyclovir is converted to acyclovir monophosphate by virus-specific thymidine kinase then further converted to acyclovir triphosphate by other cellular enzymes. Acyclovir triphosphate inhibits DNA synthesis and viral replication by competing with deoxyguanosine triphosphate for viral DNA polymerase and being incorporated into viral DNA.

Use Treatment of initial and prophylaxis of recurrent mucosal and cutaneous herpes simplex (HSV-1 and HSV-2) infections; herpes simplex encephalitis; herpes zoster; genital herpes infection; varicella-zoster infections in healthy, nonpregnant persons >13 years of age, children >12 months of age who have a chronic skin or lung disorder or are receiving long-term aspirin therapy, and immunocompromised patients; for herpes zoster, acyclovir should be started within 72 hours of the appearance of the rash to be effective; acyclovir will not prevent postherpetic neuralgias

USUAL DOSAGE

Dosing weight should be based on the smaller of lean body weight or total body weight

Treatment of herpes simplex virus infections: Children >12 years and Adults: I.V.:

Mucocutaneous HSV or severe initial herpes genitalis infection: 750 mg/m²/day divided every 8 hours or 5 mg/kg/dose every 8 hours for 5-10 days

HSV encephalitis: 1500 mg/m²/day divided every 8 hours or 10 mg/kg/dose for 10 days

Treatment of genital herpes simplex virus infections: Adults:

Oral: 200 mg every 4 hours while awake (5 times/day) for 10 days if initial episode; for 5 days if recurrence (begin at earliest signs of disease)

Topical: ½" ribbon of ointment for a 4" square surface area every 3 hours (6 times/day)

Treatment of varicella-zoster virus (chickenpox) infections:

Oral:

Children: 10-20 mg/kg/dose (up to 800 mg) 4 times/day for 5 days; begin treatment within the first 24 hours of rash onset

Adults: 600-800 mg/dose every 4 hours while awake (5 times/day) for 7-10 days or 1000 mg every 6 hours for 5 days

I.V.: Children and Adults: 1500 mg/m²/day divided every 8 hours or 10 mg/kg/dose every 8 hours for 7 days

Treatment of herpes zoster (shingles) infections:

Oral:

Children (immunocompromised): 250-600 mg/m²/dose 4-5 times/day for 7-10 days

Adults (immunocompromised): 800 mg every 4 hours (5 times/day) for 7-10 days

I.V.:

Children and Adults (immunocompromised): 10 mg/kg/dose or 500 mg/m²/dose every 8 hours

Older Adults (immunocompromised): 7.5 mg/kg/dose every 8 hours

If nephrotoxicity occurs: 5 mg/kg/dose every 8 hours

Prophylaxis in immunocompromised patients:

Varicella zoster or herpes zoster in HIV-positive patients: Adults: Oral: 400 mg every 4 hours (5 times/day) for 7-10 days

Bone marrow transplant recipients: Children and Adults: I.V.:

Allogeneic patients who are HSV seropositive: 150 mg/m²/dose (5 mg/kg) every 12 hours; with clinical symptoms of herpes simplex: 150 mg/m²/dose every 8 hours

Allogeneic patients who are CMV seropositive: 500 mg/m²/dose (10 mg/kg) every 8 hours; for clinically symptomatic CMV infection, consider replacing acyclovir with ganciclovir

Chronic suppressive therapy for recurrent genital herpes simplex virus infections:

Adults: 200 mg 3-4 times/day or 400 mg twice daily for up to 12 months, followed by re-evaluation

Dosing adjustment in renal impairment:

Oral: HSV/varicella-zoster:

Cl_{cr} 10-25 mL/minute: Administer dose every 8 hours

Cl_{cr} <10 mL/minute: Administer dose every 12 hours

I.V.:

Cl_{cr} 25-50 mL/minute: 5-10 mg/kg/dose: Administer every 12 hours

Cl_{cr} 10-25 mL/minute: 5-10 mg/kg/dose: Administer every 24 hours

Cl_{cr} <10 mL/minute: 2.5-5 mg/kg/dose: Administer every 24 hours

Hemodialysis: Dialyzable (50% to 100%); administer dose postdialysis

Peritoneal dialysis: Dose as for Cl_{cr} <10 mL/minute

Continuous arteriovenous or venovenous hemofiltration (CAVH/CAVHD) effects: Dose as for Cl_{cr} <10 mL/minute

Dosage Forms CAP: 200 mg. **POWDER for inj:** 500 mg (10 mL),1000 mg (20 mL). **OINT, top:** 5% [50 mg/g] (3 g, 15 g). **SUSP, oral** (banana flavor): 200 mg/5 mL. **TAB:** 400 mg, 800 mg

Contraindications Hypersensitivity to acyclovir

Warnings/Precautions Use with caution in patients with pre-existing renal disease or in those receiving other nephrotoxic drugs concurrently; maintain adequate urine output during the first 2 hours after I.V. infusion; use with caution in patients with underlying neurologic abnormalities, serious hepatic or electrolyte abnormalities, or substantial hypoxia

Pregnancy Risk Factor C

Adverse Reactions

>10%: Local: Inflammation at injection site

1% to 10%:

Central nervous system: Lethargy, dizziness, seizures, confusion, agitation, coma, headache

Dermatologic: Rash

Gastrointestinal: Nausea, vomiting

Neuromuscular & skeletal: Tremor

Renal: Impaired renal function

<1%: Anemia, anorexia, hallucinations, insomnia, leukopenia, LFT elevation, mental depression, sore throat, thrombocytopenia

Drug Interactions Increased CNS side effects with zidovudine and probenecid

Half-Life 3 hours (normal renal function)

Education and Monitoring Issues

Patient Education: This is not a cure for herpes (recurrences tend to appear within 3 months of original infection), nor will this medication reduce the risk of transmission to others when lesions are present. Take as directed for full course of therapy; do not discontinue even if feeling better. Maintain adequate hydration (2-3 L/day of fluids unless instructed to restrict fluid intake) to prevent renal complications. Avoid use of other topical creams, lotions, or ointments unless approved by prescriber. You may experience nausea or vomiting (small frequent meals, frequent mouth care, sucking lozenges, or chewing gum may help); lightheadedness or dizziness (use caution when driving or engaging in tasks that require alertness until response to drug is known); headache, fever, muscle pain (an analgesic may be recommended). Report persistent lethargy, acute headache, severe nausea or vomiting, confusion or hallucinations, rash, or difficulty breathing.

Monitoring Parameters: Urinalysis, BUN, serum creatinine, liver enzymes, CBC

Related Information

Treatment of Sexually Transmitted Diseases *on page 1210*

- **Adagen™** *see* Pegademase Bovine *on page 707*
- **Adalat®** *see* Nifedipine *on page 653*
- **Adalat® CC** *see* Nifedipine *on page 653*
- **Adalat PA®** *see* Nifedipine *on page 653*

Adapalene (a DAP a leen)

Pharmacologic Class Acne Products

U.S. Brand Names Differin®

Use Treatment of acne vulgaris

USUAL DOSAGE Children >12 years and Adults: Topical: Apply once daily at bedtime; therapeutic results should be noticed after 8-12 weeks of treatment

Contraindications Hypersensitivity to adapalene or any of the components in the vehicle gel

Pregnancy Risk Factor C

- **Adderall®** *see* Dextroamphetamine and Amphetamine *on page 261*
- **Adeflor®** *see* Vitamins, Multiple *on page 981*
- **Adenocard®** *see* Adenosine *on page 24*

Adenosine (a DEN oh seen)

Pharmacologic Class Antiarrhythmic Agent, Class IV

U.S. Brand Names Adenocard®

Generic Available No

Mechanism of Action Slows conduction time through the A-V node, interrupting the re-entry pathways through the A-V node, restoring normal sinus rhythm

Use Treatment of paroxysmal supraventricular tachycardia (PSVT) including that associated with accessory bypass tracts (Wolff-Parkinson-White syndrome); when clinically advisable, appropriate vagal maneuvers should be attempted prior to adenosine administration; not effective in atrial flutter, atrial fibrillation, or ventricular tachycardia; also used diagnostically as an adjunct to thallium-201 myocardial scintigraphy in patients unable to exercise adequately

USUAL DOSAGE Rapid I.V. push (over 1-2 seconds) via peripheral line:

Neonates: Initial dose: 0.05 mg/kg; if not effective within 2 minutes, increase dose by 0.05 mg/kg increments every 2 minutes to a maximum dose of 0.25 mg/kg or until termination of PSVT

Maximum single dose: 12 mg

Infants and Children: Pediatric advanced life support (PALS): Treatment of SVT: 0.1 mg/kg; if not effective, administer 0.2 mg/kg

Alternatively: Initial dose: 0.05 mg/kg; if not effective within 2 minutes, increase dose by 0.05 mg/kg increments every 2 minutes to a maximum dose of 0.25 mg/kg or until termination of PSVT; medium dose required: 0.15 mg/kg

Maximum single dose: 12 mg

Adults: 6 mg; if not effective within 1-2 minutes, 12 mg may be given; may repeat 12 mg bolus if needed

Maximum single dose: 12 mg

Hemodialysis: Significant drug removal is unlikely based on physiochemical characteristics

Peritoneal dialysis: Significant drug removal is unlikely based on physiochemical characteristics

Note: Patients who are receiving concomitant theophylline therapy may be less likely to respond to adenosine therapy

Note: Higher doses may be needed for administration via peripheral versus central vein

Dosage Forms DIAGNOSTIC use: 60 mg/20 mL and 90 mg/30 mL single-dose vials. **INJ** (preservative free): 3 mg/mL (2 mL)

Contraindications Known hypersensitivity to adenosine; second or third degree A-V block or sick-sinus syndrome (except in patients with a functioning artificial pacemaker), atrial flutter, atrial fibrillation, and ventricular tachycardia (the drug is not effective in converting these arrhythmias to sinus rhythm)

Warnings/Precautions Patients with pre-existing S-A nodal dysfunction may experience prolonged sinus pauses after adenosine; there have been reports of atrial fibrillation/flutter in patients with PSVT associated with accessory conduction pathways after adenosine; adenosine decreases conduction through the A-V node and may produce a short lasting first, second, or third degree heart block. Because of the very short half-life, the effects are generally self limiting. At the time of conversion to normal sinus rhythm, a variety of new rhythms may appear on the EKG.

A limited number of patients with asthma have received adenosine and have not experienced exacerbation of their asthma. Be alert to the possibility that adenosine could produce bronchoconstriction in patients with asthma.

Pregnancy Risk Factor C

Pregnancy Implications Clinical effects on the fetus: Case reports (4) on administration during pregnancy have indicated no adverse effects on fetus or newborn attributable to adenosine

Adverse Reactions

>10%:

Cardiovascular: Facial flushing (18%), palpitations, chest pain, hypotension

Central nervous system: Headache

Respiratory: Shortness of breath/dyspnea (12%)

Miscellaneous: Sweating

1% to 10%:

Central nervous system: Dizziness

Gastrointestinal: Nausea (3%)

Neuromuscular & skeletal: Paresthesia, numbness

Respiratory: Chest pressure (7%)

<1% (limited to important or life-threatening symptoms): Hypotension, lightheadedness, headache, dizziness, intracranial pressure, hyperventilation

Drug Interactions

Theophylline and caffeine (methylxanthines) antagonize adenosine's effects; may require increased dose of adenosine

Dipyridamole potentiates effects of adenosine; reduce dose of adenosine

Carbamazepine may increase heart block

Onset Clinical effects occur rapidly

Duration Very brief

Half-Life <10 seconds

Education and Monitoring Issues

Patient Education: Adenosine is administered in emergencies, patient education should be appropriate to the situation.

Monitoring Parameters: EKG monitoring, heart rate, blood pressure

Manufacturer Fujisawa Healthcare, Inc

Related Information

Pharmaceutical Manufacturers Directory *on page 1020*

- **Adipex-P®** *see* Phentermine *on page 726*
- **Adlone® Injection** *see* Methylprednisolone *on page 589*
- **Adrucil® Injection** *see* Fluorouracil *on page 376*
- **Adsorbocarpine® Ophthalmic** *see* Pilocarpine *on page 736*
- **Adsorbonac® Ophthalmic [OTC]** *see* Sodium Chloride *on page 858*
- **Advil® [OTC]** *see* Ibuprofen *on page 458*
- **AeroBid®-M Oral Aerosol Inhaler** *see* Flunisolide *on page 373*
- **AeroBid® Oral Aerosol Inhaler** *see* Flunisolide *on page 373*
- **Aerodine® [OTC]** *see* Povidone-Iodine *on page 756*
- **Aerolate®** *see* Theophylline Salts *on page 906*
- **Aerolate III®** *see* Theophylline Salts *on page 906*
- **Aerolate JR®** *see* Theophylline Salts *on page 906*
- **Aerolate SR®** *see* Theophylline Salts *on page 906*
- **Aerolone®** *see* Isoproterenol *on page 488*
- **Aeroseb-Dex®** *see* Dexamethasone *on page 256*
- **Aeroseb-HC®** *see* Hydrocortisone *on page 447*
- **A.F. Anacin®** *see* Acetaminophen *on page 17*
- **Afrin® Saline Mist [OTC]** *see* Sodium Chloride *on page 858*
- **Afrin® Tablet [OTC]** *see* Pseudoephedrine *on page 792*
- **Aftate® for Athlete's Foot [OTC]** *see* Tolnaftate *on page 931*
- **Aftate® for Jock Itch [OTC]** *see* Tolnaftate *on page 931*
- **Agenerase™** *see* Amprenavir *on page 61*
- **Aggrenox™** *see* Aspirin and Extended-Release Dipyridamole *on page 75*
- **Agrylin®** *see* Anagrelide *on page 63*
- **A-hydroCort®** *see* Hydrocortisone *on page 447*
- **Airbron** *see* Acetylcysteine *on page 20*
- **Airet®** *see* Albuterol *on page 27*
- **AKBeta®** *see* Levobunolol *on page 519*
- **AK-Chlor® Ophthalmic** *see* Chloramphenicol *on page 178*
- **Ak-Cide** *see* Sulfacetamide Sodium and Prednisolone *on page 876*
- **AK-Cide® Ophthalmic** *see* Sulfacetamide Sodium and Prednisolone *on page 876*
- **AK-Con®** *see* Naphazoline *on page 636*
- **AK-Dex®** *see* Dexamethasone *on page 256*
- **AK-Dilate® Ophthalmic Solution** *see* Phenylephrine *on page 727*
- **AK-Fluor** *see* Fluorescein Sodium *on page 375*
- **AK-Homatropine® Ophthalmic** *see* Homatropine *on page 438*
- **AK-NaCl® [OTC]** *see* Sodium Chloride *on page 858*
- **AK-Nefrin® Ophthalmic Solution** *see* Phenylephrine *on page 727*
- **AK-Pentolate®** *see* Cyclopentolate *on page 235*
- **AK-Poly-Bac® Ophthalmic** *see* Bacitracin and Polymyxin B *on page 90*
- **AK-Pred® Ophthalmic** *see* Prednisolone *on page 762*
- **AKPro® Ophthalmic** *see* Dipivefrin *on page 285*
- **AK-Spore H.C.® Ophthalmic Ointment** *see* Bacitracin, Neomycin, Polymyxin B, and Hydrocortisone *on page 90*
- **AK-Spore H.C.® Ophthalmic Suspension** *see* Neomycin, Polymyxin B, and Hydrocortisone *on page 644*
- **AK-Spore H.C.® Otic** *see* Neomycin, Polymyxin B, and Hydrocortisone *on page 644*
- **AK-Spore® Ophthalmic Ointment** *see* Bacitracin, Neomycin, and Polymyxin B *on page 90*
- **AK-Spore® Ophthalmic Solution** *see* Neomycin, Polymyxin B, and Gramicidin *on page 644*
- **Ak-Sulf** *see* Sulfacetamide Sodium *on page 876*
- **AK-Sulf® Ophthalmic** *see* Sulfacetamide Sodium *on page 876*
- **AK-Taine®** *see* Proparacaine *on page 782*
- **AKTob® Ophthalmic** *see* Tobramycin *on page 924*
- **AK-Tracin® Ophthalmic** *see* Bacitracin *on page 89*
- **AK-Trol®** *see* Neomycin, Polymyxin B, and Dexamethasone *on page 644*

- **Ala-Cort®** *see* Hydrocortisone *on page 447*
- **Alamast™** *see* Pemirolast *on page 707*
- **Ala-Scalp®** *see* Hydrocortisone *on page 447*
- **Alba-Dex®** *see* Dexamethasone *on page 256*
- **Albalon® Liquifilm®** *see* Naphazoline *on page 636*

Albendazole (al BEN da zole)

Pharmacologic Class Anthelmintic

U.S. Brand Names Albenza®

Generic Available No

Mechanism of Action Active metabolite, albendazole, causes selective degeneration of cytoplasmic microtubules in intestinal and tegmental cells of intestinal helminths and larvae; glycogen is depleted, glucose uptake and cholinesterase secretion are impaired, and desecratory substances accumulate intracellulary. ATP production decreases causing energy depletion, immobilization, and worm death.

Use Treatment of parenchymal neurocysticercosis and cystic hydatid disease of the liver, lung, and peritoneum; albendazole has activity against *Ascaris lumbricoides* (roundworm), *Ancylostoma duodenale* and *Necator americanus* (hookworms), *Enterobius vermicularis* (pinworm), *Hymenolepis nana* and *Taenia* sp (tapeworms), *Opisthorchis sinensis* and *Opisthorchis viverrini* (liver flukes), *Strongyloides stercoralis* and *Trichuris trichiura* (whipworm); activity has also been shown against the liver fluke *Clonorchis sinensis, Giardia lamblia, Cysticercus cellulosae, Echinococcus granulosus, Echinococcus multilocularis,* and *Toxocara* sp.

USUAL DOSAGE Oral:

Neurocysticercosis:

<60 kg: 15 mg/kg/day in 2 divided doses (maximum: 800 mg/day) with meals for 8-30 days

≥60 kg: 400 mg twice daily for 8-30 days

Note: Give concurrent anticonvulsant and steroid therapy during first week

Hydatid:

<60 kg: 15 mg/kg/day in 2 divided doses with meals (maximum: 800 mg/day) for three 28-day cycles with 14-day drug-free interval in-between

≥60 kg: 400 mg twice daily for 3 cycles as above

Strongyloidiasis/tapeworm:

≤2 years: 200 mg/day for 3 days; may repeat in 3 weeks

>2 years and Adults: 400 mg/day for 3 days; may repeat in 3 weeks

Giardiasis: Adults: 400 mg/day for 3 days

Hookworm, pinworm, roundworm:

≤2 years: 200 mg as a single dose; may repeat in 3 weeks

>2 years and Adults: 400 mg as a single dose; may repeat in 3 weeks

Dosage Forms TAB: 200 mg

Contraindications Patients with hypersensitivity to albendazole or its components; pregnant women, if possible

Warnings/Precautions Discontinue therapy if LFT elevations are significant; may restart treatment when decreased to pretreatment values. Becoming pregnant within 1 month following therapy is not advised. Corticosteroids should be administered 1-2 days before albendazole therapy in patients with neurocysticercosis to minimize inflammatory reactions and steroid and anticonvulsant therapy should be used concurrently during the first week of therapy for neurocysticercosis to prevent cerebral hypertension. If retinal lesions exist in patients with neurocysticercosis, weigh risk of further retinal damage due to albendazole-induced changes to the retinal lesion vs benefit of disease treatment.

Pregnancy Risk Factor C

Pregnancy Implications Albendazole has been shown to be teratogenic in laboratory animals and should not be used during pregnancy, if at all possible

Adverse Reactions N = neurocysticercosis; H = hydatid disease

Central nervous system: Dizziness, vertigo, fever (≤1%); headache (11% - N; 1% - H); increased intracranial pressure

Dermatologic: Alopecia/rash/urticaria (<1%)

Gastrointestinal: Abdominal pain (6% - H, 0% - N); nausea/vomiting (3% to 6%)

Hematologic: Leukopenia (reversible) (<1%); granulocytopenia/agranulocytopenia/pancytopenia (rare)

Hepatic: Increased LFTs (~15% - H, <1% - N)

Miscellaneous: Allergic reactions (<1%)

Drug Interactions May inhibit CYP1A2 enzyme (mild)

Decreased effect: Carbamazepine may accelerate albendazole metabolism

Increased effect: Dexamethasone increases plasma levels of albendazole metabolites; praziquantel may increase plasma concentrations of albendazole by 50%; albendazole inhibits hepatic CYP1A enzyme and may consequently interact by increasing the concentrations of many drugs which are metabolized by this route; food (especially fatty meals) increases the oral bioavailability by 4-5 times

Half-Life 8-12 hours

Education and Monitoring Issues

Patient Education: Take according to prescribed dosage schedule with meals. You may experience loss of hair (reversible); dizziness or headaches (use caution when driving or engaging in tasks that require alertness until response to drug is known). Report unusual fever, abdominal pain, unresolved vomiting, yellowing of skin or eyes, darkening of urine, or light colored stools.

Monitoring Parameters: Monitor fecal specimens for ova and parasites for 3 weeks after treatment; if positive, retreat; monitor LFTs, and clinical signs of hepatotoxicity; CBC at start of each 28-day cycle and every 2 weeks during therapy

Manufacturer SmithKline Beecham Pharmaceuticals

Related Information

Pharmaceutical Manufacturers Directory *on page 1020*

- ♦ **Albenza®** *see* Albendazole *on page 26*
- ♦ **Albert® Docusate** *see* Docusate *on page 290*
- ♦ **Albert® Glyburide** *see* Glyburide *on page 415*
- ♦ **Albert® Oxybutynin** *see* Oxybutynin *on page 690*
- ♦ **Albert® Pentoxifylline** *see* Pentoxifylline *on page 715*

Albumin (al BYOO min)

Pharmacologic Class Blood Product Derivative; Plasma Volume Expander, Colloid

U.S. Brand Names Albuminar®; Albumisol®; Albunex®; Albutein®; Buminate®; Plasbumin®

Use Plasma volume expansion and maintenance of cardiac output in the treatment of certain types of shock or impending shock; may be useful for burn patients, ARDS, and cardiopulmonary bypass; other uses considered by some investigators (but not proven) are retroperitoneal surgery, peritonitis, and ascites; unless the condition responsible for hypoproteinemia can be corrected, albumin can provide only symptomatic relief or supportive treatment; nutritional supplementation is not an appropriate indication for albumin

USUAL DOSAGE I.V.:

5% should be used in hypovolemic patients or intravascularly-depleted patients

25% should be used in patients in whom fluid and sodium intake must be minimized

Dose depends on condition of patient:

Children:

Emergency initial dose: 25 g

Nonemergencies: 25% to 50% of the adult dose

Adults: Usual dose: 25 g; no more than 250 g should be administered within 48 hours

Hypoproteinemia: 0.5-1 g/kg/dose; repeat every 1-2 days as calculated to replace ongoing losses

Hypovolemia: 0.5-1 g/kg/dose; repeat as needed; maximum dose: 6 g/kg/day

Contraindications Patients with severe anemia or cardiac failure, known hypersensitivity to albumin; avoid 25% concentration in preterm infants due to risk of idiopathic ventricular hypertrophy

Pregnancy Risk Factor C

- ♦ **Albuminar®** *see* Albumin *on page 27*
- ♦ **Albumisol®** *see* Albumin *on page 27*
- ♦ **Albunex®** *see* Albumin *on page 27*
- ♦ **Albutein®** *see* Albumin *on page 27*

Albuterol (al BYOO ter ole)

Pharmacologic Class $Beta_2$ Agonist

U.S. Brand Names Airet®; Proventil®; Proventil® HFA; Ventolin®; Ventolin® Rotocaps®; Volmax®

Generic Available Yes

Mechanism of Action Relaxes bronchial smooth muscle by action on $beta_2$-receptors with little effect on heart rate

Use Bronchodilator in reversible airway obstruction due to asthma or COPD

USUAL DOSAGE

Oral:

Children:

2-6 years: 0.1-0.2 mg/kg/dose 3 times/day; maximum dose not to exceed 12 mg/day (divided doses)

6-12 years: 2 mg/dose 3-4 times/day; maximum dose not to exceed 24 mg/day (divided doses)

Children >12 years and Adults: 2-4 mg/dose 3-4 times/day; maximum dose not to exceed 32 mg/day (divided doses)

Elderly: 2 mg 3-4 times/day; maximum: 8 mg 4 times/day

Inhalation MDI: 90 mcg/spray:

Children <12 years: 1-2 inhalations 4 times/day using a tube spacer

Children ≥12 years and Adults: 1-2 inhalations every 4-6 hours; maximum: 12 inhalations/day

Exercise-induced bronchospasm: 2 inhalations 15 minutes before exercising

(Continued)

Albuterol *(Continued)*

Inhalation: Nebulization: 0.01-0.05 mL/kg of 0.5% solution every 4-6 hours; intensive care patients may require more frequent administration; minimum dose: 0.1 mL; maximum dose: 1 mL diluted in 1-2 mL normal saline; continuous nebulized albuterol at 0.3 mg/kg/hour has been used safely in the treatment of severe status asthmaticus in children; continuous nebulized doses of 3 mg/kg/hour ±2.2 mg/kg/hour in children whose mean age was 20.7 months resulted in no cardiac toxicity; the optimal dosage for continuous nebulization remains to be determined.

Hemodialysis: Not removed

Peritoneal dialysis: Significant drug removal is unlikely based on physiochemical characteristics

Dosage Forms AERO: 90 mcg/dose (17 g) [200 doses]; (Proventil®, Ventolin®): 90 mcg/dose (17 g) [200 doses]; Chlorofluorocarbon-free (Proventil® HFA): 90 mcg/dose (17 g). **CAP for oral inhalation**: (Ventolin® Rotacaps®): 200 mcg [to be used with Rotahaler® inhalation device]. **SOLN, inhalation:** 0.083% (3 mL), 0.5% (20 mL); (Airet®): 0.083%; (Proventil®): 0.083% (3 mL), 0.5% (20 mL); (Ventolin®): 0.5% (20 mL). **SYR,** as sulfate: 2 mg/5 mL (480 mL); (Proventil®, Ventolin®): 2 mg/5 mL (480 mL). **TAB,** as sulfate: 2 mg, 4 mg; (Proventil®, Ventolin®): 2 mg, 4 mg; Extended release: (Proventil® Repetabs®): 4 mg; (Volmax®): 4 mg, 8 mg

Contraindications Hypersensitivity to albuterol, adrenergic amines or any ingredients

Warnings/Precautions Use with caution in patients with hyperthyroidism, diabetes mellitus, or sensitivity to sympathomimetic amines; cardiovascular disorders including coronary insufficiency or hypertension; excessive use may result in tolerance

Some adverse reactions may occur more frequently in children 2-5 years of age than in adults and older children

Because of its minimal effect on beta$_1$-receptors and its relatively long duration of action, albuterol is a rational choice in the elderly when a beta agonist is indicated. All patients should utilize a spacer device when using a metered dose inhaler. Oral use should be avoided in the elderly due to adverse effects.

Pregnancy Risk Factor C

Pregnancy Implications

Clinical effects on the fetus: Crosses the placenta. Tocolytic effects, fetal tachycardia, fetal hypoglycemia secondary to maternal hyperglycemia with oral or intravenous routes reported. Available evidence suggests safe use during pregnancy.

Breast-feeding/lactation: No data on crossing into breast milk or clinical effects on the infant

Adverse Reactions

>10%:

- Cardiovascular: Tachycardia, palpitations, pounding heartbeat
- Gastrointestinal: GI upset, nausea

1% to 10%:

- Cardiovascular: Flushing of face, hypertension or hypotension
- Central nervous system: Nervousness, CNS stimulation, hyperactivity, insomnia, dizziness, lightheadedness, drowsiness, headache
- Gastrointestinal: Xerostomia, heartburn, vomiting, unusual taste
- Genitourinary: Dysuria
- Neuromuscular & skeletal: Muscle cramping, tremor, weakness
- Respiratory: Coughing
- Miscellaneous: Diaphoresis (increased)

<1%: Chest pain, loss of appetite, paradoxical bronchospasm, unusual pallor

Drug Interactions

Decreased effect: Beta-adrenergic blockers (eg, propranolol)

Increased therapeutic effect: Inhaled ipratropium may increase duration of bronchodilation, nifedipine may increase FEV-1

Increased toxicity: Cardiovascular effects are potentiated in patients also receiving MAO inhibitors, tricyclic antidepressants, sympathomimetic agents (eg, amphetamine, dopamine, dobutamine), inhaled anesthetics (eg, enflurane)

Onset Peak effect: Oral: 2-3 hours; Nebulization/oral inhalation: Within 0.5-2 hours

Duration Oral: 4-6 hours; Nebulization/oral inhalation: 3-4 hours

Half-Life Inhalation: 3.8 hours; Oral: 3.7-5 hours

Education and Monitoring Issues

Patient Education: Use exactly as directed. Do not use more often than recommended. Maintain adequate hydration (2-3 L/day of fluids unless instructed to restrict fluid intake). You may experience nervousness, dizziness, or fatigue (use caution when driving or engaging in hazardous activities until response to drug is known); dry mouth, unpleasant taste, stomach upset (frequent small meals, frequent mouth care, chewing gum, or sucking lozenges may help); or difficulty urinating (always void before treatment). Report unresolved GI upset, dizziness or fatigue, vision changes, chest pain or palpitations, persistent inability to void, nervousness or insomnia, muscle cramping or tremor, or unusual cough.

Monitoring Parameters: Heart rate, CNS stimulation, asthma symptoms, arterial or capillary blood gases (if patients condition warrants)

Related Information

Bronchodilators Comparison *on page 1235*
Ipratropium and Albuterol *on page 484*

- **Alcaine®** *see* Proparacaine *on page 782*

Alclometasone (al kloe MET a sone)

Pharmacologic Class Corticosteroid, Topical

U.S. Brand Names Aclovate® Topical

Generic Available No

Mechanism of Action Stimulates the synthesis of enzymes needed to decrease inflammation, suppress mitotic activity, and cause vasoconstriction

Use Treats inflammation of corticosteroid-responsive dermatosis (low potency topical corticosteroid); may be used in pediatric patients ≥1 year of age, although the safety and efficacy for >3 weeks have not been established. Use in pediatric patients <1 year of age is not recommended because safety and efficacy have not been established.

USUAL DOSAGE Topical: Apply a thin film to the affected area 2-3 times/day. Therapy should be discontinued when control is achieved; if no improvement is seen, reassessment of diagnosis may be necessary.

Dosage Forms CRM: 0.05% (15 g, 45 g, 60 g). **OINT, top:** 0.05% (15 g, 45 g, 60 g)

Contraindications Viral, fungal, or tubercular skin lesions, known hypersensitivity to alclometasone or any component

Warnings/Precautions Adverse systemic effects may occur when used on large areas of the body, denuded areas, for prolonged periods of time, with an occlusive dressing, and/or in infants or small children

Pregnancy Risk Factor C

Adverse Reactions

1% to 10%:

Dermatologic: Itching, erythema, dryness papular rashes
Local: Burning, irritation

<1%: Acneiform eruptions, hypertrichosis, hypopigmentation, maceration of skin, miliaria, perioral dermatitis, skin atrophy, striae

Education and Monitoring Issues

Patient Education: Before applying, gently wash area to reduce risk of infection; apply a thin film to cleansed area and rub in gently and thoroughly until medication vanishes; avoid exposure to sunlight, severe sunburn may occur

Manufacturer GlaxoWellcome

Related Information

Pharmaceutical Manufacturers Directory *on page 1020*

- **Alcomicin** *see* Gentamicin *on page 408*
- **Alconefrin® Nasal Solution [OTC]** *see* Phenylephrine *on page 727*
- **Aldactazide®** *see* Hydrochlorothiazide and Spironolactone *on page 443*
- **Aldactone®** *see* Spironolactone *on page 867*
- **Aldara™** *see* Imiquimod *on page 464*

Aldesleukin (al des LOO kin)

Pharmacologic Class Biological Response Modulator

U.S. Brand Names Proleukin®

Mechanism of Action IL-2 promotes proliferation, differentiation, and recruitment of T and B cells, natural killer (NK) cells, and thymocytes; IL-2 also causes cytolytic activity in a subset of lymphocytes and subsequent interactions between the immune system and malignant cells; IL-2 can stimulate lymphokine-activated killer (LAK) cells and tumor-infiltrating lymphocytes (TIL) cells. LAK cells (which are derived from lymphocytes from a patient and incubated in IL-2) have the ability to lyse cells which are resistant to NK cells; TIL cells (which are derived from cancerous tissue from a patient and incubated in IL-2) have been shown to be 50% more effective than LAK cells in experimental studies.

Use Treatment of metastatic renal cell carcinoma; also, investigated in tumors known to have a response to immunotherapy, such as melanoma; has been used in conjunction with LAK cells, TIL cells, IL-1, and interferon

USUAL DOSAGE Refer to individual protocols; all orders must be written in million International units (million IU)

Adults: Metastatic renal cell carcinoma (RCC):

Treatment consists of two 5-day treatment cycles separated by a rest period. 600,000 units/kg (0.037 mg/kg)/dose administered every 8 hours by a 15-minute I.V. infusion for a total of 14 doses; following 9 days of rest, the schedule is repeated for another 14 doses, for a maximum of 28 doses per course

Dose modification: In high-dose therapy of RCC, see manufacturer's guidelines for holding and restarting therapy; hold or interrupt a dose - DO NOT DOSE REDUCE; or refer to specific protocol

Retreatment: Patients should be evaluated for response approximately 4 weeks after completion of a course of therapy and again immediately prior to the scheduled start of the next treatment course; additional courses of treatment may be given to patients

(Continued)

Aldesleukin *(Continued)*

only if there is some tumor shrinkage or stable disease following the last course and retreatment is not contraindicated. Each treatment course should be separated by a rest period of at least 7 weeks from the date of hospital discharge; tumors have continued to regress up to 12 months following the initiation of therapy

Investigational regimen: S.C.: 11 million Units (flat dose) daily x 4 days per week for 4 consecutive weeks; repeat every 6 weeks

Dosage Forms POWDER for inj, lyophilized: 22 x 10^6 international units [18 million international units/mL = 1.1 mg/mL when reconstituted]

Contraindications Known history of hypersensitivity to interleukin-2 or any component; patients with an abnormal thallium stress test or pulmonary function test; patients who have had an organ allograft; retreatment in patients who have experienced sustained ventricular tachycardia (≥5 beats), cardiac rhythm disturbances not controlled or unresponsive to management, recurrent chest pain with EKG changes (consistent with angina or myocardial infarction), intubation required >72 hours, pericardial tamponade; renal dysfunction requiring dialysis >72 hours, coma or toxic psychosis lasting >48 hours, repetitive or difficult to control seizures, bowel ischemia/perforation, GI bleeding requiring surgery

Warnings/Precautions High-dose IL-2 therapy has been associated with capillary leak syndrome (CLS); CLS results in hypotension and reduced organ perfusion which may be severe and can result in death; therapy should be restricted to patients with normal cardiac and pulmonary functions as defined by thallium stress and formal pulmonary function testing; extreme caution should be used in patients with normal thallium stress tests and pulmonary functions tests who have a history of prior cardiac or pulmonary disease. Postnephrectomy patients must have a serum creatinine of ≤1.5 mg/dL prior to treatment.

Intensive aldesleukin treatment is associated with impaired neutrophil function (reduced chemotaxis) and with an increased risk of disseminated infection, including sepsis and bacterial endocarditis, in treated patients. Consequently, pre-existing bacterial infections should be adequately treated prior to initiation of therapy. Additionally, all patients with indwelling central lines should receive antibiotic prophylaxis effective against *S. aureus*. Antibiotic prophylaxis which has been associated with a reduced incidence of staphylococcal infections in aldesleukin studies includes the use of oxacillin, nafcillin, ciprofloxacin, or vancomycin.

Standard prophylactic supportive care during high-dose IL-2 treatment includes acetaminophen to relieve constitutional symptoms and an H_2-antagonist to reduce the risk of GI ulceration and/or bleeding.

Pregnancy Risk Factor C

Adverse Reactions

>10%:

Cardiovascular: Sensory dysfunction, sinus tachycardia, arrhythmias, pulmonary congestion; hypotension (dose-limiting toxicity) which may require vasopressor support and hemodynamic changes resembling those seen in septic shock can be seen within 2 hours of administration; angina, acute myocardial infarction, SVT with hypotension has been reported, edema

Central nervous system: Dizziness, pain, fever, chills, cognitive changes, fatigue, malaise, disorientation, somnolence, paranoid delusion, and other behavioral changes; reversible and dose related; however, may continue to worsen for several days even after the infusion is stopped

Dermatologic: Pruritus, erythema, rash, dry skin, exfoliative dermatitis, macular erythema

Gastrointestinal: Nausea, vomiting, weight gain, diarrhea, stomatitis, anorexia, GI bleeding

Hematologic: Anemia, thrombocytopenia, leukopenia, eosinophilia, coagulation disorders

Hepatic: Elevated transaminase and alkaline phosphatase, jaundice

Neuromuscular & skeletal: Weakness, rigors which can be decreased or ameliorated with acetaminophen or a nonsteroidal agent and meperidine

Renal: Oliguria, anuria, proteinuria; renal failure (dose-limiting toxicity) manifested as oliguria noted within 24-48 hours of initiation of therapy; marked fluid retention, azotemia, and increased serum creatinine seen, which may return to baseline within 7 days of discontinuation of therapy; hypophosphatemia

Respiratory: Dyspnea, pulmonary edema

1% to 10%: Cardiovascular: Increase in vascular permeability: Capillary-leak syndrome manifested by severe peripheral edema, ascites, pulmonary infiltration, and pleural effusion; occurs in 2% to 4% of patients and is resolved after therapy ends

<1%: Acidosis, allergic reactions, alopecia, arthritis, coma, congestive heart failure, hypercalcemia, hypocalcemia, hypomagnesemia, hypothyroidism, increased plasma levels of stress-related hormones, muscle spasm, pancreatitis, polyuria, seizure

Drug Interactions

Decreased toxicity: Corticosteroids have been shown to decrease toxicity of IL-2, but have not been used since there is concern that they may decrease the efficacy of the lymphokine

Increased toxicity:

Aldesleukin may affect central nervous function; therefore, interactions could occur following concomitant administration of psychotropic drugs (eg, narcotics, analgesics, antiemetics, sedatives, tranquilizers)

Concomitant administration of drugs possessing nephrotoxic (eg, aminoglycosides, indomethacin), myelotoxic (eg, cytotoxic chemotherapy), cardiotoxic (eg, doxorubicin), or hepatotoxic (eg, methotrexate, asparaginase) effects with aldesleukin may ↑ toxicity in these organ systems; the safety and efficacy of aldesleukin in combination with chemotherapy agents has not been established

Beta-blockers and other antihypertensives may potentiate the hypotension seen with Proleukin®

Iodinated contrast media: Acute reactions including fever, chills, nausea, vomiting, pruritus, rash, diarrhea, hypotension, edema, and oliguria have occurred within hours of contrast infusion; this reaction may occur within 4 weeks or up to several months after IL-2 administration

Half-Life 20-120 minutes

Education and Monitoring Issues

Patient Education: This drug can only be administered by infusion. Avoid alcohol and all OTC or prescription drugs unless approved by your oncologist. You will be sensitive to sunlight; use of sunblock (15 SPF or greater), wear protective clothing, or avoid direct sun exposure. You will be susceptible to infection; avoid crowds or infected persons or persons with contagious diseases. Frequent mouth care and small frequent meals may help counteract any GI effects you may experience and will help maintain adequate nutrition and fluid intake. This drug may result in many side effects; you will be monitored and assessed closely during therapy, however, it is important that you report any changes or problems for evaluation. Report any changes in urination, unusual bruising or bleeding, chest pain or palpitations, acute dizziness, respiratory difficulty, fever or chills, changes in cognition, rash, feelings of pain or numbness in extremities, severe GI upset or diarrhea, vaginal discharge or mouth sores, yellowing of eyes or skin, or any changes in color of urine or stool.

Monitoring Parameters:

The following clinical evaluations are recommended for all patients prior to beginning treatment and then daily during drug administration:

Standard hematologic tests including CBC, differential, and platelet counts

Blood chemistries including electrolytes, renal and hepatic function tests

Chest x-rays

Daily monitoring during therapy should include vital signs (temperature, pulse, blood pressure, and respiration rate) and weight; in a patient with a decreased blood pressure, especially <90 mm Hg, constant cardiac monitoring for rhythm should be conducted. If an abnormal complex or rhythm is seen, an EKG should be performed; vital signs in these hypotension patients should be taken hourly and central venous pressure (CVP) checked.

During treatment, pulmonary function should be monitored on a regular basis by clinical examination, assessment of vital signs and pulse oximetry. Patients with dyspnea or clinical signs of respiratory impairment (tachypnea or rales) should be further assessed with arterial blood gas determination. These tests are to be repeated as often as clinically indicated.

Cardiac function is assessed daily by clinical examination and assessment of vital signs. Patients with signs or symptoms of chest pain, murmurs, gallops, irregular rhythm or palpitations should be further assessed with an EKG examination and CPK evaluation. If there is evidence of cardiac ischemia or congestive heart failure, a repeat thallium study should be done.

Manufacturer Chiron Therapeutics

Related Information

Pharmaceutical Manufacturers Directory *on page 1020*

- ♦ **Aldoclor®** *see* Chlorothiazide and Methyldopa *on page 185*
- ♦ **Aldomet®** *see* Methyldopa *on page 586*
- ♦ **Aldoril®** *see* Methyldopa and Hydrochlorothiazide *on page 587*
- ♦ **Aldoril®-15** *see* Methyldopa and Hydrochlorothiazide *on page 587*
- ♦ **Aldoril®-25** *see* Methyldopa and Hydrochlorothiazide *on page 587*

Alendronate (a LEN droe nate)

Pharmacologic Class Bisphosphonate Derivative

U.S. Brand Names Fosamax®

Mechanism of Action A bisphosphonate which inhibits bone resorption via actions on osteoclasts or on osteoclast precursors; decreases the rate of bone resorption direction, leading to an indirect decrease in bone formation

Use Treatment of osteoporosis in postmenopausal women, Paget's disease of the bone; treatment of glucocorticoid-induced osteoporosis in males and females with low bone

(Continued)

Alendronate *(Continued)*

mineral density who are receiving a daily dosage ≥7.5 mg of prednisone (or equivalent) and who have low bone mineral density

USUAL DOSAGE Oral: Alendronate must be taken with plain water first thing in the morning and ≥30 minutes before the first food, beverage, or other medication of the day. Patients should be instructed to take alendronate with a full glass of water (6-8 oz) and not lie down for at least 30 minutes to improve alendronate absorption.

Adults: Patients with osteoporosis or Paget's disease should receive supplemental calcium and vitamin D if dietary intake is inadequate

Osteoporosis in postmenopausal women:

Prophylaxis: 5 mg once daily

Treatment: 10 mg once daily

Paget's disease of bone: 40 mg once daily for 6 months

Retreatment: Relapses during the 12 months following therapy occurred in 9% of patients who responded to treatment. Specific retreatment data are not available. Retreatment with alendronate may be considered, following a 6-month post-treatment evaluation period, in patients who have relapsed based on increases in serum alkaline phosphatase, which should be measured periodically. Retreatment may also be considered in those who failed to normalize their serum alkaline phosphatase.

Treatment of glucocorticoid-induced osteoporosis: 5 mg once daily. A dose of 10 mg once daily should be used in postmenopausal women who are not receiving estrogen. Patients treated with glucocorticoids should receive adequate amounts of calcium and vitamin D.

Elderly: No dosage adjustment is necessary

Dosage adjustment in renal impairment: Cl_{cr} <35 mL/minute: Alendronate is not recommended due to lack of experience

Dosage adjustment in hepatic impairment: None necessary

Dosage Forms TAB: 5 mg, 10 mg, 40 mg

Contraindications Hypersensitivity to bisphosphonates or any component of the product; hypocalcemia; abnormalities of the esophagus which delay esophageal emptying such as stricture or achalasia; inability to stand or sit upright for at least 30 minutes

Warnings/Precautions Use caution in patients with renal impairment; hypocalcemia must be corrected before therapy initiation with alendronate; ensure adequate calcium and vitamin D intake to provide for enhanced needs in patients with Paget's disease in whom the pretreatment rate of bone turnover may be greatly elevated

Pregnancy Risk Factor C

Adverse Reactions Note: Incidence of adverse effects increases significantly in patients treated for Paget's disease at 40 mg/day, mostly GI adverse effects

1% to 10%:

Central nervous system: Headache (2.6%); pain (4.1%)

Gastrointestinal: Flatulence (2.6%); acid regurgitation (2%); esophagitis ulcer (1.5%); dysphagia, abdominal distention (1%)

<1%: erythema (rare), gastritis (0.5%), rash

Alcohol Interactions Limit use (significant consumption may increase risk of osteoporosis)

Half-Life Estimated to exceed 10 years due to release of alendronate from the skeleton

Education and Monitoring Issues

Patient Education: Take as directed, with a full glass of water. Stay in sitting or standing position for 30 minutes following administration to reduce potential for esophageal irritation. Avoid aspirin- or aspirin-containing medications. Consult prescriber to determine necessity of lifestyle changes or dietary supplements of calcium or dietary vitamin D. You may experience GI upset (eg, flatulence, bloating, nausea, acid regurgitation); small frequent meals may help. Report acute headache or gastric pain, unresolved GI upset, or acid stomach.

Monitoring Parameters: Alkaline phosphatase should be periodically measured; serum calcium, phosphorus, and possibly potassium due to its drug class; use of absorptiometry may assist in noting benefit in osteoporosis; monitor pain and fracture rate

Reference Range: Calcium (total): Adults: 9.0-11.0 mg/dL (2.05-2.54 mmol/L), may slightly decrease with aging; phosphorus: 2.5-4.5 mg/dL (0.81-1.45 mmol/L)

Manufacturer Merck & Co

Related Information

Pharmaceutical Manufacturers Directory *on page 1020*

♦ **Alesse™** *see* Ethinyl Estradiol and Levonorgestrel *on page 341*

♦ **Aleve® [OTC]** *see* Naproxen *on page 636*

♦ **Alfenta** *see* Alfentanil *on page 32*

Alfentanil (al FEN ta nil)

Pharmacologic Class Analgesic, Narcotic; General Anesthetic

U.S. Brand Names Alfenta®

Use Analgesic adjunct given by continuous infusion or in incremental doses in maintenance of anesthesia with barbiturate or N_2O or a primary anesthetic agent for the induction of anesthesia in patients undergoing general surgery in which endotracheal intubation and mechanical ventilation are required

USUAL DOSAGE Doses should be titrated to appropriate effects; wide range of doses is dependent upon desired degree of analgesia/anesthesia

Children <12 years: Dose not established

Adults: Dose should be based on ideal body weight; see table.

Alfentanil

Indication	Approx Duration of Anesthesia (min)	Induction Period (Initial Dose) (mcg/kg)	Maintenance Period (Increments/ Infusion)	Total Dose (mcg/kg)	Effects
Incremental injection	≤30	8-20	3-5 mcg/kg or 0.5-1 mcg/kg/ min	8-40	Spontaneously breathing or assisted ventilation when required.
	30-60	20-50	5-15 mcg/kg	Up to 75	Assisted or controlled ventilation required. Attenuation of response to laryngoscopy and intubation.
Continuous infusion	>45	50-75	0.5-3 mcg/kg/ min average infusion rate 1-1.5 mcg/kg/min	Dependent on duration of procedure	Assisted or controlled ventilation required. Some attenuation of response to intubation and incision, with intraoperative stability.
Anesthetic induction	>45	130-245	0.5-1.5 mcg/kg/ min or general anesthetic	Dependent on duration of procedure	Assisted or controlled ventilation required. Administer slowly (over 3 minutes). Concentration of inhalation agents reduced by 30% to 50% for initial hour.

Contraindications Hypersensitivity to alfentanil hydrochloride or narcotics; increased intracranial pressure, severe respiratory depression

Pregnancy Risk Factor C

Related Information

Lipid-Lowering Agents Comparison *on page 1243*

Narcotic Agonists Comparison *on page 1244*

♦ **Alferon® N** *see* Interferon Alfa-n3 *on page 478*

Alglucerase (al GLOO ser ase)

Pharmacologic Class Enzyme

U.S. Brand Names Ceredase®

Use Orphan drug: Treatment of Gaucher's disease

USUAL DOSAGE Usually administered as a 20-60 unit/kg I.V. infusion given with a frequency ranging from 3 times/week to once every 2 weeks

Contraindications Hypersensitivity to any component

Pregnancy Risk Factor C

Alitretinoin (a li TRET i noyn)

Pharmacologic Class Antineoplastic Agent, Miscellaneous; Retinoic Acid Derivative

U.S. Brand Names Panretin®

Mechanism of Action Binds to retinoid receptors to inhibit growth of Kaposi's sarcoma

Use Topical treatment of cutaneous lesions in AIDS-related Kaposi's sarcoma; not indicated when systemic therapy for Kaposi's sarcoma is indicated

USUAL DOSAGE Topical: Apply gel twice daily to cutaneous Kaposi's sarcoma lesions

Dosage Forms GEL: 0.1%, 60 g tube

Contraindications Hypersensitivity to alitretinoin, other retinoids, or any component of the formulation

Warnings/Precautions May cause fetal harm if absorbed by a woman who is pregnant. Patients with cutaneous T cell lymphoma have a high incidence of treatment-limiting adverse reactions. May be photosensitizing (based on experience with other retinoids); minimize sun or other UV exposure of treated areas. Do not use concurrently with topical products containing DEET (increased toxicity may result). Safety in pediatric patients or geriatric patients has not been established. Occlusive dressing should not be used.

Pregnancy Risk Factor D

Pregnancy Implications Potentially teratogenic and/or embryotoxic; limb, craniofacial, or skeletal defects have been observed in animal models. If used during pregnancy or if the patient becomes pregnant while using alitretinoin, the woman should be advised of potential harm to the fetus. Women of childbearing potential should avoid becoming pregnant. Excretion in human breast milk is unknown; women are advised to discontinue breast-feeding prior to using this medication.

(Continued)

Alitretinoin *(Continued)*

Adverse Reactions

>10%:

Central nervous system: Pain (0% to 34%)

Dermatologic: Rash (25% to 77%), pruritus (8% to 11%)

Neuromuscular & skeletal: Paresthesia (3% to 22%)

5% to 10%:

Cardiovascular: Edema (3% to 8%)

Dermatologic: Exfoliative dermatitis (3% to 9%), skin disorder (0% to 8%)

Drug Interactions Increased toxicity of DEET may occur if products containing this compound are used concurrently with alitretinoin. Due to limited absorption after topical application, interaction with systemic medications is unlikely.

Education and Monitoring Issues

Patient Education: For external use only. Use exactly as directed; do not overuse. Avoid use of any product such as insect repellants containing DEET (check with your pharmacist). Wear protective clothing and or avoid exposure to direct sun or sunlamps. Wash hands thoroughly before applying. Avoid applying skin products that contain alcohol of harsh chemicals during treatment. Do not apply occlusive dressings. Stop treatment and inform prescriber if rash, skin irritation, redness, scaling, or excessive dryness appears.

Manufacturer Ligand Pharmaceuticals, Inc

Related Information

Pharmaceutical Manufacturers Directory *on page 1020*

- **Alka-Mints® [OTC]** *see* Calcium Carbonate *on page 130*
- **Alkeran®** *see* Melphalan *on page 561*
- **Allbee® With C** *see* Vitamins, Multiple *on page 981*
- **Allegra®** *see* Fexofenadine *on page 361*
- **Allegra-D™** *see* Fexofenadine and Pseudoephedrine *on page 362*
- **Allerdryl®** *see* Diphenhydramine *on page 282*
- **Allerest® Eye Drops [OTC]** *see* Naphazoline *on page 636*
- **Allerfrin® w/Codeine** *see* Triprolidine, Pseudoephedrine, and Codeine *on page 958*
- **Allergan® Ear Drops** *see* Antipyrine and Benzocaine *on page 67*
- **AllerMax® Oral [OTC]** *see* Diphenhydramine *on page 282*
- **Allernix®** *see* Diphenhydramine *on page 282*

Allopurinol (al oh PURE i nole)

Pharmacologic Class Xanthine Oxidase Inhibitor

U.S. Brand Names Aloprim™; Zyloprim®

Generic Available Yes

Mechanism of Action Allopurinol inhibits xanthine oxidase, the enzyme responsible for the conversion of hypoxanthine to xanthine to uric acid. Allopurinol is metabolized to oxypurinol which is also an inhibitor of xanthine oxidase; allopurinol acts on purine catabolism, reducing the production of uric acid without disrupting the biosynthesis of vital purines.

Use

Oral: Prevention of attack of gouty arthritis and nephropathy; also used to treat secondary hyperuricemia which may occur during treatment of tumors or leukemia, and to prevent recurrent calcium oxalate calculi

Intravenous: Management of patients with leukemia, lymphoma, and solid tumor malignancies who are receiving cancer chemotherapy which causes elevations of serum and urinary uric acid levels and who cannot tolerate oral therapy

Adult Maintenance Doses of Allopurinol*

Creatinine Clearance (mL/min)	Maintenance Dose of Allopurinol (mg)
140	400 qd
120	350 qd
100	300 qd
80	250 qd
60	200 qd
40	150 qd
20	100 qd
10	100 q2d
0	100 q3d

*This table is based on a standard maintenance dose of 300 mg of allopurinol per day for a patient with a creatinine clearance of 100 mL/min.

USUAL DOSAGE

Oral:

Children ≤10 years: 10 mg/kg/day in 2-3 divided doses **or** 200-300 mg/m^2/day in 2-4 divided doses, maximum: 800 mg/24 hours

Alternative: <6 years: 150 mg/day in 3 divided doses; 6-10 years: 300 mg/day in 2-3 divided doses

Children >10 years and Adults: Daily doses >300 mg should be administered in divided doses

Myeloproliferative neoplastic disorders: 600-800 mg/day in 2-3 divided doses for prevention of acute uric acid nephropathy for 2-3 days starting 1-2 days before chemotherapy

Gout: Mild: 200-300 mg/day; Severe: 400-600 mg/day

Elderly: Initial: 100 mg/day, increase until desired uric acid level is obtained

Dosing adjustment in renal impairment: Oral: Must be adjusted due to accumulation of allopurinol and metabolites; removed by hemodialysis. See table.

Hemodialysis: Administer dose posthemodialysis or administer 50% supplemental dose

I.V.: Intravenous daily dose can be given as a single infusion or in equally divided doses at 6-, 8-, or 12-hour intervals. A fluid intake sufficient to yield a daily urinary output of at least 2 L in adults and the maintenance of a neutral or, preferably, slightly alkaline urine are desirable.

Children: Starting dose: 200 mg/m^2/day

Adults: 200-400 mg/m^2]/day (max: 600 mg/day)

Dosing adjustment in renal impairment: I.V.:

Cl_{cr} 10-20 mL/minute: 200 mg/day

Cl_{cr} 3-10 mL/minute: 100 mg/day

Cl_{cr} <3 mL/minute: 100 mg/day at extended intervals

Dosage Forms **INJ:** 500 mg. **TAB:** 100 mg, 300 mg

Contraindications Not to be used in pregnancy or lactation, or in patients with a previous severe allergy reaction to allopurinol or any component

Warnings/Precautions Do not use to treat asymptomatic hyperuricemia. Discontinue at first signs of rash; reduce dosage in renal insufficiency, reinstate with caution in patients who have had a previous mild allergic reaction, use with caution in children; monitor liver function and complete blood counts before initiating therapy and periodically during therapy, use with caution in patients taking diuretics concurrently. Risk of skin rash may be increased in patients receiving amoxicillin or ampicillin. The risk of hypersensitivity may be increased in patients receiving thiazides, and possibly ACE inhibitors.

Pregnancy Risk Factor C

Pregnancy Implications Clinical effects on the fetus: There are few reports describing the use of allopurinol during pregnancy; no adverse fetal outcomes attributable to allopurinol have been reported in humans

Adverse Reactions The most common adverse reaction to allopurinol is a skin rash (usually maculopapular; however, more severe reactions, including Stevens-Johnson syndrome, have also been reported). While some studies cite an incidence of these reactions as high as >10% of cases (often in association with ampicillin or amoxicillin), the product labeling cites a much lower incidence, reflected below. Allopurinol should be discontinued at the first appearance of a rash or other sign of hypersensitivity.

>1%:

Dermatologic: Rash (1.5%)

Gastrointestinal: Nausea (1.3%), vomiting (1.2%)

Renal: Renal failure/impairment (1.2%)

<1%: Acute tubular necrosis, agranulocytosis, angioedema, aplastic anemia, bronchospasm, cataracts, dyspepsia, exfoliative dermatitis, epistaxis, granuloma anulare, granulomatous hepatitis, gynecomastia, hypersensitivity syndrome, increased alkaline phosphatase or hepatic transaminases, interstitial nephritis, macular retinitis, nephrolithiasis, neuritis, pancreatitis, paresthesia, peripheral neuropathy, Steven's Johnson syndrome, TEN, toxic pustuloderma, vasculitis

Drug Interactions Hepatic enzyme inhibitor

Decreased effect: Alcohol decreases effectiveness, uricosurics

Increased toxicity:

Inhibits metabolism of azathioprine and mercaptopurine (reduce to 1/3 or 1/4 of usual dose)

Use with ampicillin or amoxicillin may increase the incidence of skin rash

Urinary acidification with large amounts of vitamin C may increase kidney stone formation

Thiazide diuretics enhance toxicity, monitor renal function; thiazide diuretics and captopril (possibly other ACE inhibitors) may increase risk of hypersensitivity

Vidarabine neurotoxicity may be enhanced

Cyclosporine levels may be increased

Hepatic iron uptake may be increased with iron supplements

Allopurinol prolongs half-life of oral anticoagulants; allopurinol increases serum half-life of theophylline; allopurinol may compete for excretion in renal tubule with chlorpropamide and increases chlorpropamide's serum half-life

Alcohol Interactions Avoid use (may decrease effectiveness)

(Continued)

Allopurinol *(Continued)*

Onset Decreases in serum uric acid occur in 1-2 days with nadir achieved in 1-2 weeks

Half-Life Parent drug: 1-3 hours; Oxypurinol: 18-30 hours; End-stage renal disease: Half-life prolonged

Education and Monitoring Issues

Patient Education: Take as directed. Maintain adequate hydration (2-3 L/day of fluids unless instructed to restrict fluid intake) to avoid possible adverse renal problems. While using this medication, do not use alcohol, other prescription or OTC medications, or vitamin substances without consulting prescriber. You may experience drowsiness (use caution when driving or engaging in tasks requiring alertness until response to drug is known); nausea, vomiting, or heartburn (small frequent meals, frequent mouth care, chewing gum, or sucking lozenges may help); hair loss (reversible). Report skin rash or lesions; painful urination or blood in urine or stool; unresolved nausea or vomiting; numbness of extremities; pain or irritation of the eyes; swelling of lips, mouth, or tongue; unusual fatigue; easy bruising or bleeding; yellowing of skin or eyes; or any change in color of urine or stool.

Monitoring Parameters: CBC, serum uric acid levels, I & O, hepatic and renal function, especially at start of therapy

Reference Range: Uric acid, serum: An increase occurs during childhood

Adults:

Male: 3.4-7 mg/dL or slightly more

Female: 2.4-6 mg/dL or slightly more

Values >7 mg/dL are sometimes arbitrarily regarded as hyperuricemia, but there is no sharp line between normals on the one hand, and the serum uric acid of those with clinical gout. Normal ranges cannot be adjusted for purine ingestion, but high purine diet increases uric acid. Uric acid may be increased with body size, exercise, and stress.

- **Almora® (Gluconate)** *see* Magnesium Salts (Other) *on page 551*
- **Alocril™** *see* Nedocromil Sodium *on page 639*
- **Alomide® Ophthalmic** *see* Lodoxamide Tromethamine *on page 536*
- **Aloprim™** *see* Allopurinol *on page 34*
- **Alor® 5/500** *see* Hydrocodone and Aspirin *on page 445*
- **Alora™ Transdermal** *see* Estradiol *on page 327*

Alosetron (a LOE se tron)

Pharmacologic Class 5-HT_3 Receptor Antagonist

U.S. Brand Names Lotronex®

Mechanism of Action Alosetron is a potent and selective antagonist of a subtype of the serotonin receptor, 5-HT_3 receptor. 5-HT_3 receptors are extensively distributed on enteric neurons in the human gastrointestinal tract, as well as other peripheral and central locations. Activation of these channels affect the regulation of visceral pain, colonic transit, and gastrointestinal secretions. In patients with irritable bowel syndrome, improvement in pain, abdominal discomfort, urgency, and diarrhea may occur.

Use Treatment of irritable bowel syndrome (IBS) in women whose predominant bowel symptom is diarrhea; use in males with IBS has not been substantiated

Investigational use: Alosetron has demonstrated effectiveness as an antiemetic for a wide variety of causes of emesis

USUAL DOSAGE

Adults: Female: Oral: 1 mg twice daily with or without food. Patients who experience constipation may need to interrupt therapy.

Dosage adjustment in renal impairment: No dosage adjustment is recommended for patients with Cl_{cr} 4-56 mL/minute; use in Cl_{cr} <4 mL/minute or hemodialysis patients has not been studied

Dosage adjustment in hepatic impairment: Specific guidelines are not available

Elderly: Dosage adjustment is not required

Dosage Forms TAB: 1 mg

Contraindications Hypersensitivity to alosetron or any component

Warnings/Precautions Constipation is a frequent, dose-related side effect. Patients who have not had a bowel movement in 3-4 days should be instructed to hold therapy until bowel movements resume. Acute ischemic colitis has been reported during alosetron treatment. Discontinue in patients who experience rectal bleeding or a sudden worsening of abdominal pain. Use with caution in patients with a history of bowel obstruction. Safety and efficacy have not been established in pediatric or male patients.

Pregnancy Risk Factor B

Pregnancy Implications No adequate and well-controlled studies have been done in pregnant women. Alosetron should be used in pregnant women only if clearly needed. Animal studies indicate that alosetron and/or metabolites are excreted in breast milk. It is not known if alosetron in excreted in human milk. Caution should be used in administering alosetron to a nursing woman.

Adverse Reactions

>10%: Gastrointestinal: Constipation (28%)

1% to 10%:

Central nervous system: Sleep disorders (3%), depression (2%)

Cardiovascular: Hypertension (2%)

Gastrointestinal: Nausea (7%), gastrointestinal discomfort and pain (5%), abdominal discomfort and pain (5%), gastrointestinal gaseous symptoms (3%), viral infections (2%), dyspepsia (3%), abdominal distention (2%), hemorrhoids (2%)

Otic: Bacterial ear infection (1%)

Respiratory: Allergic rhinitis (2%); throat and tonsil discomfort and pain (1%); bacterial ear, nose and throat infection (1%)

<1%: Elevated hepatic transaminases (0.5%), acute ischemic colitis, arrhythmias, contusions, hematomas, photophobia, proctitis, abnormal bilirubin levels, breathing disorders, cough, sedation and abnormal dreams, allergies, allergic reactions, unusual odors and taste, anxiety, menstrual disorders, sexual function disorders, acne, folliculitis, urinary infections, polyuria, diuresis

Case report: Hepatitis

Drug Interactions CYP2C9, CYP3A4, and CYP1A2 enzyme substrate; inhibits CYP1A2, 2E1 only at extremely high concentrations (no clinical significance)

Inducers or inhibitors of these enzymes theoretically may change the clearance of alosetron, but this has not been evaluated. Alosetron inhibits N-acetyltransferase which may influence the metabolism of drugs such as isoniazid, procainamide, and hydralazine but there has not been any investigation of this.

Onset 1 hour to peak effect

Duration Sufficient to permit once-daily dosing

Half-Life 1.5 hours

Education and Monitoring Issues

Patient Education: Take as directed. Discontinue medication and notify prescriber if you develop sudden cramping or abdominal pain, blood in stool, or persistent constipation. Consult prescriber if breast-feeding.

Dietary Considerations: Take with or without food

Manufacturer GlaxoWellcome

Related Information

Pharmaceutical Manufacturers Directory *on page 1020*

♦ **Alpha-Baclofen®** *see* Baclofen *on page 90*

♦ **Alphagan®** *see* Brimonidine *on page 112*

♦ **Alpha-Lac** *see* Lactulose *on page 506*

♦ **Alphamin®** *see* Hydroxocobalamin *on page 451*

♦ **Alpha-Tamoxifen®** *see* Tamoxifen *on page 890*

♦ **Alphatrex®** *see* Betamethasone *on page 103*

Alprazolam (al PRAY zoe lam)

Pharmacologic Class Benzodiazepine

U.S. Brand Names Alprazolam Intensol®; Xanax®

Generic Available No

Mechanism of Action Binds at stereospecific receptors at several sites within the central nervous system, including the limbic system, reticular formation; effects may be mediated through GABA

Use Treatment of anxiety; adjunct in the treatment of depression; management of panic attacks

USUAL DOSAGE Oral:

Children <18 years: Safety and dose have not been established

Adults:

Anxiety: Effective doses are 0.5-4 mg/day in divided doses; the manufacturer recommends starting at 0.25-0.5 mg 3 times/day; titrate dose upward; maximum: 4 mg/day

Depression: Average dose required: 2.5-3 mg/day in divided doses

Alcohol withdrawal: Usual dose: 2-2.5 mg/day in divided doses

Panic disorder: Many patients obtain relief at 2 mg/day, as much as 6 mg/day may be required

Dosing adjustment in hepatic impairment: Reduce dose by 50% to 60% or avoid in cirrhosis

Note: Treatment >4 months should be re-evaluated to determine the patient's need for the drug

Dosage Forms SOLN, oral: 1 mg/mL (30 mL), 0.5 mg/5 mL (500 mL). **TAB:** 0.25 mg, 0.5 mg, 1 mg, 2 mg

Contraindications Hypersensitivity to alprazolam or any component; there may be a cross-sensitivity with other benzodiazepines; severe uncontrolled pain, narrow-angle glaucoma, severe respiratory depression, pre-existing CNS depression; not to be used in pregnancy or lactation

Warnings/Precautions Withdrawal symptoms including seizures have occurred 18 hours to 3 days after abrupt discontinuation; when discontinuing therapy, decrease daily dose by no more than 0.5 mg every 3 days; reduce dose in patients with significant hepatic disease. Not intended for management of anxieties and minor distresses associated with everyday life.

(Continued)

Alprazolam *(Continued)*

Pregnancy Risk Factor D

Adverse Reactions

>10%:

Central nervous system: Drowsiness, fatigue, ataxia, lightheadedness, memory impairment, dysarthria, irritability

Dermatologic: Rash

Endocrine & metabolic: Decreased libido, menstrual disorders

Gastrointestinal: Xerostomia, decreased salivation, increased or decreased appetite, weight gain or loss

Genitourinary: Micturition difficulties

1% to 10%:

Cardiovascular: Hypotension

Central nervous system: Confusion, dizziness, disinhibition, akathisia, increased libido

Dermatologic: Dermatitis

Gastrointestinal: Increased salivation

Genitourinary: Sexual dysfunction, incontinence

Neuromuscular & skeletal: Rigidity, tremor, muscle cramps

Otic: Tinnitus

Respiratory: Nasal congestion

Drug Interactions CYP3A3/4 enzyme substrate

Carbamazepine, rifampin, rifabutin may enhance the metabolism of alprazolam and decrease its therapeutic effect; consider using an alternative sedative/hypnotic agent

Amprenavir, cimetidine, ciprofloxacin, clarithromycin, clozapine, CNS depressants, diltiazem, disulfiram, digoxin, erythromycin, ethanol, fluconazole, fluoxetine, fluvoxamine, isoniazid, itraconazole, ketoconazole, labetalol, levodopa, loxapine, metoprolol, metronidazole, miconazole, nefazodone, nelfinavir, omeprazole, phenytoin, rifabutin, rifampin, ritonavir, troleandomycin, valproic acid, verapamil may increase the serum level and/or toxicity of alprazolam; monitor for altered benzodiazepine response

Alcohol Interactions Avoid use (may increase central nervous system depression)

Onset Within 1 hour

Duration Variable, 8-24 hours

Half-Life 12-15 hours

Education and Monitoring Issues

Patient Education: Take exactly as directed (do not increase dose or frequency); may cause physical and/or psychological dependence. Do not use excessive alcohol, or other prescription or OTC medications (especially pain medications, sedatives, antihistamines, or hypnotics) without consulting prescriber. Maintain adequate hydration (2-3 L/day of fluids unless instructed to restrict fluid intake). You may experience drowsiness, lightheadedness, impaired coordination, dizziness, or blurred vision (use caution when driving or engaging in hazardous tasks until response to drug is known); nausea, vomiting, or dry mouth (small frequent meals, frequent mouth care, chewing gum, or sucking lozenges may help); constipation (increased exercise, fluids, or dietary fruit and fiber may help); altered sexual drive or ability (reversible); photosensitivity (use sunscreen, wear protective clothing and eyewear, avoid direct sunlight). Report persistent CNS effects (eg, confusion, depression, increased sedation, excitation, headache, agitation, insomnia or nightmares, dizziness, fatigue, impaired coordination, changes in personality, or changes in cognition); changes in urinary pattern; muscle cramping, weakness, tremors, or rigidity; ringing in ears or visual disturbances; chest pain, palpitations, or rapid heartbeat; excessive perspiration; excessive GI symptoms (cramping, constipation, vomiting, anorexia); or worsening of condition.

Dietary Considerations: Grapefruit juice: May increase serum level and/or toxicity of alprazolam

Monitoring Parameters: Respiratory and cardiovascular status

♦ **Alprazolam Intensol®** *see* Alprazolam *on page 37*

Alprostadil (al PROS ta dill)

Pharmacologic Class Prostaglandin

U.S. Brand Names Caverject® Injection; Edex™ Injection; Muse® Pellet; Prostin VR Pediatric® Injection

Use Temporary maintenance of patency of ductus arteriosus in neonates with ductal-dependent congenital heart disease until surgery can be performed. These defects include cyanotic (eg, pulmonary atresia, pulmonary stenosis, tricuspid atresia, Fallot's tetralogy, transposition of the great vessels) and acyanotic (eg, interruption of aortic arch, coarctation of aorta, hypoplastic left ventricle) heart disease; diagnosis and treatment of erectile dysfunction of vasculogenic, psychogenic, or neurogenic etiology; adjunct in the diagnosis of erectile dysfunction

Investigational: Treatment of pulmonary hypertension in infants and children with congenital heart defects with left-to-right shunts

USUAL DOSAGE

Patent ductus arteriosus (Prostin VR Pediatric®):

I.V. continuous infusion into a large vein, or alternatively through an umbilical artery catheter placed at the ductal opening: 0.05-0.1 mcg/kg/minute with therapeutic response, rate is reduced to lowest effective dosage; with unsatisfactory response, rate is increased gradually; maintenance: 0.01-0.4 mcg/kg/minute

PGE_1 is usually given at an infusion rate of 0.1 mcg/kg/minute, but it is often possible to reduce the dosage to $^1/_2$ or even $^1/_{10}$ without losing the therapeutic effect. The mixing schedule is shown in the table.

Alprostadil

Add 1 Ampul (500 mcg) to:	Concentration (mcg/mL)	Infusion Rate	
		mL/kg/min Needed to Infuse 0.1 mcg/kg/min	mL/kg/24 h
250 mL	2	0.05	72
100 mL	5	0.02	28.8
50 mL	10	0.01	14.4
25 mL	20	0.005	7.2

Therapeutic response is indicated by increased pH in those with acidosis or by an increase in oxygenation (pO_2) usually evident within 30 minutes

Erectile dysfunction

Caverject®, Edex®:

Vasculogenic, psychogenic, or mixed etiology: Individualize dose by careful titration; usual dose: 2.5-60 mcg (doses >60 mcg are not recommended); initiate dosage titration at 2.5 mcg, increasing by 2.5 mcg to a dose of 5 mcg and then in increments of 5-10 mcg depending on the erectile response until the dose produces an erection suitable for intercourse, not lasting >1 hour; if there is absolutely no response to initial 2.5 mcg dose, the second dose may increased to 7.5 mcg, followed by increments of 5-10 mcg

Neurogenic etiology (eg, spinal cord injury): Initiate dosage titration at 1.25 mcg, increasing to a doses of 2.5 mcg and then 5 mcg; increase further in increments 5 mcg until the dose is reached that produces an erection suitable for intercourse, not lasting >1 hour

Note: Patient must stay in the prescriber's office until complete detumescence occurs; if there is no response, then the next higher dose may be given within 1 hour; if there is still no response, a 1-day interval before giving the next dose is recommended; increasing the dose or concentration in the treatment of impotence results in increasing pain and discomfort

Muse® Pellet: Intraurethral: Administer as needed to achieve an erection; duration of action is about 30-60 minutes; use only two systems per 24-hour period

Contraindications Hyaline membrane disease or persistent fetal circulation and when a dominant left-to-right shunt is present; respiratory distress syndrome; hypersensitivity to the drug or components; conditions predisposing patients to priapism (sickle cell anemia, multiple myeloma, leukemia); patients with anatomical deformation of the penis, penile implants; use in men for whom sexual activity is inadvisable or contraindicated; pregnancy

Pregnancy Risk Factor X

♦ **Alrex™** *see* Loteprednol *on page 544*

♦ **Altace™** *see* Ramipril *on page 807*

Alteplase (AL te plase)

Pharmacologic Class Thrombolytic Agent

U.S. Brand Names Activase®

Generic Available No

Mechanism of Action Initiates local fibrinolysis by binding to fibrin in a thrombus (clot) and converts entrapped plasminogen to plasmin

Use Management of acute myocardial infarction for the lysis of thrombi in coronary arteries; management of acute massive pulmonary embolism (PE) in adults

Acute myocardial infarction (AMI): Chest pain ≥20 minutes, ≤12-24 hours; S-T elevation ≥0.1 mV in at least two EKG leads

Acute pulmonary embolism (APE): Age ≤75 years: As soon as possible within 5 days of thrombotic event. Documented massive pulmonary embolism by pulmonary angiography or echocardiography or high probability lung scan with clinical shock.

Acute ischemic stroke (rule out hemorrhagic courses before administering)

Unlabeled uses: Peripheral arterial occlusion treatment and central venous catheter clearance

USUAL DOSAGE

Coronary artery thrombi: I.V.: Front loading dose: Total dose is 100 mg over 1.5 hours (for patients who weigh ≤67 kg, use 1.25 mg/kg/total dose). Add this dose to a 100 mL bag of 0.9% sodium chloride for a total volume of 200 mL. Infuse 15 mg (30 mL) over 1-2

(Continued)

Alteplase *(Continued)*

minutes; infuse 50 mg (100 mL) over 30 minutes. Begin heparin 5000-10,000 unit bolus followed by continuous infusion of 1000 units/hour. Infuse the remaining 35 mg (70 mL) of alteplase over the next hour. For ≤67 kg: 15 mg I.V. bolus over 1-2 minutes. Infuse 0.75 mg/kg (not to exceed 50 mg) over next 30 minutes and then 0.5 mg/kg over next 60 minutes (not to exceed 35 mg).

Acute pulmonary embolism: 100 mg over 2 hours

Acute ischemic stroke: Doses should be given within the first 3 hours of onset of symptoms. Load with 0.09 mg/kg as a bolus, followed by 0.81 mg/kg as a continuous infusion over 60 minutes; maximum total dose should not exceed 90 mg

Unlabeled use: Central venous catheter clearance: 2 mg (1 mg/mL) retained in catheter for 2 hours

Dosage Forms POWDER for inj, lyophilized (recombinant): 20 mg [11.6 million units] (20 mL), 50 mg [29 million units] (50 mL), 100 mg [58 million units] (100 mL)

Contraindications No central venous puncture (CVP line) or noncompressible arterial sticks. BP systolic ≥185, diastolic ≥110 unresponsive to nitrate or calcium antagonist; recent (within 1 month): cerebrovascular accident, gastrointestinal bleeding, trauma or surgery, prolonged external cardiac massage; intracranial neoplasm, suspected aortic dissection, arteriovenous malformation or aneurysm, bleeding diathesis, hemostatic defects, seizure occurring at the time of stroke, suspicion of subarachnoid hemorrhage

Warnings/Precautions Doses >150 mg have been associated with an increase of intracranial hemorrhage; acute pericarditis, severe liver dysfunction, septic thrombophlebitis, patients receiving concurrent oral anticoagulants, advanced age

Pregnancy Risk Factor C

Adverse Reactions As with all drugs which may affect hemostasis, bleeding is the major adverse effect associated with alteplase. Hemorrhage may occur at virtually any site. Risk is dependent on multiple variables, including the dosage administered, concurrent use of multiple agents which alter hemostasis, and patient predisposition. Rapid lysis of coronary artery thrombi by thrombolytic agents may be associated with reperfusion-related atrial and/or ventricular arrhythmias.

1% to 10%:

Cardiovascular: Hypotension
Central nervous system: Fever
Dermatologic: Bruising (1%)
Gastrointestinal: GI hemorrhage (5%), nausea, vomiting
Local: Bleeding at catheter puncture site (15.3%, accelerated administration)
Hematologic: Bleeding (0.5% major, 7% minor: GUSTO trial)
Genitourinary: GU hemorrhage (4%)

<1% (limited to important or life-threatening symptoms): Intracranial hemorrhage (0.4% to 0.87% when dose is ≤100 mg), retroperitoneal hemorrhage, pericardial hemorrhage, gingival hemorrhage, epistaxis, allergic reactions: anaphylaxis, anaphylactoid reactions, laryngeal edema, rash, and urticaria (<0.02%).

Additional cardiovascular events associated with use in myocardial infarction: A-V block, cardiogenic shock, heart failure, cardiac arrest, recurrent ischemia/infarction, myocardial rupture, electromechanical dissociation, pericardial effusion, pericarditis, mitral regurgitation, cardiac tamponade, thromboembolism, pulmonary edema, asystole, ventricular tachycardia, bradycardia, ruptured intracranial A-V malformation, seizure, hemorrhagic bursitis, cholesterol crystal embolization

Additional events associated with use in pulmonary embolism: Pulmonary re-embolization, pulmonary edema, pleural effusion, thromboembolism

Additional events associated with use in stroke: Cerebral edema, cerebral herniation, seizure, new ischemic stroke

Drug Interactions

Aminocaproic acid (antifibrinolytic agent) may decrease effectiveness.

Drugs which affect platelet function (eg, NSAIDs, dipyridamole, ticlopidine, clopidogrel, IIb/IIIa antagonists) may potentiate the risk of hemorrhage; use with caution.

Heparin and aspirin: Use with aspirin and heparin may increase the risk of bleeding. However, aspirin and heparin were used concomitantly with alteplase in many patients in myocardial infarction or pulmonary embolism trials. This combination was prohibited in the NINDS t-PA stroke trial.

Nitroglycerin may increase the hepatic clearance of alteplase, potentially reducing lytic activity (limited clinical information).

Warfarin or oral anticoagulants: Risk of bleeding may be increased during concurrent therapy.

Duration >50% present in plasma is cleared within 5 minutes after the infusion has been terminated, and ~80% is cleared within 10 minutes

Half-Life Cleared rapidly by the liver; ~80% is cleared within 10 minutes after infusion is terminated

Education and Monitoring Issues

Patient Education: This medication can only be administered I.V. You will have a tendency to bleed easily following this medication; use caution to prevent injury - use electric razor, soft toothbrush, and use caution with sharps. Strict bedrest should be maintained to reduce the risk of bleeding. If bleeding occurs, apply pressure to bleeding spot until bleeding stops completely. Report unusual bruising or bleeding; blood in urine, stool, or vomitus; bleeding gums; changes in vision; difficulty breathing; or chest pain.

Reference Range:

Not routinely measured; literature supports therapeutic levels of 0.52-1.8 μg/mL
Fibrinogen: 200-400 mg/dL
Activated partial thromboplastin time (APTT): 22.5-38.7 seconds
Prothrombin time (PT): 10.9-12.2 seconds

Manufacturer Genentech, Inc

Related Information

Pharmaceutical Manufacturers Directory *on page 1020*

- **ALternaGEL® [OTC]** *see* Aluminum Hydroxide *on page 41*
- **Alu-Cap® [OTC]** *see* Aluminum Hydroxide *on page 41*
- **Alugel** *see* Aluminum Hydroxide *on page 41*

Aluminum Acetate and Acetic Acid

(a LOO mi num AS e tate & a SEE tik AS id)

Pharmacologic Class Otic Agent, Anti-infective

U.S. Brand Names Otic Domeboro®

Dosage Forms SOLN, otic: Aluminum acetate 10% and acetic acid 2% (60 mL)

Aluminum Hydroxide (a LOO mi num hye DROKS ide)

Pharmacologic Class Antacid; Antidote

U.S. Brand Names ALternaGEL® [OTC]; Alu-Cap® [OTC]; Alu-Tab® [OTC]; Amphojel® [OTC]; Dialume® [OTC]; Nephrox Suspension [OTC]

Generic Available Yes

Use Treatment of hyperacidity; hyperphosphatemia

USUAL DOSAGE Oral:

Peptic ulcer disease:
Children: 5-15 mL/dose every 3-6 hours or 1 and 3 hours after meals and at bedtime
Adults: 15-45 mL every 3-6 hours or 1 and 3 hours after meals and at bedtime

Prophylaxis against gastrointestinal bleeding:
Infants: 2-5 mL/dose every 1-2 hours
Children: 5-15 mL/dose every 1-2 hours
Adults: 30-60 mL/dose every hour
Titrate to maintain the gastric pH >5

Hyperphosphatemia:
Children: 50-150 mg/kg/24 hours in divided doses every 4-6 hours, titrate dosage to maintain serum phosphorus within normal range
Adults: 500-1800 mg, 3-6 times/day, between meals and at bedtime; best taken with a meal or within 20 minutes of a meal

Antacid: Adults: 30 mL 1 and 3 hours postprandial and at bedtime

Dosage Forms CAP: (Alu-Cap®): 400 mg; (Dialume®): 500 mg. **LIQ:** 600 mg/5 mL; (ALternaGEL®): 600 mg/5 mL. **SUSP, oral:** 320 mg/5 mL, 450 mg/5 mL, 675 mg/5 mL; (Amphojel®): 320 mg/5 mL. **TAB:** (Amphojel®): 300 mg, 600 mg; (Alu-Tab®): 500 mg

Contraindications Hypersensitivity to aluminum salts or drug components

Warnings/Precautions Hypophosphatemia may occur with prolonged administration or large doses; aluminum intoxication and osteomalacia may occur in patients with uremia. Use with caution in patients with congestive heart failure, renal failure, edema, cirrhosis, and low sodium diets, and patients who have recently suffered gastrointestinal hemorrhage; uremic patients not receiving dialysis may develop osteomalacia and osteoporosis due to phosphate depletion.

Elderly, due to disease and/or drug therapy, may be predisposed to constipation and fecal impaction. Careful evaluation of possible drug interactions must be done. When used as an antacid in ulcer treatment, consider buffer capacity (mEq/mL) to calculate dose; consider renal insufficiency as predisposition to aluminum toxicity.

Pregnancy Risk Factor C

Pregnancy Implications

Clinical effects on the fetus: No data available; available evidence suggests safe use during pregnancy and breast-feeding
Breast-feeding/lactation: No data available

Adverse Reactions

>10%: Gastrointestinal: Constipation, chalky taste, stomach cramps, fecal impaction
1% to 10%: Gastrointestinal: Nausea, vomiting, discoloration of feces (white speckles)
<1%: Hypomagnesemia, hypophosphatemia

Drug Interactions Decreased effect: Tetracyclines, digoxin, indomethacin, or iron salts, isoniazid, allopurinol, benzodiazepines, corticosteroids, penicillamine, phenothiazines, ranitidine, ketoconazole, itraconazole

Education and Monitoring Issues

Patient Education: Take as directed, preferably 2 hours before or 2 hours after meals and any other medications. Dilute liquid dose with water or juice and shake well. Do not increase sodium intake and maintain adequate hydration (2-3 L/day of fluids unless

(Continued)

Aluminum Hydroxide *(Continued)*

instructed to restrict fluid intake). Chew tablet thoroughly before swallowing with full glass of water. You may experience constipation (increased exercise or dietary fluids, fiber, and fruit may help). If unrelieved, contact prescriber. Report unresolved nausea, malaise, muscle weakness, blood in stool or black stool, or abdominal pain.

Monitoring Parameters: Monitor phosphorous levels periodically when patient is on chronic therapy

♦ **Alupent®** *see* Metaproterenol *on page 572*
♦ **Alu-Tab® [OTC]** *see* Aluminum Hydroxide *on page 41*

Amantadine (a MAN ta deen)

Pharmacologic Class Anti-Parkinson's Agent (Dopamine Agonist); Antiviral Agent

U.S. Brand Names Symadine®; Symmetrel®

Generic Available Yes

Mechanism of Action As an antiviral, blocks the uncoating of influenza A virus preventing penetration of virus into host; antiparkinsonian activity may be due to its blocking the reuptake of dopamine into presynaptic neurons and causing direct stimulation of postsynaptic receptors

Use Symptomatic and adjunct treatment of parkinsonism; prophylaxis and treatment of influenza A viral infection; treatment of drug-induced extrapyramidal symptoms

USUAL DOSAGE

Children:

- Influenza treatment:
  - 1-9 years: (<45 kg): 5-9 mg/kg/day in 1-2 divided doses to a maximum of 150 mg/day
  - 10-12 years: 100-200 mg/day in 1-2 divided doses
- Influenza prophylaxis: Administer for 10-21 days following exposure if the vaccine is concurrently given or for 90 days following exposure if the vaccine is unavailable or contraindicated and re-exposure is possible

Adults:

- Drug-induced extrapyramidal reactions: 100 mg twice daily; may increase to 300 mg/day, if needed
- Parkinson's disease: 100 mg twice daily as sole therapy; may increase to 400 mg/day if needed with close monitoring; initial dose: 100 mg/day if with other serious illness or with high doses of other anti-Parkinson drugs
- Influenza A viral infection: 200 mg/day in 1-2 divided doses
- Prophylaxis: Minimum 10-day course of therapy following exposure if the vaccine is concurrently given or for 90 days following exposure if the vaccine is unavailable or contraindicated and re-exposure is possible

Elderly patients should take the drug in 2 daily doses rather than a single dose to avoid adverse neurologic reactions; see Warnings/Precautions

Dosing interval in renal impairment:

- Cl_{cr} 50-60 mL/minute: Administer 200 mg alternating with 100 mg/day
- Cl_{cr} 30-50 mL/minute: Administer 100 mg/day
- Cl_{cr} 20-30 mL/minute: Administer 200 mg twice weekly
- Cl_{cr} 10-20 mL/minute: Administer 100 mg 3 times/week
- Cl_{cr} <10 mL/minute: Administer 200 mg alternating with 100 mg every 7 days

Hemodialysis: Slightly hemodialyzable (5% to 20%); no supplemental dose is needed

Peritoneal dialysis: No supplemental dose is needed

Continuous arteriovenous or venovenous hemofiltration (CAVH/CAVHD): No supplemental dose is needed

Dosage Forms CAP: 100 mg. **SYR:** 50 mg/5 mL (480 mL)

Contraindications Hypersensitivity to amantadine hydrochloride or any component

Warnings/Precautions Use with caution in patients with liver disease, a history of recurrent and eczematoid dermatitis, uncontrolled psychosis or severe psychoneurosis, seizures and in those receiving CNS stimulant drugs; reduce dose in renal disease; when treating Parkinson's disease, do not discontinue abruptly. In many patients, the therapeutic benefits of amantadine are limited to a few months. Elderly patients may be more susceptible to the CNS effects (using 2 divided daily doses may minimize this effect).

Pregnancy Risk Factor C

Adverse Reactions

1% to 10%:

- Cardiovascular: Orthostatic hypotension, peripheral edema
- Central nervous system: Insomnia, depression, anxiety, irritability, dizziness, hallucinations, ataxia, headache, somnolence, nervousness, dream abnormality, agitation, fatigue, confusion
- Dermatologic: Livedo reticularis
- Gastrointestinal: Nausea, anorexia, constipation, diarrhea, xerostomia
- Respiratory: Dry nose

<1%: Amnesia, congestive heart failure, decreased libido, dyspnea, eczematoid dermatitis, euphoria, hyperkinesis, hypertension, instances of convulsions, leukopenia, neutropenia, oculogyric episodes, psychosis, rash, slurred speech, urinary retention, visual disturbances, vomiting, weakness

Drug Interactions

Increased effect: Drugs with anticholinergic or CNS stimulant activity

Increased toxicity/levels: Hydrochlorothiazide plus triamterene, amiloride

Alcohol Interactions Avoid use (may increase central nervous system adverse effects)

Onset Onset of antidyskinetic action: Within 48 hours

Half-Life Normal renal function: 2-7 hours; End-stage renal disease: 7-10 days

Education and Monitoring Issues

Patient Education: Take as directed; do not increase dosage, take more often than prescribed, or discontinue without consulting prescriber. Maintain adequate hydration (2-3 L/day of fluids unless instructed to restrict fluid intake) and void before taking medication. Take last dose of day in the afternoon to reduce incidence of insomnia. Avoid alcohol, sedatives, or hypnotics unless consulting prescriber. You may experience decreased mental alertness or coordination (use caution when driving, climbing stairs, or engaging in tasks requiring alertness until response to drug is known); nausea, or dry mouth (small frequent meals, frequent mouth care, sucking lozenges, or chewing gum may help). Report unusual swelling of extremities, difficulty breathing or shortness of breath, change in gait or increased tremors, or changes in mentation (depression, anxiety, irritability, hallucination, slurred speech).

Monitoring Parameters: Renal function, mental status, blood pressure

Related Information

Community Acquired Pneumonia in Adults *on page 1200*

Parkinson's Disease Dosing *on page 1249*

♦ **Amaphen®** *see* Butalbital Compound *on page 123*

♦ **Amaryl®** *see* Glimepiride *on page 412*

♦ **Amatine** *see* Midodrine *on page 603*

♦ **Ambenyl® Cough Syrup** *see* Bromodiphenhydramine and Codeine *on page 114*

♦ **Ambien™** *see* Zolpidem *on page 995*

♦ **Ambi® Skin Tone [OTC]** *see* Hydroquinone *on page 450*

Amcinonide (am SIN oh nide)

Pharmacologic Class Corticosteroid, Topical

U.S. Brand Names Cyclocort®

Generic Available No

Mechanism of Action Stimulates the synthesis of enzymes needed to decrease inflammation, suppress mitotic activity, and cause vasoconstriction

Use Relief of the inflammatory and pruritic manifestations of corticosteroid-responsive dermatoses (high potency corticosteroid)

USUAL DOSAGE Adults: Topical: Apply in a thin film 2-3 times/day. Therapy should be discontinued when control is achieved; if no improvement is seen, reassessment of diagnosis may be necessary.

Dosage Forms CRM: 0.1% (15 g, 30 g, 60 g). **LOT:** 0.1% (20 mL, 60 mL). **OINT, top:** 0.1% (15 g, 30 g, 60 g)

Contraindications Hypersensitivity to amcinonide or any component; use on the face, groin, or axilla

Warnings/Precautions Adverse systemic effects may occur when used on large areas of the body, denuded areas, for prolonged periods of time, with an occlusive dressing, and/or in infants or small children; occlusive dressings should not be used in presence of infection or weeping lesions

Pregnancy Risk Factor C

Adverse Reactions

1% to 10%:

Dermatologic: Itching, maceration of skin, skin atrophy, erythema, dryness, papular rashes

Local: Burning, irritation

<1%: Acneiform eruptions, hypertrichosis, hypopigmentation, miliaria, perioral dermatitis, striae

Education and Monitoring Issues

Patient Education: Before applying, gently wash area to reduce risk of infection; apply a thin film to cleansed area and rub in gently and thoroughly until medication vanishes; avoid exposure to sunlight, severe sunburn may occur

♦ **Amcort®** *see* Triamcinolone *on page 944*

♦ **Amen®** *see* Medroxyprogesterone Acetate *on page 558*

♦ **Amerge®** *see* Naratriptan *on page 637*

♦ **Americaine® [OTC]** *see* Benzocaine *on page 98*

♦ **A-methaPred® Injection** *see* Methylprednisolone *on page 589*

♦ **Ametop®** *see* Tetracaine *on page 902*

♦ **Amgenal® Cough Syrup** *see* Bromodiphenhydramine and Codeine *on page 114*

♦ **Amicar®** *see* Aminocaproic Acid *on page 46*

Amikacin (am i KAY sin)

Pharmacologic Class Antibiotic, Aminoglycoside

U.S. Brand Names Amikin® Injection

Generic Available No

Mechanism of Action Inhibits protein synthesis in susceptible bacteria by binding to 30S ribosomal subunits

Use Treatment of serious infections due to organisms resistant to gentamicin and tobramycin including *Pseudomonas, Proteus, Serratia,* and other gram-positive bacilli (bone infections, respiratory tract infections, endocarditis, and septicemia); documented infection of mycobacterial organisms susceptible to amikacin

USUAL DOSAGE Individualization is critical because of the low therapeutic index

Use of ideal body weight (IBW) for determining the mg/kg/dose appears to be more accurate than dosing on the basis of total body weight (TBW)

In morbid obesity, dosage requirement may best be estimated using a dosing weight of IBW + 0.4 (TBW - IBW)

Initial and periodic peak and trough plasma drug levels should be determined, particularly in critically ill patients with serious infections or in disease states known to significantly alter aminoglycoside pharmacokinetics (eg, cystic fibrosis, burns, or major surgery)

Infants, Children, and Adults: I.M., I.V.: 5-7.5 mg/kg/dose every 8 hours

Some clinicians suggest a daily dose of 15-20 mg/kg for all patients with normal renal function. This dose is at least as efficacious with similar, if not less, toxicity than conventional dosing.

Dosing interval in renal impairment: Some patients may require larger or more frequent doses if serum levels document the need (ie, cystic fibrosis or febrile granulocytopenic patients)

Cl_{cr} ≥60 mL/minute: Administer every 8 hours

Cl_{cr} 40-60 mL/minute: Administer every 12 hours

Cl_{cr} 20-40 mL/minute: Administer every 24 hours

Cl_{cr} <20 mL/minute: Loading dose, then monitor levels

Hemodialysis: Dialyzable (50% to 100%); administer dose postdialysis or administer ⅔ normal dose as a supplemental dose postdialysis and follow levels

Peritoneal dialysis: Dose as Cl_{cr} <20 mL/minute: Follow levels

Continuous arteriovenous or venovenous hemodiafiltration (CAVH) effects: Dose as for Cl_{cr} 10-40 mL/minute and follow levels

Dosage Forms INJ: 50 mg/mL (2 mL, 4 mL), 250 mg/mL (2 mL, 4 mL)

Contraindications Hypersensitivity to amikacin sulfate or any component; cross-sensitivity may exist with other aminoglycosides

Warnings/Precautions Dose and/or frequency of administration must be monitored and modified in patients with renal impairment; drug should be discontinued if signs of ototoxicity, nephrotoxicity, or hypersensitivity occur; ototoxicity is proportional to the amount of drug given and the duration of treatment; tinnitus or vertigo may be indications of vestibular injury and impending bilateral irreversible damage; renal damage is usually reversible

Pregnancy Risk Factor C

Adverse Reactions

1% to 10%:

Central nervous system: Neurotoxicity

Otic: Ototoxicity (auditory), ototoxicity (vestibular)

Renal: Nephrotoxicity

<1%: Arthralgia, drowsiness, drug fever, dyspnea, eosinophilia, headache, hypotension, nausea, paresthesia, rash, vomiting, tremor, weakness

Drug Interactions

Decreased effect of aminoglycoside: High concentrations of penicillins and/or cephalosporins (*in vitro* data)

Increased toxicity of aminoglycoside: Indomethacin I.V., amphotericin, loop diuretics, vancomycin, enflurane, methoxyflurane; increased toxicity of depolarizing and nondepolarizing neuromuscular blocking agents and polypeptide antibiotics with administration of aminoglycosides

Half-Life Dependent on renal function: Normal renal function: 1.4-2.3 hours; Anuria: End-stage renal disease: 28-86 hours

Education and Monitoring Issues

Patient Education: This drug can only be administered I.V. or I.M. It is important to maintain adequate hydration (2-3 L/day of fluids unless instructed to restrict fluid intake). Report change in hearing acuity, ringing or roaring in ears, alteration in balance, vertigo, feeling of fullness in head; pain, tingling, or numbness of any body part; change in urinary pattern or decrease in urine; signs of opportunistic infection (eg, white plaques in mouth, vaginal discharge, unhealed sores, sore throat, unusual fever, chills); pain, redness, or swelling at injection site; or other adverse reactions.

Monitoring Parameters: Urinalysis, BUN, serum creatinine, appropriately timed peak and trough concentrations, vital signs, temperature, weight, I & O, hearing parameters

Reference Range:

Sample size: 0.5-2 mL blood (red top tube) or 0.1-1 mL serum (separated)

Therapeutic levels:
Peak:
Life-threatening infections: 25-30 μg/mL
Serious infections: 20-25 μg/mL
Urinary tract infections: 15-20 μg/mL
Trough:
Serious infections: 1-4 μg/mL
Life-threatening infections: 4-8 μg/mL
Toxic concentration: Peak: >35 μg/mL; Trough: >10 μg/mL
Timing of serum samples: Draw peak 30 minutes after completion of 30-minute infusion or at 1 hour following initiation of infusion or I.M. injection; draw trough within 30 minutes prior to next dose

Related Information
Antimicrobial Drugs of Choice *on page 1182*

♦ **Amikin® Injection** *see* Amikacin *on page 44*

Amiloride (a MIL oh ride)

Pharmacologic Class Diuretic, Potassium Sparing
U.S. Brand Names Midamor®
Generic Available Yes
Mechanism of Action Interferes with potassium/sodium exchange (active transport) in the distal tubule, cortical collecting tubule and collecting duct by inhibiting sodium, potassium-ATPase; decreases calcium excretion; increases magnesium loss
Use Counteracts potassium loss induced by other diuretics in the treatment of hypertension or edematous conditions including CHF, hepatic cirrhosis, and hypoaldosteronism; usually used in conjunction with more potent diuretics such as thiazides or loop diuretics
Investigational: Cystic fibrosis
USUAL DOSAGE Oral:
Children: Although safety and efficacy have not been established by the FDA in children, a dosage of 0.625 mg/kg/day has been used in children weighing 6-20 kg
Adults: 5-10 mg/day (up to 20 mg)
Elderly: Initial: 5 mg once daily or every other day
Dosing adjustment in renal impairment:
Cl_{cr} 10-50 mL/minute: Administer at 50% of normal dose
Cl_{cr} <10 mL/minute: Avoid use
Dosage Forms TAB, as hydrochloride: 5 mg
Contraindications Hyperkalemia, potassium supplementation and impaired renal function or potassium-sparing diuretics, hypersensitivity to amiloride or any component
Warnings/Precautions Use cautiously in patients with severe hepatic insufficiency; may cause hyperkalemia (serum levels >5.5 mEq/L) which, if uncorrected, is potentially fatal; medication should be discontinued if potassium level are >6.5 mEq/L
Pregnancy Risk Factor B
Adverse Reactions
1% to 10%:
Central nervous system: Headache, fatigue, dizziness
Endocrine & metabolic: Hyperkalemia, hyperchloremic metabolic acidosis, dehydration, hyponatremia, gynecomastia
Gastrointestinal: Nausea, diarrhea, vomiting, abdominal pain, gas pain, appetite changes, constipation
Genitourinary: Impotence
Neuromuscular & skeletal: Muscle cramps, weakness
Respiratory: Cough, dyspnea
<1% (limited to important or life-threatening symptoms): Orthostatic hypotension, arrhythmias, palpitations, chest pain, alopecia, GI bleeding, polyuria, bladder spasms, dysuria, jaundice, increased intraocular pressure, shortness of breath
Drug Interactions
Decreased effect of amiloride: Nonsteroidal anti-inflammatory agents
Increased risk of amiloride-associated hyperkalemia: Avoid use or use with extreme caution with triamterene, spironolactone, angiotensin-converting enzyme (ACE) inhibitors, potassium preparations, indomethacin
Increased toxicity of amantadine and lithium by reduction of renal excretion
Onset 2 hours
Duration 24 hours
Half-Life Normal renal function: 6-9 hours; End-stage renal disease: 8-144 hours
Education and Monitoring Issues
Patient Education: Take as directed, preferably early in day. Do not increase dietary intake of potassium unless instructed by prescriber (too much potassium can be as harmful as too little). You may experience dizziness or fatigue; use caution when driving or engaging in tasks that require alertness until response to drug is known. You may experience constipation (increased dietary fluid, fiber, or fruit may help), impotence (reversible), or loss of head hair (rare). Report muscle cramping or weakness, unresolved nausea or vomiting, palpitations, or difficulty breathing.
(Continued)

Amiloride *(Continued)*

Monitoring Parameters: I & O, daily weights, blood pressure, serum electrolytes, renal function

Related Information

Amiloride and Hydrochlorothiazide *on page 46*
Heart Failure Guidelines *on page 1099*

Amiloride and Hydrochlorothiazide

(a MIL oh ride & hye droe klor oh THYE a zide)

Pharmacologic Class Diuretic, Combination

U.S. Brand Names Moduretic®

Dosage Forms TAB: Amiloride hydrochloride 5 mg and hydrochlorothiazide 50 mg

Pregnancy Risk Factor B

Aminocaproic Acid (a mee noe ka PROE ik AS id)

Pharmacologic Class Hemostatic Agent

U.S. Brand Names Amicar®

Use Treatment of excessive bleeding from fibrinolysis

USUAL DOSAGE In the management of acute bleeding syndromes, oral dosage regimens are the same as the I.V. dosage regimens in adults and children

Chronic bleeding: Oral, I.V.: 5-30 g/day in divided doses at 3- to 6-hour intervals

Acute bleeding syndrome:

- Children: Oral, I.V.: 100 mg/kg or 3 g/m² during the first hour, followed by continuous infusion at the rate of 33.3 mg/kg/hour or 1 g/m²/hour; total dosage should not exceed 18 g/m²/24 hours
  - Traumatic hyphema: Oral: 100 mg/kg/dose every 6-8 hours
- Adults:
  - Oral: For elevated fibrinolytic activity, administer 5 g during first hour, followed by 1-1.25 g/hour for approximately 8 hours or until bleeding stops
  - I.V.: 4-5 g in 250 mL of diluent during first hour followed by continuous infusion at the rate of 1-1.25 g/hour in 50 mL of diluent, continue for 8 hours or until bleeding stops
  - Maximum daily dose: Oral, I.V.: 30 g

Dosing adjustment in renal impairment: Oliguria or ESRD: Reduce dose by 15% to 25%

Contraindications Disseminated intravascular coagulation, hematuria of upper urinary tract; use of factor IX concentrate of anti-inhibitor coagulant concentrate

Pregnancy Risk Factor C

♦ **Amino-Cerv™ Vaginal Cream** *see* Urea *on page 962*

Aminoglutethimide (a mee noe gloo TETH i mide)

Pharmacologic Class Antineoplastic Agent, Miscellaneous

U.S. Brand Names Cytadren®

Generic Available No

Mechanism of Action Blocks the enzymatic conversion of cholesterol to delta-5-pregnenolone, thereby reducing the synthesis of adrenal glucocorticoids, mineralocorticoids, estrogens, aldosterone, and androgens

Use Suppression of adrenal function in selected patients with Cushing's syndrome; also used successfully in postmenopausal patients with advanced breast carcinoma and in patients with metastatic prostate carcinoma as salvage (third-line hormonal agent)

USUAL DOSAGE Adults: Oral:

250 mg every 6 hours may be increased at 1- to 2-week intervals to a total of 2 g/day; administer in divided doses, 2-3 times/day to reduce incidence of nausea and vomiting. Follow adrenal cortical response by careful monitoring of plasma cortisol until the desired level of suppression is achieved.

Mineralocorticoid (fludrocortisone) replacement therapy may be necessary in up to 50% of patients. If glucocorticoid replacement therapy is necessary, 20-30 mg hydrocortisone orally in the morning will replace endogenous secretion.

Dosing adjustment in renal impairment: Dose reduction may be necessary

Dosage Forms TAB, scored: 250 mg

Contraindications Hypersensitivity to aminoglutethimide or any component and glutethimide

Warnings/Precautions Monitor blood pressure in all patients at appropriate intervals; hypothyroidism may occur; **mineralocorticoid replacement therapy may be necessary in up to 50% of patients** (ie, fludrocortisone); if glucocorticoid replacement therapy is necessary, 20-30 mg of hydrocortisone daily in the morning will replace endogenous secretion (steroid replacement regimen is controversial - high-dose versus low-dose)

Pregnancy Risk Factor D

Pregnancy Implications Suspected of causing virilization when given throughout pregnancy

Adverse Reactions Most adverse effects will diminish in incidence and severity after the first 2-6 weeks

>10%:

Central nervous system: Headache, dizziness, drowsiness, and lethargy are frequent at the start of therapy, clumsiness

Dermatologic: Skin rash

Gastrointestinal: Nausea, vomiting, anorexia

Hepatic: Cholestatic jaundice

Neuromuscular & skeletal: Myalgia

Renal: Nephrotoxicity

Respiratory: Pulmonary alveolar damage

Miscellaneous: Systemic lupus erythematosus

1% to 10%:

Cardiovascular: Hypotension and tachycardia, orthostatic hypotension

Dermatologic: Hirsutism in females

Endocrine & metabolic: Adrenocortical insufficiency

Hematologic: Rare cases of neutropenia, leukopenia, thrombocytopenia, pancytopenia, and agranulocytosis have been reported

<1%: Adrenal suppression, goiter, hyperkalemia, hypothyroidism, lipid abnormalities (hypercholesterolemia)

Drug Interactions CYP-450 hepatic microsomal enzyme inducer

Decreased effect:

Dexamethasone: Reported to increase metabolism

Digitoxin: Increases clearance of digitoxin after 3-8 weeks of aminoglutethimide therapy

Theophylline: Aminoglutethimide increases metabolism of theophylline

Warfarin: Decreases anticoagulant response to warfarin

Increased toxicity: Propranolol: Case report of enhanced aminoglutethimide toxicity (rash and lethargy)

Onset 3-5 days

Half-Life 7-15 hours; shorter following multiple administrations than following single doses (induces hepatic enzymes increasing its own metabolism)

Education and Monitoring Issues

Patient Education: May be taken with food to reduce incidence of nausea. Small frequent meals may also reduce incidence of nausea and vomiting. You may experience drowsiness or dizziness; avoid driving or engaging in tasks that require alertness until response to drug is known. Masculinization may occur and is reversible when treatment is discontinued. Report rash, unresolved nausea, vomiting, lethargy, yellowing of skin or eyes, easy bruising or bleeding, change in color of urine or stool, increased growth of facial hair, thick tongue, severe mood swings, palpitations, or respiratory difficulty.

Aminolevulinic Acid (a mee noe le vu LIN ik AS id)

Pharmacologic Class Photosensitizing Agent, Topical; Porphyrin Agent, Topical

U.S. Brand Names Levulan® Kerastick™

Mechanism of Action Aminolevulinic acid is a metabolic precursor of protoporphyrin IX (PpIX), which is a photosensitizer. Photosensitization following application of aminolevulinic acid topical solution occurs through the metabolic conversion to PpIX. When exposed to light of appropriate wavelength and energy, accumulated PpIX produces a photodynamic reaction.

Use Treatment of nonhyperkeratotic actinic keratoses of the face or scalp; to be used in conjunction with blue light illumination

USUAL DOSAGE Adults: Topical: Apply to actinic keratoses (**not** perilesional skin) followed 14-18 hours later by blue light illumination. Application/treatment may be repeated at a treatment site after 8 weeks.

Dosage Forms SOLN, top: 20% (with applicator)

Contraindications Individuals with cutaneous photosensitivity at wavelengths of 400-450 nm; porphyria; allergy to porphyrins; hypersensitivity to any component

Warnings/Precautions For external use only. Do not apply to eyes or mucous membranes. Treatment site will become photosensitive following application. Patients should be instructed to avoid exposure to sunlight, bright indoor lights, or tanning beds during the period prior to blue light treatment. Should be applied by a qualified health professional to avoid application to perilesional skin. Has not been tested in individuals with coagulation defects (acquired or inherited).

Pregnancy Risk Factor C

Pregnancy Implications No adequate or well-controlled studies in pregnant women. Should be used during pregnancy only if clearly needed; excretion in breast milk is unknown; use caution in breast-feeding.

Adverse Reactions

Transient stinging, burning, itching, erythema and edema result from the photosensitizing properties of this agent. Symptoms subside between 1 minute and 24 hours after turning off the blue light illuminator. Severe stinging or burning was reported in at least 50% of patients from at least 1 lesional site treatment.

>10%: Dermatologic: Severe stinging or burning (50%), scaling of the skin/crusted skin (64% to 71%), hyperpigmentation/hypopigmentation (22% to 36%), itching (14% to 25%), erosion (2% to 14%)

(Continued)

Aminolevulinic Acid *(Continued)*

1% to 10%:

Central nervous system: Dysesthesia (0% to 2%)

Dermatologic: Skin ulceration (2% to 4%), vesiculation (4% to 5%), pustular drug eruption (0% to 4%), skin disorder (5% to 12%)

Hematologic: Bleeding/hemorrhage (2% to 4%)

Local: Wheal/flare (2% to 7%), local pain (1%), tenderness (1%), edema (1%), scabbing (0% to 2%)

Drug Interactions Photosensitizing agent including griseofulvin, thiazide diuretics, sulfonamides, sulfonylureas, phenothiazines, and tetracyclines theoretically may increase the photosensitizing potential of aminolevulinic acid

Onset Peak fluorescence: 11 hours

Half-Life 30 hours

Education and Monitoring Issues

Patient Education: Avoid exposure to sunlight, bright indoor lights, or tanning beds during the period prior to blue light treatment. Wear a wide-brimmed hat to protect from exposure. Sunscreens do not protect against photosensitization by this agent.

Manufacturer DUSA Pharmaceuticals, Inc

Related Information

Pharmaceutical Manufacturers Directory *on page 1020*

♦ **Amino-Opti-E® [OTC]** *see* Vitamin E *on page 980*

♦ **Aminophyllin™** *see* Theophylline Salts *on page 906*

Aminosalicylate Sodium (a MEE noe sa LIS i late SOW dee um)

Pharmacologic Class Salicylate

U.S. Brand Names Sodium P.A.S.

Use Adjunctive treatment of tuberculosis used in combination with other antitubercular agents; has also been used in Crohn's disease

USUAL DOSAGE Oral:

Children: 150 mg/kg/day in 3-4 equally divided doses

Adults: 150 mg/kg/day in 2-3 equally divided doses (usually 12-14 g/day)

Dosing adjustment in renal impairment:

Cl_{cr} 10-50 mL/minute: Administer 50% to 75% of dose

Cl_{cr} <10 mL/minute: Administer 50% of dose

Administer after hemodialysis

Contraindications Hypersensitivity to aminosalicylate sodium

Pregnancy Risk Factor C

Amiodarone (a MEE oh da rone)

Pharmacologic Class Antiarrhythmic Agent, Class III

U.S. Brand Names Cordarone®; Pacerone®

Generic Available No

Mechanism of Action Class III antiarrhythmic agent which inhibits adrenergic stimulation, prolongs the action potential and refractory period in myocardial tissue; decreases A-V conduction and sinus node function

Use

Oral: Management of life-threatening recurrent ventricular fibrillation (VF) or hemodynamically unstable ventricular tachycardia (VT)

I.V.: Initiation of treatment and prophylaxis of frequency recurring VF and unstable VT in patients refractory to other therapy. Also, for patients for whom oral amiodarone is indicated but who are unable to take oral medication.

USUAL DOSAGE

Oral:

Children (calculate doses for children <1 year on body surface area): Loading dose: 10-15 mg/kg/day or 600-800 mg/1.73 m^2/day for 4-14 days or until adequate control of arrhythmia or prominent adverse effects occur (this loading dose may be given in 1-2 divided doses/day); dosage should then be reduced to 5 mg/kg/day or 200-400 mg/1.73 m^2/day given once daily for several weeks; if arrhythmia does not recur, reduce to lowest effective dosage possible; usual daily minimal dose: 2.5 mg/kg/day; maintenance doses may be given for 5 of 7 days/week

Adults: Ventricular arrhythmias: 800-1600 mg/day in 1-2 doses for 1-3 weeks, then when adequate arrhythmia control is achieved decrease to 600-800 mg/day in 1-2 doses for 1 month; maintenance: 400 mg/day; lower doses are recommended for supraventricular arrhythmias

I.V.:

First 24 hours: 1000 mg according to following regimen

Step 1: 150 mg (100 mL) over first 10 minutes (mix 3 mL in 100 mL D_5W)

Step 2: 360 mg (200 mL) over next 6 hours (mix 18 mL in 500 mL D_5W)

Step 3: 540 mg (300 mL) over next 18 hours

After the first 24 hours: 0.5 mg/minute utilizing concentration of 1-6 mg/mL

Breakthrough VF or VT: 150 mg supplemental doses in 100 mL D_5W over 10 minutes

Note: When switching from I.V. to oral therapy, use the following as a guide:
<1-week I.V. infusion → 800-1600 mg/day
1- to 3-week I.V. infusion → 600-800 mg/day
>3-week I.V. infusion → 400 mg

Recommendations for conversion to intravenous amiodarone after oral administration: During long-term amiodarone therapy (ie, ≥4 months), the mean plasma-elimination half-life of the active metabolite of amiodarone is 61 days; replacement therapy may not be necessary in such patients if oral therapy is discontinued for a period <2 weeks, since any changes in serum amiodarone concentrations during this period may **not** be clinically significant

Dosing adjustment in hepatic impairment: Probably necessary in substantial hepatic impairment

Hemodialysis: Not dialyzable (0% to 5%); supplemental dose is not necessary

Peritoneal dialysis effects: Not dialyzable (0% to 5%); supplemental dose is not necessary

Dosage Forms INJ: 50 mg/mL with benzyl alcohol (3 mL). **TAB, scored:** 200 mg

Contraindications Hypersensitivity to amiodarone; severe sinus node dysfunction, second and third degree A-V block, marked sinus bradycardia except if pacemaker is placed, pregnancy and lactation; administration with amprenavir, ritonavir, nelfinavir, or sparfloxacin

Warnings/Precautions Not considered first-line antiarrhythmic due to high incidence of significant and potentially fatal toxicity (ie, hypersensitivity pneumonitis or interstitial/alveolar pneumonitis, hepatic failure, heart block, bradycardia or exacerbated arrhythmias), especially with large doses; reserve for use in arrhythmias refractory to other therapy; hospitalize patients while loading dose is administered; use cautiously in elderly due to predisposition to toxicity; use very cautiously and with close monitoring in patients with thyroid or liver disease. Due to an extensive tissue distribution and prolonged elimination period, the time at which a life-threatening arrhythmia will recur following discontinued therapy or an interaction with subsequent treatment may occur is unpredictable; patients must be observed carefully and extreme caution taken when other antiarrhythmic agents are substituted after discontinuation of amiodarone.

Pregnancy Risk Factor D

Adverse Reactions With large dosages (>400 mg/day), adverse reactions occur in ~75% of patients and require discontinuance in 5% to 20%.

>10%:

- Cardiovascular: Hypotension (I.V.: 16%)
- Central nervous system: Between 20% and 40% of patients experience some form of neurologic adverse events (see central nervous system and neuromuscular effects: 1% to 10% frequencies).
- Gastrointestinal: Nausea, vomiting

1% to 10%:

- Cardiovascular: Congestive heart failure, arrhythmias (including atropine-resistant bradycardia, heart block, sinus arrest, ventricular tachycardia), proarrhythmic, myocardial depression, flushing, edema. Additional effects associated with I.V. administration include asystole, cardiac arrest, electromechanical dissociation, ventricular tachycardia and cardiogenic shock.
- Central nervous system: Fever, fatigue, involuntary movements, incoordination, malaise, sleep disturbances, ataxia, dizziness, headache
- Dermatologic: Photosensitivity (10%)
- Endocrine & metabolic: Hypothyroidism or hyperthyroidism (less common), decreased libido
- Gastrointestinal: Constipation, anorexia, abdominal pain, abnormal salivation, abnormal taste (oral form)
- Hematologic: Coagulation abnormalities
- Hepatic: Abnormal LFTs
- Local: Phlebitis (I.V.: with concentrations >3 mg/mL)
- Neuromuscular & skeletal: Paresthesia, tremor, muscular weakness, peripheral neuropathy
- Ocular: Visual disturbances, corneal microdeposits
- Genitourinary: noninfectious epididymitis (3% to 11%)
- Respiratory: Pulmonary toxicity has been estimated to occur at a frequency between 2% and 7% of patients (some reports indicate a frequency as high as 17%). Toxicity may present as hypersensitivity pneumonitis, pulmonary fibrosis (cough, fever, malaise), pulmonary inflammation, interstitial pneumonitis, or alveolar pneumonitis. Other rare pulmonary toxicities are listed under the <1% category.
- Miscellaneous: Abnormal smell (oral form)

<1% (limited to important or life-threatening symptoms): Hypotension (with oral form), vasculitis, atrial fibrillation, increased Q-T interval, ventricular fibrillation, nodal arrhythmia, sinus bradycardia, optic neuropathy, optic neuritis, photophobia, pseudotumor cerebri, hyperglycemia, hypertriglyceridemia, epididymitis, thrombocytopenia, pancreatitis, cirrhosis, severe hepatotoxicity (potentially fatal hepatitis), hepatitis, cholestasis, cirrhosis, increased ALT/AST, abnormal renal function, diarrhea, pulmonary edema, bronchiolitis obliterans organizing pneumonia (BOOP), pleuritis, rash, alopecia, discoloration of skin (slate-blue), Stevens-Johnson syndrome, toxic epidermal necrolysis, thrombocytopenia, pancytopenia, neutropenia, ventricular fibrillation, vomiting,

(Continued)

Amiodarone *(Continued)*

angioedema, anaphylactic shock, aplastic anemia, myoclonic jerks, jaw tremor, dyskinesias, parkinsonian symptoms, delirium, encephalopathy, brain stem dysfunction, impotence, loss of libido

Case reports: Bone marrow granuloma, leukocytoclastic vasculitis, acute intracranial hypertension (I.V.), gynecomastia, toxic epidermal necrolysis

Drug Interactions CYP3A3/4 enzyme substrate; CYP2C9, 2D6, and 3A3/4 enzyme inhibitor

Amiodarone appears to interfere with the hepatic metabolism of several drugs resulting in significantly increased plasma concentrations; see table.

Amiodarone Common Drug Interactions

Drug	Interaction
Anticoagulants, oral	The effects of the anticoagulant is increased due to inhibition of its metabolism.
β-adrenergic receptor antagonists	β-blocker effects are enhanced by amiodarone's inhibition of the β-blocker's hepatic metabolism.
Calcium channel antagonists	Additive effects of both drugs resulting in a reduction in cardiac sinus conduction, atrioventricular nodal conduction, and myocardial contractility.
Cholestyramine	Increased enterohepatic elimination of amiodarone may occur resulting in decreased serum levels and half-life.
Cimetidine	Increased amiodarone levels may result
Cyclosporine	Results in persistently elevated cyclosporine levels and elevated creatinine despite reduction in cyclosporine dosage.
Digoxin	Digoxin concentrations may be increased with resultant increases in activity and potential for toxicity.
Disopyramide	Q-T prolongation may occur in addition to arrhythmias.
Fentanyl	Concurrent use with amiodarone may result in hypotension, bradycardia, and decreased cardiac output.
Flecainide	Flecainide plasma concentrations are increased.
Methotrexate	Chronic use of amiodarone impairs MTX metabolism resulting in MTX toxicity.
Phenytoin	Phenytoin serum concentrations are increased due to reduction in phenytoin metabolism, with possible symptoms of phenytoin toxicity; amiodarone levels may be decreased.
Procainamide	Procainamide serum concentrations may be increased.
Quinidine	Quinidine serum concentrations may be increased and can potentially cause fatal cardiac dysrhythmias.
Ritonavir	Increased risk of amiodarone cardiotoxicity results.
Sparfloxacin	Risk of cardiotoxicity may be increased.
Theophylline	Increased theophylline levels and resultant toxicity may occur; effects may be delayed and may persist after amiodarone discontinuation

Onset Onset of effect: 3 days to 3 weeks after starting therapy; Peak effect: 1 week to 5 months; onset of I.V. form may be more rapid

Duration Following discontinuation of therapy: 7-50 days

Half-Life Oral chronic therapy: 40-55 days (range: 26-107 days)

Education and Monitoring Issues

Patient Education: Emergency use: Patient condition will determine amount of patient education. Oral: May be taken with food to reduce GI disturbance. Do not change dosage or discontinue drug without consulting prescriber. Regular blood work, ophthalmic exams, and cardiac assessment will be necessary while taking this medication on a long-term basis. You may experience dizziness, weakness, or insomnia (use caution when driving, climbing stairs, or engaging in tasks requiring alertness until response to drug is known); hypotension (use caution changing position - rising from sitting or lying); nausea, vomiting, loss of appetite, stomach discomfort, or abnormal taste (small frequent meals, frequent mouth care, chewing gum, or sucking lozenges may help); photosensitivity (use sunscreen, wear protective clothing and eyewear, avoid direct sunlight); or decreased libido (reversible). Report persistent dry cough or shortness of breath; chest pain, palpitations, irregular or slow heartbeat; unusual bruising or bleeding; blood in urine, feces, vomitus; pain, swelling, or warmth in calves; muscle tremor, weakness, numbness, or changes in gait; skin rash or irritation; or changes in urinary patterns.

Monitoring Parameters: Monitor heart rate (EKG) and rhythm throughout therapy; assess patient for signs of thyroid dysfunction (thyroid function tests and liver enzymes), lethargy, edema of the hands, feet, weight loss, and pulmonary toxicity (baseline pulmonary function tests)

Reference Range: Therapeutic: 0.5-2.5 mg/L (SI: 1-4 μmol/L) (parent); desethyl metabolite is active and is present in equal concentration to parent drug

- **Amitone® [OTC]** *see* Calcium Carbonate *on page 130*

Amitriptyline (a mee TRIP ti leen)

Pharmacologic Class Antidepressant, Tricyclic (Tertiary Amine)

U.S. Brand Names Elavil®; Enovil®

Generic Available Yes

Mechanism of Action Increases the synaptic concentration of serotonin and/or norepinephrine in the central nervous system by inhibition of their reuptake by the presynaptic neuronal membrane

Use Treatment of various forms of depression, often in conjunction with psychotherapy; analgesic for certain chronic and neuropathic pain, prophylaxis against migraine headaches

USUAL DOSAGE

Children: Pain management: Oral: Initial: 0.1 mg/kg at bedtime, may advance as tolerated over 2-3 weeks to 0.5-2 mg/day at bedtime

Adolescents: Oral: Initial: 25-50 mg/day; may administer in divided doses; increase gradually to 100 mg/day in divided doses

Adults:

Oral: 30-100 mg/day single dose at bedtime or in divided doses; dose may be gradually increased up to 300 mg/day; once symptoms are controlled, decrease gradually to lowest effective dose

I.M.: 20-30 mg 4 times/day

Dosing interval in hepatic impairment: Use with caution and monitor plasma levels and patient response

Hemodialysis: Nondialyzable

Dosage Forms INJ: 10 mg/mL (10 mL). **TAB:** 10 mg, 25 mg, 50 mg, 75 mg, 100 mg, 150 mg

Contraindications Hypersensitivity to amitriptyline (cross-sensitivity with other tricyclics may occur); patients receiving MAO inhibitors within past 14 days; narrow-angle glaucoma; avoid use during pregnancy and lactation

Warnings/Precautions

Amitriptyline should not be abruptly discontinued in patients receiving high doses for prolonged periods

Use with caution in patients with cardiac conduction disturbances; an EKG prior to initiation of therapy is advised; use with caution in patients with a history of hyperthyroidism, renal or hepatic impairment

The most anticholinergic and sedating of the antidepressants; pronounced effects on the cardiovascular system (hypotension), hence, many psychiatrists agree it is best to avoid in the elderly

Pregnancy Risk Factor D

Adverse Reactions Anticholinergic effects may be pronounced; moderate to marked sedation can occur (tolerance to these effects usually occurs)

Cardiovascular: Orthostatic hypotension, tachycardia, nonspecific EKG changes, changes in A-V conduction

Central nervous system: Restlessness, dizziness, insomnia, sedation, fatigue, anxiety, impaired cognitive function, seizures, extrapyramidal symptoms

Dermatologic: Allergic rash, urticaria, photosensitivity

Gastrointestinal: Weight gain, xerostomia, constipation

Genitourinary: Urinary retention

Ocular: Blurred vision, mydriasis

Miscellaneous: Diaphoresis

Drug Interactions CYP1A2, 2C9, 2C19, 2D6, and 3A3/4 enzyme substrate

Carbamazepine, phenobarbital, and rifampin may increase the metabolism of amitriptyline resulting in decreased effect of amitriptyline

Amitriptyline inhibits the antihypertensive response to bethanidine, clonidine, debrisoquin, guanadrel, guanethidine, guanabenz, guanfacine; monitor BP; consider alternate antihypertensive agent

Concurrent use of TCAs with cisapride is contraindicated; may increase risk of malignant arrhythmias

Abrupt discontinuation of clonidine may cause hypertensive crisis, amitriptyline may enhance the response

Use with altretamine may cause orthostatic hypertension

Amitriptyline may be additive with or may potentiate the action of other CNS depressants (sedatives, hypnotics, or ethanol)

With MAO inhibitors, hyperpyrexia, hypertension, tachycardia, confusion, seizures, and **deaths have been reported** (serotonin syndrome); this combination should be avoided

Amitriptyline may increase the prothrombin time in patients stabilized on warfarin

Cimetidine and methylphenidate may decrease the metabolism of amitriptyline

Additive anticholinergic effects seen with other anticholinergic agents

The SSRIs, to varying degrees, inhibit the metabolism of TCAs and clinical toxicity may result

(Continued)

Amitriptyline *(Continued)*

Use of lithium with a TCA may increase the risk for neurotoxicity
Phenothiazines may increase concentration of some TCAs and TCAs may increase concentration of phenothiazines; monitor for altered clinical response
TCAs may enhance the hypoglycemic effects of tolazamide, chlorpropamide, or insulin; monitor for changes in blood glucose levels
Cholestyramine and colestipol may bind TCAs and reduce their absorption; monitor for altered response
TCAs may enhance the effect of amphetamines; monitor for adverse CV effects
Diltiazem and verapamil appear to decrease the metabolism of imipramine and potentially other TCAs; monitor for increased TCA concentrations
The pressor response to I.V. epinephrine, norepinephrine, and phenylephrine may be enhanced in patients receiving TCAs; this combination is best avoided
Indinavir, ritonavir may inhibit the metabolism of clomipramine and potentially other TCAs; monitor for altered effects; a decrease in TCA dosage may be required
Quinidine may inhibit the metabolism of TCAs; monitor for altered effect
Combined use of anticholinergics with TCAs may produce additive anticholinergic effects
Combined use of beta-agonists with TCAs may predispose patients to cardiac arrhythmias

Alcohol Interactions Avoid use (may increase central nervous system depression)

Onset Onset of therapeutic effect: 7-21 days
Desired therapeutic effect (for depression) may take as long as 3-4 weeks, at that point dosage should be reduced to lowest effective level.
When used for migraine headache prophylaxis, therapeutic effect may take as long as 6 weeks. A higher dosage may be required in a heavy smoker, because of increased metabolism.

Half-Life 9-25 hours (15-hour average)

Education and Monitoring Issues

Patient Education: Take exactly as directed (do not increase dose or frequency); may take several weeks to achieve desired results; may cause physical and/or psychological dependence. Do not use alcohol, excess caffeine, and other prescription or OTC medications not approved by prescriber. Maintain adequate hydration (2-3 L/day of fluids unless instructed to restrict fluid intake). May turn urine blue-green (normal). You may experience drowsiness, lightheadedness, impaired coordination, dizziness, or blurred vision (use caution when driving or engaging in tasks requiring alertness until response to drug is known); constipation (increased exercise, fluids, or dietary fruit and fiber may help); urinary retention (void before taking medication); postural hypotension (use caution climbing stairs or when changing position from lying or sitting to standing); altered sexual drive or ability (reversible); or photosensitivity (use sunscreen, wear protective clothing and eyewear, avoid direct sunlight). Report persistent CNS effects (eg, nervousness, restlessness, insomnia, anxiety, excitation, headache, agitation, impaired coordination, changes in cognition); muscle cramping, weakness, tremors, or rigidity; ringing in ears or visual disturbances; chest pain, palpitations, or irregular heartbeat; blurred vision; or worsening of condition.

Dietary Considerations: Grapefruit juice may potentially inhibit the metabolism of TCAs

Monitoring Parameters: Monitor blood pressure and pulse rate prior to and during initial therapy; evaluate mental status; monitor weight

Reference Range: Therapeutic: Amitriptyline and nortriptyline 100-250 ng/mL (SI: 360-900 nmol/L); nortriptyline 50-150 ng/mL (SI: 190-570 nmol/L); Toxic: >0.5 μg/mL; plasma levels do not always correlate with clinical effectiveness

Related Information

Amitriptyline and Chlordiazepoxide *on page 52*
Amitriptyline and Perphenazine *on page 52*
Antidepressant Agents Comparison *on page 1231*

Amitriptyline and Chlordiazepoxide

(a mee TRIP ti leen & klor dye az e POKS ide)

Pharmacologic Class Antidepressant, Tricyclic (Tertiary Amine)

U.S. Brand Names Limbitrol® DS 10-25

Dosage Forms TAB: 5-12.5: Amitriptyline hydrochloride 12.5 mg and chlordiazepoxide 5 mg; 10-25: Amitriptyline hydrochloride 25 mg and chlordiazepoxide 10 mg

Pregnancy Risk Factor D

Alcohol Interactions Avoid use (may increase central nervous system depression)

Amitriptyline and Perphenazine (a mee TRIP ti leen & per FEN a zeen)

Pharmacologic Class Antidepressant, Tricyclic (Tertiary Amine)

U.S. Brand Names Etrafon®; Triavil®

Dosage Forms TAB: 2-10: Amitriptyline hydrochloride 10 mg and perphenazine 2 mg; 4-10: Amitriptyline hydrochloride 10 mg and perphenazine 4 mg; 2-25: Amitriptyline hydrochloride 25 mg and perphenazine 2 mg; 4-25: Amitriptyline hydrochloride 25 mg and perphenazine 4 mg; 4-50: Amitriptyline hydrochloride 50 mg and perphenazine 4 mg

Pregnancy Risk Factor D

Alcohol Interactions Avoid use (may increase central nervous system depression)

Amlexanox (am LEKS an oks)

Pharmacologic Class Anti-inflammatory, Locally Applied

U.S. Brand Names Aphthasol™

Generic Available No

Mechanism of Action As a benzopyrano-bipyridine carboxylic acid derivative, amlexanox has anti-inflammatory and antiallergic properties; it inhibits chemical mediatory release of the slow-reacting substance of anaphylaxis (SRS-A) and may have antagonistic effect son interleukin-3

Use Treatment of aphthous ulcers (ie, canker sores); has been investigated in many allergic disorders

USUAL DOSAGE Administer (0.5 cm - ¼") directly on ulcers 4 times/day following oral hygiene, after meals, and at bedtime

Dosage Forms PASTE: 5% (5 g)

Contraindications Hypersensitivity to amlexanox or components

Warnings/Precautions Discontinue therapy if rash or contact mucositis develops

Pregnancy Risk Factor B

Pregnancy Implications Due to lack of data, avoid use in pregnancy or lactation, if possible

Adverse Reactions

1% to 2%:

Dermatologic: Allergic contact dermatitis

Gastrointestinal: Oral irritation

<1%: Contact mucositis

Half-Life 3.5 hours

Education and Monitoring Issues

Patient Education: Apply as soon as possible and continue 4 times/day (after meals and at bedtime); wash hands after use; contact prescriber if no reduction in pain occurs within 10 days

Manufacturer Block Drug Co, Inc

Related Information

Pharmaceutical Manufacturers Directory *on page 1020*

Amlodipine (am LOE di peen)

Pharmacologic Class Calcium Channel Blocker

U.S. Brand Names Norvasc®

Generic Available No

Mechanism of Action Inhibits calcium ion from entering the "slow channels" or select voltage-sensitive areas of vascular smooth muscle and myocardium during depolarization, producing a relaxation of coronary vascular smooth muscle and coronary vasodilation; increases myocardial oxygen delivery in patients with vasospastic angina

Use Treatment of hypertension and angina (chronic stable or Prinzmetal's) with or without other therapy

USUAL DOSAGE Adults: Oral:

Hypertension: Initial dose: 2.5-5 mg once daily; usual dose: 5 mg once daily; maximum dose: 10 mg once daily; in general, titrate in 2.5 mg increments over 7-14 days

Angina: Usual dose: 10 mg; use lower doses for elderly or those with hepatic insufficiency (eg, 2.5-5 mg)

Dialysis: Hemodialysis and peritoneal dialysis does not enhance elimination; supplemental dose is not necessary

Dosage adjustment in hepatic impairment: 2.5 mg once daily

Dosage Forms TAB: 2.5 mg, 5 mg, 10 mg

Contraindications Hypersensitivity

Warnings/Precautions Use with caution and titrate dosages for patients with impaired renal or hepatic function; use caution when treating patients with congestive heart failure, sick-sinus syndrome, severe left ventricular dysfunction, hypertrophic cardiomyopathy (especially obstructive), concomitant therapy with beta-blockers or digoxin, edema, or increased intracranial pressure with cranial tumors; do not abruptly withdraw (may cause chest pain); elderly may experience hypotension and constipation more readily.

Pregnancy Risk Factor C

Pregnancy Implications Teratogenic and embryotoxic effects have been demonstrated in small animals. No well controlled studies have been conducted in pregnant women. Use in pregnancy only when clearly needed and when the benefits outweigh the potential hazard to the fetus.

Clinical effects on the fetus: No data on crossing the placenta

Breast-feeding/lactation: No data on crossing into breast milk

Adverse Reactions

>10%: Cardiovascular: Peripheral edema (1.8% to 14.6% dose-related)

(Continued)

Amlodipine *(Continued)*

1% to 10%:

Central nervous system: Flushing (0.7% to 2.6%), palpitations (0.7% to 4.5%), headache (7.3%; similar to placebo)

Dermatologic: Rash (1% to 2%), pruritus (1% to 2%)

Endocrine & metabolic: Male sexual dysfunction (1% to 2%)

Gastrointestinal: Nausea (2.9%), abdominal pain (1% to 2%), dyspepsia (1% to 2%), gingival hyperplasia

Neuromuscular & skeletal: Muscle cramps (1% to 2%), weakness (1% to 2%)

Respiratory: Shortness of breath (1% to 2%), pulmonary edema (15% from PRAISE trial, CHF population)

<1%: Hypotension, bradycardia, arrhythmias, syncope, tachycardia, nervousness, insomnia, malaise, weight gain, anorexia, diarrhea, constipation, vomiting, xerostomia, flatulence, micturition disorder, joint stiffness, paresthesia, tremor, tinnitus, chest pain, hypotension, peripheral ischemia, postural hypotension, postural dizziness, hypoesthesia, vertigo, dysphagia, back pain, hot flushes, pain, rigors, arthrosis, myalgia, female sexual dysfunction, depression, abnormal dreams, anxiety, depersonalization, epistaxis, rash erythematous, rash maculopapular, abnormal vision, conjunctivitis, diplopia, eye pain, micturition frequency, nocturia, increased sweating, thirst, purpura

<0.1% (limited to important or life-threatening symptoms): Cardiac failure, pulse irregularity, extrasystoles, skin discoloration, urticaria, skin dryness, alopecia, dermatitis, muscle weakness, twitching, ataxia, hypertonia, migraine, cold and clammy skin, apathy, agitation, amnesia, gastritis, increased appetite, loose stools, coughing, rhinitis, dysuria, polyuria, parosmia, taste perversion, abnormal visual accommodation, xerophthalmia

Case reports: Thrombocytopenia, nonthrombocytopenic purpura, leukocytoclastic vasculitis, EPS, gynecomastia, Stevens-Johnson syndrome, erythema multiforme, exfoliative dermatitis, dysosmia, phototoxicity

Drug Interactions CYP3A3/4 enzyme substrate

Increased effect:

Amlodipine and benazepril may increase hypotensive effect

Amlodipine and cyclosporine may increase cyclosporine levels

Beta-blockers in combination with calcium antagonists may result in increased cardiac depression

Severe hypotension or increased fluid volume requirements have occurred with fentanyl and calcium blockers

Onset 30-50 minutes; Peak effect: 6-12 hours

Duration 24 hours

Half-Life 30-50 hours

Education and Monitoring Issues

Patient Education: Take as prescribed; do not stop abruptly without consulting prescriber. You may experience headache (if unrelieved, consult prescriber), nausea or vomiting (frequent small meals may help), or constipation (increased dietary bulk and fluids may help). May cause drowsiness; use caution when driving or engaging in tasks that require alertness until response to drug is known. Report unrelieved headache, vomiting, constipation, palpitations, peripheral or facial swelling, weight gain >5 lb/week, or respiratory changes.

Manufacturer Pfizer U.S. Pharmaceutical Group

Related Information

Amlodipine and Benazepril *on page 54*

Calcium Channel Blocking Agents Comparison *on page 1236*

Pharmaceutical Manufacturers Directory *on page 1020*

Amlodipine and Benazepril (am LOE di peen & ben AY ze pril)

Pharmacologic Class Antihypertensive Agent, Combination

U.S. Brand Names Lotrel®

Dosage Forms CAP: Amlodipine 2.5 mg and benazepril hydrochloride 10 mg, Amlodipine 5 mg and benazepril hydrochloride 10 mg, Amlodipine 5 mg and benazepril hydrochloride 20 mg

Pregnancy Risk Factor C (first trimester); D (2nd and 3rd trimesters)

Manufacturer Novartis

Related Information

Pharmaceutical Manufacturers Directory *on page 1020*

♦ **AMO Vitrax®** *see* Sodium Hyaluronate *on page 859*

Amoxapine (a MOKS a peen)

Pharmacologic Class Antidepressant, Tricyclic (Secondary Amine)

U.S. Brand Names Asendin®

Generic Available Yes

Mechanism of Action Reduces the reuptake of serotonin and norepinephrine and blocks the response of dopamine receptors to dopamine

Use Treatment of neurotic and endogenous depression and mixed symptoms of anxiety and depression

USUAL DOSAGE Once symptoms are controlled, decrease gradually to lowest effective dose. Maintenance dose is usually given at bedtime to reduce daytime sedation. Oral:

Children: Not established in children <16 years of age

Adolescents: Initial: 25-50 mg/day; increase gradually to 100 mg/day; may administer as divided doses or as a single dose at bedtime

Adults: Initial: 25 mg 2-3 times/day, if tolerated, dosage may be increased to 100 mg 2-3 times/day; may be given in a single bedtime dose when dosage <300 mg/day

Elderly: Initial: 25 mg at bedtime increased by 25 mg weekly for outpatients and every 3 days for inpatients if tolerated; usual dose: 50-150 mg/day, but doses up to 300 mg may be necessary

Maximum daily dose:
- Inpatient: 600 mg
- Outpatient: 400 mg

Dosage Forms TAB: 25 mg, 50 mg, 100 mg, 150 mg

Contraindications Hypersensitivity to amoxapine; cross-sensitivity with other tricyclics may occur; narrow-angle glaucoma; patients receiving MAO inhibitors within past 14 days

Warnings/Precautions Use with caution in patients with seizures, cardiac conduction disturbances, cardiovascular diseases, urinary retention, hyperthyroidism, or those receiving thyroid replacement; do not discontinue abruptly in patients receiving high doses chronically; tolerance develops in 1-3 months in some patients, close medical follow-up is essential

Pregnancy Risk Factor C

Adverse Reactions

>10%:
- Central nervous system: Drowsiness
- Gastrointestinal: Xerostomia, constipation

1% to 10%:
- Central nervous system: Dizziness, headache, confusion, nervousness, restlessness, insomnia, ataxia, excitement, anxiety
- Dermatologic: Edema, skin rash
- Endocrine: Elevated prolactin levels
- Gastrointestinal: Nausea
- Neuromuscular & skeletal: Tremor, weakness
- Ocular: Blurred vision
- Miscellaneous: Diaphoresis

<1%: Abdominal pain, abnormal taste, agranulocytosis, allergic reactions, breast enlargement, delayed micturition, diarrhea, elevated liver enzymes, epigastric distress, extrapyramidal symptoms, flatulence, galactorrhea, hypertension, hypotension, impotence, incoordination, increased intraocular pressure, increased or decreased libido, lacrimation, leukopenia, menstrual irregularity, mydriasis, nasal stuffiness, neuroleptic malignant syndrome, numbness, painful ejaculation, paresthesia, photosensitivity, seizures, SIADH, syncope, tachycardia, tardive dyskinesia, testicular edema, tinnitus, urinary retention, vomiting

Drug Interactions CYP1A2, 2C9, 2C19, 2D6, and 3A3/4 enzyme substrate

Carbamazepine, phenobarbital, and rifampin may increase the metabolism of amoxapine resulting in decreased effect of amoxapine

Amoxapine inhibits the antihypertensive response to bethanidine, clonidine, debrisoquin, guanadrel, guanethidine, guanabenz, guanfacine; monitor BP; consider alternate antihypertensive agent

Abrupt discontinuation of clonidine may cause hypertensive crisis, amoxapine may enhance the response

Use with altretamine may cause orthostatic hypertension

Amoxapine may be additive with or may potentiate the action of other CNS depressants (sedatives, hypnotics, or ethanol)

With MAO inhibitors, hyperpyrexia, hypertension, tachycardia, confusion, seizures, and **deaths have been reported** (serotonin syndrome); this combination should be avoided

Amoxapine may increase the prothrombin time in patients stabilized on warfarin

Cimetidine and methylphenidate may decrease the metabolism of amoxapine; additive anticholinergic effects seen with other anticholinergic agents

The SSRIs, to varying degrees, inhibit the metabolism of TCAs and clinical toxicity may result

Use of lithium with a TCA may increase the risk for neurotoxicity

Phenothiazines may increase concentration of some TCAs and TCAs may increase concentration of phenothiazines; monitor for altered clinical response

TCAs may enhance the hypoglycemic effects of tolazamide, chlorpropamide, or insulin; monitor for changes in blood glucose levels

Cholestyramine and colestipol may bind TCAs and reduce their absorption; monitor for altered response

TCAs may enhance the effect of amphetamines; monitor for adverse CV effects

Verapamil and diltiazem appear to decrease the metabolism of imipramine and potentially other TCAs; monitor for increased TCA concentrations. The pressor response to I.V.

(Continued)

Amoxapine *(Continued)*

epinephrine, norepinephrine, and phenylephrine may be enhanced in patients receiving TCAs; this combination is best avoided.

Indinavir, ritonavir may inhibit the metabolism of clomipramine and potentially other TCAs; monitor for altered effects; a decrease in TCA dosage may be required

Quinidine may inhibit the metabolism of TCAs; monitor for altered effect

Combined use of anticholinergics with TCAs may produce additive anticholinergic effects; combined use of beta-agonists with TCAs may predispose patients to cardiac arrhythmias

Alcohol Interactions Avoid use (may increase central nervous system depression)

Onset Onset of antidepressant effect: Usually occurs after 1-2 weeks

Half-Life Parent drug: 11-16 hours; Active metabolite: 30 hours

Education and Monitoring Issues

Patient Education: Take exactly as directed (do not increase dose or frequency). Full effect may not occur for 3-5 weeks; may cause physical and/or psychological dependence. Do not use excessive alcohol or other prescription or OTC medications (especially pain medications, sedatives, antihistamines, or hypnotics) without consulting prescriber. Maintain adequate hydration (2-3 L/day of fluids unless instructed to restrict fluid intake). You may experience drowsiness, lightheadedness, impaired coordination, dizziness, or blurred vision (use caution when driving or engaging in tasks requiring alertness until response to drug is known); nausea, vomiting, increased appetite, or dry mouth (small frequent meals, frequent mouth care, chewing gum, or sucking lozenges may help); constipation (increased exercise, fluids, or dietary fruit and fiber may help); or altered sexual drive or ability (reversible). Report persistent CNS effects (confusion, restlessness, anxiety, insomnia, excitation, headache, dizziness, fatigue, impaired coordination); muscle cramping, weakness, tremors, or rigidity; visual disturbances; excessive GI symptoms (cramping, constipation, vomiting); or worsening of condition.

Dietary Considerations: Grapefruit juice may potentially inhibit the metabolism of TCAs

Monitoring Parameters: Monitor blood pressure and pulse rate prior to and during initial therapy evaluate mental status; monitor weight

Reference Range: Therapeutic: Amoxapine: 20-100 ng/mL (SI: 64-319 nmol/L); 8-OH amoxapine: 150-400 ng/mL (SI: 478-1275 nmol/L); both: 200-500 ng/mL (SI: 637-1594 nmol/L)

Related Information

Antidepressant Agents Comparison *on page 1231*

Amoxicillin (a moks i SIL in)

Pharmacologic Class Antibiotic, Penicillin

U.S. Brand Names Amoxil®; Biomox®; Polymox®; Trimox®; Wymox®

Generic Available Yes

Mechanism of Action Inhibits bacterial cell wall synthesis by binding to one or more of the penicillin binding proteins (PBPs); which in turn inhibits the final transpeptidation step of peptidoglycan synthesis in bacterial cell walls, thus inhibiting cell wall biosynthesis. Bacteria eventually lyse due to ongoing activity of cell wall autolytic enzymes (autolysins and murein hydrolases) while cell wall assembly is arrested.

Use Treatment of otitis media, sinusitis, and infections caused by susceptible organisms involving the respiratory tract, skin, and urinary tract; prophylaxis of bacterial endocarditis in patients undergoing surgical or dental procedures; approved in combination for eradication of *H. pylori*

USUAL DOSAGE Oral:

Children: 20-50 mg/kg/day in divided doses every 8 hours

Subacute bacterial endocarditis prophylaxis: 50 mg/kg 1 hour before procedure

Adults: 250-500 mg every 8 hours or 500-875 mg twice daily; maximum dose: 2-3 g/day

Endocarditis prophylaxis: 2 g 1 hour before procedure

Helicobacter pylori: 1000 mg twice daily; clinically effective treatment regimens include triple therapy with clarithromycin and ranitidine; clarithromycin and a proton pump inhibitor

Dosing interval in renal impairment:

Cl_{cr} 10-50 mL/minute: Administer every 12 hours

Cl_{cr} <10 mL/minute: Administer every 24 hours

Dialysis: Moderately dialyzable (20% to 50%) by hemo- or peritoneal dialysis; approximately 50 mg of amoxicillin per liter of filtrate is removed by continuous arteriovenous or venovenous hemofiltration (CAVH); dose as per Cl_{cr} <10 mL/minute guidelines

Dosage Forms CAP: 250 mg, 500 mg. **POWDER for oral susp:** 125 mg/5 mL (5 mL, 80 mL, 100 mL, 150 mL, 200 mL); 250 mg/5 mL (5 mL, 80 mL, 100 mL, 150 mL, 200 mL). **POWDER for oral susp, drops:** 50 mg/mL (15 mL, 30 mL). **SUSP, oral:** 200 mg/5 mL; 400 mg/5 mL. **TAB:** Chewable: 125 mg, 200 mg, 250 mg, 400 mg; Film coated: 500 mg, 875 mg

Contraindications Hypersensitivity to amoxicillin, penicillin, or any component

Warnings/Precautions In patients with renal impairment, doses and/or frequency of administration should be modified in response to the degree of renal impairment; a high percentage of patients with infectious mononucleosis have developed rash during therapy with amoxicillin; a low incidence of cross-allergy with other beta-lactams and cephalosporins exists

Pregnancy Risk Factor B

Adverse Reactions

1% to 10%:

Central nervous system: Fever

Dermatologic: Urticaria, rash

Miscellaneous: Allergic reactions (includes serum sickness, rash, angioedema, bronchospasm, hypotension, etc)

<1%: Anxiety, confusion, depression (with large doses or patients with renal dysfunction), hallucinations, interstitial nephritis, jaundice, leukopenia, nausea, neutropenia, seizures, thrombocytopenia, vomiting

Drug Interactions

Decreased effect: Efficacy of oral contraceptives may be reduced

Increased effect: Disulfiram, probenecid may increase amoxicillin levels

Increased toxicity: Allopurinol theoretically has an additive potential for amoxicillin rash

Half-Life Adults with normal renal function: 0.7-1.4 hours; Patients with Cl_{cr} <10 mL/minute: 7-21 hours

Education and Monitoring Issues

Patient Education: Take entire prescription, even if you are feeling better. Take at equal intervals around-the-clock; may be taken with milk, juice, or food. You may experience nausea or vomiting (small frequent meals, frequent mouth care, sucking lozenges, or chewing gum may help). If diabetic, drug may cause false tests with Clinitest® urine glucose monitoring; use of glucose oxidase methods (Clinistix®) or serum glucose monitoring is preferable. This drug may interfere with oral contraceptives; an alternate form of birth control should be used. Report rash; unusual diarrhea; vaginal itching, burning, or pain; unresolved vomiting or constipation; fever or chills; unusual bruising or bleeding; or if condition being treated worsens or does not improve by the time prescription is completed.

Dietary Considerations: Food: May be taken with food

Monitoring Parameters: With prolonged therapy, monitor renal, hepatic, and hematologic function periodically; assess patient at beginning and throughout therapy for infection; monitor for signs of anaphylaxis during first dose

Related Information

Animal and Human Bites Guidelines *on page 1177*

Antimicrobial Drugs of Choice *on page 1182*

Helicobacter pylori Treatment *on page 1107*

Prevention of Bacterial Endocarditis *on page 1154*

Treatment of Sexually Transmitted Diseases *on page 1210*

Amoxicillin and Clavulanate Potassium

(a moks i SIL in & klav yoo LAN ate poe TASS ee um)

Pharmacologic Class Antibiotic, Penicillin

U.S. Brand Names Augmentin®

Generic Available No

Mechanism of Action Clavulanic acid binds and inhibits beta-lactamases that inactivate amoxicillin resulting in amoxicillin having an expanded spectrum of activity. Amoxicillin inhibits bacterial cell wall synthesis by binding to one or more of the penicillin binding proteins (PBPs); which in turn inhibits the final transpeptidation step of peptidoglycan synthesis in bacterial cell walls, thus inhibiting cell wall biosynthesis. Bacteria eventually lyse due to ongoing activity of cell wall autolytic enzymes (autolysins and murein hydrolases) while cell wall assembly is arrested.

Use Treatment of otitis media, sinusitis, and infections caused by susceptible organisms involving the lower respiratory tract, skin and skin structure, and urinary tract; spectrum same as amoxicillin with additional coverage of beta-lactamase producing *B. catarrhalis*, *H. influenzae*, *N. gonorrhoeae*, and *S. aureus* (not MRSA).

USUAL DOSAGE Oral:

Children ≤40 kg: 20-40 mg (amoxicillin)/kg/day in divided doses every 8 hours or 45 mg/kg in divided doses every 12 hours

Children >40 kg and Adults: 250-500 mg every 8 hours or 875 mg every 12 hours

Note: Augmentin® 200 suspension or chewable tablets 200 mg dosed every 12 hours is considered equivalent to Augmentin® "125" dosed every 8 hours; Augmentin® 400 suspension and chewable tablets may be similarly dosed every 12 hours and are equivalent to Augmentin® "250" every 8 hours

Dosing interval in renal impairment:

Cl_{cr} 10-30 mL/minute: Administer every 12 hours

Cl_{cr} <10 mL/minute: Administer every 24 hours

Hemodialysis: Moderately dialyzable (20% to 50%)

Amoxicillin/clavulanic acid: Administer dose after dialysis

Peritoneal dialysis: Moderately dialyzable (20% to 50%)

Amoxicillin: Administer 250 mg every 12 hours

Clavulanic acid: Dose for Cl_{cr} <10 mL/minute

(Continued)

Amoxicillin and Clavulanate Potassium *(Continued)*

Continuous arteriovenous or venovenous hemofiltration (CAVH) effects:

Amoxicillin: ~50 mg of amoxicillin/L of filtrate is removed

Clavulanic acid: Dose for Cl_{cr} <10 mL/minute

Dosage Forms SUSP, oral: 125 (banana flavor): Amoxicillin trihydrate 125 mg and clavulanate potassium 31.25 mg per 5 mL (75 mL, 150 mL); 200: Amoxicillin 200 mg and clavulanate potassium 28.5 mg per 5 mL (50 mL, 75 mL, 100 mL); 250 (orange flavor): Amoxicillin trihydrate 250 mg and clavulanate potassium 62.5 mg per 5 mL (75 mL, 150 mL); 400: Amoxicillin 400 mg and clavulanate potassium 57 mg per 5 mL (50 mL, 75 mL, 100 mL). **TAB:** 250: Amoxicillin trihydrate 250 mg and clavulanate potassium 125 mg; 500: Amoxicillin trihydrate 500 mg and clavulanate potassium 125 mg; 875: Amoxicillin trihydrate 875 mg and clavulanate potassium 125 mg. **TAB, chewable:** 125: Amoxicillin trihydrate 125 mg and clavulanate potassium 31.25 mg; 200: Amoxicillin trihydrate 200 mg and clavulanate potassium 28.5 mg 250: Amoxicillin trihydrate 250 mg and clavulanate potassium 62.5 mg; 400: Amoxicillin trihydrate 400 mg and clavulanate potassium 57 mg

Contraindications Known hypersensitivity to amoxicillin, clavulanic acid, or penicillin; concomitant use of disulfiram

Warnings/Precautions In patients with renal impairment, doses and/or frequency of administration should be modified in response to the degree of renal impairment; high percentage of patients with infectious mononucleosis have developed rash during therapy; a low incidence of cross-allergy with cephalosporins exists; incidence of diarrhea is higher than with amoxicillin alone. Hepatic dysfunction, although rare, is more common in elderly and/or males, and occurs more frequently with prolonged treatment.

Pregnancy Risk Factor B

Adverse Reactions

1% to 10%:

Dermatologic: Rash, urticaria

Gastrointestinal: Nausea, vomiting, diarrhea

Genitourinary: Vaginitis

<1%: Abdominal discomfort, flatulence, headache

Drug Interactions

Decreased effect: Efficacy of oral contraceptives may be reduced

Increased effect: Disulfiram, probenecid may increase amoxicillin levels, increased effect of anticoagulants

Increased toxicity: Allopurinol theoretically has an additive potential for amoxicillin rash

Half-Life Adults with normal renal function: ~1 hour for both agents; Patients with Cl_{cr} <10 mL/minute: 7-21 hours

Education and Monitoring Issues

Patient Education: Take entire prescription, even if you are feeling better. Take at equal intervals around-the-clock; may be taken with milk, juice, or food. You may experience nausea or vomiting (small frequent meals, frequent mouth care, sucking lozenges, or chewing gum may help). If using oral contraceptives, use additional contraceptive measures; amoxicillin may reduce effectiveness of your oral contraceptive. Report rash; unusual diarrhea; vaginal itching, burning, or pain; unresolved vomiting or constipation; fever or chills; unusual bruising or bleeding; or if condition being treated worsens or does not improve by the time prescription is completed.

Monitoring Parameters: Assess patient at beginning and throughout therapy for infection; with prolonged therapy, monitor renal, hepatic, and hematologic function periodically; monitor for signs of anaphylaxis during first dose

Related Information

Animal and Human Bites Guidelines *on page 1177*

Antimicrobial Drugs of Choice *on page 1182*

♦ **Amoxil®** *see* Amoxicillin *on page 56*

Amphetamine (am FET a meen)

Pharmacologic Class Amphetamine; Central Nervous System Stimulant, Amphetamine

Use Treatment of narcolepsy; exogenous obesity; abnormal behavioral syndrome in children (minimal brain dysfunction); attention deficit/hyperactivity disorder (ADHD)

USUAL DOSAGE Oral:

Narcolepsy:

Children:

6-12 years: 5 mg/day, increase by 5 mg at weekly intervals

>12 years: 10 mg/day, increase by 10 mg at weekly intervals

Adults: 5-60 mg/day in 2-3 divided doses

Attention deficit/hyperactivity disorder: Children:

3-5 years: 2.5 mg/day, increase by 2.5 mg at weekly intervals

>6 years: 5 mg/day, increase by 5 mg at weekly intervals not to exceed 40 mg/day

Short-term adjunct to exogenous obesity: Children >12 years and Adults: 10 mg or 15 mg long-acting capsule daily, up to 30 mg/day; or 5-30 mg/day in divided doses (immediate release tablets only); see "Obesity Treatment Guidelines for Adults" in Appendix

Contraindications Patients with advanced arteriosclerosis, symptomatic cardiovascular disease, moderate to severe hypertension, hyperthyroidism, glaucoma, hypersensitivity, diabetes mellitus, agitated states, patients with a history of drug abuse, and during or within 14 days following MAO inhibitor therapy. Stimulant medications are contraindicated for use in children with attention deficit/hyperactivity disorders and concomitant Tourette's syndrome or tics.

Pregnancy Risk Factor C

♦ **Amphojel** *see* Aluminum Hydroxide *on page 41*

Ampicillin (am pi SIL in)

Pharmacologic Class Antibiotic, Penicillin

U.S. Brand Names Marcillin®; Omnipen®; Omnipen®-N; Polycillin®; Polycillin-N®; Principen®; Totacillin®; Totacillin®-N

Generic Available Yes

Mechanism of Action Inhibits bacterial cell wall synthesis by binding to one or more of the penicillin binding proteins (PBPs); which in turn inhibits the final transpeptidation step of peptidoglycan synthesis in bacterial cell walls, thus inhibiting cell wall biosynthesis. Bacteria eventually lyse due to ongoing activity of cell wall autolytic enzymes (autolysins and murein hydrolases) while cell wall assembly is arrested.

Use Treatment of susceptible bacterial infections (nonbeta-lactamase-producing organisms); susceptible bacterial infections caused by streptococci, pneumococci, nonpenicillinase-producing staphylococci, *Listeria*, meningococci; some strains of *H. influenzae*, *Salmonella*, *Shigella*, *E. coli*, *Enterobacter*, and *Klebsiella*

USUAL DOSAGE

Neonates: I.M., I.V.:

Postnatal age ≤7 days:

≤2000 g: Meningitis: 50 mg/kg/dose every 12 hours; other infections: 25 mg/kg/dose every 12 hours

>2000 g: Meningitis: 50 mg/kg/dose every 8 hours; other infections: 25 mg/kg/dose every 8 hours

Postnatal age >7 days:

<1200 g: Meningitis: 50 mg/kg/dose every 12 hours; other infections: 25 mg/kg/dose every 12 hours

1200-2000 g: Meningitis: 50 mg/kg/dose every 8 hours; other infections: 25 mg/kg/dose every 8 hours

>2000 g: Meningitis: 50 mg/kg/dose every 6 hours; other infections: 25 mg/kg/dose every 6 hours

Infants and Children: I.M., I.V.: 100-400 mg/kg/day in doses divided every 4-6 hours

Meningitis: 200 mg/kg/day in doses divided every 4-6 hours; maximum dose: 12 g/day

Children: Oral: 50-100 mg/kg/day in doses divided every 6 hours; maximum dose: 2-3 g/day

Adults:

Oral: 250-500 mg every 6 hours

I.M.: 500 mg to 1.5 g every 4-6 hours

I.V.: 500 mg to 3 g every 4-6 hours; maximum dose: 12 g/day

Sepsis/meningitis: 150-250 mg/kg/24 hours divided every 3-4 hours

Dosing interval in renal impairment:

Cl_{cr} 30-50 mL/minute: Administer every 6-8 hours

Cl_{cr} 10-30 mL/minute: Administer every 8-12 hours

Cl_{cr} <10 mL/minute: Administer every 12 hours

Hemodialysis: Moderately dialyzable (20% to 50%); administer dose after dialysis

Peritoneal dialysis: Moderately dialyzable (20% to 50%)

Administer 250 mg every 12 hours

Continuous arteriovenous or venovenous hemofiltration (CAVH) effects: Dose as for Cl_{cr} 10-50 mL/minute; ~50 mg of ampicillin per liter of filtrate is removed

Dosage Forms

Ampicillin anhydrous: **CAP:** 250 mg, 500 mg

Ampicillin sodium: **POWDER for inj:** 125 mg, 250 mg, 500 mg, 1 g, 2 g, 10 g

Ampicillin trihydrate: **CAP:** 250 mg, 500 mg; **POWDER for oral susp:** 125 mg/5 mL (5 mL unit dose, 80 mL, 100 mL, 150 mL, 200 mL); 250 mg/5 mL (5 mL unit dose, 80 mL, 100 mL, 150 mL, 200 mL); 500 mg/5 mL (5 mL unit dose, 100 mL); **POWDER for oral susp, drops:** 100 mg/mL (20 mL)

Contraindications Known hypersensitivity to ampicillin or other penicillins

Warnings/Precautions Dosage adjustment may be necessary in patients with renal impairment; a low incidence of cross-allergy with other beta-lactams exists; high percentage of patients with infectious mononucleosis have developed rash during therapy with ampicillin. Appearance of a rash should be carefully evaluated to differentiate a nonallergic ampicillin rash from a hypersensitivity reaction. Ampicillin rash occurs in 5% to 10% of children receiving ampicillin and is a generalized dull red, maculopapular rash, generally appearing 3-14 days after the start of therapy. It normally begins on the trunk and spreads over most of the body. It may be most intense at pressure areas, elbows, and knees.

Pregnancy Risk Factor B

(Continued)

Ampicillin *(Continued)*

Adverse Reactions

>10%: Local: Pain at injection site

1% to 10%:

Dermatologic: Rash (appearance of a rash should be carefully evaluated to differentiate, if possible; nonallergic ampicillin rash from hypersensitivity reaction; incidence is higher in patients with viral infections, *Salmonella* infections, lymphocytic leukemia, or patients that have hyperuricemia)

Gastrointestinal: Diarrhea, vomiting, oral candidiasis, abdominal cramps

Miscellaneous: Allergic reaction (includes serum sickness, urticaria, angioedema, bronchospasm, hypotension, etc)

<1%: Anemia, decreased lymphocytes, eosinophilia, granulocytopenia, hemolytic anemia, interstitial nephritis (rare), leukopenia, penicillin encephalopathy, seizures (with large I.V. doses or patients with renal dysfunction), thrombocytopenia, thrombocytopenic purpura

Drug Interactions

Decreased effect: Efficacy of oral contraceptives may be reduced

Increased effect: Disulfiram, probenecid may increase penicillin levels, increased effect of anticoagulants

Increased toxicity: Allopurinol theoretically has an additive potential for amoxicillin (ampicillin) rash

Half-Life 1-1.8 hours; Anuria/end-stage renal disease: 7-20 hours

Education and Monitoring Issues

Patient Education: Take entire prescription, even if you are feeling better. Take at equal intervals around-the-clock; preferably on an empty stomach with a full glass of water (1 hour before or 2 hours after meals). Maintain adequate hydration (2-3 L/day of fluids unless instructed to restrict fluid intake). You may experience nausea or vomiting (small frequent meals, frequent mouth care, sucking lozenges, or chewing gum may help). If diabetic, drug may cause false tests with Clinitest® urine glucose monitoring; use of glucose oxidase methods (Clinistix®) or serum glucose monitoring is preferable. This drug may interfere with oral contraceptives; an alternate form of birth control should be used. Report rash; unusual diarrhea; unusual vaginal discharge, itching, burning, or pain; mouth sores; unresolved vomiting or constipation; fever or chills; unusual bruising or bleeding; or if condition being treated worsens or does not improve by the time prescription is completed.

Dietary Considerations: Food: Decreases drug absorption rate; decreases drug serum concentration. Take on an empty stomach 1 hour before or 2 hours after meals.

Monitoring Parameters: With prolonged therapy monitor renal, hepatic, and hematologic function periodically; observe signs and symptoms of anaphylaxis during first dose

Related Information

Animal and Human Bites Guidelines *on page 1177*
Antibiotic Treatment of Adults With Infective Endocarditis *on page 1179*
Antimicrobial Drugs of Choice *on page 1182*
Prevention of Bacterial Endocarditis *on page 1154*

Ampicillin and Sulbactam (am pi SIL in & SUL bak tam)

Pharmacologic Class Antibiotic, Penicillin

U.S. Brand Names Unasyn®

Generic Available No

Mechanism of Action The addition of sulbactam, a beta-lactamase inhibitor, to ampicillin extends the spectrum of ampicillin to include some beta-lactamase producing organisms; inhibits bacterial cell wall synthesis by binding to one or more of the penicillin binding proteins (PBPs); which in turn inhibits the final transpeptidation step of peptidoglycan synthesis in bacterial cell walls, thus inhibiting cell wall biosynthesis. Bacteria eventually lyse due to ongoing activity of cell wall autolytic enzymes (autolysins and murein hydrolases) while cell wall assembly is arrested.

Use Treatment of susceptible bacterial infections involved with skin and skin structure, intra-abdominal infections, gynecological infections; spectrum is that of ampicillin plus organisms producing beta-lactamases such as *S. aureus*, *H. influenzae*, *E. coli*, and anaerobes

USUAL DOSAGE Unasyn® (ampicillin/sulbactam) is a combination product. Each 3 g vial contains 2 g of ampicillin and 1 g of sulbactam. Sulbactam has very little antibacterial activity by itself, but effectively extends the spectrum of ampicillin to include beta-lactamase producing strains that are resistant to ampicillin alone. Therefore, dosage recommendations for Unasyn® are based on the ampicillin component.

I.M., I.V.:

Children (3 months to 12 years): 100-200 mg ampicillin/kg/day (150-300 mg Unasyn®) divided every 6 hours; maximum dose: 8 g ampicillin/day (12 g Unasyn®)

Adults: 1-2 g ampicillin (1.5-3 g Unasyn®) every 6-8 hours; maximum dose: 8 g ampicillin/day (12 g Unasyn®)

Dosing interval in renal impairment:

Cl_{cr} 15-29 mL/minute: Administer every 12 hours

Cl_{cr} 5-14 mL/minute: Administer every 24 hours

Dosage Forms POWDER for inj: 1.5 g [ampicillin sodium 1 g and sulbactam sodium 0.5 g], 3 g [ampicillin sodium 2 g and sulbactam sodium 1 g]

Contraindications Hypersensitivity to ampicillin, sulbactam or any component, or penicillins

Warnings/Precautions Dosage adjustment may be necessary in patients with renal impairment; a low incidence of cross-allergy with other beta-lactams exists; high percentage of patients with infectious mononucleosis have developed rash during therapy with ampicillin. Appearance of a rash should be carefully evaluated to differentiate a nonallergic ampicillin rash from a hypersensitivity reaction. Ampicillin rash occurs in 5% to 10% of children receiving ampicillin and is a generalized dull red, maculopapular rash, generally appearing 3-14 days after the start of therapy. It normally begins on the trunk and spreads over most of the body. It may be most intense at pressure areas, elbows, and knees.

Pregnancy Risk Factor B

Adverse Reactions

>10%: Local: Pain at injection site (I.M.)

1% to 10%:

Dermatologic: Rash

Gastrointestinal: Diarrhea

Local: Pain at injection site (I.V.)

Miscellaneous: Allergic reaction (may include serum sickness, urticaria, bronchospasm, hypotension, etc)

<1%: Chest pain, chills, decreased hemoglobin and hematocrit, dysuria, enterocolitis, fatigue, hairy tongue, headache, increased BUN/creatinine, increased liver enzymes, interstitial nephritis (rare), itching, leukopenia, malaise, nausea, neutropenia, penicillin encephalopathy, pseudomembranous colitis, seizures (with large I.V. doses or patients with renal dysfunction), thrombocytopenia, thrombophlebitis, vaginitis, vomiting

Drug Interactions

Decreased effect: Efficacy of oral contraceptives may be reduced

Increased effect: Disulfiram, probenecid results in increased ampicillin levels

Increased toxicity: Allopurinol theoretically has an additive potential for ampicillin rash

Half-Life 1-1.8 hours

Education and Monitoring Issues

Patient Education: Take entire prescription, even if you are feeling better. Take at equal intervals around-the-clock; preferably on an empty stomach with a full glass of water (1 hour before or 2 hours after meals). Maintain adequate hydration (2-3 L/day of fluids unless instructed to restrict fluid intake). You may experience nausea or vomiting (small frequent meals, frequent mouth care, sucking lozenges, or chewing gum may help). If diabetic, drug may cause false tests with Clinitest® urine glucose monitoring; use of glucose oxidase methods (Clinistix®) or serum glucose monitoring is preferable. This drug may interfere with oral contraceptives; an alternate form of birth control should be used. Report rash; unusual diarrhea; vaginal discharge, itching, burning, or pain; mouth sores; unresolved vomiting or constipation; fever or chills; unusual bruising or bleeding; or if condition being treated worsens or does not improve by the time prescription is completed.

Monitoring Parameters: With prolonged therapy, monitor hematologic, renal, and hepatic function; monitor for signs of anaphylaxis during first dose

Manufacturer Pfizer U.S. Pharmaceutical Group

Related Information

Animal and Human Bites Guidelines *on page 1177*

Antimicrobial Drugs of Choice *on page 1182*

Community Acquired Pneumonia in Adults *on page 1200*

Pharmaceutical Manufacturers Directory *on page 1020*

♦ **Ampicin® Sodium** *see* Ampicillin *on page 59*

Amprenavir (am PRE na veer)

Pharmacologic Class Antiretroviral Agent, Protease Inhibitor

U.S. Brand Names Agenerase™

Use Treatment of HIV infections in combination with at least two other antiretroviral agents

USUAL DOSAGE Oral:

Capsules:

Children ≥4-12 years (<50 kg): 20 mg/kg twice daily or 15 mg/kg 3 times daily; maximum: 2400 mg/day

Adults and Children >13 years (>50 kg): 1200 mg twice daily

Solution: Children 4-12 years or older (up to 18 years weighing <50 kg): 22.5 mg/kg twice daily or 17 mg/kg 3 times daily; maximum: 2800 mg/day

Dosage adjustment in hepatic impairment:

Child-Pugh score between 5-8: 450 mg twice daily

Child-Pugh score between 9-12: 300 mg twice daily

Contraindications Hypersensitivity to amprenavir or any component; concurrent therapy with rifampin, bepridil, cisapride, dihydroergotamine, ergotamine, midazolam, and triazolam; severe previous allergic reaction to sulfonamides

(Continued)

Amprenavir *(Continued)*

Warnings/Precautions Because of hepatic metabolism and effect on cytochrome P-450 enzymes, amprenavir should be used with caution in combination with other agents metabolized by this system (see Contraindications and Drug Interactions). Use with caution in patients with diabetes mellitus, sulfonamide allergy, hepatic impairment, or hemophilia. Redistribution of fat may occur (eg, buffalo hump, peripheral wasting, cushingoid appearance). Additional vitamin E supplements should be avoided. Concurrent use of sildenafil should be avoided.

Pregnancy Risk Factor C

Adverse Reactions Protease inhibitors cause dyslipidemia which includes elevated cholesterol and triglycerides and a redistribution of body fat centrally to cause "protease paunch," buffalo hump, facial atrophy, and breast enlargement. These agents also cause hyperglycemia.

>10%:

Dermatologic: Rash (28%)

Endocrine & metabolic: Hyperglycemia (37% to 41%), hypertriglyceridemia (36% to 47%)

Gastrointestinal: Nausea (38% to 73%), vomiting (20% to 29%), diarrhea (33% to 56%)

Miscellaneous: Perioral tingling/numbness

1% to 10%:

Central nervous system: Depression (4% to 15%), headache, paresthesia, fatigue

Dermatologic: Stevens-Johnson syndrome (1% of total, 4% of patients who develop a rash)

Endocrine & metabolic: Hypercholesterolemia (4% to 9%)

Gastrointestinal: Taste disorders (1% to 10%)

Drug Interactions CYP3A4 inhibitor and substrate

Increased effect/toxicity: Abacavir, clarithromycin, indinavir, ritonavir, ketoconazole, and zidovudine increase the AUC of amprenavir. Nelfinavir had no effect on AUC, but increased the C_{min} of amprenavir. Amprenavir increased the AUC of ketoconazole, rifabutin, and zidovudine during concurrent therapy. Amprenavir may enhance the toxicity of bepridil, cisapride, dihydroergotamine, ergotamine, midazolam, and triazolam - concurrent therapy with these drugs and amprenavir is contraindicated. May increase serum concentration of HMGCoA reductase inhibitors (atorvastatin, cerivastatin, lovastatin, simvastatin) , increasing the risk of myopathy/rhabdomyolysis. Amprenavir may also increase the serum concentrations of diltiazem, nicardipine, nifedipine, nimodipine, alprazolam, clorazepate, diazepam, flurazepam, itraconazole, dapsone, erythromycin, loratadine, sildenafil, carbamazepine, and pimozide. May also increase the toxic effect of amiodarone, lidocaine, quinidine, warfarin, and tricyclic antidepressants. Serum concentration monitoring of these drugs is necessary.

Manufacturer GlaxoWellcome

Related Information

Antiretroviral Therapy for HIV Infection *on page 1190*
Pharmaceutical Manufacturers Directory *on page 1020*

Amrinone (AM ri none)

Pharmacologic Class Adrenergic Agonist Agent

U.S. Brand Names Inocor®

Use Short-term management of congestive heart failure; adjunctive therapy of pulmonary hypertension; normally prescribed for patients who have not responded well to therapy with digitalis, diuretics, and vasodilators

USUAL DOSAGE Dosage is based on clinical response (**Note:** Dose should not exceed 10 mg/kg/24 hours)

Children and Adults: 0.75 mg/kg I.V. bolus over 2-3 minutes followed by maintenance infusion of 5-10 mcg/kg/minute; I.V. bolus may need to be repeated in 30 minutes

Dosing adjustment in renal failure: Cl_{cr} <10 mL/minute: Administer 50% to 75% of dose

Dosage Forms INJ: 5 mg/mL (20 mL)

Contraindications Hypersensitivity to amrinone lactate or sulfites (contains sodium metabisulfite)

Warnings/Precautions Increased risk of hospitalization and death with long-term use

Pregnancy Risk Factor C

Adverse Reactions

1% to 10%:

Cardiovascular: Arrhythmias (3%, especially in high-risk patients), hypotension (1% to 2%), (may be infusion rate-related)

Gastrointestinal: Nausea (1% to 2%)

Hematologic: Thrombocytopenia (may be dose-related)

<1% (limited to important or life-threatening symptoms): Chest pain, fever, vomiting, abdominal pain, anorexia, hepatotoxicity, pain or burning at injection site, hypersensitivity, especially with prolonged therapy; contains sulfites resulting in allergic reactions in susceptible people

Drug Interactions

Furosemide: A precipitate forms on admixture with amrinone

Diuretics may cause significant hypovolemia and decrease filling pressure
Digitalis: Inotropic effects are additive

Onset I.V.: Within 2-5 minutes

Duration Dose dependent (~30 minutes low dose, ~2 hours higher doses)

Half-Life Adults, normal: 3.6 hours; Adults with CHF: 5.8 hours

- **Amvisc®** *see* Sodium Hyaluronate *on page 859*
- **Amvisc® Plus** *see* Sodium Hyaluronate *on page 859*
- **Anabolin® Injection** *see* Nandrolone *on page 635*
- **Anacin® [OTC]** *see* Aspirin *on page 72*
- **Anadrol®** *see* Oxymetholone *on page 693*
- **Anafranil®** *see* Clomipramine *on page 213*

Anagrelide (an AG gre lide)

Pharmacologic Class Platelet Reducing Agent

U.S. Brand Names Agrylin®

Mechanism of Action Anagrelide appears to inhibit cyclic nucleotide phosphodiesterase and the release of arachidonic acid from phospholipase, possibly by inhibiting phospholipase A2. It also causes a dose-related reduction in platelet production, which results from decreased megakaryocyte hypermaturation. The drug disrupts the postmitotic phase of maturation.

Use Agent for essential thrombocythemia (ET); treatment of thrombocytopenia secondary to myeloproliferative disorders

USUAL DOSAGE Adults: Oral: 0.5 mg 4 times/day or 1 mg twice daily

Maintain for ≥1 week, then adjust to the lowest effective dose to reduce and maintain platelet count <600,000 μL ideally to the normal range; the dose must not be increased by >0.5 mg/day in any 1 week; maximum dose: 10 mg/day or 2.5 mg/dose

Dosage Forms CAP: 0.5 mg, 1 mg

Contraindications Hypersensitivity to anagrelide

Warnings/Precautions Anagrelide should be used with caution in patients with known or suspected heart disease, and only if the potential benefits of therapy outweigh the potential risks. Thrombocytopenia appears to be the main dose-limiting side effect of anagrelide; palpitations, orthostatic hypotension, and headache have also been reported. Caution is warranted when anagrelide is used in patients with reduced renal function or hepatic dysfunction.

Pregnancy Risk Factor C

Pregnancy Implications Clinical effects on the fetus: The relative risks must be weighed carefully in relation to the potential benefits. Animal reproduction studies have shown an adverse effect on the fetus when anagrelide was administered during pregnancy. There are no adequate and well-controlled studies in humans; however, the potential benefits may warrant the use of this drug in pregnant women despite the potential risks.

Adverse Reactions

Cardiovascular: Palpitations (27.2%), chest pain (7.8%), tachycardia (7.3%), orthostatic hypotension, CHF, cardiomyopathy, myocardial infarction (rare), complete heart block, angina, and atrial fibrillation

Central nervous system: Headache (44%), dizziness (14.7%), bad dreams, impaired concentration ability

Hematologic: Anemia, thrombocytopenia, ecchymosis and lymphadenopathy have been reported rarely

Drug Interactions There is a single case report that suggests sucralfate may interfere with anagrelide absorption

Duration 6-24 hours

Half-Life 1.3 hours

Education and Monitoring Issues

Patient Education: Before using this drug, tell your prescriber your entire medical history, including any allergies (especially drug allergies), heart, kidney, or liver disease. Limit alcohol intake, as it may aggravate side effects. To avoid dizziness and lightheadedness when rising from a seated or lying position, get up slowly. This medication should be used only when clearly needed during pregnancy. Discuss the risks and benefits with your prescriber. It is not known whether this drug is excreted into breast milk. It is recommended to discontinue the drug or not to breast-feed, taking into account the risk to the infant. Tell your prescriber and pharmacist of all nonprescription and prescription medications you may use, especially sucralfate. Do not share this medication with others. Laboratory tests will be done to monitor the effectiveness and possible side effects of this drug.

Dietary Considerations: Food: No clinically significant effect on absorption

Monitoring Parameters: Anagrelide therapy requires close supervision of the patient. Because of the positive inotropic effects and side effects of anagrelide, a pretreatment cardiovascular examination is recommended along with careful monitoring during treatment; while the platelet count is being lowered (usually during the first 2 weeks of treatment), blood counts (hemoglobin, white blood cells), liver function test (AST, ALT) and renal function (serum creatinine, BUN) should be monitored.

(Continued)

Anagrelide *(Continued)*

Reference Range: Thrombocythemia: 60-300 ng/mL

Manufacturer Roberts Pharmaceuticals

Related Information

Pharmaceutical Manufacturers Directory *on page 1020*

- ♦ **Anandron®** *see* Nilutamide *on page 655*
- ♦ **Anapolon®** *see* Oxymetholone *on page 693*
- ♦ **Anaprox®** *see* Naproxen *on page 636*
- ♦ **Anaspaz®** *see* Hyoscyamine *on page 456*

Anastrozole (an AS troe zole)

Pharmacologic Class Antineoplastic Agent, Miscellaneous

U.S. Brand Names Arimidex®

Mechanism of Action Potent and selective nonsteroidal aromatase inhibitor. It significantly lowers serum estradiol concentrations and has no detectable effect on formation of adrenal corticosteroids or aldosterone. In postmenopausal women, the principal source of circulating estrogen is conversion of adrenally generated androstenedione to estrone by aromatase in peripheral tissues.

Use Treatment of advanced breast cancer in postmenopausal women with disease progression following tamoxifen therapy. Patients with ER-negative disease and patients who did not respond to tamoxifen therapy rarely responded to anastrozole.

USUAL DOSAGE Breast cancer: Adults: Oral (refer to individual protocols): 1 mg once daily

Dosage adjustment in renal impairment: Because only about 10% is excreted unchanged in the urine, dosage adjustment in patients with renal insufficiency is not necessary

Dosage adjustment in hepatic impairment: Plasma concentrations in subjects with hepatic cirrhosis were within the range concentrations in normal subjects across all clinical trials; therefore, no dosage adjustment is needed

Dosage Forms TAB: 1 mg

Contraindications Hypersensitivity to any component

Warnings/Precautions Use with caution in patients with hyperlipidemias; mean serum total cholesterol and LDL cholesterol occurs in patients receiving anastrozole

Pregnancy Risk Factor C

Pregnancy Implications Clinical effects on the fetus: Anastrozole can cause fetal harm when administered to a pregnant woman

Adverse Reactions

>5%:

Cardiovascular: Flushing

Gastrointestinal: Little to mild nausea (10%), vomiting

Neuromuscular & skeletal: Increased bone and tumor pain

2% to 5%:

Cardiovascular: Hypertension

Central nervous system: Somnolence, confusion, insomnia, anxiety, nervousness, fever, malaise, accidental injury

Dermatologic: Hair thinning, pruritus

Endocrine & metabolic: Breast pain

Gastrointestinal: Weight loss

Genitourinary: Urinary tract infection

Local: Thrombophlebitis

Neuromuscular & skeletal: Myalgia, arthralgia, pathological fracture, neck pain

Respiratory: Sinusitis, bronchitis, rhinitis

Miscellaneous: Flu-like syndrome, infection

Drug Interactions CYP3A3/4 enzyme substrate; CYP1A2, 2C8, 2C9, and 3A3/4 enzyme inhibitor

Anastrozole inhibited *in vitro* metabolic reactions catalyzed by CYP1A2, CYP2C8/9, and CYP3A4, but only at relatively high concentrations. It is unlikely that coadministration of anastrozole with other drugs will result in clinically significant inhibition of cytochrome P-450-mediated metabolism of other drugs.

Half-Life 50 hours

Education and Monitoring Issues

Patient Education: Take as prescribed. Maintain adequate hydration (2-3 L/day of fluids unless instructed to restrict fluid intake) and nutrition. If experiencing nausea, vomiting, or anorexia, small frequent meals, frequent mouth care, sucking lozenges, or chewing gum may help or contact prescriber for relief. This medication may cause dizziness and fatigue (use caution when driving or engaging in tasks that require alertness until response to drug is known); or increased bone pain (contact prescriber for analgesia). You will be more susceptible to infection (avoid crowds and exposure to infection, and avoid immunizations unless approved by prescriber). Report swelling of extremities, chest pain or palpitations, acute headache or dizziness, increased muscle pain or weakness, CNS changes (eg, confusion, insomnia, nervousness), breast or pelvic pain, unusual bruising or bleeding, flu-like symptoms, or respiratory difficulty.

Manufacturer AstraZeneca

Related Information

Pharmaceutical Manufacturers Directory *on page 1020*

- **Anbesol® [OTC]** *see* Benzocaine *on page 98*
- **Anbesol Baby** *see* Benzocaine *on page 98*
- **Anbesol® Maximum Strength [OTC]** *see* Benzocaine *on page 98*
- **Ancef®** *see* Cefazolin *on page 149*
- **Ancobon®** *see* Flucytosine *on page 369*
- **Ancotil®** *see* Flucytosine *on page 369*
- **Andriol** *see* Testosterone *on page 898*
- **Androderm® Transdermal System** *see* Testosterone *on page 898*
- **Andro/Fem® Injection** *see* Estradiol and Testosterone *on page 329*
- **AndroGel®** *see* Testosterone *on page 898*
- **Android®** *see* Methyltestosterone *on page 591*
- **Andro-L.A.® Injection** *see* Testosterone *on page 898*
- **Androlone®-D Injection** *see* Nandrolone *on page 635*
- **Androlone® Injection** *see* Nandrolone *on page 635*
- **Andropository® Injection** *see* Testosterone *on page 898*
- **Anergan®** *see* Promethazine *on page 779*
- **Anestacon®** *see* Lidocaine *on page 527*
- **Anexate®** *see* Flumazenil *on page 371*
- **Anexsia®** *see* Hydrocodone and Acetaminophen *on page 444*
- **Angiotensin-Related Agents Comparison** *see page 1226*
- **Animal and Human Bites Guidelines** *see page 1177*

Anisotropine (an iss oh TROE peen)

Pharmacologic Class Anticholinergic Agent

U.S. Brand Names Valpin® 50

Use Adjunctive treatment of peptic ulcer

USUAL DOSAGE Adults: Oral: 50 mg 3 times/day

Contraindications Narrow-angle glaucoma, obstructive GI tract or uropathy, severe ulcerative colitis, myasthenia gravis, intestinal atony, hepatic disease, hypersensitivity

Pregnancy Risk Factor C

Anistreplase (a NISS tre plase)

Pharmacologic Class Thrombolytic Agent

U.S. Brand Names Eminase®

Generic Available No

Mechanism of Action Activates the conversion of plasminogen to plasmin by forming a complex exposing plasminogen-activating site and cleavage of a peptide bond that converts plasminogen to plasmin; plasmin being capable of thrombolysis, by degrading fibrin, fibrinogen and other procoagulant proteins into soluble fragments, effective both outside and within the formed thrombus/embolus

Use Management of acute myocardial infarction (AMI) in adults; lysis of thrombi obstructing coronary arteries, reduction of infarct size; and reduction of mortality associated with AMI

USUAL DOSAGE Adults: I.V.: 30 units injected over 2-5 minutes as soon as possible after onset of symptoms

Dosage Forms POWDER for inj, lyophilized: 30 units

Contraindications Active internal bleeding, history of CVA, intracranial neoplasma, known hypersensitivity to anistreplase or other kinases (streptokinase); history of cerebrovascular accident; recent intracranial surgery or trauma; arteriovenous malformation or aneurysm; severe uncontrolled hypertension

Pregnancy Risk Factor C

Adverse Reactions As with all drugs which may affect hemostasis, bleeding is the major adverse effect associated with anistreplase. Hemorrhage may occur at virtually any site. Risk is dependent on multiple variables, including the dosage administered, concurrent use of multiple agents which alter hemostasis, and patient predisposition. Rapid lysis of coronary artery thrombi by thrombolytic agents may be associated with reperfusion-related atrial and/or ventricular arrhythmias.

1% to 10%:

Central nervous system: Intracranial hemorrhage (1%)
Cardiovascular: Hypotension (10.4%)
Gastrointestinal: Gastrointestinal hemorrhage (2%), gingival hemorrhage (1%)
Genitourinary: Hematuria (2.4%)
Hematologic: Hematoma (2.8%)
Local: Bleeding at puncture sites (4.6%)
Respiratory: Hemoptysis (2.2%)

(Continued)

Anistreplase *(Continued)*

<1% (limited to important or life-threatening symptoms): Anaphylactic reaction, anaphylactoid reaction, bronchospasm, angioedema, urticaria, pruritus, flushing, rash (sometimes with delayed appearance 1-2 weeks after treatment), eosinophilia, arthralgia, pedal edema, proteinuria, vasculitis, Guillain-Barré syndrome, adult respiratory distress syndrome, epistaxis, anemia, ocular hemorrhage

<10% (unknown causal relationship): Chills, fever, headache, shock, cardiac rupture, emboli, nausea, vomiting, diaphoresis, purpura, thrombocytopenia, elevated transaminases, arthralgia, agitation, dizziness, paresthesia, tremor, vertigo, dyspnea, pulmonary edema

Drug Interactions

Aminocaproic acid (antifibrinolytic agent) may decrease effectiveness

Drugs which affect platelet function (eg, NSAIDs, dipyridamole, ticlopidine, clopidogrel, IIb/IIIa antagonists) may potentiate the risk of hemorrhage; use with caution

Heparin and aspirin: Use with aspirin and heparin may increase the risk of bleeding. However, aspirin and heparin were used concomitantly with anistreplase in the majority of patients in clinical studies. Aspirin was not associated with an increased rate of hemorrhagic CVAs in clinical trials.

Warfarin or oral anticoagulants: Risk of bleeding may be increased during concurrent therapy

Duration Fibrinolytic effect persists for 4-6 hours following administration.

Half-Life 70-120 minutes

Education and Monitoring Issues

Patient Education: I.V. administration for cardiac emergencies: Patient instruction should be appropriate to situation. Following infusion, absolute bedrest is important; call for assistance changing position. You will have increased tendency to bleed; avoid razors, scissors or sharps, and use soft toothbrush or cotton swabs. Report back pain, abdominal pain, muscle cramping, acute onset headache, chest pain, or bleeding.

Manufacturer Roberts Pharmaceuticals

Related Information

Pharmaceutical Manufacturers Directory *on page 1020*

- **Anodynos-DHC®** *see* Hydrocodone and Acetaminophen *on page 444*
- **Anoquan®** *see* Butalbital Compound *on page 123*
- **Ansaid® Oral** *see* Flurbiprofen *on page 384*
- **Antabuse®** *see* Disulfiram *on page 288*
- **Antazone®** *see* Sulfinpyrazone *on page 881*
- **Anthra-Derm®** *see* Anthralin *on page 66*
- **Anthraforte®** *see* Anthralin *on page 66*

Anthralin (AN thra lin)

Pharmacologic Class Antipsoriatic Agent; Keratolytic Agent

U.S. Brand Names Anthra-Derm®; Drithocreme®; Drithocreme® HP 1%; Dritho-Scalp®; Micanol® Cream

Use Treatment of psoriasis (quiescent or chronic psoriasis)

USUAL DOSAGE Adults: Topical: Generally, apply once a day or as directed. The irritant potential of anthralin is directly related to the strength being used and each patient's individual tolerance. Always commence treatment for at least one week using the lowest strength possible.

Skin application: Apply sparingly only to psoriatic lesions and rub gently and carefully into the skin until absorbed. Avoid applying an excessive quantity which may cause unnecessary soiling and staining of the clothing or bed linen.

Scalp application: Comb hair to remove scalar debris and, after suitably parting, rub cream well into the lesions, taking care to prevent the cream from spreading onto the forehead

Remove by washing or showering; optimal period of contact will vary according to the strength used and the patient's response to treatment. Continue treatment until the skin is entirely clear (ie, when there is nothing to feel with the fingers and the texture is normal)

Contraindications Hypersensitivity to anthralin or any component, acute psoriasis (acutely or actively inflamed psoriatic eruptions); use on the face

Pregnancy Risk Factor C

- **Anthranol®** *see* Anthralin *on page 66*
- **Anthrascalp®** *see* Anthralin *on page 66*
- **AntibiOtic® Otic** *see* Neomycin, Polymyxin B, and Hydrocortisone *on page 644*
- **Antibiotic Treatment of Adults With Infective Endocarditis** *see page 1179*
- **Anticoagulation Guidelines** *see page 1068*
- **Anticonvulsants by Seizure Type Comparison** *see page 1230*
- **Antidepressant Agents Comparison** *see page 1231*
- **Antihist-1® [OTC]** *see* Clemastine *on page 207*

- **Antihist-D®** *see* Clemastine and Phenylpropanolamine *on page 207*
- **Antilirium®** *see* Physostigmine *on page 734*
- **Antimicrobial Drugs of Choice** *see page 1182*
- **Antiminth® [OTC]** *see* Pyrantel Pamoate *on page 793*

Antipyrine and Benzocaine (an tee PYE reen & BEN zoe kane)

Pharmacologic Class Otic Agent, Analgesic; Otic Agent, Cerumenolytic
U.S. Brand Names Allergan® Ear Drops; Auralgan®; Auroto®; Otocalm® Ear
Dosage Forms SOLN, otic: Antipyrine 5.4% and benzocaine 1.4% (10 mL, 15 mL)
Pregnancy Risk Factor C

Antirabies Serum (Equine) (an tee RAY beez SEER um EE kwine)

Pharmacologic Class Serum
Generic Available No
Mechanism of Action Affords passive immunity against rabies
Use Rabies prophylaxis
USUAL DOSAGE 1000 units/55 lb in a single dose, infiltrate up to 50% of dose around the wound
Dosage Forms INJ: 125 units/mL (8 mL)
Pregnancy Risk Factor C
Adverse Reactions 1% to 10%:
Central nervous system: Pain (local)
Dermatologic: Urticaria
Miscellaneous: Serum sickness

- **Antiretroviral Therapy for HIV Infection** *see page 1190*
- **Antispas® Injection** *see* Dicyclomine *on page 266*

Antithymocyte Globulin (Rabbit)

(an te THY moe site GLOB yu lin RAB bit)

Pharmacologic Class Immunosuppressant Agent
U.S. Brand Names Thymoglobulin®
Mechanism of Action May involve elimination of antigen-reactive T-lymphocytes (killer cells) in peripheral blood or alteration of T-cell function
Use Treatment of renal transplant acute rejection in conjunction with concomitant immunosuppression
USUAL DOSAGE I.V.: 1.5 mg/kg/day for 7-14 days
Dosage Forms INJ: 25 mg vials (with diluent)
Contraindications Patients with history of allergy or anaphylaxis to rabbit proteins, or who have an acute viral illness
Warnings/Precautions Infusion may produce fever and chills. To minimize, the first dose should be infused over a minimum of 6 hours into a high-flow vein. Also, premedication with corticosteroids, acetaminophen, and/or an antihistamine and/or slowing the infusion rate may reduce reaction incidence and intensity.

Prolonged use or overdosage of Thymoglobulin® in association with other immunosuppressive agents may cause over-immunosuppression resulting in severe infections and may increase the incidence of lymphoma or post-transplant lymphoproliferative disease (PTLD) or other malignancies. Appropriate antiviral, antibacterial, antiprotozoal, and/or antifungal prophylaxis is recommended.

Thymoglobulin® should only be used by prescribers experienced in immunosuppressive therapy for the treatment of renal transplant patients. Medical surveillance is required during the infusion. In rare circumstances, anaphylaxis has been reported with use. In such cases, the infusion should be terminated immediately. Medical personnel should be available to treat patients who experience anaphylaxis. Emergency treatment such as 0.3-0.5 mL aqueous epinephrine (1:1000 dilution) subcutaneously and other resuscitative measures including oxygen, intravenous fluids, antihistamines, corticosteroids, pressor amines, and airway management, as clinically indicated, should be provided. Thymoglobulin® or other rabbit immunoglobulins should not be administered again for such patients. Thrombocytopenia or neutropenia may result from cross-reactive antibodies and is reversible following dose adjustments.

Pregnancy Risk Factor C
Adverse Reactions
>10%:
Central nervous system: Fever, chills, headache
Dermatologic: Rash
Endocrine & metabolic: Hyperkalemia
Gastrointestinal: Abdominal pain, diarrhea
Hematologic: Leukopenia, thrombocytopenia
Neuromuscular & skeletal: Weakness
Respiratory: Dyspnea
Miscellaneous: Systemic infection, pain
(Continued)

Antithymocyte Globulin (Rabbit) *(Continued)*

1% to 10%:
- Gastrointestinal: Gastritis
- Respiratory: Pneumonia
- Miscellaneous: Sensitivity reactions: Anaphylaxis may be indicated by hypotension, respiratory distress, serum sickness, viral infection

Education and Monitoring Issues

Monitoring Parameters: Lymphocyte profile, CBC with differential and platelet count, vital signs during administration

♦ **Anti-Tuss® Expectorant [OTC]** *see* Guaifenesin *on page 423*
♦ **Antivert®** *see* Meclizine *on page 556*
♦ **Antrizine®** *see* Meclizine *on page 556*
♦ **Anturan®** *see* Sulfinpyrazone *on page 881*
♦ **Anturane®** *see* Sulfinpyrazone *on page 881*
♦ **Anucort-HC® Suppository** *see* Hydrocortisone *on page 447*
♦ **Anuprep HC® Suppository** *see* Hydrocortisone *on page 447*
♦ **Anusol® HC-1 [OTC]** *see* Hydrocortisone *on page 447*
♦ **Anusol® HC-2.5% [OTC]** *see* Hydrocortisone *on page 447*
♦ **Anusol-HC® Suppository** *see* Hydrocortisone *on page 447*
♦ **Anxanil®** *see* Hydroxyzine *on page 455*
♦ **Anzemet®** *see* Dolasetron *on page 292*
♦ **Apacet® [OTC]** *see* Acetaminophen *on page 17*
♦ **Aphthasol™** *see* Amlexanox *on page 53*
♦ **A.P.L.®** *see* Chorionic Gonadotropin *on page 196*
♦ **Aplisol®** *see* Tuberculin Purified Protein Derivative *on page 960*
♦ **Aplisol®** *see* Tuberculin Tests *on page 960*
♦ **Aplitest®** *see* Tuberculin Purified Protein Derivative *on page 960*
♦ **Aplitest®** *see* Tuberculin Tests *on page 960*
♦ **Apo®-Acetazolamide** *see* Acetazolamide *on page 19*
♦ **Apo®-Allopurinol** *see* Allopurinol *on page 34*
♦ **Apo®-Alpraz** *see* Alprazolam *on page 37*
♦ **Apo®-Amilzide** *see* Amiloride and Hydrochlorothiazide *on page 46*
♦ **Apo®-Amitriptyline** *see* Amitriptyline *on page 51*
♦ **Apo®-Amoxi** *see* Amoxicillin *on page 56*
♦ **Apo®-Ampi Trihydrate** *see* Ampicillin *on page 59*
♦ **Apo®-ASA** *see* Aspirin *on page 72*
♦ **Apo®-Atenol** *see* Atenolol *on page 76*
♦ **Apo® Bromocriptine** *see* Bromocriptine *on page 113*
♦ **Apo®-C** *see* Ascorbic Acid *on page 72*
♦ **Apo-Cal®** *see* Calcium Carbonate *on page 130*
♦ **Apo®-Capto** *see* Captopril *on page 134*
♦ **Apo®-Carbamazepine** *see* Carbamazepine *on page 137*
♦ **Apo®-Cefaclor** *see* Cefaclor *on page 147*
♦ **Apo®-Cephalex** *see* Cephalexin *on page 169*
♦ **Apo®-Chlorax** *see* Clidinium and Chlordiazepoxide *on page 208*
♦ **Apo®-Chlordiazepoxide** *see* Chlordiazepoxide *on page 180*
♦ **Apo®-Chlorpromazine** *see* Chlorpromazine *on page 187*
♦ **Apo®-Chlorpropamide** *see* Chlorpropamide *on page 189*
♦ **Apo®-Chlorthalidone** *see* Chlorthalidone *on page 191*
♦ **Apo®-Cimetidine** *see* Cimetidine *on page 198*
♦ **Apo®-Clomipramine** *see* Clomipramine *on page 213*
♦ **Apo®-Clonidine** *see* Clonidine *on page 216*
♦ **Apo®-Clorazepate** *see* Clorazepate *on page 218*
♦ **Apo®-Cloxi** *see* Cloxacillin *on page 220*
♦ **Apo®-Diazepam** *see* Diazepam *on page 261*
♦ **Apo®-Diclo** *see* Diclofenac *on page 263*
♦ **Apo®-Diflunisal** *see* Diflunisal *on page 271*
♦ **Apo®-Diltiaz** *see* Diltiazem *on page 278*
♦ **Apo®-Dipyridamole FC** *see* Dipyridamole *on page 285*
♦ **Apo®-Dipyridamole SC** *see* Dipyridamole *on page 285*
♦ **Apo®-Doxepin** *see* Doxepin *on page 298*
♦ **Apo®-Doxy** *see* Doxycycline *on page 300*
♦ **Apo®-Doxy Tabs** *see* Doxycycline *on page 300*
♦ **Apo®-Enalapril** *see* Enalapril *on page 309*
♦ **Apo®-Erythro E-C** *see* Erythromycin *on page 323*

- **Apo®-Famotidine** *see* Famotidine *on page 350*
- **Apo®-Fenofibrate** *see* Fenofibrate *on page 353*
- **Apo®-Fluphenazine** *see* Fluphenazine *on page 381*
- **Apo®-Flurazepam** *see* Flurazepam *on page 383*
- **Apo®-Flurbiprofen** *see* Flurbiprofen *on page 384*
- **Apo®-Fluvoxamine** *see* Fluvoxamine *on page 388*
- **Apo®-Folic** *see* Folic Acid *on page 390*
- **Apo®-Furosemide** *see* Furosemide *on page 399*
- **Apo®-Gain** *see* Minoxidil *on page 607*
- **Apo®-Gemfibrozil** *see* Gemfibrozil *on page 406*
- **Apo®-Glyburide** *see* Glyburide *on page 415*
- **Apo®-Guanethidine** *see* Guanethidine *on page 425*
- **Apo®-Hydralazine** *see* Hydralazine *on page 440*
- **Apo®-Hydro** *see* Hydrochlorothiazide *on page 442*
- **Apo®-Hydroxyzine** *see* Hydroxyzine *on page 455*
- **Apo®-Ibuprofen** *see* Ibuprofen *on page 458*
- **Apo®-Imipramine** *see* Imipramine *on page 462*
- **Apo®-Indapadmide** *see* Indapamide *on page 467*
- **Apo®-Indomethacin** *see* Indomethacin *on page 469*
- **Apo®-Ipravent** *see* Ipratropium *on page 483*
- **Apo®-ISDN** *see* Isosorbide Dinitrate *on page 490*
- **Apo®-K** *see* Potassium Chloride *on page 751*
- **Apo®-Keto** *see* Ketoprofen *on page 500*
- **Apo®-Keto-E** *see* Ketoprofen *on page 500*
- **Apo®-Levocarb** *see* Levodopa and Carbidopa *on page 521*
- **Apo®-Lisinopril** *see* Lisinopril *on page 532*
- **Apo®-Lorazepam** *see* Lorazepam *on page 541*
- **Apo®-Lovastatin** *see* Lovastatin *on page 544*
- **Apo®-Meprobamate** *see* Meprobamate *on page 565*
- **Apo®-Methazide** *see* Methyldopa and Hydrochlorothiazide *on page 587*
- **Apo®-Methyldopa** *see* Methyldopa *on page 586*
- **Apo®-Metoclop** *see* Metoclopramide *on page 592*
- **Apo®-Metoprolol (Type L)** *see* Metoprolol *on page 595*
- **Apo®-Metronidazole** *see* Metronidazole *on page 597*
- **Apo®-Minocycline** *see* Minocycline *on page 607*
- **Apo®-Nadol** *see* Nadolol *on page 628*
- **Apo®-Naproxen** *see* Naproxen *on page 636*
- **Apo®-Nifed** *see* Nifedipine *on page 653*
- **Apo®-Nitrofurantoin** *see* Nitrofurantoin *on page 658*
- **Apo®-Nizatidine** *see* Nizatidine *on page 662*
- **Apo®-Nortriptyline** *see* Nortriptyline *on page 665*
- **Apo®-Oxazepam** *see* Oxazepam *on page 686*
- **Apo®-Pentoxifylline SR** *see* Pentoxifylline *on page 715*
- **Apo®-Pen VK** *see* Penicillin V Potassium *on page 713*
- **Apo®-Peram** *see* Amitriptyline and Perphenazine *on page 52*
- **Apo®-Perphenazine** *see* Perphenazine *on page 719*
- **Apo®-Pindol** *see* Pindolol *on page 738*
- **Apo®-Piroxicam** *see* Piroxicam *on page 744*
- **Apo®-Prazo** *see* Prazosin *on page 760*
- **Apo®-Prednisone** *see* Prednisone *on page 763*
- **Apo®-Primidone** *see* Primidone *on page 766*
- **Apo®-Procainamide** *see* Procainamide *on page 769*
- **Apo®-Propranolol** *see* Propranolol *on page 786*
- **Apo®-Ranitidine** *see* Ranitidine Hydrochloride *on page 809*
- **Apo®-Salvent** *see* Albuterol *on page 27*
- **Apo®-Selegiline** *see* Selegiline *on page 843*
- **Apo®-Spirozide** *see* Hydrochlorothiazide and Spironolactone *on page 443*
- **Apo®-Sulfamethoxazole** *see* Sulfamethoxazole *on page 879*
- **Apo®-Sulfasalazine** *see* Sulfasalazine *on page 880*
- **Apo®-Sulfatrim** *see* Co-Trimoxazole *on page 230*
- **Apo®-Sulfinpyraz** *see* Sulfinpyrazone *on page 881*
- **Apo®-Sulin** *see* Sulindac *on page 883*
- **Apo®-Tamox** *see* Tamoxifen *on page 890*
- **Apo®-Temazepam** *see* Temazepam *on page 894*
- **Apo®-Tetra** *see* Tetracycline *on page 903*

- **Apothecary/Metric Equivalents** *see page 1035*
- **Apo®-Thioridazine** *see* Thioridazine *on page 912*
- **Apo®-Timol** *see* Timolol *on page 922*
- **Apo®-Timop** *see* Timolol *on page 922*
- **Apo®-Tolbutamide** *see* Tolbutamide *on page 928*
- **Apo®-Triazide** *see* Hydrochlorothiazide and Triamterene *on page 443*
- **Apo®-Triazo** *see* Triazolam *on page 948*
- **Apo®-Trihex** *see* Trihexyphenidyl *on page 952*
- **Apo®-Trimip** *see* Trimipramine *on page 955*
- **Apo®-Verap** *see* Verapamil *on page 975*
- **Apo®-Zidovudine** *see* Zidovudine *on page 991*

Apraclonidine (a pra KLOE ni deen)

Pharmacologic Class Alpha$_2$ Agonist, Ophthalmic

U.S. Brand Names Iopidine®

Use Prevention and treatment of postsurgical intraocular pressure elevation

USUAL DOSAGE Adults: Ophthalmic:

0.5%: Instill 1-2 drops in the affected eye(s) 3 times/day; since apraclonidine 0.5% will be used with other ocular glaucoma therapies, use an approximate 5-minute interval between instillation of each medication to prevent washout of the previous dose

1%: Instill 1 drop in operative eye 1 hour prior to anterior segment laser surgery, second drop in eye immediately upon completion of procedure

Dosing adjustment in renal impairment: Although the topical use of apraclonidine has not been studied in renal failure patients, structurally related clonidine undergoes a significant increase in half-life in patients with severe renal impairment; close monitoring of cardiovascular parameters in patients with impaired renal function is advised if they are candidates for topical apraclonidine therapy

Dosing adjustment in hepatic impairment: Close monitoring of cardiovascular parameters in patients with impaired liver function is advised because the systemic dosage form of clonidine is partially metabolized in the liver

Contraindications Known hypersensitivity to apraclonidine or clonidine

Pregnancy Risk Factor C

- **Apresazide®** *see* Hydralazine and Hydrochlorothiazide *on page 442*
- **Apresoline®** *see* Hydralazine *on page 440*
- **Aprodine® w/C** *see* Triprolidine, Pseudoephedrine, and Codeine *on page 958*

Aprotinin (a proe TYE nin)

Pharmacologic Class Blood Product Derivative; Hemostatic Agent

U.S. Brand Names Trasylol®

Mechanism of Action Serine protease inhibitor; inhibits plasmin, kallikrein, and platelet activation producing antifibrinolytic effects; a weak inhibitor of plasma pseudocholinesterase. It also inhibits the contact phase activation of coagulation and preserves adhesive platelet glycoproteins making them resistant to damage from increased circulating plasmin or mechanical injury occurring during bypass

Use Reduction or prevention of blood loss in patients undergoing coronary artery bypass surgery when a high risk of excessive bleeding exists; this includes open heart reoperation, pre-existing coagulopathies, operations on the great vessels, and when a patient's beliefs prohibit blood transfusions

Unlabeled use: May decrease blood loss and transfusion requirements during and after major orthopedic surgery and organ transplantation procedures

USUAL DOSAGE

Test dose: **All** patients should receive a 1 mL I.V. test dose at least 10 minutes prior to the loading dose to assess the potential for allergic reactions

Regimen A (standard dose):
- 2 million units (280 mg) loading dose I.V. over 20-30 minutes
- 2 million units (280 mg) into pump prime volume
- 500,000 units/hour (70 mg/hour) I.V. during operation

Regimen B (low dose):
- 1 million units (140 mg) loading dose I.V. over 20-30 minutes
- 1 million units (140 mg) into pump prime volume
- 250,000 units/hour (35 mg/hour) I.V. during operation

Dosage Forms INJ: 1.4 mg/mL [10,000 units/mL] (100 mL, 200 mL)

Contraindications Hypersensitivity to aprotinin or any component, patients with thromboembolic disease requiring anticoagulants or blood factor administration

Warnings/Precautions Patients with a previous exposure to aprotinin are at an increased risk of hypersensitivity reactions

Pregnancy Risk Factor B

Adverse Reactions

1% to 10%:

Cardiovascular: Atrial fibrillation, myocardial infarction, heart failure, atrial flutter, ventricular tachycardia, hypotension, supraventricular tachycardia

Central nervous system: Fever, mental confusion
Local: Phlebitis
Renal: Increased potential for postoperative renal dysfunction
Respiratory: Dyspnea, bronchoconstriction

<1% (limited to important or life-threatening symptoms): Cerebral embolism, cerebrovascular events, convulsions, hemolysis, liver damage, pulmonary edema

Drug Interactions

Heparin and aprotinin prolong ACT. The ACT becomes a poor measure of adequate anticoagulation with the concurrent use of these drugs

Fibrinolytic drugs may have poorer activity; aprotinin blocks this fibrinolytic activity; avoid concurrent use

Captopril's antihypertensive effects may be blocked; avoid concurrent use

Half-Life 150 minutes

Education and Monitoring Issues

Patient Education: You will be unaware of the effects of this drug, however, you will be closely monitored at all times.

Monitoring Parameters: Bleeding times, prothrombin time, activated clotting time, platelet count, red blood cell counts, hematocrit, hemoglobin and fibrinogen degradation products; for toxicity also include renal function tests and blood pressure

Reference Range: Antiplasmin effects occur when plasma aprotinin concentrations are 125 KIU/mL and antikallikrein effects occur when plasma levels are 250-500 KIU/mL; it remains unknown if these plasma concentrations are required for clinical benefits to occur during cardiopulmonary bypass

Manufacturer Bayer Corp (Biological and Pharmaceutical Division)

Related Information

Pharmaceutical Manufacturers Directory *on page 1020*

Ascorbic Acid (a SKOR bik AS id)

Pharmacologic Class Vitamin, Water Soluble

U.S. Brand Names Ascorbicap® [OTC]; C-Crystals® [OTC]; Cebid® Timecelles® [OTC]; Cecon® [OTC]; Cevalin® [OTC]; Cevi-Bid® [OTC]; Ce-Vi-Sol® [OTC]; Dull-C® [OTC]; Flavorcee® [OTC]; N'ice® Vitamin C Drops [OTC]; Vita-C® [OTC]

Use Prevention and treatment of scurvy and to acidify the urine

Investigational: In large doses to decrease the severity of "colds"; dietary supplementation; a 20-year study was recently completed involving 730 individuals which indicates a possible decreased risk of death by stroke when ascorbic acid at doses ≥45 mg/day was administered

USUAL DOSAGE Oral, I.M., I.V., S.C.:

Recommended daily allowance (RDA):
- <6 months: 30 mg
- 6 months to 1 year: 35 mg
- 1-3 years: 40 mg
- 4-10 years: 45 mg
- 11-14 years: 50 mg
- Women: 75 mg/day
- Men: 90 mg/day
- Adult smokers: Add an additional 35 mg/day

Children:
- Scurvy: 100-300 mg/day in divided doses for at least 2 weeks
- Urinary acidification: 500 mg every 6-8 hours
- Dietary supplement: 35-100 mg/day

Adults:
- Scurvy: 100-250 mg 1-2 times/day for at least 2 weeks
- Urinary acidification: 4-12 g/day in 3-4 divided doses
- Prevention and treatment of colds: 1-3 g/day
- Dietary supplement: 50-200 mg/day

Contraindications Large doses during pregnancy

Pregnancy Risk Factor A; C (if used in doses above RDA recommendation)

- ♦ **Ascorbicap® [OTC]** *see* Ascorbic Acid *on page 72*
- ♦ **Ascriptin® [OTC]** *see* Aspirin *on page 72*
- ♦ **Asendin®** *see* Amoxapine *on page 54*
- ♦ **Asmalix®** *see* Theophylline Salts *on page 906*
- ♦ **A-Spas® S/L** *see* Hyoscyamine *on page 456*
- ♦ **Aspergum® [OTC]** *see* Aspirin *on page 72*

Aspirin (AS pir in)

Pharmacologic Class Antiplatelet Agent; Salicylate

U.S. Brand Names Anacin® [OTC]; Arthritis Foundation® Pain Reliever [OTC]; A.S.A. [OTC]; Ascriptin® [OTC]; Aspergum® [OTC]; Asprimox® [OTC]; Bayer® Aspirin [OTC]; Bayer® Buffered Aspirin [OTC]; Bayer® Low Adult Strength [OTC]; Bufferin® [OTC]; Buffex® [OTC]; Cama® Arthritis Pain Reliever [OTC]; Easprin®; Ecotrin® [OTC]; Ecotrin® Low Adult Strength [OTC]; Empirin® [OTC]; Extra Strength Adprin-B® [OTC]; Extra Strength Bayer® Enteric 500 Aspirin [OTC]; Extra Strength Bayer® Plus [OTC]; Halfprin® 81® [OTC]; Regular Strength Bayer® Enteric 500 Aspirin [OTC]; St Joseph® Adult Chewable Aspirin [OTC]; ZORprin®

Generic Available Yes

Mechanism of Action Inhibits prostaglandin synthesis, acts on the hypothalamus heat-regulating center to reduce fever, blocks prostaglandin synthetase action which prevents formation of the platelet-aggregating substance thromboxane A_2

Use Treatment of mild to moderate pain, inflammation, and fever; may be used as a prophylaxis of myocardial infarction and transient ischemic episodes; management of rheumatoid arthritis, rheumatic fever, osteoarthritis, and gout (high dose)

USUAL DOSAGE

Children:
- Analgesic and antipyretic: Oral, rectal: 10-15 mg/kg/dose every 4-6 hours, up to a total of 60-80 mg/kg/24 hours
- Anti-inflammatory: Oral: Initial: 60-90 mg/kg/day in divided doses; usual maintenance: 80-100 mg/kg/day divided every 6-8 hours, maximum dose: 3.6 g/day; monitor serum concentrations
- Kawasaki disease: Oral: 80-100 mg/kg/day divided every 6 hours; after fever resolves: 8-10 mg/kg/day once daily; monitor serum concentrations
- Antirheumatic: Oral: 60-100 mg/kg/day in divided doses every 4 hours

Adults:
- Analgesic and antipyretic: Oral, rectal: 325-650 mg every 4-6 hours up to 4 g/day
- Anti-inflammatory: Oral: Initial: 2.4-3.6 g/day in divided doses; usual maintenance: 3.6-5.4 g/day; monitor serum concentrations
- TIA: Oral: 1.3 g/day in 2-4 divided doses
- Myocardial infarction prophylaxis: 160-325 mg/day

Dosing adjustment in renal impairment: Cl_{cr} <10 mL/minute: Avoid use

Hemodialysis: Dialyzable (50% to 100%)

Dosing adjustment in hepatic disease: Avoid use in severe liver disease

Dosage Forms CAP: 356.4 mg and caffeine 30 mg. **GUM:** 227.5 mg; Timed release: 650 mg. **SUPP, rectal:** 60 mg, 120 mg, 125 mg, 130 mg, 195 mg, 200 mg, 300 mg, 325 mg, 600 mg, 650 mg, 1.2 g. **TAB:** 65 mg, 75 mg, 81 mg, 325 mg, 500 mg; With caffeine: 400 mg and caffeine 32 mg; Buffered: 325 mg and magnesium-aluminum hydroxide 150 mg, 325 mg, magnesium hydroxide 75 mg, aluminum hydroxide 75 mg, buffered with calcium carbonate, 325 mg and magnesium-aluminum hydroxide 75 mg; Chewable: 81 mg; Controlled release: 800 mg; Delayed release: 81 mg; Enteric coated: 81 mg, 325 mg, 500 mg, 650 mg, 975 mg

Contraindications Bleeding disorders (factor VII or IX deficiencies), hypersensitivity to salicylates or other NSAIDs, tartrazine dye and asthma

Warnings/Precautions Use with caution in patients with platelet and bleeding disorders, renal dysfunction, erosive gastritis, or peptic ulcer disease, previous nonreaction does not guarantee future safe taking of medication; do not use aspirin in children <16 years of age for chickenpox or flu symptoms due to the association with Reye's syndrome

Otic: Discontinue use if dizziness, tinnitus, or impaired hearing occurs; surgical patients: avoid ASA if possible, for 1 week prior to surgery because of the possibility of postoperative bleeding; use with caution in impaired hepatic function

Elderly are a high-risk population for adverse effects from nonsteroidal anti-inflammatory agents. As much as 60% of elderly with GI complications to NSAIDs can develop peptic ulceration and/or hemorrhage asymptomatically. Also, concomitant disease and drug use contribute to the risk for GI adverse effects. Use lowest effective dose for shortest period possible. Consider renal function decline with age. Use of NSAIDs can compromise existing renal function especially when Cl_{cr} is <30 mL/minute. Tinnitus may be a difficult and unreliable indication of toxicity due to age-related hearing loss or eighth cranial nerve damage. CNS adverse effects such as confusion, agitation, and hallucination are generally seen in overdose or high-dose situations, but elderly may demonstrate these adverse effects at lower doses than younger adults.

Pregnancy Risk Factor C; D (if full-dose aspirin in 3rd trimester)

Adverse Reactions As with all drugs which may affect hemostasis, bleeding is associated with aspirin. Hemorrhage may occur at virtually any site. Risk is dependent on multiple variables including dosage, concurrent use of multiple agents which alter hemostasis, and patient susceptibility. Many adverse effects of aspirin are dose-related, and are rare at low dosages. Other serious reactions are idiosyncratic, related to allergy or individual sensitivity. Accurate estimation of frequencies is not possible. The reactions listed below have been reported for aspirin.

Central nervous system: Fatigue, insomnia, nervousness, agitation, confusion, dizziness, headache, lethargy, cerebral edema, hyperthermia, coma

Cardiovascular: Hypotension, tachycardia, dysrhythmias, edema

Dermatologic: Rash, angioedema, urticaria

Endocrine and metabolic: Acidosis, hyperkalemia, dehydration, hypoglycemia (children), hyperglycemia, hypernatremia (buffered forms)

Gastrointestinal: Nausea, vomiting, dyspepsia, epigastric discomfort, heartburn, stomach pains, gastrointestinal ulceration (6% to 31%), gastric erosions, gastric erythema, duodenal ulcers

Hematologic: Anemia, disseminated intravascular coagulation, prolongation of prothrombin times, coagulopathy, thrombocytopenia, hemolytic anemia, bleeding, iron deficiency anemia

Hepatic: Hepatotoxicity, increased transaminases, hepatitis (reversible)

Neuromuscular and skeletal: Rhabdomyolysis, weakness, acetabular bone destruction (OA)

Otic: Hearing loss, tinnitus

Renal: Interstitial nephritis, papillary necrosis, proteinuria, renal impairment, renal failure (including cases caused by rhabdomyolysis), increased BUN, increased serum creatinine

Respiratory: Asthma, bronchospasm, dyspnea, laryngeal edema, hyperpnea, tachypnea, respiratory alkalosis, noncardiogenic pulmonary edema

Miscellaneous: Anaphylaxis, prolonged pregnancy and labor, stillbirths, low birth weight, peripartum bleeding, Reye's syndrome

Case reports: Colonic ulceration, esophageal stricture, esophagitis with esophageal ulcer, esophageal hematoma, oral mucosal ulcers (aspirin-containing chewing gum), coronary artery spasm, conduction defect and atrial fibrillation (toxicity), delirium, ischemic brain infarction, colitis, rectal stenosis (suppository), cholestatic jaundice, periorbital edema, rhinosinusitis

Drug Interactions

ACE inhibitors: The effects of ace inhibitors may be blunted by aspirin administration, particularly at higher dosages.

Buspirone increases aspirin's free % *in vitro.*

Carbonic anhydrase inhibitors and corticosteroids have been associated with alteration in salicylate serum concentrations.

Heparin and low molecular weight heparins: Concurrent use may increase the risk of bleeding.

(Continued)

Aspirin *(Continued)*

Methotrexate serum levels may be increased; consider discontinuing aspirin 2-3 days before high-dose methotrexate treatment or avoid concurrent use.
NSAIDs may increase the risk of gastrointestinal adverse effects and bleeding. Serum concentrations of some NSAIDs may be decreased by aspirin.
Platelet inhibitors (IIb/IIa antagonists): Risk of bleeding may be increased.
Probenecid effects may be antagonized by aspirin.
Sulfonylureas: The effects of older sulfonylurea agents (tolazamide, tolbutamide) may be potentiated due to displacement from plasma proteins. This effect does not appear to be clinically significant for newer sulfonylurea agents (glyburide, glipizide, glimepiride).
Valproic acid may be displaced from its binding sites which can result in toxicity.
Verapamil may potentiate the prolongation of bleeding time associated with aspirin.
Warfarin and oral anticoagulants may increase the risk of bleeding.

Alcohol Interactions Avoid use (may enhance gastric mucosal irritation)

Onset Peak in 1-2 hours

Duration 4-6 hours

Half-Life Dose dependent; 3 hours at low dose, up to 10 hours at higher doses

Education and Monitoring Issues

Patient Education: Use exactly as directed (do not increase dose or frequency); adverse reactions can occur with overuse. Take with food or milk. Do not use aspirin with strong vinegary odor. Do not crush or chew extended release products. While using this medication, avoid alcohol, excessive amounts of vitamin C, or salicylate-containing foods (curry powder, prunes, raisins, tea, or licorice), other prescription or OTC medications containing aspirin or salicylate, or other NSAIDs without consulting prescriber. Maintain adequate hydration (2-3 L/day of fluids unless instructed to restrict fluid intake). You may experience nausea, vomiting, gastric discomfort (frequent mouth care, small frequent meals, sucking lozenges, or chewing gum may help). GI bleeding, ulceration, or perforation can occur with or without pain. May discolor stool (pink/red). Stop taking aspirin and report ringing in ears; persistent pain in stomach; unresolved nausea or vomiting; difficulty breathing or shortness of breath; unusual bruising or bleeding (mouth, urine, stool); or skin rash.

Dietary Considerations:

Food: May decrease the rate but not the extent of oral absorption. Drug may cause GI upset, bleeding, ulceration, perforation. Take with food or large volume of water or milk to minimize GI upset.

Folic acid: Hyperexcretion of folate; folic acid deficiency may result, leading to macrocytic anemia. Supplement with folic acid if necessary.

Iron: With chronic aspirin use and at doses of 3-4 g/day, iron deficiency anemia may result; supplement with iron if necessary

Sodium: Hypernatremia resulting from buffered aspirin solutions or sodium salicylate containing high sodium content. Avoid or use with caution in CHF or any condition where hypernatremia would be detrimental.

Curry powder, paprika, licorice, Benedictine liqueur, prunes, raisins, tea and gherkins: Potential salicylate accumulation. These foods contain 6 mg salicylate/100 g. An ordinarily American diet contains 10-200 mg/day of salicylate. Foods containing salicylates may contribute to aspirin hypersensitivity. Patients at greatest risk for aspirin hypersensitivity include those with asthma, nasal polyposis or chronic urticaria.

Fresh fruits containing vitamin C: Displaces drug from binding sites, resulting in increased urinary excretion of aspirin. Educate patients regarding the potential for a decreased analgesic effect of aspirin with consumption of foods high in vitamin C.

Reference Range: Timing of serum samples: Peak levels usually occur 2 hours after ingestion. Salicylate serum concentrations correlate with the pharmacological actions and adverse effects observed. See table.

Serum Salicylate: Clinical Correlations

Serum Salicylate Concentration (mcg/mL)	Desired Effects	Adverse Effects/Intoxication
~100	Antiplatelet Antipyresis Analgesia	GI intolerance and bleeding, hypersensitivity, hemostatic defects
150-300	Anti-inflammatory	Mild salicylism
250-400	Treatment of rheumatic fever	Nausea/vomiting, hyperventilation, salicylism, flushing, sweating, thirst, headache, diarrhea, and tachycardia
>400-500		Respiratory alkalosis, hemorrhage, excitement, confusion, asterixis, pulmonary edema, convulsions, tetany, metabolic acidosis, fever, coma, cardiovascular collapse, renal and respiratory failure

Related Information

Aspirin and Codeine *on page 75*
Aspirin and Meprobamate *on page 76*
Carisoprodol and Aspirin *on page 142*
Carisoprodol, Aspirin, and Codeine *on page 142*
Methocarbamol and Aspirin *on page 582*
Orphenadrine, Aspirin, and Caffeine *on page 681*
Propoxyphene and Aspirin *on page 786*

Aspirin and Codeine (AS pir in & KOE deen)

Pharmacologic Class Analgesic, Combination (Narcotic)

U.S. Brand Names Empirin® With Codeine

Use Relief of mild to moderate pain

Dosage Forms TAB: #2: Aspirin 325 mg and codeine phosphate 15 mg, #3: Aspirin 325 mg and codeine phosphate 30 mg, #4: Aspirin 325 mg and codeine phosphate 60 mg

Pregnancy Risk Factor D

Aspirin and Extended-Release Dipyridamole

(AS pir in & dye peer ID a mole)

Pharmacologic Class Antiplatelet Agent

U.S. Brand Names Aggrenox™

Mechanism of Action The antithrombotic action results from additive antiplatelet effects. Dipyridamole inhibits the uptake of adenosine into platelets, endothelial cells, and erythrocytes. Aspirin inhibits platelet aggregation by irreversible inhibition of platelet cyclooxygenase and thus inhibits the generation of thromboxane A2.

Use Reduction in the risk of stroke in patients who have had transient ischemia of the brain or completed ischemic stroke due to thrombosis

USUAL DOSAGE Adults: Oral: 1 capsule (200 mg dipyridamole, 25 mg aspirin) twice daily.

Dosage adjustment in renal impairment: Avoid use in patients with severe renal dysfunction (Cl_{cr} <10 mL/minute). Studies have not been done in patients with renal impairment.

Dosage adjustment in hepatic impairment: Avoid use in patients with severe hepatic impairment; studies have not been done in patients with varying degrees of hepatic impairment

Elderly: Plasma concentrations were 40% higher, but specific dosage adjustments have not been recommended

Dosage Forms CAP: 200 mg dipyridamole, 25 mg aspirin

Contraindications Hypersensitivity to dipyridamole, aspirin, or any component; allergy to NSAIDs; patients with asthma, rhinitis, and nasal polyps; bleeding disorders (factor VII or IX deficiencies); children <16 years of age with viral infections; pregnancy (especially 3rd trimester)

Warnings/Precautions Patients who consume ≥3 alcoholic drinks per day are at risk of bleeding. Cautious use in patients with inherited or acquired bleeding disorders including those of liver disease or vitamin K deficiency. Watch for signs and symptoms of GI ulcers and bleeding. Avoid use in patients with active peptic ulcer disease. Discontinue use if dizziness, tinnitus, or impaired hearing occurs. Stop 1-2 weeks before elective surgical procedures to avoid bleeding. Use caution in the elderly who are at high risk for adverse events. Cautious use in patients with hypotension, patients with unstable angina, recent MI, and hepatic dysfunction. Avoid in patients with severe renal failure. Safety and efficacy in children have not been established.

Pregnancy Risk Factor B (dipyridamole); D (aspirin)

Pregnancy Implications Aggrenox™ should be used in pregnancy only if the benefit justifies the potential risk to the fetus. It should not be used in the third trimester of pregnancy.

Adverse Reactions

>10%:

Central nervous system: Headache (38.2%)

Gastrointestinal: Dyspepsia, abdominal pain (17.5%), nausea (16%), diarrhea (12.7%)

1% to 10%:

Central nervous system: Pain (6.4%), seizures (1.7%), fatigue (5.8%), malaise (1.6%), syncope (1%), amnesia (2.4%), confusion (1.1%), somnolence (1.2%)

Cardiovascular: Cardiac failure (1.6%)

Dermatologic: Purpura (1.4%)

Gastrointestinal: Vomiting (8.4%), bleeding (4.1%), rectal bleeding 1.6%, hemorrhoids (1%), hemorrhage 1.2%, anorexia (1.2%)

Hematologic: Anemia (1.6%)

Neuromuscular & skeletal: Back pain (4.6%), weakness (1.8%), arthralgia (5.5%), arthritis (2.1%), arthrosis (1.1%), myalgia (1.2%)

Respiratory: Cough (1.5%), upper respiratory tract infections (1%), epistaxis (2.4%)

<1% (limited to life-threatening or important symptoms): Intracranial hemorrhage (0.6%), allergic reaction, fever, hypotension, coma, dizziness, paresthesia, cerebral hemorrhage, subarachnoid hemorrhage, gastritis, ulceration, perforation, tinnitus, deafness,

(Continued)

Aspirin and Extended-Release Dipyridamole *(Continued)*

tachycardia, palpitations, arrhythmia, supraventricular tachycardia, cholelithiasis, jaundice, hepatic function abnormality, hyperglycemia, thirst, hematoma, gingival bleeding, agitation, uterine hemorrhage, hyperpnea, asthma, bronchospasm, hemoptysis, pulmonary edema, taste loss, pruritus, urticaria, renal insufficiency and failure, hematuria, flushing, hypothermia, chest pain, angina pectoris, cerebral edema, pancreatitis, Reye's syndrome, hematemesis, hearing impairment, anaphylaxis, laryngeal edema, hepatitis, hepatic failure, rhabdomyolysis, hypoglycemia, dehydration, prolonged PT time, disseminated intravascular coagulation, coagulopathy, thrombocytopenia, prolonged pregnancy and labor, stillbirths, lower weight infants, antepartum and postpartum bleeding, tachypnea, dyspnea, rash, alopecia, angioedema, Stevens-Johnson syndrome, interstitial nephritis, papillary necrosis, proteinuria, allergic vasculitis, anemia (aplastic), pancytopenia, thrombocytosis

Drug Interactions

Increased effects: Plasma levels and cardiovascular effects of adenosine are increased; decrease adenosine dose. Use of aspirin-dipyridamole with anticoagulants (heparin, low molecular weight heparins, warfarin) or antiplatelet agents (NSAIDs, IIb/IIIa antagonists) may increase the risk of bleeding. Serum concentrations and and toxicity of methotrexate may be increased when used concurrently with aspirin; avoid concurrent use. Serum concentrations of acetazolamide, phenytoin or valproic acid may be increased with aspirin. Concurrent use of verapamil may prolong bleeding times.

Decreased effect: Angiotensin-converting enzyme inhibitors may have diminished pharmacologic effect with aspirin (at higher dosages). The effect of cholinesterase inhibitors may be reduced with concurrent aspirin-dipyridamole therapy; avoid concurrent use. Aspirin may diminish the effect of diuretics, probenecid, and sulfinpyrazone.

Education and Monitoring Issues

Patient Education: Take exactly as directed (do not increase dose or frequency). Swallow capsule whole without chewing or crushing; may be taken with food to reduce GI upset. Avoid alcohol, aspirin or aspirin-containing medication and other OTC medications unless approved by prescriber. May cause dizziness, confusion, or blurred vision (avoid driving or engaging in tasks that require alertness until response to drug is known) or nausea, vomiting, anorexia (take medication with food, eating small frequent meals, and using good mouth care may help). Watch closely for signs of stroke (weakness, acute headache, numbness or loss of strength in any part of the body, disturbances in speech) and notify prescriber immediately. GI bleeding, ulceration, or perforation can occur with or without pain. Report unusual signs of bleeding or bruising, weakness, back or muscle pain, chest pain, cough, skin rash, or persistent diarrhea,

Monitoring Parameters: Hemoglobin, hematocrit, signs or symptoms of bleeding, signs or symptoms of stroke

Manufacturer Boehringer Ingelheim, Inc

Related Information

Pharmaceutical Manufacturers Directory *on page 1020*

Aspirin and Meprobamate (AS pir in & me proe BA mate)

Pharmacologic Class Antianxiety Agent, Miscellaneous

U.S. Brand Names Equagesic®

Dosage Forms TAB: Aspirin 325 mg and meprobamate 200 mg

Pregnancy Risk Factor D

- **Aspirin Backache** *see* Methocarbamol and Aspirin *on page 582*
- **Aspirin Free Anacin® Maximum Strength [OTC]** *see* Acetaminophen *on page 17*
- **Asprimox® [OTC]** *see* Aspirin *on page 72*
- **Astelin® Nasal Spray** *see* Azelastine *on page 85*
- **Asthma Guidelines** *see page 1077*
- **Astramorph™ PF Injection** *see* Morphine Sulfate *on page 618*
- **Atacand™** *see* Candesartan *on page 133*
- **Atamet®** *see* Levodopa and Carbidopa *on page 521*
- **Atarax®** *see* Hydroxyzine *on page 455*
- **Atasol®** *see* Acetaminophen *on page 17*
- **Atasol® 8, 15, 30 With Caffeine** *see* Acetaminophen and Codeine *on page 18*

Atenolol (a TEN oh lole)

Pharmacologic Class Beta Blocker, $Beta_1$ Selective

U.S. Brand Names Tenormin®

Generic Available Yes

Mechanism of Action Competitively blocks response to beta-adrenergic stimulation, selectively blocks $beta_1$-receptors with little or no effect on $beta_2$-receptors except at high doses

Use Treatment of hypertension, alone or in combination with other agents; management of angina pectoris, postmyocardial infarction patients

Unlabeled use: Acute alcohol withdrawal, supraventricular and ventricular arrhythmias, and migraine headache prophylaxis

USUAL DOSAGE

Oral:

Children: 1-2 mg/kg/dose given daily

Adults:

Hypertension: 50 mg once daily, may increase to 100 mg/day; doses >100 mg are unlikely to produce any further benefit

Angina pectoris: 50 mg once daily, may increase to 100 mg/day; some patients may require 200 mg/day

Postmyocardial infarction: Follow I.V. dose with 100 mg/day or 50 mg twice daily for 6-9 days postmyocardial infarction

I.V.: Postmyocardial infarction: Early treatment: 5 mg slow I.V. over 5 minutes; may repeat in 10 minutes; if both doses are tolerated, may start oral atenolol 50 mg every 12 hours or 100 mg/day for 6-9 days postmyocardial infarction

Dosing interval for oral atenolol in renal impairment:

Cl_{cr} 15-35 mL/minute: Administer 50 mg/day maximum

Cl_{cr} <15 mL/minute: Administer 50 mg every other day maximum

Hemodialysis: Moderately dialyzable (20% to 50%) via hemodialysis; administer dose postdialysis or administer 25-50 mg supplemental dose

Peritoneal dialysis: Elimination is not enhanced; supplemental dose is not necessary

Dosage Forms INJ: 0.5 mg/mL (10 mL). **TAB:** 25 mg, 50 mg, 100 mg

Contraindications Hypersensitivity to beta-blocking agents, pulmonary edema, cardiogenic shock, bradycardia, heart block without a pacemaker, uncompensated congestive heart failure, sinus node dysfunction, A-V conduction abnormalities

Warnings/Precautions Safety and efficacy in children have not been established; administer with caution to patients (especially the elderly) with bronchospastic disease, CHF, renal dysfunction, severe peripheral vascular disease, myasthenia gravis, diabetes mellitus, hyperthyroidism. **Abrupt withdrawal of the drug should be avoided**, drug should be discontinued over 1-2 weeks; may potentiate hypoglycemia in a diabetic patient and mask signs and symptoms; modify dosage in patients with renal impairment.

Pregnancy Risk Factor D

Pregnancy Implications

Clinical effects on the fetus: Crosses the placenta; persistent beta-blockade, bradycardia, IUGR; IUGR probably related to maternal hypertension. Available evidence suggest safe use during pregnancy and breast-feeding. Monitor breast-fed infant for symptoms of beta-blockade.

Breast-feeding/lactation: Crosses into breast milk. American Academy of Pediatrics considers **compatible** with breast-feeding.

Clinical effects on the infant: Symptoms have been reported of beta-blockade including cyanosis, hypothermia, bradycardia.

Adverse Reactions

1% to 10%:

Cardiovascular: Persistent bradycardia (3%), hypotension (4%), second or third degree A-V block (0.7% to 1.7%), Raynaud's phenomenon (rare)

Central nervous system: Dizziness (4% to 13%), fatigue (3% to 6%), lethargy (1% to 3%), confusion (rare), mental impairment (rare)

Gastrointestinal: Diarrhea (2% to 3%), nausea (3% to 4%)

Genitourinary: Impotence (rare)

Respiratory: Dyspnea (especially with large doses), wheezing (0% to 3%)

Miscellaneous: Cold extremities (<10%)

<1%: Depression, headache, nightmares

Drug Interactions

Alpha-blockers (prazosin, terazosin): Concurrent use of beta-blockers may increase risk of orthostasis

Ampicillin, in single doses of 1 gram, decrease atenolol's pharmacologic actions

Antacids (magnesium-aluminum, calcium antacids or salts) may reduce the bioavailability of atenolol

Clonidine: Hypertensive crisis after or during withdrawal of either agent

Drugs which slow A-V conduction (digoxin): Effects may be additive with beta-blockers

Glucagon: Atenolol may blunt the hyperglycemic action of glucagon

Insulin and oral hypoglycemics: Atenolol masks the tachycardia that usually accompanies hypoglycemia

NSAIDs (ibuprofen, indomethacin, naproxen, piroxicam) may reduce the antihypertensive effects of beta-blockers

Salicylates may reduce the antihypertensive effects of beta-blockers

Sulfonylureas: Beta-blockers may alter response to hypoglycemic agents

Verapamil or diltiazem may have synergistic or additive pharmacological effects when taken concurrently with beta-blockers

Alcohol Interactions Limit use (may increase risk of hypotension or dizziness)

Onset Peak concentrations in 1-2 hours with oral; more rapid with I.V.

Duration 12-24 hours in normal renal function

Half-Life Normal renal function: 6-9 hours, longer in those with renal impairment; End-stage renal disease: 15-35 hours

(Continued)

Atenolol *(Continued)*

Education and Monitoring Issues

Patient Education: Take exactly as directed. Do not increase, decrease, or adjust dosage without consulting prescriber. Take pulse daily, prior to medication and follow prescriber's instruction about holding medication. Do not take with antacids. Do not use alcohol or OTC medications (eg, cold remedies) without consulting prescriber. If diabetic, monitor serum sugars closely (may alter glucose tolerance or mask signs of hypoglycemia). May cause fatigue, dizziness, or postural hypotension; use caution when changing position from lying or sitting to standing, when driving, or when climbing stairs until response to medication is known. May cause alteration in sexual performance (reversible). Report unresolved swelling of extremities, difficulty breathing or new cough, unresolved fatigue, unusual weight gain, unresolved constipation, or unusual muscle weakness.

Monitoring Parameters: Monitor blood pressure, apical and radial pulses, fluid I & O, daily weight, respirations, and circulation in extremities before and during therapy

Related Information

Atenolol and Chlorthalidone *on page 78*
Beta-Blockers Comparison *on page 1233*

Atenolol and Chlorthalidone (a TEN oh lole & klor THAL i done)

Pharmacologic Class Antihypertensive Agent, Combination

U.S. Brand Names Tenoretic®

Dosage Forms TAB: 50: Atenolol 50 mg and chlorthalidone 25 mg; 100: Atenolol 100 mg and chlorthalidone 25 mg

Pregnancy Risk Factor D

♦ **Atgam®** *see* Lymphocyte Immune Globulin *on page 548*
♦ **Ativan®** *see* Lorazepam *on page 541*
♦ **Atolone®** *see* Triamcinolone *on page 944*

Atorvastatin (a TORE va sta tin)

Pharmacologic Class Antilipemic Agent (HMG-CoA Reductase Inhibitor)

U.S. Brand Names Lipitor®

Mechanism of Action Inhibitor of 3-hydroxy-3-methylglutaryl coenzyme A (HMG-CoA) reductase, the rate limiting enzyme in cholesterol synthesis (reduces the production of mevalonic acid from HMG-CoA); this then results in a compensatory increase in the expression of LDL receptors on hepatocyte membranes and a stimulation of LDL catabolism

Use Adjunct to diet for the reduction of elevated total and LDL cholesterol levels and to increase high-density lipoprotein cholesterol (HDL-C) in patients with hypercholesterolemia (types IIa, IIb, and IIc); used in hypercholesterolemic patients without clinically evident heart disease to reduce the risk of myocardial infarction, to reduce the risk for revascularization, and reduce the risk of death due to cardiovascular causes; adjunct to diet for Fredrickson type IV/Fredrickson type II who do not respond to diet

USUAL DOSAGE Adults: Oral: Initial: 10 mg once daily, titrate up to 80 mg/day if needed

Dosing adjustment in renal impairment: No dosage adjustment necessary

Dosing adjustment in hepatic impairment: Decrease dosage with severe disease (eg, chronic alcoholic liver disease)

Dosage Forms TAB: 10 mg, 20 mg, 40 mg

Contraindications Hypersensitivity to atorvastatin or its components; patients with active liver disease; pregnancy or lactation

Warnings/Precautions Discontinue therapy if symptoms of myopathy or renal failure due to rhabdomyolysis develop. Use with caution in patients with history of liver disease or who consume excessive amounts of alcohol. It is recommended that liver function tests (LFTs) be performed prior to and at 12 weeks following both the initiation of therapy and any elevation in dose, and periodically (eg, semiannually) thereafter.

Pregnancy Risk Factor X

Adverse Reactions

>10%: Central nervous system: Headache (2.5% to 16.7%)

2% to 10%:

Central nervous system: Weakness (0% to 3.8%), insomnia, dizziness

Cardiovascular: Chest pain, peripheral edema

Dermatologic: Rash (1.1% to 3.9%)

Gastrointestinal: Abdominal pain (0% to 3.8%), constipation (0% to 2.5%), diarrhea (0% to 3.85), dyspepsia (1.3% to 2.85), flatulence (1.1% to 2.8%), nausea

Genitourinary: Urinary tract infection

Neuromuscular & skeletal: Arthralgia (0% to 5.1%), myalgia (0% to 5.6%), back pain (0% to 3.8%), arthritis

Miscellaneous: Infection (2% to 10%), flu-like syndrome (0% to 3.2%), allergic reaction (0% to 2.8%)

Respiratory: Sinusitis (0% to 6.4%), pharyngitis (0% to 2.5%), bronchitis, rhinitis

<2% (limited to important or life-threatening symptoms): Pneumonia, dyspnea, epistaxis, face edema, fever, photosensitivity, malaise, edema, gastroenteritis, elevated transaminases, colitis, vomiting, gastritis, xerostomia, rectal hemorrhage, esophagitis, eructation, glossitis, stomatitis, anorexia, increased appetite, biliary pain, cheilitis, duodenal ulcer, dysphagia, enteritis, melena, gingival hemorrhage, tenesmus, hepatitis, pancreatitis, cholestatic jaundice, paresthesia, somnolence, abnormal dreams, decreased libido, emotional lability, incoordination, peripheral neuropathy, torticollis, facial paralysis, hyperkinesia, depression, hypesthesia, hypertonia, leg cramps, bursitis, myasthenia, myositis, tendinous contracture, pruritus, alopecia, dry skin, urticaria, acne, eczema, seborrhea, skin ulcer, cystitis, hematuria, impotence, dysuria, nocturia, epididymitis, fibrocystic breast disease, vaginal hemorrhage, nephritis, abnormal urination, amblyopia, tinnitus, deafness, glaucoma, taste loss, taste perversion, palpitation, vasodilation, syncope, migraine, postural hypotension, phlebitis, arrhythmia, angina, hypertension, hyperglycemia, gout, weight gain, hypoglycemia, ecchymosis, anemia, lymphadenopathy, thrombocytopenia, petechiae, pharyngitis, rhinitis, myopathy

Postmarketing reports have included anaphylaxis, angioneurotic edema, bullous rashes, erythema multiforme, toxic epidermal necrolysis, Stevens-Johnson syndrome, and rhabdomyolysis.

Additional class-related events or case reports (not necessarily reported with atorvastatin therapy): Myopathy, increased CPK (>10x normal), rhabdomyolysis, renal failure (secondary to rhabdomyolysis), alteration in taste, impaired extraocular muscle movement, facial paresis, tremor, memory loss, vertigo, paresthesia, peripheral neuropathy, peripheral nerve palsy, anxiety, depression, psychic disturbance, hypersensitivity reaction, angioedema, anaphylaxis, systemic lupus erythematosus-like syndrome, polymyalgia rheumatica, dermatomyositis, vasculitis, purpura, thrombocytopenia, leukopenia, hemolytic anemia, positive ANA, increased ESR, eosinophilia, arthritis, urticaria, photosensitivity, fever, chills, flushing, malaise, dyspnea, rash, toxic epidermal necrolysis, erythema multiforme, Stevens-Johnson syndrome, pancreatitis, hepatitis, cholestatic jaundice, fatty liver, cirrhosis, fulminant hepatic necrosis, hepatoma, anorexia, vomiting, alopecia, nodules, skin discoloration, dryness of skin/mucous membranes, nail changes, gynecomastia, decreased libido, erectile dysfunction, impotence, cataracts, ophthalmoplegia, elevated transaminases, increased alkaline phosphatase, increased GGT, hyperbilirubinemia, thyroid dysfunction

Drug Interactions CYP3A3/4 enzyme substrate

Increased toxicity: Gemfibrozil (musculoskeletal effects such as myopathy, myalgia and/or muscle weakness accompanied by markedly elevated CK concentrations, rash and/or pruritus); clofibrate, niacin (myopathy), erythromycin, cyclosporine, oral anticoagulants (elevated PT)

Protease inhibitors (amprenavir, nelfinavir, ritonavir) may increase serum concentrations of atorvastatin, increasing the risk of myopathy/rhabdomyolysis

Increased effect/toxicity of levothyroxine

Concurrent use of erythromycin and atorvastatin may result in rhabdomyolysis

Onset Maximal reduction in plasma cholesterol and triglycerides in 2 weeks; initial changes in 3-5 days

Half-Life 14 hours (parent)

Education and Monitoring Issues

Patient Education: May take with meals at any time of day. Maintain adequate hydration (2-3 L/day of fluids unless instructed to restrict fluid intake). You will need laboratory evaluation during therapy. May cause headache (mild analgesic may help); diarrhea (yogurt or buttermilk may help); euphoria, giddiness, confusion (use caution when driving or engaging in tasks that require alertness until response to medication is known). Report unresolved diarrhea, excessive or acute muscle cramping or weakness, changes in mood or memory, yellowing of skin or eyes, easy bruising or bleeding, and unusual fatigue.

Monitoring Parameters: Lipid levels after 2-4 weeks; LFTs, CPK

It is recommended that liver function tests (LFTs) be performed prior to and at 12 weeks following both the initiation of therapy and any elevation in dose, and periodically (eg, semiannually) thereafter

Manufacturer Parke-Davis

Related Information

Pharmaceutical Manufacturers Directory *on page 1020*

Atovaquone (a TOE va kwone)

Pharmacologic Class Antiprotozoal

U.S. Brand Names Mepron™

Mechanism of Action Has not been fully elucidated; may inhibit electron transport in mitochondria inhibiting metabolic enzymes

Use Acute oral treatment of mild to moderate *Pneumocystis carinii* pneumonia (PCP) in patients who are intolerant to co-trimoxazole; prophylaxis of PCP in patients intolerant to co-trimoxazole; treatment/suppression of *Toxoplasma gondii* encephalitis, primary prophylaxis of HIV-infected persons at high risk for developing *Toxoplasma gondii* encephalitis

(Continued)

Atovaquone *(Continued)*

USUAL DOSAGE Adults: Oral: 750 mg twice daily with food for 21 days

Dosage Forms SUSP, oral (citrus flavor): 750 mg/5 mL (210 mL)

Contraindications Life-threatening allergic reaction to the drug or formulation

Warnings/Precautions Has only been indicated in mild to moderate PCP; use with caution in elderly patients due to potentially impaired renal, hepatic, and cardiac function

Pregnancy Risk Factor C

Adverse Reactions Note: Adverse reaction statistics have been compiled from studies including patients with advanced HIV disease; consequently, it is difficult to distinguish reactions attributed to atovaquone from those caused by the underlying disease or a combination, thereof.

>10%:

- Central nervous system: Headache, fever, insomnia, anxiety
- Dermatologic: Rash
- Gastrointestinal: Nausea, diarrhea, vomiting
- Respiratory: Cough

1% to 10%:

- Central nervous system: Dizziness
- Dermatologic: Pruritus
- Endocrine & metabolic: Hypoglycemia, hyponatremia
- Gastrointestinal: Abdominal pain, constipation, anorexia, dyspepsia, increased amylase
- Hematologic: Anemia, neutropenia, leukopenia
- Hepatic: Elevated liver enzymes
- Neuromuscular & skeletal: Weakness
- Renal: Elevated BUN/creatinine
- Miscellaneous: Oral moniliasis

Drug Interactions

Decreased effect: Rifamycins used concurrently decrease the steady-state plasma concentrations of atovaquone

Note: Possible increased toxicity with other highly protein bound drugs

Half-Life 2.9 days

Education and Monitoring Issues

Patient Education: Take as directed. Take with high-fat meals. You may experience dizziness or lightheadedness; use caution when driving or engaging in tasks that require alertness until response to drug is known. Small meals may help reduce nausea. Report unresolved diarrhea, fever, mouth sores (use good mouth care), unresolved headache or vomiting.

Dietary Considerations: Administer with food

Manufacturer GlaxoWellcome

Related Information

Pharmaceutical Manufacturers Directory *on page 1020*

♦ **Atozine®** *see* Hydroxyzine *on page 455*

♦ **Atridox™** *see* Doxycycline *on page 300*

♦ **Atrohist® Plus** *see* Chlorpheniramine, Phenylephrine, Phenylpropanolamine, and Belladonna Alkaloids *on page 187*

♦ **Atromid-S®** *see* Clofibrate *on page 211*

♦ **Atropair® Ophthalmic** *see* Atropine *on page 80*

Atropine (A troe peen)

Pharmacologic Class Anticholinergic Agent; Anticholinergic Agent, Ophthalmic; Antidote; Antispasmodic Agent, Gastrointestinal; Ophthalmic Agent, Mydriatic

U.S. Brand Names Atropair® Ophthalmic; Atropine-Care® Ophthalmic; Atropisol® Ophthalmic; Isopto® Atropine Ophthalmic; I-Tropine® Ophthalmic; Ocu-Tropine® Ophthalmic

Generic Available Yes

Mechanism of Action Blocks the action of acetylcholine at parasympathetic sites in smooth muscle, secretory glands and the CNS; increases cardiac output, dries secretions, antagonizes histamine and serotonin

Use Preoperative medication to inhibit salivation and secretions; treatment of sinus bradycardia; management of peptic ulcer; treat exercise-induced bronchospasm; antidote for organophosphate pesticide poisoning; produce mydriasis and cycloplegia for examination of the retina and optic disc and accurate measurement of refractive errors; uveitis

USUAL DOSAGE Note: Doses <0.1 mg have been associated with paradoxical bradycardia

Neonates, Infants, and Children:

Preanesthetic: Oral, I.M., I.V., S.C.:

- <5 kg: 0.02 mg/kg/dose 30-60 minutes preop then every 4-6 hours as needed; use of a minimum dosage of 0.1 mg in neonates <5 kg will result in dosages >0.02 mg/kg; there is no documented minimum dosage in this age group
- >5 kg: 0.01-0.02 mg/kg/dose to a maximum 0.4 mg/dose 30-60 minutes preop; minimum dose: 0.1 mg

Bradycardia: I.V., intratracheal: 0.02 mg/kg, minimum dose 0.1 mg, maximum single dose: 0.5 mg in children and 1 mg in adolescents; may repeat in 5-minute intervals to a maximum total dose of 1 mg in children or 2 mg in adolescents. (**Note:** For intratracheal administration, the dosage must be diluted with normal saline to a total volume of 1-2 mL); when treating bradycardia in neonates, reserve use for those patients unresponsive to improved oxygenation and epinephrine.

Children:

Bronchospasm: Inhalation: 0.03-0.05 mg/kg/dose 3-4 times/day

Preprocedure: Ophthalmic: 0.5% solution: Instill 1-2 drops twice daily for 1-3 days before the procedure

Uveitis: Ophthalmic: 0.5% solution: Instill 1-2 drops up to 3 times/day

Adults (doses <0.5 mg have been associated with paradoxical bradycardia):

Asystole: I.V.: 1 mg; may repeat every 3-5 minutes as needed

Preanesthetic: I.M., I.V., S.C.: 0.4-0.6 mg 30-60 minutes preop and repeat every 4-6 hours as needed

Bradycardia: I.V.: 0.5-1 mg every 5 minutes, not to exceed a total of 2 mg or 0.04 mg/kg; may give intratracheal in 1 mg/10 mL dilution only, intratracheal dose should be 2-2.5 times the I.V. dose

Neuromuscular blockade reversal: I.V.: 25-30 mcg/kg 30 seconds before neostigmine or 10 mcg/kg 30 seconds before edrophonium

Organophosphate or carbamate poisoning: I.V.: 1-2 mg/dose every 10-20 minutes until atropine effect (dry flushed skin, tachycardia, mydriasis, fever) is observed, then every 1-4 hours for at least 24 hours; up to 50 mg in first 24 hours and 2 g over several days may be given in cases of severe intoxication

Bronchospasm: Inhalation: 0.025-0.05 mg/kg/dose every 4-6 hours as needed (maximum: 5 mg/dose)

Ophthalmic solution: 1%:

Preprocedure: Instill 1-2 drops 1 hour before the procedure

Uveitis: Instill 1-2 drops 4 times/day

Ophthalmic ointment: Apply a small amount in the conjunctival sac up to 3 times/day; compress the lacrimal sac by digital pressure for 1-3 minutes after instillation

Dosage Forms **INJ:** 0.1 mg/mL (5 mL, 10 mL); 0.3 mg/mL (1 mL, 30 mL); 0.4 mg/mL (1 mL, 20 mL, 30 mL); 0.5 mg/mL (1 mL, 5 mL, 30 mL); 0.8 mg/mL (0.5 mL, 1 mL); 1 mg/mL (1 mL, 10 mL). **OINT, ophth:** 0.5%, 1% (3.5 g). **SOLN, ophth:** 0.5% (1 mL, 5 mL); 1% (1 mL, 2 mL, 5 mL, 15 mL); 2% (1 mL, 2 mL); 3% (5 mL). **TAB:** 0.4 mg

Contraindications Hypersensitivity to atropine sulfate or any component; narrow-angle glaucoma; tachycardia; thyrotoxicosis; obstructive disease of the GI tract; obstructive uropathy

Warnings/Precautions Use with caution in children with spastic paralysis; use with caution in elderly patients. Low doses cause a paradoxical decrease in heart rates. Some commercial products contain sodium metabisulfite, which can cause allergic-type reactions. May accumulate with multiple inhalational administration, particularly in the elderly. Heat prostration may occur in hot weather. Use with caution in patients with autonomic neuropathy, prostatic hypertrophy, hyperthyroidism, congestive heart failure, cardiac arrhythmias, chronic lung disease, biliary tract disease; anticholinergic agents are generally not well tolerated in the elderly and their use should be avoided when possible; atropine is rarely used except as a preoperative agent or in the acute treatment of bradyarrhythmias.

Pregnancy Risk Factor C

Adverse Reactions

>10%:

Dermatologic: Dry, hot skin

Gastrointestinal: Impaired GI motility, constipation, dry throat, xerostomia

Local: Irritation at injection site

Respiratory: Dry nose

Miscellaneous: Diaphoresis (decreased)

1% to 10%:

Dermatologic: Increased sensitivity to light

Endocrine & metabolic: Decreased flow of breast milk

Gastrointestinal: Dysphagia

<1%: Ataxia, confusion, delirium, drowsiness, fatigue, headache, loss of memory, orthostatic hypotension, palpitations, restlessness, tachycardia, ventricular fibrillation; the elderly may be at increased risk for confusion and hallucinations, rash, bloated feeling, nausea, vomiting, dysuria, tremor, weakness, increased intraocular pain, blurred vision, mydriasis

Drug Interactions

Decreased effect: Phenothiazines, levodopa, antihistamines with cholinergic mechanisms decrease anticholinergic effects of atropine

Increased toxicity: Amantadine increases anticholinergic effects, thiazides increase effect

Onset I.V.: Rapid onset

Half-Life 2-3 hours

Education and Monitoring Issues

Patient Education: Take exactly as directed, 30 minutes before meals. Maintain adequate hydration (2-3 L/day of fluids unless instructed to restrict fluid intake). Void

(Continued)

Atropine *(Continued)*

before taking medication. You may experience dizziness, blurred vision, sensitivity to light (use caution when driving or engaging in tasks requiring alertness until response to drug is known); dry mouth, nausea, or vomiting (small frequent meals, frequent mouth care, sucking lozenges, or chewing gum may help); orthostatic hypotension (use caution when climbing stairs and when rising from lying or sitting position); constipation (increased exercise, fluid, or dietary fiber may reduce constipation, if not effective consult prescriber); increased sensitivity to heat and decreased perspiration (avoid extremes of heat, reduce exercise in hot weather); decreased milk if breast-feeding. Report hot, dry, flushed skin; blurred vision or vision changes; difficulty swallowing; chest pain, palpitations, or rapid heartbeat; painful or difficult urination; increased confusion, depression, or loss of memory; rapid or difficult respirations; muscle weakness or tremors; or eye pain.

Ophthalmic: Instill as often as recommended. Wash hands before using. Sit or lie down, open eye, look at ceiling, and instill prescribed amount of solution. Do not blink for 30 seconds, close eye and roll eye in all directions, and apply gentle pressure to inner corner of eye for 1-2 minutes. Do not let tip of applicator touch eye or contaminate tip of applicator. Temporary stinging or blurred vision may occur.

Monitoring Parameters: Heart rate, blood pressure, pulse, mental status; intravenous administration requires a cardiac monitor

Related Information

Difenoxin and Atropine *on page 270*

Hyoscyamine, Atropine, Scopolamine, Kaolin, Pectin, and Opium *on page 457*

- **Atropine-Care® Ophthalmic** *see* Atropine *on page 80*
- **Atropisol® Ophthalmic** *see* Atropine *on page 80*
- **Atrovent®** *see* Ipratropium *on page 483*
- **Augmentin®** *see* Amoxicillin and Clavulanate Potassium *on page 57*
- **Auralgan®** *see* Antipyrine and Benzocaine *on page 67*

Auranofin (au RANE oh fin)

Pharmacologic Class Gold Compound

U.S. Brand Names Ridaura®

Generic Available No

Mechanism of Action The exact mechanism of action of gold is unknown; gold is taken up by macrophages which results in inhibition of phagocytosis and lysosomal membrane stabilization; other actions observed are decreased serum rheumatoid factor and alterations in immunoglobulins. Additionally, complement activation is decreased, prostaglandin synthesis is inhibited, and lysosomal enzyme activity is decreased.

Use Management of active stage of classic or definite rheumatoid arthritis in patients that do not respond to or tolerate other agents; psoriatic arthritis; adjunctive or alternative therapy for pemphigus

USUAL DOSAGE Oral:

Children: Initial: 0.1 mg/kg/day divided daily; usual maintenance: 0.15 mg/kg/day in 1-2 divided doses; maximum: 0.2 mg/kg/day in 1-2 divided doses

Adults: 6 mg/day in 1-2 divided doses; after 3 months may be increased to 9 mg/day in 3 divided doses; if still no response after 3 months at 9 mg/day, discontinue drug

Dosing adjustment in renal impairment:

Cl_{cr} 50-80 mL/minute: Reduce dose to 50%

Cl_{cr} <50 mL/minute: Avoid use

Dosage Forms CAP: 3 mg [gold 29%]

Contraindications Renal disease, history of blood dyscrasias, congestive heart failure, exfoliative dermatitis, necrotizing enterocolitis, history of anaphylactic reactions

Warnings/Precautions NSAIDs and corticosteroids may be discontinued after starting gold therapy; therapy should be discontinued if platelet count falls to <100,000/mm^3; WBC <4000, granulocytes <1500/mm^3, explain possibility of adverse effects and their manifestations; use with caution in patients with renal or hepatic impairment

Pregnancy Risk Factor C

Adverse Reactions

>10%:

Dermatologic: Itching, rash

Gastrointestinal: Stomatitis

Ocular: Conjunctivitis

Renal: Proteinuria

1% to 10%:

Dermatologic: Urticaria, alopecia

Gastrointestinal: Glossitis

Hematologic: Eosinophilia, leukopenia, thrombocytopenia

Renal: Hematuria

<1%: Agranulocytosis, anemia, angioedema, aplastic anemia, dysphagia, GI hemorrhage, gingivitis, hepatotoxicity, interstitial pneumonitis, metallic taste, peripheral neuropathy, ulcerative enterocolitis

Drug Interactions Increased toxicity: Penicillamine, antimalarials, hydroxychloroquine, cytotoxic agents, immunosuppressants

Onset Delayed; may require as long as 3 months

Duration Prolonged

Half-Life 21-31 days

Education and Monitoring Issues

Patient Education: Minimize exposure to sunlight; benefits from drug therapy may take as long as 3 months to appear; notify prescriber of pruritus, rash, sore mouth; metallic taste may occur; take shortly after a meal or light snack, can be given as bedtime dose if drowsiness occurs; optimum effect may take 2-4 weeks to be achieved; avoid alcohol; be aware of possible photosensitivity reaction; may cause painful erections; avoid sudden changes in position

Monitoring Parameters: Monitor urine for protein; CBC and platelets; monitor for mouth ulcers and skin reactions; may monitor auranofin serum levels

Reference Range: Gold: Normal: 0-0.1 μg/mL (SI: 0-0.0064 μmol/L); Therapeutic: 1-3 μg/mL (SI: 0.06-0.18 μmol/L); Urine: <0.1 μg/24 hours

♦ **Auro® Ear Drops [OTC]** *see* Carbamide Peroxide *on page 139*

♦ **Aurolate®** *see* Gold Sodium Thiomalate *on page 418*

Aurothioglucose (aur oh thye oh GLOO kose)

Pharmacologic Class Gold Compound

U.S. Brand Names Solganal®

Generic Available No

Mechanism of Action Unknown, may decrease prostaglandin synthesis or may alter cellular mechanisms by inhibiting sulfhydryl systems

Use Adjunctive treatment in adult and juvenile active rheumatoid arthritis; alternative or adjunct in treatment of pemphigus; psoriatic patients who do not respond to NSAIDs

USUAL DOSAGE I.M.: Doses should initially be given at weekly intervals

Children 6-12 years: Initial: 0.25 mg/kg/dose first week; increment at 0.25 mg/kg/dose increasing with each weekly dose; maintenance: 0.75-1 mg/kg/dose weekly not to exceed 25 mg/dose to a total of 20 doses, then every 2-4 weeks

Adults: 10 mg first week; 25 mg second and third week; then 50 mg/week until 800 mg to 1 g cumulative dose has been given; if improvement occurs without adverse reactions, administer 25-50 mg every 2-3 weeks, then every 3-4 weeks

Dosage Forms INJ, suspension: 50 mg/mL [gold 50%] (10 mL)

Contraindications Renal disease, history of blood dyscrasias, congestive heart failure, exfoliative dermatitis, hepatic disease, SLE, history of hypersensitivity

Warnings/Precautions Use with caution in patients with impaired renal or hepatic function; NSAIDs and corticosteroids may be discontinued over time after initiating gold therapy; explain the possibility of adverse reactions before initiating therapy; pregnancy should be ruled out before therapy is started; therapy should be discontinued if platelet counts fall to <100,000/mm^3, WBC <4000/mm^3, granulocytes <1500/mm^3

Pregnancy Risk Factor C

Adverse Reactions

>10%:

Dermatologic: Itching, rash, exfoliative dermatitis, reddened skin

Gastrointestinal: Gingivitis, glossitis, metallic taste, stomatitis

1% to 10%: Renal: Proteinuria

<1%: Agranulocytosis, allergic reaction (severe), alopecia, anaphylactic shock, aplastic anemia, bronchitis, conjunctivitis, corneal ulcers, EEG abnormalities, encephalitis, eosinophilia, fever, glomerulitis, hematuria, hepatotoxicity, interstitial pneumonitis, iritis, leukopenia, nephrotic syndrome, peripheral neuropathy, pharyngitis, pulmonary fibrosis, thrombocytopenia, ulcerative enterocolitis, vaginitis

Drug Interactions Increased toxicity: Penicillamine, antimalarials, hydroxychloroquine, cytotoxic agents, immunosuppressants

Education and Monitoring Issues

Patient Education: Minimize exposure to sunlight; benefits from drug therapy may take as long as 3 months to appear; notify prescriber of pruritus, rash, sore mouth; metallic taste may occur

Monitoring Parameters: CBC with differential, platelet count, urinalysis, baseline renal and liver function tests

Reference Range: Gold: Normal: 0-0.1 μg/mL (SI: 0-0.0064 μmol/L); Therapeutic: 1-3 μg/mL (SI: 0.06-0.18 μmol/L); Urine: <0.1 μg/24 hours

♦ **Auroto®** *see* Antipyrine and Benzocaine *on page 67*

♦ **Avalide®** *see* Irbesartan and Hydrochlorothiazide *on page 485*

♦ **Avandia®** *see* Rosiglitazone *on page 834*

♦ **Avapro®** *see* Irbesartan *on page 484*

♦ **AVC™ Cream** *see* Sulfanilamide *on page 880*

♦ **AVC™ Suppository** *see* Sulfanilamide *on page 880*

♦ **Avelox™** *see* Moxifloxacin *on page 620*

♦ **Aventyl® Hydrochloride** *see* Nortriptyline *on page 665*

- **Avirax®** *see* Acyclovir *on page 22*
- **Avita®** *see* Tretinoin, Topical *on page 944*
- **Avitene®** *see* Microfibrillar Collagen Hemostat *on page 601*
- **Avlosulfon®** *see* Dapsone *on page 248*
- **Avonex™** *see* Interferon Beta-1a *on page 479*
- **Axid®** *see* Nizatidine *on page 662*
- **Axid® AR [OTC]** *see* Nizatidine *on page 662*
- **Axotal®** *see* Butalbital Compound *on page 123*
- **Ayercillin®** *see* Penicillin G Procaine *on page 712*
- **Ayr® Saline [OTC]** *see* Sodium Chloride *on page 858*
- **Azactam®** *see* Aztreonam *on page 88*

Azatadine (a ZA ta deen)

Pharmacologic Class Antihistamine

U.S. Brand Names Optimine®

Generic Available No

Mechanism of Action Azatadine is a piperidine-derivative antihistamine; has both anticholinergic and antiserotonin activity; has been demonstrated to inhibit mediator release from human mast cells *in vitro*; mechanism of this action is suggested to prevent calcium entry into the mast cell through voltage-dependent calcium channels

Use Treatment of perennial and seasonal allergic rhinitis and chronic urticaria

USUAL DOSAGE Children >12 years and Adults: Oral: 1-2 mg twice daily

Dosage Forms TAB: 1 mg

Contraindications Hypersensitivity to azatadine or to other related antihistamines including cyproheptadine; patients taking monoamine oxidase inhibitors should not use azatadine

Warnings/Precautions Sedation and somnolence are the most commonly reported adverse effects

Pregnancy Risk Factor B

Adverse Reactions

>10%:

Central nervous system: Slight to moderate drowsiness

Respiratory: Thickening of bronchial secretions

1% to 10%:

Central nervous system: Headache, fatigue, nervousness, dizziness

Gastrointestinal: Appetite increase, weight gain, nausea, diarrhea, abdominal pain, xerostomia

Neuromuscular & skeletal: Arthralgia

Respiratory: Pharyngitis

<1%: Angioedema, bronchospasm, depression, edema, epistaxis, hepatitis, myalgia, palpitations, paresthesia, photosensitivity, rash

Drug Interactions Increased effect/toxicity: Procarbazine, CNS depressants, tricyclic antidepressants, alcohol

Alcohol Interactions Avoid use (may increase central nervous system depression)

Onset 1-2 hours

Half-Life ~8.7 hours

Education and Monitoring Issues

Patient Education: Take as directed; do not exceed recommended dose. Avoid use of other depressants, alcohol, or sleep-inducing medications unless approved by prescriber. You may experience drowsiness or dizziness (use caution when driving or engaging in tasks requiring alertness until response to drug is known); or dry mouth, abdominal pain, or nausea (frequent small meals, frequent mouth care, chewing gum, or sucking hard candy may help). Report persistent sore throat, difficulty breathing, or expectorating (thick secretions); excessive sedation or mental stimulation; frequent nosebleeds; unusual joint or muscle pain; or lack of improvement or worsening of condition.

Related Information

Azatadine and Pseudoephedrine *on page 84*

Azatadine and Pseudoephedrine (a ZA ta deen & soo doe e FED rin)

Pharmacologic Class Antihistamine/Decongestant Combination

U.S. Brand Names Rynatan®; Trinalin®

Dosage Forms TAB: Azatadine maleate 1 mg and pseudoephedrine sulfate 120 mg

Pregnancy Risk Factor C

Azathioprine (ay za THYE oh preen)

Pharmacologic Class Immunosuppressant Agent

U.S. Brand Names Imuran®

Generic Available Yes

Mechanism of Action Antagonizes purine metabolism and may inhibit synthesis of DNA, RNA, and proteins; may also interfere with cellular metabolism and inhibit mitosis

Use Adjunct with other agents in prevention of rejection of solid organ transplants; also used in severe active rheumatoid arthritis unresponsive to other agents; other autoimmune diseases (ITP, SLE, MS, Crohn's Disease); **azathioprine is an imidazolyl derivative of 6-mercaptopurine**

USUAL DOSAGE I.V. dose is equivalent to oral dose (dosing should be based on ideal body weight):

Children and Adults: Solid organ transplantation: Oral, I.V.: 2-5 mg/kg/day to start, then 1-2 mg/kg/day maintenance

Adults: Rheumatoid arthritis: Oral: 1 mg/kg/day for 6-8 weeks; increase by 0.5 mg/kg every 4 weeks until response or up to 2.5 mg/kg/day

Dosing adjustment in renal impairment:

Cl_{cr} 10-50 mL/minute: Administer 75% of normal dose daily

Cl_{cr} <10 mL/minute: Administer 50% of normal dose daily

Hemodialysis: Slightly dialyzable (5% to 20%)

Administer dose posthemodialysis

CAPD effects: Unknown

CAVH effects: Unknown

Dosage Forms INJ: 100 mg (20 mL). **TAB, scored:** 50 mg

Contraindications Hypersensitivity to azathioprine or any component; pregnancy and lactation

Warnings/Precautions Chronic immunosuppression increases the risk of neoplasia; has mutagenic potential to both men and women and with possible hematologic toxicities; use with caution in patients with liver disease, renal impairment; monitor hematologic function closely

Pregnancy Risk Factor D

Adverse Reactions Dose reduction or temporary withdrawal allows reversal

>10%:

Central nervous system: Fever, chills

Gastrointestinal: Nausea, vomiting, anorexia, diarrhea

Hematologic: Thrombocytopenia, leukopenia, anemia

Miscellaneous: Secondary infection

1% to 10%:

Dermatologic: Rash

Hematologic: Pancytopenia

Hepatic: Hepatotoxicity

<1%: Alopecia, aphthous stomatitis, arthralgias (which include myalgias), dyspnea, hypotension, maculopapular rash, rare hypersensitivity reactions, retinopathy, rigors

Drug Interactions Increased toxicity: Allopurinol (decreases azathioprine dose to $^1/_3$ to $^1/_4$ of normal dose)

Half-Life Parent drug: 12 minutes; 6-mercaptopurine: 0.7-3 hours; End-stage renal disease: Slightly prolonged

Education and Monitoring Issues

Patient Education: Take as prescribed (may take in divided doses or with food if GI upset occurs).

Rheumatoid arthritis: Response may not occur for up to 3 months; do not discontinue without consulting prescriber.

Organ transplant: Azathioprine will usually be prescribed with other antirejection medications.

You will be susceptible to infection (avoid vaccinations unless approved by prescriber) and avoid crowds or infected persons or persons with contagious diseases. You may experience nausea, vomiting, loss of appetite (small frequent meals, frequent mouth care, chewing gum, or sucking lozenges may help). Report abdominal pain and unresolved gastrointestinal upset (eg, persistent vomiting or diarrhea); unusual fever or chills, bleeding or bruising, sore throat, unhealed sores, or signs of infection; yellowing of skin or eyes; or change in color of urine or stool.

Monitoring Parameters: CBC, platelet counts, total bilirubin, alkaline phosphatase

♦ **Azdone®** *see* Hydrocodone and Aspirin *on page 445*

Azelaic Acid (a zeh LAY ik AS id)

Pharmacologic Class Topical Skin Product, Acne

U.S. Brand Names Azelex®

Use *Acne vulgaris*: Topical treatment of mild to moderate inflammatory acne vulgaris

USUAL DOSAGE Adults: Topical: After skin is thoroughly washed and patted dry, gently but thoroughly massage a thin film of azelaic acid cream into the affected areas twice daily, in the morning and evening. The duration of use can vary and depends on the severity of the acne. In the majority of patients with inflammatory lesions, improvement of the condition occurs within 4 weeks.

Contraindications Known hypersensitivity to any of components

Pregnancy Risk Factor B

Azelastine (a ZEL as teen)

Pharmacologic Class Antihistamine

U.S. Brand Names Astelin® Nasal Spray

(Continued)

Azelastine *(Continued)*

Mechanism of Action Competes with histamine for H_1-receptor sites on effector cells in the blood vessels and respiratory tract; reduces hyper-reactivity of the airways; increases the motility of bronchial epithelial cilia, improving mucociliary transport

Use Treatment of the symptoms of seasonal allergic rhinitis such as rhinorrhea, sneezing, and nasal pruritus in adults and children >12 years of age

USUAL DOSAGE Children ≥12 years and Adults: 2 sprays (137 mcg/spray) each nostril twice daily. Before initial use, the delivery system should be primed with 4 sprays or until a fine mist appears. If 3 or more days have elapsed since last use, the delivery system should be reprimed.

Dosage Forms SOLN, nasal: 1 mg/mL [137 mcg/actuation] (17 mL)

Contraindications Hypersensitivity to azelastine or any component

Warnings/Precautions Use with caution in asthmatics; patients with hepatic or renal dysfunction may require lower doses

Pregnancy Risk Factor C

Adverse Reactions

>10%:

- Central nervous system: Headache (14.8%), somnolence (11.5%)
- Gastrointestinal: Bitter taste (19.7%)

2% to 10%:

- Central nervous system: Dizziness (2%), fatigue (2.3%)
- Gastrointestinal: Nausea (2.8%), weight increase (2%), dry mouth (2.8%)
- Respiratory: Nasal burning (4.1%), pharyngitis (3.8%), paroxysmal sneezing (3.1%), rhinitis (2.3%), epistaxis (2%)

<2%:

- Body as a whole: Allergic reactions, back pain, viral infections, malaise, extremity pain, abdominal pain
- Cardiovascular: Flushing, hypertension, tachycardia
- Central nervous system: Drowsiness, fatigue, vertigo, depression, nervousness, hypoesthesia
- Dermatologic: Contact dermatitis, eczema, hair and follicle infection, furunculosis
- Gastrointestinal: Constipation, gastroenteritis, glossitis, increased appetite, ulcerative stomatitis, vomiting, increased ALT, aphthous stomatitis
- Genitourinary: Urinary frequency, hematuria, albuminuria, amenorrhea
- Neuromuscular & skeletal: Myalgia, vertigo, temporomandibular dislocation, hypoesthesia, hyperkinesia
- Ocular: Conjunctivitis, watery eyes, eye pain
- Respiratory: Bronchospasm, coughing, throat burning, laryngitis
- Psychological: Anxiety, depersonalization, sleep disorder, abnormal thinking

Drug Interactions May cause additive sedation when concomitantly administered with other CNS depressant medications; cimetidine can increase the AUC and C_{max} of azelastine by as much as 65%

Onset 3 hours

Duration 12 hours

Half-Life 22 hours

Education and Monitoring Issues

Patient Education: Causes drowsiness and may impair ability to perform hazardous activities requiring mental alertness or physical coordination; avoid spraying in eyes

♦ **Azelex®** *see* Azelaic Acid *on page 85*

Azithromycin (az ith roe MYE sin)

Pharmacologic Class Antibiotic, Macrolide

U.S. Brand Names Zithromax™

Generic Available No

Mechanism of Action Inhibits RNA-dependent protein synthesis at the chain elongation step; binds to the 50S ribosomal subunit resulting in blockage of transpeptidation

Use

Children: Treatment of acute otitis media due to *H. influenzae*, *M. catarrhalis*, or *S. pneumoniae*; pharyngitis/tonsillitis due to *S. pyogenes*

Adults:

- Treatment of mild to moderate upper and lower respiratory tract infections, infections of the skin and skin structure, and sexually transmitted diseases due to susceptible strains of *C. trachomatis*, *M. catarrhalis*, *H. influenzae*, *S. aureus*, *S. pneumoniae*, *Mycoplasma pneumoniae*, and *C. psittaci*; community-acquired pneumonia, pelvic inflammatory disease (PID)
- For preventing or delaying the onset of infection with *Mycobacterium avium* complex (MAC)
- Prophylaxis of bacterial endocarditis in patients who are allergic to penicillin and undergoing surgical or dental procedures

USUAL DOSAGE

Oral:

Children ≥6 months: Otitis media and community-acquired pneumonia: 10 mg/kg on day 1 (maximum: 500 mg/day) followed by 5 mg/kg/day once daily on days 2-5 (maximum: 250 mg/day)

Children ≥2 years: Pharyngitis, tonsillitis: 12 mg/kg/day once daily for 5 days (maximum: 500 mg/day)

Children: *M. avium*-infected patients with acquired immunodeficiency syndrome: Not currently FDA approved for use; 10-20 mg/kg/day once daily (maximum: 40 mg/kg/day) has been used in clinical trials; prophylaxis for first episode of MAC: 5-12 mg/kg/day once daily (maximum: 500 mg/day)

Adolescents ≥16 years and Adults:

Respiratory tract, skin and soft tissue infections: 500 mg on day 1 followed by 250 mg/day on days 2-5 (maximum: 500 mg/day)

Uncomplicated chlamydial urethritis/cervicitis or chancroid: Single 1 g dose

Gonococcal urethritis/cervicitis: Single 2 g dose

Prophylaxis of disseminated *M. avium* complex disease in patient with advanced HIV infection: 1200 mg once weekly (may be combined with rifabutin)

Prophylaxis for bacterial endocarditis: 500 mg 1 hour prior to the procedure

I.V.: Adults:

Community-acquired pneumonia: 500 mg as a single dose for at least 2 days, follow I.V. therapy by the oral route with a single daily dose of 500 mg to complete a 7-10 day course of therapy

Pelvic inflammatory disease (PID): 500 mg as a single dose for 1-2 days, follow I.V. therapy by the oral route with a single daily dose of 250 mg to complete a 7 day course of therapy

Dosage Forms POWDER for injection: 500 mg. **POWDER for oral susp:** 100 mg/5 mL (15 mL); 200 mg/5 mL (15 mL, 22.5 mL); 1 g (single-dose packet). **TAB:** 250 mg, 600 mg

Contraindications Hepatic impairment, known hypersensitivity to azithromycin, other macrolide antibiotics, or any azithromycin components; use with pimozide

Warnings/Precautions Use with caution in patients with hepatic dysfunction; hepatic impairment with or without jaundice has occurred chiefly in older children and adults; it may be accompanied by malaise, nausea, vomiting, abdominal colic, and fever; discontinue use if these occur; may mask or delay symptoms of incubating gonorrhea or syphilis, so appropriate culture and susceptibility tests should be performed prior to initiating azithromycin; pseudomembranous colitis has been reported with use of macrolide antibiotics; safety and efficacy have not been established in children <6 months of age with acute otitis media and in children <2 years of age with pharyngitis/tonsillitis

Pregnancy Risk Factor B

Adverse Reactions

1% to 10%: Gastrointestinal: Diarrhea, nausea, abdominal pain, cramping, vomiting (especially with high single-dose regimens)

<1%: Allergic reactions, angioedema, cholestatic jaundice, dizziness, elevated LFTs, eosinophilia, fever, headache, hypertrophic pyloric stenosis, nephritis, ototoxicity, rash, thrombophlebitis, vaginitis, ventricular arrhythmias

Drug Interactions May inhibit CYP3A3/4 enzyme (mild)

Decreased peak serum levels: Aluminum- and magnesium-containing antacids by 24% but not total absorption

Increased effect/toxicity: Azithromycin may increase levels of tacrolimus, phenytoin, ergot alkaloids, alfentanil, terfenadine, bromocriptine, carbamazepine, cyclosporine, digoxin, disopyramide, and triazolam; azithromycin did not affect the response to warfarin or theophylline although caution is advised when administered together

Avoid use with pimozide due to significant risk of cardiotoxicity

Half-Life 68 hours

Education and Monitoring Issues

Patient Education: Take as directed. Take all of prescribed medication. Do not discontinue until prescription is completed. Take suspension 1 hour before or 2 hours after meals; tablet form may be taken with meals to decrease GI effects. Do not take with aluminum- or magnesium-containing antacids. May cause transient abdominal distress, diarrhea, headache. Report signs of additional infections (eg, sores in mouth or vagina, vaginal discharge, unresolved fever, severe vomiting, or diarrhea).

Dietary Considerations: Food: Azithromycin suspension has significantly increased rate of absorption (46%) with food

Monitoring Parameters: Liver function tests, CBC with differential

Manufacturer Pfizer U.S. Pharmaceutical Group

Related Information

Antimicrobial Drugs of Choice *on page 1182*

Community Acquired Pneumonia in Adults *on page 1200*

Pharmaceutical Manufacturers Directory *on page 1020*

Prevention of Bacterial Endocarditis *on page 1154*

Treatment of Sexually Transmitted Diseases *on page 1210*

♦ **Azmacort™** *see* Triamcinolone *on page 944*

♦ **Azo Gantrisin** *see* Sulfisoxazole and Phenazopyridine *on page 882*

- **Azopt™** *see* Brinzolamide *on page 113*
- **Azo-Standard® [OTC]** *see* Phenazopyridine *on page 721*
- **Azo-Sulfisoxazole** *see* Sulfisoxazole and Phenazopyridine *on page 882*

Aztreonam (AZ tree oh nam)

Pharmacologic Class Antibiotic, Miscellaneous

U.S. Brand Names Azactam®

Generic Available No

Mechanism of Action Inhibits bacterial cell wall synthesis by binding to one or more of the penicillin binding proteins (PBPs); which in turn inhibits the final transpeptidation step of peptidoglycan synthesis in bacterial cell walls, thus inhibiting cell wall biosynthesis. Bacteria eventually lyse due to ongoing activity of cell wall autolytic enzymes (autolysins and murein hydrolases) while cell wall assembly is arrested. Monobactam structure makes cross-allergenicity with beta-lactams unlikely.

Use Treatment of patients with urinary tract infections, lower respiratory tract infections, septicemia, skin/skin structure infections, intra-abdominal infections, and gynecological infections caused by susceptible gram-negative bacilli; often useful in patients with allergies to penicillins or cephalosporins

USUAL DOSAGE

Neonates: I.M., I.V.:

- Postnatal age ≤7 days:
  - <2000 g: 30 mg/kg/dose every 12 hours
  - >2000 g: 30 mg/kg/dose every 8 hours
- Postnatal age >7 days:
  - <1200 g: 30 mg/kg/dose every 12 hours
  - 1200-2000 g: 30 mg/kg/dose every 8 hours
  - >2000 g: 30 mg/kg/dose every 6 hours

Children >1 month: I.M., I.V.: 90-120 mg/kg/day divided every 6-8 hours

- Cystic fibrosis: 50 mg/kg/dose every 6-8 hours (ie, up to 200 mg/kg/day); maximum: 6-8 g/day

Adults:

- Urinary tract infection: I.M., I.V.: 500 mg to 1 g every 8-12 hours
- Moderately severe systemic infections: 1 g I.V. or I.M. or 2 g I.V. every 8-12 hours
- Severe systemic or life-threatening infections (especially caused by *Pseudomonas aeruginosa*): I.V.: 2 g every 6-8 hours; maximum: 8 g/day

Dosing adjustment in renal impairment: Adults:

- Cl_{cr} >50 mL/minute: 500 mg to 1 g every 6-8 hours
- Cl_{cr} 10-50 mL/minute: 50% to 75% of usual dose given at the usual interval
- Cl_{cr} <10 mL/minute: 25% of usual dosage given at the usual interval

Hemodialysis: Moderately dialyzable (20% to 50%); administer dose postdialysis or supplemental dose of 500 mg after dialysis

Peritoneal dialysis: Administer as for Cl_{cr} <10 mL/minute

Continuous arteriovenous or venovenous hemofiltration (CAVH/CAVHD): Dose as for Cl_{cr} 10-50 mL/minute

Dosage Forms POWDER for inj: 500 mg (15 mL, 100 mL), 1 g (15 mL, 100 mL), 2 g (15 mL, 100 mL)

Contraindications Hypersensitivity to aztreonam or any component

Warnings/Precautions Rare cross-allergenicity to penicillins and cephalosporins; requires dosing adjustment in renal impairment

Pregnancy Risk Factor B

Adverse Reactions

1% to 10%:

- Dermatologic: Rash
- Gastrointestinal: Diarrhea, nausea, vomiting
- Local: Thrombophlebitis, pain at injection site

<1%: Abnormal taste, anaphylaxis, aphthous ulcer, breast tenderness, confusion, diplopia, dizziness, elevated liver enzymes, eosinophilia, fever, halitosis, headache, hepatitis, hypotension, insomnia, jaundice, leukopenia, myalgia, neutropenia, numb tongue, pseudomembranous colitis, seizures, sneezing, thrombocytopenia, tinnitus, vaginitis, vertigo, weakness

Half-Life Normal renal function: 1.7-2.9 hours; End-stage renal disease: 6-8 hours

Education and Monitoring Issues

Patient Education: This medication can only be administered I.M. or I.V. You may experience nausea or GI distress. Frequent mouth care, frequent small meals, sucking lozenges, or chewing gum may help relieve these symptoms. May cause false readings with urine glucose testing. Diabetics should use alternate means of monitoring glucose. Report any unrelieved diarrhea or vomiting, pain at injection sites, unresolved fever, unhealed or new sores in mouth or vagina, vaginal discharge, or acute onset of respiratory difficulty.

Monitoring Parameters: Periodic liver function test; monitor for signs of anaphylaxis during first dose

Manufacturer Bristol-Myers Squibb Company (Pharmaceutical Division)

Related Information
Antimicrobial Drugs of Choice *on page 1182*
Pharmaceutical Manufacturers Directory *on page 1020*

- **Azulfidine®** *see* Sulfasalazine *on page 880*
- **Azulfidine® EN-tabs®** *see* Sulfasalazine *on page 880*
- **B6-250** *see* Pyridoxine *on page 796*
- **Babee® Teething® [OTC]** *see* Benzocaine *on page 98*
- **Baby Orajel** *see* Benzocaine *on page 98*
- **B-A-C®** *see* Butalbital Compound *on page 123*

Bacampicillin (ba kam pi SIL in)

Pharmacologic Class Penicillin
U.S. Brand Names Spectrobid®
Use Treatment of susceptible bacterial infections involving the urinary tract, skin structure, upper and lower respiratory tract; activity is identical to that of ampicillin
USUAL DOSAGE Oral:
Children <25 kg: 25-50 mg/kg/day in divided doses every 12 hours
Children >25 kg and Adults: 400-800 mg every 12 hours
Dosing interval in renal impairment:
Cl_{cr} 10-30 mL/minute: Administer every 24 hours
Cl_{cr} <10 mL/minute: Administer every 36 hours
Contraindications Hypersensitivity to bacampicillin or any component or penicillins
Pregnancy Risk Factor B

- **Bacid® [OTC]** *see Lactobacillus acidophilus* and *Lactobacillus bulgaricus on page 505*
- **Baciguent® Topical [OTC]** *see* Bacitracin *on page 89*
- **Baci-IM® Injection** *see* Bacitracin *on page 89*
- **Bacitin** *see* Bacitracin *on page 89*

Bacitracin (bas i TRAY sin)

Pharmacologic Class Antibiotic, Ophthalmic; Antibiotic, Topical; Antibiotic, Miscellaneous
U.S. Brand Names AK-Tracin® Ophthalmic; Baciguent® Topical [OTC]; Baci-IM® Injection
Generic Available Yes
Mechanism of Action Inhibits bacterial cell wall synthesis by preventing transfer of mucopeptides into the growing cell wall
Use Treatment of susceptible bacterial infections mainly has activity against gram-positive bacilli; due to toxicity risks, systemic and irrigant uses of bacitracin should be limited to situations where less toxic alternatives would not be effective; oral administration has been successful in antibiotic-associated colitis and has been used for enteric eradication of vancomycin-resistant enterococci (VRE)
USUAL DOSAGE Children and Adults **(do not administer I.V.)**:
Infants: I.M.:
≤2.5 kg: 900 units/kg/day in 2-3 divided doses
>2.5 kg: 1000 units/kg/day in 2-3 divided doses
Children: I.M.: 800-1200 units/kg/day divided every 8 hours
Adults: Antibiotic-associated colitis: Oral: 25,000 units 4 times/day for 7-10 days
Topical: Apply 1-5 times/day
Ophthalmic, ointment: Instill 1/4" to 1/2" ribbon every 3-4 hours into conjunctival sac for acute infections, or 2-3 times/day for mild to moderate infections for 7-10 days
Irrigation, solution: 50-100 units/mL in normal saline, lactated Ringer's, or sterile water for irrigation; soak sponges in solution for topical compresses 1-5 times/day or as needed during surgical procedures
Dosage Forms INJ: 50,000 units. **OINT:** Ophth: 500 units/g (1 g, 3.5 g, 3.75 g); (AK-Tracin®): 500 units/g (3.5 g); Topical: 500 units/g (1.5 g, 3.75 g, 15 g, 30 g, 120 g, 454 g)
Contraindications Hypersensitivity to bacitracin or any component; I.M. use is contraindicated in patients with renal impairment
Warnings/Precautions Prolonged use may result in overgrowth of nonsusceptible organisms; I.M. use may cause renal failure due to tubular and glomerular necrosis; **do not administer intravenously** because severe thrombophlebitis occurs
Pregnancy Risk Factor C
Adverse Reactions 1% to 10%:
Cardiovascular: Hypotension, edema of the face/lips, tightness of chest
Central nervous system: Pain
Dermatologic: Rash, itching
Gastrointestinal: Anorexia, nausea, vomiting, diarrhea, rectal itching
Hematologic: Blood dyscrasias
Miscellaneous: Diaphoresis
Drug Interactions Increased toxicity: Nephrotoxic drugs, neuromuscular blocking agents, and anesthetics (↑ neuromuscular blockade)
Duration 6-8 hours
(Continued)

Bacitracin *(Continued)*

Education and Monitoring Issues

Patient Education:

Oral, I.M.: Maintain adequate hydration (2-3 L/day of fluids unless instructed to restrict fluid intake). Report rash, redness, or itching; change in urinary pattern; acute dizziness; swelling of face or lips; chest pain or tightness; acute nausea or vomiting; or loss of appetite (small frequent meals or frequent mouth care may help).

Ophthalmic: Instill as many times per day as directed. Wash hands before using. Gently pull lower eyelid forward, instill prescribed amount of ointment into lower eyelid. Close eye and roll eyeball in all directions. May cause blurred vision; use caution when driving or engaging in tasks that require clear vision. Report any adverse reactions such as rash or itching, swelling of face or lips, burning or pain in eye, worsening of condition, or if condition does not improve.

Topical: Apply a thin film as many times as day as prescribed to the affected area. May cover with porous sterile bandage (avoid occlusive dressings). Do not use longer than 1 week unless advised by healthcare provider.

Monitoring Parameters: I.M.: Urinalysis, renal function tests

Related Information

Antimicrobial Drugs of Choice *on page 1182*
Bacitracin and Polymyxin B *on page 90*
Bacitracin, Neomycin, and Polymyxin B *on page 90*
Bacitracin, Neomycin, Polymyxin B, and Hydrocortisone *on page 90*

Bacitracin and Polymyxin B (bas i TRAY sin & pol i MIKS in bee)

Pharmacologic Class Antibiotic, Ophthalmic; Antibiotic, Topical

U.S. Brand Names AK-Poly-Bac® Ophthalmic; Betadine® First Aid Antibiotics + Moisturizer [OTC]; Polysporin® Ophthalmic; Polysporin® Topical

Use Treatment of superficial infections caused by susceptible organisms

Dosage Forms OINT: Ophth: Bacitracin 500 units and polymyxin B sulfate 10,000 units per g (3.5 g); Topical: Bacitracin 500 units and polymyxin B sulfate 10,000 units per g in white petrolatum (15 g, 30 g). **POWDER:** Bacitracin 500 units and polymyxin B sulfate 10,000 units per g (10 g)

Pregnancy Risk Factor C

Bacitracin, Neomycin, and Polymyxin B

(bas i TRAY sin, nee oh MYE sin, & pol i MIKS in bee)

Pharmacologic Class Antibiotic, Ophthalmic; Antibiotic, Topical

U.S. Brand Names AK-Spore® Ophthalmic Ointment; Medi-Quick® Topical Ointment [OTC]; Mycitracin® Topical [OTC]; Neomixin® Topical [OTC]; Neosporin® Ophthalmic Ointment; Neosporin® Topical Ointment [OTC]; Ocutricin® Topical Ointment; Septa® Topical Ointment [OTC]; Triple Antibiotic® Topical

Use Helps prevent infection in minor cuts, scrapes and burns; short-term treatment of superficial external ocular infections caused by susceptible organisms

Dosage Forms OINT: Ophth: Bacitracin 400 units, neomycin sulfate 3.5 mg, and polymyxin B sulfate 10,000 units and per g; Topical: Bacitracin 400 units, neomycin sulfate 3.5 mg, and polymyxin B sulfate 5000 units per g

Pregnancy Risk Factor C

Bacitracin, Neomycin, Polymyxin B, and Hydrocortisone

(bas i TRAY sin, nee oh MYE sin, pol i MIKS in bee, & hye droe KOR ti sone)

Pharmacologic Class Antibiotic, Ophthalmic; Antibiotic, Otic; Antibiotic, Topical; Corticosteroid, Ophthalmic; Corticosteroid, Otic; Corticosteroid, Topical

U.S. Brand Names AK-Spore H.C.® Ophthalmic Ointment; Cortisporin® Ophthalmic Ointment; Cortisporin® Topical Ointment; Neotricin HC® Ophthalmic Ointment

Use Prevention and treatment of susceptible superficial topical infections

Dosage Forms OINT: Ophth: Bacitracin 400 units, neomycin sulfate 3.5 mg, polymyxin B sulfate 10,000 units, and hydrocortisone 10 mg per g (3.5 g); Topical: Bacitracin 400 units, neomycin sulfate 3.5 mg, polymyxin B sulfate 10,000 units, and hydrocortisone 10 mg per g (15 g)

Pregnancy Risk Factor C

Baclofen (BAK loe fen)

Pharmacologic Class Skeletal Muscle Relaxant

U.S. Brand Names Lioresal®

Generic Available No

Mechanism of Action Inhibits the transmission of both monosynaptic and polysynaptic reflexes at the spinal cord level, possibly by hyperpolarization of primary afferent fiber terminals, with resultant relief of muscle spasticity

Use Treatment of reversible spasticity associated with multiple sclerosis or spinal cord lesions

Unlabeled use: Intractable hiccups, intractable pain relief, and bladder spasticity

USUAL DOSAGE

Oral (avoid abrupt withdrawal of drug):

Children:

2-7 years: Initial: 10-15 mg/24 hours divided every 8 hours; titrate dose every 3 days in increments of 5-15 mg/day to a maximum of 40 mg/day

≥8 years: Maximum: 60 mg/day in 3 divided doses

Adults: 5 mg 3 times/day, may increase 5 mg/dose every 3 days to a maximum of 80 mg/day

Hiccups: Adults: Usual effective dose: 10-20 mg 2-3 times/day

Intrathecal:

Test dose: 50-100 mcg, doses >50 mcg should be given in 25 mcg increments, separated by 24 hours

Maintenance: After positive response to test dose, a maintenance intrathecal infusion can be administered via an implanted intrathecal pump. Initial dose via pump: Infusion at a 24-hour rate dosed at twice the test dose.

Dosing adjustment in renal impairment: It is necessary to reduce dosage in renal impairment but there are no specific guidelines available

Hemodialysis: Poor water solubility allows for accumulation during chronic hemodialysis. Low-dose therapy is recommended. There have been several case reports of accumulation of baclofen resulting in toxicity symptoms (organic brain syndrome, myoclonia, deceleration and steep potentials in EEG) in patients with renal failure who have received normal doses of baclofen.

Dosage Forms **INJ, intrathecal** (preservative free): 500 mcg/mL (20 mL); 2000 mcg/mL (5 mL). **TAB:** 10 mg, 20 mg

Contraindications Hypersensitivity to baclofen or any component

Warnings/Precautions Use with caution in patients with seizure disorder, impaired renal function; avoid abrupt withdrawal of the drug; elderly are more sensitive to the effects of baclofen and are more likely to experience adverse CNS effects at higher doses.

Pregnancy Risk Factor C

Adverse Reactions

>10%:

Central nervous system: Drowsiness, vertigo, psychiatric disturbances, insomnia, slurred speech, ataxia, hypotonia

Neuromuscular & skeletal: Weakness

1% to 10%:

Cardiovascular: Hypotension

Central nervous system: Fatigue, confusion, headache

Dermatologic: Rash

Gastrointestinal: Nausea, constipation

Genitourinary: Polyuria

<1%: Abdominal pain, abnormal taste, anorexia, chest pain, depression, diarrhea, dyspnea, dysuria, enuresis, euphoria, excitement, hallucinations, hematuria, impotence, inability to ejaculate, nocturia, palpitations, paresthesia, syncope, urinary retention, vomiting, xerostomia

Drug Interactions

Increased effect: Opiate analgesics, benzodiazepines, hypertensive agents

Increased toxicity: CNS depressants and alcohol (sedation), tricyclic antidepressants (short-term memory loss), clindamycin (neuromuscular blockade), guanabenz (sedation), MAO inhibitors (decrease blood pressure, CNS, and respiratory effects)

Alcohol Interactions Avoid use (may increase central nervous system depression)

Onset Muscle relaxation effect requires 3-4 days; Peak effect: Maximal clinical effect is not seen for 5-10 days

Half-Life 3.5 hours

Education and Monitoring Issues

Patient Education: Take this drug as prescribed. Do not discontinue without consulting prescriber (abrupt discontinuation may cause hallucinations). Do not take any prescription or OTC sleep-inducing drugs, sedatives, antispasmodics without consulting prescriber. Avoid alcohol use. You may experience transient drowsiness, lethargy, or dizziness; use caution when driving or engaging in tasks requiring alertness until response to drug is known. Frequent small meals or lozenges may reduce GI upset. Report unresolved insomnia, painful urination, change in urinary patterns, constipation, or persistent confusion.

- **Bacticort® Otic** *see* Neomycin, Polymyxin B, and Hydrocortisone *on page 644*
- **Bactocill®** *see* Oxacillin *on page 683*
- **BactoShield® Topical [OTC]** *see* Chlorhexidine Gluconate *on page 181*
- **Bactrim™** *see* Co-Trimoxazole *on page 230*
- **Bactrim™ DS** *see* Co-Trimoxazole *on page 230*
- **Bactroban®** *see* Mupirocin *on page 622*
- **Bactroban® Nasal** *see* Mupirocin *on page 622*
- **Baldex®** *see* Dexamethasone *on page 256*
- **Balminil® Decongestant** *see* Pseudoephedrine *on page 792*
- **Balminil® Expectorant** *see* Guaifenesin *on page 423*

- **Balsulph** *see* Sulfacetamide Sodium *on page 876*
- **Bancap®** *see* Butalbital Compound *on page 123*
- **Bancap HC®** *see* Hydrocodone and Acetaminophen *on page 444*
- **Banophen® Oral [OTC]** *see* Diphenhydramine *on page 282*
- **Bapadin®** *see* Bepridil *on page 101*
- **Barbidonna®** *see* Hyoscyamine, Atropine, Scopolamine, and Phenobarbital *on page 456*
- **Barbilixir®** *see* Phenobarbital *on page 723*
- **Barbita®** *see* Phenobarbital *on page 723*
- **Barc™ Liquid [OTC]** *see* Pyrethrins *on page 795*
- **Baridium® [OTC]** *see* Phenazopyridine *on page 721*
- **Barophen®** *see* Hyoscyamine, Atropine, Scopolamine, and Phenobarbital *on page 456*
- **Barriere-HC** *see* Hydrocortisone *on page 447*
- **Basaljel** *see* Aluminum Hydroxide *on page 41*

Basiliximab (ba si LIKS i mab)

Pharmacologic Class Immunosuppressant Agent; Monoclonal Antibody

U.S. Brand Names Simulect®

Mechanism of Action Chimeric (murine/human) monoclonal antibody which blocks the alpha-chain of the interleukin-2 (IL-2) receptor complex; this receptor is expressed on activated T lymphocytes and is a critical pathway for activating cell-mediated allograft rejection

Use Prophylaxis of acute organ rejection in renal transplantation

USUAL DOSAGE I.V.:

Children 2-15 years of age: 12 mg/m^2 (maximum: 20 mg) within 2 hours prior to transplant surgery, followed by a second dose of 12 mg/m^2 (maximum: 20 mg/dose) 4 days after transplantation

Adults: 20 mg within 2 hours prior to transplant surgery, followed by a second 20 mg dose 4 days after transplantation

Dosing adjustment/comments in renal or hepatic impairment: No specific dosing adjustment recommended

Dosage Forms POWDER for inj: 20 mg

Contraindications Known hypersensitivity to murine proteins or any component of this product

Warnings/Precautions To be used as a component of immunosuppressive regimen which includes cyclosporine and corticosteroids. Only prescribers experienced in transplantation and immunosuppression should prescribe, and patients should receive the drug in a facility with adequate equipment and staff capable of providing the laboratory and medical support required for transplantation.

The incidence of lymphoproliferative disorders and/or opportunistic infections may be increased by immunosuppressive therapy. Hypersensitivity reactions have not been observed in clinical trials. However, similar medications have been associated with reactions including urticaria, dyspnea, and hypotension. Discontinue the drug if a reaction occurs. Medications for the treatment of hypersensitivity reactions should be available for immediate use. Effects of readministration have not been evaluated in humans. Treatment may result in the development of human antimurine antibodies (HAMA); however, limited evidence suggesting the use of muromonab-CD3 or other murine products is not precluded.

Pregnancy Risk Factor B

Pregnancy Implications IL-2 receptors play an important role in the development of the immune system. Use in pregnant women only when benefit exceeds potential risk to the fetus. Women of childbearing potential should use effective contraceptive measures before beginning treatment and for 2 months after completion of therapy with this agent.

It is not known whether basiliximab is excreted in human milk. Because many immunoglobulins are secreted in milk and the potential for serious adverse reactions exists, a decision should be made whether to discontinue nursing or discontinue the drug, taking into account the importance of the drug to the mother.

Adverse Reactions Administration of basiliximab did not appear to increase the incidence or severity of adverse effects in clinical trials. Adverse events were reported in 99% of both the placebo and basiliximab groups.

>10%:

Cardiovascular: Edema, peripheral edema, hypertension
Central nervous system: Fever, headache, dizziness, insomnia
Dermatologic: Wound complications, acne
Endocrine and metabolic: Hypokalemia, hyperkalemia, hyperglycemia, hyperuricemia, hypophosphatemia, hypocalcemia, hypercholesterolemia, acidosis
Gastrointestinal: Constipation, nausea, diarrhea, abdominal pain, vomiting, dyspepsia, moniliasis, weight gain
Genitourinary: Dysuria, urinary tract infection
Hematologic: Anemia
Neuromuscular and skeletal: Leg pain, back pain, tremor

Respiratory: Dyspnea, infection (upper respiratory), coughing, rhinitis, pharyngitis
Miscellaneous: Viral infection, asthenia

3% to 10%:

Cardiovascular: Chest pain, cardiac failure, hypotension, arrhythmia, tachycardia, vascular disorder, generalized edema

Central nervous system: Hypoesthesia, neuropathy, agitation, anxiety, depression, malaise, fatigue, rigors

Dermatologic: Cyst, herpes infection, hypertrichosis, pruritus, rash, skin disorder, skin ulceration

Endocrine and metabolic: Dehydration, diabetes mellitus, fluid overload, hypercalcemia, hyperlipidemia, hypoglycemia, hypomagnesemia

Gastrointestinal: Flatulence, gastroenteritis, GI hemorrhage, gingival hyperplasia, melena, esophagitis, stomatitis

Genitourinary: Impotence, genital edema, albuminuria, bladder disorder, hematuria, urinary frequency, oliguria, abnormal renal function, renal tubular necrosis, ureteral disorder, urinary retention

Hematologic: Hematoma, hemorrhage, purpura, thrombocytopenia, thrombosis, polycythemia

Neuromuscular and skeletal: Arthralgia, arthropathy, cramps, fracture, hernia, myalgia, paresthesia

Ocular: Cataract, conjunctivitis, abnormal vision

Renal: Increased BUN

Respiratory: Bronchitis, bronchospasm, pneumonia, pulmonary edema, sinusitis

Miscellaneous: Accidental trauma, facial edema, sepsis, infection, increased glucocorticoids

Drug Interactions Basiliximab is an immunoglobulin; specific drug interactions have not been evaluated, but are not anticipated

Duration Mean: 36 days (determined by IL-2R alpha saturation)

Half-Life Mean: 7.2 days

Education and Monitoring Issues

Patient Education: This medication, which may help to reduce transplant rejection, can only be given by infusion. You will be monitored and assessed closely during infusion and thereafter, however, it is important that you report any changes or problems for evaluation. You will be susceptible to infection; avoid crowds or infected persons or persons with contagious diseases. Frequent mouth care and small frequent meals may help counteract any GI effects you may experience and will help maintain adequate nutrition and fluid intake. Report any changes in urination; unusual bruising or bleeding; chest pain or palpitations; acute dizziness; respiratory difficulty; fever or chills; changes in cognition; rash; feelings of pain or numbness in extremities; severe GI upset or diarrhea; unusual back or leg pain or muscle tremors; vision changes; or any sign of infection (chills, fever, sore throat, easy bruising or bleeding, mouth sores, unhealed sores, vaginal discharge).

Monitoring Parameters: Signs and symptoms of acute rejection

Manufacturer Novartis

Related Information

Pharmaceutical Manufacturers Directory *on page 1020*

- **Baxedin** *see* Chlorhexidine Gluconate *on page 181*
- **Baycol™** *see* Cerivastatin *on page 171*
- **Bayer® Aspirin [OTC]** *see* Aspirin *on page 72*
- **Bayer® Buffered Aspirin [OTC]** *see* Aspirin *on page 72*
- **Bayer® Low Adult Strength [OTC]** *see* Aspirin *on page 72*

Becaplermin (be KAP ler min)

Pharmacologic Class Topical Skin Product

U.S. Brand Names Regranex®

Mechanism of Action Recombinant B-isoform homodimer of human platelet-derived growth factor (rPDGF-BB) which enhances formation of new granulation tissue, induces fibroblast proliferation, and differentiation to promote wound healing

Use Debridement adjunct for the treatment of diabetic ulcers that occur on the lower limbs and feet

USUAL DOSAGE Adults: Topical:

Diabetic ulcers: Apply appropriate amount of gel once daily with a cotton swab or similar tool, as a coating over the ulcer

The amount of becaplermin to be applied will vary depending on the size of the ulcer area. To calculate the length of gel to apply to the ulcer, measure the greatest length of the ulcer by the greatest width of the ulcer in inches. Refer to following table to calculate the length of gel to administer.

Note: If the ulcer does not decrease in size by ~30% after 10 weeks of treatment or complete healing has not occurred in 20 weeks, continued treatment with becaplermin gel should be reassessed.

(Continued)

Becaplermin *(Continued)*

Formula to Calculate Length of Gel in Inches to Be Applied Daily

Tube Size	Formula
15 or 7.5 g tube	length x width x 0.6
2 g tube	length x width x 1.3

Dosage Forms GEL, top: 0.01% (2 g, 7.5 g, 15 g)

Contraindications Hypersensitivity to becaplermin or any component of its formulation; known neoplasm(s) at the site(s) of application; active infection at ulcer site

Warnings/Precautions Concurrent use of corticosteroids, cancer chemotherapy, or other immunosuppressive agents; ulcer wounds related to arterial or venous insufficiency. Thermal, electrical, or radiation burns at wound site. Malignancy (potential for tumor proliferation, although unproven; topical absorption is minimal). Should not be used in wounds that close by primary intention. For external use only.

Pregnancy Risk Factor C

Adverse Reactions <1%: Erythema with purulent discharge, exuberant granulation tissue, local pain, skin ulceration, tunneling of ulcer, ulcer infection

Onset 8-10 weeks to complete healing

Education and Monitoring Issues

Patient Education:

Hands should be washed thoroughly before applying. The tip of the tube should not come into contact with the ulcer or any other surface; the tube should be recapped tightly after each use. A cotton swab, tongue depressor, or other application aid should be used to apply gel.

Step-by-step instructions for application:

Squeeze the calculated length of gel on to a clean, firm, nonabsorbable surface (wax paper)

With a clean cotton swab, tongue depressor, or similar application aid, spread the measured gel over the ulcer area to obtain an even layer

Cover with a saline-moistened gauze dressing. After ~12 hours, the ulcer should be gently rinsed with saline or water to remove residual gel and covered with a saline-moistened gauze dressing (**without** gel).

Monitoring Parameters: Ulcer volume (pressure ulcers); wound area; evidence of closure; drainage (diabetic ulcers); signs/symptoms of toxicity (erythema, local infections)

Manufacturer Ortho-McNeil Pharmaceutical

Related Information

Pharmaceutical Manufacturers Directory *on page 1020*

- **Beclodisk®** *see* Beclomethasone *on page 94*
- **Becloforte®** *see* Beclomethasone *on page 94*

Beclomethasone (be kloe METH a sone)

Pharmacologic Class Corticosteroid, Oral Inhaler; Corticosteroid, Nasal

U.S. Brand Names Beclovent® Oral Inhaler; Beconase AQ® Nasal Inhaler; Beconase® Nasal Inhaler; Vancenase® AQ Inhaler; Vancenase® Nasal Inhaler; Vanceril® Oral Inhaler

Generic Available No

Mechanism of Action Controls the rate of protein synthesis, depresses the migration of polymorphonuclear leukocytes, fibroblasts, reverses capillary permeability, and lysosomal stabilization at the cellular level to prevent or control inflammation

Use

Oral inhalation: Treatment of bronchial asthma in patients who require chronic administration of corticosteroids

Nasal aerosol: Symptomatic treatment of seasonal or perennial rhinitis and nasal polyposis

USUAL DOSAGE Nasal inhalation and oral inhalation dosage forms are not to be used interchangeably

Aqueous inhalation, nasal:

Vancenase® AQ, Beconase® AQ: Children ≥6 years and Adults: 1-2 inhalations each nostril twice daily

Vancenase® AQ 84 mcg: Children ≥6 years and Adults: 1-2 inhalations in each nostril once daily

Intranasal (Vancenase®, Beconase®):

Children 6-12 years: 1 inhalation in each nostril 3 times/day

Children ≥12 years and Adults: 1 inhalation in each nostril 2-4 times/day or 2 inhalations each nostril twice daily; usual maximum maintenance: 1 inhalation in each nostril 3 times/day

Oral inhalation (doses should be titrated to the lowest effective dose once asthma is controlled):

Beclovent®, Vanceril®:

Children 6-12 years: 1-2 inhalations 3-4 times/day (alternatively: 2-4 inhalations twice daily); maximum dose: 10 inhalations/day

Children ≥12 years and Adults: 2 inhalations 3-4 times/day (alternatively: 4 inhalations twice daily); maximum dose: 20 inhalations/day; patients with severe asthma: Initial: 12-16 inhalations/day (divided 3-4 times/day); dose should be adjusted downward according to patient's response

Vanceril® 84 mcg double strength:

Children 6-12 years: 2 inhalations twice daily; maximum dose: 5 inhalations/day

Children ≥12 years and Adults: 2 inhalations twice daily; maximum dose: 10 inhalations/day; patients with severe asthma: Initial: 6-8 inhalations/day (divided twice daily); dose should be adjusted downward according to patient's response

NIH Guidelines (NIH, 1997) (give in divided doses):

Children:

"Low" dose: 84-336 mcg/day (42 mcg/puff: 2-8 puffs/day or 84 mcg/puff: 1-4 puffs/day)

"Medium" dose: 336-672 mcg/day (42 mcg/puff: 8-16 puffs/day or 84 mcg/puff: 4-8 puffs/day)

"High" dose: >672 mcg/day (42 mcg/puff: >16 puffs/day or 84 mcg/puff >8 puffs/day)

Adults:

"Low" dose: 168-504 mcg/day (42 mcg/puff: 4-12 puffs/day or 84 mcg/puff: 2-6 puffs/day)

"Medium" dose: 504-840 mcg/day (42 mcg/puff: 12-20 puffs/day or 84 mcg/puff: 6-10 puffs/day)

"High" dose: >840 mcg/day (42 mcg/puff: >20 puffs/day or 84 mcg/puff: >10 puffs/day)

Dosage Forms NASAL: Inhalation: (Beconase®, Vancenase®): 42 mcg/inhalation [200 metered doses] (16.8 g); Spray, (Vancenase® AQ Nasal): 0.084% [120 actuations] (19 g); Spray, aqueous, nasal, (Beconase® AQ, Vancenase® AQ): 42 mcg/inhalation [≥200 metered doses] (25 g), 84 mcg/inhalation [≥200 metered doses] (25 g). **ORAL:** Inhalation: (Beclovent®, Vanceril®): 42 mcg/inhalation [200 metered doses] (16.8 g); (Vanceril® Double Strength): 84 mcg/inhalation (5.4 g - 40 metered doses, 12.2 g - 120 metered doses)

Contraindications Status asthmaticus; hypersensitivity to the drug or fluorocarbons, oleic acid in the formulation, systemic fungal infections

Warnings/Precautions Not to be used in status asthmaticus; safety and efficacy in children <6 years of age have not been established; avoid using higher than recommended dosages since suppression of hypothalamic, pituitary, or adrenal function may occur

Controlled clinical studies have shown that inhaled and intranasal corticosteroids may cause a reduction in growth velocity in pediatric patients. Growth velocity provides a means of comparing the rate of growth among children of the same age.

In studies involving inhaled corticosteroids, the average reduction in growth velocity was approximately 1 cm (about 1/3 of an inch) per year. It appears that the reduction is related to dose and how long the child takes the drug.

Long-term effects of this reduction in growth velocity on final adult height are unknown. Likewise, it also has not yet been determined whether patients' growth will "catch up" if treatment in discontinued. Drug manufacturers will continue to monitor these drugs to learn more about long-term effects. Children are prescribed inhaled corticosteroids to treat asthma. Intranasal corticosteroids are generally used to prevent and treat allergy-related nasal symptoms.

Patients are advised not to stop using their inhaled or intranasal corticosteroids without first speaking to their healthcare providers about the benefits of these drugs compared to their risks.

Pregnancy Risk Factor C

Pregnancy Implications Data does not support an association between drug and congenital defects in humans

Clinical effects on fetus: No data on crossing the placenta or effects on the fetus
Breast-feeding/lactation: No data on crossing into breast milk or effects on the infant

Adverse Reactions

>10%:

Local: Growth of *Candida* in the mouth, irritation and burning of the nasal mucosa
Respiratory: Cough, hoarseness

1% to 10%:

Gastrointestinal: Xerostomia
Local: Nasal ulceration
Respiratory: Epistaxis

<1%: Bronchospasm, dysphagia, headache, nasal congestion, nasal septal perforations, rash, rhinorrhea, sneezing

Onset Therapeutic effect: Within 1-4 weeks of use

(Continued)

Beclomethasone *(Continued)*

Half-Life Oral: Initial: 3 hours; Terminal: 15 hours

Education and Monitoring Issues

Patient Education: Use as directed; do not increase dosage or discontinue abruptly without consulting prescriber. It may take 1-4 weeks for you to realize full effects of treatment. Review use of inhaler or spray with prescriber or follow package insert for directions. Keep oral inhaler clean and unobstructed. Always rinse mouth and throat after use of inhaler to prevent opportunistic infection. If you are also using an inhaled bronchodilator, wait 10 minutes before using this steroid aerosol. Report adverse effects such as skin redness, rash, or irritation; pain or burning of nasal mucosa; white plaques in mouth or fuzzy tongue; unresolved headache; or worsening of condition or lack of improvement.

Manufacturer GlaxoWellcome

Related Information

Asthma Guidelines *on page 1077*
Pharmaceutical Manufacturers Directory *on page 1020*

♦ **Beclovent® Oral Inhaler** *see* Beclomethasone *on page 94*
♦ **Beconase AQ® Nasal Inhaler** *see* Beclomethasone *on page 94*
♦ **Beconase® Nasal Inhaler** *see* Beclomethasone *on page 94*
♦ **Becotin® Pulvules®** *see* Vitamins, Multiple *on page 981*
♦ **Beepen-VK®** *see* Penicillin V Potassium *on page 713*
♦ **Belix® Oral [OTC]** *see* Diphenhydramine *on page 282*

Belladonna and Opium (bel a DON a & OH pee um)

Pharmacologic Class Analgesic, Combination (Narcotic); Antispasmodic Agent, Urinary

U.S. Brand Names B&O Supprettes®

Use Relief of moderate to severe pain associated with rectal or bladder tenesmus that may occur in postoperative states and neoplastic situations; pain associated with ureteral spasms not responsive to non-narcotic analgesics and to space intervals between injections of opiates

USUAL DOSAGE Adults: Rectal: 1 suppository 1-2 times/day, up to 4 doses/day

Contraindications Glaucoma, severe renal or hepatic disease, bronchial asthma, respiratory depression, convulsive disorders, acute alcoholism, premature labor

Pregnancy Risk Factor C

Belladonna, Phenobarbital, and Ergotamine Tartrate

(bel a DON a, fee noe BAR bi tal, & er GOT a meen TAR trate)

Pharmacologic Class Ergot Derivative

U.S. Brand Names Bellergal-S®; Bel-Phen-Ergot S®; Phenerbel-S®

Dosage Forms TAB, sustained release: l-alkaloids of belladonna 0.2 mg, phenobarbital 40 mg, and ergotamine tartrate 0.6 mg

Pregnancy Risk Factor X

Half-Life Ergotamine: 21 hours

Education and Monitoring Issues

Patient Education: Take as directed; do not take more than recommended dose. Maintain adequate nutritional and fluid intake (2-3 L/day of fluids unless instructed to restrict fluid intake) to prevent constipation. May cause drowsiness or dizziness (use caution when driving or engaging in tasks that require alertness until response to drug is known); dry throat or mouth (frequent mouth care or sucking on lozenges may help); dry nose (use humidifier); photosensitivity (use sunblock, wear protective clothing and eyewear, avoid direct sunlight); nausea or vomiting (small frequent meals, frequent mouth care, sucking lozenges, or chewing gum may help); dry skin (mild skin lotion may help); or orthostatic hypotension (use caution when rising from sitting or lying position or climbing stairs). Report any signs of numbness in extremities (fingers and toes), unusual leg pain or cyanosis of extremities; difficulty swallowing; persistent muscle pain or weakness; pain in eye or vision changes; or chest pain, rapid heartbeat, or palpitations.

♦ **Bellergal®** *see* Belladonna, Phenobarbital, and Ergotamine Tartrate *on page 96*
♦ **Bellergal-S®** *see* Belladonna, Phenobarbital, and Ergotamine Tartrate *on page 96*
♦ **Bellergal® Spacetabs®** *see* Belladonna, Phenobarbital, and Ergotamine Tartrate *on page 96*
♦ **Bel-Phen-Ergot S®** *see* Belladonna, Phenobarbital, and Ergotamine Tartrate *on page 96*
♦ **Benadryl® Injection** *see* Diphenhydramine *on page 282*
♦ **Benadryl® Oral [OTC]** *see* Diphenhydramine *on page 282*
♦ **Benadryl® Topical** *see* Diphenhydramine *on page 282*
♦ **Ben-Allergin-50® Injection** *see* Diphenhydramine *on page 282*

Benazepril (ben AY ze pril)

Pharmacologic Class Angiotensin-Converting Enzyme (ACE) Inhibitors

U.S. Brand Names Lotensin®

Generic Available No

Mechanism of Action Competitive inhibition of angiotensin I being converted to angiotensin II, a potent vasoconstrictor, through the angiotensin I-converting enzyme (ACE) activity, with resultant lower levels of angiotensin II which causes an increase in plasma renin activity and a reduction in aldosterone secretion

Use Treatment of hypertension, either alone or in combination with other antihypertensive agents

Unlabeled use: Congestive heart failure, postmyocardial infarction, nephropathy

USUAL DOSAGE Adults: Oral: 20-40 mg/day as a single dose or 2 divided doses; base dosage adjustments on peak (2-6 hours after dosing) and trough responses

Dosing interval in renal impairment: Cl_{cr} <30 mL/minute: Administer 5 mg/day initially; maximum daily dose: 40 mg

Hemodialysis: Moderately dialyzable (20% to 50%); administer dose postdialysis or administer 25% to 35% supplemental dose

Peritoneal dialysis: Supplemental dose is not necessary

Dosage Forms TAB: 5 mg, 10 mg, 20 mg, 40 mg

Contraindications Hypersensitivity to benazepril or any component or other ACE inhibitors

Warnings/Precautions Use with caution in patients with collagen vascular disease, hypovolemia, valvular stenosis, hyperkalemia, recent anesthesia; modify dosage in patients with renal impairment (especially renal artery stenosis), severe congestive heart failure, or with coadministered diuretic therapy; experience in children is limited; severe hypotension may occur in patients who are sodium and/or volume depleted; initiate lower doses and monitor closely when starting therapy in these patients

Pregnancy Risk Factor C (1st trimester); D (2nd and 3rd trimesters)

Pregnancy Implications It is not known whether benazepril is excreted in human milk

Clinical effects on the fetus: No data available on crossing the placenta. Cranial defects, hypocalvaria/acalvaria, oligohydramnios, persistent anuria following delivery, hypotension, renal defects, renal dysgenesis/dysplasia, renal failure, pulmonary hypoplasia, limb contractures secondary to oligohydramnios and stillbirth reported. ACE inhibitors should be avoided during pregnancy.

Breast-feeding/lactation: Crosses into breast milk. American Academy of Pediatrics considers **compatible** with breast-feeding.

Adverse Reactions

1% to 10%:

- Cardiovascular: Postural dizziness (1.5%)
- Central nervous system: Headache (6.2%), dizziness (3.6%), fatigue (2.4%), somnolence (1.6%)
- Endocrine & metabolic: Hyperkalemia (1%), increased uric acid
- Gastrointestinal: Nausea (1.3%)
- Renal: Increased serum creatinine (2%), worsening of renal function may occur in patients with bilateral renal artery stenosis or hypovolemia
- Respiratory: Cough (1.2% to 10%)

<1% (limited to important or life-threatening symptoms): Hypotension, postural hypotension (0.3%), syncope, angina, palpitation, peripheral edema, angioedema, laryngeal edema, shock, Stevens-Johnson syndrome, pemphigus, hypersensitivity, dermatitis, rash, pruritus, photosensitivity, flushing, pancreatitis, constipation, gastritis, vomiting, melena, thrombocytopenia, hemolytic anemia, anxiety, decreased libido, hypertonia, insomnia, nervousness, paresthesia, asthma, bronchitis, dyspnea, sinusitis, urinary tract infection, arthritis, impotence, alopecia, arthralgia, myalgia, asthenia, sweating, gynecomastia

Eosinophilic pneumonitis, neutropenia, anaphylaxis, renal insufficiency and renal failure have been reported with other ACE inhibitors. In addition, a syndrome including fever, myalgia, arthralgia, interstitial nephritis, vasculitis, rash, eosinophilia, and elevated ESR has been reported to be associated with ACE inhibitors.

Drug Interactions

Alpha$_1$ blockers: Hypotensive effect increased.

Aspirin and NSAIDs may decrease ACE inhibitor efficacy.

Diuretics: Hypovolemia due to diuretics may precipitate acute hypotensive events or acute renal failure.

Insulin: Risk of hypoglycemia may be increased.

Lithium: Risk of lithium toxicity may be increased; monitor lithium levels.

Potassium-sparing diuretics or potassium supplements (amiloride, potassium, spironolactone, triamterene): Increased risk of hyperkalemia.

Trimethoprim (high dose) may increase the risk of hyperkalemia.

Alcohol Interactions Avoid use (may increase risk of hypotension or dizziness)

Onset

Reduction in plasma angiotensin-converting enzyme activity: Oral: Peak effect: 1-2 hours after administration of 2-20 mg dose

(Continued)

Benazepril *(Continued)*

Reduction in blood pressure: Peak effect after single oral dose: 2-6 hours; Maximum response with continuous therapy: 2 weeks

Duration >90% inhibition for 24 hours has been observed after 5-20 mg dose

Half-Life Parent drug: 0.6 hour; Metabolite elimination: 22 hours (from 24 hours after dosing onward); Metabolite: 1.5-2 hours after fasting or 2-4 hours after a meal

Education and Monitoring Issues

Patient Education: Take exactly as directed; do not discontinue without consulting prescriber. Take first dose at bedtime. Take all doses on an empty stomach (30 minutes before or 2 hours after meals). This drug does not eliminate need for diet or exercise regimen as recommended by prescriber. May cause dizziness, fainting, lightheadedness (use caution when driving or engaging in tasks that require alertness until response to drug is known); postural hypotension (use caution when rising from lying or sitting position or climbing stairs); nausea, vomiting, abdominal pain, dry mouth, or transient loss of appetite (small frequent meals, frequent mouth care, sucking lozenges, or chewing gum may help) - report if these persist. Report mouth sores; fever or chills; swelling of extremities, face, mouth, or tongue; difficulty in breathing or unusual cough; or other persistent adverse reactions.

Manufacturer Novartis

Related Information

Amlodipine and Benazepril *on page 54*
Angiotensin-Related Agents Comparison *on page 1226*
Benazepril and Hydrochlorothiazide *on page 98*
Pharmaceutical Manufacturers Directory *on page 1020*

Benazepril and Hydrochlorothiazide

(ben AY ze pril & hye droe klor oh THYE a zide)

Pharmacologic Class Antihypertensive Agent, Combination

U.S. Brand Names Lotensin® HCT

Dosage Forms TAB: Benazepril 5 mg and hydrochlorothiazide 6.25 mg; Benazepril 10 mg and hydrochlorothiazide 12.5 mg; Benazepril 20 mg and hydrochlorothiazide 12.5 mg; Benazepril 20 mg and hydrochlorothiazide 25 mg

Pregnancy Risk Factor C (1st trimester); D (2nd and 3rd trimesters)

Manufacturer Ciba-Geigy Pharmaceuticals

Related Information

Pharmaceutical Manufacturers Directory *on page 1020*

- **Benemid®** *see* Probenecid *on page 768*

Bentoquatam (ben to KWA tam)

Pharmacologic Class Protectant, Topical

U.S. Brand Names IvyBlock®

Use Skin protectant for the prevention of allergic contact dermatitis to poison oak, ivy, and sumac

USUAL DOSAGE Children >6 years and Adults: Topical: Apply to skin 15 minutes prior to potential exposure to poison ivy, poison oak, or poison sumac, and reapply every 4 hours

Contraindications Hypersensitivity to bentoquatam

- **Bentyl® Hydrochloride Injection** *see* Dicyclomine *on page 266*
- **Bentyl® Hydrochloride Oral** *see* Dicyclomine *on page 266*
- **Bentylol®** *see* Dicyclomine *on page 266*
- **Benuryl®** *see* Probenecid *on page 768*
- **Benylin® Codeine** *see* Guaifenesin, Pseudoephedrine, and Codeine *on page 425*
- **Benylin® Cough Syrup [OTC]** *see* Diphenhydramine *on page 282*
- **Benylin® DM-E** *see* Guaifenesin and Dextromethorphan *on page 424*
- **Benylin® Expectorant [OTC]** *see* Guaifenesin and Dextromethorphan *on page 424*
- **Benzamycin®** *see* Erythromycin and Benzoyl Peroxide *on page 325*

Benzocaine (BEN zoe kane)

Pharmacologic Class Local Anesthetic

U.S. Brand Names Americaine® [OTC]; Anbesol® [OTC]; Anbesol® Maximum Strength [OTC]; Babee® Teething® [OTC]; Benzocol® [OTC]; Benzodent® [OTC]; Chigger-Tox® [OTC]; Cylex® [OTC]; Dermoplast® [OTC]; Foille® [OTC]; Foille® Medicated First Aid [OTC]; Hurricaine®; Lanacane® [OTC]; Maximum Strength Anbesol® [OTC]; Maximum Strength Orajel® [OTC]; Mycinettes® [OTC]; Numzitdent® [OTC]; Numzit Teething® [OTC]; Orabase®-B [OTC]; Orabase®-O [OTC]; Orajel® Brace-Aid Oral Anesthetic [OTC]; Orajel® Maximum Strength [OTC]; Orajel® Mouth-Aid [OTC]; Orasept® [OTC]; Orasol® [OTC]; Oratect™ [OTC]; Rhulicaine® [OTC]; Rid-A-Pain® [OTC]; Slim-Mint® [OTC]; Solarcaine® [OTC]; Spec-T® [OTC]; Tanac® [OTC]; Trocaine® [OTC]; Unguentine® [OTC]; Vicks® Children's Chloraseptic® [OTC]; Vicks® Chloraseptic® Sore Throat [OTC]; Zilactin®-B Medicated [OTC]

Use Temporary relief of pain associated with local anesthetic for pruritic dermatosis, pruritus, minor burns, acute congestive and serous otitis media, swimmer's ear, otitis externa, toothache, minor sore throat pain, canker sores, hemorrhoids, rectal fissures, anesthetic lubricant for passage of catheters and endoscopic tubes; nonprescription diet aide

USUAL DOSAGE

Children and Adults:

Mucous membranes: Dosage varies depending on area to be anesthetized and vascularity of tissues

Oral mouth/throat preparations: Do not administer for >2 days or in children <2 years of age, unless directed by a prescriber; refer to specific package labeling

Topical: Apply to affected area as needed

Adults: Nonprescription diet aid: 6-15 mg just prior to food consumption, not to exceed 45 mg/day

Contraindications Children <1 year of age; secondary bacterial infection of area; ophthalmic use; known hypersensitivity to benzocaine or other ester type local anesthetics

Pregnancy Risk Factor C

Related Information

Antipyrine and Benzocaine *on page 67*

Benzocaine, Butyl Aminobenzoate, Tetracaine, and Benzalkonium Chloride *on page 99*

Benzocaine, Butyl Aminobenzoate, Tetracaine, and Benzalkonium Chloride

(BEN zoe kane, BYOO til a meen oh BENZ oh ate, TET ra kane, & benz al KOE nee um KLOR ide)

Pharmacologic Class Local Anesthetic

U.S. Brand Names Cetacaine®

Dosage Forms AERO: Benzocaine 14%, butyl aminobenzoate 2%, tetracaine 2%, and benzalkonium chloride 0.5% (56 g)

Pregnancy Risk Factor C

Education and Monitoring Issues

Patient Education: This spray may help control pain or gagging. If mouth or throat is numb, use caution with food and fluids. Your sensation to heat may be disturbed, your ability to swallow may be disturbed; use caution when swallowing to prevent choking.

- **Benzocol® [OTC]** *see* Benzocaine *on page 98*
- **Benzodent® [OTC]** *see* Benzocaine *on page 98*

Benzonatate (ben ZOE na tate)

Pharmacologic Class Antitussive

U.S. Brand Names Tessalon® Perles

Generic Available No

Mechanism of Action Tetracaine congener with antitussive properties; suppresses cough by topical anesthetic action on the respiratory stretch receptors

Use Symptomatic relief of nonproductive cough

USUAL DOSAGE Children >10 years and Adults: Oral: 100 mg 3 times/day or every 4 hours up to 600 mg/day

Dosage Forms CAP: 100 mg

Contraindications Known hypersensitivity to benzonatate or related compounds (such as tetracaine)

Pregnancy Risk Factor C

Adverse Reactions 1% to 10%:

Central nervous system: Sedation, headache, dizziness

Dermatologic: Rash

Gastrointestinal: GI upset

Neuromuscular & skeletal: Numbness in chest

Ocular: Burning sensation in eyes

Respiratory: Nasal congestion

Onset Therapeutic: Within 15-20 minutes

Duration 3-8 hours

Education and Monitoring Issues

Patient Education: Take only as prescribed; do not exceed prescribed dose or frequency. Do not break or chew capsule. Maintain adequate hydration (2-3 L/day of fluids unless instructed to restrict fluid intake). Avoid use of other depressants, alcohol, or sleep-inducing medications unless approved by prescriber. You may experience drowsiness, impaired coordination, blurred vision, or increased anxiety (use caution when driving or engaging in tasks requiring alertness until response to drug is known); or upset stomach or nausea (frequent small meals, frequent mouth care, chewing gum, or sucking hard candy may help). Report persistent CNS changes (dizziness, sedation, tremor, or agitation), numbness in chest or feeling of chill, visual changes or burning in

(Continued)

Benzonatate *(Continued)*

eyes, numbness of mouth or difficulty swallowing, or lack of improvement or worsening of condition.

Monitoring Parameters: Monitor patient's chest sounds and respiratory pattern

Benzoyl Peroxide and Hydrocortisone

(BEN zoe il peer OKS ide & hye droe KOR ti sone)

Pharmacologic Class Acne Products

U.S. Brand Names Vanoxide-HC®

Dosage Forms LOT: Benzoyl peroxide 5% and hydrocortisone alcohol 0.5% (25 mL)

Pregnancy Risk Factor C

Benztropine (BENZ troe peen)

Pharmacologic Class Anticholinergic Agent; Anti-Parkinson's Agent (Anticholinergic)

U.S. Brand Names Cogentin®

Generic Available Yes: Tablet

Mechanism of Action Thought to partially block striatal cholinergic receptors to help balance cholinergic and dopaminergic activity

Use Adjunctive treatment of Parkinson's disease; also used in treatment of drug-induced extrapyramidal effects (except tardive dyskinesia) and acute dystonic reactions

USUAL DOSAGE Use in children <3 years of age should be reserved for life-threatening emergencies

Drug-induced extrapyramidal reaction: Oral, I.M., I.V.:
- Children >3 years: 0.02-0.05 mg/kg/dose 1-2 times/day
- Adults: 1-4 mg/dose 1-2 times/day

Acute dystonia: Adults: I.M., I.V.: 1-2 mg

Parkinsonism: Oral:
- Adults: 0.5-6 mg/day in 1-2 divided doses; if one dose is greater, administer at bedtime; titrate dose in 0.5 mg increments at 5- to 6-day intervals
- Elderly: Initial: 0.5 mg once or twice daily; increase by 0.5 mg as needed at 5-6 days; maximum: 6 mg/day

Dosage Forms INJ: 1 mg/mL (2 mL). **TAB:** 0.5 mg, 1 mg, 2 mg

Contraindications Children <3 years of age, use with caution in older children (dosage not established); patients with narrow-angle glaucoma; hypersensitivity to any component; pyloric or duodenal obstruction, stenosing peptic ulcers; bladder neck obstructions; achalasia; myasthenia gravis

Warnings/Precautions Use with caution in hot weather or during exercise. Elderly patients frequently develop increased sensitivity and require strict dosage regulation - side effects may be more severe in elderly patients with atherosclerotic changes. Use with caution in patients with tachycardia, cardiac arrhythmias, hypertension, hypotension, prostatic hypertrophy (especially in the elderly) or any tendency toward urinary retention, liver or kidney disorders and obstructive disease of the GI or GU tract. When given in large doses or to susceptible patients, may cause weakness and inability to move particular muscle groups.

Pregnancy Risk Factor C

Adverse Reactions

>10%:
- Dermatologic: Dry skin
- Gastrointestinal: Constipation, dry throat, xerostomia
- Respiratory: Dry nose
- Miscellaneous: Diaphoresis (decreased)

1% to 10%:
- Dermatologic: Increased sensitivity to light
- Endocrine & metabolic: Decreased flow of breast milk
- Gastrointestinal: Dysphagia

<1%: Ataxia, bloated feeling, blurred vision, coma, drowsiness, dysuria, fatigue, hallucinations, headache, increased intraocular pain, loss of memory, mydriasis, nausea, nervousness, orthostatic hypotension, palpitations, rash, tachycardia, ventricular fibrillation, vomiting, weakness; the elderly may be at increased risk for confusion and hallucinations

Drug Interactions

Decreased effect: May increase gastric degradation of levodopa and decrease the amount of levodopa absorbed by delaying gastric emptying; the opposite may be true for digoxin

Therapeutic effects of cholinergic agents (tacrine, donepezil) and neuroleptics may be antagonized

Increased toxicity: Central and/or peripheral anticholinergic syndrome can occur when administered with amantadine, rimantadine, narcotic analgesics, phenothiazines and other antipsychotics (especially with high anticholinergic activity), tricyclic antidepressants, quinidine and some other antiarrhythmics, and antihistamines

Alcohol Interactions Avoid use (may increase central nervous system depression)

Onset Oral: Within 1 hour; Parenteral: Within 15 minutes

Duration 6-48 hours (wide range)

Education and Monitoring Issues

Patient Education: Take exactly as directed; do not increase, decrease, or discontinue without consulting prescriber. Take at the same time each day. Do not use alcohol and all prescription or OTC sedatives or CNS depressants without consulting prescriber. You may experience drowsiness, dizziness, confusion, and blurred vision (use caution when driving, climbing stairs, or engaging in tasks requiring alertness until response to drug is known); increased susceptibility to heat stroke, decreased perspiration (use caution in hot weather - maintain adequate fluids and reduce exercise activity); constipation (increased exercise, fluids, or dietary fruit and fiber may help). Report unresolved nausea, vomiting, or gastric disturbances; rapid or pounding heartbeat, chest pain or palpitation; difficulty breathing; CNS changes (hallucination, loss of memory, nervousness, etc); eye pain; prolonged fever; painful or difficult urination; unresolved constipation; increased muscle spasticity or rigidity; skin rash; or significant worsening of condition.

Related Information

Parkinson's Disease Dosing *on page 1249*

Benzylpenicilloyl-polylysine (BEN zil pen i SIL oyl pol i LIE seen)

Pharmacologic Class Diagnostic Agent

U.S. Brand Names Pre-Pen®

Use Adjunct in assessing the risk of administering penicillin (penicillin or benzylpenicillin) in adults with a history of clinical penicillin hypersensitivity

USUAL DOSAGE PPL is administered by a scratch technique or by intradermal injection. For initial testing, PPL should always be applied via the scratch technique. **Do not administer intradermally to patients who have positive reactions to a scratch test.** PPL test alone does not identify those patients who react to a minor antigenic determinant and does not appear to predict reliably the occurrence of late reactions.

Scratch test: Use scratch technique with a 20-gauge needle to make 3-5 mm nonbleeding scratch on epidermis, apply a small drop of solution to scratch, rub in gently with applicator or toothpick. A positive reaction consists of a pale wheal surrounding the scratch site which develops within 10 minutes and ranges from 5-15 mm or more in diameter.

Intradermal test: Use intradermal test with a tuberculin syringe with a 26- to 30-gauge short bevel needle; a dose of 0.01-0.02 mL is injected intradermally. A control of 0.9% sodium chloride should be injected at least 1.5" from the PPL test site. Most skin responses to the intradermal test will develop within 5-15 minutes.

Interpretation:

(-) Negative: No reaction

(±) Ambiguous: Wheal only slightly larger than original bleb with or without erythematous flare and larger than control site

(+) Positive: Itching and marked increase in size of original bleb

Control site should be reactionless

Contraindications Patients known to be extremely hypersensitive to penicillin

Pregnancy Risk Factor C

Bepridil (BE pri dil)

Pharmacologic Class Calcium Channel Blocker

U.S. Brand Names Vascor®

Generic Available No

Mechanism of Action Bepridil, a type 4 calcium antagonist, possesses characteristics of the traditional calcium antagonists, inhibiting calcium ion from entering the "slow channels" or select voltage-sensitive areas of vascular smooth muscle and myocardium during depolarization and producing a relaxation of coronary vascular smooth muscle and coronary vasodilation. However, bepridil may also inhibit fast sodium channels (inward), which may account for some of its side effects (eg, arrhythmias); a direct bradycardia effect of bepridil has been postulated via direct action on the S-A node.

Use Treatment of chronic stable angina; due to side effect profile, reserve for patients who have been intolerant of other antianginal therapy; bepridil may be used alone or in combination with nitrates or beta-blockers

USUAL DOSAGE Adults: Oral: Initial: 200 mg/day, then adjust dose at 10-day intervals until optimal response is achieved; usual dose: 300 mg/day; maximum daily dose: 400 mg

Dosage Forms TAB: 200 mg, 300 mg, 400 mg

Contraindications History of serious ventricular or atrial arrhythmias (especially tachycardia or those associated with accessory conduction pathways), uncompensated cardiac insufficiency, congenital Q-T interval prolongation, patients taking other drugs that prolong the Q-T interval, history of hypersensitivity to bepridil or any component, calcium channel blockers, or adenosine; concurrent administration with amprenavir, ritonavir or sparfloxacin

Warnings/Precautions Use with great caution in patients with history of IHSS, second or third degree A-V block, cardiogenic shock; reserve for patients in whom other antianginals have failed. Carefully titrate dosages for patients with impaired renal or hepatic function; use caution when treating patients with congestive heart failure, significant hypotension,

(Continued)

Bepridil *(Continued)*

severe left ventricular dysfunction, hypertrophic cardiomyopathy (especially obstructive), concomitant therapy with beta-blockers or digoxin, edema, or increased intracranial pressure with cranial tumors; do not abruptly withdraw (may cause chest pain); elderly may experience hypotension and constipation more readily.

If dosage reduction does not maintain the Q-T within a safe range (not to exceed 0.52 seconds during therapy), discontinue the medication; has class I antiarrhythmic properties and can induce new arrhythmias, including VT/VF; it can also cause torsade de pointes type ventricular tachycardia due to its ability to prolong the Q-T interval; avoid use in patients in the immediate period postinfarction.

Pregnancy Risk Factor C

Adverse Reactions

>10%:

- Central nervous system: Dizziness
- Gastrointestinal: Nausea, dyspepsia

1% to 10%:

- Cardiovascular: Bradycardia, edema, palpitations
- Central nervous system: Nervousness, headache (7% to 13%), drowsiness, psychiatric disturbances (<2%), insomnia (2% to 3%)
- Dermatologic: Rash (≤2%)
- Endocrine & metabolic: Sexual dysfunction
- Gastrointestinal: Diarrhea, anorexia, xerostomia, constipation, abdominal pain, dyspepsia, flatulence
- Neuromuscular & skeletal: Weakness (6.5% to 14%), tremor (<9%), paresthesia (2.5%)
- Ocular: Blurred vision
- Otic: Tinnitus
- Respiratory: Rhinitis, dyspnea (≤8.7%), cough (≤2%)
- Miscellaneous (≤2%): Flu syndrome, diaphoresis

<1%: Abnormal taste, akathisia, altered behavior, arthritis, fever, hypertension, pharyngitis, prolonged Q-T intervals, syncope, ventricular premature contractions

Drug Interactions CYP3A3/4 enzyme substrate

Increased toxicity/effect/levels:

- Bepridil and cyclosporine may increase cyclosporine levels (other calcium channel blockers have been shown to interact)
- Bepridil and digitalis glycoside may increase digitalis glycoside levels
- Use with amprenavir, ritonavir, sparfloxacin (possibly also gatifloxacin and moxifloxacin) may increase risk of bepridil toxicity, especially its cardiotoxicity
- Coadministration with beta-blocking agents may result in increased depressant effects on myocardial contractility or A-V conduction
- Severe hypotension or increased fluid volume requirements may occur with concomitant fentanyl

Use with cisapride may increase the risk of malignant arrhythmias, concurrent use is contraindicated

Onset 1 hour

Half-Life 24 hours

Education and Monitoring Issues

Patient Education: Take as directed (may be taken with food to reduce gastric side effects). Do not discontinue without consulting prescriber. Regular EKGs and follow-up with prescriber may be required. If taking potassium supplements or potassium-sparing diuretics, serum potassium monitoring will be required. May cause dizziness, shakiness, visual disturbances, or headache; use caution when driving or engaging in tasks that require alertness until response to drug is known. Report irregular or pounding heartbeat, respiratory difficulty, swelling of hands or feet, unresolved headache, dizziness, constipation, or any unusual bleeding or bruising.

Monitoring Parameters: EKG and serum electrolytes, blood pressure, signs and symptoms of congestive heart failure; elderly may need very close monitoring due to underlying cardiac and organ system defects

Reference Range: 1-2 ng/mL

Manufacturer Ortho-McNeil Pharmaceutical

Related Information

Calcium Channel Blocking Agents Comparison *on page 1236*
Pharmaceutical Manufacturers Directory *on page 1020*

Beractant (ber AKT ant)

Pharmacologic Class Lung Surfactant

U.S. Brand Names Survanta®

Generic Available No

Mechanism of Action Replaces deficient or ineffective endogenous lung surfactant in neonates with respiratory distress syndrome (RDS) or in neonates at risk of developing RDS. Surfactant prevents the alveoli from collapsing during expiration by lowering surface tension between air and alveolar surfaces.

Use Prevention and treatment of respiratory distress syndrome (RDS) in premature infants

Prophylactic therapy: Body weight <1250 g in infants at risk for developing or with evidence of surfactant deficiency

Rescue therapy: Treatment of infants with RDS confirmed by x-ray and requiring mechanical ventilation (administer as soon as possible - within 8 hours of age)

USUAL DOSAGE

Prophylactic treatment: Administer 100 mg phospholipids (4 mL/kg) intratracheal as soon as possible; as many as 4 doses may be administered during the first 48 hours of life, no more frequently than 6 hours apart. The need for additional doses is determined by evidence of continuing respiratory distress; if the infant is still intubated and requiring at least 30% inspired oxygen to maintain a $PaO_2 \leq 80$ torr.

Rescue treatment: Administer 100 mg phospholipids (4 mL/kg) as soon as the diagnosis of RDS is made; may repeat if needed, no more frequently than every 6 hours to a maximum of 4 doses

Dosage Forms SUSP: 200 mg (8 mL)

Warnings/Precautions Rapidly affects oxygenation and lung compliance and should be restricted to a highly supervised use in a clinical setting with immediate availability of clinicians experienced with intubation and ventilatory management of premature infants. If transient episodes of bradycardia and decreased oxygen saturation occur, discontinue the dosing procedure and initiate measures to alleviate the condition; produces rapid improvements in lung oxygenation and compliance that may require immediate reductions in ventilator settings and FiO_2.

Adverse Reactions During the dosing procedure:

>10%: Cardiovascular: Transient bradycardia

1% to 10%: Respiratory: Oxygen desaturation

<1%: Apnea, endotracheal tube blockage, hypercarbia, hypertension, hypocarbia, hypotension, increased probability of post-treatment nosocomial sepsis, pallor, pulmonary air leaks, pulmonary interstitial emphysema, vasoconstriction

Education and Monitoring Issues

Monitoring Parameters: Continuous EKG and transcutaneous O_2 saturation should be monitored during administration; frequent arterial blood gases are necessary to prevent postdosing hyperoxia and hypocarbia

Manufacturer Ross Laboratories

Related Information

Pharmaceutical Manufacturers Directory *on page 1020*

- **Berocca®** *see* Vitamin B Complex With Vitamin C and Folic Acid *on page 979*
- **Berubigen®** *see* Cyanocobalamin *on page 233*
- **Beta-2®** *see* Isoetharine *on page 486*
- **Beta-Blockers Comparison** *see page 1233*

Beta-Carotene (BAY tah-KARE oh teen)

Pharmacologic Class Vitamin, Fat Soluble

U.S. Brand Names Solatene®

Use Reduces severity of photosensitivity reactions in patients with erythropoietic protoporphyria (EPP)

Unlabeled use: Prophylaxis and treatment of polymorphous light eruption and prophylaxis against photosensitivity reactions in erythropoietic protoporphyria

USUAL DOSAGE Oral:

Children <14 years: 30-150 mg/day

Adults: 30-300 mg/day

Contraindications Hypersensitivity to beta-carotene

Pregnancy Risk Factor C

- **Betachron E-R®** *see* Propranolol *on page 786*
- **Betadine® [OTC]** *see* Povidone-Iodine *on page 756*
- **Betadine® First Aid Antibiotics + Moisturizer [OTC]** *see* Bacitracin and Polymyxin B *on page 90*
- **Betagan® [OTC]** *see* Povidone-Iodine *on page 756*
- **Betagan® Liquifilm®** *see* Levobunolol *on page 519*
- **Betaloc®** *see* Metoprolol *on page 595*
- **Betaloc® Durules®** *see* Metoprolol *on page 595*

Betamethasone (bay ta METH a sone)

Pharmacologic Class Corticosteroid, Oral; Corticosteroid, Parenteral; Corticosteroid, Topical

U.S. Brand Names Alphatrex®; Betatrex®; Beta-Val®; Celestone®; Celestone® Soluspan®; Cel-U-Jec®; Diprolene®; Diprolene® AF; Diprosone®; Luxiq™; Maxivate®; Psorion® Cream; Teladar®; Valisone®

Generic Available Yes

Mechanism of Action Controls the rate of protein synthesis, depresses the migration of polymorphonuclear leukocytes, fibroblasts, reverses capillary permeability, and lysosomal stabilization at the cellular level to prevent or control inflammation

(Continued)

Betamethasone *(Continued)*

Use Inflammatory dermatoses such as seborrheic or atopic dermatitis, neurodermatitis, anogenital pruritus, psoriasis, inflammatory phase of xerosis

USUAL DOSAGE Base dosage on severity of disease and patient response

Children: Use lowest dose listed as initial dose for adrenocortical insufficiency (physiologic replacement)

I.M.: 0.0175-0.125 mg base/kg/day divided every 6-12 hours **or** 0.5-7.5 mg base/m²/day divided every 6-12 hours

Oral: 0.0175-0.25 mg/kg/day divided every 6-8 hours **or** 0.5-7.5 mg/m²/day divided every 6-8 hours

Adolescents and Adults:

Oral: 2.4-4.8 mg/day in 2-4 doses; range: 0.6-7.2 mg/day

I.M.: Betamethasone sodium phosphate and betamethasone acetate: 0.6-9 mg/day (generally, 1/3 to 1/2 of oral dose) divided every 12-24 hours

Foam: Apply twice daily, once in the morning and once at night

Dosing adjustment in hepatic impairment: Adjustments may be necessary in patients with liver failure because betamethasone is extensively metabolized in the liver

Intrabursal, intra-articular, intradermal: 0.25-2 mL

Intralesional: Rheumatoid arthritis/osteoarthritis:

Very large joints: 1-2 mL

Large joints: 1 mL

Medium joints: 0.5-1 mL

Small joints: 0.25-0.5 mL

Topical: Apply thin film 2-4 times/day. Therapy should be discontinued when control is achieved; if no improvement is seen, reassessment of diagnosis may be necessary.

Dosage Forms

Betamethasone base (Celestone®), Oral: **SYR:** 0.6 mg/5 mL (118 mL). **TAB:** 0.6 mg

Betamethasone dipropionate (Diprosone®): **AERO:** 0.1% (85 g). **CRM:** 0.05% (15 g, 45 g). **LOT:** 0.05% (20 mL, 30 mL, 60 mL). **OINT:** 0.05% (15 g, 45 g)

Betamethasone dipropionate augmented (Diprolene®): **CRM:** 0.05% (15 g, 45 g). **GEL:** 0.05% (15 g, 45 g). **LOT:** 0.05% (30 mL, 60 mL). **OINT, top:** 0.05% (15 g, 45 g)

Betamethasone valerate (Betatrex®, Valisone®): **CRM:** 0.01% (15 g, 60 g); 0.1% (15 g, 45 g, 110 g, 430 g). **LOT:** 0.1% (20 mL, 60 mL). **OINT:** 0.1% (15 g, 45 g). (Beta-Val®): **CRM:** 0.01% (15 g, 60 g), 0.1% (15 g, 45 g, 110 g, 430 g); **LOT:** 0.1% (20 mL, 60 mL). (Luxiq™): **FOAM:** 100 g aluminum can (box of 1)

INJ: Sodium phosphate (Celestone® Phosphate, Cel-U-Jec®): 4 mg betamethasone phosphate/mL (equivalent to 3 mg betamethasone/mL) (5 mL) **INJ, susp:** Sodium phosphate and acetate (Celestone® Soluspan®): 6 mg/mL (3 mg of betamethasone sodium phosphate and 3 mg of betamethasone acetate per mL) (5 mL)

Contraindications Systemic fungal infections; hypersensitivity to betamethasone or any component

Warnings/Precautions Fatalities have occurred due to adrenal insufficiency in asthmatic patients during and after transfer from systemic corticosteroids to aerosol steroids; several months may be required for recovery of this syndrome; during this period, aerosol steroids do **not** provide the systemic steroid needed to treat patients having trauma, surgery, or infections; use with caution in patients with hypothyroidism, cirrhosis, ulcerative colitis; do not use occlusive dressings on weeping or exudative lesions and general caution with occlusive dressings should be observed; discontinue if skin irritation or contact dermatitis should occur; do not use in patients with decreased skin circulation

Pregnancy Risk Factor C

Pregnancy Implications Clinical effects on the fetus: There are no reports linking the use of betamethasone with congenital defects in the literature; betamethasone is often used in patients with premature labor [26-34 weeks gestation] to stimulate fetal lung maturation

Adverse Reactions

>10%:

Central nervous system: Insomnia

Gastrointestinal: Increased appetite, indigestion

Ocular: Temporary mild blurred vision

1% to 10%:

Dermatologic: Erythema, itching

Endocrine & metabolic: Diabetes mellitus

Local: Dryness, irritation, papular rashes, burning

Ocular: Cataracts

<1%: Acneiform eruptions, confusion, convulsions, cushingoid state, glaucoma, headache, hyperpigmentation or hypertrichosis, hypertension, hypopigmentation, impaired wound healing, maceration of skin, miliaria, myalgia, osteoporosis, peptic ulcer, perioral dermatitis, skin atrophy, sodium retention, sterile abscess, striae, sudden blindness, thin fragile skin, vertigo

Drug Interactions CYP3A enzyme substrate

Decreased effect (corticosteroid) by barbiturates, phenytoin, rifampin

Alcohol Interactions Avoid use (may enhance gastric mucosal irritation)

Half-Life 6.5 hours

Education and Monitoring Issues

Patient Education: Take exactly as directed; do not increase dose or discontinue abruptly, consult prescriber. Take oral medication with or after meals. Limit intake of caffeine or stimulants. Prescriber may recommend increased dietary vitamins, minerals, or iron. Diabetics should monitor glucose levels closely (antidiabetic medication may need to be adjusted). Inform prescriber if you are experiencing greater than normal levels of stress (medication may need adjustment). Some forms of this medication may cause GI upset (oral medication may be taken with meals to reduce GI upset; small frequent meals and frequent mouth care may reduce GI upset). You may be more susceptible to infection (avoid crowds and persons with contagious or infective conditions). Report promptly excessive nervousness or sleep disturbances; signs of infection (sore throat, unhealed injuries); excessive growth of body hair or loss of skin color; changes in vision; excessive or sudden weight gain (>3 lb/week); swelling of face or extremities; difficulty breathing; muscle weakness; change in color of stools (tarry) or persistent abdominal pain; or worsening of condition or failure to improve.

Topical: For external use only, Not for eyes or mucous membranes or open wounds. Apply in a thin layer (may rub in lightly). Apply light dressing (if necessary) to area being treated. Do not use occlusive dressing unless so advised by prescriber. Avoid prolonged or excessive use around sensitive tissues, genital, or rectal areas. Inform prescriber if condition worsens (redness, swelling, irritation, open sores) or fails to improve.

Manufacturer Schering-Plough Corp

Related Information

Betamethasone and Clotrimazole *on page 105*
Corticosteroids Comparison *on page 1237*
Pharmaceutical Manufacturers Directory *on page 1020*

Betamethasone and Clotrimazole

(bay ta METH a sone & kloe TRIM a zole)

Pharmacologic Class Antifungal Agent, Topical

U.S. Brand Names Lotrisone®

Dosage Forms CRM: Betamethasone dipropionate 0.05% and clotrimazole 1% (15 g, 45 g)

Pregnancy Risk Factor C

♦ **Betapace®** *see* Sotalol *on page 863*
♦ **Betapace AF®** *see* Sotalol *on page 863*
♦ **Betapen®-VK** *see* Penicillin V Potassium *on page 713*
♦ **Betasept® [OTC]** *see* Chlorhexidine Gluconate *on page 181*
♦ **Betaseron®** *see* Interferon Beta-1b *on page 480*
♦ **Betatrex®** *see* Betamethasone *on page 103*
♦ **Beta-Val®** *see* Betamethasone *on page 103*
♦ **Betaxin®** *see* Thiamine *on page 911*

Betaxolol (be TAKS oh lol)

Pharmacologic Class Beta Blocker, Beta$_1$ Selective; Ophthalmic Agent, Antiglaucoma

U.S. Brand Names Betoptic® Ophthalmic; Betoptic® S Ophthalmic; Kerlone® Oral

Generic Available No

Mechanism of Action Competitively blocks beta$_1$-receptors, with little or no effect on beta$_2$-receptors; ophthalmic reduces intraocular pressure by reducing the production of aqueous humor

Use Treatment of chronic open-angle glaucoma and ocular hypertension; management of hypertension

USUAL DOSAGE Adults:

Ophthalmic: Instill 1 drop twice daily

Oral: 10 mg/day; may increase dose to 20 mg/day after 7-14 days if desired response is not achieved; initial dose in elderly patients: 5 mg/day

Dosage Forms SOLN, ophth (Betoptic®): 0.5% (2.5 mL, 5 mL, 10 mL). **SUSP, ophth** (Betoptic® S): 0.25% (2.5 mL, 10 mL, 15 mL). **TAB** (Kerlone®): 10 mg, 20 mg

Contraindications Bronchial asthma, sinus bradycardia, second and third degree A-V block, cardiac failure (unless a functioning pacemaker present), cardiogenic shock, hypersensitivity to betaxolol or any component

Warnings/Precautions Some products contain sulfites which can cause allergic reactions; diminished response occurs over time; use with caution in patients with decreased renal or hepatic function (dosage adjustment required); patients with a history of asthma, congestive heart failure, diabetes mellitus, or bradycardia appear to be at a higher risk for adverse effects

Pregnancy Risk Factor C (per manufacturer); D (2nd and 3rd trimesters, based on expert analysis)

Adverse Reactions

1% to 10%:

Cardiovascular: Bradycardia, palpitations, edema, congestive heart failure

Central nervous system: Dizziness, fatigue, lethargy, headache

(Continued)

Betaxolol *(Continued)*

Dermatologic: Erythema, itching

Ocular: Mild ocular stinging and discomfort, tearing, photophobia, decreased corneal sensitivity, keratitis

Miscellaneous: Cold extremities

<1%: Chest pain, depression, hallucinations, nervousness, thrombocytopenia

Drug Interactions CYP1A2 and 2D6 enzyme substrate

Alpha-blockers (prazosin, terazosin): Concurrent use of beta-blockers may increase risk of orthostasis

Clonidine; Hypertensive crisis after or during withdrawal of either agent

Drugs which slow A-V conduction (digoxin): Effects may be additive with beta-blockers

Glucagon: Betaxolol may blunt the hyperglycemic action of glucagon

Insulin and oral hypoglycemics: May mask tachycardia from hypoglycemia

NSAIDs (ibuprofen, indomethacin, naproxen, piroxicam) may reduce the antihypertensive effects of beta-blockers

Salicylates may reduce the antihypertensive effects of beta-blockers

Sulfonylureas: Beta-blockers may alter response to hypoglycemic agents

Verapamil or diltiazem may have synergistic or additive pharmacological effects when taken concurrently with beta-blockers

Alcohol Interactions Limit use (may increase risk of hypotension or dizziness)

Onset Ophthalmic: 30 minutes; Oral: 1-1.5 hours

Duration Ophthalmic: 12 hours

Half-Life Oral: 12-22 hours

Education and Monitoring Issues

Patient Education: Oral: Use as directed; do not increase dose unless directed by prescriber. You may experience dizziness or blurred vision (use caution when driving engaging in tasks requiring alertness until response to drug is known); nausea or vomiting (small frequent meals, frequent mouth care, sucking lozenges, or chewing gum may help). Report persistent GI response (nausea, vomiting, diarrhea, or constipation); chest pain or palpitations; unusual cough, difficulty breathing, swelling or coolness of extremities; or unusual mental depression.

Monitoring Parameters: Ophthalmic: Intraocular pressure. Systemic: Blood pressure, pulse

Related Information

Beta-Blockers Comparison *on page 1233*

♦ **Betaxon®** *see* Levobetaxolol *on page 518*

Bethanechol (be THAN e kole)

Pharmacologic Class Cholinergic Agonist

U.S. Brand Names Duvoid®; Myotonachol™; Urabeth®; Urecholine®

Generic Available Yes: Tablet

Mechanism of Action Stimulates cholinergic receptors in the smooth muscle of the urinary bladder and gastrointestinal tract resulting in increased peristalsis, increased GI and pancreatic secretions, bladder muscle contraction, and increased ureteral peristaltic waves

Use Nonobstructive urinary retention and retention due to neurogenic bladder; treatment and prevention of bladder dysfunction caused by phenothiazines; diagnosis of flaccid or atonic neurogenic bladder; gastroesophageal reflux

USUAL DOSAGE

Children:

Oral:

Abdominal distention or urinary retention: 0.6 mg/kg/day divided 3-4 times/day

Gastroesophageal reflux: 0.1-0.2 mg/kg/dose given 30 minutes to 1 hour before each meal to a maximum of 4 times/day

S.C.: 0.15-0.2 mg/kg/day divided 3-4 times/day

Adults:

Oral: 10-50 mg 2-4 times/day

S.C.: 2.5-5 mg 3-4 times/day, up to 7.5-10 mg every 4 hours for neurogenic bladder

Dosage Forms INJ: 5 mg/mL (1 mL). **TAB:** 5 mg, 10 mg, 25 mg, 50 mg

Contraindications Hypersensitivity to bethanechol; do not use in patients with mechanical obstruction of the GI or GU tract or when the strength or integrity of the GI or bladder wall is in question. It is also contraindicated in patients with hyperthyroidism, peptic ulcer disease, epilepsy, obstructive pulmonary disease, bradycardia, vasomotor instability, atrioventricular conduction defects, hypotension, or parkinsonism; **contraindicated for I.M. or I.V. use due to a likely severe cholinergic reaction**

Warnings/Precautions Potential for reflux infection if the sphincter fails to relax as bethanechol contracts the bladder; use with caution when administering to nursing women, as it is unknown if the drug is excreted in breast milk; safety and efficacy in children <5 years of age have not been established; syringe containing atropine should be readily available for treatment of serious side effects; for S.C. injection only; do not administer I.M. or I.V.

Pregnancy Risk Factor C

Adverse Reactions
Oral: <1%: Hypotension, cardiac arrest, flushed skin, abdominal cramps, diarrhea, nausea, vomiting, salivation, bronchial constriction, diaphoresis, vasomotor response
Subcutaneous: 1% to 10%:
Cardiovascular: Hypotension, cardiac arrest, flushed skin
Gastrointestinal: Abdominal cramps, diarrhea, nausea, vomiting, salivation
Respiratory: Bronchial constriction
Miscellaneous: Diaphoresis, vasomotor response

Drug Interactions
Decreased effect: Procainamide, quinidine
Increased toxicity: Bethanechol and ganglionic blockers → critical fall in blood pressure; cholinergic drugs or anticholinesterase agents

Onset Oral: 30-90 minutes; S.C.: 5-15 minutes

Duration Oral: Up to 6 hours; S.C.: 2 hours

Education and Monitoring Issues
Patient Education: Oral: Take as directed, on an empty stomach to avoid nausea or vomiting. Do not discontinue without consulting prescriber. Maintain adequate hydration (2-3 L/day of fluids unless instructed to restrict fluid intake). May cause dizziness or hypotension (rise slowly from sitting or lying position and use caution when driving or climbing stairs); vomiting or loss of appetite (frequent small meals, frequent mouth care, sucking lozenges, or chewing gum may help). Report persistent abdominal discomfort; significantly increased salivation, sweating, tearing, or urination; flushed skin; chest pain or palpitations; acute headache; unresolved diarrhea; excessive fatigue, insomnia, dizziness, or depression; increased muscle, joint, or body pain; vision changes or blurred vision; or respiratory difficulty or wheezing.
Monitoring Parameters: Observe closely for side effects

- **Betimol® Ophthalmic** *see* Timolol *on page 922*
- **Betnesol® [Disodium Phosphate]** *see* Betamethasone *on page 103*
- **Betoptic® Ophthalmic** *see* Betaxolol *on page 105*
- **Betoptic® S Ophthalmic** *see* Betaxolol *on page 105*
- **Bewon®** *see* Thiamine *on page 911*
- **Bexophene®** *see* Propoxyphene and Aspirin *on page 786*
- **Biaxin™** *see* Clarithromycin *on page 206*
- **Biaxin™ XL** *see* Clarithromycin *on page 206*

Bicalutamide (bye ka LOO ta mide)

Pharmacologic Class Androgen

U.S. Brand Names Casodex®

Mechanism of Action Pure nonsteroidal antiandrogen that binds to androgen receptors; specifically a competitive inhibitor for the binding of dihydrotestosterone and testosterone; prevents testosterone stimulation of cell growth in prostate cancer

Use In combination therapy with LHRH agonist analogues in treatment of advanced prostatic carcinoma

USUAL DOSAGE Adults: Oral: 50 mg once daily (morning or evening), with or without food. It is recommended that bicalutamide be taken at the same time each day; start treatment with bicalutamide at the same time as treatment with an LHRH analog.
Dosage adjustment in renal impairment: None necessary as renal impairment has no significant effect on elimination
Dosage adjustment in liver impairment: Limited data in subjects with severe hepatic impairment suggest that excretion of bicalutamide may be delayed and could lead to further accumulation. Use with caution in patients with moderate to severe hepatic impairment.

Dosage Forms TAB: 50 mg

Contraindications Known hypersensitivity to drug or any components of the product; pregnancy

Pregnancy Risk Factor X

Adverse Reactions
>10%: Endocrine & metabolic: Hot flashes (49%)
≥2% to <5%:
Cardiovascular: Angina pectoris, congestive heart failure, edema
Central nervous system: Anxiety, depression, confusion, somnolence, nervousness, fever, chills
Dermatologic: Dry skin, pruritus, alopecia
Endocrine & metabolic: Breast pain, diabetes mellitus, decreased libido, dehydration, gout
Gastrointestinal: Anorexia, dyspepsia, rectal hemorrhage, xerostomia, melena, weight gain
Genitourinary: Polyuria, urinary impairment, dysuria, urinary retention, urinary urgency
Hepatic: Alkaline phosphatase increased
Neuromuscular & skeletal: Myasthenia, arthritis, myalgia, leg cramps, pathological fracture, neck pain, hypertonia, neuropathy
Renal: Creatinine increased
(Continued)

Bicalutamide *(Continued)*

Respiratory: Cough increased, pharyngitis, bronchitis, pneumonia, rhinitis, lung disorder

Miscellaneous: Sepsis, neoplasma

<1%: Diarrhea (0.5%)

Half-Life Active enantiomer is 5.8 days

Education and Monitoring Issues

Patient Education: Take as directed and do not alter dose or discontinue without consulting prescriber. Take at the same time each day with or without food. Void before taking medication. Diabetics should monitor serum glucose closely and notify prescriber of changes. You may lose your hair and experience impotency. May cause dizziness, confusion, or drowsiness (use caution when driving or engaging in tasks that require alertness until response to drug is known); nausea or vomiting (small frequent meals, frequent mouth care, sucking lozenges, or chewing gum may help); or constipation (increased dietary fiber, fruit, or fluid and increased exercise may help). Report easy bruising or bleeding; yellowing of skin or eyes; change in color of urine or stool; unresolved changes in CNS (nervousness, chills, insomnia, somnolence); skin rash, redness, or irritation; chest pain or palpitations; difficulty breathing; urinary retention or inability to void; muscle weakness, tremors, or pain; persistent nausea, vomiting, diarrhea, or constipation; or other unusual signs or adverse reactions.

Monitoring Parameters: Serum prostate-specific antigen, alkaline phosphatase, acid phosphatase, or prostatic acid phosphatase; prostate gland dimensions; skeletal survey; liver scans; chest x-rays; physical exam every 3 months; bone scan every 3-6 months; CBC, LFTs, EKG, echocardiograms, and serum testosterone and luteinizing hormone (periodically)

Manufacturer AstraZeneca

Related Information

Pharmaceutical Manufacturers Directory *on page 1020*

- **Bicillin® C-R** *see* Penicillin G Benzathine and Procaine Combined *on page 710*
- **Bicillin® C-R 900/300** *see* Penicillin G Benzathine and Procaine Combined *on page 710*
- **Bicillin® L-A** *see* Penicillin G Benzathine, Parenteral *on page 710*
- **Bicitra®** *see* Sodium Citrate and Citric Acid *on page 859*
- **Biltricide®** *see* Praziquantel *on page 759*
- **Biocal** *see* Calcium Carbonate *on page 130*
- **Biocef** *see* Cephalexin *on page 169*
- **Bioderm®** *see* Bacitracin and Polymyxin B *on page 90*
- **Biodine [OTC]** *see* Povidone-Iodine *on page 756*
- **Biohist®-LA** *see* Carbinoxamine and Pseudoephedrine *on page 140*
- **Biolon** *see* Sodium Hyaluronate *on page 859*
- **Biomox®** *see* Amoxicillin *on page 56*
- **Bio-Tab® Oral** *see* Doxycycline *on page 300*
- **Biozyme-C®** *see* Collagenase *on page 227*
- **Biquin** *see* Quinidine *on page 802*
- **Bismatrol® [OTC]** *see* Bismuth *on page 108*

Bismuth (BIZ muth)

Pharmacologic Class Antidiarrheal

U.S. Brand Names Bismatrol® [OTC]; Devrom® [OTC]; Pepto-Bismol® [OTC]; Pink Bismuth® [OTC]

Generic Available Yes

Mechanism of Action Bismuth subsalicylate exhibits both antisecretory and antimicrobial action. This agent may provide some anti-inflammatory action as well. The salicylate moiety provides antisecretory effect and the bismuth exhibits antimicrobial directly against bacterial and viral gastrointestinal pathogens. Bismuth has some antacid properties.

Use Symptomatic treatment of mild, nonspecific diarrhea; indigestion, nausea, control of traveler's diarrhea (enterotoxigenic *Escherichia coli*); an adjunct with other agents such as metronidazole, tetracycline, and an H_2-antagonist in the treatment of *Helicobacter pylori*-associated duodenal ulcer disease

USUAL DOSAGE Oral:

Nonspecific diarrhea: Subsalicylate:

Children: Up to 8 doses/24 hours:

3-6 years: $^1/_3$ tablet or 5 mL every 30 minutes to 1 hour as needed

6-9 years: $^2/_3$ tablet or 10 mL every 30 minutes to 1 hour as needed

9-12 years: 1 tablet or 15 mL every 30 minutes to 1 hour as needed

Adults: 2 tablets or 30 mL every 30 minutes to 1 hour as needed up to 8 doses/24 hours

Prevention of traveler's diarrhea: 2.1 g/day or 2 tablets 4 times/day before meals and at bedtime

Subgallate: 1-2 tablets 3 times/day with meals

Helicobacter pylori: Chew 2 tablets 4 times/day with meals and at bedtime with other agents in selected regimen (eg, an H_2-antagonist, tetracycline and metronidazole) for 14 days

Dosing adjustment in renal impairment: Should probably be avoided in patients with renal failure

Dosage Forms LIQ, as subsalicylate (Pepto-Bismol®, Bismatrol®): 262 mg/15 mL (120 mL, 240 mL, 360 mL, 480 mL); 524 mg/15 mL (120 mL, 240 mL, 360 mL). **TAB:** Chewable, as subsalicylate (Pepto-Bismol®, Bismatrol®): 262 mg; Chewable, as subgallate (Devrom®): 200 mg

Contraindications Do not use subsalicylate in patients with influenza or chickenpox because of risk of Reye's syndrome; do not use in patients with known hypersensitivity to salicylates; history of severe GI bleeding; history of coagulopathy

Warnings/Precautions Subsalicylate should be used with caution if patient is taking aspirin; use with caution in children, especially those <3 years of age and those with viral illness; may be neurotoxic with very large doses

Pregnancy Risk Factor C; D (3rd trimester)

Adverse Reactions

>10%: Gastrointestinal: Discoloration of the tongue (darkening), grayish black stools

<1%: Anxiety, confusion, headache, hearing loss, impaction may occur in infants and debilitated patients, mental depression, muscle spasms, slurred speech, tinnitus, weakness

Drug Interactions

Decreased effect: Tetracyclines and uricosurics

Increased toxicity: Aspirin, warfarin, hypoglycemics

Education and Monitoring Issues

Patient Education: Chew tablet well or shake suspension well before using; may darken stools; if diarrhea persists for more than 2 days, consult a prescriber; can turn tongue black; tinnitus may indicate toxicity and use should be discontinued

Related Information

Antimicrobial Drugs of Choice *on page 1182*
Bismuth Subsalicylate, Metronidazole, and Tetracycline *on page 109*
Helicobacter pylori Treatment *on page 1107*

Bismuth Subsalicylate, Metronidazole, and Tetracycline

(BIZ muth sub sa LIS i late, me troe NI da zole, & tet ra SYE kleen)

Pharmacologic Class Antidiarrheal

U.S. Brand Names Helidac™

Use In combination with an H_2 antagonist, used to treat and decrease rate of recurrence of active duodenal ulcer associated with *H. pylori* infection

Dosage Forms CAP: Tetracycline: 500 mg. **TAB:** Bismuth subsalicylate: Chewable: 262.4 mg; Metronidazole: 250 mg

Manufacturer Procter & Gamble Co

Related Information

Pharmaceutical Manufacturers Directory *on page 1020*

Bisoprolol (bis OH proe lol)

Pharmacologic Class Beta Blocker, $Beta_1$ Selective

U.S. Brand Names Zebeta®

Mechanism of Action Selective inhibitor of $beta_1$-adrenergic receptors; competitively blocks $beta_1$-receptors, with little or no effect on $beta_2$-receptors at doses <10 mg

Use Treatment of hypertension, alone or in combination with other agents

Unlabeled use: Angina pectoris, supraventricular arrhythmias, PVCs, NY heart class II/III congestive heart failure

USUAL DOSAGE Oral:

Adults: 5 mg once daily, may be increased to 10 mg, and then up to 20 mg once daily, if necessary

Elderly: Initial dose: 2.5 mg/day; may be increased by 2.5-5 mg/day; maximum recommended dose: 20 mg/day

Dosing adjustment in renal/hepatic impairment: Cl_{cr} <40 mL/minute: Initial: 2.5 mg/day; increase cautiously

Hemodialysis: Not dialyzable

Dosage Forms TAB: 5 mg, 10 mg

Contraindications Hypersensitivity to beta-blocking agents, uncompensated congestive heart failure; cardiogenic shock; bradycardia or heart block; sinus node dysfunction; A-V conduction abnormalities. Although bisoprolol primarily blocks $beta_1$-receptors, high doses can result in $beta_2$-receptor blockage. Therefore, use with caution in patients (especially elderly) with bronchospastic lung disease and renal dysfunction.

Warnings/Precautions Use with caution in patients with inadequate myocardial function, bronchospastic disease, hyperthyroidism, undergoing anesthesia; and in those with impaired hepatic function; acute withdrawal may exacerbate symptoms (gradually taper over a 2-week period)

Pregnancy Risk Factor C (per manufacturer); D (2nd and 3rd trimesters, based on expert analysis)

(Continued)

Bisoprolol *(Continued)*

Adverse Reactions

>10%: Central nervous system: Fatigue, lethargy

1% to 10%:

Cardiovascular: Hypotension, chest pain, heart failure, Raynaud's phenomenon, heart block, edema, bradycardia

Central nervous system: Headache, dizziness, insomnia, confusion, depression, abnormal dreams

Dermatologic: Rash

Gastrointestinal: Constipation, diarrhea, dyspepsia, nausea, flatulence, anorexia

Genitourinary: Polyuria, impotence, urinary retention

Hepatic: Increased LFTs

Neuromuscular & skeletal: Arthralgia, myalgia

Ocular: Abnormal vision

Respiratory: Dyspnea, rhinitis, cough

Drug Interactions CYP2D6 enzyme substrate

Alpha-blockers (prazosin, terazosin): Concurrent use of beta-blockers may increase risk of orthostasis

Clonidine: Hypertensive crisis after or during withdrawal of either agent

Drugs which slow A-V conduction (digoxin): Effects may be additive with beta-blockers

Glucagon: Bisoprolol may blunt the hyperglycemic action of glucagon

Insulin: Bisoprolol may mask tachycardia from hypoglycemia

NSAIDs (ibuprofen, indomethacin, naproxen, piroxicam) may reduce the antihypertensive effects of beta-blockers

Salicylates may reduce the antihypertensive effects of beta-blockers

Sulfonylureas: Beta-blockers may alter response to hypoglycemic agents

Onset 1-2 hours

Half-Life 9-12 hours

Education and Monitoring Issues

Patient Education: Take exactly as directed. Do not increase, decrease, or adjust dosage without consulting prescriber. Do not take with antacids and do not use alcohol or OTC medications (eg, cold remedies) without consulting prescriber. If diabetic, monitor serum sugars closely (may alter glucose tolerance or mask signs of hypoglycemia). May cause fatigue, dizziness, or postural hypotension; use caution when changing position from lying or sitting to standing, or when driving or climbing stairs until response to medication is known. May cause alteration in sexual performance (reversible). Report palpitations, unresolved swelling of extremities, difficulty breathing or new cough, unresolved fatigue, unusual weight gain, unresolved constipation, or unusual muscle weakness.

Monitoring Parameters: Blood pressure, EKG, neurologic status

Manufacturer Lederle Laboratories

Related Information

Beta-Blockers Comparison *on page 1233*

Bisoprolol and Hydrochlorothiazide *on page 110*

Pharmaceutical Manufacturers Directory *on page 1020*

Bisoprolol and Hydrochlorothiazide

(bis OH proe lol & hye droe klor oh THYE a zide)

Pharmacologic Class Antihypertensive Agent, Combination

U.S. Brand Names Ziac™

Dosage Forms TAB: Bisoprolol fumarate 2.5 mg and hydrochlorothiazide 6.25 mg; Bisoprolol fumarate 5 mg and hydrochlorothiazide 6.25 mg; Bisoprolol fumarate 10 mg and hydrochlorothiazide 6.25 mg

Pregnancy Risk Factor C; D (2nd and 3rd trimesters)

Manufacturer Lederle Laboratories

Related Information

Pharmaceutical Manufacturers Directory *on page 1020*

Bitolterol (bye TOLE ter ole)

Pharmacologic Class $Beta_2$ Agonist

U.S. Brand Names Tornalate®

Generic Available No

Mechanism of Action Selectively stimulates $beta_2$-adrenergic receptors in the lungs producing bronchial smooth muscle relaxation; minor $beta_1$ activity

Use Prevention and treatment of bronchial asthma and bronchospasm

USUAL DOSAGE Children >12 years and Adults:

Bronchospasm: 2 inhalations at an interval of at least 1-3 minutes, followed by a third inhalation if needed

Prevention of bronchospasm: 2 inhalations every 8 hours; do not exceed 3 inhalations every 6 hours or 2 inhalations every 4 hours

Dosage Forms AERO, oral: 0.8% [370 mcg/metered spray, 300 inhalations] (15 mL). **SOLN, inh:** 0.2% (10 mL, 30 mL, 60 mL)

Contraindications Known hypersensitivity to bitolterol

Warnings/Precautions Use with caution in patients with unstable vasomotor symptoms, diabetes, hyperthyroidism, prostatic hypertrophy or a history of seizures; also use caution in the elderly and those patients with cardiovascular disorders such as coronary artery disease, arrhythmias, and hypertension; excessive use may result in cardiac arrest and death; do not use concurrently with other sympathomimetic bronchodilators

Pregnancy Risk Factor C

Adverse Reactions

>10%: Neuromuscular & skeletal: Trembling

1% to 10%:

Cardiovascular: Flushing of face, hypertension, pounding heartbeat
Central nervous system: Dizziness, lightheadedness, nervousness
Gastrointestinal: Xerostomia, nausea, unpleasant taste
Respiratory: Bronchial irritation, coughing

<1%: Arrhythmias, chest pain, insomnia, paradoxical bronchospasm, tachycardia

Drug Interactions

Decreased effect: Beta-adrenergic blockers (eg, propranolol)

Increased effect: Inhaled ipratropium may increase duration of bronchodilation, nifedipine may increase FEV-1

Increased toxicity: MAO inhibitors, tricyclic antidepressants, sympathomimetic agents (eg, amphetamine, dopamine, dobutamine), inhaled anesthetics (eg, enflurane)

Onset Rapid

Duration 4-8 hours

Half-Life 3 hours

Education and Monitoring Issues

Patient Education: Use exactly as directed. Do not use more often than recommended. Maintain adequate hydration (2-3 L/day of fluids unless instructed to restrict fluid intake). You may experience nervousness, dizziness, or fatigue (use caution when driving or engaging in tasks requiring alertness until response to drug is known); or dry mouth, stomach upset (frequent small meals, frequent mouth care, chewing gum, or sucking hard candy may help). Report unresolved GI upset; dizziness or fatigue; vision changes; chest pain, rapid heartbeat, or palpitations; nervousness or insomnia; muscle cramping or tremor; or unusual cough.

Monitoring Parameters: Assess lung sounds, pulse, and blood pressure before administration and during peak of medication; observe patient for wheezing after administration

Manufacturer Dura Pharmaceuticals

Related Information

Bronchodilators Comparison *on page 1235*
Pharmaceutical Manufacturers Directory *on page 1020*

♦ **Bleph®-10 Liquifilm** *see* Sulfacetamide Sodium *on page 876*
♦ **Bleph®-10 Ophthalmic** *see* Sulfacetamide Sodium *on page 876*
♦ **Blephamide®** *see* Sulfacetamide Sodium and Prednisolone *on page 876*
♦ **Blephamide® Ophthalmic** *see* Sulfacetamide Sodium and Prednisolone *on page 876*
♦ **Blis-To-Sol® [OTC]** *see* Tolnaftate *on page 931*
♦ **Blocadren® Oral** *see* Timolol *on page 922*
♦ **Body Surface Area of Adults and Children** *see page 1037*
♦ **Bonamine** *see* Meclizine *on page 556*
♦ **Bonine® [OTC]** *see* Meclizine *on page 556*
♦ **B&O Supprettes®** *see* Belladonna and Opium *on page 96*
♦ **Botox®** *see* Botulinum Toxin Type A *on page 111*

Botulinum Toxin Type A (BOT yoo lin num TOKS in type aye)

Pharmacologic Class Ophthalmic Agent, Toxin

U.S. Brand Names Botox®

Use Treatment of strabismus and blepharospasm associated with dystonia (including benign essential blepharospasm or VII nerve disorders in patients ≥12 years of age)

Unlabeled use: Treatment of hemifacial spasms, spasmodic torticollis (ie, cervical dystonia, clonic twisting of the head), oromandibular dystonia, spasmodic dysphonia (laryngeal dystonia) and other dystonias (ie, writer's cramp, focal task-specific dystonias)

Orphan drug: Treatment of dynamic muscle contracture in pediatric cerebral palsy patients

USUAL DOSAGE

Strabismus: 1.25-5 units (0.05-0.15 mL) injected into any one muscle

Subsequent doses for residual/recurrent strabismus: Re-examine patients 7-14 days after each injection to assess the effect of that dose. Subsequent doses for patients experiencing incomplete paralysis of the target may be increased up to two fold the previously administered dose. Maximum recommended dose as a single injection for any one muscle is 25 units.

Blepharospasm: 1.25-2.5 units (0.05-0.10 mL) injected into the orbicularis oculi muscle

(Continued)

Botulinum Toxin Type A *(Continued)*

Subsequent doses: Each treatment lasts approximately 3 months. At repeat treatment sessions, the dose may be increased up to twofold if the response from the initial treatment is considered insufficient (usually defined as an effect that does not last >2 months). There appears to be little benefit obtainable from injecting >5 units per site. Some tolerance may be found if treatments are given any more frequently than every 3 months.

The cumulative dose should not exceed 200 units in a 30-day period

Contraindications Hypersensitivity to botulinum A toxin; relative contraindications to botulinum toxin therapy include diseases of neuromuscular transmission and coagulopathy, including anticoagulant therapy; injections into the central area of the upper eyelid (rapid diffusion of toxin into the levator can occur resulting in a marked ptosis).

Pregnancy Risk Factor C

- **Breathe Free® [OTC]** *see* Sodium Chloride *on page 858*
- **Breezee® Mist Antifungal [OTC]** *see* Miconazole *on page 600*
- **Breezee® Mist Antifungal [OTC]** *see* Tolnaftate *on page 931*
- **Breonesin® [OTC]** *see* Guaifenesin *on page 423*
- **Brethaire® Inhalation Aerosol** *see* Terbutaline *on page 897*
- **Brethine® Injection** *see* Terbutaline *on page 897*
- **Brethine® Oral** *see* Terbutaline *on page 897*
- **Brevicon®** *see* Ethinyl Estradiol and Norethindrone *on page 342*
- **Bricanyl® Injection** *see* Terbutaline *on page 897*
- **Bricanyl® Oral** *see* Terbutaline *on page 897*

Brimonidine (bri MOE ni deen)

Pharmacologic Class $Alpha_2$ Agonist, Ophthalmic

U.S. Brand Names Alphagan®

Mechanism of Action Selective for $alpha_2$-receptors; appears to result in reduction of aqueous humor formation and increase uveoscleral outflow

Use Lowering of intraocular pressure in patients with open-angle glaucoma or ocular hypertension

USUAL DOSAGE Adults: Ophthalmic: Instill 1 drop in affected eye(s) 3 times/day (approximately every 8 hours)

Dosage Forms SOLN, ophth: 0.2% (5 mL, 10 mL)

Contraindications Known hypersensitivity to brimonidine tartrate or any component of this medication; patients receiving monoamine oxidase (MAO) inhibitor therapy

Warnings/Precautions Exercise caution in treating patients with severe cardiovascular disease. Use with caution in patients with depression, cerebral or coronary insufficiency, Raynaud's phenomenon, orthostatic hypotension or thromboangiitis obliterans.

The preservative in brimonidine tartrate, benzalkonium chloride, may be absorbed by soft contact lenses; instruct patients wearing soft contact lenses to wait at least 15 minutes after instilling brimonidine tartrate to insert soft contact lenses

Use with caution in patients with hepatic or renal impairment

Loss of effect in some patients may occur. The IOP-lowering efficacy observed with brimonidine tartrate during the first of month of therapy may not always reflect the long term-level of IOP reduction. Routinely monitor IOP.

Agitation, apnea, bradycardia, convulsions, cyanosis, depression, dyspnea, emotional instability, hypotension, hypothermia, hypotonia, hypoventilation, irritability, lethargy, somnolence, and stupor have been reported in pediatric patients - safety and effectiveness have not been established in pediatric patients.

Pregnancy Risk Factor B

Adverse Reactions

>10%:

Central nervous system: Headache, fatigue/drowsiness

Gastrointestinal: Xerostomia

Ocular: Ocular hyperemia, burning and stinging, blurring, foreign body sensation, conjunctival follicles, ocular allergic reactions and ocular pruritus

1% to 10%:

Central nervous system: Dizziness

Ocular: Corneal staining/erosion, photophobia, eyelid erythema, ocular ache/pain, ocular dryness, tearing, eyelid edema, conjunctival edema, blepharitis, ocular irritation, conjunctival blanching, abnormal vision, lid crusting, conjunctival hemorrhage, abnormal taste, conjunctival discharge

Respiratory: Upper respiratory symptoms

<1%: Allergic response, some systemic effects have also been reported including GI, CNS, and cardiovascular symptoms (arrhythmias)

Drug Interactions
Increased effect:
CNS depressants (eg, alcohol, barbiturates, opiates, sedatives, anesthetics): Additive or potentiating effect
Topical beta-blockers, pilocarpine → additive decreased intraocular pressure, antihypertensives, cardiac glycosides
Decreased effect: Tricyclic antidepressants can affect the metabolism and uptake of circulating amines

Onset 1-4 hours

Duration 12 hours

Education and Monitoring Issues
Patient Education: Do not touch dropper to the eyes or face
Monitoring Parameters: Closely monitor patients who develop fatigue or drowsiness

Brinzolamide (brin ZOH la mide)

Pharmacologic Class Carbonic Anhydrase Inhibitor

U.S. Brand Names Azopt™

Use Lowers intraocular pressure to treat glaucoma in patients with ocular hypertension or open-angle glaucoma

USUAL DOSAGE Adults: Ophthalmic: Instill 1 drop in affected eye(s) 3 times/day

Contraindications Hypersensitivity to brinzolamide or any component

Pregnancy Risk Factor C

♦ **Brioschi** *see* Sodium Bicarbonate *on page 856*
♦ **Bromanate® DC** *see* Brompheniramine, Phenylpropanolamine, and Codeine *on page 114*
♦ **Bromanyl® Cough Syrup** *see* Bromodiphenhydramine and Codeine *on page 114*

Bromocriptine (broe moe KRIP teen)

Pharmacologic Class Anti-Parkinson's Agent (Dopamine Agonist); Ergot Derivative

U.S. Brand Names Parlodel®

Generic Available No

Mechanism of Action Semisynthetic ergot alkaloid derivative with dopaminergic properties; inhibits prolactin secretion and can improve symptoms of Parkinson's disease by directly stimulating dopamine receptors in the corpus stratum

Use
Usually used with levodopa or levodopa/carbidopa to treat Parkinson's disease - treatment of parkinsonism in patients unresponsive or allergic to levodopa
Prolactin-secreting pituitary adenomas
Acromegaly
Amenorrhea/galactorrhea secondary to hyperprolactinemia in the absence of primary tumor
The indication for prevention of postpartum lactation has been withdrawn voluntarily by Sandoz Pharmaceuticals Corporation

USUAL DOSAGE Oral:
Children 11-15 years: Prolactin-secreting adenomas: 1.25-2.5 mg/day; daily range: 2.5-10 mg
Adults:
Parkinsonism: 1.25 mg 2 times/day, increased by 2.5 mg/day in 2- to 4-week intervals (usual dose range is 30-90 mg/day in 3 divided doses), though elderly patients can usually be managed on lower doses
Hyperprolactinemia: 2.5 mg 2-3 times/day
Acromegaly: Initial: 1.25-2.5 mg increasing as necessary every 3-7 days; usual dose: 20-30 mg/day
Dosing adjustment in hepatic impairment: No guidelines are available, however, may be necessary

Dosage Forms CAP: 5 mg. **TAB:** 2.5 mg

Contraindications Hypersensitivity to bromocriptine or any component, severe ischemic heart disease or peripheral vascular disorders, pregnancy

Warnings/Precautions Use with caution in patients with impaired renal or hepatic function

Pregnancy Risk Factor B

Adverse Reactions Incidence of adverse effects is high, especially at beginning of treatment and with dosages >20 mg/day

1% to 10%:
Cardiovascular: Hypotension, Raynaud's phenomenon
Central nervous system: Mental depression, confusion, hallucinations
Gastrointestinal: Nausea, constipation, anorexia
Neuromuscular & skeletal: Leg cramps
Respiratory: Nasal congestion
<1%: Abdominal cramps, dizziness, drowsiness, fatigue, headache, hypertension, insomnia, myocardial infarction, seizures, syncope, vomiting

Drug Interactions CYP3A3/4 enzyme substrate
Decreased effect: Antipsychotics may inhibit bromocriptine's ability to lower prolactin
(Continued)

Bromocriptine *(Continued)*

Increased toxicity: Isometheptene add phenylpropanolamine (and other sympathomimetics) should be avoided in patients receiving bromocriptine; may increase risk of hypertension and seizure

Erythromycin, fluvoxamine, and nefazodone may increase bromocriptine concentrations

Alcohol Interactions Avoid use (may increase gastrointestinal side effects or alcohol intolerance)

Onset Peak serum concentrations: 1-2 hours

Half-Life Half-life (biphasic): Initial: 6-8 hours; Terminal: 50 hours

Education and Monitoring Issues

Patient Education: Take exactly as directed (may be prescribed in conjunction with levodopa/carbidopa); do not change dosage or discontinue without consulting prescriber. Therapeutic effects may take several weeks or months to achieve and you may need frequent monitoring during first weeks of therapy. Take with meals if GI upset occurs, before meals if dry mouth occurs, after eating if drooling or if nausea occurs. Take at the same time each day. Maintain adequate hydration (2-3 L/day of fluids unless instructed to restrict fluid intake); void before taking medication. Do not use alcohol and prescription or OTC sedatives or CNS depressants without consulting prescriber. Urine or perspiration may appear darker. You may experience drowsiness, dizziness, confusion, or vision changes (use caution when driving, climbing stairs, or engaging in tasks requiring alertness until response to drug is known); orthostatic hypotension (use caution when changing position - rising to standing from sitting or lying); constipation (increased exercise, fluids, or dietary fruit and fiber may help); nasal congestion (consult prescriber for appropriate relief); nausea, vomiting, loss of appetite, or stomach discomfort (small frequent meals, frequent mouth care, chewing gum, or sucking lozenges may help). Report unresolved constipation or vomiting; chest pain or irregular heartbeat; acute headache or dizziness; CNS changes (hallucination, loss of memory, seizures, acute headache, nervousness, etc); painful or difficult urination; increased muscle spasticity, rigidity, or involuntary movements; skin rash; or significant worsening of condition.

Monitoring Parameters: Monitor blood pressure closely as well as hepatic, hematopoietic, and cardiovascular function

Related Information

Parkinson's Disease Dosing *on page 1249*

Bromodiphenhydramine and Codeine

(brome oh dye fen HYE dra meen & KOE deen)

Pharmacologic Class Antihistamine/Antitussive

U.S. Brand Names Ambenyl® Cough Syrup; Amgenal® Cough Syrup; Bromanyl® Cough Syrup; Bromotuss® w/Codeine Cough Syrup

Dosage Forms LIQ: Bromodiphenhydramine hydrochloride 12.5 mg and codeine phosphate 10 mg per 5 mL

Pregnancy Risk Factor C

♦ **Bromotuss® w/Codeine Cough Syrup** *see* Bromodiphenhydramine and Codeine *on page 114*

♦ **Bromphen® DC w/Codeine** *see* Brompheniramine, Phenylpropanolamine, and Codeine *on page 114*

Brompheniramine, Phenylpropanolamine, and Codeine

(brome fen IR a meen, fen il proe pa NOLE a meen, & KOE deen)

Pharmacologic Class Antihistamine/Decongestant/Antitussive

U.S. Brand Names Bromanate® DC; Bromphen® DC w/Codeine; Dimetane®-DC; Myphetane DC®; Poly-Histine CS®

Dosage Forms LIQ: Brompheniramine maleate 2 mg, phenylpropanolamine hydrochloride 12.5 mg, and codeine phosphate 10 mg per 5 mL with alcohol 0.95% (480 mL)

Pregnancy Risk Factor C

Alcohol Interactions Avoid use (may increase central nervous system depression)

♦ **Bronalide®** *see* Flunisolide *on page 373*

♦ **Bronchial®** *see* Theophylline and Guaifenesin *on page 906*

♦ **Bronchodilators Comparison** *see page 1235*

♦ **Bronkodyl®** *see* Theophylline Salts *on page 906*

♦ **Bronkometer®** *see* Isoetharine *on page 486*

♦ **Bronkosol®** *see* Isoetharine *on page 486*

♦ **Brontex® Liquid** *see* Guaifenesin and Codeine *on page 424*

♦ **Brontex® Tablet** *see* Guaifenesin and Codeine *on page 424*

♦ **Bucladin®-S Softab®** *see* Buclizine *on page 114*

Buclizine (BYOO kli zeen)

Pharmacologic Class Antihistamine

U.S. Brand Names Bucladin®-S Softab®; Vibazine®

Generic Available Yes

Mechanism of Action Buclizine acts centrally to suppress nausea and vomiting. It is a piperazine antihistamine closely related to cyclizine and meclizine. It also has CNS depressant, anticholinergic, antispasmodic, and local anesthetic effects, and suppresses labyrinthine activity and conduction in vestibular-cerebellar nerve pathways.

Use Prevention and treatment of motion sickness; symptomatic treatment of vertigo

USUAL DOSAGE Adults: Oral:

Motion sickness (prophylaxis): 50 mg 30 minutes prior to traveling; may repeat 50 mg after 4-6 hours

Vertigo: 50 mg twice daily, up to 150 mg/day

Dosage Forms TAB, chewable: 50 mg

Contraindications Known hypersensitivity to buclizine

Warnings/Precautions Product contains tartrazine; use with caution in patients with angle-closure glaucoma, peptic ulcer, urinary tract obstruction, hyperthyroidism; some preparations contain sodium bisulfite; syrup contains alcohol

Pregnancy Risk Factor C

Adverse Reactions

>10%: Central nervous system: Drowsiness

<1%: Blurred vision, dizziness, fatigue, hypotension, insomnia, nausea, palpitations, paradoxical excitement, sedation, tremor, urinary retention, vomiting

Drug Interactions Increased toxicity: CNS depressants, MAO inhibitors, tricyclic antidepressants

Education and Monitoring Issues

Patient Education: Take as directed. Do not increase dose or take more often than recommended. May cause drowsiness; use caution when driving or engaging in tasks that require alertness until response to drug is known. May cause dry mouth; lozenges, gum, or liquids may help. May cause headache or feelings of jitteriness or anxiety; these will go away when drug is discontinued.

Budesonide (byoo DES oh nide)

Pharmacologic Class Corticosteroid, Oral Inhaler; Corticosteroid, Nasal; Corticosteroid, Topical

U.S. Brand Names Pulmicort® Turbuhaler®; Rhinocort®; Rhinocort® Aqua™

Mechanism of Action Controls the rate of protein synthesis, depresses the migration of polymorphonuclear leukocytes, fibroblasts, reverses capillary permeability, and lysosomal stabilization at the cellular level to prevent or control inflammation

Use

Intranasal: Children and Adults: Management of symptoms of seasonal or perennial rhinitis

Oral inhalation: Maintenance and prophylactic treatment of asthma; includes patients who require corticosteroids and those who may benefit from systemic dose reduction/elimination

USUAL DOSAGE

Children <6 years: Not recommended

Aerosol inhalation: Children ≥6 years and Adults:

Rhinocort®: Nasal: Initial: 8 sprays (4 sprays/nostril) per day (256 mcg/day), given as either 2 sprays in each nostril in the morning and evening or as 4 sprays in each nostril in the morning; after symptoms decrease (usually by 3-7 days), reduce dose slowly every 2-4 weeks to the smallest amount needed to control symptoms

Rhinocort® Aqua™: 64 mcg/day as a single 32 mcg spray in each nostril. Some patients who do not achieve adequate control may benefit from increased dosage. A reduced dosage may be effective after initial control is achieved.

Maximum dose: Children <12 years: 129 mcg/day; Adults: 256 mcg/day

Oral inhalation:

Children ≥6 years:

Previous therapy of bronchodilators alone: 200 mcg twice initially which may be increased up to 400 mcg twice daily

Previous therapy of inhaled corticosteroids: 200 mcg twice initially which may be increased up to 400 mcg twice daily

Previous therapy of oral corticosteroids: The highest recommended dose in children is 400 mcg twice daily

Adults:

Previous therapy of bronchodilators alone: 200-400 mcg twice initially which may be increased up to 400 mcg twice daily

Previous therapy of inhaled corticosteroids: 200-400 mcg twice initially which may be increased up to 800 mcg twice daily

Previous therapy of oral corticosteroids: 400-800 mcg twice daily which may be increased up to 800 mcg twice daily

NIH Guidelines (NIH, 1997) (give in divided doses twice daily):

Children:

"Low" dose: 100-200 mcg/day

"Medium" dose: 200-400 mcg/day (1-2 inhalations/day)

"High" dose: >400 mcg/day (>2 inhalation/day)

(Continued)

Budesonide *(Continued)*

Adults:
"Low" dose: 200-400 mcg/day (1-2 inhalations/day)
"Medium" dose: 400-600 mcg/day (2-3 inhalations/day)
"High" dose: >600 mcg/day (>3 inhalation/day)

Dosage Forms AERO: 50 mcg released per actuation to deliver ~32 mcg to patient via nasal adapter [200 metered doses] (7 g); (Rhinocort® Aqua™): 32 mcg (60, 120 metered sprays); 64 mcg (120 metered sprays). **POWDER** (Turbuhaler): ~160 mcg delivered (200 mcg released) with each actuation (200 doses/inhaler)

Warnings/Precautions Controlled clinical studies have shown that inhaled and intranasal corticosteroids may cause a reduction in growth velocity in pediatric patients. Growth velocity provides a means of comparing the rate of growth among children of the same age.

In studies involving inhaled corticosteroids, the average reduction in growth velocity was approximately 1 cm (about 1/3 of an inch) per year. It appears that the reduction is related to dose and how long the child takes the drug.

FDA's Pulmonary and Allergy Drugs and Metabolic and Endocrine Drugs advisory committees discussed this issue at a July 1998 meeting. They recommended that the agency develop class-wide labeling to inform healthcare providers so they would understand this potential side effect and monitor growth routinely in pediatric patients who are treated with inhaled corticosteroids, intranasal corticosteroids or both.

Long-term effects of this reduction in growth velocity on final adult height are unknown. Likewise, it also has not yet been determined whether patients' growth will "catch up" if treatment in discontinued. Drug manufacturers will continue to monitor these drugs to learn more about long-term effects. Children are prescribed inhaled corticosteroids to treat asthma. Intranasal corticosteroids are generally used to prevent and treat allergy-related nasal symptoms.

Patients are advised not to stop using their inhaled or intranasal corticosteroids without first speaking to their healthcare providers about the benefits of these drugs compared to their risks.

Pregnancy Risk Factor C

Adverse Reactions

>10%:
Cardiovascular: Pounding heartbeat
Central nervous system: Nervousness, headache, dizziness
Dermatologic: Itching, rash
Gastrointestinal: GI irritation, bitter taste, oral candidiasis
Respiratory: Coughing, upper respiratory tract infection, bronchitis, hoarseness
Miscellaneous: Increased susceptibility to infections, diaphoresis

1% to 10%:
Central nervous system: Insomnia, psychic changes
Dermatologic: Acne, urticaria
Endocrine & metabolic: Menstrual problems
Gastrointestinal: Anorexia, increase in appetite, xerostomia, dry throat, loss of taste perception
Ocular: Cataracts
Respiratory: Epistaxis
Miscellaneous: Loss of smell

<1%: Abdominal fullness, bronchospasm, shortness of breath

Drug Interactions CYP3A3/4 enzyme substrate

Although there have been no reported drug interactions to date, one would expect budesonide could potentially interact with drugs known to interact with other corticosteroids

Half-Life 2-3 hours

Education and Monitoring Issues

Patient Education: Use as directed; do not increase dosage or discontinue abruptly without consulting prescriber. It may take several days for you to realize full effects of treatment. If you are also using an inhaled bronchodilator, wait 10 minutes before using this steroid aerosol. You may experience dizziness, anxiety, or blurred vision (rise slowly from sitting or lying position and use caution when driving or engaging in tasks requiring alertness until response to drug is known); or taste disturbance or aftertaste (frequent mouth care and mouth rinses may help). Report pounding heartbeat or chest pain; acute nervousness or inability to sleep; severe sneezing or nosebleed; difficulty breathing, sore throat, hoarseness, or bronchitis; respiratory difficulty or bronchospasms; disturbed menstrual pattern; vision changes; loss of taste or smell perception; or worsening of condition or lack of improvement.

Manufacturer AstraZeneca

Related Information

Asthma Guidelines *on page 1077*
Pharmaceutical Manufacturers Directory *on page 1020*

♦ **Bufferin® [OTC]** *see* Aspirin *on page 72*

♦ **Buffex® [OTC]** *see* Aspirin *on page 72*

Bumetanide (byoo MET a nide)

Pharmacologic Class Diuretic, Loop

U.S. Brand Names Bumex®

Generic Available No

Mechanism of Action Inhibits reabsorption of sodium and chloride in the ascending loop of Henle and proximal renal tubule, interfering with the chloride-binding cotransport system, thus causing increased excretion of water, sodium, chloride, magnesium, phosphate and calcium; it does not appear to act on the distal tubule

Use Management of edema secondary to congestive heart failure or hepatic or renal disease including nephrotic syndrome; may be used alone or in combination with antihypertensives in the treatment of hypertension; can be used in furosemide-allergic patients; (1 mg = 40 mg furosemide)

USUAL DOSAGE

Children (not FDA-approved for use in children <18 years of age):
- <6 months: Dose not established
- >6 months:
  - Oral: Initial: 0.015 mg/kg/dose once daily or every other day; maximum dose: 0.1 mg/kg/day
  - I.M., I.V.: Dose not established

Adults:
- Oral: 0.5-2 mg/dose 1-2 times/day; maximum: 10 mg/day
- I.M., I.V.: 0.5-1 mg/dose; maximum: 10 mg/day
- Continuous I.V. infusions of 0.9-1 mg/hour may be more effective than bolus dosing

Dosage Forms INJ: 0.25 mg/mL (2 mL, 4 mL, 10 mL). **TAB:** 0.5 mg, 1 mg, 2 mg

Contraindications Hypersensitivity to bumetanide or any component; in anuria or increasing azotemia

Warnings/Precautions Profound diuresis with fluid and electrolyte loss is possible; close medical supervision and dose evaluation is required; use caution when dosing in patients with hepatic failure

Pregnancy Risk Factor C (per manufacturer); D (based on expert analysis)

Adverse Reactions

>10%:
- Endocrine & metabolic: Hyperuricemia (18%), hypochloremia (14.9%), hypokalemia (14.7%)
- Renal: Azotemia (10.6%)

1% to 10%:
- Neuromuscular & skeletal: Muscle cramps (1.1%)
- Central nervous system: Dizziness (1.1%)
- Endocrine & metabolic: Hyponatremia (9.2%), hyperglycemia (6.6%), variations in phosphorus (4.5%), CO_2 content (4.3%), bicarbonate (3.1%), and calcium (2.4%)
- Renal: Increased serum creatinine (7.4%)
- Otic: Ototoxicity (1.1%)

<1% (limited to important or life-threatening symptoms): Hypotension, orthostatic hypotension, headache, nausea, encephalopathy (in patients with pre-existing liver disease), impaired hearing, pruritus, weakness, hives, abdominal pain, arthritic pain, musculoskeletal pain, rash, vomiting, vertigo, chest pain, ear discomfort, fatigue, dehydration, sweating, hyperventilation, dry mouth, upset stomach, renal failure, asterixis, itching, nipple tenderness, diarrhea, premature ejaculation

Drug Interactions

ACE inhibitors: Hypotensive effects and/or renal effects are potentiated by hypovolemia

Antidiabetic agents: Glucose tolerance may be decreased

Antihypertensive agents: Hypotensive effects may be enhanced

Cholestyramine or colestipol may reduce bioavailability of bumetanide

Digoxin: Ethacrynic acid-induced hypokalemia may predispose to digoxin toxicity; monitor potassium

Indomethacin (and other NSAIDs) may reduce natriuretic and hypotensive effects of diuretics

Lithium: Renal clearance may be reduced; isolated reports of lithium toxicity have occurred; monitor lithium levels

NSAIDs: Risk of renal impairment may increase when used in conjunction with diuretics

Ototoxic drugs (aminoglycosides, cis-platinum): Concomitant use of bumetanide may increase risk of ototoxicity, especially in patients with renal dysfunction

Peripheral adrenergic-blocking drugs or ganglionic blockers: Effects may be increased

Salicylates (high-dose) with diuretics may predispose patients to salicylate toxicity due to reduced renal excretion or alter renal function

Sparfloxacin, gatifloxacin, and moxifloxacin: Risk of hypokalemia and cardiotoxicity may be increased; avoid use

Thiazides: Synergistic diuretic effects occur

Alcohol Interactions Limit use (may increase risk of dizziness or lightheadedness)

Onset Oral, I.M.: 0.5-1 hour I.V.: 2-3 minutes

Duration 6 hours

(Continued)

Bumetanide *(Continued)*

Half-Life Adults: 1-1.5 hours

Education and Monitoring Issues

Patient Education: May be taken with food to reduce GI effects. Take single dose early in day (single dose) or last dose early in afternoon (twice daily) to prevent sleep interruptions. Include orange juice or bananas (or other sources of potassium-rich foods) in your daily diet but do not take supplemental potassium without consulting prescriber. You may experience dizziness, hypotension, lightheadedness, or weakness; use caution when changing position (rising from sitting or lying position), when driving, exercising, climbing stairs, or performing hazardous tasks, and avoid excessive exercise in hot weather. Report swelling of ankles or feet, weight increase or decrease more than 3 pounds in any one day, increased fatigue, muscle cramps or trembling, and any changes in hearing.

Monitoring Parameters: Blood pressure, serum electrolytes, renal function

Related Information

Heart Failure Guidelines *on page 1099*

- **Bumex®** *see* Bumetanide *on page 117*
- **Buminate®** *see* Albumin *on page 27*
- **Buphenyl®** *see* Sodium Phenylbutyrate *on page 859*

Bupivacaine (byoo PIV a kane)

Pharmacologic Class Local Anesthetic

U.S. Brand Names Marcaine®; Sensorcaine®; Sensorcaine®-MPF

Generic Available Yes

Mechanism of Action Blocks both the initiation and conduction of nerve impulses by decreasing the neuronal membrane's permeability to sodium ions, which results in inhibition of depolarization with resultant blockade of conduction

Use Local anesthetic (injectable) for peripheral nerve block, infiltration, sympathetic block, caudal or epidural block, retrobulbar block

USUAL DOSAGE Dose varies with procedure, depth of anesthesia, vascularity of tissues, duration of anesthesia and condition of patient. Metabisulfites (in epinephrine-containing injection); do not use solutions containing preservatives for caudal or epidural block.

Caudal block (with or without epinephrine):
- Children: 1-3.7 mg/kg
- Adults: 15-30 mL of 0.25% or 0.5%

Epidural block (other than caudal block):
- Children: 1.25 mg/kg/dose
- Adults: 10-20 mL of 0.25% or 0.5%

Peripheral nerve block: 5 mL dose of 0.25% or 0.5% (12.5-25 mg); maximum: 2.5 mg/kg (plain); 3 mg/kg (with epinephrine); up to a maximum of 400 mg/day

Sympathetic nerve block: 20-50 mL of 0.25% (no epinephrine) solution

Dosage Forms INJ: 0.25% (10 mL, 20 mL, 30 mL, 50 mL); 0.5% (10 mL, 20 mL, 30 mL, 50 mL); 0.75% (2 mL, 10 mL, 20 mL, 30 mL). **INJ with epinephrine** (1:200,000): 0.25% (10 mL, 30 mL, 50 mL); 0.5% (1.8 mL, 3 mL, 5 mL, 10 mL, 30 mL, 50 mL); 0.75% (30 mL)

Contraindications Hypersensitivity to bupivacaine hydrochloride or any component, para-aminobenzoic acid or parabens

Warnings/Precautions Use with caution in patients with liver disease. Some commercially available formulations contain sodium metabisulfite, which may cause allergic-type reactions. Pending further data, should not be used in children <12 years of age and the solution for spinal anesthesia should not be used in children <18 years of age. **Do not use solutions containing preservatives for caudal or epidural block**; convulsions due to systemic toxicity leading to cardiac arrest have been reported, presumably following unintentional intravascular injection. 0.75% is **not** recommended for obstetrical anesthesia.

Pregnancy Risk Factor C

Adverse Reactions 1% to 10% (dose related):
- Cardiovascular: Cardiac arrest, hypotension, bradycardia, palpitations
- Central nervous system: Seizures, restlessness, anxiety, dizziness
- Gastrointestinal: Nausea, vomiting
- Neuromuscular & skeletal: Weakness
- Ocular: Blurred vision
- Otic: Tinnitus
- Respiratory: Apnea

Drug Interactions
- Increased effect: Hyaluronidase
- Increased toxicity: Beta-blockers, ergot-type oxytocics, MAO inhibitors, TCAs, phenothiazines, vasopressors

Onset Onset of anesthesia (dependent on route administered): Within 4-10 minutes generally

Duration 1.5-8.5 hours

Half-Life 1.5-5.5 hours

Education and Monitoring Issues

Patient Education: This medication is given to reduce sensation in the injected area. You will experience decreased sensation to pain, heat, or cold in the area and/or decreased muscle strength (depending on area of application) until the effects wear off; use necessary caution to reduce incidence of possible injury until full sensation returns. If used in mouth, do not eat or drink until full sensation returns. Immediately report chest pain or palpitations; increased restlessness, anxiety, or dizziness; skeletal or muscle weakness; difficulty breathing; ringing in ears; or changes in vision.

Monitoring Parameters: Monitor fetal heart rate during paracervical anesthesia

Manufacturer AstraZeneca

Related Information

Pharmaceutical Manufacturers Directory *on page 1020*

♦ **Buprenex®** *see* Buprenorphine *on page 119*

Buprenorphine (byoo pre NOR feen)

Pharmacologic Class Analgesic, Narcotic

U.S. Brand Names Buprenex®

Generic Available No

Mechanism of Action Opiate agonist/antagonist that produces analgesia by binding to kappa and mu opiate receptors in the CNS

Use Management of moderate to severe pain

USUAL DOSAGE I.M., slow I.V.:

Children ≥13 years and Adults: 0.3-0.6 mg every 6 hours as needed

Elderly: 0.15 mg every 6 hours; elderly patients are more likely to suffer from confusion and drowsiness compared to younger patients

Long-term use is not recommended

Dosage Forms INJ: 0.3 mg/mL (1 mL)

Contraindications Hypersensitivity to buprenorphine or any component

Warnings/Precautions Use with caution in patients with hepatic dysfunction or possible neurologic injury; may precipitate abstinence syndrome in narcotic-dependent patients; tolerance or drug dependence may result from extended use

Pregnancy Risk Factor C

Adverse Reactions

>10%: Central nervous system: Sedation

1% to 10%:

Cardiovascular: Hypotension

Central nervous system: Respiratory depression, dizziness, headache

Gastrointestinal: Vomiting, nausea

Ocular: Miosis

Miscellaneous: Diaphoresis

<1%: Blurred vision, bradycardia, confusion, constipation, cyanosis, depression, diplopia, dyspnea, euphoria, hypertension, nervousness, paresthesia, pruritus, slurred speech, tachycardia, urinary retention, xerostomia

Drug Interactions

Barbiturate anesthetics may produce additive respiratory and CNS depression

Respiratory and CV collapse was reported in a patient who received diazepam and buprenorphine

Alcohol Interactions Avoid use (may increase central nervous system depression)

Onset Onset of analgesia: Within 10-30 minutes

Duration 6-8 hours

Half-Life 2.2-3 hours (range: 1.2-7.2 hours)

Education and Monitoring Issues

Patient Education: If self-administered, use exactly as directed (do not increase dose or frequency). While using this medication, do not use alcohol and other prescription or OTC medications (especially sedatives, tranquilizers, antihistamines, or pain medications) without consulting prescriber. May cause dizziness, drowsiness, confusion, or blurred vision (use caution when driving, climbing stairs, or changing position - rising from sitting or lying to standing, or when engaging in tasks requiring alertness until response to drug is known). You may experience nausea or vomiting (frequent mouth care, small frequent meals, sucking lozenges, or chewing gum may help). Report unresolved nausea or vomiting; difficulty breathing or shortness of breath; excessive sedation or unusual weakness; rapid heartbeat or palpitations.

Monitoring Parameters: Pain relief, respiratory and mental status, CNS depression, blood pressure

Manufacturer Reckitt & Colman

Related Information

Lipid-Lowering Agents Comparison *on page 1243*

Narcotic Agonists Comparison *on page 1244*

Pharmaceutical Manufacturers Directory *on page 1020*

Bupropion (byoo PROE pee on)

Pharmacologic Class Antidepressant, Dopamine-Reuptake Inhibitor

U.S. Brand Names Wellbutrin®; Wellbutrin® SR; Zyban™

Generic Available No

Mechanism of Action Antidepressant structurally different from all other previously marketed antidepressants; like other antidepressants the mechanism of bupropion's activity is not fully understood; weak blocker of serotonin and norepinephrine re-uptake, inhibits neuronal dopamine re-uptake and is **not** a monoamine oxidase A or B inhibitor

Use Treatment of depression; adjunct in smoking cessation

Unlabeled uses: Adjunct for cocaine abuse, ADHD, and bipolar disease

USUAL DOSAGE Oral:

Adults:

Depression: 100 mg 3 times/day; begin at 100 mg twice daily; may increase to a maximum dose of 450 mg/day

Smoking cessation: Initiate with 150 mg once daily for 3 days; increase to 150 mg twice daily; treatment should continue for 7-12 weeks

Elderly: Depression: 50-100 mg/day, increase by 50-100 mg every 3-4 days as tolerated; there is evidence that the elderly respond at 150 mg/day in divided doses, but some may require a higher dose

Dosing adjustment/comments in renal or hepatic impairment: Patients with renal or hepatic failure should receive a reduced dosage initially and be closely monitored

Dosage Forms TAB: 75 mg, 100 mg; Sustained release: 100 mg, 150 mg; (Zyban™): 150 mg

Contraindications Seizure disorder, prior diagnosis of bulimia or anorexia nervosa, known hypersensitivity to bupropion, concurrent use of a monoamine oxidase (MAO) inhibitor

Warnings/Precautions The estimated seizure potential is increased many fold in doses in the 450-600 mg/day range; giving a single dose <150 mg will lessen the seizure potential; use in patients with renal or hepatic impairment increases possible toxic effects

Pregnancy Risk Factor B

Adverse Reactions

>10%:

Cardiovascular: Tachycardia
Central nervous system: Agitation, insomnia, headache, dizziness, sedation
Gastrointestinal: Nausea, vomiting, xerostomia, constipation
Neuromuscular & skeletal: Tremor
Ocular: Blurred vision
Respiratory: Rhinitis
Miscellaneous: Diaphoresis

1% to 10%:

Cardiovascular: Hypertension, palpitations
Central nervous system: Anxiety, nervousness, confusion, hostility, abnormal dreams
Dermatologic: Rash, acne, dry skin
Endocrine & metabolic: Hyper- or hypoglycemia
Gastrointestinal: Anorexia, diarrhea, dyspepsia
Neuromuscular & skeletal: Arthralgia, myalgia
Otic: Tinnitus

Drug Interactions CYP2B6 and 2D6 enzyme substrate, CYP3A3/4 enzyme substrate (minor)

Monitor for treatment-emergent hypertension in patients treated with bupropion and nicotine patch

Carbamazepine, cimetidine, phenobarbital, and phenytoin may increase the metabolism (decrease clinical effect) of bupropion

Cimetidine may inhibit the metabolism (increase clinical/adverse effects) of bupropion

Toxicity of bupropion is enhanced by levodopa and phenelzine (MAOI)

Use with caution in individuals receiving other agents that may lower seizure threshold (antipsychotics, antidepressants, theophylline, abrupt discontinuation of benzodiazepines, systemic steroids)

Alcohol Interactions Avoid use (may increase central nervous system depression)

Onset >2 weeks to therapeutic effect

Half-Life 14 hours

Education and Monitoring Issues

Patient Education:

Depression: Take as directed, in equally divided doses, do not take in larger dose or more often than recommended. Do not discontinue without consulting prescriber. Do not use excessive alcohol or OTC medications not approved by prescriber. May cause drowsiness, clouded sensorium, restlessness, or agitation (use caution when driving or engaging in tasks requiring alertness until response to drug is known); nausea, vomiting, or dry mouth (small frequent meals, frequent mouth care, chewing gum, or sucking lozenges may help); constipation (increased exercise, fluids, or dietary fruit and fiber may help); or impotence (reversible). Report persistent CNS effects (agitation, confusion, anxiety, restlessness, insomnia, psychosis, hallucinations, seizures); muscle weakness or tremor; skin rash or irritation; chest pain or palpitations, abdominal pain or blood in stools; yellowing of skin or eyes; difficulty breathing, bronchitis, or unusual cough.

Smoking cessation: Use as directed, do not take extra doses. Do not combine narcotic patches with use of Zyban™ unless approved by prescriber. May cause dry mouth and insomnia (these may resolve with continued use). Report any difficulty breathing, unusual cough, dizziness, or muscle tremors.

Monitoring Parameters: Monitor body weight

Reference Range: Therapeutic levels (trough, 12 hours after last dose): 50-100 ng/mL

Manufacturer GlaxoWellcome

Related Information

Antidepressant Agents Comparison *on page 1231*

Pharmaceutical Manufacturers Directory *on page 1020*

- **Burinex®** *see* Bumetanide *on page 117*
- **Buscopan** *see* Scopolamine *on page 842*
- **BuSpar®** *see* Buspirone *on page 121*

Buspirone (byoo SPYE rone)

Pharmacologic Class Antianxiety Agent, Miscellaneous

U.S. Brand Names BuSpar®

Generic Available No

Mechanism of Action The mechanism of action of buspirone is unknown; it differs from typical benzodiazepine anxiolytics in that it does not exert anticonvulsant or muscle relaxant effects; it also lacks the prominent sedative effect that is associated with more typical anxiolytics; *in vitro* preclinical studies have shown that buspirone has a high affinity for serotonin (5-HT_{1A}) receptors; buspirone has no significant affinity for benzodiazepine receptors and does not affect GABA binding *in vitro* or *in vivo* when tested in preclinical models; buspirone has moderate affinity for brain D_2-dopamine receptors; some studies do suggest that buspirone may have indirect effects on other neurotransmitter systems

Use Management of anxiety; has shown little potential for abuse

USUAL DOSAGE Adults: Oral: 15 mg/day (5 mg 3 times/day); may increase in increments of 5 mg/day every 2-4 days to a maximum of 60 mg/day

Note: The safety and efficacy profile of buspirone in elderly patients has been demonstrated to be similar to those in younger patients; there were no effects of age on its pharmacokinetics

Dosing adjustment in renal or hepatic impairment: Dosage should be decreased in patients with severe hepatic insufficiency; in anuric patients, doses should be reduced by 25% to 50% of usual dose

Dosage Forms TAB: 5 mg, 7.5 mg, 10 mg, 15 mg

Contraindications Hypersensitivity to buspirone or any component

Warnings/Precautions Safety and efficacy not established in children <18 years of age; use in hepatic or renal impairment is not recommended; does not prevent or treat withdrawal from benzodiazepines

Pregnancy Risk Factor B

Adverse Reactions

>10%:

Central nervous system: Dizziness, lightheadedness, headache, restlessness

Gastrointestinal: Nausea

1% to 10%: Central nervous system: Drowsiness

<1%: Ataxia, blurred vision, chest pain, confusion, diarrhea, disorientation, eosinophilia, excitement, fever, flatulence, insomnia, leukopenia, muscle weakness, nightmares, rash, sedation, tachycardia, tinnitus urticaria, vomiting, xerostomia

Drug Interactions CYP3A3/4 enzyme substrate

Concurrent use of buspirone with SSRIs or trazodone may cause serotonin syndrome

Erythromycin, clarithromycin, itraconazole, and ketoconazole may result in large increases in buspirone concentrations (dizziness, sedation)

Enzyme inducers (carbamazepine, rifampin) may reduce serum concentrations of buspirone resulting in loss of efficacy

Buspirone should not be used concurrently with an MAO inhibitor due to reports of increased blood pressure

Diltiazem and verapamil may increase serum concentrations of buspirone; consider a dihydropyridine calcium channel blocker

Alcohol Interactions Avoid use (may increase central nervous system depression)

Onset Peak serum concentration: Within 1 hour

Half-Life 2-3 hours

Education and Monitoring Issues

Patient Education: Take only as directed; do not increase dose or take more often than prescribed. May take 2-3 weeks to see full effect; do not discontinue without consulting prescriber. Do not use excessive alcohol or other prescription or OTC medications (especially pain medications, sedatives, antihistamines, or hypnotics) without consulting prescriber. Maintain adequate hydration (2-3 L/day of fluids unless instructed to restrict fluid intake). You may experience drowsiness, lightheadedness, impaired coordination, dizziness, or blurred vision (use caution when driving or engaging in tasks

(Continued)

Buspirone *(Continued)*

requiring alertness until response to drug is known); or upset stomach, nausea (small frequent meals, frequent mouth care, chewing gum, or sucking lozenges may help). Report persistent vomiting, chest pain or rapid heartbeat, persistent CNS effects (eg, confusion, restlessness, anxiety, insomnia, excitation, headache, dizziness, fatigue, impaired coordination), or worsening of condition.

Dietary Considerations: Grapefruit juice may result in large increases in buspirone concentrations (dizziness, sedation)

Monitoring Parameters: Mental status, symptoms of anxiety; monitor for benzodiazepine withdrawal

Manufacturer Bristol-Myers Squibb Company (Pharmaceutical Division)

Related Information

Pharmaceutical Manufacturers Directory *on page 1020*

Busulfan (byoo SUL fan)

Pharmacologic Class Antineoplastic Agent, Alkylating Agent

U.S. Brand Names Myleran®

Generic Available No

Mechanism of Action Reacts with N-7 position of guanosine and interferes with DNA replication and transcription of RNA. Busulfan has a more marked effect on myeloid cells (and is, therefore, useful in the treatment of CML) than on lymphoid cells. The drug is also very toxic to hematopoietic stem cells (thus its usefulness in high doses in BMT preparative regimens). Busulfan exhibits little immunosuppressive activity. Interferes with the normal function of DNA by alkylation and cross-linking the strands of DNA.

Use

Oral: Chronic myelogenous leukemia and bone marrow disorders, such as polycythemia vera and myeloid metaplasia, conditioning regimens for bone marrow transplantation

I.V.: Combination therapy with cyclophosphamide as a conditioning regimen prior to allogeneic hematopoietic progenitor cell transplantation for chronic myelogenous leukemia

USUAL DOSAGE Busulfan should be based on adjusted ideal body weight because actual body weight, ideal body weight, or other factors can produce significant differences in busulfan clearance among lean, normal, and obese patients

Oral (refer to individual protocols):

Children:

For remission induction of CML: 0.06-0.12 mg/kg/day **OR** 1.8-4.6 mg/m^2/day; titrate dosage to maintain leukocyte count above 40,000/mm^3; reduce dosage by 50% if the leukocyte count reaches 30,000-40,000/mm^3; discontinue drug if counts fall to ≤20,000/mm^3

BMT marrow-ablative conditioning regimen: 1 mg/kg/dose (ideal body weight) every 6 hours for 16 doses

Adults:

BMT marrow-ablative conditioning regimen: 1 mg/kg/dose (ideal body weight) every 6 hours for 16 doses

Remission: Induction of CML: 4-8 mg/day (may be as high as 12 mg/day); Maintenance doses: Controversial, range from 1-4 mg/day to 2 mg/week; treatment is continued until WBC reaches 10,000-20,000 cells/mm^3 at which time drug is discontinued; when WBC reaches 50,000/mm^3, maintenance dose is resumed

Unapproved uses:

Polycythemia vera: 2-6 mg/day

Thrombocytosis: 4-6 mg/day

I.V.: 0.8 mg/kg (ideal body weight or actual body weight, whichever is lower) every 6 hours for 4 days (a total of 16 doses)

I.V. dosing in morbidly obese patients: Dosing should be based on adjusted ideal body weight (AIBW) which should be calculated as ideal body weight (IBW) + 0.25 times (actual weight minus ideal body weight)

AIBW = IBW + 0.25 x (AW - IBW)

Cyclophosphamide, in combination with busulfan, is given on each of two days as a 1-hour infusion at a dose of 160 mg/m^2 beginning on day 3, 6 hours following the 16th dose of busulfan

Dosage Forms INJ: 60 mg/10 mL ampuls. **TAB:** 2 mg

Contraindications Failure to respond to previous courses; should not be used in pregnancy or lactation; hypersensitivity to busulfan or any component

Warnings/Precautions The U.S. Food and Drug Administration (FDA) currently recommends that procedures for proper handling and disposal of antineoplastic agents be considered. May induce severe bone marrow hypoplasia; reduce or discontinue dosage at first sign, as reflected by an abnormal decrease in any of the formed elements of the blood; use with caution in patients recently given other myelosuppressive drugs or radiation treatment. If white blood count is high, hydration and allopurinol should be employed to prevent hyperuricemia.

Pregnancy Risk Factor D

Adverse Reactions

>10%:

Dermatologic: Urticaria, erythema, alopecia

Endocrine & metabolic: Ovarian suppression, amenorrhea, sterility

Genitourinary: Azospermia, testicular atrophy; malignant tumors have been reported in patients on busulfan therapy

Hematologic: Severe pancytopenia, leukopenia, thrombocytopenia, anemia, and bone marrow suppression are common and patients should be monitored closely while on therapy; since this is a delayed effect (busulfan affects the stem cells), the drug should be discontinued temporarily at the first sign of a large or rapid fall in any blood element; some patients may develop bone marrow fibrosis or chronic aplasia which is probably due to the busulfan toxicity; in large doses, busulfan is myeloablative and is used for this reason in BMT

Myelosuppressive:

WBC: Moderate

Platelets: Moderate

Onset (days): 7-10

Nadir (days): 14-21

Recovery (days): 28

1% to 10%:

Dermatologic: Skin hyperpigmentation (busulfan tan)

Gastrointestinal: Nausea, vomiting, diarrhea; drug has little effect on the GI mucosal lining

Emetic potential: Low (<10%)

Hepatic: Elevated LFTs

Neuromuscular & skeletal: Weakness

Ocular: Cataracts

<1%: Adrenal suppression, blurred vision, cataracts, endocardial fibrosis, generalized or myoclonic seizures and loss of consciousness have been associated with high-dose busulfan (4 mg/kg/day), gynecomastia, hepatic dysfunction, hyperuricemia, isolated cases of hemorrhagic cystitis have been reported; after long-term or high-dose therapy, a syndrome known as busulfan lung may occur; this syndrome is manifested by a diffuse interstitial pulmonary fibrosis and persistent cough, fever, rales, and dyspnea; may be relieved by corticosteroids.

Drug Interactions CYP3A3/4 enzyme substrate

Duration 28 days

Half-Life After first dose: 3.4 hours; After last dose: 2.3 hours

Education and Monitoring Issues

Patient Education: Take oral medication as directed with chilled liquids. Maintain adequate hydration (2-3 L/day of fluids unless instructed to restrict fluid intake) to help prevent kidney complications. Avoid alcohol, acidic or spicy foods, aspirin or OTC medications unless approved by prescriber. Brush teeth with soft toothbrush or cotton swab. You may lose hair or experience darkening of skin color (reversible when medication is discontinued), amenorrhea, sterility, or skin rash. You may experience nausea, vomiting, anorexia, or constipation (small frequent meals, increased exercise, and increased dietary fruit or fiber may help). You will be more susceptible to infection (avoid crowds or contagious persons, and do not receive any vaccinations unless approved by prescriber). Report palpitations or chest pain, excessive dizziness, confusion, respiratory difficulty, numbness or tingling of extremities, unusual bruising or bleeding, pain or changes in urination, or other adverse effects.

Monitoring Parameters: CBC with differential and platelet count, hemoglobin, liver function tests

Manufacturer GlaxoWellcome

Related Information

Pharmaceutical Manufacturers Directory *on page 1020*

♦ **Butace®** *see* Butalbital Compound *on page 123*

Butalbital Compound (byoo TAL bi tal KOM pound)

Pharmacologic Class Analgesic, Non-narcotic; Barbiturate

U.S. Brand Names Amaphen®; Anoquan®; Axotal®; B-A-C®; Bancap®; Butace®; Endolor®; Esgic®; Femcet®; Fiorgen PF®; Fioricet®; Fiorinal®; G-1®; Isollyl® Improved; Lanorinal®; Margesic®; Marnal®; Medigesic®; Phrenilin®; Phrenilin® Forte; Repan®; Sedapap-10®; Triad®; Triapin®; Two-Dyne®

Generic Available Yes

Mechanism of Action Butalbital, like other barbiturates, has a generalized depressant effect on the central nervous system (CNS). Barbiturates have little effect on peripheral nerves or muscle at usual therapeutic doses. However, at toxic doses serious effects on the cardiovascular system and other peripheral systems may be observed. These effects may result in hypotension or skeletal muscle weakness. While all areas of the central nervous system are acted on by barbiturates, the mesencephalic reticular activating system is extremely sensitive to their effects. Barbiturates act at synapses where gamma-aminobenzoic acid is a neurotransmitter, but they may act in other areas as well.

Use Relief of symptomatic complex of tension or muscle contraction headache

(Continued)

Butalbital Compound *(Continued)*

USUAL DOSAGE Adults: Oral: 1-2 tablets or capsules every 4 hours; not to exceed 6/day

Dosing interval in renal or hepatic impairment: Should be reduced

Dosage Forms CAP, with acetaminophen: (Amaphen®, Anoquan®, Butace®, Endolor®, Esgic®, Femcet®, G-1®, Margesic®, Medigesic®, Repan®, Triad®, Two-Dyne®): Butalbital 50 mg, caffeine 40 mg, and acetaminophen 325 mg; (Bancap®, Triapin®): Butalbital 50 mg and acetaminophen 325 mg; (Phrenilin® Forte): Butalbital 50 mg and acetaminophen 650 mg. **CAP, with aspirin:** (Fiorgen PF®, Fiorinal®, Isollyl® Improved, Lanorinal®, Marnal®): Butalbital 50 mg, caffeine 40 mg, and aspirin 325 mg. **TAB, with acetaminophen:** (Esgic®, Fioricet®, Repan®): Butalbital 50 mg, caffeine 40 mg, and acetaminophen 325 mg; (Phrenilin®): Butalbital 50 mg and acetaminophen 325 mg; (Sedapap-10®): Butalbital 50 mg and acetaminophen 650 mg. **TAB, with aspirin:** (Axotal®): Butalbital 50 mg and aspirin 650 mg; (B-A-C®): Butalbital 50 mg, caffeine 40 mg, and aspirin 650 mg; (Fiorinal®, Isollyl® Improved, Lanorinal®, Marnal®): Butalbital 50 mg, caffeine 40 mg, and aspirin 325 mg

Contraindications Patients with porphyria, known hypersensitivity to butalbital or any component

Warnings/Precautions Children and teenagers should not use for chickenpox or flu symptoms before a prescriber is consulted about Reye's syndrome (Fiorinal®)

Pregnancy Risk Factor D

Adverse Reactions

>10%:

Central nervous system: Dizziness, lightheadedness, drowsiness, "hangover" effect

Gastrointestinal: Nausea, heartburn, stomach pains, dyspepsia, epigastric discomfort

1% to 10%:

Central nervous system: Confusion, mental depression, unusual excitement, nervousness, faint feeling, headache, insomnia, nightmares, fatigue

Dermatologic: Rash

Gastrointestinal: Constipation, vomiting, gastrointestinal ulceration

Hematologic: Hemolytic anemia

Neuromuscular & skeletal: Weakness

Respiratory: Dyspnea

Miscellaneous: Anaphylactic shock

<1%: Agranulocytosis, bronchospasm, exfoliative dermatitis, hallucinations, hepatotoxicity, hypotension, impaired renal function, iron deficiency anemia, jitters, leukopenia, megaloblastic anemia, occult bleeding, prolongation of bleeding time, respiratory depression, Stevens-Johnson syndrome, thrombocytopenia, thrombophlebitis

Drug Interactions

Decreased effect: Phenothiazines, haloperidol, quinidine, cyclosporine, TCAs, corticosteroids, theophylline, ethosuximide, warfarin, oral contraceptives, chloramphenicol, griseofulvin, doxycycline, beta-blockers

Increased effect/toxicity: Propoxyphene, benzodiazepines, CNS depressants, valproic acid, methylphenidate, chloramphenicol

Alcohol Interactions Avoid use (may increase central nervous system depression)

Education and Monitoring Issues

Patient Education: Children and teenagers should not use this product; may cause drowsiness, avoid alcohol or other CNS depressants, may impair judgment and coordination; may cause physical and psychological dependence with prolonged use; do not exceed recommended dose

Butenafine (byoo TEN a fine)

Pharmacologic Class Antifungal Agent

U.S. Brand Names Mentax®

Use Topical treatment of tinea pedis (athlete's foot) and tinea cruris (jock itch)

USUAL DOSAGE Children >12 years and Adults: Topical: Apply once daily for 4 weeks to the affected area and surrounding skin

Contraindications Hypersensitivity to butenafine or components

Pregnancy Risk Factor B

Butoconazole (byoo toe KOE na zole)

Pharmacologic Class Antifungal Agent

U.S. Brand Names Femstat®

Use Local treatment of vulvovaginal candidiasis

USUAL DOSAGE Adults:

Nonpregnant: Insert 1 applicatorful (~5 g) intravaginally at bedtime as a single dose; therapy may extend for up to 6 days, if necessary, as directed by prescriber

Pregnant: **Use only during 2nd or 3rd trimester**

Contraindications Known hypersensitivity to butoconazole

Pregnancy Risk Factor C (for use only in 2nd or 3rd trimester)

Related Information

Treatment of Sexually Transmitted Diseases *on page 1210*

Butorphanol (byoo TOR fa nole)

Pharmacologic Class Analgesic, Narcotic

U.S. Brand Names Stadol®; Stadol® NS

Generic Available No

Mechanism of Action Mixed narcotic agonist-antagonist with central analgesic actions; binds to opiate receptors in the CNS, causing inhibition of ascending pain pathways, altering the perception of and response to pain; produces generalized CNS depression

Use Management of moderate to severe pain; injection also for preoperative or preanesthetic supplement to balanced anesthesia; relief of labor pain

Unlabeled use: Nasal spray: Acute relief of migraine headaches

USUAL DOSAGE Adults:

I.M.: 1-4 mg every 3-4 hours as needed

I.V.: 0.5-2 mg every 3-4 hours as needed

Nasal spray: Headache: 1 spray in 1 nostril; if adequate pain relief is not achieved within 60-90 minutes, an additional 1 spray in 1 nostril may be given (each spray gives ~1 mg of butorphanol); may repeat in 3-4 hours after the last dose as needed

Dosing adjustment in renal impairment:

Cl_{cr} 10-50 mL/minute: Administer 75% of dose

Cl_{cr} <10 mL/minute: Administer 50% of dose

Dosage Forms INJ: 1 mg/mL (1 mL), 2 mg/mL (1 mL, 2 mL, 10 mL). **SPRAY, nasal:** 10 mg/mL [14-15 doses] (2.5 mL)

Contraindications Hypersensitivity to butorphanol or any component; avoid use in opiate-dependent patients who have not been detoxified, may precipitate opiate withdrawal

Warnings/Precautions Use with caution in patients with hepatic/renal dysfunction, may elevate CSF pressure, may increase cardiac workload; tolerance of drug dependence may result from extended use

Pregnancy Risk Factor C; D (if used for prolonged periods or in high doses at term)

Adverse Reactions

>10%:

Central nervous system: Drowsiness, dizziness, insomnia (Stadol® NS), nasal congestion (Stadol® NS)

Gastrointestinal: Nausea, vomiting (13%)

1% to 10%:

Cardiovascular: Vasodilation, palpitations

Central nervous system: Lightheadedness, headache

Dermatologic: Pruritus

Gastrointestinal: Anorexia, unpleasant taste (Stadol® NS), constipation, xerostomia

Neuromuscular & skeletal: Weakness, tremor (Stadol® NS)

Ocular: Blurred vision

Otic: Ear pain/tinnitus (Stadol® NS)

Respiratory (Stadol® NS): Bronchitis, cough, dyspnea, epistaxis, nasal irritation, pharyngitis, rhinitis

Miscellaneous: Diaphoresis (increased)

<1%: Blurred vision, bradycardia, CNS depression, confusion, constipation, dependence with prolonged use, dyspnea, false sense of well being, hallucinations, hypertension, malaise, mental depression, nightmares, painful urination, paradoxical CNS stimulation, rash, respiratory depression, restlessness, shortness of breath, stomach cramps, tachycardia, tinnitus, weakness, decreased urination, hypotension, syncope

Drug Interactions Increased toxicity: CNS depressants, phenothiazines, barbiturates, skeletal muscle relaxants, alfentanil, guanabenz, MAO inhibitors

Alcohol Interactions Avoid use (may increase central nervous system depression)

Onset I.M.: 5-10 minutes; I.V.: <10 minutes; Nasal: Within 15 minutes

Duration I.M./I.V.: 3-4 hours; Nasal: 4-5 hours

Half-Life 2.5-4 hours

Education and Monitoring Issues

Patient Education: If self-administered, use exactly as directed (do not increase dose or frequency); may cause physical and/or psychological dependence. While using this medication, do not use alcohol and other prescription or OTC medications (especially sedatives, tranquilizers, antihistamines, or pain medications) without consulting prescriber. May cause dizziness, drowsiness, confusion, or blurred vision (use caution when driving, climbing stairs, or changing position - rising from sitting or lying to standing, or when engaging in tasks requiring alertness until response to drug is known); nausea or vomiting, or loss of appetite (frequent mouth care, small frequent meals, sucking lozenges, or chewing gum may help). Report unresolved nausea or vomiting; difficulty breathing or shortness of breath; restlessness, insomnia, euphoria, or nightmares; excessive sedation or unusual weakness; facial flushing, rapid heartbeat, or palpitations; urinary difficulty; or vision changes.

Monitoring Parameters: Pain relief, respiratory and mental status, blood pressure

Reference Range: 0.7-1.5 ng/mL

Related Information

Lipid-Lowering Agents Comparison *on page 1243*

Narcotic Agonists Comparison *on page 1244*

- **Byclomine® Injection** *see* Dicyclomine *on page 266*
- **Bydramine® Cough Syrup [OTC]** *see* Diphenhydramine *on page 282*

Cabergoline (ca BER go leen)

Pharmacologic Class Ergot-like Derivative

U.S. Brand Names Dostinex®

Mechanism of Action Cabergoline is a long-acting dopamine receptor agonist with a high affinity for D_2 receptors; prolactin secretion by the anterior pituitary is predominantly under hypothalamic inhibitory control exerted through the release of dopamine

Use Treatment of hyperprolactinemic disorders, either idiopathic or due to pituitary adenomas

Unlabeled use: Adjunct for the treatment of Parkinson's disease

USUAL DOSAGE Initial dose: Oral: 0.25 mg twice weekly; the dose may be increased by 0.25 mg twice weekly up to a maximum of 1 mg twice weekly according to the patient's serum prolactin level. Dosage increases should not occur more rapidly than every 4 weeks. Once a normal serum prolactin level is maintained for 6 months, the dose may be discontinued and prolactin levels monitored to determine if cabergoline is still required. The durability of efficacy beyond 24 months of therapy has not been established.

Dosage Forms TAB: 0.5 mg

Contraindications Patients with uncontrolled hypertension or hypersensitivity to ergot derivatives

Warnings/Precautions Initial doses >1 mg may cause orthostatic hypotension. Use caution when patients are receiving other medications which may reduce blood pressure. Not indicated for the inhibition or suppression of physiologic lactation since it has been associated with cases of hypertension, stroke, and seizures. Because cabergoline is extensively metabolized by the liver, careful monitoring in patients with hepatic impairment is warranted. Female patients should instruct the prescriber if they are pregnant, become pregnant, or intend to become pregnant. Should not be used in patients with pregnancy-induced hypertension unless benefit outweighs potential risk. Do not give to postpartum women who are breast-feeding or planning to breast-feed. In all patients, prolactin concentrations should be monitored monthly until normalized.

Pregnancy Risk Factor B

Adverse Reactions

>10%:

Central nervous system: Headache (26%), dizziness (17%)

Gastrointestinal: Nausea (29%)

1% to 10%:

Body as whole: Asthenia (6%), fatigue (5%), syncope (1%), influenza-like symptoms (1%), malaise (1%), periorbital edema (1%), peripheral edema (1%)

Cardiovascular: Hot flashes (3%), hypotension (1%), dependent edema (1%), palpitations (1%)

Central nervous system: Vertigo (4%), depression (3%), somnolence (2%), anxiety (1%), insomnia (1%), impaired concentration (1%), nervousness (1%)

Dermatologic: Acne (1%), pruritus (1%)

Endocrine: Breast pain (2%), dysmenorrhea (1%)

Gastrointestinal: Constipation (7%), abdominal pain (5%), dyspepsia (5%), vomiting (4%), xerostomia (2%), diarrhea (2%), flatulence (2%), throat irritation (1%), toothache (1%), anorexia (1%)

Neuromuscular & skeletal: Pain (2%), arthralgia (1%), paresthesias (2%)

Ocular: Abnormal vision (1%)

Respiratory: Rhinitis (1%)

Drug Interactions

Additive hypotensive effects may occur when cabergoline is administered with antihypertensive medications; dosage adjustment of the antihypertensive medication may be required

Decreased effect: Dopamine antagonists (eg, phenothiazines, butyrophenones, thioxanthenes, or metoclopramide) may reduce the therapeutic effects of cabergoline and should not be used concomitantly

Half-Life 63-69 hours

Education and Monitoring Issues

Patient Education: Patient should be instructed to notify prescriber if she suspects she is pregnant, becomes pregnant, or intends to become pregnant during therapy with cabergoline. A pregnancy test should be done if there is any suspicion of pregnancy and continuation of treatment should be discussed with prescriber.

Manufacturer Pharmacia & Upjohn

Related Information

Parkinson's Disease Dosing *on page 1249*

Pharmaceutical Manufacturers Directory *on page 1020*

- **Cafatine®** *see* Ergotamine *on page 323*
- **Cafatine-PB®** *see* Ergotamine *on page 323*
- **Cafergot®** *see* Ergotamine *on page 323*
- **Cafetrate®** *see* Ergotamine *on page 323*

Caffeine and Sodium Benzoate (KAF een & SOW dee um BEN zoe ate)

Pharmacologic Class Diuretic, Miscellaneous

Dosage Forms INJ: Caffeine 125 mg and sodium benzoate 125 mg per mL (2 mL)

Pregnancy Risk Factor C

- **Cal-500** *see* Calcium Carbonate *on page 130*
- **Calan®** *see* Verapamil *on page 975*
- **Calan® SR** *see* Verapamil *on page 975*
- **Cal Carb-HD® [OTC]** *see* Calcium Carbonate *on page 130*
- **Calci-Chew™ [OTC]** *see* Calcium Carbonate *on page 130*
- **Calciday-667® [OTC]** *see* Calcium Carbonate *on page 130*

Calcifediol (kal si fe DYE ole)

Pharmacologic Class Vitamin D Analog

U.S. Brand Names Calderol®

Generic Available No

Mechanism of Action Vitamin D analog that (along with calcitonin and parathyroid hormone) regulates serum calcium homeostasis by promoting absorption of calcium and phosphorus in the small intestine; promotes renal tubule resorption of phosphate; increases rate of accretion and resorption in bone minerals

Use Treatment and management of metabolic bone disease associated with chronic renal failure or hypocalcemia in patients on chronic renal dialysis

USUAL DOSAGE Oral: Hepatic osteodystrophy:

Infants: 5-7 mcg/kg/day

Children and Adults: Usual dose: 20-100 mcg/day or 20-200 mcg every other day; titrate to obtain normal serum calcium/phosphate levels; increase dose at 4-week intervals; initial dose: 300-350 mcg/week, administered daily or on alternate days

Dosage Forms CAP: 20 mcg, 50 mcg

Contraindications Hypercalcemia; known hypersensitivity to calcifediol; malabsorption syndrome; hypervitaminosis D; significantly decreased renal function

Warnings/Precautions Adequate (supplemental) dietary calcium is necessary for clinical response to vitamin D; calcium-phosphate product (serum calcium times phosphorus) must not exceed 70; avoid hypercalcemia

Pregnancy Risk Factor C (per manufacturer); A/D (if dosage exceeds RDA, based on expert analysis)

Adverse Reactions Percentage unknown: Anorexia, bone pain, cardiac arrhythmias, conjunctivitis, constipation, elevated LFTs, headache, hypercalcemia, hypermagnesemia, hypertension, hypotension, irritability, metallic taste, myalgia, nausea, pancreatitis, photophobia, polydipsia, polyuria, pruritus, seizures (rare), somnolence, vomiting, xerostomia

Drug Interactions

Decreased effect: Cholestyramine, colestipol

Increased effect: Thiazide diuretics

Additive effect: Antacids (magnesium)

Onset Time to peak serum concentration: 4 hours

Half-Life 12-22 days

Education and Monitoring Issues

Patient Education: Take exact dose as prescribed; do not increase dose. Maintain recommended diet and calcium supplementation. Avoid taking magnesium-containing antacids. You may experience nausea, vomiting, or metallic taste (frequent small meals, frequent mouth care, chewing gum, or sucking lozenges may help) or hypotension (use caution when rising from sitting or lying position or when climbing stairs or bending over). Report chest pain or palpitations, acute headache, skin rash, change in vision or eye irritation, CNS changes, weakness or lethargy.

Manufacturer Organon, Inc

Related Information

Pharmaceutical Manufacturers Directory *on page 1020*

- **Calciferol™ Injection** *see* Ergocalciferol *on page 321*
- **Calciferol™ Oral** *see* Ergocalciferol *on page 321*
- **Calciject** *see* Calcium Chloride *on page 131*
- **Calcijex™** *see* Calcitriol *on page 129*
- **Calcilean** *see* Heparin *on page 433*
- **Calcimar® Injection** *see* Calcitonin *on page 128*
- **Calci-Mix™ [OTC]** *see* Calcium Carbonate *on page 130*

Calcipotriene (kal si POE try een)

Pharmacologic Class Topical Skin Product; Vitamin, Fat Soluble

U.S. Brand Names Dovonex®

Mechanism of Action Synthetic vitamin D_3 analog which regulates skin cell production and proliferation

Use Treatment of moderate plaque psoriasis

(Continued)

Calcipotriene *(Continued)*

USUAL DOSAGE Adults: Topical: Apply in a thin film to the affected skin twice daily and rub in gently and completely

Dosage Forms CRM: 0.005% (30 g, 60 g, 100 g). **OINT, top:** 0.005% (30 g, 60 g, 100 g). **SOLN, top:** 0.005%

Contraindications Hypersensitivity to any components of the preparation; patients with demonstrated hypercalcemia or evidence of vitamin D toxicity; use on the face

Warnings/Precautions Use may cause irritations of lesions and surrounding uninvolved skin. If irritation develops, discontinue use. Transient, rapidly reversible elevation of serum calcium has occurred during use. If elevation in serum calcium occurs above the normal range, discontinue treatment until calcium levels are normal. For external use only; not for ophthalmic, oral or intravaginal use.

Pregnancy Risk Factor C

Adverse Reactions

>10%: Dermatologic: Burning, itching, skin irritation, erythema, dry skin, peeling, rash, worsening of psoriasis

1% to 10%: Dermatologic: Dermatitis

<1%: Folliculitis, hypercalcemia, hyperpigmentation, skin atrophy

Education and Monitoring Issues

Patient Education: For external use only. Use exactly as directed; do not overuse. Before using, wash and dry area gently. Wear gloves to apply a thin film to affected area and rub in gently. If dressing is necessary, use a porous dressing. Avoid contact with eyes. Avoid exposing treated area to direct sunlight; sunburn can occur. Report increased swelling, redness, rash, itching, signs of infection, worsening of condition, or lack of healing.

Manufacturer Westwood Squibb Pharmaceuticals

Related Information

Pharmaceutical Manufacturers Directory *on page 1020*

♦ **Calcite** *see* Calcium Carbonate *on page 130*

Calcitonin (kal si TOE nin)

Pharmacologic Class Antidote

U.S. Brand Names Calcimar® Injection; Cibacalcin® Injection; Miacalcin® Injection; Miacalcin® Nasal Spray; Osteocalcin® Injection; Salmonine® Injection

Generic Available No

Mechanism of Action Structurally similar to human calcitonin; it directly inhibits osteoclastic bone resorption; promotes the renal excretion of calcium, phosphate, sodium, magnesium and potassium by decreasing tubular reabsorption; increases the jejunal secretion of water, sodium, potassium, and chloride

Use

Calcitonin (salmon): Treatment of Paget's disease of bone and as adjunctive therapy for hypercalcemia; also used in postmenopausal osteoporosis and osteogenesis imperfecta

Calcitonin (human): Treatment of Paget's disease of bone

USUAL DOSAGE

Children: Dosage not established

Adults:

Paget's disease:

Salmon calcitonin: I.M., S.C.: 100 units/day to start, 50 units/day or 50-100 units every 1-3 days maintenance dose

Human calcitonin: S.C.: Initial: 0.5 mg/day (maximum: 0.5 mg twice daily); maintenance: 0.5 mg 2-3 times/week or 0.25 mg/day

Hypercalcemia: Initial: Salmon calcitonin: I.M., S.C.: 4 units/kg every 12 hours; may increase up to 8 units/kg every 12 hours to a maximum of every 6 hours

Osteogenesis imperfecta: Salmon calcitonin: I.M., S.C.: 2 units/kg 3 times/week

Postmenopausal osteoporosis: Salmon calcitonin:

I.M., S.C.: 100 units/day

Intranasal: 200 units (1 spray)/day

Dosage Forms INJ: Human (Cibacalcin®): 0.5 mg/vial; Salmon: 200 units/mL (2 mL). **SPRAY, nasal:** 200 units/activation (0.09 mL/dose) (2 mL glass bottle with pump)

Contraindications Hypersensitivity to salmon protein or gelatin diluent

Warnings/Precautions A skin test should be performed prior to initiating therapy of calcitonin salmon; have epinephrine immediately available for a possible hypersensitivity reaction

Pregnancy Risk Factor C

Adverse Reactions

>10%:

Cardiovascular: Facial flushing

Gastrointestinal: Nausea, diarrhea, anorexia

Local: Edema at injection site

1% to 10%: Genitourinary: Polyuria

<1%: Chills, dizziness, edema, headache, nasal congestion, paresthesia, rash, shortness of breath, urticaria, weakness

Onset Hypercalcemia: Onset of reduction in calcium: 2 hours

Duration Hypercalcemia: 6-8 hours

Half-Life S.C.: 1.2 hours

Education and Monitoring Issues

Patient Education: When this drug is given subcutaneously or I.M. it will be necessary for you or a significant other to learn to prepare and give the injections (keep drug vials in a refrigerator - do not freeze). Report significant nasal irritation if using calcitonin nasal spray. Follow directions exactly. Increased warmth and flushing may be experienced with this drug and should only last about 1 hour after administration (taking drug in the evening may minimize these discomforts). Immediately report twitching, muscle spasm, dark colored urine, hives, significant skin rash, palpitations, or difficulty breathing.

Monitoring Parameters: Serum electrolytes and calcium; alkaline phosphatase and 24-hour urine collection for hydroxyproline excretion (Paget's disease); serum calcium

Reference Range: Therapeutic: <19 pg/mL (SI: 19 ng/L) basal, depending on the assay

Calcitriol (kal si TRYE ole)

Pharmacologic Class Vitamin D Analog

U.S. Brand Names Calcijex™; Rocaltrol®

Generic Available No

Mechanism of Action Promotes absorption of calcium in the intestines and retention at the kidneys thereby increasing calcium levels in the serum; decreases excessive serum phosphatase levels, parathyroid hormone levels, and decreases bone resorption; increases renal tubule phosphate resorption

Use Management of hypocalcemia in patients on chronic renal dialysis; reduce elevated parathyroid hormone levels

Unlabeled use: Decrease severity of psoriatic lesions in psoriatic vulgaris; vitamin D resistant rickets

USUAL DOSAGE Individualize dosage to maintain calcium levels of 9-10 mg/dL

Renal failure:
- Children:
  - Oral: 0.25-2 mcg/day have been used (with hemodialysis); 0.014-0.041 mcg/kg/day (not receiving hemodialysis); increases should be made at 4- to 8-week intervals
  - I.V.: 0.01-0.05 mcg/kg 3 times/week if undergoing hemodialysis
- Adults:
  - Oral: 0.25 mcg/day or every other day (may require 0.5-1 mcg/day); increases should be made at 4- to 8-week intervals
  - I.V.: 0.5 mcg/day 3 times/week (may require from 0.5-3 mcg/day given 3 times/week) if undergoing hemodialysis

Hypoparathyroidism/pseudohypoparathyroidism: Oral (evaluate dosage at 2- to 4-week intervals):
- Children:
  - <1 year: 0.04-0.08 mcg/kg once daily
  - 1-5 years: 0.25-0.75 mcg once daily
- Children >6 years and Adults: 0.5-2 mcg once daily

Vitamin D-dependent rickets: Children and Adults: Oral: 1 mcg once daily

Vitamin D-resistant rickets (familial hypophosphatemia): Children and Adults: Oral: Initial: 0.015-0.02 mcg/kg once daily; maintenance: 0.03-0.06 mcg/kg once daily; maximum dose: 2 mcg once daily

Hypocalcemia in premature infants: Oral: 1 mcg once daily for 5 days

Hypocalcemic tetany in premature infants: I.V.: 0.05 mcg/kg once daily for 5-12 days

Dosage Forms CAP: 0.25 mcg, 0.5 mcg. **INJ:** 1 mcg/mL (1 mL); 2 mcg/mL (1 mL). **SOLN, oral:** 1 mcg/mL

Contraindications Hypercalcemia; vitamin D toxicity; abnormal sensitivity to the effects of vitamin D; malabsorption syndrome

Warnings/Precautions Adequate dietary (supplemental) calcium is necessary for clinical response to vitamin D; maintain adequate fluid intake; calcium-phosphate product (serum calcium times phosphorus) must not exceed 70; avoid hypercalcemia or use with renal function impairment and secondary hyperparathyroidism

Pregnancy Risk Factor C (per manufacturer); A/D (if dosage exceeds RDA, based on expert analysis)

Adverse Reactions

Percentage unknown: Anorexia, bone pain, cardiac arrhythmias, conjunctivitis, constipation, elevated LFTs, headache, hypermagnesemia, hypertension, hypotension, irritability, metallic taste, myalgia, nausea, pancreatitis, photophobia, polydipsia, polyuria, pruritus, seizures (rare), somnolence, vomiting, xerostomia

>10%: Endocrine & metabolic: Hypercalcemia (33%)

Drug Interactions

Decreased effect/absorption: Cholestyramine, colestipol

Increased effect: Thiazide diuretics

Additive effect: Magnesium-containing antacids

(Continued)

Calcitriol *(Continued)*

Onset ~2-6 hours

Duration 3-5 days

Half-Life 3-8 hours

Education and Monitoring Issues

Patient Education: Take exact dose as prescribed; do not increase dose. Maintain recommended diet and calcium supplementation. Avoid taking magnesium-containing antacids. You may experience nausea, vomiting, loss of appetite, or metallic taste (frequent small meals, frequent mouth care, chewing gum, or sucking lozenges may help); or hypotension (use caution when rising from sitting or lying position or when climbing stairs or bending over). Report chest pain or palpitations; acute headache; skin rash; change in vision or eye irritation; CNS changes; unusual weakness or fatigue; persistent nausea, vomiting, cramps, or diarrhea; or muscle or bone pain.

Monitoring Parameters: Monitor symptoms of hypercalcemia (weakness, fatigue, somnolence, headache, anorexia, dry mouth, metallic taste, nausea, vomiting, cramps, diarrhea, muscle pain, bone pain and irritability)

Reference Range: Calcium (serum) 9-10 mg/dL (4.5-5 mEq/L) but do not include the I.V. dosages; phosphate: 2.5-5 mg/dL

Calcium Acetate (KAL see um AS e tate)

Pharmacologic Class Electrolyte Supplement, Oral

U.S. Brand Names Calphron®; Phos-Ex® 125; PhosLo®

Use

Oral: Control of hyperphosphatemia in end-stage renal failure; calcium acetate binds to phosphorus in the GI tract better than other calcium salts due to its lower solubility and subsequent reduced absorption and increased formation of calcium phosphate; calcium acetate does not promote aluminum absorption

I.V.: Calcium supplementation in parenteral nutrition therapy

USUAL DOSAGE

Oral: Adults, on dialysis: Initial: 2 tablets with each meal, can be increased gradually to 3-4 tablets with each meal to bring the serum phosphate value <6 mg/dL as long as hypercalcemia does not develop

I.V.: Dose is dependent on the requirements of the individual patient; in central venous total parental nutrition (TPN), calcium is administered at a concentration of 5 mEq (10 mL)/L of TPN solution; the additive maintenance dose in neonatal TPN is 0.5 mEq calcium/kg/day (1.0 mL/kg/day)

Neonates: 70-200 mg/kg/day

Infants and Children: 70-150 mg/kg/day

Adolescents: 18-35 mg/kg/day

Contraindications Hypercalcemia, renal calculi, hypophosphatemia

Pregnancy Risk Factor C

Calcium Carbonate (KAL see um KAR bun ate)

Pharmacologic Class Antacid; Electrolyte Supplement, Oral

U.S. Brand Names Alka-Mints® [OTC]; Amitone® [OTC]; Cal Carb-HD® [OTC]; Calci-Chew™ [OTC]; Calciday-667® [OTC]; Calci-Mix™ [OTC]; Cal-Plus® [OTC]; Caltrate® 600 [OTC]; Caltrate, Jr.® [OTC]; Chooz® [OTC]; Dicarbosil® [OTC]; Equilet® [OTC]; Florical® [OTC]; Gencalc® 600 [OTC]; Mallamint® [OTC]; Nephro-Calci® [OTC]; Os-Cal® 500 [OTC]; Oyst-Cal 500 [OTC]; Oystercal® 500; Rolaids® Calcium Rich [OTC]; Tums® [OTC]; Tums® E-X Extra Strength Tablet [OTC]; Tums® Extra Strength Liquid [OTC]

Use As an antacid, and treatment and prevention of calcium deficiency or hyperphosphatemia (eg, osteoporosis, osteomalacia, mild/moderate renal insufficiency, hypoparathyroidism, postmenopausal osteoporosis, rickets); has been used to bind phosphate

USUAL DOSAGE Oral (dosage is in terms of elemental calcium):

Adequate intakes:

0-6 months: 210 mg/day
7-12 months: 270 mg/day
1-3 years: 500 mg/day
4-8 years: 800 mg/day
Adults, male/female:
- 9-18 years: 1300 mg/day
- 19-50 years: 1000 mg/day
- >51 years: 1200 mg/day

Female: Pregnancy:
- ≤18 years: 1300 mg/day
- >19 years: 1000 mg/day

Female: Lactating:
- ≤18 years: 1300 mg/day
- >19 years: 1000 mg/day

Hypocalcemia (dose depends on clinical condition and serum calcium level): Dose expressed in mg of **elemental calcium**

Neonates: 50-150 mg/kg/day in 4-6 divided doses; not to exceed 1 g/day

Children: 45-65 mg/kg/day in 4 divided doses

Adults: 1-2 g or more/day in 3-4 divided doses

Adults:

Dietary supplementation: 500 mg to 2 g divided 2-4 times/day

Antacid: 2 tablets or 10 mL every 2 hours, up to 12 times/day

Adults >51 years of age: Osteoporosis: 1200 mg/day

Dosing adjustment in renal impairment: Cl_{cr} <25 mL/minute: Dosage adjustments may be necessary depending on the serum calcium levels

Contraindications Hypercalcemia, renal calculi, hypophosphatemia

Pregnancy Risk Factor C

Related Information

Calcium Carbonate and Magnesium Carbonate *on page 131*

Calcium Carbonate and Magnesium Carbonate

(KAL see um KAR bun ate & mag NEE zhum KAR bun ate)

Pharmacologic Class Antacid

U.S. Brand Names Mylanta® Gelcaps®

♦ **Calcium Channel Blocking Agents Comparison** *see page 1236*

Calcium Chloride (KAL see um KLOR ide)

Pharmacologic Class Electrolyte Supplement, Oral

Use Cardiac resuscitation when epinephrine fails to improve myocardial contractions, cardiac disturbances of hyperkalemia, hypocalcemia, or calcium channel blocking agent toxicity; emergent treatment of hypocalcemic tetany, treatment of hypermagnesemia

USUAL DOSAGE Note: Calcium chloride is 3 times as potent as calcium gluconate

Cardiac arrest in the presence of hyperkalemia or hypocalcemia, magnesium toxicity, or calcium antagonist toxicity: I.V.:

Infants and Children: 20 mg/kg; may repeat in 10 minutes if necessary

Adults: 2-4 mg/kg (10% solution), repeated every 10 minutes if necessary

Hypocalcemia: I.V.:

Infants and Children: 10-20 mg/kg/dose (infants <1 mEq; children 1-7 mEq), repeat every 4-6 hours if needed

Adults: 500 mg to 1 g (7-14 mEq)/dose repeated every 4-6 hours if needed

Hypocalcemic tetany: I.V.:

Infants and Children: 10 mg/kg (0.5-0.7 mEq/kg) over 5-10 minutes; may repeat after 6-8 hours or follow with an infusion with a maximum dose of 200 mg/kg/day

Adults: 1 g over 10-30 minutes; may repeat after 6 hours

Hypocalcemia secondary to citrated blood transfusion: I.V.:

Neonates: Give 0.45 mEq **elemental** calcium for each 100 mL citrated blood infused

Adults: 1.35 mEq calcium with each 100 mL of citrated blood infused

Dosing adjustment in renal impairment: Cl_{cr} <25 mL/minute: Dosage adjustments may be necessary depending on the serum calcium levels

Contraindications In ventricular fibrillation during cardiac resuscitation, hypercalcemia, and in patients with risk of digitalis toxicity, renal or cardiac disease

Pregnancy Risk Factor C

Calcium Glubionate (KAL see um gloo BYE oh nate)

Pharmacologic Class Electrolyte Supplement, Oral

U.S. Brand Names Neo-Calglucon® [OTC]

Use Adjunct in treatment and prevention of postmenopausal osteoporosis; treatment and prevention of calcium depletion or hyperphosphatemia (eg, osteoporosis, osteomalacia, mild/moderate renal insufficiency, hypoparathyroidism, rickets)

USUAL DOSAGE Dosage is in terms of **elemental** calcium

Adequate intakes:

0-6 months: 210 mg/day

7-12 months: 270 mg/day

1-3 years: 500 mg/day

4-8 years: 800 mg/day

Adults, male/female:

9-18 years: 1300 mg/day

19-50 years: 1000 mg/day

>51 years: 1200 mg/day

Female: Pregnancy:

≤18 years: 1300 mg/day

>19 years: 1000 mg/day

Female: Lactating:

≤18 years: 1300 mg/day

>19 years: 1000 mg/day

Syrup is a hyperosmolar solution; dosage is in terms of calcium glubionate, elemental calcium is in parentheses

Neonatal hypocalcemia: 1200 mg (77 mg Ca^{++})/kg/day in 4-6 divided doses

Maintenance: Infants and Children: 600-2000 mg (38-128 mg Ca^{++})/kg/day in 4 divided doses up to a maximum of 9 g (575 mg Ca^{++})/day

Adults: 6-18 g (~0.5-1 g Ca^{++})/day in divided doses

(Continued)

Calcium Glubionate *(Continued)*

Dosing adjustment in renal impairment: Cl_{cr} <25 mL/minute: Dosage adjustments may be necessary depending on the serum calcium levels

Contraindications Hypercalcemia, renal calculi, ventricular fibrillation

Pregnancy Risk Factor C

Calcium Gluceptate (KAL see um gloo SEP tate)

Pharmacologic Class Electrolyte Supplement, Oral

Use Treatment of cardiac disturbances of hyperkalemia, hypocalcemia, or calcium channel blocker toxicity; cardiac resuscitation when epinephrine fails to improve myocardial contractions; treatment of hypermagnesemia and hypocalcemia

USUAL DOSAGE Dose expressed in mg of calcium gluceptate (elemental calcium is in parentheses)

Cardiac resuscitation in the presence of hypocalcemia, hyperkalemia, magnesium toxicity, or calcium channel blocker toxicity: I.V.:
- Children: 110 mg (9 mg Ca^{++})/kg/dose
- Adults: 1.1-1.5 g (90-123 mg Ca^{++})

Hypocalcemia:
- I.M.:
  - Children: 200-500 mg (16.4-41 mg Ca^{++})/kg/day divided every 6 hours
  - Adults: 500 mg to 1.1 g/dose as needed
- I.V.: Adults: 1.1-4.4 g (90-360 mg Ca^{++}) administered slowly as needed (≤2 mL/minute)

After citrated blood administration: Children and Adults: I.V.: 0.45 mEq Ca^{++}/100 mL blood infused

Dosing adjustment in renal impairment: Cl_{cr} <25 mL/minute: Dosage adjustments may be necessary depending on the serum calcium levels

Calcium Gluconate (KAL see um GLOO koe nate)

Pharmacologic Class Electrolyte Supplement, Oral

U.S. Brand Names Kalcinate®

Use Treatment and prevention of hypocalcemia; treatment of tetany, cardiac disturbances of hyperkalemia, cardiac resuscitation when epinephrine fails to improve myocardial contractions, hypocalcemia, or calcium channel blocker toxicity; calcium supplementation

USUAL DOSAGE Dosage is in terms of **elemental** calcium

Adequate intakes:
- 0-6 months: 210 mg/day
- 7-12 months: 270 mg/day
- 1-3 years: 500 mg/day
- 4-8 years: 800 mg/day
- Adults, male/female:
  - 9-18 years: 1300 mg/day
  - 19-50 years: 1000 mg/day
  - >51 years: 1200 mg/day
- Female: Pregnancy:
  - ≤18 years: 1300 mg/day
  - >19 years: 1000 mg/day
- Female: Lactating:
  - ≤18 years: 1300 mg/day
  - >19 years: 1000 mg/day

Dosage expressed in terms of **calcium gluconate**

Hypocalcemia: I.V.:
- Neonates: 200-800 mg/kg/day as a continuous infusion or in 4 divided doses
- Infants and Children: 200-500 mg/kg/day as a continuous infusion or in 4 divided doses
- Adults: 2-15 g/24 hours as a continuous infusion or in divided doses

Hypocalcemia: Oral:
- Children: 200-500 mg/kg/day divided every 6 hours
- Adults: 500 mg to 2 g 2-4 times/day
- Osteoporosis/bone loss: Oral: 1000-1500 mg in divided doses/day

Hypocalcemia secondary to citrated blood infusion: I.V.: Give 0.45 mEq **elemental** calcium for each 100 mL citrated blood infused

Hypocalcemic tetany: I.V.:
- Neonates: 100-200 mg/kg/dose, may follow with 500 mg/kg/day in 3-4 divided doses or as an infusion
- Infants and Children: 100-200 mg/kg/dose (0.5-0.7 mEq/kg/dose) over 5-10 minutes; may repeat every 6-8 hours **or** follow with an infusion of 500 mg/kg/day
- Adults: 1-3 g (4.5-16 mEq) may be administered until therapeutic response occurs

Calcium antagonist toxicity, magnesium intoxication or cardiac arrest in the presence of hyperkalemia or hypocalcemia: Calcium chloride is recommended calcium salt: I.V.:
- Infants and Children: 100 mg/kg/dose (maximum: 3 g/dose)
- Adults: 500-800 mg; maximum: 3 g/dose

Maintenance electrolyte requirements for total parenteral nutrition: I.V.: Daily requirements: Adults: 8-16 mEq/1000 kcal/24 hours

Dosing adjustment in renal impairment: Cl_{cr} <25 mL/minute: Dosage adjustments may be necessary depending on the serum calcium levels

Contraindications In ventricular fibrillation during cardiac resuscitation; patients with risk of digitalis toxicity, renal or cardiac disease, hypercalcemia, renal calculi, hypophosphatemia

Pregnancy Risk Factor C

- **Calcium-Sandoz** *see* Calcium Carbonate *on page 130*
- **Calcium-Sandoz** *see* Calcium Glubionate *on page 131*
- **CaldeCORT®** *see* Hydrocortisone *on page 447*
- **CaldeCORT® Anti-Itch Spray** *see* Hydrocortisone *on page 447*
- **Calderol®** *see* Calcifediol *on page 127*
- **Cal-Mag** *see* Calcium Carbonate and Magnesium Carbonate *on page 131*
- **Calmylin Codeine D-E** *see* Guaifenesin, Pseudoephedrine, and Codeine *on page 425*
- **Calmylin Expectorant** *see* Guaifenesin *on page 423*
- **Calphron®** *see* Calcium Acetate *on page 130*
- **Cal-Plus® [OTC]** *see* Calcium Carbonate *on page 130*
- **Calsan** *see* Calcium Carbonate *on page 130*
- **Caltine®** *see* Calcitonin *on page 128*
- **Caltrate** *see* Calcium Carbonate *on page 130*
- **Caltrate® 600 [OTC]** *see* Calcium Carbonate *on page 130*
- **Caltrate, Jr.® [OTC]** *see* Calcium Carbonate *on page 130*
- **Cama® Arthritis Pain Reliever [OTC]** *see* Aspirin *on page 72*

Candesartan (kan de SAR tan)

Pharmacologic Class Angiotensin II Antagonists

U.S. Brand Names Atacand™

Mechanism of Action Candesartan is an angiotensin receptor antagonist. Angiotensin II acts as a vasoconstrictor. In addition to causing direct vasoconstriction, angiotensin II also stimulates the release of aldosterone. Once aldosterone is released, sodium as well as water are reabsorbed. The end result is an elevation in blood pressure. Candesartan binds to the AT1 angiotensin II receptor. This binding prevents angiotensin II from binding to the receptor thereby blocking the vasoconstriction and the aldosterone secreting effects of angiotensin II.

Use Alone or in combination with other antihypertensive agents in treating essential hypertension; may have an advantage over losartan due to minimal metabolism requirements and consequent use in mild to moderate hepatic impairment

USUAL DOSAGE Adults: Oral: Usual dose is 4-32 mg once daily; dosage must be individualized; blood pressure response is dose-related over the range of 2-32 mg; the usual recommended starting dose of 16 mg once daily when it is used as monotherapy in patients who are not volume depleted; it can be administered once or twice daily with total daily doses ranging from 8-32 mg; larger doses do not appear to have a greater effect and there is relatively little experience with such doses

No initial dosage adjustment is necessary for elderly patients (although higher concentrations (C_{max}) and AUC were observed in these populations), for patients with mildly impaired renal function, or for patients with mildly impaired hepatic function.

Dosage Forms TAB: 4 mg, 8 mg, 16 mg, 32 mg

Contraindications Hypersensitivity to candesartan or any component; sensitivity to other A-II receptor antagonists; pregnancy; hyperaldosteronism (primary); renal artery stenosis (bilateral)

Warnings/Precautions Avoid use or use smaller dose in volume-depleted patients. Drugs which alter renin-angiotensin system have been associated with deterioration in renal function, including oliguria, acute renal failure and progressive azotemia. Use with caution in patients with renal artery stenosis (unilateral or bilateral) to avoid decrease in renal function; use caution in patients with pre-existing renal insufficiency (may decrease renal perfusion).

Pregnancy Risk Factor C (1st trimester); D (2nd and 3rd trimesters)

Pregnancy Implications Avoid use in the nursing mother, if possible, since candesartan may be excreted in breast milk. The drug should be discontinued as soon as possible when pregnancy is detected. Drugs which act directly on renin-angiotensin can cause fetal and neonatal morbidity and death.

Adverse Reactions May be associated with worsening of renal function in patients dependent on renin-angiotensin-aldosterone system.

Cardiovascular: Flushing, chest pain, peripheral edema, tachycardia, palpitations, angina, myocardial infarction,

Central nervous system: Dizziness, lightheadedness, drowsiness, fatigue, headache, vertigo, anxiety, depression, somnolence, fever

Dermatologic: Angioedema, rash (>0.5%)

Endocrine & metabolic: Hyperglycemia, hypertriglyceridemia

Gastrointestinal: Nausea, diarrhea, vomiting, dyspepsia, gastroenteritis

Genitourinary: Hyperuricemia, hematuria

(Continued)

Candesartan *(Continued)*

Neuromuscular & skeletal: Back pain, arthralgia, paresthesias, increased CPK, myalgia, weakness

Respiratory: Upper respiratory tract infection, pharyngitis, rhinitis, bronchitis, cough, sinusitis, epistaxis, dyspnea

Miscellaneous: Diaphoresis (increased)

Drug Interactions

Lithium: Risk of toxicity may be increased by candesartan; monitor lithium levels

Potassium-sparing diuretics (amiloride, spironolactone, triamterene): Increased risk of hyperkalemia

Potassium supplements may increase the risk of hyperkalemia

Trimethoprim (high dose) may increase the risk of hyperkalemia

Onset 2-3 hours; peak effect: 6-8 hours

Duration >24 hours

Half-Life Dose-dependent: 5-9 hours

Education and Monitoring Issues

Patient Education: Take exactly as directed; do not miss doses, alter dosage, or discontinue without consulting prescriber. Do not alter salt or potassium intake without consulting prescriber. May cause hypotension (change position slowly when rising from sitting or lying or when climbing stairs); transient drowsiness, dizziness, or headache (avoid driving or engaging in tasks requiring alertness until response to drug is known); or nausea or vomiting (small frequent meals may help). Report unusual weight gain or swelling of ankles and hands; persistent fatigue; unusual flu or cold symptoms or dry cough; difficulty breathing; chest pain or palpitations; swelling of eyes, face, or lips; skin rash; muscle pain or weakness; unusual bleeding (in urine, stool, or gums); or excessive sweating.

Dietary Considerations: Food reduces the time to maximal concentration and increases the C_{max}

Monitoring Parameters: Supine blood pressure, electrolytes, serum creatinine, BUN, urinalysis, symptomatic hypotension, and tachycardia

Reference Range: Therapeutic blood concentration: 34-183 ng/mL

Manufacturer AstraZeneca

Related Information

Angiotensin-Related Agents Comparison *on page 1226*

Pharmaceutical Manufacturers Directory *on page 1020*

♦ **Canesten** *see* Clotrimazole *on page 220*

♦ **Capastat®** *see* Capreomycin *on page 134*

♦ **Capastat® Sulfate** *see* Capreomycin *on page 134*

♦ **Capital® and Codeine** *see* Acetaminophen and Codeine *on page 18*

♦ **Capoten®** *see* Captopril *on page 134*

♦ **Capozide®** *see* Captopril and Hydrochlorothiazide *on page 136*

Capreomycin (kap ree oh MYE sin)

Pharmacologic Class Antibiotic, Miscellaneous

U.S. Brand Names Capastat® Sulfate

Use Treatment of tuberculosis in conjunction with at least one other antituberculosis agent

USUAL DOSAGE I.M.:

Infants and Children: 15 mg/kg/day, up to 1 g/day maximum

Adults: 15-20 mg/kg/day up to 1 g/day for 60-120 days, followed by 1 g 2-3 times/week

Dosing interval in renal impairment: Adults:

Cl_{cr} >100 mL/minute: Administer 13-15 mg/kg every 24 hours

Cl_{cr} 80-100 mL/minute: Administer 10-13 mg/kg every 24 hours

Cl_{cr} 60-80 mL/minute: Administer 7-10 mg/kg every 24 hours

Cl_{cr} 40-60 mL/minute: Administer 11-14 mg/kg every 48 hours

Cl_{cr} 20-40 mL/minute: Administer 10-14 mg/kg every 72 hours

Cl_{cr} <20 mL/minute: Administer 4-7 mg/kg every 72 hours

Contraindications Known hypersensitivity to capreomycin sulfate

Pregnancy Risk Factor C

Related Information

Antimicrobial Drugs of Choice *on page 1182*

Tuberculosis Treatment Guidelines *on page 1213*

Captopril (KAP toe pril)

Pharmacologic Class Angiotensin-Converting Enzyme (ACE) Inhibitors

U.S. Brand Names Capoten®

Generic Available Yes

Mechanism of Action Competitive inhibitor of angiotensin-converting enzyme (ACE); prevents conversion of angiotensin I to angiotensin II, a potent vasoconstrictor; results in lower levels of angiotensin II which causes an increase in plasma renin activity and a reduction in aldosterone secretion

Use Management of hypertension and treatment of congestive heart failure; left ventricular dysfunction after myocardial infarction (MI), diabetic nephropathy

Unlabeled use: Hypertensive crisis, rheumatoid arthritis, diagnosis of anatomic renal artery stenosis, hypertension secondary to scleroderma renal crisis, diagnosis of aldosteronism, idiopathic edema, Bartter's syndrome, increase circulation in Raynaud's phenomenon

USUAL DOSAGE Note: Dosage must be titrated according to patient's response; use lowest effective dose. Oral:

Infants: Initial: 0.15-0.3 mg/kg/dose; titrate dose upward to maximum of 6 mg/kg/day in 1-4 divided doses; usual required dose: 2.5-6 mg/kg/day

Children: Initial: 0.5 mg/kg/dose; titrate upward to maximum of 6 mg/kg/day in 2-4 divided doses

Older Children: Initial: 6.25-12.5 mg/dose every 12-24 hours; titrate upward to maximum of 6 mg/kg/day

Adolescents: Initial: 12.5-25 mg/dose given every 8-12 hours; increase by 25 mg/dose to maximum of 450 mg/day

Adults:

Hypertension:

Initial dose: 12.5-25 mg 2-3 times/day; may increase by 12.5-25 mg/dose at 1- to 2-week intervals up to 50 mg 3 times/day; add diuretic before further dosage increases

Maximum dose: 150 mg 3 times/day

Congestive heart failure:

Initial dose: 6.25-12.5 mg 3 times/day in conjunction with cardiac glycoside and diuretic therapy; initial dose depends upon patient's fluid/electrolyte status

Target dose: 50 mg 3 times/day

Maximum dose: 150 mg 3 times/day

LVD after MI: Initial dose: 6.25 mg followed by 12.5 mg 3 times/day; then increase to 25 mg 3 times/day during next several days and then over next several weeks to target dose of 50 mg 3 times/day

Diabetic nephropathy: 25 mg 3 times/day; other antihypertensives often given concurrently

Dosing adjustment in renal impairment:

Cl_{cr} 10-50 mL/minute: Administer at 75% of normal dose

Cl_{cr} <10 mL/minute: Administer at 50% of normal dose

Note: Smaller dosages given every 8-12 hours are indicated in patients with renal dysfunction; renal function and leukocyte count should be carefully monitored during therapy

Hemodialysis: Moderately dialyzable (20% to 50%); administer dose postdialysis or administer 25% to 35% supplemental dose

Peritoneal dialysis: Supplemental dose is not necessary

Dosage Forms TAB: 12.5 mg, 25 mg, 50 mg, 100 mg

Contraindications Hypersensitivity to captopril, other ACE inhibitors, or any component

Warnings/Precautions Use with caution and decrease dosage in patients with renal impairment (especially renal artery stenosis), severe congestive heart failure, or with coadministered diuretic therapy; experience in children is limited. Severe hypotension may occur in patients who are sodium and/or volume depleted, initiate lower doses and monitor closely when starting therapy in these patients; ACE inhibitors may be preferred agents in elderly patients with congestive heart failure and diabetes mellitus (diabetic proteinuria is reduced, minimal CNS effects, and enhanced insulin sensitivity); however due to decreased renal function, tolerance must be carefully monitored.

Pregnancy Risk Factor C (1st trimester); D (2nd and 3rd trimesters)

Pregnancy Implications

Clinical effects on the fetus: No data available on crossing the placenta. Cranial defects, hypocalvaria/acalvaria, oligohydramnios, persistent anuria following delivery, hypotension, renal defects, renal dysgenesis/dysplasia, renal failure, pulmonary hypoplasia, limb contractures secondary to oligohydramnios and stillbirth reported. ACE inhibitors should be avoided during pregnancy.

Breast-feeding/lactation: Crosses into breast milk. American Academy of Pediatrics considers **compatible** with breast-feeding.

Adverse Reactions

1% to 10%:

Cardiovascular: Hypotension (1% to 2.5%), tachycardia (1%), chest pain (1%), palpitation (1%)

Dermatologic: Rash (maculopapular or urticarial) (4% to 7%), pruritus, (2%); In patients with rash, a positive ANA and/or eosinophilia has been noted in 7% to 10%

Endocrine & metabolic: Hyperkalemia (1% to 11%)

Renal: Proteinuria (1%), increased serum creatinine, worsening of renal function (may occur in patients with bilateral renal artery stenosis or hypovolemia)

Respiratory: Cough (0.5% to 2%)

Miscellaneous: Hypersensitivity reactions (rash, pruritus, fever, arthralgia, and eosinophilia) have occurred in 4% to 7% of patients (depending on dose and renal function); dysgeusia - loss of taste or diminished perception (2% to 4%)

(Continued)

Captopril *(Continued)*

Neutropenia may occur in up to 3.7% of patients with renal insufficiency or collagen-vascular disease.

Incidence not determined: Angioedema, renal insufficiency, renal failure, nephrotic syndrome, polyuria, oliguria, urinary frequency, anemia, thrombocytopenia, pancytopenia, agranulocytosis, flushing, pallor, angina, myocardial infarction, Raynaud's syndrome, congestive heart failure, increased serum transaminases, increased serum bilirubin, increased alkaline phosphatase, anaphylactoid reactions, asthenia, gynecomastia, cardiac arrest, cerebrovascular insufficiency, rhythm disturbances, orthostatic hypotension, syncope, bullous pemphigus, erythema multiforme, Stevens-Johnson syndrome, exfoliative dermatitis, pancreatitis, glossitis, dyspepsia, anemia, anemia, jaundice, hepatitis, hepatic necrosis (rare), cholestasis, hyponatremia (symptomatic), myalgia, myasthenia, ataxia, confusion, depression, nervousness, somnolence, bronchospasm, eosinophilic pneumonitis, rhinitis, blurred vision, impotence

<1% (frequency ≤ to placebo) (limited to important or life-threatening symptoms): Gastric irritation, abdominal pain, nausea, vomiting, diarrhea, anorexia, constipation, aphthous ulcers, peptic ulcer, dizziness, headache, malaise, fatigue, insomnia, xerostomia, dyspnea, alopecia, paresthesia, angina, glomerulonephritis, cholestatic jaundice, psoriasis, hyperthermia, myalgia, arthralgia

Case reports: Aplastic anemia, hemolytic anemia, bronchospasm, alopecia, systemic lupus erythematosus, Kaposi's sarcoma, pericarditis, exacerbations of Huntington's disease, Guillain-Barré syndrome, seizures (in premature infants). A syndrome which may include fever, myalgia, arthralgia, interstitial nephritis, vasculitis, rash, eosinophilia, and elevated ESR has been reported for captopril and other ACE inhibitors.

Drug Interactions CYP2D6 enzyme substrate

Allopurinol: Case reports (rare) indicate a possible increased risk of Stevens-Johnson syndrome when combined with captopril

Alpha$_1$ blockers: Hypotensive effect increased

Aspirin and NSAIDs may decrease ACE inhibitor efficacy and/or increase adverse renal effects

Diuretics: Hypovolemia due to diuretics may precipitate acute hypotensive events or acute renal failure

Insulin: Risk of hypoglycemia may be increased

Lithium: Risk of lithium toxicity may be increased; monitor lithium levels, especially the first 4 weeks of therapy

Mercaptopurine: Risk of neutropenia may be increased

Potassium-sparing diuretics (amiloride, potassium, spironolactone, triamterene): Increased risk of hyperkalemia

Potassium supplements may increase the risk of hyperkalemia

Trimethoprim (high dose) may increase the risk of hyperkalemia

Alcohol Interactions Avoid use (may increase risk of hypotension or dizziness)

Onset Maximal decrease in blood pressure 1-1.5 hours after dose

Duration Dose related, may require several weeks of therapy before full hypotensive effect is seen

Half-Life Dependent upon renal and cardiac function: Adults, normal: 1.9 hours; Congestive heart failure: 2.06 hours; Anuria: 20-40 hours

Education and Monitoring Issues

Patient Education: Take exactly as directed; do not discontinue without consulting prescriber. Take first dose at bedtime. Take all doses on an empty stomach (30 minutes before or 2 hours after meals). This drug does not eliminate need for diet or exercise regimen as recommended by prescriber. Do not use potassium supplements or salt substitutes containing potassium without consulting prescriber. May cause dizziness, fainting, lightheadedness (use caution when driving or engaging in tasks that require alertness until response to drug is known); postural hypotension (use caution when rising from lying or sitting position or climbing stairs); nausea, vomiting, abdominal pain, dry mouth, or transient loss of appetite (small frequent meals, frequent mouth care, sucking lozenges, or chewing gum may help) - report if these persist. Report chest pain or palpitations; mouth sores; fever or chills; swelling of extremities, face, mouth, or tongue; skin rash; numbness, tingling, or pain in muscles; difficulty in breathing or unusual cough; other persistent adverse reactions.

Monitoring Parameters: BUN, serum creatinine, urine dipstick for protein, complete leukocyte count, and blood pressure

Related Information

Angiotensin-Related Agents Comparison *on page 1226*
Captopril and Hydrochlorothiazide *on page 136*
Heart Failure Guidelines *on page 1099*

Captopril and Hydrochlorothiazide

(KAP toe pril & hye droe klor oh THYE a zide)

Pharmacologic Class Antihypertensive Agent, Combination

U.S. Brand Names Capozide®

Dosage Forms TAB: 25/15: Captopril 25 mg and hydrochlorothiazide 15 mg; 25/25: Captopril 25 mg and hydrochlorothiazide 25 mg; 50/15: Captopril 50 mg and hydrochlorothiazide 15 mg; 50/25: Captopril 50 mg and hydrochlorothiazide 25 mg

Pregnancy Risk Factor C; D (2nd and 3rd trimesters)

Alcohol Interactions Avoid use (may increase risk of hypotension or dizziness)

♦ **Carafate®** *see* Sucralfate *on page 874*

Caramiphen and Phenylpropanolamine

(kar AM i fen & fen il proe pa NOLE a meen)

Pharmacologic Class Antihistamine

U.S. Brand Names Ordrine AT® Extended Release Capsule; Rescaps-D® S.R. Capsule; Tuss-Allergine® Modified T.D. Capsule; Tussogest® Extended Release Capsule

Dosage Forms CAP, timed release: Caramiphen edisylate 40 mg and phenylpropanolamine hydrochloride 75 mg. **LIQ:** Caramiphen edisylate 6.7 mg and phenylpropanolamine hydrochloride 12.5 mg per 5 mL

Pregnancy Risk Factor C

Carbachol (KAR ba kole)

Pharmacologic Class Cholinergic Agonist

U.S. Brand Names Carbastat® Ophthalmic; Carboptic® Ophthalmic; Isopto® Carbachol Ophthalmic; Miostat® Intraocular

Use Lowers intraocular pressure in the treatment of glaucoma; cause miosis during surgery

USUAL DOSAGE Adults:

Ophthalmic: Instill 1-2 drops up to 3 times/day

Intraocular: 0.5 mL instilled into anterior chamber before or after securing sutures

Contraindications Acute iritis, acute inflammatory disease of the anterior chamber, hypersensitivity to carbachol or any component

Pregnancy Risk Factor C

Carbamazepine (kar ba MAZ e peen)

Pharmacologic Class Anticonvulsant, Miscellaneous

U.S. Brand Names Carbatrol®; Epitol®; Tegretol®; Tegretol®-XR

Generic Available Yes

Mechanism of Action In addition to anticonvulsant effects, carbamazepine has anticholinergic, antineuralgic, antidiuretic, muscle relaxant and antiarrhythmic properties; may depress activity in the nucleus ventralis of the thalamus or decrease synaptic transmission or decrease summation of temporal stimulation leading to neural discharge by limiting influx of sodium ions across cell membrane or other unknown mechanisms; stimulates the release of ADH and potentiates its action in promoting reabsorption of water; chemically related to tricyclic antidepressants

Use Prophylaxis of generalized tonic-clonic, partial (especially complex partial), and mixed partial or generalized seizure disorder; pain relief of trigeminal neuralgia

Unlabeled use: Treat bipolar disorders and other affective disorders; resistant schizophrenia, alcohol withdrawal, restless leg syndrome, and psychotic behavior associated with dementia

USUAL DOSAGE Oral (adjust dose according to patient's response and serum concentrations):

Children:

<6 years: Initial: 5 mg/kg/day; dosage may be increased every 5-7 days to 10 mg/kg/day; then up to 20 mg/kg/day if necessary; administer in 2-4 divided doses/day

6-12 years: Initial: 100 mg twice daily or 10 mg/kg/day in 2 divided doses; increase by 100 mg/day at weekly intervals depending upon response; usual maintenance: 20-30 mg/kg/day in 2-4 divided doses/day; maximum dose: 1000 mg/day

Children >12 years and Adults: 200 mg twice daily to start, increase by 200 mg/day at weekly intervals until therapeutic levels achieved; usual dose: 800-1200 mg/day in 3-4 divided doses; some patients have required up to 1.6-2.4 g/day

Trigeminal or glossopharyngeal neuralgia: Initial: 100 mg twice daily with food, gradually increasing in increments of 100 mg twice daily as needed; usual maintenance: 400-800 mg daily in 2 divided doses

Dosing adjustment in renal impairment: Cl_{cr} <10 mL/minute: Administer 75% of dose

Dosage Forms CAP, extended release: 200 mg, 300 mg. **SUSP, oral** (citrus-vanilla flavor): 100 mg/5 mL (450 mL). **TAB:** 200 mg; Chewable: 100 mg; Extended release: 100 mg, 200 mg, 400 mg

Contraindications Hypersensitivity to carbamazepine or any component; **may have cross-sensitivity with tricyclic antidepressants**; should not be used in any patient with bone marrow suppression, MAO inhibitor use; the oral suspension should not be administered simultaneously with other liquid medicinal agents or diluents

Warnings/Precautions MAO inhibitors should be discontinued for a minimum of 14 days before carbamazepine is begun; administer with caution to patients with history of cardiac damage or hepatic disease; potentially fatal blood cell abnormalities have been reported following treatment; early detection of hematologic change is important; advise patients of early signs and symptoms including fever, sore throat, mouth ulcers, infections, easy

(Continued)

Carbamazepine *(Continued)*

bruising, petechial or purpuric hemorrhage; carbamazepine is not effective in absence, myoclonic or akinetic seizures; exacerbation of certain seizure types have been seen after initiation of carbamazepine therapy in children with mixed seizure disorders. Elderly may have increased risk of SIADH-like syndrome.

Pregnancy Risk Factor D

Pregnancy Implications

Clinical effects on the fetus: Crosses the placenta. Dysmorphic facial features, cranial defects, cardiac defects, spina bifida, IUGR, and multiple other malformations reported. Epilepsy itself, number of medications, genetic factors, or a combination of these probably influence the teratogenicity of anticonvulsant therapy. Benefit:risk ratio usually favors continued use during pregnancy and breast-feeding.

Breast-feeding/lactation: Crosses into breast milk. American Academy of Pediatrics considers **compatible** with breast-feeding.

Adverse Reactions

Dermatologic: Rash; but does not necessarily mean the drug should not be stopped

>10%:

Central nervous system: Sedation, dizziness, fatigue, ataxia, confusion
Gastrointestinal: Nausea, vomiting
Ocular: Blurred vision, nystagmus

1% to 10%:

Dermatologic: Stevens-Johnson syndrome, toxic epidermal necrolysis
Endocrine & metabolic: Hyponatremia, SIADH
Gastrointestinal: Diarrhea
Miscellaneous: Diaphoresis

<1%: Agranulocytosis, aplastic anemia, arrhythmias, A-V block, bone marrow suppression, bradycardia, congestive heart failure, diplopia, edema, eosinophilia, hepatitis, hypersensitivity, hypertension or hypotension, hypocalcemia, hyponatremia, leukopenia, mental depression, neutropenia (can be transient), pancytopenia, peripheral neuritis, sexual problems in males, slurred speech, swollen glands, syncope, thrombocytopenia, urinary retention

Drug Interactions CYP2C8 and 3A3/4 enzyme substrate; CYP1A2, 2C, and 3A3/4 inducer

Carbamazepine (CBZ) is a heteroinducer. It induces its own metabolism as well as the metabolism of other drugs. If CBZ is added to a drug regimen, serum concentrations may decrease. Conversely, if CBZ is part of an ongoing regimen and it is discontinued, elevated concentrations of the other drugs may result.

Carbamazepine may induce the metabolism of benzodiazepines, citalopram, clozapine, corticosteroids, cyclosporine, doxycycline, ethosuximide, felbamate, felodipine, haloperidol, mebendazole, methadone, oral contraceptives, phenytoin, tacrolimus, theophylline, thyroid hormones, tricyclic antidepressants, valproic acid, warfarin; monitor for altered response; dose adjustment may be needed

Cimetidine, clarithromycin, **danazol**, **diltiazem**, erythromycin, felbamate, fluoxetine, fluvoxamine, isoniazid, lamotrigine, metronidazole, **propoxyphene**, **verapamil**, fluconazole, itraconazole, and ketoconazole may inhibit hepatic metabolism of carbamazepine with resultant increase of carbamazepine serum concentrations and toxicity

Protease inhibitors (amprenavir, ritonavir, nelfinavir) may increase the serum levels of carbamazepine

CBZ may enhance hepatotoxic potential of acetaminophen

Neurotoxicity may result in patients receiving lithium and CBZ concurrently

Carbamazepine suspension is incompatible with chlorpromazine solution and thioridazine liquid. Schedule carbamazepine suspension at least 1-2 hours apart from other liquid medicinals.

Alcohol Interactions Avoid use (may increase central nervous system depression)

Onset Requires several days to reach steady-state concentrations; absorption is errative and slow

Half-Life Initial: 18-55 hours; Multiple dosing: 12-17 hours

Education and Monitoring Issues

Patient Education: Take exactly as directed (do not increase dose or frequency or discontinue without consulting prescriber). While using this medication, do not use alcohol and other prescription or OTC medications (especially pain medications, sedatives, antihistamines, or hypnotics) without consulting prescriber. Maintain adequate hydration (2-3 L/day of fluids unless instructed to restrict fluid intake). You may experience drowsiness, dizziness, or blurred vision (use caution when driving or engaging in tasks requiring alertness until response to drug is known); nausea, vomiting, loss of appetite, or dry mouth (small frequent meals, frequent mouth care, chewing gum, or sucking lozenges may help). Wear identification of epileptic status and medications. Report CNS changes, mentation changes, or changes in cognition; muscle cramping, weakness, tremors, changes in gait; persistent GI symptoms (cramping, constipation, vomiting, anorexia); rash or skin irritations; unusual bruising or bleeding (mouth, urine, stool); worsening of seizure activity, or loss of seizure control.

Dietary Considerations:

Food: Drug may cause GI upset, take with large amount of water or food to decrease GI upset. May need to split doses to avoid GI upset.

Sodium: SIADH and water intoxication; monitor fluid status; may need to restrict fluid

Reference Range:

Timing of serum samples: Absorption is slow, peak levels occur 6-8 hours after ingestion of the first dose; the half-life ranges from 8-60 hours, therefore, steady-state is achieved in 2-5 days

Therapeutic levels: 6-12 μg/mL (SI: 25-51 μmol/L)

Toxic concentration: >15 μg/mL; patients who require higher levels of 8-12 μg/mL (SI: 34-51 μmol/L) should be watched closely. Side effects including CNS effects occur commonly at higher dosage levels. If other anticonvulsants are given therapeutic range is 4-8 μg/mL.

Related Information

Anticonvulsants by Seizure Type Comparison *on page 1230*

Epilepsy Guidelines *on page 1091*

Carbamide Peroxide (KAR ba mide per OKS ide)

Pharmacologic Class Anti-infective Agent, Oral; Otic Agent, Cerumenolytic

U.S. Brand Names Auro® Ear Drops [OTC]; Debrox® Otic [OTC]; E•R•O Ear [OTC]; Gly-Oxide® Oral [OTC]; Mollifene® Ear Wax Removing Formula [OTC]; Murine® Ear Drops [OTC]; Orajel® Perioseptic® [OTC]; Proxigel® Oral [OTC]

Use Relief of minor inflammation of gums, oral mucosal surfaces and lips including canker sores and dental irritation; emulsify and disperse ear wax

USUAL DOSAGE Children and Adults:

Gel: Gently massage on affected area 4 times/day; do not drink or rinse mouth for 5 minutes after use

Oral solution (should not be used for >7 days): Oral preparation should not be used in children <3 years of age; apply several drops undiluted on affected area 4 times/day after meals and at bedtime; expectorate after 2-3 minutes **or** place 10 drops onto tongue, mix with saliva, swish for several minutes, expectorate

Otic:

Children <12 years: Tilt head sideways and individualize the dose according to patient size; 3 drops (range: 1-5 drops) twice daily for up to 4 days, tip of applicator should not enter ear canal; keep drops in ear for several minutes by keeping head tilted and placing cotton in ear

Children ≥12 years and Adults: Tilt head sideways and instill 5-10 drops twice daily up to 4 days, tip of applicator should not enter ear canal; keep drops in ear for several minutes by keeping head tilted and placing cotton in ear

Contraindications Otic preparation should not be used in patients with a perforated tympanic membrane; ear drainage, ear pain or rash in the ear; do not use in the eye; do not use otic preparation longer than 4 days; oral preparation should not be used in children <3 years

Pregnancy Risk Factor C

- **Carbastat® Ophthalmic** *see* Carbachol *on page 137*
- **Carbatrol®** *see* Carbamazepine *on page 137*

Carbenicillin (kar ben i SIL in)

Pharmacologic Class Antibiotic, Penicillin

U.S. Brand Names Geocillin®

Use Treatment of serious urinary tract infections and prostatitis caused by susceptible gram-negative aerobic bacilli

USUAL DOSAGE Oral:

Children: 30-50 mg/kg/day divided every 6 hours; maximum dose: 2-3 g/day

Adults: 1-2 tablets every 6 hours for urinary tract infections or 2 tablets every 6 hours for prostatitis

Dosing interval in renal impairment: Adults:

Cl_{cr} 10-50 mL/minute: Administer 382-764 mg every 12-24 hours

Cl_{cr} <10 mL/minute: Administer 382-764 mg every 24-48 hours

Moderately dialyzable (20% to 50%)

Contraindications Hypersensitivity to carbenicillin or any component or penicillins

Pregnancy Risk Factor B

Carbidopa (kar bi DOE pa)

Pharmacologic Class Anti-Parkinson's Agent; Dopaminergic Agent (Antiparkinson's)

U.S. Brand Names Lodosyn®

Use Given with levodopa in the treatment of parkinsonism to enable a lower dosage of levodopa to be used and a more rapid response to be obtained and to decrease side-effects; for details of administration and dosage, see Levodopa; has no effect without levodopa

USUAL DOSAGE Adults: Oral: 70-100 mg/day; maximum daily dose: 200 mg

Contraindications Hypersensitivity to carbidopa or levodopa

(Continued)

Carbidopa *(Continued)*

Pregnancy Risk Factor C

Carbinoxamine and Pseudoephedrine

(kar bi NOKS a meen & soo doe e FED rin)

Pharmacologic Class Adrenergic Agonist Agent; Antihistamine, H_1 Blocker; Decongestant

U.S. Brand Names Biohist®-LA; Carbiset® Tablet; Carbiset-TR® Tablet; Carbodec® Syrup; Carbodec® Tablet; Carbodec TR® Tablet; Cardec-S® Syrup; Palgic-D® [OTC]; Rondec® Drops; Rondec® Filmtab®; Rondec® Syrup; Rondec-TR®

Generic Available Yes

Mechanism of Action Carbinoxamine competes with histamine for H_1-receptor sites on effector cells in the gastrointestinal tract, blood vessels, and respiratory tract

Use Temporary relief of nasal congestion, running nose, sneezing, itching of nose or throat, and itchy, watery eyes due to the common cold, hay fever, or other respiratory allergies

USUAL DOSAGE Oral:

Children:

Drops: 1-18 months: 0.25-1 mL 4 times/day

Syrup:

18 months to 6 years: 2.5 mL 3-4 times/day

>6 years: 5 mL 2-4 times/day

Adults:

Liquid: 5 mL 4 times/day

Tablets: 1 tablet 4 times/day

Dosage Forms DROPS: Carbinoxamine maleate 2 mg and pseudoephedrine hydrochloride 25 mg per mL (30 mL with dropper). **SYR:** Carbinoxamine maleate 4 mg and pseudoephedrine hydrochloride 60 mg per 5 mL (120 mL, 480 mL). **TAB:** Film-coated: Carbinoxamine maleate 4 mg and pseudoephedrine hydrochloride 60 mg; Extended release: Carbinoxamine maleate 8 mg and pseudoephedrine hydrochloride 90 mg; Sustained release: Carbinoxamine maleate 8 mg and pseudoephedrine hydrochloride 120 mg

Contraindications Hypersensitivity to carbinoxamine or pseudoephedrine or any component; severe hypertension or coronary artery disease, MAO inhibitor therapy, GI or GU obstruction, narrow-angle glaucoma; avoid use in premature or term infants due to a possible association with SIDS

Warnings/Precautions Narrow-angle glaucoma, bladder neck obstruction, symptomatic prostatic hypertrophy, asthmatic attack, and stenosing peptic ulcer

Pregnancy Risk Factor C

Adverse Reactions

>10%:

Central nervous system: Slight to moderate drowsiness

Respiratory: Thickening of bronchial secretions

1% to 10%:

Central nervous system: Headache, fatigue, nervousness, dizziness

Gastrointestinal: Appetite increase, weight gain, nausea, diarrhea, abdominal pain, xerostomia

Neuromuscular & skeletal: Arthralgia

Respiratory: Pharyngitis

<1%: Angioedema, bronchospasm, depression, edema, epistaxis, hepatitis, myalgia, palpitations, paresthesia, photosensitivity, rash

Drug Interactions Increased toxicity: Barbiturates, TCAs, MAO inhibitors, ethanolamine antihistamines

Education and Monitoring Issues

Patient Education: Take as directed; do not exceed recommended dose. Maintain adequate hydration (2-3 L/day of fluids unless instructed to restrict fluid intake). Avoid use of other depressants, alcohol, or sleep-inducing medications unless approved by prescriber. You may experience drowsiness, impaired coordination, blurred vision, or increased anxiety (use caution when driving or engaging in tasks requiring alertness until response to drug is known); or dry mouth or nausea (frequent small meals, frequent mouth care, chewing gum, or sucking hard candy may help). Report persistent dizziness, sedation, or agitation; difficulty breathing or increased cough; changes in urinary pattern; muscle weakness; or lack of improvement or worsening of condition.

Carbinoxamine, Pseudoephedrine, and Dextromethorphan

(kar bi NOKS a meen, soo doe e FED rin, & deks troe meth OR fan)

Pharmacologic Class Antihistamine/Decongestant/Antitussive

U.S. Brand Names Carbodec DM®; Cardec DM®; Pseudo-Car® DM; Rondamine-DM® Drops; Rondec®-DM; Tussafed® Drops

Dosage Forms DROPS: Carbinoxamine maleate 2 mg, pseudoephedrine hydrochloride 25 mg, and dextromethorphan hydrobromide 4 mg per mL (30 mL). **SYR:** Carbinoxamine maleate 4 mg, pseudoephedrine hydrochloride 60 mg, and dextromethorphan hydrobromide 15 mg per 5 mL (120 mL, 480 mL, 4000 mL)

Pregnancy Risk Factor C

- **Carbiset® Tablet** *see* Carbinoxamine and Pseudoephedrine *on page 140*
- **Carbiset-TR® Tablet** *see* Carbinoxamine and Pseudoephedrine *on page 140*
- **Carbocaine®** *see* Mepivacaine *on page 565*
- **Carbodec DM®** *see* Carbinoxamine, Pseudoephedrine, and Dextromethorphan *on page 140*
- **Carbodec® Syrup** *see* Carbinoxamine and Pseudoephedrine *on page 140*
- **Carbodec® Tablet** *see* Carbinoxamine and Pseudoephedrine *on page 140*
- **Carbodec TR® Tablet** *see* Carbinoxamine and Pseudoephedrine *on page 140*

Carboprost Tromethamine (KAR boe prost tro METH a meen)

Pharmacologic Class Abortifacient; Prostaglandin

U.S. Brand Names Hemabate™

Generic Available No

Mechanism of Action Carboprost tromethamine is a prostaglandin similar to prostaglandin F_2 alpha (dinoprost) except for the addition of a methyl group at the C-15 position. This substitution produces longer duration of activity than dinoprost; carboprost stimulates uterine contractility which usually results in expulsion of the products of conception and is used to induce abortion between 13-20 weeks of pregnancy. Hemostasis at the placenta-tion site is achieved through the myometrial contractions produced by carboprost.

Use Termination of pregnancy and refractory postpartum uterine bleeding

Investigational: Hemorrhagic cystitis

USUAL DOSAGE Adults: I.M.:

Abortion: Initial: 250 mcg, then 250 mcg at 1½-hour to 3½-hour intervals depending on uterine response; a 500 mcg dose may be given if uterine response is not adequate after several 250 mcg doses; do not exceed 12 mg total dose or continuous administration for >2 days

Refractory postpartum uterine bleeding: Initial: 250 mcg; may repeat at 15- to 90-minute intervals to a total dose of 2 mg

Bladder irrigation for hemorrhagic cystitis (refer to individual protocols): [0.4-1.0 mg/dL as solution] 50 mL instilled into bladder 4 times/day for 1 hour

Dosage Forms INJ: Carboprost 250 mcg and tromethamine 83 mcg per mL (1 mL)

Contraindications Hypersensitivity to carboprost tromethamine or any component; acute pelvic inflammatory disease; pregnancy

Warnings/Precautions Use with caution in patients with history of asthma, hypotension or hypertension, cardiovascular, adrenal, renal or hepatic disease, anemia, jaundice, diabetes, epilepsy or compromised uteri

Pregnancy Risk Factor X

Adverse Reactions

>10%: Gastrointestinal: Nausea (33%)

1% to 10%: Cardiovascular: Flushing (7%)

<1%: Abnormal taste, asthma, bladder spasms, blurred vision, breast tenderness, coughing, diarrhea, drowsiness, dystonia, fever, headache, hematemesis, hiccups, hypertension, hypotension, myalgia, nervousness, respiratory distress, septic shock, vasovagal syndrome, vertigo, vomiting, xerostomia

Drug Interactions Increased toxicity: Oxytocic agents

Education and Monitoring Issues

Patient Education: This medication is used to stimulate expulsion of uterine contents (fetal tissue) or stimulate uterine contractions to reduce uterine bleeding. Report increased blood loss, acute abdominal cramping, persistent elevation of temperature, foul-smelling vaginal discharge. Increased temperature (elevated temperature) may occur 1-16 hours after therapy and last for several hours.

- **Carboptic® Ophthalmic** *see* Carbachol *on page 137*
- **Cardec DM®** *see* Carbinoxamine, Pseudoephedrine, and Dextromethorphan *on page 140*
- **Cardec-S® Syrup** *see* Carbinoxamine and Pseudoephedrine *on page 140*
- **Cardem®** *see* Celiprolol *on page 168*
- **Cardene®** *see* Nicardipine *on page 649*
- **Cardene® I.V.** *see* Nicardipine *on page 649*
- **Cardene® SR** *see* Nicardipine *on page 649*
- **Cardioquin®** *see* Quinidine *on page 802*
- **Cardizem® CD** *see* Diltiazem *on page 278*
- **Cardizem® Injectable** *see* Diltiazem *on page 278*
- **Cardizem® SR** *see* Diltiazem *on page 278*
- **Cardizem® Tablet** *see* Diltiazem *on page 278*
- **Cardura®** *see* Doxazosin *on page 297*

Carisoprodol (kar i soe PROE dole)

Pharmacologic Class Skeletal Muscle Relaxant

U.S. Brand Names Rela®; Sodol®; Soma®; Soprodol®; Soridol®

Generic Available Yes

(Continued)

Carisoprodol *(Continued)*

Mechanism of Action Precise mechanism is not yet clear, but many effects have been ascribed to its central depressant actions

Use Skeletal muscle relaxant

USUAL DOSAGE Adults: Oral: 350 mg 3-4 times/day; take last dose at bedtime; compound: 1-2 tablets 4 times/day

Dosage Forms TAB: 350 mg

Contraindications Acute intermittent porphyria, hypersensitivity to carisoprodol, meprobamate or any component

Warnings/Precautions Use with caution in renal and hepatic dysfunction

Pregnancy Risk Factor C

Adverse Reactions

>10%: Central nervous system: Drowsiness

1% to 10%:

- Cardiovascular: Tachycardia, tightness in chest, flushing of face, syncope
- Central nervous system: Mental depression, allergic fever, dizziness, lightheadedness, headache, paradoxical CNS stimulation
- Dermatologic: Angioedema
- Gastrointestinal: Nausea, vomiting, stomach cramps
- Neuromuscular & skeletal: Trembling
- Ocular: Burning eyes
- Respiratory: Shortness of breath
- Miscellaneous: Hiccups

<1%: Aplastic anemia, ataxia, blurred vision, eosinophilia, erythema multiforme, leukopenia, rash, urticaria

Drug Interactions CYP2C19 enzyme substrate

Increased toxicity: Alcohol, CNS depressants, phenothiazines

Alcohol Interactions Avoid use (may increase central nervous system depression)

Onset Within 30 minutes

Duration 4-6 hours

Half-Life 8 hours

Education and Monitoring Issues

Patient Education: Take exactly as directed with food. Do not increase dose or discontinue without consulting prescriber. Do not use alcohol, prescriptive or OTC antidepressants, sedatives, and pain medications without consulting prescriber. You may experience drowsiness, dizziness, lightheadedness (avoid driving or engaging in tasks requiring alertness until response to drug is known); nausea, vomiting, or cramping (small, frequent meals, frequent mouth care, or sucking hard candy may help); or postural hypotension (change position slowly when rising from sitting or lying or when climbing stairs). Report excessive drowsiness or mental agitation; palpitations, rapid heartbeat, or chest pain; skin rash; muscle cramping or tremors; or respiratory difficulty.

Monitoring Parameters: Look for relief of pain and/or muscle spasm and avoid excessive drowsiness

Related Information

Carisoprodol and Aspirin *on page 142*
Carisoprodol, Aspirin, and Codeine *on page 142*

Carisoprodol and Aspirin (kar i soe PROE dole & AS pir in)

Pharmacologic Class Skeletal Muscle Relaxant

U.S. Brand Names Soma® Compound

Dosage Forms TAB: Carisoprodol 200 mg and aspirin 325 mg

Pregnancy Risk Factor C

Alcohol Interactions Avoid use (may increase central nervous system depression)

Carisoprodol, Aspirin, and Codeine

(kar i soe PROE dole, AS pir in, and KOE deen)

Pharmacologic Class Skeletal Muscle Relaxant

U.S. Brand Names Soma® Compound w/Codeine

Dosage Forms TAB: Carisoprodol 200 mg, aspirin 325 mg, and codeine phosphate 16 mg

Pregnancy Risk Factor C

Alcohol Interactions Avoid use (may increase central nervous system depression)

♦ **Carmol-HC® Topical** *see* Urea and Hydrocortisone *on page 963*
♦ **Carmol® Topical [OTC]** *see* Urea *on page 962*
♦ **Carnitor® Injection** *see* Levocarnitine *on page 519*
♦ **Carnitor® Oral** *see* Levocarnitine *on page 519*

Carteolol (KAR tee oh lole)

Pharmacologic Class Beta Blocker (with Intrinsic Sympathomimetic Activity); Ophthalmic Agent, Antiglaucoma

U.S. Brand Names Cartrol® Oral; Ocupress® Ophthalmic

Generic Available No

Mechanism of Action Blocks both $beta_1$- and $beta_2$-receptors and has mild intrinsic sympathomimetic activity; has negative inotropic and chronotropic effects and can significantly slow A-V nodal conduction

Use Management of hypertension; treatment of chronic open-angle glaucoma and intraocular hypertension

USUAL DOSAGE Adults:

Oral: 2.5 mg as a single daily dose, with a maintenance dose normally 2.5-5 mg once daily; doses >10 mg do not increase response and may in fact decrease effect

Ophthalmic: Instill 1 drop in affected eye(s) twice daily

Dosing interval in renal impairment:

Cl_{cr} >60 mL/minute/1.73 m^2: Administer every 24 hours

Cl_{cr} 20-60 mL/minute/1.73 m^2: Administer every 48 hours

Cl_{cr} <20 mL/minute/1.73 m^2: Administer every 72 hours

Dosage Forms SOLN, ophth (Ocupress®): 1% (5 mL, 10 mL). **TAB** (Cartrol®): 2.5 mg, 5 mg

Contraindications Bronchial asthma, sinus bradycardia, second and third degree A-V block, cardiac failure (unless a functioning pacemaker present), cardiogenic shock, hypersensitivity to betaxolol or any component

Warnings/Precautions Some products contain sulfites which can cause allergic reactions; diminished response over time; may increase muscle weaknesses; use with a miotic in angle-closure glaucoma; use with caution in patients with decreased renal or hepatic function (dosage adjustment required) or patients with a history of asthma, congestive heart failure, or bradycardia; severe CNS, cardiovascular, and respiratory adverse effects have been seen following ophthalmic use

Pregnancy Risk Factor C (per manufacturer); D (2nd and 3rd trimesters, based on expert analysis)

Adverse Reactions

Ophthalmic:

>10%: Ocular: Conjunctival hyperemia

1% to 10%:

Ocular: Anisocoria, corneal punctate keratitis, corneal staining, decreased corneal sensitivity, eye pain, vision disturbances

Systemic:

>10%:

Central nervous system: Drowsiness, insomnia

Endocrine & metabolic: Decreased sexual ability

1% to 10%:

Cardiovascular: Bradycardia, palpitations, edema, congestive heart failure, reduced peripheral circulation

Central nervous system: Mental depression

Gastrointestinal: Diarrhea or constipation, nausea, vomiting, stomach discomfort

Respiratory: Bronchospasm

Miscellaneous: Cold extremities

<1% (limited to important or life-threatening symptoms): Chest pain, arrhythmias, orthostatic hypotension, nervousness, headache, depression, hallucinations, confusion (especially in the elderly), psoriasiform eruption, itching, polyuria, thrombocytopenia, leukopenia, shortness of breath

Drug Interactions

Albuterol (and other $beta_2$ agonists): Effects may be blunted by nonspecific beta-blockers.

Alpha-blockers (prazosin, terazosin): Concurrent use of beta-blockers may increase risk of orthostasis.

Carteolol causes hypertension when used with local anesthetics (tetracaine, lidocaine, or bupivacaine) containing epinephrine.

Clonidine: Hypertensive crisis after or during withdrawal of either agent.

Drugs which slow A-V conduction (digoxin): Effects may be additive with beta-blockers.

Glucagon: Carteolol may blunt the hyperglycemic action of glucagon.

Insulin: Carteolol may mask tachycardia from hypoglycemia.

NSAIDs (ibuprofen, indomethacin, naproxen, piroxicam) may reduce the antihypertensive effects of beta-blockers.

Salicylates may reduce the antihypertensive effects of beta-blockers.

Sulfonylureas: Beta-blockers may alter response to hypoglycemic agents.

Verapamil or diltiazem may have synergistic or additive pharmacological effects when taken concurrently with beta-blockers.

Alcohol Interactions Limit use (may increase risk of hypotension or dizziness)

Onset Onset of effect: Oral: 1-1.5 hours; Peak effect: 2 hours

Duration 12 hours

Half-Life 6 hours

Education and Monitoring Issues

Patient Education:

Oral: Take exactly as directed. Do not increase, decrease, or adjust dosage without consulting prescriber. Take pulse daily, prior to medication; follow prescriber's instruction about holding medication. Do not take with antacids and avoid alcohol or OTC medications (eg, cold remedies) without consulting prescriber. If diabetic,

(Continued)

Carteolol *(Continued)*

monitor serum blood glucose closely (may alter glucose tolerance or mask signs of hypoglycemia). May cause fatigue, dizziness, or postural hypotension; use caution when changing position from lying or sitting to standing, when driving, or climbing stairs until response to medication is known. May cause alteration in sexual performance (reversible). Report unresolved swelling of extremities, difficulty breathing or new cough, unresolved fatigue, unusual weight gain, unresolved constipation, or unusual muscle weakness.

Ophthalmic: Wash hands before instilling. Sit or lie down to instill. Open eye, look at ceiling, and instill prescribed amount of medication. Close eye and apply gentle pressure to inner corner of eye. Do not let tip of applicator touch eye or contaminate tip of applicator. Temporary stinging or burning may occur. Report persistent pain, burning, vision disturbances, swelling, itching, or worsening of condition.

Monitoring Parameters: Ophthalmic: Intraocular pressure; Systemic: Blood pressure, pulse, CNS status

Manufacturer Abbott Laboratories (Pharmaceutical Product Division)

Related Information

Beta-Blockers Comparison *on page 1233*
Pharmaceutical Manufacturers Directory *on page 1020*

♦ **Cartia® XT** *see* Diltiazem *on page 278*

♦ **Cartrol® Oral** *see* Carteolol *on page 142*

Carvedilol (KAR ve dil ole)

Pharmacologic Class Alpha-/Beta- Blocker; Beta Blocker, Nonselective

U.S. Brand Names Coreg®

Mechanism of Action As a racemic mixture, carvedilol has nonselective beta-adrenoreceptor and alpha-adrenergic blocking activity at equal potency. No intrinsic sympathomimetic activity has been documented. Associated effects include reduction of cardiac output, exercise- or beta agonist-induced tachycardia, reduction of reflex orthostatic tachycardia, vasodilation, decreased peripheral vascular resistance (especially in standing position), decreased renal vascular resistance, reduced plasma renin activity, and increased levels of atrial natriuretic peptide.

Use Management of hypertension; can be used alone or in combination with other agents, especially thiazide-type diuretics; treatment of mild or moderate congestive heart failure of ischemia or cardiomyopathic origin in conjunction with digitalis, diuretics, and ACE inhibitors to reduce the progression of disease as evidenced by cardiovascular death, cardiovascular hospitalizations, or the need to adjust other heart failure medications

Unlabeled use: Appears to be effective in the treatment of angina and idiopathic cardiomyopathy

USUAL DOSAGE Adults: Oral:

Hypertension: 6.25 mg twice daily; if tolerated, dose should be maintained for 1-2 weeks, then increased to 12.5 mg twice daily; dosage may be increased to a maximum of 25 mg twice daily after 1-2 weeks; reduce dosage if heart rate drops to <55 beats/minute

Congestive heart failure: 3.125 mg twice daily for 2 weeks; if this dose is tolerated, may increase to 6.25 mg twice daily. Double the dose every 2 weeks to the highest dose tolerated by patient. (Prior to initiating therapy, other heart failure medications should be stabilized.)

Maximum recommended dose:

<85 kg: 25 mg twice daily

>85 kg: 50 mg twice daily

Angina pectoris (unlabeled use): 25-50 mg twice daily

Idiopathic cardiomyopathy (unlabeled use): 6.25-25 mg twice daily

Dosing adjustment in renal impairment: None necessary

Dosing adjustment in hepatic impairment: Use is contraindicated in liver dysfunction

Dosage Forms TAB: 3.125 mg, 6.25 mg, 12.5 mg, 25 mg

Contraindications Uncompensated congestive heart failure (NYHA Class IV), asthma or bronchospastic disease (status asthmaticus may result), cardiogenic shock, severe bradycardia or second or third degree heart block, and symptomatic hepatic disease; hypersensitivity to any component

Warnings/Precautions Use with caution in patients with congestive heart failure treated with digitalis, diuretic, or ACE inhibitor since A-V conduction may be slowed; discontinue therapy if any evidence of liver injury occurs; use caution in patients with peripheral vascular disease, those undergoing anesthesia, in hyperthyroidism and diabetes mellitus. If no other antihypertensive is tolerated, very small doses may be cautiously used in patients with bronchospastic disease. Abrupt withdrawal of the drug should be avoided, drug should be discontinued over 1-2 weeks; do not use in pregnant or nursing women; may potentiate hypoglycemia in a diabetic patient and mask signs and symptoms; safety and efficacy in children have not been established.

Pregnancy Risk Factor C (per manufacturer); D (2nd and 3rd trimesters, based on expert analysis)

Pregnancy Implications

Clinical effects on the fetus: Use during pregnancy only if the potential benefit justifies the risk

Breast-feeding/lactation: Possible excretion in breast milk; avoid administration in lactating women, if possible

Adverse Reactions Note: Frequency ranges include data from hypertension and heart failure trials. Higher rates of adverse reactions have generally been noted in patients with congestive heart failure. However, the frequency of adverse effects associated with placebo is also increased in this population. Events occurring at a frequency > placebo in clinical trials:

>10%:

Cardiovascular: Chest pain (14.4%)

Central nervous system: Dizziness (6.2% to 32.4%), fatigue (4.3% to 23.9%)

Endocrine & metabolic: Hyperglycemia (12.2%)

Gastrointestinal: Diarrhea (11.8%)

Respiratory: Upper respiratory tract infection (18.3%)

1% to 10%:

Cardiovascular: Bradycardia (2.1% to 8.8%), hypotension (8.5%), generalized edema (5.1%), syncope (3.4%), hypertension (2.9%), A-V block (2.9%), lower extremity edema (1.4% to 2.2%), angina (aggravated) (2.0%), postural hypotension (1.8%)

Central nervous system: Pain (8.6%), headache (8.1%), fever (3.1%), paresthesia (2.0%), somnolence (1.8%), insomnia (1.6%), malaise, hypesthesia, vertigo

Endocrine & metabolic: Weight gain (9.7%), gout (6.3%), hypercholesterolemia (4.1%), dehydration (2.1%), hypervolemia (2.0%), hypertriglyceridemia (1.2%), hyperuricemia, hypoglycemia, hyponatremia

Gastrointestinal: Nausea (8.5%), abdominal pain (1.4% to 7.2%), vomiting (6.3%), diarrhea (2.2%), melena, periodontitis

Genitourinary: Urinary tract infection (1.8% to 3.1%), hematuria (2.9%), impotence

Hematologic: Thrombocytopenia (1.1% to 2.0%), decreased prothrombin, purpura

Hepatic: Increased transaminases, increased alkaline phosphatase

Neuromuscular & skeletal: Back pain (2.3% to 6.9%), arthralgia (6.4%), myalgia (3.4%)

Ocular: Abnormal vision (5.0%)

Renal: Increased BUN (6.0%), abnormal renal function, albuminuria, glycosuria

Respiratory: Sinusitis (5.4%), bronchitis (5.4%), pharyngitis (1.5% to 3.1%), rhinitis (2.1%), dyspnea (1.4%)

Miscellaneous: Infection (2.2%), injury (2.9% to 5.9%), increased sweating (2.9%), viral infection (1.8%), allergy, sudden death

<1% (limited to important or life-threatening symptoms): Peripheral ischemia, tachycardia, hypokinesis, bilirubinemia, elevated hepatic enzymes (hypertension: 0.2%; congestive heart failure: 0.4%), nervousness, sleep disorder, aggravated depression, impaired concentration, abnormal thinking, paranoia, emotional lability, asthma, decreased libido (male), pruritus, erythematous rash, maculopapular rash, psoriaform rash, photosensitivity, tinnitus, micturition frequency, xerostomia, increased sweating, hypokalemia, diabetes mellitus, hypertriglyceridemia, anemia, leukopenia, A-V block (complete), bundle branch block, myocardial ischemia, cerebrovascular disorder, convulsion, migraine, neuralgia, paresis, anaphylactoid reaction, alopecia, exfoliative dermatitis, amnesia, GI hemorrhage, bronchospasm, pulmonary edema, decreased hearing, respiratory alkalosis, increased BUN, decreased HDL cholesterol, pancytopenia, atypical lymphocytes.

Additional events from clinical trials in heart failure patients occurring at a frequency >2% but equal to or less than the frequency reported in patients receiving placebo: Asthenia, cardiac failure, flatulence, dyspepsia, palpitation, hyperkalemia, arthritis, depression, anemia, coughing, rash, leg cramps, chest pain, dyspepsia, headache, nausea, pain, sinusitis, upper respiratory infection.

Postmarketing case reports: Aplastic anemia (rare): All events occurred in patients receiving other medications capable of causing this effect; Stevens-Johnson syndrome.

Drug Interactions CYP2C, 2C9, 2D6 substrate

Inhibitors of CYP2D6 including quinidine, paroxetine, and propafenone are likely to increase blood levels of carvedilol

Alpha-blockers (prazosin, terazosin): Concurrent use of beta-blockers may increase risk of orthostasis

Clonidine: Hypertensive crisis after or during withdrawal of either agent

Cyclosporin blood levels may be increased by carvedilol

Digoxin blood levels may be increased

Fluoxetine may increase carvedilol blood levels

Paroxetine may increase carvedilol blood levels

Rifampin may decrease in carvedilol blood concentration

Insulin and oral hypoglycemics: Carvedilol may masks symptoms of hypoglycemia

Salicylates may reduce the antihypertensive effects of beta-blockers

NSAIDs (ibuprofen, indomethacin, naproxen, piroxicam) may reduce the antihypertensive effects of beta-blockers

Verapamil or diltiazem may have synergistic or additive pharmacological effects when taken concurrently with beta-blockers

Glucagon: Carvedilol may blunt the hyperglycemic action of glucagon

(Continued)

Carvedilol *(Continued)*

Sulfonylureas: Beta-blockers may alter response to hypoglycemic agents

Drugs which slow A-V conduction (digoxin): Effects may be additive with beta-blockers

Onset Within 1-2 hours

Half-Life 7-10 hours

Education and Monitoring Issues

Patient Education: Take exactly as directed. Do not increase, decrease, or adjust dosage without consulting prescriber. Take pulse daily, prior to medication; follow prescriber's instruction about holding medication. Do not take with antacids and avoid alcohol or OTC medications (eg, cold remedies) without consulting prescriber. If diabetic, monitor serum glucose closely (may alter glucose tolerance or mask signs of hypoglycemia). May cause fatigue, dizziness, or postural hypotension; use caution when changing position from lying or sitting to standing, when driving, or climbing stairs until response to medication is known. May cause alteration in sexual performance (reversible). Report unresolved swelling of extremities, difficulty breathing or new cough, unresolved fatigue, unusual weight gain, unresolved constipation, or unusual muscle weakness.

Monitoring Parameters: Heart rate, blood pressure (base need for dosage increase on trough blood pressure measurements and for tolerance on standing systolic pressure 1 hour after dosing)

Manufacturer SmithKline Beecham Pharmaceuticals

Related Information

Beta-Blockers Comparison *on page 1233*

Pharmaceutical Manufacturers Directory *on page 1020*

Cascara Sagrada (kas KAR a sah GRAH dah)

Pharmacologic Class Laxative, Stimulant

Use Temporary relief of constipation; sometimes used with milk of magnesia ("black and white" mixture)

USUAL DOSAGE Note: Cascara sagrada fluid extract is 5 times more potent than cascara sagrada aromatic fluid extract

Oral (aromatic fluid extract):

- Infants: 1.25 mL/day (range: 0.5-1.5 mL) as needed
- Children 2-11 years: 2.5 mL/day (range: 1-3 mL) as needed
- Children ≥12 years and Adults: 5 mL/day (range: 2-6 mL) as needed at bedtime (1 tablet as needed at bedtime)

Contraindications Nausea, vomiting, abdominal pain, fecal impaction, intestinal obstruction, GI bleeding, appendicitis, congestive heart failure

Pregnancy Risk Factor C

♦ **Casodex®** *see* Bicalutamide *on page 107*

♦ **Cataflam® Oral** *see* Diclofenac *on page 263*

♦ **Catapres® Oral** *see* Clonidine *on page 216*

♦ **Catapres-TTS® Transdermal** *see* Clonidine *on page 216*

♦ **Caverject®** *see* Alprostadil *on page 38*

♦ **Caverject® Injection** *see* Alprostadil *on page 38*

Cayenne

Pharmacologic Class Herb

Mechanism of Action Capsaicin selectively activates certain populations of unmyelinated primary afferent sensory neurons (type "C"). Many of cayenne's positive effects on the cardiovascular system can be attributed to its excitation of a distinct population of these neurons in the vagus nerve. Topically, capsaicin is reportedly effective in postherpetic neuralgia, postmastectomy pain syndrome, osteo and rheumatoid arthritis, painful diabetic neuropathy, psoriasis, and pruritus. Both the gastric and duodenal mucosa are thought to contain capsaicin-sensitive areas that protect against acid and drug induced ulcers when stimulated by capsaicin. It increases mucosal blood flow and/or vascular permeability; may inhibit gastric motility, and may activate duodenal motility.

Use

Cardiovascular circulatory support (Newall, 1996)

Digestive stimulant (Newall, 1996)

Inflammation and pain (topical) (Magnusson, 1996; Rains, 1995; Tandan, 1992; Nagy 1982)

USUAL DOSAGE

Oral: 400 mg 3 times/day, standardized to contain ≥0.25% capsaicin content per dose; may also be standardized to Scoville heat units, with 150,000 being average

Topical: Apply as directed by manufacturer

Contraindications Use with caution in individuals with GI ulceration (based on case reports). Due to pharmacological activity, may interfere with MAO inhibitors and antihypertensive therapies due to increased catecholamine secretion (Newall, 1996).

Warnings/Precautions Use all herbal supplements with extreme caution in children <2 years of age and in pregnancy or lactation. Some herbs are contraindicated in pregnancy or lactation; make sure to observe warnings. Use with caution in individuals on medication and with pre-existing medical conditions. Always review for potential herb-drug interactions (HDIs) and other warnings. Large and prolonged doses may increase the potential for adverse effects. Herbs may cause transient adverse effects such as nausea, vomiting, and GI distress due to a variety of chemical constituents. Caution should be used in individuals having known allergies to plants.

Drug Interactions Antihypertensives, aspirin or aspirin-containing compounds, MAO inhibitors

- **C-Crystals® [OTC]** *see* Ascorbic Acid *on page 72*
- **Cebid® Timecelles® [OTC]** *see* Ascorbic Acid *on page 72*
- **Ceclor®** *see* Cefaclor *on page 147*
- **Ceclor® CD** *see* Cefaclor *on page 147*
- **Cecon® [OTC]** *see* Ascorbic Acid *on page 72*
- **Cedax®** *see* Ceftibuten *on page 162*
- **Cedocard®-SR** *see* Isosorbide Dinitrate *on page 490*
- **CeeNU** *see* Lomustine *on page 537*

Cefaclor (SEF a klor)

Pharmacologic Class Antibiotic, Cephalosporin (Second Generation)

U.S. Brand Names Ceclor®; Ceclor® CD

Generic Available No

Mechanism of Action Inhibits bacterial cell wall synthesis by binding to one or more of the penicillin-binding proteins (PBPs) which in turn inhibits the final transpeptidation step of peptidoglycan synthesis in bacterial cell walls, thus inhibiting cell wall biosynthesis. Bacteria eventually lyse due to ongoing activity of cell wall autolytic enzymes (autolysins and murein hydrolases) while cell wall assembly is arrested.

Use Infections caused by susceptible organisms including *Staphylococcus aureus* and *H. influenzae*; treatment of otitis media, sinusitis, and infections involving the respiratory tract, skin and skin structure, bone and joint, and urinary tract

USUAL DOSAGE Oral:

Children >1 month: 20-40 mg/kg/day divided every 8-12 hours; maximum dose: 2 g/day (total daily dose may be divided into two doses for treatment of otitis media or pharyngitis)

Adults: 250-500 mg every 8 hours

Extended release tablets: 500 mg every 12 hours for 7 days for acute bacterial exacerbations of or secondary infections with chronic bronchitis or 375 mg every 12 hour for 10 days for pharyngitis or tonsillitis or for uncomplicated skin and skin structure infections

Dosing adjustment in renal impairment: Cl_{cr} <50 mL/minute: Administer 50% of dose

Hemodialysis: Moderately dialyzable (20% to 50%)

Dosage Forms CAP: 250 mg, 500 mg. **POWDER for oral susp** (strawberry flavor): 125 mg/5 mL (75 mL, 150 mL); 187 mg/5 mL (100 mL); 250 mg/5 mL (75 mL, 150 mL); 375 mg/5 mL (100 mL). **TAB, extended release:** 375 mg, 500 mg

Contraindications Hypersensitivity to cefaclor, any component, or cephalosporins

Warnings/Precautions Modify dosage in patients with severe renal impairment; prolonged use may result in superinfection; a low incidence of cross-hypersensitivity to penicillins exists

Pregnancy Risk Factor B

Adverse Reactions

1% to 10%:

Gastrointestinal: Diarrhea (1.5%)

Hematologic: Eosinophilia (2%)

Hepatic: Elevated transaminases (2.5%)

Dermatologic: Rash (maculopapular, erythematous, or morbilliform) (1% to 1.5%)

<1%: Agitation, anaphylaxis, angioedema, arthralgia, cholestatic jaundice, CNS irritability, confusion, dizziness, hallucinations, hemolytic anemia, hepatitis, hyperactivity, insomnia, interstitial nephritis, nausea, nervousness, neutropenia, prolonged PT, pruritus, pseudomembranous colitis, seizures, serum-sickness, somnolence, Stevens-Johnson syndrome, urticaria, vaginitis, vomiting

Reactions reported with other cephalosporins include fever, abdominal pain, superinfection, renal dysfunction, toxic nephropathy, hemorrhage, cholestasis

Drug Interactions

Increased effect: Probenecid may decrease cephalosporin elimination

Increased toxicity: Furosemide, aminoglycosides may be a possible additive to nephrotoxicity

Half-Life 0.5-1 hour, prolonged with renal impairment

Education and Monitoring Issues

Patient Education: Take as directed, at regular intervals around-the-clock (with or without food). Chilling oral suspension improves flavor (do not freeze). Do not chew or crush extended release tablets. Complete full course of medication, even if you feel better. Drink 2-3 L fluid/day. Small frequent meals, frequent mouth care, sucking

(Continued)

Cefaclor *(Continued)*

lozenges, or chewing gum may reduce nausea or vomiting. If diarrhea occurs, yogurt or buttermilk may help. May cause false-positive test with Clinitest®; use another form of testing. May interfere with oral contraceptives; additional contraceptive measures are necessary. Report severe, unresolved diarrhea; abdominal pain; vaginal itching or drainage; sores in mouth; blood, pus, or mucus in stool or urine; easy bleeding or bruising; unusual fever or chills; rash; or respiratory difficulty.

Monitoring Parameters: Assess patient at beginning and throughout therapy for infection; monitor for signs of anaphylaxis during first dose

Related Information

Antimicrobial Drugs of Choice *on page 1182*

Cefadroxil (sef a DROKS il)

Pharmacologic Class Antibiotic, Cephalosporin (First Generation)

U.S. Brand Names Duricef®; Ultracef®

Generic Available No

Mechanism of Action Inhibits bacterial cell wall synthesis by binding to one or more of the penicillin-binding proteins (PBPs) which in turn inhibits the final transpeptidation step of peptidoglycan synthesis in bacterial cell walls, thus inhibiting cell wall biosynthesis. Bacteria eventually lyse due to ongoing activity of cell wall autolytic enzymes (autolysins and murein hydrolases) while cell wall assembly is arrested.

Use Treatment of susceptible gram-positive bacilli and cocci (not enterococcus); some gram-negative bacilli including *E. coli, Proteus*, and *Klebsiella* may be susceptible

USUAL DOSAGE Oral:

Children: 30 mg/kg/day divided twice daily up to a maximum of 2 g/day

Adults: 1-2 g/day in 2 divided doses

Prophylaxis against bacterial endocarditis: 2 g 1 hour prior to the procedure

Dosing interval in renal impairment:

Cl_{cr} 10-25 mL/minute: Administer every 24 hours

Cl_{cr} <10 mL/minute: Administer every 36 hours

Dosage Forms CAP: 500 mg. **SUSP, oral:** 125 mg/5 mL, 250 mg/5 mL, 500 mg/5 mL (50 mL, 100 mL). **TAB:** 1 g

Contraindications Hypersensitivity to cefadroxil or other cephalosporins

Warnings/Precautions Modify dosage in patients with severe renal impairment; prolonged use may result in superinfection; use with caution in patients with a history of penicillin allergy especially IgE-mediated reactions (eg, anaphylaxis, urticaria); may cause antibiotic-associated colitis or colitis secondary to *C. difficile*

Pregnancy Risk Factor B

Adverse Reactions

1% to 10%: Gastrointestinal: Diarrhea

<1%: Abdominal pain, agranulocytosis, anaphylaxis, angioedema, arthralgia, cholestasis, dyspepsia, elevated transaminases, erythema multiforme, fever, nausea, neutropenia, pruritus, pseudomembranous colitis, rash (maculopapular and erythematous), serum sickness, Stevens-Johnson syndrome, thrombocytopenia, urticaria, vaginitis, vomiting

Reactions reported with other cephalosporins include abdominal pain, aplastic anemia, eosinophilia, hemolytic anemia, hemorrhage, increased BUN, increased creatinine, pancytopenia, prolonged prothrombin time, renal dysfunction, seizures, superinfection. toxic epidermal necrolysis, toxic nephropathy

Drug Interactions

Increased effect: Probenecid may decrease cephalosporin elimination

Increased toxicity: Furosemide, aminoglycosides may be a possible additive to nephrotoxicity

Half-Life 1-2 hours; 20-24 hours in renal failure

Education and Monitoring Issues

Patient Education: Take as directed, at regular intervals around-the-clock (with or without food). Chilling oral suspension improves flavor (do not freeze). Complete full course of medication, even if you feel better. Drink 2-3 L fluid/day. If diarrhea occurs, yogurt or buttermilk may help. May cause false-positive test with Clinitest®; use another form of testing. May interfere with oral contraceptives; additional contraceptive measures are necessary. Report severe, unresolved diarrhea; abdominal pain; vaginal itching or drainage; sores in mouth; blood, pus, or mucus in stool or urine; easy bleeding or bruising; unusual fever or chills; rash; or respiratory difficulty.

Monitoring Parameters: Observe for signs and symptoms of anaphylaxis during first dose

Related Information

Prevention of Bacterial Endocarditis *on page 1154*

♦ **Cefadyl®** *see* Cephapirin *on page 170*

Cefamandole (sef a MAN dole)

Pharmacologic Class Antibiotic, Cephalosporin (Second Generation)

U.S. Brand Names Mandol®

Use Treatment of susceptible bacterial infection; mainly respiratory tract, skin and skin structure, bone and joint, urinary tract and gynecologic, septicemia; surgical prophylaxis. Active against methicillin-sensitive staphylococci, many streptococci, and various gram-negative bacilli including *E. coli*, some *Klebsiella*, *P. mirabilis*, *H. influenzae*, and *Moraxella*.

USUAL DOSAGE I.M., I.V.:

Children: 50-150 mg/kg/day in divided doses every 4-8 hours

Adults: Usual dose: 500-1000 mg every 4-8 hours; in life-threatening infections: 2 g every 4 hours may be needed

Dosing interval in renal impairment:

Cl_{cr} 25-50 mL/minute: 1-2 g every 8 hours

Cl_{cr} 10-25 mL/minute: 1 g every 8 hours

Cl_{cr} <10 mL/minute: 1 g every 12 hours

Hemodialysis: Moderately dialyzable (20% to 50%)

Contraindications Hypersensitivity to cefamandole nafate, any component, or cephalosporins

Pregnancy Risk Factor B

Cefazolin (sef A zoe lin)

Pharmacologic Class Antibiotic, Cephalosporin (First Generation)

U.S. Brand Names Ancef®; Kefzol®; Zolicef®

Generic Available Yes

Mechanism of Action Inhibits bacterial cell wall synthesis by binding to one or more of the penicillin-binding proteins (PBPs) which in turn inhibits the final transpeptidation step of peptidoglycan synthesis in bacterial cell walls, thus inhibiting cell wall biosynthesis. Bacteria eventually lyse due to ongoing activity of cell wall autolytic enzymes (autolysins and murein hydrolases) while cell wall assembly is arrested.

Use Treatment of gram-positive bacilli and cocci (except enterococcus); some gram-negative bacilli including *E. coli*, *Proteus*, and *Klebsiella* may be susceptible

USUAL DOSAGE I.M., I.V.:

Children >1 month: 25-100 mg/kg/day divided every 6-8 hours; maximum: 6 g/day

Adults: 250 mg to 2 g every 6-12 (usually 8) hours, depending on severity of infection; maximum dose: 12 g/day

Dosing adjustment in renal impairment:

Cl_{cr} 10-30 mL/minute: Administer every 12 hours

Cl_{cr} <10 mL/minute: Administer every 24 hours

Hemodialysis: Moderately dialyzable (20% to 50%); administer dose postdialysis or administer supplemental dose of 0.5-1 g after dialysis

Peritoneal dialysis: Administer 0.5 g every 12 hours

Continuous arteriovenous or venovenous hemofiltration (CAVH/CAVHD): Dose as for Cl_{cr} 10-30 mL/minute; removes 30 mg of cefazolin per liter of filtrate per day

Dosage Forms INF premixed in D_5W (frozen) (Ancef®): 500 mg (50 mL); 1 g (50 mL). **INJ** (Kefzol®): 500 mg, 1 g. **POWDER for inj** (Ancef®, Zolicef®): 250 mg, 500 mg, 1 g, 5 g, 10 g, 20 g

Contraindications Hypersensitivity to cefazolin sodium, any component, or cephalosporins

Warnings/Precautions Modify dosage in patients with severe renal impairment; prolonged use may result in superinfection; use with caution in patients with a history of penicillin allergy especially IgE-mediated reactions (eg, anaphylaxis, urticaria); may cause antibiotic-associated colitis or colitis secondary to *C. difficile*

Pregnancy Risk Factor B

Adverse Reactions

1% to 10%:

Gastrointestinal: Diarrhea

Local: Pain at injection site

<1%: Abdominal cramps, anaphylaxis, anorexia, elevated transaminases, eosinophilia, fever, leukopenia, nausea, neutropenia, oral candidiasis, phlebitis, pruritus, pseudomembranous colitis, rash, seizures, Stevens-Johnson syndrome, thrombocytopenia, thrombocytosis, vaginitis, vomiting

Other reactions with cephalosporins include abdominal pain, aplastic anemia, cholestasis, hemolytic anemia, hemorrhage, pancytopenia, prolonged prothrombin time, renal dysfunction, superinfection, toxic epidermal necrolysis, toxic nephropathy

Drug Interactions

Increased effect: High-dose probenecid decreases clearance

Increased toxicity: Aminoglycosides increase nephrotoxic potential

Half-Life 90-150 minutes (prolonged with renal impairment); End-stage renal disease: 40-70 hours

Education and Monitoring Issues

Patient Education: This drug is administered I.V. or I.M. Drink 2-3 L fluid/day. If diarrhea occurs, yogurt or buttermilk may help. May cause false-positive test with Clinitest®; use another form of testing. May interfere with oral contraceptives; additional contraceptive measures are necessary. Report severe, unresolved diarrhea; abdominal

(Continued)

Cefazolin *(Continued)*

pain; vaginal itching or drainage; sores in mouth; blood, pus, or mucus in stool or urine; easy bleeding or bruising; unusual fever or chills; rash; or respiratory difficulty.

Monitoring Parameters: Renal function periodically when used in combination with other nephrotoxic drugs, hepatic function tests, CBC; monitor for signs of anaphylaxis during first dose

Related Information

Animal and Human Bites Guidelines *on page 1177*
Antibiotic Treatment of Adults With Infective Endocarditis *on page 1179*
Prevention of Bacterial Endocarditis *on page 1154*

Cefdinir (SEF di ner)

Pharmacologic Class Antibiotic, Cephalosporin (Third Generation)

U.S. Brand Names Omnicef®

Mechanism of Action Inhibits bacterial cell wall synthesis by binding to one or more of the penicillin-binding proteins (PBPs) which in turn inhibits the final transpeptidation step of peptidoglycan synthesis in bacterial cell walls, thus inhibiting cell wall biosynthesis. Bacteria eventually lyse due to ongoing activity of cell wall autolytic enzymes (autolysins and murein hydrolases) while cell wall assembly is arrested.

Use Treatment of community-acquired pneumonia, acute exacerbations of chronic bronchitis, acute bacterial otitis media, acute maxillary sinusitis, pharyngitis/tonsillitis, and uncomplicated skin and skin structure infections

USUAL DOSAGE Oral:

Children: 7 mg/kg/dose twice daily or 14 mg/kg/dose once daily for 10 days (maximum: 600 mg/day)

Acute otitis: 7 mg/kg twice daily for 5 days

Adolescents and Adults: 300 mg twice daily or 600 mg once daily for 10 days

Chronic bronchitis, acute exacerbation: 300 mg twice daily for 5 days

Dosing adjustment in renal impairment: Cl_{cr} <30 mL/minute: 300 mg once daily

Hemodialysis removes cefdinir; recommended initial dose: 300 mg (or 7 mg/kg/dose) every other day. At the conclusion of each hemodialysis session, 300 mg (or 7 mg/kg/dose) should be given. Subsequent doses (300 mg or 7 mg/kg/dose) should be administered every other day.

Dosage Forms CAP: 300 mg. **SUSP, oral:** 125 mg/5 mL (60 mL, 100 mL)

Contraindications Hypersensitivity to cephalosporins or related antibiotics

Warnings/Precautions Administer cautiously to penicillin-sensitive patients. There is evidence of partial cross-allergenicity and cephalosporins cannot be assumed to be an absolutely safe alternative to penicillin in the penicillin-allergic patient. Serum sickness-like reactions have been reported. Signs and symptoms occur after a few days of therapy and resolve a few days after drug discontinuation with no serious sequelae. Pseudomembranous colitis occurs; consider its diagnosis in patients who develop diarrhea with antibiotic use.

Pregnancy Risk Factor B

Adverse Reactions

>1%: Gastrointestinal: Diarrhea

<1%: Arthralgia, candidiasis, cholestatic jaundice, eosinophilia, headache, hemolytic anemia, interstitial nephritis, nausea, nephrotoxicity with transient elevations of BUN/creatinine, nervousness, neutropenia, positive Coombs' test, pruritus, pseudomembranous colitis, rash, seizures (with high doses and renal dysfunction), serum sickness, slightly increased AST/ALT, Stevens-Johnson syndrome, thrombocytopenia, urticaria, vomiting

Drug Interactions

Decreased effect: Coadministration with iron or antacids reduces the rate and extent of cefdinir absorption

Increased effect: Probenecid increases the effects of cephalosporins by decreasing the renal elimination in those which are secreted by tubular secretion

Increased toxicity: Anticoagulant effects may be increased when administered with cephalosporins

Half-Life 2-4 hours

Education and Monitoring Issues

Patient Education: Take as directed, at regular intervals around-the-clock (with or without food). Chilling oral suspension improves flavor (do not freeze). Complete full course of medication, even if you feel better. Drink 2-3 L fluid/day. If diarrhea occurs, yogurt or buttermilk may help. May cause false-positive test with Clinitest®; use another form of testing. May interfere with oral contraceptives; additional contraceptive measures are necessary. Report severe, unresolved diarrhea; abdominal pain; vaginal itching or drainage; sores in mouth; blood, pus, or mucus in stool or urine; easy bleeding or bruising; unusual fever or chills; rash; or respiratory difficulty.

Monitoring Parameters: Observe for signs and symptoms of anaphylaxis during first dose

Manufacturer Parke-Davis

Related Information

Pharmaceutical Manufacturers Directory *on page 1020*

Cefepime (SEF e pim)

Pharmacologic Class Antibiotic, Cephalosporin (Fourth Generation)

U.S. Brand Names Maxipime®

Mechanism of Action Inhibits bacterial cell wall synthesis by binding to one or more of the penicillin-binding proteins (PBPs) which in turn inhibits the final transpeptidation step of peptidoglycan synthesis in bacterial cell walls, thus inhibiting cell wall biosynthesis. Bacterial eventually lyse due to ongoing activity of cell wall autolytic enzymes (autolysis and murein hydrolases) while cell wall assembly is arrested.

Use Treatment of uncomplicated and complicated urinary tract infections, including pyelonephritis caused by typical urinary tract pathogens; monotherapy for febrile neutropenia; uncomplicated skin and skin structure infections caused by *Streptococcus pyogenes*; moderate to severe pneumonia caused by pneumococcus, *Pseudomonas aeruginosa*, and other gram-negative organisms; complicated intra-abdominal infections (in combination with metronidazole). Also active against methicillin-susceptible staphylococci, *Enterobacter* sp, and many other gram-negative bacilli.

Pediatrics (2 months to 16 years of age): Empiric therapy of febrile neutropenia patients, uncomplicated skin/soft tissue infections, pneumonia, and uncomplicated/complicated urinary tract infections.

USUAL DOSAGE I.V.:

Children:

Febrile neutropenia: 50 mg/kg every 8 hours for 7-10 days

Uncomplicated skin/soft tissue infections, pneumonia, and complicated/uncomplicated UTI: 50 mg/kg twice daily

Adults:

Most infections: 1-2 g every 12 hours for 5-10 days; higher doses or more frequent administration may be required in pseudomonal infections

Urinary tract infections, uncomplicated: 500 mg every 12 hours

Monotherapy for febrile neutropenic patients: 2 g every 8 hours for 7 days or until the neutropenia resolves

Dosing adjustment in renal impairment:

Cefepime Hydrochloride

Creatinine Clearance (mL/minute)	Recommended Maintenance Schedule		
>60 Normal recommended dosing schedule	500 mg every 12 hours	1 g every 12 hours	2 g every 12 hours
30-60	500 mg every 24 hours	1 g every 24 hours	1 g every 24 hours
11-29	500 mg every 24 hours	500 mg every 24 hours	1 g every 24 hours
<10	250 mg every 24 hours	250 mg every 24 hours	500 mg every 24 hours

Hemodialysis: Removed by dialysis; administer supplemental dose of 250 mg after each dialysis session

Peritoneal dialysis: Removed to a lesser extent than hemodialysis; administer 250 mg every 48 hours

Continuous arteriovenous or venovenous hemofiltration (CAVH/CAVHD): Dose as normal Cl_{cr} (eg, >30 mL/minute)

Dosage Forms INF, piggy-back: 1 g (100 mL), 2 g (100 mL); (ADD-Vantage®): 1 g. **INJ:** 500 mg, 1 g, 2 g

Contraindications Hypersensitivity to cefepime or its components, or other cephalosporins

Warnings/Precautions Modify dosage in patients with severe renal impairment; prolonged use may result in superinfection; use with caution in patients with a history of penicillin or cephalosporin allergy, especially IgE-mediated reactions (eg, anaphylaxis, urticaria); may cause antibiotic-associated colitis or colitis secondary to *C. difficile*

Pregnancy Risk Factor B

Adverse Reactions

>10%: Hematologic: Positive Coombs' test without hemolysis

1% to 10%:

Dermatologic: Rash, pruritus

Gastrointestinal: : Diarrhea, nausea, vomiting

Central nervous system: Fever (1%), headache (1%)

Local: Pain, erythema at injection site

<1%: Agranulocytosis, encephalopathy, leukopenia, myoclonus, neuromuscular excitability, neutropenia, seizures, thrombocytopenia

Other reactions with cephalosporins include aplastic anemia, erythema multiforme, hemolytic anemia, hemorrhage, pancytopenia, prolonged PT, renal dysfunction, Stevens-

(Continued)

Cefepime *(Continued)*

Johnson syndrome, superinfection, toxic epidermal necrolysis, toxic nephropathy, vaginitis

Drug Interactions

Increased effect: High-dose probenecid decreases clearance

Increased toxicity: Aminoglycosides increase nephrotoxic potential

Half-Life 2 hours; prolonged in renal impairment

Education and Monitoring Issues

Patient Education: This drug is administered I.V. or I.M. Drink 2-3 L fluid/day. If diarrhea occurs, yogurt or buttermilk may help. May cause false-positive test with Clinitest®; use another form of testing. May interfere with oral contraceptives; additional contraceptive measures are necessary. Report severe, unresolved diarrhea; abdominal pain; vaginal itching or drainage; sores in mouth; blood, pus, or mucus in stool or urine; easy bleeding or bruising; unusual fever or chills; rash; or respiratory difficulty.

Monitoring Parameters: Obtain specimen for culture and sensitivity prior to the first dose; monitor for signs of anaphylaxis during first dose

Manufacturer Bristol-Myers Squibb Company (Pharmaceutical Division)

Related Information

Antimicrobial Drugs of Choice *on page 1182*

Pharmaceutical Manufacturers Directory *on page 1020*

Cefixime (sef IKS eem)

Pharmacologic Class Antibiotic, Cephalosporin (Third Generation)

U.S. Brand Names Suprax®

Generic Available No

Mechanism of Action Inhibits bacterial cell wall synthesis by binding to one or more of the penicillin binding proteins (PBPs); which in turn inhibits the final transpeptidation step of peptidoglycan synthesis in bacterial cell walls, thus inhibiting cell wall biosynthesis. Bacteria eventually lyse due to ongoing activity of cell wall autolytic enzymes (autolysins and murein hydrolases) while cell wall assembly is arrested.

Use Treatment of urinary tract infections, otitis media, respiratory infections due to susceptible organisms including *S. pneumoniae* and *S. pyogenes*, *H. influenzae* and many Enterobacteriaceae; documented poor compliance with other oral antimicrobials; outpatient therapy of serious soft tissue or skeletal infections due to susceptible organisms; single-dose oral treatment of uncomplicated cervical/urethral gonorrhea due to *N. gonorrhoeae*

USUAL DOSAGE Oral:

Children: 8 mg/kg/day divided every 12-24 hours

Adolescents and Adults: 400 mg/day divided every 12-24 hours

Uncomplicated cervical/urethral gonorrhea due to *N. gonorrhoeae*: 400 mg as a single dose

For *S. pyogenes* infections, treat for 10 days; use suspension for otitis media due to increased peak serum levels as compared to tablet form

Dosing adjustment in renal impairment:

Cl_{cr} 21-60 mL/minute or with renal hemodialysis: Administer 75% of the standard dose

Cl_{cr} <20 mL/minute or with CAPD: Administer 50% of the standard dose

Moderately dialyzable (10%)

Dosage Forms POWDER for oral susp (strawberry flavor): 100 mg/5 mL (50 mL, 100 mL). **TAB, film coated:** 200 mg, 400 mg

Contraindications Hypersensitivity to cefixime or cephalosporins

Warnings/Precautions Prolonged use may result in superinfection; modify dosage in patients with renal impairment; use with caution in patients with a history of penicillin allergy especially IgE-mediated reactions (eg, anaphylaxis, urticaria); may cause antibiotic-associated colitis or colitis secondary to *C. difficile*

Pregnancy Risk Factor B

Adverse Reactions

>10%: Gastrointestinal: Diarrhea (16%)

1% to 10%: Gastrointestinal: Abdominal pain, nausea, dyspepsia, flatulence

<1%: Candidiasis, dizziness, eosinophilia, erythema multiforme, fever, headache, increased BUN, increased creatinine, leukopenia, prolonged PT, pruritus, pseudomembranous colitis, rash, serum sickness-like reaction, Stevens-Johnson syndrome, thrombocytopenia, transaminase elevations, urticaria, vaginitis, vomiting

Other reactions with cephalosporins include agranulocytosis, anaphylaxis, aplastic anemia, cholestasis, colitis, hemolytic anemia, hemorrhage, interstitial nephritis, neutropenia, pancytopenia, renal dysfunction, seizures, superinfection, toxic epidermal necrolysis, toxic nephropathy

Drug Interactions

Increased effect: Probenecid may decrease cephalosporin elimination

Increased toxicity: Furosemide, aminoglycosides may be a possible additive to nephrotoxicity

Half-Life Normal renal function: 3-4 hours; Renal failure: Up to 11.5 hours

Education and Monitoring Issues

Patient Education: Take as directed, at regular intervals around-the-clock (with or without food). Chilling oral suspension improves flavor (do not freeze). Complete full course of medication, even if you feel better. Drink 2-3 L fluid/day. If diarrhea occurs, yogurt or buttermilk may help. May cause false-positive test with Clinitest®; use another form of testing. May interfere with oral contraceptives; additional contraceptive measures are necessary. Report severe, unresolved diarrhea; abdominal pain; vaginal itching or drainage; sores in mouth; blood, pus, or mucus in stool or urine; easy bleeding or bruising; unusual fever or chills,; rash; or respiratory difficulty.

Monitoring Parameters: With prolonged therapy, monitor renal and hepatic function periodically; observe for signs and symptoms of anaphylaxis during first dose

Manufacturer Lederle Laboratories

Related Information

Antimicrobial Drugs of Choice *on page 1182*
Pharmaceutical Manufacturers Directory *on page 1020*
Treatment of Sexually Transmitted Diseases *on page 1210*

♦ **Cefizox®** *see* Ceftizoxime *on page 163*

Cefmetazole (sef MET a zole)

Pharmacologic Class Antibiotic, Cephalosporin (Second Generation)

U.S. Brand Names Zefazone®

Generic Available No

Mechanism of Action Inhibits bacterial cell wall synthesis by binding to one or more of the penicillin-binding proteins (PBPs) which in turn inhibits the final transpeptidation step of peptidoglycan synthesis in bacterial cell walls, thus inhibiting cell wall biosynthesis. Bacteria eventually lyse due to ongoing activity of cell wall autolytic enzymes (autolysins and murein hydrolases) while cell wall assembly is arrested.

Use Second generation cephalosporin, useful for susceptible aerobic and anaerobic gram-positive and gram-negative bacteria; surgical prophylaxis, specifically colorectal and OB-GYN

USUAL DOSAGE Adults: I.V.:

Infections: 2 g every 6-12 hours for 5-14 days

Prophylaxis: 2 g 30-90 minutes before surgery **or** 1 g 30-90 minutes before surgery; repeat 8 and 16 hours later

Dosing interval in renal impairment:

Cl_{cr} 50-90 mL/minute: Administer every 12 hours

Cl_{cr} 10-50 mL/minute: Administer every 16-24 hours

Cl_{cr} <10 mL/minute: Administer every 48 hours

Dosage Forms POWDER for inj: 1 g, 2 g

Contraindications Hypersensitivity to cefmetazole or any component or cephalosporins

Warnings/Precautions Modify dosage in patients with severe renal impairment; prolonged use may result in superinfection; use with caution in patients with a history of penicillin allergy especially IgE-mediated reactions (eg, anaphylaxis, urticaria); may cause antibiotic-associated colitis or colitis secondary to *C. difficile*

Pregnancy Risk Factor B

Adverse Reactions Contains MTT side chain which may lead to increased risk of hypoprothrombinemia and bleeding.

1% to 10%:

Dermatologic: Rash

Gastrointestinal: Diarrhea

<1%: Bleeding, candidiasis, dyspnea, epigastric pain, epistaxis, fever, headache, hot flashes, hypotension, pain at injection site, phlebitis, pseudomembranous colitis, respiratory distress, shock, vaginitis

Other reactions with cephalosporins include agranulocytosis, anaphylaxis, aplastic anemia, cholestasis, colitis, erythema multiforme, hemolytic anemia, hemorrhage, interstitial nephritis, neutropenia, pancytopenia, renal dysfunction, seizures, Stevens-Johnson syndrome, superinfection, toxic epidermal necrolysis, toxic nephropathy

Drug Interactions

Increased effect: Probenecid may decrease cephalosporin elimination

Increased toxicity: Furosemide, aminoglycosides may be a possible additive to nephrotoxicity

Alcohol Interactions Avoid use (may cause a disulfiram-like reaction; symptoms include headache, nausea, vomiting, chest or abdominal pain)

Half-Life 72 minutes; prolonged in renal impairment

Education and Monitoring Issues

Patient Education: This drug is administered I.V. or I.M. Drink 2-3 L fluid/day. Avoid alcohol during therapy and for 72 hours after last dose (may cause severe disulfiram-like reactions). If diarrhea occurs, yogurt or buttermilk may help. May cause false-positive test with Clinitest®; use another form of testing. May interfere with oral contraceptives; additional contraceptive measures are necessary. Report severe, unresolved diarrhea; vaginal itching or drainage; sores in mouth; blood, pus, or mucus in stool or urine; easy bleeding or bruising; unusual fever or chills; rash; or respiratory difficulty.

(Continued)

Cefmetazole *(Continued)*

Monitoring Parameters: Monitor prothrombin times; observe for signs and symptoms of anaphylaxis during first dose

Related Information

Antimicrobial Drugs of Choice *on page 1182*

- **Cefobid®** *see* Cefoperazone *on page 155*
- **Cefol® Filmtab®** *see* Vitamins, Multiple *on page 981*

Cefonicid (se FON i sid)

Pharmacologic Class Antibiotic, Cephalosporin (Second Generation)

U.S. Brand Names Monocid®

Generic Available No

Mechanism of Action Inhibits bacterial cell wall synthesis by binding to one or more of the penicillin-binding proteins (PBPs) which in turn inhibits the final transpeptidation step of peptidoglycan synthesis in bacterial cell walls, thus inhibiting cell wall biosynthesis. Bacteria eventually lyse due to ongoing activity of cell wall autolytic enzymes (autolysins and murein hydrolases) while cell wall assembly is arrested.

Use Treatment of susceptible bacterial infection; mainly respiratory tract, skin and skin structure, bone and joint, urinary tract and gynecologic, septicemia; active against methicillin-sensitive staphylococci, many streptococci, and various gram-negative bacilli including *E. coli*, some *Klebsiella*, *P. mirabilis*, *H. influenzae*, and *Moraxella*.

USUAL DOSAGE Adults: I.M., I.V.: 0.5-2 g every 24 hours

Prophylaxis: Preop: 1 g/hour

Dosing interval in renal impairment: See table.

Cefonicid Sodium

Cl_{cr} (mL/min/1.73 m^2)	Dose (mg/kg) for Each Dosing Interval
60-79	10-24 q24h
40-59	8-20 q24h
20-39	4-15 q24h
10-19	4-15 q48h
5-9	4-15 q3-5d
<5	3-4 q3-5d

Dosage Forms POWDER for inj: 500 mg, 1 g, 10 g

Contraindications Hypersensitivity to cefonicid sodium, any component, or cephalosporins

Warnings/Precautions Modify dosage in patients with severe renal impairment; prolonged use may result in superinfection; use with caution in patients with a history of penicillin allergy especially IgE-mediated reactions (eg, anaphylaxis, urticaria); may cause antibiotic-associated colitis or colitis secondary to *C. difficile*

Pregnancy Risk Factor B

Adverse Reactions

1% to 10%:

Hematologic: Increased eosinophils (2.9%), increased platelets (1.7%)

Hepatic: Altered liver function tests (increased transaminases, LDH, alkaline phosphatase) (1.6%)

Local: Pain, burning at injection site (5.7%)

<1%: Abdominal pain, anaphylactoid reactions, decreased WBC, diarrhea, erythema, fever, increased BUN, increased creatinine, increased transaminases, interstitial nephritis, neutropenia, pruritus, pseudomembranous colitis, rash, thrombocytopenia

Other reactions with cephalosporins include agranulocytosis, anaphylaxis, aplastic anemia, cholestasis, colitis, hemolytic anemia, hemorrhage, pancytopenia, renal dysfunction, seizures, Stevens-Johnson syndrome, superinfection, toxic epidermal necrolysis, toxic nephropathy

Drug Interactions

Increased effect: Probenecid may decrease cephalosporin elimination

Increased toxicity: Furosemide, aminoglycosides may be a possible additive to nephrotoxicity

Half-Life 6-7 hours; prolonged in renal impairment

Education and Monitoring Issues

Patient Education: This medication is administered I.M. or I.V. Drink 2-3 L fluid/day. If diarrhea occurs, yogurt or buttermilk may help. May cause false-positive test with Clinitest®; use another form of testing. May interfere with oral contraceptives; additional contraceptive measures are necessary. Report severe, unresolved diarrhea; abdominal pain; vaginal itching or drainage; sores in mouth; blood, pus, or mucus in stool or urine; easy bleeding or bruising; unusual fever or chills; rash; or respiratory difficulty.

Monitoring Parameters: Observe for signs and symptoms of anaphylaxis during first dose

Cefoperazone (sef oh PER a zone)

Pharmacologic Class Antibiotic, Cephalosporin (Third Generation)

U.S. Brand Names Cefobid®

Generic Available No

Mechanism of Action Inhibits bacterial cell wall synthesis by binding to one or more of the penicillin-binding proteins (PBPs) which in turn inhibits the final transpeptidation step of peptidoglycan synthesis in bacterial cell walls, thus inhibiting cell wall biosynthesis. Bacteria eventually lyse due to ongoing activity of cell wall autolytic enzymes (autolysins and murein hydrolases) while cell wall assembly is arrested.

Use Treatment of susceptible bacterial infection; mainly respiratory tract, skin and skin structure, bone and joint, urinary tract and gynecologic as well as septicemia. Active against a variety of gram-negative bacilli, some gram-positive cocci, and has some activity against *Pseudomonas aeruginosa.*

USUAL DOSAGE I.M., I.V.:

Children (not approved): 100-150 mg/kg/day divided every 8-12 hours; up to 12 g/day

Adults: 2-4 g/day in divided doses every 12 hours; up to 12 g/day

Dosing adjustment in hepatic impairment: Reduce dose 50% in patients with advanced liver cirrhosis; maximum daily dose: 4 g

Dosage Forms INJ, premixed (frozen): 1 g (50 mL); 2 g (50 mL). **POWDER for inj:** 1 g, 2 g

Contraindications Hypersensitivity to cefoperazone or any component or cephalosporins

Warnings/Precautions Modify dosage in patients with severe renal or hepatic impairment; prolonged use may result in superinfection; although rare, cefoperazone may interfere with hemostasis via destruction of vitamin K-producing intestinal bacteria, prevention of activation of prothrombin by the attachment of a methyltetrazolethiol side chain, and by an immune-mediated thrombocytopenia; use with caution in patients with a history of penicillin allergy especially IgE-mediated reactions (eg, anaphylaxis, urticaria); may cause antibiotic-associated colitis or colitis secondary to *C. difficile*

Pregnancy Risk Factor B

Adverse Reactions Contains MTT side chain which may lead to increased risk of hypoprothrombinemia and bleeding.

1% to 10%:

Dermatologic: Rash (maculopapular or erythematous) (2%)

Gastrointestinal: Diarrhea (3%)

Hematologic: Decreased neutrophils (2%), decreased hemoglobin or hematocrit (5%), eosinophilia (10%)

Hepatic: Increased transaminases (5% to 10%)

<1%: Bleeding, drug fever, elevated BUN, elevated creatinine, hypoprothrombinemia, induration at injection site, nausea, pain at injection site, phlebitis, pseudomembranous colitis, vomiting

Other reactions with cephalosporins include agranulocytosis, anaphylaxis, aplastic anemia, cholestasis, colitis, hemolytic anemia, pancytopenia, renal dysfunction, seizures, Stevens-Johnson syndrome, superinfection, toxic epidermal necrolysis, toxic nephropathy

Drug Interactions

Disulfiram-like reaction has been reported when taken within 72 hours of alcohol consumption

Increased nephrotoxicity: Aminoglycosides, furosemide

Alcohol Interactions Avoid use (may cause a disulfiram-like reaction; symptoms include headache, nausea, vomiting, chest or abdominal pain)

Half-Life 2 hours, higher with hepatic disease or biliary obstruction

Education and Monitoring Issues

Patient Education: This drug is administered I.M. or I.V. Drink 2-3 L fluid/day. Avoid alcohol during therapy and for 72 hours after last dose (may cause severe disulfiram-like reactions). If diarrhea occurs, yogurt or buttermilk may help. May cause false-positive test with Clinitest®; use another form of testing. May interfere with oral contraceptives; additional contraceptive measures are necessary. Report severe, unresolved diarrhea; abdominal pain; vaginal itching or drainage; sores in mouth; blood, pus, or mucus in stool or urine; easy bleeding or bruising; unusual fever or chills; rash; or respiratory difficulty.

Monitoring Parameters: Monitor for coagulation abnormalities and diarrhea; observe for signs and symptoms of anaphylaxis during first dose

Manufacturer Pfizer U.S. Pharmaceutical Group

Related Information

Pharmaceutical Manufacturers Directory *on page 1020*

♦ **Cefotan®** *see* Cefotetan *on page 157*

Cefotaxime (sef oh TAKS eem)

Pharmacologic Class Antibiotic, Cephalosporin (Third Generation)

U.S. Brand Names Claforan®

Generic Available No

Mechanism of Action Inhibits bacterial cell wall synthesis by binding to one or more of the penicillin-binding proteins (PBPs) which in turn inhibits the final transpeptidation step of peptidoglycan synthesis in bacterial cell walls, thus inhibiting cell wall biosynthesis. Bacteria eventually lyse due to ongoing activity of cell wall autolytic enzymes (autolysins and murein hydrolases) while cell wall assembly is arrested.

Use Treatment of susceptible infection in respiratory tract, skin and skin structure, bone and joint, urinary tract, gynecologic as well as septicemia, and documented or suspected meningitis. Active against most gram-negative bacilli (not *Pseudomonas*) and gram-positive cocci (not enterococcus). Active against many penicillin-resistant pneumococci.

USUAL DOSAGE

Neonates: I.V.:
- 0-1 week: 50 mg/kg every 12 hours
- 1-4 weeks: 50 mg/kg every 8 hours

Infants and Children 1 month to 12 years: I.M., I.V.: <50 kg: 50-180 mg/kg/day in divided doses every 4-6 hours
- Meningitis: 200 mg/kg/day in divided doses every 6 hours

Children >12 years and Adults:
- Gonorrhea: I.M.: 1 g as a single dose
- Uncomplicated infections: I.M., I.V.: 1 g every 12 hours
- Moderate/severe infections: I.M., I.V.: 1-2 g every 8 hours
- Infections commonly needing higher doses (eg, septicemia): I.V.: 2 g every 6-8 hours
- Life-threatening infections: I.V.: 2 g every 4 hours
- Preop: I.M., I.V.: 1 g 30-90 minutes before surgery
- C-section: 1 g as soon as the umbilical cord is clamped, then 1 g I.M., I.V. at 6- and 12-hours intervals

Dosing interval in renal impairment:
- Cl_{cr} 10-50 mL/minute: Administer every 8-12 hours
- Cl_{cr} <10 mL/minute: Administer every 24 hours

Hemodialysis: Moderately dialyzable

Dosing adjustment in hepatic impairment: Moderate dosage reduction is recommended in severe liver disease

Continuous arteriovenous or venovenous hemodiafiltration (CAVH) effects: Administer 1 g every 12 hour

Dosage Forms INF, premixed in D_5W (frozen): 1 g (50 mL); 2 g (50 mL). **POWDER for inj:** 500 mg, 1 g, 2 g, 10 g

Contraindications Hypersensitivity to cefotaxime, any component, or cephalosporins

Warnings/Precautions Modify dosage in patients with severe renal impairment; prolonged use may result in superinfection; a potentially life-threatening arrhythmia has been reported in patients who received a rapid bolus injection via central line. Use caution in patients with colitis; minimize tissue inflammation by changing infusion sites when needed. Use with caution in patients with a history of penicillin allergy especially IgE-mediated reactions (eg, anaphylaxis, urticaria); may cause antibiotic-associated colitis or colitis secondary to *C. difficile*.

Pregnancy Risk Factor B

Adverse Reactions

1% to 10%:
- Dermatologic: Rash, pruritus
- Gastrointestinal: Diarrhea, nausea, vomiting, colitis
- Local: Pain at injection site

<1%: Anaphylaxis, arrhythmias (after rapid IV injection via central catheter), candidiasis, eosinophilia, fever, headache, increased BUN, increased creatinine, increased transaminases, interstitial nephritis, neutropenia, phlebitis, pseudomembranous colitis, thrombocytopenia, transaminase elevations, urticaria, vaginitis

Other reactions with cephalosporins include agranulocytosis, aplastic anemia, cholestasis, colitis, hemolytic anemia, hemorrhage, pancytopenia, renal dysfunction, seizures, Stevens-Johnson syndrome, superinfection, toxic epidermal necrolysis, toxic nephropathy

Drug Interactions

Increased effect: Probenecid may decrease cephalosporin elimination

Increased toxicity: Furosemide, aminoglycosides may be a possible additive to nephrotoxicity

Half-Life

Cefotaxime: 1-1.5 hours (prolonged with renal and/or hepatic impairment)

Desacetylcefotaxime: 1.5-1.9 hours (prolonged with renal impairment)

Education and Monitoring Issues

Patient Education: This medication is administered I.M. or I.V. Drink 2-3 L fluid/day. If diarrhea occurs, yogurt or buttermilk may help. May cause false-positive test with Clinitest®; use another form of testing. May interfere with oral contraceptives; additional contraceptive measures are necessary. Report severe, unresolved diarrhea;abdominal pain; vaginal itching or drainage; sores in mouth; blood, pus, or mucus in stool or urine; easy bleeding or bruising; unusual fever or chills; rash; or respiratory difficulty.

Monitoring Parameters: Observe for signs and symptoms of anaphylaxis during first dose; CBC with differential (especially with long courses)

Manufacturer Hoechst-Marion Roussel

Related Information

Antibiotic Treatment of Adults With Infective Endocarditis *on page 1179*
Antimicrobial Drugs of Choice *on page 1182*
Community Acquired Pneumonia in Adults *on page 1200*
Pharmaceutical Manufacturers Directory *on page 1020*
Treatment of Sexually Transmitted Diseases *on page 1210*

Cefotetan (SEF oh tee tan)

Pharmacologic Class Antibiotic, Cephalosporin (Second Generation)

U.S. Brand Names Cefotan®

Generic Available No

Mechanism of Action Inhibits bacterial cell wall synthesis by binding to one or more of the penicillin-binding proteins (PBPs) which in turn inhibits the final transpeptidation step of peptidoglycan synthesis in bacterial cell walls, thus inhibiting cell wall biosynthesis. Bacteria eventually lyse due to ongoing activity of cell wall autolytic enzymes (autolysins and murein hydrolases) while cell wall assembly is arrested.

Use Less active against staphylococci and streptococci than first generation cephalosporins, but active against anaerobes including *Bacteroides fragilis*; active against gram-negative enteric bacilli including *E. coli*, *Klebsiella*, and *Proteus*; used predominantly for respiratory tract, skin and skin structure, bone and joint, urinary tract and gynecologic as well as septicemia; surgical prophylaxis; intra-abdominal infections and other mixed infections

USUAL DOSAGE I.M., I.V.:

Children: 20-40 mg/kg/dose every 12 hours

Adults: 1-6 g/day in divided doses every 12 hours; usual dose: 1-2 g every 12 hours for 5-10 days; 1-2 g may be given every 24 hours for urinary tract infection

Dosing interval in renal impairment:

Cl_{cr} 10-30 mL/minute: Administer every 24 hours

Cl_{cr} <10 mL/minute: Administer every 48 hours

Hemodialysis: Slightly dialyzable (5% to 20%)

Continuous arteriovenous or venovenous hemodiafiltration (CAVH) effects: Administer 750 mg every 12 hours

Dosage Forms POWDER for inj: 1 g (10 mL, 100 mL), 2 g (20 mL, 100 mL), 10 g (100 mL)

Contraindications Hypersensitivity to cefotetan, any component, or cephalosporins

Warnings/Precautions Modify dosage in patients with severe renal impairment; prolonged use may result in superinfection; although cefotetan contains the methyltetrazolethiol side chain, bleeding has not been a significant problem; use with caution in patients with a history of penicillin allergy especially IgE-mediated reactions (eg, anaphylaxis, urticaria); may cause antibiotic-associated colitis or colitis secondary to *C. difficile*

Pregnancy Risk Factor B

Adverse Reactions Contains MTT side chain which may lead to increased risk of hypoprothrombinemia and bleeding.

1% to 10%:

Gastrointestinal: Diarrhea (1.3%)

Hepatic: Increased transaminases (1.2%)

Miscellaneous: Hypersensitivity reactions (1.2%)

<1%: Agranulocytosis, anaphylaxis, bleeding, elevated BUN, elevated creatinine, eosinophilia, fever, hemolytic anemia, leukopenia, nausea, nephrotoxicity, phlebitis, prolonged PT, pruritus, pseudomembranous colitis, rash, thrombocytopenia, thrombocytosis, urticaria, vomiting

Other reactions with cephalosporins include agranulocytosis, aplastic anemia, cholestasis, colitis, hemolytic anemia, hemorrhage, pancytopenia, renal dysfunction, seizures, Stevens-Johnson syndrome, superinfection, toxic epidermal necrolysis, toxic nephropathy

Drug Interactions

Disulfiram-like reaction has been reported when taken within 72 hours of alcohol consumption

Increased cephalosporin plasma levels: Probenecid

Increased nephrotoxicity: Aminoglycosides, furosemide

Alcohol Interactions Avoid use (may cause a disulfiram-like reaction; symptoms include headache, nausea, vomiting, chest or abdominal pain)

Half-Life 1.5-3 hours; prolonged in severe renal impairment

Education and Monitoring Issues

Patient Education: This medication is administered I.V. or I.M. Drink 2-3 L fluid/day. Avoid alcohol during therapy and for 72 hours after last dose (may cause severe

(Continued)

Cefotetan *(Continued)*

disulfiram-like reactions). If diarrhea occurs, yogurt or buttermilk may help. May cause false-positive test with Clinitest®; use another form of testing. May interfere with oral contraceptives; additional contraceptive measures are necessary. Report severe, unresolved diarrhea; abdominal pain; vaginal itching or drainage; sores in mouth; blood, pus, or mucus in stool or urine; easy bleeding or bruising; unusual fever or chills; rash; or respiratory difficulty.

Monitoring Parameters: Observe for signs and symptoms of anaphylaxis during first dose

Manufacturer AstraZeneca

Related Information

Animal and Human Bites Guidelines *on page 1177*
Antimicrobial Drugs of Choice *on page 1182*
Pharmaceutical Manufacturers Directory *on page 1020*
Treatment of Sexually Transmitted Diseases *on page 1210*

Cefoxitin (se FOKS i tin)

Pharmacologic Class Antibiotic, Cephalosporin (Second Generation)

U.S. Brand Names Mefoxin®

Generic Available No

Mechanism of Action Inhibits bacterial cell wall synthesis by binding to one or more of the penicillin-binding proteins (PBPs) which in turn inhibits the final transpeptidation step of peptidoglycan synthesis in bacterial cell walls, thus inhibiting cell wall biosynthesis. Bacteria eventually lyse due to ongoing activity of cell wall autolytic enzymes (autolysins and murein hydrolases) while cell wall assembly is arrested.

Use Less active against staphylococci and streptococci than first generation cephalosporins, but active against anaerobes including *Bacteroides fragilis*; active against gram-negative enteric bacilli including *E. coli*, *Klebsiella*, and *Proteus*; used predominantly for respiratory tract, skin and skin structure, bone and joint, urinary tract and gynecologic as well as septicemia; surgical prophylaxis; intra-abdominal infections and other mixed infections

USUAL DOSAGE I.M., I.V.:

Infants >3 months and Children:
- Mild to moderate infection: 80-100 mg/kg/day in divided doses every 4-6 hours
- Severe infection: 100-160 mg/kg/day in divided doses every 4-6 hours
- Maximum dose: 12 g/day

Adults: 1-2 g every 6-8 hours (I.M. injection is painful); up to 12 g/day

Dosing interval in renal impairment:
- Cl_{cr} 30-50 mL/minute: Administer every 8-12 hours
- Cl_{cr} 10-30 mL/minute: Administer every 12-24 hours
- Cl_{cr} <10 mL/minute: Administer every 24-48 hours

Hemodialysis: Moderately dialyzable (20% to 50%)

Continuous arteriovenous or venovenous hemodiafiltration (CAVH) effects: Dose as for Cl_{cr} 10-50 mL/minute

Dosage Forms INF, premixed in D_5W (frozen): 1 g (50 mL); 2 g (50 mL). **POWDER for inj:** 1 g, 2 g, 10 g

Contraindications Hypersensitivity to cefoxitin, any component, or cephalosporins

Warnings/Precautions Use with caution in patients with history of colitis; cefoxitin may increase resistance of organisms by inducing beta-lactamase; modify dosage in patients with severe renal impairment; prolonged use may result in superinfection; use with caution in patients with a history of penicillin allergy especially IgE-mediated reactions (eg, anaphylaxis, urticaria); may cause antibiotic-associated colitis or colitis secondary to *C. difficile*

Pregnancy Risk Factor B

Adverse Reactions

1% to 10%: Gastrointestinal: Diarrhea

<1%: Anaphylaxis, angioedema, bone marrow suppression, dyspnea, eosinophilia, exacerbation of myasthenia gravis, exfoliative dermatitis, fever, hemolytic anemia, hypotension, increased BUN, increased creatinine, increased nephrotoxicity (with aminoglycosides), increased transaminases, interstitial nephritis, jaundice, leukopenia, nausea, phlebitis, prolonged PT, pruritus, pseudomembranous colitis, rash, thrombocytopenia, thrombophlebitis, toxic epidermal necrolysis, vomiting

Other reactions with cephalosporins include agranulocytosis, aplastic anemia, cholestasis, colitis, erythema multiforme, hemolytic anemia, hemorrhage, pancytopenia, renal dysfunction, seizures, serum-sickness reactions, Stevens-Johnson syndrome, superinfection, toxic epidermal necrolysis, toxic nephropathy, urticaria, vaginitis

Drug Interactions

Increased effect: Probenecid may decrease cephalosporin elimination

Increased toxicity: Furosemide, aminoglycosides may be a possible additive to nephrotoxicity

Half-Life 45-60 minutes, increases significantly with renal insufficiency

Education and Monitoring Issues

Patient Education: This medication is administered I.M. or I.V. Drink 2-3 L fluid/day. If diarrhea occurs, yogurt or buttermilk may help. May cause false-positive test with Clinitest®; use another form of testing. May interfere with oral contraceptives; additional contraceptive measures are necessary. Report severe, unresolved diarrhea; abdominal pain; vaginal itching or drainage; sores in mouth; blood, pus, or mucus in stool or urine; easy bleeding or bruising; unusual fever or chills; rash; or respiratory difficulty.

Monitoring Parameters: Monitor renal function periodically when used in combination with other nephrotoxic drugs; observe for signs and symptoms of anaphylaxis during first dose

Related Information

Antimicrobial Drugs of Choice *on page 1182*

Treatment of Sexually Transmitted Diseases *on page 1210*

Cefpodoxime (sef pode OKS eem)

Pharmacologic Class Antibiotic, Cephalosporin (Second Generation)

U.S. Brand Names Vantin®

Generic Available No

Mechanism of Action Inhibits bacterial cell wall synthesis by binding to one or more of the penicillin-binding proteins (PBPs) which in turn inhibits the final transpeptidation step of peptidoglycan synthesis in bacterial cell walls, thus inhibiting cell wall biosynthesis. Bacteria eventually lyse due to ongoing activity of cell wall autolytic enzymes (autolysins and murein hydrolases) while cell wall assembly is arrested.

Use Treatment of susceptible acute, community-acquired pneumonia caused by *S. pneumoniae* or nonbeta-lactamase producing *H. influenzae*; acute uncomplicated gonorrhea caused by *N. gonorrhoeae*; uncomplicated skin and skin structure infections caused by *S. aureus* or *S. pyogenes*; acute otitis media caused by *S. pneumoniae, H. influenzae*, or *M. catarrhalis*; pharyngitis or tonsillitis; and uncomplicated urinary tract infections caused by *E. coli, Klebsiella*, and *Proteus*

USUAL DOSAGE Oral:

Children >5 months to 12 years:

Acute otitis media: 10 mg/kg/day as a single dose or divided every 12 hours (400 mg/day)

Pharyngitis/tonsillitis: 10 mg/kg/day in 2 divided doses (maximum: 200 mg/day)

Children ≥13 years and Adults:

Acute community-acquired pneumonia and bacterial exacerbations of chronic bronchitis: 200 mg every 12 hours for 14 days and 10 days, respectively

Skin and skin structure: 400 mg every 12 hours for 7-14 days

Uncomplicated gonorrhea (male and female) and rectal gonococcal infections (female): 200 mg as a single dose

Pharyngitis/tonsillitis: 100 mg every 12 hours for 10 days

Uncomplicated urinary tract infection: 100 mg every 12 hours for 7 days

Dosing adjustment in renal impairment: Cl_{cr} <30 mL/minute: Administer every 24 hours

Dosage Forms GRANULES for oral susp (lemon creme flavor): 50 mg/5 mL (100 mL); 100 mg/5 mL (100 mL). **TAB, film coated:** 100 mg, 200 mg

Contraindications Hypersensitivity to cefpodoxime or cephalosporins

Warnings/Precautions Modify dosage in patients with severe renal impairment; prolonged use may result in superinfection; a low incidence of cross-hypersensitivity to penicillins exists

Pregnancy Risk Factor B

Adverse Reactions

>10%:

Dermatologic: Diaper rash (12.1%)

Gastrointestinal: Diarrhea in infants and toddlers (15.4%)

1% to 10%:

Central nervous system: Headache (1.1%)

Dermatologic: Rash (1.4%)

Gastrointestinal: Diarrhea (7.2%), nausea (3.8%), abdominal pain (1.6%), vomiting (1.1% to 2.1%)

Genitourinary: Vaginal infections (3.1%)

<1%: Anaphylaxis, anxiety, chest pain, cough, decreased appetite, decreased salivation, dizziness, epistaxis, eye itching, fatigue, fever, flatulence, flushing, fungal skin infection, hypotension, insomnia, malaise, nightmares, pruritus, purpuric nephritis, pseudomembranous colitis, taste alteration, tinnitus, vaginal candidiasis, weakness

Other reactions with cephalosporins include agranulocytosis, aplastic anemia, cholestasis, colitis, erythema multiforme, hemolytic anemia, hemorrhage, interstitial nephritis, pancytopenia, renal dysfunction, seizures, serum-sickness reactions, Stevens-Johnson syndrome, superinfection, toxic epidermal necrolysis, toxic nephropathy, urticaria, vaginitis

Drug Interactions

Decreased effect: Antacids and H_2-receptor antagonists (reduce absorption and serum concentration of cefpodoxime)

Increased effect: Probenecid may decrease cephalosporin elimination

(Continued)

Cefpodoxime *(Continued)*

Increased toxicity: Furosemide, aminoglycosides may be a possible additive to nephrotoxicity

Half-Life 2.2 hours (prolonged with renal impairment)

Education and Monitoring Issues

Patient Education: Take as directed, at regular intervals around-the-clock (with or without food). Chilling oral suspension improves flavor (do not freeze). Complete full course of medication, even if you feel better. Drink 2-3 L fluid/day. If diarrhea occurs, yogurt or buttermilk may help. May cause false-positive test with Clinitest®; use another form of testing. May interfere with oral contraceptives; additional contraceptive measures are necessary. Report severe, unresolved diarrhea; abdominal pain; vaginal itching or drainage; sores in mouth; blood, pus, or mucus in stool or urine; easy bleeding or bruising; unusual fever or chills; rash; or respiratory difficulty.

Monitoring Parameters: Observe for signs and symptoms of anaphylaxis during first dose

Manufacturer Pharmacia & Upjohn

Related Information

Antimicrobial Drugs of Choice *on page 1182*
Community Acquired Pneumonia in Adults *on page 1200*
Pharmaceutical Manufacturers Directory *on page 1020*
Treatment of Sexually Transmitted Diseases *on page 1210*

Cefprozil (sef PROE zil)

Pharmacologic Class Antibiotic, Cephalosporin (Second Generation)

U.S. Brand Names Cefzil®

Generic Available No

Mechanism of Action Inhibits bacterial cell wall synthesis by binding to one or more of the penicillin-binding proteins (PBPs) which in turn inhibits the final transpeptidation step of peptidoglycan synthesis in bacterial cell walls, thus inhibiting cell wall biosynthesis. Bacteria eventually lyse due to ongoing activity of cell wall autolytic enzymes (autolysins and murein hydrolases) while cell wall assembly is arrested.

Use Treatment of otitis media and infections involving the respiratory tract and skin and skin structure; Active against methicillin-sensitive staphylococci, many streptococci, and various gram-negative bacilli including *E. coli*, some *Klebsiella*, *P. mirabilis*, *H. influenzae*, and *Moraxella*.

USUAL DOSAGE Oral:

Infants and Children >6 months to 12 years: Otitis media: 15 mg/kg every 12 hours for 10 days

Pharyngitis/tonsillitis:

Children 2-12 years: 7.5 -15 mg/kg/day divided every 12 hours for 10 days (administer for >10 days if due to *S. pyogenes*); maximum: 1 g/day

Children >13 years and Adults: 500 mg every 24 hours for 10 days

Uncomplicated skin and skin structure infections:

Children 2-12 years: 20 mg/kg every 24 hours for 10 days; maximum: 1 g/day

Children >13 years and Adults: 250 mg every 12 hours, or 500 mg every 12-24 hours for 10 days

Secondary bacterial infection of acute bronchitis or acute bacterial exacerbation of chronic bronchitis: 500 mg every 12 hours for 10 days

Dosing adjustment in renal impairment: Cl_{cr} <30 mL/minute: Reduce dose by 50%

Hemodialysis: Reduced by hemodialysis; administer dose after the completion of hemodialysis

Dosage Forms POWDER for oral susp, as anhydrous: 125 mg/5 mL (50 mL, 75 mL, 100 mL); 250 mg/5 mL (50 mL, 75 mL, 100 mL). **TAB,** as anhydrous: 250 mg, 500 mg

Contraindications Hypersensitivity to cefprozil or any component or cephalosporins

Warnings/Precautions Modify dosage in patients with severe renal impairment; prolonged use may result in superinfection; use with caution in patients with a history of penicillin allergy especially IgE-mediated reactions (eg, anaphylaxis, urticaria); may cause antibiotic-associated colitis or colitis secondary to *C. difficile*

Pregnancy Risk Factor B

Adverse Reactions

1% to 10%:

Central nervous system: Dizziness (1%)
Dermatologic: Diaper rash (1.5%)
Gastrointestinal: Diarrhea (2.9%), nausea (3.5%), vomiting (1%), abdominal pain (1%)
Genitourinary: Vaginitis, genital pruritus (1.6%)
Hepatic: Increased transaminases (2%)
Miscellaneous: Superinfection

<1%: Anaphylaxis, angioedema, arthralgia, cholestatic jaundice, confusion, elevated BUN, elevated creatinine, eosinophilia, erythema multiforme, fever, headache, hyperactivity, insomnia, leukopenia, pseudomembranous colitis, rash, serum sickness, somnolence, Stevens-Johnson syndrome, thrombocytopenia, urticaria

Other reactions with cephalosporins include agranulocytosis, aplastic anemia, colitis, hemolytic anemia, hemorrhage, interstitial nephritis, pancytopenia, renal dysfunction, seizures, superinfection, toxic epidermal necrolysis, toxic nephropathy, vaginitis

Drug Interactions

Increased effect: Probenecid may decrease cephalosporin elimination

Increased toxicity: Furosemide, aminoglycosides may be a possible additive to nephrotoxicity

Half-Life 1.3 hours (normal renal function)

Education and Monitoring Issues

Patient Education: Take as directed, at regular intervals around-the-clock (with or without food). Chilling oral suspension improves flavor (do not freeze). Complete full course of medication, even if you feel better. Drink 2-3 L fluid/day. If diarrhea occurs, yogurt or buttermilk may help. May cause false-positive test with Clinitest®; use another form of testing. May interfere with oral contraceptives; additional contraceptive measures are necessary. Report severe, unresolved diarrhea; abdominal pain; vaginal itching or drainage; sores in mouth; blood, pus, or mucus in stool or urine; easy bleeding or bruising; unusual fever or chills; rash; or respiratory difficulty.

Monitoring Parameters: Assess patient at beginning and throughout therapy for infection; monitor for signs of anaphylaxis during first dose

Manufacturer Bristol-Myers Squibb Company (Pharmaceutical Division)

Related Information

Community Acquired Pneumonia in Adults *on page 1200*
Pharmaceutical Manufacturers Directory *on page 1020*

Ceftazidime (SEF tay zi deem)

Pharmacologic Class Antibiotic, Cephalosporin (Third Generation)

U.S. Brand Names Ceptaz™; Fortaz®; Tazicef®; Tazidime®

Generic Available No

Mechanism of Action Inhibits bacterial cell wall synthesis by binding to one or more of the penicillin-binding proteins (PBPs) which in turn inhibits the final transpeptidation step of peptidoglycan synthesis in bacterial cell walls, thus inhibiting cell wall biosynthesis. Bacteria eventually lyse due to ongoing activity of cell wall autolytic enzymes (autolysins and murein hydrolases) while cell wall assembly is arrested.

Use Treatment of documented susceptible *Pseudomonas aeruginosa* infection and infections due to other susceptible aerobic gram-negative organisms; empiric therapy of a febrile, granulocytopenic patient

USUAL DOSAGE

Neonates 0-4 weeks: I.V.: 30 mg/kg every 12 hours

Infants and Children 1 month to 12 years: I.V.: 30-50 mg/kg/dose every 8 hours; maximum dose: 6 g/day

Adults: I.M., I.V.: 500 mg to 2 g every 8-12 hours

Urinary tract infections: 250-500 mg every 12 hours

Dosing interval in renal impairment:

Cl_{cr} 30-50 mL/minute: Administer every 12 hours

Cl_{cr} 10-30 mL/minute: Administer every 24 hours

Cl_{cr} <10 mL/minute: Administer every 48-72 hours

Hemodialysis: Dialyzable (50% to 100%)

Continuous arteriovenous or venovenous hemodiafiltration (CAVH) effects: Dose as for Cl_{cr} 30-50 mL/minute

Dosage Forms INF, premixed (frozen) (Fortaz®): 1 g (50 mL); 2 g (50 mL). **POWDER for inj:** 500 mg, 1 g, 2 g, 6 g

Contraindications Hypersensitivity to ceftazidime, any component, or cephalosporins

Warnings/Precautions Modify dosage in patients with severe renal impairment; prolonged use may result in superinfection; use with caution in patients with a history of penicillin allergy especially IgE-mediated reactions (eg, anaphylaxis, urticaria); may cause antibiotic-associated colitis or colitis secondary to *C. difficile*

Pregnancy Risk Factor B

Adverse Reactions

1% to 10%:

Gastrointestinal: Diarrhea (1.3%)

Local: Pain at injection site (1.4%)

Miscellaneous: Hypersensitivity reactions (2%)

<1%: Anaphylaxis, angioedema, asterixis, candidiasis, dizziness, elevated transaminases, encephalopathy, eosinophilia, erythema multiforme, fever, headache, hemolytic anemia, increased BUN, increased creatinine, leukopenia, nausea, neuromuscular excitability, paresthesia, phlebitis, pruritus, pseudomembranous colitis, rash, Stevens-Johnson syndrome, toxic epidermal necrolysis, thrombocytosis, vaginitis, vomiting

Other reactions with cephalosporins include agranulocytosis, aplastic anemia, cholestasis, colitis, elevated BUN, elevated creatinine, hemolytic anemia, hemorrhage, interstitial nephritis, pancytopenia, prolonged PT, renal dysfunction, seizures, serum-sickness reactions, superinfection, toxic nephropathy, urticaria

(Continued)

Ceftazidime *(Continued)*

Drug Interactions

Increased effect: Probenecid may decrease cephalosporin elimination; aminoglycosides: *in vitro* studies indicate additive or synergistic effect against some strains of Enterobacteriaceae and *Pseudomonas aeruginosa*

Increased toxicity: Furosemide, aminoglycosides may be a possible additive to nephrotoxicity

Half-Life 1-2 hours (prolonged with renal impairment)

Education and Monitoring Issues

Patient Education: This medication is administered I.M. or I.V. Drink 2-3 L fluid/day. If diarrhea occurs, yogurt or buttermilk may help. May cause false-positive test with Clinitest®; use another form of testing. May interfere with oral contraceptives; additional contraceptive measures are necessary. Report severe, unresolved diarrhea; abdominal pain; vaginal itching or drainage; sores in mouth; blood, pus, or mucus in stool or urine; easy bleeding or bruising; unusual fever or chills; rash; or respiratory difficulty.

Monitoring Parameters: Observe for signs and symptoms of anaphylaxis during first dose

Related Information

Antimicrobial Drugs of Choice *on page 1182*

Ceftibuten (sef TYE byoo ten)

Pharmacologic Class Antibiotic, Cephalosporin (Third Generation)

U.S. Brand Names Cedax®

Mechanism of Action Inhibits bacterial cell wall synthesis by binding to one or more of the penicillin-binding proteins (PBPs) which in turn inhibits the final transpeptidation step of peptidoglycan synthesis in bacterial cell walls, thus inhibiting cell wall biosynthesis. Bacteria eventually lyse due to ongoing activity of cell wall autolytic enzymes (autolysins and murein hydrolases) while cell wall assembly is arrested.

Use Oral cephalosporin for bronchitis, otitis media, and pharyngitis/tonsillitis due to *H. influenzae* and *M. catarrhalis*, both beta-lactamase-producing and nonproducing strains, as well as *S. pneumoniae* (weak) and *S. pyogenes*

USUAL DOSAGE Oral:

Children <12 years: 9 mg/kg/day for 10 days; maximum daily dose: 400 mg

Children ≥12 years and Adults: 400 mg once daily for 10 days; maximum: 400 mg

Dosage adjustment in renal impairment:

Cl_{cr} 30-49 mL//minute: Administer 4.5 mg/kg or 200 mg every 24 hours

Cl_{cr} <29 mL/minute: Administer 2.25 mg/kg or 100 mg every 24 hours

Dosage Forms CAP: 400 mg. **POWDER for oral susp** (cherry flavor): 90 mg/5 mL (30 mL, 60 mL, 120 mL); 180 mg/5 mL (30 mL, 60 mL, 120 mL)

Contraindications In patients with known allergy to the cephalosporin group of antibiotics

Warnings/Precautions Modify dosage in patients with severe renal impairment, prolonged use may result in superinfection; use with caution in patients with a history of penicillin allergy, especially IgE-mediated reactions (eg, anaphylaxis, urticaria); may cause antibiotic-associated colitis or colitis secondary to *C. difficile*

Pregnancy Risk Factor B

Adverse Reactions

1% to 10%:

Central nervous system: Headache (3%), dizziness (1%)

Gastrointestinal: Nausea (4%), diarrhea (3%), dyspepsia (2%), vomiting (1%), abdominal pain (1%)

Hematologic: Increased eosinophils (3%), decreased hemoglobin (2%), thrombocytosis

Hepatic: Increased ALT (1%), increased bilirubin (1%)

Renal: Increased BUN (4%)

<1%: Agitation, anorexia, candidiasis, constipation, diaper rash, dry mouth, dyspnea, dysuria, fatigue, increased creatinine, increased transaminases, insomnia, irritability, leukopenia, nasal congestion, paresthesia, rash, rigors, urticaria

Other reactions with cephalosporins include agranulocytosis, anaphylaxis, angioedema, aplastic anemia, asterixis, candidiasis, cholestasis, colitis, encephalopathy, erythema multiforme, fever, hemolytic anemia, hemorrhage, interstitial nephritis, neuromuscular excitability, pancytopenia, paresthesia, prolonged PT, pruritus, pseudomembranous colitis, renal dysfunction, seizures, serum-sickness reactions, Stevens-Johnson syndrome, superinfection, toxic epidermal necrolysis, toxic nephropathy, vaginitis

Drug Interactions

Increased effect: High-dose probenecid decreases clearance

Increased toxicity: Aminoglycosides increase nephrotoxic potential

Half-Life 2 hours

Education and Monitoring Issues

Patient Education: Take as directed, at regular intervals around-the-clock (with or without food). Chilling oral suspension improves flavor (do not freeze). Complete full course of medication, even if you feel better. Drink 2-3 L fluid/day. If diarrhea occurs, yogurt or buttermilk may help. May cause false-positive test with Clinitest®; use another form of testing. May interfere with oral contraceptives; additional contraceptive measures are necessary. Report severe, unresolved diarrhea; abdominal pain; vaginal itching or drainage; sores in mouth; blood, pus, or mucus in stool or urine; easy bleeding or bruising; unusual fever or chills; rash; or respiratory difficulty.

Monitoring Parameters: Observe for signs and symptoms of anaphylaxis during first dose; with prolonged therapy, monitor renal, hepatic, and hematologic function periodically

Manufacturer Schering-Plough Corp

Related Information

Pharmaceutical Manufacturers Directory *on page 1020*

♦ **Ceftin® Oral** *see* Cefuroxime *on page 165*

Ceftizoxime (sef ti ZOKS eem)

Pharmacologic Class Antibiotic, Cephalosporin (Third Generation)

U.S. Brand Names Cefizox®

Generic Available No

Mechanism of Action Inhibits bacterial cell wall synthesis by binding to one or more of the penicillin-binding proteins (PBPs) which in turn inhibits the final transpeptidation step of peptidoglycan synthesis in bacterial cell walls, thus inhibiting cell wall biosynthesis. Bacteria eventually lyse due to ongoing activity of cell wall autolytic enzymes (autolysins and murein hydrolases) while cell wall assembly is arrested.

Use Treatment of susceptible bacterial infection, mainly respiratory tract, skin and skin structure, bone and joint, urinary tract and gynecologic, as well as septicemia; active against many gram-negative bacilli (not *Pseudomonas*), some gram-positive cocci (not *Enterococcus*), and some anaerobes

USUAL DOSAGE I.M., I.V.:

Children ≥6 months: 150-200 mg/kg/day divided every 6-8 hours (maximum of 12 g/24 hours)

Adults: 1-2 g every 8-12 hours, up to 2 g every 4 hours or 4 g every 8 hours for life-threatening infections

Dosing adjustment in renal impairment: Adults:

Cl_{cr} 10-30 mL/minute: Administer 1 g every 12 hours

Cl_{cr} <10 mL/minute: Administer 1 g every 24 hours

Moderately dialyzable (20% to 50%)

Continuous arteriovenous or venovenous hemodiafiltration (CAVH) effects: Dose as for Cl_{cr} 10-50 mL/minute

Dosage Forms INJ in D_5W (frozen): 1 g (50 mL); 2 g (50 mL). **POWDER for inj:** 500 mg, 1 g, 2 g, 10 g

Contraindications Hypersensitivity to ceftizoxime, any component, or cephalosporins

Warnings/Precautions Modify dosage in patients with severe renal impairment, prolonged use may result in superinfection; use with caution in patients with a history of penicillin allergy, especially IgE-mediated reactions (eg, anaphylaxis, urticaria); may cause antibiotic-associated colitis or colitis secondary to *C. difficile*

Pregnancy Risk Factor B

Adverse Reactions

1% to 10%:

Central nervous system: Fever

Dermatologic: Rash, pruritus

Hematologic: Eosinophilia, thrombocytosis

Hepatic: Elevated transaminases, alkaline phosphatase

Local: Pain, burning at injection site

<1%: Anaphylaxis, anemia, diarrhea, increased bilirubin, increased BUN, increased creatinine, injection site reactions, leukopenia, nausea, neutropenia, numbness, paresthesia, phlebitis, thrombocytopenia, vaginitis, vomiting

Other reactions reported with cephalosporins include agranulocytosis, angioedema, aplastic anemia, asterixis, candidiasis, cholestasis, colitis, encephalopathy, erythema multiforme, hemolytic anemia, hemorrhage, interstitial nephritis, neuromuscular excitability, pancytopenia, prolonged PT, pseudomembranous colitis, renal dysfunction, seizures, serum-sickness reactions, Stevens-Johnson syndrome, superinfection, toxic epidermal necrolysis, toxic nephropathy

Drug Interactions

Increased effect: Probenecid may decrease cephalosporin elimination

Increased toxicity: Furosemide, aminoglycosides may be a possible additive to nephrotoxicity

Half-Life 1.6 hours, increases to 25 hours when Cl_{cr} falls to <10 mL/minute

Education and Monitoring Issues

Patient Education: This medication is administered I.M. or I.V. Drink 2-3 L fluid/day. If diarrhea occurs, yogurt or buttermilk may help. May cause false-positive test with Clinitest®; use another form of testing. May interfere with oral contraceptives; additional contraceptive measures are necessary. Report severe, unresolved diarrhea; abdominal pain; vaginal itching or drainage; sores in mouth; blood, pus, or mucus in stool or urine; easy bleeding or bruising; unusual fever or chills; rash; or respiratory difficulty.

(Continued)

Ceftizoxime *(Continued)*

Monitoring Parameters: Observe for signs and symptoms of anaphylaxis during first dose

Manufacturer Fujisawa Healthcare, Inc

Related Information

Antimicrobial Drugs of Choice *on page 1182*
Pharmaceutical Manufacturers Directory *on page 1020*
Treatment of Sexually Transmitted Diseases *on page 1210*

Ceftriaxone (sef trye AKS one)

Pharmacologic Class Antibiotic, Cephalosporin (Third Generation)

U.S. Brand Names Rocephin®

Generic Available No

Mechanism of Action Inhibits bacterial cell wall synthesis by binding to one or more of the penicillin-binding proteins (PBPs) which in turn inhibits the final transpeptidation step of peptidoglycan synthesis in bacterial cell walls, thus inhibiting cell wall biosynthesis. Bacteria eventually lyse due to ongoing activity of cell wall autolytic enzymes (autolysins and murein hydrolases) while cell wall assembly is arrested.

Use Treatment of lower respiratory tract infections, skin and skin structure infections, bone and joint infections, intra-abdominal and urinary tract infections, sepsis and meningitis due to susceptible organisms; documented or suspected infection due to susceptible organisms in home care patients and patients without I.V. line access; treatment of documented or suspected gonococcal infection or chancroid; emergency room management of patients at high risk for bacteremia, periorbital or buccal cellulitis, salmonellosis or shigellosis, and pneumonia of unestablished etiology (<5 years of age); treatment of Lyme disease, depends on the stage of the disease (used in Stage II and Stage III, but not stage I; doxycycline is the drug of choice for Stage I)

USUAL DOSAGE I.M., I.V.:

Neonates:

- Postnatal age ≤7 days: 50 mg/kg/day given every 24 hours
- Postnatal age >7 days:
  - ≤2000 g: 50 mg/kg/day given every 24 hours
  - >2000 g: 50-75 mg/kg/day given every 24 hours
- Gonococcal prophylaxis: 25-50 mg/kg as a single dose (dose not to exceed 125 mg)
- Gonococcal infection: 25-50 mg/kg/day (maximum dose: 125 mg) given every 24 hours for 10-14 days

Infants and Children: 50-75 mg/kg/day in 1-2 divided doses every 12-24 hours; maximum: 2 g/24 hours

- Meningitis: 100 mg/kg/day divided every 12-24 hours, up to a maximum of 4 g/24 hours; loading dose of 75 mg/kg/dose may be given at start of therapy
- Otitis media: Single I.M. injection
- Uncomplicated gonococcal infections, sexual assault, and STD prophylaxis: I.M.: 125 mg as a single dose plus doxycycline
- Complicated gonococcal infections:
  - Infants: I.M., I.V.: 25-50 mg/kg/day in a single dose (maximum: 125 mg/dose); treat for 7 days for disseminated infection and 7-14 days for documented meningitis
  - <45 kg: 50 mg/kg/day once daily; maximum: 1 g/day; for ophthalmia, peritonitis, arthritis, or bacteremia: 50-100 mg/kg/day divided every 12-24 hours; maximum: 2 g/day for meningitis or endocarditis
  - >45 kg: 1 g/day once daily for disseminated gonococcal infections; 1-2 g dose every 12 hours for meningitis or endocarditis
- Acute epididymitis: I.M.: 250 mg in a single dose

Adults: 1-2 g every 12-24 hours (depending on the type and severity of infection); maximum dose: 2 g every 12 hours for treatment of meningitis

- Uncomplicated gonorrhea: I.M.: 250 mg as a single dose
- Surgical prophylaxis: 1 g 30 minutes to 2 hours before surgery

Dosing adjustment in renal or hepatic impairment: No change necessary

Hemodialysis: Not dialyzable (0% to 5%); administer dose postdialysis

Peritoneal dialysis: Administer 750 mg every 12 hours

Continuous arteriovenous or venovenous hemofiltration (CAVH/CAVHD): Removes 10 mg of ceftriaxone per liter of filtrate per day

Dosage Forms INF, premixed (frozen): 1 g in $D_{3.8}W$ (50 mL); 2 g in $D_{2.4}W$ (50 mL). **POWDER for inj:** 250 mg, 500 mg, 1 g, 2 g, 10 g

Contraindications Hypersensitivity to ceftriaxone sodium, any component, or cephalosporins; **do not use in hyperbilirubinemic neonates**, particularly those who are premature since ceftriaxone is reported to displace bilirubin from albumin binding sites

Warnings/Precautions Modify dosage in patients with severe renal impairment, prolonged use may result in superinfection; use with caution in patients with a history of penicillin allergy, especially IgE-mediated reactions (eg, anaphylaxis, urticaria); may cause antibiotic-associated colitis or colitis secondary to *C. difficile*

Pregnancy Risk Factor B

Adverse Reactions

1% to 10%:

Dermatologic: Rash (1.7%)

Gastrointestinal: Diarrhea (2.7%)

Hematologic: Eosinophilia (6%), thrombocytosis (5.1%), leukopenia (2.1%)

Hepatic: Elevated transaminases (3.1% to 3.3%)

Local: Pain, induration at injection site (1%)

Renal: Increased BUN (1.2%)

<1%: Anemia, candidiasis, chills, diaphoresis, dizziness, dysgeusia, fever, flushing, headache, hemolytic anemia, increased alkaline phosphatase, increased bilirubin, increased creatinine, lymphopenia, nausea, neutropenia, phlebitis, prolonged PT, pruritus, thrombocytopenia, urinary casts, vaginitis, vomiting

Other reactions with cephalosporins include agranulocytosis, anaphylaxis, angioedema, aplastic anemia, asterixis, cholestasis, colitis, encephalopathy, erythema multiforme, hemolytic anemia, hemorrhage, interstitial nephritis, neuromuscular excitability, pancytopenia, paresthesia, pseudomembranous colitis, renal dysfunction, seizures, serum-sickness reactions, Stevens-Johnson syndrome, superinfection, toxic epidermal necrolysis, toxic nephropathy

Drug Interactions

Increased effect:

Aminoglycosides may result in synergistic antibacterial activity

High-dose probenecid decreases clearance

Increased toxicity: Aminoglycosides increase nephrotoxic potential

Half-Life Normal renal and hepatic function: 5-9 hours

Education and Monitoring Issues

Patient Education: This medication is administered I.M. or I.V. Drink 2-3 L fluid/day. If diarrhea occurs, yogurt or buttermilk may help. May cause false-positive test with Clinitest®; use another form of testing. May interfere with oral contraceptives; additional contraceptive measures are necessary. Report severe, unresolved diarrhea; abdominal pain; vaginal itching or drainage; sores in mouth; blood, pus, or mucus in stool or urine; easy bleeding or bruising; unusual fever or chills; rash; or respiratory difficulty.

Monitoring Parameters: Observe for signs and symptoms of anaphylaxis

Manufacturer Roche Laboratories

Related Information

Animal and Human Bites Guidelines *on page 1177*

Antibiotic Treatment of Adults With Infective Endocarditis *on page 1179*

Antimicrobial Drugs of Choice *on page 1182*

Community Acquired Pneumonia in Adults *on page 1200*

Pharmaceutical Manufacturers Directory *on page 1020*

Treatment of Sexually Transmitted Diseases *on page 1210*

Cefuroxime (se fyoor OKS eem)

Pharmacologic Class Antibiotic, Cephalosporin (Second Generation)

U.S. Brand Names Ceftin® Oral; Kefurox® Injection; Zinacef® Injection

Generic Available No

Mechanism of Action Inhibits bacterial cell wall synthesis by binding to one or more of the penicillin-binding proteins (PBPs) which in turn inhibits the final transpeptidation step of peptidoglycan synthesis in bacterial cell walls, thus inhibiting cell wall biosynthesis. Bacteria eventually lyse due to ongoing activity of cell wall autolytic enzymes (autolysins and murein hydrolases) while cell wall assembly is arrested.

Use Treatment of infections caused by staphylococci, group B streptococci, *H. influenzae* (types A and B), *E. coli*, *Enterobacter*, *Salmonella*, and *Klebsiella*; treatment of susceptible infections of the lower respiratory tract, otitis media, urinary tract, skin and soft tissue, bone and joint, sepsis and gonorrhea, acute bacterial maxillary sinusitis

USUAL DOSAGE

Children:

Pharyngitis, tonsillitis: Oral:

Suspension: 20 mg/kg/day (maximum: 500 mg/day) in 2 divided doses

Tablet: 125 mg every 12 hours

Acute otitis media, impetigo: Oral:

Suspension: 30 mg/kg/day (maximum: 1 g/day) in 2 divided doses

Tablet: 250 mg every 12 hours

I.M., I.V.: 75-150 mg/kg/day divided every 8 hours; maximum dose: 6 g/day

Meningitis: Not recommended (doses of 200-240 mg/kg/day divided every 6-8 hours have been used); maximum dose: 9 g/day

Acute bacterial maxillary sinusitis: 30 mg/kg/day divided twice daily for 10 days; maximum daily dose: 100 mg

Adults:

Oral: 250-500 mg twice daily

Uncomplicated urinary tract infection: 125-250 mg every 12 hours

Acute bacterial maxillary sinusitis: 250 mg twice daily for 10 days

I.M., I.V.: 750 mg to 1.5 g/dose every 8 hours or 100-150 mg/kg/day in divided doses every 6-8 hours; maximum: 6 g/24 hours

(Continued)

Cefuroxime *(Continued)*

Dosing adjustment in renal impairment:

Cl_{cr} 10-20 mL/minute: Administer every 12 hours

Cl_{cr} <10 mL/minute: Administer every 24 hours

Hemodialysis: Dialyzable (25%)

Note: Cefuroxime axetil film-coated tablets and oral suspension are not bioequivalent and are not substitutable on a mg/mg basis

Continuous arteriovenous or venovenous hemodiafiltration (CAVH) effects: Dose as for Cl_{cr} 10-20 mL/minute

Dosage Forms

Cefuroxime sodium: **Inf, premixed** (frozen) (Zinacef®): 750 mg (50 mL), 1.5 g (50 mL). **POWDER for inj:** 750 mg, 1.5 g, 7.5 g; (Kefurox®, Zinacef®): 750 mg, 1.5 g, 7.5 g

Cefuroxime axetil: **POWDER for oral susp** (tutti-frutti flavor) (Ceftin®): 125 mg/5 mL (50 mL, 100 mL, 200 mL); 250 mg/5 ml (50 mL, 100 mL). **TAB** (Ceftin®): 125 mg, 250 mg, 500 mg

Contraindications Hypersensitivity to cefuroxime, any component, or cephalosporins

Warnings/Precautions Modify dosage in patients with severe renal impairment, prolonged use may result in superinfection; use with caution in patients with a history of penicillin allergy, especially IgE-mediated reactions (eg, anaphylaxis, urticaria); may cause antibiotic-associated colitis or colitis secondary to *C. difficile*

Pregnancy Risk Factor B

Adverse Reactions

1% to 10%:

Hematologic: Eosinophilia (7%), decreased hemoglobin and hematocrit (10%)

Hepatic: Increased transaminases (4%), increased alkaline phosphatase (2%)

Local: Thrombophlebitis (1.7%)

<1%: Anaphylaxis, angioedema, colitis, diarrhea, dizziness, erythema multiforme, fever, GI bleeding, headache, increased BUN, increased creatinine, interstitial nephritis, leukopenia, nausea, neutropenia, pain at injection site, pseudomembranous colitis, rash, seizures, stomach cramps, toxic epidermal necrolysis, vaginitis, vomiting,

Other reactions with cephalosporins include agranulocytosis, aplastic anemia, asterixis, cholestasis, colitis, encephalopathy, hemolytic anemia, hemorrhage, neuromuscular excitability, pancytopenia, prolonged PT, serum-sickness reactions, superinfection, toxic nephropathy

Drug Interactions

Increased effect: High-dose probenecid decreases clearance

Increased toxicity: Aminoglycosides increase nephrotoxic potential

Half-Life 1-2 hours (prolonged in renal impairment)

Education and Monitoring Issues

Patient Education: Take as directed, at regular intervals around-the-clock (with or without food). Chilling oral suspension improves flavor (do not freeze). Complete full course of medication, even if you feel better. Drink 2-3 L fluid/day. If diarrhea occurs, yogurt or buttermilk may help. May cause false-positive test with Clinitest®; use another form of testing. May interfere with oral contraceptives; additional contraceptive measures are necessary. Report severe, unresolved diarrhea; abdominal pain; vaginal itching or drainage; sores in mouth; blood, pus, or mucus in stool or urine; easy bleeding or bruising; unusual fever or chills; rash; or respiratory difficulty.

Monitoring Parameters: Observe for signs and symptoms of anaphylaxis during first dose; with prolonged therapy, monitor renal, hepatic, and hematologic function periodically

Manufacturer GlaxoWellcome

Related Information

Antimicrobial Drugs of Choice *on page 1182*

Community Acquired Pneumonia in Adults *on page 1200*

Pharmaceutical Manufacturers Directory *on page 1020*

♦ **Cefzil®** *see* Cefprozil *on page 160*

♦ **Celebrex™** *see* Celecoxib *on page 166*

Celecoxib (ce le COX ib)

Pharmacologic Class Nonsteroidal Anti-Inflammatory Agent (NSAID)

U.S. Brand Names Celebrex™

Mechanism of Action Inhibits prostaglandin synthesis by decreasing the activity of the enzyme, cyclo-oxygenase-2 (COX-2), which results in decreased formation of prostaglandin precursors. Celecoxib does not inhibit cyclo-oxygenase-1 (COX-1) at therapeutic concentrations.

Use Relief of the signs and symptoms of osteoarthritis; relief of the signs and symptoms of rheumatoid arthritis in adults; reduces the number of adenomatous colorectal polyps in familial adenomatous polyposis patients as adjunct to usual care

USUAL DOSAGE Adults: Oral:

Osteoarthritis: 200 mg/day as a single dose or in divided dose twice daily

Rheumatoid arthritis: 100-200 mg twice daily

Familial adenomatous polyposis (FAP): 400 mg twice daily

Dosing adjustment in renal impairment: No specific dosage adjustment is recommended

Dosing adjustment in hepatic impairment: Reduced dosage is recommended (AUC may be increased by 40% to 180%)

Dosing adjustment for elderly: No specific adjustment is recommended. However, the AUC in elderly patients may be increased by 50% as compared to younger subjects. Use the lowest recommended dose in patients weighing <50 kg.

Dosage Forms CAP: 100 mg, 200 mg

Contraindications Hypersensitivity to celecoxib or any component, sulfonamides, aspirin, or other nonsteroidal anti-inflammatory drugs (NSAIDs)

Warnings/Precautions Gastrointestinal irritation, ulceration, bleeding, and perforation may occur with NSAIDs (it is unclear whether celecoxib is associated with rates of these events which are similar to nonselective NSAIDs). Use with caution in patients with a history of GI disease (bleeding or ulcers), decreased renal function, hepatic disease, congestive heart failure, hypertension, or asthma. Anaphylactoid reactions may occur, even with no prior exposure to celecoxib. Use caution in patients with known or suspected deficiency of CYP2C9 isoenzyme.

Pregnancy Risk Factor C; D (after 34 weeks gestation or close to delivery)

Pregnancy Implications In late pregnancy may cause premature closure of the ductus arteriosus. In animal studies, celecoxib has been found to be excreted in milk; it is not known whether celecoxib is excreted in human milk. Because many drugs are excreted in milk, and the potential for serious adverse reactions exists, a decision should be made whether to discontinue nursing or discontinue the drug, taking into account the importance of the drug to the mother.

Adverse Reactions

>10%: Central nervous system: Headache (15.8%)

2% to 10%:

- Cardiovascular: Peripheral edema (2.1%)
- Central nervous system: Insomnia (2.3%), dizziness (2%)
- Dermatologic: Skin rash (2.2%)
- Gastrointestinal: Dyspepsia (8.8%), diarrhea (5.6%), abdominal pain (4.1%), nausea (3.5%), flatulence (2.2%)
- Neuromuscular & skeletal: Back pain (2.8%)
- Respiratory: Upper respiratory tract infection (8.1%), sinusitis (5%), pharyngitis (2.3%), rhinitis (2%)
- Miscellaneous: Accidental injury (2.9%)

0.1% to 2%:

- Cardiovascular: Hypertension (aggravated), chest pain, myocardial infarction, palpitation, tachycardia, facial edema, peripheral edema
- Central nervous system: Migraine, vertigo, hypoesthesia, fatigue, fever, pain, hypotonia, anxiety, depression, nervousness, somnolence
- Dermatologic: Alopecia, dermatitis, photosensitivity, pruritus, rash (maculopapular), rash (erythematous), dry skin, urticaria
- Endocrine & metabolic: Hot flashes, diabetes mellitus, hyperglycemia, hypercholesterolemia, breast pain, dysmenorrhea, menstrual disturbances, hypokalemia
- Gastrointestinal: Constipation, tenesmus, diverticulitis, eructation, esophagitis, gastroenteritis, vomiting, gastroesophageal reflux, hemorrhoids, hiatal hernia, melena, stomatitis, anorexia, increased appetite, taste disturbance, dry mouth, tooth disorder, weight gain
- Genitourinary: Prostate disorder, vaginal bleeding, vaginitis, monilial vaginitis, dysuria, cystitis, urinary frequency, incontinence, urinary tract infection,
- Hepatic: Elevated transaminases, increased alkaline phosphatase
- Hematologic: Anemia, thrombocytopenia, ecchymosis
- Neuromuscular & skeletal: Leg cramps, increased CPK, neck stiffness, arthralgia, myalgia, bone disorder, fracture, synovitis, tendonitis, neuralgia, paresthesia, neuropathy, weakness
- Ocular: Glaucoma, blurred vision, cataract, conjunctivitis, eye pain
- Otic: Deafness, tinnitus, earache, otitis media
- Renal: Increased BUN, increased creatinine, albuminuria, hematuria, renal calculi
- Respiratory: Bronchitis, bronchospasm, cough, dyspnea, laryngitis, pneumonia, epistaxis
- Miscellaneous: Allergic reactions, flu-like syndrome, breast cancer, herpes infection, bacterial infection, moniliasis, viral infection, increased diaphoresis

<0.1% (limited to severe): Acute renal failure, ataxia, cerebrovascular accident, colitis, congestive heart failure, esophageal perforation, gangrene, gastrointestinal bleeding, intestinal obstruction, intestinal perforation, pancreatitis, pulmonary embolism, sepsis, sudden death, syncope, thrombocytopenia, thrombophlebitis, ventricular fibrillation

Drug Interactions CYP2C9 substrate; CYP2D6 inhibitor

Decreased effect: Efficacy of thiazide diuretics, loop diuretics (furosemide), or ACE-inhibitors may be diminished by celecoxib; aluminum and magnesium-containing antacids may decrease AUC and C_{max} of celecoxib 10% and 37% respectively

Increased effect: Inhibitors of isoenzyme 2C9 may result in significant increases in celecoxib concentrations. Coadministration of drugs by 2D6 may result in increased

(Continued)

Celecoxib *(Continued)*

serum concentrations of these agents. Fluconazole increases celecoxib concentrations two-fold. Lithium concentrations may be increased by celecoxib. Celecoxib may be used with low-dose aspirin, however rates of gastrointestinal bleeding may be increased with coadministration. Celecoxib may increase INR when added to warfarin therapy (case reports).

Half-Life 11 hours

Education and Monitoring Issues

Patient Education: Do not take more than recommended dose. May be taken with food to reduce GI upset. Do not take with antacids. Avoid alcohol, aspirin, or OTC medication unless approved by prescriber. You may experience dizziness, confusion, or blurred vision (avoid driving or engaging in tasks requiring alertness until response to drug is known); anorexia, nausea, vomiting, taste disturbance, gastric distress (small frequent meals, frequent mouth care, sucking lozenges, or chewing gum may help). GI bleeding, ulceration, or perforation can occur with or without pain; it is unclear whether celecoxib has rates of these events which are similar to nonselective NSAIDs. Stop taking medication and report immediately stomach pain or cramping, unusual bleeding or bruising, or blood in vomitus, stool, or urine. Report persistent insomnia; skin rash; unusual fatigue or easy bruising or bleeding; muscle pain, tremors, or weakness; sudden weight gain; changes in hearing (ringing in ears); changes in vision; changes in urination pattern; or respiratory difficulty.

Dietary Considerations: Peak concentrations are delayed and AUC is increased by 10% to 20% when taken with a high-fat meal; celecoxib may be taken without regard to meals

Monitoring Parameters: Periodic LFTs

Manufacturer Searle

Related Information

Nonsteroidal Anti-Inflammatory Agents Comparison *on page 1248*
Pharmaceutical Manufacturers Directory *on page 1020*

♦ **Celectol®** *see* Celiprolol *on page 168*
♦ **Celestone®** *see* Betamethasone *on page 103*
♦ **Celestone® Soluspan®** *see* Betamethasone *on page 103*
♦ **Celexa™** *see* Citalopram *on page 203*

Celiprolol (SEE li proe lole)

Pharmacologic Class Beta Blocker

U.S. Brand Names Cardem®; Celectol®; Corliprol®; Selecor®; Selectol®

Mechanism of Action Selective $beta_1$-adrenergic blocking agent with weak $alpha_2$ receptor blocking activity; $beta_2$-adrenergic agonist and intrinsic sympathomimetic activity

USUAL DOSAGE Oral: 200-600 mg once daily; no dosage alteration needed the in elderly

Dosage adjustment in renal impairment: Adjustment may be needed

Contraindications Hypersensitivity to celiprolol or other beta-blocking agents; sinus bradycardia; heart block greater than first-degree (except in patients with a functioning artificial pacemaker); cardiogenic shock; uncompensated cardiac failure

Warnings/Precautions Administer cautiously in compensated heart failure and monitor for a worsening of the condition. Avoid abrupt discontinuation in patients with a history of CAD; slowly wean while monitoring for signs and symptoms of ischemia. Use caution with concurrent use of beta-blockers and either verapamil or diltiazem; bradycardia or heart block can occur. In general, beta-blockers should be avoided in patients with bronchospastic disease. Use cautiously in PVD (can exacerbate arterial insufficiency). Can mask signs of thyrotoxicosis. Dosage adjustment is required in patients with renal dysfunction. Use care with anesthetic agents that decrease myocardial function.

Adverse Reactions

Cardiovascular: Bradycardia, A-V block, Raynaud's syndrome, congestive heart failure, sinus bradycardia, myocardial depression

Central nervous system: Insomnia, dizziness, headache, depression

Gastrointestinal: Nausea, diarrhea, xerostomia

Neuromuscular & skeletal: Tremors

Drug Interactions Expected interactions:

Alpha-blockers (prazosin, terazosin): Concurrent use of beta-blockers may increase risk of orthostasis

Ampicillin, in single doses of 1 gram, decrease celiprolol's pharmacologic actions

Antacids (magnesium-aluminum, calcium antacids or salts) may reduce the bioavailability of celiprolol

Clonidine: Hypertensive crisis after or during withdrawal of either agent

Drugs which slow A-V conduction (digoxin): Effects may be additive with beta-blockers

Glucagon: Celiprolol may blunt the hyperglycemic action of glucagon

Insulin and oral hypoglycemics: Celiprolol masks the tachycardia that usually accompanies hypoglycemia

NSAIDs (ibuprofen, indomethacin, naproxen, piroxicam) may reduce the antihypertensive effects of beta-blockers

Salicylates may reduce the antihypertensive effects of beta-blockers

Sulfonylureas: Beta-blockers may alter response to hypoglycemic agents
Verapamil or diltiazem may have synergistic or additive pharmacological effects when taken concurrently with beta-blockers

Half-Life 4-10 hours

Education and Monitoring Issues

Monitoring Parameters: Monitor blood pressure, apical and radial pulses, I & O, daily weight, respirations, and circulation in extremities before and during therapy

- **CellCept®** *see* Mycophenolate *on page 624*
- **Cel-U-Jec®** *see* Betamethasone *on page 103*
- **Cenafed® [OTC]** *see* Pseudoephedrine *on page 792*
- **Cena-K®** *see* Potassium Chloride *on page 751*
- **Cenestin™** *see* Estrogens, Conjugated (Synthetic) *on page 332*
- **Cenolate®** *see* Sodium Ascorbate *on page 856*
- **Centratuss DM Expectorant** *see* Guaifenesin and Dextromethorphan *on page 424*

Cephalexin (sef a LEKS in)

Pharmacologic Class Antibiotic, Cephalosporin (First Generation)

U.S. Brand Names Biocef; Keflex®; Keftab®

Generic Available Yes

Mechanism of Action Inhibits bacterial cell wall synthesis by binding to one or more of the penicillin-binding proteins (PBPs) which in turn inhibits the final transpeptidation step of peptidoglycan synthesis in bacterial cell walls, thus inhibiting cell wall biosynthesis. Bacteria eventually lyse due to ongoing activity of cell wall autolytic enzymes (autolysins and murein hydrolases) while cell wall assembly is arrested.

Use Treatment of susceptible bacterial infections, including those caused by group A beta-hemolytic *Streptococcus, Staphylococcus, Klebsiella pneumoniae, E. coli, Proteus mirabilis*, and *Shigella*; predominantly used for lower respiratory tract, urinary tract, skin and soft tissue, and bone and joint; prophylaxis against bacterial endocarditis in high-risk patients undergoing surgical or dental procedures who are allergic to penicillin

USUAL DOSAGE Oral:

Children: 25-50 mg/kg/day every 6 hours; severe infections: 50-100 mg/kg/day in divided doses every 6 hours; maximum: 3 g/24 hours

Adults: 250-1000 mg every 6 hours; maximum: 4 g/day

Prophylaxis of bacterial endocarditis: 2 g 1 hour prior to the procedure

Dosing adjustment in renal impairment: Adults:

Cl_{cr} 10-40 mL/minute: 250-500 mg every 8-12 hours

Cl_{cr} <10 mL/minute: 250 mg every 12-24 hours

Hemodialysis: Moderately dialyzable (20% to 50%)

Dosage Forms

Cephalexin monohydrate: **CAP:** 250 mg, 500 mg. **POWDER, for oral susp:** 125 mg/5 mL (5 mL unit dose, 60 mL, 100 mL, 200 mL); 250 mg/5 mL (5 mL unit dose, 100 mL, 200 mL). **SUSP, oral, pediatric:** 100 mg/mL [5 mg/drop] (10 mL). **TAB:** 250 mg, 500 mg, 1 g

Cephalexin hydrochloride: **TAB:** 500 mg

Contraindications Hypersensitivity to cephalexin, any component, or cephalosporins

Warnings/Precautions Modify dosage in patients with severe renal impairment, prolonged use may result in superinfection; use with caution in patients with a history of penicillin allergy, especially IgE-mediated reactions (eg, anaphylaxis, urticaria); may cause antibiotic-associated colitis or colitis secondary to *C. difficile*

Pregnancy Risk Factor B

Adverse Reactions

1% to 10%: Gastrointestinal: Diarrhea

<1%: Abdominal pain, agitation, anaphylaxis, anemia, angioedema, arthralgia, cholestasis, confusion, dizziness, dyspepsia, eosinophilia, erythema multiforme, fatigue, gastritis, hallucinations, headache, hepatitis, increased transaminases, interstitial nephritis, nausea, neutropenia, pseudomembranous colitis, rash, serum-sickness reaction, Stevens-Johnson syndrome, thrombocytopenia, toxic epidermal necrolysis, urticaria, vomiting

Other reactions with cephalosporins include agranulocytosis, anaphylaxis, aplastic anemia, asterixis, colitis, encephalopathy, hemolytic anemia, hemorrhage, neuromuscular excitability, pancytopenia, prolonged PT, seizures, superinfection

Drug Interactions

Increased effect: High-dose probenecid decreases clearance

Increased toxicity: Aminoglycosides increase nephrotoxic potential

Half-Life 0.5-1.2 hours (prolonged with renal impairment)

Education and Monitoring Issues

Patient Education: Take as directed, at regular intervals around-the-clock (with or without food). Chilling oral suspension improves flavor (do not freeze). Complete full course of medication, even if you feel better. Drink 2-3 L fluid/day. If diarrhea occurs, yogurt or buttermilk may help. May cause false-positive test with Clinitest®; use another form of testing. May interfere with oral contraceptives; additional contraceptive

(Continued)

Cephalexin *(Continued)*

measures are necessary. Report severe, unresolved diarrhea; abdominal pain; vaginal itching or drainage; sores in mouth; blood, pus, or mucus in stool or urine; easy bleeding or bruising; unusual fever or chills; rash; or respiratory difficulty.

Dietary Considerations: Food: Peak antibiotic serum concentration is lowered and delayed, but total drug absorbed is not affected; take on an empty stomach. If GI distress, take with food.

Monitoring Parameters: With prolonged therapy monitor renal, hepatic, and hematologic function periodically; monitor for signs of anaphylaxis during first dose

Related Information

Animal and Human Bites Guidelines *on page 1177*
Prevention of Bacterial Endocarditis *on page 1154*

Cephalothin (sef A loe thin)

Pharmacologic Class Cephalosporin (First Generation)

Use Treatment of infections when caused by susceptible strains in respiratory, genitourinary, gastrointestinal, skin and soft tissue, bone and joint infections; septicemia; treatment of susceptible gram-positive bacilli and cocci (never enterococcus); some gram-negative bacilli including *E. coli, Proteus*, and *Klebsiella* may be susceptible

USUAL DOSAGE I.M., I.V.:

Neonates:
- Postnatal age <7 days:
  - <2000 g: 20 mg every 12 hours
  - >2000 g: 20 mg every 8 hours
- Postnatal age >7 days:
  - <2000 g: 20 mg every 8 hours
  - >2000 g: 20 mg every 6 hours

Children: 75-125 mg/kg/day divided every 4-6 hours; maximum dose: 10 g in a 24-hour period

Adults: 500 mg to 2 g every 4-6 hours

Dosing interval in renal impairment:
- Cl_{cr} 10-50 mL/minute: Administer every 6-8 hours
- Cl_{cr} <10 mL/minute: Administer every 12 hours

Continuous arteriovenous or venovenous hemodiafiltration (CAVH) effects: Administer 1 g every 8 hours

Contraindications Hypersensitivity to cephalothin or cephalosporins

Pregnancy Risk Factor B

Cephapirin (sef a PYE rin)

Pharmacologic Class Antibiotic, Cephalosporin (First Generation)

U.S. Brand Names Cefadyl®

Use Treatment of infections when caused by susceptible strains in respiratory, genitourinary, gastrointestinal, skin and soft tissue, bone and joint infections, septicemia; treatment of susceptible gram-positive bacilli and cocci (never enterococcus); some gram-negative bacilli including *E. coli, Proteus*, and *Klebsiella* may be susceptible

USUAL DOSAGE I.M., I.V.:

Children: 10-20 mg/kg/dose every 6 hours up to 4 g/24 hours

Adults: 500 mg to 1 g every 6 hours up to 12 g/day

Perioperative prophylaxis: 1-2 g 30 minutes to 1 hour prior to surgery and every 6 hours as needed for 24 hours following

Dosing interval in renal impairment:
- Cl_{cr} 10-50 mL/minute: Administer every 6-8 hours
- Cl_{cr} <10 mL/minute: Administer every 12 hours

Continuous arteriovenous or venovenous hemodiafiltration (CAVH) effects: Administer 1 g every 8 hours

Contraindications Hypersensitivity to cephapirin sodium, any component, or cephalosporins

Pregnancy Risk Factor B

Cephradine (SEF ra deen)

Pharmacologic Class Antibiotic, Cephalosporin (First Generation)

U.S. Brand Names Velosef®

Generic Available Yes

Mechanism of Action Inhibits bacterial cell wall synthesis by binding to one or more of the penicillin-binding proteins (PBPs) which in turn inhibits the final transpeptidation step of peptidoglycan synthesis in bacterial cell walls, thus inhibiting cell wall biosynthesis. Bacteria eventually lyse due to ongoing activity of cell wall autolytic enzymes (autolysins and murein hydrolases) while cell wall assembly is arrested.

Use Treatment of infections when caused by susceptible strains in respiratory, genitourinary, gastrointestinal, skin and soft tissue, bone and joint infections; treatment of susceptible gram-positive bacilli and cocci (never enterococcus); some gram-negative bacilli including *E. coli, Proteus*, and *Klebsiella* may be susceptible

USUAL DOSAGE Oral:

Children ≥9 months: 25-50 mg/kg/day in divided doses every 6 hours

Adults: 250-500 mg every 6-12 hours

Dosing adjustment in renal impairment: Adults:

Cl_{cr} 10-50 mL/minute: 250 mg every 6 hours

Cl_{cr} <10 mL/minute: 125 mg every 6 hours

Dosage Forms CAP: 250 mg, 500 mg. **POWDER for inj:** 250 mg, 500 mg, 1 g, 2 g (in ready-to-use infusion bottles). **POWDER for oral susp:** 125 mg/5 mL (5 mL, 100 mL, 200 mL); 250 mg/5 mL (5 mL, 100 mL, 200 mL)

Contraindications Hypersensitivity to cephradine, any component, or cephalosporins

Warnings/Precautions Modify dosage in patients with severe renal impairment, prolonged use may result in superinfection; use with caution in patients with a history of penicillin allergy, especially IgE-mediated reactions (eg, anaphylaxis, urticaria); may cause antibiotic-associated colitis or colitis secondary to *C. difficile*

Pregnancy Risk Factor B

Adverse Reactions

1% to 10%: Gastrointestinal: Diarrhea

<1%: Increased BUN, increased creatinine, nausea, pseudomembranous colitis, rash, vomiting

Other reactions with cephalosporins include agranulocytosis, anaphylaxis, angioedema, aplastic anemia, asterixis, cholestasis, dizziness, encephalopathy, erythema multiforme, fever, headache, hemolytic anemia, hemorrhage, interstitial nephritis, leukopenia, neuromuscular excitability, neutropenia, pancytopenia, prolonged PT, seizures, serum-sickness reactions, Stevens-Johnson syndrome, superinfection, toxic epidermal necrolysis, toxic nephropathy, vaginitis

Drug Interactions

Increased effect: High-dose probenecid decreases clearance

Increased toxicity: Aminoglycosides increase nephrotoxic potential

Half-Life 1-2 hours; prolonged in renal impairment

Education and Monitoring Issues

Patient Education: Oral: Take as directed, at regular intervals around-the-clock (with or without food). Chilling oral suspension improves flavor (do not freeze). Complete full course of medication, even if you feel better. Drink 2-3 L fluid/day. If diarrhea occurs, yogurt or buttermilk may help. May cause false-positive test with Clinitest®; use another form of testing. May interfere with oral contraceptives; additional contraceptive measures are necessary. Report severe, unresolved diarrhea; abdominal pain; vaginal itching or drainage; sores in mouth; blood, pus, or mucus in stool or urine; easy bleeding or bruising; unusual fever or chills; rash; or respiratory difficulty.

Monitoring Parameters: Observe for signs and symptoms of anaphylaxis during first dose

- **Cephulac®** *see* Lactulose *on page 506*
- **Ceporacin** *see* Cephalothin *on page 170*
- **Ceptaz™** *see* Ceftazidime *on page 161*
- **Ceredase®** *see* Alglucerase *on page 33*

Cerivastatin (se ree va STAT in)

Pharmacologic Class Antilipemic Agent (HMG-CoA Reductase Inhibitor)

U.S. Brand Names Baycol™

Mechanism of Action As an HMG-CoA reductase inhibitor, cerivastatin competitively inhibits 3-hydroxyl-3-methylglutaryl coenzyme A (HMG-CoA) reductase, the enzyme that catalyzes the rate-limiting step in cholesterol biosynthesis

Use Adjunct to dietary therapy to for the reduction of elevated total and LDL cholesterol levels in patients with primary hypercholesterolemia and mixed dyslipidemia when the response to dietary restriction of saturated fat and cholesterol and other nonpharmacological measures alone has been inadequate

USUAL DOSAGE Adults: Oral: 0.3 mg once daily in the evening; may be taken with or without food

Dosing adjustment with renal impairment: Moderate to severe impairment (<60 mL/minute): Starting dose: 0.2 mg

Dosing adjustment in hepatic impairment: Avoidance suggested; no guidelines for dosage reduction available

Dosage Forms TAB: 0.2 mg, 0.3 mg, 0.4 mg

Contraindications Hypersensitivity or severe adverse reactions to cerivastatin or other statins; active hepatic disease, pregnancy

Warnings/Precautions Use with caution in patients with history of liver disease, those who are breast-feeding, and those predisposed to renal failure

Pregnancy Risk Factor X

Pregnancy Implications Breast-feeding/lactation: Breast-feeding is not recommended by manufacturer

(Continued)

Cerivastatin *(Continued)*

Adverse Reactions

1% to 10%:

Central nervous system: Weakness (3.1%), insomnia (2%), headache (0.4% to 5.7%)
Cardiovascular: Chest pain (2%), peripheral edema (2%)
Gastrointestinal: Abdominal pain (1.4% to 3.4%), diarrhea (1.5% to 3.8%)
Neuromuscular & skeletal: Arthralgia (4.4%), myalgia (2.3%)
Respiratory: Cough (2.4%)

<1% (including class-related events not necessarily reported with cerivastatin therapy and postmarketing case reports): Myopathy, muscle cramps, increased CPK (>10x normal), rhabdomyolysis, renal failure (secondary to rhabdomyolysis), blurred vision, alteration in taste, impaired extraocular muscle movement, facial paresis, tremor, dizziness, memory loss, vertigo, paresthesia, peripheral neuropathy, peripheral nerve palsy, anxiety, depression, psychic disturbance, hypersensitivity reaction, angioedema, anaphylaxis, rash, systemic lupus erythematosus-like syndrome, polymyalgia rheumatica, dermatomyositis, vasculitis, purpura, thrombocytopenia, leukopenia, hemolytic anemia, positive ANA, increased ESR, eosinophilia, arthritis, urticaria, photosensitivity, fever, chills, flushing, malaise, dyspnea, toxic epidermal necrolysis, erythema multiforme, Stevens-Johnson syndrome, pancreatitis, hepatitis, cholestatic jaundice, fatty liver, cirrhosis, fulminant hepatic necrosis, hepatoma, anorexia, vomiting, alopecia, pruritus, nodules, skin discoloration, dryness of skin/mucous membranes, nail changes, gynecomastia, decreased libido, erectile dysfunction, impotence, cataracts, ophthalmoplegia, elevated transaminases, increased alkaline phosphatase, increased GGT, hyperbilirubinemia, thyroid dysfunction

Drug Interactions CYP3A3/4 enzyme substrate

Inhibitors of CYP3A3/4 (amprenavir, clarithromycin, cyclosporine, danazol, diltiazem, fluvoxamine, erythromycin, fluconazole, indinavir, itraconazole, ketoconazole, miconazole, nefazodone, nelfinavir, ritonavir, saquinavir, troleandomycin, and verapamil) increase cerivastatin blood levels; may increase the risk of cerivastatin-induced myopathy and rhabdomyolysis

Cholestyramine reduces cerivastatin absorption. Separate administration times by at least 4 hours

Cholestyramine and colestipol (bile acid sequestrants): Cholesterol-lowering effects are additive

Clofibrate and fenofibrate may increase the risk of myopathy and rhabdomyolysis

Gemfibrozil: Increased risk of myopathy and rhabdomyolysis

Niacin may increase the risk of myopathy and rhabdomyolysis

Onset Maximal reductions in ~2 weeks

Half-Life 2-3 hours

Education and Monitoring Issues

Patient Education: Take prescribed dose in the evening (with or without food). You will need laboratory evaluation during therapy. Maintain adequate hydration (2-3 L/day of fluids unless instructed to restrict fluid intake). May cause headache (mild analgesic may help); drowsiness, dizziness, or blurred vision (use caution when driving or engaging in tasks that require alertness until response to medication is known). Report chest pain; swelling of extremities; weight gain (>5 lb/week); respiratory difficulty; persistent vomiting or abdominal pain; muscle weakness or pain; persistent cough; swelling of mouth, lips, or face; unusual bruising or bleeding; or skin rash.

Dietary Considerations: Grapefruit juice may inhibit metabolism of cerivastatin via CYP3A3/4; avoid high dietary intakes of grapefruit juice

Monitoring Parameters: Serum total cholesterol, LDL, HDL, triglycerides, apolipoprotein B, diet, weight, LFTs

Manufacturer Bayer Corp (Biological and Pharmaceutical Division)

Related Information

Pharmaceutical Manufacturers Directory *on page 1020*

- **Cerumenex® Otic** *see* Triethanolamine Polypeptide Oleate-Condensate *on page 949*
- **Cervidil® Vaginal Insert** *see* Dinoprostone *on page 281*
- **C.E.S.®** *see* Estrogens, Conjugated *on page 331*
- **Cetacaine®** *see* Benzocaine, Butyl Aminobenzoate, Tetracaine, and Benzalkonium Chloride *on page 99*
- **Cetacort®** *see* Hydrocortisone *on page 447*
- **Cetamide® Ophthalmic** *see* Sulfacetamide Sodium *on page 876*
- **Cetapred® Ophthalmic** *see* Sulfacetamide Sodium and Prednisolone *on page 876*

Cetirizine (se TI ra zeen)

Pharmacologic Class Antihistamine

U.S. Brand Names Zyrtec®

Mechanism of Action Competes with histamine for H_1-receptor sites on effector cells in the gastrointestinal tract, blood vessels, and respiratory tract

Use Perennial and seasonal allergic rhinitis and other allergic symptoms including urticaria

USUAL DOSAGE Children ≥6 years and Adults: Oral: 5-10 mg once daily, depending upon symptom severity

Dosing interval in renal/hepatic impairment: Cl_{cr} ≤31 mL/minute: Administer 5 mg once daily

Dosage Forms SYR: 5 mg/5 mL (120 mL). **TAB:** 5 mg, 10 mg

Contraindications Hypersensitivity to cetirizine, hydroxyzine, or any component

Warnings/Precautions Cetirizine should be used cautiously in patients with hepatic or renal dysfunction, the elderly and in nursing mothers. Doses >10 mg/day may cause significant drowsiness

Pregnancy Risk Factor B

Adverse Reactions

>10%: Central nervous system: Headache has been reported to occur in 10% to 12% of patients, drowsiness has been reported in as much as 26% of patients on high doses

1% to 10%:

Central nervous system: Somnolence, fatigue, dizziness

Gastrointestinal: Xerostomia

<1%: Depression

Drug Interactions Increased toxicity: CNS depressants, anticholinergics

Alcohol Interactions Avoid use (may increase central nervous system depression)

Onset Within 15-30 minutes

Half-Life 8-11 hours

Education and Monitoring Issues

Patient Education: Take as directed; do not exceed recommended dose. Avoid use of other depressants, alcohol, or sleep-inducing medications unless approved by prescriber. You may experience drowsiness or dizziness (use caution when driving or engaging in tasks requiring alertness until response to drug is known); or dry mouth (frequent small meals, frequent mouth care, chewing gum, or sucking hard candy may help). Report persistent sedation, confusion, or agitation; persistent nausea or vomiting; changes in urinary pattern; blurred vision; chest pain or palpitations; or lack of improvement or worsening of condition.

Monitoring Parameters: Relief of symptoms, sedation and anticholinergic effects

Manufacturer Pfizer U.S. Pharmaceutical Group

Related Information

Pharmaceutical Manufacturers Directory *on page 1020*

♦ **Cevalin® [OTC]** *see* Ascorbic Acid *on page 72*

♦ **Cevi-Bid® [OTC]** *see* Ascorbic Acid *on page 72*

Cevimeline (se vi ME leen)

Pharmacologic Class Cholinergic Agonist

U.S. Brand Names Evoxac®

Mechanism of Action Binds to muscarinic (cholinergic) receptors, causing an increase in secretion of exocrine glands (including salivary glands)

Use Treatment of symptoms of dry mouth in patients with Sjögren's syndrome

USUAL DOSAGE Adults: Oral: 30 mg 3 times/day

Dosage adjustment in renal/hepatic impairment: Not studied; no specific dosage adjustment is recommended

Elderly: No specific dosage adjustment is recommended; however, use caution when initiating due to potential for increased sensitivity

Dosage Forms CAP: 30 mg

Contraindications Known hypersensitivity to cevimeline; uncontrolled asthma; narrow-angle glaucoma; acute iritis; other conditions where miosis is undesirable

Warnings/Precautions May alter cardiac conduction and/or heart rate; use caution in patients with significant cardiovascular disease, including angina, myocardial infarction, or conduction disturbances. Cevimeline has the potential to increase bronchial smooth muscle tone, airway resistance, and bronchial secretions; use with caution in patients with controlled asthma, COPD, or chronic bronchitis. May cause decreased visual acuity (particularly at night and in patients with central lens changes) and impaired depth perception. Patients should be cautioned about driving at night or performing hazardous activities in reduced lighting. May cause a variety of parasympathomimetic effects, which may be particularly dangerous in elderly patients; excessive sweating may lead to dehydration in some patients.

Use with caution in patients with a history of biliary stones or nephrolithiasis; cevimeline may induce smooth muscle spasms, precipitating cholangitis, cholecystitis, biliary obstruction, renal colic, or ureteral reflux in susceptible patients. Patients with a known or suspected deficiency of CYP2D6 may be at higher risk of adverse effects. Safety and efficacy has not been established in pediatric patients.

Pregnancy Risk Factor C

Pregnancy Implications There are no adequate or well-controlled studies in pregnant women. Use only if potential benefit justifies potential risk to the fetus. Excretion in breast milk is unknown/not recommended.

(Continued)

Cevimeline *(Continued)*

Adverse Reactions

>10%:

Central nervous system: Headache (14%; placebo 20%)
Gastrointestinal: Nausea (14%), diarrhea (10%)
Respiratory: Rhinitis (11%), sinusitis (12%), upper respiratory infection (11%)
Miscellaneous: Increased sweating (19%)

1% to 10%:

Cardiovascular: Peripheral edema, chest pain, edema, palpitation
Central nervous system: Dizziness (4%), fatigue (3%), pain (3%), insomnia (2%), anxiety (1%), fever, depression, migraine, hypoesthesia, vertigo
Dermatologic: Rash (4%; placebo 6%), pruritus, skin disorder, erythematous rash
Endocrine & metabolic: Hot flashes (2%)
Gastrointestinal: Dyspepsia (8%; placebo 9%), abdominal pain (8%), vomiting (5%), excessive salivation (2%), constipation, salivary gland pain, dry mouth, sialoadenitis, gastroesophageal reflux, flatulence, ulcerative stomatitis, eructation, increased amylase, anorexia, tooth disorder
Genitourinary: Urinary tract infection (6%), vaginitis, cystitis
Hematologic: Anemia
Local: Abscess
Neuromuscular & skeletal: back pain (5%), arthralgia (4%), skeletal pain (3%), rigors (1%), hypertonia, tremor, myalgia, hyporeflexia, leg cramps
Ocular: Conjunctivitis (4%), abnormal vision, eye pain, eye abnormality, xerophthalmia
Otic: Ear ache, otitis media
Respiratory: Coughing (6%), bronchitis (4%), pneumonia, epistaxis
Miscellaneous: Flu-like syndrome, infection, fungal infection, allergy, hiccups

<1% (limited to important or life-threatening symptoms): Syncope, malaise, substernal chest pain, abnormal ECG, hypertension, hypotension, arrhythmia, T wave inversion, angina, myocardial infarction, pericarditis, pulmonary embolism, peripheral ischemia, thrombophlebitis, vasculitis, dysphagia, enterocolitis, gastric ulcer, gastrointestinal hemorrhage, ileus, melena, mucositis, esophageal stricture, esophagitis, peptic ulcer, stomatitis, tongue discoloration, tongue ulceration, hypothyroidism, thrombocytopenic purpura, thrombocytopenia, anemia, eosinophilia, granulocytopenia, leukopenia, leukocytosis, lymphadenopathy, cholelithiasis, increased transaminases, arthropathy, avascular necrosis (femoral head), bursitis, costochondritis, synovitis, tendonitis, tenosynovitis, coma, dyskinesia, dysphonia, aggravated multiple sclerosis, neuralgia, neuropathy, paresthesia, agitation, confusion, depersonalization, emotional lability, manic reaction, paranoia, somnolence, hyperkinesia, hallucination, fall, sepsis, bronchospasm, nasal ulcer, pleural effusion, pulmonary fibrosis, systemic lupus erythematosus, alopecia, dermatitis, eczema, photosensitivity reaction, dry skin, skin ulceration, bullous eruption, deafness, motion sickness, parosmia, taste perversion, blepharitis, cataract, corneal ulceration, diplopia, glaucoma, anterior chamber hemorrhage, retinal disorder, scleritis, tinnitus, epididymitis, menstrual disorder, genital pruritus, dysuria, hematuria, renal calculus, abnormal renal function, decreased urine flow, postural hypotension, aphasia, convulsions, paralysis, gingival hyperplasia, intestinal obstruction, bundle branch block, increased CPK, electrolyte abnormality, aggressive behavior, delirium, impotence, apnea, oliguria, urinary retention, lymphocytosis

Drug Interactions CYP2D6 and CYP3A3/4 substrate

Increased effect: Drugs which inhibit CYP2D6 (including amiodarone, fluoxetine, paroxetine, quinidine, ritonavir) or CYP3A3/4 (including diltiazem, erythromycin, itraconazole, ketoconazole, verapamil) may increase levels of cevimeline. The effects of other cholinergic agents may be increased during concurrent administration with cevimeline. Concurrent use of cevimeline and beta-blockers may increase the potential for conduction disturbances.

Decreased effect: Anticholinergic agents (atropine, TCA's, phenothiazines) may antagonize the effects of cevimeline

Onset 1.5-2 hours

Half-Life 5 hours

Education and Monitoring Issues

Patient Education: May be taken with or without food; take with food if medicine causes upset stomach. May cause decreased visual acuity (particularly at night and in patients with central lens changes) and impaired depth perception; patients should be cautioned about driving at night or performing hazardous activities in reduced lighting.

Dietary Considerations: Take with or without food

Manufacturer Daiichi Pharmaceutical Corp

Related Information

Pharmaceutical Manufacturers Directory *on page 1020*

♦ **Ce-Vi-Sol® [OTC]** *see* Ascorbic Acid *on page 72*

Chamomile

Pharmacologic Class Herbal

Mechanism of Action Pharmacologic activities include antispasmodic, anti-inflammatory, antiulcer, and antibacterial effects; a sedative effect has also been documented

Use Has been used for indigestion and its hypnotic properties; topical anti-inflammatory agent; used for hemorrhoids, irritable bowel, eczema, mastitis and leg ulcers; used to flavor cigarette tobacco

USUAL DOSAGE

Tea: ±150 mL H_2O poured over heaping tablespoon (±3 g) of chamomile, covered and steeped 5-10 minutes; tea used 3-4 times/day for G.I. upset

Liquid extract: 1-4 mL 3 times/day

Contraindications Known hypersensitivity to *Asteraceae/Compositae* family

Warnings/Precautions Use with caution in asthmatics; cross sensitivity may occur in individuals allergic to ragweed pollens, asters, or chrysanthemums

Pregnancy Implications Excessive use should be avoided due to potential teratogenicity

Adverse Reactions

Dermatologic: Contact dermatitis, immunologic contact urticaria

Gastrointestinal: Emesis (from dried flowering heads)

Miscellaneous: Anaphylaxis

While the toxicity of its main chemical constituent (Bisabolol) is low, the tea is essentially prepared from various allergens (ie, pollen-laden flower heads) which can cause hypersensitivity reactions especially in atopic individuals; contains various flavonoids (apigenin, herniarin)

Drug Interactions May increase effect of coumarin-type anticoagulants at high dosages

♦ **Charac** *see* Charcoal *on page 175*

♦ **Charcoaid® [OTC]** *see* Charcoal *on page 175*

Charcoal (CHAR kole)

Pharmacologic Class Antidiarrheal; Antidote; Antiflatulent

U.S. Brand Names Actidose-Aqua® [OTC]; Actidose® With Sorbitol [OTC]; Charcoaid® [OTC]; Charcocaps® [OTC]; Insta-Char® [OTC]; Liqui-Char® [OTC]

Generic Available Yes

Mechanism of Action Adsorbs toxic substances or irritants, thus inhibiting GI absorption; adsorbs intestinal gas; the addition of sorbitol results in hyperosmotic laxative action causing catharsis

Use Emergency treatment in poisoning by drugs and chemicals; repetitive doses for gastric dialysis in uremia to adsorb various waste products, and repetitive doses have proven useful to enhance the elimination of certain drugs (eg, theophylline, phenobarbital, and aspirin)

USUAL DOSAGE Oral:

Acute poisoning:

Charcoal with sorbitol: Single-dose:

- Children 1-12 years: 1-2 g/kg/dose or 15-30 g or approximately 5-10 times the weight of the ingested poison; 1 g adsorbs 100-1000 mg of poison; the use of repeat oral charcoal with sorbitol doses is not recommended. In young children, sorbitol should be repeated no more than 1-2 times/day.
- Adults: 30-100 g

Charcoal in water:

- Single-dose:
  - Infants <1 year: 1 g/kg
  - Children 1-12 years: 15-30 g or 1-2 g/kg
  - Adults: 30-100 g or 1-2 g/kg
- Multiple-dose:
  - Infants <1 year: 0.5 g/kg every 4-6 hours
  - Children 1-12 years: 20-60 g or 0.5-1 g/kg every 2-6 hours until clinical observations, serum drug concentration have returned to a subtherapeutic range, or charcoal stool apparent
  - Adults: 20-60 g or 0.5-1 g/kg every 2-6 hours

Gastric dialysis: Adults: 20-50 g every 6 hours for 1-2 days

Intestinal gas, diarrhea, GI distress: Adults: 520-975 mg after meals or at first sign of discomfort; repeat as needed to a maximum dose of 4.16 g/day

Dosage Forms CAP (Charcocaps®): 260 mg. **LIQ, activated:** (Actidose-Aqua®): 12.5 g (60 mL), 25 g (120 mL); (Liqui-Char®): 12.5 g (60 mL), 15 g (75 mL), 25 g (120 mL), 30 g (120 mL), 50 g (240 mL); (SuperChar®): 30 g (240 mL). **LIQ, activated,** with propylene glycol: 12.5 g (60 mL), 25 g (120 mL); With sorbitol: (Actidose® With Sorbitol): 25 g (120 mL), 50 g (240 mL); (Charcoaid®): 30 g (150 mL); (SuperChar®): 30 g (240 mL). **POWDER for susp, activated:** 15 g, 30 g, 40 g, 120 g, 240 g; (SuperChar®): 30 g

Contraindications Not effective for cyanide, mineral acids, caustic alkalis, organic solvents, iron, ethanol, methanol poisoning, lithium; do not use charcoal with sorbitol in patients with fructose intolerance; charcoal with sorbitol is not recommended in children <1 year.

Warnings/Precautions When using ipecac with charcoal, induce vomiting with ipecac before administering activated charcoal since charcoal adsorbs ipecac syrup; charcoal may cause vomiting which is hazardous in petroleum distillate and caustic ingestions; if charcoal in sorbitol is administered, doses should be limited to prevent excessive fluid and electrolyte losses; do not mix charcoal with milk, ice cream, or sherbet

Pregnancy Risk Factor C

(Continued)

Charcoal *(Continued)*

Adverse Reactions

>10%:

Gastrointestinal: Vomiting, diarrhea with sorbitol, constipation

Miscellaneous: Stools will turn black

<1%: Swelling of abdomen

Drug Interactions Do not administer concomitantly with syrup of ipecac; do not mix with milk, ice cream, or sherbet

Education and Monitoring Issues

Patient Education: Charcoal will cause your stools to turn black. Do not self-administer as an antidote before calling the poison control center, hospital emergency room, or prescriber for instructions (charcoal is not the antidote for all poisons).

- **Charcocaps® [OTC]** *see* Charcoal *on page 175*
- **Charcodote Aqueous** *see* Charcoal *on page 175*
- **Chealamide®** *see* Edetate Disodium *on page 305*
- **Chelated Manganese® [OTC]** *see* Manganese *on page 554*
- **Chenix®** *see* Chenodiol *on page 176*

Chenodiol (kee noe DYE ole)

Pharmacologic Class Bile Acid

U.S. Brand Names Chenix®

Use Oral dissolution of cholesterol gallstones in selected patients

USUAL DOSAGE Adults: Oral: 13-16 mg/kg/day in 2 divided doses, starting with 250 mg twice daily the first 2 weeks and increasing by 250 mg/day each week thereafter until the recommended or maximum tolerated dose is achieved

Dosing comments in hepatic impairment: Contraindicated for use in presence of known hepatocyte dysfunction or bile ductal abnormalities

Contraindications Presence of known hepatocyte dysfunction or bile ductal abnormalities; a gallbladder confirmed as nonvisualizing after two consecutive single doses of dye; radiopaque stones; gallstone complications or compelling reasons for gallbladder surgery; inflammatory bowel disease or active gastric or duodenal ulcer; pregnancy

Pregnancy Risk Factor X

- **Cheracol®** *see* Guaifenesin and Codeine *on page 424*
- **Cheracol® D [OTC]** *see* Guaifenesin and Dextromethorphan *on page 424*
- **Chibroxin™ Ophthalmic** *see* Norfloxacin *on page 663*
- **Chigger-Tox® [OTC]** *see* Benzocaine *on page 98*
- **Children's Advil® Oral Suspension [OTC]** *see* Ibuprofen *on page 458*
- **Children's Motrin® Oral Suspension [OTC]** *see* Ibuprofen *on page 458*
- **Children's Silapap® [OTC]** *see* Acetaminophen *on page 17*
- **Children's Silfedrine® [OTC]** *see* Pseudoephedrine *on page 792*

Chloral Hydrate (KLOR al HYE drate)

Pharmacologic Class Hypnotic, Miscellaneous

U.S. Brand Names Aquachloral® Supprettes®

Generic Available Yes

Mechanism of Action Central nervous system depressant effects are due to its active metabolite trichloroethanol, mechanism unknown

Use Short-term sedative and hypnotic (<2 weeks), sedative/hypnotic for dental and diagnostic procedures; sedative prior to EEG evaluations

USUAL DOSAGE

Children:

Sedation, anxiety: Oral, rectal: 5-15 mg/kg/dose every 8 hours, maximum: 500 mg/dose

Prior to EEG: Oral, rectal: 20-25 mg/kg/dose, 30-60 minutes prior to EEG; may repeat in 30 minutes to maximum of 100 mg/kg or 2 g total

Hypnotic: Oral, rectal: 20-40 mg/kg/dose up to a maximum of 50 mg/kg/24 hours or 1 g/dose or 2 g/24 hours

Sedation, nonpainful procedure: Oral: 50-75 mg/kg/dose 30-60 minutes prior to procedure; may repeat 30 minutes after initial dose if needed, to a total maximum dose of 120 mg/kg or 1 g total

Adults: Oral, rectal:

Sedation, anxiety: 250 mg 3 times/day

Hypnotic: 500-1000 mg at bedtime or 30 minutes prior to procedure, not to exceed 2 g/24 hours

Dosing adjustment/comments in renal impairment: Cl_{cr} <50 mL/minute: Avoid use

Hemodialysis: Dialyzable (50% to 100%); supplemental dose is not necessary

Dosing adjustment/comments in hepatic impairment: Avoid use in patients with severe hepatic impairment

Dosage Forms SUPP, rectal: 324 mg, 500 mg, 648 mg. **SYR:** 250 mg/5 mL (10 mL); 500 mg/5 mL (5 mL, 10 mL, 480 mL)

Contraindications Hypersensitivity to chloral hydrate or any component; hepatic or renal impairment; gastritis or ulcers; severe cardiac disease

Warnings/Precautions Use with caution in patients with porphyria; use with caution in neonates, drug may accumulate with repeated use, prolonged use in neonates associated with hyperbilirubinemia; tolerance to hypnotic effect develops, therefore, not recommended for use >2 weeks; taper dosage to avoid withdrawal with prolonged use; trichloroethanol (TCE), a metabolite of chloral hydrate, is a carcinogen in mice; there is no data in humans. Chloral hydrate is considered a second line hypnotic agent in the elderly. Recent interpretive guidelines from the Health Care Financing Administration (HCFA) discourage the use of chloral hydrate in residents of long-term care facilities.

Pregnancy Risk Factor C

Adverse Reactions

Central nervous system: Ataxia, disorientation, sedation, excitement (paradoxical), dizziness, fever, headache, confusion, lightheadedness, nightmares, hallucinations, drowsiness, "hangover" effect

Dermatologic: Rash, urticaria

Gastrointestinal: Gastric irritation, nausea, vomiting, diarrhea, flatulence

Hematologic: Leukopenia, eosinophilia, acute intermittent porphyria

Miscellaneous: Physical and psychological dependence may occur with prolonged use of large doses

Drug Interactions

Chloral hydrate and ethanol (and other CNS depressants) have additive CNS depressant effects; monitor for CNS depression

Chloral hydrate's metabolite may displace warfarin from its protein binding sites resulting in an increase in the hypoprothrombinemic response to warfarin; warfarin dosages may need to be adjusted

Diaphoresis, flushing, and hypertension have occurred in patients who received I.V. furosemide within 24 hours after administration of chloral hydrate; consider using a benzodiazepine

Alcohol Interactions Avoid use (may increase central nervous system depression)

Onset 0.5-1 hour

Duration 4-8 hours

Half-Life Active metabolite: 8-11 hours

Education and Monitoring Issues

Patient Education: Use exactly as directed (do not increase dose or frequency or discontinue without consulting prescriber); may cause physical and/or psychological dependence. While using this medication, do not use alcohol and other prescription or OTC medications (especially, pain medications, sedatives, antihistamines, or hypnotics) without consulting prescriber. Maintain adequate hydration (2-3 L/day of fluids unless instructed to restrict fluid intake). You may experience drowsiness, dizziness, or blurred vision (use caution when driving or engaging in tasks requiring alertness until response to drug is known); nausea, vomiting, unpleasant taste (small frequent meals, frequent mouth care, chewing gum, or sucking lozenges may help); diarrhea (buttermilk, boiled milk, yogurt may help). Report skin rash or irritation, CNS changes (confusion, depression, increased sedation, excitation, headache, insomnia, or nightmares), unresolved gastrointestinal distress, chest pain or palpitations, or ineffectiveness of medication.

Monitoring Parameters: Vital signs, O_2 saturation and blood pressure with doses used for conscious sedation

Chlorambucil (klor AM byoo sil)

Pharmacologic Class Antineoplastic Agent, Alkylating Agent

U.S. Brand Names Leukeran®

Generic Available No

Mechanism of Action Chlorambucil is a nitrogen mustard derivative that appears to work as a bifunctional alkylating agent. It probably forms intrastrand cross-links, interfering with DNA replication and RNA transcription and translation. Chlorambucil appears to be cell-cycle nonspecific.

Use Management of chronic lymphocytic leukemia, Hodgkin's and non-Hodgkin's lymphoma; breast and ovarian carcinoma; Waldenström's macroglobulinemia, testicular carcinoma, thrombocythemia, choriocarcinoma

USUAL DOSAGE Oral (refer to individual protocols):

Children:

General short courses: 0.1-0.2 mg/kg/day **OR** 4.5 mg/m^2/day for 3-6 weeks for remission induction (usual: 4-10 mg/day); maintenance therapy: 0.03-0.1 mg/kg/day (usual: 2-4 mg/day)

Nephrotic syndrome: 0.1-0.2 mg/kg/day every day for 5-15 weeks with low-dose prednisone

Chronic lymphocytic leukemia (CLL):

Biweekly regimen: Initial: 0.4 mg/kg/dose every 2 weeks; increase dose by 0.1 mg/kg every 2 weeks until a response occurs and/or myelosuppression occurs

Monthly regimen: Initial: 0.4 mg/kg, increase dose by 0.2 mg/kg every 4 weeks until a response occurs and/or myelosuppression occurs

(Continued)

Chlorambucil *(Continued)*

Malignant lymphomas:

Non-Hodgkin's lymphoma: 0.1 mg/kg/day

Hodgkin's lymphoma: 0.2 mg/kg/day

Adults: 0.1-0.2 mg/kg/day **OR** 3-6 mg/m^2/day for 3-6 weeks, then adjust dose on basis of blood counts. Pulse dosing has been used in CLL as intermittent, biweekly, or monthly doses of 0.4 mg/kg and increased by 0.1 mg/kg until the disease is under control or toxicity ensues. An alternate regimen is 14 mg/m^2/day for 5 days, repeated every 21-28 days.

Hemodialysis: Supplemental dosing is not necessary

Peritoneal dialysis: Supplemental dosing is not necessary

Dosage Forms TAB, sugar coated: 2 mg

Contraindications Previous resistance; hypersensitivity to chlorambucil or any component or other alkylating agents

Warnings/Precautions The U.S. Food and Drug Administration (FDA) currently recommends that procedures for proper handling and disposal of antineoplastic agents be considered. Use with caution in patients with seizure disorder and bone marrow suppression; reduce initial dosage if patient has received radiation therapy, myelosuppressive drugs or has a depressed baseline leukocyte or platelet count within the previous 4 weeks. Can severely suppress bone marrow function; affects human fertility; carcinogenic in humans and probably mutagenic and teratogenic as well; chromosomal damage has been documented; secondary AML may be associated with chronic therapy.

Pregnancy Risk Factor D

Pregnancy Implications Clinical effects on the fetus: Carcinogenic and mutagenic in humans

Adverse Reactions

>10%:

Hematologic: Myelosuppressive: Use with caution when receiving radiation; bone marrow suppression frequently occurs and occasionally bone marrow failure has occurred; blood counts should be monitored closely while undergoing treatment; leukopenia, thrombocytopenia, anemia

WBC: Moderate

Platelets: Moderate

Onset (days): 7

Nadir (days): 10-14

Recovery (days): 28

1% to 10%:

Dermatologic: Skin rashes

Endocrine & metabolic: Hyperuricemia, menstrual changes

Gastrointestinal: Nausea, vomiting, diarrhea, oral ulceration are all infrequent

Emetic potential: Low (<10%)

<1%: Agitation, ataxia, confusion, drug fever, hallucination; rarely generalized or focal seizures, rash, fertility impairment; has caused chromosomal damage in men, both reversible and permanent sterility have occurred in both sexes; can produce amenorrhea in females, oral ulceration, oligospermia, hepatotoxicity, hepatic necrosis, weakness, tremors, muscular twitching, peripheral neuropathy, pulmonary fibrosis, secondary malignancies; Increased incidence of AML; skin hypersensitivity

Duration ~4 weeks

Half-Life 90 minutes to 2 hours

Education and Monitoring Issues

Patient Education: Take exactly as directed (may be taken with chilled liquids). Maintain adequate hydration (2-3 L/day of fluids unless instructed to restrict fluid intake). Avoid alcohol, acidic, spicy, or hot foods, aspirin, or OTC medications unless approved by prescriber. You may experience menstrual irregularities and/or sterility. You will be more susceptible to infection (avoid crowds or contagious persons, and do not receive any vaccinations unless approved by prescriber). Frequent mouth care with soft toothbrush or cotton swab may reduce occurrence of mouth sores. Report easy bruising or bleeding; fever or chills; numbness, pain, or tingling of extremities; muscle cramping or weakness; unusual swelling of extremities; menstrual irregularities; or any difficulty breathing.

Monitoring Parameters: Liver function tests, CBC, leukocyte counts, platelets, serum uric acid

Manufacturer GlaxoWellcome

Related Information

Pharmaceutical Manufacturers Directory *on page 1020*

Chloramphenicol (klor am FEN i kole)

Pharmacologic Class Antibiotic, Ophthalmic; Antibiotic, Otic; Antibiotic, Miscellaneous

U.S. Brand Names AK-Chlor® Ophthalmic; Chloromycetin®; Chloroptic® Ophthalmic

Generic Available Yes

Mechanism of Action Reversibly binds to 50S ribosomal subunits of susceptible organisms preventing amino acids from being transferred to growing peptide chains thus inhibiting protein synthesis

Use Treatment of serious infections due to organisms resistant to other less toxic antibiotics or when its penetrability into the site of infection is clinically superior to other antibiotics to which the organism is sensitive; useful in infections caused by *Bacteroides*, *H. influenzae*, *Neisseria meningitidis*, *Salmonella*, and *Rickettsia*; active against many vancomycin-resistant enterococci

USUAL DOSAGE

Meningitis: I.V.: Infants >30 days and Children: 50-100 mg/kg/day divided every 6 hours

Other infections: I.V.:

Infants >30 days and Children: 50-75 mg/kg/day divided every 6 hours; maximum daily dose: 4 g/day

Adults: 50-100 mg/kg/day in divided doses every 6 hours; maximum daily dose: 4 g/day

Ophthalmic: Children and Adults: Instill 1-2 drops or 1.25 cm (1/2" of ointment every 3-4 hours); increase interval between applications after 48 hours to 2-3 times/day

Otic solution: Instill 2-3 drops into ear 3 times/day

Topical: Gently rub into the affected area 1-4 times/day

Dosing adjustment/comments in hepatic impairment: Avoid use in severe liver impairment as increased toxicity may occur

Hemodialysis: Slightly dialyzable (5% to 20%) via hemo- and peritoneal dialysis; no supplemental doses needed in dialysis or continuous arteriovenous or veno-venous hemofiltration (CAVH/CAVHD)

Dosage Forms CAP: 250 mg. **OINT, ophth:** 1% [10 mg/g] (3.5 g); (AK-Chlor®, Chloromycetin®, Chloroptic® S.O.P.®): 1% [10 mg/g] (3.5 g). **POWDER for inj,** as sodium succinate: 1 g. **POWDER for ophth soln** (Chloromycetin®): 25 mg/vial (15 mL). **SOLN:** 0.5% [5 mg/mL] (7.5 mL, 15 mL). **OPHTH** (AK-Chlor®, Chloroptic®): 0.5% [5 mg/mL] (2.5 mL, 7.5 mL, 15 mL). **OTIC** (Chloromycetin®): 0.5% (15 mL)

Contraindications Hypersensitivity to chloramphenicol or any component

Warnings/Precautions Use with caution in patients with impaired renal or hepatic function and in neonates; reduce dose with impaired liver function; use with care in patients with glucose 6-phosphate dehydrogenase deficiency. Serious and fatal blood dyscrasias have occurred after both short-term and prolonged therapy; should not be used when less potentially toxic agents are effective; prolonged use may result in superinfection.

Pregnancy Risk Factor C

Adverse Reactions <1%: Aplastic anemia, bone marrow suppression, diarrhea, enterocolitis, gray syndrome, headache, nausea, nightmares, optic neuritis, peripheral neuropathy, rash, stomatitis, vomiting

Three (3) major toxicities associated with chloramphenicol include:

Aplastic anemia, an idiosyncratic reaction which can occur with any route of administration; usually occurs 3 weeks to 12 months after initial exposure to chloramphenicol

Bone marrow suppression is thought to be dose-related with serum concentrations >25 μg/mL and reversible once chloramphenicol is discontinued; anemia and neutropenia may occur during the first week of therapy

Gray syndrome is characterized by circulatory collapse, cyanosis, acidosis, abdominal distention, myocardial depression, coma, and death; reaction appears to be associated with serum levels ≥50 μg/mL; may result from drug accumulation in patients with impaired hepatic or renal function

Drug Interactions CYP2C9 enzyme inhibitor

Decreased effect: Phenobarbital and rifampin may decrease concentration of chloramphenicol

Increased toxicity: Chloramphenicol inhibits the metabolism of chlorpropamide, phenytoin, oral anticoagulants

Alcohol Interactions Use with caution (may cause a mild disulfiram-like reaction; symptoms include headache, nausea, vomiting, chest or abdominal pain)

Half-Life Prolonged with markedly reduced liver function or combined liver/kidney dysfunction; Normal renal function: 1.6-3.3 hours; End-stage renal disease: 3-7 hours; Cirrhosis: 10-12 hours

Education and Monitoring Issues

Patient Education:

Oral: Take as directed, at regular intervals around-the-clock, with a large glass of water. Maintain adequate hydration (2-3 L/day of fluids unless instructed to restrict fluid intake). During I.V. administration, a bitter taste may occur; this will pass. Diabetics: Drug may cause false-positive test with Clinitest® glucose monitoring; use alternative glucose monitoring. This drug may interfere with effectiveness of oral contraceptives. You may experience nausea, vomiting (frequent small meals, frequent mouth care, sucking lozenges, or chewing gum may help). Report persistent rash, diarrhea; pain, burning, or numbness of extremities; petechiae; sore throat; fatigue; unusual bleeding or bruising; vaginal itching or discharge; mouth sores; yellowing of skin or eyes; dark urine or stool discoloration (blue); CNS disturbances (nightmares acute headache); or lack or improvement or worsening of condition.

Ophthalmic: Wash hands before instilling. Sit or lie down to instill. Open eye, look at ceiling, and instill prescribed amount of medication. Close eye and apply gentle

(Continued)

Chloramphenicol *(Continued)*

pressure to inner corner of eye. Do not let tip of applicator touch eye or contaminate tip of applicator. Temporary stinging or burning may occur. Report persistent pain, burning, vision disturbances, swelling, itching, rash, or worsening of condition.

Otic: Wash hands before instilling. Tilt head with affected ear upward. Gently grasp ear lobe and lift back and upward. Instill prescribed drops into ear canal. Do not push dropper into ear. Remain with head tilted for 2 minutes. Report ringing in ears, discharge, or worsening of condition.

Topical: Wash hands before applying or wear gloves. Apply thin film to affected area. May apply porous dressing. Report persistent burning, swelling, itching, or worsening of condition.

Dietary Considerations: Folic acid, iron salts, vitamin B_{12}: May decrease intestinal absorption of vitamin B_{12}; may have increased dietary need for riboflavin, pyridoxine, and vitamin B_{12}; monitor hematological status

Monitoring Parameters: CBC with reticulocyte and platelet counts, periodic liver and renal function tests, serum drug concentration

Reference Range:

Therapeutic levels: 15-20 μg/mL; Toxic concentration: >40 μg/mL; Trough: 5-10 μg/mL

Timing of serum samples: Draw levels 1.5 hours and 3 hours after completion of I.V. or oral dose; trough levels may be preferred; should be drawn ≤1 hour prior to dose

Related Information

Antimicrobial Drugs of Choice *on page 1182*
Chloramphenicol and Prednisolone *on page 180*
Chloramphenicol, Polymyxin B, and Hydrocortisone *on page 180*

Chloramphenicol and Prednisolone

(klor am FEN i kole & pred NIS oh lone)

Pharmacologic Class Antibiotic/Corticosteroid, Ophthalmic

U.S. Brand Names Chloroptic-P® Ophthalmic

Dosage Forms OINT, ophth: Chloramphenicol 1% and prednisolone 0.5% (3.5 g)

Pregnancy Risk Factor C

Chloramphenicol, Polymyxin B, and Hydrocortisone

(klor am FEN i kole, pol i MIKS in bee, & hye droe KOR ti sone)

Pharmacologic Class Antibiotic/Corticosteroid, Ophthalmic

Dosage Forms SOLN, ophth: Chloramphenicol 1%, polymyxin B sulfate 10,000 units, and hydrocortisone acetate 0.5% per g (3.75 g)

Pregnancy Risk Factor C

Chlordiazepoxide (klor dye az e POKS ide)

Pharmacologic Class Benzodiazepine

U.S. Brand Names Libritabs®; Librium®; Mitran® Oral; Reposans-10® Oral

Generic Available Yes

Use Approved for anxiety, may be useful for acute alcohol withdrawal symptoms

USUAL DOSAGE

Children:
- <6 years: Not recommended
- >6 years: Anxiety: Oral, I.M.: 0.5 mg/kg/24 hours divided every 6-8 hours

Adults:
- Anxiety:
  - Oral: 15-100 mg divided 3-4 times/day
  - I.M., I.V.: Initial: 50-100 mg followed by 25-50 mg 3-4 times/day as needed
- Preoperative anxiety: I.M.: 50-100 mg prior to surgery
- Alcohol withdrawal symptoms: Oral, I.V.: 50-100 mg to start, dose may be repeated in 2-4 hours as necessary to a maximum of 300 mg/24 hours

Dosing adjustment in renal impairment: Cl_{cr} <10 mL/minute: Administer 50% of dose

Hemodialysis: Not dialyzable (0% to 5%)

Dosing adjustment/comments in hepatic impairment: Avoid use

Dosage Forms CAP: 5 mg, 10 mg, 25 mg. **POWDER for inj:** 100 mg. **TAB:** 5 mg, 10 mg, 25 mg

Contraindications Hypersensitivity to chlordiazepoxide or any component, pre-existing CNS depression, severe uncontrolled pain

Warnings/Precautions Use with caution in patients with respiratory depression, CNS impairment, liver dysfunction, or a history of drug dependence

Pregnancy Risk Factor D

Adverse Reactions

>10%:
- Central nervous system: Drowsiness, fatigue, ataxia, lightheadedness, memory impairment, dysarthria, irritability
- Dermatologic: Rash
- Endocrine & metabolic: Decreased libido, menstrual disorders

Gastrointestinal: Xerostomia, decreased salivation, increased or decreased appetite, weight gain or loss
Genitourinary: Micturition difficulties

1% to 10%:
Cardiovascular: Hypotension
Central nervous system: Confusion, dizziness, disinhibition, akathisia, increased libido
Dermatologic: Dermatitis
Gastrointestinal: Increased salivation
Genitourinary: Sexual dysfunction, incontinence
Neuromuscular & skeletal: Rigidity, tremor, muscle cramps
Otic: Tinnitus
Respiratory: Nasal congestion

Drug Interactions CYP3A3/4 enzyme substrate

Decreased therapeutic effect: Carbamazepine, rifampin, rifabutin may enhance the metabolism of alprazolam and decrease its therapeutic effect; consider using an alternative sedative/hypnotic agent

Increased toxicity: Cimetidine, ciprofloxacin, clarithromycin, clozapine, CNS depressants, diltiazem, disulfiram, digoxin, erythromycin, ethanol, fluconazole, fluoxetine, fluvoxamine, isoniazid, itraconazole, ketoconazole, labetalol, levodopa, loxapine, metoprolol, metronidazole, miconazole, nefazodone, omeprazole, phenytoin, rifabutin, rifampin, troleandomycin, valproic acid, verapamil may increase the serum level and/or toxicity of alprazolam; monitor for altered benzodiazepine response

Alcohol Interactions Avoid use (may increase central nervous system depression)

Onset Peak concentrations in ~2 hours

Duration 48 hours to 1 week

Half-Life 6.6-25 hours; End-stage renal disease: 5-30 hours; Cirrhosis: 30-63 hours

Education and Monitoring Issues

Patient Education: Oral: Take exactly as directed (do not increase dose or frequency); may cause physical and/or psychological dependence. Do not use excessive alcohol or other prescription or OTC medications (especially pain medications, sedatives, antihistamines, or hypnotics) without consulting prescriber. Maintain adequate hydration (2-3 L/day of fluids unless instructed to restrict fluid intake). You may experience drowsiness, lightheadedness, impaired coordination, dizziness, or blurred vision (use caution when driving or engaging in tasks requiring alertness until response to drug is known); or dry mouth (small frequent meals, frequent mouth care, chewing gum, or sucking lozenges may help); constipation (increased exercise, fluids, or dietary fruit and fiber may help); or altered sexual drive or ability (reversible). Report persistent CNS effects (eg, euphoria, confusion, increased sedation, depression); chest pain, palpitations, or rapid heartbeat; muscle cramping, weakness, tremors, rigidity, or altered gait; or worsening of condition.

Dietary Considerations: Grapefruit juice may increase serum levels and/or toxicity

Monitoring Parameters: Respiratory and cardiovascular status, mental status, check for orthostasis

Reference Range: Therapeutic: 0.1-3 μg/mL (SI: 0-10 μmol/L); Toxic: >23 μg/mL (SI: >77 μmol/L)

Related Information

Amitriptyline and Chlordiazepoxide *on page 52*
Clidinium and Chlordiazepoxide *on page 208*

Chlorhexidine Gluconate (klor HEKS i deen GLOO koe nate)

Pharmacologic Class Antibiotic, Oral Rinse; Antibiotic, Topical

U.S. Brand Names BactoShield® Topical [OTC]; Betasept® [OTC]; Dyna-Hex® Topical [OTC]; Exidine® Scrub [OTC]; Hibiclens® Topical [OTC]; Hibistat® Topical [OTC]; Peridex® Oral Rinse; PerioChip®; PerioGard®

Use Skin cleanser for surgical scrub, cleanser for skin wounds, germicidal hand rinse, and as antibacterial dental rinse. Chlorhexidine is active against gram-positive and gram-negative organisms, facultative anaerobes, aerobes, and yeast.

USUAL DOSAGE Adults:

Oral rinse (Peridex®):

Precede use of solution by flossing and brushing teeth; completely rinse toothpaste from mouth. Swish 15 mL undiluted oral rinse around in mouth for 30 seconds, then expectorate. Caution patient not to swallow the medicine. Avoid eating for 2-3 hours after treatment. (The cap on bottle of oral rinse is a measure for 15 mL.)

When used as a treatment of gingivitis, the regimen begins with oral prophylaxis. Patient treats mouth with 15 mL chlorhexidine, swishes for 30 seconds, then expectorates. This is repeated twice daily (morning and evening). Patient should have a re-evaluation followed by a dental prophylaxis every 6 months.

Cleanser:

Surgical scrub: Scrub 3 minutes and rinse thoroughly, wash for an additional 3 minutes
Hand wash: Wash for 15 seconds and rinse
Hand rinse: Rub 15 seconds and rinse

(Continued)

Chlorhexidine Gluconate *(Continued)*

Periodontal chip: Adults: One chip is inserted into a periodontal pocket with a probing pocket depth ≥5 mm. Up to 8 chips may be inserted in a single visit. Treatment is recommended every 3 months in pockets with a remaining depth ≥5 mm. If dislodgment occurs 7 days or more after placement, the subject is considered to have had the full course of treatment. If dislodgment occurs within 48 hours, a new chip should be inserted.

Insertion of periodontal chip: Pocket should be isolated and surrounding area dried prior to chip insertion. The chip should be grasped using forceps with the rounded edges away from the forceps. The chip should be inserted into the periodontal pocket to its maximum depth. It may be maneuvered into position using the tips of the forceps or a flat instrument. The chip biodegrades completely and does not need to be removed. Patients should avoid dental floss at the site of PerioChip® insertion for 10 days after placement because flossing might dislodge the chip.

Contraindications Known hypersensitivity to chlorhexidine gluconate

Pregnancy Risk Factor B

- **Chlorhexseptic** *see* Chlorhexidine Gluconate *on page 181*
- **Chloromycetin®** *see* Chloramphenicol *on page 178*

Chloroprocaine (klor oh PROE kane)

Pharmacologic Class Local Anesthetic

U.S. Brand Names Nesacaine®; Nesacaine®-MPF

Generic Available No

Mechanism of Action Chloroprocaine HCl is benzoic acid, 4-amino-2-chloro-2-(diethylamino) ethyl ester monohydrochloride. Chloroprocaine is an ester-type local anesthetic, which stabilizes the neuronal membranes and prevents initiation and transmission of nerve impulses thereby affecting local anesthetic actions. Local anesthetics including chloroprocaine, reversibly prevent generation and conduction of electrical impulses in neurons by decreasing the transient increase in permeability to sodium. The differential sensitivity generally depends on the size of the fiber; small fibers are more sensitive than larger fibers and require a longer period for recovery. Sensory pain fibers are usually blocked first, followed by fibers that transmit sensations of temperature, touch, and deep pressure. High concentrations block sympathetic somatic sensory and somatic motor fibers. The spread of anesthesia depends upon the distribution of the solution. This is primarily dependent on the volume of drug injected.

Use Infiltration anesthesia and peripheral and epidural anesthesia

USUAL DOSAGE Dosage varies with anesthetic procedure, the area to be anesthetized, the vascularity of the tissues, depth of anesthesia required, degree of muscle relaxation required, and duration of anesthesia; range: 1.5-25 mL of 2% to 3% solution; single adult dose should not exceed 800 mg

Infiltration and peripheral nerve block: 1% to 2%

Infiltration, peripheral and central nerve block, including caudal and epidural block: 2% to 3%, without preservatives

Dosage Forms INJ: Preservative free (Nesacaine®-MPF): 2% (30 mL), 3% (30 mL); With preservative (Nesacaine®): 1% (30 mL), 2% (30 mL)

Contraindications Known hypersensitivity to chloroprocaine, or other ester type anesthetics; myasthenia gravis; concurrent use of bupivacaine; do not use for subarachnoid administration

Warnings/Precautions Use with caution in patients with cardiac disease, renal disease, and hyperthyroidism; convulsions and cardiac arrest have been reported presumably due to intravascular injection

Pregnancy Risk Factor C

Adverse Reactions <1%: Anaphylactoid reactions, anxiety, blurred vision, bradycardia, cardiovascular collapse, chills, confusion, disorientation, drowsiness, edema, hypotension, myocardial depression, nausea, respiratory arrest, restlessness, seizures, shivering, tinnitus, transient stinging or burning at injection site, tremor, unconsciousness, urticaria, vomiting

Onset 6-12 minutes

Duration 30-60 minutes

Education and Monitoring Issues

Patient Education: This medication is given to reduce sensation in the injected area. You will experience decreased sensation to pain, heat, or cold in the area and/or decreased muscle strength (depending on area of application) until the effects wear off; use necessary caution to reduce incidence of possible injury until full sensation returns. Immediately report chest pain or palpitations; increased restlessness, confusion, anxiety, or dizziness; difficulty breathing; chills, shivering, or tremors; ringing in ears; or changes in vision.

- **Chloroptic® Ophthalmic** *see* Chloramphenicol *on page 178*
- **Chloroptic-P® Ophthalmic** *see* Chloramphenicol and Prednisolone *on page 180*

Chloroquine and Primaquine (KLOR oh kwin & PRIM a kween)

Pharmacologic Class Antimalarial Agent

U.S. Brand Names Aralen® Phosphate With Primaquine Phosphate

Generic Available No

Mechanism of Action Chloroquine concentrates within parasite acid vesicles and raises internal pH resulting in inhibition of parasite growth; may involve aggregates of ferriprotoporphyrin IX acting as chloroquine receptors causing membrane damage; may also interfere with nucleoprotein synthesis. Primaquine eliminates the primary tissue exoerythrocytic forms of *P. falciparum*; disrupts mitochondria and binds to DNA.

Use Prophylaxis of malaria, regardless of species, in all areas where the disease is endemic

USUAL DOSAGE Oral: Start at least 1 day before entering the endemic area; continue for 8 weeks after leaving the endemic area

Children: For suggested weekly dosage (based on body weight), see table:

Weight		Chloroquine Base (mg)	Primaquine Base (mg)	Dose* (mL)
lb	kg			
10-15	4.5-6.8	20	3	2.5
16-25	7.3-11.4	40	6	5
26-35	11.8-15.9	60	9	7.5
36-45	16.4-20.5	80	12	10
46-55	20.9-25	100	15	12.5
56-100	25.4-45.4	150	22.5	½ tablet
100+	>45.4	300	45	1 tablet

*Dose based on liquid containing approximately 40 mg of chloroquine base and 6 mg primaquine base per 5 mL, prepared from chloroquine phosphate with primaquine phosphate tablets.

Adults: 1 tablet/week on the same day each week

Dosage Forms TAB: Chloroquine phosphate 500 mg [base 300 mg] and primaquine phosphate 79 mg [base 45 mg]

Contraindications Retinal or visual field changes, known hypersensitivity to chloroquine or primaquine

Warnings/Precautions Use with caution in patients with psoriasis, porphyria, hepatic dysfunction, G-6-PD deficiency

Pregnancy Risk Factor C

Adverse Reactions

1% to 10%: Gastrointestinal: Diarrhea, nausea

<1%: Anorexia, blood dyscrasias, blurred vision, EKG changes, fatigue, hair bleaching, headache, hypotension, personality changes, pruritus, retinopathy, stomatitis, vomiting

Drug Interactions

Decreased absorption if administered concomitantly with kaolin and magnesium trisilicate

Increased toxicity/levels with cimetidine

Education and Monitoring Issues

Monitoring Parameters: Periodic CBC, examination for muscular weakness, and ophthalmologic examination in patients receiving prolonged therapy

Chloroquine Phosphate (KLOR oh kwin FOS fate)

Pharmacologic Class Aminoquinoline (Antimalarial)

U.S. Brand Names Aralen® Phosphate

Generic Available Yes

Mechanism of Action Binds to and inhibits DNA and RNA polymerase; interferes with metabolism and hemoglobin utilization by parasites; inhibits prostaglandin effects; chloroquine concentrates within parasite acid vesicles and raises internal pH resulting in inhibition of parasite growth; may involve aggregates of ferriprotoporphyrin IX acting as chloroquine receptors causing membrane damage; may also interfere with nucleoprotein synthesis

Use Suppression or chemoprophylaxis of malaria; treatment of uncomplicated or mild to moderate malaria; extraintestinal amebiasis

Unlabeled use: Rheumatoid arthritis; discoid lupus erythematosus, scleroderma, pemphigus

USUAL DOSAGE Oral (**dosage expressed in terms of mg of base**):

Suppression or prophylaxis of malaria:

Children: Administer 5 mg base/kg/week on the same day each week (not to exceed 300 mg base/dose); begin 1-2 weeks prior to exposure; continue for 4-6 weeks after leaving endemic area; if suppressive therapy is not begun prior to exposure, double the initial loading dose to 10 mg base/kg and administer in 2 divided doses 6 hours apart, followed by the usual dosage regimen

Adults: 300 mg/week (base) on the same day each week; begin 1-2 weeks prior to exposure; continue for 4-6 weeks after leaving endemic area; if suppressive therapy

(Continued)

Chloroquine Phosphate *(Continued)*

is not begun prior to exposure, double the initial loading dose to 600 mg base and administer in 2 divided doses 6 hours apart, followed by the usual dosage regimen

Acute attack:

Oral:

Children: 10 mg/kg on day 1, followed by 5 mg/kg 6 hours later and 5 mg/kg on days 2 and 3

Adults: 600 mg on day 1, followed by 300 mg 6 hours later, followed by 300 mg on days 2 and 3

I.M. (as hydrochloride):

Children: 5 mg/kg, repeat in 6 hours

Adults: Initial: 160-200 mg, repeat in 6 hours if needed; maximum: 800 mg first 24 hours; begin oral dosage as soon as possible and continue for 3 days until 1.5 g has been given

Extraintestinal amebiasis:

Children: Oral: 10 mg/kg once daily for 2-3 weeks (up to 300 mg base/day)

Adults:

Oral: 600 mg base/day for 2 days followed by 300 mg base/day for at least 2-3 weeks

I.M., as hydrochloride: 160-200 mg/day for 10 days; resume oral therapy as soon as possible

Dosing adjustment in renal impairment: Cl_{cr} <10 mL/minute: Administer 50% of dose

Hemodialysis: Minimally removed by hemodialysis

Dosage Forms INJ: 50 mg [40 mg base]/mL (5 mL). **TAB:** 250 mg [150 mg base]; 500 mg [300 mg base]

Contraindications Retinal or visual field changes; patients with psoriasis; known hypersensitivity to chloroquine

Warnings/Precautions Use with caution in patients with liver disease, G-6-PD deficiency, alcoholism or in conjunction with hepatotoxic drugs, psoriasis, porphyria may be exacerbated; retinopathy (irreversible) has occurred with long or high-dose therapy; discontinue drug if any abnormality in the visual field or if muscular weakness develops during treatment

Pregnancy Risk Factor C

Adverse Reactions

>1%: Gastrointestinal: Nausea, diarrhea

<1%: Anorexia, blood dyscrasias, blurred vision, EKG changes, fatigue, hair bleaching, headache, hypotension, personality changes, pruritus, retinopathy, stomatitis, vomiting

Drug Interactions

Chloroquine and other 4-aminoquinolones may be decreased due to GI binding with kaolin or magnesium trisilicate

Increased effect: Cimetidine increases levels of chloroquine and probably other 4-aminoquinolones

Half-Life 3-5 days

Education and Monitoring Issues

Patient Education: It is important to complete full course of therapy which may take up to 6 months for full effect. May be taken with meals to decrease GI upset and bitter aftertaste. Avoid alcohol. You should have regular ophthalmic exams (every 4-6 months) if using this medication over extended periods. You may experience skin discoloration (blue/black), hair bleaching, or skin rash. If you have psoriasis, you may experience exacerbation. May turn urine black/brown (normal). You may experience nausea, vomiting, or loss of appetite (small frequent meals, frequent mouth care, sucking lozenges, or chewing gum may help) or increased sensitivity to sunlight (wear dark glasses and protective clothing, use sunblock, and avoid direct exposure to sunlight). Report vision changes, rash or itching, persistent diarrhea or GI disturbances, change in hearing acuity or ringing in the ears, chest pain or palpitation, CNS changes, unusual fatigue, easy bruising or bleeding, or any other persistent adverse reactions.

Monitoring Parameters: Periodic CBC, examination for muscular weakness, and ophthalmologic examination in patients receiving prolonged therapy

Chlorothiazide (klor oh THYE a zide)

Pharmacologic Class Diuretic, Thiazide

U.S. Brand Names Diurigen®; Diuril®

Use Management of mild to moderate hypertension, or edema associated with congestive heart failure, pregnancy, or nephrotic syndrome in patients unable to take oral hydrochlorothiazide, when a thiazide is the diuretic of choice

USUAL DOSAGE

Infants <6 months:

Oral: 20-40 mg/kg/day in 2 divided doses

I.V.: 2-8 mg/kg/day in 2 divided doses

Infants >6 months and Children:

Oral: 20 mg/kg/day in 2 divided doses

I.V.: 4 mg/kg/day

Adults:

Oral: 500 mg to 2 g/day divided in 1-2 doses

I.V.: 100-500 mg/day (for edema only)

Elderly: Oral: 500 mg once daily **or** 1 g 3 times/week

Contraindications Hypersensitivity to chlorothiazide or any component; cross-sensitivity with other thiazides or sulfonamides; do not use in anuric patients.

Pregnancy Risk Factor C (per manufacturer); D (based on expert analysis)

Related Information

Chlorothiazide and Methyldopa *on page 185*

Chlorothiazide and Reserpine *on page 185*

Chlorothiazide and Methyldopa (klor oh THYE a zide & meth il DOE pa)

Pharmacologic Class Antihypertensive Agent, Combination

U.S. Brand Names Aldoclor®

Dosage Forms TAB: 150: Chlorothiazide 150 mg and methyldopa 250 mg; 250: Chlorothiazide 250 mg and methyldopa 250 mg

Pregnancy Risk Factor D

Chlorothiazide and Reserpine (klor oh THYE a zide & re SER peen)

Pharmacologic Class Antihypertensive Agent, Combination

Dosage Forms TAB: 250: Chlorothiazide 250 mg and reserpine 0.125 mg; 500: Chlorothiazide 500 mg and reserpine 0.125 mg

Pregnancy Risk Factor D

Chlorotrianisene (klor oh trye AN i seen)

Pharmacologic Class Estrogen Derivative

U.S. Brand Names TACE®

Generic Available No

Mechanism of Action Diethylstilbestrol derivative with similar estrogenic actions

Use Treat inoperable prostatic cancer; management of atrophic vaginitis, female hypogonadism, vasomotor symptoms of menopause

USUAL DOSAGE Adults: Oral:

Atrophic vaginitis: 12-25 mg/day in 28-day cycles (21 days on and 7 days off)

Female hypogonadism: 12-25 mg cyclically for 21 days. May be followed by I.M. progesterone 100 mg or 5 days of oral progestin; next course may begin on day 5 of induced uterine bleeding.

Postpartum breast engorgement: 12 mg 4 times/day for 7 days or 50 mg every 6 hours for 6 doses; administer first dose within 8 hours after delivery

Vasomotor symptoms associated with menopause: 12-25 mg cyclically for 30 days; one or more courses may be prescribed

Prostatic cancer (inoperable/progressing): 12-25 mg/day

Dosage Forms CAP: 12 mg, 25 mg

Contraindications Thrombophlebitis, breast cancer, undiagnosed abnormal vaginal bleeding, known or suspected pregnancy

Warnings/Precautions Estrogens have been reported to increase the risk of endometrial carcinoma; do not use estrogens during pregnancy

Pregnancy Risk Factor X

Adverse Reactions

>10%:

Cardiovascular: Peripheral edema

Endocrine & metabolic: Enlargement of breasts (female and male), breast tenderness

Gastrointestinal: Nausea, anorexia, bloating

1% to 10%:

Central nervous system: Headache

Endocrine & metabolic: Increased libido (female), decreased libido (male)

Gastrointestinal: Vomiting, diarrhea

<1%: Alterations in frequency and flow of menses, amenorrhea, anxiety, breast tumors, chloasma, cholestatic jaundice, decreased glucose tolerance, depression, dizziness, edema, GI distress, hypertension, increased susceptibility to *Candida* infection, increased triglycerides and LDL, intolerance to contact lenses, melasma, myocardial infarction, nausea, rash, stroke, thromboembolism

Onset Commonly occurs within 14 days of therapy

Education and Monitoring Issues

Patient Education: Take as directed. May cause enlargement of breast (male/female), menstrual irregularity, increased libido (female), decreased libido (male), nausea or vomiting (small frequent meals, frequent mouth care, sucking lozenges, or chewing gum may help), or acute headache (mild analgesic may help). Report persistent diarrhea; swelling of feet, hands, or legs; sudden severe headache; disturbance of speech or vision; warmth, swelling, or pain in calves; severe abdominal pain; rash; emotional lability; chest pain or palpitations; or signs of vaginal infection.

Chlorpheniramine and Phenylephrine

(klor fen IR a meen & fen il EF rin)

Pharmacologic Class Antihistamine/Decongestant Combination

U.S. Brand Names Dallergy-D® Syrup; Ed A-Hist® Liquid; Histatab® Plus Tablet [OTC]; Histor-D® Syrup; Rolatuss® Plain Liquid; Ru-Tuss® Liquid

Dosage Forms CAP, sustained release: Chlorpheniramine maleate 8 mg and phenylephrine hydrochloride 20 mg. **LIQ:** (Dallergy-D®, Histor-D®, Rolatuss® Plain, Ru-Tuss®): Chlorpheniramine maleate 2 mg and phenylephrine hydrochloride 5 mg per 5 mL; (Ed A-Hist® Liquid): Chlorpheniramine maleate 4 mg and phenylephrine hydrochloride 10 mg per 5 mL. **TAB** (Histatab® Plus): Chlorpheniramine maleate 2 mg and phenylephrine hydrochloride 5 mg

Pregnancy Risk Factor C

Alcohol Interactions Avoid use (may increase central nervous system depression)

Chlorpheniramine, Ephedrine, Phenylephrine, and Carbetapentane

(klor fen IR a meen, e FED rin, fen il EF rin, & kar bay ta PEN tane)

Pharmacologic Class Antihistamine/Decongestant/Antitussive

U.S. Brand Names Rentamine®; Rynatuss® Pediatric Suspension; Tri-Tannate Plus®

Dosage Forms LIQ: Carbetapentane tannate 30 mg, ephedrine tannate 5 mg, phenylephrine tannate 5 mg, and chlorpheniramine tannate 4 mg per 5 mL

Pregnancy Risk Factor C

Alcohol Interactions Avoid use (may increase central nervous system depression)

Chlorpheniramine, Phenindamine, and Phenylpropanolamine

(klor fen IR a meen, fen IN dah meen, & fen il proe pa NOLE a meen)

Pharmacologic Class Antihistamine/Decongestant Combination

U.S. Brand Names Nolamine®

Dosage Forms TAB, timed release: Chlorpheniramine maleate 4 mg, phenindamine tartrate 24 mg, and phenylpropanolamine hydrochloride 50 mg

Alcohol Interactions Avoid use (may increase central nervous system depression)

Chlorpheniramine, Phenylephrine, and Codeine

(klor fen IR a meen, fen il EF rin, & KOE deen)

Pharmacologic Class Antihistamine/Decongestant/Antitussive

U.S. Brand Names Pediacof®; Pedituss®

Dosage Forms LIQ: Chlorpheniramine maleate 0.75 mg, phenylephrine hydrochloride 2.5 mg, and codeine phosphate 5 mg with potassium iodide 75 mg per 5 mL

Alcohol Interactions Avoid use (may increase central nervous system depression)

Chlorpheniramine, Phenylephrine, and Methscopolamine

(klor fen IR a meen, fen il EF rin, & meth skoe POL a meen)

Pharmacologic Class Antihistamine/Decongestant/Anticholinergic

U.S. Brand Names D.A.II® Tablet; Dallergy®; Dura-Vent/DA®; Extendryl® SR; Histor-D® Timecelles®

Dosage Forms CAP, sustained release: Chlorpheniramine maleate 8 mg, phenylephrine hydrochloride 20 mg, and methscopolamine nitrate 2.5 mg; Chlorpheniramine maleate 8 mg, phenylephrine hydrochloride 10 mg, and methscopolamine nitrate 2.5 mg. **SYR:** Chlorpheniramine maleate 2 mg, phenylephrine hydrochloride 10 mg, and methscopolamine nitrate 0.625 mg per 5 mL. **TAB:** Chlorpheniramine maleate 4 mg, phenylephrine hydrochloride 10 mg, and methscopolamine nitrate 1.25 mg

Alcohol Interactions Avoid use (may increase central nervous system depression)

Chlorpheniramine, Phenylephrine, and Phenylpropanolamine

(klor fen IR a meen, fen il EF rin, & fen il proe pa NOLE a meen)

Pharmacologic Class Antihistamine/Decongestant Combination

U.S. Brand Names Hista-Vadrin® Tablet

Dosage Forms TAB: Chlorpheniramine maleate 6 mg, phenylephrine hydrochloride 5 mg, and phenylpropanolamine hydrochloride 40 mg

Pregnancy Risk Factor C

Alcohol Interactions Avoid use (may increase central nervous system depression)

Chlorpheniramine, Phenylephrine, and Phenyltoloxamine

(klor fen IR a meen, fen il EF rin, & fen il tole LOKS a meen)

Pharmacologic Class Antihistamine/Decongestant Combination

U.S. Brand Names Comhist®; Comhist® LA

Dosage Forms CAP, sustained release (Comhist® LA): Chlorpheniramine maleate 4 mg, phenylephrine hydrochloride 20 mg, and phenyltoloxamine citrate 50 mg. **TAB** (Comhist®): Chlorpheniramine maleate 2 mg, phenylephrine hydrochloride 10 mg, and phenyltoloxamine citrate 25 mg

Pregnancy Risk Factor C
Alcohol Interactions Avoid use (may increase central nervous system depression)

Chlorpheniramine, Phenylephrine, Phenylpropanolamine, and Belladonna Alkaloids

(klor fen IR a meen, fen il EF rin, fen il proe pa NOLE a meen, & bel a DON a AL ka loydz)

Pharmacologic Class Cold Preparation
U.S. Brand Names Atrohist® Plus; Phenahist-TR®; Phenchlor® S.H.A.; Ru-Tuss®; Stahist®
Dosage Forms TAB, sustained release: Chlorpheniramine 8 mg, phenylephrine 25 mg, phenylpropanolamine 50 mg, hyoscyamine 0.19 mg, atropine 0.04 mg, and scopolamine 0.01 mg
Pregnancy Risk Factor C
Alcohol Interactions Avoid use (may increase central nervous system depression)

Chlorpheniramine, Phenyltoloxamine, Phenylpropanolamine, and Phenylephrine

(klor fen IR a meen, fen il tole LOKS a meen, fen il proe pa NOLE a meen, & fen il EF rin)

Pharmacologic Class Antihistamine/Decongestant Combination
U.S. Brand Names Naldecon®; Naldelate®; Nalgest®; Nalspan®; New Decongestant®; Par Decon®; Tri-Phen-Chlor®; Uni-Decon®
Dosage Forms DROPS, pediatric: Chlorpheniramine maleate 0.5 mg, phenyltoloxamine citrate 2 mg, phenylpropanolamine hydrochloride 5 mg, and phenylephrine hydrochloride 1.25 mg per mL. **SYR:** Chlorpheniramine maleate 2.5 mg, phenyltoloxamine citrate 7.5 mg, phenylpropanolamine hydrochloride 20 mg, and phenylephrine hydrochloride 5 mg per 5 mL. **SYR, pediatric:** Chlorpheniramine maleate 0.5 mg, phenyltoloxamine citrate 2 mg, phenylpropanolamine hydrochloride 5 mg, and phenylephrine hydrochloride 1.25 mg per 5 mL. **TAB, sustained release:** Chlorpheniramine maleate 5 mg, phenyltoloxamine citrate 15 mg, phenylpropanolamine hydrochloride 40 mg, and phenylephrine hydrochloride 10 mg
Pregnancy Risk Factor C
Alcohol Interactions Avoid use (may increase central nervous system depression)

Chlorpheniramine, Pseudoephedrine, and Codeine

(klor fen IR a meen, soo doe e FED rin, & KOE deen)

Pharmacologic Class Antihistamine/Decongestant/Antitussive
U.S. Brand Names Codehist® DH; Decohistine® DH; Dihistine® DH; Ryna-C® Liquid
Dosage Forms LIQ: Chlorpheniramine maleate 2 mg, pseudoephedrine hydrochloride 30 mg, and codeine phosphate 10 mg (120 mL, 480 mL)
Pregnancy Risk Factor C
Alcohol Interactions Avoid use (may increase central nervous system depression)

Chlorpheniramine, Pyrilamine, and Phenylephrine

(klor fen IR a meen, pye RIL a meen, & fen il EF rin)

Pharmacologic Class Antihistamine/Decongestant Combination
U.S. Brand Names Rhinatate® Tablet; R-Tannamine® Tablet; R-Tannate® Tablet; Rynatan® Pediatric Suspension; Rynatan® Tablet; Tanoral® Tablet; Triotann® Tablet; Tri-Tannate® Tablet
Dosage Forms LIQ: Chlorpheniramine tannate 2 mg, pyrilamine tannate 12.5 mg, and phenylephrine tannate 5 mg per 5 mL. **TAB:** Chlorpheniramine tannate 8 mg, pyrilamine maleate 12.5 mg, and phenylephrine tannate 25 mg
Pregnancy Risk Factor C
Alcohol Interactions Avoid use (may increase central nervous system depression)

Chlorpheniramine, Pyrilamine, Phenylephrine, and Phenylpropanolamine

(klor fen IR a meen, pye RIL a meen, fen il EF rin, & fen il proe pa NOLE a meen)

Pharmacologic Class Antihistamine/Decongestant Combination
U.S. Brand Names Histalet Forte® Tablet
Dosage Forms TAB: Chlorpheniramine maleate 4 mg, pyrilamine maleate 25 mg, phenylephrine hydrochloride 10 mg, and phenylpropanolamine hydrochloride 50 mg
Pregnancy Risk Factor C
Alcohol Interactions Avoid use (may increase central nervous system depression)

♦ **Chlorprom®** *see* Chlorpromazine *on page 187*

Chlorpromazine (klor PROE ma zeen)

Pharmacologic Class Antipsychotic Agent, Phenothiazine, Aliphatic
U.S. Brand Names Ormazine; Thorazine®
Generic Available Yes
(Continued)

Chlorpromazine *(Continued)*

Mechanism of Action Blocks postsynaptic mesolimbic dopaminergic receptors in the brain; exhibits a strong alpha-adrenergic blocking effect and depresses the release of hypothalamic and hypophyseal hormones; believed to depress the reticular activating system, thus affecting basal metabolism, body temperature, wakefulness, vasomotor tone, and emesis

Use Treatment of nausea and vomiting; psychoses; Tourette's syndrome; mania; intractable hiccups (adults); behavioral problems (children)

USUAL DOSAGE

Children >6 months:

Psychosis:

Oral: 0.5-1 mg/kg/dose every 4-6 hours; older children may require 200 mg/day or higher

I.M., I.V.: 0.5-1 mg/kg/dose every 6-8 hours; maximum dose for <5 years (22.7 kg): 40 mg/day; maximum for 5-12 years (22.7-45.5 kg): 75 mg/day

Nausea and vomiting:

Oral: 0.5-1 mg/kg/dose every 4-6 hours as needed

I.M., I.V.: 0.5-1 mg/kg/dose every 6-8 hours; maximum dose for <5 years (22.7 kg): 40 mg/day; maximum for 5-12 years (22.7-45.5 kg): 75 mg/day

Rectal: 1 mg/kg/dose every 6-8 hours as needed

Adults:

Psychosis:

Oral: Range: 30-800 mg/day in 1-4 divided doses, initiate at lower doses and titrate as needed; usual dose: 200 mg/day; some patients may require 1-2 g/day

I.M., I.V.: Initial: 25 mg, may repeat (25-50 mg) in 1-4 hours, gradually increase to a maximum of 400 mg/dose every 4-6 hours until patient is controlled; usual dose: 300-800 mg/day

Intractable hiccups: Oral, I.M.: 25-50 mg 3-4 times/day

Nausea and vomiting:

Oral: 10-25 mg every 4-6 hours

I.M., I.V.: 25-50 mg every 4-6 hours

Rectal: 50-100 mg every 6-8 hours

Elderly (nonpsychotic patient; dementia behavior): Initial: 10-25 mg 1-2 times/day; increase at 4- to 7-day intervals by 10-25 mg/day. Increase dose intervals (bid, tid, etc) as necessary to control behavior response or side effects; maximum daily dose: 800 mg; gradual increases (titration) may prevent some side effects or decrease their severity.

Hemodialysis: Not dialyzable (0% to 5%)

Dosing adjustment/comments in hepatic impairment: Avoid use in severe hepatic dysfunction

Dosage Forms CAP, sustained action: 30 mg, 75 mg, 150 mg, 200 mg, 300 mg. **CONC, oral:** 30 mg/mL (120 mL); 100 mg/mL (60 mL, 240 mL). **INJ:** 25 mg/mL (1 mL, 2 mL, 10 mL). **SUPP, rectal,** as base: 25 mg, 100 mg. **SYR:** 10 mg/5 mL (120 mL). **TAB:** 10 mg, 25 mg, 50 mg, 100 mg, 200 mg

Contraindications Hypersensitivity to chlorpromazine hydrochloride or any component; cross-sensitivity with other phenothiazines may exist; avoid use in patients with narrow-angle glaucoma

Warnings/Precautions Safety in children <6 months of age has not been established; use with caution in patients with seizures, bone marrow suppression, or severe liver disease

Significant hypotension may occur, especially when the drug is administered parenterally; injection contains benzyl alcohol; injection also contains sulfites which may cause allergic reaction

Tardive dyskinesia: Prevalence rate may be 40% in elderly; development of the syndrome and the irreversible nature are proportional to duration and total cumulative dose over time. May be reversible if diagnosed early in therapy.

Extrapyramidal reactions are more common in elderly with up to 50% developing these reactions after 60 years of age. Drug-induced **Parkinson's syndrome** occurs often. **Akathisia** is the most common extrapyramidal reaction in elderly.

Increased confusion, memory loss, psychotic behavior, and agitation frequently occur as a consequence of anticholinergic effects

Orthostatic hypotension is due to alpha-receptor blockade, the elderly are at greater risk for orthostatic hypotension

Antipsychotic associated sedation in nonpsychotic patients is extremely unpleasant due to feelings of depersonalization, derealization, and dysphoria

Life-threatening arrhythmias have occurred at therapeutic doses of antipsychotics

Pregnancy Risk Factor C

Adverse Reactions

Cardiovascular: Postural hypotension, tachycardia, dizziness, nonspecific Q-T changes

Central nervous system: Drowsiness, dystonias, akathisia, pseudoparkinsonism, tardive dyskinesia, neuroleptic malignant syndrome, seizures

Dermatologic: Photosensitivity, dermatitis, skin pigmentation (slate gray)

Endocrine & metabolic: Lactation, breast engorgement, false-positive pregnancy test, amenorrhea, gynecomastia, hyper- or hypoglycemia

Gastrointestinal: Xerostomia, constipation, nausea

Genitourinary: Urinary retention, ejaculatory disorder, impotence

Hematologic: Agranulocytosis, eosinophilia, leukopenia, hemolytic anemia, aplastic anemia, thrombocytopenic purpura

Hepatic: Jaundice

Ocular: Blurred vision, corneal and lenticular changes, epithelial keratopathy, pigmentary retinopathy

Drug Interactions CYP1A2, 2D6, and 3A3/4 enzyme substrate; CYP2D6 enzyme inhibitor

Phenothiazines inhibit the ability of bromocriptine to lower serum prolactin concentrations

Benztropine (and other anticholinergics) may inhibit the therapeutic response to CPZ and excess anticholinergic effects may occur

Chloroquine may increase CPZ concentrations

Cigarette smoking may enhance the hepatic metabolism of CPZ. Larger doses may be required compared to a nonsmoker.

Concurrent use of CPZ with an antihypertensive may produce additive hypotensive effects

Antihypertensive effects of guanethidine and guanadrel may be inhibited by CPZ

Concurrent use with TCA may produce increased toxicity or altered therapeutic response

CPZ may inhibit the antiparkinsonian effect of levodopa; avoid this combination

CPZ plus lithium may rarely produce neurotoxicity

Barbiturates may reduce CPZ concentrations

Propranolol may increase CPZ concentrations

Sulfadoxine-pyrimethamine may increase CPZ concentrations

CPZ and possibly other low potency antipsychotics may reverse the pressor effects of epinephrine

CPZ and CNS depressants (ethanol, narcotics) may produce additive CNS depressant effects

CPZ and trazodone may produce additive hypotensive effects

Alcohol Interactions Avoid use (may increase central nervous system depression)

Onset Peak concentration after oral dose: 1-2 hours

Half-Life Half-life, biphasic: Initial: 2 hours; Terminal: 30 hours

Education and Monitoring Issues

Patient Education: Use exactly as directed (do not increase dose or frequency); may cause physical and/or psychological dependence. Do not discontinue without consulting prescriber. Tablets/capsules may be taken with food. Mix oral solution with 2-4 ounces of liquid (eg, juice, milk, water). Do not take within 2 hours of any antacid. Store away from light. Avoid excess alcohol or caffeine and other prescription or OTC medications not approved by prescriber. Maintain adequate hydration (2-3 L/day of fluids unless instructed to restrict fluid intake). May turn urine red-brown (normal). You may experience excess drowsiness, lightheadedness, dizziness, or blurred vision (use caution driving or when engaging in tasks requiring alertness until response to drug is known); dry mouth, upset stomach, nausea, vomiting, anorexia (small frequent meals, frequent mouth care, sucking lozenges, or chewing gum may help); constipation (increased exercise, fluids, or dietary fruit and fiber may help); postural hypotension (use caution climbing stairs or when changing position from lying or sitting to standing); urinary retention (void before taking medication); ejaculatory dysfunction (reversible); decreased perspiration (avoid strenuous exercise in hot environments); or photosensitivity (use sunscreen, wear protective clothing and eyewear, avoid direct sunlight). Report persistent CNS effects (trembling fingers, altered gait or balance, excessive sedation, seizures, unusual movements, anxiety, abnormal thoughts, confusion, personality changes); chest pain, palpitations, rapid heartbeat, or severe dizziness; unresolved urinary retention or changes in urinary pattern; altered menstrual pattern, change in libido, swelling or pain in breasts (male or female); vision changes, skin rash, irritation, or changes in color of skin (gray-blue); or worsening of condition.

Monitoring Parameters: Orthostatic blood pressures; tremors, gait changes, abnormal movement in trunk, neck, buccal area, or extremities; monitor target behaviors for which the agent is given; watch for hypotension when administering I.M. or I.V.

Reference Range:

Therapeutic: 50-300 ng/mL (SI: 157-942 nmol/L)

Toxic: >750 ng/mL (SI: >2355 nmol/L); serum concentrations poorly correlate with expected response

Chlorpropamide (klor PROE pa mide)

Pharmacologic Class Antidiabetic Agent, Oral

U.S. Brand Names Diabinese®

Generic Available Yes

Mechanism of Action Stimulates insulin release from the pancreatic beta cells; reduces glucose output from the liver; insulin sensitivity is increased at peripheral target sites

Use Control blood sugar in adult onset, noninsulin-dependent diabetes (type II)

Unlabeled use: Neurogenic diabetes insipidus

USUAL DOSAGE Oral: The dosage of chlorpropamide is variable and should be individualized based upon the patient's response

(Continued)

Chlorpropamide *(Continued)*

Initial dose:

Adults: 250 mg/day in mild to moderate diabetes in middle-aged, stable diabetic

Elderly: 100-125 mg/day in older patients

Subsequent dosages may be increased or decreased by 50-125 mg/day at 3- to 5-day intervals

Maintenance dose: 100-250 mg/day; severe diabetics may require 500 mg/day; avoid doses >750 mg/day

Dosing adjustment/comments in renal impairment: Cl_{cr} <50 mL/minute: Avoid use

Hemodialysis: Removed with hemoperfusion

Peritoneal dialysis: Supplemental dose is not necessary

Dosing adjustment in hepatic impairment: Dosage reduction is recommended. Conservative initial and maintenance doses are recommended in patients with liver impairment because chlorpropamide undergoes extensive hepatic metabolism.

Dosage Forms TAB: 100 mg, 250 mg

Contraindications Cross-sensitivity may exist with other hypoglycemics or sulfonamides; do not use with type I diabetes or with severe renal, hepatic, thyroid, or other endocrine disease

Warnings/Precautions

Patients should be properly instructed in the early detection and treatment of hypoglycemia; long half-life may complicate recovery from excess effects

Because of chlorpropamide's long half-life, duration of action, and the increased risk for hypoglycemia, it is not considered a hypoglycemic agent of choice in the elderly; see Pharmacodynamics/Kinetics

Pregnancy Risk Factor C

Pregnancy Implications

Clinical effects on the fetus: Crosses the placenta. Hypoglucemia; ear defects reported; other malformations reported but may have been secondary to poor maternal glucose control/diabetes. Insulin is the drug of choice for the control of diabetes mellitus during pregnancy.

Breast-feeding/lactation: Crosses into breast milk

Adverse Reactions

>10%:

Central nervous system: Headache, dizziness

Gastrointestinal: Anorexia, constipation, heartburn, epigastric fullness, nausea, vomiting, diarrhea

1% to 10%: Dermatologic: Skin rash, urticaria, photosensitivity

<1%: Agranulocytosis, aplastic anemia, blood dyscrasias, bone marrow suppression, cholestatic jaundice, edema, hemolytic anemia, hypoglycemia, hyponatremia, SIADH, thrombocytopenia

Drug Interactions

Decreased effect: Thiazides and hydantoins (eg, phenytoin) decrease chlorpropamide effectiveness may increase blood glucose

Increased toxicity:

Increases alcohol-associated disulfiram reactions

Increases oral anticoagulant effects

Salicylates may increase chlorpropamide effects may decrease blood glucose

Sulfonamides may decrease sulfonylureas clearance

Alcohol Interactions Avoid use (may cause hypoglycemia). Chlorpropamide inhibits alcohol's usual metabolism. Patients can have a disulfiram-like reaction (headache, nausea, vomiting, chest or abdominal pain) if they drink alcohol concurrently.

Onset Oral: Within 6-8 hours

Half-Life 30-42 hours; prolonged in the elderly or with renal disease; End-stage renal disease: 50-200 hours

Education and Monitoring Issues

Patient Education: Avoid alcohol; take at the same time each day; avoid hypoglycemia, eat regularly, do not skip meals; carry a quick source of sugar

Dietary Considerations:

Food: Chlorpropamide may cause GI upset; take with food. Take at the same time each day; eat regularly and do not skip meals.

Glucose: Decreases blood glucose concentration; hypoglycemia may occur. Educate patients how to detect and treat hypoglycemia. Monitor for signs and symptoms of hypoglycemia. Administer glucose if necessary. Evaluate patient's diet and exercise regimen. May need to decrease or discontinue dose of sulfonylurea.

Sodium: Reports of hyponatremia and SIADH. Those at increased risk include patients on medications or who have medical conditions that predispose them to hyponatremia. Monitor sodium serum concentration and fluid status. May need to restrict water intake.

Monitoring Parameters: Fasting blood glucose, normal Hgb A_{1c} or fructosamine levels; monitor for signs and symptoms of hypoglycemia, (fatigue, sweating, numbness of extremities); monitor urine for glucose and ketones

Reference Range: Target range: Adults:

Fasting blood glucose: <120 mg/dL

Glycosylated hemoglobin: <7%

Related Information

Hypoglycemic Drugs and Thiazolidinedione Information *on page 1240*

Chlorthalidone (klor THAL i done)

Pharmacologic Class Diuretic, Thiazide

U.S. Brand Names Hygroton®; Thalitone®

Generic Available Yes

Mechanism of Action Sulfonamide-derived diuretic that inhibits sodium and chloride reabsorption in the cortical-diluting segment of the ascending loop of Henle

Use Management of mild to moderate hypertension, used alone or in combination with other agents; treatment of edema associated with congestive heart failure, nephrotic syndrome, or pregnancy. Recent studies have found chlorthalidone effective in the treatment of isolated systolic hypertension in the elderly.

USUAL DOSAGE Oral:

Children (nonapproved): 2 mg/kg/dose 3 times/week or 1-2 mg/kg/day

Adults:

- Edema: 50-100 mg/day or 100 mg every other day; may increase to 200 mg but greater doses do not usually result in increased response
- Hypertension: Initial: 25 mg/day, increase slowly to 100 mg/day or add additional antihypertensives

Elderly: Initial: 12.5-25 mg/day or every other day; there is little advantage to using doses >25 mg/day

Note: Thalidone 30 mg = chlorthalidone 25 mg

Dosing interval in renal impairment: Cl_{cr} <10 mL/minute: Administer every 48 hours

Dosage Forms TAB: 25 mg, 50 mg, 100 mg; (Hygroton®): 25 mg, 50 mg, 100 mg; (Thalitone®): 15 mg, 25 mg

Contraindications Hypersensitivity to chlorthalidone or any component, cross-sensitivity with other thiazides or sulfonamides; do not use in anuric patients

Warnings/Precautions Use with caution in patients with hypokalemia, renal disease, hepatic disease, gout, lupus erythematosus, diabetes mellitus; use with caution in severe renal diseases

Pregnancy Risk Factor B (per manufacturer); D (based on expert analysis)

Adverse Reactions

1% to 10%:

- Endocrine & metabolic: Hypokalemia
- Dermatologic: Photosensitivity
- Gastrointestinal: Anorexia, epigastric distress

<1% (limited to important or life-threatening symptoms): Dizziness, headache, weakness, restlessness, insomnia, purpura, rash, urticaria, necrotizing angiitis, vasculitis, cutaneous vasculitis, hyperuricemia or gout, hyponatremia, sexual ability (decreased), hyperglycemia, glycosuria, nausea, vomiting, cholecystitis, pancreatitis, diarrhea or constipation, polyuria, aplastic anemia, leukopenia, agranulocytosis, thrombocytopenia, hepatic function impairment, paresthesia, muscle cramps or spasm

Drug Interactions

Angiotensin-converting enzyme inhibitors: Increased hypotension if aggressively diuresed with a thiazide diuretic

Beta-blockers increase hyperglycemic effects in type 2 diabetes mellitus

Cyclosporine and thiazides can increase the risk of gout or renal toxicity; avoid concurrent use

Digoxin toxicity can be exacerbated if a thiazide induces hypokalemia or hypomagnesemia

Lithium toxicity can occur by reducing renal excretion of lithium; monitor lithium concentration and adjust as needed

Neuromuscular blocking agents can prolong blockade; monitor serum potassium and neuromuscular status

NSAIDs can decrease the efficacy of thiazides reducing the diuretic and antihypertensive effects

Onset Peak effect: 2-6 hours

Half-Life 35-55 hours; may be prolonged with renal impairment, with anuria: 81 hours

Education and Monitoring Issues

Patient Education: Take prescribed dose with food early in the day. Include orange juice, bananas, or other food rich in potassium in your diet, but do not take potassium supplements without consulting prescriber. You may experience postural hypotension (use caution when rising from lying or sitting position, when climbing stairs, or when driving); photosensitivity (use sunblock, wear protective clothing and eyewear, avoid direct sunlight); decreased accommodation to heat (avoid excessive exercise in hot weather). Report muscle weakness, tremors, or cramping; persistent nausea or vomiting; swelling of extremities; significant increase in weight; respiratory difficulty; rash; unusual weakness or fatigue; or easy bruising or bleeding.

Monitoring Parameters: Assess weight, I & O records daily to determine fluid loss; blood pressure, serum electrolytes, renal function

(Continued)

Chlorthalidone *(Continued)*

Related Information

Atenolol and Chlorthalidone *on page 78*
Clonidine and Chlorthalidone *on page 217*
Heart Failure Guidelines *on page 1099*

♦ **Chlor-Tripolon® N.D.** *see* Loratadine and Pseudoephedrine *on page 541*

Chlorzoxazone (klor ZOKS a zone)

Pharmacologic Class Skeletal Muscle Relaxant

U.S. Brand Names Flexaphen®; Paraflex®; Parafon Forte™ DSC

Generic Available Yes

Mechanism of Action Acts on the spinal cord and subcortical levels by depressing polysynaptic reflexes

Use Symptomatic treatment of muscle spasm and pain associated with acute musculoskeletal conditions

USUAL DOSAGE Oral:

Children: 20 mg/kg/day or 600 mg/m^2/day in 3-4 divided doses
Adults: 250-500 mg 3-4 times/day up to 750 mg 3-4 times/day

Dosage Forms CAPLET (Parafon Forte™ DSC): 500 mg. **CAP** (Flexaphen®, Mus-Lax®): 250 mg with acetaminophen 300 mg. **TAB** Paraflex®: 250 mg

Contraindications Known hypersensitivity to chlorzoxazone; impaired liver function

Pregnancy Risk Factor C

Adverse Reactions

>10%: Central nervous system: Drowsiness

1% to 10%:

- Cardiovascular: Tachycardia, tightness in chest, flushing of face, syncope
- Central nervous system: Mental depression, allergic fever, dizziness, lightheadedness, headache, paradoxical stimulation
- Dermatologic: Angioedema
- Gastrointestinal: Nausea, vomiting, stomach cramps
- Neuromuscular & skeletal: Trembling
- Ocular: Burning of eyes
- Respiratory: Shortness of breath
- Miscellaneous: Hiccups

<1%: Aplastic anemia, ataxia, blurred vision, eosinophilia, erythema multiforme, leukopenia, rash, urticaria

Drug Interactions CYP2E1 enzyme substrate

Increased effect/toxicity: Alcohol, CNS depressants

Alcohol Interactions Avoid use (may increase central nervous system depression)

Onset Within 1 hour

Duration 6-12 hours

Education and Monitoring Issues

Patient Education: Take exactly as directed, with food. Do not increase dose or discontinue without consulting prescriber. Do not use alcohol, prescriptive or OTC antidepressants, sedatives, or pain medications without consulting prescriber. May turn urine orange or red (normal). You may experience drowsiness, dizziness, lightheadedness (avoid driving or engaging in tasks that require alertness until response to drug is known); nausea, vomiting, or cramping (small, frequent meals, frequent mouth care, or sucking hard candy may help); postural hypotension (change position slowly when rising from sitting or lying or when climbing stairs); or constipation (increased dietary fluids and fibers or increased exercise may help). Report excessive drowsiness or mental agitation; palpitations, rapid heartbeat, or chest pain; skin rash or swelling of mouth or face; persistent diarrhea or constipation; or unusual weakness or bleeding.

Monitoring Parameters: Periodic liver functions tests

♦ **Cholac®** *see* Lactulose *on page 506*

♦ **Choledyl®** *see* Theophylline Salts *on page 906*

Cholestyramine Resin (koe LES tir a meen REZ in)

Pharmacologic Class Antilipemic Agent (Bile Acid Seqestrant)

U.S. Brand Names LoCHOLEST®; LoCHOLEST® Light; Prevalite®; Questran®; Questran® Light

Generic Available Yes

Mechanism of Action Forms a nonabsorbable complex with bile acids in the intestine, releasing chloride ions in the process; inhibits enterohepatic reuptake of intestinal bile salts and thereby increases the fecal loss of bile salt-bound low density lipoprotein cholesterol

Use Adjunct in the management of primary hypercholesterolemia; pruritus associated with elevated levels of bile acids; diarrhea associated with excess fecal bile acids; binding toxicologic agents; pseudomembraneous colitis

USUAL DOSAGE Oral (dosages are expressed in terms of anhydrous resin):

Powder:

Children: 240 mg/kg/day in 3 divided doses; need to titrate dose depending on indication

Adults: 4 g 1-2 times/day to a maximum of 24 g/day and 6 doses/day

Tablet: Adults: Initial: 4 g once or twice daily; maintenance: 8-16 g/day in 2 divided doses

Dialysis: Not removed by hemo- or peritoneal dialysis; supplemental doses not necessary with dialysis or continuous arteriovenous or venovenous hemofiltration effects

Dosage Forms POWDER: 4 g of resin/9 g of powder (9 g, 378 g); For oral susp: With aspartame: 4 g of resin/5 g of powder (5 g, 210 g); With phenylalanine: 4 g of resin/5.5 g of powder (60s)

Contraindications Avoid using in complete biliary obstruction; hypersensitive to cholestyramine or any component; hyperlipoproteinemia types III, IV, V

Warnings/Precautions Use with caution in patients with constipation (GI dysfunction); caution patients with phenylketonuria (Questran® Light contains aspartame); overdose may result in GI obstruction

Pregnancy Risk Factor C

Adverse Reactions

>10%: Gastrointestinal: Constipation, heartburn, nausea, vomiting, stomach pain

1% to 10%:

Central nervous system: Headache

Gastrointestinal: Belching, bloating, diarrhea

<1% (limited to important or life-threatening symptoms): Hyperchloremic acidosis, gallstones or pancreatitis, GI bleeding, peptic ulcer, steatorrhea or malabsorption syndrome, hypoprothrombinemia (secondary to vitamin K deficiency)

Drug Interactions

Cholestyramine can reduce the absorption of numerous medications when used concurrently. Give other medications 1 hour before or 4 hours after giving cholestyramine. Medications which may be affected include HMG-CoA reductase inhibitors, thiazide diuretics, propranolol (and potentially other beta-blockers), corticosteroids, thyroid hormones, digoxin, valproic acid, NSAIDs, loop diuretics, sulfonylureas

Warfarin and other oral anticoagulants: Hypoprothrombinemic effects may be reduced by cholestyramine. Separate administration times (as detailed above) and monitor INR closely when initiating or discontinuing.

Onset Peak effect: 21 days

Education and Monitoring Issues

Patient Education: Take once or twice a day as directed. Do not take the powder in its dry form; mix with fluid, applesauce, pudding, or jello. Chew bars thoroughly. Take other medications 2 hours before or 4 hours after cholestyramine. Ongoing medical follow-up and laboratory tests may be required. You may experience GI effects (these should resolve after continued use); nausea and vomiting (small frequent meals, frequent mouth care, sucking lozenges, or chewing gum may help); constipation (increased exercise, dietary fluid, fiber, or fruit may help - consult prescriber about use of stool softener or laxative). Report unusual stomach cramping, pain or blood in stool; unresolved nausea, vomiting, or constipation.

Choline Magnesium Trisalicylate

(KOE leen mag NEE zhum trye sa LIS i late)

Pharmacologic Class Salicylate

U.S. Brand Names Tricosal®; Trilisate®

Generic Available No

Mechanism of Action Inhibits prostaglandin synthesis; acts on the hypothalamus heat-regulating center to reduce fever; blocks the generation of pain impulses

Use Management of osteoarthritis, rheumatoid arthritis, and other arthritis; salicylate salts may not inhibit platelet aggregation and, therefore, should not be substituted for aspirin in the prophylaxis of thrombosis

USUAL DOSAGE Oral (based on total salicylate content):

Children <37 kg: 50 mg/kg/day given in 2 divided doses

Adults: 500 mg to 1.5 g 2-3 times/day; usual maintenance dose: 1-4.5 g/day

Dosing adjustment/comments in renal impairment: Avoid use in severe renal impairment

Dosage Forms LIQ: 500 mg/5 mL [choline salicylate 293 mg and magnesium salicylate 362 mg per 5 mL] (237 mL). **TAB:** 500 mg: Choline salicylate 293 mg and magnesium salicylate 362 mg; 750 mg: Choline salicylate 440 mg and magnesium salicylate 544 mg; 1000 mg: Choline salicylate 587 mg and magnesium salicylate 725 mg

Contraindications Bleeding disorders; hypersensitivity to salicylates or other nonacetylated salicylates or other NSAIDs; tartrazine dye hypersensitivity, asthma

Warnings/Precautions Use with caution in patients with impaired renal function, erosive gastritis, or peptic ulcer; avoid use in patients with suspected varicella or influenza (salicylates have been associated with Reye's syndrome in children <16 years of age when used to treat symptoms of chickenpox or the flu). Tinnitus or impaired hearing may indicate toxicity; discontinue use 1 week prior to surgical procedures.

(Continued)

Choline Magnesium Trisalicylate *(Continued)*

Elderly are a high-risk population for adverse effects from nonsteroidal anti-inflammatory agents. As much as 60% of elderly can develop peptic ulceration and/or hemorrhage asymptomatically. Use lowest effective dose for shortest period possible. Tinnitus may be a difficult and unreliable indication of toxicity due to age-related hearing loss or eighth cranial nerve damage. CNS adverse effects may be observed in the elderly at lower doses than younger adults.

Pregnancy Risk Factor C; D (3rd trimester or near term)

Adverse Reactions

>10%: Gastrointestinal: Nausea, heartburn, stomach pains, dyspepsia, epigastric discomfort

1% to 10%:

- Central nervous system: Fatigue
- Dermatologic: Rash
- Gastrointestinal: Gastrointestinal ulceration
- Hematologic: Hemolytic anemia
- Neuromuscular & skeletal: Weakness
- Respiratory: Dyspnea
- Miscellaneous: Anaphylactic shock

<1%: Bronchospasm, hepatotoxicity, impaired renal function, increased uric acid, insomnia, iron deficiency anemia, jitters, leukopenia, nervousness, occult bleeding, prolongation of bleeding time, thrombocytopenia

Drug Interactions

Decreased effect: Antacids + Trilisate® may decrease salicylate concentration

Increased toxicity: Warfarin + Trilisate® may possibly increase hypoprothrombinemic effect

Alcohol Interactions Avoid use (may enhance gastric mucosal irritation)

Onset Peak concentrations in ~2 hours after oral dose

Half-Life Dose-dependent ranging from 2-3 hours at low doses to 30 hours at high doses

Education and Monitoring Issues

Patient Education: If self-administered, use exactly as directed (do not increase dose or frequency); adverse reactions can occur with overuse. Take with food or milk. While using this medication, do not use alcohol, excessive amounts of vitamin C, or salicylate-containing foods (curry powder, prunes, raisins, tea, or licorice), other prescription or OTC medications containing aspirin or salicylate, or other NSAIDs without consulting prescriber. Maintain adequate hydration (2-3 L/day of fluids unless instructed to restrict fluid intake). You may experience nausea, vomiting, gastric discomfort (frequent mouth care, small frequent meals, sucking lozenges, or chewing gum may help). GI bleeding, ulceration, or perforation can occur with or without pain. Stop taking medication and report ringing in ears; persistent pain in stomach; unresolved nausea or vomiting; difficulty breathing or shortness of breath; unusual bruising or bleeding (mouth, urine, stool); or skin rash.

Dietary Considerations:

Food: May decrease the rate but not the extent of oral absorption. Drug may cause GI upset, bleeding, ulceration, perforation. Take with food or or large volume of water or milk to minimize GI upset.

Folic acid: Hyperexcretion of folate; folic acid deficiency may result, leading to macrocytic anemia. Supplement with folic acid if necessary.

Iron: With chronic use and at doses of 3-4 g/day, iron deficiency anemia may result; supplement with iron if necessary

Magnesium: Hypermagnesemia resulting from magnesium salicylate; avoid or use with caution in renal insufficiency

Sodium: Hypernatremia resulting from buffered aspirin solutions or sodium salicylate containing high sodium content. Avoid or use with caution in CHF or any condition where hypernatremia would be detrimental.

Curry powder, paprika, licorice, Benedictine liqueur, prunes, raisins, tea and gherkins: Potential salicylate accumulation. These foods contain 6 mg salicylate/100 g. An ordinary American diet contains 10-200 mg/day of salicylate. Foods containing salicylates may contribute to aspirin hypersensitivity. Patients at greatest risk for aspirin hypersensitivity include those with asthma, nasal polyposis, or chronic urticaria.

Monitoring Parameters: Serum magnesium with high dose therapy or in patients with impaired renal function; serum salicylate levels, renal function, hearing changes or tinnitus, abnormal bruising, weight gain and response (ie, pain)

Reference Range: Salicylate blood levels for anti-inflammatory effect: 150-300 µg/mL; analgesia and antipyretic effect: 30-50 µg/mL

Manufacturer Purdue Frederick Co

Related Information

Pharmaceutical Manufacturers Directory *on page 1020*

Choline Salicylate (KOE leen sa LIS i late)

Pharmacologic Class Analgesic, Non-narcotic; Nonsteroidal Anti-inflammatory Drug (NSAID)

U.S. Brand Names Arthropan® [OTC]

Generic Available No

Mechanism of Action Inhibits prostaglandin synthesis; acts on the hypothalamus heat-regulating center to reduce fever; blocks the generation of pain impulses

Use Temporary relief of pain of rheumatoid arthritis, rheumatic fever, osteoarthritis, and other conditions for which oral salicylates are recommended; useful in patients in which there is difficulty in administering doses in a tablet or capsule dosage form, because of the liquid dosage form

USUAL DOSAGE

Children >12 years and Adults: Oral: 5 mL (870 mg) every 3-4 hours, if necessary, but not more than 6 doses in 24 hours

Rheumatoid arthritis: 870-1740 mg (5-10 mL) up to 4 times/day

Dosing adjustment/comments in renal impairment: Avoid use in severe renal impairment

Dosage Forms LIQ (mint flavor): 870 mg/5 mL (240 mL, 480 mL)

Contraindications Hypersensitivity to salicylates or any component or other nonacetylated salicylates

Warnings/Precautions Use with caution in patients with impaired renal function, erosive gastritis, or peptic ulcer; avoid use in patients with suspected varicella or influenza (salicylates have been associated with Reye's syndrome in children <16 years of age when used to treat symptoms of chickenpox or the flu)

Pregnancy Risk Factor C

Adverse Reactions

>10%: Gastrointestinal: Nausea, heartburn, stomach pains, dyspepsia, epigastric discomfort

1% to 10%:

Central nervous system: Fatigue
Dermatologic: Rash
Gastrointestinal: Gastrointestinal ulceration
Hematologic: Hemolytic anemia
Neuromuscular & skeletal: Weakness
Respiratory: Dyspnea
Miscellaneous: Anaphylactic shock

<1%: Bronchospasm, hepatotoxicity, impaired renal function, insomnia, iron deficiency anemia, jitters, leukopenia, nervousness, occult bleeding, prolongation of bleeding time, thrombocytopenia

Drug Interactions

Decreased effect with antacids
Increased effect of warfarin

Onset Peak concentration: 2 hours

Half-Life 2-30 hours

Education and Monitoring Issues

Patient Education: Take with food; do not take with antacids; watch for bleeding gums or any signs of GI bleeding; take with food or milk to minimize GI distress, notify prescriber if ringing in ears or persistent GI pain occurs

Chondroitin Sulfate

Pharmacologic Class Nutraceutical

Mechanism of Action Cartilage tissue is a mixture of glycosaminoglycans (GAGs). One of the primary GAGs is chondroitin sulfate. Chondroitin sulfate also inhibits synovial enzymes (elastase, hyaluronidase) which may contribute to cartilage destruction and loss of joint function. Although studies are not conclusive, chondroitin has been reported to act synergistically with glucosamine to support the maintenance of joint cartilage in osteoarthritis.

Use Osteoarthritis (Uebelhart, 1998)

USUAL DOSAGE Oral: Dosage range: 300-1500 mg/day

Dosage Forms Chondroitin sulfate (CS), as chondroitin-4-sulphate and chondroitin-6-sulphate, found naturally combined with type II collagen

Adverse Reactions

Drug/Nutrient Interactions: None known

Nutrient/Nutrient Interactions: No adverse interactions have been reported either with CS or in combination with glucosamine/galactosamine

Chondroitin Sulfate-Sodium Hyaluronate

(kon DROY tin SUL fate-SOW de um hye al yoor ON ate)

Pharmacologic Class Ophthalmic Agent, Viscoelastic

U.S. Brand Names Duovisc® With Kit; Viscoat®

Use Surgical aid in anterior segment procedures, protects corneal endothelium and coats intraocular lens thus protecting it

USUAL DOSAGE Carefully introduce (using a 27-gauge needle or cannula) into anterior chamber after thoroughly cleaning the chamber with a balanced salt solution

Contraindications Hypersensitivity to hyaluronate

Pregnancy Risk Factor C

- **Chooz® [OTC]** *see* Calcium Carbonate *on page 130*
- **Chorex®** *see* Chorionic Gonadotropin *on page 196*

Chorionic Gonadotropin (kor ee ON ik goe NAD oh troe pin)

Pharmacologic Class Ovulation Stimulator

U.S. Brand Names A.P.L.®; Chorex®; Choron®; Follutein®; Glukor®; Gonic®; Pregnyl®; Profasi® HP

Generic Available Yes

Mechanism of Action Stimulates production of gonadal steroid hormones by causing production of androgen by the testis; as a substitute for luteinizing hormone (LH) to stimulate ovulation

Use Induces ovulation and pregnancy in anovulatory, infertile females; treatment of hypogonadotropic hypogonadism, prepubertal cryptorchidism

USUAL DOSAGE I.M.:

Children:

Prepubertal cryptorchidism: 1000-2000 units/m^2/dose 3 times/week for 3 weeks **OR** 4000 units 3 times/week for 3 weeks **OR** 5000 units every second day for 4 injections **OR** 500 units 3 times/week for 4-6 weeks

Hypogonadotropic hypogonadism: 500-1000 units 3 times/week for 3 weeks, followed by the same dose twice weekly for 3 weeks **OR** 1000-2000 units 3 times/week **OR** 4000 units 3 times/week for 6-9 months; reduce dosage to 2000 units 3 times/week for additional 3 months

Adults: Induction of ovulation: 5000-10,000 units one day following last dose of menotropins

Dosage Forms POWDER for inj, human origin: 200 units/mL (10 mL, 25 mL), 500 units/mL (10 mL), 1000 units/mL (10 mL), 2000 units/mL (10 mL)

Contraindications Hypersensitivity to chorionic gonadotropin or any component; precocious puberty, prostatic carcinoma or similar neoplasms

Warnings/Precautions Use with caution in asthma, seizure disorders, migraine, cardiac or renal disease; **not** effective in the treatment of obesity

Pregnancy Risk Factor C

Adverse Reactions

1% to 10%:

Central nervous system: Mental depression, fatigue

Endocrine & metabolic: Pelvic pain, ovarian cysts, enlargement of breasts, precocious puberty

Local: Pain at the injection site

Neuromuscular & skeletal: Premature closure of epiphyses

<1%: Gynecomastia, headache, irritability, ovarian hyperstimulation syndrome, peripheral edema, restlessness

Half-Life Half-life, biphasic: Initial: 11 hours; Terminal: 23 hours

Education and Monitoring Issues

Patient Education: Discontinue immediately if possibility of pregnancy

Reference Range: Depends on application and methodology; <3 mIU/mL (SI: <3 units/L) usually normal (nonpregnant)

- **Choron®** *see* Chorionic Gonadotropin *on page 196*
- **Chromagen® OB [OTC]** *see* Vitamins, Multiple *on page 981*

Chromium

Pharmacologic Class Herbal

Mechanism of Action Chromium picolinate is the only active form of chromium. It appears that chromium, in its trivalent form, increases insulin sensitivity and improves glucose transport into cells. The mechanism by which this happens could include one or more of the following:

Increase the number of insulin receptors

Enhance insulin binding to target tissues

Promote activation of insulin-receptor tyrosine kinase activity

Enhance beta cell sensitivity in the pancreas

Use Improves glycemic control; increases lean body mass; reduces obesity; improves lipid profile by decreasing total cholesterol and triglycerides, increasing HDL

USUAL DOSAGE 50-600 mcg/day

Adverse Reactions Gastrointestinal: Nausea, loose stools, flatulence, changes in appetite

Isolated reports of anemia, cognitive impairment, renal failure

Drug Interactions Any medications that may also affect blood sugars; (eg, beta-blockers, thiazides, any medications prescribed to treat diabetes); discuss chromium use prior to initiating

- **Chronulac®** *see* Lactulose *on page 506*
- **Cibacalcin® Injection** *see* Calcitonin *on page 128*

Ciclopirox (sye kloe PEER oks)

Pharmacologic Class Antifungal Agent

U.S. Brand Names Loprox®; Penlac™

Use

Cream/lotion: Treatment of tinea pedis (athlete's foot), tinea cruris (jock itch), tinea corporis (ringworm), cutaneous candidiasis, and tinea versicolor (pityriasis)

Lacquer: Topical treatment of mild to moderate onychomycosis of the fingernails and toenails due to *Trichophyton rubrum*

USUAL DOSAGE Children >10 years and Adults:

Cream/lotion: Apply twice daily, gently massage into affected areas; if no improvement after 4 weeks of treatment, re-evaluate the diagnosis

Lacquer: Apply to affected nails daily (as a part of a comprehensive management program for onychomycosis)

Contraindications Known hypersensitivity to ciclopirox or any of its components; avoid occlusive wrappings or dressings

Pregnancy Risk Factor B

Cidofovir (si DOF o veer)

Pharmacologic Class Antiviral Agent

U.S. Brand Names Vistide®

Use Treatment of cytomegalovirus (CMV) retinitis in patients with acquired immunodeficiency syndrome (AIDS). **Note:** Should be administered with probenecid.

USUAL DOSAGE

Induction: 5 mg/kg I.V. over 1 hour once weekly for 2 consecutive weeks

Maintenance: 5 mg/kg over 1 hour once every other week

Administer with probenecid - 2 g orally 3 hours prior to each cidofovir dose and 1 g at 2 and 8 hours after completion of the infusion (total: 4 g)

Hydrate with 1 L of 0.9% NS I.V. prior to cidofovir infusion; a second liter may be administered over a 1- to 3-hour period immediately following infusion, if tolerated

Dosing adjustment in renal impairment:

Cl_{cr} 41-55 mL/minute: 2 mg/kg

Cl_{cr} 30-40 mL/minute: 1.5 mg/kg

Cl_{cr} 20-29 mL/minute: 1 mg/kg

Cl_{cr} <19 mL/minute: 0.5 mg/kg

If the creatinine increases by 0.3-0.4 mg/dL, reduce the cidofovir dose to 3 mg/kg; discontinue therapy for increases ≥0.5 mg/dL or development of ≥3+ proteinuria

Contraindications Patients with hypersensitivity to cidofovir and in patients with a history of clinically severe hypersensitivity to probenecid or other sulfa-containing medications

Pregnancy Risk Factor C

♦ **Cidomycin** *see* Gentamicin *on page 408*

Cilostazol (sil OH sta zol)

Pharmacologic Class Antiplatelet Agent

U.S. Brand Names Pletal®

Mechanism of Action Cilostazol and its metabolites are inhibitors of phosphodiesterase III. As a result cyclic AMP is increased leading to inhibition of platelet aggregation and vasodilation. Other effects of phosphodiesterase III inhibition include increased cardiac contractility, accelerated A-V nodal conduction, increased ventricular automaticity, heart rate, and coronary blood flow.

Use Symptomatic management of peripheral vascular disease, primarily intermittent claudication; currently being investigated for the treatment of acute coronary syndromes and for graft patency improvement in percutaneous coronary interventions with or without stenting

USUAL DOSAGE Adults: Oral: 100 mg twice daily taken at least one-half hour before or 2 hours after breakfast and dinner; dosage should be reduced to 50 mg twice daily during concurrent therapy with inhibitors of CYP3A4 or CYP2C19 (see Drug Interactions)

Dosage Forms TAB: 50 mg, 100 mg

Contraindications Hypersensitivity to cilostazol or any component of the formulation; heart failure (of any severity)

Warnings/Precautions Use with caution in patients receiving platelet aggregation inhibitors (effects are unknown), hepatic impairment (not studied). Use with caution in patients receiving inhibitors of CYP3A4 (such as ketoconazole or erythromycin) or inhibitors of CYP2C19 (such as omeprazole); use with caution in severe underlying heart disease; use is not recommended in nursing mothers

Pregnancy Risk Factor C

Pregnancy Implications In animal studies, abnormalities of the skeletal, renal and cardiovascular system were increased. In addition, the incidence of stillbirth and decreased birth weights were increased. It is not known whether cilostazol is excreted in human milk. Because of the potential risk to nursing infants, a decision to discontinue the drug or discontinue nursing should be made.

(Continued)

Cilostazol *(Continued)*

Adverse Reactions

>10%:

Central nervous system: Headache (27% to 34%)

Gastrointestinal: Abnormal stools (12% to 15%), diarrhea (12% to 19%)

Miscellaneous: Infection (10% to 14%)

2% to 10%:

Cardiovascular: Peripheral edema (7% to 9%), palpitation (5% to 10%), tachycardia (4%)

Central nervous system: Dizziness (9% to 10%)

Gastrointestinal: Dyspepsia (6%), nausea (6% to 7%), abdominal pain (4% to 5%), flatulence (2% to 3%)

Neuromuscular & skeletal: Back pain (6% to 7%), myalgia (2% to 3%)

Respiratory: Rhinitis (7% to 12%), pharyngitis (7% to 10%), cough (3% to 4%)

<2%: Albuminuria, amblyopia, anemia, anorexia, anxiety, arthralgia, blindness, bone pain, bursitis, cardiac arrest, cerebral infarction/ischemia, chills, cholelithiasis, colitis, congestive heart failure, conjunctivitis, cystitis, diabetes mellitus, diplopia, dry skin, duodenal ulcer, duodenitis, ecchymosis, edema, esophageal hemorrhage, esophagitis, facial edema, fever, gastritis, gout, hematemesis, hemorrhage, hyperlipidemia, hyperuricemia, hypotension, increased creatinine, insomnia, malaise, melena, myocardial infarction/ischemia, neuralgia, nuchal rigidity, pelvic pain, peptic ulcer, polycythemia, postural hypotension, purpura, retinal hemorrhage, retroperitoneal hemorrhage, supraventricular arrhythmia, syncope, tongue edema, urinary frequency, urticaria, vaginal hemorrhage, vaginitis, ventricular arrhythmia

Drug Interactions CYP3A4 and CYP2C19 cytochrome enzyme substrate

Increased effect/toxicity: Increased concentrations of cilostazol have been observed during concurrent therapy with omeprazole, an inhibitor of CYP2C19 and during concurrent therapy with inhibitors of CYP3A4 such as clarithromycin, erythromycin, itraconazole, fluconazole, miconazole, fluvoxamine, fluoxetine, nefazodone, sertraline, and diltiazem. Platelet aggregation with aspirin is further inhibited when coadministered with cilostazol, it remains unclear whether concurrent oral anticoagulants or other antiplatelet drugs can increase cilostazol toxicity.

Onset 2-4 weeks

Half-Life 11-13 hours

Education and Monitoring Issues

Patient Education: Use exactly as directed; do not discontinue without consulting prescriber. Beneficial effect may take between 2-12 weeks. Take on an empty stomach (30 minutes before or 2 hours after meals). Do not take with grapefruit juice. You may experience nervousness, dizziness, or fatigue (use caution when driving or engaging in tasks requiring alertness until response to treatment is known); nausea, vomiting, or flatulence (frequent small meals, frequent mouth care, chewing gum or sucking hard candy may help); or postural hypotension (change position slowly when rising from sitting or lying position or climbing stairs). Report chest pain, palpitations, unusual heart beat, or swelling of extremities; unusual bleeding; unresolved GI upset or pain; dizziness, nervousness, sleeplessness, or fatigue; muscle cramping or tremor; unusual cough; or other adverse effects.

Dietary Considerations: Avoid concurrent ingestion of grapefruit juice due to the potential to inhibit CYP3A4. Avoid administration with meals. Taking cilostazol with a high-fat meal increases the AUC by 25% and the peak concentration may be increased by 90%; it is best to take cilostazol 30 minutes before or 2 hours after meals.

Manufacturer Otsuka America Pharmaceutical

Related Information

Pharmaceutical Manufacturers Directory *on page 1020*

♦ **Ciloxan™ Ophthalmic** *see* Ciprofloxacin *on page 199*

Cimetidine (sye MET i deen)

Pharmacologic Class Histamine H_2 Antagonist

U.S. Brand Names Tagamet®; Tagamet® HB [OTC]

Generic Available No

Mechanism of Action Competitive inhibition of histamine at H_2-receptors of the gastric parietal cells resulting in reduced gastric acid secretion, gastric volume and hydrogen ion concentration reduced

Use Short-term treatment of active duodenal ulcers and benign gastric ulcers; long-term prophylaxis of duodenal ulcer; gastric hypersecretory states; gastroesophageal reflux; prevention of upper GI bleeding in critically ill patients.

USUAL DOSAGE

Children: Oral, I.M., I.V.: 20-40 mg/kg/day in divided doses every 4 hours

Adults: Short-term treatment of active ulcers:

Oral: 300 mg 4 times/day or 800 mg at bedtime or 400 mg twice daily for up to 8 weeks

I.M., I.V.: 300 mg every 6 hours or 37.5 mg/hour by continuous infusion; I.V. dosage should be adjusted to maintain an intragastric pH ≥5

Patients with an active bleed: Administer cimetidine as a continuous infusion (see above)

Duodenal ulcer prophylaxis: Oral: 400-800 mg at bedtime
Gastric hypersecretory conditions: Oral, I.M., I.V.: 300-600 mg every 6 hours; dosage not to exceed 2.4 g/day

Dosing adjustment/interval in renal impairment: Children and Adults:
Cl_{cr} 20-40 mL/minute: Administer every 8 hours or 75% of normal dose
Cl_{cr} 0-20 mL/minute: Administer every 12 hours or 50% of normal dose

Hemodialysis: Slightly dialyzable (5% to 20%)

Dosing adjustment/comments in hepatic impairment: Usual dose is safe in mild liver disease but use with caution and in reduced dosage in severe liver disease; increased risk of CNS toxicity in cirrhosis suggested by enhanced penetration of CNS

Dosage Forms INF, in NS: 300 mg (50 mL). **INJ:** 150 mg/mL (2 mL, 8 mL). **LIQ, oral** (mint-peach flavor): 300 mg/5 mL with alcohol 2.8% (5 mL, 240 mL). **TAB:** 100 mg, 200 mg, 300 mg, 400 mg, 800 mg

Contraindications Hypersensitivity to cimetidine, other component, or other H_2-antagonists

Warnings/Precautions Adjust dosages in renal/hepatic impairment or patients receiving drugs metabolized through the P-450 system

Pregnancy Risk Factor B

Adverse Reactions

1% to 10%:
Central nervous system: Dizziness, agitation, headache, drowsiness
Gastrointestinal: Diarrhea, nausea, vomiting

<1%: Agranulocytosis, bradycardia, confusion, decreased sexual ability, edema of the breasts, elevated creatinine, fever, gynecomastia, hypotension, increased AST/ALT, myalgia, neutropenia, rash, tachycardia, thrombocytopenia

Drug Interactions CYP3A3/4 enzyme substrate; CYP1A2, 2C9, 2C18, 2C19, 2D6, and 3A3/4 enzyme inhibitor

Increased toxicity: Decreased elimination of lidocaine, theophylline, phenytoin, metronidazole, triamterene, procainamide, quinidine, and propranolol

Inhibition of warfarin metabolism, tricyclic antidepressant metabolism, diazepam elimination and cyclosporine elimination

Alcohol Interactions Avoid use (may increase central nervous system depression and enhance gastric mucosal irritation)

Onset 1 hour; peak serum concentrations ~1 hour after oral dose

Duration 6 hours

Half-Life Normal renal function: 2 hours

Education and Monitoring Issues

Patient Education: Take with meals. Limit xanthine-containing foods and beverages which may decrease iron absorption. To be effective, continue to take for the prescribed time (possibly 4-8 weeks) even though symptoms may have improved. Smoking decreases the effectiveness of cimetidine; stop smoking if possible. Avoid use of caffeine or aspirin products. Report diarrhea, black tarry stools, coffee ground like emesis, dizziness, confusion, rash, unusual bleeding or bruising, sore throat, and fever.

Monitoring Parameters: Blood pressure with I.V. push administration, CBC, gastric pH, signs and symptoms of peptic ulcer disease, occult blood with GI bleeding, monitor renal function to correct dose; monitor for side effects

♦ **Cinobac® Pulvules®** *see* Cinoxacin *on page 199*

Cinoxacin (sin OKS a sin)

Pharmacologic Class Quinolone

U.S. Brand Names Cinobac® Pulvules®

Use Treatment of urinary tract infections

USUAL DOSAGE Children >12 years and Adults: Oral: 1 g/day in 2-4 doses for 7-14 days

Dosing interval in renal impairment:
Cl_{cr} 20-50 mL/minute: 250 mg twice daily
Cl_{cr} <20 mL/minute: 250 mg/day

Contraindications History of convulsive disorders, hypersensitivity to cinoxacin or any component or other quinolones

Pregnancy Risk Factor B

♦ **Cipro** *see* Ciprofloxacin *on page 199*

Ciprofloxacin (sip roe FLOKS a sin)

Pharmacologic Class Antibiotic, Ophthalmic; Antibiotic, Quinolone

U.S. Brand Names Ciloxan™ Ophthalmic; Cipro®; Cipro® I.V.

Generic Available No

Mechanism of Action Inhibits DNA-gyrase in susceptible organisms; inhibits relaxation of supercoiled DNA and promotes breakage of double-stranded DNA

Use Treatment of documented or suspected infections of the lower respiratory tract, sinuses, skin and skin structure, bone/joints, and urinary tract including prostatitis, due to susceptible bacterial strains; especially indicated for *Pseudomonal* infections and those due to multidrug resistant gram-negative organisms, chronic bacterial prostatitis, infectious diarrhea, complicated gram-negative and anaerobic intra-abdominal infections (with

(Continued)

Ciprofloxacin *(Continued)*

metronidazole) due to *E. coli* (enteropathic strains), *B. fragilis, P. mirabilis, K. pneumoniae, P. aeruginosa, Campylobacter jejuni* or *Shigella*; approved for acute sinusitis caused by *H. influenzae* or *M. catarrhalis*; also used to treat typhoid fever due to *Salmonella typhi* (although eradication of the chronic typhoid carrier state has not been proven), osteomyelitis when parenteral therapy is not feasible, and sexually transmitted diseases such as uncomplicated cervical and urethral gonorrhea due to *Neisseria gonorrhoeae*; used ophthalmologically for superficial ocular infections (corneal ulcers, conjunctivitis) due to susceptible strains

USUAL DOSAGE

Children (see Warnings/Precautions):

- Oral: 20-30 mg/kg/day in 2 divided doses; maximum: 1.5 g/day
  - Cystic fibrosis: 20-40 mg/kg/day divided every 12 hours
- I.V.: 15-20 mg/kg/day divided every 12 hours
  - Cystic fibrosis: 15-30 mg/kg/day divided every 8-12 hours

Adults: Oral:

- Urinary tract infection: 250-500 mg every 12 hours for 7-10 days, depending on severity of infection and susceptibility; (3 investigations (n=975) indicate the minimum effective dose for women with acute, uncomplicated urinary tract infection may be 100 mg twice daily for 3 days)
- Lower respiratory tract, skin/skin structure infections: 500-750 mg twice daily for 7-14 days depending on severity and susceptibility
- Bone/joint infections: 500-750 mg twice daily for 4-6 weeks, depending on severity and susceptibility
- Infectious diarrhea: 500 mg every 12 hours for 5-7 days
- Typhoid fever: 500 mg every 12 hours for 10 days
- Urethral/cervical gonococcal infections: 250-500 mg as a single dose (CDC recommends concomitant doxycycline or azithromycin due to developing resistance; avoid use in Asian or Western Pacific travelers)
- Disseminated gonococcal infection: 500 mg twice daily to complete 7 days of therapy (initial treatment with ceftriaxone 1 g I.M./I.V. daily for 24-48 hours after improvement begins)
- Chancroid: 500 mg twice daily for 3 days
- Mild to moderate sinusitis: 500 mg every 12 hours for 10 days

Adults: I.V.

- Urinary tract infection: 200-400 mg every 12 hours for 7-10 days
- Lower respiratory tract, skin/skin structure infection (mild to moderate): 400 mg every 12 hours for 7-14 days

Ophthalmic: Instill 1-2 drops in eye(s) every 2 hours while awake for 2 days and 1-2 drops every 4 hours while awake for the next 5 days

Dosing adjustment in renal impairment:

- Cl_{cr} <30 mL/minute:
  - 500 mg every 24 hours or
  - 750 mg every 24 hours

Dialysis: Only small amounts of ciprofloxacin are removed by hemo- or peritoneal dialysis (<10%); usual dose: 250-500 mg every 24 hours following dialysis

Continuous arteriovenous or venovenous hemodiafiltration (CAVH) effects: Administer 200-400 mg I.V. every 12 hours

Dosage Forms INF: In D_5W: 400 mg (200 mL); In NS or D_5W: 200 mg (100 mL). **INJ:** 200 mg (20 mL); 400 mg (40 mL). **SOLN, ophth:** 3.5 mg/mL (2.5 mL, 5 mL). **SUSP, oral:** 250 mg/5 mL (100 mL); 500 mg/5 mL (100 mL). **TAB:** 100 mg, 250 mg, 500 mg, 750 mg

Contraindications Hypersensitivity to ciprofloxacin, any component or other quinolones

Warnings/Precautions Not recommended in children <18 years of age; has caused transient arthropathy in children; CNS stimulation may occur (tremor, restlessness, confusion, and very rarely hallucinations or seizures); use with caution in patients with known or suspected CNS disorder; green discoloration of teeth in newborns has been reported; prolonged use may result in superinfection; may rarely cause inflamed or ruptured tendons (discontinue use immediately with signs of inflammation or tendon pain)

Pregnancy Risk Factor C

Adverse Reactions

1% to 10%:

- Central nervous system: Headache, restlessness
- Gastrointestinal: Nausea, diarrhea, vomiting, abdominal pain
- Dermatologic: Rash

<1%: Acute renal failure, anemia, arthralgia, confusion, dizziness, increased liver enzymes, ruptured tendons, seizures, tremor

Drug Interactions CYP1A2 enzyme inhibitor

Decreased effect:

- Enteral feedings may decrease plasma concentrations of ciprofloxacin probably by >30% inhibition of absorption. Ciprofloxacin should not be administered with enteral feedings. The feeding would need to be discontinued for 1-2 hours prior to and after ciprofloxacin administration. Nasogastric administration produces a greater loss of ciprofloxacin bioavailability than does nasoduodenal administration.

Aluminum/magnesium products, didanosine, and sucralfate may decrease absorption of ciprofloxacin by ≥90% if administered concurrently

RECOMMENDATION: Administer ciprofloxacin 2 hours before dose OR administer ciprofloxacin at least 4 hours and preferably 6 hours after the dose of these agents OR change to an H_2-antagonist or omeprazole

Calcium, iron, zinc, and multivitamins with minerals products may decrease absorption of ciprofloxacin significantly if administered concurrently

RECOMMENDATION: Administer ciprofloxacin 2 hours before dose OR administer ciprofloxacin at least 2 hours after the dose of these agents

Increased toxicity:

Caffeine and theophylline → CNS stimulation when concurrent with ciprofloxacin

Cyclosporine may increase serum creatinine levels

Half-Life Adults with normal renal function: 3-5 hours

Education and Monitoring Issues

Patient Education: Take as directed, preferably on an empty stomach (30 minutes before or 2 hours after meals). Take entire prescription even if feeling better. Maintain adequate hydration (2-3 L/day of fluids unless instructed to restrict fluid intake) to avoid concentrated urine and crystal formation. You may experience nausea, vomiting, or anorexia (small frequent meals, frequent mouth care, sucking lozenges, or chewing gum may help). Report immediately any signs of skin rash, joint or back pain, or difficulty breathing. Report unusual fever or chills; vaginal itching or foul-smelling vaginal discharge; easy bruising or bleeding; or pain, inflammation, or rupture of a tendon.

Dietary Considerations:

Food: Decreases rate, but not extent, of absorption. Drug may cause GI upset; take without regard to meals (manufacturer prefers that drug is taken 2 hours after meals)

Dairy products, oral multivitamins, and mineral supplements: Absorption decreased by divalent and trivalent cations. These cations bind to and form insoluble complexes with quinolones. Avoid taking these substrates with ciprofloxacin. The manufacturer states that the usual dietary intake of calcium has not been shown to interfere with ciprofloxacin absorption.

Caffeine: Possible exaggerated or prolonged effects of caffeine. Ciprofloxacin reduces total body clearance of caffeine. Patients consuming regular large quantities of caffeinated beverages may need to restrict caffeine intake if excessive cardiac or CNS stimulation occurs.

Monitoring Parameters: Patients receiving concurrent ciprofloxacin, theophylline, or cyclosporine should have serum levels monitored

Reference Range: Therapeutic: 2.6-3 µg/mL; Toxic: >5 µg/mL

Manufacturer Bayer Corp (Biological and Pharmaceutical Division)

Related Information

Antimicrobial Drugs of Choice *on page 1182*
Ciprofloxacin and Hydrocortisone *on page 201*
Pharmaceutical Manufacturers Directory *on page 1020*
Treatment of Sexually Transmitted Diseases *on page 1210*
Tuberculosis Treatment Guidelines *on page 1213*

Ciprofloxacin and Hydrocortisone

(sip roe FLOKS a sin & hye droe KOR ti sone)

Pharmacologic Class Antibiotic/Corticosteroid, Otic

U.S. Brand Names Cipro® HC Otic

Dosage Forms SUSP, otic: Ciprofloxacin hydrochloride 0.2% and hydrocortisone 1%

Manufacturer Bayer Corp (Biological and Pharmaceutical Division)

Related Information

Pharmaceutical Manufacturers Directory *on page 1020*

♦ **Cipro® HC Otic** *see* Ciprofloxacin and Hydrocortisone *on page 201*

♦ **Cipro® I.V.** *see* Ciprofloxacin *on page 199*

Cisapride (SIS a pride)

Pharmacologic Class Gastrointestinal Agent, Prokinetic

U.S. Brand Names Propulsid®

Mechanism of Action Enhances the release of acetylcholine at the myenteric plexus. *In vitro* studies have shown cisapride to have serotonin-4 receptor agonistic properties which may increase gastrointestinal motility and cardiac rate; increases lower esophageal sphincter pressure and lower esophageal peristalsis; accelerates gastric emptying of both liquids and solids.

Use Treatment of nocturnal symptoms of gastroesophageal reflux disease (GERD), also demonstrated effectiveness for gastroparesis, refractory constipation, and nonulcer dyspepsia

USUAL DOSAGE A 12-lead EKG should be performed prior to administration of cisapride. Treatment with cisapride should not be initiated if the QT_c value exceeds 450 milliseconds. Serum electrolytes (potassium, calcium, and magnesium) and creatinine (Continued)

TO BE WITHDRAWN FROM U.S. MARKET IN 2000

Cisapride *(Continued)*

should be assessed prior to administration of cisapride and whenever conditions develop that may affect electrolyte balance or renal function.

Oral:

Children: 0.15-0.3 mg/kg/dose 3-4 times/day; maximum: 10 mg/dose

Adults: Initial: 10 mg 4 times/day at least 15 minutes before meals and at bedtime; in some patients the dosage will need to be increased to 20 mg to obtain a satisfactory result

Dosage Forms SUSP, oral (cherry cream flavor): 1 mg/mL (450 mL). **TAB, scored:** 10 mg, 20 mg

Contraindications Hypersensitivity to cisapride or any of its components; GI hemorrhage, mechanical obstruction, GI perforation, or other situations when GI motility stimulation is dangerous

Serious cardiac arrhythmias including ventricular tachycardia, ventricular fibrillation, torsade de pointes, and Q-T prolongation have been reported in patients taking cisapride with other drugs that inhibit CYP3A4. Some of these events have been fatal. Concomitant oral or intravenous administration of the following drugs with cisapride may lead to elevated cisapride blood levels and is contraindicated:

Antibiotics: Oral or I.V. erythromycin, clarithromycin, troleandomycin

Antidepressants: Nefazodone, maprotiline

Antifungals: Oral or I.V. fluconazole, itraconazole, miconazole, oral ketoconazole

Phenothiazines: Prochlorperazine, promethazine

Protease inhibitors: Amprenavir, indinavir, ritonavir

Cisapride is also contraindicated for patients with history of prolonged electrocardiographic Q-T intervals, known family history of congenital long Q-T syndrome; clinically significant bradycardia, renal failure, history of ventricular arrhythmias, ischemic heart disease, and congestive heart failure; uncorrected electrolyte disorders (hypokalemia, hypomagnesemia); respiratory failure; and concomitant medications known to prolong the Q-T interval and increase the risk of arrhythmia, such as certain antiarrhythmics, certain antipsychotics, certain antidepressants, bepridil, sparfloxacin, and terodiline. The preceding list of drugs is not comprehensive (see Drug Interactions). Cisapride should not be used in patients with uncorrected hypokalemia or hypomagnesemia, or who might experience rapid reduction of plasma potassium such as those administered potassium-wasting diuretics and/or insulin in acute settings.

A 12-lead EKG should be performed prior to administration of cisapride. Treatment with cisapride should not be initiated if the QT_c value exceeds 450 milliseconds. Serum electrolytes (potassium, calcium, and magnesium) and creatinine should be assessed prior to administration of cisapride and whenever conditions develop that may affect electrolyte balance or renal function.

Warnings/Precautions Serious cardiac arrhythmias including ventricular tachycardia, ventricular fibrillation, torsade de pointes, and Q-T prolongation have been reported in patients taking this drug. Many of these patients also took drugs expected to increase cisapride blood levels by inhibiting the CYP3A4 enzymes that metabolize cisapride. These drugs include clarithromycin, erythromycin, troleandomycin, nefazodone, fluconazole, itraconazole, ketoconazole, indinavir and ritonavir. Some of these events have been fatal. Cisapride is contraindicated in patients taking any of these drugs. **Q-T prolongation, torsade de pointes (sometimes with syncope), cardiac arrest and sudden death have been reported in patients taking cisapride without the above-mentioned contraindicated drugs.** Most patients had disorders that may have predisposed them to arrhythmias with cisapride. Cisapride is contraindicated for those patients with: history of prolonged electrocardiographic Q-T intervals; renal failure; history of ventricular arrhythmias, ischemic heart disease, and congestive heart failure; uncorrected electrolyte disorders (hypokalemia, hypomagnesemia); respiratory failure; and concomitant medications known to prolong the Q-T interval and increase the risk of arrhythmia, such as certain antiarrhythmics, including those of Class 1A (such as quinidine and procainamide) and Class III (such as sotalol); tricyclic antidepressants (such as amitriptyline); certain tetracyclic antidepressants (such as maprotiline); certain antipsychotic medications (such as certain phenothiazines and sertindole), bepridil, sparfloxacin and terodiline. (The preceding lists of drugs are not comprehensive.) Recommended doses of cisapride should not be exceeded.

Potential benefits should be weighed against risks prior administration of cisapride to patients who have or may develop prolongation of cardiac conduction intervals, particularly QT_c. These include patients with conditions that could predispose them to the development of serious arrhythmias, such as multiple organ failure, COPD, apnea and advanced cancer. Cisapride should not be used in patients with uncorrected hypokalemia or hypomagnesemia, such as those with severe dehydration, vomiting or malnutrition, or those taking potassium-wasting diuretics. Cisapride should not be used in patients who might experience rapid reduction of plasma potassium, such as those administered potassium-wasting diuretics and/or insulin in acute settings.

Pregnancy Risk Factor C

Adverse Reactions

>5%:

Central nervous system: Headache

Dermatologic: Rash

Gastrointestinal: Diarrhea, GI cramping, dyspepsia, flatulence, nausea, xerostomia

Respiratory: Rhinitis

<5%:

Cardiovascular: Tachycardia

Central nervous system: Extrapyramidal effects, somnolence, fatigue, seizures, insomnia, anxiety

Hematologic: Thrombocytopenia, increased LFTs, pancytopenia, leukopenia, granulocytopenia, aplastic anemia

Respiratory: Sinusitis, coughing, upper respiratory tract infection, increased incidence of viral infection

Drug Interactions CYP3A3/4 enzyme substrate

Azole antifungals (fluconazole, itraconazole, ketoconazole, miconazole) increase cisapride's concentration. Pre-existing cardiovascular disease or electrolyte imbalances increase the risk of malignant arrhythmias; concurrent use is contraindicated.

Nefazodone and maprotiline may increase the risk of malignant arrhythmias; concurrent use is contraindicated

Protease inhibitors (amprenavir, indinavir, nelfinavir, ritonavir) increase cisapride's concentration. Increased risk of malignant arrhythmias; concurrent use is contraindicated.

Cimetidine increases the bioavailability of cisapride; use an alternative H_2 antagonist

Macrolides (clarithromycin, erythromycin, troleandomycin) increase cisapride. Risk of arrhythmias; concurrent use is contraindicated.

Sertindole may increase the risk of malignant arrhythmias; concurrent use is contraindicated

Phenothiazines (prochlorperazine, promethazine) may increase the risk of malignant arrhythmias; concurrent use is contraindicated

Class Ia (quinidine, procainamide) and Class III (amiodarone, sotalol) antiarrhythmics increase the risk of malignant arrhythmias; concurrent use is contraindicated

TCAs increase the risk of malignant arrhythmias; concurrent use is contraindicated

Bepridil increases the risk of malignant arrhythmias; concurrent use is contraindicated

Quinolone antibiotics: Sparfloxacin, gatifloxacin, moxifloxacin increase the risk of malignant arrhythmias; concurrent use is contraindicated

Warfarin: Isolated cases of increased INR; monitor closely

Alcohol Interactions Avoid or limit use (cisapride may increase absorption of alcohol)

Onset 0.5-1 hour

Half-Life 6-12 hours

Education and Monitoring Issues

Patient Education: Take before meals. Avoid alcohol and other CNS depressants. May cause increased sedation. Report severe abdominal pain, prolonged diarrhea, weight loss, or extreme fatigue.

Dietary Considerations: Concomitant use with grapefruit juice should be avoided as it increases the bioavailability of cisapride

Manufacturer Janssen Pharmaceutical, Inc

Related Information

Pharmaceutical Manufacturers Directory *on page 1020*

Citalopram (sye TAL oh pram)

Pharmacologic Class Antidepressant, Selective Serotonin Reuptake Inhibitor

U.S. Brand Names Celexa™

Mechanism of Action Inhibits CNS neuronal reuptake of serotonin, which enhances serotonergic activity. Activity as an antidepressant has been presumed to be associated with this effect. Has limited or no affinity for histamine, dopamine, acetylcholine (muscarinic), GABA, benzodiazepine, and adrenergic (alpha- and beta-) receptors. Antagonism of these receptors is believed to be associated with sedative, anticholinergic and cardiovascular adverse effects of tricyclic antidepressants.

Use Treatment of depression; currently being evaluated for use in the treatment of dementia, smoking cessation, alcohol abuse, obsessive-compulsive disorder, and diabetic neuropathy

USUAL DOSAGE Oral: 20 mg once daily, in the morning or evening. Dose is generally increased to 40 mg once daily. Doses should be increased by 20 mg at intervals of not less than 1 week. Doses >40 mg/day are not generally recommended, although some patients may respond to doses up to 60 mg/day.

Elderly or hepatically impaired patients: Initial dose of 20 mg is recommended; increase dose to 40 mg/day only in nonresponders

Maintenance: Generally, patients are maintained on the dose required for acute stabilization. If side effects are bothersome, dose reduction by 20 mg/day may be considered.

Dosing adjustment in renal impairment: None necessary in mild to moderate renal impairment; best avoided in severely impaired renal function (Cl_{cr} <20 mL/minute)

(Continued)

Citalopram *(Continued)*

Dosage Forms SOLN, oral: 10 mg/5 mL. **TAB**, as hydrobromide: 20 mg, 40 mg, 60 mg

Contraindications Known hypersensitivity to citalopram; hypersensitivity or other adverse sequelae during therapy with other SSRIs; concomitant use with MAO inhibitors or within 2 weeks of discontinuing MAO inhibitors. Potential for severe reaction when used with MAO inhibitors - serotonin syndrome (hyperthermia, muscular rigidity, mental status changes/agitation, autonomic instability) may occur, possibly resulting in death. Do not use citalopram and MAO inhibitors within 14 days of each other.

Warnings/Precautions As with all antidepressants, use with caution in patients with a history of mania (may activate hypomania/mania). Use with caution in patients with a history of seizures and patients at high risk of suicide. Has potential to impair cognitive/ motor performance - should use caution operating hazardous machinery. Elderly and patients with hepatic insufficiency should receive lower dosages. Use with caution in renal insufficiency and other concomitant illness (due to limited drug experience). May cause hyponatremia/SIADH.

Pregnancy Risk Factor C

Pregnancy Implications Animal reproductive studies have revealed adverse effects on fetal and postnatal development (at doses higher than human therapeutic doses). Should be used in pregnancy only if potential benefit justifies potential risk. Citalopram is excreted in human milk; a decision should be made whether to continue or discontinue nursing or discontinue the drug.

Adverse Reactions

>10%:

Central nervous system: Somnolence, insomnia
Gastrointestinal: Nausea, xerostomia
Miscellaneous: Diaphoresis

<10%:

Central nervous system: Anxiety, anorexia, agitation, yawning
Dermatologic: Rash, pruritus
Gastrointestinal: Diarrhea, dyspepsia, vomiting, abdominal pain
Endocrine & metabolic: Sexual dysfunction
Neuromuscular & skeletal: Tremor, arthralgia, myalgia
Respiratory: Cough, rhinitis, sinusitis

Drug Interactions CYP3A3/4 and CYP2C19 enzyme substrate; CYP2D6, 1A2, and 2C19 enzyme inhibitor (weak)

Carbamazepine may enhance the metabolism of citalopram
Cimetidine may inhibit the metabolism of citalopram
The combined use of citalopram with buspirone, MAO inhibitors, moclobemide, nefazodone, or tramadol may result in serotonin syndrome
Citalopram may increase plasma level of metoprolol

Alcohol Interactions Avoid use (may increase central nervous system depression)

Onset Usually >2 weeks

Half-Life 24-48 hours (average 35 hours - doubled in patients with hepatic impairment)

Education and Monitoring Issues

Patient Education: The effects of this medication may take up to 3 weeks. Take as directed; do not alter dose or frequency without consulting prescriber. Avoid alcohol, caffeine, and CNS stimulants. You may experience sexual dysfunction (reversible). May cause dizziness, anxiety, or blurred vision (rise slowly from sitting or lying position and use caution when driving or engaging in tasks requiring alertness until response to drug is known); nausea or dry mouth (frequent small meals, frequent mouth care, chewing gum, or sucking lozenges may help). Report confusion or impaired concentration, severe headache, palpitations, rash, insomnia or nightmares, changes in personality, muscle weakness or tremors, altered gait pattern, signs and symptoms of respiratory infection, or excessive perspiration.

Monitoring Parameters: Monitor patient periodically for symptom resolution, heart rate, blood pressure, liver function tests, and CBC with continued therapy

Manufacturer Forest Pharmaceutical, Inc

Related Information

Antidepressant Agents Comparison *on page 1231*
Pharmaceutical Manufacturers Directory *on page 1020*

♦ **Citro-Mag** *see* Magnesium Citrate *on page 550*

Cladribine (KLA dri been)

Pharmacologic Class Antineoplastic Agent, Antimetabolite

U.S. Brand Names Leustatin™

Mechanism of Action A purine antimetabolite, cladribine is a prodrug that is activated via phosphorylation by deoxycytidine kinase to a 5′-triphosphate form, and incorporated into DNA, inducing DNA strand breaks, shutdown of DNA synthesis, and depletion of nicotinamide adenine dinucleotide (NAD), and adenosine triphosphate (ATP). Effects are seen in resting (G_0) as well as dividing cells. Cladribine's mechanism for killing slowly dividing cells is uncertain, but may be related to ATP depletion and/or deoxycytidine kinase activity.

Use Treatment of hairy cell leukemia (HCL) and chronic lymphocytic leukemias

USUAL DOSAGE I.V.:

Children:

Acute leukemia: The safety and effectiveness of cladribine in children have not been established; in a phase I study involving patients 1-21 years of age with relapsed acute leukemia, cladribine was administered by CIV at doses ranging from 3-10.7 mg/m²/day for 5 days (0.5-2 times the dose recommended in HCL). Investigators reported beneficial responses in this study; the dose-limiting toxicity was severe myelosuppression with profound neutropenia and thrombocytopenia.

CIV: 15-18 mg/m²/day for 5 days

Adults:

Hairy cell leukemia:

CIV: 0.09-0.1 mg/kg/day continuous infusion for 7 consecutive days, one cycle, or repeated every 28-35 days

CIV: 4 mg/m²/day for 7 days

Non-Hodgkin's lymphoma: CIV: 0.1 mg/kg/day for 7 days

Dosage Forms INJ (preservative free): 1 mg/mL (10 mL)

Contraindications Patients with a prior history of hypersensitivity to cladribine

Warnings/Precautions The U.S. Food and Drug Administration (FDA) currently recommends that procedures for proper handling and disposal of antineoplastic agents be considered. Because of its myelosuppressive properties, cladribine should be used with caution in patients with pre-existing hematologic or immunologic abnormalities; prophylactic administration of allopurinol should be considered in patients receiving cladribine because of the potential for hyperuricemia secondary to tumor lysis; appropriate antibiotic therapy should be administered promptly in patients exhibiting signs and symptoms of neutropenia and infection.

Pregnancy Risk Factor D

Adverse Reactions

>10%:

Bone marrow suppression: Commonly observed in patients treated with cladribine, especially at high doses; at the initiation of treatment, however, most patients in clinical studies had hematologic impairment as a result of HCL. During the first 2 weeks after treatment initiation, mean platelet counts decline and subsequently increased with normalization of mean counts by day 12. Absolute neutrophil counts and hemoglobin declined and subsequently increased with normalization of mean counts by week 5 and week 6. CD4 counts nadir at approximately 270, 4-6 months after treatments. Mean CD4 counts after 15 months were <500/mm³. Patients should be considered immunosuppressed for up to one year after cladribine therapy.

Central nervous system: Fatigue, headache

Fever: Temperature ≥101°F has been associated with the use of cladribine in approximately 66% of patients in the first month of therapy. Although 69% of patients developed fevers, <33% of febrile events were associated with documented infection.

Dermatologic: Rash

Gastrointestinal: Nausea and vomiting are not severe with cladribine at any dose level. Most cases of nausea were mild, not accompanied by vomiting and did not require treatment with antiemetics. In patients requiring antiemetics, nausea was easily controlled most often by chlorpromazine.

Local: Injection site reactions

1% to 10%:

Cardiovascular: Edema, tachycardia

Central nervous system: Dizziness, insomnia, pain, chills, malaise

Dermatologic: Pruritus, erythema

Gastrointestinal: Constipation, abdominal pain

Neuromuscular & skeletal: Myalgia, arthralgia, weakness

Miscellaneous: Diaphoresis, trunk pain

Half-Life Half-life: Biphasic: Alpha: 25 minutes; Beta: 6.7 hours; Terminal, mean (normal renal function): 5.4 hours

Education and Monitoring Issues

Patient Education: This drug can only be administered by infusion. Do not use alcohol, aspirin-containing products, or OTC medications without consulting prescriber. It is important to maintain adequate hydration (2-3 L/day of fluids unless instructed to restrict fluid intake) and nutrition during therapy; frequent small meals may help. You may experience nausea or vomiting (frequent small meals, frequent mouth care, sucking lozenges, or chewing gum may help). You will be more susceptible to infection (avoid crowds and exposure to infection, and avoid immunization unless approved by prescriber). You may experience muscle weakness or pain (mild analgesics may help). Frequent mouth care with soft toothbrush or cotton swabs and frequent mouth rinses may help relieve mouth sores. Report rash; fever; chills; unusual bruising or bleeding; signs of infection; excessive fatigue; yellowing of eyes or skin; change in color of urine or stool; swelling, warmth, or pain in extremities; or difficult respirations.

Manufacturer Ortho Biotech, Inc

Related Information

Pharmaceutical Manufacturers Directory *on page 1020*

♦ **Claforan®** *see* Cefotaxime *on page 156*
♦ **Claripex®** *see* Clofibrate *on page 211*

Clarithromycin (kla RITH roe mye sin)

Pharmacologic Class Antibiotic, Macrolide

U.S. Brand Names Biaxin™; Biaxin™ XL

Generic Available No

Mechanism of Action Exerts its antibacterial action by binding to 50S ribosomal subunit resulting in inhibition of protein synthesis. The 14-OH metabolite of clarithromycin is twice as active as the parent compound against certain organisms.

Use In adults, for treatment of pharyngitis/tonsillitis, acute maxillary sinusitis, acute exacerbation of chronic bronchitis, pneumonia, uncomplicated skin/skin structure infections due to susceptible *S. pyogenes*, *S. pneumoniae*, *S. agalactiae*, viridans *Streptococcus*, *M. catarrhalis*, *C. trachomatis*, *Legionella* sp, *Mycoplasma pneumoniae*,*S. aureus*, *H. influenzae*; has activity against *M. avium* and *M. intracellulare* infection and is indicated for treatment of and prevention of disseminated mycobacterial infections due to *M. avium* complex disease (eg, patients with advanced HIV infection); indicated for the treatment of duodenal ulcer disease due to *H. pylori* in regimens with other drugs including amoxicillin and lansoprazole or omeprazole, ranitidine, bismuth citrate, bismuth subsalicylate, tetracycline and/or an H_2-antagonist (see index); also indicated for prophylaxis of bacterial endocarditis in patients who are allergic to penicillin and undergoing surgical or dental procedures

In children, for treatment of pharyngitis/tonsillitis, acute maxillary sinusitis, acute otitis media, uncomplicated skin/skin structure infections due to the above organisms; treatment of and prevention of disseminated mycobacterial infections due to *M. avium* complex disease (eg, patients with advanced HIV infection)

Exhibits the same spectrum of *in vitro* activity as erythromycin, but with significantly increased potency against those organisms

USUAL DOSAGE Safe use in children has not been established

Children ≥6 months: 15 mg/kg/day divided every 12 hours; dosages of 7.5 mg/kg twice daily up to 500 mg twice daily children with AIDS and disseminated MAC infection

Adults: Oral:
- Usual dose: 250-500 mg every 12 hours **or** 1000 mg (2 x 500 mg extended release tablets) once daily for for 7-14 days
- Upper respiratory tract: 250-500 mg every 12 hours for 10-14 days
- Pharyngitis/tonsillitis: 250 mg every 12 hours for 10 days
- Acute maxillary sinusitis: 500 mg every 12 hours **or** 1000 mg (2 x 500 mg extended release tablets) once daily for 14 days

Lower respiratory tract: 250-500 mg every 12 hours for 7-14 days
- Acute exacerbation of chronic bronchitis due to:
  - *M. catarrhalis* and *S. pneumoniae*: 250 mg every 12 hours **or** 1000 mg (2 x 500 mg extended release tablets) once daily for 7-14 days
  - *H. influenzae*: 500 mg every 12 hours for 7-14 days
- Pneumonia due to *M. pneumoniae* and *S. pneumoniae*: 250 mg every 12 hours for 7-14 days
- Mycobacterial infection (prevention and treatment): 500 mg twice daily (use with other antimycobacterial drugs, eg, ethambutol, clofazimine, or rifampin)

Prophylaxis of bacterial endocarditis: 500 mg 1 hour prior to procedure

Uncomplicated skin and skin structure: 250 mg every 12 hours for 7-14 days

Helicobacter pylori: Combination regimen with bismuth subsalicylate, tetracycline, clarithromycin, and an H_2-receptor antagonist; or combination of omeprazole and clarithromycin; 250 mg twice daily to 500 mg 3 times/day

Dosing adjustment in renal impairment: Adults: Oral:
- Cl_{cr} <30 mL/minute: 500 mg loading dose, then 250 mg once or twice daily

Dosing adjustment in severe renal impairment: Decreased doses or prolonged dosing intervals are recommended

Dosage Forms GRANULES for oral susp: 125 mg/5 mL (50 mL, 100 mL); 250 mg/5 mL (50 mL, 100 mL). **TAB, film coated:** 250 mg, 500 mg; Extended release: 500 mg

Contraindications Hypersensitivity to clarithromycin, erythromycin, or any macrolide antibiotic; use with pimozide, astemizole, cisapride, terfenadine

Warnings/Precautions In presence of severe renal impairment with or without coexisting hepatic impairment, decreased dosage or prolonged dosing interval may be appropriate; antibiotic-associated colitis has been reported with use of clarithromycin; elderly patients have experienced increased incidents of adverse effects due to known age-related decreases in renal function

Pregnancy Risk Factor C

Adverse Reactions

1% to 10%:
- Central nervous system: Headache
- Gastrointestinal: Diarrhea, nausea, abnormal taste, heartburn, abdominal pain

<1% (limited to important or life-threatening symptoms): Ventricular tachycardia, QT prolongation, torsade de pointes, *Clostridium difficile* colitis, decreased white blood

count, elevated prothrombin time, thrombocytopenia; elevated AST, alkaline phosphatase, and bilirubin; elevated BUN/serum creatinine, shortness of breath, leukopenia, neutropenia, manic behavior, tremor, hypoglycemia, anaphylaxis, Stevens-Johnson syndrome, anxiety, hallucinations

Drug Interactions CYP3A3/4 enzyme substrate; CYP1A2 and 3A3/4 enzyme inhibitor

Increased levels:

Clarithromycin increases serum theophylline levels by as much as 20%

Increased concentration of HMG CoA-reductase inhibitors (lovastatin and simvastatin)

Amprenavir AUC is increase by clarithromycin

Significantly increases carbamazepine levels and those of cyclosporine, digoxin, ergot alkaloid, tacrolimus, omeprazole and triazolam; increases levels of cisapride - concurrent use is contraindicated

Peak levels (but not AUC) of zidovudine are often increased; terfenadine and astemizole should be avoided with use of clarithromycin since plasma levels may be increased by >3 times; serious arrhythmias have occurred with cisapride and other drugs which inhibit CYP3A4 enzymes (eg, clarithromycin)

Fluconazole increases clarithromycin levels and AUC by ~25%; death has been reported with administration of pimozide and clarithromycin

Pimozide's serum concentration may be elevated; concurrent use is contraindicated

Ritonavir increases clarithromycin serum concentrations

Note: While other drug interactions (bromocriptine, disopyramide, lovastatin, phenytoin, and valproate) known to occur with erythromycin have not been reported in clinical trials with clarithromycin, concurrent use of these drugs should be monitored closely

Alcohol Interactions Use with caution (alcohol may increase central nervous system depression)

Half-Life 5-7 hours

Education and Monitoring Issues

Patient Education: Take full course of therapy; do not discontinue without consulting prescriber. Maintain adequate hydration (2-3 L/day of fluids unless instructed to restrict fluid intake). You may experience nausea (small frequent meals, or sucking lozenges may help); abnormal taste (frequent mouth care or chewing gum may help); diarrhea, headache, or abdominal cramps (medication may be ordered). Report persistent fever or chills, easy bruising or bleeding, or joint pain. Report severe persistent diarrhea, skin rash, sores in mouth, foul-smelling urine, rapid heartbeat or palpitations, or difficulty breathing. Do not refrigerate oral suspension (more palatable at room temperature).

Manufacturer Abbott Laboratories (Pharmaceutical Product Division)

Related Information

Antimicrobial Drugs of Choice *on page 1182*

Community Acquired Pneumonia in Adults *on page 1200*

Helicobacter pylori Treatment *on page 1107*

Pharmaceutical Manufacturers Directory *on page 1020*

Prevention of Bacterial Endocarditis *on page 1154*

- **Claritin®** *see* Loratadine *on page 540*
- **Claritin-D®** *see* Loratadine and Pseudoephedrine *on page 541*
- **Claritin-D® 24-Hour** *see* Loratadine and Pseudoephedrine *on page 541*
- **Claritin® Extra** *see* Loratadine and Pseudoephedrine *on page 541*
- **Clavulin®** *see* Amoxicillin and Clavulanate Potassium *on page 57*
- **Clear Eyes® [OTC]** *see* Naphazoline *on page 636*
- **Clear Tussin® 30** *see* Guaifenesin and Dextromethorphan *on page 424*

Clemastine (KLEM as teen)

Pharmacologic Class Antihistamine

U.S. Brand Names Antihist-1® [OTC]; Tavist®; Tavist®-1 [OTC]

Use Perennial and seasonal allergic rhinitis and other allergic symptoms including urticaria

USUAL DOSAGE Oral:

Children <12 years: 0.4-1 mg twice daily

Children >12 years and Adults: 1.34 mg twice daily to 2.68 mg 3 times/day; do not exceed 8.04 mg/day; lower doses should be considered in patients >60 years

Contraindications Narrow-angle glaucoma, hypersensitivity to clemastine or any component

Pregnancy Risk Factor C

Related Information

Clemastine and Phenylpropanolamine *on page 207*

Clemastine and Phenylpropanolamine

(KLEM as teen & fen il proe pa NOLE a meen)

Pharmacologic Class Antihistamine/Decongestant Combination

U.S. Brand Names Antihist-D®; Tavist-D®

Dosage Forms TAB: Clemastine fumarate 1.34 mg and phenylpropanolamine hydrochloride 75 mg

Pregnancy Risk Factor B

Alcohol Interactions Avoid use (may increase central nervous system depression)

- **Cleocin 3®** *see* Clindamycin *on page 208*
- **Cleocin HCl®** *see* Clindamycin *on page 208*
- **Cleocin Pediatric®** *see* Clindamycin *on page 208*
- **Cleocin Phosphate®** *see* Clindamycin *on page 208*
- **Cleocin T®** *see* Clindamycin *on page 208*

Clidinium and Chlordiazepoxide (kli DI nee um & klor dye az e POKS ide)

Pharmacologic Class Antispasmodic Agent, Gastrointestinal

U.S. Brand Names Clindex®; Librax®

Dosage Forms CAP: Clidinium bromide 2.5 mg and chlordiazepoxide hydrochloride 5 mg

Pregnancy Risk Factor D

Education and Monitoring Issues

Patient Education: Take as directed before meals; do not increase dose and do not discontinue without consulting prescriber first. Avoid alcohol and other CNS depressant medications (antihistamines, sleeping aids, antidepressants) unless approved by prescriber. Void before taking medication. This drug may impair mental alertness (use caution when driving or engaging in tasks that require alertness until response to drug is known). Report excessive and persistent anticholinergic effects (blurred vision, headache, flushing, tachycardia, nervousness, constipation, dizziness, insomnia, mental confusion or excitement, dry mouth, altered taste perception, dysphagia, palpitations, bradycardia, urinary hesitancy or retention, impotence, decreased sweating), or change in color of urine or stools.

- **Climara® Transdermal** *see* Estradiol *on page 327*
- **Clinda-Derm® Topical Solution** *see* Clindamycin *on page 208*

Clindamycin (klin da MYE sin)

Pharmacologic Class Antibiotic, Miscellaneous

U.S. Brand Names Cleocin 3®; Cleocin HCl®; Cleocin Pediatric®; Cleocin Phosphate®; Cleocin T®; Clinda-Derm® Topical Solution; Clindets®; C/T/S® Topical Solution

Generic Available Yes: Injection

Mechanism of Action Reversibly binds to 50S ribosomal subunits preventing peptide bond formation thus inhibiting bacterial protein synthesis; bacteriostatic or bactericidal depending on drug concentration, infection site, and organism

Use Treatment against aerobic and anaerobic streptococci (except enterococci), most staphylococci, *Bacteroides* sp and *Actinomyces*; used topically in treatment of severe acne, vaginally for *Gardnerella vaginalis*, alternate treatment for toxoplasmosis; prophylaxis in the prevention of bacterial endocarditis in high-risk patients undergoing surgical or dental procedures in patients allergic to penicillin; may be useful in PCP

USUAL DOSAGE Avoid in neonates (contains benzyl alcohol)

Infants and Children:

Oral: 8-20 mg/kg/day as hydrochloride; 8-25 mg/kg/day as palmitate in 3-4 divided doses; minimum dose of palmitate: 37.5 mg 3 times/day

I.M., I.V.:

<1 month: 15-20 mg/kg/day

>1 month: 20-40 mg/kg/day in 3-4 divided doses

Children and Adults: Topical: Apply a thin film twice daily

Adults:

Oral: 150-450 mg/dose every 6-8 hours; maximum dose: 1.8 g/day

I.M., I.V.: 1.2-1.8 g/day in 2-4 divided doses; maximum dose: 4.8 g/day

Bacterial endocarditis prophylaxis: 600 mg 1 hour prior to the procedure

Pelvic inflammatory disease: I.V.: 900 mg every 8 hours with gentamicin 2 mg/kg, then 1.5 mg/kg every 8 hours; continue after discharge with doxycycline 100 mg twice daily or oral clindamycin 450 mg 5 times/day for 10-14 days

Pneumocystis carinii pneumonia:

Oral: 300-450 mg 4 times/day with primaquine

I.M., I.V.: 1200-2400 mg/day with pyrimethamine

I.V.: 600 mg 4 times/day with primaquine

Vaginal: One full applicator (100 mg) inserted intravaginally once daily before bedtime for 3 or 7 consecutive days

Intravaginal suppositories: Insert one ovule (100 mg clindamycin) daily into vagina at bedtime for 3 days

Dosing adjustment in hepatic impairment: Adjustment recommended in patients with severe hepatic disease

Dosage Forms

Clindamycin hydrochloride: **CAP:** 75 mg, 150 mg, 300 mg

Clindamycin palmitate: **GRANULES for oral soln:** 75 mg/5 mL (100 mL)

Clindamycin phosphate: **CRM, vag:** 2% (40 g). **GEL, top:** 1% [10 mg/g] (7.5 g, 30 g). **INF** in D_5W: 300 mg (50 mL); 600 mg (50 mL). **INJ:** 150 mg/mL (2 mL, 4 mL, 6 mL, 50 mL, 60 mL). **LOT, top:** 1% [10 mg/mL] (60 mL). **PLEDGETS:** 1%. **SOLN, top:** 1% [10 mg/mL] (30 mL, 60 mL, 480 mL)

SUPP, vag: 2.5 g (clindamycin 100 mg)

Contraindications Hypersensitivity to clindamycin or any component; previous pseudomembranous colitis, hepatic impairment

Warnings/Precautions Dosage adjustment may be necessary in patients with severe hepatic dysfunction; can cause severe and possibly fatal colitis; use with caution in patients with a history of pseudomembranous colitis; discontinue drug if significant diarrhea, abdominal cramps, or passage of blood and mucus occurs

Pregnancy Risk Factor B

Adverse Reactions

>10%: Gastrointestinal: Diarrhea

1% to 10%:

Dermatologic: Rashes

Gastrointestinal: Pseudomembranous colitis (more common with oral form), nausea, vomiting

<1%: Elevated liver enzymes, eosinophilia, granulocytopenia, hypotension, neutropenia, polyarthritis, rare renal dysfunction, sterile abscess at I.M. injection site, Stevens-Johnson syndrome, thrombocytopenia, thrombophlebitis, urticaria

Drug Interactions CYP3A3/4 enzyme substrate

Increased duration of neuromuscular blockade from tubocurarine, pancuronium

Half-Life 1.6-5.3 hours, average: 2-3 hours

Education and Monitoring Issues

Patient Education:

Oral: Take each dose with a full glass of water. Complete full prescription, even if feeling better. You may experience nausea or vomiting (small frequent meals, frequent mouth care, chewing gum, or sucking lozenges may help). Report dizziness; persistent gastrointestinal effects (pain, diarrhea, vomiting); skin redness, rash, or burning; fever; chills; unusual bruising or bleeding; signs of infection; excessive fatigue; yellowing of eyes or skin; change in color of urine or blackened stool; swelling, warmth, or pain in extremities; difficult respirations; bloody or fatty stool (do not take antidiarrheal without consulting prescriber); or lack or improvement or worsening of condition.

Topical: Wash hands before applying or wear gloves. Apply thin film of gel, lotion, or solution to affected area. May apply porous dressing. Report persistent burning, swelling, itching, or worsening of condition.

Vaginal: Wash hands before using. At bedtime, gently insert full applicator into vagina and expel cream. Wash applicator with soap and water following use. Remain lying down for 30 minutes following administration. Avoid intercourse during 7 days of therapy. Report adverse reactions (dizziness, nausea, vomiting, stomach cramps, or headache) or lack of improvement or worsening of condition.

Monitoring Parameters: Observe for changes in bowel frequency, monitor for colitis and resolution of symptoms; during prolonged therapy monitor CBC, liver and renal function tests periodically

Related Information

Animal and Human Bites Guidelines *on page 1177*
Antimicrobial Drugs of Choice *on page 1182*
Community Acquired Pneumonia in Adults *on page 1200*
Prevention of Bacterial Endocarditis *on page 1154*
Treatment of Sexually Transmitted Diseases *on page 1210*

♦ **Clindets®** *see* Clindamycin *on page 208*
♦ **Clindex®** *see* Clidinium and Chlordiazepoxide *on page 208*
♦ **Clinoril®** *see* Sulindac *on page 883*

Clioquinol (klye oh KWIN ole)

Pharmacologic Class Antifungal Agent

U.S. Brand Names Vioform® [OTC]

Use Topically in the treatment of tinea pedis, tinea cruris, and skin infections caused by dermatophytic fungi (ringworm)

USUAL DOSAGE Children and Adults: Topical: Apply 2-3 times/day; do not use for longer than 7 days

Contraindications Not effective in the treatment of scalp or nail fungal infections; children <2 years of age, hypersensitivity to any component

Pregnancy Risk Factor C

Related Information

Clioquinol and Hydrocortisone *on page 209*

Clioquinol and Hydrocortisone (klye oh KWIN ole & hye droe KOR ti sone)

Pharmacologic Class Antifungal Agent, Topical

U.S. Brand Names Corque® Topical; Pedi-Cort V® Creme

Dosage Forms CRM: Clioquinol 3% and hydrocortisone 1% (20 g)

Pregnancy Risk Factor C

Clobetasol (kloe BAY ta sol)

Pharmacologic Class Corticosteroid, Topical

U.S. Brand Names Temovate® Topical

Generic Available Yes

Mechanism of Action Stimulates the synthesis of enzymes needed to decrease inflammation, suppress mitotic activity, and cause vasoconstriction

Use Short-term relief of inflammation of moderate to severe corticosteroid-responsive dermatosis (very high potency topical corticosteroid)

USUAL DOSAGE Adults: Topical: Apply twice daily for up to 2 weeks with no more than 50 g/week. Therapy should be discontinued when control is achieved; if no improvement is seen, reassessment of diagnosis may be necessary.

Dosage Forms CRM: 0.05% (15 g, 30 g, 45 g); In emollient base: 0.05% (15 g, 30 g, 60 g). **GEL:** 0.05% (15 g, 30 g, 45 g). **OINT, top:** 0.05% (15 g, 30 g, 45 g). **SCALP application:** 0.05% (25 mL, 50 mL)

Contraindications Known hypersensitivity to clobetasol; viral, fungal, or tubercular skin lesions

Warnings/Precautions Adrenal suppression can occur if used for >14 days

Pregnancy Risk Factor C

Adverse Reactions

1% to 10%:

Dermatologic: Itching, erythema

Local: Burning, dryness, irritation, papular rashes

<1%: Acneiform eruptions, hypertrichosis, hypopigmentation, maceration of skin, miliaria, perioral dermatitis, skin atrophy, striae

Education and Monitoring Issues

Patient Education: A thin film of cream or ointment is effective; do not overuse; do not use tight-fitting diapers or plastic pants on children being treated in the diaper area; use only as prescribed and for no longer than the period prescribed; apply sparingly in light film; rub in lightly; avoid contact with eyes; notify prescriber if condition being treated persists or worsens

♦ **Clocort® Maximum Strength** *see* Hydrocortisone *on page 447*

Clocortolone (kloe KOR toe lone)

Pharmacologic Class Corticosteroid, Topical

U.S. Brand Names Cloderm® Topical

Generic Available No

Mechanism of Action Stimulates the synthesis of enzymes needed to decrease inflammation, suppress mitotic activity, and cause vasoconstriction

Use Inflammation of corticosteroid-responsive dermatoses (medium potency topical corticosteroid)

USUAL DOSAGE Adults: Apply sparingly and gently; rub into affected area from 1-4 times/day. Therapy should be discontinued when control is achieved; if no improvement is seen, reassessment of diagnosis may be necessary.

Dosage Forms CRM: 0.1% (15 g, 45 g)

Contraindications Known hypersensitivity to clocortolone; viral, fungal, or tubercular skin lesions

Warnings/Precautions Adrenal suppression can occur if used for >14 days

Pregnancy Risk Factor C

Adverse Reactions

1% to 10%:

Dermatologic: Itching, erythema

Local: Burning, dryness, irritation, papular rashes

<1%: Acneiform eruptions, hypertrichosis, hypopigmentation, maceration of skin, miliaria, perioral dermatitis, skin atrophy, striae

Education and Monitoring Issues

Patient Education: A thin film of cream or ointment is effective; do not overuse; do not use tight-fitting diapers or plastic pants on children being treated in the diaper area; use only as prescribed, and for no longer than the period prescribed; apply sparingly in light film; rub in lightly; avoid contact with eyes; notify prescriber if condition being treated persists or worsens

♦ **Cloderm® Topical** *see* Clocortolone *on page 210*

Clofazimine (kloe FA zi meen)

Pharmacologic Class Leprostatic Agent

U.S. Brand Names Lamprene®

Generic Available No

Mechanism of Action Binds preferentially to mycobacterial DNA to inhibit mycobacterial growth; also has some anti-inflammatory activity through an unknown mechanism

Use Orphan drug: Treatment of dapsone-resistant leprosy; multibacillary dapsone-sensitive leprosy; erythema nodosum leprosum; *Mycobacterium avium-intracellulare* (MAI) infections

USUAL DOSAGE Oral:

Children: Leprosy: 1 mg/kg/day every 24 hours in combination with dapsone and rifampin

Adults:

Dapsone-resistant leprosy: 100 mg/day in combination with one or more antileprosy drugs for 3 years; then alone 100 mg/day

Dapsone-sensitive multibacillary leprosy: 100 mg/day in combination with two or more antileprosy drugs for at least 2 years and continue until negative skin smears are obtained, then institute single drug therapy with appropriate agent

Erythema nodosum leprosum: 100-200 mg/day for up to 3 months or longer then taper dose to 100 mg/day when possible

Pyoderma gangrenosum: 300-400 mg/day for up to 12 months

Dosing adjustment in hepatic impairment: Should be considered in severe hepatic dysfunction

Dosage Forms CAP: 50 mg

Contraindications Hypersensitivity to clofazimine or any component

Warnings/Precautions Use with caution in patients with GI problems; dosages >100 mg/day should be used for as short a duration as possible; skin discoloration may lead to depression

Pregnancy Risk Factor C

Adverse Reactions

>10%:

Dermatologic: Dry skin

Gastrointestinal: Abdominal pain, nausea, vomiting, diarrhea

Miscellaneous: Pink to brownish-black discoloration of the skin and conjunctiva

1% to 10%:

Dermatologic: Rash, pruritus

Endocrine & metabolic: Elevated blood sugar

Gastrointestinal: Fecal discoloration

Genitourinary: Discoloration of urine

Ocular: Irritation of the eyes

Miscellaneous: Discoloration of sputum, sweat

<1%: Acneiform eruptions, anemia, anorexia, bone pain, bowel obstruction, constipation, cystitis, diminished vision, dizziness, drowsiness, edema, enlarged liver, eosinophilia, eosinophilic enteritis, erythroderma, fatigue, fever, GI bleeding, giddiness, headache, hepatitis, hypokalemia, increased albumin/serum bilirubin/AST, jaundice, lymphadenopathy, monilial cheilosis, neuralgia, phototoxicity, taste disorder, vascular pain, weight loss

Drug Interactions Decreased effect with dapsone (unconfirmed)

Half-Life Terminal: 8 days; Tissue: 70 days

Education and Monitoring Issues

Patient Education: May be taken with meals. Drug may cause a pink to brownish-black discoloration of the skin, conjunctiva, tears, sweat, urine, feces, and nasal secretions. Although reversible, it may take months to years for skin discoloration to disappear after therapy is complete. Report promptly bone or joint pain, GI disturbance, or vision disturbances.

Manufacturer Novartis

Related Information

Antimicrobial Drugs of Choice *on page 1182*
Pharmaceutical Manufacturers Directory *on page 1020*
Tuberculosis Treatment Guidelines *on page 1213*

Clofibrate (kloe FYE brate)

Pharmacologic Class Antilipemic Agent (Fibric Acid)

U.S. Brand Names Atromid-S®

Generic Available Yes

Mechanism of Action Mechanism is unclear but thought to reduce cholesterol synthesis and triglyceride hepatic-vascular transference

Use Adjunct to dietary therapy in the management of hyperlipidemias associated with high triglyceride levels (types III, IV, V); primarily lowers triglycerides and very low density lipoprotein

USUAL DOSAGE Adults: Oral: 500 mg 4 times/day; some patients may respond to lower doses

Dosing interval in renal impairment:

Cl_{cr} >50 mL/minute: Administer every 6-12 hours

Cl_{cr} 10-50 mL/minute: Administer every 12-18 hours

Cl_{cr} <10 mL/minute: Avoid use

Hemodialysis: Elimination is not enhanced via hemodialysis; supplemental dose is not necessary

Dosage Forms CAP: 500 mg

Contraindications Hypersensitivity to clofibrate or any component, severe hepatic or renal impairment, primary biliary cirrhosis

(Continued)

Clofibrate *(Continued)*

Warnings/Precautions Clofibrate has been shown to be tumorigenic in animal studies; increased risk of cholelithiasis, cholecystitis; discontinue if lipid response is not obtained; no evidence substantiates a beneficial effect on cardiovascular mortality

Pregnancy Risk Factor C

Adverse Reactions

Common: Gastrointestinal: Nausea, diarrhea

Less common:

Central nervous system: Headache, dizziness, fatigue

Gastrointestinal: Vomiting, loose stools, heartburn, flatulence, abdominal distress, epigastric pain

Neuromuscular & skeletal: Muscle cramping, aching, weakness, myalgia

Frequency unknown: Fever, chest pain, cardiac arrhythmias, rash, urticaria, pruritus, alopecia, dry,brittle hair, toxic epidermal necrolysis, erythema multiforme, Stevens-Johnson syndrome, weight gain, polyphagia, gynecomastia, hyperkalemia, stomatitis, gallstones, pancreatitis, gastritis, peptic ulcer, weight gain, impotence, decreased libido, leukopenia, anemia, eosinophilia, agranulocytosis, thrombocytopenic purpura, increased liver function test, hepatomegaly, jaundice, dysuria, hematuria, proteinuria, renal toxicity, (allergic), rhabdomyolysis-induced renal failure, myalgia, myopathy, myositis, arthralgia, rhabdomyolysis, increased creatinine phosphokinase (CPK), rheumatoid arthritis, tremor, thrombophlebitis, photophobic, flu-like syndrome, increased sweating, systemic lupus erythematosus

Drug Interactions

Chlorpropamide: May increase risk of hypoglycemia

Furosemide: Increased blood levels of both in hypoalbuminemia

HMG-CoA reductase inhibitors (atorvastatin, cerivastatin, fluvastatin, lovastatin, pravastatin, simvastatin) may increase the risk of myopathy and rhabdomyolysis. The manufacturer warns against the concomitant use. However, combination therapy with statins has been used in some patients with resistant hyperlipidemias (with great caution)

Insulin: Hypoglycemic effects may be potentiated by an unknown mechanism

Probenecid may decrease the clearance of clofibrate

Rifampin: Decreased clofibrate blood levels

Sulfonylureas (including glyburide, glipizide): Hypoglycemic effects may be potentiated by an unknown mechanism

Warfarin: Increased hypoprothrombinemic response; monitor INRs closely when clofibrate is initiated or discontinued

Half-Life 6-24 hours, increases significantly with reduced renal function; with anuria: 110 hours

Education and Monitoring Issues

Patient Education: This drug will have to be taken long-term and ongoing follow-up is essential. Adherence to a cardiac risk reduction program, including adherence to prescribed diet, is of major importance. This drug may cause stomach upset; if this occurs, take medication with food or milk. Report chest pain, shortness of breath, irregular heartbeat, palpitations, severe stomach pain with nausea and vomiting, persistent fever, sore throat, or unusual bleeding or bruising.

Monitoring Parameters: Serum lipids, cholesterol and triglycerides, LFTs, CBC

Manufacturer Wyeth-Ayerst Laboratories

Related Information

Pharmaceutical Manufacturers Directory *on page 1020*

♦ **Clomid®** *see* Clomiphene *on page 212*

Clomiphene (KLOE mi feen)

Pharmacologic Class Ovulation Stimulator

U.S. Brand Names Clomid®; Milophene®; Serophene®

Generic Available No

Mechanism of Action Induces ovulation by stimulating the release of pituitary gonadotropins

Use Treatment of ovulatory failure in patients desiring pregnancy

Unlabeled use: Male infertility

USUAL DOSAGE Adults: Oral:

Male (infertility): 25 mg/day for 25 days with 5 days rest, or 100 mg every Monday, Wednesday, Friday

Female (ovulatory failure): 50 mg/day for 5 days (first course); start the regimen on or about the fifth day of cycle. The dose should be increased only in those patients who do not ovulate in response to cyclic 50 mg Clomid®. A low dosage or duration of treatment course is particularly recommended if unusual sensitivity to pituitary gonadotropin is suspected, such as in patients with polycystic ovary syndrome.

If ovulation does not appear to occur after the first course of therapy, a second course of 100 mg/day (two 50 mg tablets given as a single daily dose) for 5 days should be given. This course may be started as early as 30 days after the previous one after precautions are taken to exclude the presence of pregnancy. Increasing the dosage or duration of therapy beyond 100 mg/day for 5 days is not recommended. The majority of patients who are going to ovulate will do so after the first course of therapy. If ovulation does not occur after 3 courses of therapy, further treatment is not recommended and the patient should be re-evaluated. If 3 ovulatory responses occur, but pregnancy has not been achieved, further treatment is not recommended. If menses does not occur after an ovulatory response, the patient should be re-evaluated. Long-term cyclic therapy is not recommended beyond a total of about 6 cycles.

Dosage Forms TAB: 50 mg

Contraindications Hypersensitivity or allergy to clomiphene citrate or any of its components; liver disease, abnormal uterine bleeding, suspected pregnancy, enlargement or development of ovarian cyst, uncontrolled thyroid or adrenal dysfunction in the presence of an organic intracranial lesion such as pituitary tumor

Warnings/Precautions Patients unusually sensitive to pituitary gonadotropins (eg, polycystic ovary disease); multiple pregnancies, blurring or other visual symptoms can occur, ovarian hyperstimulation syndrome, and abdominal pain

Pregnancy Risk Factor X

Adverse Reactions

>10%: Endocrine & metabolic: Hot flashes, ovarian enlargement

1% to 10%:

- Cardiovascular: Thromboembolism
- Central nervous system: Mental depression, headache
- Endocrine & metabolic: Breast enlargement (males), breast discomfort (females), abnormal menstrual flow
- Gastrointestinal: Distention, bloating, nausea, vomiting, hepatotoxicity
- Ocular: Blurring of vision, diplopia, floaters, after-images, phosphenes, photophobia

<1%: Alopecia (reversible), fatigue, insomnia, polyuria, weight gain

Half-Life 5-7 days

Education and Monitoring Issues

Patient Education: Follow recommended schedule of dosing. You may experience hot flashes (cool clothes and cool environment may help). Report acute sudden headache; difficulty breathing; warmth, pain, redness, or swelling in calves; breast enlargement (male) or breast discomfort (female); abnormal menstrual bleeding; vision changes (blurring, diplopia, photophobia, floaters); acute abdominal discomfort; or fever.

Reference Range: FSH and LH are expected to peak 5-9 days after completing clomiphene; ovulation assessed by basal body temperature or serum progesterone 2 weeks after last clomiphene dose

Clomipramine (kloe MI pra meen)

Pharmacologic Class Antidepressant, Tricyclic (Tertiary Amine)

U.S. Brand Names Anafranil®

Generic Available No

Mechanism of Action Clomipramine appears to affect serotonin uptake while its active metabolite, desmethylclomipramine, affects norepinephrine uptake

Use Treatment of obsessive-compulsive disorder (OCD); may also relieve depression, panic attacks, and chronic pain

USUAL DOSAGE Oral: Initial:

Children >10 years of age: 25 mg/day and gradually increase, as tolerated, to a maximum of 3 mg/kg/day or 200 mg/day, whichever is smaller

The safety and efficacy of clomipramine in pediatric patients <10 years of age have not been established and, therefore, dosing recommendations cannot be made

Adults: 25 mg/day and gradually increase, as tolerated, to 100 mg/day the first 2 weeks, may then be increased to a total of 250 mg/day maximum

Dosage Forms CAP: 25 mg, 50 mg, 75 mg

Contraindications Patients in acute recovery stage of recent myocardial infarction; not to be used within 14 days of MAO inhibitors

Warnings/Precautions Seizures are likely and are dose-related; can be additive when coadministered with other drugs that can lower the seizure threshold; use with caution in patients with asthma, bladder outlet destruction, narrow-angle glaucoma

Pregnancy Risk Factor C

Adverse Reactions

>10%:

- Central nervous system: Dizziness, drowsiness, headache, insomnia, nervousness
- Endocrine & metabolic: Libido changes
- Gastrointestinal: Xerostomia, constipation, increased appetite, nausea, weight gain, dyspepsia, anorexia, abdominal pain
- Neuromuscular & skeletal: Fatigue, tremor, myoclonus
- Miscellaneous: Increased diaphoresis

1% to 10%:

- Cardiovascular: Hypotension, palpitations, tachycardia
- Central nervous system: Confusion, hypertonia, sleep disorder, yawning, speech disorder, abnormal dreaming, paresthesia, memory impairment, anxiety, twitching, impaired coordination, agitation, migraine, depersonalization, emotional lability, flushing, fever
- Dermatologic: Rash, pruritus, dermatitis

(Continued)

Clomipramine *(Continued)*

Gastrointestinal: Diarrhea, vomiting
Genitourinary: Difficult urination
Ocular: Blurred vision, eye pain

<1%: Abnormal accommodation, alopecia, breast enlargement, decreased lower esophageal sphincter tone may cause GE reflux, galactorrhea, hyperacusis, increased liver enzymes, marrow depression, photosensitivity, prostatic disorder, seizures, SIADH, trouble with gums

Drug Interactions CYP1A2, 2C19, 2D6, and 3A3/4 enzyme substrate; CYP2D6 enzyme inhibitor

Carbamazepine, phenobarbital, and rifampin may increase the metabolism of clomipramine resulting in decreased effect of clomipramine

Clomipramine inhibits the antihypertensive response to bethanidine, clonidine, debrisoquin, guanadrel, guanethidine, guanabenz, guanfacine; monitor BP; consider alternate antihypertensive agent

Abrupt discontinuation of clonidine may cause hypertensive crisis, clomipramine may enhance the response

Use with altretamine may cause orthostatic hypertension

Clomipramine may be additive with or may potentiate the action of other CNS depressants (sedatives, hypnotics, or ethanol)

With MAO inhibitors, hyperpyrexia, hypertension, tachycardia, confusion, seizures, and **deaths have been reported** (serotonin syndrome); this combination should be avoided

Clomipramine may increase the prothrombin time in patients stabilized on warfarin

Cimetidine and methylphenidate may decrease the metabolism of clomipramine

Additive anticholinergic effects seen with other anticholinergic agents

The SSRIs, to varying degrees, inhibit the metabolism of TCAs and clinical toxicity may result

Use of lithium with a TCA may increase the risk for neurotoxicity

Phenothiazines may increase concentration of some TCAs and TCAs may increase concentration of phenothiazines; monitor for altered clinical response

TCAs may enhance the hypoglycemic effects of tolazamide, chlorpropamide, or insulin; monitor for changes in blood glucose levels

Cholestyramine and colestipol may bind TCAs and reduce their absorption; monitor for altered response

TCAs may enhance the effect of amphetamines; monitor for adverse CV effects

Diltiazem and verapamil appear to decrease the metabolism of imipramine and potentially other TCAs; monitor for increased TCA concentrations

The pressor response to I.V. epinephrine, norepinephrine, and phenylephrine may be enhanced in patients receiving TCAs; this combination is best avoided

Indinavir, ritonavir may inhibit the metabolism of clomipramine and potentially other TCAs; monitor for altered effects; a decrease in TCA dosage may be required

Quinidine may inhibit the metabolism of TCAs; monitor for altered effect

Combined use of anticholinergics with TCAs may produce additive anticholinergic effects

Combined use of beta-agonists with TCAs may predispose patients to cardiac arrhythmias

Alcohol Interactions Avoid use (may increase central nervous system depression)

Onset Usually >2 weeks to therapeutic effect

Half-Life 20-30 hours

Education and Monitoring Issues

Patient Education: Take multiple dose medication with meals to reduce side effects. Take single daily dose at bedtime to reduce daytime sedation. The effect of this drug may take several weeks to appear. Do not use excessive alcohol, caffeine, and other prescriptive or OTC medications without consulting prescriber. May cause dizziness, drowsiness, headache, or seizures (use caution when driving or engaging in tasks that require alertness until response to drug is known); dry mouth or unpleasant aftertaste (sucking lozenges and frequent mouth care may help); constipation (increased fluids, dietary fiber and fruits, or exercise may help); or orthostatic hypotension (use caution when rising from lying or sitting to standing position or when climbing stairs). Report unresolved constipation or GI upset, unusual muscle weakness, palpitations, or persistent CNS disturbances (hallucinations, delirium, insomnia, or impaired gait).

Dietary Considerations: Grapefruit juice may potentially inhibit the metabolism of TCAs

Related Information

Antidepressant Agents Comparison *on page 1231*

Clonazepam (kloe NA ze pam)

Pharmacologic Class Benzodiazepine

U.S. Brand Names Klonopin™

Generic Available No

Mechanism of Action Suppresses the spike-and-wave discharge in absence seizures by depressing nerve transmission in the motor cortex

Use Prophylaxis of petit mal, petit mal variant (Lennox-Gastaut), akinetic, and myoclonic seizures

Unlabeled use: Restless legs syndrome, neuralgia, multifocal tic disorder, parkinsonian dysarthria, acute manic episodes, adjunct therapy for schizophrenia

USUAL DOSAGE Oral:

Children <10 years or 30 kg:

Initial daily dose: 0.01-0.03 mg/kg/day (maximum: 0.05 mg/kg/day) given in 2-3 divided doses; increase by no more than 0.5 mg every third day until seizures are controlled or adverse effects seen

Usual maintenance dose: 0.1-0.2 mg/kg/day divided 3 times/day; not to exceed 0.2 mg/kg/day

Adults:

Initial daily dose not to exceed 1.5 mg given in 3 divided doses; may increase by 0.5-1 mg every third day until seizures are controlled or adverse effects seen

Usual maintenance dose: 0.05-0.2 mg/kg; do not exceed 20 mg/day

Hemodialysis: Supplemental dose is not necessary

Dosage Forms TAB: 0.5 mg, 1 mg, 2 mg

Contraindications Hypersensitivity to clonazepam, any component, or other benzodiazepines; severe liver disease, acute narrow-angle glaucoma

Warnings/Precautions Use with caution in patients with chronic respiratory disease or impaired renal function; abrupt discontinuance may precipitate withdrawal symptoms, status epilepticus or seizures, in patients with a history of substance abuse; clonazepam-induced behavioral disturbances may be more frequent in mentally handicapped patients

Pregnancy Risk Factor D

Pregnancy Implications

Clinical effects on the fetus: Two reports of cardiac defects; respiratory depression, lethargy, hypotonia may be observed in newborns exposed near time of delivery. Epilepsy itself, number of medications, genetic factors, or a combination of these probably influence the teratogenicity of anticonvulsant therapy. Benefit:risk ratio usually favors continued use during pregnancy and breast-feeding.

Breast-feeding/lactation: Crosses into breast milk

Clinical effects on the infant: CNS depression, respiratory depression reported. No recommendation from the American Academy of Pediatrics.

Adverse Reactions

>10%: Central nervous system: Drowsiness

1% to 10%:

Central nervous system: Dizziness, abnormal coordination, ataxia, dysarthria, depression, memory disturbance, fatigue

Dermatologic: Dermatitis, allergic reactions

Endocrine & metabolic: Decreased libido

Gastrointestinal: Anorexia, constipation, diarrhea, xerostomia

Respiratory: Upper respiratory tract infection, sinusitis, rhinitis, coughing

<1%: Blood dyscrasias, menstrual irregularities

Drug Interactions CYP3A3/4 enzyme substrate

Disulfiram may inhibit the metabolism of clonazepam

The combined use of clonazepam and valproic acid has been associated with absence seizures

Carbamazepine, rifampin, rifabutin may enhance the metabolism of clonazepam and decrease its therapeutic effect; consider using an alternative sedative/hypnotic agent

Cimetidine, ciprofloxacin, clarithromycin, clozapine, CNS depressants, diltiazem, disulfiram, digoxin, erythromycin, ethanol, fluconazole, fluoxetine, fluvoxamine, isoniazid, itraconazole, ketoconazole, labetalol, levodopa, loxapine, metoprolol, metronidazole, miconazole, nefazodone, omeprazole, phenytoin, rifabutin, rifampin, troleandomycin, verapamil may increase the serum level and/or toxicity of clonazepam; monitor for altered benzodiazepine response

Alcohol Interactions Avoid use (may increase central nervous system depression)

Onset 20-60 minutes

Duration Up to 12 hours

Half-Life 19-50 hours

Education and Monitoring Issues

Patient Education: Take exactly as directed (do not increase dose or frequency); may cause physical and/or psychological dependence. While using this medication, do not use alcohol and other prescription or OTC medications (especially pain medications, sedatives, antihistamines, or hypnotics) without consulting prescriber. Maintain adequate hydration (2-3 L/day of fluids unless instructed to restrict fluid intake). You may experience drowsiness, dizziness, or blurred vision (use caution when driving or engaging in tasks requiring alertness until response to drug is known); nausea, vomiting, loss of appetite, or dry mouth (small frequent meals, frequent mouth care, chewing gum, or sucking lozenges may help); constipation (increased exercise, fluids, or dietary fruit and fiber may help). If medication is used to control seizures, wear identification that you are taking an antiepileptic medication. Report excessive drowsiness, dizziness, fatigue, or impaired coordination; CNS changes (confusion, depression, increased sedation, excitation, headache, agitation, insomnia, or nightmares) or changes in cognition; difficulty breathing or shortness of breath; changes in urinary pattern, changes in sexual activity; muscle cramping, weakness, tremors, or rigidity;

(Continued)

Clonazepam *(Continued)*

ringing in ears or visual disturbances, excessive perspiration, or excessive GI symptoms (cramping, constipation, vomiting, anorexia); worsening of seizure activity, or loss of seizure control.

Dietary Considerations: Grapefruit juice may increase serum levels and/or toxicity

Reference Range: Relationship between serum concentration and seizure control is not well established

Timing of serum samples: Peak serum levels occur 1-3 hours after oral ingestion; the half-life is 20-40 hours; therefore, steady-state occurs in 5-7 days

Therapeutic levels: 20-80 ng/mL; Toxic concentration: >80 ng/mL

Related Information

Anticonvulsants by Seizure Type Comparison *on page 1230*

Epilepsy Guidelines *on page 1091*

Clonidine (KLOE ni deen)

Pharmacologic Class Alpha$_2$ Agonist

U.S. Brand Names Catapres® Oral; Catapres-TTS® Transdermal; Duraclon® Injection

Generic Available Yes: Tablet

Mechanism of Action Stimulates alpha$_2$-adrenoceptors in the brain stem, thus activating an inhibitory neuron, resulting in reduced sympathetic outflow, producing a decrease in vasomotor tone and heart rate; epidural clonidine may produce pain relief at spinal presynaptic and postjunctional alpha$_2$-adrenoceptors by preventing pain signal transmission; pain relief occurs only for the body regions innervated by the spinal segments where analgesic concentrations of clonidine exist

Use Management of mild to moderate hypertension; either used alone or in combination with other antihypertensives; not recommended for first-line therapy for hypertension; as a second-line agent for decreasing heroin or nicotine withdrawal symptoms in patients with severe symptoms; indicated by the epidural route, in combination with opiates, for treatment of severe pain in refractory cancer patients (most effective in patients with neuropathic pain); other uses may include prophylaxis of migraines, glaucoma, and diabetes-associated diarrhea

USUAL DOSAGE

Oral:

Children: Initial: 5-10 mcg/kg/day in divided doses every 8-12 hours; increase gradually at 5- to 7-day intervals to 25 mcg/kg/day in divided doses every 6 hours; maximum: 0.9 mg/day

Clonidine tolerance test (test of growth hormone release from pituitary): 0.15 mg/m^2 or 4 mcg/kg as single dose

Adults: Initial dose: 0.1 mg twice daily, usual maintenance dose: 0.2-1.2 mg/day in 2-4 divided doses; maximum recommended dose: 2.4 mg/day

Nicotine withdrawal symptoms: 0.1 mg twice daily to maximum of 0.4 mg/day for 3-4 weeks

Elderly: Initial: 0.1 mg once daily at bedtime, increase gradually as needed

Transdermal: Apply once every 7 days; for initial therapy start with 0.1 mg and increase by 0.1 mg at 1- to 2-week intervals; dosages >0.6 mg do not improve efficacy

Epidural infusion: Starting dose: 30 mcg/hour; titrate as required for relief of pain or presence of side effects; minimal experience with doses >40 mcg/hour; should be considered an adjunct to intraspinal opiate therapy

Dosing adjustment in renal impairment: Cl_{cr} <10 mL/minute: Administer 50% to 75% of normal dose initially

Dialysis: Not dialyzable (0% to 5%) via hemo- or peritoneal dialysis; supplemental dose not necessary

Dosage Forms INJ (preservative free): 100 mcg/mL (10 mL). **PATCH, transdermal:** 1, 2, and 3 (0.1, 0.2, 0.3 mg/day, 7-day duration). **TAB:** 0.1 mg, 0.2 mg, 0.3 mg

Contraindications Hypersensitivity to clonidine hydrochloride or any component

Warnings/Precautions Use with caution in cerebrovascular disease, coronary insufficiency, renal impairment, sinus node dysfunction; do not abruptly discontinue as rapid increase in blood pressure and symptoms of sympathetic overactivity (ie, increased heart rate, tremor, agitation, anxiety, insomnia, sweating, palpitations) may occur; **if need to discontinue, taper dose gradually over 1 week or more (2-4 days with epidural product)**; adjust dosage in patients with renal dysfunction (especially the elderly); not recommended for obstetrical, postpartum or perioperative pain management or in those with severe hemodynamic instability due to unacceptable risk of hypotension and bradycardia; clonidine injection should be administered via a continuous epidural infusion device

Pregnancy Risk Factor C

Pregnancy Implications

Clinical effects on the fetus: Crosses the placenta. Caution should be used with this drug due to the potential of rebound hypertension with abrupt discontinuation.

Breast-feeding/lactation: Crosses into breast milk. American Academy of Pediatrics has NO RECOMMENDATION.

Adverse Reactions

>10%:

Central nervous system: Drowsiness, dizziness

Gastrointestinal: Xerostomia

1% to 10%:

Cardiovascular: Chest pain, orthostatic hypotension, palpitations, tachycardia, bradycardia, EKG abnormalities

Central nervous system: Mental depression, headache, fatigue, nervousness, agitation, insomnia

Dermatologic: Rash

Endocrine & metabolic: Decreased sexual activity, loss of libido

Gastrointestinal: vomiting, constipation, nausea, anorexia, malaise, weight gain

Genitourinary: Nocturia, impotence

Neuromuscular & skeletal: Weakness

<1%: Abdominal pain, abnormal liver function tests, alopecia, anxiety, blurred vision, burning eyes, congestive heart failure, constipation, delirium, micturition difficulty, nightmares, pruritus, Raynaud's phenomenon, restlessness, syncope, thrombocytopenia, urinary retention, urticaria, visual and auditory hallucinations, vivid dreams

Drug Interactions

Concurrent use with antipsychotics (especially low potency) or nitroprusside may produce additive hypotensive effects

Clonidine may decrease the symptoms of hypoglycemia; monitor patients receiving antidiabetic agents

Clonidine may increase cyclosporine (and perhaps tacrolimus) serum concentrations; cyclosporine dosage adjustment may be needed

Tricyclic antidepressants antagonize hypotensive effects of clonidine; best to avoid this combination; consider an alternative agent

Increased toxicity: Beta-blockers may potentiate bradycardia in patients receiving clonidine and may increase the rebound hypertension of withdrawal; discontinue beta-blocker several days before clonidine is tapered

Tricyclic antidepressants may enhance the hypertensive response associated with abrupt clonidine withdrawal

Narcotic analgesics may potentiate hypotensive effects of clonidine

Alcohol and barbiturates may increase the CNS depression; epidural clonidine may prolong the sensory and motor blockade of local anesthetics

Alcohol Interactions Avoid use (may increase central nervous system depression)

Onset Oral: 0.5-1 hour; T_{max}: 2-4 hours

Duration >24 hours

Half-Life Normal renal function: 6-20 hours; Renal impairment: 18-41 hours

Education and Monitoring Issues

Patient Education: Take as directed, at bedtime. Do not skip doses or discontinue without consulting prescriber. If using patch, check daily for correct placement. Do not use OTC medications which may affect blood pressure (eg, cough or cold remedies, diet pills, stay-awake medications) without consulting prescriber. This medication may cause drowsiness, dizziness, or impaired judgment (use caution when driving or engaging in tasks that require alertness until response is known); decreased libido or sexual function (will resolve when drug is discontinued); postural hypotension (use caution when rising from sitting or lying position or when climbing stairs); constipation (increase roughage, bulk in diet); or dry mouth or nausea (frequent mouth care or sucking lozenges may help). Report difficulty, pain, or burning on urination; increased nervousness or depression; sudden weight gain (weigh yourself in the same clothes at the same time of day once a week); unusual or persistent swelling of ankles, feet, or extremities; wet cough or respiratory difficulty; chest pain or palpitations; muscle weakness, fatigue, or pain; or other persistent side effects.

Monitoring Parameters: Blood pressure, standing and sitting/supine, respiratory rate and depth, pain relief, mental status, heart rate (bradycardia may be treated with atropine)

Reference Range: Therapeutic: 1-2 ng/mL (SI: 4.4-8.7 nmol/L)

Related Information

Clonidine and Chlorthalidone *on page 217*

Clonidine and Chlorthalidone (KLOE ni deen & klor THAL i done)

Pharmacologic Class Antihypertensive Agent, Combination

U.S. Brand Names Combipres®

Dosage Forms TAB: 0.1: Clonidine 0.1 mg and chlorthalidone 15 mg; 0.2: Clonidine 0.2 mg and chlorthalidone 15 mg; 0.3: Clonidine 0.3 mg and chlorthalidone 15 mg

Pregnancy Risk Factor C

Clopidogrel (kloh PID oh grel)

Pharmacologic Class Antiplatelet Agent

U.S. Brand Names Plavix®

Mechanism of Action Blocks the ADP receptors, which prevent fibrinogen binding at that site and thereby reduce the possibility of platelet adhesion and aggregation

(Continued)

Clopidogrel *(Continued)*

Use The reduction of atherosclerotic events (myocardial infarction, stroke, vascular deaths) in patients with atherosclerosis documented by recent myocardial infarctions, recent stroke or established peripheral arterial disease

USUAL DOSAGE Adults: Oral: 75 mg once daily

Dosing adjustment in renal impairment and elderly: None necessary

Dosage Forms TAB: 75 mg

Contraindications In patients with active bleeding (eg, peptic ulcer disease, intracranial hemorrhage), patients with coagulation disorders, or patients who have demonstrated hypersensitivity to the drug or any components of the drug product

Warnings/Precautions Patients receiving anticoagulants or other antiplatelet drugs concurrently, liver disease, patients having a previous hypersensitivity or other untoward effects related to ticlopidine, hypertension, renal impairment, history of bleeding or hemostatic disorders or drug-related hematologic disorders, and consider discontinuing in patients scheduled for major surgery, 7 days prior to that surgery

Pregnancy Risk Factor B

Adverse Reactions As with all drugs which may affect hemostasis, bleeding is associated with clopidogrel. Hemorrhage may occur at virtually any site. Risk is dependent on multiple variables, including the concurrent use of multiple agents which alter hemostasis and patient susceptibility.

>10%:

Gastrointestinal: The overall incidence of gastrointestinal events (including abdominal pain, vomiting, dyspepsia, gastritis and constipation) has been documented to be 27.1% compared to 29.8% in patients receiving aspirin.

2.5% to 10%:

Cardiovascular: Chest pain (8.3%), edema (4.1%), hypertension (4.3%)

Central nervous system: Headache (7.6%), dizziness (6.2%), depression (3.6%), fatigue (3.3%), general pain (6.4%)

Dermatologic: Rash (4.2%), pruritus (3.3%)

Endocrine and metabolic: Hypercholesterolemia (4.0%)

Gastrointestinal: Abdominal pain (5.6%), dyspepsia (5.2%), diarrhea (4.5%), nausea (3.4%), hemorrhage (2%)

Genitourinary: Urinary tract infection (3.1%)

Hematologic: Purpura (5.3%), epistaxis (2.9%)

Hepatic: Liver function test abnormalities (<3%; discontinued in 0.11%)

Neuromuscular and skeletal: Arthralgia (6.3%), back pain (5.8%)

Respiratory: Dyspnea (4.5%), rhinitis (4.2%), bronchitis (3.7%), coughing (3.1%), upper respiratory infections (8.7%)

Miscellaneous: Flu-like syndrome (7.5%)

1% to 2.5%: Syncope, palpitation, weakness, cardiac failure, leg cramps, neuralgia, paresthesia, vertigo, atrial fibrillation, hyperuricemia, gout, arthritis, GI hemorrhage, hematoma, anxiety, insomnia, anemia, eczema, cystitis, cataract, conjunctivitis

<1% (limited to important or life-threatening symptoms): Allergic reaction, ischemic necrosis, bilirubinemia, fatty liver, hematuria, hemoptysis, intracranial hemorrhage (0.4%), retroperitoneal bleeding, hepatitis, ocular hemorrhage, pulmonary hemorrhage, purpura, thrombocytopenia, aplastic anemia, hypochromic anemia, menorrhagia, hemothorax, bullous eruption, maculopapular rash, urticaria, agranulocytosis, granulocytopenia, leukopenia, neutropenia (0.05%)

Drug Interactions Increased effect/toxicity: When used with other drugs that can increase bleeding risk such as heparins, warfarins, NSAIDs and other antiplatelet drugs

Onset Maximum effect: 3-7 days

Half-Life 7-8 hours

Education and Monitoring Issues

Patient Education: Take as directed. May cause headache or dizziness; use caution when driving or engaging in tasks that require alertness until response to drug is known. Small frequent meals, frequent mouth care, sucking lozenges, or chewing gum may reduce nausea or vomiting. Mild analgesics may reduce arthralgia or back pain. Report immediately unusual or acute chest pain or respiratory difficulties, skin rash, unresolved diarrhea or gastrointestinal distress, nosebleed, or acute headache.

Dietary Considerations: Food: May be taken without regard to meals

Monitoring Parameters: Signs of bleeding

Manufacturer Sanofi Winthrop Pharmaceuticals

Related Information

Pharmaceutical Manufacturers Directory *on page 1020*

♦ **Clopra®** *see* Metoclopramide *on page 592*

Clorazepate (klor AZ e pate)

Pharmacologic Class Benzodiazepine

U.S. Brand Names Gen-XENE®; Tranxene®

Generic Available Yes

Mechanism of Action Facilitates gamma aminobutyric acid (GABA)-mediated transmission inhibitory neurotransmitter action, depresses subcortical levels of CNS

Use Treatment of generalized anxiety and panic disorders; management of alcohol withdrawal; adjunct anticonvulsant in management of partial seizures

USUAL DOSAGE Oral:

Children 9-12 years: Anticonvulsant: Initial: 3.75-7.5 mg/dose twice daily; increase dose by 3.75 mg at weekly intervals, not to exceed 60 mg/day in 2-3 divided doses

Children >12 years and Adults: Anticonvulsant: Initial: Up to 7.5 mg/dose 2-3 times/day; increase dose by 7.5 mg at weekly intervals; not to exceed 90 mg/day

Adults:

Anxiety: 7.5-15 mg 2-4 times/day, or given as single dose of 11.25 or 22.5 mg at bedtime

Alcohol withdrawal: Initial: 30 mg, then 15 mg 2-4 times/day on first day; maximum daily dose: 90 mg; gradually decrease dose over subsequent days

Dosage Forms CAP: 3.75 mg, 7.5 mg, 15 mg. **TAB:** 3.75 mg, 7.5 mg, 15 mg; Single dose: 11.25 mg, 22.5 mg

Contraindications Hypersensitivity to clorazepate dipotassium or any component; cross-sensitivity with other benzodiazepines may exist; avoid using in patients with pre-existing CNS depression, severe uncontrolled pain, or narrow-angle glaucoma

Warnings/Precautions Use with caution in patients with hepatic or renal disease; abrupt discontinuation may cause withdrawal symptoms or seizures

Pregnancy Risk Factor D

Adverse Reactions

Cardiovascular: Hypotension

Central nervous system: Drowsiness, fatigue, ataxia, lightheadedness, memory impairment, insomnia, anxiety, headache, depression, slurred speech, confusion, nervousness, dizziness, irritability

Dermatologic: Rash

Endocrine & metabolic: Decreased libido

Gastrointestinal: Xerostomia, constipation, diarrhea, decreased salivation, nausea, vomiting, increased or decreased appetite

Neuromuscular & skeletal: Dysarthria, tremor

Ocular: Blurred vision, diplopia

Drug Interactions

Carbamazepine, rifampin, rifabutin may enhance the metabolism of clorazepate and decrease its therapeutic effect; consider using an alternative sedative/hypnotic agent

Amprenavir, cimetidine, ciprofloxacin, clarithromycin, clozapine, CNS depressants, diltiazem, disulfiram, digoxin, erythromycin, ethanol, fluconazole, fluoxetine, fluvoxamine, isoniazid, itraconazole, ketoconazole, labetalol, levodopa, loxapine, metoprolol, metronidazole, miconazole, nefazodone, nelfinavir, omeprazole, phenytoin, rifabutin, rifampin, ritonavir, troleandomycin, valproic acid, verapamil may increase the serum level and/or toxicity of clorazepate; monitor for altered benzodiazepine response

Alcohol Interactions Avoid use (may increase central nervous system depression)

Onset ~1 hour

Duration Variable, 8-24 hours

Half-Life Desmethyldiazepam: 48-96 hours; Oxazepam: 6-8 hours

Education and Monitoring Issues

Patient Education: Take exactly as directed (do not increase dose or frequency); may cause physical and/or psychological dependence. Do not use excessive alcohol and other prescription or OTC medications (especially pain medications, sedatives, antihistamines, or hypnotics) without consulting prescriber. Maintain adequate hydration (2-3 L/day of fluids unless instructed to restrict fluid intake). You may experience drowsiness, lightheadedness, impaired coordination, dizziness, or blurred vision (use caution when driving or engaging in tasks requiring alertness until response to drug is known); nausea, vomiting, or dry mouth (small frequent meals, frequent mouth care, chewing gum, or sucking lozenges may help); constipation (increased exercise, fluids, or dietary fruit and fiber may help); altered sexual drive or ability (reversible); or photosensitivity (use sunscreen, wear protective clothing and eyewear, avoid direct sunlight). Report persistent CNS effects (eg, confusion, depression, increased sedation, excitation, headache, agitation, insomnia or nightmares, dizziness, fatigue, impaired coordination, changes in personality, or changes in cognition); changes in urinary pattern; muscle cramping, weakness, tremors, or rigidity; ringing in ears or visual disturbances; chest pain, palpitations, or rapid heartbeat; excessive perspiration; excessive GI symptoms (cramping, constipation, vomiting, anorexia); or worsening of condition.

Dietary Considerations: Grapefruit juice may increase serum levels and/or toxicity

Monitoring Parameters: Respiratory and cardiovascular status, excess CNS depression

Reference Range: Therapeutic: 0.12-1 μg/mL (SI: 0.36-3.01 μmol/L)

Related Information

Epilepsy Guidelines *on page 1091*

♦ **Clotrimaderm** *see* Clotrimazole *on page 220*

Clotrimazole (kloe TRIM a zole)

Pharmacologic Class Antifungal Agent, Oral Nonabsorbed; Antifungal Agent, Topical; Antifungal Agent, Vaginal

U.S. Brand Names Femizole-7® [OTC]; Fungoid® Solution; Gyne-Lotrimin® [OTC]; Gynix®; Lotrimin®; Lotrimin® AF Cream [OTC]; Lotrimin® AF Lotion [OTC]; Lotrimin® AF Solution [OTC]; Mycelex®; Mycelex®-7; Mycelex®-G

Generic Available No

Mechanism of Action Binds to phospholipids in the fungal cell membrane altering cell wall permeability resulting in loss of essential intracellular elements

Use Treatment of susceptible fungal infections, including oropharyngeal, candidiasis, dermatophytoses, superficial mycoses, and cutaneous candidiasis, as well as vulvovaginal candidiasis; limited data suggest that clotrimazole troches may be effective for prophylaxis against oropharyngeal candidiasis in neutropenic patients

USUAL DOSAGE

Children >3 years and Adults:

Oral:

Prophylaxis: 10 mg troche dissolved 3 times/day for the duration of chemotherapy or until steroids are reduced to maintenance levels

Treatment: 10 mg troche dissolved slowly 5 times/day for 14 consecutive days

Topical: Apply twice daily; if no improvement occurs after 4 weeks of therapy, reevaluate diagnosis

Children >12 years and Adults:

Vaginal:

Cream: Insert 1 applicatorful of 1% vaginal cream daily (preferably at bedtime) for 7 consecutive days

Tablet: Insert 100 mg/day for 7 days or 500 mg single dose

Topical: Apply to affected area twice daily (morning and evening) for 7 consecutive days

Dosage Forms COMBINATION pack (Mycelex-7®): Vag tab 100 mg (7's) and vag crm 1% (7 g). **CRM:** Topical (Lotrimin®, Lotrimin® AF, Mycelex®, Mycelex® OTC): 1% (15 g, 30 g, 45 g, 90 g); Vag (Femizole-7®, Gyne-Lotrimin®, Mycelex®-G): 1% (45 g, 90 g). **LOT** (Lotrimin®): 1% (30 mL). **SOLN, top** (Fungoid®, Lotrimin®, Lotrimin® AF, Mycelex®, Mycelex® OTC): 1% (10 mL, 30 mL). **TAB, vag** (Gyne-Lotrimin®, Gynix®; Mycelex®-G): 100 mg (7s), 500 mg (1s). **TROCHE** (Mycelex®): 10 mg. **TWIN pack** (Mycelex®): Vag tab 500 mg (1's) and vag crm 1% (7 g)

Contraindications Hypersensitivity to clotrimazole or any component

Warnings/Precautions Clotrimazole should not be used for treatment of systemic fungal infection; safety and effectiveness of clotrimazole lozenges (troches) in children <3 years of age have not been established

Pregnancy Risk Factor B; C (oral)

Adverse Reactions

>10%: Hepatic: Abnormal LFTs, causal relationship between troches and elevated LFTs not clearly established

1% to 10%:

Gastrointestinal: Nausea and vomiting may occur in patients on clotrimazole troches

Local: Mild burning, irritation, stinging to skin or vaginal area

Drug Interactions CYP3A3/4 and 3A5-7 enzyme inhibitor

Education and Monitoring Issues

Patient Education:

Oral: Do not swallow oral medication whole; allow to dissolve slowly in mouth. You may experience nausea or vomiting (small frequent meals, frequent mouth care, chewing gum, or sucking lozenges may help). Report signs of opportunistic infection (eg, white plaques in mouth, fever, chills, perianal itching or vaginal discharge, fatigue, unhealed wounds or sores).

Topical: Wash hands before applying or wear gloves. Apply thin film of gel, lotion, or solution to affected area. May apply porous dressing. Report persistent burning, swelling, itching, worsening of condition, or lack of response to therapy.

Vaginal: Wash hands before using. Insert full applicator into vagina gently and expel cream, or insert tablet into vagina, at bedtime. Wash applicator with soap and water following use. Remain lying down for 30 minutes following administration. Avoid intercourse during therapy (sexual partner may experience penile burning or itching). Report adverse reactions (eg, vulvular itching, frequent urination), worsening of condition, or lack of response to therapy.

Monitoring Parameters: Periodic liver function tests during oral therapy with clotrimazole lozenges

Related Information

Betamethasone and Clotrimazole *on page 105*
Treatment of Sexually Transmitted Diseases *on page 1210*

Cloxacillin (kloks a SIL in)

Pharmacologic Class Penicillin

U.S. Brand Names Cloxapen®; Tegopen®

Use Treatment of susceptible bacterial infections, notably penicillinase-producing staphylococci causing respiratory tract, skin and skin structure, bone and joint, urinary tract infections

USUAL DOSAGE Oral:

Children >1 month (<20 kg): 50-100 mg/kg/day in divided doses every 6 hours; up to a maximum of 4 g/day

Children (>20 kg) and Adults: 250-500 mg every 6 hours

Hemodialysis: Not dialyzable (0% to 5%)

Contraindications Hypersensitivity to cloxacillin or any component, or penicillins

Pregnancy Risk Factor B

♦ **Cloxapen®** *see* Cloxacillin *on page 220*

Clozapine (KLOE za peen)

Pharmacologic Class Antipsychotic Agent, Dibenzodiazepine

U.S. Brand Names Clozaril®

Generic Available No

Mechanism of Action Clozapine is a weak dopamine$_1$ and dopamine$_2$ receptor blocker; in addition, it blocks the serotonin$_2$, alpha-adrenergic, and histamine H_1 central nervous system receptors

Use Management of schizophrenic patients

USUAL DOSAGE Adults: Oral: 25 mg once or twice daily initially and increased, as tolerated to a target dose of 300-450 mg/day after 2 weeks, but may require doses as high as 600-900 mg/day

Dosage Forms TAB: 25 mg, 100 mg

Contraindications In patients with WBC ≤3500 cells/mm^3 before therapy; if WBC falls to <3000 cells/mm^3 during therapy the drug should be withheld until signs and symptoms of infection disappear and WBC rises to >3000 cells/mm^3

Warnings/Precautions Medication should not be stopped abruptly; taper off over 1-2 weeks. WBC testing should occur weekly for the first 6 months of therapy; thereafter, if acceptable WBC counts are maintained (WBC ≥3000/mm^3, ANC ≥1500/mm^3) then WBC counts can be monitored every other week. WBCs must be monitored weekly for the first 4 weeks after therapy discontinuation. Significant risk of agranulocytosis, potentially life-threatening. Use with caution in patients receiving other marrow suppressive agents.

Pregnancy Risk Factor B

Adverse Reactions

>10%:

Cardiovascular: Tachycardia

Central nervous system: Drowsiness, dizziness

Gastrointestinal: Constipation, unusual weight gain, diarrhea, sialorrhea

Genitourinary: Urinary incontinence

1% to 10%:

Cardiovascular: EKG changes, hypertension, hypotension, syncope

Central nervous system: Akathisia, seizures, headache, nightmares, akinesia, confusion, insomnia, fatigue, myoclonic jerks

Dermatologic: Rash

Gastrointestinal: Abdominal discomfort, heartburn, xerostomia, nausea, vomiting

Hematologic: Eosinophilia, leukopenia

Neuromuscular & skeletal: Tremor

Miscellaneous: Diaphoresis (increased), fever

<1%: Agranulocytosis, arrhythmias, blurred vision, congestive heart failure, difficult urination, granulocytopenia, impotence, myocardial infarction, myocarditis, neuroleptic malignant syndrome, pericardial effusion, pericarditis, rigidity, tardive dyskinesia, thrombocytopenia

Drug Interactions CYP1A2, 2C (minor), 2E1, 3A3/4 enzyme substrate, CYP2D6 enzyme substrate (minor)

Benzodiazepines in combination with clozapine may produce respiratory depression and hypotension, especially during the first few weeks of therapy; monitor for altered response

Carbamazepine, phenytoin, and primidone increase the hepatic metabolism of clozapine; monitor for altered response

Cigarette smoking may enhance the metabolism of clozapine; larger doses may be required compared to nonsmokers

Clarithromycin, cimetidine, erythromycin, fluoxetine, fluvoxamine, paroxetine, sertraline, and troleandomycin may inhibit the metabolism of clozapine; monitor for altered clozapine effect; use alternative agents

Clozapine may reverse the pressor effect of epinephrine

Valproic acid may cause reductions in clozapine concentrations; monitor for altered response

Alcohol Interactions Avoid use (may increase central nervous system depression)

Half-Life Mean half-life: 12 hours (range: 4-66 hours)

Education and Monitoring Issues

Patient Education: Use exactly as directed (do not increase dose or frequency); may cause physical and/or psychological dependence. Do not discontinue without

(Continued)

Clozapine *(Continued)*

consulting prescriber. Avoid excess alcohol or caffeine and other prescription or OTC medications not approved by prescriber. Maintain adequate hydration (2-3 L/day of fluids unless instructed to restrict fluid intake). You may experience headache, excess drowsiness, dizziness, or blurred vision (use caution driving or when engaging in tasks requiring alertness until response to drug is known); dry mouth, nausea, vomiting (small frequent meals, frequent mouth care, sucking lozenges, or chewing gum may help); or postural hypotension (use caution climbing stairs or when changing position from lying or sitting to standing). Report persistent CNS effects (insomnia, depression, altered consciousness); palpitations, rapid heartbeat, severe dizziness; vision changes; hypersalivation, tearing, sweating; difficulty breathing; or worsening of condition.

♦ **Clozaril®** *see* Clozapine *on page 221*
♦ **CoActifed** *see* Triprolidine, Pseudoephedrine, and Codeine *on page 958*
♦ **Cobex®** *see* Cyanocobalamin *on page 233*

Cocaine (koe KANE)

Pharmacologic Class Local Anesthetic

Generic Available Yes

Mechanism of Action Ester local anesthetic blocks both the initiation and conduction of nerve impulses by decreasing the neuronal membrane's permeability to sodium ions, which results in inhibition of depolarization with resultant blockade of conduction; interferes with the uptake of norepinephrine by adrenergic nerve terminals producing vasoconstriction

Use Topical anesthesia (ester derivative) for mucous membranes

USUAL DOSAGE Dosage depends on the area to be anesthetized, tissue vascularity, technique of anesthesia, and individual patient tolerance; use the lowest dose necessary to produce adequate anesthesia should be used, not to exceed 1 mg/kg. Use reduced dosages for children, elderly, or debilitated patients.

Topical application (ear, nose, throat, bronchoscopy): Concentrations of 1% to 4% are used; concentrations >4% are not recommended because of potential for increased incidence and severity of systemic toxic reactions

Dosage Forms POWDER: 5 g, 25 g. **SOLN, top:** 4% [40 mg/mL] (2 mL, 4 mL, 10 mL); 10% [100 mg/mL] (4 mL, 10 mL); Viscous: 4% [40 mg/mL] (4 mL, 10 mL); 10% [100 mg/mL] (4 mL, 10 mL). **TAB, soluble, for top soln:** 135 mg

Contraindications Systemic use, hypersensitivity to cocaine or any component; pregnancy if nonmedicinal use

Warnings/Precautions Use with caution in patients with hypertension, severe cardiovascular disease, or thyrotoxicosis; use with caution in patients with severely traumatized mucosa and sepsis in the region of intended application. Repeated topical application can result in psychic dependence and tolerance. May cause cornea to become clouded or pitted, therefore, normal saline should be used to irrigate and protect cornea during surgery; not for injection.

Pregnancy Risk Factor C; X (if nonmedicinal use)

Adverse Reactions

>10%:

Central nervous system: CNS stimulation

Gastrointestinal: Loss of taste perception

Respiratory: Chronic rhinitis, nasal congestion

Miscellaneous: Loss of smell

1% to 10%:

Cardiovascular: Decreased heart rate with low doses, increased heart rate with moderate doses, hypertension, tachycardia, cardiac arrhythmias

Central nervous system: Nervousness, restlessness, euphoria, excitement, hallucination, seizures

Gastrointestinal: Vomiting

Neuromuscular & skeletal: Tremors and clonic-tonic reactions

Ocular: Sloughing of the corneal epithelium, ulceration of the cornea

Respiratory: Tachypnea, respiratory failure

Drug Interactions CYP3A3/4 enzyme substrate

Increased toxicity: MAO inhibitors

Onset Onset of action: Within 1 minute; Peak action: Within 5 minutes

Duration ≥30 minutes, depending on dosage administered

Half-Life Following topical administration to mucosa: 75 minutes

Education and Monitoring Issues

Patient Education: When used orally, do not take anything by mouth until full sensation returns. Ocular: Use caution when driving or engaging in tasks that require alert vision (mydriasis may last for several hours). At time of use or immediately thereafter, report any unusual cardiovascular, CNS, or respiratory symptoms immediately. Following use, report skin irritation or eruption; alterations in vision, eye pain or irritation; persistent gastrointestinal effects; muscle or skeletal tremors, numbness, or rigidity; urinary or genital problems; or persistent fatigue. When used orally, do not take anything by mouth until full sensation returns.

Monitoring Parameters: Vital signs

Reference Range: Therapeutic: 100-500 ng/mL (SI: 330 nmol/L); Toxic: >1000 ng/mL (SI: >3300 nmol/L)

- **Codafed® Expectorant** *see* Guaifenesin, Pseudoephedrine, and Codeine *on page 425*
- **Codamine®** *see* Hydrocodone and Phenylpropanolamine *on page 446*
- **Codamine® Pediatric** *see* Hydrocodone and Phenylpropanolamine *on page 446*
- **Codehist® DH** *see* Chlorpheniramine, Pseudoephedrine, and Codeine *on page 187*

Codeine (KOE deen)

Pharmacologic Class Analgesic, Narcotic; Antitussive

Generic Available Yes

Mechanism of Action Binds to opiate receptors in the CNS, causing inhibition of ascending pain pathways, altering the perception of and response to pain; causes cough supression by direct central action in the medulla; produces generalized CNS depression

Use Treatment of mild to moderate pain; antitussive in lower doses; dextromethorphan has equivalent antitussive activity but has much lower toxicity in accidental overdose

USUAL DOSAGE Doses should be titrated to appropriate analgesic effect; when changing routes of administration, note that oral dose is $^2/_3$ as effective as parenteral dose

Analgesic:
- Children: Oral, I.M., S.C.: 0.5-1 mg/kg/dose every 4-6 hours as needed; maximum: 60 mg/dose
- Adults: Oral, I.M., I.V., S.C.: 30 mg/dose; range: 15-60 mg every 4-6 hours as needed

Antitussive: Oral (for nonproductive cough):
- Children: 1-1.5 mg/kg/day in divided doses every 4-6 hours as needed: Alternative dose according to age:
  - 2-6 years: 2.5-5 mg every 4-6 hours as needed; maximum: 30 mg/day
  - 6-12 years: 5-10 mg every 4-6 hours as needed; maximum: 60 mg/day
- Adults: 10-20 mg/dose every 4-6 hours as needed; maximum: 120 mg/day

Dosing adjustment in renal impairment:
- Cl_{cr} 10-50 mL/minute: Administer 75% of dose
- Cl_{cr} <10 mL/minute: Administer 50% of dose

Dosing adjustment in hepatic impairment: Probably necessary in hepatic insufficiency

Dosage Forms

Codeine phosphate: **INJ:** 30 mg (1 mL, 2 mL); 60 mg (1 mL, 2 mL). **TAB, soluble:** 30 mg, 60 mg

Codeine sulfate: **TAB:** 15 mg, 30 mg, 60 mg; Soluble: 15 mg, 30 mg, 60 mg **SOLN, oral:** 15 mg/5 mL

Contraindications Hypersensitivity to codeine or any component

Warnings/Precautions Use with caution in patients with hypersensitivity reactions to other phenanthrene derivative opioid agonists (morphine, hydrocodone, hydromorphone, levorphanol, oxycodone, oxymorphone); respiratory diseases including asthma, emphysema, COPD, or severe liver or renal insufficiency; some preparations contain sulfites which may cause allergic reactions; tolerance or drug dependence may result from extended use

Not recommended for use for cough control in patients with a productive cough; not recommended as an antitussive for children <2 years of age; the elderly may be particularly susceptible to the CNS depressant and confusion as well as constipating effects of narcotics

Pregnancy Risk Factor C; D (if used for prolonged periods or in high doses at term)

Adverse Reactions

Percentage unknown: Increased AST, ALT

>10%:
- Central nervous system: Drowsiness
- Gastrointestinal: Constipation

1% to 10%:
- Cardiovascular: Tachycardia or bradycardia, hypotension
- Central nervous system: Dizziness, lightheadedness, false feeling of well being, malaise, headache, restlessness, paradoxical CNS stimulation, confusion
- Dermatologic: Rash, urticaria
- Gastrointestinal: Xerostomia, anorexia, nausea, vomiting,
- Genitourinary: Decreased urination, ureteral spasm
- Hepatic: Increased LFTs
- Local: Burning at injection site
- Ocular: Blurred vision
- Neuromuscular & skeletal: Weakness
- Respiratory: Shortness of breath, dyspnea
- Miscellaneous: Histamine release

<1%: Biliary spasm, convulsions, hallucinations, insomnia, mental depression, muscle rigidity, nightmares, paralytic ileus, stomach cramps, trembling

Drug Interactions CYP2D6 and 3A3/4 enzyme substrate; CYP2D6 enzyme inhibitor

(Continued)

Codeine *(Continued)*

Decreased effect with cigarette smoking

Increased toxicity: CNS depressants, phenothiazines, TCAs, other narcotic analgesics, guanabenz, MAO inhibitors, neuromuscular blockers

Alcohol Interactions Avoid use (may increase central nervous system depression)

Onset

Onset of action: Oral: 0.5-1 hour; I.M.: 10-30 minutes

Peak action: Oral: 1-1.5 hours; I.M.: 0.5-1 hour

Duration 4-6 hours

Half-Life 2.5-3.5 hours

Education and Monitoring Issues

Patient Education: If self-administered, use exactly as directed (do not increase dose or frequency); may cause physical and/or psychological dependence. While using this medication, do not use alcohol and other prescription or OTC medications (especially sedatives, tranquilizers, antihistamines, or pain medications) without consulting prescriber. Maintain adequate hydration (2-3 L/day of fluids unless instructed to restrict fluid intake). May cause dizziness, drowsiness, confusion, agitation, impaired coordination, or blurred vision (use caution when driving, climbing stairs, or changing position - rising from sitting or lying to standing, or when engaging in tasks requiring alertness until response to drug is known); nausea or vomiting, or loss of appetite (frequent mouth care, small frequent meals, sucking lozenges, or chewing gum may help); constipation (increased exercise, fluids, or dietary fruit and fiber may help - if constipation remains an unresolved problem, consult prescriber about use of stool softeners). Report confusion, insomnia, excessive nervousness, excessive sedation or drowsiness, or shakiness; acute GI upset; difficulty breathing or shortness of breath; facial flushing, rapid heartbeat or palpitations; urinary difficulty; unusual muscle weakness; or vision changes.

Dietary Considerations: Food: Glucose may cause hyperglycemia; monitor blood glucose concentrations

Monitoring Parameters: Pain relief, respiratory and mental status, blood pressure, heart rate

Reference Range: Therapeutic: Not established; Toxic: >1.1 µg/mL

Related Information

Aspirin and Codeine *on page 75*
Bromodiphenhydramine and Codeine *on page 114*
Brompheniramine, Phenylpropanolamine, and Codeine *on page 114*
Carisoprodol, Aspirin, and Codeine *on page 142*
Chlorpheniramine, Phenylephrine, and Codeine *on page 186*
Chlorpheniramine, Pseudoephedrine, and Codeine *on page 187*
Guaifenesin and Codeine *on page 424*
Guaifenesin, Pseudoephedrine, and Codeine *on page 425*
Lipid-Lowering Agents Comparison *on page 1243*
Narcotic Agonists Comparison *on page 1244*
Promethazine and Codeine *on page 780*
Promethazine, Phenylephrine, and Codeine *on page 780*
Terpin Hydrate and Codeine *on page 898*
Triprolidine, Pseudoephedrine, and Codeine *on page 958*

- **Codeine Contin®** *see* Codeine *on page 223*
- **Codiclear® DH** *see* Hydrocodone and Guaifenesin *on page 445*
- **Codoxy®** *see* Oxycodone and Aspirin *on page 692*
- **Codroxomin®** *see* Hydroxocobalamin *on page 451*
- **Cogentin®** *see* Benztropine *on page 100*
- **Co-Gesic®** *see* Hydrocodone and Acetaminophen *on page 444*
- **Cognex®** *see* Tacrine *on page 886*
- **Colace® [OTC]** *see* Docusate *on page 290*
- **Colax-C®** *see* Docusate *on page 290*

Colchicine (KOL chi seen)

Pharmacologic Class Colchicine

Generic Available Yes: Tablet

Mechanism of Action Decreases leukocyte motility, decreases phagocytosis in joints and lactic acid production, thereby reducing the deposition of urate crystals that perpetuates the inflammatory response

Use Treat acute gouty arthritis attacks and prevent recurrences of such attacks, management of familial Mediterranean fever

USUAL DOSAGE

Prophylaxis of familial Mediterranean fever: Oral:

Children:

≤5 years: 0.5 mg/day

>5 years: 1-1.5 mg/day in 2-3 divided doses

Adults: 1-2 mg/day in 2-3 divided doses

Gouty arthritis, acute attacks: Adults:
Oral: Initial: 0.5-1.2 mg, then 0.5-0.6 mg every 1-2 hours or 1-1.2 mg every 2 hours until relief or GI side effects (nausea, vomiting, or diarrhea) occur to a maximum total dose of 8 mg; wait 3 days before initiating another course of therapy
I.V.: Initial: 1-3 mg, then 0.5 mg every 6 hours until response, not to exceed 4 mg/day; if pain recurs, it may be necessary to administer a daily dose of 1-2 mg for several days, however, do not administer more colchicine by any route for at least 7 days after a full course of I.V. therapy (4 mg), transfer to oral colchicine in a dose similar to that being given I.V.
Gouty arthritis, prophylaxis of recurrent attacks: Adults: Oral: 0.5-0.6 mg/day or every other day
Dosing adjustment in renal impairment:
Cl_{cr} <50 mL/minute: Avoid chronic use or administration
Cl_{cr} <10 mL/minute: Decrease dose by 50% for treatment of acute attacks
Hemodialysis: Not dialyzable (0% to 5%); supplemental dose is not necessary
Peritoneal dialysis: Supplemental dose is not necessary

Dosage Forms INJ: 0.5 mg/mL (2 mL). **TAB:** 0.5 mg, 0.6 mg

Contraindications Hypersensitivity to colchicine or any component; serious renal, gastrointestinal, hepatic, or cardiac disorders; blood dyscrasias

Warnings/Precautions Severe local irritation can occur following S.C. or I.M. administration; use with caution in debilitated patients or elderly patients or patients with severe GI, renal, or liver disease

Pregnancy Risk Factor C (oral); D (parenteral)

Adverse Reactions
>10%: Gastrointestinal: Nausea, vomiting, diarrhea, abdominal pain
1% to 10%:
Dermatologic: Alopecia
Gastrointestinal: Anorexia
<1%: Agranulocytosis, aplastic anemia, azoospermia, bone marrow suppression, hepatotoxicity, myopathy, peripheral neuritis, rash

Drug Interactions
Decreased effect: Vitamin B_{12} absorption may be decreased
Increased toxicity:
Sympathomimetic agents
CNS depressant effects are enhanced

Alcohol Interactions Avoid use (may cause increased stomach irritation)

Onset Oral: Relief of pain and inflammation occurs after 24-48 hours; I.V.: 6-12 hours

Half-Life 12-30 minutes; End-stage renal disease: 45 minutes

Education and Monitoring Issues
Patient Education: Take as directed; do not exceed recommended dosage. Consult prescriber about a low-purine diet. Maintain adequate hydration (2-3 L/day of fluids unless instructed to restrict fluid intake). Do not use alcohol or aspirin-containing medication without consulting prescriber. You may experience nausea, vomiting, or anorexia (small frequent meals, frequent mouth care, chewing gum, or sucking lozenges may help); hair loss (reversible). Stop medication and report to prescriber if severe vomiting, watery or bloody diarrhea, or abdominal pain occurs. Report muscle tremors or weakness; fatigue; easy bruising or bleeding; yellowing of eyes or skin; or pale stool or dark urine.
Dietary Considerations: Food: Cyanocobalamin (Vitamin B_{12}): Malabsorption of the substrate. May result in macrocytic anemia or neurologic dysfunction. May need to supplement with Vitamin B_{12}.
Monitoring Parameters: CBC and renal function test

Related Information
Colchicine and Probenecid *on page 225*

Colchicine and Probenecid (KOL chi seen & proe BEN e sid)

Pharmacologic Class Antigout Agent

Dosage Forms TAB: Colchicine 0.5 mg and probenecid 0.5 g

Pregnancy Risk Factor C (oral); D (parenteral)

Alcohol Interactions Avoid use (may cause increased stomach irritation)

♦ **Colestid®** *see* Colestipol *on page 225*

Colestipol (koe LES ti pole)

Pharmacologic Class Antilipemic Agent (Bile Acid Seqestrant)

U.S. Brand Names Colestid®

Generic Available No

Mechanism of Action Binds with bile acids to form an insoluble complex that is eliminated in feces; it thereby increases the fecal loss of bile acid-bound low density lipoprotein cholesterol

Use Adjunct in management of primary hypercholesterolemia; regression of arteriolosclerosis; relief of pruritus associated with elevated levels of bile acids; possibly used to decrease plasma half-life of digoxin in toxicity
(Continued)

Colestipol *(Continued)*

USUAL DOSAGE Adults: Oral:

Granules: 5-30 g/day given once or in divided doses 2-4 times/day; initial dose: 5 g 1-2 times/day; increase by 5 g at 1- to 2-month intervals

Tablets: 2-16 g/day; initial dose: 2 g 1-2 times/day; increase by 2 g at 1- to 2-month intervals

Dosage Forms GRANULES: 5 g packet, 300 g, 500 g. **TAB:** 1 g

Contraindications Hypersensitivity to colestipol or any component; avoid using in complete biliary obstruction

Warnings/Precautions Avoid in patients with high triglycerides, GI dysfunction (constipation); may be associated with increased bleeding tendency as a result of hypothrombinemia secondary to vitamin K deficiency; may cause depletion of vitamins A, D, E

Pregnancy Risk Factor C

Adverse Reactions

>10%: Gastrointestinal: Constipation

1% to 10%:

Central nervous system: Headache, dizziness, anxiety, vertigo, drowsiness, fatigue

Gastrointestinal: Abdominal pain and distention, belching, flatulence, nausea, vomiting, diarrhea

<1% (limited to important or life-threatening symptoms): Peptic ulceration, gallstones, GI irritation and bleeding, anorexia, steatorrhea or malabsorption syndrome, cholelithiasis, cholecystitis, shortness of breath

Drug Interactions

Colestipol can reduce the absorption of numerous medications when used concurrently. Give other medications 1 hour before or 4 hours after giving colestipol. Medications which may be affected include HMG-CoA reductase inhibitors, thiazide diuretics, propranolol (and potentially other beta-blockers), corticosteroids, thyroid hormones, digoxin, valproic acid, NSAIDs, loop diuretics, sulfonylureas

Warfarin and other oral anticoagulants: Absorption is reduced by cholestyramine, may also be reduced by colestipol. Separate administration times (as detailed above) and monitor INR closely when initiating or discontinuing.

Education and Monitoring Issues

Patient Education: Take with 38-45 ounces of water or fruit juice. Rinse glass with small amount of water to ensure full dose is taken. Other medications should be taken 2 hours before or 2 hours after colestipol. You may experience constipation (increased exercise, increased dietary fluids, fruit, fiber, or stool softener may help) or drowsiness or dizziness (use caution when driving or engaging in tasks that require alertness until response to drug is known). Report acute gastric pain, tarry stools, or difficulty breathing.

Manufacturer Pharmacia & Upjohn

Related Information

Pharmaceutical Manufacturers Directory *on page 1020*

Colfosceril Palmitate (kole FOS er il PALM i tate)

Pharmacologic Class Lung Surfactant

U.S. Brand Names Exosurf® Neonatal

Generic Available No

Mechanism of Action Replaces deficient or ineffective endogenous lung surfactant in neonates with respiratory distress syndrome (RDS) or in neonates at risk of developing RDS; reduces surface tension and stabilizes the alveoli from collapsing

Use Neonatal respiratory distress syndrome:

Prophylactic therapy: Body weight <1350 g in infants at risk for developing RDS; body weight >1350 g in infants with evidence of pulmonary immaturity

Rescue therapy: Treatment of infants with RDS based on respiratory distress not attributable to any other causes and chest radiographic findings consistent with RDS

USUAL DOSAGE For intratracheal use only. Neonates:

Prophylactic treatment: Administer 5 mL/kg (as two 2.5 mL/kg half-doses) as soon as possible; the second and third doses should be administered at 12 and 24 hours later to those infants remaining on ventilators

Rescue treatment: Administer 5 mL/kg (as two 2.5 mL/kg half-doses) as soon as the diagnosis of RDS is made; the second 5 mL/kg (as two 2.5 mL/kg half-doses) dose should be administered 12 hours later

Dosage Forms POWDER for inj, lyophilized: 108 mg (10 mL)

Warnings/Precautions Pulmonary hemorrhaging may occur especially in infants <700 g. Mucous plugs may have formed in the endotracheal tube in those infants whose ventilation was markedly impaired during or shortly after dosing. If chest expansion improves substantially, the ventilator PIP setting should be reduced immediately. Hyperoxia and hypocarbia (hypocarbia can decrease blood flow to the brain) may occur requiring appropriate ventilator adjustments.

Adverse Reactions 1% to 10%: Respiratory: Pulmonary hemorrhage, apnea, mucous plugging, decrease in transcutaneous O_2 of >20%

Education and Monitoring Issues

Monitoring Parameters: Continuous EKG and transcutaneous O_2 saturation should be monitored during administration; frequent ABG sampling is necessary to prevent postdosing hyperoxia and hypocarbia

Manufacturer GlaxoWellcome

Related Information

Pharmaceutical Manufacturers Directory *on page 1020*

Colistin, Neomycin, and Hydrocortisone

(koe LIS tin, nee oh MYE sin, & hye droe KOR ti sone)

Pharmacologic Class Antibiotic/Corticosteroid, Otic

U.S. Brand Names Coly-Mycin® S Otic Drops; Cortisporin-TC® Otic

Dosage Forms SUSP, otic: (Coly-Mycin® S Otic Drops): Colistin sulfate 0.3%, neomycin sulfate 0.47%, and hydrocortisone acetate 1% (5 mL, 10 mL); (Cortisporin-TC®): Colistin sulfate 0.3%, neomycin sulfate 0.33%, and hydrocortisone acetate 1% (5 mL, 10 mL)

Pregnancy Risk Factor C

Collagenase (KOL la je nase)

Pharmacologic Class Enzyme, Topical Debridement

U.S. Brand Names Biozyme-C®; Santyl®

Use Promotes debridement of necrotic tissue in dermal ulcers and severe burns

USUAL DOSAGE Topical: Apply once daily (or more frequently if the dressing becomes soiled)

Contraindications Known hypersensitivity to collagenase

Pregnancy Risk Factor C

- ♦ **Colovage®** *see* Polyethylene Glycol-Electrolyte Solution *on page 747*
- ♦ **Coly-Mycin® S Otic Drops** *see* Colistin, Neomycin, and Hydrocortisone *on page 227*
- ♦ **Colyte®** *see* Polyethylene Glycol-Electrolyte Solution *on page 747*
- ♦ **Comalose-R** *see* Lactulose *on page 506*
- ♦ **Combantrin** *see* Pyrantel Pamoate *on page 793*
- ♦ **Combipres®** *see* Clonidine and Chlorthalidone *on page 217*
- ♦ **Combivent** *see* Ipratropium and Albuterol *on page 484*
- ♦ **Combivir™** *see* Zidovudine and Lamivudine *on page 992*
- ♦ **Comfort® [OTC]** *see* Naphazoline *on page 636*
- ♦ **Comhist®** *see* Chlorpheniramine, Phenylephrine, and Phenyltoloxamine *on page 186*
- ♦ **Comhist® LA** *see* Chlorpheniramine, Phenylephrine, and Phenyltoloxamine *on page 186*
- ♦ **Community Acquired Pneumonia in Adults** *see page 1200*
- ♦ **Compazine®** *see* Prochlorperazine *on page 773*
- ♦ **Compoz® Gel Caps [OTC]** *see* Diphenhydramine *on page 282*
- ♦ **Compoz® Nighttime Sleep Aid [OTC]** *see* Diphenhydramine *on page 282*
- ♦ **Comtan®** *see* Entacapone *on page 314*
- ♦ **Comvax™** *see Haemophilus* b Conjugate and Hepatitis b Vaccine *on page 426*
- ♦ **Congest** *see* Estrogens, Conjugated *on page 331*
- ♦ **Constant-T®** *see* Theophylline Salts *on page 906*
- ♦ **Constilac®** *see* Lactulose *on page 506*
- ♦ **Constulose®** *see* Lactulose *on page 506*
- ♦ **Contac® Cough Formula Liquid [OTC]** *see* Guaifenesin and Dextromethorphan *on page 424*
- ♦ **Control® [OTC]** *see* Phenylpropanolamine *on page 729*
- ♦ **Copaxone®** *see* Glatiramer Acetate *on page 412*
- ♦ **Cophene XP®** *see* Hydrocodone, Pseudoephedrine, and Guaifenesin *on page 446*
- ♦ **Coptin®** *see* Sulfadiazine *on page 877*
- ♦ **Coradur®** *see* Isosorbide Dinitrate *on page 490*
- ♦ **Corax®** *see* Chlordiazepoxide *on page 180*
- ♦ **Cordarone®** *see* Amiodarone *on page 48*
- ♦ **Cordema** *see* Sodium Chloride *on page 858*
- ♦ **Cordran®** *see* Flurandrenolide *on page 382*
- ♦ **Cordran® SP** *see* Flurandrenolide *on page 382*
- ♦ **Coreg®** *see* Carvedilol *on page 144*
- ♦ **Corgard®** *see* Nadolol *on page 628*
- ♦ **Corium®** *see* Clidinium and Chlordiazepoxide *on page 208*
- ♦ **Corliprol®** *see* Celiprolol *on page 168*
- ♦ **Corque® Topical** *see* Clioquinol and Hydrocortisone *on page 209*
- ♦ **Cortacet** *see* Hydrocortisone *on page 447*
- ♦ **CortaGel® [OTC]** *see* Hydrocortisone *on page 447*
- ♦ **Cortaid® Maximum Strength [OTC]** *see* Hydrocortisone *on page 447*
- ♦ **Cortaid® With Aloe [OTC]** *see* Hydrocortisone *on page 447*

- **Cortamed** *see* Hydrocortisone *on page 447*
- **Cortate** *see* Hydrocortisone *on page 447*
- **Cortatrigen® Otic** *see* Neomycin, Polymyxin B, and Hydrocortisone *on page 644*
- **Cort-Dome®** *see* Hydrocortisone *on page 447*
- **Cortef®** *see* Hydrocortisone *on page 447*
- **Cortef® Feminine Itch** *see* Hydrocortisone *on page 447*
- **Cortenema®** *see* Hydrocortisone *on page 447*
- **Corticaine® Topical** *see* Dibucaine and Hydrocortisone *on page 263*
- **Corticosteroids Comparison** *see page 1237*
- **Corticreme** *see* Hydrocortisone *on page 447*
- **Cortifoam®** *see* Hydrocortisone *on page 447*
- **Cortiment** *see* Hydrocortisone *on page 447*

Cortisone Acetate (KOR ti sone AS e tate)

Pharmacologic Class Adrenal Corticosteroid

U.S. Brand Names Cortone® Acetate

Generic Available Yes

Mechanism of Action Decreases inflammation by suppression of migration of polymorphonuclear leukocytes and reversal of increased capillary permeability

Use Management of adrenocortical insufficiency

USUAL DOSAGE If possible, administer glucocorticoids before 9 AM to minimize adrenocortical suppression; dosing depends upon the condition being treated and the response of the patient; supplemental doses may be warranted during times of stress in the course of withdrawing therapy

Children:
- Anti-inflammatory or immunosuppressive: Oral: 2.5-10 mg/kg/day **or** 20-300 mg/m^2/day in divided doses every 6-8 hours
- Physiologic replacement: Oral: 0.5-0.75 mg/kg/day **or** 20-25 mg/m^2/day in divided doses every 8 hours

Adults: Oral: 25-300 mg/day in divided doses every 12-24 hours

Hemodialysis: Supplemental dose is not necessary

Peritoneal dialysis: Supplemental dose is not necessary

Dosage Forms TAB: 5 mg, 10 mg, 25 mg

Contraindications Serious infections, except septic shock or tuberculous meningitis; administration of live virus vaccines

Warnings/Precautions Use with caution in patients with hypothyroidism, cirrhosis, hypertension, congestive heart failure, ulcerative colitis, thromboembolic disorders, osteoporosis, convulsive disorders, peptic ulcer, diabetes mellitus, myasthenia gravis; prolonged therapy (>5 days) of pharmacologic doses of corticosteroids may lead to hypothalamic-pituitary-adrenal suppression, the degree of adrenal suppression varies with the degree and duration of glucocorticoid therapy; this must be taken into consideration when taking patients off steroids

Pregnancy Risk Factor D

Adverse Reactions

>10%:
- Central nervous system: Insomnia, nervousness
- Gastrointestinal: Increased appetite, indigestion

1% to 10%:
- Dermatologic: Hirsutism
- Endocrine & metabolic: Diabetes mellitus
- Neuromuscular & skeletal: Arthralgia
- Ocular: Cataracts, glaucoma
- Respiratory: Epistaxis

<1%: Abdominal distention, acne, alkalosis, amenorrhea, bruising, Cushing's syndrome, delirium, edema, euphoria, fractures, glucose intolerance, growth suppression, hallucinations, headache, hyperglycemia, hyperpigmentation, hypersensitivity reactions, hypertension, hypokalemia, mood swings, muscle wasting, myalgia, nausea, osteoporosis, pancreatitis, peptic ulcer, pituitary-adrenal axis suppression, pseudotumor cerebri, psychoses, seizures, skin atrophy, sodium and water retention, ulcerative esophagitis, vertigo, vomiting

Drug Interactions CYP3A3/4 enzyme substrate

Decreased effect:
- Barbiturates, phenytoin, rifampin may decrease cortisone effects
- Live virus vaccines
- Anticholinesterase agents may decrease effect
- Cortisone may decrease warfarin effects
- Cortisone may decrease effects of salicylates

Increased effect: Estrogens (increase cortisone effects)

Increased toxicity:
- Cortisone + NSAIDs may increase ulcerogenic potential
- Cortisone may increase potassium deletion due to diuretics

Alcohol Interactions Avoid use (may enhance gastric mucosal irritation)

Onset Peak effect: Oral: Within 2 hours; I.M.: Within 20-48 hours

Half-Life 30 minutes to 2 hours; End-stage renal disease: 3.5 hours

Education and Monitoring Issues

Patient Education: Take with meals or take with food or milk; do not discontinue drug without notifying prescriber

Related Information

Corticosteroids Comparison *on page 1237*

- **Cortisporin** *see* Bacitracin, Neomycin, Polymyxin B, and Hydrocortisone *on page 90*
- **Cortisporin** *see* Neomycin, Polymyxin B, and Hydrocortisone *on page 644*
- **Cortisporin® Ophthalmic Ointment** *see* Bacitracin, Neomycin, Polymyxin B, and Hydrocortisone *on page 90*
- **Cortisporin® Ophthalmic Suspension** *see* Neomycin, Polymyxin B, and Hydrocortisone *on page 644*
- **Cortisporin® Otic** *see* Neomycin, Polymyxin B, and Hydrocortisone *on page 644*
- **Cortisporin-TC® Otic** *see* Colistin, Neomycin, and Hydrocortisone *on page 227*
- **Cortisporin® Topical Cream** *see* Neomycin, Polymyxin B, and Hydrocortisone *on page 644*
- **Cortisporin® Topical Ointment** *see* Bacitracin, Neomycin, Polymyxin B, and Hydrocortisone *on page 90*
- **Cortizone®-5 [OTC]** *see* Hydrocortisone *on page 447*
- **Cortizone®-10 [OTC]** *see* Hydrocortisone *on page 447*
- **Cortoderm** *see* Hydrocortisone *on page 447*
- **Cortone** *see* Cortisone Acetate *on page 228*
- **Cortone® Acetate** *see* Cortisone Acetate *on page 228*
- **Cortrosyn®** *see* Cosyntropin *on page 229*
- **Corvert®** *see* Ibutilide *on page 459*
- **Coryphen® Codeine** *see* Aspirin and Codeine *on page 75*
- **CoSudafed Expectorant** *see* Guaifenesin, Pseudoephedrine, and Codeine *on page 425*

Cosyntropin (koe sin TROE pin)

Pharmacologic Class Diagnostic Agent

U.S. Brand Names Cortrosyn®

Generic Available No

Mechanism of Action Stimulates the adrenal cortex to secrete adrenal steroids (including hydrocortisone, cortisone), androgenic substances, and a small amount of aldosterone

Use Diagnostic test to differentiate primary adrenal from secondary (pituitary) adrenocortical insufficiency

USUAL DOSAGE

Adrenocortical insufficiency: I.M., I.V. (over 2 minutes): Peak plasma cortisol concentrations usually occur 45-60 minutes after cosyntropin administration

Neonates: 0.015 mg/kg/dose

Children <2 years: 0.125 mg

Children >2 years and Adults: 0.25-0.75 mg

When greater cortisol stimulation is needed, an I.V. infusion may be used:

Children >2 years and Adults: 0.25 mg administered at 0.04 mg/hour over 6 hours

Congenital adrenal hyperplasia evaluation: 1 mg/m^2/dose up to a maximum of 1 mg

Dosage Forms POWDER for inj: 0.25 mg

Contraindications Known hypersensitivity to cosyntropin

Warnings/Precautions Use with caution in patients with pre-existing allergic disease or a history of allergic reactions to corticotropin

Pregnancy Risk Factor C

Adverse Reactions

1% to 10%:

Cardiovascular: Flushing

Central nervous system: Mild fever

Dermatologic: Pruritus

Gastrointestinal: Chronic pancreatitis

<1%: Hypersensitivity reactions

Education and Monitoring Issues

Reference Range: Normal baseline cortisol; increase in serum cortisol after cosyntropin injection of >7 μg/dL or peak response >18 μg/dL; plasma cortisol concentrations should be measured immediately before and exactly 30 minutes after a dose

Manufacturer Organon, Inc

Related Information

Pharmaceutical Manufacturers Directory *on page 1020*

- **Cotazym®** *see* Pancrelipase *on page 698*
- **Cotazym-S®** *see* Pancrelipase *on page 698*
- **Cotridin** *see* Triprolidine, Pseudoephedrine, and Codeine *on page 958*
- **Cotrifed** *see* Triprolidine, Pseudoephedrine, and Codeine *on page 958*

- **Cotrim®** *see* Co-Trimoxazole *on page 230*
- **Cotrim® DS** *see* Co-Trimoxazole *on page 230*

Co-Trimoxazole (koe-trye MOKS a zole)

Pharmacologic Class Antibiotic, Sulfonamide Derivative

U.S. Brand Names Bactrim™; Bactrim™ DS; Cotrim®; Cotrim® DS; Septra®; Septra® DS; Sulfatrim®

Generic Available Yes

Mechanism of Action Sulfamethoxazole interferes with bacterial folic acid synthesis and growth via inhibition of dihydrofolic acid formation from para-aminobenzoic acid; trimethoprim inhibits dihydrofolic acid reduction to tetrahydrofolate resulting in sequential inhibition of enzymes of the folic acid pathway

Use

Oral treatment of urinary tract infections due to *E. coli*, *Klebsiella* and *Enterobacter* sp, *P. morganii*, *P. mirabilis* and *P. vulgaris*; acute otitis media in children and acute exacerbations of chronic bronchitis in adults due to susceptible strains of *H. influenzae* or *S. pneumoniae*; prophylaxis of *Pneumocystis carinii* pneumonitis (PCP), traveler's diarrhea due to enterotoxigenic *E. coli* or *Cyclospora*

I.V. treatment or severe or complicated infections when oral therapy is not feasible, for documented PCP, empiric treatment of PCP in immune compromised patients; treatment of documented or suspected shigellosis, typhoid fever, *Nocardia asteroides* infection, or other infections caused by susceptible bacteria

Unlabeled use: Cholera and salmonella-type infections and nocardiosis; chronic prostatitis; as prophylaxis in neutropenic patients with *P. carinii* infections, in leukemics, and in patients following renal transplantation, to decrease incidence of gram-negative rod infections

USUAL DOSAGE Dosage recommendations are based on the trimethoprim component

Children >2 months:

- Mild to moderate infections: Oral, I.V.: 8 mg TMP/kg/day in divided doses every 12 hours
- Serious infection/*Pneumocystis*: I.V.: 20 mg TMP/kg/day in divided doses every 6 hours
- Urinary tract infection prophylaxis: Oral: 2 mg TMP/kg/dose daily
- Prophylaxis of *Pneumocystis*: Oral, I.V.: 10 mg TMP/kg/day or 150 mg TMP/m^2/day in divided doses every 12 hours for 3 days/week; dose should not exceed 320 mg trimethoprim and 1600 mg sulfamethoxazole 3 days/week

Adults:

- Urinary tract infection/chronic bronchitis: Oral: 1 double strength tablet every 12 hours for 10-14 days
- Sepsis: I.V.: 20 TMP/kg/day divided every 6 hours
- *Pneumocystis carinii*:
  - Prophylaxis: Oral: 1 double strength tablet daily or 3 times/week
  - Treatment: Oral, I.V.: 15-20 mg TMP/kg/day in 3-4 divided doses

Dosing adjustment in renal impairment: Adults:

- I.V.:
  - Cl_{cr} 15-30 mL/minute: Administer 2.5-5 mg/kg every 12 hours
  - Cl_{cr} <15 mL/minute: Administer 2.5-5 mg/kg every 24 hours
- Oral:
  - Cl_{cr} 15-30 mL/minute: Administer 1 double strength tablet every 24 hours or 1 single strength tablet every 12 hours
  - Cl_{cr} <15 mL/minute: Not recommended

Dosage Forms The 5:1 ratio (SMX to TMP) remains constant in all dosage forms. **INJ:** Sulfamethoxazole 80 mg and trimethoprim 16 mg per mL (5 mL, 10 mL, 20 mL, 30 mL, 50 mL). **SUSP, oral:** Sulfamethoxazole 200 mg and trimethoprim 40 mg per 5 mL (20 mL, 100 mL, 150 mL, 200 mL, 480 mL). **TAB:** Sulfamethoxazole 400 mg and trimethoprim 80 mg; Double strength: Sulfamethoxazole 800 mg and trimethoprim 160 mg

Contraindications Hypersensitivity to any sulfa drug or any component; porphyria; megaloblastic anemia due to folate deficiency; infants <2 months of age; marked hepatic damage

Warnings/Precautions Use with caution in patients with G-6-PD deficiency, impaired renal or hepatic function; maintain adequate hydration to prevent crystalluria; adjust dosage in patients with renal impairment. Injection vehicle contains benzyl alcohol and sodium metabisulfite. Fatalities associated with severe reactions including Stevens-Johnson syndrome, toxic epidermal necrolysis, hepatic necrosis, agranulocytosis, aplastic anemia and other blood dyscrasias; discontinue use at first sign of rash. Elderly patients appear at greater risk for more severe adverse reactions. May cause hypoglycemia, particularly in malnourished, or patients with renal or hepatic impairment. Use with caution in patients with porphyria or thyroid dysfunction. Slow acetylators may be more prone to adverse reactions.

Pregnancy Risk Factor C (per manufacturer); D (if near term, based on expert analysis)

Pregnancy Implications Do not use at term to avoid kernicterus in the newborn and use during pregnancy only if risks outweigh the benefits since folic acid metabolism may be affected

Adverse Reactions

>10%:

Dermatologic: Allergic skin reactions including rashes and urticaria, photosensitivity

Gastrointestinal: Nausea, vomiting, anorexia

1% to 10%:

Dermatologic: Stevens-Johnson syndrome, toxic epidermal necrolysis (rare)

Hematologic: Blood dyscrasias

Hepatic: Hepatitis

<1%: Aplastic anemia, ataxia, cholestatic jaundice, confusion, depression, diarrhea, erythema multiforme, fever, granulocytopenia, hallucinations, hemolysis (with G-6-PD deficiency), interstitial nephritis, kernicterus in neonates, megaloblastic anemia, pancreatitis, pancytopenia, pseudomembranous colitis, rhabdomyolysis, seizures, serum sickness, stomatitis, thrombocytopenia

Drug Interactions CYP2C9 enzyme inhibitor

Decreased effect: Cyclosporines

Increased effect/toxicity: Phenytoin, cyclosporines (nephrotoxicity), methotrexate (displaced from binding sites), dapsone, sulfonylureas, and oral anticoagulants; may compete for renal secretion of methotrexate; digoxin concentrations increased

Half-Life SMX: 9 hours; TMP: 6-17 hours, both are prolonged in renal failure

Education and Monitoring Issues

Patient Education: Take oral medication with 8 oz of water on an empty stomach (1 hour before or 2 hours after meals) for best absorption. Finish all medication; do not skip doses. You may experience increased sensitivity to sunlight; use sunblock, wear protective clothing and dark glasses, or avoid direct exposure to sunlight. Small frequent meals, frequent mouth care, sucking lozenges, or chewing gum may reduce nausea or vomiting. Report skin rash, sore throat, blackened stool, or unusual bruising or bleeding immediately.

Related Information

Animal and Human Bites Guidelines *on page 1177*

Antimicrobial Drugs of Choice *on page 1182*

♦ **Cough Syrup** *see* Guaifenesin, Pseudoephedrine, and Codeine *on page 425*

♦ **Cough Syrup DM-E** *see* Guaifenesin and Dextromethorphan *on page 424*

♦ **Cough Syrup DM Expectorant** *see* Guaifenesin and Dextromethorphan *on page 424*

♦ **Cough Syrup with Guaifenesin** *see* Guaifenesin and Dextromethorphan *on page 424*

♦ **Coumadin®** *see* Warfarin *on page 982*

♦ **Covera-HS®** *see* Verapamil *on page 975*

♦ **Coversyl** *see* Perindopril Erbumine *on page 717*

♦ **Cozaar®** *see* Losartan *on page 542*

♦ **Creatinine Clearance Estimating Methods in Patients With Stable Renal Function** *see page 1047*

♦ **Creon® 10** *see* Pancrelipase *on page 698*

♦ **Creon® 20** *see* Pancrelipase *on page 698*

♦ **Crixivan®** *see* Indinavir *on page 468*

♦ **Crolom® Ophthalmic Solution** *see* Cromolyn Sodium *on page 231*

Cromolyn Sodium (KROE moe lin SOW dee um)

Pharmacologic Class Mast Cell Stabilizer; Ophthalmic Agent

U.S. Brand Names Crolom® Ophthalmic Solution; Gastrocrom® Oral; Intal® Nebulizer Solution; Intal® Oral Inhaler; Nasalcrom® Nasal Solution

Generic Available No

Mechanism of Action Prevents the mast cell release of histamine, leukotrienes and slow-reacting substance of anaphylaxis by inhibiting degranulation after contact with antigens

Use Adjunct in the prophylaxis of allergic disorders, including rhinitis, giant papillary conjunctivitis, and asthma; inhalation product may be used for prevention of exercise-induced bronchospasm; systemic mastocytosis, food allergy, and treatment of inflammatory bowel disease; **cromolyn is a prophylactic drug with no benefit for acute situations**

USUAL DOSAGE

Oral:

Systemic mastocytosis:

Neonates and preterm Infants: Not recommended

Infants and Children <2 years: 20 mg/kg/day in 4 divided doses; may increase in patients 6 months to 2 years of age if benefits not seen after 2-3 weeks; do not exceed 30 mg/kg/day

Children 2-12 years: 100 mg 4 times/day; not to exceed 40 mg/kg/day

Children >12 years and Adults: 200 mg 4 times/day

Food allergy and inflammatory bowel disease:

Children <2 years: Not recommended

Children 2-12 years: Initial dose: 100 mg 4 times/day; may double the dose if effect is not satisfactory within 2-3 weeks; not to exceed 40 mg/kg/day

(Continued)

Cromolyn Sodium *(Continued)*

Children >12 years and Adults: Initial dose: 200 mg 4 times/day; may double the dose if effect is not satisfactory within 2-3 weeks; up to 400 mg 4 times/day

Once desired effect is achieved, dose may be tapered to lowest effective dose

Inhalation:

For chronic control of asthma, taper frequency to the lowest effective dose (ie, 4 times/day to 3 times/day to twice daily):

Nebulization solution: Children >2 years and Adults: Initial: 20 mg 4 times/day; usual dose: 20 mg 3-4 times/day

Metered spray:

Children 5-12 years: Initial: 2 inhalations 4 times/day; usual dose: 1-2 inhalations 3-4 times/day

Children ≥12 years and Adults: Initial: 2 inhalations 4 times/day; usual dose: 2-4 inhalations 3-4 times/day

Prevention of allergen- or exercise-induced bronchospasm: Administer 10-15 minutes prior to exercise or allergen exposure but no longer than 1 hour before:

Nebulization solution: Children >2 years and Adults: Single dose of 20 mg

Metered spray: Children >5 years and Adults: Single dose of 2 inhalations

Dosage Forms INH, oral (Intal®): 800 mcg/spray (8.1 g). **SOLN:** For nebulization: 10 mg/mL (2 mL); (Intal®): 10 mg/mL (2 mL); As sodium, oral (Gastrocrom®): 100 mg/5 mL. **NASAL** (Nasalcrom®): 40 mg/mL (13 mL). **OPHTH** (Crolom®): 4% (2.5 mL, 10 mL)

Contraindications Hypersensitivity to cromolyn or any component; acute asthma attacks

Warnings/Precautions Severe anaphylactic reactions may occur rarely; cromolyn is a prophylactic drug with no benefit for acute situations; do not use in patients with severe renal or hepatic impairment; caution should be used when withdrawing the drug or tapering the dose as symptoms may reoccur; use with caution in patients with a history of cardiac arrhythmias

Pregnancy Risk Factor B

Pregnancy Implications

Clinical effects on the fetus: No data on whether cromolyn crosses the placenta or clinical effects on the fetus. Available evidence suggests safe use during pregnancy.

Breast-feeding/lactation: No data on whether cromolyn crosses into breast milk or clinical effects on the infant

Adverse Reactions

>10%:

Gastrointestinal: Unpleasant taste (inhalation aerosol)

Respiratory: Hoarseness, coughing

1% to 10%:

Dermatologic: Angioedema

Gastrointestinal: Xerostomia

Genitourinary: Dysuria

Respiratory: Sneezing, nasal congestion

<1%: Anaphylactic reactions, arthralgia, diarrhea, dizziness, eosinophilic pneumonia, headache, lacrimation, nasal burning, nausea, ocular stinging, pulmonary infiltrates, rash, throat irritation, urticaria, vomiting, wheezing

Onset Maximal effect requires weeks

Half-Life 80-90 minutes

Education and Monitoring Issues

Patient Education: Oral: Use as directed; do not increase dosage or discontinue abruptly without consulting prescriber. You may experience dizziness or nervousness (use caution when driving or engaging in tasks requiring alertness until response to drug is known); diarrhea (boiled milk, yogurt, or buttermilk may help); or headache or muscle pain (mild analgesic may offer relief). Report persistent insomnia; skin rash or irritation; abdominal pain or difficulty swallowing; unusual cough, bronchospasm, or difficulty breathing; decreased urination; or if condition worsens or fails to improve.

Nebulizer: Store nebulizer solution away from light. Prepare nebulizer according to package instructions. Clear as much mucus as possible before use. Rinse mouth following each use to prevent opportunistic infection and reduce unpleasant after-taste. Report if symptoms worsen or condition fails to improve.

Nasal: Instill 1 spray into each nostril 3-4 times a day. You may experience unpleasant taste (rinsing mouth and frequent oral care may help); or headache (mild analgesic may help). Report increased sneezing, burning, stinging, or irritation inside of nose; sore throat, hoarseness, nosebleed; anaphylactic reaction (skin rash, fever, chills, backache, difficulty breathing, chest pain); or worsening of condition or lack of improvement.

Ophthalmic: For ophthalmic use only. Wash hands before using. Tilt head back and look upward. Put drops of suspension or apply thin ribbon of ointment inside lower eyelid. Close eye and roll eyeball in all directions. Do not blink for ½ minute. apply gentle pressure to inner corner of eye for 30 seconds. Do not use any other eye preparation for at least 10 minutes. Do not let tip of applicator touch eye or contaminate tip of applicator. Do not share medication with anyone else. Temporary stinging or blurred vision may occur. Inform prescriber if condition worsens or fails to improve or if you experience eye pain, redness, burning, watering, dryness, double vision, puffiness around eye, vision disturbances, or other adverse eye response; or worsening of condition or lack of improvement.

Monitoring Parameters: Periodic pulmonary function tests

Crotamiton (kroe TAM i tonn)

Pharmacologic Class Scabicidal Agent

U.S. Brand Names Eurax® Topical

Use Treatment of scabies (*Sarcoptes scabiei*) and symptomatic treatment of pruritus

USUAL DOSAGE Topical:

Scabicide: Children and Adults: Wash thoroughly and scrub away loose scales, then towel dry; apply a thin layer and massage drug onto skin of the entire body from the neck to the toes (with special attention to skin folds, creases, and interdigital spaces). Repeat application in 24 hours. Take a cleansing bath 48 hours after the final application. Treatment may be repeated after 7-10 days if live mites are still present.

Pruritus: Massage into affected areas until medication is completely absorbed; repeat as necessary

Contraindications Hypersensitivity to crotamiton or other components; patients who manifest a primary irritation response to topical medications

Pregnancy Risk Factor C

- **Crystamine®** *see* Cyanocobalamin *on page 233*
- **Crysti 1000®** *see* Cyanocobalamin *on page 233*
- **Crysticillin® A.S.** *see* Penicillin G Procaine *on page 712*
- **Crystodigin®** *see* Digitoxin *on page 272*
- **C/T/S® Topical Solution** *see* Clindamycin *on page 208*
- **Cuprimine®** *see* Penicillamine *on page 708*
- **Curretab®** *see* Medroxyprogesterone Acetate *on page 558*
- **Cutivate™** *see* Fluticasone *on page 386*

Cyanocobalamin (sye an oh koe BAL a min)

Pharmacologic Class Vitamin, Water Soluble

U.S. Brand Names Berubigen®; Cobex®; Crystamine®; Crysti 1000®; Cyanoject®; Cyomin®; Ener-B® [OTC]; Kaybovite-1000®; Nascobal®; Redisol®; Rubramin-PC®; Sytobex®

Generic Available Yes

Mechanism of Action Coenzyme for various metabolic functions, including fat and carbohydrate metabolism and protein synthesis, used in cell replication and hematopoiesis

Use Treatment of pernicious anemia; vitamin B_{12} deficiency; increased B_{12} requirements due to pregnancy, thyrotoxicosis, hemorrhage, malignancy, liver or kidney disease

USUAL DOSAGE

Recommended daily allowance (RDA):
- Children: 0.3-2 mcg
- Adults: 2 mcg

Nutritional deficiency: Oral: 25-250 mcg/day

Anemias: I.M. or deep S.C. (oral is not generally recommended due to poor absorption and I.V. is not recommended due to more rapid elimination):

Pernicious anemia, congenital (if evidence of neurologic involvement): 1000 mcg/day for at least 2 weeks; maintenance: 50-100 mcg/month or 100 mcg for 6-7 days; if there is clinical improvement, give 100 mcg every other day for 7 doses, then every 3-4 days for 2-3 weeks; follow with 100 mcg/month for life. Administer with folic acid if needed.

Children: 30-50 mcg/day for 2 or more weeks (to a total dose of 1000-5000 mcg), then follow with 100 mcg/month as maintenance dosage

Adults: 100 mcg/day for 6-7 days; if improvement, administer same dose on alternate days for 7 doses; then every 3-4 days for 2-3 weeks; once hematologic values have returned to normal, maintenance dosage: 100 mcg/month. **Note:** Use only parenteral therapy as oral therapy is not dependable.

Vitamin B_{12} deficiency:

Children:

Neurologic signs: 100 mcg/day for 10-15 days (total dose of 1-1.5 mg), then once or twice weekly for several months; may taper to 60 mcg every month

Hematologic signs: 10-50 mcg/day for 5-10 days, followed by 100-250 mcg/dose every 2-4 weeks

Adults: Initial: 30 mcg/day for 5-10 days; maintenance: 100-200 mcg/month

Schilling test: I.M.: 1000 mcg

Dosage Forms GEL, nasal: (Ener-B®): 400 mcg/0.1 mL; (Nascobal®): 500 mcg/0.1 mL (5 mL). **INJ:** 30 mcg/mL (30 mL), 100 mcg/mL (1 mL, 10 mL, 30 mL), 1000 mcg/mL (1 mL, 10 mL, 30 mL). **TAB** [OTC]: 25 mcg, 50 mcg, 100 mcg, 250 mcg, 500 mcg, 1000 mcg

Contraindications Hypersensitivity to cyanocobalamin or any component, cobalt; patients with hereditary optic nerve atrophy

Warnings/Precautions I.M. route used to treat pernicious anemia; vitamin B_{12} deficiency for >3 months results in irreversible degenerative CNS lesions; treatment of vitamin B_{12} megaloblastic anemia may result in severe hypokalemia, sometimes, fatal, when anemia

(Continued)

Cyanocobalamin *(Continued)*

corrects due to cellular potassium requirements. B_{12} deficiency masks signs of polycythemia vera; vegetarian diets may result in B_{12} deficiency; pernicious anemia occurs more often in gastric carcinoma than in general population.

Pregnancy Risk Factor A; C (if dose exceeds RDA recommendation)

Adverse Reactions

1% to 10%:

Dermatologic: Itching

Gastrointestinal: Diarrhea

<1%: Anaphylaxis, peripheral vascular thrombosis, urticaria

Education and Monitoring Issues

Patient Education: Use exactly as directed. Pernicious anemia may require monthly injections for life. Report skin rash; swelling, pain, or redness of extremities; or acute persistent diarrhea.

Monitoring Parameters: Serum potassium, erythrocyte and reticulocyte count, hemoglobin, hematocrit

Reference Range: Normal range of serum B_{12} is 150-750 pg/mL; this represents 0.1% of total body content. Metabolic requirements are 2-5 µg/day; years of deficiency required before hematologic and neurologic signs and symptoms are seen. Occasional patients with significant neuropsychiatric abnormalities may have no hematologic abnormalities and normal serum cobalamin levels, 200 pg/mL (SI: >150 pmol/L), or more commonly between 100-200 pg/mL (SI: 75-150 pmol/L). There exists evidence that people, particularly elderly whose serum cobalamin concentrations <300 pg/mL, should receive replacement parenteral therapy; this recommendation is based upon neuropsychiatric disorders and cardiovascular disorders associated with lower sodium cobalamin concentrations.

- **Cyanoject®** *see* Cyanocobalamin *on page 233*
- **Cyclen** *see* Ethinyl Estradiol and Norgestimate *on page 344*

Cyclobenzaprine (sye kloe BEN za preen)

Pharmacologic Class Skeletal Muscle Relaxant

U.S. Brand Names Flexeril®

Generic Available Yes

Mechanism of Action Centrally acting skeletal muscle relaxant pharmacologically related to tricyclic antidepressants; reduces tonic somatic motor activity influencing both alpha and gamma motor neurons

Use Treatment of muscle spasm associated with acute painful musculoskeletal conditions; supportive therapy in tetanus

USUAL DOSAGE Oral: **Note:** Do not use longer than 2-3 weeks

Children: Dosage has not been established

Adults: 20-40 mg/day in 2-4 divided doses; maximum dose: 60 mg/day

Dosage Forms TAB: 10 mg

Contraindications Hypersensitivity to cyclobenzaprine or any component; do not use concomitantly or within 14 days of MAO inhibitors; hyperthyroidism, congestive heart failure, arrhythmias

Warnings/Precautions Cyclobenzaprine shares the toxic potentials of the tricyclic antidepressants and the usual precautions of tricyclic antidepressant therapy should be observed; use with caution in patients with urinary hesitancy or angle-closure glaucoma

Pregnancy Risk Factor B

Adverse Reactions

>10%:

Central nervous system: Drowsiness, dizziness, lightheadedness

Gastrointestinal: Xerostomia

1% to 10%:

Cardiovascular: Edema of the face/lips, syncope

Gastrointestinal: Bloated feeling

Genitourinary: Problems in urinating, polyuria

Hepatic: Hepatitis

Neuromuscular & skeletal: Problems in speaking, muscle weakness

Ocular: Blurred vision

Otic: Tinnitus

<1%: Arrhythmia, ataxia, confusion, constipation, dermatitis, dyspepsia, fatigue, headache, hypotension, nausea, nervousness, rash, stomach cramps, tachycardia, unpleasant taste

Drug Interactions CYP1A2, 2D6 and 3A3/4 enzyme substrate

Increased toxicity:

Do not use concomitantly or within 14 days after MAO inhibitors

Because of similarities to the tricyclic antidepressants, may have additive toxicities

Anticholinergics: Because of cyclobenzaprine's anticholinergic action, use with caution in patients receiving these agents

Alcohol, barbiturates, and other CNS depressants: Effects may be enhanced by cyclobenzaprine

Alcohol Interactions Avoid use (may increase central nervous system depression)

Onset Commonly occurs within 1 hour

Duration 8 to >24 hours

Half-Life 1-3 days

Education and Monitoring Issues

Patient Education: Take exactly as directed. Do not increase dose or discontinue without consulting prescriber. Do not use alcohol, prescriptive or OTC antidepressants, sedatives, or pain medications without consulting prescriber. You may experience drowsiness, dizziness, lightheadedness (avoid driving or engaging in tasks that require alertness until response to drug is known); or urinary retention (void before taking medication). Report excessive drowsiness or mental agitation, chest pain, skin rash, swelling of mouth/face, difficulty speaking, ringing in ears, or blurred vision.

- **Cyclocort®** *see* Amcinonide *on page 43*
- **Cyclogyl®** *see* Cyclopentolate *on page 235*
- **Cyclomen®** *see* Danazol *on page 246*
- **Cyclomydril® Ophthalmic** *see* Cyclopentolate and Phenylephrine *on page 235*

Cyclopentolate (sye kloe PEN toe late)

Pharmacologic Class Anticholinergic Agent

U.S. Brand Names AK-Pentolate®; Cyclogyl®; I-Pentolate®

Use Diagnostic procedures requiring mydriasis and cycloplegia

USUAL DOSAGE

Infants: Instill 1 drop of 0.5% into each eye 5-10 minutes before examination

Children: Instill 1 drop of 0.5%, 1%, or 2% in eye followed by 1 drop of 0.5% or 1% in 5 minutes, if necessary

Adults: Instill 1 drop of 1% followed by another drop in 5 minutes; 2% solution in heavily pigmented iris

Contraindications Narrow-angle glaucoma, known hypersensitivity to drug

Pregnancy Risk Factor C

Related Information

Cyclopentolate and Phenylephrine *on page 235*

Cyclopentolate and Phenylephrine (sye kloe PEN toe late & fen il EF rin)

Pharmacologic Class Anticholinergic/Adrenergic Agonist

U.S. Brand Names Cyclomydril® Ophthalmic

Dosage Forms SOLN, ophth: Cyclopentolate hydrochloride 0.2% and phenylephrine hydrochloride 1% (2 mL, 5 mL)

Pregnancy Risk Factor C

Cyclophosphamide (sye kloe FOS fa mide)

Pharmacologic Class Antineoplastic Agent, Alkylating Agent

U.S. Brand Names Cytoxan® Injection; Cytoxan® Oral; Neosar® Injection

Generic Available No

Mechanism of Action Cyclophosphamide is an alkylating agent that prevents cell division by cross-linking DNA strands and decreasing DNA synthesis. It is a cell cycle phase nonspecific agent. Cyclophosphamide also possesses potent immunosuppressive activity. Cyclophosphamide is a prodrug that must be metabolized to active metabolites in the liver.

Use Treatment of Hodgkin's and non-Hodgkin's lymphoma, Burkitt's lymphoma, chronic lymphocytic leukemia, chronic granulocytic leukemia, AML, ALL, mycosis fungoides, breast cancer, multiple myeloma, neuroblastoma, retinoblastoma, rhabdomyosarcoma, Ewing's sarcoma; testicular, endometrium and ovarian, and lung cancer, and as a conditioning regimen for BMT; prophylaxis of rejection for kidney, heart, liver, and BMT transplants, severe rheumatoid disorders, nephrotic syndrome, Wegener's granulomatosis, idiopathic pulmonary hemosideroses, myasthenia gravis, multiple sclerosis, systemic lupus erythematosus, lupus nephritis, autoimmune hemolytic anemia, idiopathic thrombocytic purpura, macroglobulinemia, and antibody-induced pure red cell aplasia

USUAL DOSAGE Refer to individual protocols

Patients with compromised bone marrow function may require a 33% to 50% reduction in initial loading dose

Children:

SLE: I.V.: 500-750 mg/m^2 every month; maximum dose: 1 g/m^2

JRA/vasculitis: I.V.: 10 mg/kg every 2 weeks

Children and Adults:

Oral: 50-100 mg/m^2/day as continuous therapy or 400-1000 mg/m^2 in divided doses over 4-5 days as intermittent therapy

I.V.:

Single Doses: 400-1800 mg/m^2 (30-50 mg/kg) per treatment course (1-5 days) which can be repeated at 2-4 week intervals

MAXIMUM SINGLE DOSE WITHOUT BMT is 7 g/m^2 (190 mg/kg) SINGLE AGENT THERAPY

Continuous daily doses: 60-120 mg/m^2 (1-2.5 mg/kg) per day

(Continued)

Cyclophosphamide *(Continued)*

Autologous BMT: IVPB: 50 mg/kg/dose x 4 days or 60 mg/kg/dose for 2 days; total dose is usually divided over 2-4 days

Nephrotic syndrome: Oral: 2-3 mg/kg/day every day for up to 12 weeks when corticosteroids are unsuccessful

Dosing adjustment in renal impairment: A large fraction of cyclophosphamide is eliminated by hepatic metabolism

Some authors recommend no dose adjustment unless severe renal insufficiency (Cl_{cr} <20 mL/minute)

Cl_{cr} >10 mL/minute: Administer 100% of normal dose

Cl_{cr} <10 mL/minute: Administer 75% of normal dose

Hemodialysis: Moderately dialyzable (20% to 50%); administer dose posthemodialysis or administer supplemental 50% dose

CAPD effects: Unknown

CAVH effects: Unknown

Dosing adjustment in hepatic impairment: Some authors recommend dosage reductions (of up to 30%); however, the pharmacokinetics of cyclophosphamide are not significantly altered in the presence of hepatic insufficiency. Cyclophosphamide undergoes hepatic transformation in the liver to its 4-hydroxycyclophosphamide, which breaks down to its active form, phosphoramide mustard.

Dosage Forms POWDER for inj: 100 mg, 200 mg, 500 mg, 1 g, 2 g; Lyophilized: 100 mg, 200 mg, 500 mg, 1 g, 2 g. **TAB:** 25 mg, 50 mg

Contraindications Hypersensitivity to cyclophosphamide or any component

Warnings/Precautions The U.S. Food and Drug Administration (FDA) currently recommends that procedures for proper handling and disposal of antineoplastic agents be considered. Possible dosage adjustment needed for renal or hepatic failure; use with caution in patients with bone marrow suppression.

Pregnancy Risk Factor D

Adverse Reactions

>10%:

Dermatologic: Alopecia is frequent, but hair will regrow although it may be of a different color or texture; alopecia usually occurs 3 weeks after therapy

Endocrine & metabolic: Fertility: May cause sterility; interferes with oogenesis and spermatogenesis; may be irreversible in some patients; gonadal suppression (amenorrhea)

Gastrointestinal: Nausea and vomiting occur more frequently with larger doses, usually beginning 6-10 hours after administration; also seen are anorexia, diarrhea, stomatitis; mucositis

Emetic potential:

Oral: Low (<10%)

<1 g: Moderate (30% to 60%)

≥1 g: High (>90%)

Time course of nausea/vomiting: Onset: 6-8 hours; Duration: 8-24 hours

Hepatic: Jaundice seen occasionally

1% to 10%:

Central nervous system: Headache

Dermatologic: Skin rash, facial flushing

Hematologic: Myelosuppressive: Thrombocytopenia occurs less frequently than with mechlorethamine, anemia

WBC: Moderate

Platelets: Moderate

Onset (days): 7

Nadir (days): 10-14

Recovery (days): 21

<1%: Anaphylactic reactions; high-dose therapy may cause cardiac dysfunction manifested as congestive heart failure; cardiac necrosis or hemorrhagic myocarditis has occurred rarely, but is fatal. Cyclophosphamide may also potentiate the cardiac toxicity of anthracyclines.

Dizziness, darkening of skin/fingernails, hyperglycemia, hypokalemia, distortion, hyperuricemia, SIADH has occurred with I.V. doses >50 mg/kg, stomatitis, acute hemorrhagic cystitis is believed to be a result of chemical irritation of the bladder by acrolein, a cyclophosphamide metabolite. Acute hemorrhagic cystitis occurs in 7% to 12% of patients, and has been reported in up to 40% of patients. Hemorrhagic cystitis can be severe and even fatal. Patients should be encouraged to drink plenty of fluids (3-4 L/day) during therapy, void frequently, and avoid taking the drug at nighttime. If large I.V. doses are being administered, I.V. hydration should be given during therapy. The administration of mesna or continuous bladder irrigation may also be warranted.

Hepatic toxicity, renal tubular necrosis has occurred, but usually resolves after the discontinuation of therapy, nasal congestion occurs when given in large I.V. doses via 30-60 minute infusion; patients experience runny eyes, nasal burning, rhinorrhea, sinus congestion, and sneezing during or immediately after the infusion; interstitial pulmonary fibrosis with prolonged high dosage has occurred; secondary malignancy has developed with cyclophosphamide alone or in combination with other antineoplastics; both bladder carcinoma and acute leukemia are well documented; rare instances of anaphylaxis have been reported

Drug Interactions CYP2B6, 2D6, and 3A3/4 enzyme substrate

Decreased effect: Digoxin: Cyclophosphamide may decrease digoxin serum levels

Increased toxicity:

Allopurinol may cause increase in bone marrow depression and may result in significant elevations of cyclophosphamide cytotoxic metabolites

Anesthetic agents: Cyclophosphamide reduces serum pseudocholinesterase concentrations and may prolong the neuromuscular blocking activity of succinylcholine; use with caution with halothane, nitrous oxide, and succinylcholine

Chloramphenicol results in prolonged cyclophosphamide half-life to increase toxicity

Cimetidine inhibits hepatic metabolism of drugs and may decrease or increase the activation of cyclophosphamide

Doxorubicin: Cyclophosphamide may enhance cardiac toxicity of anthracyclines

Phenobarbital and phenytoin induce hepatic enzymes and cause a more rapid production of cyclophosphamide metabolites with a concurrent decrease in the serum half-life of the parent compound

Tetrahydrocannabinol results in enhanced immunosuppression in animal studies

Thiazide diuretics: Leukopenia may be prolonged

Half-Life 4-6.5 hours

Education and Monitoring Issues

Patient Education: Tablets should be taken early in the day on an empty stomach. If GI distress occurs, may be taken with food. Maintain adequate fluid balance (2-3 L/day of fluids unless instructed to restrict fluid intake). Void frequently and report any difficulty or pain with urination or blood in urine. May cause hair loss (reversible after treatment) or sterility or amenorrhea (sometimes reversible). If you are diabetic, you will need to monitor serum glucose closely to avoid hypoglycemia. You may be more susceptible to infection; avoid crowds and unnecessary exposure to infection. Do not receive immunizations unless approved by prescriber. Report unusual bleeding or bruising; persistent fever or sore throat; stool (black stool), or vomitus; delayed healing of any wounds; skin rash; yellowing of skin or eyes; or changes in color of urine or stool.

Monitoring Parameters: CBC with differential and platelet count, BUN, UA, serum electrolytes, serum creatinine

Manufacturer Bristol-Myers Squibb Company (Pharmaceutical Division)

Related Information

Pharmaceutical Manufacturers Directory *on page 1020*

Cycloserine (sye kloe SER een)

Pharmacologic Class Antibiotic, Miscellaneous; Antitubercular Agent

U.S. Brand Names Seromycin® Pulvules®

Use Adjunctive treatment in pulmonary or extrapulmonary tuberculosis; has been studied for use in Gaucher's disease

USUAL DOSAGE Some of the neurotoxic effects may be relieved or prevented by the concomitant administration of pyridoxine

Tuberculosis: Oral:

Children: 10-20 mg/kg/day in 2 divided doses up to 1000 mg/day for 18-24 months

Adults: Initial: 250 mg every 12 hours for 14 days, then administer 500 mg to 1 g/day in 2 divided doses for 18-24 months (maximum daily dose: 1 g)

Dosing interval in renal impairment:

Cl_{cr} 10-50 mL/minute: Administer every 24 hours

Cl_{cr} <10 mL/minute: Administer every 36-48 hours

Contraindications Known hypersensitivity to cycloserine

Pregnancy Risk Factor C

Related Information

Antimicrobial Drugs of Choice *on page 1182*

Tuberculosis Treatment Guidelines *on page 1213*

Cyclosporine (SYE kloe spor een)

Pharmacologic Class Immunosuppressant Agent

U.S. Brand Names Neoral® Oral; Sandimmune® Injection; Sandimmune® Oral; Sang® CyA

Generic Available No

Mechanism of Action Inhibition of production and release of interleukin II and inhibits interleukin II-induced activation of resting T-lymphocytes

Use Immunosuppressant which may be used with azathioprine and/or corticosteroids to prolong organ and patient survival in kidney, liver, heart, and bone marrow transplants; severe psoriasis; also used in some cases of severe autoimmune disease that are resistant to corticosteroids and other therapy.

USUAL DOSAGE Children and Adults (oral dosage is ~3 times the I.V. dosage); dosage should be based on ideal body weight:

(Continued)

Cyclosporine *(Continued)*

I.V.:

Initial: 5-6 mg/kg/day beginning 4-12 hours prior to organ transplantation; patients should be switched to oral cyclosporine as soon as possible; dose should be infused over 2-24 hours

Maintenance: 2-10 mg/kg/day in divided doses every 8-12 hours; dose should be adjusted to maintain whole blood FPIA trough concentrations in the reference range

Oral: Solution or soft gelatin capsule (Sandimmune®):

Initial: 14-18 mg/kg/day, beginning 4-12 hours prior to organ transplantation

Maintenance: 5-15 mg/kg/day divided every 12-24 hours; maintenance dose is usually tapered to 3-10 mg/kg/day

Focal segmental glomerulosclerosis: Initial: 3 mg/kg/day divided every 12 hours

Autoimmune diseases: 1-3 mg/kg/day

Dosing considerations of cyclosporine, see table.

Cyclosporine

Condition	Cyclosporine
Switch from I.V. to oral therapy	Threefold increase in dose
T-tube clamping	Decrease dose; increase availability of bile facilitates absorption of CsA
Pediatric patients	About 2-3 times higher dose compared to adults
Liver dysfunction	Decrease I.V. dose; increase oral dose
Renal dysfunction	Decrease dose to decrease levels if renal dysfunction is related to the drug
Dialysis	Not removed
Inhibitors of hepatic metabolism	Decrease dose
Inducers of hepatic metabolism	Monitor drug level; may need to increase dose

Oral: **Solution or soft gelatin capsule in a microemulsion (Neoral®):** Based on the organ transplant population:

Initial: Same as the initial dose for solution or soft gelatin capsule (listed above) **or**

Renal: 9 mg/kg/day (range: 6-12 mg/kg/day)

Liver: 8 mg/kg/day (range: 4-12 mg/kg/day)

Heart: 7 mg/kg/day (range: 4-10 mg/kg/day)

Note: A 1:1 ratio conversion from Sandimmune® to Neoral® has been recommended initially; however, lower doses of Neoral® may be required after conversion to prevent overdose. Total daily doses should be adjusted based on the cyclosporine trough blood concentration and clinical assessment of organ rejection. CsA blood trough levels should be determined prior to conversion. After conversion to Neoral®, CsA trough levels should be monitored every 4-7 days. **Neoral® and Sandimmune® are not bioequivalent and cannot be used interchangeably.**

Hemodialysis: Supplemental dose is not necessary

Peritoneal dialysis: Supplemental dose is not necessary

Dosing adjustment in hepatic impairment: Probably necessary, monitor levels closely

Dosing adjustment recommendations for renal impairment during cyclosporine therapy for severe psoriasis:

Serum creatinine levels ≥25% above pretreatment levels: Take another sample within 2 weeks. If the level remains ≥25% above pretreatment levels, decrease dosage of cyclosporine microemulsion by 25% to 50%. If 2 dosage adjustments do not reverse the increase in serum creatinine levels, treatment should be discontinued.

Serum creatinine ≥50% above pretreatment levels: Decrease cyclosporine dosage by 25% to 50%. If 2 dosage adjustments do not reverse the increase in serum creatinine levels, treatment should be discontinued.

Note: Increase the frequency of blood pressure monitoring after each alteration in dosage of cyclosporine. Cyclosporine dosage should be decreased by 25% to 50% in patients with no history of hypertension who develop sustained hypertension during therapy and, if hypertension persists, treatment with cyclosporine should be discontinued.

Dosage Forms CAP (Sandimmune®): 25 mg, 100 mg. **SOFT GEL:** 25 mg, 100 mg; (Sandimmune®): 50 mg; For microemulsion (Neoral®): 25 mg, 100 mg. **INJ** (Sandimmune®): 50 mg/mL (5 mL). **SOLN:** Oral (Sandimmune®): 100 mg/mL (50 mL); Oral for microemulsion (Neoral®): 100 mg/mL (50 mL)

Contraindications

Hypersensitivity to cyclosporine, Cremaphor EL® (I.V. solution), or any other I.V. component (ie, polyoxyl 35 castor oil is an ingredient of the parenteral formulation and polyoxyl 40 hydrogenated castor oil is an ingredient of the cyclosporine capsules and solution for microemulsion)

Use in severe psoriasis therapy: Concomitant treatment of cyclosporine with other psoriasis treatments such as psoralens + ultraviolet A (UVA) light PUVA, UVB therapy, other radiation therapy or other immunosuppressive agents may result in excessive immunosuppression and increased risk of malignancies. Concomitant treatment of cyclosporine with methotrexate or coal tar. The risk of skin malignancies is increased in patients who have previously been treated with these other psoriasis therapies prior to cyclosporine therapy.

Warnings/Precautions Infection and possible development of lymphoma may result. Make dose adjustments to avoid toxicity or possible organ rejection using cyclosporine blood levels because absorption is erratic and elimination is highly variable. Adjustment of dose should only be made under the direct supervision of an experienced prescriber; reserve the use of I.V. for use only in patients who cannot take oral; adequate airway and other supportive measures and agents for treating anaphylaxis should be present when I.V. drug is given. Nephrotoxic, if possible avoid concomitant use of other potentially nephrotoxic drugs (eg, acyclovir, aminoglycoside antibiotics, amphotericin B, ciprofloxacin). Can cause systemic hypertension or nephrotoxicity when used with other psoriasis therapies.

Pregnancy Risk Factor C

Pregnancy Implications Clinical effects on the fetus: Based on small numbers of patients, the use of cyclosporine during pregnancy apparently does not pose a major risk to the fetus

Adverse Reactions

>10%:

- Cardiovascular: Hypertension
- Dermatologic: Hirsutism
- Endocrine & metabolic: Hypomagnesemia, hypokalemia
- Gastrointestinal: Gingival hypertrophy
- Neuromuscular & skeletal: Tremor
- Renal: Nephrotoxicity

1% to 10%:

- Central nervous system: Seizure, headache
- Dermatologic: Acne
- Gastrointestinal: Abdominal discomfort, nausea, vomiting
- Neuromuscular & skeletal: Leg cramps

<1%: Anaphylaxis, flushing, hepatotoxicity, hyperkalemia, hyperuricemia, hypomagnesemia, hypotension, increased susceptibility to infection, myositis, pancreatitis, paresthesias, respiratory distress, sensitivity to temperature extremes, sinusitis, tachycardia, warmth

Drug Interactions CYP3A3/4 enzyme substrate

Decreased effect: Drugs that decrease cyclosporine concentrations: Carbamazepine, phenobarbital, phenytoin, rifampin, isoniazid

Increased toxicity:

- Drugs that increase cyclosporine concentrations: Azithromycin, clarithromycin, diltiazem, erythromycin, fluconazole, itraconazole, ketoconazole, nicardipine, verapamil
- Drugs that enhance nephrotoxicity of cyclosporine: Aminoglycosides, amphotericin B, acyclovir
- Lovastatin: Myositis, myalgias, rhabdomyolysis, acute renal failure
- Nifedipine: Increases risk of gingival hyperplasia

Drug-Herb interactions: Ginkgo (ginkgo biloba) was reported to protect liver cells from damage caused by cyclosporine in an *in vitro* experiment; however, human trials have not been reported. Avoid St John's wort, significantly reduces cyclosporine levels.

Half-Life

Solution or soft gelatin capsule (Sandimmune®): Biphasic, alpha phase: 1.4 hours and terminal phase 6-24 hours

Solution or soft gelatin capsule in a microemulsion (Neoral®): 8.4 hours

Education and Monitoring Issues

Patient Education: Use glass container for liquid solution (do not use plastic or styrofoam cup). Mixing with milk, chocolate milk, or orange juice at room temperature improves flavor. Mix thoroughly and drink at once. Take dose at the same time each day. You will be susceptible to infection; avoid crowds and exposure to any infectious diseases. Do not have any vaccinations without consulting prescriber. Practice good oral hygiene to reduce gum inflammation; see dentist regularly during treatment. Report acute headache; unusual hair growth or deepening of voice; mouth sores or swollen gums; persistent nausea, vomiting, or abdominal pain; muscle pain or cramping; unusual swelling of extremities, weight gain, or change in urination; or chest pain or rapid heartbeat.

Dietary Considerations: Grapefruit juice increases cyclosporine concentrations

Monitoring Parameters:

Cyclosporine trough levels, serum electrolytes, renal function, hepatic function, blood pressure, serum cholesterol

Psoriasis therapy: Biweekly monitoring of blood pressure, complete blood count, and levels of BUN, uric acid, potassium, lipids and magnesium during the first three months of treatment for psoriasis. Monthly monitoring is recommended after this initial period.

(Continued)

Cyclosporine *(Continued)*

Reference Range: Reference ranges are method dependent and specimen dependent; use the same analytical method consistently; trough levels should be obtained immediately prior to next dose

Method-dependent and specimen-dependent

Trough levels should be obtained:

Oral: 12-18 hours after dose (chronic usage)

I.V.: 12 hours after dose **or** immediately prior to next dose

Therapeutic range: Not absolutely defined, dependent on organ transplanted, time after transplant, organ function and CsA toxicity

General range of 100-400 ng/mL

Toxic level: Not well defined, nephrotoxicity may occur at any level

- **Cycofed® Pediatric** *see* Guaifenesin, Pseudoephedrine, and Codeine *on page 425*
- **Cycrin®** *see* Medroxyprogesterone Acetate *on page 558*
- **Cylert®** *see* Pemoline *on page 708*
- **Cylex® [OTC]** *see* Benzocaine *on page 98*
- **Cyomin®** *see* Cyanocobalamin *on page 233*

Cyproheptadine (si proe HEP ta deen)

Pharmacologic Class Antihistamine

U.S. Brand Names Periactin®

Generic Available Yes

Mechanism of Action A potent antihistamine and serotonin antagonist, competes with histamine for H_1-receptor sites on effector cells in the gastrointestinal tract, blood vessels, and respiratory tract

Use Perennial and seasonal allergic rhinitis and other allergic symptoms including urticaria

Unlabeled use: Appetite stimulation, blepharospasm, cluster headaches, migraine headaches, Nelson's syndrome, pruritus, schizophrenia, spinal cord damage associated spasticity, and tardive dyskinesia

USUAL DOSAGE Oral:

Children: 0.25 mg/kg/day in 2-3 divided doses or 8 mg/m²/day in 2-3 divided doses

2-6 years: 2 mg every 8-12 hours (not to exceed 12 mg/day)

7-14 years: 4 mg every 8-12 hours (not to exceed 16 mg/day)

Adults: 4-20 mg/day divided every 8 hours (not to exceed 0.5 mg/kg/day)

Dosing adjustment in hepatic impairment: Dosage should be reduced in patients with significant hepatic dysfunction

Dosage Forms SYR: 2 mg/5 mL with alcohol 5% (473 mL). **TAB:** 4 mg

Contraindications Hypersensitivity to cyproheptadine or any component; narrow-angle glaucoma, bladder neck obstruction, acute asthmatic attack, stenosing peptic ulcer, GI tract obstruction, those on MAO inhibitors; avoid use in premature and term newborns due to potential association with SIDS

Warnings/Precautions Do not use in neonates, safety and efficacy have not been established in children <2 years of age; symptomatic prostate hypertrophy; antihistamines are more likely to cause dizziness, excessive sedation, syncope, toxic confusion states, and hypotension in the elderly. In case reports, cyproheptadine has promoted weight gain in anorexic adults, though it has not been specifically studied in the elderly. All cases of weight loss or decreased appetite should be adequately assessed.

Pregnancy Risk Factor B

Adverse Reactions

>10%:

Central nervous system: Slight to moderate drowsiness

Respiratory: Thickening of bronchial secretions

1% to 10%:

Central nervous system: Headache, fatigue, nervousness, dizziness

Gastrointestinal: Appetite stimulation, nausea, diarrhea, abdominal pain, xerostomia

Neuromuscular & skeletal: Arthralgia

Respiratory: Pharyngitis

<1%: Allergic reactions, angioedema, bronchospasm, CNS stimulation, depression, edema, epistaxis, hemolytic anemia, hepatitis, leukopenia, myalgia, palpitations, paresthesia, photosensitivity, rash, sedation, seizures, tachycardia, thrombocytopenia

Drug Interactions Increased toxicity: MAO inhibitors → hallucinations

Alcohol Interactions Avoid use (may increase central nervous system depression)

Education and Monitoring Issues

Patient Education: Take as directed; do not exceed recommended dose. Avoid use of other depressants, alcohol, or sleep-inducing medications unless approved by prescriber. You may experience drowsiness or dizziness (use caution when driving or engaging in tasks requiring alertness until response to drug is known); or dry mouth, nausea, or abdominal pain (frequent small meals, frequent mouth care, chewing gum, or sucking hard candy may help). Report persistent sedation, confusion, or agitation; changes in urinary pattern; blurred vision; chest pain or palpitations; sore throat difficulty breathing or expectorating (thick secretions); or lack of improvement or worsening of condition.

♦ **Cystagon®** *see* Cysteamine *on page 241*

Cysteamine (sis TEE a meen)

Pharmacologic Class Anticystine Agent; Urinary Tract Product

U.S. Brand Names Cystagon®

Mechanism of Action Reacts with cystine in the lysosome to convert it to cysteine and to a cysteine-cysteamine mixed disulfide, both of which can then exit the lysosome in patients with cystinosis, an inherited defect of lysosomal transport

Use Orphan drug: Management of nephropathic cystinosis

USUAL DOSAGE Initiate therapy with 1/4 to 1/8 of maintenance dose; titrate slowly upward over 4-6 weeks

Children <12 years: Oral: Maintenance: 1.3 g/m²/day divided into 4 doses

Children >12 years and Adults (>110 lbs): 2 g/day in 4 divided doses; dosage may be increased to 1.95 g/m²/day if cystine levels are <1 nmol/1/2 cystine/mg protein, although intolerance and incidence of adverse events may be increased

Dosage Forms CAP: 50 mg, 150 mg

Contraindications Hypersensitivity to cysteamine or penicillamine

Warnings/Precautions Withhold cysteamine if a mild rash develops; restart at a lower dose and titrate to therapeutic dose; adjust cysteamine dose if CNS symptoms due to the drug develop, rather than the disease; adjust cysteamine dose downward if severe GI symptoms develop (most common during initiation of therapy)

Pregnancy Risk Factor C

Pregnancy Implications

Clinical effects on the fetus: Use only when the potential benefits outweigh the potential hazards to the fetus; in animal studies, cysteamine reduced the fertility of rats and offspring survival at very large doses

Breast-feeding/lactation: It is unknown whether cysteamine is excreted in breast milk; discontinue nursing or discontinue drug during lactation

Adverse Reactions

>5%:

Central nervous system: Fever, lethargy (11%)

Dermatologic: Rash (7%)

Gastrointestinal: Vomiting (35%), anorexia (31%), diarrhea (16%)

<5%:

Cardiovascular: Hypertension

Central nervous system: Somnolence, encephalopathy, headache, seizures, ataxia, confusion, dizziness, jitteriness, nervousness, impaired cognition, emotional changes, hallucinations, nightmares

Dermatologic: Urticaria

Endocrine & metabolic: Dehydration

Gastrointestinal: Bad breath, abdominal pain, dyspepsia, constipation, gastroenteritis, duodenitis, duodenal ulceration

Hematologic: Anemia, leukopenia

Hepatic: Abnormal LFTs

Neuromuscular & skeletal: Tremor, hyperkinesia

Otic: Decreased hearing

Education and Monitoring Issues

Patient Education: Take as directed. Maintain adequate hydration (2-3 L/day of fluids unless instructed to restrict fluid intake). It may be necessary to include other medication in treatment regimen. Periodic blood tests will need to be performed. You may experience dizziness, confusion, or lethargy; use caution with tasks that require alertness until response to drug is known. Report fever, gastric disturbances, or rash.

Monitoring Parameters: Blood counts and LFTs during therapy; monitor leukocyte cystine measurements every 3 months to determine adequate dosage and compliance (measure 5-6 hours after administration); monitor more frequently when switching salt forms

Reference Range: Leukocyte cystine: <1 nmol/1/2 cystine/mg protein

♦ **Cystistat** *see* Sodium Hyaluronate *on page 859*

♦ **Cystospaz®** *see* Hyoscyamine *on page 456*

♦ **Cystospaz-M®** *see* Hyoscyamine *on page 456*

♦ **Cytadren®** *see* Aminoglutethimide *on page 46*

♦ **CytoGam™** *see* Cytomegalovirus Immune Globulin (Intravenous-Human) *on page 241*

Cytomegalovirus Immune Globulin (Intravenous-Human)

(sye toe meg a low VYE rus i MYUN GLOB yoo lin in tra VEE nus-HYU man)

Pharmacologic Class Immune Globulin

U.S. Brand Names CytoGam™

Generic Available No

Mechanism of Action CMV-IGIV is a preparation of immunoglobulin G derived from pooled healthy blood donors with a high titer of CMV antibodies; administration provides a passive source of antibodies against cytomegalovirus

(Continued)

Cytomegalovirus Immune Globulin (Intravenous-Human) *(Continued)*

Use Attenuation of primary CMV disease associated with immunosuppressed recipients of kidney transplantation; especially indicated for CMV-negative recipients of CMV-positive donor; has been used as adjunct therapy in the treatment of CMV disease in immunocompromised patients

USUAL DOSAGE I.V.:

Dosing schedule:

Initial dose (within 72 hours after transplant): 150 mg/kg/dose

2, 4, 6, 8 weeks after transplant: 100 mg/kg/dose

12 and 16 weeks after transplant: 50 mg/kg/dose

Severe CMV pneumonia: Regimens of 400 mg/kg on days 1, 2, 7 or 8, followed by 200 mg/kg have been used

Administration rate: Administer at 15 mg/kg/hour initially, then increase to 30 mg/kg/hour after 30 minutes if no untoward reactions, then increase to 60 mg/kg/hour after another 30 minutes; volume not to exceed 75 mL/hour

Dosage Forms POWDER for inj, lyophilized, detergent treated: 2500 mg ±250 mg (50 mL)

Contraindications Hypersensitivity to any component, patients with selective immunoglobulin A deficiency (↑ potential for anaphylaxis); persons with IgA deficiency

Warnings/Precautions Studies indicate that product carries little or no risk for transmission of HIV; give with caution to patients with prior allergic reactions to human immunoglobulin preparations; do not perform skin testing

Pregnancy Risk Factor C

Adverse Reactions

1% to 10%:

Cardiovascular: Flushing of face

Gastrointestinal: Nausea, vomiting

Neuromuscular & skeletal: Muscle cramps, back pain

Respiratory: Wheezing

Miscellaneous: Diaphoresis

<1%: Aseptic meningitis syndrome, chills, dizziness, fever, headache, hypersensitivity reactions, tightness in the chest

Drug Interactions May inactivate live virus vaccines (eg, measles, mumps, rubella); if IGIV administration within 3 months of vaccination with live virus products, revaccinate

Education and Monitoring Issues

Patient Education: This medication can only be administered by infusion. You will be monitored closely during the infusion. If you experience nausea ask for assistance, do not get up alone. Do not have any vaccination for the next 3 months without consulting prescriber. Immediately report chills, muscle cramping, low back pain, chest pain or tightness, or difficulty breathing.

- **Cytotec®** *see* Misoprostol *on page 610*
- **Cytovene®** *see* Ganciclovir *on page 402*
- **Cytoxan® Injection** *see* Cyclophosphamide *on page 235*
- **Cytoxan® Oral** *see* Cyclophosphamide *on page 235*

Daclizumab (da KLIK su mab)

Pharmacologic Class Immunosuppressant Agent

U.S. Brand Names Zenapax®

Mechanism of Action Inhibits the binding of IL-2 to the high affinity IL-2 receptor, thus suppressing T cell activity against allografts. Its active ingredient, daclizumab, a humanized monoclonal antibody, binds to the alpha subunit of the high affinity interleukin-2 receptor (IL-2R) which is expressed on activated T cells.

Use Prophylaxis of acute organ rejection in patients receiving renal transplants; used as part of an immunosuppressive regimen that includes cyclosporine and corticosteroids

USUAL DOSAGE Children and Adults: IVPB: 1 mg/kg, used as part of an immunosuppressive regimen that includes cyclosporine and corticosteroids for a total of 5 doses; give the first dose ≤24 hours before transplantation. The 4 remaining doses should be administered at intervals of 14 days.

Dosing adjustment in renal impairment: None necessary

Dosage Forms INJ: 5 mg/mL (5 mL)

Contraindications Hypersensitivity to any component of the product

Warnings/Precautions Only prescribers experienced in immunosuppressive therapy and management of organ transplant patients should prescribe daclizumab. Manage patients receiving the drug in facilities equipped and staffed with adequate laboratory and supportive medical resources. Readministration of daclizumab after an initial course of therapy has not been studied in humans. The potential risks of such readministration, specifically those associated with immunosuppression or the occurrence of anaphylaxis/anaphylactoid reactions, are not known.

Pregnancy Risk Factor C

Adverse Reactions

>10%: Endocrine & metabolic: Hyperglycemia (32%)

1% to 10%:

Cardiovascular: Peripheral edema, hypertension, hypotension, aggravated hypertension, tachycardia, thrombosis, bleeding, chest pain

Central nervous system: Headache, dizziness, prickly sensation, depression, anxiety, fever, fatigue, insomnia, shivering, generalized weakness

Dermatologic: Impaired wound healing without infection, acne, pruritus, hirsutism, rash

Endocrine & metabolic: Fluid overload, diabetes mellitus, dehydration, edema

Gastrointestinal: Constipation, nausea, diarrhea, vomiting, abdominal pain, pyrosis, dyspepsia, abdominal distention, epigastric pain (not food-related), flatulence, gastritis, hemorrhoids

Genitourinary: Dysuria, urinary tract disorder, urinary retention

Hematologic: Urinary tract bleeding

Local: Injection site pain

Neuromuscular & skeletal: Tremor, musculoskeletal pain, back pain, arthralgia, leg cramps, myalgia, pain

Ocular: Blurred vision

Renal: Oliguria, renal tubular necrosis, renal damage, hydronephrosis, renal insufficiency

Respiratory: Dyspnea, pulmonary edema, coughing, atelectasis, congestion, rhinitis, pharyngitis, hypoxia, rales, abnormal breath sounds, pleural effusion

Miscellaneous: Increased diaphoresis, night sweats, post-traumatic pain

Half-Life 20 days

Manufacturer Roche Laboratories

Related Information

Pharmaceutical Manufacturers Directory *on page 1020*

- **D.A.II® Tablet** *see* Chlorpheniramine, Phenylephrine, and Methscopolamine *on page 186*
- **Dalacin® C [Hydrochloride]** *see* Clindamycin *on page 208*
- **Dalalone D.P.®** *see* Dexamethasone *on page 256*
- **Dalalone L.A.®** *see* Dexamethasone *on page 256*
- **Dallergy®** *see* Chlorpheniramine, Phenylephrine, and Methscopolamine *on page 186*
- **Dallergy-D® Syrup** *see* Chlorpheniramine and Phenylephrine *on page 186*
- **Dalmane®** *see* Flurazepam *on page 383*

Dalteparin (dal TE pa rin)

Pharmacologic Class Low Molecular Weight Heparin

U.S. Brand Names Fragmin®

Mechanism of Action Low molecular weight heparin analog with a molecular weight of 4000-6000 daltons; the commercial product contains 3% to 15% heparin with a molecular weight <3000 daltons, 65% to 78% with a molecular weight of 3000-8000 daltons and 14% to 26% with a molecular weight >8000 daltons; while dalteparin has been shown to inhibit both factor Xa and factor IIa (thrombin), the antithrombotic effect of dalteparin is characterized by a higher ratio of antifactor Xa to antifactor IIa activity (ratio = 4)

Use Prevention of deep vein thrombosis which may lead to pulmonary embolism, in patients requiring hip arthroplasty or abdominal surgery who are at risk for thromboembolism complications (ie, patients >40 years of age, obese patients, patients with malignancy, history of deep vein thrombosis or pulmonary embolism, and surgical procedures requiring general anesthesia and lasting >30 minutes); medical stabilization of patients with unstable coronary artery disease, such as unstable angina or non-Q-wave myocardial infarction

USUAL DOSAGE Adults: S.C.:

Low-moderate risk patients undergoing abdominal surgery: 2500 units 1-2 hours prior to surgery, then once daily for 5-10 days postoperatively

High risk patients undergoing abdominal surgery: 5000 units 1-2 hours prior to surgery and then once daily for 5-10 days postoperatively

Patients undergoing total hip surgery: 2500 units 1-2 hours prior to surgery, then 2500 units 6 hours after surgery (evening of the day of surgery), followed by 5000 units once daily for 7-10 days

Treatment of DVT: 100 units/kg twice daily or 200 units/kg once daily

Patients with unstable angina or non-Q-wave myocardial infarction: 120 units/kg body weight (maximum dose: 10,000 units) every 12 hours for 5-8 days with concurrent aspirin therapy; discontinue dalteparin once patient is clinically stable

Dosage Forms INJ: Prefilled syringe: Antifactor Xa 2500 units per 0.2 mL; Antifactor Xa 5000 units per 0.2 mL; Multidose vial: 95,000 international units

Contraindications Hypersensitivity to dalteparin or other low-molecular weight heparins; cerebrovascular disease or other active hemorrhage; cerebral aneurysm; severe uncontrolled hypertension

Warnings/Precautions Use with caution in patients with pre-existing thrombocytopenia, recent childbirth, subacute bacterial endocarditis, peptic ulcer disease, pericarditis or pericardial effusion, liver or renal function impairment, recent lumbar puncture, vasculitis, concurrent use of aspirin (increased bleeding risk), previous hypersensitivity to heparin,

(Continued)

Dalteparin *(Continued)*

heparin-associated thrombocytopenia. Patients should be observed closely for bleeding if dalteparin is administered during or immediately following diagnostic lumbar puncture, epidural anesthesia, or spinal anesthesia. If thromboembolism develops despite dalteparin prophylaxis, dalteparin should be discontinued and appropriate treatment should be initiated.

Pregnancy Risk Factor B

Adverse Reactions

1% to 10%

Hematologic: Bleeding (2.7% to 4.6%), wound hematoma (0.1% to 3.4%)

Local: Pain at injection site (up to 12%), injection site hematoma (0.2% to 7.1%)

<1% (limited to important or life-threatening symptoms): Thrombocytopenia (including heparin-induced thrombocytopenia), allergic reaction (fever, pruritus, rash, injections site reaction, bullous eruption), anaphylactoid reaction, injection site hematoma, operative site bleeding, gastrointestinal bleeding, skin necrosis. Spinal or epidural hematomas can occur following neuraxial anesthesia or spinal puncture, resulting in paralysis. Risk is increased in patients with indwelling epidural catheters or concomitant use of other drugs affecting hemostasis, osteoporosis (3-6 month use).

Drug Interactions

Drugs which affect platelet function (eg, aspirin, NSAIDs, dipyridamole, ticlopidine, clopidogrel) may potentiate the risk of hemorrhage

Thrombolytic agents increase the risk of hemorrhage

Warfarin: Risk of bleeding may be increased during concurrent therapy Dalteparin is commonly continued during the initiation of warfarin therapy to assure anticoagulation and to protect against possible transient hypercoagulability

Onset 1-2 hours

Duration >12 hours

Half-Life 2-5 hours

Education and Monitoring Issues

Patient Education: This drug can only be administered by injection. You may have a tendency to bleed easily while taking this drug; brush teeth with soft brush, floss with waxed floss, use electric razor, avoid scissors or sharp knives and potentially harmful activities. Report unusual fever; unusual bleeding or bruising (bleeding gums, nosebleed, blood in urine, dark stool); pain in joints or back; severe head pain; skin rash; or redness, swelling, or pain at injection site.

Monitoring Parameters: Periodic CBC including platelet count; stool occult blood tests; monitoring of PT and PTT is not necessary

Reference Range: Therapeutic plasma anti-Xa levels (antifactor Xa): 0.1-0.6 units/mL (antithrombotic activity); activated partial thromboplastin time (APTT) is not considered useful for dalteparin monitoring

Manufacturer Pharmacia & Upjohn

Related Information

Pharmaceutical Manufacturers Directory *on page 1020*

♦ **Damason-P®** *see* Hydrocodone and Aspirin *on page 445*

Danaparoid (da NAP a roid)

Pharmacologic Class Anticoagulant; Low Molecular Weight Heparin

U.S. Brand Names Orgaran®

Use Prevention of postoperative deep vein thrombosis following elective hip replacement surgery

Unlabeled use: Systemic anticoagulation for patients with heparin-induced thrombocytopenia: Factor Xa inhibition is used to monitor degree of anticoagulation if necessary

USUAL DOSAGE S.C.:

Children: Safety and effectiveness have not been established

Adults: 750 anti-Xa units twice daily; beginning 1-4 hours before surgery and then not sooner than 2 hours after surgery and every 12 hours until the risk of DVT has diminished, the average duration of therapy is 7-10 days

Treatment: See table.

Dosing adjustment in elderly and severe renal impairment: Adjustment may be necessary; patients with serum creatinine levels ≥2.0 mg/dL should be carefully monitored

Hemodialysis: See table

Dosage Forms INJ: 750 anti-Xa units/0.6 mL

Contraindications Patients with severe hemorrhagic diathesis including active major bleeding, hemorrhagic stroke in the acute phase, hemophilia and idiopathic thrombocytopenic purpura; type II thrombocytopenia associated with a positive *in vitro* test for antiplatelet antibody in the presence of danaparoid, hypersensitivity to danaparoid or known hypersensitivity to pork products

Adult Danaparoid Treatment Dosing Regimens

	Body Weight (kg)	I.V. Bolus aFXaU	Long–Term Infusion aFXaU	Level of aFXaU/mL	Monitoring
Deep Vein Thrombosis OR Acute Pulmonary Embolism	<55 55-90 >90	1250 2500 3750	400 units/h over 4 h then 300 units/h over 4 h, then 150-200 units/h maintenance dose	0.5-0.8	Days 1-3 daily, then every alternate day
Deep Vein Thrombosis OR Pulmonary Embolism >5 d old	<90 >90	1250 1250	S.C.: 3 x 750/d S.C.: 3 x 1250/d	<0.5	Not necessary
Embolectomy	<90 >90 and high risk	2500 preoperatively 2500 preoperatively	S.C.: 2 x 1250/d postoperatively 750 units/20 mL NaCl perioperatively, arterial irrigation if necessary	<0.4 0.5-0.8	Not necessary Days 1-3 daily, then every alternate day
Peripheral Arterial Bypass		2500 preoperatively	150-200 units/h	0.5-0.8	Days 1-3 daily, then every alternate day
Cardiac Catheter	<90 >90	2500 preoperatively 3750 preoperatively			
Surgery (excluding vascular)			S.C.: 750, 1-4 h preoperatively S.C.: 750, 2-5 h postoperatively, then 2 x 750/d	<0.35	Not necessary

Haemodialysis With Danaparoid Sodium

Dialysis on alternate days	**Dosage prior to dialysis in aFXaU (dosage for body wt <55 kg)**	
First dialysis	3750 (2500)	
Second dialysis	3750 (2000)	
Further dialysis:		
aFXa level before dialysis (eg, day 5)	**Bolus before next dialysis, aFXaU (eg, day 7)**	**aFXa level during dialysis**
<0.3	3000 (<55 kg 2000)	0.5-0.8
0.3-0.35	2500 (2000)	
0.35-0.4	2000 (1500)	
>0.4	0	
	if fibrin strands occur, 1500 aFXaU I.V.	
Monitoring: 30 minutes before dialysis and after 4 hours of dialysis		
Daily Dialysis		
First dialysis	3750 (2500)	
Second dialysis	2500 (2000)	
Further dialyses	See above	
As with "dialysis on alternate days", always take the aFXa activity preceding the previous dialysis as a basis for the current dosage.		

Warnings/Precautions Do not administer intramuscularly; use with extreme caution in patients with a history of bacterial endocarditis, hemorrhagic stroke, recent CNS or ophthalmological surgery, bleeding diathesis, uncontrolled arterial hypertension, or a history of recent gastrointestinal ulceration and hemorrhage. Danaparoid shows a low cross-sensitivity with antiplatelet antibodies in individuals with type II heparin-induced thrombocytopenia. This product contains sodium sulfite which may cause allergic-type reactions, including anaphylactic symptoms and life-threatening asthmatic episodes in susceptible people; this is seen more frequently in asthmatics.

Carefully monitor patients receiving low molecular weight heparins or heparinoids. These drugs, when used concurrently with spinal or epidural anesthesia or spinal puncture, may cause bleeding or hematomas within the spinal column. Increased pressure on the spinal cord may result in permanent paralysis if not detected and treated immediately.
(Continued)

Danaparoid *(Continued)*

Note: Danaparoid is **not** effectively antagonized by protamine sulfate. No other antidote is available, so extreme caution is needed in monitoring dose given and resulting Xa inhibition effect.

Pregnancy Risk Factor B

Adverse Reactions As with all anticoagulants, bleeding is the major adverse effect of danaparoid. Hemorrhage may occur at virtually any site. Risk is dependent on multiple variables.

>10%:
- Central nervous system: Fever (22.2%)
- Gastrointestinal: Nausea (4.1% to 14.3%), constipation (3.5% to 11.3%)

1% to 10%:
- Central nervous system: Insomnia (3.1%), headache (2.6%), asthenia (2.3%), dizziness (2.3%), pain (8.7%)
- Cardiovascular: Peripheral edema (3.3%), edema (2.6%)
- Dermatologic: Rash (2.1% to 4.8%), pruritus (3.9%)
- Gastrointestinal: Vomiting (2.9%)
- Genitourinary: Urinary tract infection (2.6% to 4.0%), urinary retention (2.0%)
- Hematologic: Anemia (2.2%)
- Local: Injection site pain (7.6% to 13.7%), injection site hematoma (5%)
- Neuromuscular & skeletal: Joint disorder (2.6%)
- Miscellaneous: Infection (2.1%)

<1% (limited to important or life-threatening symptoms): Spinal or epidural hematomas can occur following neuraxial anesthesia or spinal puncture, resulting in paralysis. Risk is increased in patients with indwelling epidural catheters or concomitant use of other drugs affecting hemostasis, thrombocytopenia, hyperkalemia, wound infection, skin rash, allergic reaction.

Drug Interactions
- Drugs which affect platelet function (eg, aspirin, NSAIDs, dipyridamole, ticlopidine, clopidogrel) may potentiate the risk of hemorrhage
- Thrombolytic agents increase the risk of hemorrhage
- Warfarin (and other oral anticoagulants) may increase the risk of bleeding with danaparoid

Onset Maximum antifactor Xa and antithrombin (antifactor IIa) activities occur 2-5 hours after S.C. administration

Half-Life Plasma: Mean terminal half-life: ~24 hours

Education and Monitoring Issues

Patient Education: This drug can only be administered by injection. You may have a tendency to bleed easily while taking this drug; brush teeth with soft brush, floss with waxed floss, use electric razor, avoid scissors or sharp knives and potentially harmful activities. Report unusual swelling of extremities or sudden increase in weight; unusual fever; persistent nausea, vomiting, or GI upset; unusual bleeding or bruising (bleeding gums, nosebleed, blood in urine, dark stool); pain in joints or back; pain or itching on urination; skin rash; or redness, swelling, or pain at injection site.

Monitoring Parameters: Platelets, occult blood, and anti-Xa activity, if available; the monitoring of PT and/or PTT is not necessary

Manufacturer Organon, Inc

Related Information

Pharmaceutical Manufacturers Directory *on page 1020*

Danazol (DA na zole)

Pharmacologic Class Androgen

U.S. Brand Names Danocrine®

Generic Available No

Mechanism of Action Suppresses pituitary output of follicle-stimulating hormone and luteinizing hormone that causes regression and atrophy of normal and ectopic endometrial tissue; decreases rate of growth of abnormal breast tissue; reduces attacks associated with hereditary angioedema by increasing levels of C4 component of complement

Use Treatment of endometriosis, fibrocystic breast disease, and hereditary angioedema

USUAL DOSAGE Adults: Oral:
- Female: Endometriosis: Initial: 200-400 mg/day in 2 divided doses for mild disease; individualize dosage. Usual maintenance dose: 800 mg/day in 2 divided doses to achieve amenorrhea and rapid response to painful symptoms. Continue therapy uninterrupted for 3-6 months (up to 9 months).
- Female: Fibrocystic breast disease: Range: 10-400 mg/day in 2 divided doses
- Male/Female: Hereditary angioedema: Initial: 200 mg 2-3 times/day; after favorable response, decrease the dosage by 50% or less at intervals of 1-3 months or longer if the frequency of attacks dictates. If an attack occurs, increase the dosage by up to 200 mg/day.

Dosage Forms CAP: 50 mg, 100 mg, 200 mg

Contraindications Undiagnosed genital bleeding, hypersensitivity to danazol or any component; pregnancy

Warnings/Precautions Use with caution in patients with seizure disorders, migraine, or conditions influenced by edema; impaired hepatic, renal, or cardiac disease, pregnancy, lactation

Pregnancy Risk Factor X

Adverse Reactions

>10%:

Cardiovascular: Edema

Dermatologic: Oily skin, acne, hirsutism

Endocrine & metabolic: Fluid retention, breakthrough bleeding, irregular menstrual periods, decreased breast size

Gastrointestinal: Weight gain

Hepatic: Hepatic impairment

Miscellaneous: Voice deepening

1% to 10%:

Endocrine & metabolic: Virilization, androgenic effects, amenorrhea, hypoestrogenism

Neuromuscular & skeletal: Weakness

<1%: Benign intracranial hypertension, bleeding gums, carpal tunnel syndrome, cholestatic jaundice, dizziness, enlarged clitoris, headache, monilial vaginitis, pancreatitis, photosensitivity, skin rashes, testicular atrophy

Drug Interactions CYP3A3/4 enzyme inhibitor

Increased toxicity: Decreased insulin requirements; warfarin may increase anticoagulant effects

Onset Within 4 weeks following daily doses

Half-Life 4.5 hours (variable)

Education and Monitoring Issues

Patient Education: Take as directed; do not discontinue without consulting prescriber. Therapy may take up to several months depending on purpose for therapy. Diabetics should monitor serum glucose closely and notify prescriber of changes; this medication can alter glycemic response. You may experience acne, growth of body hair, deepening of voice, loss of libido, impotence, or menstrual irregularity (usually reversible). Report changes in menstrual pattern; deepening of voice or unusual growth of body hair; persistent penile erections; fluid retention (swelling of ankles, feet, or hands, difficulty breathing, or sudden weight gain); change in color of urine or stool; yellowing of eyes or skin; unusual bruising or bleeding; or other adverse reactions.

Manufacturer Sanofi Winthrop Pharmaceuticals

Related Information

Pharmaceutical Manufacturers Directory *on page 1020*

♦ **Danocrine®** *see* Danazol *on page 246*

♦ **Dantrium®** *see* Dantrolene *on page 247*

Dantrolene (DAN troe leen)

Pharmacologic Class Skeletal Muscle Relaxant

U.S. Brand Names Dantrium®

Generic Available No

Mechanism of Action Acts directly on skeletal muscle by interfering with release of calcium ion from the sarcoplasmic reticulum; prevents or reduces the increase in myoplasmic calcium ion concentration that activates the acute catabolic processes associated with malignant hyperthermia

Use Treatment of spasticity associated with spinal cord injury, stroke, cerebral palsy, or multiple sclerosis; also used as treatment of malignant hyperthermia

USUAL DOSAGE

Spasticity: Oral:

Children: Initial: 0.5 mg/kg/dose twice daily, increase frequency to 3-4 times/day at 4- to 7-day intervals, then increase dose by 0.5 mg/kg to a maximum of 3 mg/kg/dose 2-4 times/day up to 400 mg/day

Adults: 25 mg/day to start, increase frequency to 2-4 times/day, then increase dose by 25 mg every 4-7 days to a maximum of 100 mg 2-4 times/day or 400 mg/day

Malignant hyperthermia: Children and Adults:

Oral: 4-8 mg/kg/day in 4 divided doses

Preoperative prophylaxis: Begin 1-2 days prior to surgery with last dose 3-4 hours prior to surgery

I.V.: 1 mg/kg; may repeat dose up to cumulative dose of 10 mg/kg (mean effective dose is 2.5 mg/kg), then switch to oral dosage

Preoperative: 2.5 mg/kg ~1¼ hours prior to anesthesia and infused over 1 hour with additional doses as needed and individualized

Dosage Forms CAP: 25 mg, 50 mg, 100 mg. **POWDER for inj:** 20 mg

Contraindications Active hepatic disease; should not be used where spasticity is used to maintain posture or balance

Warnings/Precautions Use with caution in patients with impaired cardiac function or impaired pulmonary function; has potential for hepatotoxicity; overt hepatitis has been most frequently observed between the third and twelfth month of therapy; hepatic injury appears to be greater in females and in patients >35 years of age

(Continued)

Dantrolene *(Continued)*

Pregnancy Risk Factor C

Adverse Reactions

>10%:

Central nervous system: Drowsiness, dizziness, lightheadedness, fatigue

Dermatologic: Rash

Gastrointestinal: Diarrhea (mild), nausea, vomiting

Neuromuscular & skeletal: Muscle weakness

1% to 10%:

Cardiovascular: Pleural effusion with pericarditis

Central nervous system: Chills, fever, headache, insomnia, nervousness, mental depression

Gastrointestinal: Diarrhea (severe), constipation, anorexia, stomach cramps

Ocular: Blurred vision

Respiratory: Respiratory depression

<1%: Confusion, hepatitis, seizures

Drug Interactions Increased toxicity: Estrogens (hepatotoxicity), CNS depressants (sedation), MAO inhibitors, phenothiazines, clindamycin (increased neuromuscular blockade), verapamil (hyperkalemia and cardiac depression), warfarin, clofibrate and tolbutamide

Alcohol Interactions Avoid use (may increase central nervous system depression)

Half-Life 8.7 hours

Education and Monitoring Issues

Patient Education: Take exactly as directed. Do not increase dose or discontinue without consulting prescriber. Do not use alcohol, prescriptive or OTC antidepressants, sedatives, or pain medications without consulting prescriber. You may experience drowsiness, dizziness, lightheadedness (avoid driving or engaging in tasks that require alertness until response to drug is known); nausea or vomiting (small, frequent meals, frequent mouth care, or sucking hard candy may help); or diarrhea (buttermilk, boiled milk, or yogurt may help). Report excessive confusion; drowsiness or mental agitation; chest pain, palpitations, or difficulty breathing; skin rash; or vision disturbances.

Monitoring Parameters: Motor performance should be monitored for therapeutic outcomes; nausea, vomiting, and liver function tests should be monitored for potential hepatotoxicity; intravenous administration requires cardiac monitor and blood pressure monitor

Manufacturer Proctor & Gamble Co

Related Information

Pharmaceutical Manufacturers Directory *on page 1020*

Dapiprazole (DA pi pray zole)

Pharmacologic Class Alpha$_1$ Blockers

U.S. Brand Names Rēv-Eyes™

Use Reverse dilation due to drugs (adrenergic or parasympathomimetic) after eye exams

USUAL DOSAGE Adults: Administer 2 drops followed 5 minutes later by an additional 2 drops applied to the conjunctiva of each eye; should not be used more frequently than once a week in the same patient

Contraindications Contraindicated in the presence of conditions where miosis is unacceptable, such as acute iritis and in patients with a history of hypersensitivity to any component of the formulation

Pregnancy Risk Factor B

Dapsone (DAP sone)

Pharmacologic Class Antibiotic, Miscellaneous

U.S. Brand Names Avlosulfon®

Generic Available No

Mechanism of Action Competitive antagonist of para-aminobenzoic acid (PABA) and prevents normal bacterial utilization of PABA for the synthesis of folic acid

Use Treatment of leprosy and dermatitis herpetiformis (infections caused by *Mycobacterium leprae*)

Prophylaxis of toxoplasmosis in severely immunocompromised patients; alternative agent for *Pneumocystis carinii* pneumonia prophylaxis (given alone) and treatment (given with trimethoprim)

May be useful in relapsing polychondritis, prophylaxis of malaria, inflammatory bowel disorders, leishmaniasis, rheumatic/connective tissue disorders, brown recluse spider bites

USUAL DOSAGE Oral:

Leprosy:

Children: 1-2 mg/kg/24 hours, up to a maximum of 100 mg/day

Adults: 50-100 mg/day for 3-10 years

Dermatitis herpetiformis: Adults: Start at 50 mg/day, increase to 300 mg/day, or higher to achieve full control, reduce dosage to minimum level as soon as possible

Prophylaxis of *Pneumocystis carinii* pneumonia:

Children >1 month: 1 mg/kg/day; maximum: 100 mg

Adults: 100 mg/day

Treatment of *Pneumocystis carinii* pneumonia: Adults: 100 mg/day in combination with trimethoprim (15-20 mg/kg/day) for 21 days

Dosing in renal impairment: No specific guidelines are available

Dosage Forms TAB: 25 mg, 100 mg

Contraindications Hypersensitivity to dapsone or any component

Warnings/Precautions Use with caution in patients with severe anemia, G-6-PD, methemoglobin reductase or hemoglobin M deficiency; hypersensitivity to other sulfonamides; aplastic anemia, agranulocytosis and other severe blood dyscrasias have resulted in death; monitor carefully; treat severe anemia prior to therapy; serious dermatologic reactions (including toxic epidermal necrolysis) are rare but potential occurrences; sulfone reactions may also occur as potentially fatal hypersensitivity reactions; these, but not leprosy reactional states, require drug discontinuation; dapsone is carcinogenic in small animals

Pregnancy Risk Factor C

Adverse Reactions

1% to 10%: Hematologic: Hemolysis, methemoglobinemia

<1%: Reactional states (ie, abrupt changes in clinical activity occurring during any leprosy treatment; classified as reversal of erythema nodosum leprosum reactions); agranulocytosis, anemia, blurred vision, cholestatic jaundice, exfoliative dermatitis, headache, hepatitis, insomnia, leukopenia, nausea, peripheral neuropathy (usually in nonleprosy patients), photosensitivity, SLE, tinnitus, vomiting

Drug Interactions CYP2C9, 2E1, and 3A3/4 enzyme substrate

Decreased effect/levels: Para-aminobenzoic acid, didanosine, and rifampin decrease dapsone effects

Increased toxicity: Folic acid antagonists may increase the risk of hematologic reactions of dapsone; probenecid decreases dapsone excretion; trimethoprim with dapsone may increase toxic effects of both drugs

Levels may be increased by protease inhibitors (amprenavir, nelfinavir, ritonavir)

Half-Life 30 hours (range: 10-50 hours)

Education and Monitoring Issues

Patient Education: Take as directed, for full term of therapy (treatment for leprosy may take 3-10 years). Do not take with antacids, alkaline foods, or drugs (may decrease dapsone absorption). Frequent blood tests may be required during therapy. Discontinue if rash develops and notify prescriber. Report persistent sore throat, fever, chills; constant fatigue; yellowing of skin or eyes; or easy bruising or bleeding.

Monitoring Parameters: Monitor patient for signs of jaundice and hemolysis; CBC weekly for first month, monthly for 6 months, and semiannually thereafter

Related Information

Antimicrobial Drugs of Choice *on page 1182*

- **Daraprim®** *see* Pyrimethamine *on page 797*
- **Darvocet-N®** *see* Propoxyphene and Acetaminophen *on page 786*
- **Darvocet-N® 100** *see* Propoxyphene and Acetaminophen *on page 786*
- **Darvon®** *see* Propoxyphene *on page 784*
- **Darvon® Compound-65 Pulvules®** *see* Propoxyphene and Aspirin *on page 786*
- **Darvon-N®** *see* Propoxyphene *on page 784*
- **Darvon-N® Compound (contains caffeine)** *see* Propoxyphene and Aspirin *on page 786*
- **Darvon-N® With ASA** *see* Propoxyphene and Aspirin *on page 786*
- **Daskil®** *see* Terbinafine *on page 896*
- **Daypro™** *see* Oxaprozin *on page 685*
- **DC 240® Softgels® [OTC]** *see* Docusate *on page 290*
- **DDAVP® Nasal Spray** *see* Desmopressin Acetate *on page 254*
- **Debrisan® [OTC]** *see* Dextranomer *on page 259*
- **Debrox® Otic [OTC]** *see* Carbamide Peroxide *on page 139*
- **Decaderm®** *see* Dexamethasone *on page 256*
- **Decadron®** *see* Dexamethasone *on page 256*
- **Decadron®-LA** *see* Dexamethasone *on page 256*
- **Decadron® Turbinaire®** *see* Dexamethasone *on page 256*
- **Deca-Durabolin® Injection** *see* Nandrolone *on page 635*
- **Decaject-L.A.®** *see* Dexamethasone *on page 256*
- **Decaspray®** *see* Dexamethasone *on page 256*
- **Declomycin®** *see* Demeclocycline *on page 251*
- **Decofed® Syrup [OTC]** *see* Pseudoephedrine *on page 792*
- **Decohistine® DH** *see* Chlorpheniramine, Pseudoephedrine, and Codeine *on page 187*
- **Decohistine® Expectorant** *see* Guaifenesin, Pseudoephedrine, and Codeine *on page 425*
- **Deconsal® Sprinkle®** *see* Guaifenesin and Phenylephrine *on page 425*
- **Degest® 2 [OTC]** *see* Naphazoline *on page 636*

- **Dehydral®** *see* Methenamine *on page 579*
- **Dekasol-L.A.®** *see* Dexamethasone *on page 256*
- **Deladumone® Injection** *see* Estradiol and Testosterone *on page 329*
- **Delatest® Injection** *see* Testosterone *on page 898*
- **Delatestryl® Injection** *see* Testosterone *on page 898*

Delavirdine (de la VIR deen)

Pharmacologic Class Antiretroviral Agent, Reverse Transcriptase Inhibitor (Non-Nucleoside)

U.S. Brand Names Rescriptor®

Use Treatment of HIV-1 infection in combination with at least two additional antiretroviral agents

USUAL DOSAGE Adults: Oral: 400 mg 3 times/day

Contraindications Known hypersensitivity to delavirdine or any components

Warnings/Precautions Avoid use with terfenadine, astemizole, benzodiazepines, clarithromycin, dapsone, cisapride, rifabutin, rifampin; use with caution in patients with hepatic or renal dysfunction; due to rapid emergence of resistance, delavirdine should not be used as monotherapy; cross-resistance may be conferred to other non-nucleoside reverse transcriptase inhibitors, although potential for cross-resistance with protease inhibitors is low. Long-term effects of delavirdine are not known. Safety and efficacy have not been established in children. Rash, which occurs frequently, may require discontinuation of therapy; usually occurs within 1-3 weeks and lasts <2 weeks. Most patients may resume therapy following a treatment interruption.

Pregnancy Risk Factor C

Adverse Reactions >2%:

Central nervous system: Headache, fatigue
Dermatologic: Rash, pruritus
Gastrointestinal: Nausea, diarrhea, vomiting
Metabolic: Increased ALT/AST

Drug Interactions CYP2D6 and 3A3/4 enzyme substrate; CYP2D6 and 3A3/4 enzyme inhibitor

Increased plasma concentrations of delavirdine: Clarithromycin, ketoconazole, fluoxetine

Decreased plasma concentrations of delavirdine: Carbamazepine, phenobarbital, phenytoin, rifabutin, rifampin, didanosine, saquinavir

Decreased absorption of delavirdine: Antacids, histamine-2 receptor antagonists, didanosine

Delavirdine increases plasma concentrations of: Indinavir, saquinavir, terfenadine, astemizole, clarithromycin, dapsone, rifabutin, ergot derivatives, alprazolam, midazolam, triazolam, dihydropyridines, cisapride, quinidine, warfarin, sildenafil, amphotericin, antiarrhythmics, nonsedating antihistamines, sedative-hypnotics, calcium channel blockers, amprenavir

Delavirdine decreases plasma concentrations of: Didanosine

Manufacturer Pharmacia & Upjohn

Related Information

Antiretroviral Therapy for HIV Infection *on page 1190*
Pharmaceutical Manufacturers Directory *on page 1020*

- **Delaxin®** *see* Methocarbamol *on page 581*
- **Delcort®** *see* Hydrocortisone *on page 447*
- **Delestrogen® Injection** *see* Estradiol *on page 327*
- **Delta-Cortef® Oral** *see* Prednisolone *on page 762*
- **Deltasone®** *see* Prednisone *on page 763*
- **Delta-Tritex®** *see* Triamcinolone *on page 944*
- **Del-Vi-A®** *see* Vitamin A *on page 978*
- **Demadex®** *see* Torsemide *on page 934*

Demecarium (dem e KARE ee um)

Pharmacologic Class Cholinesterase Inhibitor

U.S. Brand Names Humorsol® Ophthalmic

Use Management of chronic simple glaucoma, chronic and acute angle-closure glaucoma; strabismus

USUAL DOSAGE Children/Adults: Ophthalmic:

Glaucoma: Instill 1 drop into eyes twice weekly to a maximum dosage of 1 or 2 drops twice daily for up to 4 months

Strabismus:

Diagnosis: Instill 1 drop daily for 2 weeks, then 1 drop every 2 days for 2-3 weeks. If eyes become straighter, an accommodative factor is demonstrated.

Therapy: Instill not more than 1 drop at a time in both eyes every day for 2-3 weeks. Then reduce dosage to 1 drop every other day for 3-4 weeks and re-evaluate. Continue at 1 drop every 2 days to 1 drop twice a week and evaluate the patient's condition every 4-12 weeks. If improvement continues, reduce dose to 1 drop once a week and eventually off of medication. Discontinue therapy after 4 months if control of the condition still requires 1 drop every 2 days.

Contraindications Hypersensitivity to demecarium or any component, acute inflammatory disease of anterior chamber; pregnancy

Pregnancy Risk Factor C

Demeclocycline (dem e kloe SYE kleen)

Pharmacologic Class Antibiotic, Tetracycline Derivative

U.S. Brand Names Declomycin®

Generic Available No

Mechanism of Action Inhibits protein synthesis by binding with the 30S and possibly the 50S ribosomal subunit(s) of susceptible bacteria; may also cause alterations in the cytoplasmic membrane; inhibits the action of ADH in patients with chronic SIADH

Use Treatment of susceptible bacterial infections (acne, gonorrhea, pertussis and urinary tract infections) caused by both gram-negative and gram-positive organisms; used when penicillin is contraindicated (other agents are preferred); treatment of chronic syndrome of inappropriate secretion of antidiuretic hormone (SIADH)

USUAL DOSAGE Oral:

Children ≥8 years: 8-12 mg/kg/day divided every 6-12 hours

Adults: 150 mg 4 times/day or 300 mg twice daily

Uncomplicated gonorrhea (penicillin sensitive): 600 mg stat, 300 mg every 12 hours for 4 days (3 g total)

SIADH: 900-1200 mg/day or 13-15 mg/kg/day divided every 6-8 hours initially, then decrease to 600-900 mg/day

Dosing adjustment/comments in renal/hepatic impairment: Should be avoided in patients with renal/hepatic dysfunction

Dosage Forms CAP: 150 mg. **TAB:** 150 mg, 300 mg

Contraindications Hypersensitivity to demeclocycline, tetracyclines, or any component

Warnings/Precautions Do not administer to children <9 years of age; photosensitivity reactions occur frequently with this drug, avoid prolonged exposure to sunlight, do not use tanning equipment

Pregnancy Risk Factor D

Adverse Reactions

1% to 10%:

Dermatologic: Photosensitivity

Gastrointestinal: Nausea, diarrhea

<1%: Abdominal cramps, acute renal failure, anaphylaxis, anorexia, azotemia, bulging fontanels in infants, dermatologic effects, diabetes insipidus syndrome, esophagitis, exfoliative dermatitis, increased intracranial pressure, paresthesia, pericarditis, pigmentation of nails, pruritus, superinfections, vomiting

Drug Interactions

Decreased effect with antacids (aluminum, calcium, zinc, or magnesium), bismuth salts, sodium bicarbonate, barbiturates, carbamazepine, hydantoins

Decreased effect of oral contraceptives

Increased effect of warfarin

Drug-Herb interactions: Berberine is a chemical extracted from **goldenseal** (*Hydrastis canadensis*), **barberry** (*Berberis vulgaris*), and **Oregon grape** (*Berberis aquifolium*), which has been shown to have antibacterial activity. One double-blind study found that giving berberine concurrently with tetracycline reduced the efficacy of tetracycline in the treatment of cholera. Berberine may decrease absorption of tetracycline. Another double-blind trial did not find that berberine interfered with tetracycline in cholera patients. Until more studies are completed, berberine-containing herbs should not be taken concomitantly with tetracyclines.

Onset Onset of action for diuresis in SIADH: Several days

Half-Life Reduced renal function: 10-17 hours

Education and Monitoring Issues

Patient Education: Preferable to take on an empty stomach (1 hour before or 2 hours after meals). Take at regularly scheduled times around-the-clock. Avoid antacids, iron, or dairy products within 2 hours of taking demeclocycline. You may experience photosensitivity (use sunscreen, wear protective clothing and eyewear, avoid direct sunlight); dizziness or lightheadedness (use caution when driving or engaging in tasks that require alertness until response to drug is known); nausea/vomiting (frequent small meals, frequent mouth care, sucking lozenges, or chewing gum may help); or diarrhea (buttermilk, yogurt, or boiled milk may help). If diabetic, drug may cause false tests with Clinitest® urine glucose monitoring; use of glucose oxidase methods (Clinistix®) or serum glucose monitoring is preferable. Report rash or intense itching; yellowing of skin or eyes; change in color of urine or stools; fever or chills; dark urine or pale stools; vaginal itching or discharge; foul-smelling stools; excessive thirst or urination; acute headache; unresolved diarrhea; or difficulty breathing.

Monitoring Parameters: CBC, renal and hepatic function

Manufacturer Lederle Laboratories

(Continued)

Demeclocycline *(Continued)*

Related Information

Pharmaceutical Manufacturers Directory *on page 1020*

- **Demerol®** *see* Meperidine *on page 563*
- **Demulen®** *see* Ethinyl Estradiol and Ethynodiol Diacetate *on page 341*
- **Denavir™** *see* Penciclovir *on page 708*
- **Depacon™** *see* Valproic Acid and Derivatives *on page 967*
- **Depakene®** *see* Valproic Acid and Derivatives *on page 967*
- **Depakote®** *see* Valproic Acid and Derivatives *on page 967*
- **depAndrogyn® Injection** *see* Estradiol and Testosterone *on page 329*
- **depAndro® Injection** *see* Testosterone *on page 898*
- **Depen®** *see* Penicillamine *on page 708*
- **depGynogen® Injection** *see* Estradiol *on page 327*
- **depMedalone® Injection** *see* Methylprednisolone *on page 589*
- **Depo®-Estradiol Injection** *see* Estradiol *on page 327*
- **Depogen® Injection** *see* Estradiol *on page 327*
- **Depoject® Injection** *see* Methylprednisolone *on page 589*
- **Depo-Medrol® Injection** *see* Methylprednisolone *on page 589*
- **Deponit® Patch** *see* Nitroglycerin *on page 659*
- **Depopred® Injection** *see* Methylprednisolone *on page 589*
- **Depo-Provera® Injection** *see* Medroxyprogesterone Acetate *on page 558*
- **Depo-Testadiol® Injection** *see* Estradiol and Testosterone *on page 329*
- **Depotest® Injection** *see* Testosterone *on page 898*
- **Depotestogen® Injection** *see* Estradiol and Testosterone *on page 329*
- **Depo®-Testosterone Injection** *see* Testosterone *on page 898*
- **Depression Guidelines** *see page 1087*
- **Deproic** *see* Valproic Acid and Derivatives *on page 967*
- **Deproist® Expectorant With Codeine** *see* Guaifenesin, Pseudoephedrine, and Codeine *on page 425*
- **Dermacort®** *see* Hydrocortisone *on page 447*
- **Dermaflex® Gel** *see* Lidocaine *on page 527*
- **Dermarest Dricort®** *see* Hydrocortisone *on page 447*
- **Derma-Smoothe** *see* Fluocinolone *on page 374*
- **Derma-Smoothe/FS®** *see* Fluocinolone *on page 374*
- **Dermasone** *see* Clobetasol *on page 210*
- **Dermatop®** *see* Prednicarbate *on page 761*
- **Dermazin®** *see* Silver Sulfadiazine *on page 852*
- **DermiCort®** *see* Hydrocortisone *on page 447*
- **Dermolate® [OTC]** *see* Hydrocortisone *on page 447*
- **Dermoplast® [OTC]** *see* Benzocaine *on page 98*
- **Dermovate** *see* Clobetasol *on page 210*
- **Dermtex® HC With Aloe** *see* Hydrocortisone *on page 447*
- **Deronil** *see* Dexamethasone *on page 256*

Desipramine (des IP ra meen)

Pharmacologic Class Antidepressant, Tricyclic (Secondary Amine)

U.S. Brand Names Norpramin®

Mechanism of Action Traditionally believed to increase the synaptic concentration of norepinephrine in the central nervous system by inhibition of its reuptake by the presynaptic neuronal membrane. However, additional receptor effects have been found including desensitization of adenyl cyclase, down regulation of beta-adrenergic receptors, and down regulation of serotonin receptors.

Use Treatment of various forms of depression, often in conjunction with psychotherapy; analgesic adjunct in chronic pain

Unlabeled use: Peripheral neuropathies

USUAL DOSAGE Oral:

Children 6-12 years: 10-30 mg/day or 1-5 mg/kg/day in divided doses; do not exceed 5 mg/kg/day

Adolescents: Initial: 25-50 mg/day; gradually increase to 100 mg/day in single or divided doses; maximum: 150 mg/day

Adults: Initial: 75 mg/day in divided doses; increase gradually to 150-200 mg/day in divided or single dose; maximum: 300 mg/day

Elderly: Initial dose: 10-25 mg/day; increase by 10-25 mg every 3 days for inpatients and every week for outpatients if tolerated; usual maintenance dose: 75-100 mg/day, but doses up to 150 mg/day may be necessary

Hemodialysis/peritoneal dialysis: Supplemental dose is not necessary

Dosage Forms TAB: 10 mg, 25 mg, 50 mg, 75 mg, 100 mg, 150 mg

Contraindications Hypersensitivity to desipramine (cross-sensitivity with other tricyclic antidepressants may occur); patients receiving MAO inhibitors within past 14 days; narrow-angle glaucoma; use immediately postmyocardial infarction

Warnings/Precautions Use with caution in patients with cardiovascular disease, conduction disturbances, urinary retention, seizure disorders, hyperthyroidism or those receiving thyroid replacement; do not discontinue abruptly in patients receiving long-term high-dose therapy

Pregnancy Risk Factor C

Adverse Reactions

Cardiovascular: Arrhythmias, hypotension, hypertension, palpitations, heart block, tachycardia

Central nervous system: Dizziness, drowsiness, headache, confusion, delirium, hallucinations, nervousness, restlessness, parkinsonian syndrome, insomnia, disorientation, anxiety, agitation, hypomania, exacerbation of psychosis, incoordination, seizures, extrapyramidal symptoms

Dermatologic: Alopecia, photosensitivity, skin rash, urticaria

Endocrine & metabolic: Breast enlargement, galactorrhea, SIADH

Gastrointestinal: Xerostomia, decreased lower esophageal sphincter tone may cause GE reflux, constipation, nausea, unpleasant taste, weight gain, anorexia, abdominal cramps, weight loss, diarrhea, heartburn

Genitourinary: Difficult urination, sexual dysfunction, testicular edema

Hematologic: Agranulocytosis, eosinophilia, purpura, thrombocytopenia

Hepatic: Cholestatic jaundice, increased liver enzyme

Neuromuscular & skeletal: Fine muscle tremors, weakness, numbness, tingling, paresthesia of extremities, ataxia

Ocular: Blurred vision, disturbances of accommodation, mydriasis, increased intraocular pressure

Miscellaneous: Diaphoresis (excessive), allergic reactions

Drug Interactions CYP1A2 and 2D6 enzyme substrate; CYP2D6 inhibitor CYP1A2, 2C9, 2C19, 2D6, and 3A3/4 enzyme substrate

Carbamazepine, phenobarbital, and rifampin may increase the metabolism of desipramine resulting in decreased effect of desipramine

Desipramine inhibits the antihypertensive response to bethanidine, clonidine, debrisoquin, guanadrel, guanethidine, guanabenz, guanfacine; monitor BP; consider alternate antihypertensive agent

Abrupt discontinuation of clonidine may cause hypertensive crisis, desipramine may enhance the response

Use with altretamine may cause orthostatic hypertension

Desipramine may be additive with or may potentiate the action of other CNS depressants (sedatives, hypnotics, or ethanol)

With MAO inhibitors, hyperpyrexia, hypertension, tachycardia, confusion, seizures, and **deaths have been reported** (serotonin syndrome); this combination should be avoided

Desipramine may increase the prothrombin time in patients stabilized on warfarin

Cimetidine and methylphenidate may decrease the metabolism of desipramine

Additive anticholinergic effects seen with other anticholinergic agents

The SSRIs, to varying degrees, inhibit the metabolism of TCAs and clinical toxicity may result

Use of lithium with a TCA may increase the risk for neurotoxicity

Phenothiazines may increase concentration of some TCAs and TCAs may increase concentration of phenothiazines; monitor for altered clinical response

TCAs may enhance the hypoglycemic effects of tolazamide, chlorpropamide, or insulin; monitor for changes in blood glucose levels

Cholestyramine and colestipol may bind TCAs and reduce their absorption; monitor for altered response

TCAs may enhance the effect of amphetamines; monitor for adverse CV effects

Verapamil and diltiazem appear to decrease the metabolism of imipramine and potentially other TCAs; monitor for increased TCA concentrations. The pressor response to I.V. epinephrine, norepinephrine, and phenylephrine may be enhanced in patients receiving TCAs, this combination is best avoided.

Protease inhibitors: Indinavir and ritonavir inhibit the metabolism of clomipramine, desipramine and potentially other TCAs; monitor for altered effects; a decrease in TCA dosage may be required

Quinidine may inhibit the metabolism of TCAs, monitor for altered effect

Combined use of anticholinergics with TCAs may produce additive anticholinergic effects; combined use of beta-agonists with TCAs may predispose patients to cardiac arrhythmias

Alcohol Interactions Avoid use (may increase central nervous system depression)

Onset 1-3 weeks (maximum antidepressant effects: after >2 weeks)

Half-Life 7-60 hours

Education and Monitoring Issues

Patient Education: Take exactly as directed (do not increase dose or frequency); may take several weeks to achieve desired results; may cause physical and/or psychological dependence. Avoid excessive alcohol, excess caffeine, and other prescription or OTC

(Continued)

Desipramine *(Continued)*

medications not approved by prescriber. Maintain adequate hydration (2-3 L/day of fluids unless instructed to restrict fluid intake). You may experience drowsiness, lightheadedness, impaired coordination, dizziness, or blurred vision (use caution when driving or engaging in tasks requiring alertness until response to drug is known); constipation (increased exercise, fluids, or dietary fruit and fiber may help); urinary retention (void before taking medication); postural hypotension (use caution climbing stairs or when changing position from lying or sitting to standing); altered sexual drive or ability (reversible); or photosensitivity (use sunscreen, wear protective clothing and eyewear, avoid direct sunlight). Report persistent CNS effects (eg, nervousness, restlessness, insomnia, anxiety, excitation, headache, agitation, impaired coordination, changes in cognition); muscle cramping, weakness, tremors, or rigidity; chest pain, palpitations, or irregular heartbeat; blurred vision or eye pain; yellowing of skin or eyes; or worsening of condition.

Dietary Considerations: Grapefruit juice may potentially inhibit the metabolism of TCAs

Monitoring Parameters: Monitor blood pressure and pulse rate prior to and during initial therapy; evaluate mental status; monitor weight

Reference Range:

Plasma levels do not always correlate with clinical effectiveness

Timing of serum samples: Draw trough just before next dose

Therapeutic: 50-300 ng/mL

In elderly patients the response rate is greatest with steady-state plasma concentrations >115 ng/mL

Possible toxicity: >300 ng/mL

Toxic: >1000 ng/mL

Related Information

Antidepressant Agents Comparison *on page 1231*

Desmopressin Acetate (des moe PRES in AS e tate)

Pharmacologic Class Vasopressin Analog, Synthetic

U.S. Brand Names DDAVP® Nasal Spray; Stimate™ Nasal

Generic Available No

Mechanism of Action Enhances reabsorption of water in the kidneys by increasing cellular permeability of the collecting ducts; possibly causes smooth muscle constriction with resultant vasoconstriction; raises plasma levels of von Willebrand factor and factor VIII

Use Treatment of diabetes insipidus and controlling bleeding in mild hemophilia, von Willebrand disease, and thrombocytopenia (eg, uremia), nocturnal enuresis

USUAL DOSAGE

Children:

Diabetes insipidus: 3 months to 12 years: Intranasal (using 100 mcg/mL nasal solution): Initial: 5 mcg/day (0.05 mL/day) divided 1-2 times/day; range: 5-30 mcg/day (0.05-0.3 mL/day) divided 1-2 times/day; adjust morning and evening doses separately for an adequate diurnal rhythm of water turnover

Hemophilia: >3 months: I.V. 0.3 mcg/kg; may repeat dose if needed; begin 30 minutes before procedure; dilute I.V. dose in 50 mL 0.9% sodium chloride and infuse over 15-30 minutes

Nocturnal enuresis: ≥6 years: Intranasal (using 100 mcg/mL nasal solution): Initial: 20 mcg (0.2 mL) at bedtime; range: 10-40 mcg; it is recommended that 1/2 of the dose be given in each nostril

Children 12 years and Adults:

Diabetes insipidus:

I.V., S.C.: 2-4 mcg/day in 2 divided doses or 1/10 of the maintenance intranasal dose; dilute I.V. dose in 50 mL 0.9% sodium chloride and infuse over 15-30 minutes

Intranasal (using 100 mcg/mL nasal solution): 5-40 mcg/day (0.05-0.4 mL) divided 1-3 times/day; adjust morning and evening doses separately for an adequate diurnal rhythm of water turnover. **Note:** The nasal spray pump can only deliver doses of 10 mcg (0.1 mL) or multiples of 10 mcg (0.1 mL), if doses other than this are needed, the rhinal tube delivery system is preferred.

Hemophilia/uremic bleeding:

I.V.: 0.3 mcg/kg by slow infusion, begin 30 minutes before procedure; dilute I.V. dose in 50 mL 0.9% sodium chloride and infuse over 15-30 minutes

Nasal spray: Using high concentration spray: <50 kg: 150 mcg (1 spray); >50 kg: 300 mcg (1 spray each nostril); repeat use is determined by the patient's clinical condition and laboratory work; if using preoperatively, administer 2 hours before surgery

Oral: Begin therapy 12 hours after the last intranasal dose for patients previously on intranasal therapy

Children: Initial: 0.05 mg; fluid restrictions are required in children to prevent hyponatremia and water intoxication

Adults: 0.05 mg twice daily; adjust individually to optimal therapeutic dose. Total daily dose should be increased or decreased (range: 0.1-1.2 mg divided 2-3 times/day) as needed to obtain adequate antidiuresis.

Dosage Forms INJ (DDAVP®): 4 mcg/mL (1 mL). **SOLN, nasal:** (DDAVP®): 100 mcg/mL (2.5 mL, 5 mL); (Stimate™): 1.5 mg/mL (2.5 mL). **TAB** (DDAVP®): 0.1 mg, 0.2 mg

Contraindications Hypersensitivity to desmopressin or any component; avoid using in patients with type IIB or platelet-type von Willebrand disease, patients with <5% factor VIII activity level

Warnings/Precautions Avoid overhydration especially when drug is used for its hemostatic effect

Pregnancy Risk Factor B

Adverse Reactions

1% to 10%:

Cardiovascular: Facial flushing
Central nervous system: Headache, dizziness
Gastrointestinal: Nausea, abdominal cramps
Genitourinary: Vulval pain
Local: Pain at the injection site
Respiratory: Nasal congestion

<1%: Hyponatremia, increase in blood pressure, water intoxication

Drug Interactions

Decreased effect: Demeclocycline, lithium may decrease ADH effects
Increased effect: Chlorpropamide, fludrocortisone may increase ADH response

Alcohol Interactions Avoid use (may decrease desmopressin's antidiuretic effect)

Onset

Intranasal administration: Onset of ADH effects: Within 1 hour; Peak effect: Within 1-5 hours

I.V. infusion: Onset of increased factor VIII activity: Within 15-30 minutes; Peak effect: 90 minutes to 3 hours

Duration Intranasal administration: 5-21 hours

Half-Life I.V. infusion: Elimination (terminal): 75 minutes

Education and Monitoring Issues

Patient Education: Use specific product as directed. Diabetes insipidus: Avoid overhydration. Weigh yourself daily at the same time in the same clothes. Report increased weight or swelling of extremities. If using intranasal product, inspect nasal membranes regularly. Report swelling or increased nasal congestion. All uses: Report unresolved headache, difficulty breathing, acute heartburn or nausea, abdominal cramping, or vulval pain.

Monitoring Parameters: Blood pressure and pulse should be monitored during I.V. infusion

Diabetes insipidus: Fluid intake, urine volume, specific gravity, plasma and urine osmolality, serum electrolytes

Hemophilia: Factor VIII antigen levels, APTT, bleeding time (for von Willebrand disease and thrombocytopathies)

- **Desocort** *see* Desonide *on page 255*
- **Desogen®** *see* Ethinyl Estradiol and Desogestrel *on page 341*

Desonide (DES oh nide)

Pharmacologic Class Corticosteroid, Topical

U.S. Brand Names DesOwen® Topical; Tridesilon® Topical

Generic Available No

Mechanism of Action Stimulates the synthesis of enzymes needed to decrease inflammation, suppress mitotic activity, and cause vasoconstriction

Use Adjunctive therapy for inflammation in acute and chronic corticosteroid responsive dermatosis (low potency corticosteroid)

USUAL DOSAGE Children and Adults: Topical: Apply 2-4 times/day sparingly. Therapy should be discontinued when control is achieved; if no improvement is seen, reassessment of diagnosis may be necessary.

Dosage Forms CRM, top: 0.05% (15 g, 60 g). **LOT:** 0.05% (60 mL, 120 mL). **OINT, top:** 0.05% (15 g, 60 g)

Contraindications Known hypersensitivity to desonide, fungal infections, tuberculosis of skin, herpes simplex

Warnings/Precautions Use with caution in patients with impaired circulation, skin infections

Pregnancy Risk Factor C

Adverse Reactions <1%: Acneiform eruptions, allergic contact dermatitis, dry skin, folliculitis, hypertrichosis, hypopigmentation, irritation, itching, local burning, miliaria, perioral dermatitis, secondary infection, skin atrophy, skin maceration, striae

Onset Commonly noted within 7 days of continued therapy

Education and Monitoring Issues

Patient Education: A thin film of cream or ointment is effective, do not overuse; rub in lightly; do not use tight-fitting diapers or plastic pants on children being treated in the

(Continued)

Desonide *(Continued)*

diaper area; use only as prescribed and for no longer than the period prescribed; avoid contact with eyes; notify prescriber if condition being treated persists or worsens

- **DesOwen® Topical** *see* Desonide *on page 255*

Desoximetasone (des oks i MET a sone)

Pharmacologic Class Corticosteroid, Topical

U.S. Brand Names Topicort®; Topicort®-LP

Generic Available Yes

Mechanism of Action Stimulates the synthesis of enzymes needed to decrease inflammation, suppress mitotic activity, and cause vasoconstriction; high potency, fluorinated topical corticosteroid

Use Relieves inflammation and pruritic symptoms of corticosteroid-responsive dermatosis [medium to high potency topical corticosteroid]

USUAL DOSAGE Desoximetasone is a potent fluorinated topical corticosteroid. All of the preparations are considered high potency. Therapy should be discontinued when control is achieved; if no improvement is seen, reassessment of diagnosis may be necessary.

Children: Apply sparingly in a very thin film to affected area 1-2 times/day
Adults: Apply sparingly in a thin film twice daily

Dosage Forms CRM, top: (Topicort®): 0.25% (15 g, 60 g, 120 g); (Topicort®-LP): 0.05% (15 g, 60 g). **GEL, top:** 0.05% (15 g, 60 g). **OINT, top** (Topicort®): 0.25% (15 g, 60 g)

Contraindications Known hypersensitivity to desoximetasone, topical fungal infections, tuberculosis of skin herpes simplex

Warnings/Precautions Use with caution in patients with impaired circulation; skin infections

Pregnancy Risk Factor C

Adverse Reactions <1%: Acneiform eruptions, allergic contact dermatitis, dry skin, folliculitis, hypertrichosis, hypopigmentation, irritation, itching, local burning, miliaria, perioral dermatitis, secondary infection skin atrophy, skin maceration, striae

Education and Monitoring Issues

Patient Education: A thin film of cream or ointment is effective, do not overuse; rub in lightly; do not use tight-fitting diapers or plastic pants on children being treated in the diaper area; use only as prescribed and for no longer than the period prescribed; avoid contact with eyes; notify prescriber if condition being treated persists or worsens

- **Desoxyn®** *see* Methamphetamine *on page 577*
- **Desoxyn Gradumet®** *see* Methamphetamine *on page 577*
- **Desyrel®** *see* Trazodone *on page 941*
- **Detensol®** *see* Propranolol *on page 786*
- **Detrol™** *see* Tolterodine *on page 931*
- **Detussin® Expectorant** *see* Hydrocodone, Pseudoephedrine, and Guaifenesin *on page 446*
- **Detussin® Liquid** *see* Hydrocodone and Pseudoephedrine *on page 446*
- **Devrom® [OTC]** *see* Bismuth *on page 108*
- **Dexacidin®** *see* Neomycin, Polymyxin B, and Dexamethasone *on page 644*
- **Dexair®** *see* Dexamethasone *on page 256*

Dexamethasone (deks a METH a sone)

Pharmacologic Class Corticosteroid, Oral; Corticosteroid, Oral Inhaler; Corticosteroid, Nasal; Corticosteroid, Ophthalmic; Corticosteroid, Parenteral; Corticosteroid, Topical

U.S. Brand Names Aeroseb-Dex®; AK-Dex®; Alba-Dex®; Baldex®; Dalalone D.P.®; Dalalone L.A.®; Decaderm®; Decadron®; Decadron®-LA; Decadron® Turbinaire®; Decaject-L.A.®; Decaspray®; Dekasol-L.A.®; Dexair®; Dexasone L.A.®; Dexone®; Dexone L.A.®; Dezone®; Hexadrol®; I-Methasone®; Maxidex®; Ocu-Dex®; Solurex L.A.®

Generic Available Yes

Mechanism of Action Decreases inflammation by suppression of migration of polymorphonuclear leukocytes and reversal of increased capillary permeability; suppresses normal immune response

Use Systemically and locally for chronic inflammation, allergic, hematologic, neoplastic, and autoimmune diseases; may be used in management of cerebral edema, septic shock, as a diagnostic agent, antiemetic

USUAL DOSAGE

Neonates:

Airway edema or extubation: I.V.: Usual: 0.25 mg/kg/dose given 4 hours prior to scheduled extubation and then every 8 hours for 3 doses total; range: 0.25-1 mg/kg/dose for 1-3 doses; maximum dose: 1 mg/kg/day. **Note:** A longer duration of therapy may be needed with more severe cases.

Bronchopulmonary dysplasia (to facilitate ventilator weaning): Oral:, I.V.: Numerous dosing schedules have been proposed; range: 0.5-0.6 mg/kg/day given in divided doses every 12 hours for 3-7 days, then taper over 1-6 weeks

Children:

Antiemetic (prior to chemotherapy): I.V. (should be given as sodium phosphate): 10 mg/m^2/dose (maximum: 20 mg) for first dose then 5 mg/m^2/dose every 6 hours as needed

Anti-inflammatory immunosuppressant: Oral, I.M., I.V. (injections should be given as sodium phosphate): 0.08-0.3 mg/kg/day **or** 2.5-10 mg/m^2/day in divided doses every 6-12 hours

Extubation or airway edema: Oral, I.M., I.V. (injections should be given as sodium phosphate): 0.5-2 mg/kg/day in divided doses every 6 hours beginning 24 hours prior to extubation and continuing for 4-6 doses afterwards

Cerebral edema: I.V. (should be given as sodium phosphate): Loading dose: 1-2 mg/kg/dose as a single dose; maintenance: 1-1.5 mg/kg/day (maximum: 16 mg/day) in divided doses every 4-6 hours for 5 days then taper for 5 days, then discontinue

Bacterial meningitis in infants and children >2 months: I.V. (should be given as sodium phosphate): 0.6 mg/kg/day in 4 divided doses every 6 hours for the first 4 days of antibiotic treatment; start dexamethasone at the time of the first dose of antibiotic

Physiologic replacement: Oral, I.M., I.V.: 0.03-0.15 mg/kg/day or 0.6-0.75 mg/m^2/day in divided doses every 6-12 hours

Adults:

Acute nonlymphoblastic leukemia (ANLL) protocol: I.V.: 2 mg/m^2/dose every 8 hours for 12 doses

Antiemetic (prior to chemotherapy): Oral/I.V. (should be given as sodium phosphate): 10 mg/m^2/dose (usually 20 mg) for first dose then 5 mg/m^2/dose every 6 hours as needed

Anti-inflammatory:

Oral, I.M., I.V. (injections should be given as sodium phosphate): 0.75-9 mg/day in divided doses every 6-12 hours

I.M. (as acetate): 8-16 mg; may repeat in 1-3 weeks

Intralesional (as acetate): 0.8-1.6 mg

Intra-articular/soft tissue (as acetate): 4-16 mg; may repeat in 1-3 weeks

Intra-articular, intralesional, or soft tissue (as sodium phosphate): 0.4-6 mg/day

Cerebral edema: I.V. 10 mg stat, 4 mg I.M./I.V. (should be given as sodium phosphate) every 6 hours until response is maximized, then switch to oral regimen, then taper off if appropriate; dosage may be reduced after 24 days and gradually discontinued over 5-7 days

Diagnosis for Cushing's syndrome: Oral: 1 mg at 11 PM, draw blood at 8 AM the following day for plasma cortisol determination

Physiological replacement: Oral, I.M., I.V. (should be given as sodium phosphate): 0.03-0.15 mg/kg/day **OR** 0.6-0.75 mg/m^2/day in divided doses every 6-12 hours

Shock therapy:

Addisonian crisis/shock (ie, adrenal insufficiency/responsive to steroid therapy): I.V. (given as sodium phosphate): 4-10 mg as a single dose, which may be repeated if necessary

Unresponsive shock (ie, unresponsive to steroid therapy): I.V. (given as sodium phosphate): 1-6 mg/kg as a single I.V. dose or up to 40 mg initially followed by repeat doses every 2-6 hours while shock persists

Hemodialysis: Supplemental dose is not necessary

Peritoneal dialysis: Supplemental dose is not necessary

Ophthalmic:

Ointment: Apply thin coating into conjunctival sac 3-4 times/day; gradually taper dose to discontinue

Suspension: Instill 2 drops into conjunctival sac every hour during the day and every other hour during the night; gradually reduce dose to every 3-4 hours, then to 3-4 times/day

Topical: Apply 1-4 times/day. Therapy should be discontinued when control is achieved; if no improvement is seen, reassessment of diagnosis may be necessary.

Dosage Forms

Dexamethasone acetate: **INJ:** 8 mg/mL (1 mL, 5 mL); 16 mg/mL (1 mL, 5 mL)

Dexamethasone base: **AERO, top:** 0.01% (58 g), 0.04% (25 g). **ELIX:** 0.5 mg/5 mL (5 mL, 20 mL, 100 mL, 120 mL, 237 mL, 240 mL, 500 mL). **SOLN, oral:** 0.5 mg/5 mL (5 mL, 20 mL, 500 mL). **SOLN, oral concentrate:** 0.5 mg/0.5 mL (30 mL) (30% alcohol). **SUSP, ophth:** 0.1% (5 mL, 15 mL). **TAB:** 0.25 mg, 0.5 mg, 0.75 mg, 1 mg, 1.5 mg, 2 mg, 4 mg, 6 mg. **THERAPEUTIC pack:** Six 1.5 mg tabs and eight 0.75 mg tabs

Dexamethasone sodium phosphate: **AERO, nasal:** 84 mcg/activation (12.6 g); Oral: 84 mcg/activation (12.6 g). **CRM:** 0.1% (15 g, 30 g). **INJ:** 4 mg/mL (1 mL, 5 mL, 10 mL, 25 mL, 30 mL); 10 mg/mL (1 mL, 10 mL); 20 mg/mL (5 mL); 24 mg/mL (5 mL, 10 mL). **OINT, ophth:** 0.05% (3.5 g)

Contraindications Active untreated infections; use in ophthalmic viral, fungal, or tuberculosis diseases of the eye

Warnings/Precautions Fatalities have occurred due to adrenal insufficiency in asthmatic patients during and after transfer from systemic corticosteroids to aerosol steroids; aerosol steroids do **not** provide the systemic steroid needed to treat patients having trauma, surgery, or infections; use with caution in patients with hypothyroidism, cirrhosis, hypertension, congestive heart failure, ulcerative colitis, thromboembolic disorders. (Continued)

Dexamethasone *(Continued)*

Because of the risk of adverse effects, systemic corticosteroids should be used cautiously in the elderly in the smallest possible dose and for the shortest possible time.

Controlled clinical studies have shown that inhaled and intranasal corticosteroids may cause a reduction in growth velocity in pediatric patients. Growth velocity provides a means of comparing the rate of growth among children of the same age.

In studies involving inhaled corticosteroids, the average reduction in growth velocity was approximately 1 cm (about 1/3 of an inch) per year. It appears that the reduction is related to dose and how long the child takes the drug.

FDA's Pulmonary and Allergy Drugs and Metabolic and Endocrine Drugs advisory committees discussed this issue at a July 1998 meeting. They recommended that the agency develop class-wide labeling to inform healthcare providers so they would understand this potential side effect and monitor growth routinely in pediatric patients who are treated with inhaled corticosteroids, intranasal corticosteroids or both.

Long-term effects of this reduction in growth velocity on final adult height are unknown. Likewise, it also has not yet been determined whether patients' growth will "catch up" if treatment in discontinued. Drug manufacturers will continue to monitor these drugs to learn more about long-term effects. Children are prescribed inhaled corticosteroids to treat asthma. Intranasal corticosteroids are generally used to prevent and treat allergy-related nasal symptoms.

Patients are advised not to stop using their inhaled or intranasal corticosteroids without first speaking to their healthcare providers about the benefits of these drugs compared to their risks.

Pregnancy Risk Factor C

Pregnancy Implications Dexamethasone has been used in patients with premature labor (26-34 weeks gestation) to stimulate fetal lung maturation

Clinical effects on the fetus: Crosses the placenta; transient leukocytosis reported. Available evidence suggests safe use during pregnancy

Breast-feeding/lactation: No data on crossing into breast milk or effects on the infant

Adverse Reactions

Systemic:

>10%:

Central nervous system: Insomnia, nervousness

Gastrointestinal: Increased appetite, indigestion

1% to 10%:

Dermatologic: Hirsutism

Endocrine & metabolic: Diabetes mellitus

Neuromuscular & skeletal: Arthralgia

Ocular: Cataracts

Respiratory: Epistaxis

<1%: Abdominal distention, acne, amenorrhea, bone growth suppression, bruising, Cushing's syndrome, delirium, euphoria, hallucinations, headache, hyperglycemia, hyperpigmentation, hypersensitivity reactions, mood swings, muscle wasting, pancreatitis, seizures, skin atrophy, sodium and water retention, ulcerative esophagitis

Topical: <1%: Acneiform eruptions, allergic contact dermatitis, dryness, folliculitis, hypertrichosis, hypopigmentation, irritation, itching, local burning, miliaria, perioral dermatitis, secondary infection, skin atrophy, skin maceration, striae

Drug Interactions CYP3A3/4 enzyme substrate; CYP3A3/4 enzyme inducer; CYP3A3/4 enzyme inhibitor

Decreased effect: Barbiturates, phenytoin, rifampin may decrease dexamethasone effects; dexamethasone decreases effect of salicylates, vaccines, toxoids

Alcohol Interactions Avoid use (may enhance gastric mucosal irritation)

Duration Duration of metabolic effect: Can last for 72 hours; acetate is a long-acting repository preparation with a prompt onset of action.

Half-Life Normal renal function: 1.8-3.5 hours; Biological half-life: 36-54 hours

Education and Monitoring Issues

Patient Education: Take exactly as directed; do not increase dose or discontinue abruptly without consulting prescriber. Take oral medication with or after meals. Limit intake of caffeine or stimulants. Prescriber may recommend increased dietary vitamins, minerals, or iron. Diabetics should monitor glucose levels closely (antidiabetic medication may need to be adjusted). Inform prescriber if you are experiencing greater than normal levels of stress (medication may need adjustment). Some forms of this medication may cause GI upset (oral medication may be taken with meals to reduce GI upset; small frequent meals and frequent mouth care may reduce GI upset). You may be more susceptible to infection (avoid crowds and persons with contagious or infective conditions). Report promptly excessive nervousness or sleep disturbances; any signs of infection (sore throat, unhealed injuries); excessive growth of body hair or loss of skin color; changes in vision; excessive or sudden weight gain (>3 lb/week); swelling of face or extremities; difficulty breathing; muscle weakness; change in color of stools (tarry) or persistent abdominal pain; or worsening of condition or failure to improve.

Ophthalmic: For ophthalmic use only. Wash hands before using. Tilt head back and look upward. Put drops of suspension or apply thin ribbon of ointment inside lower eyelid. Close eye and roll eyeball in all directions. Do not blink for 1/2 minute. Apply gentle pressure to inner corner of eye for 30 seconds. Do not use any other eye preparation for at least 10 minutes. Do not touch tip of applicator to eye or contaminate tip of applicator. Do not share medication with anyone else. Wear sunglasses when in sunlight; you may be more sensitive to bright light. Inform prescriber if condition worsens or fails to improve or if you experience eye pain, disturbances of vision, or other adverse eye response.

Topical: For external use only. Not for eyes or mucous membranes or open wounds. Apply in very thin layer to occlusive dressing. Apply dressing to area being treated. Avoid prolonged or excessive use around sensitive tissues, genital, or rectal areas. Inform prescriber if condition worsens (swelling, redness, irritation, pain, open sores) or fails to improve.

Aerosol: Not for use during acute asthmatic attack. Follow directions that accompany product. Rinse mouth and throat after use to prevent candidiasis. Do not use intranasal product if you have a nasal infection, nasal injury, or recent nasal surgery. If using two products, consult prescriber in which order to use the two products. Inform prescriber if condition worsens or does not improve.

Monitoring Parameters: Hemoglobin, occult blood loss, serum potassium, and glucose

Reference Range: Dexamethasone suppression test, overnight: 8 AM cortisol <6 µg/100 mL (dexamethasone 1 mg); plasma cortisol determination should be made on the day after giving dose

Related Information

Corticosteroids Comparison *on page 1237*
Neomycin and Dexamethasone *on page 643*
Neomycin, Polymyxin B, and Dexamethasone *on page 644*
Tobramycin and Dexamethasone *on page 925*

♦ **Dexasone L.A.®** *see* Dexamethasone *on page 256*
♦ **Dexasporin®** *see* Neomycin, Polymyxin B, and Dexamethasone *on page 644*
♦ **Dexatrim® Pre-Meal [OTC]** *see* Phenylpropanolamine *on page 729*
♦ **Dexchlor®** *see* Dexchlorpheniramine *on page 259*

Dexchlorpheniramine (deks klor fen EER a meen)

Pharmacologic Class Antihistamine

U.S. Brand Names Dexchlor®; Poladex®; Polaramine®

Use Perennial and seasonal allergic rhinitis and other allergic symptoms including urticaria

USUAL DOSAGE Oral:

Children:
- 2-5 years: 0.5 mg every 4-6 hours (do not use timed release)
- 6-11 years: 1 mg every 4-6 hours or 4 mg timed release at bedtime

Adults: 2 mg every 4-6 hours or 4-6 mg timed release at bedtime or every 8-10 hours

Contraindications Narrow-angle glaucoma, hypersensitivity to dexchlorpheniramine or any component

Pregnancy Risk Factor B

♦ **Dexedrine®** *see* Dextroamphetamine *on page 260*
♦ **Dexferrum®** *see* Iron Dextran Complex *on page 485*
♦ **Dexone®** *see* Dexamethasone *on page 256*
♦ **Dexone L.A.®** *see* Dexamethasone *on page 256*

Dexpanthenol (deks PAN the nole)

Pharmacologic Class Gastrointestinal Agent, Stimulant

U.S. Brand Names Ilopan®; Ilopan-Choline®; Panthoderm® [OTC]

Use Prophylactic use to minimize paralytic ileus, treatment of postoperative distention

USUAL DOSAGE

Children and Adults: Relief of itching and aid in skin healing: Topical: Apply to affected area 1-2 times/day

Adults:
- Relief of gas retention: Oral: 2-3 tablets 3 times/day
- Prevention of postoperative ileus: I.M.: 250-500 mg stat, repeat in 2 hours, followed by doses every 6 hours until danger passes
- Paralyzed ileus: I.M.: 500 mg stat, repeat in 2 hours, followed by doses every 6 hours, if needed

Contraindications Hemophilia; mechanical obstruction of ileus

Pregnancy Risk Factor C

Dextranomer (deks TRAN oh mer)

Pharmacologic Class Topical Skin Product

U.S. Brand Names Debrisan® [OTC]

(Continued)

Dextranomer *(Continued)*

Use Clean exudative ulcers and wounds such as venous stasis ulcers, decubitus ulcers, and infected traumatic and surgical wounds; no controlled studies have found dextranomer to be more effective than conventional therapy

USUAL DOSAGE Debride and clean wound prior to application; apply to affected area once or twice daily in a 1/4" layer; apply a dressing and seal on all four sides; removal should be done by irrigation

Contraindications Deep fistulas, sinus tracts, hypersensitivity to any component

Pregnancy Risk Factor C

Dextroamphetamine (deks troe am FET a meen)

Pharmacologic Class Stimulant

U.S. Brand Names Dexedrine®; Dextrostat®

Generic Available Yes

Mechanism of Action Blocks reuptake of dopamine and norepinephrine from the synapse, thus increases the amount of circulating dopamine and norepinephrine in cerebral cortex to reticular activating system; inhibits the action of monoamine oxidase and causes catecholamines to be released

Use Narcolepsy, exogenous obesity, abnormal behavioral syndrome in children (minimal brain dysfunction), attention deficit/hyperactivity disorder (ADHD)

USUAL DOSAGE Oral:

- Children:
  - Narcolepsy: 6-12 years: Initial: 5 mg/day, may increase at 5 mg increments in weekly intervals until side effects appear; maximum dose: 60 mg/day
  - Attention deficit/hyperactivity disorder:
    - 3-5 years: Initial: 2.5 mg/day given every morning; increase by 2.5 mg/day in weekly intervals until optimal response is obtained, usual range: 0.1-0.5 mg/kg/dose every morning with maximum of 40 mg/day
    - ≥6 years: 5 mg once or twice daily; increase in increments of 5 mg/day at weekly intervals until optimal response is reached, usual range: 0.1-0.5 mg/kg/dose every morning (5-20 mg/day) with maximum of 40 mg/day
- Children >12 years and Adults:
  - Narcolepsy: Initial: 10 mg/day, may increase at 10 mg increments in weekly intervals until side effects appear; maximum: 60 mg/day
  - Exogenous obesity: 5-30 mg/day in divided doses of 5-10 mg 30-60 minutes before meals

Dosage Forms CAP, sustained release: 5 mg, 10 mg, 15 mg. **ELIX:** 5 mg/5 mL (480 mL). **TAB:** 5 mg, 10 mg (5 mg tabs contain tartrazine)

Contraindications Hypersensitivity to dextroamphetamine or any component; advanced arteriosclerosis, hypertension, hyperthyroidism, glaucoma, MAO inhibitors

Warnings/Precautions Use with caution in patients with psychopathic personalities, cardiovascular disease, HTN, angina, and glaucoma; has high potential for abuse; use in weight reduction programs only when alternative therapy has been ineffective; prolonged administration may lead to drug dependence

Pregnancy Risk Factor C

Adverse Reactions

- >10%:
  - Cardiovascular: Arrhythmia
  - Central nervous system: False feeling of well being, nervousness, restlessness, insomnia
- 1% to 10%:
  - Cardiovascular: Hypertension
  - Central nervous system: Mood or mental changes, dizziness, lightheadedness, headache
  - Endocrine & metabolic: Changes in libido
  - Gastrointestinal: Diarrhea, nausea, vomiting, stomach cramps, constipation, anorexia, weight loss, xerostomia
  - Ocular: Blurred vision
  - Miscellaneous: Diaphoresis (increased)
- <1%: Chest pain, CNS stimulation (severe), hyperthermia, paranoia, rash, seizures, tolerance and withdrawal with prolonged use, Tourette's syndrome, urticaria

Drug Interactions

- Decreased effect: Methyldopa decreased antihypertensive efficacy; ethosuximide; decreased effect with acidifiers, psychotropics
- Increased toxicity: May precipitate hypertensive crisis in patients receiving MAO inhibitors and arrhythmias in patients receiving general anesthetics
- Increased effect/toxicity of TCAs, phenytoin, phenobarbital, propoxyphene, norepinephrine and meperidine

Onset 1-1.5 hours

Half-Life 34 hours (urine pH dependent)

Education and Monitoring Issues

Patient Education: Take exactly as directed (do not increase dose or frequency without consulting prescriber); may cause physical and/or psychological dependence. Take early in day to avoid sleep disturbance, 30 minutes before meals. Avoid alcohol, caffeine, or OTC medications that act as stimulants. You may experience restlessness, false sense of euphoria, or impaired judgment (use caution when driving or engaging in tasks requiring alertness until response to drug is known); dry mouth (frequent mouth care, sucking lozenges, or chewing gum may help); nausea or vomiting (small frequent meals, frequent mouth care may help); constipation (increased exercise, dietary fiber, fruit, or fluid may help); diarrhea (buttermilk, boiled milk, or yogurt may help); or altered libido (reversible). Diabetics need to monitor serum glucose closely (may alter antidiabetic medication requirements). Report chest pain, palpitations, or irregular heartbeat; extreme fatigue or depression; CNS changes (aggressiveness, restlessness, euphoria, sleep disturbances); severe unremitting abdominal distress or cramping; blackened stool; changes in sexual activity; or blurred vision.

Monitoring Parameters: Growth in children and CNS activity in all

Related Information

Dextroamphetamine and Amphetamine *on page 261*

Dextroamphetamine and Amphetamine

(deks troe am FET a meen & am FET a meen)

Pharmacologic Class Amphetamine

U.S. Brand Names Adderall®

Dosage Forms TAB: 10 mg [dextroamphetamine sulfate 2.5 mg, dextroamphetamine saccharate 2.5 mg and amphetamine aspartate 2.5 mg, amphetamine sulfate 2.5 mg]; 30 mg [dextroamphetamine sulfate 7.5 mg, dextroamphetamine saccharate 7.5 mg and amphetamine aspartate 7.55 mg, amphetamine sulfate 7.5 mg]

Pregnancy Risk Factor C

- **Dextrostat®** *see* Dextroamphetamine *on page 260*
- **Dey-Dose® Isoproterenol** *see* Isoproterenol *on page 488*
- **Dey-Dose® Metaproterenol** *see* Metaproterenol *on page 572*
- **Dey-Drop® Ophthalmic Solution** *see* Silver Nitrate *on page 851*
- **Dey-Lute® Isoetharine** *see* Isoetharine *on page 486*
- **Dezone®** *see* Dexamethasone *on page 256*
- **DHC Plus®** *see* Dihydrocodeine Compound *on page 276*
- **D.H.E. 45® Injection** *see* Dihydroergotamine *on page 277*
- **DHT™** *see* Dihydrotachysterol *on page 277*
- **Diaβeta®** *see* Glyburide *on page 415*
- **Diabetes Mellitus Treatment** *see page 1089*
- **Diabetic Tussin DM® [OTC]** *see* Guaifenesin and Dextromethorphan *on page 424*
- **Diabetic Tussin EX® [OTC]** *see* Guaifenesin *on page 423*
- **Diabinese®** *see* Chlorpropamide *on page 189*
- **Dialose® [OTC]** *see* Docusate *on page 290*
- **Dialume® [OTC]** *see* Aluminum Hydroxide *on page 41*
- **Diamox®** *see* Acetazolamide *on page 19*
- **Diamox Sequels®** *see* Acetazolamide *on page 19*
- **Diapid® Nasal Spray** *see* Lypressin *on page 549*
- **Diar-Aid® [OTC]** *see* Loperamide *on page 538*
- **Diastat® Rectal Delivery System** *see* Diazepam *on page 261*
- **Diazemuls®** *see* Diazepam *on page 261*
- **Diazemuls® Injection** *see* Diazepam *on page 261*

Diazepam (dye AZ e pam)

Pharmacologic Class Benzodiazepine

U.S. Brand Names Diastat® Rectal Delivery System; Diazemuls® Injection; Diazepam Intensol®; Dizac® Injectable Emulsion; Valium® Injection; Valium® Oral

Generic Available Yes

Mechanism of Action Depresses all levels of the CNS, including the limbic and reticular formation, probably through the increased action of gamma-aminobutyric acid (GABA), which is a major inhibitory neurotransmitter in the brain

Use Management of general anxiety disorders, panic disorders, and provide preoperative sedation, light anesthesia, and amnesia; treatment of status epilepticus, alcohol withdrawal symptoms; used as a skeletal muscle relaxant

USUAL DOSAGE Oral absorption is more reliable than I.M.

Children:

Conscious sedation for procedures: Oral: 0.2-0.3 mg/kg (maximum: 10 mg) 45-60 minutes prior to procedure

Sedation or muscle relaxation or anxiety:

Oral: 0.12-0.8 mg/kg/day in divided doses every 6-8 hours

(Continued)

Diazepam *(Continued)*

I.M., I.V.: 0.04-0.3 mg/kg/dose every 2-4 hours to a maximum of 0.6 mg/kg within an 8-hour period if needed

Status epilepticus:

Infants 30 days to 5 years: I.V.: 0.05-0.3 mg/kg/dose given over 2-3 minutes, every 15-30 minutes to a maximum total dose of 5 mg; repeat in 2-4 hours as needed **or** 0.2-0.5 mg/dose every 2-5 minutes to a maximum total dose of 5 mg

>5 years: I.V.: 0.05-0.3 mg/kg/dose given over 2-3 minutes every 15-30 minutes to a maximum total dose of 10 mg; repeat in 2-4 hours as needed **or** 1 mg/dose given over 2-3 minutes, every 2-5 minutes to a maximum total dose of 10 mg

Rectal: 0.5 mg/kg, then 0.25 mg/kg in 10 minutes if needed

Adolescents: Conscious sedation for procedures:

Oral: 10 mg

I.V.: 5 mg, may repeat with 1/2 dose if needed

Adults:

Anxiety/sedation/skeletal muscle relaxation:

Oral: 2-10 mg 2-4 times/day

I.M., I.V.: 2-10 mg, may repeat in 3-4 hours if needed

Status epilepticus: I.V.: 5-10 mg every 10-20 minutes, up to 30 mg in an 8-hour period; may repeat in 2-4 hours if necessary

Elderly: Oral: Initial:

Anxiety: 1-2 mg 1-2 times/day; increase gradually as needed, rarely need to use >10 mg/day

Skeletal muscle relaxant: 2-5 mg 2-4 times/day

Hemodialysis: Not dialyzable (0% to 5%); supplemental dose is not necessary

Dosing adjustment in hepatic impairment: Reduce dose by 50% in cirrhosis and avoid in severe/acute liver disease

Dosage Forms GEL, rectal delivery system (Diastat®): Pediatric rectal tip (4.4 cm): 5 mg/mL (2.5 mg, 5 mg, 10 mg) [twin packs]; Adult rectal tip (6 cm): 5 mg/mL (10 mg, 15 mg, 20 mg) [twin packs]. **INJ:** 5 mg/mL (1 mL, 2 mL, 5 mL, 10 mL); Emulsified: (Dizac®): 5 mg/mL (3 mL); (Diazemuls®): 5 mg/mL (2 mL). **SOLN, oral** (wintergreen-spice flavor): 5 mg/5 mL (5 mL, 10 mL, 500 mL); Oral concentrate (Diazepam Intensol®): 5 mg/mL (30 mL). **TAB:** 2 mg, 5 mg, 10 mg

Contraindications Hypersensitivity to diazepam or any component; there may be a cross-sensitivity with other benzodiazepines; do not use in a comatose patient, in those with pre-existing CNS depression, respiratory depression, narrow-angle glaucoma, or severe uncontrolled pain; do not use in pregnant women

Warnings/Precautions Use with caution in patients receiving other CNS depressants, patients with low albumin, hepatic dysfunction, and in the elderly and young infants. Due to its long-acting metabolite, diazepam is not considered a drug of choice in the elderly; long-acting benzodiazepines have been associated with falls in the elderly.

Pregnancy Risk Factor D

Pregnancy Implications

Clinical effects on the fetus: Crosses the placenta. Oral clefts reported, however, more recent data does not support an association between drug and oral clefts; inguinal hernia, cardiac defects, spina bifida, dysmorphic facial features, skeletal defects, multiple other malformations reported; hypotonia and withdrawal symptoms reported following use near time of delivery

Breast-feeding/lactation: Crosses into breast milk

Clinical effects on the infant: Sedation; American Academy of Pediatrics reports that USE MAY BE OF CONCERN.

Adverse Reactions

>10%:

Cardiovascular: Cardiac arrest, bradycardia, cardiovascular collapse, tachycardia, chest pain

Central nervous system: Drowsiness, ataxia, amnesia, slurred speech, paradoxical excitement or rage, fatigue, lightheadedness, insomnia, memory impairment, headache, anxiety, depression

Dermatologic: Rash

Endocrine & metabolic: Decreased libido

Gastrointestinal: Xerostomia, changes in salivation, constipation, nausea, vomiting, diarrhea, increased or decreased appetite

Local: Phlebitis, pain with injection

Neuromuscular & skeletal: Dysarthria

Ocular: Blurred vision, diplopia

Respiratory: Decrease in respiratory rate, apnea, laryngospasm

Miscellaneous: Diaphoresis

1% to 10%:

Cardiovascular: Syncope, hypotension

Central nervous system: Confusion, nervousness, dizziness, akathisia

Dermatologic: Dermatitis

Gastrointestinal: Weight gain or loss

Neuromuscular & skeletal: Rigidity, tremor, muscle cramps

Otic: Tinnitus
Respiratory: Nasal congestion, hyperventilation
Miscellaneous: Hiccups

<1%: Blood dyscrasias, menstrual irregularities, physical and psychological dependence with prolonged use reflex slowing

Drug Interactions CYP1A2 and 2C8 enzyme substrate, CYP3A3/4 enzyme substrate (minor), and diazepam and desmethyldiazepam are CYP2C19 enzyme substrates

Carbamazepine, rifampin, rifabutin may enhance the metabolism of diazepam and decrease its therapeutic effect; consider using an alternative sedative/hypnotic agent

Amprenavir, cimetidine, ciprofloxacin, clarithromycin, clozapine, CNS depressants, diltiazem, disulfiram, digoxin, erythromycin, ethanol, fluconazole, fluoxetine, fluvoxamine, isoniazid, itraconazole, ketoconazole, labetalol, levodopa, loxapine, metoprolol, metronidazole, miconazole, nefazodone, nelfinavir, omeprazole, phenytoin, rifabutin, rifampin, ritonavir, troleandomycin, valproic acid, verapamil may increase the serum level and/or toxicity of diazepam; monitor for altered benzodiazepine response

Alcohol Interactions Avoid use (may increase central nervous system depression)

Onset I.V. for status epilepticus: Almost immediate

Duration I.V. for status epilepticus: Short, 20-30 minutes

Half-Life

Parent drug: 20-50 hours; increased half-life in the elderly and those with severe hepatic disorders

Active major metabolite (desmethyldiazepam): 50-100 hours

Education and Monitoring Issues

Patient Education: Take exactly as directed (do not increase dose or frequency); may cause physical and/or psychological dependence. While using this medication, do not use alcohol and other prescription or OTC medications (especially pain medications, sedatives, antihistamines, or hypnotics) without consulting prescriber. Maintain adequate hydration (2-3 L/day of fluids unless instructed to restrict fluid intake). You may experience drowsiness, dizziness, or blurred vision (use caution when driving or engaging in tasks requiring alertness until response to drug is known); nausea, vomiting, loss of appetite, or dry mouth (small frequent meals, frequent mouth care, chewing gum, or sucking lozenges may help); constipation (increased exercise, fluids, or dietary fruit and fiber may help). If medication is used to control seizures, wear identification that you are taking an antiepileptic medication. Report CNS changes (confusion, depression, increased sedation, excitation, headache, agitation, insomnia or nightmares, dizziness, fatigue, or impaired coordination) or changes in cognition; difficulty breathing or shortness of breath; changes in urinary pattern; changes in sexual activity; muscle cramping, weakness, tremors, or rigidity; ringing in ears or visual disturbances, excessive perspiration, or excessive GI symptoms (cramping, constipation, vomiting, anorexia); worsening of seizure activity, or loss of seizure control.

Dietary Considerations: Grapefruit juice may increase serum levels and/or toxicity

Monitoring Parameters: Respiratory rate, heart rate, blood pressure with I.V. use

Reference Range: Therapeutic: Diazepam: 0.2-1.5 μg/mL (SI: 0.7-5.3 μmol/L); N-desmethyldiazepam (nordiazepam): 0.1-0.5 μg/mL (SI: 0.35-1.8 μmol/L)

Related Information

Anticonvulsants by Seizure Type Comparison *on page 1230*

♦ **Diazepam Intensol®** *see* Diazepam *on page 261*

♦ **Dibent® Injection** *see* Dicyclomine *on page 266*

Dibucaine and Hydrocortisone (DYE byoo kane & hye droe KOR ti sone)

Pharmacologic Class Anesthetic/Corticosteroid

U.S. Brand Names Corticaine® Topical

Dosage Forms CRM: Dibucaine 5% and hydrocortisone 5%

Pregnancy Risk Factor C

♦ **Dicarbosil® [OTC]** *see* Calcium Carbonate *on page 130*

Dichlorodifluoromethane and Trichloromonofluoromethane

(dye klor oh dye flor oh METH ane & tri klor oh mon oh flor oh METH ane)

Pharmacologic Class Analgesic, Topical

U.S. Brand Names Fluori-Methane® Topical Spray

Dosage Forms SPRAY, top: Dichlorodifluoromethane 15% and trichloromonofluoromethane 85%

Diclofenac (dye KLOE fen ak)

Pharmacologic Class Nonsteroidal Anti-Inflammatory Agent (NSAID); Ophthalmic Agent

U.S. Brand Names Cataflam® Oral; Voltaren® Ophthalmic; Voltaren® Oral; Voltaren®-XR Oral

Generic Available No

Mechanism of Action Inhibits prostaglandin synthesis by decreasing the activity of the enzyme, cyclo-oxygenase, which results in decreased formation of prostaglandin precursors

(Continued)

Diclofenac *(Continued)*

Use Acute treatment of mild to moderate pain; acute and chronic treatment of rheumatoid arthritis, ankylosing spondylitis, and osteoarthritis; used for juvenile rheumatoid arthritis, gout, dysmenorrhea; ophthalmic solution for postoperative inflammation after cataract extraction

USUAL DOSAGE Adults:

Oral:

Analgesia: Starting dose: 50 mg 3 times/day

Rheumatoid arthritis: 150-200 mg/day in 2-4 divided doses (100 mg/day of sustained release product)

Osteoarthritis: 100-150 mg/day in 2-3 divided doses (100-200 mg/day of sustained release product)

Ankylosing spondylitis: 100-125 mg/day in 4-5 divided doses

Ophthalmic: Instill 1 drop into affected eye 4 times/day beginning 24 hours after cataract surgery and continuing for 2 weeks

Dosage Forms

Diclofenac sodium: **SOLN, ophth** (Voltaren®): 0.1% (2.5 mL, 5 mL). **TAB** Delayed release (Voltaren®): 25 mg, 50 mg, 75 mg; Enteric coated: 25 mg, 50 mg, 75 mg; Extended release (Voltaren®-XR):100 mg

Diclofenac potassium: **TAB** (Cataflam®): 50 mg

Contraindications Known hypersensitivity to diclofenac, any component, aspirin or other nonsteroidal anti-inflammatory drugs (NSAIDs); porphyria

Warnings/Precautions Use with caution in patients with congestive heart failure, hypertension, decreased renal or hepatic function, history of GI disease, or those receiving anticoagulants

Pregnancy Risk Factor B; D (3rd trimester)

Adverse Reactions

>10%:

Dermatologic: Rash

Gastrointestinal: Abdominal cramps, heartburn, indigestion, nausea

1% to 10%:

Cardiovascular: Angina pectoris, arrhythmias

Central nervous system: Dizziness, nervousness

Dermatologic: Itching

Gastrointestinal: GI ulceration, vomiting

Genitourinary: Vaginal bleeding

Otic: Tinnitus

<1%: Agranulocytosis, anaphylaxis, anemia, angioedema, blurred vision, change in vision, chest pain, congestive heart failure, convulsions, cystitis, decreased hearing, diaphoresis (increased), drowsiness, epistaxis, erythema multiforme, exfoliative dermatitis, forgetfulness, hepatitis, hypertension, insomnia, interstitial nephritis, laryngeal edema, leukopenia, mental depression, nephrotic syndrome, pancytopenia, peripheral neuropathy, renal impairment, shortness of breath, Stevens-Johnson syndrome, stomatitis, tachycardia, thrombocytopenia, trembling, urticaria, weakness, wheezing

Drug Interactions CYP2C8 and 2C9 enzyme substrate; CYP2C9 enzyme inhibitor

Decreased effect with aspirin; decreased effect of thiazides, furosemide

Increased toxicity of digoxin, methotrexate, cyclosporine, lithium, insulin, sulfonylureas, potassium-sparing diuretics, aspirin, warfarin

Alcohol Interactions Avoid use (may enhance gastric mucosal irritation)

Onset Cataflam® has a more rapid onset of action than does the sodium salt (Voltaren®), because it is absorbed in the stomach instead of the duodenum.

Half-Life 2 hours

Education and Monitoring Issues

Patient Education:

Oral: Take this medication exactly as directed; do not increase dose without consulting prescriber. Do not crush or chew tablets. Take with 8 ounces of water, along with food or milk products to reduce GI distress. Maintain adequate fluid intake (2-3 L/day of fluids unless instructed to restrict fluid intake). Avoid excessive alcohol, aspirin and aspirin-containing medication, and all other anti-inflammatory medications unless consulting prescriber. You may experience dizziness, nervousness, or headache (use caution when driving or engaging in tasks requiring alertness until response to drug is known); nausea, vomiting, dry mouth, or heartburn (frequent small meals, frequent mouth care, sucking lozenges, or chewing gum may help); or constipation (increased exercise, fluids, or dietary fruit and fiber may help). GI bleeding, ulceration, or perforation can occur with or without pain; discontinue medication and contact prescriber if persistent abdominal pain or cramping, or blood in stool occurs. Report chest pain or palpitations; breathlessness or difficulty breathing; unusual bruising/bleeding or blood in urine, stool, mouth, or vomitus; unusual fatigue; skin rash or itching; unusual weight gain or swelling of extremities; change in urinary pattern; change in vision or hearing; or ringing in ears.

Ophthalmic: For ophthalmic use only. Apply prescribed amount as often as directed. Wash hands before using and do not let tip of applicator touch eye or contaminate tip of applicator. Tilt head back and look upward. Gently pull down lower lid and put drop(s) in inner corner of eye. Close eye and roll eyeball in all directions. Do not blink for 1/2 minute. Apply gentle pressure to inner corner of eye for 30 seconds. Wipe away excess from skin around eye. Do not use any other eye preparation for at least 10 minutes. Do not touch tip of applicator to eye or contaminate tip of applicator. Do not share medication with anyone else. May cause sensitivity to bright light (dark glasses may help); temporary stinging or blurred vision may occur. Inform prescriber if you experience eye pain, redness, burning, watering, dryness, double vision, puffiness around eye, vision disturbances, or other adverse eye response; worsening of condition or lack of improvement. Consult prescriber if pregnant or breast-feeding.

Monitoring Parameters: Monitor CBC, liver enzymes; monitor urine output and BUN/serum creatinine in patients receiving diuretics; occult blood loss

Related Information

Nonsteroidal Anti-Inflammatory Agents Comparison *on page 1248*

Diclofenac and Misoprostol (dye KLOE fen ak & mye soe PROST ole)

Pharmacologic Class Nonsteroidal Anti-Inflammatory Agent (NSAID); Prostaglandin

U.S. Brand Names Arthrotec®

Use The diclofenac component is indicated for the treatment of osteoarthritis and rheumatoid arthritis; the misoprostol component is indicated for the prophylaxis of NSAID-induced gastric and duodenal ulceration

Dosage Forms TAB: Diclofenac 50 mg and misoprostol 200 mcg, diclofenac 75 mg and misoprostol 200 mcg

Pregnancy Risk Factor X

Alcohol Interactions Avoid use (may enhance gastric mucosal irritation)

Manufacturer Searle

Related Information

Pharmaceutical Manufacturers Directory *on page 1020*

Dicloxacillin (dye kloks a SIL in)

Pharmacologic Class Antibiotic, Penicillin

U.S. Brand Names Dycill®; Dynapen®; Pathocil®

Generic Available Yes

Mechanism of Action Inhibits bacterial cell wall synthesis by binding to one or more of the penicillin binding proteins (PBPs); which in turn inhibits the final transpeptidation step of peptidoglycan synthesis in bacterial cell walls, thus inhibiting cell wall biosynthesis. Bacteria eventually lyse due to ongoing activity of cell wall autolytic enzymes (autolysins and murein hydrolases) while cell wall assembly is arrested.

Use Treatment of systemic infections such as pneumonia, skin and soft tissue infections, and osteomyelitis caused by penicillinase-producing staphylococci

USUAL DOSAGE Oral:

Use in newborns not recommended

Children <40 kg: 12.5-25 mg/kg/day divided every 6 hours; doses of 50-100 mg/kg/day in divided doses every 6 hours have been used for therapy of osteomyelitis

Children >40 kg and Adults: 125-250 mg every 6 hours

Dosage adjustment in renal impairment: Not necessary

Hemodialysis: Not dialyzable (0% to 5%); supplemental dosage not necessary

Peritoneal dialysis: Supplemental dosage not necessary

Continuous arteriovenous or venovenous hemofiltration (CAVH/CAVHD): Supplemental dosage not necessary

Dosage Forms CAP: 125 mg, 250 mg, 500 mg. **POWDER for oral susp:** 62.5 mg/5 mL (80 mL, 100 mL, 200 mL)

Contraindications Known hypersensitivity to dicloxacillin, penicillin, or any components

Warnings/Precautions Monitor PT if patient concurrently on warfarin; elimination of drug is slow in neonates; use with caution in patients allergic to cephalosporins; bad taste of suspension may make compliance difficult

Pregnancy Risk Factor B

Adverse Reactions

1% to 10%: Gastrointestinal: Nausea, diarrhea, abdominal pain

<1%: Agranulocytosis, anemia, eosinophilia, fever, hematuria, hemolytic anemia, hepatotoxicity, hypersensitivity, increased BUN/creatinine, interstitial nephritis, leukopenia, neutropenia, prolonged PT, pseudomembranous colitis, rash (maculopapular to exfoliative), seizures with extremely high doses and/or renal failure, serum sickness-like reactions, thrombocytopenia, transient elevated LFTs, vaginitis, vomiting

Drug Interactions

Decreased effect: Efficacy of oral contraceptives may be reduced; decreased effect of warfarin

Increased effect: Disulfiram, probenecid may increase penicillin levels

Half-Life 0.6-0.8 hours; slightly prolonged in patients with renal impairment

Education and Monitoring Issues

Patient Education: Take medication as directed, with a large glass of water 1 hour before or 2 hours after meals. Take at regular intervals around-the-clock and take for length of time prescribed. You may experience some gastric distress (small frequent meals may help) and diarrhea (if this persists, consult prescriber). If diabetic, drug may

(Continued)

Dicloxacillin *(Continued)*

cause false tests with Clinitest® urine glucose monitoring; use of glucose oxidase methods (Clinistix®) or serum glucose monitoring is preferable. This drug may interfere with oral contraceptives; an alternate form of birth control should be used. Report fever, vaginal itching, sores in the mouth, loose foul-smelling stools, yellowing of skin or eyes, and change in color of urine or stool.

Dietary Considerations: Food: Decreases drug absorption rate; decreases drug serum concentration. Administer on an empty stomach 1 hour before or 2 hours after meals.

Monitoring Parameters: Monitor prothrombin time if patient concurrently on warfarin; monitor for signs of anaphylaxis during first dose

Related Information

Animal and Human Bites Guidelines *on page 1177*

Dicyclomine (dye SYE kloe meen)

Pharmacologic Class Anticholinergic Agent

U.S. Brand Names Antispas® Injection; Bentyl® Hydrochloride Injection; Bentyl® Hydrochloride Oral; Byclomine® Injection; Dibent® Injection; Dilomine® Injection; Di-Spaz® Injection; Di-Spaz® Oral; Or-Tyl® Injection

Generic Available Yes

Mechanism of Action Blocks the action of acetylcholine at parasympathetic sites in smooth muscle, secretory glands and the CNS

Use Treatment of functional disturbances of GI motility such as irritable bowel syndrome

Unlabeled use: Urinary incontinence

USUAL DOSAGE

Oral:

Infants >6 months: 5 mg/dose 3-4 times/day

Children: 10 mg/dose 3-4 times/day

Adults: Begin with 80 mg/day in 4 equally divided doses, then increase up to 160 mg/day

I.M. **(should not be used I.V.)**: Adults: 80 mg/day in 4 divided doses (20 mg/dose)

Dosage Forms CAP: 10 mg, 20 mg. **INJ:** 10 mg/mL (2 mL, 10 mL). **SYR:** 10 mg/5 mL (118 mL, 473 mL, 946 mL). **TAB:** 20 mg

Contraindications Hypersensitivity to any anticholinergic drug; narrow-angle glaucoma, myasthenia gravis; should not be used in infants <6 months of age; nursing mothers

Warnings/Precautions Use with caution in patients with hepatic or renal disease, ulcerative colitis, hyperthyroidism, cardiovascular disease, hypertension, tachycardia, GI obstruction, obstruction of the urinary tract. The elderly are at increased risk for anticholinergic effects, confusion and hallucinations.

Pregnancy Risk Factor B

Adverse Reactions Adverse reactions are included here that have been reported for pharmacologically similar drugs with anticholinergic/antispasmodic action

Cardiovascular: Syncope, tachycardia, palpitations

Central nervous system: Dizziness, lightheadedness, tingling, headache, drowsiness, nervousness, numbness, mental confusion and/or excitement, dyskinesia, lethargy, speech disturbance, insomnia

Dermatologic: Rash, urticaria, itching, and other dermal manifestations; severe allergic reaction or drug idiosyncrasies including anaphylaxis

Endocrine & metabolic: Suppression of lactation

Gastrointestinal: Xerostomia, nausea, vomiting, constipation, bloated feeling, abdominal pain, taste loss, anorexia

Genitourinary: Urinary hesitancy, urinary retention, impotence

Neuromuscular & skeletal: Weakness

Ocular: Blurred vision, diplopia, mydriasis, cycloplegia, increased ocular tension

Respiratory: Dyspnea, apnea, asphyxia, nasal stuffiness or congestion, sneezing, throat congestion

Miscellaneous: Decreased diaphoresis

Drug Interactions

Decreased effect: Phenothiazines, anti-Parkinson's drugs, haloperidol, sustained release dosage forms; decreased effect with antacids

Increased toxicity: Anticholinergics, amantadine, narcotic analgesics, type I antiarrhythmics, antihistamines, phenothiazines, TCAs

Alcohol Interactions Limit use (may increase central nervous system depression)

Onset 1-2 hours

Duration Up to 4 hours

Half-Life Initial phase: 1.8 hours; Terminal phase: 9-10 hours

Education and Monitoring Issues

Patient Education: Take as directed before meals; do not increase dose and do not discontinue without consulting prescriber. Avoid alcohol and other CNS depressant medications (antihistamines, sleeping aids, antidepressants) unless approved by prescriber. Void before taking medication. This drug may impair mental alertness (use caution when driving or engaging in tasks that require alertness until response to drug is known); constipation (increased dietary fluid, fruit, or fiber and increased exercise may help). Report excessive and persistent anticholinergic effects (blurred vision, headache, flushing, tachycardia, nervousness, dizziness, insomnia, mental confusion or excitement, dry mouth, altered taste perception, dysphagia, palpitations, bradycardia, urinary hesitancy or retention, impotence, decreased sweating), change in color of urine or stools, or irritation or redness at injection site.

Monitoring Parameters: Pulse, anticholinergic effect, urinary output, GI symptoms

Didanosine (dye DAN oh seen)

Pharmacologic Class Antiretroviral Agent, Reverse Transcriptase Inhibitor (Nucleoside)

U.S. Brand Names Videx®

Use Treatment of HIV infection; always to be used in combination with at least two other antiretroviral agents

USUAL DOSAGE Oral (administer on an empty stomach):

Children: 180 mg/m²/day divided every 12 hours **or** dosing is based on body surface area (m²): See table.

Didanosine — Pediatric Dosing

Body Surface Area (m²)	Dosing (Tablets) (mg bid)
≤0.4	25
0.5-0.7	50
0.8-1	75
1.1-1.4	100

Adults: Dosing is based on patient weight: See table.

Didanosine — Adult Dosing

Patient Weight (kg)	Dosing	
	Tablet	Buffered Powder*
≥60	400 mg qd or 200 mg bid**	250 mg bid
<60	250 mg qd or 125 mg bid	167 mg bid

*Not suitable for qd dosing except for patients with renal impairment

**The 200 mg strength tablet should only be used as a component of the 400 mg once-daily regimen

Note: Children >1 year and Adults should receive 2 tablets per dose and children <1 year should receive 1 tablet per dose for adequate buffering and absorption; tablets should be chewed; didanosine has also been used as 300 mg once daily

Dosing adjustment in renal impairment: See table.

Recommended Dose (mg) of Didanosine by Body Weight

Creatinine Clearance (mL/min)	≥60 kg		<60 kg	
	Tablet[a] (mg)	Buffered Powder[b] (mg)	Tablet[a] (mg)	Buffered Powder[b] (mg)
≥60	400 qd or 200 bid	250 bid	250 qd or 125 bid	167 bid
30-59	200 qd or 100 bid	100 bid	150 qd or 75 bid	100 bid
10-29	150 qd	167 qd	100 qd	100 qd
<10	100 qd	100 qd	75 qd	100 qd

[a] Chewable/dispersible buffered tablet; 2 tablets must be taken with each dose; different strengths of tablets may be combined to yield the recommended dose.

[b] Buffered powder for oral solution

Hemodialysis: Removed by hemodialysis (40% to 60%)

Dosing adjustment in hepatic impairment: Should be considered

Contraindications Hypersensitivity to any component

Warnings/Precautions Peripheral neuropathy occurs in ~35% of patients receiving the drug; pancreatitis (sometimes fatal) occurs in ~9%; risk factors for developing pancreatitis include a previous history of the condition, concurrent cytomegalovirus or *Mycobacterium avium-intracellulare* infection, and concomitant use of pentamidine or co-trimoxazole; discontinue didanosine if clinical signs of pancreatitis occur. Didanosine may cause retinal depigmentation in children receiving doses >300 mg/m²/day. Patients should undergo retinal examination every 6-12 months. Use with caution in patients with decreased renal or hepatic function, phenylketonuria, sodium-restricted diets, or with edema, congestive heart failure or hyperuricemia; in high concentrations, didanosine is mutagenic. Lactic

(Continued)

Didanosine *(Continued)*

acidosis and severe hepatomegaly have occurred with antiretroviral nucleoside analogues.

Pregnancy Risk Factor B

Adverse Reactions

>10%:

Central nervous system: Anxiety, headache, irritability, insomnia, restlessness
Gastrointestinal: Abdominal pain, nausea, diarrhea
Neuromuscular & skeletal: Peripheral neuropathy

1% to 10%:

Central nervous system: Depression
Dermatologic: Rash, pruritus
Gastrointestinal: Pancreatitis (2% to 3%)

<1%: Alopecia, anaphylactoid reaction, anemia, diabetes mellitus, granulocytopenia, hepatitis, hypersensitivity, lactic acidosis/hepatomegaly, leukopenia, optic neuritis, renal impairment, retinal depigmentation, seizures, thrombocytopenia

Drug Interactions Drugs whose absorption depends on the level of acidity in the stomach such as ketoconazole, itraconazole, and dapsone should be administered at least 2 hours prior to didanosine

Decreased effect: Didanosine may decrease absorption of quinolones or tetracyclines, didanosine should be held during PCP treatment with pentamidine; didanosine may decrease levels of indinavir

Increased toxicity: Concomitant administration of other drugs which have the potential to cause peripheral neuropathy or pancreatitis may increase the risk of these toxicities

Manufacturer Bristol-Myers Squibb Company (Pharmaceutical Division)

Related Information

Antiretroviral Therapy for HIV Infection *on page 1190*
Pharmaceutical Manufacturers Directory *on page 1020*

♦ **Didronel®** *see* Etidronate Disodium *on page 346*

Dienestrol (dye en ES trole)

Pharmacologic Class Estrogen Derivative

U.S. Brand Names DV® Vaginal Cream; Ortho® Dienestrol Vaginal

Generic Available No

Mechanism of Action Increases the synthesis of DNA, RNA, and various proteins in target tissues; reduces the release of gonadotropin-releasing hormone from the hypothalamus; reduces FSH and LH release from the pituitary

Use Symptomatic management of atrophic vaginitis or kraurosis vulvae in postmenopausal women

USUAL DOSAGE Adults: Vaginal: Insert 1 applicatorful once or twice daily for 1-2 weeks and then ½ of that dose for 1-2 weeks; maintenance dose: 1 applicatorful 1-3 times/week for 3-6 months

Dosage Forms CRM, vag: 0.01% (30 g, 78 g)

Contraindications Pregnancy; should not be used during lactation or undiagnosed vaginal bleeding

Warnings/Precautions Use with caution in patients with a history of thromboembolism, stroke, myocardial infarction (especially age >40 who smoke), liver tumor, hypertension, cardiac, renal or hepatic insufficiency

Pregnancy Risk Factor X

Adverse Reactions

1% to 10%:

Cardiovascular: Peripheral edema
Gastrointestinal: Anorexia, abdominal cramping

<1%: Alterations in frequency and flow of menses, anxiety, breast tenderness or enlargement, chloasma, cholestatic jaundice, decreased glucose tolerance, depression, dizziness, GI distress, headache, hypertension, increased susceptibility to *Candida* infection, increased triglycerides and LDL, melasma, migraine, myocardial infarction, nausea, rash, stroke, thromboembolism

Education and Monitoring Issues

Patient Education: Use as directed. Insert cream high in vagina. Remain lying down for 30 minutes following insertion. Use of sanitary napkin following administration will protect clothing; do not use a tampon. May cause breast tenderness or enlargement (consult prescriber for relief). Discontinue use and report promptly any pain, redness, warmth, or swelling in calves; sudden onset difficulty breathing; headache; loss of vision; difficulty speaking; sharp or sudden chest pain; severe abdominal pain; or unusual bleeding.

Diethylpropion (dye eth il PROE pee on)

Pharmacologic Class Anorexiant

U.S. Brand Names Tenuate®; Tenuate® Dospan®

Generic Available Yes

Mechanism of Action Diethylpropion is used as an anorexiant agent possessing pharmacological and chemical properties similar to those of amphetamines. The mechanism of action of diethylpropion in reducing appetite appears to be secondary to CNS effects, specifically stimulation of the hypothalamus to release catecholamines into the central nervous system; anorexiant effects are mediated via norepinephrine and dopamine metabolism. An increase in physical activity and metabolic effects (inhibition of lipogenesis and enhancement of lipolysis) may also contribute to weight loss.

Use Short-term adjunct in exogenous obesity

USUAL DOSAGE Adults: Oral:

Tablet: 25 mg 3 times/day before meals or food

Tablet, controlled release: 75 mg at midmorning

See "Obesity Treatment Guidelines for Adults" in Appendix

Dosage Forms TAB: 25 mg; Controlled release: 75 mg

Contraindications Known hypersensitivity to diethylpropion; during or within 14 days following administration of MAO inhibitors (hypertensive crises may result)

Warnings/Precautions Prolonged administration may lead to dependence; use with caution in patients with mental illness or diabetes mellitus, advanced arteriosclerosis, cardiovascular disease, nephritis, angina pectoris, hypertension, glaucoma, and patients with a history of drug abuse

Pregnancy Risk Factor B

Adverse Reactions

Cardiovascular: Hypertension, palpitations, tachycardia, chest pain, T-wave changes, arrhythmias, pulmonary hypertension, valvalopathy

Central nervous system: Euphoria, nervousness, insomnia, restlessness, dizziness, anxiety, headache, agitation, confusion, mental depression, psychosis, CVA, seizure

Dermatologic: Alopecia, urticaria, skin rash, ecchymosis, erythema

Endocrine & metabolic: Changes in libido, gynecomastia, menstrual irregularities, porphyria

Gastrointestinal: Nausea, vomiting, abdominal cramps, constipation, xerostomia, metallic taste

Genitourinary: Impotence

Hematologic: Bone marrow depression, agranulocytosis, leukopenia

Neuromuscular & skeletal: Tremor

Ocular: Blurred vision, mydriasis

Drug Interactions

Diethylpropion may displace guanethidine from the neuron and antagonize its antihypertensive effects; discontinue diethylpropion or use alternative antihypertensive

Concurrent use or use within 14 days following the administration of a MAOI is contraindicated (hypertensive crisis)

Concurrent use of sibutramine and diethylpropion is contraindicated (severe hypertension, tachycardia)

Concurrent use with TCA may result in hypertension and CNS stimulation; best to avoid this combination

Concurrent use with other anorectic agents may cause serious cardiac problems and is contraindicated

Alcohol Interactions Avoid use

Onset 1 hour

Duration 12-24 hours

Education and Monitoring Issues

Patient Education: Take exactly as directed (do not increase dose or frequency without consulting prescriber); may cause physical and/or psychological dependence. Do not crush or chew extended release tablets. Take early in day to avoid sleep disturbance, 1 hour before meals. Avoid alcohol, caffeine, or OTC medications that act as stimulants. You may experience restlessness, false sense of euphoria, or impaired judgment (use caution when driving or engaging in tasks requiring alertness until response to drug is known); dry mouth (frequent mouth care, sucking lozenges, or chewing gum may help); nausea or vomiting (small frequent meals, frequent mouth care may help); constipation (increased exercise, dietary fiber, fruit, or fluid may help); diarrhea (buttermilk, boiled milk, or yogurt may help); or altered libido (reversible). Diabetics need to monitor serum glucose closely (may alter antidiabetic medication requirements). Report chest pain, palpitations, or irregular heartbeat; muscle weakness or tremors; extreme fatigue or depression; CNS changes (aggressiveness, restlessness, euphoria, sleep disturbances); severe unremitting abdominal distress or cramping; changes in sexual activity; changes in urinary pattern; or blurred vision.

Monitoring Parameters: Monitor CNS

Diethylstilbestrol (dye eth il stil BES trole)

Pharmacologic Class Estrogen Derivative

U.S. Brand Names Stilphostrol®

Generic Available Yes

Mechanism of Action Competes with estrogenic and androgenic compounds for binding onto tumor cells and thereby inhibits their effects on tumor growth

(Continued)

Diethylstilbestrol *(Continued)*

Use Palliative treatment of inoperable metastatic prostatic carcinoma and postmenopausal inoperable, progressing breast cancer

USUAL DOSAGE Adults:

Male:

Prostate carcinoma (inoperable, progressing): Oral: 1-3 mg/day

Diphosphate: (inoperable, progressing): Oral: 50 mg 3 times/day; increase up to 200 mg or more 3 times/day; maximum daily dose: 1 g

I.V.: Administer 0.5 g, dissolved in 250 mL of saline or D_5W, administer slowly the first 10-15 minutes then adjust rate so that the entire amount is given in 1 hour; repeat for ≥5 days depending on patient response, then repeat 0.25-0.5 g 1-2 times for one week or change to oral therapy

Female: Postmenopausal (inoperable, progressing) breast carcinoma: Oral: 15 mg/day

Dosage Forms

Diethylstilbestrol base: **TAB:** 1 mg, 2.5 mg, 5 mg

Diethylstilbestrol diphosphate sodium: **INJ** (Stilphostrol®): 0.25 g (5 mL). **TAB** (Stilphostrol®): 50 mg

Contraindications Undiagnosed vaginal bleeding, during pregnancy; breast cancer except in select patients with metastatic disease

Warnings/Precautions Use with caution in patients with a history of thromboembolism, stroke, myocardial infarction (especially >40 years of age who smoke), liver tumor, hypertension, cardiac, renal or hepatic insufficiency; estrogens have been reported to increase the risk of endometrial carcinoma; do not use estrogens during pregnancy

Pregnancy Risk Factor X

Adverse Reactions

>10%:

Cardiovascular: Peripheral edema

Endocrine & metabolic: Enlargement of breasts (female and male), breast tenderness

Gastrointestinal: Anorexia, bloating

1% to 10%:

Central nervous system: Headache

Endocrine & metabolic: Increased libido (female), decreased libido (male)

Gastrointestinal: Vomiting, diarrhea

<1%: Alterations in frequency and flow of menses, amenorrhea, anxiety, breast tumors, chloasma, cholestatic jaundice, decreased glucose tolerance, depression, dizziness, edema, GI distress, hypertension, increased LDL, increased susceptibility to *Candida* infection, increased triglycerides, intolerance to contact lenses, melasma, myocardial infarction, nausea, rash, stroke, thromboembolism

Education and Monitoring Issues

Patient Education: Use as directed with or after meals (sustained release may be taken at midmorning - do not crush or chew). May cause breast tenderness or enlargement (consult prescriber for relief). You may be more sensitive to sunlight; use sunblock, wear protective clothing and dark glasses, or avoid direct exposure to sunlight. If you are diabetic, monitor serum glucose closely; antidiabetic agent may need to be adjusted. Discontinue use and report promptly any pain, redness, warmth, or swelling in calves; sudden onset difficulty breathing; headache; loss of vision; difficulty speaking; sharp or sudden chest pain; severe abdominal pain; or unusual bleeding or speech.

Difenoxin and Atropine (dye fen OKS in & A troe peen)

Pharmacologic Class Antidiarrheal

U.S. Brand Names Motofen®

Dosage Forms TAB: Difenoxin hydrochloride 1 mg and atropine sulfate 0.025 mg

Pregnancy Risk Factor C

Education and Monitoring Issues

Patient Education: Take as directed; do not exceed recommended dose. If no relief in 48 hours, contact prescriber. Avoid alcohol. Keep out of reach of children; can cause severe and fatal respiratory depression if accidentally ingested. You may experience lightheadedness, depression, dizziness, or weakness; use caution when driving or engaging in tasks that require alertness until response to drug is known. Report acute dizziness, headache, or gastrointestinal symptoms.

♦ **Differin®** *see* Adapalene *on page 23*

Diflorasone (dye FLOR a sone)

Pharmacologic Class Corticosteroid, Topical

U.S. Brand Names Florone®; Florone E®; Maxiflor®; Psorcon™ E

Generic Available No

Mechanism of Action Decreases inflammation by suppression of migration of polymorphonuclear leukocytes and reversal of increased capillary permeability

Use Relieves inflammation and pruritic symptoms of corticosteroid-responsive dermatosis (high to very high potency topical corticosteroid)

Maxiflor®: High potency topical corticosteroid

Psorcon™: Very high potency topical corticosteroid

USUAL DOSAGE Topical: Apply ointment sparingly 1-3 times/day; apply cream sparingly 2-4 times/day. Therapy should be discontinued when control is achieved; if no improvement is seen, reassessment of diagnosis may be necessary.

Dosage Forms CRM: 0.05% (15 g, 30 g, 60 g). **OINT, top:** 0.05% (15 g, 30 g, 60 g)

Contraindications Known hypersensitivity to diflorasone

Warnings/Precautions Use with caution in patients with impaired circulation; skin infections

Pregnancy Risk Factor C

Adverse Reactions <1%: Arthralgia, burning, dryness, folliculitis, itching, maceration, muscle atrophy, secondary infection

Education and Monitoring Issues

Patient Education: A thin film of cream or ointment is effective; do not overuse; do not use tight-fitting diapers or plastic pants on children being treated in the diaper area; use only as prescribed, and for no longer than the period prescribed; apply sparingly in light film; rub in lightly; avoid contact with eyes; notify prescriber if condition being treated persists or worsens

♦ **Diflucan®** *see* Fluconazole *on page 368*

Diflunisal (dye FLOO ni sal)

Pharmacologic Class Nonsteroidal Anti-Inflammatory Agent (NSAID)

U.S. Brand Names Dolobid®

Generic Available No

Mechanism of Action Inhibits prostaglandin synthesis by decreasing the activity of the enzyme, cyclo-oxygenase, which results in decreased formation of prostaglandin precursors

Use Management of inflammatory disorders usually including rheumatoid arthritis and osteoarthritis; can be used as an analgesic for treatment of mild to moderate pain

USUAL DOSAGE Adults: Oral:

Pain: Initial: 500-1000 mg followed by 250-500 mg every 8-12 hours; maximum daily dose: 1.5 g

Inflammatory condition: 500-1000 mg/day in 2 divided doses; maximum daily dose: 1.5 g

Dosing adjustment in renal impairment: Cl_{cr} <50 mL/minute: Administer 50% of normal dose

Dosage Forms TAB: 250 mg, 500 mg

Contraindications Hypersensitivity to diflunisal or any component, may be a cross-sensitivity with other nonsteroidal anti-inflammatory agents including aspirin; should not be used in patients with active GI bleeding

Warnings/Precautions Peptic ulceration and GI bleeding have been reported; platelet function and bleeding time are inhibited; ophthalmologic effects; impaired renal function, use lower dosage; peripheral edema; possibility of Reye's syndrome; elevation in liver tests

Pregnancy Risk Factor C; D (3rd trimester)

Adverse Reactions

>10%:

Central nervous system: Headache

Endocrine & metabolic: Fluid retention

1% to 10%:

Cardiovascular: Angina pectoris, arrhythmias

Central nervous system: Dizziness

Dermatologic: Rash

Gastrointestinal: GI ulceration

Genitourinary: Vaginal bleeding

Otic: Tinnitus

<1%: Agranulocytosis, anaphylaxis, angioedema, blurred vision, change in vision, chest pain, convulsions, cystitis, decreased hearing, diaphoresis (increased), drowsiness, erythema multiforme, esophagitis or gastritis, exfoliative dermatitis, hallucinations, hemolytic anemia, hepatitis, insomnia, interstitial nephritis, itching, mental depression, nephrotic syndrome, nervousness, peripheral neuropathy, renal impairment, shortness of breath, Stevens-Johnson syndrome, stomatitis, tachycardia, thrombocytopenia, toxic epidermal necrolysis, trembling, urticaria, vasculitis, weakness, wheezing

Drug Interactions

Decreased effect with antacids

Increased effect/toxicity of digoxin, methotrexate, anticoagulants, phenytoin, sulfonylureas, sulfonamides, lithium, indomethacin, hydrochlorothiazide, acetaminophen (levels)

Alcohol Interactions Avoid use (may enhance gastric mucosal irritation)

Onset Onset of analgesia: Within 1 hour

Duration 8-12 hours

Half-Life 8-12 hours; prolonged with renal impairment

Education and Monitoring Issues

Patient Education: If self-administered, use exactly as directed (do not increase dose or frequency); adverse reactions can occur with overuse. Do not take longer than 3

(Continued)

Diflunisal *(Continued)*

days for fever, or 10 days for pain without consulting medical advisor. Take with food or milk. While using this medication, do not use alcohol, excessive amounts of vitamin C, or salicylate-containing foods (curry powder, prunes, raisins, tea, or licorice), other prescription or OTC medications containing aspirin or salicylate, or other NSAIDs without consulting prescriber. Maintain adequate hydration (2-3 L/day of fluids unless instructed to restrict fluid intake). You may experience nausea, vomiting, gastric discomfort (frequent mouth care, small frequent meals, chewing gum, or sucking lozenges may help). GI bleeding, ulceration, or perforation can occur with or without pain. Stop taking medication and report ringing in ears; persistent pain in stomach; unresolved nausea or vomiting; difficulty breathing or shortness of breath; unusual bruising or bleeding (mouth, urine, stool); skin rash; unusual swelling of extremities; chest pain; or palpitations.

- **Digess** *see* Pancrelipase *on page 698*
- **Digibind®** *see* Digoxin Immune Fab *on page 275*
- **Digitaline** *see* Digitoxin *on page 272*

Digitoxin (di ji TOKS in)

Pharmacologic Class Antiarrhythmic Agent, Miscellaneous; Cardiac Glycoside

U.S. Brand Names Crystodigin®

Use Treatment of congestive heart failure, atrial fibrillation, atrial flutter, paroxysmal atrial tachycardia, and cardiogenic shock

USUAL DOSAGE Oral:

Children: Doses are very individualized; **when recommended**, digitalizing dose is as follows:

<1 year: 0.045 mg/kg
1-2 years: 0.04 mg/kg
>2 years: 0.03 mg/kg which is equivalent to 0.75 mg/m^2
Maintenance: Approximately $^1/_{10}$ of the digitalizing dose

Adults: Oral:

Rapid loading dose: Initial: 0.6 mg followed by 0.4 mg and then 0.2 mg at intervals of 4-6 hours
Slow loading dose: 0.2 mg twice daily for a period of 4 days followed by a maintenance dose
Maintenance: 0.05-0.3 mg/day
Most common dose: 0.15 mg/day

Dosing adjustment in renal impairment: Cl_{cr} <10 mL/minute: Administer 50% to 75% of normal dose

Hemodialysis: Not dialyzable (0% to 5%)

Dosing adjustment in hepatic impairment: Dosage reduction is necessary in severe liver disease

Digoxin (di JOKS in)

Pharmacologic Class Antiarrhythmic Agent, Class IV; Cardiac Glycoside

U.S. Brand Names Lanoxicaps®; Lanoxin®

Generic Available Yes: Tablet

Mechanism of Action

Congestive heart failure: Inhibition of the sodium/potassium ATPase pump which acts to increase the intracellular sodium-calcium exchange to increase intracellular calcium leading to increased contractility

Supraventricular arrhythmias: Direct suppression of the A-V node conduction to increase effective refractory period and decrease conduction velocity - positive inotropic effect, enhanced vagal tone, and decreased ventricular rate to fast atrial arrhythmias. Atrial fibrillation may decrease sensitivity and increase tolerance to higher serum digoxin concentrations.

Use Treatment of congestive heart failure and to slow the ventricular rate in tachyarrhythmias such as atrial fibrillation, atrial flutter, and supraventricular tachycardia (paroxysmal atrial tachycardia); cardiogenic shock; may not slow progression of heart failure or affect survival but proven to relieve signs and symptoms of heart failure.

USUAL DOSAGE When changing from oral (tablets or liquid) or I.M. to I.V. therapy, dosage should be reduced by 20% to 25%. See table.

Dosing adjustment/interval in renal impairment:

Cl_{cr} 10-50 mL/minute: Administer 25% to 75% of dose or every 36 hours
Cl_{cr} <10 mL/minute: Administer 10% to 25% of dose or every 48 hours
Reduce loading dose by 50% in ESRD

Hemodialysis: Not dialyzable (0% to 5%)

Dosage Forms CAP: 50 mcg, 100 mcg, 200 mcg. **ELIX:** 50 mcg/mL with alcohol 10% (60 mL). **INJ:** 250 mcg/mL (1 mL, 2 mL); Pediatric: 100 mcg/mL (1 mL). **TAB:** 125 mcg, 250 mcg, 500 mcg

Contraindications Hypersensitivity to digoxin or any component; A-V block, idiopathic hypertrophic subaortic stenosis, or constrictive pericarditis

Dosage Recommendations for Digoxin

Age	Total Digitalizing Dose† (mcg/kg*)		Daily Maintenance Dose‡ (mcg/kg*)	
	P.O.	I.V. or I.M.	P.O.	I.V. or I.M.
Preterm infant*	20-30	15-25	5-7.5	4-6
Full-term infant*	25-35	20-30	6-10	5-8
1 mo - 2 y*	35-60	30-50	10-15	7.5-12
2-5 y*	30-40	25-35	7.5-10	6-9
5-10 y*	20-35	15-30	5-10	4-8
>10 y*	10-15	8-12	2.5-5	2-3
Adults	0.75-1.5 mg	0.5-1 mg	0.125-0.5 mg	0.1-0.4 mg

*Based on lean body weight and normal renal function for age. Decrease dose in patients with ↓ renal function; digitalizing dose often not recommended in infants and children.

†Give one-half of the total digitalizing dose (TDD) in the initial dose, then give one-quarter of the TDD in each of two subsequent doses at 8- to 12-hour intervals. Obtain EKG 6 hours after each dose to assess potential toxicity.

‡Divided every 12 hours in infants and children <10 years of age. Given once daily to children >10 years of age and adults.

Warnings/Precautions Use with caution in patients with hypoxia, myxedema, hypothyroidism, acute myocarditis; patients with incomplete A-V block (Stokes-Adams attack) may progress to complete block with digitalis drug administration; use with caution in patients with acute myocardial infarction, severe pulmonary disease, advanced heart failure, idiopathic hypertrophic subaortic stenosis, Wolff-Parkinson-White syndrome, sick-sinus syndrome (bradyarrhythmias), amyloid heart disease, and constrictive cardiomyopathies; adjust dose with renal impairment; elderly and neonates may develop exaggerated serum/tissue concentrations due to age-related alterations in clearance and pharmacodynamic differences; exercise will reduce serum concentrations of digoxin due to increased skeletal muscle uptake; recent studies indicate photopsia, chromatopsia and decreased visual acuity may occur even with therapeutic serum drug levels

Pregnancy Risk Factor C

Adverse Reactions Incidence of reactions are not always reported.

Cardiovascular: Heart block; first-, second- (Wenckebach), or third-degree heart block; asystole; atrial tachycardia with block; A-V dissociation; accelerated junctional rhythm; ventricular tachycardia or ventricular fibrillation; PR prolongation; ST segment depression

Central nervous system: Visual disturbances (blurred or yellow vision), headache (3.2%), weakness, dizziness (4.9%), apathy, confusion, mental disturbances (4.1%), anxiety, depression, delirium, hallucinations, fever

Dermatologic: Maculopapular rash (1.6%), erythematous, scarlatiniform, papular, vesicular or bullous rashes, urticaria, pruritus, facial, angioneurotic or laryngeal edema, shedding of fingernails or toenails, alopecia

Gastrointestinal: Nausea (3.2%), vomiting (1.6%), diarrhea (3.2%), abdominal pain

<1% (limited to important or life-threatening symptoms): Gynecomastia, thrombocytopenia, palpitations, unifocal or multiform ventricular premature contractions (especially bigeminy or trigeminy), anorexia, abdominal pain, intestinal ischemia, hemorrhagic necrosis of the intestines, increase plasma estrogen and decreased serum luteinizing hormone in men and postmenopausal women and decreased plasma testosterone in men, vaginal cornification, eosinophilia, sexual dysfunction, sweating

Children are more likely to experience cardiac arrhythmias as a sign of excessive dosing. The most common are conduction disturbances or tachyarrhythmias (atrial tachycardia with or without block) and junctional tachycardia. Ventricular tachyarrhythmias are less common. In infants, sinus bradycardia may be a sign of digoxin toxicity. Any arrhythmia seen in a child on digoxin should be considered as digoxin toxicity. The gastrointestinal and central nervous system symptoms are not frequently seen in children.

Drug Interactions

Amiloride may reduce the inotropic response to digoxin

Cholestyramine, colestipol, kaolin-pectin may reduce digoxin absorption; separate administration

Levothyroxine (and other thyroid supplements) may decrease digoxin blood levels

Metoclopramide may reduce the absorption of digoxin tablets

Penicillamine has been associated with reductions in digoxin blood levels

Amiodarone reduces renal and nonrenal clearance of digoxin and may have additive effects on heart rate. Reduce digoxin dose by 50% with start of amiodarone.

Benzodiazepines (alprazolam, diazepam) have been associated with isolated reports of digoxin toxicity

Beta-blocking agents (propranolol) may have additive effects on heart rate

Calcium preparations: Rare cases of acute digoxin toxicity have been associated with parenteral calcium (bolus) administration

Carvedilol may increase digoxin blood levels in addition to potentiating its effects on heart rate

(Continued)

Digoxin *(Continued)*

Cyclosporine may increase digoxin levels, possibly due to reduced renal clearance
Erythromycin, clarithromycin, and tetracyclines may increase digoxin (not capsule form) blood levels in a subset of patients
Indomethacin has been associated with isolated reports of increased digoxin blood levels/toxicity
Itraconazole may increase digoxin blood levels in some patients; monitor
Moricizine may increase the toxicity of digoxin (mechanism undefined)
Propafenone increases digoxin blood levels. Effects are highly variable; monitor closely.
Propylthiouracil (and methimazole) may increase digoxin blood levels by reducing thyroid hormone
Quinidine increases digoxin blood levels substantially. Effect is variable (33% to 50%). Monitor digoxin blood levels/effect closely. Reduce digoxin dose by 50% with start of quinidine. Other related agents (hydroxychloroquine, quinine) should be used with caution.
Spironolactone may interfere with some digoxin assays, but may also increase blood levels directly. However, spironolactone may attenuate the inotropic effect of digoxin. Monitor effects of digoxin closely.
Succinylcholine administration to patients on digoxin has been associated with an increased risk of arrhythmias.
Verapamil diltiazem, bepridil, and nitrendipine increased serum digoxin concentrations. Other calcium channel blocking agents do not appear to share this effect. Reduce digoxin's dose with the start of verapamil.
Drugs which cause hypokalemia (thiazide and loop diuretics, amphotericin B): Hypokalemia may potentiate digoxin toxicity
These medications have been associated with reduced digoxin blood levels which appear to be of limited clinical significance: Aminoglutethimide, aminosalicylic acid, aluminum-containing antacids, sucralfate, sulfasalazine, neomycin, ticlopidine
These medications have been associated with increased digoxin blood levels which appear to be of limited clinical significance: Famciclovir, flecainide, ibuprofen, fluoxetine, nefazodone, cimetidine, famotidine, ranitidine, omeprazole, trimethoprim

Onset Oral: 1-2 hours; I.V.: 5-30 minutes; Peak effect: Oral: 2-8 hours; I.V.: 1-4 hours

Duration 3-4 days both forms

Half-Life

Dependent upon age, renal and cardiac function: Adults: 38-48 hours; Adults, anephric: 4-6 days
Half-life: Parent drug: 38 hours; Metabolites: Digoxigenin: 4 hours; Monodigitoxoside: 3-12 hours

Education and Monitoring Issues

Patient Education: Take as directed; do not discontinue without consulting prescriber. Maintain adequate dietary intake of potassium (do not increase without consulting prescriber). Adequate dietary potassium will reduce risk of digoxin toxicity. Take pulse at the same time each day; follow prescriber instructions for holding medication if pulse is below 50. Notify prescriber of acute changes in pulse. Report loss of appetite, nausea, vomiting, persistent diarrhea, swelling of extremities, palpitations, "yellowing" or blurred vision, mental confusion or depression, or unusual fatigue.

Monitoring Parameters:

When to draw serum digoxin concentrations: Digoxin serum concentrations are monitored because digoxin possesses a narrow therapeutic serum range; the therapeutic endpoint is difficult to quantify and digoxin toxicity may be life-threatening. Digoxin serum levels should be drawn **at least 4 hours after an intravenous dose** and **at least 6 hours after an oral dose (optimally 12-24 hours after a dose).**

Initiation of therapy:

If a loading dose is given: Digoxin serum concentration may be drawn within 12-24 hours after the initial loading dose administration. Levels drawn this early may confirm the relationship of digoxin plasma levels and response but are of little value in determining maintenance doses.

If a loading dose is not given: Digoxin serum concentration should be obtained after 3-5 days of therapy

Maintenance therapy:

Trough concentrations should be followed just prior to the next dose or at a minimum of 4 hours after an I.V. dose and at least 6 hours after an oral dose

Digoxin serum concentrations should be obtained within 5-7 days (approximate time to steady-state) after any dosage changes. Continue to obtain digoxin serum concentrations 7-14 days after any change in maintenance dose. **Note:** In patients with end-stage renal disease, it may take 15-20 days to reach steady-state.

Additionally, patients who are receiving potassium-depleting medications such as diuretics, should be monitored for potassium, magnesium, and calcium levels

Digoxin serum concentrations should be obtained whenever any of the following conditions occur:

Questionable patient compliance or to evaluate clinical deterioration following an initial good response
Changing renal function

Suspected digoxin toxicity
Initiation or discontinuation of therapy with drugs (amiodarone, quinidine, verapamil) which potentially interact with digoxin; if quinidine therapy is started; digoxin levels should be drawn within the first 24 hours after starting quinidine therapy, then 7-14 days later or empirically skip one day's digoxin dose and decrease the daily dose by 50%
Any disease changes (hypothyroidism)
Heart rate and rhythm should be monitored along with periodic EKGs to assess both desired effects and signs of toxicity
Follow closely (especially in patients receiving diuretics or amphotericin) for decreased serum potassium and magnesium or increased calcium, all of which predispose to digoxin toxicity
Assess renal function
Be aware of drug interactions

Reference Range:

Digoxin therapeutic serum concentrations:
Congestive heart failure: 0.8-2 ng/mL
Arrhythmias: 1.5-2.5 ng/mL

Adults: <0.5 ng/mL; probably indicates underdigitalization unless there are special circumstances
Toxic: >2.5 ng/mL; tachyarrhythmias commonly require levels >2 ng/mL
Digoxin-like immunoreactive substance (DLIS) may cross-react with digoxin immunoassay. DLIS has been found in patients with renal and liver disease, congestive heart failure, neonates, and pregnant women (3rd trimester).

Related Information
Heart Failure Guidelines *on page 1099*

Digoxin Immune Fab (di JOKS in i MYUN fab)

Pharmacologic Class Antidote
U.S. Brand Names Digibind®
Generic Available No
Mechanism of Action Binds with molecules of digoxin or digitoxin and then is excreted by the kidneys and removed from the body
Use Digoxin immune Fab are specific antibodies for the treatment of digitalis intoxication in carefully selected patients; use in life-threatening ventricular arrhythmias secondary to digoxin, acute digoxin ingestion (ie, >10 mg in adults or >4 mg in children), hyperkalemia (serum potassium >5 mEq/L) in the setting of digoxin toxicity
USUAL DOSAGE Each vial of Digibind® 40 mg will bind ~0.6 mg of digoxin or digitoxin

Estimation of the dose is based on the body burden of digitalis. This may be calculated if the amount ingested is known or the postdistribution serum drug level is known.

Tablets Ingested	Fab Dose	
(0.25 mg)	(mg)	(vials)
5	68	1.7
10	136	3.4
25	340	8.5
50	680	17
75	1000	25
100	1360	34
150	2000	50

Fab dose based on serum drug level postdistribution:
Digoxin:
No. of vials = level (ng/mL) x body weight (kg) divided by 100
Digitoxin:
No. of vials = digitoxin (ng/mL) x body weight (kg) divided by 1000
If neither amount ingested nor drug level are known, dose empirically with 10 and 5 vials for acute and chronic toxicity, respectively

Dosage Forms POWDER for inj, lyophilized: 38 mg
Contraindications Hypersensitivity to sheep products
Warnings/Precautions Use with caution in renal or cardiac failure; allergic reactions possible (sheep product)-skin testing not routinely recommended; epinephrine should be immediately available, Fab fragments may be eliminated more slowly in patients with renal failure, heart failure may be exacerbated as digoxin level is reduced; total serum digoxin concentration may rise precipitously following administration of Digibind®, but this will be almost entirely bound to the Fab fragment and not able to react with receptors in the body; Digibind® will interfere with digitalis immunoassay measurements - this will result in clinically misleading serum digoxin concentrations until the Fab fragment is eliminated from the body (several days to >1 week after Digibind® administration). Hypokalemia has been reported to occur following reversal of digitalis intoxication as has
(Continued)

Digoxin Immune Fab *(Continued)*

exacerbation of underlying heart failure. Serum digoxin levels drawn prior to therapy may be difficult to evaluate if 6-8 hours have not elapsed after the last dose of digoxin (time to equilibration between serum and tissue); redigitalization should not be initiated until Fab fragments have been eliminated from the body, which may occur over several days or greater than a week in patients with impaired renal function.

Pregnancy Risk Factor C

Adverse Reactions <1% (limited to important or life-threatening symptoms): Worsening of low cardiac output or congestive heart failure, rapid ventricular response in patients with atrial fibrillation as digoxin is withdrawn, facial edema and redness, hypokalemia

Drug Interactions Decreased potassium; increased digoxin levels

Onset I.V.: Improvement in signs or symptoms occur within 2-30 minutes

Half-Life 15-20 hours; prolonged in patients with renal impairment

Education and Monitoring Issues

Patient Education: Patient education and instruction will be determined by patient condition and ability to understand. Immediately report dizziness, palpitations, cramping, or difficulty breathing.

Monitoring Parameters: Serum potassium, serum digoxin concentration prior to first dose of digoxin immune Fab; **digoxin levels will greatly increase with Digibind® use and are not an accurate determination of body stores**

Manufacturer GlaxoWellcome

Related Information

Pharmaceutical Manufacturers Directory *on page 1020*

- **Dihistine® DH** *see* Chlorpheniramine, Pseudoephedrine, and Codeine *on page 187*
- **Dihistine® Expectorant** *see* Guaifenesin, Pseudoephedrine, and Codeine *on page 425*
- **Dihydrex® Injection** *see* Diphenhydramine *on page 282*

Dihydrocodeine Compound (dye hye droe KOE deen KOM pound)

Pharmacologic Class Analgesic, Narcotic

U.S. Brand Names DHC Plus®; Synalgos®-DC

Generic Available Yes

Mechanism of Action Binds to opiate receptors in the CNS, causing inhibition of ascending pain pathways, altering the perception of and response to pain; causes cough suppression by direct central action in the medulla; produces generalized CNS depression

Use Management of mild to moderate pain that requires relaxation

USUAL DOSAGE Adults: Oral: 1-2 capsules every 4-6 hours as needed for pain

Dosage Forms CAP: (DHC Plus®): Dihydrocodeine bitartrate 16 mg, acetaminophen 356.4 mg, and caffeine 30 mg; (Synalgos®-DC): Dihydrocodeine bitartrate 16 mg, aspirin 356.4 mg, and caffeine 30 mg

Contraindications Hypersensitivity to dihydrocodeine or any component

Warnings/Precautions Use with caution in patients with hypersensitivity reactions to other phenanthrene derivative opioid agonists (morphine, hydrocodone, hydromorphone, levorphanol, oxycodone, oxymorphone); respiratory diseases including asthma, emphysema, COPD, or severe liver or renal insufficiency; some preparations contain sulfites which may cause allergic reactions; dextromethorphan has equivalent antitussive activity but has much lower toxicity in accidental overdose; tolerance of drug dependence may result from extended use

Pregnancy Risk Factor B; D (if used for prolonged periods or in high doses at term)

Adverse Reactions

>10%:

Central nervous system: Lightheadedness, dizziness, drowsiness, sedation
Dermatologic: Pruritus, skin reactions
Gastrointestinal: Nausea, vomiting, constipation

1% to 10%:

Cardiovascular: Hypotension, palpitations, bradycardia, peripheral vasodilation
Central nervous system: Increased intracranial pressure
Endocrine & metabolic: Antidiuretic hormone release
Gastrointestinal: Biliary tract spasm
Genitourinary: Urinary tract spasm
Ocular: Miosis
Respiratory: Respiratory depression
Miscellaneous: Histamine release, physical and psychological dependence with prolonged use

Drug Interactions CYP2D6 enzyme substrate

Increased toxicity: MAO inhibitors may increase adverse symptoms

Alcohol Interactions Avoid use (may increase central nervous system depression)

Onset 4-5 hours

Half-Life 3.5-4.5 hours

Education and Monitoring Issues

Patient Education: If self-administered, use exactly as directed (do not increase dose or frequency); may cause physical and/or psychological dependence. While using this medication, do not use alcohol and other prescription or OTC medications (especially sedatives, tranquilizers, antihistamines, or pain medications) without consulting prescriber. Maintain adequate hydration (2-3 L/day of fluids unless instructed to restrict fluid intake). May cause dizziness, drowsiness, impaired coordination, or blurred vision (use caution when driving, climbing stairs, or changing position - rising from sitting or lying to standing or when engaging in tasks requiring alertness until response to drug is known); nausea or vomiting (frequent mouth care, small frequent meals, chewing gum, or sucking lozenges may help); constipation (increased exercise, fluids, or dietary fruit and fiber may help - if constipation remains an unresolved problem, consult prescriber about use of stool softeners). Report chest pain or rapid heartbeat; acute headache; swelling of extremities or unusual weight gain; changes in urinary elimination; acute headache; back or flank pain or spasms; or other adverse reactions.

Dihydroergotamine (dye hye droe er GOT a meen)

Pharmacologic Class Ergot Derivative

U.S. Brand Names D.H.E. 45® Injection; Migranal® Nasal Spray

Generic Available Yes

Mechanism of Action Ergot alkaloid alpha-adrenergic blocker directly stimulates vascular smooth muscle to vasoconstrict peripheral and cerebral vessels; also has effects on serotonin receptors

Use Aborts or prevents vascular headaches; also as an adjunct for DVT prophylaxis for hip surgery, for orthostatic hypotension, xerostomia secondary to antidepressant use, and pelvic congestion with pain

USUAL DOSAGE Adults:

I.M.: 1 mg at first sign of headache; repeat hourly to a maximum dose of 3 mg total

I.V.: Up to 2 mg maximum dose for faster effects; maximum dose: 6 mg/week

Intranasal: 1 spray (0.5 mg) of nasal spray should be administered into each nostril; repeat as needed within 15 minutes, up to a total of 6 sprays in any 24-hour period and no more than 8 sprays in a week

Dosing adjustment in hepatic impairment: Dosage reductions are probably necessary but specific guidelines are not available

Dosage Forms INJ: 1 mg/mL (1 mL). **SPRAY nasal:** 4 mg/mL [0.5 mg/spray] (1 mL)

Contraindications High-dose aspirin therapy, hypersensitivity to dihydroergotamine or any component. DHE should not be used within 24 hours of sumatriptan, zolmitriptan, other serotonin agonists or ergot-like agents. DHE should be avoided during or within 2 weeks of discontinuing MAO inhibitors. Avoid concurrent use with amprenavir, ritonavir, nelfinavir and other protease inhibitors. Pregnancy is contraindicated.

Warnings/Precautions Use with caution in hypertension, angina, peripheral vascular disease, impaired renal or hepatic function; avoid pregnancy

Pregnancy Risk Factor X

Adverse Reactions

>10%:

Cardiovascular: Localized edema, peripheral vascular effects (numbness and tingling of fingers and toes)

Central nervous system: Drowsiness, dizziness

Gastrointestinal: Xerostomia, diarrhea, nausea, vomiting

1% to 10%:

Cardiovascular: Precordial distress and pain, transient tachycardia or bradycardia

Neuromuscular & skeletal: Muscle pain in the extremities, weakness in the legs

Drug Interactions

Increased effect of heparin

Increased toxicity with erythromycin, clarithromycin, nitroglycerin, propranolol, troleandomycin

Amprenavir, ritonavir, nelfinavir (and possibly other protease inhibitors) enhance the toxicity of ergot alkaloids - concurrent use should be avoided

Alcohol Interactions Avoid use (may cause or worsen headaches)

Onset Within 15-30 minutes

Duration 3-4 hours

Half-Life 1.3-3.9 hours

Education and Monitoring Issues

Patient Education: Take this drug as rapidly as possible when first symptoms occur. Rare feelings of numbness or tingling of fingers, toes, or face may occur; use caution and avoid injury. May cause drowsiness; avoid activities requiring alertness until effects of medication are known. Report heart palpitations, severe nausea or vomiting, or severe numbness of fingers or toes.

Reference Range: Minimum concentration for vasoconstriction is reportedly 0.06 ng/mL

Dihydrotachysterol (dye hye droe tak IS ter ole)

Pharmacologic Class Vitamin D Analog

U.S. Brand Names DHT™; Hytakerol®

(Continued)

Dihydrotachysterol *(Continued)*

Generic Available Yes

Mechanism of Action Synthetic analogue of vitamin D with a faster onset of action; stimulates calcium and phosphate absorption from the small intestine, promotes secretion of calcium from bone to blood; promotes renal tubule resorption of phosphate

Use Treatment of hypocalcemia associated with hypoparathyroidism; prophylaxis of hypocalcemic tetany following thyroid surgery

USUAL DOSAGE Oral:

Hypoparathyroidism:

Infants and young Children: Initial: 1-5 mg/day for 4 days, then 0.1-0.5 mg/day

Older Children and Adults: Initial: 0.8-2.4 mg/day for several days followed by maintenance doses of 0.2-1 mg/day

Nutritional rickets: 0.5 mg as a single dose or 13-50 mcg/day until healing occurs

Renal osteodystrophy: Maintenance: 0.25-0.6 mg/24 hours adjusted as necessary to achieve normal serum calcium levels and promote bone healing

Dosage Forms CAP (Hytakerol®):0.125 mg. **SOLN:** Oral concentrate (DHT™): 0.2 mg/mL (30 mL); Oral, in oil (Hytakerol®): 0.25 mg/mL (15 mL). **TAB** (DHT™): 0.125 mg, 0.2 mg, 0.4 mg

Contraindications Hypercalcemia, known hypersensitivity to dihydrotachysterol

Warnings/Precautions Calcium-phosphate product (serum calcium and phosphorus) must not exceed 70; avoid hypercalcemia; use with caution in coronary artery disease, decreased renal function (especially with secondary hyperparathyroidism), renal stones, and elderly

Pregnancy Risk Factor A; D (if used in doses above the recommended daily allowance)

Adverse Reactions

>10%:

Endocrine & metabolic: Hypercalcemia

Renal: Elevated serum creatinine, hypercalciuria

<1%: Anemia, anorexia, convulsions, metastatic calcification, nausea, polydipsia, polyuria, renal damage, vomiting, weakness, weight loss

Drug Interactions

Decreased effect/levels of vitamin D: Cholestyramine, colestipol, mineral oil; phenytoin and phenobarbital may inhibit activation may decrease effectiveness

Increased toxicity: Thiazide diuretics increase calcium

Onset Peak hypercalcemic effect: Within 2-4 weeks

Duration Can be as long as 9 weeks

Education and Monitoring Issues

Patient Education: Take exact dose prescribed; do not take more than recommended. Your prescriber may recommend a special diet. Do not increase calcium intake without consulting prescriber. Avoid magnesium supplements or magnesium-containing antacids. You may experience nausea, vomiting, or metallic taste (frequent small meals, frequent mouth care, or sucking hard candy may help); or hypotension (use caution when rising from sitting or lying position or when climbing stairs or bending over). Report chest pain or palpitations; acute headache, dizziness, or feeling of weakness; unresolved nausea or vomiting; persistent metallic taste; unrelieved muscle or bone pain; or CNS irritability.

Monitoring Parameters: Monitor renal function, serum calcium, and phosphate concentrations; if hypercalcemia is encountered, discontinue agent until serum calcium returns to normal

Reference Range: Calcium (serum): 9-10 mg/dL (4.5-5 mEq/L)

- **Dilacor™ XR** *see* Diltiazem *on page 278*
- **Dilantin®** *see* Phenytoin *on page 730*
- **Dilatrate®-SR** *see* Isosorbide Dinitrate *on page 490*
- **Dilaudid®** *see* Hydromorphone *on page 449*
- **Dilaudid-5®** *see* Hydromorphone *on page 449*
- **Dilaudid-HP®** *see* Hydromorphone *on page 449*
- **Dilocaine®** *see* Lidocaine *on page 527*
- **Dilomine® Injection** *see* Dicyclomine *on page 266*

Diloxanide Furoate (dye LOKS ah nide FYOOR oh ate)

Pharmacologic Class Amebicide

U.S. Brand Names Furamide®

Generic Available No

Use Treatment of amebiasis (asymptomatic cyst passers)

- **Diltia XT®** *see* Diltiazem *on page 278*

Diltiazem (dil TYE a zem)

Pharmacologic Class Calcium Channel Blocker

U.S. Brand Names Cardizem® CD; Cardizem® Injectable; Cardizem® SR; Cardizem® Tablet; Cartia® XT; Dilacor™ XR; Diltia XT®; Tiamate®; Tiazac™

Generic Available Yes

Mechanism of Action Inhibits calcium ion from entering the "slow channels" or select voltage-sensitive areas of vascular smooth muscle and myocardium during depolarization, producing a relaxation of coronary vascular smooth muscle and coronary vasodilation; increases myocardial oxygen delivery in patients with vasospastic angina

Use

Capsule: Essential hypertension (alone or in combination) - sustained release only; chronic stable angina or angina from coronary artery spasm

Injection: Atrial fibrillation or atrial flutter; paroxysmal supraventricular tachycardia (PSVT)

Unlabeled use: Prevention of reinfarction of non-Q-wave myocardial infarction, dyskinesia, and Raynaud's syndrome

USUAL DOSAGE Adults:

Angina: Oral: Usual starting dose: 30 mg 4 times/day; sustained release: 120-180 mg once daily; dosage should be increased gradually at 1- to 2-day intervals until optimum response is obtained. Doses up to 360 mg/day have been effectively used. Hypertension is controllable with single daily doses of sustained release products, or divided daily doses of regular release products, in the range of 240-360 mg/day

Sustained-release capsules:

Cardizem® SR: Initial: 60-120 mg twice daily; adjust to maximum antihypertensive effect (usually within 14 days); usual range: 240-360 mg/day

Cardizem® CD, Tiazac™: Hypertension: Total daily dose of short-acting administered once daily or initially 180 or 240 mg once daily; adjust to maximum effect (usually within 14 days); maximum: 480 mg/day; usual range: 240-360 mg/day

Cardizem® CD: Angina: Initial: 120-180 mg once daily; maximum: 480 mg once/day

Dilacor™ XR:

Hypertension: 180-240 mg once daily; maximum: 540 mg/day; usual range: 180-480 mg/day; use lower dose in elderly

Angina: Initial: 120 mg/day; titrate slowly over 7-14 days up to 480 mg/day, as needed

I.V. (requires an infusion pump): See table.

Diltiazem — I.V. Dosage and Administration

Initial Bolus Dose	0.25 mg/kg actual body weight over 2 min (average adult dose: 20 mg)
Repeat Bolus Dose May be administered after 15 min if the response is inadequate.	0.35 mg/kg actual body weight over 2 min (average adult dose: 25 mg)
Continuous Infusion Infusions >24 h or infusion rates >15 mg/h are not recommended.	Initial infusion rate of 10 mg/h; rate may be increased in 5 mg/h increments up to 15 mg/h as needed; some patients may respond to an initial rate of 5 mg/h.

If Cardizem® injectable is administered by continuous infusion for >24 hours, the possibility of decreased diltiazem clearance, prolonged elimination half-life, and increased diltiazem and/or diltiazem metabolite plasma concentrations should be considered

Conversion from I.V. diltiazem to oral diltiazem: Start oral approximately 3 hours after bolus dose

Oral dose (mg/day) is approximately equal to [rate (mg/hour) x 3 + 3] x 10

3 mg/hour = 120 mg/day
5 mg/hour = 180 mg/day
7 mg/hour = 240 mg/day
11 mg/hour = 360 mg/day

Dosing comments in renal/hepatic impairment: Use with caution as extensively metabolized by the liver and excreted in the kidneys and bile

Dialysis: Not removed by hemo- or peritoneal dialysis; supplemental dose is not necessary

Dosage Forms CAP, sustained release: 60 mg, 90 mg, 120 mg, 180 mg, 240 mg, 300 mg; (Cardizem® CD): 120 mg, 180 mg, 240 mg, 300 mg, 360 mg; (Cardizem® SR): 60 mg, 90 mg, 120 mg; (Cartia® XT): 120 mg, 180 mg, 240 mg, 300 mg; (Dilacor™ XR): 180 mg, 240 mg; (Diltia XT®): 120 mg, 180 mg, 240 mg; (Tiazac™): 120 mg, 180 mg, 240 mg, 300 mg, 360 mg, 420 mg. **INJ:** 5 mg/mL (5 mL, 10 mL); (Cardizem®): 5 mg/mL (5 mL, 10 mL). **TAB:** (Cardizem®): 30 mg, 60 mg, 90 mg, 120 mg; Extended release (Tiamate®): 120 mg, 180 mg, 240 mg

Contraindications Severe hypotension (<90 mm Hg systolic) or second and third degree heart block except with a functioning pacemaker; hypersensitivity to diltiazem; sick sinus syndrome, acute myocardial infarction, and pulmonary congestion

Warnings/Precautions Use with caution and titrate dosages for patients with hypotension or patients taking antihypertensives, impaired renal or hepatic function, or when treating patients with congestive heart failure. Use caution with concomitant therapy with beta-blockers or digoxin. Monitor LFTs during therapy since these enzymes may rarely be

(Continued)

Diltiazem *(Continued)*

increased and symptoms of hepatic injury may occur; usually reverses with drug discontinuation; avoid abrupt withdrawal of calcium blockers since rebound angina is theoretically possible.

Pregnancy Risk Factor C

Pregnancy Implications

Clinical effects on the fetus: Teratogenic and embryotoxic effects have been demonstrated in small animals given doses 5-10 times the adult dose (mg/kg)

Breast-feeding/lactation: Freely diffuses into breast milk; however, the American Academy of Pediatrics considers diltiazem to be **compatible** with breast-feeding. Available evidence suggest safe use during breast-feeding.

Adverse Reactions

>10%: Gastrointestinal: Gingival hyperplasia (21%)

1% to 10%:

Cardiovascular: Sinus bradycardia (1.5% to 6%), first-degree A-V block (1.8% to 7.6%), EKG abnormality (4.1%), peripheral edema (dose-related 5.4% to 8%), flushing (1.9% to 3%), hypotension (1%), palpitations (1.3%)

Central nervous system: Dizziness (3.4% to 7%), headache (4.5% to 12%), somnolence (1.3%), insomnia (1%)

Gastrointestinal: Nausea (1.3% to 1.6%), constipation (1.6%), dyspepsia (1.3%)

Neuromuscular & skeletal: Weakness (2.8% to 5%)

Dermatological: Rash (1& to 1.5%)

Renal: Polyuria (1.3%)

<1% (limited to important or life-threatening symptoms): Angina, arrhythmia, second- or third-degree A-V block, bundle branch block, congestive heart failure, syncope, tachycardia, ventricular extrasystoles, abnormal dreams, amnesia, depression, gait abnormalities, hallucinations, nervousness, paresthesia, personality change, tremor, anorexia, diarrhea, dry mouth, dysgeusia, thirst, vomiting, weight gain, petechiae, photosensitivity, pruritus, urticaria, amblyopia, dyspnea, epistaxis, eye irritation, hyperglycemia, hyperuricemia, impotence, muscle cramps, nasal congestion, nocturia, osteoarticular pain, sexual difficulties, myoclonus, tinnitus

Case reports: Agranulocytosis, leukocytopenia (overdose), thrombocytopenia, akathisia, mania, psychosis, Parkinsonian-like syndrome, TEN, Stevens-Johnson syndrome, erythema multiforme, exfoliative dermatitis, gynecomastia

Drug Interactions CYP3A3/4 enzyme substrate; CYP1A2, 2D6, and 3A3/4 enzyme inhibitor

Decreased effect: Moricizine has decreased diltiazem concentrations and decreased its half-life

Increased toxicity:

Diltiazem has increased peak plasma moricizine levels and decreased oral clearance; side effect frequency increases

Diltiazem and amiodarone may cause increased bradycardia and decreased cardiac output

Diltiazem and cimetidine may cause increased bioavailability of diltiazem

Severe hypotension possible with concurrent administration with fentanyl

Both increased and decreased lithium levels have occurred with diltiazem; use caution with coadministration

Diltiazem and cyclosporine may cause increased cyclosporine levels and subsequent renal toxicity

Diltiazem and digoxin may cause increased digoxin levels and additive effects

Diltiazem and beta-blockers may result in increased cardiac depression

Cisapride toxicity (Q-T prolongation) may be increased with diltiazem

Protease inhibitors (amprenavir, ritonavir, nelfinavir) may increase the serum levels of diltiazem

Theophylline effects possibly enhanced with diltiazem

Diltiazem with carbamazepine may result in increased carbamazepine levels and possible toxic effects

Alcohol Interactions Avoid use

Onset Oral: 30-60 minutes (including sustained release)

Half-Life 4-6 hours, may increase with renal impairment; 5-7 hours with sustained release

Education and Monitoring Issues

Patient Education: Oral: Take as directed; do not alter dosage or discontinue therapy without consulting prescriber. Do not crush or chew extended release form. Avoid (or limit) alcohol and caffeine. You may experience dizziness or lightheadedness (use caution when driving or engaging in tasks requiring alertness until response to drug is known); nausea or vomiting (small frequent meals, frequent mouth care, chewing gum, or sucking lozenges may help); constipation (increased exercise, dietary fiber, fruit, or fluid may help); diarrhea (buttermilk, boiled milk, or yogurt may help). Report chest pain, palpitations, irregular heartbeat, unusual cough, difficulty breathing, swelling of extremities, muscle tremors or weakness, confusion or acute lethargy, or skin rash.

Monitoring Parameters: Liver function tests, blood pressure, EKG

Related Information

Calcium Channel Blocking Agents Comparison *on page 1236*

Enalapril and Diltiazem *on page 311*

- **Dimetane®-DC** *see* Brompheniramine, Phenylpropanolamine, and Codeine *on page 114*

Dinoprostone (dye noe PROST one)

Pharmacologic Class Abortifacient; Prostaglandin

U.S. Brand Names Cervidil® Vaginal Insert; Prepidil® Vaginal Gel; Prostin E_2® Vaginal Suppository

Generic Available No

Mechanism of Action A synthetic prostaglandin E_2 abortifacient that stimulates uterine contractions similar to those seen during natural labor

Use

Gel: Promote cervical ripening prior to labor induction; usage for gel include any patient undergoing induction of labor with an unripe cervix, most commonly for pre-eclampsia, eclampsia, postdates, diabetes, intrauterine growth retardation, and chronic hypertension

Suppositories: Terminate pregnancy from 12th through 28th week of gestation; evacuate uterus in cases of missed abortion or intrauterine fetal death; manage benign hydatidiform mole

USUAL DOSAGE

Abortifacient: Insert 1 suppository high in vagina, repeat at 3- to 5-hour intervals until abortion occurs up to 240 mg (maximum dose); continued administration for longer than 2 days is not advisable

Cervical ripening:

Gel:

Intracervical: 0.25-1 mg

Intravaginal: 2.5 mg

Suppositories: Intracervical: 2-3 mg

Dosage Forms INSERT, vag (Cervidil®): 10 mg. **GEL, endocervical:** 0.5 mg in 3 g syringes [each package contains a 10-mm and 20-mm shielded catheter]. **SUPP, vag:** 20 mg

Contraindications

Gel: Hypersensitivity to prostaglandins or any constituents of the cervical gel, history of asthma, contracted pelvis, malpresentation of the fetus

Gel: The following are "relative" contraindications and should only be considered by the prescriber under these circumstances: Patients in whom vaginal delivery is not indicated (ie, herpes genitalia with a lesion at the time of delivery), prior uterine surgery, breech presentation, multiple gestation, polyhydramnios, premature rupture of membranes

Suppository: Known hypersensitivity to dinoprostone, acute pelvic inflammatory disease, uterine fibroids, cervical stenosis

Warnings/Precautions Dinoprostone should be used only by medically trained personnel in a hospital; caution in patients with cervicitis, infected endocervical lesions, acute vaginitis, compromised (scarred) uterus or history of asthma, hypertension or hypotension, epilepsy, diabetes mellitus, anemia, jaundice, or cardiovascular, renal, or hepatic disease. Oxytocin should not be used simultaneously with Prepidil® (>6 hours of the last dose of Prepidil®).

Pregnancy Risk Factor C

Adverse Reactions

>10%:

Central nervous system: Headache

Gastrointestinal: Vomiting, diarrhea, nausea

1% to 10%:

Cardiovascular: Bradycardia

Central nervous system: Fever

Neuromuscular & skeletal: Back pain

<1%: Bronchospasm, cardiac arrhythmias, chills, coughing, dizziness, dyspnea, flushing, hot flashes, hypotension, pain, shivering, syncope, tightness of the chest, vasomotor and vasovagal reactions, wheezing

Drug Interactions Increased effect of oxytocics

Onset Onset of effect (uterine contractions): Within 10 minutes

Duration Up to 2-3 hours

Education and Monitoring Issues

Patient Education: Nausea and vomiting, cramping or uterine pain, or fever may occur. Report acute pain, respiratory difficulty, or skin rash. Closely monitor for vaginal discharge for several days. Report vaginal bleeding, itching, malodorous or bloody discharge, or severe cramping.

- **Diocaine** *see* Proparacaine *on page 782*
- **Diochloram** *see* Chloramphenicol *on page 178*
- **Diocto® [OTC]** *see* Docusate *on page 290*
- **Diocto-K® [OTC]** *see* Docusate *on page 290*
- **Diodex** *see* Dexamethasone *on page 256*
- **Diodoquin®** *see* Iodoquinol *on page 480*

- **Dioeze® [OTC]** *see* Docusate *on page 290*
- **Diofluor** *see* Fluorescein Sodium *on page 375*
- **Dioflur-P** *see* Proparacaine and Fluorescein *on page 783*
- **Diogent** *see* Gentamicin *on page 408*
- **Diomycin** *see* Erythromycin *on page 323*
- **Dionephrine** *see* Phenylephrine *on page 727*
- **Diopentolate** *see* Cyclopentolate *on page 235*
- **Diopticon** *see* Naphazoline *on page 636*
- **Dioptimyd** *see* Sulfacetamide Sodium and Prednisolone *on page 876*
- **Dioptrol** *see* Neomycin, Polymyxin B, and Dexamethasone *on page 644*
- **Diospor HC** *see* Neomycin, Polymyxin B, and Hydrocortisone *on page 644*
- **Diosporin** *see* Neomycin, Polymyxin B, and Gramicidin *on page 644*
- **Diosulf** *see* Sulfacetamide Sodium *on page 876*
- **Diotrope** *see* Tropicamide *on page 958*
- **Dioval® Injection** *see* Estradiol *on page 327*
- **Diovan™** *see* Valsartan *on page 968*
- **Diovan™ HCT** *see* Valsartan and Hydrochlorothiazide *on page 969*
- **Dipentum®** *see* Olsalazine *on page 674*
- **Diphenacen-50® Injection** *see* Diphenhydramine *on page 282*
- **Diphen® Cough [OTC]** *see* Diphenhydramine *on page 282*
- **Diphenhist [OTC]** *see* Diphenhydramine *on page 282*

Diphenhydramine (dye fen HYE dra meen)

Pharmacologic Class Antihistamine

U.S. Brand Names AllerMax® Oral [OTC]; Banophen® Oral [OTC]; Belix® Oral [OTC]; Benadryl® Injection; Benadryl® Oral [OTC]; Benadryl® Topical; Ben-Allergin-50® Injection; Benylin® Cough Syrup [OTC]; Bydramine® Cough Syrup [OTC]; Compoz® Gel Caps [OTC]; Compoz® Nighttime Sleep Aid [OTC]; Dihydrex® Injection; Diphenacen-50® Injection; Diphen® Cough [OTC]; Diphenhist [OTC]; Dormarex® 2 Oral [OTC]; Dormin® Oral [OTC]; Genahist® Oral; Hydramyn® Syrup [OTC]; Hyrexin-50® Injection; Maximum Strength Nytol® [OTC]; Miles Nervine® Caplets [OTC]; Nordryl® Injection; Nordryl® Oral; Nytol® Oral [OTC]; Phendry® Oral [OTC]; Siladryl® Oral [OTC]; Silphen® Cough [OTC]; Sleep-eze 3® Oral [OTC]; Sleepinal® [OTC]; Sleepwell 2-nite® [OTC]; Sominex® Oral [OTC]; Tusstat® Syrup; Twilite® Oral [OTC]; Uni-Bent® Cough Syrup; 40 Winks® [OTC]

Generic Available Yes

Mechanism of Action Competes with histamine for H_1-receptor sites on effector cells in the gastrointestinal tract, blood vessels, and respiratory tract

Use Symptomatic relief of allergic symptoms caused by histamine release which include nasal allergies and allergic dermatosis; can be used for mild nighttime sedation; prevention of motion sickness and as an antitussive; has antinauseant and topical anesthetic properties; treatment of phenothiazine-induced dystonic reactions

USUAL DOSAGE

Children:

Oral: (>10 kg): 12.5-25 mg 3-4 times/day; maximum daily dose: 300 mg

I.M., I.V.: 5 mg/kg/day or 150 mg/m^2/day in divided doses every 6-8 hours, not to exceed 300 mg/day

Adults:

Oral: 25-50 mg every 6-8 hours

Nighttime sleep aid: 50 mg at bedtime

I.M., I.V.: 10-50 mg in a single dose every 2-4 hours, not to exceed 400 mg/day

Topical: For external application, not longer than 7 days

Dosage Forms CAP: 25 mg, 50 mg. **CRM:** 1%, 2%. **ELIX:** 12.5 mg/5 mL (5 mL, 10 mL, 20 mL, 120 mL, 480 mL, 3780 mL). **INJ:** 10 mg/mL (10 mL, 30 mL); 50 mg/mL (1 mL, 10 mL). **LOT:** 1% (75 mL). **SOLN, top spray:** 1% (60 mL). **SYR:** 12.5 mg/5 mL (5 mL, 120 mL, 240 mL, 480 mL, 3780 mL). **TAB:** 25 mg, 50 mg

Contraindications Hypersensitivity to diphenhydramine or any component; should not be used in acute attacks of asthma

Warnings/Precautions Use with caution in patients with angle-closure glaucoma, peptic ulcer, urinary tract obstruction, hyperthyroidism; some preparations contain sodium bisulfite; syrup contains alcohol; diphenhydramine has high sedative and anticholinergic properties, so it may not be considered the antihistamine of choice for prolonged use in the elderly

Pregnancy Risk Factor B

Adverse Reactions

Cardiovascular: Hypotension, palpitations, tachycardia

Central nervous system: Sedation, sleepiness, dizziness, disturbed coordination, headache, fatigue, nervousness, paradoxical excitement, insomnia, euphoria, confusion

Dermatologic: Photosensitivity, rash, angioedema, urticaria

Gastrointestinal: Nausea, vomiting, diarrhea, abdominal pain, xerostomia, appetite increase, weight gain, dry mucous membranes, anorexia

Genitourinary: Urinary retention, urinary frequency, difficult urination

Hematologic: Hemolytic anemia, thrombocytopenia, agranulocytosis
Neuromuscular & skeletal: Tremor, paresthesia
Ocular: blurred vision
Respiratory: Thickening of bronchial secretions

Drug Interactions CYP2D6 enzyme substrate

May increase gastric degradation of levodopa and decrease the amount of levodopa absorbed by delaying gastric emptying; the opposite may be true for digoxin

Therapeutic effects of cholinergic agents (tacrine, donepezil) and neuroleptics may be antagonized

Central and/or peripheral anticholinergic syndrome can occur when administered with amantadine, rimantadine, narcotic analgesics, phenothiazines and other antipsychotics (especially with high anticholinergic activity), tricyclic antidepressants, quinidine and some other antiarrhythmics, and antihistamines

Syrup should not be given to patients taking drugs that can cause disulfiram reactions (ie, metronidazole, chlorpropamide) due to high alcohol content

Alcohol Interactions Avoid use (may increase central nervous system depression)

Onset Maximum sedative effect: 1-3 hours; I.V. more rapid

Duration 4-7 hours

Half-Life 2-8 hours; elderly: 13.5 hours

Education and Monitoring Issues

Patient Education: Take as directed; do not exceed recommended dose. Avoid use of other depressants, alcohol, or sleep-inducing medications unless approved by prescriber. You may experience drowsiness or dizziness (use caution when driving or engaging in tasks requiring alertness until response to drug is known); or dry mouth, nausea, or vomiting (frequent small meals, frequent mouth care, chewing gum, or sucking hard candy may help). Report persistent sedation, confusion, or agitation; changes in urinary pattern; blurred vision; sore throat, difficulty breathing, or expectorating (thick secretions); or lack of improvement or worsening of condition.

Reference Range:

Antihistamine effects at levels >25 ng/mL
Drowsiness at levels 30-40 ng/mL
Mental impairment at levels >60 ng/mL
Therapeutic: Not established
Toxic: >0.1 μg/mL

Diphenoxylate and Atropine (dye fen OKS i late & A troe peen)

Pharmacologic Class Antidiarrheal

U.S. Brand Names Lofene®; Logen®; Lomanate®; Lomodix®; Lomotil®; Lonox®; Low-Quel®

Generic Available Yes

Mechanism of Action Diphenoxylate inhibits excessive GI motility and GI propulsion; commercial preparations contain a subtherapeutic amount of atropine to discourage abuse

Use Treatment of diarrhea

USUAL DOSAGE Oral:

Children (use with caution in young children due to variable responses): Liquid: 0.3-0.4 mg of diphenoxylate/kg/day in 2-4 divided doses **or**

<2 years: Not recommended
2-5 years: 2 mg of diphenoxylate 3 times/day
5-8 years: 2 mg of diphenoxylate 4 times/day
8-12 years: 2 mg of diphenoxylate 5 times/day

Adults: 15-20 mg/day of diphenoxylate in 3-4 divided doses; maintenance: 5-15 mg/day in 2-3 divided doses

Dosage Forms SOLN, oral: Diphenoxylate hydrochloride 2.5 mg and atropine sulfate 0.025 mg per 5 mL (4 mL, 10 mL, 60 mL). **TAB:** Diphenoxylate hydrochloride 2.5 mg and atropine sulfate 0.025 mg

Contraindications Hypersensitivity to diphenoxylate, atropine or any component; severe liver disease, jaundice, dehydrated patient, and narrow-angle glaucoma; it should not be used for children <2 years of age

Warnings/Precautions High doses may cause physical and psychological dependence with prolonged use; use with caution in patients with ulcerative colitis, dehydration, and hepatic dysfunction; reduction of intestinal motility may be deleterious in diarrhea resulting from *Shigella*, *Salmonella*, toxigenic strains of *E. coli*, and from pseudomembranous enterocolitis associated with broad spectrum antibiotics; children may develop signs of atropinism (dryness of skin and mucous membranes, thirst, hyperthermia, tachycardia, urinary retention, flushing) even at the recommended dosages; if there is no response with 48 hours, the drug is unlikely to be effective and should be discontinued; if chronic diarrhea is not improved symptomatically within 10 days at maximum dosage of 20 mg/day, control is unlikely with further use.

Pregnancy Risk Factor C

(Continued)

Diphenoxylate and Atropine *(Continued)*

Adverse Reactions

1% to 10%:

Central nervous system: Nervousness, restlessness, dizziness, drowsiness, headache, mental depression

Gastrointestinal: Paralytic ileus, xerostomia

Genitourinary: Urinary retention and dysuria

Ocular: Blurred vision

Respiratory: Respiratory depression

<1%: Abdominal discomfort, diaphoresis (increased), euphoria, hyperthermia, muscle cramps, nausea, pancreatitis, pruritus, sedation, stomach cramps, tachycardia, urticaria, vomiting, weakness

Drug Interactions Increased toxicity: MAO inhibitors (hypertensive crisis), CNS depressants, antimuscarinics (paralytic ileus); may prolong half-life of drugs metabolized in liver

Alcohol Interactions Avoid use (may increase central nervous system depression)

Onset Onset of action: Within 45-60 minutes; Peak effect: Within 2 hours

Duration 3-4 hours

Half-Life Diphenoxylate: 2.5 hours

Education and Monitoring Issues

Patient Education: Take as directed; do not exceed recommended dosage. If no response within 48 hours, notify prescriber. Avoid alcohol or other prescriptive or OTC sedatives or depressants. You may experience drowsiness, blurred vision, impaired coordination; use caution when driving or engaging in tasks that require alertness until response to drug is known. Sucking on lozenges or chewing gum may reduce dry mouth. Report difficulty urinating, persistent diarrhea, respiratory difficulties, fever, or palpitations.

Monitoring Parameters: Watch for signs of atropinism (dryness of skin and mucous membranes, tachycardia, thirst, flushing); monitor number and consistency of stools; observe for signs of toxicity, fluid and electrolyte loss, hypotension, and respiratory depression

♦ **Diphenylan Sodium®** *see* Phenytoin *on page 730*

Diphtheria and Tetanus Toxoid (dif THEER ee a & TET a nus TOKS oyd)

Pharmacologic Class Toxoid

Generic Available Yes

Use Active immunity against diphtheria and tetanus when pertussis vaccine is contraindicated; tetanus prophylaxis in wound management

DT: Infants and children through 6 years of age

Td: Children and adults ≥7 years of age

USUAL DOSAGE I.M.:

Infants and Children (DT):

6 weeks to 1 year: Three 0.5 mL doses at least 4 weeks apart; administer a reinforcing dose 6-12 months after the third injection

1-6 years: Two 0.5 mL doses at least 4 weeks apart; reinforcing dose 6-12 months after second injection; if final dose is given after seventh birthday, use adult preparation

4-6 years (booster immunization): 0.5 mL; not necessary if all 4 doses were given after fourth birthday - routinely administer booster doses at 10-year intervals with the adult preparation

Children >7 years and Adults: Should receive Td; 2 primary doses of 0.5 mL each, given at an interval of 4-6 weeks; third (reinforcing) dose of 0.5 mL 6-12 months later; boosters every 10 years

Tetanus Prophylaxis in Wound Management

Number of Prior Tetanus Toxoid Doses	Clean, Minor Wounds		All Other Wounds	
	Td*	TIG†	Td*	TIG†
Unknown or <3	Yes	No	Yes	Yes
≥3‡	No#	No	No¶	No

*Adult tetanus and diphtheria toxoids; use pediatric preparations (DT or DTP) if the patient is <7 years old.

†Tetanus immune globulin.

‡If only three doses of fluid tetanus toxoid have been received, a fourth dose of toxoid, preferably an adsorbed toxoid, should be given.

#Yes, if >10 years since last dose.

¶Yes, if >5 years since last dose.

Adapted from Report of the Committee on Infectious Diseases, American Academy of Pediatrics, Elk Grove Village, IL: American Academy of Pediatrics, 1986.

Dosage Forms INJ:

Pediatric use: Diphtheria 6.6 Lf units and tetanus 5 Lf units per 0.5 mL (5 mL); Diphtheria 10 Lf units and tetanus 5 Lf units per 0.5 mL (0.5 mL, 5 mL); Diphtheria 12.5 Lf units and tetanus 5 Lf units per 0.5 mL (5 mL); Diphtheria 15 Lf units and tetanus 10 Lf units per 0.5 mL (5 mL)

Adult use: Diphtheria 1.5 Lf units and tetanus 5 Lf units per 0.5 mL (0.5 mL, 5 mL); Diphtheria 2 Lf units and tetanus 5 Lf units per 0.5 mL (5 mL); Diphtheria 2 Lf units and tetanus 10 Lf units per 0.5 mL (5 mL)

Contraindications Patients receiving immunosuppressive agents, prior anaphylactic, allergic, or systemic reactions; hypersensitivity to diphtheria and tetanus toxoid or any component; acute respiratory infection or other active infection

Warnings/Precautions History of a neurologic reaction or immediate hypersensitivity reaction following a previous dose. History of severe local reaction (Arthus-type) following previous dose (such individuals should not be given further routine or emergency doses of tetanus and diphtheria toxoids for 10 years). Do not confuse pediatric DT with adult diphtheria and tetanus toxoid (Td), absorbed (Td) is used in patients >7 years of age; primary immunization should be postponed until the second year of life due to possibility of CNS damage or convulsion; have epinephrine 1:1000 available.

Pregnancy Risk Factor C

Pregnancy Implications Clinical effects on the fetus: Td and T vaccines are not known to cause special problems for pregnant women or their unborn babies. While prescribers do not usually recommend giving any drugs or vaccines to pregnant women, a pregnant women who needs Td vaccine should get it; wait until 2nd trimester if possible.

Adverse Reactions Severe adverse reactions must be reported to the FDA

>10%: Central nervous system: Fretfulness, drowsiness

1% to 10%:

Central nervous system: Persistent crying

Gastrointestinal: Anorexia, vomiting

<1%: Arthus-type hypersensitivity reactions, convulsions (rarely), edema, hypotension, pain, pruritus, redness, tachycardia, tenderness, transient fever, urticaria

Drug Interactions Decreased effect with immunosuppressive agents, immunoglobulins if given within 1 month (eg, concomitant administration with tetanus immune globulin decreased the immune response to Td)

Education and Monitoring Issues

Patient Education: DT, Td and T vaccines cause few problems (mild fever or soreness, swelling, and redness/knot at the injection site); these problems usually last 1-2 days, but this does not happen nearly as often as with DTP vaccine

Related Information

Animal and Human Bites Guidelines *on page 1177*

Dipivefrin (dye PI ve frin)

Pharmacologic Class Adrenergic Agonist Agent

U.S. Brand Names AKPro® Ophthalmic; Propine® Ophthalmic

Use Reduces elevated intraocular pressure in chronic open-angle glaucoma; also used to treat ocular hypertension, low tension, and secondary glaucomas

USUAL DOSAGE Adults: Ophthalmic: Instill 1 drop every 12 hours into the eyes

Contraindications Hypersensitivity to dipivefrin, ingredients in the formulation, or epinephrine; contraindicated in patients with angle-closure glaucoma

Pregnancy Risk Factor B

♦ **Diprivan®** *see* Propofol *on page 783*

♦ **Diprolene®** *see* Betamethasone *on page 103*

♦ **Diprolene® AF** *see* Betamethasone *on page 103*

♦ **Diprolene® Glycol [Dipropionate]** *see* Betamethasone *on page 103*

♦ **Diprosone®** *see* Betamethasone *on page 103*

Dipyridamole (dye peer ID a mole)

Pharmacologic Class Antiplatelet Agent; Vasodilator

U.S. Brand Names Persantine®

Generic Available Yes

Mechanism of Action Inhibits the activity of adenosine deaminase and phosphodiesterase, which causes an accumulation of adenosine, adenine nucleotides, and cyclic AMP; these mediators then inhibit platelet aggregation and may cause vasodilation; may also stimulate release of prostacyclin or PGD_2; causes coronary vasodilation

Use Maintains patency after surgical grafting procedures including coronary artery bypass; used with warfarin to decrease thrombosis in patients after artificial heart valve replacement; used with aspirin to prevent coronary artery thrombosis; in combination with aspirin or warfarin to prevent other thromboembolic disorders. Dipyridamole may also be given 2 days prior to open heart surgery to prevent platelet activation by extracorporeal bypass pump and as a diagnostic agent in CAD; also approved as an alternative to exercise during Thallium myocardial perfusion imaging for the evaluation of coronary artery disease in patients who cannot exercise adequately

USUAL DOSAGE

Children: Oral: 3-6 mg/kg/day in 3 divided doses

Doses of 4-10 mg/kg/day have been used investigationally to treat proteinuria in pediatric renal disease

(Continued)

Dipyridamole *(Continued)*

Mechanical prosthetic heart valves: Oral: 2-5 mg/kg/day (used in combination with an oral anticoagulant in children who have systemic embolism despite adequate oral anticoagulant therapy, and used in combination with low-dose oral anticoagulation (INR 2-3) plus aspirin in children in whom full-dose oral anticoagulation is contraindicated)

Adults:

Oral: 75-400 mg/day in 3-4 divided doses

Evaluation of coronary artery disease: I.V.: 0.14 mg/kg/minute for 4 minutes; maximum dose: 60 mg

Hemodialysis: Significant drug removal is unlikely based on physiochemical characteristics

Dosage Forms INJ: 10 mg/2 mL. **TAB:** 25 mg, 50 mg, 75 mg

Contraindications Hypersensitivity to dipyridamole or any component

Warnings/Precautions Safety and effectiveness in children <12 years of age have not been established; may further decrease blood pressure in patients with hypotension due to peripheral vasodilation; use with caution in patients taking other drugs which affect platelet function or coagulation and in patients with hemostatic defects. Since evidence suggests that clinically used doses are ineffective for prevention of platelet aggregation, consideration for low-dose aspirin (81-325 mg/day) alone may be necessary; this will decrease cost as well as inconvenience.

Pregnancy Risk Factor B

Adverse Reactions

>10%:

Cardiovascular: Exacerbation of angina pectoris (19.7% - I.V.)

Central nervous system: Dizziness (13.6% - P.O.), headache (12.2% - I.V.)

1% to 10%:

Cardiovascular: Hypotension (4.6%), hypertension (1.5%), blood pressure lability (1.6%), EKG abnormalities(ST-T changes, extrasystoles),chest pain, tachycardia (3.2% - I.V.)

Central nervous system: Headache (2.3% - I.V.), flushing (3.4% - I.V.), fatigue (1.2% - I.V.)

Dermatologic: Rash (2.3% - P.O.)

Gastrointestinal: Abdominal distress (6.1% - P.O.), nausea (4.6% - I.V.)

Respiratory: Dyspnea (2.6% - I.V.)

Neuromuscular & Skeletal: Paresthesia (1.3% - I.V.)

<1% (limited to important or life-threatening symptoms):

I.V.: EKG abnormalities, arrhythmias (ventricular tachycardia, bradycardia, A-V block, SVT, atrial fibrillation, asystole), palpitations, MI, syncope, orthostatic hypotension, cardiomyopathy, edema, hypertonia, tremor, abnormal coordination, vertigo, dyspepsia, dry mouth, abdominal pain, flatulence, vomiting, eructation, dysphagia, tenesmus, increased appetite, pharyngitis, bronchospasm, hyperventilation, rhinitis, coughing, pleural pain, myalgia, back pain, injection site reaction, diaphoresis, asthenia, malaise, arthralgia, rigor, dysgeusia, leg cramping, earache, tinnitus, vision abnormalities, thirst, depersonalization, renal pain, perineal pain, breast pain, intermittent claudication.

P.O.: Diarrhea, vomiting, flushing, pruritus, angina pectoris, liver dysfunction.

Case reports: Rapidly progressive glomerulonephritis, thrombotic thrombocytopenic purpura, esophageal hematoma, gallstones, epistaxis, pharyngeal bleeding, respiratory arrest (I.V.)

Drug Interactions

Increased toxicity: Heparin may increase anticoagulation

Decreased hypotensive effect (I.V.): Theophylline

Half-Life 10-12 hours

Education and Monitoring Issues

Patient Education: Oral: Take exactly as directed, with or without food. You may experience mild headache, transient diarrhea, or temporary dizziness (sit or lie down when taking medication). You may have a tendency to bleed easy; use caution with sharps, needles, or razors. Report any unusual bleeding (eg, gums, urine, stool) chest pain, acute abdominal cramping or severe diarrhea, acute and persistent headache or dizziness, rash, difficulty breathing, or swelling of extremities.

Dirithromycin (dye RITH roe mye sin)

Pharmacologic Class Antibiotic, Macrolide

U.S. Brand Names Dynabac®

Use Treatment of mild to moderate upper and lower respiratory tract infections due to *Moraxella catarrhalis, Streptococcus pneumoniae, Legionella pneumophila, H. influenzae,* or *S. pyogenes* ie, acute exacerbation of chronic bronchitis, secondary bacterial infection of acute bronchitis, community-acquired pneumonia, pharyngitis/tonsillitis, and uncomplicated infections of the skin and skin structure due to *Staphylococcus aureus*

USUAL DOSAGE Adults: Oral: 500 mg once daily for 5-14 days (14 days required for treatment of community-acquired pneumonia due to *Legionella, Mycoplasma,* or *S. pneumoniae*; 10 days is recommended for treatment of *S. pyogenes* pharyngitis/tonsillitis)

Dosing adjustment in renal impairment: None necessary

Dosing adjustment in hepatic impairment: None needed in mild dysfunction; not studied in moderate to severe dysfunction

Contraindications Hypersensitivity to any macrolide or component of dirithromycin; use with pimozide

Pregnancy Risk Factor C

- **Disalcid®** *see* Salsalate *on page 837*
- **Disipal** *see* Orphenadrine *on page 681*
- **Disonate® [OTC]** *see* Docusate *on page 290*

Disopyramide (dye soe PEER a mide)

Pharmacologic Class Antiarrhythmic Agent, Class I-A

U.S. Brand Names Norpace®

Generic Available Yes

Mechanism of Action Class IA antiarrhythmic: Decreases myocardial excitability and conduction velocity; reduces disparity in refractory between normal and infarcted myocardium; possesses anticholinergic, peripheral vasoconstrictive, and negative inotropic effects

Use Suppression and prevention of unifocal and multifocal premature, ventricular premature complexes, coupled ventricular tachycardia; effective in the conversion of atrial fibrillation, atrial flutter, and paroxysmal atrial tachycardia to normal sinus rhythm and prevention of the reoccurrence of these arrhythmias after conversion by other methods

USUAL DOSAGE Oral:

Children:

- <1 year: 10-30 mg/kg/24 hours in 4 divided doses
- 1-4 years: 10-20 mg/kg/24 hours in 4 divided doses
- 4-12 years: 10-15 mg/kg/24 hours in 4 divided doses
- 12-18 years: 6-15 mg/kg/24 hours in 4 divided doses

Adults:

- <50 kg: 100 mg every 6 hours or 200 mg every 12 hours (controlled release)
- >50 kg: 150 mg every 6 hours or 300 mg every 12 hours (controlled release); if no response, may increase to 200 mg every 6 hours; maximum dose required for patients with severe refractory ventricular tachycardia is 400 mg every 6 hours

Dosing adjustment in renal impairment: 100 mg (nonsustained release) given at the following intervals: See table.

Disopyramide Phosphate

Creatinine Clearance (mL/min)	Dosage Interval
30-40	q8h
15-30	q12h
<15	q24h

or alter the dose as follows:

- Cl_{cr} 30-<40 mL/minute: Reduce dose 50%
- Cl_{cr} 15-30 mL/minute: Reduce dose 75%

Dialysis: Not dialyzable (0% to 5%) by hemo- or peritoneal methods; supplemental dose not necessary

Dosing interval in hepatic impairment: 100 mg every 6 hours or 200 mg every 12 hours (controlled release)

Dosage Forms CAP: 100 mg, 150 mg; Sustained action: 100 mg, 150 mg

Contraindications Pre-existing second or third degree A-V block, cardiogenic shock, or known hypersensitivity to the drug; coadministration with sparfloxacin

Warnings/Precautions Pre-existing urinary retention, family history, or existing angle-closure glaucoma, myasthenia gravis, hypotension during initiation of therapy, congestive heart failure unless caused by an arrhythmias, widening of QRS complex during therapy or Q-T interval (>25% to 50% of baseline QRS complex or Q-T interval), sick-sinus syndrome or WPW, renal or hepatic impairment require decrease in dosage; disopyramide ineffective in hypokalemia and potentially toxic with hyperkalemia. Due to changes in total clearance (decreased) in elderly, monitor closely; the anticholinergic action may be intolerable and require discontinuation.

Pregnancy Risk Factor C

Adverse Reactions The most common adverse effects are related to cholinergic blockade. The most serious adverse effects of disopyramide are hypotension and congestive heart failure.

>10%:

- Gastrointestinal: Xerostomia (32%), constipation (11%)
- Genitourinary: Urinary hesitancy (14% to 23%)

1% to 10%:

- Cardiovascular: Congestive heart failure, hypotension, cardiac conduction disturbance, edema, syncope, chest pain

(Continued)

Disopyramide *(Continued)*

Central nervous system: Fatigue, headache, malaise, dizziness, nervousness
Dermatologic: Rash, generalized dermatoses, pruritus
Endocrine & metabolic: Weight gain, hypokalemia, elevated cholesterol, elevated triglycerides
Gastrointestinal: Dry throat, nausea, abdominal distension, flatulence, abdominal bloating, anorexia, diarrhea, vomiting
Genitourinary: Urinary retention, urinary frequency, urinary urgency, impotence (1% to 3%)
Neuromuscular & skeletal: Muscle weakness, muscular pain
Ocular: Blurred vision, dry eyes
Respiratory: Dyspnea

<1% (limited to important or life-threatening symptoms): New or worsened arrhythmias (proarrhythmic effect), hypoglycemia, cholestatic jaundice, fever, respiratory distress, thrombocytopenia, agranulocytosis, gynecomastia, psychotic reaction, depression, insomnia, dysuria, numbness, tingling, paresthesia, elevated transaminases, A-V block, increased serum creatinine, increased BUN, elevated creatinine, decreased hemoglobin, decreased hematocrit, hepatotoxicity. Rare cases of lupus have been reported (generally in patients previously receiving procainamide).

Case reports: Peripheral neuropathy, psychosis, pupillary dilation, toxic cutaneous blisters

Drug Interactions CYP3A3/4 enzyme substrate

Inhibitors of CYP3A3/4 may increase blood levels
Beta-blockers may cause additive/excessive negative inotropic activity
Enzyme inducers (phenobarbital, phenytoin, rifampin) decrease disopyramide blood levels
Erythromycin and clarithromycin increase disopyramide blood levels; may cause QRS widening and/or Q-T interval prolongation
Procainamide, quinidine, propafenone, or flecainide can cause increased/excessive negative inotropic effects or prolonged conduction
Drugs which may prolong the Q-T interval - amiodarone, amitriptyline, bepridil, cisapride, disopyramide, erythromycin, haloperidol, imipramine, pimozide, quinidine, sotalol, and thioridazine may be additive with disopyramide; use with caution
Sparfloxacin, gatifloxacin, and moxifloxacin may result in additional prolongation of the Q-T interval; concurrent use is contraindicated

Onset 0.5-3.5 hours

Duration 1.5-8.5 hours

Half-Life 4-10 hours, increased half-life with hepatic or renal disease

Education and Monitoring Issues

Patient Education: Take as directed, at regular intervals around-the-clock. Do not alter dosage or discontinue therapy without consulting prescriber. Do not crush or chew extended release form. Avoid (or limit) alcohol and caffeine. You may experience dizziness or blurred vision (use caution when driving or engaging in tasks requiring alertness until response to drug is known); or dry mouth (frequent mouth care or sucking on lozenges may help). Report any change in urinary pattern or difficulty urinating; chest pain, palpitations, irregular heartbeat; unusual cough, difficulty breathing, swelling of extremities; muscle tremors or weakness; confusion or acute lethargy; or skin rash.

Monitoring Parameters: EKG, blood pressure, disopyramide drug level, urinary retention, CNS anticholinergic effects (confusion, agitation, hallucinations, etc)

Reference Range:

Therapeutic concentration:
Atrial arrhythmias: 2.8-3.2 μg/mL
Ventricular arrhythmias 3.3-7.5 μg/mL
Toxic concentration: >7 μg/mL

- **Disotate®** *see* Edetate Disodium *on page 305*
- **Di-Spaz® Injection** *see* Dicyclomine *on page 266*
- **Di-Spaz® Oral** *see* Dicyclomine *on page 266*
- **Dispos-a-Med® Isoproterenol** *see* Isoproterenol *on page 488*

Disulfiram (dye SUL fi ram)

Pharmacologic Class Aldehyde Dehydrogenase Inhibitor

U.S. Brand Names Antabuse®

Generic Available Yes

Mechanism of Action Disulfiram is a thiuram derivative which interferes with aldehyde dehydrogenase. When taken concomitantly with alcohol, there is an increase in serum acetaldehyde levels. High acetaldehyde causes uncomfortable symptoms including flushing, nausea, thirst, palpitations, chest pain, vertigo, and hypotension. This reaction is the basis for disulfiram use in postwithdrawal long-term care of alcoholism.

Use Management of chronic alcoholism

USUAL DOSAGE Adults: Oral: Do not administer until the patient has abstained from alcohol for at least 12 hours

Initial: 500 mg/day as a single dose for 1-2 weeks; maximum daily dose is 500 mg

Average maintenance dose: 250 mg/day; range: 125-500 mg; duration of therapy is to continue until the patient is fully recovered socially and a basis for permanent self control has been established; maintenance therapy may be required for months or even years

Dosage Forms TAB: 250 mg, 500 mg; (Antabuse®): 250 mg

Contraindications Severe myocardial disease and coronary occlusion, hypersensitivity to disulfiram or any component, patient receiving alcohol, paraldehyde, alcohol-containing preparations like cough syrup or tonics

Warnings/Precautions Use with caution in patients with diabetes, hypothyroidism, seizure disorders, hepatic cirrhosis, or insufficiency; should never be administered to a patient when he/she is in a state of alcohol intoxication, or without his/her knowledge

Pregnancy Risk Factor C

Adverse Reactions

Central nervous system: Drowsiness, headache, fatigue, psychosis
Dermatologic: Rash, acneiform eruptions, allergic dermatitis
Gastrointestinal: Metallic or garlic-like aftertaste
Genitourinary: Impotence
Hepatic: Hepatitis
Neuromuscular & skeletal: Peripheral neuritis, polyneuritis, peripheral neuropathy
Ocular: Optic neuritis

Drug Interactions CYP2C9 and 2E1 enzyme inhibitor, both disulfiram and diethyldithiocarbamate (disulfiram metabolite) are CYP3A3/4 enzyme inhibitors

Disulfiram may increase serum concentrations of benzodiazepines that undergo oxidative metabolism (all but oxazepam, lorazepam, temazepam)

Disulfiram increases phenytoin and theophylline serum concentrations; toxicity may occur

Disulfiram inhibits the metabolism of warfarin resulting in an increased hypoprothombinemic response

Disulfiram results in severe ethanol intolerance (Antabuse® reaction) secondary to disulfiram's ability to inhibit aldehyde dehydrogenase; this combination should be avoided

Combined use with isoniazid, metronidazole, or MAOIs may result in adverse CNS effects; this combination should be avoided

Intravenous trimethoprim-sulfamethoxazole contains 10% ethanol as a solubilizing agent and may interact with disulfiram; monitor for Antabuse® reaction

Alcohol Interactions Disulfiram inhibits alcohol's usual metabolism. Patients can have a disulfiram reaction (headache, nausea, vomiting, chest or abdominal pain) if they drink alcohol concurrently. Avoid all alcohol, cough syrups, elixirs, vinegars, cider, extracts, or foods with alcohol in it while taking disulfiram and for 2 weeks after it is stopped.

Onset Full effect: 12 hours

Duration May persist for 1-2 weeks after last dose

Education and Monitoring Issues

Patient Education: Tablets can be crushed or mixed with water or juice. Metallic aftertaste may occur; this will go away. Do not drink any alcohol, including products containing alcohol (cough and cold syrups), or use alcohol-containing skin products while taking this medication or for at least 3 days and preferably 14 days after stopping this medication. Drowsiness, tiredness, or visual changes may occur; use care when driving or engaging in tasks requiring alertness until response to drug is known. You may experience impotence; this will reverse when medication is discontinued. Report yellow color in eyes or skin and any respiratory difficulty.

- **Ditropan®** *see* Oxybutynin *on page 690*
- **Ditropan XL®** *see* Oxybutynin *on page 690*
- **Diuchlor®** *see* Hydrochlorothiazide *on page 442*
- **Diurigen®** *see* Chlorothiazide *on page 184*
- **Diuril®** *see* Chlorothiazide *on page 184*
- **Dixarit®** *see* Clonidine *on page 216*
- **Dizac® Injectable Emulsion** *see* Diazepam *on page 261*
- **Dizmiss® [OTC]** *see* Meclizine *on page 556*
- **D-Med® Injection** *see* Methylprednisolone *on page 589*
- **DM E Suppressant Expectorant** *see* Guaifenesin and Dextromethorphan *on page 424*
- **DM Plus Expectorant** *see* Guaifenesin and Dextromethorphan *on page 424*

Dobutamine (doe BYOO ta meen)

Pharmacologic Class Adrenergic Agonist Agent; Sympathomimetic

U.S. Brand Names Dobutrex® Injection

Generic Available No

Mechanism of Action Stimulates $beta_1$-adrenergic receptors, causing increased contractility and heart rate, with little effect on $beta_2$- or alpha-receptors

Use Increase cardiac output in the short-term treatment of patients with cardiac decompensation caused by depressed contractility from organic heart disease, cardiac surgical procedures, or acute MI

USUAL DOSAGE I.V. infusion:

Neonates and Children: 2.5-15 mcg/kg/minute, titrate to desired response

(Continued)

Dobutamine *(Continued)*

Adults: 2.5-15 mcg/kg/minute; maximum: 40 mcg/kg/minute, titrate to desired response

Infusion Rates of Various Dilutions of Dobutamine

Desired Delivery Rate (mcg/kg/min)	Infusion Rate(mL/kg/min)	
	500 mcg/mL*	1000 mcg/mL†
2.5	0.005	0.0025
5.0	0.01	0.005
7.5	0.015	0.0075
10.0	0.02	0.01
12.5	0.025	0.0125
15.0	0.03	0.015

* 500 mg per liter or 250 mg per 500 mL of diluent.

†1000 mg per liter or 250 mg per 250 mL of diluent.

Dosage Forms INF: 12.5 mg/mL (20 mL)

Contraindications Hypersensitivity to sulfites (commercial preparation contains sodium bisulfite); patients with idiopathic hypertrophic subaortic stenosis

Warnings/Precautions Hypovolemia should be corrected prior to use; infiltration causes local inflammatory changes, extravasation may cause dermal necrosis; use with extreme caution following myocardial infarction; potent drug, must be diluted prior to use

Pregnancy Risk Factor B

Adverse Reactions

>10%: Cardiovascular: Ectopic heartbeats, increased heart rate, chest pain, angina, palpitations, hypertension; in higher doses, ventricular tachycardia or arrhythmias may be seen; patients with atrial fibrillation or flutter are at risk of developing a rapid ventricular response

1% to 10%:
- Cardiovascular: Premature ventricular beats, chest pain, angina, palpitations
- Central nervous system: Headache
- Gastrointestinal: Nausea, vomiting
- Neuromuscular & skeletal: Mild leg cramps, paresthesia
- Respiratory: Dyspnea

Drug Interactions

Decreased effect: Beta-adrenergic blockers may antagonize the cardiac effects of dobutamine, resulting in predominantly alpha-adrenergic effects and increased peripheral resistance

Increased toxicity: General anesthetics (ie, halothane or cyclopropane) and usual doses of dobutamine have resulted in ventricular arrhythmias in animals

Onset I.V.: 1-10 minutes; Peak effect: Within 10-20 minutes

Half-Life 2 minutes

Education and Monitoring Issues

Patient Education: When administered in emergencies, patient education should be appropriate to the situation. If patient is aware, instruct to promptly report chest pain, palpitations, rapid heartbeat, headache, nervousness, or restlessness, nausea or vomiting, or difficulty breathing.

Monitoring Parameters: Blood pressure, EKG, heart rate, CVP, RAP, MAP, urine output; if pulmonary artery catheter is in place, monitor CI, PCWP, and SVR; also monitor serum potassium

♦ **Dobutrex® Injection** *see* Dobutamine *on page 289*

Docusate (DOK yoo sate)

Pharmacologic Class Stool Softener

U.S. Brand Names Colace® [OTC]; DC 240® Softgels® [OTC]; Dialose® [OTC]; Diocto® [OTC]; Diocto-K® [OTC]; Dioeze® [OTC]; Disonate® [OTC]; DOK® [OTC]; DOS® Softgel® [OTC]; D-S-S® [OTC]; Kasof® [OTC]; Modane® Soft [OTC]; Pro-Cal-Sof® [OTC]; Regulax SS® [OTC]; Sulfalax® [OTC]; Surfak® [OTC]

Use Stool softener in patients who should avoid straining during defecation and constipation associated with hard, dry stools; prophylaxis for straining (Valsalva) following myocardial infarction. A safe agent to be used in elderly; some evidence that doses <200 mg are ineffective; stool softeners are unnecessary if stool is well hydrated or "mushy" and soft; shown to be ineffective used long-term.

USUAL DOSAGE Docusate salts are interchangeable; the amount of sodium, calcium, or potassium per dosage unit is clinically insignificant

Infants and Children <3 years: Oral: 10-40 mg/day in 1-4 divided doses

Children: Oral:
- 3-6 years: 20-60 mg/day in 1-4 divided doses
- 6-12 years: 40-150 mg/day in 1-4 divided doses

Adolescents and Adults: Oral: 50-500 mg/day in 1-4 divided doses

Older Children and Adults: Rectal: Add 50-100 mg of docusate liquid to enema fluid (saline or water); administer as retention or flushing enema

Contraindications Concomitant use of mineral oil; intestinal obstruction, acute abdominal pain, nausea, vomiting; hypersensitivity to docusate or any component

Pregnancy Risk Factor C

Dofetilide doe FET il ide

Pharmacologic Class Antiarrhythmic Agent, Class III

U.S. Brand Names Tikosyn™

Mechanism of Action Vaughan Williams Class III antiarrhythmic activity. Blockade of the cardiac ion channel carrying the rapid component of the delayed rectifier potassium current. Dofetilide has no effect on sodium channels, adrenergic alpha-receptors, or adrenergic beta-receptors. It increases the monophasic action potential duration due to delayed repolarization. The increase in the Q-T interval is a function of prolongation of both effective and functional refractory periods in the His-Purkinje system and the ventricles. Changes in cardiac conduction velocity and sinus node function have not been observed in patients with or without structural heart disease. PR and QRS width remain the same in patients with pre-existing heart block and or sick sinus syndrome.

Use Maintenance of normal sinus rhythm in patients with atrial fibrillation/atrial flutter of greater than 1 week's duration who have been converted to normal sinus rhythm; conversion of atrial fibrillation and atrial flutter to normal sinus rhythm

USUAL DOSAGE Adults: Sustained tachycardia (ventricular): Oral: 0.25-1 mg twice daily; lower dose in patients with renal insufficiency

Dosage adjustment in renal impairment:

Cl_{cr} >60 mL/minute: Administer 500 mcg twice daily.

Cl_{cr} 40-60 mL/minute: Administer 250 mcg twice daily.

Cl_{cr} 20-39 mL/minute: Administer 125 mcg twice daily.

Cl_{cr} <20 mL/minute: Contraindicated in this group.

Dosage Forms CAP: 125 mcg, 250 mcg, 500 mcg

Contraindications Patients with paroxysmal atrial fibrillation; patients with congenital or acquired long Q-T syndromes, do not use if a baseline Q-T interval or QT_c is >440 msec (500 msec in patients with ventricular conduction abnormalities); severe renal impairment (estimated Cl_{cr} <20 mL/minute); concurrent use with verapamil, cimetidine, trimethoprim (alone or in combination with sulfamethoxazole), ketoconazole, prochlorperazine, or megestrol; known hypersensitivity to dofetilide, baseline heart rate <50 beats/minute; other drugs that prolong Q-T intervals (phenothiazines, cisapride, bepridil, tricyclic antidepressants, certain oral macrolides: sparfloxacin, gatifloxacin, moxifloxacin); hypokalemia or hypomagnesemia; concurrent amiodarone

Warnings/Precautions Note: Must be initiated (or reinitiated) in a setting with continuous monitoring and staff familiar with the recognition and treatment of life-threatening arrhythmias. Patients must be monitored with continuous EKG for a minimum of 3 days, or for a minimum of 12 hours after electrical or pharmacological cardioversion to normal sinus rhythm, whichever is greater. Patients should be readmitted for continuous monitoring if dosage is later increased.

Reserve for patients who are highly symptomatic with atrial fibrillation/atrial flutter; torsade de pointes significantly increases with doses >500 mcg twice daily; hold Class Ia or Class II antiarrhythmics for at least three half-lives prior to starting dofetilide; use in patients on amiodarone therapy only if serum amiodarone level is <0.3 mg/L or if amiodarone was stopped for >3 months previously; correct hypokalemia or hypomagnesemia before initiating dofetilide and maintain within normal limits during treatment.

Patients with sick sinus syndrome or with second or third-degree heart block should not receive dofetilide unless a functional pacemaker is in place. Defibrillation threshold is reduced in patients with ventricular tachycardia or ventricular fibrillation undergoing implantation of a cardioverter-defibrillator device. Safety and efficacy in children (<18 years old) have not been established. Use with caution in renal impairment; not recommended in patients receiving drugs which may compete for renal secretion via cationic transport. Use with caution in patients with severe hepatic impairment.

Pregnancy Risk Factor C

Adverse Reactions

Supraventricular arrhythmia patients (incidence > placebo)

>10%: Central nervous system: Headache (11%)

2% to 10%:

Central nervous system: Dizziness (8%), insomnia (4%)

Cardiovascular: Ventricular tachycardia (2.6% to 3.7%), chest pain (10%), torsade de pointes (3.3% in CHF patients and 0.9% in patients with a recent MI; up to 10.5% in patients receiving doses in excess of those recommended). Torsade de pointes occurs most frequently within the first 3 days of therapy.

Dermatologic: Rash (3%)

Gastrointestinal: Nausea (5%), diarrhea (3%), abdominal pain (3%)

Neuromuscular & skeletal: Back pain (3%)

Respiratory: Dyspnea (6%), respiratory tract infection (7%)

Miscellaneous: Flu syndrome (4%)

(Continued)

Dofetilide *(Continued)*

<2%:

Central nervous system: CVA, facial paralysis, flaccid paralysis, migraine, paralysis

Cardiovascular: A-V block (0.4% to 1.5%), ventricular fibrillation (0% to 0.4%), bundle branch block, heart block, edema, heart arrest, myocardial infarct, sudden death, syncope

Dermatologic: Angioedema

Gastrointestinal: Liver damage

Neuromuscular & skeletal: Paresthesia

Respiratory: Cough

>2% (incidence ≤ placebo): Anxiety, pain, angina, atrial fibrillation, hypertension, palpitation, supraventricular tachycardia, peripheral edema, urinary tract infection, weakness, arthralgia, sweating

Drug Interactions CYP3A3/4 enzyme substrate (minor)

Inhibitors of CYP3A3/4 (erythromycin, clarithromycin, azole antifungal agents, protease inhibitors, serotonin reuptake inhibitors, amiodarone, cannabinoids, diltiazem, nefazodone, norfloxacin, quinine, zafirlukast) should be used cautiously as they may increase dofetilide levels.

Cimetidine, a cation transport system inhibitor, inhibits dofetilide's elimination and can cause a 58% increase in dofetilide's plasma levels; concomitant use is contraindicated.

Drugs which prolong Q-T interval (including bepridil, cisapride, erythromycin, tricyclic antidepressants, phenothiazines, sparfloxacin, gatifloxacin, moxifloxacin): Use is contraindicated.

Verapamil causes an increase in dofetilide's peak plasma levels by 42%. In the supraventricular arrhythmia and a higher incidence of torsade de pointes was seen in patients on verapamil; concomitant use is contraindicated.

Ketoconazole increases dofetilide's C_{max} (53% males, 97% females) and the AUC (41% males, 69% females) when used concurrently; concomitant use is contraindicated.

Trimethoprim (alone or in combination with sulfamethoxazole) increases dofetilide's C_{max} (103%) and AUC (93%); concomitant use is contraindicated.

Renal cationic transport inhibitors (including triamterene, metformin, amiloride, prochlorperazine, megestrol) may increase dofetilide levels; coadminister with caution.

Diuretics and other drugs (aminoglycosides) which deplete potassium or magnesium may increase dofetilide toxicity (torsade de pointes).

Drugs which have been reported **not** to affect dofetilide include digoxin, amlodipine, phenytoin, glyburide, ranitidine, omeprazole, hormone replacement therapy (conjugated estrogens/medroxyprogesterone), antacid (aluminum/magnesium hydroxide), and theophylline.

Half-Life 10 hours

Education and Monitoring Issues

Patient Education: This medication can only be administered I.V. and you must be monitored continuously during therapy and for some length of time following therapy. Report immediately any chest pain or palpitations; headache, confusion, or agitation; nausea, abdominal or back pain; swelling around mouth, face, tongue, or throat; cough or flu-like symptoms; or other unusual reactions.

Dietary Considerations: Grapefruit juice may increase dofetilide levels

Monitoring Parameters: EKG monitoring with attention to QT_c and occurrence of ventricular arrhythmias, baseline serum creatinine and changes in serum creatinine. Check serum potassium and magnesium levels if on medications where these electrolyte disturbances can occur, or if patient has a history of hypokalemia or hypomagnesemia.

Manufacturer Pfizer U.S. Pharmaceutical Group

Related Information

Pharmaceutical Manufacturers Directory *on page 1020*

- **DOK® [OTC]** *see* Docusate *on page 290*
- **Doktors® Nasal Solution [OTC]** *see* Phenylephrine *on page 727*
- **Dolacet®** *see* Hydrocodone and Acetaminophen *on page 444*

Dolasetron (dol A se tron)

Pharmacologic Class Selective 5-HT_3 Receptor Antagonist

U.S. Brand Names Anzemet®

Mechanism of Action Dolasetron is a pseudopelletierine-derived serotonin antagonist. Serotonin antagonists block the serotonin receptors in the chemoreceptor trigger zone and in the gastrointestinal tract. Once the receptor site is blocked, antagonism of vomiting occurs.

Use Prevention of nausea and vomiting associated with emetogenic cancer chemotherapy, including initial and repeat courses; prevention of postoperative nausea and vomiting and treatment of postoperative nausea and vomiting (injectable form only)

USUAL DOSAGE

Children <2 years: Not recommended for use

Nausea and vomiting associated with chemotherapy (including initial and repeat courses):
Children 2-16 years:
Oral: 1.8 mg/kg within 1 hour before chemotherapy; maximum: 100 mg/dose
I.V.: 1.8 mg/kg ~30 minutes before chemotherapy; maximum: 100 mg/dose
Adults:
Oral: 100 mg within 1 hour before chemotherapy
I.V.: 1.8 mg/kg ~30 minutes before chemotherapy or may give 100 mg
Prevention of postoperative nausea and vomiting:
Children 2-16 years:
Oral: 1.2 mg within 2 hours before surgery; maximum: 100 mg/dose
I.V.: 0.35 mg/kg (maximum: 12.5 mg) ~15 minutes before stopping anesthesia
Adults:
Oral: 100 mg within 2 hours before surgery
I.V.: 12.5 mg ~15 minutes before stopping anesthesia
Treatment of postoperative nausea and vomiting: I.V. only:
Children 2-16 years: 0.35 mg/kg as soon as needed
Adults: 12.5 mg as soon as needed

Dosing adjustment for elderly, renal/hepatic impairment: No dosage adjustment is recommended

Dosage Forms **INJ:** 20 mg/mL (0.625 mL, 5 mL). **TAB:** 50 mg, 100 mg

Contraindications Patients known to have hypersensitivity to the drug

Warnings/Precautions Dolasetron should be administered with caution in patients who have or may develop prolongation of cardiac conduction intervals, particularly QT_c intervals. These include patients with hypokalemia or hypomagnesemia, patients taking diuretics with potential for inducing electrolyte abnormalities, patients with congenital Q-T syndrome, patients taking antiarrhythmic drugs or other drugs which lead to Q-T prolongation, and cumulative high-dose anthracycline therapy.

Pregnancy Risk Factor B

Adverse Reactions Dolasetron can cause electrocardiographic interval changes, which are related in frequency and magnitude to blood levels of the metabolite, hydrodolasetron

>2%:
Cardiovascular: Hypertension
Central nervous system: Headache, fatigue, dizziness, fever, chills and shivering
Gastrointestinal: Diarrhea, abdominal pain
Genitourinary: Urinary retention
Hepatic: Transient increases in liver enzymes

Drug Interactions CYP2D6 and 3A3/4 enzyme substrate

Blood levels of the active metabolite are increased when dolasetron is coadministered with cimetidine, decreased with rifampin. Clearance of hydrodolasetron decreases when dolasetron is given with atenolol.

Half-Life Dolasetron: <10 minutes; hydrodolasetron 7.3 hours

Education and Monitoring Issues

Patient Education: This drug is given to reduce the incidence of nausea and vomiting. You may experience headache, drowsiness, or dizziness; request assistance when getting up or changing position and do not perform activities requiring alertness. Report immediately unusual pain, chills, or fever; severe headache or diarrhea; chest pain, palpitations, or tightness; swelling of throat or feeling of tightness in throat; or difficulty urinating.

Monitoring Parameters: Liver function tests, blood pressure and pulse, and EKG in patients with cardiovascular disease

Manufacturer Hoechst-Marion Roussel

Related Information

Pharmaceutical Manufacturers Directory *on page 1020*

♦ **Dolene®** *see* Propoxyphene *on page 784*
♦ **Dolobid®** *see* Diflunisal *on page 271*
♦ **Dolophine®** *see* Methadone *on page 576*

Donepezil (don EH pa zil)

Pharmacologic Class Acetylcholinesterase Inhibitor (Central)

U.S. Brand Names Aricept®

Mechanism of Action Alzheimer's disease is characterized by cholinergic deficiency in the cortex and basal forebrain, which contributes to cognitive deficits. Donepezil reversibly and noncompetitively inhibits centrally-active acetylcholinesterase, the enzyme responsible for hydrolysis of acetylcholine. This appears to result in increased concentrations of acetylcholine available for synaptic transmission in the central nervous system.

Use Treatment of mild to moderate dementia of the Alzheimer's type

USUAL DOSAGE Adults: Initial: 5 mg/day at bedtime; may increase to 10 mg/day at bedtime after 4-6 weeks

Dosage Forms **TAB:** 5 mg, 10 mg

Contraindications Patients who are hypersensitive to donepezil or piperidine derivatives

(Continued)

Donepezil *(Continued)*

Warnings/Precautions Use with caution in patients with sick sinus syndrome or other supraventricular cardiac conduction abnormalities, in patients with seizures or asthma; avoid use in nursing mothers

Pregnancy Risk Factor C

Adverse Reactions

>10%:

Central nervous system: Headache

Gastrointestinal: Nausea, diarrhea

1% to 10%:

Cardiovascular: Syncope, chest pain, hypertension, atrial fibrillation, hypotension, hot flashes

Central nervous system: Fatigue, insomnia, dizziness, depression, abnormal dreams, somnolence

Dermatologic: Bruising

Gastrointestinal: Anorexia, vomiting, weight loss, fecal incontinence, GI bleeding, bloating, epigastric pain

Genitourinary: Frequent urination

Neuromuscular & skeletal: Muscle cramps, arthritis, body pain

Drug Interactions CYP2D6 and 3A3/4 enzyme substrate

Ketoconazole and quinidine inhibit donepezil's metabolism *in vitro*; monitor for altered clinical response

Phenytoin, carbamazepine, dexamethasone, rifampin, and phenobarbital may increase the rate of elimination of donepezil; monitor for altered clinical response

Anticholinergic agents (benztropine) may inhibit the effects of donepezil

A synergistic effect may be seen with concurrent administration of succinylcholine or cholinergic agonists (bethanechol)

Onset May require extended treatment

Duration May be prolonged, particularly in older patients

Half-Life 70 hours

Education and Monitoring Issues

Patient Education: This medication will not cure the disease, but may help reduce symptoms. Use as directed; do not increase dose or discontinue without consulting prescriber. Maintain adequate hydration (2-3 L/day of fluids unless instructed to restrict fluid intake). May cause dizziness, sedation, or hypotension (rise slowly from sitting or lying position and use caution when driving or climbing stairs); vomiting or loss of appetite (frequent small meals, frequent mouth care, chewing gum, or sucking lozenges may help); or diarrhea (boiled milk, yogurt, or buttermilk may help). Report persistent abdominal discomfort; significantly increased salivation, sweating, tearing, or urination; flushed skin; chest pain or palpitations; acute headache; unresolved diarrhea; excessive fatigue, insomnia, dizziness, or depression; increased muscle, joint, or body pain; vision changes or blurred vision; or shortness of breath or wheezing.

Manufacturer Pfizer U.S. Pharmaceutical Group

Related Information

Pharmaceutical Manufacturers Directory *on page 1020*

- **Donnagel®-PG Capsule** *see* Kaolin and Pectin With Opium *on page 498*
- **Donnagel®-PG Suspension** *see* Kaolin and Pectin With Opium *on page 498*
- **Donnamar®** *see* Hyoscyamine *on page 456*
- **Donnapectolin-PG®** *see* Hyoscyamine, Atropine, Scopolamine, Kaolin, Pectin, and Opium *on page 457*
- **Donnapine®** *see* Hyoscyamine, Atropine, Scopolamine, and Phenobarbital *on page 456*
- **Donna-Sed®** *see* Hyoscyamine, Atropine, Scopolamine, and Phenobarbital *on page 456*
- **Donnatal®** *see* Hyoscyamine, Atropine, Scopolamine, and Phenobarbital *on page 456*
- **Dopamet®** *see* Methyldopa *on page 586*

Dopamine (DOE pa meen)

Pharmacologic Class Adrenergic Agonist Agent; Sympathomimetic

U.S. Brand Names Intropin® Injection

Generic Available Yes

Mechanism of Action Stimulates both adrenergic and dopaminergic receptors, lower doses are mainly dopaminergic stimulating and produce renal and mesenteric vasodilation, higher doses also are both dopaminergic and $beta_1$-adrenergic stimulating and produce cardiac stimulation and renal vasodilation; large doses stimulate alpha-adrenergic receptors

Use Increase cardiac output, blood pressure, and urine flow as an adjunct in the treatment of shock persisting after adequate fluid volume replacement; increase cardiac output and blood pressure during cardiopulmonary resuscitation

USUAL DOSAGE I.V. infusion (administration requires the use of an infusion pump):

Neonates: 1-20 mcg/kg/minute continuous infusion, titrate to desired response

Children: 1-20 mcg/kg/minute, maximum: 50 mcg/kg/minute continuous infusion, titrate to desired response

Adults: 1-5 mcg/kg/minute up to 50 mcg/kg/minute, titrate to desired response; infusion may be increased by 1-4 mcg/kg/minute at 10- to 30-minute intervals until optimal response is obtained

If dosages >20-30 mcg/kg/minute are needed, a more direct-acting pressor may be more beneficial (ie, epinephrine, norepinephrine)

The hemodynamic effects of dopamine are dose-dependent:

Low-dose: 1-3 mcg/kg/minute, increased renal blood flow and urine output

Intermediate-dose: 3-10 mcg/kg/minute, increased renal blood flow, heart rate, cardiac contractility, and cardiac output

High-dose: >10 mcg/kg/minute, alpha-adrenergic effects begin to predominate, vasoconstriction, increased blood pressure

Dosage Forms INF in D_5W: 0.8 mg/mL (250 mL, 500 mL); 1.6 mg/mL (250 mL, 500 mL); 3.2 mg/mL (250 mL, 500 mL). **INJ:** 40 mg/mL (5 mL, 10 mL, 20 mL); 80 mg/mL (5 mL, 20 mL); 160 mg/mL (5 mL)

Contraindications Hypersensitivity to sulfites (commercial preparation contains sodium bisulfite); pheochromocytoma or ventricular fibrillation

Warnings/Precautions Safety in children has not been established; hypovolemia should be corrected by appropriate plasma volume expanders before administration; extravasation may cause tissue necrosis (treat extravasation with phentolamine); potent drug, must be diluted prior to use; patient's hemodynamic status should be monitored; use with caution in patients with cardiovascular disease or cardiac arrhythmias or patients with occlusive vascular disease (due to potential gangrene of extremities)

Pregnancy Risk Factor C

Adverse Reactions

>10%:

Cardiovascular: Ectopic heartbeats, tachycardia, vasoconstriction, hypotension, cardiac conduction abnormalities, widened QRS complex, ventricular arrhythmias

Central nervous system: Headache

Gastrointestinal: Nausea, vomiting

Respiratory: Dyspnea

1% to 10%: Cardiovascular: Bradycardia, gangrene of the extremities, hypertension

<1%: Anxiety, azotemia, decreased urine output, piloerection

Drug Interactions Increased effect: Dopamine's effects are prolonged and intensified by MAO inhibitors, alpha- and beta-adrenergic blockers, general anesthetics, phenytoin

Beta-blockers (nonselective ones) may increase hypertensive effect; avoid concurrent use.

Cocaine may cause malignant arrhythmias; avoid concurrent use.

Guanethidine's hypotensive effects may only be partially reversed; may need to use a direct-acting sympathomimetic.

MAO inhibitors potentiate hypertension and hypertensive crisis; avoid concurrent use.

Methyldopa can increase the pressor response; be aware of patient's drug regimen.

Reserpine increases the pressor response; be aware of patient's drug regimen.

TCAs increase the pressor response; be aware of patient's drug regimen.

Onset 5 minutes

Duration <10 minutes

Half-Life 2 minutes

Education and Monitoring Issues

Patient Education: When administered in emergencies, patient education should be appropriate to the situation. If patient is aware, instruct to promptly report chest pain, palpitations, rapid heartbeat, headache, nervousness or restlessness, nausea or vomiting, or difficulty breathing.

Monitoring Parameters: Blood pressure, EKG, heart rate, CVP, RAP, MAP, urine output; if pulmonary artery catheter is in place, monitor CI, PCWP, SVR, and PVR

- **Dopar®** *see* Levodopa *on page 520*
- **Dopram® Injection** *see* Doxapram *on page 296*
- **Doral®** *see* Quazepam *on page 798*
- **Dormarex® 2 Oral [OTC]** *see* Diphenhydramine *on page 282*
- **Dormin® Oral [OTC]** *see* Diphenhydramine *on page 282*
- **Doryx®** *see* Doxycycline *on page 300*

Dorzolamide (dor ZOLE a mide)

Pharmacologic Class Carbonic Anhydrase Inhibitor

U.S. Brand Names Trusopt®

Mechanism of Action Reversible inhibition of the enzyme carbonic anhydrase resulting in reduction of hydrogen ion secretion at renal tubule and an increased renal excretion of sodium, potassium, bicarbonate, and water to decrease production of aqueous humor; also inhibits carbonic anhydrase in central nervous system to retard abnormal and excessive discharge from CNS neurons

Use Lowers intraocular pressure to treat glaucoma in patients with ocular hypertension or open-angle glaucoma

USUAL DOSAGE Adults: Glaucoma: Instill 1 drop in the affected eye(s) 3 times/day

(Continued)

Dorzolamide *(Continued)*

Dosage Forms SOLN, ophth: 2%

Contraindications Hypersensitivity to any component of the product; contains benzalkonium chloride as a preservative

Warnings/Precautions

Although administered topically, systemic absorption occurs. Same types of adverse reactions attributed to sulfonamides may occur with topical administration.

Because dorzolamide and its metabolite are excreted predominantly by the kidney, it is not recommended for use in patients with severe renal impairment (Cl_{cr} <30 mL/minute); use with caution in patients with hepatic impairment

Local ocular adverse effects (conjunctivitis and lid reactions) were reported with chronic administration. Many resolved with discontinuation of drug therapy. If such reactions occur, discontinue dorzolamide.

There is a potential for an additive effect in patients receiving an oral carbonic anhydrase inhibitor and dorzolamide. The concomitant administration of dorzolamide and oral carbonic anhydrase inhibitors is not recommended.

Benzalkonium chloride is the preservative in dorzolamide which may be absorbed by soft contact lenses. Dorzolamide should not be administered while wearing soft contact lenses.

Pregnancy Risk Factor C

Adverse Reactions

>10%:

- Gastrointestinal: Bitter taste following administration (25%)
- Ocular: Burning, stinging or discomfort immediately following administration (33%); superficial punctate keratitis (10% to 15%); signs and symptoms of ocular allergic reaction (10%)

5% to 10% Ocular: Blurred vision, tearing, dryness, photophobia

<1%: Fatigue, headache, iridocyclitis, nausea, rashes, urolithiasis, weakness

Drug Interactions Increased toxicity: Salicylates use may result in carbonic anhydrase inhibitor accumulation and toxicity including CNS depression and metabolic acidosis

Onset Peak effect: 2 hours

Duration 8-12 hours

Half-Life Terminal RBC half-life of 147 days

Education and Monitoring Issues

Patient Education:

If serious or unusual reactions or signs of hypersensitivity occur, discontinue use of the product

If any ocular reactions, particularly conjunctivitis and lid reactions, discontinue use and seek prescriber's advice. If an intercurrent ocular condition (eg, trauma, ocular surgery, infection) occur, immediately seek your prescriber's advice concerning the continued use of the present multidose container.

Avoid allowing the tip of the dispensing container to contact the eye or surround structures

Monitoring Parameters: Monitor serum electrolyte levels (potassium) and blood pH levels; Ophthalmic exams and IOP periodically

Manufacturer Merck & Co

Related Information

Pharmaceutical Manufacturers Directory *on page 1020*

♦ **DOS® Softgel® [OTC]** *see* Docusate *on page 290*

♦ **Dostinex®** *see* Cabergoline *on page 126*

♦ **Dovonex®** *see* Calcipotriene *on page 127*

Doxapram (DOKS a pram)

Pharmacologic Class Respiratory Stimulant

U.S. Brand Names Dopram® Injection

Use Respiratory and CNS stimulant; stimulates respiration in patients with drug-induced CNS depression or postanesthesia respiratory depression; in hospitalized patients with COPD associated with acute hypercapnia

USUAL DOSAGE Not for use in newborns since doxapram contains a significant amount of benzyl alcohol (0.9%)

Neonatal apnea (apnea of prematurity): I.V.:

- Initial: 1-1.5 mg/kg/hour
- Maintenance: 0.5-2.5 mg/kg/hour, titrated to the lowest rate at which apnea is controlled

Adults: Respiratory depression following anesthesia: I.V.:

- Initial: 0.5-1 mg/kg; may repeat at 5-minute intervals; maximum total dose: 2 mg/kg
- I.V. infusion: Initial: 5 mg/minute until adequate response or adverse effects seen; decrease to 1-3 mg/minute; usual total dose: 0.5-4 mg/kg; maximum: 300 mg

Hemodialysis: Not dialyzable

Dosage Forms INJ: 20 mg/mL (20 mL)

Contraindications Hypersensitivity to doxapram or any component; epilepsy, cerebral edema, head injury, severe pulmonary disease, pheochromocytoma, cardiovascular disease, hypertension, hyperthyroidism

Pregnancy Risk Factor B

Onset Respiratory stimulation begins: I.V.: Within 20-40 seconds; Peak effect: Within 1-2 minutes

Duration 5-12 minutes

Half-Life 3.4 hours (mean half-life)

Doxazosin (doks AYE zoe sin)

Pharmacologic Class Alpha$_1$ Blockers

U.S. Brand Names Cardura®

Generic Available No

Mechanism of Action Competitively inhibits postsynaptic alpha-adrenergic receptors which results in vasodilation of veins and arterioles and a decrease in total peripheral resistance and blood pressure; approximately 50% as potent on a weight by weight basis as prazosin

Use Treatment of hypertension alone or in conjunction with diuretics, cardiac glycosides, ACE inhibitors or calcium antagonists (particularly appropriate for those with hypertension and other cardiovascular risk factors such as hypercholesterolemia and diabetes mellitus); treatment of urinary outflow obstruction and/or obstructive and irritative symptoms associated with benign prostatic hyperplasia (particularly useful in patients with troublesome symptoms who are unable or unwilling to undergo invasive procedures, but who require rapid symptomatic relief)

USUAL DOSAGE Oral:

Adults: 1 mg once daily in morning or evening; may be increased to 2 mg once daily; thereafter titrate upwards, if needed, over several weeks, balancing therapeutic benefit with doxazosin-induced postural hypotension; maximum dose for hypertension: 16 mg/day, for BPH: 8 mg/day

Elderly: Initial: 0.5 mg once daily

Dosage Forms TAB: 1 mg, 2 mg, 4 mg, 8 mg

Contraindications Hypersensitivity to doxazosin or any component

Warnings/Precautions Use with caution in patients with renal impairment. Can cause marked hypotension and syncope with sudden loss of consciousness with the first dose. Anticipate a similar effect if therapy is interrupted for a few days, if dosage is increased rapidly, or if another antihypertensive drug is introduced.

Pregnancy Risk Factor C

Adverse Reactions

>10%: Central nervous system: Dizziness (16% to 19%), headache (10% to 14%)

1% to 10%:

- Cardiovascular: Orthostatic hypotension (dose-related; 0.3% up to 10%), edema (2.7% to 4%), hypotension (1.7%), palpitation (1.2% to 2%), chest pain (1.2% to 2%), arrhythmia (1%), syncope (2%), flushing (1%)
- Central nervous system: Fatigue (8% to 12%), somnolence (3% to 5%), nervousness (2%), pain (2%), vertigo (2%), insomnia (1% to 1.2%), anxiety (1.1%), paresthesia (1%), movement disorder (1%), ataxia (1%), hypertonia (1%), depression (1%), weakness (1%)
- Dermatologic: Rash (1%), pruritus (1%)
- Endocrine & metabolic: Sexual dysfunction (2%)
- Gastrointestinal: Abdominal pain (2.4%), diarrhea (2% to 2.3%), dyspepsia (1% to 1.7%), nausea (1.5% to 3%) xerostomia (1.4% to 2%), constipation (1%), flatulence (1%)
- Genitourinary: Urinary tract infection (1.4%), impotence (1.1%), polyuria (2%), incontinence (1%)
- Neuromuscular & skeletal: Back pain (1.8%), arthritis (1%), muscle weakness (1%), myalgia (1%), muscle cramps (1%)
- Ocular: Abnormal vision (1.4% to 2%), conjunctivitis (1%)
- Otic: Tinnitus (1%)
- Respiratory: Rhinitis (3%), dyspnea (1% to 2.6%), respiratory disorder (1.1%), epistaxis (1%)
- Miscellaneous: Flu-like syndrome (1.1%), increased sweating (1.1%)

<1% (limited to important or life-threatening symptoms): Tachycardia, bradycardia, peripheral ischemia, syncope, hypoesthesia, increased sweating, agitation, weight gain, angina, myocardial infarction, stroke, pallor, thirst, gout, hypokalemia, lymphadenopathy, purpura, breast pain, alopecia, dry skin, eczema, paresis, twitching, confusion, migraine, impaired concentration, paranoia, amnesia, emotional lability, abnormal thinking, depersonalization, parosmia, earache, taste perversion, photophobia, abnormal lacrimation, increased appetite, anorexia, fecal incontinence, gastroenteritis, bronchospasm, sinusitis, coughing, pharyngitis, renal calculus, hot flashes, infection, fever, rigors, weight loss

Case reports: Leukopenia, cataplexy, enuresis, systemic lupus erythematosus

(Continued)

Doxazosin *(Continued)*

Drug Interactions

NSAIDs may reduce antihypertensive efficacy

ACE inhibitors: Hypotensive effect may be increased

Beta-blockers: Hypotensive effect may be increased

Calcium channel blockers: Hypotensive effect may be increased

Alcohol Interactions Use with caution (may increase risk of hypotension or dizziness)

Onset Peak serum concentration: 1-2 hours

Duration >24 hours

Half-Life 22 hours

Education and Monitoring Issues

Patient Education: Take as directed, at bedtime. Do not skip dose or discontinue without consulting prescriber. Follow recommended diet and exercise program. Do not use OTC medications which may affect blood pressure (eg, cough or cold remedies, diet pills, stay-awake medications) without consulting prescriber. This medication may cause drowsiness, dizziness, or impaired judgment (use caution when driving or engaging in tasks that require alertness until response to drug is known); postural hypotension (use caution when rising from sitting or lying position or when climbing stairs); or dry mouth or nausea (frequent mouth care or sucking lozenges may help). Report increased nervousness or depression; sudden weight gain (weigh yourself in the same clothes at the same time of day once a week); unusual or persistent swelling of ankles, feet, or extremities; palpitations or rapid heartbeat; muscle weakness, fatigue, or pain; or other persistent side effects.

Monitoring Parameters: Blood pressure, standing and sitting/supine

Manufacturer Pfizer U.S. Pharmaceutical Group

Related Information

Pharmaceutical Manufacturers Directory *on page 1020*

Doxepin (DOKS e pin)

Pharmacologic Class Antidepressant, Tricyclic (Tertiary Amine); Topical Skin Product

U.S. Brand Names Sinequan® Oral; Zonalon® Topical Cream

Generic Available Yes

Mechanism of Action Increases the synaptic concentration of serotonin and/or norepinephrine in the central nervous system by inhibition of their reuptake by the presynaptic neuronal membrane

Use

Oral: Treatment of various forms of depression, usually in conjunction with psychotherapy; treatment of anxiety disorders

Unlabeled use: Analgesic for certain chronic and neuropathic pain

Topical: Short-term (<8 days) management of moderate pruritus in adults with atopic dermatitis or lichen simplex chronicus

USUAL DOSAGE

Oral (entire daily dose may be given at bedtime):

Adolescents: Initial: 25-50 mg/day in single or divided doses; gradually increase to 100 mg/day

Adults: Initial: 30-150 mg/day at bedtime or in 2-3 divided doses; may gradually increase up to 300 mg/day; single dose should not exceed 150 mg; select patients may respond to 25-50 mg/day

Dosing adjustment in hepatic impairment: Use a lower dose and adjust gradually

Topical: Adults: Apply a thin film 4 times/day with at least 3- to 4-hour interval between applications

Dosage Forms CAP: 10 mg, 25 mg, 50 mg, 75 mg, 100 mg, 150 mg. **CONC, oral:** 10 mg/mL (120 mL). **CRM:** 5% (30 g)

Contraindications Hypersensitivity to doxepin or any component (cross-sensitivity with other tricyclic antidepressants may occur); narrow-angle glaucoma

Warnings/Precautions Use with caution in patients with cardiovascular disease, conduction disturbances, seizure disorders, urinary retention, hyperthyroidism, or those receiving thyroid replacement; avoid use during lactation; use with caution in pregnancy; do not discontinue abruptly in patients receiving chronic high-dose therapy

Pregnancy Risk Factor C

Adverse Reactions

Cardiovascular: Hypotension, hypertension, tachycardia

Central nervous system: Drowsiness, dizziness, headache, disorientation, ataxia, confusion, seizure

Dermatologic: Alopecia, photosensitivity, rash, pruritus

Endocrine & metabolic: Breast enlargement, galactorrhea, SIADH, increase or decrease in blood sugar, increased or decreased libido

Gastrointestinal: Xerostomia, constipation, vomiting, indigestion, anorexia, aphthous stomatitis, nausea, unpleasant taste, weight gain, diarrhea, trouble with gums, decreased lower esophageal sphincter tone may cause GE reflux

Genitourinary: Urinary retention, testicular edema

Hematologic: Agranulocytosis, leukopenia, eosinophilia, thrombocytopenia, purpura

Neuromuscular & skeletal: Weakness, tremors, numbness, paresthesia, extrapyramidal symptoms, tardive dyskinesia

Ocular: Blurred vision

Otic: Tinnitus

Miscellaneous: Diaphoresis (excessive), allergic reactions

Drug Interactions CYP2D6 enzyme substrate

Decreased effect of bretylium, guanethidine, clonidine, levodopa; decreased effect with ascorbic acid, cholestyramine

Increased effect/toxicity of carbamazepine, amphetamines, thyroid preparations, sympathomimetics

Increased toxicity with fluoxetine (seizures), thyroid preparations, MAO inhibitors, albuterol, CNS depressants (ie, benzodiazepines, opiate analgesics, phenothiazines, alcohol), anticholinergics, cimetidine

Alcohol Interactions Avoid use (may increase central nervous system depression)

Onset Peak antidepressant effect: Usually more than 2 weeks; anxiolytic effects may occur sooner

Half-Life 6-8 hours

Education and Monitoring Issues

Patient Education: Oral: Take exactly as directed (do not increase dose or frequency); may take several weeks to achieve desired results; may cause physical and/or psychological dependence. Avoid excessive alcohol, caffeine, and other prescription or OTC medications not approved by prescriber. Maintain adequate hydration (2-3 L/day of fluids unless instructed to restrict fluid intake). You may experience drowsiness, lightheadedness, impaired coordination, dizziness, or blurred vision (use caution when driving or engaging in tasks requiring alertness until response to drug is known); constipation (increased exercise, fluids, or dietary fruit and fiber may help); urinary retention (void before taking medication); postural hypotension (use caution climbing stairs or when changing position from lying or sitting to standing); altered sexual drive or ability (reversible); or photosensitivity (use sunscreen, wear protective clothing and eyewear, avoid direct sunlight). Report persistent CNS effects (eg, nervousness, restlessness, insomnia, anxiety, excitation, headache, agitation, impaired coordination, changes in cognition); muscle cramping, weakness, tremors, or rigidity; chest pain, palpitations, or irregular heartbeat; blurred vision or eye pain; yellowing of skin or eyes; or worsening of condition.

Monitoring Parameters: Monitor blood pressure and pulse rate prior to and during initial therapy; monitor mental status, weight

Reference Range: Therapeutic: 30-150 ng/mL; Toxic: >500 ng/mL; utility of serum level monitoring is controversial

Related Information

Antidepressant Agents Comparison *on page 1231*

Doxercalciferol (dox er kal si fe FEER ole)

Pharmacologic Class Vitamin D Analog

U.S. Brand Names Hectorol®

Mechanism of Action Doxercalciferol is metabolized to the active form of vitamin D. The active form of vitamin D controls the intestinal absorption of dietary calcium, the tubular reabsorption of calcium by the kidneys, and in conjunction with PTH, the mobilization of calcium from the skeleton.

Use Reduction of elevated intact parathyroid hormone (iPTH) in the management of secondary hyperparathyroidism in patients on chronic hemodialysis

USUAL DOSAGE

Adults: Oral:

If the iPTH >400 pg/mL, then the initial dose is 10 mcg 3 times/week at dialysis. The dose is adjusted at 8-week intervals based upon the iPTH levels.

If the iPTH level is decreased by 50% and >300 pg/mL, then the dose can be increased to 12.5 mcg 3 times/week for 8 more weeks. This titration process can continue at 8-week intervals up to a maximum dose of 20 mcg 3 times/week. Each increase should be by 2.5 mcg/dose.

If the iPTH is between 150-300 pg/mL, maintain the current dose.

If the iPTH is <100 pg/mL, then suspend the drug for 1 week. Resume doxercalciferol at a reduced dose. Decrease each dose (not weekly dose) by at least 2.5 mcg.

Dosage adjustment in renal impairment: No adjustment required

Dosage adjustment in hepatic impairment: Use caution in these patients; no guidelines for dosage adjustment

Dosage Forms CAP: 2.5 mcg

Contraindications History of hypercalcemia or evidence of vitamin D toxicity; hyperphosphatemia should be corrected before initiating therapy

Warnings/Precautions Other forms of vitamin D should be discontinued when doxercalciferol is started. Overdose from vitamin D is dangerous and needs to be avoided. Careful dosage titration and monitoring can minimize risk. Hyperphosphatemia exacerbates secondary hyperparathyroidism, diminishing the effect of doxercalciferol. Hyperphosphatemia needs to be corrected for best results. Use with caution in patients with hepatic impairment. Safety and efficacy have not been established in pediatrics.

(Continued)

Doxercalciferol *(Continued)*

Pregnancy Risk Factor B

Pregnancy Implications Reproduction in animals (usual and high dose) do not reveal teratogenic or fetotoxic effects. Studies in humans are lacking. Excretion in breast milk is unknown. Other vitamin D derivatives are excreted in breast milk and are compatible with breast-feeding.

Adverse Reactions Some of the signs and symptoms of hypercalcemia include anorexia, nausea, vomiting, constipation, polyuria, weakness, fatigue, confusion, stupor, and coma.

>10%:
- Central nervous system: Headache (28%), malaise (28%), dizziness (11.5%)
- Cardiovascular: Edema (34.4%)
- Gastrointestinal: Nausea/vomiting (34%)
- Respiratory: Dyspnea (11.5%)

1% to 10%:
- Central nervous system: Sleep disorder (3.3%)
- Cardiovascular: Bradycardia (6.6%)
- Neuromuscular & skeletal: Arthralgia (4.9%)
- Gastrointestinal: Anorexia (4.9%), constipation (3.3%), dyspepsia (4.9%)
- Dermatologic: Pruritus (8.2%)
- Miscellaneous: Abscess (3.3%)

Drug Interactions

Decreased effect: Cholestyramine, mineral oil (both reduce absorption)

Increased toxicity: Concurrent use of other vitamin D supplements, magnesium containing antacids and supplements (hypermagnesemia)

Half-Life 32-37 hours

Education and Monitoring Issues

Patient Education: Take exactly as directed (do not miss doses). Follow diet recommended by prescriber. Avoid other vitamin D products, magnesium-containing antacids, or OTC products unless approved by prescriber. Report nausea, vomiting, loss of appetite, unresolved constipation, feelings of fatigue or weakness, confusion or inability to sleep, difficulty breathing or unusual heart beat, change in urinary pattern, or skin rash.

Monitoring Parameters: Before initiating, check iPTH, serum calcium and phosphorus. Check weekly thereafter until stable. Serum iPTH, calcium, phosphorus, and alkaline phosphatase should be monitored.

Reference Range: Serum calcium times phosphorus product should be less than 70

- ♦ **Doxy®** *see* Doxycycline *on page 300*
- ♦ **Doxychel®** *see* Doxycycline *on page 300*
- ♦ **Doxycin** *see* Doxycycline *on page 300*

Doxycycline (doks i SYE kleen)

Pharmacologic Class Antibiotic, Tetracycline Derivative

U.S. Brand Names Atridox™; Bio-Tab® Oral; Doryx®; Doxy®; Doxychel®; Periostat®; Vibramycin®; Vibramycin® IV; Vibra-Tabs®

Generic Available Yes

Mechanism of Action Inhibits protein synthesis by binding with the 30S and possibly the 50S ribosomal subunit(s) of susceptible bacteria; may also cause alterations in the cytoplasmic membrane

Use Principally in the treatment of infections caused by susceptible *Rickettsia*, *Chlamydia*, and *Mycoplasma* along with uncommon susceptible gram-negative and gram-positive organisms; alternative to mefloquine for malaria prophylaxis; treatment for syphilis in penicillin-allergic patients; often active against vancomycin-resistant enterococci; used for community-acquired pneumonia and other common infections due to susceptible organisms; sclerosing agent for pleural effusions

USUAL DOSAGE Oral, I.V.:

Children ≥8 years (<45 kg): 2-5 mg/kg/day in 1-2 divided doses, not to exceed 200 mg/day

Children >8 years (>45 kg) and Adults: 100-200 mg/day in 1-2 divided doses

- Acute gonococcal infection: 200 mg immediately, then 100 mg at bedtime on the first day followed by 100 mg twice daily for 3 days **OR** 300 mg immediately followed by 300 mg in 1 hour
- Primary and secondary syphilis: 300 mg/day in divided doses for ≥10 days
- Uncomplicated chlamydial infections: 100 mg twice daily for ≥7 days
- Endometritis, salpingitis, parametritis, or peritonitis: 100 mg I.V. twice daily with cefoxitin 2 g every 6 hours for 4 days and for ≥48 hours after patient improves; then continue with oral therapy 100 mg twice daily to complete a 10- to 14-day course of therapy
- Sclerosing agent for pleural effusion injection: 500 mg as a single dose in 30-50 mL of NS or SWI

Dosing adjustment in renal impairment: Cl_{cr} <10 mL/minute: 100 mg every 24 hours

Dialysis: Not dialyzable; 0% to 5% by hemo- and peritoneal methods or by continuous arteriovenous or venovenous hemofiltration (CAVH/CAVHD); no supplemental dosage necessary

Dosage Forms

Doxycycline calcium: **SYR** (raspberry-apple flavor) (Vibramycin®): 50 mg/5 mL (30 mL, 473 mL)

Doxycycline hyclate; **CAP:** (Periostat®): 20 mg; (Doxychel®, Vibramycin®): 50 mg; (Doxy®, Doxychel®, Vibramycin®): 100 mg. **CAP, coated pellets** (Doryx®): 100 mg. **GEL, for subgingival application** (Atridox™): 50 mg in each 500 mg of blended formulation; 2-syringe system contains doxycycline syringe (50 mg) and delivery system syringe (450 mg) along with a blunt cannula. **POWDER for inj** (Doxy®, Doxychel®, Vibramycin® IV): 100 mg, 200 mg. **TAB:** (Doxychel®): 50 mg; (Bio-Tab®, Doxychel®, Vibra-Tabs®): 100 mg

Doxycycline monohydrate: **CAP** (Monodox®): 50 mg, 100 mg. **POWDER for oral susp** (raspberry flavor) (Vibramycin®): 25 mg/5 mL (60 mL)

Contraindications Hypersensitivity to doxycycline, tetracycline or any component; children <8 years of age; severe hepatic dysfunction

Warnings/Precautions Use of tetracyclines during tooth development may cause permanent discoloration of the teeth and enamel hypoplasia; prolonged use may result in superinfection; photosensitivity reaction may occur with this drug; avoid prolonged exposure to sunlight or tanning equipment. Do not administer to children ≤8 years of age.

Pregnancy Risk Factor D

Adverse Reactions

>10%: Miscellaneous: Discoloration of teeth in children

1% to 10%: Gastrointestinal: Esophagitis

<1%: Bulging fontanels in infants, diarrhea, eosinophilia, hepatotoxicity, increased intracranial pressure, phlebitis, photosensitivity, nausea, neutropenia, rash

Drug Interactions CYP3A3/4 enzyme substrate

Decreased effect with antacids containing aluminum, calcium, or magnesium

Iron and bismuth subsalicylate may decrease doxycycline bioavailability

Barbiturates, phenytoin, and carbamazepine decrease doxycycline's half-life

Increased effect of warfarin

Drug-Herb interactions: Berberine is a chemical extracted from **goldenseal** (*Hydrastis canadensis*), **barberry** (*Berberis vulgaris*), and **Oregon grape** (*Berberis aquifolium*), which has been shown to have antibacterial activity. One double-blind study found that giving berberine concurrently with tetracycline reduced the efficacy of tetracycline in the treatment of cholera. Berberine may decrease absorption of tetracycline. Another double-blind trial did not find that berberine interfered with tetracycline in cholera patients. Until more studies are completed, berberine-containing herbs should not be taken concomitantly with tetracyclines.

Alcohol Interactions Chronic alcohol ingestion may reduce the serum concentration of doxycycline. Alcohol absorption and levels are increased in acute alcohol ingestion.

Half-Life 12-15 hours (usually increases to 22-24 hours with multiple dosing); End-stage renal disease: 18-25 hours

Education and Monitoring Issues

Patient Education: Take as directed, for the entire prescription, even if you are feeling better. Avoid alcohol and maintain adequate hydration (2-3 L/day of fluids unless instructed to restrict fluid intake). You may be very sensitive to sunlight; use sunblock, wear protective clothing and eyewear, or avoid exposure to direct sunlight. You may experience lightheadedness, dizziness, or drowsiness (use caution when driving or engaging in tasks that require alertness until response to drug is known); nausea or vomiting (small frequent meals, frequent mouth care, sucking lozenges, or chewing gum may help); or diarrhea (buttermilk, boiled milk, or yogurt may help). If diabetic, drug may cause false tests with Clinitest® urine glucose monitoring; use of glucose oxidase methods (Clinistix®) or serum glucose monitoring is preferable. Report any burning or pain at infusion site immediately. Report skin rash or itching, easy bruising or bleeding, yellowing of skin or eyes, pale stool or dark urine, unhealed sores of mouth, itching or vaginal discharge, fever or chills, or unusual cough.

Related Information

Animal and Human Bites Guidelines *on page 1177*

Antimicrobial Drugs of Choice *on page 1182*

Community Acquired Pneumonia in Adults *on page 1200*

Treatment of Sexually Transmitted Diseases *on page 1210*

♦ **Doxytec** *see* Doxycycline *on page 300*

♦ **Dramamine® II [OTC]** *see* Meclizine *on page 556*

♦ **Drenison** *see* Flurandrenolide *on page 382*

♦ **Drisdol® Oral** *see* Ergocalciferol *on page 321*

♦ **Dristan® Saline Spray [OTC]** *see* Sodium Chloride *on page 858*

♦ **Drithocreme®** *see* Anthralin *on page 66*

♦ **Drithocreme® HP 1%** *see* Anthralin *on page 66*

♦ **Dritho-Scalp®** *see* Anthralin *on page 66*

♦ **Drixoral® Non-Drowsy [OTC]** *see* Pseudoephedrine *on page 792*

Dronabinol (droe NAB i nol)

Pharmacologic Class Antiemetic

U.S. Brand Names Marinol®

Generic Available Yes

Mechanism of Action Not well defined, probably inhibits the vomiting center in the medulla oblongata

Use When conventional antiemetics fail to relieve the nausea and vomiting associated with cancer chemotherapy, AIDS-related anorexia

USUAL DOSAGE Oral:

Children: NCI protocol recommends 5 mg/m² starting 6-8 hours before chemotherapy and every 4-6 hours after to be continued for 12 hours after chemotherapy is discontinued

Adults: 5 mg/m² 1-3 hours before chemotherapy, then administer 5 mg/m²/dose every 2-4 hours after chemotherapy for a total of 4-6 doses/day; dose may be increased up to a maximum of 15 mg/m²/dose if needed (dosage may be increased by 2.5 mg/m² increments)

Appetite stimulant (AIDS-related): Initial: 2.5 mg twice daily (before lunch and dinner); titrate up to a maximum of 20 mg/day

Dosage Forms CAP: 2.5 mg, 5 mg, 10 mg

Contraindications Use only for cancer chemotherapy-induced nausea; should not be used in patients with a history of schizophrenia or in patients with known hypersensitivity to dronabinol or any component

Warnings/Precautions Use with caution in patients with heart disease, hepatic disease, or seizure disorders; reduce dosage in patients with severe hepatic impairment

Pregnancy Risk Factor C

Adverse Reactions

>10%: Central nervous system: Drowsiness, dizziness, detachment, anxiety, difficulty concentrating, mood change

1% to 10%:

Cardiovascular: Orthostatic hypotension, tachycardia

Central nervous system: Ataxia, depression, headache, vertigo, hallucinations, memory lapse

Gastrointestinal: Xerostomia

Neuromuscular & skeletal: Paresthesia, weakness

<1%: Diaphoresis, diarrhea, myalgia, nightmares, speech difficulties, syncope, tinnitus

Drug Interactions CYP2C18 and 3A3/4 enzyme substrate

Increased toxicity (drowsiness) with alcohol, barbiturates, benzodiazepines

Alcohol Interactions Avoid use (may increase central nervous system depression)

Onset Within 1 hour

Half-Life 19-24 hours

Education and Monitoring Issues

Patient Education: Take exactly as directed; do not increase dose or take more often than prescribed. Do not use alcohol or other depressant medications without consulting prescriber. You may experience psychotic reaction, impaired coordination or judgment, faintness, dizziness, or drowsiness (do not drive or engage in activities that require alertness and coordination until response to drug is known); clumsiness, unsteadiness, or muscular weakness (change position slowly and use caution when climbing stairs). Report excessive or persistent CNS changes (euphoria, anxiety, depression, memory lapse, bizarre though patterns, excitability, inability to control thoughts or behavior, fainting), respiratory difficulties, rapid heartbeat, or other adverse reactions.

Monitoring Parameters: CNS effects, heart rate, blood pressure

Reference Range: Antinauseant effects: 5-10 ng/mL

Manufacturer Roxane Laboratories, Inc

Related Information

Pharmaceutical Manufacturers Directory *on page 1020*

Droperidol (droe PER i dole)

Pharmacologic Class Antiemetic; Antipsychotic Agent, Butyrophenone

U.S. Brand Names Inapsine®

Generic Available Yes

Mechanism of Action Alters the action of dopamine in the CNS, at subcortical levels, to produce sedation; reduces emesis by blocking dopamine stimulation of the chemotrigger zone

Use Tranquilizer and antiemetic in surgical and diagnostic procedures; antiemetic for cancer chemotherapy; preoperative medication; has good antiemetic effect as well as sedative and antianxiety effects

USUAL DOSAGE Titrate carefully to desired effect

Children 2-12 years:

Premedication: I.M.: 0.1-0.15 mg/kg; smaller doses may be sufficient for control of nausea or vomiting

Adjunct to general anesthesia: I.V. induction: 0.088-0.165 mg/kg

Nausea and vomiting: I.M., I.V.: 0.05-0.06 mg/kg/dose every 4-6 hours as needed

Adults:
Premedication: I.M.: 2.5-10 mg 30 minutes to 1 hour preoperatively
Adjunct to general anesthesia: I.V. induction: 0.22-0.275 mg/kg; maintenance: 1.25-2.5 mg/dose
Alone in diagnostic procedures: I.M.: Initial: 2.5-10 mg 30 minutes to 1 hour before; then 1.25-2.5 mg if needed
Nausea and vomiting: I.M., I.V.: 2.5-5 mg/dose every 3-4 hours as needed

Dosage Forms INJ: 2.5 mg/mL (1 mL, 2 mL, 5 mL, 10 mL)

Contraindications Hypersensitivity to droperidol or any component

Warnings/Precautions Safety in children <6 months of age has not been established; use with caution in patients with seizures, bone marrow suppression, or severe liver disease

Significant hypotension may occur, especially when the drug is administered parenterally; injection contains benzyl alcohol; injection also contains sulfites which may cause allergic reaction

Tardive dyskinesia: Prevalence rate may be 40% in elderly; development of the syndrome and the irreversible nature are proportional to duration and total cumulative dose over time. May be reversible if diagnosed early in therapy.

Extrapyramidal reactions are more common in elderly with up to 50% developing these reactions after 60 years of age. Drug-induced **Parkinson's syndrome** occurs often. **Akathisia** is the most common extrapyramidal reaction in elderly.

Increased confusion, memory loss, psychotic behavior, and agitation frequently occur as a consequence of anticholinergic effects

Orthostatic hypotension is due to alpha-receptor blockade, the elderly are at greater risk for orthostatic hypotension

Antipsychotic associated sedation in nonpsychotic patients is extremely unpleasant due to feelings of depersonalization, derealization, and dysphoria

Life-threatening arrhythmias have occurred at therapeutic doses of antipsychotics

Pregnancy Risk Factor C

Pregnancy Implications
Clinical effects on the fetus: Crosses the placenta
Breast-feeding/lactation: No data available

Adverse Reactions
Cardiovascular: Mild to moderate hypotension, tachycardia, hypertension, dizziness, chills, postoperative hallucinations
Central nervous system: Postoperative drowsiness, extrapyramidal reactions, shivering
Respiratory: Respiratory depression, apnea, muscular rigidity, laryngospasm, bronchospasm

Drug Interactions Increased toxicity: CNS depressants, fentanyl and other analgesics increased blood pressure; conduction anesthesia decreased blood pressure; epinephrine decreased blood pressure; atropine, lithium

Onset Following parenteral administration: Peak effect: Within 30 minutes

Duration Following parenteral administration: 2-4 hours, may extend to 12 hours

Half-Life 2.3 hours

Education and Monitoring Issues

Patient Education: This drug may cause you to feel very sleepy; do not attempt to get up without assistance. Immediately report any difficulty breathing, confusion, loss of thought processes, or palpitations.

Monitoring Parameters: Blood pressure, heart rate, respiratory rate; observe for dystonias, extrapyramidal side effects, and temperature changes

Related Information
Droperidol and Fentanyl *on page 303*

Droperidol and Fentanyl (droe PER i dole & FEN ta nil)

Pharmacologic Class Analgesic, Combination (Narcotic)

U.S. Brand Names Innovar®

Dosage Forms INJ: Droperidol 2.5 mg and fentanyl 50 mcg per mL (2 mL, 5 mL)

Pregnancy Risk Factor C

- **Drotic® Otic** *see* Neomycin, Polymyxin B, and Hydrocortisone *on page 644*
- **Droxia™** *see* Hydroxyurea *on page 453*
- **Dr Scholl's Athlete's Foot [OTC]** *see* Tolnaftate *on page 931*
- **Dr Scholl's® Cracked Heel Relief Cream [OTC]** *see* Lidocaine *on page 527*
- **Dr Scholl's Maximum Strength Tritin [OTC]** *see* Tolnaftate *on page 931*
- **Drug Products No Longer Available in the U.S.** *see page 1009*
- **D-S-S® [OTC]** *see* Docusate *on page 290*
- **Dull-C® [OTC]** *see* Ascorbic Acid *on page 72*
- **DuoCet™** *see* Hydrocodone and Acetaminophen *on page 444*
- **Duo-Cyp® Injection** *see* Estradiol and Testosterone *on page 329*
- **Duofilm® Solution** *see* Salicylic Acid and Lactic Acid *on page 836*
- **Duogex LA** *see* Estradiol and Testosterone *on page 329*
- **Duo-Medihaler®** *see* Isoproterenol and Phenylephrine *on page 490*

- **Duo-Medihaler® Aerosol** *see* Isoproterenol and Phenylephrine *on page 490*
- **Duo-Trach®** *see* Lidocaine *on page 527*
- **Duovisc® With Kit** *see* Chondroitin Sulfate-Sodium Hyaluronate *on page 195*
- **Duphalac®** *see* Lactulose *on page 506*
- **Durabolin® Injection** *see* Nandrolone *on page 635*
- **Duraclon® Injection** *see* Clonidine *on page 216*
- **Duradyne DHC®** *see* Hydrocodone and Acetaminophen *on page 444*
- **Dura-Estrin® Injection** *see* Estradiol *on page 327*
- **Duragen® Injection** *see* Estradiol *on page 327*
- **Duragesic® Transdermal** *see* Fentanyl *on page 355*
- **Duralone® Injection** *see* Methylprednisolone *on page 589*
- **Duramorph® Injection** *see* Morphine Sulfate *on page 618*
- **Duranest®** *see* Etidocaine *on page 346*
- **Duraphyl™** *see* Theophylline Salts *on page 906*
- **Duratest® Injection** *see* Testosterone *on page 898*
- **Duratestrin® Injection** *see* Estradiol and Testosterone *on page 329*
- **Durathate® Injection** *see* Testosterone *on page 898*
- **Duratuss-G®** *see* Guaifenesin *on page 423*
- **Dura-Vent/DA®** *see* Chlorpheniramine, Phenylephrine, and Methscopolamine *on page 186*
- **Duricef®** *see* Cefadroxil *on page 148*
- **Durrax®** *see* Hydroxyzine *on page 455*
- **Duvoid®** *see* Bethanechol *on page 106*
- **DV® Vaginal Cream** *see* Dienestrol *on page 268*
- **Dyazide®** *see* Hydrochlorothiazide and Triamterene *on page 443*
- **Dycill®** *see* Dicloxacillin *on page 265*
- **Dyclone®** *see* Dyclonine *on page 304*

Dyclonine (DYE kloe neen)

Pharmacologic Class Local Anesthetic; Local Anesthetic, Oral

U.S. Brand Names Dyclone®; Sucrets® [OTC]

Use Local anesthetic prior to laryngoscopy, bronchoscopy, or endotracheal intubation; use topically for temporary relief of pain associated with oral mucosa or anogenital lesions

USUAL DOSAGE Use the lowest dose needed to provide effective anesthesia

Children and Adults: Topical solution:

Mouth sores: 5-10 mL of 0.5% or 1% to oral mucosa (swab or swish and then spit) 3-4 times/day as needed; maximum single dose: 200 mg (40 mL of 0.5% solution or 20 mL of 1% solution)

Bronchoscopy: Use 2 mL of the 1% solution or 4 mL of the 0.5% solution sprayed onto the larynx and trachea every 5 minutes until the reflex has been abolished

Contraindications Contraindicated in patients allergic to chlorobutanol (preservative used in dyclonine) or dyclonine

Pregnancy Risk Factor C

- **Dynabac®** *see* Dirithromycin *on page 286*
- **Dynacin® Oral** *see* Minocycline *on page 607*
- **DynaCirc®** *see* Isradipine *on page 494*
- **Dyna-Hex® Topical [OTC]** *see* Chlorhexidine Gluconate *on page 181*
- **Dynapen®** *see* Dicloxacillin *on page 265*
- **Dyrenium®** *see* Triamterene *on page 947*
- **Ear-Eze® Otic** *see* Neomycin, Polymyxin B, and Hydrocortisone *on page 644*
- **Easprin®** *see* Aspirin *on page 72*
- **E-Base®** *see* Erythromycin *on page 323*

Echinacea

Pharmacologic Class Herbal

Mechanism of Action Contains a caffeic acid glycoside named echinacoside (0.1% concentration) which is bactericidal. Other caffeic acid glycosides and isolutylamides associated with the plant can cause immune stimulation by increasing leukocyte phagocytosis and promoting T-cell activation. Also has an antihyaluronidase and anti-inflammatory activity; constituents have been associated with antitumor, antispasmodic effects

Use Prophylaxis and treatment of cold and flu; also used as an immunostimulant in herbal medicine; used to treat minor upper respiratory tract infections, urinary tract infections, wound/skin infections, arthritis, vaginal yeast infections

USUAL DOSAGE Continuous use should not exceed 8 weeks

Per Commission E: Expressed juice (of fresh herb): 6-9 mL/day

Capsule/tablet or tea form: 500 mg to 2 g 3 times/day

Liquid extract: 0.25-1 mL 3 times/day

Tincture: 1-2 mL 3 times/day

May be applied topically

Contraindications Autoimmune diseases, such as collagen vascular disease (Lupus, RA), multiple sclerosis; allergy to sunflowers, daisies, ragweed; tuberculosis, HIV, AIDS, pregnancy, breast-feeding; parenteral administration only contraindicated per Commission E; oral use of Echinacea not contraindicated during pregnancy by Commission E

Warnings/Precautions May alter immunosuppression; persons allergic to sunflowers may display cross-allergy potential

Adverse Reactions May become immunosuppressive with continuous use over 6-8 weeks

Gastrointestinal: Tingling sensation of tongue

Miscellaneous: Allergic reactions (rarely)

Per Commission E: None known for oral and external use

Drug Interactions Theoretically may alter response to immunosuppressive therapy

Echothiophate Iodide (ek oh THYE oh fate EYE oh dide)

Pharmacologic Class Cholinesterase Inhibitor

U.S. Brand Names Phospholine Iodide® Ophthalmic

Use Reverse toxic CNS effects caused by anticholinergic drugs; used as miotic in treatment of open-angle glaucoma; may be useful in specific case of narrow-angle glaucoma; accommodative esotropia

USUAL DOSAGE Adults:

Ophthalmic: Glaucoma: Instill 1 drop twice daily into eyes with 1 dose just prior to bedtime; some patients have been treated with 1 dose daily or every other day

Accommodative esotropia:

Diagnosis: Instill 1 drop of 0.125% once daily into both eyes at bedtime for 2-3 weeks

Treatment: Use lowest concentration and frequency which gives satisfactory response, with a maximum dose of 0.125% once daily, although more intensive therapy may be used for short periods of time

Contraindications Hypersensitivity to echothiophate or any component; most cases of angle-closure glaucoma; active uveal inflammation or any inflammatory disease of the iris or ciliary body, glaucoma associated with iridocyclitis

Pregnancy Risk Factor C

♦ **E-Complex-600® [OTC]** *see* Vitamin E *on page 980*

Econazole (e KONE a zole)

Pharmacologic Class Antifungal Agent, Topical

U.S. Brand Names Spectazole™ Topical

Use Topical treatment of tinea pedis (athlete's foot), tinea cruris (jock itch), tinea corporis (ringworm), tinea versicolor, and cutaneous candidiasis

USUAL DOSAGE Children and Adults: Topical:

Tinea pedis, tinea cruris, tinea corporis, tinea versicolor: Apply sufficient amount to cover affected areas once daily

Cutaneous candidiasis: Apply sufficient quantity twice daily (morning and evening)

Duration of treatment: Candidal infections and tinea cruris, versicolor, and corporis should be treated for 2 weeks and tinea pedis for 1 month; occasionally, longer treatment periods may be required

Contraindications Known hypersensitivity to econazole or any component

Pregnancy Risk Factor C

♦ **Econopred® Ophthalmic** *see* Prednisolone *on page 762*

♦ **Econopred® Plus Ophthalmic** *see* Prednisolone *on page 762*

♦ **Ecostatin®** *see* Econazole *on page 305*

♦ **Ecotrin® [OTC]** *see* Aspirin *on page 72*

♦ **Ecotrin® Low Adult Strength [OTC]** *see* Aspirin *on page 72*

♦ **Ed A-Hist® Liquid** *see* Chlorpheniramine and Phenylephrine *on page 186*

♦ **Edecrin®** *see* Ethacrynic Acid *on page 338*

Edetate Disodium (ED e tate dye SOW dee um)

Pharmacologic Class Chelating Agent

U.S. Brand Names Chealamide®; Disotate®; Endrate®

Generic Available Yes

Mechanism of Action Chelates with divalent or trivalent metals to form a soluble complex that is then eliminated in urine

Use Emergency treatment of hypercalcemia; control digitalis-induced cardiac dysrhythmias (ventricular arrhythmias)

USUAL DOSAGE Hypercalcemia: I.V.:

Children: 40-70 mg/kg/day slow infusion over 3-4 hours or more to a maximum of 3 g/24 hours; administer for 5 days and allow 5 days between courses of therapy

Adults: 50 mg/kg/day over 3 or more hours to a maximum of 3 g/24 hours; a suggested regimen of 5 days followed by 2 days without drug and repeated courses up to 15 total doses

(Continued)

Edetate Disodium *(Continued)*

Dosage Forms INJ: 150 mg/mL (20 mL)

Contraindications Severe renal failure or anuria

Warnings/Precautions Use of this drug is recommended only when the severity of the clinical condition justifies the aggressive measures associated with this type of therapy; use with caution in patients with renal dysfunction, intracranial lesions, seizure disorders, coronary or peripheral vascular disease

Pregnancy Risk Factor C

Adverse Reactions Rapid I.V. administration or excessive doses may cause a sudden drop in serum calcium concentration which may lead to hypocalcemic tetany, seizures, arrhythmias, and death from respiratory arrest. Do **not** exceed recommended dosage and rate of administration.

1% to 10%: Gastrointestinal: Nausea, vomiting, abdominal cramps, diarrhea

<1%: Acute tubular necrosis, anemia, arrhythmias, back pain, chills, death from respiratory arrest, dermatologic lesions, eruptions, fever, headache, hypokalemia, hypomagnesemia, muscle cramps, nephrotoxicity, pain at the site of injection, paresthesia may occur, seizures, tetany, thrombophlebitis, transient hypotension

Drug Interactions Increased effect of insulin (edetate disodium may decrease blood glucose concentrations and reduce insulin requirements in diabetic patients treated with insulin)

Half-Life 20-60 minutes

Education and Monitoring Issues

Monitoring Parameters: Cardiac function (EKG monitoring); blood pressure during infusion; renal function should be assessed before and during therapy; monitor calcium, magnesium, and potassium levels; cardiac monitor required

♦ **Edex™ Injection** *see* Alprostadil *on page 38*

Edrophonium (ed roe FOE nee um)

Pharmacologic Class Antidote; Cholinergic Agonist; Diagnostic Agent, Myasthenia Gravis

U.S. Brand Names Enlon® Injection; Reversol® Injection; Tensilon® Injection

Generic Available No

Mechanism of Action Inhibits destruction of acetylcholine by acetylcholinesterase. This facilitates transmission of impulses across myoneural junction and results in increased cholinergic responses such as miosis, increased tonus of intestinal and skeletal muscles, bronchial and ureteral constriction, bradycardia, and increased salivary and sweat gland secretions.

Use Diagnosis of myasthenia gravis; differentiation of cholinergic crises from myasthenia crises; reversal of nondepolarizing neuromuscular blockers; treatment of paroxysmal atrial tachycardia

USUAL DOSAGE Usually administered I.V., however, if not possible, I.M. or S.C. may be used:

Infants:

I.M.: 0.5-1 mg

I.V.: Initial: 0.1 mg, followed by 0.4 mg if no response; total dose = 0.5 mg

Children:

Diagnosis: Initial: 0.04 mg/kg over 1 minute followed by 0.16 mg/kg if no response, to a maximum total dose of 5 mg for children <34 kg, or 10 mg for children >34 kg

I.M.:

<34 kg: 1 mg

>34 kg: 5 mg

Titration of oral anticholinesterase therapy: 0.04 mg/kg once given 1 hour after oral intake of the drug being used in treatment; if strength improves, an increase in neostigmine or pyridostigmine dose is indicated

Adults:

Diagnosis:

I.V.: 2 mg test dose administered over 15-30 seconds; 8 mg given 45 seconds later if no response is seen; test dose may be repeated after 30 minutes

I.M.: Initial: 10 mg; if no cholinergic reaction occurs, administer 2 mg 30 minutes later to rule out false-negative reaction

Titration of oral anticholinesterase therapy: 1-2 mg given 1 hour after oral dose of anticholinesterase; if strength improves, an increase in neostigmine or pyridostigmine dose is indicated

Reversal of nondepolarizing neuromuscular blocking agents (neostigmine with atropine usually preferred): I.V.: 10 mg over 30-45 seconds; may repeat every 5-10 minutes up to 40 mg

Termination of paroxysmal atrial tachycardia: I.V. rapid injection: 5-10 mg

Differentiation of cholinergic from myasthenic crisis: I.V.: 1 mg; may repeat after 1 minute. **Note:** Intubation and controlled ventilation may be required if patient has cholinergic crisis

Dosing adjustment in renal impairment: Dose may need to be reduced in patients with chronic renal failure

Dosage Forms INJ: 10 mg/mL (1 mL, 10 mL, 15 mL)

Contraindications Hypersensitivity to edrophonium or any component, GI or GU obstruction, hypersensitivity to sulfite agents

Warnings/Precautions Use with caution in patients with bronchial asthma and those receiving a cardiac glycoside; atropine sulfate should always be readily available as an antagonist. Overdosage can cause cholinergic crisis which may be fatal. I.V. atropine should be readily available for treatment of cholinergic reactions.

Pregnancy Risk Factor C

Adverse Reactions

>10%:

Gastrointestinal: Nausea, vomiting, diarrhea, excessive salivation, stomach cramps

Miscellaneous: Diaphoresis (increased)

1% to 10%:

Genitourinary: Polyuria

Ocular: Small pupils, lacrimation

Respiratory: Increased bronchial secretions

<1%: A-V block, bradycardia, bronchospasm, diplopia, drowsiness, dysphoria, headache, hyper-reactive cholinergic responses, hypersensitivity, laryngospasm, miosis, muscle cramps, muscle spasms, respiratory paralysis, seizures, thrombophlebitis, weakness

Drug Interactions

Increased toxicity of neostigmine and/or pyridostigmine

Decreased effect: Atropine or glycopyrrolate, nondepolarizing muscle relaxants, procainamide, quinidine

Increased effect of succinylcholine, digoxin may increase the sensitivity of the heart to edrophonium

Onset I.M.: Within 2-10 minutes; I.V.: Within 30-60 seconds

Duration I.M.: 5-30 minutes; I.V.: 10 minutes

Half-Life 1.8 hours

♦ **ED-SPAZ®** *see* Hyoscyamine *on page 456*

♦ **E.E.S.®** *see* Erythromycin *on page 323*

♦ **EFA Steri** *see* Sodium Chloride *on page 858*

Efavirenz (e FAV e renz)

Pharmacologic Class Antiretroviral Agent, Reverse Transcriptase Inhibitor (Non-Nucleoside)

U.S. Brand Names Sustiva™

Use Treatment of HIV-1 infections in combination with at least two other antiretroviral agents. Also has some activity against hepatitis B virus and herpes viruses.

USUAL DOSAGE Oral: Dosing at bedtime is recommended to limit central nervous system effects; should not be used as single-agent therapy

Children: Dosage is based on body weight

10 kg to <15 kg: 200 mg once daily

15 kg to <20 kg: 250 mg once daily

20 kg to <25 kg: 300 mg once daily

25 kg to <32.5 kg: 350 mg once daily

32.5 kg to <40 kg: 400 mg once daily

≥40 kg: 600 mg once daily

Adults: 600 mg once daily

Dosing adjustment in renal impairment: None recommended

Dosing comments in hepatic impairment: Limited clinical experience, use with caution

Contraindications Clinically significant hypersensitivity to any component of the formulation

Warnings/Precautions Do not use as single-agent therapy; avoid pregnancy; women of childbearing potential should undergo pregnancy testing prior to initiation of therapy; do not administer with other agents metabolized by CYP3A4 isoenzyme including astemizole, cisapride, midazolam, triazolam or ergot alkaloids (potential for life-threatening adverse effects); history of mental illness/drug abuse (predisposition to psychological reactions); may cause depression and/or other psychiatric symptoms including impaired concentration, dizziness or drowsiness (avoid potentially hazardous tasks such as driving or operating machinery if these effects are noted); discontinue if severe rash (involving blistering, desquamation, mucosal involvement or fever) develops. Caution in patients with known or suspected hepatitis B or C infection (monitoring of liver function is recommended); hepatic impairment. Persistent elevations of serum transaminases >5 times the upper limit of normal should prompt evaluation - benefit of continued therapy should be weighed against possible risk of hepatotoxicity. Children are more susceptible to development of rash - prophylactic antihistamines may be used.

Pregnancy Risk Factor C

(Continued)

Efavirenz *(Continued)*

Adverse Reactions

2% to 10%:

Central nervous system: Dizziness (2% to 10%), inability to concentrate (0% to 9%), insomnia (0% to 7%), headache (5% to 6%) abnormal dreams (0% to 4%), somnolence (0% to 3%), depression (0% to 2%), anorexia (0% to 5%), nervousness (0% to 2%), fatigue (2% to 7%), hypoesthesia (1% to 2%)

Dermatologic: Rash (5% to 20%), pruritus (0% to 2%)

Gastrointestinal: Nausea (0% to 12%), vomiting (0% to 7%), diarrhea (2% to 12%), dyspepsia (0% to 4%), elevated transaminases (2% to 3%), abdominal pain (0% to 3%)

Miscellaneous: Increased sweating (0% to 2%)

<2%: Abnormal vision, agitation, alcohol intolerance, allergic reaction, alopecia, amnesia, anxiety, apathy, arthralgia, asthenia, asthma, ataxia, confusion, depersonalization, depression, diplopia, dry mouth, eczema, edema (peripheral), emotional lability, euphoria, fever, flatulence, flushing, folliculitis, hallucinations, hematuria, hepatitis, hot flashes, impaired coordination, increased cholesterol and triglycerides, malaise, migraine, myalgia, neuralgia, pain, palpitations, pancreatitis, paresthesia, parosmia, peripheral neuropathy, psychosis, renal calculus, seizures, skin exfoliation, speech disorder, syncope, tachycardia, taste disturbance, thrombophlebitis, tinnitus, tremor, urticaria, vertigo

Pediatric patients: Rash (40%), diarrhea (39%), fever (26%), cough (25%), nausea/vomiting (16%), central nervous system reactions (9%)

Drug Interactions

Increased effect: CYP3A4, 2C9, 2C19 inhibitor; CYP3A4 inducer; coadministration with medications metabolized by these enzymes may lead to increased concentration-related effects. Astemizole, cisapride, midazolam, triazolam and ergot alkaloids may result in life-threatening toxicities. The AUC of nelfinavir is increased (20%); AUC of both ritonavir and efavirenz are increased by 20% during concurrent therapy. The AUC of ethinyl estradiol is increased 37% by efavirenz (clinical significance unknown). May increase effect of warfarin.

Decreased effect: Other inducers of this enzyme (including phenobarbital, rifampin and rifabutin) may decrease serum concentrations of efavirenz. Concentrations of indinavir may be reduced; dosage increase to 1000 mg 3 times/day is recommended. Concentrations of saquinavir may be decreased (use as sole protease inhibitor is not recommended). Plasma concentrations of clarithromycin are decreased (clinical significance unknown). May decrease effect of warfarin.

Manufacturer DuPont Merck Pharmaceutical

Related Information

Antiretroviral Therapy for HIV Infection *on page 1190*
Pharmaceutical Manufacturers Directory *on page 1020*

♦ **Effer-K™** *see* Potassium Bicarbonate and Potassium Citrate, Effervescent *on page 751*
♦ **Effer-Syllium® [OTC]** *see* Psyllium *on page 793*
♦ **Effexor®** *see* Venlafaxine *on page 973*
♦ **Effexor® XR** *see* Venlafaxine *on page 973*
♦ **Efidac/24® [OTC]** *see* Pseudoephedrine *on page 792*

Eflornithine (ee FLOR ni theen)

Pharmacologic Class Antiprotozoal

U.S. Brand Names Ornidyl®

Use Treatment of meningoencephalitic stage of *Trypanosoma brucei gambiense* infection (sleeping sickness)

Investigational use: Slowing of excessive facial hair growth

USUAL DOSAGE Adults: I.V. infusion: 100 mg/kg/dose given every 6 hours (over at least 45 minutes) for 14 days

Dosing adjustment in renal impairment: Dose should be adjusted although no specific guidelines are available

Contraindications Hypersensitivity to eflornithine or any component

Pregnancy Risk Factor C

♦ **Efodine® [OTC]** *see* Povidone-Iodine *on page 756*
♦ **Efudex® Topical** *see* Fluorouracil *on page 376*
♦ **Elase-Chloromycetin® Topical** *see* Fibrinolysin and Desoxyribonuclease *on page 362*
♦ **Elase® Topical** *see* Fibrinolysin and Desoxyribonuclease *on page 362*
♦ **Elavil®** *see* Amitriptyline *on page 51*
♦ **Elavil Plus®** *see* Amitriptyline and Perphenazine *on page 52*
♦ **Eldecort®** *see* Hydrocortisone *on page 447*
♦ **Eldepryl®** *see* Selegiline *on page 843*
♦ **Eldercaps® [OTC]** *see* Vitamins, Multiple *on page 981*
♦ **Eldopaque® [OTC]** *see* Hydroquinone *on page 450*

- ♦ **Eldopaque Forte®** *see* Hydroquinone *on page 450*
- ♦ **Eldoquin® [OTC]** *see* Hydroquinone *on page 450*
- ♦ **Eldoquin® Forte®** *see* Hydroquinone *on page 450*
- ♦ **Elimite™ Cream** *see* Permethrin *on page 719*
- ♦ **Elixophyllin®** *see* Theophylline Salts *on page 906*
- ♦ **Elixophyllin® SR** *see* Theophylline Salts *on page 906*
- ♦ **Elocom®** *see* Mometasone Furoate *on page 615*
- ♦ **Elocon® Topical** *see* Mometasone Furoate *on page 615*
- ♦ **Eltor®** *see* Pseudoephedrine *on page 792*
- ♦ **Eltroxin®** *see* Levothyroxine *on page 526*
- ♦ **Emcyt®** *see* Estramustine *on page 329*
- ♦ **Eminase®** *see* Anistreplase *on page 65*
- ♦ **Emla** *see* Lidocaine and Prilocaine *on page 529*
- ♦ **EMLA® Anesthetic Disc** *see* Lidocaine and Prilocaine *on page 529*
- ♦ **EMLA® Cream** *see* Lidocaine and Prilocaine *on page 529*
- ♦ **Emo-Cort** *see* Hydrocortisone *on page 447*
- ♦ **Empirin® [OTC]** *see* Aspirin *on page 72*
- ♦ **Empirin® With Codeine** *see* Aspirin and Codeine *on page 75*
- ♦ **Empracet® 30, 60** *see* Acetaminophen and Codeine *on page 18*
- ♦ **Emtec-30®** *see* Acetaminophen and Codeine *on page 18*
- ♦ **E-Mycin®** *see* Erythromycin *on page 323*

Enalapril (e NAL a pril)

Pharmacologic Class Angiotensin-Converting Enzyme (ACE) Inhibitors

U.S. Brand Names Vasotec®; Vasotec® I.V.

Generic Available No

Mechanism of Action Competitive inhibitor of angiotensin-converting enzyme (ACE); prevents conversion of angiotensin I to angiotensin II, a potent vasoconstrictor; results in lower levels of angiotensin II which causes an increase in plasma renin activity and a reduction in aldosterone secretion

Use Management of mild to severe hypertension and congestive heart failure; believed to prolong survival in heart failure

Unlabeled use: Hypertensive crisis, diabetic nephropathy, rheumatoid arthritis, diagnosis of anatomic renal artery stenosis, hypertension secondary to scleroderma renal crisis, diagnosis of aldosteronism, idiopathic edema, Bartter's syndrome, postmyocardial infarction for prevention of ventricular failure

USUAL DOSAGE Use lower listed initial dose in patients with hyponatremia, hypovolemia, severe congestive heart failure, decreased renal function, or in those receiving diuretics

Infants and Children:

Investigational initial oral doses of **enalapril**: 0.1 mg/kg/day increasing as needed over 2 weeks to 0.5 mg/kg/day have been used to treat severe congestive heart failure in infants

Investigational I.V. doses of **enalaprilat**: 5-10 mcg/kg/dose administered every 8-24 hours have been used for the treatment of neonatal hypertension; monitor patients carefully; select patients may require higher doses

Adults:

Oral: **Enalapril**

Hypertension: 2.5-5 mg/day then increase as required, usual therapeutic dose for hypertension: 10-40 mg/day in 1-2 divided doses. **Note:** Initiate with 2.5 mg if patient taking diuretic which cannot be discontinued; may add a diuretic if blood pressure cannot be controlled with enalapril alone

Heart failure: As adjunct with diuretics and digitalis, initiate with 2.5 mg once or twice daily (usual range: 5-20 mg/day in 2 divided doses; maximum: 40 mg)

Asymptomatic left ventricular dysfunction: 2.5 mg twice daily, titrated as tolerated to 20 mg/day

I.V.: **Enalaprilat**

Hypertension: 1.25 mg/dose, given over 5 minutes every 6 hours; doses as high as 5 mg/dose every 6 hours have been tolerated for up to 36 hours. **Note:** If patients are concomitantly receiving diuretic therapy, begin with 0.625 mg I.V. over 5 minutes; if the effect is not adequate after 1 hour, repeat the dose and administer 1.25 mg at 6-hour intervals thereafter; if adequate, administer 0.625 mg I.V. every 6 hours

Conversion from I.V. to oral therapy if not concurrently on diuretics: 5 mg once daily; subsequent titration as needed; if concurrently receiving diuretics and responding to 0.625 mg I.V. every 6 hours, initiate with 2.5 mg/day

Dosing adjustment in renal impairment:

Oral: Enalapril:

Cl_{cr} 30-80 mL/minute: Administer 5 mg/day titrated upwards to maximum of 40 mg

Cl_{cr} <30 mL/minute: Administer 2.5 mg day; titrated upward until blood pressure is controlled

For heart failure patients with sodium <130 mEq/L or serum creatinine >1.6 mg/dL, initiate dosage with 2.5 mg/day, increasing to twice daily as needed; increase

(Continued)

Enalapril *(Continued)*

further in increments of 2.5 mg/dose at >4-day intervals to a maximum daily dose of 40 mg

I.V.: Enalaprilat:

Cl_{cr} >30 mL/minute: Initiate with 1.25 mg every 6 hours and increase dose based on response

Cl_{cr} <30 mL/minute: Initiate with 0.625 mg every 6 hours and increase dose based on response

Hemodialysis: Moderately dialyzable (20% to 50%); administer dose postdialysis (eg, 0.625 mg I.V. every 6 hours) or administer 20% to 25% supplemental dose following dialysis; Clearance: 62 mL/minute

Peritoneal dialysis: Supplemental dose is not necessary, although some removal of drug occurs

Dosing adjustment in hepatic impairment: Hydrolysis of enalapril to enalaprilat may be delayed and/or impaired in patients with severe hepatic impairment, but the pharmacodynamic effects of the drug do not appear to be significantly altered; no dosage adjustment

Dosage Forms Enalaprilat: **INJ:** 1.25 mg/mL (1 mL, 2 mL). Enalapril maleate: **TAB:** 2.5 mg, 5 mg, 10 mg, 20 mg

Contraindications Hypersensitivity to enalapril, enalaprilat, other ACE inhibitors, or any component

Warnings/Precautions Use with caution and modify dosage in patients with renal impairment (especially renal artery stenosis), severe congestive heart failure, or with coadministered diuretic therapy, valvular stenosis, hyperkalemia (>5.7 mEq/L); experience in children is limited. Severe hypotension may occur in patients who are sodium and/or volume depleted; initiate lower doses and monitor closely when starting therapy in these patients.

Pregnancy Risk Factor C (1st trimester); D (2nd and 3rd trimesters)

Pregnancy Implications

Clinical effects on the fetus: No data available on crossing the placenta. Cranial defects, hypocalvaria/acalvaria, oligohydramnios, persistent anuria following delivery, hypotension, renal defects, renal dysgenesis/dysplasia, renal failure, pulmonary hypoplasia, limb contractures secondary to oligohydramnios and stillbirth reported. ACE inhibitors should be avoided during pregnancy.

Breast-feeding/lactation: Crosses into breast milk. Detectable levels but appears clinically insignificant. American Academy of Pediatrics considers **compatible** with breast-feeding.

Adverse Reactions Note: Frequency ranges include data from hypertension and heart failure trials. Higher rates of adverse reactions have generally been noted in patients with congestive heart failure. However, the frequency of adverse effects associated with placebo is also increased in this population.

1% to 10%:

Cardiovascular: Hypotension (0.9% to 6.7%), chest pain (2%), syncope (0.5% to 2%), orthostasis (2%), orthostatic hypotension (2%)

Central nervous system: Headache (2% to 5%), dizziness (4% to 8%), fatigue (2% to 3%), weakness (2%)

Dermatologic: Rash (1.5%) Gastrointestinal: Abnormal taste, abdominal pain, vomiting, nausea, diarrhea, anorexia, constipation

Neuromuscular & skeletal: Weakness

Renal: Increased serum creatinine (0.2% to 20%), worsening of renal function (in patients with bilateral renal artery stenosis or hypovolemia)

Respiratory (1% to 2%): Bronchitis, cough, dyspnea

<1% (limited to important or life-threatening symptoms): Angina pectoris, pulmonary edema, palpitations, arrest, CVA, myocardial infarction, rhythm, insomnia, ataxia, drowsiness, confusion, depression, nervousness, vertigo, alopecia, erythema multiforme, pruritus, Stevens-Johnson syndrome, urticaria, angioedema, pemphigus, hypoglycemia, hyperkalemia, gynecomastia, stomatitis, xerostomia, dyspepsia, glossitis, pancreatitis, ileus, urinary tract infection. impotence, agranulocytosis, neutropenia, anemia, hemolysis with G-6-PD, jaundice, hepatitis, paresthesia, blurred vision, conjunctivitis, tinnitus, oliguria, renal dysfunction, asthma, bronchospasm, URI, diaphoresis. Worsening of renal function may occur in patients with bilateral renal artery stenosis or in hypovolemic patients.

Case reports: Schönlein-Henoch purpura, toxic pustuloderma, toxic epidermal necrolysis, exfoliative dermatitis, pemphigus foliaceus, photosensitivity, sicca syndrome, systemic lupus erythematosus, giant cell arteritis, depression, hallucinations, psychosis, lichenform reaction, ototoxicity. A syndrome which may include fever, myalgia, arthralgia, interstitial nephritis, vasculitis, rash, eosinophilia and positive ANA, and elevated ESR has been reported for enalapril and other ACE inhibitors.

Drug Interactions CYP3A3/4 enzyme substrate

$Alpha_1$ blockers: Hypotensive effect increased

Aspirin and NSAIDs may decrease ACE inhibitor efficacy and/or increase risk of renal adverse effects

Diuretics: Hypovolemia due to diuretics may precipitate acute hypotensive events or acute renal failure
Insulin: Risk of hypoglycemia may be increased
Lithium: Risk of lithium toxicity may be increased; monitor lithium levels, especially in the first 4 weeks of therapy
Mercaptopurine: Risk of neutropenia may be increased
Potassium-sparing diuretics (amiloride, spironolactone, triamterene): Increased risk of hyperkalemia
Potassium supplements may increase the risk of hyperkalemia
Trimethoprim (high dose) may increase the risk of hyperkalemia

Alcohol Interactions Avoid or limit use (may increase risk of hypotension or dizziness)

Onset Oral: ~1 hour

Duration Oral: 12-24 hours

Half-Life
Enalapril: Healthy: 2 hours; With congestive heart failure: 3.4-5.8 hours
Enalaprilat: 35-38 hours

Education and Monitoring Issues

Patient Education: Take exactly as directed; do not discontinue without consulting prescriber. Take first dose at bedtime. Take all doses on an empty stomach (30 minutes before or 2 hours after meals). This drug does not eliminate need for diet or exercise regimen as recommended by prescriber. Do not use potassium supplements or salt substitutes containing potassium without consulting prescriber. May cause dizziness, fainting, lightheadedness (use caution when driving or engaging in tasks that require alertness until response to drug is known); postural hypotension (use caution when rising from lying or sitting position or climbing stairs); nausea, vomiting, abdominal pain, dry mouth, or transient loss of appetite (small frequent meals, frequent mouth care, sucking lozenges, or chewing gum may help) - report if these persist. Report chest pain or palpitations; mouth sores; fever or chills; swelling of extremities, face, mouth, or tongue; skin rash; numbness, tingling, or pain in muscles; difficulty in breathing or unusual cough; or other persistent adverse reactions.

Monitoring Parameters: Blood pressure, renal function, WBC, serum potassium; blood pressure monitor required during intravenous administration

Manufacturer Merck & Co

Related Information
Angiotensin-Related Agents Comparison *on page 1226*
Enalapril and Diltiazem *on page 311*
Enalapril and Felodipine *on page 311*
Enalapril and Hydrochlorothiazide *on page 311*
Heart Failure Guidelines *on page 1099*
Pharmaceutical Manufacturers Directory *on page 1020*

Enalapril and Diltiazem (e NAL a pril & dil TYE a zem)

Pharmacologic Class Antihypertensive Agent, Combination

U.S. Brand Names Teczem®

Dosage Forms TAB, extended release: Enalapril maleate 5 mg and diltiazem maleate 180 mg

Pregnancy Risk Factor C (1st trimester); D (2nd and 3rd trimesters)

Alcohol Interactions Avoid or limit use (may increase risk of hypotension or dizziness)

Manufacturer Hoechst-Marion Roussel

Related Information
Pharmaceutical Manufacturers Directory *on page 1020*

Enalapril and Felodipine (e NAL a pril & fe LOE di peen)

Pharmacologic Class Antihypertensive Agent, Combination

U.S. Brand Names Lexxel™

Dosage Forms TAB, extended release: Enalapril maleate 5 mg and felodipine 5 mg

Pregnancy Risk Factor C (1st trimester); D (2nd and 3rd trimesters)

Alcohol Interactions Avoid or limit use (may increase risk of hypotension or dizziness)

Manufacturer AstraZeneca

Related Information
Pharmaceutical Manufacturers Directory *on page 1020*

Enalapril and Hydrochlorothiazide

(e NAL a pril & hye droe klor oh THYE a zide)

Pharmacologic Class Antihypertensive Agent, Combination

U.S. Brand Names Vaseretic® 10-25

Dosage Forms TAB: Enalapril maleate 5 mg and hydrochlorothiazide 12.5 mg, Enalapril maleate 10 mg and hydrochlorothiazide 25 mg

Pregnancy Risk Factor C (first trimester); D (second and third trimesters)

Alcohol Interactions Avoid or limit use (may increase risk of hypotension or dizziness)

Manufacturer Merck & Co

(Continued)

Enalapril and Hydrochlorothiazide *(Continued)*

Related Information

Pharmaceutical Manufacturers Directory *on page 1020*

- **Enbrel®** *see* Etanercept *on page 336*
- **Endal®** *see* Guaifenesin and Phenylephrine *on page 425*
- **Endantadine®** *see* Amantadine *on page 42*
- **End Lice® Liquid [OTC]** *see* Pyrethrins *on page 795*
- **Endocet®** *see* Oxycodone and Acetaminophen *on page 692*
- **Endocodone®** *see* Oxycodone *on page 691*
- **Endodan®** *see* Oxycodone and Aspirin *on page 692*
- **Endolor®** *see* Butalbital Compound *on page 123*
- **Endrate®** *see* Edetate Disodium *on page 305*
- **Ener-B® [OTC]** *see* Cyanocobalamin *on page 233*
- **Enlon® Injection** *see* Edrophonium *on page 306*
- **Enovil®** *see* Amitriptyline *on page 51*

Enoxacin (en OKS a sin)

Pharmacologic Class Quinolone

U.S. Brand Names Penetrex™

Use Treatment of complicated and uncomplicated urinary tract infections caused by susceptible gram-negative and gram-positive bacteria and uncomplicated urethral or cervical gonorrhea due to *N. gonorrhoeae*

USUAL DOSAGE Adults: Oral:

Complicated urinary tract infection: 400 mg twice daily for 14 days

Cystitis: 200 mg twice daily for 7 days

Uncomplicated gonorrhea: 400 mg as single dose

Dosing adjustment in renal impairment: Cl_{cr} <50 mL/minute: Administer 50% of dose

Contraindications Hypersensitivity to enoxacin, any component, or other quinolones

Pregnancy Risk Factor C

Enoxaparin (ee noks a PA rin)

Pharmacologic Class Anticoagulant; Low Molecular Weight Heparin

U.S. Brand Names Lovenox® Injection

Mechanism of Action Standard heparin consists of components with molecular weights ranging from 4000-30,000 daltons with a mean of 16,000 daltons. Heparin acts as an anticoagulant by enhancing the inhibition rate of clotting proteases by antithrombin III impairing normal hemostasis and inhibition of factor Xa. Low molecular weight heparins have a small effect on the activated partial thromboplastin time and strongly inhibit factor Xa. Enoxaparin is derived from porcine heparin that undergoes benzylation followed by alkaline depolymerization. The average molecular weight of enoxaparin is 4500 daltons which is distributed as (≤20%) 2000 daltons, (≥68%) 2000-8000 daltons, and (≤15%) >8000 daltons. Enoxaparin has a higher ratio of antifactor Xa to antifactor IIa activity than unfractionated heparin.

Use

Prophylaxis of thromboembolic disorders (deep vein thrombosis) which may lead to pulmonary embolism following hip replacement therapy or total knee replacement

Prophylaxis of thromboembolic disorders (deep vein thrombosis) which may lead to pulmonary embolism in high-risk patients who are undergoing abdominal surgery. High-risk patients include those with one or more of the following risk factors: >40 years of age, obese, general anesthesia lasting >30 minutes, malignancy, history of deep vein thrombosis or pulmonary embolism.

Prevention of ischemic complications of unstable angina and non-Q-wave myocardial infarction when concurrently administered with aspirin

Treatment of thromboembolic disorders (deep vein thrombosis with or without pulmonary embolism)

USUAL DOSAGE S.C.:

Prophylaxis of DVT following abdominal, hip replacement or knee replacement surgery:

Children: Safety and effectiveness have not been established

Adults:

DVT prophylaxis in hip replacement:

30 mg twice daily: First dose within 12-24 hours after surgery and every 12 hours until risk of deep vein thrombosis has diminished or the patient is adequately anticoagulated on warfarin. Average duration of therapy: 7-10 days

Patients who weigh <100 lbs or are ≥65 years of age: Some clinicians recommend 0.5 mg/kg/dose every 12 hours to reduce the risk of bleeding

40 mg once daily: First dose within 9-15 hours before surgery and daily until risk of deep vein thrombosis has diminished or the patient is adequately anticoagulated on warfarin. Average duration of therapy: 7-10 days unless warfarin is not given concurrently, then 40 mg S.C. once daily should be continued for 3 more weeks (4 weeks total)

DVT prophylaxis in knee replacement:

30 mg twice daily: First dose within 12-24 hours after surgery and every 12 hours until risk of deep vein thrombosis has diminished. Average duration of therapy: 7-10 days; maximum course: 14 days

Patients who weigh <100 lbs or are ≥65 years of age: Some clinicians recommend 0.5 mg/kg/dose every 12 hours to reduce the risk of bleeding

DVT prophylaxis in high-risk patients undergoing abdominal surgery: 40 mg once daily, with initial dose given 2 hours prior to surgery; usual duration: 7-10 days and up to 12 days has been tolerated in clinical trials

Treatment of acute proximal DVT: Start warfarin within 72 hours and continue enoxaparin until INR is between 2.0 and 3.0 (usually 7 days)

Inpatient treatment of DVT with or without pulmonary embolism: Adults: S.C. 1 mg/kg/dose every 12 hours or 1.5 mg/kg once daily

Outpatient treatment of DVT without pulmonary embolism: Adults: S.C.: 1 mg/kg/dose every 12 hours

Prevention of ischemic complications with unstable angina or non-Q-wave myocardial infarction: S.C.: 1 mg/kg twice daily in conjunction with oral aspirin therapy (100-325 mg once daily); treatment should be continued for a minimum of 2 days and continued until clinical stabilization (usually 2-8 days)

Dosing adjustment in renal impairment: Total clearance is lower and elimination is delayed in patients with renal failure; adjustment may be necessary in elderly and patients with severe renal impairment

Hemodialysis: Supplemental dose is not necessary

Peritoneal dialysis: Significant drug removal is unlikely based on physiochemical characteristics

Dosage Forms INJ (preservative free): Prefilled syringes: 30 mg/0.3 mL, 40 mg/0.4 mL; Grad prefilled syringe: 60 mg/0.6 mL, 80 mg/0.8 mL, 100 mg/1.0 mL; Ampul: 30 mg/0.3 mL

Contraindications Patients with active major bleeding, thrombocytopenia associated with a positive *in vitro* test for antiplatelet antibody or enoxaparin-induced platelet aggregation; hypersensitivity to enoxaparin; known hypersensitivity to heparin or pork products

Warnings/Precautions Do not administer intramuscularly; use with extreme caution in patients with a history of heparin-induced thrombocytopenia; bacterial endocarditis, hemorrhagic stroke, recent CNS or ophthalmological surgery, bleeding diathesis, uncontrolled arterial hypertension, or a history of recent gastrointestinal ulceration and hemorrhage. Elderly and patients with renal insufficiency may show delayed elimination of enoxaparin; avoid use in lactation. Patients should be observed closely for bleeding if enoxaparin is administered during or immediately following diagnostic lumbar puncture, epidural anesthesia, or spinal anesthesia. If thromboembolism develops despite enoxaparin prophylaxis, enoxaparin should be discontinued and appropriate treatment should be initiated.

Carefully monitor patients receiving low molecular weight heparins or heparinoids. These drugs, when used concurrently with spinal or epidural anesthesia or spinal puncture, may cause bleeding or hematomas within the spinal column. Increased pressure on the spinal cord may result in permanent paralysis if not detected and treated immediately.

Pregnancy Risk Factor B

Adverse Reactions As with all anticoagulants, bleeding is the major adverse effect of enoxaparin. Hemorrhage may occur at virtually any site. Risk is dependent on multiple variables. At the recommended doses, single injections of enoxaparin do not significantly influence platelet aggregation or affect global clotting time (ie, PT or APTT).

1% to 10%:

Central nervous system: Fever (5% to 8%), confusion, pain

Dermatologic: Erythema, bruising

Gastrointestinal: Nausea (3%), increased ALT/AST (5.9% to 6.1%)

Hematologic: Hemorrhage (5% to 13%), thrombocytopenia (2%), hypochromic anemia (2%)

Local: Injection site hematoma (9%), local reactions (irritation, pain, ecchymosis, erythema)

<1% (limited to important or life-threatening symptoms): Hyperlipidemia, hypertriglyceridemia, pruritus, allergic reaction, urticaria, anaphylactoid reaction, vesicobullous rash, purpura, thrombocytosis. Spinal or epidural hematomas can occur following neuraxial anesthesia or spinal puncture, resulting in paralysis. Risk is increased in patients with indwelling epidural catheters or concomitant use of other drugs affecting hemostasis.

Case reports: Skin necrosis, eczematous plaques, itchy erythematous patches

Drug Interactions

Drugs which affect platelet function (eg, aspirin, NSAIDs, dipyridamole, ticlopidine, clopidogrel) may potentiate the risk of hemorrhage

Thrombolytic agents increase the risk of hemorrhage

Warfarin: Risk of bleeding may be increased during concurrent therapy Enoxaparin is commonly continued during the initiation of warfarin therapy to assure anticoagulation and to protect against possible transient hypercoagulability

Onset Maximum antifactor Xa and antithrombin (antifactor IIa) activities occur 3-5 hours after S.C. administration.

(Continued)

Enoxaparin *(Continued)*

Duration Following a 40 mg dose, significant antifactor Xa activity persists in plasma for ~12 hours.

Half-Life Half-life, plasma: Low molecular weight heparin is 2-4 times longer than standard heparin independent of the dose.

Education and Monitoring Issues

Patient Education: This drug can only be administered by injection. You may have a tendency to bleed easily while taking this drug; brush teeth with soft brush, floss with waxed floss, use electric razor, avoid scissors or sharp knives, and potentially harmful activities. Report chest pain; persistent constipation; persistent erection; unusual bleeding or bruising (bleeding gums, nosebleed, blood in urine, dark stool); pain in joints or back; or numbness, tingling, swelling, or pain at injection site.

Monitoring Parameters: Platelets, occult blood, and anti-Xa activity, if available; the monitoring of PT and/or PTT is not necessary

Manufacturer Rhone-Poulenc Rorer Pharmaceuticals, Inc

Related Information

Pharmaceutical Manufacturers Directory *on page 1020*

Entacapone (en TA ka pone)

Pharmacologic Class Anti-Parkinson's Agent

U.S. Brand Names Comtan®

Mechanism of Action Entacapone is a reversible and selective inhibitor of catechol-O-methyltransferase (COMT). When entacapone is taken with levodopa, the pharmacokinetics are altered, resulting in more sustained levodopa serum levels compared to levodopa taken alone. The resulting levels of levodopa provide for increased concentrations available for absorption across the blood-brain barrier, thereby providing for increased CNS levels of dopamine, the active metabolite of levodopa.

Use Adjunct to levodopa/carbidopa therapy in patients with idiopathic Parkinson's disease who experience "wearing-off" symptoms at the end of a dosing interval

USUAL DOSAGE

Adults: Oral: 200 mg dose, up to a maximum of 8 times/day; maximum daily dose: 1600 mg/day. Always administer with levodopa/carbidopa. To optimize therapy, the levodopa/carbidopa dosage must be reduced, usually by 25%. This reduction is usually necessary when the patient is taking more than 800 mg of levodopa daily.

Dosage adjustment in hepatic impairment: Treat with caution and monitor carefully; AUC and C_{max} can be possibly doubled

Dosage Forms TAB: 200 mg

Contraindications Hypersensitivity to the drug or any of its components

Warnings/Precautions Patient should not be treated concomitantly with entacapone and a nonselective MAO inhibitor. Orthostatic hypotension may be increased in patients on dopaminergic therapy in Parkinson's disease.

Pregnancy Risk Factor C

Pregnancy Implications Not recommended

Adverse Reactions

>10%:

Gastrointestinal: Nausea (14%)

Neuromuscular & skeletal: Dyskinesia (25%), placebo (15%)

1% to 10%:

Central nervous system: Dizziness (8%), fatigue (6%), hallucinations (4%), anxiety (2%), somnolence (2%), agitation (1%)

Cardiovascular: Orthostatic hypotension (4.3%), syncope (1.2%)

Dermatologic: Purpura (2%)

Gastrointestinal: Diarrhea (10%), abdominal pain (8%), constipation (6%), vomiting (4%), dry mouth (3%), dyspepsia (2%), flatulence (2%), gastritis (1%), taste perversion (1%)

Genitourinary: Brown-orange urine discoloration (10%)

Neuromuscular & skeletal: Hyperkinesia (10%), hypokinesia (9%), back pain (4%), weakness (2%)

Miscellaneous: Increased sweating (2%), bacterial infection (1%)

Respiratory: Dyspnea (3%)

<1%: Hyperpyrexia and confusion (resembling neuroleptic malignant syndrome), pulmonary fibrosis, rhabdomyolysis, retroperitoneal fibrosis

Note: Approximately 14% of the 603 patients given entacapone in the double-blind, placebo-controlled trials discontinued treatment due to adverse events compared to 9% of the 400 patients who received placebo.

Drug Interactions CYP1A2 inhibitor (high dose); CYP2A6 inhibitor (high dose); CYP2C9 inhibitor (high dose); CYP2C19 inhibitor (high dose); CYP2D6 inhibitor (high dose); CYP2E1 inhibitor (high dose); CYP3A3/4 inhibitor (high dose)

Cardiac effects with drugs metabolized by COMT (eg, epinephrine, isoproterenol, dopamine, apomorphine, bitolterol, dobutamine, methyldopa) increased other CNS depressants; nonselective MAOIs are not recommended; chelates iron. Caution with drugs that interfere with glucuronidation, intestinal, biliary excretion, intestinal beta-glucuronidase (eg, probenecid, cholestyramine, erythromycin, chloramphenicol, rifampicin, ampicillin).

Onset 1 hour

Half-Life 2.4 hours

Education and Monitoring Issues

Patient Education: Take exactly as directed; do not alter dosage or discontinue without consulting prescriber. May be taken with food. Notify prescriber if any other prescription medications you are taking. Avoid all alcohol or OTC medications unless approved by your prescriber. Orange-brown urine is normal with this medication. You may experience dizziness, fatigue, or sleepiness (use caution when driving or engaging in tasks requiring alertness until response to drug is known); postural hypotension (rise slowly when getting up from chair or bed, when climbing stairs); unusual taste, nausea, vomiting, flatulence, or upset stomach (small frequent meals, good mouth care, chewing gum, or sucking hard candy may help). Report any increased or abnormal skeletal movements or pain; unresolved sedation, nausea, diarrhea, constipation, or gastrointestinal distress; signs of infection; persistent dizziness or sleepiness; or other unusual responses.

Dietary Considerations: Can take with or without food

Monitoring Parameters: Signs and symptoms of Parkinson's disease; liver function tests, blood pressure, patient's mental status

Manufacturer Novartis

Related Information

Parkinson's Disease Dosing *on page 1249*
Pharmaceutical Manufacturers Directory *on page 1020*

♦ **Entacyl** *see* Piperazine *on page 742*
♦ **Entocort®** *see* Budesonide *on page 115*
♦ **Entrophen®** *see* Aspirin *on page 72*
♦ **Entuss-D® Liquid** *see* Hydrocodone and Pseudoephedrine *on page 446*
♦ **Enulose®** *see* Lactulose *on page 506*
♦ **Enzone®** *see* Pramoxine and Hydrocortisone *on page 758*
♦ **E Pam®** *see* Diazepam *on page 261*

Ephedrine (e FED rin)

Pharmacologic Class Alpha/Beta Agonist

U.S. Brand Names Kondon's Nasal® [OTC]; Pretz-D® [OTC]

Generic Available Yes

Mechanism of Action Releases tissue stores of epinephrine and thereby produces an alpha- and beta-adrenergic stimulation; longer-acting and less potent than epinephrine

Use Treatment of mild bronchial asthma; nasal congestion; acute bronchospasm (less effective than epinephrine); idiopathic orthostatic hypotension (response variable); hypotension during anesthesia, especially spinal anesthesia

USUAL DOSAGE

Children:

Oral, S.C.: 3 mg/kg/day or 25-100 mg/m^2/day in 4-6 divided doses every 4-6 hours

I.M., slow I.V. push: 0.2-0.3 mg/kg/dose every 4-6 hours

Adults:

Oral: 25-50 mg every 3-4 hours as needed

I.M., S.C.: 25-50 mg, parenteral adult dose should not exceed 150 mg in 24 hours

I.V.: 5-25 mg/dose slow I.V. push repeated after 5-10 minutes as needed, then every 3-4 hours not to exceed 150 mg/24 hours

Dosage Forms CAP: 25 mg, 50 mg. **INJ:** 25 mg/mL (1 mL); 50 mg/mL (1 mL, 10 mL). **JELLY** (Kondon's Nasal®): 1% (20 g). **SPRAY** (Pretz-D®): 0.25% (15 mL)

Contraindications Hypersensitivity to ephedrine or any component, angle-closure glaucoma

Warnings/Precautions Blood volume depletion should be corrected before ephedrine therapy is instituted; use caution in patients with unstable vasomotor symptoms, diabetes, hyperthyroidism, prostatic hypertrophy, a history of seizures or those on other sympathomimetic agents; also use caution in the elderly and those patients with cardiovascular disorders such as coronary artery disease, arrhythmias, and hypertension. Ephedrine may cause hypertension resulting in intracranial hemorrhage. Long-term use may cause anxiety and symptoms of paranoid schizophrenia. Avoid as a bronchodilator; generally not used as a bronchodilator since new beta$_2$ agents are less toxic. Use with caution in the elderly, since it crosses the blood-brain barrier and may cause confusion.

Pregnancy Risk Factor C

Adverse Reactions

>10%: Central nervous system: CNS stimulating effects, nervousness, anxiety, apprehension, fear, tension, agitation, excitation, restlessness, irritability, insomnia, hyperactivity

1% to 10%:

Cardiovascular: Hypertension, tachycardia, palpitations, elevation or depression of blood pressure, unusual pallor

Central nervous system: Dizziness, headache

(Continued)

Ephedrine *(Continued)*

Gastrointestinal: Xerostomia, nausea, anorexia, GI upset, vomiting
Genitourinary: Painful urination
Neuromuscular & skeletal: Trembling, tremor (more common in the elderly), weakness
Miscellaneous: Diaphoresis (increased)

<1%: Arrhythmias, chest pain, dyspnea

Drug Interactions

Decreased effect: Alpha- and beta-adrenergic blocking agents decrease ephedrine vasopressor and cardiac/bronchodilating effects, respectively

Increased toxicity: Additive cardiostimulation with other sympathomimetic agents; theophylline may lead to cardiostimulation; MAO inhibitors or atropine may increase blood pressure; cardiac glycosides or halogenated general anesthetics may increase cardiac stimulation

Onset Oral: Onset of bronchodilation: Within 0.25-1 hour

Duration Oral: 3-6 hours

Half-Life 2.5-3.6 hours

Education and Monitoring Issues

Patient Education: Use this medication exactly as directed; do not take more than recommended dosage. Avoid other stimulant prescriptive or OTC medications to avoid serious overdose reactions. Store this medication away from light. You may experience dizziness, blurred vision, restlessness (use caution when driving or engaging in tasks requiring alertness until response to drug is known); or difficulty urinating (empty bladder immediately before taking this medication). Report excessive nervousness or excitation, inability to sleep, facial flushing, pounding heartbeat, muscle tremors or weakness, chest pain or palpitations, bronchial irritation or coughing, or increased sweating.

Monitoring Parameters: Blood pressure, pulse, urinary output, mental status; cardiac monitor and blood pressure monitor required

Related Information

Chlorpheniramine, Ephedrine, Phenylephrine, and Carbetapentane *on page 186*
Theophylline, Ephedrine, and Hydroxyzine *on page 906*
Theophylline, Ephedrine, and Phenobarbital *on page 906*

♦ **Epilepsy Guidelines** *see page 1091*
♦ **E-Pilo®** *see* Pilocarpine and Epinephrine *on page 736*
♦ **E-Pilo-x® Ophthalmic** *see* Pilocarpine and Epinephrine *on page 736*
♦ **Epimorph®** *see* Morphine Sulfate *on page 618*
♦ **Epitol®** *see* Carbamazepine *on page 137*
♦ **Epivir®** *see* Lamivudine *on page 506*
♦ **Epivir® HBV** *see* Lamivudine *on page 506*

Epoetin Alfa (e POE e tin AL fa)

Pharmacologic Class Colony Stimulating Factor

U.S. Brand Names Epogen®; Procrit®

Generic Available No

Mechanism of Action Induces erythropoiesis by stimulating the division and differentiation of committed erythroid progenitor cells; induces the release of reticulocytes from the bone marrow into the bloodstream, where they mature to erythrocytes. There is a dose response relationship with this effect. This results in an increase in reticulocyte counts followed by a rise in hematocrit and hemoglobin levels.

Use

Treatment of anemia associated with chronic renal failure, including patients on dialysis (end-stage renal disease) and patients not on dialysis

Treatment of anemia related to zidovudine therapy in HIV-infected patients; in patients when the endogenous erythropoietin level is ≤500 mIU/mL and the dose of zidovudine is ≤4200 mg/week

Treatment of anemia in cancer patients on chemotherapy; in patients with nonmyeloid malignancies where anemia is caused by the effect of the concomitantly administered chemotherapy; to decrease the need for transfusions in patients who will be receiving chemotherapy for a minimum of 2 months

Reduction of allogeneic block transfusion in surgery patients scheduled to undergo elective, noncardiac, nonvascular surgery

USUAL DOSAGE

Chronic renal failure patients: I.V., S.C.:

Initial dose: 50-100 units/kg 3 times/week

Reduce dose by 25 units/kg when
1) hematocrit approaches 36% **or**
2) when hematocrit increases >4 points in any 2-week period

Increase dose if hematocrit does not increase by 5-6 points after 8 weeks of therapy and hematocrit is below suggested target range

Suggested target hematocrit range: 30% to 36%

Maintenance dose: Individualize to target range

Dialysis patients: Median dose: 75 units/kg 3 times/week
Nondialysis patients: Doses of 75-150 units/kg

Zidovudine-treated, HIV-infected patients: Patients with erythropoietin levels >500 mIU/mL are **unlikely** to respond

Initial dose: I.V., S.C.: 100 units/kg 3 times/week for 8 weeks

Increase dose by 50-100 units/kg 3 times/week if response is not satisfactory in terms of reducing transfusion requirements or increasing hematocrit after 8 weeks of therapy

Evaluate response every 4-8 weeks thereafter and adjust the dose accordingly by 50-100 units/kg increments 3 times/week

If patients have not responded satisfactorily to a 300 unit/kg dose 3 times/week, it is unlikely that they will respond to higher doses

Stop dose if hematocrit exceeds 40% and resume treatment at a 25% dose reduction when hematocrit drops to 36%

Cancer patients on chemotherapy: Treatment of patients with erythropoietin levels >200 mU/mL is **not recommended**

Initial dose: S.C.: 150 units/kg 3 times/week

Dose adjustment: If response is not satisfactory in terms of reducing transfusion requirement or increasing hematocrit after 8 weeks of therapy, the dose may be increased up to 300 units/kg 3 times/week. If patients do not respond, it is unlikely that they will respond to higher doses.

If hematocrit exceeds 40%, hold the dose until it falls to 36% and reduce the dose by 25% when treatment is resumed

Surgery patients: Prior to initiating treatment, obtain a hemoglobin to establish that is is >10 mg/dL or ≤13 mg/dL

Initial dose: S.C.: 300 units/kg/day for 10 days before surgery, on the day of surgery, and for 4 days after surgery

Alternative dose: S.C.: 600 units/kg in once-weekly doses (21, 14, and 7 days before surgery) plus a fourth dose on the day of surgery

Dosage Forms 1 mL single-dose vials (preservative-free soln): 2000 units/mL, 3000 units/mL, 4000 units/mL, 10,000 units/mL, 20,000 units/mL, 40,000 units/mL. **2 mL multidose vials** (preserved soln): 10,000 units/mL

Contraindications Known hypersensitivity to albumin (human) or mammalian cell-derived products; uncontrolled hypertension

Warnings/Precautions Use with caution in patients with porphyria, hypertension, or a history of seizures; prior to and during therapy, iron stores must be evaluated. It is recommended that the epoetin dose be decreased if the hematocrit increase exceeds 4 points in any 2-week period.

Pretherapy parameters:

Serum ferritin >100 ng/dL

Transferrin saturation (serum iron/iron binding capacity x 100) of 20% to 30%

Iron supplementation (usual oral dosing of 325 mg 2-3 times/day) should be given during therapy to provide for increased requirements during expansion of the red cell mass secondary to marrow stimulation by EPO unless iron stores are already in excess

For patients with endogenous serum EPO levels which are inappropriately low for hemoglobin level, documentation of the serum EPO level will help indicate which patients may benefit from EPO therapy. Serum EPO levels can be ordered routinely from Clinical Chemistry (red top serum separator tube). Refer to "Reference Range" for information on interpretation of EPO levels.

See table:

Factors Limiting Response to Epoetin Alfa

Factor	Mechanism
Iron deficiency	Limits hemoglobin synthesis
Blood loss/hemolysis	Counteracts epoetin alfa-stimulated erythropoiesis
Infection/inflammation	Inhibits iron transfer from storage to bone marrow Suppresses erythropoiesis through activated macrophages
Aluminum overload	Inhibits iron incorporation into heme protein
Bone marrow replacement Hyperparathyroidsm Metastatic, neoplastic	Limits bone marrow volume
Folic acid/vitamin B_{12} deficiency	Limits hemoglobin synthesis
Patient compliance	Self-administered epoetin alfa or iron therapy

Increased mortality has occurred when aggressive dosing is used in CHF or anginal patients undergoing hemodialysis. An Amgen-funded study determined that when patients were targeted for a hematocrit of 42% versus a less aggressive 30%, mortality was higher (35% versus 29%).

Pregnancy Risk Factor C

(Continued)

Epoetin Alfa *(Continued)*

Pregnancy Implications Clinical effect on the fetus: Epoetin alfa has been shown to have adverse effects in rats when given in doses 5X the human dose. There are no adequate and well-controlled studies in pregnant women. Epoetin alfa should be used only if potential benefit justifies the potential risk to the fetus.

Adverse Reactions

>10%:

Cardiovascular: Hypertension

Central nervous system: Fatigue, headache, fever

1% to 10%:

Cardiovascular: Edema, chest pain

Gastrointestinal: Nausea, vomiting, diarrhea

Hematologic: Clotted access

Neuromuscular & skeletal: Arthralgias, asthenia

<1%: CVA/TIA, hypersensitivity reactions, myocardial infarction, rash

Onset Several days; Peak effect: 2-3 weeks

Half-Life Circulating: 4-13 hours in patients with chronic renal failure; 20% shorter in patients with normal renal function

Education and Monitoring Issues

Patient Education: You will require frequent blood tests to determine appropriate dosage. Do not take other medications, vitamin or iron supplements, or make significant changes in your diet without consulting prescriber. Report signs or symptoms of edema (eg, swollen extremities, difficulty breathing, rapid weight gain), onset of severe headache, acute back pain, chest pain, or muscular tremors or seizure activity.

Monitoring Parameters:

Careful monitoring of blood pressure is indicated; problems with hypertension have been noted especially in renal failure patients treated with rHuEPO. Other patients are less likely to develop this complication.

See table.

Test	Initial Phase Frequency	Maintenance Phase Frequency
Hematocrit/hemoglobin	2 x/week	2-4 x/month
Blood pressure	3 x/week	3 x/week
Serum ferritin	Monthly	Quarterly
Transferrin saturation	Monthly	Quarterly
Serum chemistries including CBC with differential, creatinine, blood urea nitrogen, potassium, phosphorous	Regularly per routine	Regularly per routine

Hematocrit should be determined twice weekly until stabilization within the target range (30% to 36%), and twice weekly for at least 2 to 6 weeks after a dose increase

Reference Range: Guidelines should be based on the following figure or published literature

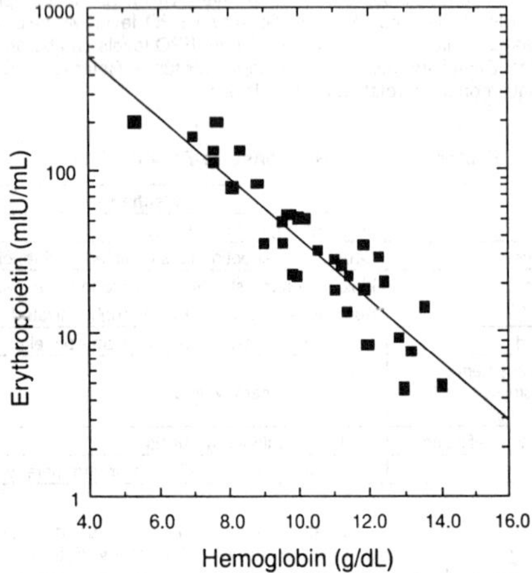

Use Treatment of primary pulmonary hypertension in NYHA Class III and IV patients

Unapproved uses: Other potential uses include pulmonary hypertension associated with ARDS, SLE, or CHF, neonatal pulmonary hypertension, cardiopulmonary bypass

Guidelines for estimating appropriateness of endogenous EPO levels for varying levels of anemia via the EIA assay method: See figure. The reference range for erythropoietin in serum, for subjects with normal hemoglobin and hematocrit, is 4.1-22.2 mIU/mL by the EIA method. Erythropoietin levels are typically inversely related to hemoglobin (and hematocrit) levels in anemias not attributed to impaired erythropoietin production.

Zidovudine-treated HIV patients: Available evidence indicates patients with endogenous serum erythropoietin levels >500 mIU/mL are unlikely to respond

Cancer chemotherapy patients: Treatment of patients with endogenous serum erythropoietin levels >200 mIU/mL is not recommended

Manufacturer Amgen, Inc

Related Information

Pharmaceutical Manufacturers Directory *on page 1020*

♦ **Epogen®** *see* Epoetin Alfa *on page 316*

Epoprostenol (e poe PROST en ole)

Pharmacologic Class Plasma Volume Expander, Colloid; Prostaglandin

U.S. Brand Names Flolan® Injection

Mechanism of Action Epoprostenol is also known as prostacyclin and PGI_2. It is a strong vasodilator of all vascular beds. In addition, it is a potent endogenous inhibitor of platelet aggregation. The reduction in platelet aggregation results from epoprostenol's activation of intracellular adenylate cyclase and the resultant increase in cyclic adenosine monophosphate concentrations within the platelets. Additionally, it is capable of decreasing thrombogenesis and platelet clumping in the lungs by inhibiting platelet aggregation.

surgery, hemodialysis, atherosclerosis, peripheral vascular disorders, and neonatal purpura fulminans

USUAL DOSAGE I.V.: The drug is administered by continuous intravenous infusion via a central venous catheter using an ambulatory infusion pump; during dose ranging it may be administered peripherally

Acute dose ranging: The initial infusion rate should be 2 ng/kg/minute by continuous I.V. and increased in increments of 2 ng/kg/minute every 15 minutes or longer until dose-limiting effects are elicited (such as chest pain, anxiety, dizziness, changes in heart rate, dyspnea, nausea, vomiting, headache, hypotension and/or flushing)

Continuous chronic infusion: Initial: 4 ng/kg/minute **less** than the maximum-tolerated infusion rate determined during acute dose ranging

If maximum-tolerated infusion rate is <5 ng/kg/minute, the chronic infusion rate should be ½ the maximum-tolerated acute infusion rate

Dosage adjustments: Dose adjustments in the chronic infusion rate should be based on persistence, recurrence, or worsening of patient symptoms of pulmonary hypertension

If symptoms persist or recur after improving, the infusion rate should be increased by 1-2 ng/kg/minute increments, every 15 minutes or greater; following establishment of a new chronic infusion rate, the patient should be observed and vital signs monitored.

Preparation of Infusion

To make 100 mL of solution with concentration:	Directions
3000 ng/mL	Dissolve one 0.5 mg vial with 5 mL supplied diluent, withdraw 3 mL, and add to sufficient diluent to make a total of 100 mL.
5000 ng/mL	Dissolve one 0.5 mg vial with 5 mL supplied diluent, withdraw entire vial contents, and add a sufficient volume of diluent to make a total of 100 mL.
10,000 ng/mL	Dissolve two 0.5 mg vials each with 5 mL supplied diluent, withdraw entire vial contents, and add a sufficient volume of diluent to make a total of 100 mL.
15,000 ng/mL	Dissolve one 1.5 mg vial with 5 mL supplied diluent, withdraw entire vial contents, and add a sufficient volume of diluent to make a total of 100 mL.

Elderly: In general, in patients ≥65 years of age dose selection should be cautious, usually starting at the low end of the dosing range, reflecting the greater frequency of decreased hepatic, renal or cardiac function in this patient population

Dosage Forms INJ: 0.5 mg/vial and 1.5 mg/vial, each supplied with 50 mL of sterile diluent

Contraindications Chronic use in patients with CHF due to severe left ventricular systolic dysfunction; hypersensitivity to epoprostenol or to structurally-related compounds

Warnings/Precautions Abrupt interruptions or large sudden reductions in dosage may result in rebound pulmonary hypertension; some patients with primary pulmonary hypertension have developed pulmonary edema during dose ranging, which may be associated with pulmonary veno-occlusive disease; during chronic use, unless contraindicated, anticoagulants should be coadministered to reduce the risk of thromboembolism. Clinical studies of epoprostenol in pulmonary hypertension did not include sufficient numbers of

(Continued)

Epoprostenol *(Continued)*

patients ≥65 years of age to substantiate its safety and efficacy in the geriatric population. As a result, in general, dose selection for an elderly patient should be cautious usually starting at the low end of the dosing range.

Pregnancy Risk Factor B

Adverse Reactions

>10%:

Cardiovascular: Flushing, tachycardia, shock, syncope, heart failure

Central nervous system: Fever, chills, anxiety, nervousness, dizziness, headache, hyperesthesia, pain

Gastrointestinal: Diarrhea, nausea, vomiting

Neuromuscular & skeletal: Jaw pain, myalgia, tremor, paresthesia

Respiratory: Hypoxia

Miscellaneous: Sepsis, flu-like symptoms

1% to 10%:

Cardiovascular: Bradycardia, hypotension, angina pectoris, edema, arrhythmias, pallor, cyanosis, palpitations, cerebrovascular accident, myocardial ischemia, chest pain

Central nervous system: Seizures, confusion, depression, insomnia

Dermatologic: Pruritus, rash

Endocrine & metabolic: Hypokalemia, weight change

Gastrointestinal: Abdominal pain, anorexia, constipation

Hematologic: Hemorrhage

Hepatic: Ascites

Neuromuscular & skeletal: Arthralgias, bone pain, weakness

Hematologic: Disseminated intravascular coagulation

Ocular: Amblyopia

Respiratory: Cough increase, dyspnea, epistaxis, pleural effusion

Miscellaneous: Diaphoresis

Drug Interactions Increased toxicity: The hypotensive effects of epoprostenol may be exacerbated by other vasodilators, diuretics, or by using acetate in dialysis fluids. Patients treated with anticoagulants and epoprostenol should be monitored for increased bleeding risk because of shared effects on platelet aggregation.

Half-Life 2.7-6 minute; steady-state levels are reached in about 15 minutes with continuous infusions

Education and Monitoring Issues

Patient Education: Therapy on this drug will probably be prolonged, possibly for years. You may experience mild headache, nausea or vomiting, and some muscular pains (use of a mild analgesia may be recommended by your prescriber). Report immediately any signs or symptoms of acute or severe headache, back pain, increased difficult breathing, flushing, fever or chills, any unusual bleeding or bruising, or any onset of unresolved diarrhea.

Monitoring Parameters: Monitor for improvements in pulmonary function, decreased exertional dyspnea, fatigue, syncope and chest pain, pulmonary vascular resistance, pulmonary arterial pressure and quality of life. In addition, the pump device and catheters should be monitored frequently to avoid "system" related failure.

Manufacturer GlaxoWellcome

Related Information

Pharmaceutical Manufacturers Directory *on page 1020*

♦ **Eprex®** *see* Epoetin Alfa *on page 316*

Eprosartan (ep roe SAR tan)

Pharmacologic Class Angiotensin II Antagonists

U.S. Brand Names Teveten®

Mechanism of Action Eprosartan is an angiotensin receptor antagonist. Angiotensin II acts as a vasoconstrictor. In addition to causing direct vasoconstriction, angiotensin II also stimulates the release of aldosterone. Once aldosterone is released, sodium, as well as water, are reabsorbed. The end result is an elevation in blood pressure. Eprosartan binds to the AT1 angiotensin II receptor. This binding prevents angiotensin II from binding to the receptor, thereby blocking the vasoconstriction and the aldosterone-secreting effects of angiotensin II.

Use Treatment of hypertension; may be used alone or in combination with other antihypertensives

USUAL DOSAGE Adults: Oral: Dosage must be individualized. Can administer once or twice daily with total daily doses of 400-800 mg. Usual starting dose is 600 mg once daily as monotherapy in patients who are euvolemic. Limited clinical experience with doses >800 mg.

Dosage adjustment in renal impairment: No starting dosage adjustment is necessary; however, carefully monitor the patient.

Dosage adjustment in hepatic impairment: No starting dosage adjustment is necessary; however, carefully monitor the patient.

Elderly: No starting dosage adjustment is necessary; however, carefully monitor the patient.

Dosage Forms TAB: 400 mg (scored), 600 mg

Contraindications Hypersensitivity to eprosartan or any component; sensitivity to other A-II receptor antagonists; bilateral renal artery stenosis; primary hyperaldosteronism; pregnancy (2nd and 3rd trimester)

Warnings/Precautions Avoid use or use a smaller dose in patients who are volume depleted; correct depletion first. Deterioration in renal function can occur with initiation. Use with caution in unilateral renal artery stenosis and pre-existing renal insufficiency; significant aortic/mitral stenosis. Safety and efficacy not established in pediatric patients.

Pregnancy Risk Factor C (1st trimester); D (2nd and 3rd trimester)

Pregnancy Implications Drugs that directly act on the renin-angiotensin system can cause fetal and neonatal morbidity and mortality when administered to pregnant women. When pregnancy is detected, drug should be discontinued as soon as possible. Women of childbearing potential should avoid pregnancy while taking this drug.

Adverse Reactions

1% to 10%:

Central nervous system: Fatigue (2%), depression (1%)

Endocrine & metabolic: Hypertriglyceridemia (1%)

Gastrointestinal: Abdominal pain (2%)

Genitourinary: Urinary tract infection (1%)

Respiratory: Upper respiratory tract infection (8%), rhinitis (4%), pharyngitis (4%), cough (4%)

Miscellaneous: Viral infection (2%), injury (2%)

<1% (limited to important or life-threatening symptoms): Alcohol intolerance, weakness, substernal chest pain, facial edema, peripheral edema, fatigue, fever, hot flashes, influenza-like symptoms, malaise, rigors, pain, angina pectoris, bradycardia, abnormal EKG, extrasystoles, atrial fibrillation, hypotension, tachycardia, palpitations, anorexia, constipation, dry mouth, esophagitis, flatulence, gastritis, gastroenteritis, gingivitis, nausea, periodontitis, toothache, vomiting, anemia, purpura, increased transaminases, increased creatine phosphokinase, diabetes mellitus, glycosuria, gout, hypercholesterolemia, hyperglycemia, hyperkalemia, hypokalemia, hyponatremia, arthritis, aggravated arthritis, arthrosis, skeletal pain, tendonitis, back pain, anxiety, ataxia, insomnia, migraine, neuritis, nervousness, paresthesia, somnolence, tremor, vertigo, herpes simplex, otitis externa, otitis media, asthma, epistaxis, eczema, furunculosis, pruritus, rash, maculopapular rash, increased sweating, conjunctivitis, abnormal vision, xerophthalmia, tinnitus, albuminuria, cystitis, hematuria, micturition frequency, polyuria, renal calculus, urinary incontinence, leg cramps, peripheral ischemia, increases in BUN or creatinine, leukopenia, neutropenia, thrombocytopenia

Drug Interactions

Lithium: Risk of toxicity may be increased by eprosartan; monitor lithium levels

Potassium-sparing diuretics (amiloride, potassium, spironolactone, triamterene): Increased risk of hyperkalemia

Potassium supplements may increase the risk of hyperkalemia

Trimethoprim (high dose) may increase the risk of hyperkalemia

Half-Life 5-7 hours

Education and Monitoring Issues

Patient Education: Take exactly as directed with food, at same time each day; do not increase or alter dosage or discontinue without consulting prescriber. Follow diet and exercise plan provided by prescriber. You may experience hypotension (rise slowly from sitting or lying position, use caution when climbing stairs, or driving until response to medication is known). Report respiratory infection, cold symptoms, unusual cough; chest pain, palpitations, or unusual heart beat; swelling of face, tongue, lips, or extremities; changes in urinary pattern; or extreme fatigue or other adverse response.

Monitoring Parameters: Baseline and periodic renal and liver function tests, urinalysis, electrolyte panels; symptoms of hypotension, tachycardia, or drug hypersensitivity

Manufacturer SmithKline Beecham Pharmaceuticals

Related Information

Angiotensin-Related Agents Comparison *on page 1226*

Pharmaceutical Manufacturers Directory *on page 1020*

♦ **Equagesic®** *see* Aspirin and Meprobamate *on page 76*

♦ **Equanil®** *see* Meprobamate *on page 565*

♦ **Equilet® [OTC]** *see* Calcium Carbonate *on page 130*

♦ **Eramycin®** *see* Erythromycin *on page 323*

♦ **Ercaf®** *see* Ergotamine *on page 323*

♦ **Ergamisol®** *see* Levamisole *on page 516*

Ergocalciferol (er goe kal SIF e role)

Pharmacologic Class Vitamin D Analog

U.S. Brand Names Calciferol™ Injection; Calciferol™ Oral; Drisdol® Oral

Use Treatment of refractory rickets, hypophosphatemia, hypoparathyroidism

USUAL DOSAGE Oral dosing is preferred; I.M. therapy required with GI, liver, or biliary disease associated with malabsorption

(Continued)

Ergocalciferol *(Continued)*

Dietary supplementation (each mcg = 40 USP units):
- Premature infants: 10-20 mcg/day (400-800 units), up to 750 mcg/day (30,000 units)
- Infants and healthy Children: 10 mcg/day (400 units)
- Adults: 10 mcg/day (400 units)

Renal failure:
- Children: 100-1000 mcg/day (4000-40,000 units)
- Adults: 500 mcg/day (20,000 units)

Hypoparathyroidism:
- Children: 1.25-5 mg/day (50,000-200,000 units) and calcium supplements
- Adults: 625 mcg to 5 mg/day (25,000-200,000 units) and calcium supplements

Vitamin D-dependent rickets:
- Children: 75-125 mcg/day (3000-5000 units); maximum: 1500 mcg/day
- Adults: 250 mcg to 1.5 mg/day (10,000-60,000 units)

Nutritional rickets and osteomalacia:
- Children and Adults (with normal absorption): 25-125 mcg/day (1000-5000 units)
- Children with malabsorption: 250-625 mcg/day (10,000-25,000 units)
- Adults with malabsorption: 250-7500 mcg (10,000-300,000 units)

Vitamin D-resistant rickets:
- Children: Initial: 1000-2000 mcg/day (40,000-80,000 units) with phosphate supplements; daily dosage is increased at 3- to 4-month intervals in 250-500 mcg (10,000-20,000 units) increments
- Adults: 250-1500 mcg/day (10,000-60,000 units) with phosphate supplements

Familial hypophosphatemia: 10,000-80,000 units daily plus 1-2 g/day elemental phosphorus

Osteoporosis prophylaxis: Adults:
- 51-70 years of age: 400 units/day
- >70 years of age: 600 units/day
- Maximum daily dose: 2000 units/day

Contraindications Hypercalcemia, hypersensitivity to ergocalciferol or any component; malabsorption syndrome; evidence of vitamin D toxicity

Pregnancy Risk Factor A; C (if dose exceeds RDA recommendation)

Ergoloid Mesylates (ER goe loid MES i lates)

Pharmacologic Class Ergot Alkaloid

U.S. Brand Names Germinal®; Hydergine®; Hydergine® LC

Use Treatment of cerebrovascular insufficiency in primary progressive dementia, Alzheimer's dementia, and senile onset

USUAL DOSAGE Adults: Oral: 1 mg 3 times/day up to 4.5-12 mg/day; up to 6 months of therapy may be necessary

Dosage Forms CAP, liq (Hydergine® LC): 1 mg. **LIQ** (Hydergine®): 1 mg/mL (100 mL). **TAB:** Oral: 0.5 mg; (Gerimal®, Hydergine®): 1 mg; Sublingual: (Gerimal®, Hydergine®): 0.5 mg, 1 mg

Contraindications Acute or chronic psychosis, hypersensitivity to ergot or any component

Pregnancy Risk Factor C

Half-Life 3.5 hours

♦ **Ergomar®** *see* Ergotamine *on page 323*

Ergonovine (er goe NOE veen)

Pharmacologic Class Ergot Derivative

U.S. Brand Names Ergotrate® Maleate

Generic Available No

Mechanism of Action Ergot alkaloid alpha-adrenergic agonist directly stimulates vascular smooth muscle to vasoconstrict peripheral and cerebral vessels; may also have antagonist effects on serotonin

Use Prevention and treatment of postpartum and postabortion hemorrhage caused by uterine atony or subinvolution

Unlabeled use: Migraine headaches, diagnostically to identify Prinzmetal's angina

USUAL DOSAGE Adults: I.M., I.V. (I.V. should be reserved for emergency use only): 0.2 mg, repeat dose in 2-4 hours as needed

Dosage Forms INJ: 0.2 mg/mL (1 mL)

Contraindications Induction of labor, threatened spontaneous abortion, hypersensitivity to ergonovine or any component

Warnings/Precautions Use with caution in patients with sepsis, heart disease, hypertension, or with hepatic or renal impairment; restore uterine responsiveness in calcium-deficient patients who do not respond to ergonovine by I.V. calcium administration; avoid prolonged use; discontinue if ergotism develops

Pregnancy Risk Factor X

Adverse Reactions

1% to 10%: Gastrointestinal: Nausea, vomiting

<1%: Bradycardia, cerebrovascular accidents, diaphoresis, dizziness, dyspnea, ergotism, headache, hypertension (sometimes extreme - treat with I.V. chlorpromazine), myocardial infarction, palpitations, seizures, shock, thrombophlebitis, tinnitus, transient chest pain

Onset Oral: Within 5-15 minutes; I.M.: Within 2-5 minutes

Duration Uterine effects persist for 3 hours, except when given I.V., then effects persist for ~45 minutes.

Education and Monitoring Issues

Patient Education: For angina diagnosis cardiologist will instruct patient about what to expect. For postpartum hemorrhage (an emergency situation) patient needs to know why the drug is being given and what side effects she might experience (eg, mild nausea and vomiting, dizziness, headache, ringing ears) and instructed to report difficulty breathing, acute headache, or numbness and cold feeling in extremities, or severe abdominal cramping.

Ergotamine (er GOT a meen)

Pharmacologic Class Ergot Derivative

U.S. Brand Names Cafatine®; Cafatine-PB®; Cafergot®; Cafetrate®; Ercaf®; Ergomar®; Wigraine®

Use Abort or prevent vascular headaches, such as migraine or cluster

USUAL DOSAGE Adults:

Oral:

Cafergot®: 2 tablets at onset of attack; then 1 tablet every 30 minutes as needed; maximum: 6 tablets per attack; do not exceed 10 tablets/week

Ergomar®: 1 tablet under tongue at first sign, then 1 tablet every 30 minutes, 3 tablets/24 hours, 5 tablets/week

Rectal (Cafergot® suppositories, Wigraine® suppositories, Cafatine® suppositories): 1 at first sign of an attack; follow with second dose after 1 hour, if needed; maximum dose: 2 per attack; do not exceed 5/week

Contraindications Hypersensitivity to ergotamine, caffeine, or any component; peripheral vascular disease, hepatic or renal disease, hypertension, peptic ulcer disease, sepsis; concurrent use of ritonavir (and possibly other protease inhibitors); avoid during pregnancy

Pregnancy Risk Factor X

Related Information

Belladonna, Phenobarbital, and Ergotamine Tartrate *on page 96*

- **Ergotrate** *see* Ergonovine *on page 322*
- **Ergotrate® Maleate** *see* Ergonovine *on page 322*
- **E•R•O Ear [OTC]** *see* Carbamide Peroxide *on page 139*
- **Erybid®** *see* Erythromycin *on page 323*
- **Eryc®** *see* Erythromycin *on page 323*
- **EryPed®** *see* Erythromycin *on page 323*
- **Ery-Tab®** *see* Erythromycin *on page 323*
- **Erythro-Base®** *see* Erythromycin *on page 323*
- **Erythrocin®** *see* Erythromycin *on page 323*

Erythromycin (er ith roe MYE sin)

Pharmacologic Class Antibiotic, Macrolide; Antibiotic, Ophthalmic

U.S. Brand Names E-Base®; E.E.S.®; E-Mycin®; Eramycin®; Eryc®; EryPed®; Ery-Tab®; Erythrocin®; Ilosone®; PCE®

Generic Available Yes

Mechanism of Action Inhibits RNA-dependent protein synthesis at the chain elongation step; binds to the 50S ribosomal subunit resulting in blockage of transpeptidation

Use Treatment of susceptible bacterial infections including *S. pyogenes*, some *S. pneumoniae*, some *S. aureus*, *M. pneumoniae*, *Legionella pneumophila*, diphtheria, pertussis, chancroid, *Chlamydia*, erythrasma, *N. gonorrhoeae*, *E. histolytica*, syphilis and nongonococcal urethritis, and *Campylobacter* gastroenteritis; used in conjunction with neomycin for decontaminating the bowel; treatment of gastroparesis

USUAL DOSAGE

Infants and Children (Note: 400 mg ethylsuccinate = 250 mg base, stearate, or estolate salts):

Oral: 30-50 mg/kg/day divided every 6-8 hours; may double doses in severe infections

Preop bowel preparation: 20 mg/kg erythromycin base at 1, 2, and 11 PM on the day before surgery combined with mechanical cleansing of the large intestine and oral neomycin

I.V.: Lactobionate: 20-40 mg/kg/day divided every 6 hours

Adults:

Oral:

Base: 250-500 mg every 6-12 hours

Ethylsuccinate: 400-800 mg every 6-12 hours

(Continued)

Erythromycin *(Continued)*

Preop bowel preparation: Oral: 1 g erythromycin base at 1, 2, and 11 PM on the day before surgery combined with mechanical cleansing of the large intestine and oral neomycin

I.V.: Lactobionate: 15-20 mg/kg/day divided every 6 hours or 500 mg to 1 g every 6 hours, or given as a continuous infusion over 24 hours (maximum: 4 g/24 hours)

Children and Adults: Ophthalmic: Instill ½" (1.25 cm) 2-8 times/day depending on the severity of the infection

Dialysis: Slightly dialyzable (5% to 20%); no supplemental dosage necessary in hemo or peritoneal dialysis or in continuous arteriovenous or venovenous hemofiltration (CAVH/CAVHD)

Erythromycin has been used as a prokinetic agent to improve gastric emptying time and intestinal motility. In adults, 200 mg was infused I.V. initially followed by 250 mg orally 3 times/day 30 minutes before meals. In children, erythromycin 3 mg/kg I.V. has been infused over 60 minutes initially followed by 20 mg/kg/day orally in 3-4 divided doses before meals or before meals and at bedtime

Dosage Forms

Oint, ophth: 0.55 mg (3.5 g)

Erythromycin base: **CAP:** Delayed release: 250 mg; Delayed release, enteric coated pellets (Eryc®): 250 mg. **TAB:** Delayed release: 333 mg; Enteric coated (E-Mycin®, Ery-Tab®, E-Base®): 250 mg, 333 mg, 500 mg; Film coated: 250 mg, 500 mg; Polymer coated particles (PCE®): 333 mg, 500 mg

Erythromycin estolate: **CAP:** 250 mg. **SUSP, oral:** 125 mg/5 mL (480 mL); 250 mg/5 mL (480 mL).

Erythromycin ethylsuccinate: **GRANULES for oral susp** (EryPed®): 400 mg/5 mL (60 mL, 100 mL, 200 mL). **POWDER for oral susp** (E.E.S.®): 200 mg/5 mL (100 mL, 200 mL). **SUSP:** Oral (E.E.S.®, EryPed®): 200 mg/5 mL (5 mL, 100 mL, 200 mL, 480 mL); 400 mg/5 mL (5 mL, 60 mL, 100 mL, 200 mL, 480 mL); Oral, drops (EryPed®): 100 mg/2.5 mL (50 mL). **TAB** (E.E.S.®): 400 mg; Chewable (EryPed®): 200 mg

Erythromycin gluceptate: **INJ:** 1000 mg (30 mL)

Erythromycin lactobionate: **POWDER for inj:** 500 mg, 1000 mg

Erythromycin stearate: **TAB, film coated** (Eramycin®, Erythrocin®): 250 mg, 500 mg

Contraindications Hepatic impairment, known hypersensitivity to erythromycin or its components; pre-existing liver disease (erythromycin estolate); concomitant use with pimozide, terfenadine, astemizole, or cisapride

Warnings/Precautions Hepatic impairment with or without jaundice has occurred, it may be accompanied by malaise, nausea, vomiting, abdominal colic, and fever; discontinue use if these occur; avoid using erythromycin lactobionate in neonates since formulations may contain benzyl alcohol which is associated with toxicity in neonates; observe for superinfections

Pregnancy Risk Factor B

Adverse Reactions

>10%: Gastrointestinal: Abdominal pain, cramping, nausea, vomiting

1% to 10%:

- Gastrointestinal: Oral candidiasis
- Hepatic: Cholestatic jaundice
- Local: Phlebitis at the injection site
- Miscellaneous: Hypersensitivity reactions

<1%: Allergic reactions, cholestatic jaundice (most common with estolate), diarrhea, eosinophilia, fever, hypertrophic pyloric stenosis, rash, pseudomembranous colitis, thrombophlebitis, ventricular arrhythmias

Drug Interactions CYP3A3/4 enzyme substrate; CYP1A2 and 3A3/4 enzyme inhibitor

Increased toxicity:

- Erythromycin decreases clearance of carbamazepine, cyclosporine, and triazolam, alfentanil, bromocriptine, digoxin (~10% of patients), disopyramide, ergot alkaloids, methylprednisolone; may decrease clearance of protease inhibitors
- Erythromycin may decrease theophylline clearance and increase theophylline's half-life by up to 60% (patients on high-dose theophylline and erythromycin or who have received erythromycin for >5 days may be at higher risk)
- Decreases metabolism of terfenadine, cisapride, and astemizole resulting in an increase in Q-T interval and potential heart failure
- Inhibits felodipine (and other dihydropyridine calcium antagonist) metabolism in the liver resulting in a twofold increase in levels and consequent toxicity
- Pimozide's serum concentration is elevated with concurrent use; death has been reported by potentiation of pimozide's cardiotoxicity when given concurrently with erythromycin; concurrent use is contraindicated
- May potentiate anticoagulant effect of warfarin and decrease metabolism of vinblastine
- Concurrent use of erythromycin and lovastatin and simvastatin may result in significantly increased levels and rhabdomyolysis
- Protease inhibitors (amprenavir, ritonavir, nelfinavir) may increase the serum levels of erythromycin

Alcohol Interactions Avoid use (may decrease absorption of erythromycin or enhance alcohol effects)

Half-Life 1.5-2 hours (peak); End-stage renal disease: 5-6 hours

Education and Monitoring Issues

Patient Education: Take as directed, around-the-clock, with a full glass of water (not juice or milk), preferably on an empty stomach (1 hour before or 2 hours after meals). Take complete prescription even if you are feeling better. You may experience nausea, vomiting, or mouth sores (small frequent meals, frequent mouth care may help). Report skin rash or itching; easy bruising or bleeding; unhealed sores of mouth; itching or vaginal discharge; watery or bloody diarrhea; unresolved vomiting; yellowing of skin or eyes; easy fatigue; pale stool or dark urine; skin rash or itching; white plaques, sores, or fuzziness in mouth; or any change in hearing.

Ophthalmic: Wash hands before applying. Pull down lower eyelid gently, instill thin ribbon of ointment into lower lid, close eye, roll eyeball in all directions. Blurred vision and stinging is temporary. Report persistent pain, burning, vision disturbances, swelling, itching, or worsening of condition.

Dietary Considerations: Food: Increased drug absorption with meals. Drug may cause GI upset; may take with food.

Related Information

Animal and Human Bites Guidelines *on page 1177*
Antimicrobial Drugs of Choice *on page 1182*
Community Acquired Pneumonia in Adults *on page 1200*
Erythromycin and Benzoyl Peroxide *on page 325*
Prophylaxis for Patients Exposed to Common Communicable Diseases *on page 1161*
Treatment of Sexually Transmitted Diseases *on page 1210*

Erythromycin and Benzoyl Peroxide

(er ith roe MYE sin & BEN zoe il per OKS ide)

Pharmacologic Class Acne Products

U.S. Brand Names Benzamycin®

Dosage Forms GEL: Erythromycin 30 mg and benzoyl peroxide 50 mg per g

Pregnancy Risk Factor C

Erythromycin and Sulfisoxazole (er ith roe MYE sin & sul fi SOKS a zole)

Pharmacologic Class Antibiotic, Macrolide Combination; Antibiotic, Macrolide; Antibiotic, Sulfonamide Derivative

U.S. Brand Names Eryzole®; Pediazole®

Generic Available Yes

Mechanism of Action Erythromycin inhibits bacterial protein synthesis; sulfisoxazole competitively inhibits bacterial synthesis of folic acid from para-aminobenzoic acid

Use Treatment of susceptible bacterial infections of the upper and lower respiratory tract, otitis media in children caused by susceptible strains of *Haemophilus influenzae*, and many other infections in patients allergic to penicillin

USUAL DOSAGE Oral (dosage recommendation is based on the product's erythromycin content):

Children ≥2 months: 50 mg/kg/day erythromycin and 150 mg/kg/day sulfisoxazole in divided doses every 6 hours; not to exceed 2 g erythromycin/day or 6 g sulfisoxazole/day for 10 days

Adults >45 kg: 400 mg erythromycin and 1200 mg sulfisoxazole every 6 hours

Dosing adjustment in renal impairment (sulfisoxazole must be adjusted in renal impairment):

Cl_{cr} 10-50 mL/minute: Administer every 8-12 hours

Cl_{cr} <10 mL/minute: Administer every 12-24 hours

Dosage Forms SUSP, oral: Erythromycin ethylsuccinate 200 mg and sulfisoxazole acetyl 600 mg per 5 mL (100 mL, 150 mL, 200 mL, 250 mL)

Contraindications Hepatic dysfunction, known hypersensitivity to erythromycin or sulfonamides; infants <2 months of age (sulfas compete with bilirubin for binding sites); patients with porphyria; concurrent use with pimozide, terfenadine, astemizole, or cisapride

Warnings/Precautions Use with caution in patients with impaired renal or hepatic function, G-6-PD deficiency (hemolysis may occur)

Pregnancy Risk Factor C

Adverse Reactions

>10%: Gastrointestinal: Abdominal pain, cramping, nausea, vomiting

1% to 10%:

Gastrointestinal: Oral candidiasis

Local: Phlebitis at the injection site

Miscellaneous: Hypersensitivity reactions

<1%: Agranulocytosis, aplastic anemia, cholestatic jaundice, crystalluria, diarrhea, eosinophilia, fever, headache, hepatic necrosis, hypertrophic pyloric stenosis, pseudomembranous colitis, rash, Stevens-Johnson syndrome, thrombophlebitis, toxic epidermal necrolysis, toxic nephrosis, ventricular arrhythmias

(Continued)

Erythromycin and Sulfisoxazole *(Continued)*

Drug Interactions

Increased effect/toxicity/levels with erythromycin/sulfisoxazole on alfentanil, astemizole, terfenadine (resulting in potentially life-threatening prolonged Q-T interval), bromocriptine, carbamazepine, cyclosporine, digoxin, disopyramide, theophylline, triazolam, lovastatin/simvastatin, ergots, methylprednisolone, cisapride, pimozide, felodipine, phenytoin, barbiturate anesthetics, methotrexate, sulfonylureas, uricosuric agents, and warfarin; may inhibit metabolism of protease inhibitors

Increased toxicity of sulfonamides occurs with concurrent diuretics, indomethacin, methenamine, probenecid, and salicylates

Education and Monitoring Issues

Monitoring Parameters: CBC and periodic liver function test

- **Eryzole®** *see* Erythromycin and Sulfisoxazole *on page 325*
- **Esclim® Transdermal** *see* Estradiol *on page 327*
- **Esgic®** *see* Butalbital Compound *on page 123*
- **Esidrix®** *see* Hydrochlorothiazide *on page 442*
- **Eskalith®** *see* Lithium *on page 534*
- **Eskalith CR®** *see* Lithium *on page 534*
- **Esoterica® Facial [OTC]** *see* Hydroquinone *on page 450*
- **Esoterica® Regular [OTC]** *see* Hydroquinone *on page 450*
- **Esoterica® Sensitive Skin Formula [OTC]** *see* Hydroquinone *on page 450*
- **Esoterica® Sunscreen [OTC]** *see* Hydroquinone *on page 450*

Estazolam (es TA zoe lam)

Pharmacologic Class Benzodiazepine

U.S. Brand Names ProSom™

Generic Available No

Mechanism of Action Benzodiazepines may exert their pharmacologic effect through potentiation of the inhibitory activity of GABA. Benzodiazepines do not alter the synthesis, release, reuptake, or enzymatic degradation of GABA.

Use Short-term management of insomnia; there has been little experience with this drug in the elderly, but because of its lack of active metabolites, it is a reasonable choice when a benzodiazepine hypnotic is indicated

USUAL DOSAGE Adults: Oral: 1 mg at bedtime, some patients may require 2 mg; start at doses of 0.5 mg in debilitated or small elderly patients

Dosing adjustment in hepatic impairment: May be necessary

Dosage Forms TAB: 1 mg, 2 mg

Contraindications Pregnancy; hypersensitivity to estazolam, cross-sensitivity with other benzodiazepines may occur, pre-existing CNS depression, sleep apnea, narrow-angle glaucoma

Warnings/Precautions Abrupt discontinuance may precipitate withdrawal or rebound insomnia; use with caution in patients receiving other CNS depressants, patients with low albumin, hepatic dysfunction, and in the elderly; do not use in pregnant women; may cause drug dependency; safety and efficacy have not been established in children <15 years of age, not recommended in nursing mothers

Pregnancy Risk Factor X

Adverse Reactions

>10%:

Central nervous system: Somnolence

Neuromuscular & skeletal: Weakness

1% to 10%:

Cardiovascular: Flushing, palpitations

Central nervous system: Anxiety, confusion, dizziness, hypokinesia, abnormal coordination, hangover, agitation, amnesia, apathy, emotional lability, euphoria, hostility, seizure, sleep disorder, stupor, twitch

Dermatologic: Dermatitis, pruritus, rash, urticaria

Gastrointestinal: Xerostomia, constipation, decreased appetite, flatulence, gastritis, increased appetite, perverse taste

Genitourinary: Frequent urination, menstrual cramps, urinary hesitancy, urinary frequency, vaginal discharge/itching

Neuromuscular & skeletal: Paresthesia

Otic: Photophobia, eye pain, eye swelling

Respiratory: Cough, dyspnea, asthma, rhinitis, sinusitis

Miscellaneous: Diaphoresis

<1%: Allergic reactions, chills, drug dependence, fever, muscle spasm, myalgia, neck pain

Drug Interactions

Carbamazepine, rifampin, rifabutin may enhance the metabolism of estazolam and decrease its therapeutic effect; consider using an alternative sedative/hypnotic agent

Cimetidine, ciprofloxacin, clarithromycin, clozapine, CNS depressants, diltiazem, disulfiram, digoxin, erythromycin, ethanol, fluconazole, fluoxetine, fluvoxamine, isoniazid, itraconazole, ketoconazole, labetalol, levodopa, loxapine, metoprolol, metronidazole, miconazole, nefazodone, omeprazole, phenytoin, rifabutin, rifampin, troleandomycin, valproic acid, verapamil may increase the serum level and/or toxicity of estazolam

Alcohol Interactions Avoid use (may increase central nervous system depression)

Onset Within 1 hour

Duration Variable

Half-Life 10-24 hours

Education and Monitoring Issues

Patient Education: Use exactly as directed (do not increase dose or frequency or discontinue without consulting prescriber); may cause physical and/or psychological dependence. While using this medication, do not use alcohol or other prescription or OTC medications (especially, pain medications, sedatives, antihistamines, or hypnotics) without consulting prescriber. Maintain adequate hydration (2-3 L/day of fluids unless instructed to restrict fluid intake). You may experience drowsiness, dizziness, or blurred vision (use caution when driving or engaging in tasks requiring alertness until response to drug is known); GI upset (take with water or milk). Report CNS changes (confusion, depression, increased sedation, excitation, headache, abnormal thinking, insomnia, or nightmares), altered voiding patterns or blood in urine, difficulty breathing, chest pain or palpitations, altered gait pattern, or ineffectiveness of medication.

Dietary Considerations: Grapefruit juice may increase serum levels and/or toxicity

Monitoring Parameters: Respiratory and cardiovascular status

- **Estinyl®** *see* Ethinyl Estradiol *on page 340*
- **Estivin® II [OTC]** *see* Naphazoline *on page 636*
- **Estrace® Oral** *see* Estradiol *on page 327*
- **Estraderm®** *see* Estradiol *on page 327*
- **Estraderm® Transdermal** *see* Estradiol *on page 327*
- **Estra-D® Injection** *see* Estradiol *on page 327*

Estradiol (es tra DYE ole)

Pharmacologic Class Estrogen Derivative

U.S. Brand Names Alora™ Transdermal; Climara® Transdermal; Delestrogen® Injection; depGynogen® Injection; Depo®-Estradiol Injection; Depogen® Injection; Dioval® Injection; Dura-Estrin® Injection; Duragen® Injection; Esclim® Transdermal; Estrace® Oral; Estraderm® Transdermal; Estra-D® Injection; Estra-L® Injection; Estring®; Estro-Cyp® Injection; Estroject-L.A.® Injection; FemPatch® Transdermal; Gynodiol® Oral; Gynogen L.A.® Injection; Innofem®; Vagifem®; Valergen® Injection; Vivelle® Transdermal

Generic Available Yes

Mechanism of Action Increases the synthesis of DNA, RNA, and various proteins in target tissues; reduces the release of gonadotropin-releasing hormone from the hypothalamus; reduces FSH and LH release from the pituitary

Use Treatment of atrophic vaginitis, atrophic dystrophy of vulva, menopausal symptoms, female hypogonadism, ovariectomy, primary ovarian failure, inoperable breast cancer, inoperable prostatic cancer, mild to severe vasomotor symptoms associated with menopause

USUAL DOSAGE All dosage needs to be adjusted based upon the patient's response

Male:

- Prostate cancer: Valerate: I.M.: ≥30 mg or more every 1-2 weeks
- Prostate cancer (androgen-dependent, inoperable, progressing): Oral: 10 mg 3 times/day for at least 3 months

Female:

- Oral:
  - Breast cancer (inoperable, progressing): 10 mg 3 times/day for at least 3 months
  - Osteoporosis prevention: 0.5 mg/day in a cyclic regimen (3 weeks on and 1 week off)
  - Hypogonadism, moderate to severe vasomotor symptoms: 1-2 mg/day in a cyclic regimen for 3 weeks on drug, then 1 week off
  - Treatment of moderate to severe vasomotor symptoms associated with menopause: 1-2 mg/day, adjusted as necessary to limit symptoms; administration should be cyclic (3 weeks on, 1 week off). Patients should be re-evaluated at 3- to 6-month intervals to determine if treatment is still necessary.
- I.M.
  - Moderate to severe vasomotor symptoms associated with menopause: Cypionate: 1-5 mg every 3-4 weeks; Valerate: 10-20 mg every 4 weeks
  - Postpartum breast engorgement: Valerate: 10-25 mg at end of first stage of labor
- Transdermal twice-weekly patch (Alora™, Esclim®, Estraderm®, Vivelle®):
  - Moderate to severe vasomotor symptoms associated with menopause, vulvar/vaginal atrophy, hypogonadism: Apply 0.05 mg patch initially (titrate dosage to response) applied twice weekly in a cyclic regimen, for 3 weeks on and 1 week off drug in patients with an intact uterus and continuously in patients without a uterus. Re-

(Continued)

Estradiol *(Continued)*

evaluate postmenopausal therapy at 3- to 6-month intervals to determine if treatment is still necessary.

Transdermal once-weekly patch (Climara®, Fempatch®):

Moderate to severe vasomotor symptoms associated with menopause: Apply 0.025-0.05 mg/day patch once weekly. Adjust dose as necessary to control symptoms. Patients should be re-evaluated at 3- to 6-month intervals to determine if treatment is still necessary.

Prevention of osteoporosis in postmenopausal women (approved indication for Climara®): Apply patch once weekly; minimum effective dose 0.025 mg/day; adjust response to therapy by biochemical markers and bone mineral density

Vaginal cream:

Atrophic vaginitis, kraurosis vulvae: Vaginal: Insert 2-4 g/day for 2 weeks then gradually reduce to 1/2 the initial dose for 2 weeks followed by a maintenance dose of 1 g 1-3 times/week

Vaginal ring (Estring®):

Postmenopausal vaginal atrophy, urogenital symptoms: Following insertion, Estring® should remain in place for 90 days

Vaginal tablets (Vagifem®):

Atrophic vaginitis: Initial: Insert 1 tablet once daily for 2 weeks; Maintenance: Insert 1 tablet twice weekly; attempts to discontinue or taper medication should be made at 3- to 6-month intervals

Dosage Forms

Estradiol base: **CRM, vag** (Estrace®): 0.1 mg/g (42.5 g). **TAB, micronized** (Estrace®): 1 mg, 2 mg. **TRANSDERMAL system:** (Alora™): 0.05 mg/24 hours [18 cm^2], total estradiol 1.5 mg; 0.075 mg/24 hours [27 cm^2], total estradiol 2.3 mg; 0.1 mg/24 hours [36 cm^2], total estradiol 3 mg; (Climara®): 0.05 mg/24 hours [12.5 cm^2], total estradiol 3.9 mg; 0.075 mg/24 hours [18.75 cm^2], total estradiol 5.85 mg; 0.1 mg/24 hours [25 cm^2], total estradiol 7.8 mg; (Esclim®): 0.025 mg/24 hours; 0.0375 mg/24 hours; 0.05 mg/24 hours; 0.075 mg/24 hours; 0.1 mg/24 hours; (Estraderm®): 0.05 mg/24 hours [10 cm^2], total estradiol 4 mg; 0.1 mg/24 hours [20 cm^2], total estradiol 8 mg; (Vivelle®): 0.0375 mg/day, 0.05 mg/day, 0.075 mg/day, 0.1 mg/day. **VAG ring** (Estring®): 2 mg gradually released over 90 days

Estradiol cypionate: **INJ** (depGynogen®, Depo®-Estradiol, Depogen®, Dura-Estrin®, Estra-D®, Estro-Cyp®, Estroject-L.A.®): 5 mg/mL (5 mL, 10 mL)

Estradiol valerate: **INJ:** (Valergen®): 10 mg/mL (5 mL, 10 mL), 20 mg/mL (1 mL, 5 mL, 10 mL), 40 mg/mL (5 mL, 10 mL); (Dioval®, Duragen®, Estra-L®, Gynogen L.A.®): 20 mg/mL (10 mL), 40 mg/mL (10 mL). **TAB:**, micronized: (Gynodiol®): 0.5 mg, 1 mg, 1.5 mg, 2 mg

Contraindications Hypersensitivity to estradiol or any component; known or suspected pregnancy; porphyria; abnormal genital bleeding of unknown etiology; known or suspected carcinoma of the breast (except in patients treated for metastatic disease); estrogen-dependent tumors; history of thrombophlebitis, thrombosis, or thromboembolic disorders associated with estrogen use

Warnings/Precautions Use with caution in patients with renal or hepatic insufficiency. Estrogens may cause premature closure of epiphyses in young individuals, in patients with a history of thromboembolism, stroke, myocardial infarction (especially >40 years of age who smoke), liver tumor, or hypertension.

Gallbladder disease may be increased by estrogens. In addition, estrogens may increase blood pressure or alter glucose regulation. Use with caution in patients with diseases which may be exacerbated by fluid retention, including asthma, epilepsy, migraine, CHF, and renal dysfunction. Estrogens have been associated with severe hypercalcemia in patients with bone metastases, and may cause severe elevations of triglycerides in patients with familial dyslipidemias. Use with caution in women with a history of pregnancy-associated jaundice or metabolic bone disease. May increase the risk of benign hepatic adenoma, which may cause significant consequences in the event of rupture.

Use vaginal tablets with caution in patients with severely atrophic vaginal mucosa or following gynecological surgery due to possible trauma from the applicator.

Estrogens have been reported to increase the risk of endometrial carcinoma; do not use estrogens during pregnancy. Before prescribing estrogen therapy to postmenopausal women, the risks and benefits must be weighed for each patient. Women should be informed of these risks and benefits, as well as possible side effects and the return of menstrual bleeding (when cycled with a progestin), and be involved in the decision to prescribe. Oral therapy may be more convenient for vaginal atrophy and stress incontinence.

Pregnancy Risk Factor X

Adverse Reactions

>10%:

Cardiovascular: Peripheral edema

Endocrine & metabolic: Enlargement of breasts (female and male), breast tenderness

Gastrointestinal: Nausea, anorexia, bloating

1% to 10%:
Central nervous system: Headache
Endocrine & metabolic: Increased libido (female), decreased libido (male)
Gastrointestinal: Vomiting, diarrhea

<1%: Amenorrhea, anxiety, breast tumors, change in menstrual flow, chloasma, cholestatic jaundice, decreased glucose tolerance, depression, dizziness, edema, folate deficiency, GI distress, hypercalcemia, increase in blood pressure, increased susceptibility to *Candida* infection, increased triglycerides and LDL, intolerance to contact lenses, melasma, myocardial infarction, pain at injection site, rash, stroke, thromboembolic disorders,

Vaginal: Trauma from applicator insertion may occur in women with severely atrophic vaginal mucosa

Drug Interactions CYP1A2 and 3A3/4 enzyme substrate

Decreased effect: Rifampin decreases estrogen serum concentrations

Increased toxicity: Hydrocortisone increases corticosteroid toxic potential; increased potential for thromboembolic events with anticoagulants

Alcohol Interactions Avoid use (routine use increases estrogen level and risk of breast cancer)

Half-Life 50-60 minutes

Education and Monitoring Issues

Patient Education: Use this drug in cycles or term as prescribed. Periodic gynecologic exam and breast exams are important. You may experience nausea or vomiting (small frequent meals may help); dizziness or mental depression (use caution when driving); photosensitivity (use sunscreen, wear protective clothing and eyewear, avoid direct sunlight); rash; loss of hair; enlargement/tenderness of breasts; increased/decreased libido. Report sudden acute pain in legs or calves, chest, or abdomen; shortness of breath; severe headache or vomiting; weakness or numbness of arms or legs; unusual vaginal bleeding; yellowing of skin or eyes; change in color of urine or stool; or easy bruising or bleeding.

Transdermal patch: Apply to clean dry skin. Do not apply transdermal patch to breasts. Apply to trunk of body (preferably abdomen). Rotate application sites. Aerosol topical corticosteroids may reduce allergic skin reaction; report persistent skin reaction.

Intravaginal cream: Insert high in vagina. Wash hands and applicator before and after use.

Reference Range:

Children: <10 pg/mL (SI: <37 pmol/L)
Male: 10-50 pg/mL (SI: 37-184 pmol/L)
Female:
Premenopausal: 30-400 pg/mL (SI: 110-1468 pmol/L)
Postmenopausal: 0-30 pg/mL (SI: 0-110 pmol/L)

Related Information

Estradiol and Testosterone *on page 329*

Estradiol and Testosterone (es tra DYE ole & tes TOS ter one)

Pharmacologic Class Estrogen and Androgen Combination

U.S. Brand Names Andro/Fem® Injection; Deladumone® Injection; depAndrogyn® Injection; Depo-Testadiol® Injection; Depotestogen® Injection; Duo-Cyp® Injection; Duratestrin® Injection; Valertest No.1® Injection

Dosage Forms INJ: (Andro/Fem®, depAndrogyn®, Depo-Testadiol®, Depotestogen®, Duo-Cyp®, Duratestrin®): Estradiol cypionate 2 mg and testosterone cypionate 50 mg per mL in cottonseed oil (1 mL, 10 mL); (Androgyn L.A.®, Deladumone®, Estra-Testrin®, Valertest No.1®): Estradiol valerate 4 mg and testosterone enanthate 90 mg per mL in sesame oil (5 mL, 10 mL)

Pregnancy Risk Factor X

♦ **Estra-L® Injection** *see* Estradiol *on page 327*

Estramustine (es tra MUS teen)

Pharmacologic Class Antineoplastic Agent, Alkylating Agent

U.S. Brand Names Emcyt®

Generic Available No

Mechanism of Action Estramustine's exact mechanism of action is unclear. It appears to bind to microtubule proteins, preventing normal tubulin function. Theoretically, the estrogen component serves as a carrier to estrogen-dependent tissues. Whether estramustine actually dissociates to an alkylating moiety in target tissues is speculative; the antitumor effect may be due solely to estrogenic effect. Estramustine causes a marked decrease in plasma testosterone levels, and increase in estrogen levels.

Use Palliative treatment of prostatic carcinoma (progressive or metastatic)

USUAL DOSAGE Adults: Oral: 14 mg/kg/day (range: 10-16 mg/kg/day) in 3-4 divided doses for 30-90 days; some patients have been maintained for >3 years on therapy

Dosage Forms CAP: 140 mg

Contraindications Active thrombophlebitis or thromboembolic disorders, hypersensitivity to estramustine or any component, estradiol or nitrogen mustard

(Continued)

Estramustine *(Continued)*

Warnings/Precautions The U.S. Food and Drug Administration (FDA) currently recommends that procedures for proper handling and disposal of antineoplastic agents be considered. Glucose tolerance may be decreased; elevated blood pressure may occur; exacerbation of peripheral edema or congestive heart disease may occur; use with caution in patients with impaired liver function, renal insufficiency, or metabolic bone diseases.

Pregnancy Risk Factor C

Adverse Reactions

>10%:

- Cardiovascular: Edema
- Gastrointestinal: Diarrhea, nausea, mild increases in AST (SGOT) or LDH
- Endocrine & metabolic: Decreased libido, breast tenderness, breast enlargement
- Respiratory: Dyspnea

1% to 10%:

- Cardiovascular: Myocardial infarction
- Central nervous system: Insomnia, lethargy
- Gastrointestinal: Anorexia, flatulence
- Hematologic: Leukopenia
- Local: Thrombophlebitis
- Neuromuscular & skeletal: Leg cramps
- Respiratory: Pulmonary embolism

<1%: Cardiac arrest, depression, hypercalcemia, hot flashes, night sweats, pigment changes, tinnitus

Drug Interactions Decreased effect: Milk products and calcium-rich foods/drugs may impair the oral absorption of estramustine phosphate sodium

Half-Life 20 hours

Education and Monitoring Issues

Patient Education: It may take several weeks to manifest effects of this medication. Store capsules in refrigerator. Do not take with milk, milk products, or other substances high in calcium. Preferable to take on an empty stomach (1 hour before or 2 hours after meals). Small frequent meals, frequent mouth care may reduce incidence of nausea or vomiting. You may experience flatulence, diarrhea, decreased libido (reversible), breast tenderness or enlargement. Report sudden acute pain or cramping in legs or calves, chest pain, shortness of breath, weakness or numbness of arms or legs, difficulty breathing, or edema (increased weight, swelling of legs or feet).

Manufacturer Pharmacia & Upjohn

Related Information

Pharmaceutical Manufacturers Directory *on page 1020*

- **Estrand** *see* Estradiol and Testosterone *on page 329*
- **Estratab®** *see* Estrogens, Esterified *on page 333*
- **Estratest®** *see* Estrogens and Methyltestosterone *on page 330*
- **Estratest® H.S.** *see* Estrogens and Methyltestosterone *on page 330*
- **Estring®** *see* Estradiol *on page 327*
- **Estro-Cyp® Injection** *see* Estradiol *on page 327*

Estrogens and Medroxyprogesterone

(ES troe jenz & me DROKS ee proe JES te rone)

Pharmacologic Class Estrogen Derivative

U.S. Brand Names Premphase™; Prempro™

Dosage Forms Premphase™: Two separate tabs in therapy pack: Conjugated estrogens 0.625 mg [Premarin®] (28s) taken orally for 28 days and medroxyprogesterone acetate [Cycrin®] 5 mg (14s) which are taken orally with a Premarin® tab on days 15 through 28; **Prempro™:** Conjugated estrogens 0.625 mg and medroxyprogesterone acetate 2.5 mg (14s)

Pregnancy Risk Factor X

Education and Monitoring Issues

Patient Education: Take this as prescribed; maintain schedule. If also taking supplemental calcium as part of osteoporosis prevention, consult prescriber for recommended amounts. Periodic gynecologic exam and breast exams are important. You may experience nausea or vomiting (small frequent meals may help); dizziness or mental depression (use caution when driving); rash, loss of hair, enlargement/tenderness of breasts, or increased/decreased libido. Report significant swelling of extremities; sudden acute pain in legs or calves, chest or abdomen; shortness of breath; severe headache or vomiting; sudden blindness; weakness or numbness of arm or leg; unusual vaginal bleeding; yellowing of skin or eyes; or unusual bruising or bleeding.

Estrogens and Methyltestosterone

(ES troe jenz & meth il tes TOS te rone)

Pharmacologic Class Estrogen and Androgen Combination

U.S. Brand Names Estratest®; Estratest® H.S.; Premarin® With Methyltestosterone

Dosage Forms TAB: (Estratest®, Menogen®): Esterified estrogen 1.25 mg and methyltestosterone 2.5 mg; (Estratest® H.S., Menogen H.S.®): Esterified estrogen 0.625 mg and methyltestosterone 1.25 mg; (Premarin® With Methyltestosterone): Conjugated estrogen 0.625 mg and methyltestosterone 5 mg; conjugated estrogen 1.25 mg and methyltestosterone 10 mg

Pregnancy Risk Factor X

Estrogens, Conjugated (ES troe jenz, KON joo gate ed)

Pharmacologic Class Estrogen Derivative

U.S. Brand Names Premarin®

Generic Available No

Mechanism of Action Increases the synthesis of DNA, RNA, and various proteins in target tissues; reduces the release of gonadotropin-releasing hormone from the hypothalamus; reduces FSH and LH release from the pituitary

Use Atrophic vaginitis; hypogonadism; primary ovarian failure; vasomotor symptoms of menopause; prostatic carcinoma; osteoporosis prophylactic; estrogen compounds are generally associated with positive lipid effects (increased HDL cholesterol, reduced LDL cholesterol); estrogens have also been associated with elevated triglycerides; however, clinically significant effects of this elevation (eg, pancreatitis) are not clearly documented

USUAL DOSAGE Adolescents and Adults:

Male: Prostate cancer: Oral: 1.25-2.5 mg 3 times/day

Female:

Osteoporosis in postmenopausal women: Oral: 0.625 mg/day, cyclically (3 weeks on, 1 week off)

Dysfunctional uterine bleeding:

Stable hematocrit: Oral: 1.25 mg twice daily for 21 days; if bleeding persists after 48 hours, increase to 2.5 mg twice daily; if bleeding persists after 48 more hours, increase to 2.5 mg 4 times/day; some recommend starting at 2.5 mg 4 times/day. (**Note:** Medroxyprogesterone acetate 10 mg/day is also given on days 17-21.)

Unstable hematocrit: Oral: I.V.: 5 mg 2-4 times/day; if bleeding is profuse, 20-40 mg every 4 hours up to 24 hours may be used. **Note:** A progestational-weighted contraception pill should also be given (eg, Ovral® 2 tablets stat and 1 tablet 4 times/day or medroxyprogesterone acetate 5-10 mg 4 times/day)

Alternatively: I.V.: 25 mg every 6-12 hours until bleeding stops

Hypogonadism: Oral: 2.5-7.5 mg/day for 20 days, off 10 days and repeat until menses occur. If bleeding does not occur by the end of this period, repeat dosage schedule. If bleeding occurs before the end of the 10-day period, begin a 20-day estrogen-progestin cyclic regimen with 2.5-7.5 mg estrogen daily in divided doses for 1-20 days. During the last 5 days of estrogen therapy, give an oral progestin. If bleeding occurs before this regimen is concluded, discontinue therapy and resume on day 5 of bleeding.

Moderate to severe vasomotor symptoms: Oral: 1.25 mg/day if patient has not menstruated in ≥2 months, start cyclic administration arbitrarily. If patient is menstruating, begin administration on day 5 of bleeding.

Postpartum breast engorgement: Oral: 3.75 mg every 4 hours for 5 doses, then 1.25 mg every 4 hours for 5 days

Atrophic vaginitis, kraurosis vulvae:

Oral: 0.3-1.25 mg or more daily depending on tissue response of the patient; administer cyclically (3 weeks of daily estrogen and 1 week off)

Vaginal: 2-4 g instilled/day 3 weeks on and 1 week off

Female castration and primary ovarian failure: Oral: 1.25 mg/day cyclically (3 weeks on, 1 week off). Adjust according to severity of symptoms and patient response. For maintenance, adjust to the lowest effective dose.

Male/Female: Uremic bleeding: I.V.: 0.6 mg/kg/dose daily for 5 days

Dosing adjustment in hepatic impairment:

Mild to moderate liver impairment: Dosage reduction of estrogens is recommended

Severe liver impairment: **Not recommended**

Dosage Forms CRM, vag: 0.625 mg/g (42.5 g). **INJ:** 25 mg (5 mL). **TAB:** 0.3 mg, 0.625 mg, 0.9 mg, 1.25 mg, 2.5 mg

Contraindications Undiagnosed vaginal bleeding; hypersensitivity to estrogens or any component; thrombophlebitis, liver disease, known or suspected pregnancy, carcinoma of the breast, estrogen dependent tumor

Warnings/Precautions Use with caution in patients with asthma, epilepsy, migraine, diabetes, cardiac or renal dysfunction; estrogens may cause premature closure of the epiphyses in young individuals; safety and efficacy in children have not been established; estrogens have been reported to increase the risk of endometrial carcinoma; do not use estrogens during pregnancy

Pregnancy Risk Factor X

Adverse Reactions Estrogen compounds are generally associated with lipid effects such as increased triglycerides (**Note:** Increased triglycerides with pancreatitis is extremely rare and has not been documented in the current literature in association with estrogen use), increased HDL cholesterol, and decreased LDL cholesterol

>10%:

Cardiovascular: Peripheral edema

(Continued)

Estrogens, Conjugated *(Continued)*

Endocrine & metabolic: Breast tenderness, hypercalcemia, enlargement of breasts
Gastrointestinal: Nausea, anorexia, bloating

1% to 10%:
Central nervous system: Headache
Endocrine & metabolic: Increased libido
Gastrointestinal: Vomiting, diarrhea
Local: Pain at injection site

<1%: Alterations in frequency and flow of menses, amenorrhea, anxiety, breast tumors, chloasma, cholestatic jaundice, decreased glucose tolerance, depression, dizziness, edema, GI distress, hypertension, increase in blood pressure, increased susceptibility to *Candida* infection, intolerance to contact lenses, melasma, myocardial infarction, rash, stroke, thromboembolic disorder

Drug Interactions CYP1A2 enzyme inducer
Decreased effect: Rifampin decreases estrogen serum concentrations
Increased toxicity:
Hydrocortisone increases corticosteroid toxic potential
Increased potential for thromboembolic events with anticoagulants

Alcohol Interactions Avoid use (routine use increases estrogen level and risk of breast cancer)

Education and Monitoring Issues

Patient Education: Follow prescribed schedule and dose. Periodic gynecologic exam and breast exams are important with long-term use. Consult prescriber for specific dietary recommendations. You may experience nausea or vomiting (small frequent meals may help); dizziness or mental depression (use caution when driving); photosensitivity (use sunscreen, wear protective clothing and eyewear, avoid direct sunlight); rash, loss of hair (reversible); enlargement/tenderness of breasts (both male and female); increased (female)/decreased (male) libido; or headache (use of mild analgesic may help). Report swelling of extremities or unusual weight gain; chest pain or palpitations; sudden acute pain, warmth, or weakness in legs or calves; shortness of breath; severe headache or vomiting; or unusual vaginal bleeding, amenorrhea, or alterations in frequency and flow of menses.

Intravaginal cream: Insert high in vagina; wash hands and applicator before and after application.

Reference Range:
Children: <10 μg/24 hours (SI: <35 μmol/day) (values at Mayo Medical Laboratories)
Adults:
Male: 15-40 μg/24 hours (SI: 52-139 μmol/day)
Female:
Menstruating: 15-80 μg/24 hours (SI: 52-277 μmol/day)
Postmenopausal: <20 μg/24 hours (SI: <69 μmol/day)

Estrogens, Conjugated (Synthetic)

(ES troe jenz, KON joo gate ed, sin THET ik)

Pharmacologic Class Estrogen Derivative

U.S. Brand Names Cenestin™

Mechanism of Action Increases the synthesis of DNA, RNA, and various proteins in target tissues; reduces the release of gonadotropin-releasing hormone from the hypothalamus; reduces FSH and LH release from the pituitary

Use Treatment of moderate to severe vasomotor symptoms of menopause

USUAL DOSAGE Adolescents and Adults: Moderate to severe vasomotor symptoms: Oral: 0.625 mg/day; may be titrated up to 1.25 mg/day. Attempts to discontinue medication should be made at 3- to 6-month intervals.

Dosage Forms TAB: 0.625 mg, 0.9 mg, 1.25 mg

Contraindications Undiagnosed vaginal bleeding; hypersensitivity to estrogens or any component; thrombophlebitis, liver disease, known or suspected pregnancy, carcinoma of the breast, estrogen dependent tumor, thromboembolic disorders

Warnings/Precautions Use with caution in patients with a history of hypercalcemia, cardiac disease, and gallbladder disease. The addition of progestins may attenuate estrogen's effects on raising HDL and lowering LDL cholesterol. May increase blood pressure and serum triglycerides (in patients with familial dyslipidemias). Use caution in patients with hepatic disease or renal dysfunction; may increase risk of venous thromboembolism; estrogens have been reported to increase the risk of endometrial carcinoma and may increase the risk of breast cancer; safety and efficacy in children have not been established; do not use estrogens during pregnancy.

Pregnancy Risk Factor X

Adverse Reactions

>10%:
Cardiovascular: Palpitation (21%), peripheral edema (10%)
Endocrine & metabolic: Breast pain (29%), menorrhagia (14%)
Central nervous system; Headache (68%), insomnia (42%), nervousness (28%), depression (28%), pain (11%), dizziness (11%)

Gastrointestinal: Abdominal pain (28%), flatulence (29%), nausea (18%), dyspepsia (10%)

Neuromuscular & skeletal: Myalgia (28%), arthralgia (25%), back pain (14%), paresthesia (33%)

Miscellaneous: Weakness (33%), infection (14%)

1% to 10%:

Gastrointestinal: Vomiting (7%), constipation (6%), diarrhea (6%)

Central nervous system: Hypertonia (6%), fever (1%)

Musculoskeletal: Leg cramps (10%)

Respiratory: Pharyngitis (8%), rhinitis (8%), cough (6%)

Additional adverse reactions associated with estrogen therapy include: Aggravation of porphyria, alopecia, alterations in frequency and flow of menses, amenorrhea, anxiety, breast enlargement, breast tenderness, breast tumors, changes in cervical secretions, changes in corneal curvature, changes in libido, chloasma, cholestatic jaundice, chorea, decreased glucose tolerance, erythema multiforme, erythema nodosum, GI distress, hirsutism, hypercalcemia, hypertension, increase in blood pressure, increased susceptibility to *Candida* infection, increased triglycerides and LDL, intolerance to contact lenses, melasma, myocardial infarction, pancreatitis, rash, stroke, thromboembolic disorder, weight gain, weight loss

Drug Interactions Specific drug interactions have not been conducted for the synthetic preparation; however, the following interactions have been noted for conjugated estrogens

Decreased effect: Rifampin decreases estrogen serum concentrations (other enzyme inducers may share this effect)

Increased toxicity:

Hydrocortisone increases corticosteroid toxic potential

Increased potential for thromboembolic events with anticoagulants

Alcohol Interactions Avoid use (routine use increases estrogen level and risk of breast cancer)

Education and Monitoring Issues

Patient Education: Follow prescribed schedule and dose. Periodic gynecologic exam and breast exams are important with long-term use. Consult prescriber for specific dietary recommendations. You may experience nausea or vomiting (small frequent meals may help); dizziness or mental depression (use caution when driving); photosensitivity (use sunscreen, wear protective clothing and eyewear, avoid direct sunlight); rash, loss of hair (reversible); enlargement/tenderness of breasts (both male and female); increased (female)/decreased (male) libido; or headache (use of mild analgesic may help). Report swelling of extremities or unusual weight gain; chest pain or palpitations; sudden acute pain, warmth, or weakness in legs or calves; shortness of breath; severe headache or vomiting; or unusual vaginal bleeding, amenorrhea, or alterations in frequency and flow of menses.

Manufacturer Duramed Pharmaceuticals

Related Information

Pharmaceutical Manufacturers Directory *on page 1020*

Estrogens, Esterified (ES troe jenz, es TER i fied)

Pharmacologic Class Estrogen Derivative

U.S. Brand Names Estratab®; Menest®

Generic Available No

Mechanism of Action Primary effects on the interphase DNA-protein complex (chromatin) by binding to a receptor (usually located in the cytoplasm of a target cell) and initiating translocation of the hormone-receptor complex to the nucleus

Use Atrophic vaginitis; hypogonadism; primary ovarian failure; vasomotor symptoms of menopause; prostatic carcinoma; osteoporosis prophylactic

USUAL DOSAGE Adults: Oral:

Male: Prostate cancer (inoperable, progressing): 1.25-2.5 mg 3 times/day

Female:

Hypogonadism: 2.5-7.5 mg of estrogen daily for 20 days followed by a 10-day rest period. Administer cyclically (3 weeks on and 1 week off). If bleeding does not occur by the end of the 10-day period, begin an estrogen-progestin cyclic regimen of 2.5-7.5 mg/day in divided doses for 20 days. During the last days of estrogen therapy, give an oral progestin. If bleeding occurs before this regimen is concluded, discontinue therapy and resume on the fifth day of bleeding.

Moderate to severe vasomotor symptoms: 1.25 mg/day administered cyclically (3 weeks on and 1 week off). If patient has not menstruated within the last 2 months or more, cyclic administration is started arbitrary. If the patient is menstruating, cyclical administration is started on day 5 of the bleeding. For short-term use only and should be discontinued as soon as possible. Re-evaluate at 3- to 6-month intervals for tapering or discontinuation of therapy.

Atopic vaginitis and kraurosis vulvae: 0.3 to ≥1.25 mg/day, depending on the tissue response of the individual patient. Administer cyclically. For short-term use only and should be discontinued as soon as possible. Re-evaluate at 3- to 6-month intervals for tapering or discontinuation of therapy.

Breast cancer (inoperable, progressing): 10 mg 3 times/day for at least 3 months

(Continued)

Estrogens, Esterified *(Continued)*

Osteoporosis, in postmenopausal women: Initial: 0.3 mg/day and increase to a maximum daily dose of 1.25 mg/day; initiate therapy as soon as possible after menopause; cyclical therapy is recommended

Female castration and primary ovarian failure: 1.25 mg/day, cyclically. Adjust dosage up- or downward according to the severity of symptoms and patient response. For maintenance, adjust dosage to lowest level that will provide effective control.

Dosing adjustment in hepatic impairment:

Mild to moderate liver impairment: Dosage reduction of estrogens is recommended

Severe liver impairment: **Not recommended**

Dosage Forms TAB: 0.3 mg, 0.625 mg, 1.25 mg, 2.5 mg

Contraindications Known or suspected cancer of the breast, except in appropriately selected patients being treated for metastatic disease; known or suspected estrogen-dependent neoplasia; known or suspected pregnancy; undiagnosed abnormal genital bleeding; active thrombophlebitis or thromboembolic disorders; past history of thrombophlebitis, thrombosis, or thromboembolic disorders associated with previous estrogen use except when used in the treatment of breast or prostatic malignancy

Warnings/Precautions Use with caution in patients with asthma, epilepsy, migraine, diabetes, cardiac or renal dysfunction; estrogens may cause premature closure of the epiphyses in young individuals; safety and efficacy in children have not been established; estrogens have been reported to increase the risk of endometrial carcinoma, do not use estrogens during pregnancy

Pregnancy Risk Factor X

Adverse Reactions

>10%:

Cardiovascular: Peripheral edema

Endocrine & metabolic: Enlargement of breasts, breast tenderness

Gastrointestinal: Nausea, anorexia, bloating

1% to 10%:

Central nervous system: Headache

Endocrine & metabolic: Increased libido

Gastrointestinal: Vomiting, diarrhea

<1%: Alterations in frequency and flow of menses, amenorrhea, anxiety, breast tumors, chloasma, cholestatic jaundice, decreased glucose tolerance, depression, dizziness, edema, GI distress, hypertension, increased susceptibility to *Candida* infection, increased triglycerides and LDL, intolerance to contact lenses, melasma, myocardial infarction, rash, stroke, thromboembolism

Drug Interactions

Decreased effect: Rifampin decreases estrogen serum concentrations

Increased toxicity:

Hydrocortisone increases corticosteroid toxic potential

Anticoagulants: Increases potential for thromboembolic events with anticoagulants

Carbamazepine, tricyclic antidepressants, and corticosteroids; increased thromboembolic potential with oral anticoagulants

Alcohol Interactions Avoid use (routine use increases estrogen level and risk of breast cancer)

Education and Monitoring Issues

Patient Education: Use this drug in cycles or term as prescribed. Take each day at the same time with food. Periodic gynecologic exam and breast exams are important. You may experience nausea or vomiting (small frequent meals may help); dizziness or mental depression (use caution when driving); rash; loss of hair; enlargement/tenderness of breasts; or increased/decreased libido. Report significant swelling of extremities, sudden acute pain in legs or calves, chest, or abdomen; shortness of breath; severe headache or vomiting; weakness or numbness of arms or legs; or unusual vaginal bleeding.

♦ **Estroject-L.A.® Injection** *see* Estradiol *on page 327*

Estrone (ES trone)

Pharmacologic Class Estrogen Derivative

U.S. Brand Names Aquest®; Kestrone®

Generic Available Yes

Mechanism of Action Estrone is a natural ovarian estrogenic hormone that is available as an aqueous mixture of water insoluble estrone and water soluble estrone potassium sulfate; all estrogens, including estrone, act in a similar manner; there is no evidence that there are biological differences among various estrogen preparations other than their ability to bind to cellular receptors inside the target cells

Use Hypogonadism; primary ovarian failure; vasomotor symptoms of menopause; prostatic carcinoma; inoperable breast cancer, kraurosis vulvae, abnormal uterine bleeding due to hormone imbalance

USUAL DOSAGE Adults: I.M.:

Male: Prostatic carcinoma: 2-4 mg 2-3 times/week

Female:

Senile vaginitis and kraurosis vulvae: 0.1-0.5 mg 2-3 times/week; cyclical (3 weeks on and 1 week off)

Breast cancer (inoperable, progressing): 5 mg 3 or more times/week

Primary ovarian failure, hypogonadism: 0.1-1 mg/week, up to 2 mg/week in single or divided doses; cyclical (3 weeks on and 1 week off)

Abnormal uterine bleeding: Brief courses of intensive therapy: 2-5 mg/day for several days

Dosing adjustment in hepatic impairment:

Mild to moderate liver impairment: Dosage reduction of estrogens is recommended

Severe liver impairment: **Not recommended**

Dosage Forms INJ: 2 mg/mL (10 mL, 30 mL), 5 mg/mL (10 mL)

Contraindications Thrombophlebitis, undiagnosed vaginal bleeding, hypersensitivity to estrogens or any component, pregnancy

Warnings/Precautions Use with caution in patients with asthma, epilepsy, migraine, diabetes, cardiac or renal dysfunction; estrogens may cause premature closure of the epiphyses in young individuals; safety and efficacy in children have not been established; estrogens have been reported to increase the risk of endometrial carcinoma, do not use estrogens during pregnancy

Pregnancy Risk Factor X

Adverse Reactions

>10%:

Cardiovascular: Peripheral edema

Endocrine & metabolic: Enlargement of breasts, breast tenderness

Gastrointestinal: Nausea, anorexia, bloating

1% to 10%:

Central nervous system: Headache

Endocrine & metabolic: Increased libido

Gastrointestinal: Vomiting, diarrhea

<1%: Alterations in frequency and flow of menses, amenorrhea, anxiety, breast tumors, chloasma, cholestatic jaundice, decreased glucose tolerance, depression, dizziness, edema, GI distress, hypertension, increased susceptibility to *Candida* infection, increased triglycerides and LDL, intolerance to contact lenses, melasma, myocardial infarction, rash, stroke, thromboembolism

Drug Interactions

Decreased effect: Rifampin decreases estrogen serum concentrations

Increased toxicity:

Hydrocortisone increases corticosteroid toxic potential

Anticoagulants: Increases potential for thromboembolic events with anticoagulants

Carbamazepine, tricyclic antidepressants, and corticosteroids; increased thromboembolic potential with oral anticoagulants

Education and Monitoring Issues

Patient Education: This drug can only be given I.M. It is important to maintain schedule of drug days and drug-free days. Periodic gynecologic exam and breast exams are important. You may experience nausea or vomiting (small frequent meals may help); dizziness or mental depression (use caution when driving); rash; loss of hair; enlargement/tenderness of breasts; or increased/decreased libido. Report significant swelling of extremities, sudden acute pain in legs or calves, chest, or abdomen; shortness of breath; severe headache or vomiting; weakness or numbness of arms or legs; or unusual vaginal bleeding.

Estropipate (ES troe pih pate)

Pharmacologic Class Estrogen Derivative

U.S. Brand Names Ogen® Oral; Ogen® Vaginal; Ortho-Est® Oral

Generic Available No

Mechanism of Action Crystalline estrone that has been solubilized as the sulfate and stabilized with piperazine. Primary effects on the interphase DNA-protein complex (chromatin) by binding to a receptor (usually located in the cytoplasm of a target cell) and initiating translocation of the hormone receptor complex to the nucleus.

Use Atrophic vaginitis; hypogonadism; primary ovarian failure; vasomotor symptoms of menopause; osteoporosis prophylactic

USUAL DOSAGE Adults: Female:

Moderate to severe vasomotor symptoms: Oral: Usual dosage range: 0.75-6 mg estropipate daily. Use the lowest dose and regimen that will control symptoms, and discontinue as soon as possible. Attempt to discontinue or taper medication at 3- to 6-month intervals. If a patient with vasomotor symptoms has not menstruated within the last ≥2 months, start the cyclic administration arbitrarily. If the patient has menstruated, start cyclic administration on day 5 of bleeding.

Hypogonadism or primary ovarian failure: Oral: 1.5-9 mg/day for the first 3 weeks, followed by a rest period of 8-10 days. Repeat if bleeding does not occur by the end of the rest period. The duration of therapy necessary to product the withdrawal bleeding will vary according to the responsiveness of the endometrium. If satisfactory withdrawal

(Continued)

Estropipate *(Continued)*

bleeding does not occur, give an oral progestin in addition to estrogen during the third week of the cycle.

Osteoporosis prevention: Oral: 0.625 mg/day for 25 days of a 31-day cycle

Atrophic vaginitis or kraurosis vulvae: Vaginal: Instill 2-4 g/day 3 weeks on and 1 week off

Dosing adjustment in hepatic impairment:

Mild to moderate liver impairment: Dosage reduction of estrogens is recommended

Severe liver impairment: **Not recommended**

Dosage Forms CRM, vag: 0.15% [estropipate 1.5 mg/g] (42.5 g tube). **TAB:** 0.625 mg [estropipate 0.75 mg], 1.25 mg [estropipate 1.5 mg], 2.5 mg [estropipate 3 mg], 5 mg [estropipate 6 mg]

Contraindications Thrombophlebitis, undiagnosed vaginal bleeding, hypersensitivity to estrogens or any component; pregnancy

Warnings/Precautions Use with caution in patients with asthma, epilepsy, migraine, diabetes, cardiac or renal dysfunction; estrogens may cause premature closure of the epiphyses in young individuals; safety and efficacy in children have not been established; estrogens have been reported to increase the risk of endometrial carcinoma, do not use estrogens during pregnancy

Pregnancy Risk Factor X

Adverse Reactions

>10%:

Cardiovascular: Peripheral edema

Endocrine & metabolic: Enlargement of breasts, breast tenderness

Gastrointestinal: Nausea, anorexia, bloating

1% to 10%:

Central nervous system: Headache

Endocrine & metabolic: Increased libido

Gastrointestinal: Vomiting, diarrhea

<1%: Alterations in frequency and flow of menses, amenorrhea, anxiety, breast tumors, chloasma, cholestatic jaundice, decreased glucose tolerance, depression, dizziness, edema, GI distress, hypertension, increased susceptibility to *Candida* infection, increased triglycerides and LDL, intolerance to contact lenses, melasma, myocardial infarction, rash, stroke, thromboembolism

Drug Interactions

Decreased effect: Rifampin decreases estrogen serum concentrations

Increased toxicity:

Hydrocortisone increases corticosteroid toxic potential

Anticoagulants: Increases potential for thromboembolic events with anticoagulants

Carbamazepine, tricyclic antidepressants, and corticosteroids; increased thromboembolic potential with oral anticoagulants

Alcohol Interactions Avoid use (routine use increases estrogen level and risk of breast cancer)

Education and Monitoring Issues

Patient Education: It is important to maintain schedule of drug days and drug-free days. Periodic gynecologic exam and breast exams are important. You may experience nausea or vomiting (small frequent meals may help); dizziness or mental depression (use caution when driving); rash; loss of hair; enlargement/tenderness of breasts; or increased/decreased libido. Report significant swelling of extremities, sudden acute pain in legs or calves, chest or abdomen; shortness of breath; severe headache or vomiting; weakness or numbness of arms or legs; or unusual vaginal bleeding.

Intravaginal cream: Insert high in vagina, wash hands and applicator before and after application.

♦ **Estrostep® 21** *see* Ethinyl Estradiol and Norethindrone *on page 342*

♦ **Estrostep® Fe** *see* Ethinyl Estradiol and Norethindrone *on page 342*

♦ **Estrouis®** *see* Estropipate *on page 335*

Etanercept (et a NER cept)

Pharmacologic Class Antirheumatic, Disease Modifying

U.S. Brand Names Enbrel®

Mechanism of Action Etanercept is a recombinant DNA-derived protein composed of tumor necrosis factor receptor (TNFR) linked to the Fc portion of human IgG1. Etanercept binds tumor necrosis factor (TNF) and blocks its interaction with cell surface receptors. TNF plays an important role in the inflammatory processes of rheumatoid arthritis (RA) and the resulting joint pathology.

Use Reduction in signs and symptoms of moderately to severely active rheumatoid arthritis in patients who have had an inadequate response to one or more disease-modifying antirheumatic drugs (DMARDs).

USUAL DOSAGE S.C.:

Children: 0.4 mg/kg (maximum: 25 mg dose)

Adult: 25 mg given twice weekly; if the prescriber determines that it is appropriate, patients may self-inject after proper training in injection technique

Elderly: Although greater sensitivity of some elderly patients cannot be ruled out, no overall differences in safety or effectiveness were observed

Dosage Forms POWDER for inj: 25 mg

Contraindications Etanercept should not be administered to patients with any active infections including chronic or local infections. Do not administer etanercept to patients with active infections including chronic or local ones. Do not administer to patients with known hypersensitivity to etanercept or any of its components.

Warnings/Precautions Etanercept may affect defenses against infections and malignancies. Safety and efficacy in patients with immunosuppression or chronic infections have not been evaluated. Discontinue administration if patient develops a serious infection. Do not start drug administration in patients with an active infection.

Impact on the development and course of malignancies is not fully defined. Treatment may result in the formation of autoimmune antibodies; cases of autoimmune disease have not been described. Non-neutralizing antibodies to etanercept may also be formed. No correlation of antibody development to clinical response or adverse events has been observed. The long-term immunogenicity, carcinogenic potential, or effect on fertility are unknown. No evidence of mutagenic activity has been observed *in vitro* or *in vivo*. The safety of etanercept has not been studied in children <4 years of age.

Allergic reactions may occur (<0.5%), but anaphylaxis has not been observed. If an anaphylactic reaction or other serious allergic reaction occurs, administration of etanercept should be discontinued immediately and appropriate therapy initiated.

Patients should be brought up to date with all immunizations before initiating therapy. No data are available concerning the effects of etanercept on vaccination. Live vaccines should not be given concurrently. No data are available concerning secondary transmission of live vaccines in patients receiving etanercept. Patients with a significant exposure to varicella virus should temporarily discontinue etanercept. Treatment with varicella zoster immune globulin should be considered.

Pregnancy Risk Factor B

Pregnancy Implications Developmental toxicity studies performed in animals have revealed no evidence of harm to the fetus. There are no studies in pregnant women; this drug should be used during pregnancy only if clearly needed.

It is not known whether etanercept is excreted in human milk or absorbed systemically after ingestion. Because many immunoglobulins are excreted in human milk, and because of the potential for serious adverse reactions in nursing infants from etanercept, a decision should be made whether to discontinue nursing or to discontinue the drug.

Adverse Reactions Events reported include those >3% with incidence higher than placebo

>10%:

- Central nervous system: Headache (17%)
- Local: Injection site reaction (37%)
- Respiratory: Respiratory tract infection (38%), upper respiratory tract infection (29%), rhinitis (12%)
- Miscellaneous: Infection (35%), positive ANA (11%), positive anti-double stranded DNA antibodies (15% by RIA, 3% by *Crithidia lucilae* assay)

>3% to 10%:

- Central nervous system: Dizziness (7%)
- Dermatologic: Rash (5%)
- Gastrointestinal: Abdominal pain (5%), dyspepsia (4%)
- Neuromuscular and skeletal: Weakness (5%)
- Respiratory: Pharyngitis (7%), respiratory disorder (5%), sinusitis (3%)

<3%: Malignancies, serious infection, heart failure, myocardial infarction, myocardial ischemia, cerebral ischemia, hypertension, hypotension, cholecystitis, pancreatitis, gastrointestinal hemorrhage, bursitis, depression, dyspnea

Pediatric patients (JRA): The percentages of patients reporting abdominal pain (17%) and vomiting (14.5%) was higher than in adult RA. Two patients developed varicella infection associated with aseptic meningitis which resolved without complications (see Warnings/Precautions).

Drug Interactions Specific drug interaction studies have not been conducted with etanercept

Onset Within 2-3 weeks

Half-Life 115 hours (98-300 hours)

Education and Monitoring Issues

Patient Education: If self-injecting, follow instructions for injection and disposal of needles exactly. If redness, swelling, or irritation appears at the injection site, contact prescriber. Do not have any vaccinations while using this medication without consulting prescriber first. You may experience headache or dizziness (use caution when driving or engaging in tasks requiring alertness until response to drug is known). If stomach pain or cramping, unusual bleeding or bruising, blood in vomitus, stool, or urine occurs, stop taking medication and contact prescriber. Report skin rash, unusual muscle or bone weakness, or signs of respiratory flu or other infection (eg, chills, fever, sore throat, easy bruising or bleeding, mouth sores, unhealed sores).

Manufacturer Immunex Corp

(Continued)

Etanercept *(Continued)*

Related Information

Pharmaceutical Manufacturers Directory *on page 1020*

Ethacrynic Acid (eth a KRIN ik AS id)

Pharmacologic Class Diuretic, Loop

U.S. Brand Names Edecrin®

Generic Available No

Mechanism of Action Inhibits reabsorption of sodium and chloride in the ascending loop of Henle and distal renal tubule, interfering with the chloride-binding cotransport system, thus causing increased excretion of water, sodium, chloride, magnesium, and calcium

Use Management of edema associated with congestive heart failure; hepatic cirrhosis or renal disease; short-term management of ascites due to malignancy, idiopathic edema, and lymphedema

USUAL DOSAGE I.V. formulation should be diluted in D_5W or NS (1 mg/mL) and infused over several minutes

Children: Oral: 1 mg/kg/dose once daily; increase at intervals of 2-3 days as needed, to a maximum of 3 mg/kg/day

Adults:

Oral: 50-200 mg/day in 1-2 divided doses; may increase in increments of 25-50 mg at intervals of several days; doses up to 200 mg twice daily may be required with severe, refractory edema

I.V.: 0.5-1 mg/kg/dose (maximum: 100 mg/dose); repeat doses not routinely recommended; however, if indicated, repeat doses every 8-12 hours

Dosing adjustment/comments in renal impairment: Cl_{cr} <10 mL/minute: Avoid use

Dialysis: Not removed by hemo- or peritoneal dialysis; supplemental dose is not necessary

Dosage Forms POWDER for inj, as ethacrynate sodium: 50 mg (50 mL). **TAB:** 25 mg, 50 mg

Contraindications Hypersensitivity to ethacrynic acid or any component; anuria, hypotension, dehydration with low serum sodium concentrations; metabolic alkalosis with hypokalemia, or history of severe, watery diarrhea from ethacrynic acid

Warnings/Precautions Use with caution in patients with advanced hepatic cirrhosis, diabetes mellitus, hypotension, dehydration, history of watery diarrhea from ethacrynic acid, hearing impairment; ototoxicity occurs more frequently than with other loop diuretics; safety and efficacy in infants have not been established

Pregnancy Risk Factor B

Pregnancy Implications

Clinical effects on the fetus: No data available. Generally, use of diuretics during pregnancy is avoided due to risk of decreased placental perfusion.

Breast-feeding/lactation: No data available

Adverse Reactions

Incidence of adverse events is not reported.

Endocrine & metabolic: Hyponatremia, hyperglycemia, variations in phosphorus, CO_2 content, bicarbonate, and calcium

Gastrointestinal: Anorexia, malaise, abdominal discomfort or pain, dysphagia, nausea, vomiting, and diarrhea, gastrointestinal bleeding, acute pancreatitis (rare)

Renal: Increased serum creatinine

<1% (limited to important or life-threatening symptoms): Reversible hyperuricemia, gout, hyperglycemia, hypoglycemia (occurred in two uremic patients who received doses above those recommended), jaundice, abnormal liver function tests, agranulocytosis, severe neutropenia, thrombocytopenia, Henoch-Schönlein purpura (in patient with rheumatic heart disease), deafness, tinnitus, temporary or permanent deafness, vertigo, blurred vision, headache, fatigue, apprehension, confusion, skin rash, fever, chills, hematuria, local irritation and pain, thrombophlebitis (with intravenous use), encephalopathy (patients with pre-existing liver disease)

Drug Interactions

ACE inhibitors: Hypotensive effects and/or renal effects are potentiated by hypovolemia

Antidiabetic agents: Glucose tolerance may be decreased

Antihypertensive agents: Hypotensive effects may be enhanced

Cephaloridine or cephalexin: Nephrotoxicity may occur

Cholestyramine or colestipol may reduce bioavailability of ethacrynic acid

Clofibrate: Protein binding may be altered in hypoalbuminemic patients receiving ethacrynic acid, potentially increasing toxicity

Digoxin: Ethacrynic acid-induced hypokalemia may predispose to digoxin toxicity; monitor potassium

Indomethacin (and other NSAIDs) may reduce natriuretic and hypotensive effects of diuretics

Lithium: Renal clearance may be reduced. Isolated reports of lithium toxicity have occurred; monitor lithium levels.

NSAIDs: Risk of renal impairment may increase when used in conjunction with diuretics

Ototoxic drugs (aminoglycosides, cis-platinum): Concomitant use of ethacrynic acid may increase risk of ototoxicity, especially in patients with renal dysfunction

Peripheral adrenergic-blocking drugs or ganglionic blockers: Effects may be increased

Salicylates (high-dose) with diuretics may predispose patients to salicylate toxicity due to reduced renal excretion or alter renal function

Sparfloxacin, gatifloxacin, and moxifloxacin: Risk of cardiotoxicity may be increased; avoid use

Thiazides: Synergistic diuretic effects occur

Onset

Onset of diuretic effect: Oral: Within 30 minutes; I.V.: 5 minutes

Peak effect: Oral: 2 hours; I.V.: 30 minutes

Duration Oral: 12 hours; I.V.: 2 hours

Half-Life Normal renal function: 2-4 hours

Education and Monitoring Issues

Patient Education: Take prescribed dose with food early in day. Include orange juice or bananas (or other potassium-rich foods) in your diet, but do not take potassium supplements without consulting prescriber. You may experience postural hypotension (use caution when rising from lying or sitting position, when climbing stairs, or when driving); lightheadedness, dizziness, or drowsiness (use caution driving or when engaging in hazardous activities); diarrhea (buttermilk, boiled milk, or yogurt may help); or decreased accommodation to heat (avoid excessive exercise in hot weather). Diabetics should monitor serum glucose closely (this medication may interfere with antidiabetic medications). Report changes in hearing or ringing in ears, persistent headache, unusual confusion or nervousness, abdominal pain or blood stool (black stool), palpitations, chest pain, rapid heartbeat, joint or muscle soreness or weakness, flu-like symptoms, skin rash or itching, or blurred vision. Report swelling of ankles or feet, weight changes of more than 3 lb/day, increased fatigue, or muscle cramping or trembling.

Monitoring Parameters: Blood pressure, renal function, serum electrolytes, and fluid status closely, including weight and I & O daily; hearing

Manufacturer Merck & Co

Related Information

Heart Failure Guidelines *on page 1099*

Pharmaceutical Manufacturers Directory *on page 1020*

Ethambutol (e THAM byoo tole)

Pharmacologic Class Antitubercular Agent

U.S. Brand Names Myambutol®

Generic Available No

Mechanism of Action Suppresses mycobacteria multiplication by interfering with RNA synthesis

Use Treatment of tuberculosis and other mycobacterial diseases in conjunction with other antituberculosis agents

USUAL DOSAGE Oral:

Ethambutol is generally not recommended in children whose visual acuity cannot be monitored. However, ethambutol should be considered for all children with organisms resistant to other drugs, when susceptibility to ethambutol has been demonstrated, or susceptibility is likely.

Note: A four-drug regimen (isoniazid, rifampin, pyrazinamide, and either streptomycin or ethambutol) is preferred for the initial, empiric treatment of TB. When the drug susceptibility results are available, the regimen should be altered as appropriate.

Children and Adults:

Daily therapy: 15-25 mg/kg/day (maximum: 2.5 g/day)

Directly observed therapy (DOT): Twice weekly: 50 mg/kg (maximum: 2.5 g)

DOT: 3 times/week: 25-30 mg/kg (maximum: 2.5 g)

Dosing interval in renal impairment:

Cl_{cr} 10-50 mL/minute: Administer every 24-36 hours

Cl_{cr} <10 mL/minute: Administer every 48 hours

Hemodialysis: Slightly dialyzable (5% to 20%); Administer dose postdialysis

Peritoneal dialysis: Dose for Cl_{cr} <10 mL/minute

Continuous arteriovenous or venovenous hemofiltration: Administer every 24-36 hours

Dosage Forms TAB: 100 mg, 400 mg

Contraindications Hypersensitivity to ethambutol or any component; optic neuritis

Warnings/Precautions Use only in children whose visual acuity can accurately be determined and monitored (not recommended for use in children <13 years of age unless the benefit outweighs the risk); dosage modification required in patients with renal insufficiency

Pregnancy Risk Factor B

Adverse Reactions

1% to 10%:

Central nervous system: Headache, confusion, disorientation

Endocrine & metabolic: Acute gout or hyperuricemia

Gastrointestinal: Abdominal pain, anorexia, nausea, vomiting

(Continued)

Ethambutol *(Continued)*

<1%: Abnormal LFTs, anaphylaxis, fever, malaise, mental confusion, optic neuritis, peripheral neuritis, pruritus, rash

Drug Interactions Decreased absorption with aluminum salts

Half-Life 2.5-3.6 hours; End-stage renal disease: 7-15 hours

Education and Monitoring Issues

Patient Education: Take as scheduled, with meals. Avoid missing doses and do not discontinue without consulting prescriber. You may experience GI distress (frequent small meals and good oral care may help), dizziness, disorientation, drowsiness (avoid driving or engaging in tasks that require alertness until response to drug is known). You will need to have frequent ophthalmic exams and periodic medical check-ups to evaluate drug effects. Report changes in vision, numbness or tingling of extremities, or persistent loss of appetite.

Monitoring Parameters: Periodic visual testing in patients receiving more than 15 mg/kg/day; periodic renal, hepatic, and hematopoietic tests

Related Information

Antimicrobial Drugs of Choice *on page 1182*
Tuberculosis Test Recommendations and Prophylaxis *on page 1163*
Tuberculosis Treatment Guidelines *on page 1213*

♦ **Ethamolin®** *see* Ethanolamine Oleate *on page 340*

Ethanolamine Oleate (ETH a nol a meen OH lee ate)

Pharmacologic Class Sclerosing Agent

U.S. Brand Names Ethamolin®

Use Mild sclerosing agent used for bleeding esophageal varices

USUAL DOSAGE Adults: 1.5-5 mL per varix, up to 20 mL total or 0.4 mL/kg for a 50 kg patient; doses should be decreased in patients with severe hepatic dysfunction and should receive less than recommended maximum dose

Contraindications Hypersensitivity to agent or oleic acid

Pregnancy Risk Factor C

Ethchlorvynol (eth klor VI nole)

Pharmacologic Class Hypnotic, Miscellaneous

U.S. Brand Names Placidyl®

Use Short-term management of insomnia

USUAL DOSAGE Adults: Oral: 500-1000 mg at bedtime

Dosing adjustment in renal impairment: Cl_{cr} <50 mL/minute: Avoid use

Contraindications Porphyria, hypersensitivity to ethchlorvynol or any component

Pregnancy Risk Factor C

Ethinyl Estradiol (ETH in il es tra DYE ole)

Pharmacologic Class Estrogen Derivative

U.S. Brand Names Estinyl®

Generic Available No

Mechanism of Action Increases the synthesis of DNA, RNA, and various proteins in target tissues; reduces the release of gonadotropin-releasing hormone from the hypothalamus; reduces FSH and LH release from the pituitary

Use Hypogonadism; primary ovarian failure; vasomotor symptoms of menopause; prostatic carcinoma; breast cancer

USUAL DOSAGE Adults: Oral:

Male: Prostatic cancer (inoperable, progressing): 0.15-2 mg/day for palliation

Female:

Hypogonadism: 0.05 mg 1-3 times/day during the first 2 weeks of a theoretical menstrual cycle. Follow with a progesterone during the last half of the arbitrary cycle. Continue for 3-6 months. The patient should not be treated for the following 2 months.

Vasomotor symptoms: Usual dosage range: 0.02-0.05 mg/day; give cyclically for short-term use only and use the lowest dose that will control symptoms. Discontinue as soon as possible and administer cyclically (3 weeks on and 1 week off). Attempt to discontinue or taper medication at 3- to 6-month intervals.

Breast cancer (inoperable, progressing): 1 mg 3 times/day for palliation

Dosing adjustment in hepatic impairment:

Mild to moderate liver impairment: Dosage reduction of estrogens is recommended

Severe liver impairment: **Not recommended**

Dosage Forms TAB: 0.02 mg, 0.05 mg, 0.25 mg, 0.5 mg

Contraindications Thrombophlebitis, undiagnosed vaginal bleeding, hypersensitivity to ethinyl estradiol or any component, pregnancy, estrogen-dependent neoplasia

Warnings/Precautions Use with caution in patients with asthma, seizure disorders, migraine, cardiac, renal or hepatic impairment, cerebrovascular disorders or history of breast cancer, past or present thromboembolic disease, smokers >35 years of age

Pregnancy Risk Factor X

Adverse Reactions

>10%:

Cardiovascular: Peripheral edema

Endocrine & metabolic: Enlargement of breasts, breast tenderness, bloating

Gastrointestinal: Nausea, anorexia

1% to 10%:

Central nervous system: Headache

Endocrine & metabolic: Increased libido

Gastrointestinal: Vomiting, diarrhea

<1%: Alterations in frequency and flow of menses, amenorrhea, anxiety, breast tumors, chloasma, cholestatic jaundice, decreased glucose tolerance, depression, dizziness, edema, GI distress, hypertension, increased susceptibility to *Candida* infection, increased triglycerides and LDL, intolerance to contact lenses, melasma, myocardial infarction, rash, stroke, thromboembolism

Drug Interactions CYP3A3/4 and 3A5-7 enzyme substrate; CYP1A2 enzyme inhibitor

Increased toxicity:

Carbamazepine, tricyclic antidepressants, and corticosteroids

Increased thromboembolic potential with oral anticoagulants

Decreased effect: Nelfinavir, ritonavir

Alcohol Interactions Avoid use (routine use increases estrogen level and risk of breast cancer)

Education and Monitoring Issues

Patient Education: Take according to recommended schedule. It is important to maintain schedule of drug days and drug-free days. Periodic gynecologic exam and breast exams for females are important. You may experience nausea or vomiting (small frequent meals may help); dizziness or mental depression (use caution when driving); rash; loss of hair; enlargement/tenderness of breasts; or increased/decreased libido. Report significant swelling in extremities, sudden acute pain in legs or calves, chest, or abdomen; shortness of breath; severe headache or vomiting; weakness or numbness of arms or legs; or unusual vaginal bleeding.

Related Information

Ethinyl Estradiol and Desogestrel *on page 341*

Ethinyl Estradiol and Desogestrel

(ETH in il es tra DYE ole & des oh JES trel)

Pharmacologic Class Contraceptive, Oral

U.S. Brand Names Desogen®; Ortho-Cept®

Pregnancy Risk Factor X

Ethinyl Estradiol and Ethynodiol Diacetate

(ETH in il es tra DYE ole & e thye noe DYE ole dye AS e tate)

Pharmacologic Class Contraceptive, Oral

U.S. Brand Names Demulen®; Zovia®

Use Prevention of pregnancy; treatment of hypermenorrhea, endometriosis, female hypogonadism

USUAL DOSAGE Adults: Female: Oral:

For 21-tablet cycle packs, with 21 active tablets (28-day packs have 21 active tablets and 7 inert tablets): Take 1 tablet daily starting on the fifth day of menstrual cycle, with day 1 being the first day of menstruation; begin taking a new cycle pack on the eighth day after taking the last tablet from the previous pack

With 28-tablet packages, dosage is 1 tablet daily without interruption; extra tablets are placebos or contain iron. If next menstrual period does not begin on schedule, rule out pregnancy before starting new dosing cycle. If menstrual period begins, start new dosing cycle 7 days after last tablet was taken. If all doses have been taken on schedule and one menstrual period is missed, continue dosing cycle. If two consecutive menstrual periods are missed, pregnancy test is required before new dosing cycle is started.

One dose missed: Take as soon as remembered or take 2 tablets next day

Two doses missed: Take 2 tablets as soon as remembered or 2 tablets next 2 days

Three doses missed: Begin new compact of tablets starting on day 1 of next cycle

Contraindications Known or suspected pregnancy, undiagnosed genital bleeding, carcinoma of the breast, estrogen-dependent tumor

Pregnancy Risk Factor X

Ethinyl Estradiol and Levonorgestrel

(ETH in il es tra DYE ole & LEE voe nor jes trel)

Pharmacologic Class Contraceptive, Oral

U.S. Brand Names Alesse™; Levlen®; Levlite®; Levora®; Nordette®; Preven™; Tri-Levlen®; Triphasil®

Use Prevention of pregnancy; treatment of hypermenorrhea, endometriosis, female hypogonadism

Note: Preven™ is **not** recommended as a form of regular contraception but is indicated as an emergency contraceptive kit

(Continued)

Ethinyl Estradiol and Levonorgestrel *(Continued)*

USUAL DOSAGE Adults: Female: Oral:

Contraception: 1 tablet daily, beginning on day 5 of menstrual cycle (first day of menstrual flow is day 1). With 20-tablet and 21-tablet packages, new dosing cycle begins 7 days after last tablet taken. With 28-tablet packages, dosage is 1 tablet daily without interruption; extra tablets are placebos or contain iron. If next menstrual period does not begin on schedule, rule out pregnancy before starting new dosing cycle. If menstrual period begins, start new dosing cycle 7 days after last tablet was taken. If all doses have been taken on schedule and one menstrual period is missed, continue dosing cycle. If two consecutive menstrual periods are missed, pregnancy test is required before new dosing cycle is started.

One dose missed: Take as soon as remembered or take 2 tablets next day

Two doses missed: Take 2 tablets as soon as remembered or 2 tablets next 2 days

Three doses missed: Begin new compact of tablets starting on day 1 of next cycle

Triphasic oral contraceptive (Tri-Levlen®, Triphasil®): 1 tablet/day in the sequence specified by the manufacturer

Emergency contraception (Preven™): Initial: 2 pills as soon as possible but within 72 hours of unprotected intercourse. This is followed by a second dose of 2 pills 12 hours later.

Contraindications Thrombophlebitis, undiagnosed vaginal bleeding, hypersensitivity to ethinyl estradiol or any component, known or suspected pregnancy, carcinoma of the breast, estrogen-dependent tumor

Pregnancy Risk Factor X

Ethinyl Estradiol and Norethindrone

(ETH in il es tra DYE ole & nor eth IN drone)

Pharmacologic Class Contraceptive, Oral

U.S. Brand Names Brevicon®; Estrostep® 21; Estrostep® Fe; FemHrt™; Genora® 0.5/35; Genora® 1/35; Jenest-28™; Loestrin®; Modicon™; N.E.E.® 1/35; Nelova™ 0.5/35E; Nelova™ 10/11; Norethin™ 1/35E; Norinyl® 1+35; Ortho-Novum® 1/35; Ortho-Novum® 7/7/7; Ortho-Novum® 10/11; Ovcon® 35; Ovcon® 50; Tri-Norinyl®

Generic Available Yes

Mechanism of Action Combination oral contraceptives inhibit ovulation via a negative feedback mechanism on the hypothalamus, which alters the normal pattern of gonadotropin secretion of a follicle-stimulating hormone (FSH) and luteinizing hormone by the anterior pituitary. The follicular phase FSH and midcycle surge of gonadotropins are inhibited. In addition, oral contraceptives produce alterations in the genital tract, including changes in the cervical mucus, rendering it unfavorable for sperm penetration even if ovulation occurs. Changes in the endometrium may also occur, producing an unfavorable environment for nidation. Oral contraceptive drugs may alter the tubal transport of the ova through the fallopian tubes. Progestational agents may also alter sperm fertility.

Use Prevention of pregnancy; treatment of hypermenorrhea, endometriosis, female hypogonadism, moderate to severe vasomotor symptoms associated with menopause; prevention of osteoporosis

USUAL DOSAGE Adults: Female: Oral:

For 21-tablet cycle packs, with 21 active tablets (28-day packs have 21 active tablets and 7 inert tablets): Take 1 tablet daily starting on the fifth day of menstrual cycle, with day 1 being the first day of menstruation; begin taking a new cycle pack on the eighth day after taking the last tablet from the previous pack

With 28-tablet packages, dosage is 1 tablet daily without interruption; extra tablets are placebos or contain iron. If next menstrual period does not begin on schedule, rule out pregnancy before starting new dosing cycle. If menstrual period begins, start new dosing cycle 7 days after last tablet was taken. If all doses have been taken on schedule and one menstrual period is missed, continue dosing cycle. If two consecutive menstrual periods are missed, pregnancy test is required before new dosing cycle is started.

One dose missed: Take as soon as remembered or take 2 tablets next day

Two doses missed: Take 2 tablets as soon as remembered or 2 tablets next 2 days

Three doses missed: Begin new compact of tablets starting on day 1 of next cycle

Biphasic oral contraceptive (Jenest™-28, Ortho-Novum™ 10/11, Nelova™ 10/11): 1 color tablet/day for 10 days, then next color tablet for 11 days

Triphasic oral contraceptive (Ortho-Novum™ 7/7/7, Tri-Norinyl®, Triphasil®): 1 tablet/day in the sequence specified by the manufacturer

Moderate to severe vasomotor symptoms associated with menopause: 1 tablet daily (1 mg norethindrone and 5 mg ethinyl estradiol); patients should be re-evaluated at 3- to 6-month intervals to determine if treatment is still necessary

Prevention of osteoporosis: 1 tablet daily (1 mg norethindrone and 5 mg ethinyl estradiol)

Dosage Forms TAB:

Brevicon®, Genora® 0.5/35, Modicon™, Nelova™ 0.5/35E: Ethinyl estradiol 0.035 mg and norethindrone 0.5 mg (21s, 28s)

Estrostep®: Triangular tablet (white): Ethinyl estradiol 0.02 mg and norethindrone acetate 1 mg, Square tablet (white): Ethinyl estradiol 0.03 mg and norethindrone acetate 1 mg, Round tablet (white): Ethinyl estradiol 0.035 mg and norethindrone acetate 1 mg

Estrostep® Fe: Triangular tablet (white): Ethinyl estradiol 0.02 mg and norethindrone acetate 1 mg, Square tablet (white): Ethinyl estradiol 0.03 mg and norethindrone acetate 1 mg, Round tablet (white): Ethinyl estradiol 0.035 mg and norethindrone acetate 1 mg, Brown tablet: Ferrous fumarate 75 mg

Loestrin® 1.5/30: Ethinyl estradiol 0.03 mg and norethindrone acetate 1.5 mg (21s); (Loestrin® Fe 1.5/30): Ethinyl estradiol 0.03 mg and norethindrone acetate 1.5 mg with ferrous fumarate 75 mg in 7 inert tablets (28s); (Loestrin® 1/20): Ethinyl estradiol 0.02 mg and norethindrone acetate 1 mg (21s); (Loestrin® Fe 1/20): Ethinyl estradiol 0.02 mg and norethindrone acetate 1 mg with ferrous fumarate 75 mg in 7 inert tablets (28s)

Genora® 1/35, N.E.E.® 1/35, Nelova® 1/35E, Norethin™ 1/35E, Norinyl® 1+35, Ortho-Novum® 1/35: Ethinyl estradiol 0.035 mg and norethindrone 1 mg (21s, 28s)

Jenest-28™: Phase 1 (7 white tablets): Ethinyl estradiol 0.035 mg and norethindrone 0.5 mg; Phase 2 (14 peach tablets): Ethinyl estradiol 0.035 mg and norethindrone 1 mg and 7 green inert tablets (28s)

Ortho-Novum® 7/7/7: Phase 1 (7 white tablets): Ethinyl estradiol 0.035 mg and norethindrone 0.5 mg; Phase 2 (7 light peach tablets): Ethinyl estradiol 0.035 mg and norethindrone 0.75 mg; Phase 3 (7 peach tablets): Ethinyl estradiol 0.035 mg and norethindrone 1 mg (21s, 28s)

Ortho-Novum® 10/11: Phase 1 (10 white tablets): Ethinyl estradiol 0.035 mg and norethindrone 0.5 mg; Phase 2 (11 dark yellow tablets): Ethinyl estradiol 0.035 mg and norethindrone 1 mg (21s, 28s)

Ovcon® 35: Ethinyl estradiol 0.035 mg and norethindrone 0.4 mg (21s, 28s)

Ovcon® 50: Ethinyl estradiol 0.050 mg and norethindrone 1 mg (21s, 28s)

Tri-Norinyl®: Phase 1 (7 blue tablets): Ethinyl estradiol 0.035 mg and norethindrone 0.5 mg; Phase 2 (9 green tablets): Ethinyl estradiol 0.035 mg and norethindrone 1 mg; Phase 3 (5 blue tablets): Ethinyl estradiol 0.035 mg and norethindrone 0.5 mg (21s, 28s)

Contraindications Thrombophlebitis, cerebral vascular disease, coronary artery disease, known or suspected breast carcinoma, undiagnosed abnormal genital bleeding, hypersensitivity to any component; pregnancy

Warnings/Precautions Use of any progestin during the first 4 months of pregnancy is not recommended; in patients with a history of thromboembolism, stroke, myocardial infarction (especially >40 years of age who smoke), liver tumor, hypertension, cardiac, renal or hepatic insufficiency; risk of cardiovascular side effects increases in those women who smoke cigarettes and in women >35 years of age. Products containing 50 mcg of estrogen should be used only when medically indicated (dose-related risk of vascular disease).

Pregnancy Risk Factor X

Adverse Reactions

>10%:

Cardiovascular: Peripheral edema

Endocrine & metabolic: Enlargement of breasts, breast tenderness

Gastrointestinal: Nausea, anorexia, bloating

1% to 10%:

Central nervous system: Headache

Endocrine & metabolic: Increased libido

Gastrointestinal: Vomiting, diarrhea

<1%: Alterations in frequency and flow of menses, amenorrhea, anxiety, breast tumors, chloasma, cholestatic jaundice, decreased glucose tolerance, depression, dizziness, edema, GI distress, hypertension, increased susceptibility to *Candida* infection, increased triglycerides and LDL, intolerance to contact lenses, melasma, myocardial infarction, rash, stroke, thromboembolism

Minimize these effects by adjusting the estrogen/progestin balance or dosage. The table categorizes products by both their estrogenic and progestational potencies; because overall activity is influenced by the interaction of components, it is difficult to precisely classify products; placement in the table is only approximate. Differences between products within a group are probably not clinically significant. See tables.

Achieving Proper Hormonal Balance in an Oral Contraceptive

Estrogen		Progestin	
Excess	**Deficiency**	**Excess**	**Deficiency**
Nausea, bloating	Early or midcycle breakthrough bleeding	Increased appetite	Late breakthrough bleeding
Cervical mucorrhea, polyposis	Increased spotting	Weight gain	Amenorrhea
Melasma	Hypomenorrhea	Tiredness, fatigue	Hypermenorrhea
Migraine headache		Hypomenorrhea	
Breast fullness or tenderness		Acne, oily scalp*	
Edema		Hair loss, hirsutism*	
Hypertension		Depression	
		Monilial vaginitis	
		Breast regression	

*Result of androgenic activity of progestins.

(Continued)

Ethinyl Estradiol and Norethindrone *(Continued)*

Pharmacological Effects of Progestins Used in Oral Contraceptives

	Progestin	Estrogen	Antiestrogen	Androgen
Norgestrel/levonorgestrel	+++	0	++	+++
Ethynodiol diacetate	++	+*	+*	+
Norethindrone acetate	+	+	+++	+
Norethindrone	+	+*	+*	+
Norethynodrel	+	+++	0	0

*Has estrogenic effect at low doses; may have antiestrogenic effect at higher doses.

+++ = pronounced effect

++ = moderate effect

+ = slight effect

0 = no effect

Drug Interactions Ethinyl estradiol is a CYP3A3/4 and 3A5-7 enzyme substrate; CYP1A2 enzyme inhibitor

Decreased effect:

Potential contraceptive failure with barbiturates, hydantoins, and rifampin

Concomitant penicillins or tetracyclines may lead to contraceptive failure

Nelfinavir decreases concentrations os norethindrone and ethinyl estradiol (may result in failure)

Increased toxicity:

Increased toxicity of carbamazepine, tricyclic antidepressants, and corticosteroids

Increased thromboembolic potential with oral anticoagulants

Alcohol Interactions Avoid use (routine use increases estrogen level)

Education and Monitoring Issues

Patient Education: Take exactly as directed; use additional method of birth control during first week of administration of first cycle; photosensitivity may occur. Women should inform their prescribers if signs or symptoms of any of the following occur thromboembolic or thrombotic disorders including sudden severe headache or vomiting, disturbance of vision or speech, loss of vision, numbness or weakness in an extremity, sharp or crushing chest pain, calf pain, shortness of breath, severe abdominal pain or mass, mental depression, or unusual bleeding.

When any doses are missed, alternative contraceptive methods should be used for the next 2 days or until 2 days into the new cycle

Women should discontinue taking the medication if they suspect they are pregnant or become pregnant

Ethinyl Estradiol and Norgestimate

(ETH in il es tra DYE ole & nor JES ti mate)

Pharmacologic Class Contraceptive, Oral

U.S. Brand Names Ortho-Cyclen®:; Ortho-Prefest®; Ortho Tri-Cyclen®

Use Prevention of pregnancy, treatment of moderate to severe vasomotor symptoms associated with menopause, prevention of osteoporosis, treatment of vulvar and vaginal atrophy

USUAL DOSAGE

Contraception: Oral: 1 tablet daily, beginning on day 5 of menstrual cycle (first day of menstrual flow is day 1). With 21-tablet packages, new dosing cycle begins 7 days after last tablet taken. With 28-tablet packages, dosage is 1 tablet daily without interruption; extra tablets are placebos or contain iron. If next menstrual period does not begin on schedule, rule out pregnancy before starting new dosing cycle. If menstrual period begins, start new dosing cycle 7 days after last tablet was taken. If all doses have been taken on schedule and one menstrual period is missed, continue dosing cycle. If two consecutive menstrual periods are missed, pregnancy test is required before new dosing cycle is started.

One dose missed: Take as soon as remembered or take 2 tablets next day

Two doses missed: Take 2 tablets as soon as remembered or 2 tablets next 2 days

Three doses missed: Begin new compact of tablets starting on day 1 of next cycle

Triphasic oral contraceptive: 1 tablet/day in the sequence specified by the manufacturer

Treatment of moderate to severe vasomotor symptoms associated with menopause, treatment of vulvar and vaginal atrophy, prevention of osteoporosis: 1 tablet daily; begin with first tablet in first row of blister card (place weekday sticker to identify the first day taken)

Contraindications Thrombophlebitis, undiagnosed vaginal bleeding, hypersensitivity to ethinyl estradiol or any component, known or suspected pregnancy, carcinoma of the breast, estrogen-dependent tumor

Pregnancy Risk Factor X

Ethinyl Estradiol and Norgestrel (ETH in il es tra DYE ole & nor JES trel)

Pharmacologic Class Contraceptive, Oral

U.S. Brand Names Lo/Ovral®; Low-Ogestrel-21®; Low-Ogestrel-28®; Ovral®

Use Prevention of pregnancy; oral: postcoital contraceptive or "morning after" pill; treatment of hypermenorrhea, endometriosis, female hypogonadism

USUAL DOSAGE Female: Oral: Contraceptive: 1 tablet daily, beginning on day 5 of menstrual cycle (first day of menstrual flow is day 1). With 20-tablet and 21-tablet packages, new dosing cycle begins 7 days after last tablet taken; with 28-tablet packages, dosage is 1 tablet daily without interruption; extra tablets are placebos or contain iron. If next menstrual period does not begin on schedule, rule out pregnancy before starting new dosing cycle; if menstrual period begins, start new dosing cycle 7 days after last tablet was taken; if all doses have been taken on schedule and one menstrual period is missed, continue dosing cycle; if two consecutive menstrual periods are missed, pregnancy test is required before new dosing cycle is started.

One dose missed: Take as soon as remembered or take 2 tablets next day

Two doses missed: Take 2 tablets as soon as remembered or 2 tablets next 2 days

Three doses missed: Begin new compact of tablets starting on day 1 of next cycle

Postcoital contraception or "morning after" pill: Oral (50 mcg ethinyl estradiol and 0.5 mg norgestrel): 2 tablets at initial visit and 2 tablets 12 hours later

Contraindications Thromboembolic disorders, cerebrovascular or coronary artery disease; known or suspected breast cancer; undiagnosed abnormal vaginal bleeding; women smokers >35 years of age; all women >40 years of age, hypersensitivity to drug or components; pregnancy

Pregnancy Risk Factor X

Ethionamide (e thye on AM ide)

Pharmacologic Class Antitubercular Agent

U.S. Brand Names Trecator®-SC

Generic Available No

Mechanism of Action Inhibits peptide synthesis

Use Treatment of tuberculosis and other mycobacterial diseases, in conjunction with other antituberculosis agents, when first-line agents have failed or resistance has been demonstrated

USUAL DOSAGE Oral:

Children: 15-20 mg/kg/day in 2 divided doses, not to exceed 1 g/day

Adults: 500-1000 mg/day in 1-3 divided doses

Dosing adjustment in renal impairment: Cl_{cr} <50 mL/minute: Administer 50% of dose

Dosage Forms TAB, sugar coated: 250 mg

Contraindications Contraindicated in patients with severe hepatic impairment or in patients who are sensitive to the drug

Warnings/Precautions Use with caution in patients receiving cycloserine or isoniazid, in diabetics

Pregnancy Risk Factor C

Adverse Reactions

>10%: Gastrointestinal: Anorexia, nausea, vomiting

1% to 10%:

- Cardiovascular: Postural hypotension
- Central nervous system: Psychiatric disturbances, drowsiness
- Gastrointestinal: Metallic taste, diarrhea
- Hepatic: Hepatitis (5%), jaundice
- Neuromuscular & skeletal: Weakness

<1%: Abdominal pain, alopecia, blurred vision, dizziness, gynecomastia, headache, hypoglycemia, hypothyroidism or goiter, olfactory disturbances, optic neuritis, peripheral neuritis, rash, seizures, stomatitis, thrombocytopenia

Half-Life 2-3 hours

Education and Monitoring Issues

Patient Education: Take this medication as prescribed; avoid missing doses and do not discontinue without contacting prescriber. You will need to schedule regular medical checkups which will include blood tests. You may experience GI upset (small frequent meals may help), metallic taste and increased salivation (lozenges, frequent mouth care), dizziness, blurred vision (use caution when driving or engaging in tasks that require alertness until response to drug is known), postural hypotension (change position slowly), impotence and/or menstrual difficulties (these will go away when drug is discontinued). Report acute unresolved GI upset, changes in vision, numbness or pain in extremities, or unusual bleeding or bruising.

Monitoring Parameters: Initial and periodic serum ALT and AST

Manufacturer Wyeth-Ayerst Laboratories

Related Information

Antimicrobial Drugs of Choice *on page 1182*

Pharmaceutical Manufacturers Directory *on page 1020*

Tuberculosis Test Recommendations and Prophylaxis *on page 1163*

Tuberculosis Treatment Guidelines *on page 1213*

♦ **Ethmozine®** *see* Moricizine *on page 617*

Ethosuximide (eth oh SUKS i mide)

Pharmacologic Class Anticonvulsant, Succinimide

U.S. Brand Names Zarontin®

Use Management of absence (petit mal) seizures, myoclonic seizures, and akinetic epilepsy; considered to be drug of choice for simple absence seizures

USUAL DOSAGE Oral:

Children 3-6 years: Initial: 250 mg/day (or 15 mg/kg/day) in 2 divided doses; increase every 4-7 days; usual maintenance dose: 15-40 mg/kg/day in 2 divided doses

Children >6 years and Adults: Initial: 250 mg twice daily; increase by 250 mg as needed every 4-7 days up to 1.5 g/day in 2 divided doses; usual maintenance dose: 20-40 mg/kg/day in 2 divided doses

Contraindications Known hypersensitivity to ethosuximide

Pregnancy Risk Factor C

Related Information

Anticonvulsants by Seizure Type Comparison *on page 1230*

Epilepsy Guidelines *on page 1091*

Ethyl Chloride and Dichlorotetrafluoroethane

(ETH il KLOR ide & dye klor oh te tra floo or oh ETH ane)

Pharmacologic Class Local Anesthetic

U.S. Brand Names Fluro-Ethyl® Aerosol

Dosage Forms AERO: Ethyl chloride 25% and dichlorotetrafluoroethane 75% (225 g)

Pregnancy Risk Factor C

♦ **Etibi®** *see* Ethambutol *on page 339*

Etidocaine (e TI doe kane)

Pharmacologic Class Local Anesthetic

U.S. Brand Names Duranest®

Generic Available No

Mechanism of Action Blocks nerve conduction through the stabilization of neuronal membranes. By preventing the transient increase in membrane permeability to sodium, the ionic fluxes necessary for initiation and transmission of electrical impulses are inhibited and local anesthesia is induced. Local anesthetics reversibly prevent generation and conduction of electrical impulses in neurons by decreasing the transient increase in permeability to sodium. The differential sensitivity generally depends on the size of the fiber; small fibers are more sensitive than larger fibers and require a longer period for recovery. Sensory pain fibers are usually blocked first, followed by fibers that transmit sensations of temperature, touch, and deep pressure. High concentrations block sympathetic somatic sensory and somatic motor fibers. The spread of anesthesia depends upon the distribution of the solution. This is primarily dependent on the volume of drug injected.

Use Infiltration anesthesia; peripheral nerve blocks; central neural blocks

USUAL DOSAGE Varies with procedure; use 1% for peripheral nerve block, central nerve block, lumbar peridural caudal; use 1.5% for maxillary infiltration or inferior alveolar nerve block; use 1% or 1.5% for intra-abdominal or pelvic surgery, lower limb surgery, or caesarean section

Dosage Forms INJ: 1% [10 mg/mL] (30 mL); With epinephrine 1:200,000: 1% [10 mg/mL] (30 mL), 1.5% [15 mg/mL] (20 mL)

Contraindications Heart block, severe hemorrhage, severe hypotension, known hypersensitivity to etidocaine or other amide local anesthetics

Warnings/Precautions Do not use for spinals; use with caution in patients with cardiac disease; fetal bradycardia may occur up to 20% of the time; use with caution in areas of inflammation or sepsis, in debilitated or elderly patients, and those with severe cardiovascular disease or hepatic dysfunction; some products may contain sulfites; not recommended as an epidural for obstetrics

Pregnancy Risk Factor B

Adverse Reactions <1%: Anaphylactoid reactions, anxiety, blurred vision, bradycardia, cardiovascular collapse, chills, confusion, disorientation, drowsiness, hypotension, myocardial depression, nausea, respiratory arrest, restlessness, seizures, shivering, tinnitus, transient stinging or burning at injection site, tremor, unconsciousness, urticaria, vomiting

Onset 2-5 minutes

Duration 4-10 hours

Education and Monitoring Issues

Reference Range: Toxic concentration: >0.1 µg/mL

Etidronate Disodium (e ti DROE nate dye SOW dee um)

Pharmacologic Class Bisphosphonate Derivative

U.S. Brand Names Didronel®

Generic Available No

Mechanism of Action Binds to hydroxyapatite and inhibits osteoclastic bone resorption; higher doses and/or prolonged use of etidronate are associated with inhibition of osteoblastic activity resulting in inhibition of bone mineralization; inhibition of bone mineralization is not usually a relevant concern in the treatment of patients with cancer-associated hypercalcemia

Use Symptomatic treatment of Paget's disease and heterotopic ossification due to spinal cord injury or after total hip replacement, hypercalcemia associated with malignancy

USUAL DOSAGE Adults: Oral formulation should be taken on an empty stomach 2 hours before any meal.

Paget's disease: Oral

Initial: 5-10 mg/kg/day (not to exceed 6 months) or 11-20 mg/kg/day (not to exceed 3 months). Doses >10 mg/kg/day are **not** recommended.

Retreatment: Initiate only after etidronate-free period ≥90 days. Monitor patients every 3-6 months. Retreatment regimens are the same as for initial treatment.

Heterotopic ossification: Oral:

Caused by spinal cord injury: 20 mg/kg/day for 2 weeks, then 10 mg/kg/day for 10 weeks; total treatment period: 12 weeks

Complicating total hip replacement: 20 mg/kg/day for 1 month preoperatively then 20 mg/kg/day for 3 months postoperatively; total treatment period is 4 months

Hypercalcemia associated with malignancy:

I.V. (dilute dose in at least 250 mL NS): 7.5 mg/kg/day for 3 days; there should be at least 7 days between courses of treatment

Oral: Start 20 mg/kg/day on the last day of infusion and continue for 30-90 days

Dosing adjustment in renal impairment:

S_{cr} 2.5-5 mg/dL: Use with caution

S_{cr} >5 mg/dL: **Not recommended**

Dosage Forms INJ: 50 mg/mL (6 mL). **TAB:** 200 mg, 400 mg

Contraindications Patients with serum creatinine >5 mg/dL; hypersensitivity to bisphosphonates

Warnings/Precautions Use with caution in patients with restricted calcium and vitamin D intake; dosage modification required in renal impairment; I.V. form may be nephrotoxic and should be used with caution, if at all, in patients with impaired renal function (serum creatinine: 2.5-4.9 mg/dL)

Pregnancy Risk Factor B (oral); C (parenteral)

Adverse Reactions

1% to 10%:

Central nervous system: Fever, convulsions

Endocrine & metabolic: Hypophosphatemia, hypomagnesemia, fluid overload

Neuromuscular & skeletal: Bone pain

Respiratory: Dyspnea

<1%: Abnormal taste, angioedema, hypersensitivity reactions, increased risk of fractures, nephrotoxicity, occult blood in stools, pain, rash

Onset I.V.: 1-2 days; oral: 1-3 months

Duration Up to 12 months

Education and Monitoring Issues

Patient Education: Maintain adequate intake of calcium and vitamin D; take medicine on an empty stomach 2 hours before meals

Monitoring Parameters: Serum calcium and phosphorous; serum creatinine and BUN

Reference Range: Calcium (total): Adults: 9.0-11.0 mg/dL

Etodolac (ee toe DOE lak)

Pharmacologic Class Nonsteroidal Anti-Inflammatory Agent (NSAID)

U.S. Brand Names Lodine®; Lodine® XL

Generic Available Yes

Mechanism of Action Inhibits prostaglandin synthesis by decreasing the activity of the enzyme, cyclo-oxygenase, which results in decreased formation of prostaglandin precursors

Use Acute and long-term use in the management of signs and symptoms of osteoarthritis and management of pain

Unapproved use: Rheumatoid arthritis

USUAL DOSAGE Single dose of 76-100 mg is comparable to the analgesic effect of aspirin 650 mg; in patients ≥65 years, no substantial differences in the pharmacokinetics or side-effects profile were seen compared with the general population

Adults: Oral:

Acute pain: 200-400 mg every 6-8 hours, as needed, not to exceed total daily doses of 1200 mg; for patients weighing <60 kg, total daily dose should not exceed 20 mg/kg/day

Osteoarthritis: Initial: 800-1200 mg/day given in divided doses: 400 mg 2 or 3 times/day; 300 mg 2, 3 or 4 times/day; 200 mg 3 or 4 times/day; total daily dose should not exceed 1200 mg; for patients weighing <60 kg, total daily dose should not exceed 20 mg/kg/day

(Continued)

Etodolac *(Continued)*

Dosage Forms CAP (Lodine®): 200 mg, 300 mg. **TAB:** (Lodine®): 400 mg, 500 mg; Extended release (Lodine® XL): 400 mg, 500 mg, 600 mg

Contraindications Hypersensitivity to etodolac, aspirin, or other NSAIDs

Warnings/Precautions Use with caution in patients with congestive heart failure, hypertension, decreased renal or hepatic function, history of GI disease, or those receiving anticoagulants

Pregnancy Risk Factor C; D (3rd trimester)

Adverse Reactions

>10%:
- Central nervous system: Dizziness
- Dermatologic: Rash
- Gastrointestinal: Abdominal cramps, heartburn, indigestion, nausea

1% to 10%:
- Central nervous system: Headache, nervousness
- Dermatologic: Itching
- Endocrine & metabolic: Fluid retention
- Gastrointestinal: Vomiting
- Otic: Tinnitus

<1%: Acute renal failure, agranulocytosis, allergic rhinitis, anemia, angioedema, arrhythmia, aseptic meningitis, bone marrow suppression, blurred vision, confusion, congestive heart failure, conjunctivitis, cystitis, decreased hearing, drowsiness, dry eyes, epistaxis, erythema multiforme, gastritis, GI ulceration, hallucinations, hemolytic anemia, hepatitis, hot flashes, hypertension, insomnia, leukopenia, mental depression, peripheral neuropathy, polydipsia, polyuria, shortness of breath, Stevens-Johnson syndrome, tachycardia, thrombocytopenia, toxic amblyopia, toxic epidermal necrolysis, urticaria

Drug Interactions

Decreased effect with aspirin

Increased effect/toxicity with aspirin (GI irritation), probenecid; increased effect/toxicity of lithium, methotrexate, digoxin, cyclosporin (nephrotoxicity), warfarin (bleeding)

Alcohol Interactions Avoid use (may enhance gastric mucosal irritation)

Onset Analgesia: 2-4 hours; Anti-inflammatory: A few days

Half-Life 7 hours

Education and Monitoring Issues

Patient Education: Take this medication exactly as directed; do not increase dose without consulting prescriber. Do not crush tablets or break capsules. Take with food or milk to reduce GI distress. Maintain adequate fluid intake (2-3 L/day of fluids unless instructed to restrict fluid intake). Do not use alcohol, aspirin, or aspirin-containing medication, and all other anti-inflammatory medications without consulting prescriber. You may experience anorexia, nausea, vomiting, or heartburn (frequent small meals, frequent mouth care, sucking lozenges, or chewing gum may help); drowsiness, dizziness, nervousness, or headache (use caution when driving or engaging in tasks requiring alertness until response to drug is known); fluid retention (weigh yourself weekly and report unusual (3-5 lb/week) weight gain). GI bleeding, ulceration, or perforation can occur with or without pain; discontinue medication and contact prescriber if persistent abdominal pain or cramping, or blood in stool occurs. Report breathlessness, difficulty breathing, or unusual cough; chest pain, rapid heartbeat, palpitations; unusual bruising/bleeding; blood in urine, stool, mouth, or vomitus; swollen extremities; skin rash or itching; acute fatigue; or changes in hearing or ringing in ears.

Monitoring Parameters: Monitor CBC, liver enzymes; in patients receiving diuretics, monitor urine output and BUN/serum creatinine

Related Information

Nonsteroidal Anti-Inflammatory Agents Comparison *on page 1248*

♦ **Etrafon®** *see* Amitriptyline and Perphenazine *on page 52*

Etretinate (e TRET i nate)

Pharmacologic Class Antipsoriatic Agent

U.S. Brand Names Tegison®

Generic Available No

Mechanism of Action Unknown; related to retinoic acid and retinol (vitamin A)

Use Treatment of severe recalcitrant psoriasis in patients intolerant of or unresponsive to standard therapies

USUAL DOSAGE Adults: Oral: Individualized; Initial: 0.75-1 mg/kg/day in divided doses, increase by 0.25 mg/kg/day at weekly intervals up to 1.5 mg/kg/day; maintenance dose established after 8-10 weeks of therapy 0.5-0.75 mg/kg/day

Dosage Forms CAP: 10 mg, 25 mg

Contraindications Pregnancy, known hypersensitivity to etretinate; because of the high likelihood of long lasting teratogenic effects, do not prescribe etretinate for women who are or who are likely to become pregnant while or after using the drug

Warnings/Precautions Not to be used in severe obesity or women of childbearing potential unless woman is capable of complying with effective contraceptive measures; therapy is normally begun on the second or third day of next normal menstrual period; effective contraception must be used for at least 1 month before beginning therapy, during therapy, and for 1 month after discontinuation of therapy; pregnancy test must be performed prior to starting therapy

Pregnancy Risk Factor X

Adverse Reactions

>10%:

Central nervous system: Fatigue, headache, fever
Dermatologic: Chapped lips, alopecia
Endocrine & metabolic: Hypercholesterolemia, hypertriglyceridemia
Gastrointestinal: Nausea, appetite change, xerostomia, sore tongue
Neuromuscular & skeletal: Hyperostosis, bone pain, arthralgia
Ocular: Eye irritation
Respiratory: Epistaxis

1% to 10%:

Cardiovascular: Edema
Central nervous system: Dizziness, lethargy
Hepatic: Hepatitis
Neuromuscular & skeletal: Myalgia
Ocular: Blurred vision
Otic: Otitis externa
Respiratory: Dyspnea

<1%: Amnesia, confusion, constipation, depression, diarrhea, dysuria, ear infection, flatulence, gingival bleeding, gout, hyperkinesia, hypertonia, kidney stones, mouth ulcers, phlebitis, photophobia, polyuria, pseudotumor cerebri, rhinorrhea, syncope, urticaria, weight loss

Drug Interactions

Increased effect: Milk increases absorption of etretinate
Increased toxicity: Additive toxicity with vitamin A

Alcohol Interactions Avoid or limit use (may increase triglyceride levels if taken in excess and increase risk of hepatotoxicity)

Half-Life 4-8 days (with multiple doses)

Education and Monitoring Issues

Patient Education: Take with food. Do not take additional vitamin A supplements. You may experience dizziness, blurred vision, or fatigue; use caution when driving or engaging in tasks that require alertness until response to drug is known. Report persistent severe nausea, abdominal pain, visual disturbances, yellowing of skin or eyes, unusual bruising or bleeding, muscle pain or cramping, or unusual nosebleeds.

Manufacturer Roche Laboratories

Related Information

Pharmaceutical Manufacturers Directory *on page 1020*

- **Euglucon®** *see* Glyburide *on page 415*
- **Eulexin®** *see* Flutamide *on page 385*
- **Eurax®** *see* Crotamiton *on page 233*
- **Eurax® Topical** *see* Crotamiton *on page 233*
- **Evac-Q-Mag® [OTC]** *see* Magnesium Citrate *on page 550*
- **Evalose®** *see* Lactulose *on page 506*
- **Everone® Injection** *see* Testosterone *on page 898*
- **Evista®** *see* Raloxifene *on page 806*
- **E-Vitamin® [OTC]** *see* Vitamin E *on page 980*
- **Evoxac®** *see* Cevimeline *on page 173*
- **Excedrin® IB [OTC]** *see* Ibuprofen *on page 458*
- **Exelderm®** *see* Sulconazole *on page 875*
- **Exidine® Scrub [OTC]** *see* Chlorhexidine Gluconate *on page 181*
- **Exosurf®** *see* Colfosceril Palmitate *on page 226*
- **Exosurf® Neonatal** *see* Colfosceril Palmitate *on page 226*
- **Exsel®** *see* Selenium Sulfide *on page 845*
- **Extendryl® SR** *see* Chlorpheniramine, Phenylephrine, and Methscopolamine *on page 186*
- **Extra Action Cough Syrup [OTC]** *see* Guaifenesin and Dextromethorphan *on page 424*
- **Extra Strength Adprin-B® [OTC]** *see* Aspirin *on page 72*
- **Extra Strength Bayer® Enteric 500 Aspirin [OTC]** *see* Aspirin *on page 72*
- **Extra Strength Bayer® Plus [OTC]** *see* Aspirin *on page 72*
- **Eye-Sed® [OTC]** *see* Zinc Supplements *on page 993*
- **Eyestil®** *see* Sodium Hyaluronate *on page 859*
- **Ezide®** *see* Hydrochlorothiazide *on page 442*
- **Factrel®** *see* Gonadorelin *on page 419*

Famciclovir (fam SYE kloe veer)

Pharmacologic Class Antiviral Agent

U.S. Brand Names Famvir™

Mechanism of Action After undergoing rapid biotransformation to the active compound, penciclovir, famciclovir is phosphorylated by viral thymidine kinase in HSV-1, HSV-2, and VZV-infected cells to a monophosphate form; this is then converted to penciclovir triphosphate and competes with deoxyguanosine triphosphate to inhibit HSV-2 polymerase (ie, herpes viral DNA synthesis/replication is selectively inhibited)

Use Management of acute herpes zoster (shingles) and recurrent episodes of genital herpes; treatment of recurrent herpes simplex in immunocompetent patients

USUAL DOSAGE Adults: Oral:

Acute herpes zoster: 500 mg every 8 hours for 7 days

Recurrent herpes simplex in immunocompetent patients: 125 mg twice daily for 5 days

Genital herpes:

Recurrent episodes: 125 mg twice daily for 5 days

Prophylaxis: 250 mg twice daily

Dosing interval in renal impairment:

Cl_{cr} 40-59 mL/minute: Administer 500 mg every 12 hours

Cl_{cr} 20-39 mL/minute: Administer 500 mg every 24 hours

Cl_{cr} <20 mL/minute: Unknown

Dosage Forms TAB: 125 mg, 250 mg, 500 mg

Contraindications Hypersensitivity to famciclovir

Warnings/Precautions Has not been studied in immunocompromised patients or patients with ophthalmic or disseminated zoster; dosage adjustment is required in patients with renal insufficiency (Cl_{cr} <60 mL/minute) and in patients with noncompensated hepatic disease; safety and efficacy have not been established in children <18 years of age; animal studies indicated increases in incidence of carcinomas, mutagenic changes, and decreases in fertility with extremely large doses

Pregnancy Risk Factor B

Pregnancy Implications

Clinical effects on the fetus: Use only if the benefit to the patient clearly exceeds the potential risk to the fetus

Breast-feeding/lactation: Due to potential for excretion of famciclovir in breast milk and for its associated tumorigenicity, discontinue nursing or discontinue the drug during lactation

Adverse Reactions

1% to 10%:

Central nervous system: Fatigue (4% to 6%), fever (1% to 3%), dizziness (3% to 5%), somnolence (1% to 2%), headache

Dermatologic: Pruritus (1% to 4%)

Gastrointestinal: Diarrhea (4% to 8%), vomiting (1% to 5%), constipation (1% to 5%), anorexia (1% to 3%), abdominal pain (1% to 4%), nausea

Neuromuscular & skeletal: Paresthesia (1% to 3%)

Respiratory: Sinusitis/pharyngitis (2%)

<1%: Arthralgia, rigors, upper respiratory infection

Drug Interactions Increased effect/toxicity:

Cimetidine: Penciclovir AUC may increase due to impaired metabolism

Digoxin: C_{max} of digoxin increases by ~19%

Probenecid: Penciclovir serum levels significantly increase

Theophylline: Penciclovir AUC/C_{max} may increase and renal clearance decrease, although not clinically significant

Half-Life Penciclovir: 2-3 hours (10, 20, and 7 hours in HSV-1, HSV-2, and VZV-infected cells); linearly decreased with reductions in renal failure

Education and Monitoring Issues

Patient Education: Take for prescribed length of time, even if condition improves. Inform prescriber at the first sign or symptom of eruption to initiate therapy. Do not discontinue without consulting prescriber. This is not a cure for genital herpes. You may experience mild GI disturbances (eg, nausea, vomiting, constipation, or diarrhea), fatigue, headaches, or muscle aches and pains. If these are severe, contact prescriber.

Manufacturer SmithKline Beecham Pharmaceuticals

Related Information

Pharmaceutical Manufacturers Directory *on page 1020*

Famotidine (fa MOE ti deen)

Pharmacologic Class Histamine H_2 Antagonist

U.S. Brand Names Mylanta AR® [OTC]; Pepcid®; Pepcid® AC Acid Controller [OTC]; Pepcid RPD™

Generic Available No

Mechanism of Action Competitive inhibition of histamine at H_2 receptors of the gastric parietal cells, which inhibits gastric acid secretion

Use

Pepcid®: Therapy and treatment of duodenal ulcer, gastric ulcer, control gastric pH in critically ill patients, symptomatic relief in gastritis, gastroesophageal reflux, active benign ulcer, and pathological hypersecretory conditions

Pepcid® AC Acid Controller: Relieves heartburn, acid indigestion and sour stomach

USUAL DOSAGE

Children: Oral, I.V.: Doses of 1-2 mg/kg/day have been used; maximum dose: 40 mg

Adults:

Oral:

Duodenal ulcer, gastric ulcer: 40 mg/day at bedtime for 4-8 weeks

Hypersecretory conditions: Initial: 20 mg every 6 hours, may increase up to 160 mg every 6 hours

GERD: 20 mg twice daily for 6 weeks

I.V.: 20 mg every 12 hours

Dosing adjustment in renal impairment:

Cl_{cr} <10 mL/minute: Administer every 24 hours or 50% of dose

Dosage Forms GELCAP: 10 mg; **INF, premixed in NS:** 20 mg (50 mL). **INJ:** 10 mg/mL (2 mL, 4 mL). **POWDER for oral susp** (cherry-banana-mint flavor): 40 mg/5 mL (50 mL). **TAB:** Chewable: 10 mg; Film coated: 20 mg, 40 mg; Disintegrating: 20 mg, 40 mg; Mylanta AR®: 10 mg; Pepcid® AC Acid Controller: 10 mg

Contraindications Hypersensitivity to famotidine or other H_2-antagonists

Warnings/Precautions Modify dose in patients with renal impairment

Pregnancy Risk Factor B

Pregnancy Implications

Clinical effects on the fetus: Crosses the placenta. No data on effects on the fetus (insufficient data).

Breast-feeding/lactation: Crosses into breast milk. American Academy of Pediatrics has NO RECOMMENDATIONS.

Adverse Reactions

1% to 10%:

Central nervous system: Dizziness, headache

Gastrointestinal: Constipation, diarrhea

<1%: Abdominal discomfort, acne, agranulocytosis, allergic reaction, anorexia, belching, bradycardia, bronchospasm, drowsiness, dry skin, fatigue, fever, flatulence, hypertension, increased AST/ALT, increased BUN/creatinine, insomnia, neutropenia, palpitations, paresthesia, proteinuria, pruritus, seizures, tachycardia, thrombocytopenia, urticaria, weakness

Drug Interactions Decreased effect of ketoconazole, itraconazole

Alcohol Interactions Avoid use (may enhance gastric mucosal irritation)

Onset Onset of GI effect: Oral: Within 1 hour

Duration 10-12 hours

Half-Life 2.5-3.5 hours; increases with renal impairment, oliguric patient: 20 hours

Education and Monitoring Issues

Patient Education: Take as directed, for full dose as prescribed, even if feeling better. Avoid alcohol and smoking (smoking decreases effectiveness of medication). You may experience some drowsiness or dizziness; use caution when driving or engaging in tasks that require alertness until response to drug is known. Increased exercise, increased dietary fluids, fruits, or fiber may reduce constipation; yogurt or buttermilk may help relieve diarrhea. Report acute headache, unresolved constipation or diarrhea, palpitations, black tarry stools, abdominal pain, rash, worsening of condition being treated, or recurrence of symptoms after therapy is completed.

Manufacturer Merck & Co

Related Information

Pharmaceutical Manufacturers Directory *on page 1020*

♦ **Famvir™** *see* Famciclovir *on page 350*

♦ **Fansidar®** *see* Sulfadoxine and Pyrimethamine *on page 878*

♦ **Fareston®** *see* Toremifene *on page 933*

♦ **Fastin®** *see* Phentermine *on page 726*

Fat Emulsion (fat e MUL shun)

Pharmacologic Class Caloric Agent

U.S. Brand Names Intralipid®; Liposyn®; Nutrilipid®; Soyacal®

Generic Available Yes

Mechanism of Action Essential for normal structure and function of cell membranes

Use Source of calories and essential fatty acids for patients requiring parenteral nutrition of extended duration

USUAL DOSAGE Fat emulsion should not exceed 60% of the total daily calories

Premature Infants: Initial dose: 0.25-0.5 g/kg/day, increase by 0.25-0.5 g/kg/day to a maximum of 3 g/kg/day depending on needs/nutritional goals; limit to 1 g/kg/day if on phototherapy; maximum rate of infusion: 0.15 g/kg/hour (0.75 mL/kg/hour of 20% solution)

(Continued)

Fat Emulsion *(Continued)*

Infants and Children: Initial dose: 0.5-1 g/kg/day, increase by 0.5 g/kg/day to a maximum of 3 g/kg/day depending on needs/nutritional goals; maximum rate of infusion: 0.25 g/kg/hour (1.25 mL/kg/hour of 20% solution)

Adolescents and Adults: Initial dose: 1 g/kg/day, increase by 0.5-1 g/kg/day to a maximum of 2.5 g/kg/day of 10% and 3 g/kg/day of 20% depending on needs/nutritional goals; maximum rate of infusion: 0.25 g/kg/hour (1.25 mL/kg/hour of 20% solution); do not exceed 50 mL/hour (20%) or 100 mL/hour (10%)

Prevention of essential fatty acid deficiency (8% to 10% of total caloric intake): 0.5-1 g/kg/24 hours

Children: 5-10 mL/kg/day at 0.1 mL/minute then up to 100 mL/hour

Adults: 500 mL (10%) twice weekly at rate of 1 mL/minute for 30 minutes, then increase to 42 mL/hour (500 mL over 12 hours)

Note: At the onset of therapy, the patient should be observed for any immediate allergic reactions such as dyspnea, cyanosis, and fever; slower initial rates of infusion may be used for the first 10-15 minutes of the infusion (eg, 0.1 mL/minute of 10% or 0.05 mL/minute of 20% solution)

Dosage Forms INJ: 10% [100 mg/mL] (100 mL, 250 mL, 500 mL), 20% [200 mg/mL] (100 mL, 250 mL, 500 mL)

Contraindications Pathologic hyperlipidemia, lipoid nephrosis, known hypersensitivity to fat emulsion and severe egg or legume (soybean) allergies, pancreatitis with hyperlipemia

Warnings/Precautions Use caution in patients with severe liver damage, pulmonary disease, anemia, or blood coagulation disorder; use with caution in jaundiced, premature, and low birth weight children

Pregnancy Risk Factor B/C

Adverse Reactions

>10%: Local: Thrombophlebitis

1% to 10%: Endocrine & metabolic: Hyperlipemia

<1%: Chest pain, cyanosis, diarrhea, dyspnea, flushing, hepatomegaly, nausea, sepsis, vomiting

Half-Life 0.5-1 hour

Education and Monitoring Issues

Patient Education: Report pain at infusion site, difficulty breathing, chest pain, calf pain, or excessive sweating.

Monitoring Parameters: Serum triglycerides; before initiation of therapy and at least weekly during therapy

♦ **Feldene®** *see* Piroxicam *on page 744*

Felodipine (fe LOE di peen)

Pharmacologic Class Calcium Channel Blocker

U.S. Brand Names Plendil®

Generic Available No

Mechanism of Action Inhibits calcium ions from entering the "slow channels" or select voltage-sensitive areas of vascular smooth muscle and myocardium during depolarization, producing a relaxation of coronary vascular smooth muscle and coronary vasodilation; increases myocardial oxygen delivery in patients with vasospastic angina

Use Treatment of hypertension, congestive heart failure

USUAL DOSAGE

Adults: Oral: 2.5-10 mg once daily; usual initial dose: 5 mg; increase by 5 mg at 2-week intervals, as needed; maximum: 10 mg

Elderly: Begin with 2.5 mg/day

Dosing adjustment/comments in hepatic impairment: Begin with 2.5 mg/day; do not use doses >10 mg/day

Dosage Forms TAB, extended release: 2.5 mg, 5 mg, 10 mg

Contraindications Hypersensitivity to felodipine or any component or other calcium channel blocker; severe hypotension or second and third degree heart block

Warnings/Precautions Use with caution and titrate dosages for patients with impaired renal or hepatic function; use caution when treating patients with congestive heart failure, sick-sinus syndrome, severe left ventricular dysfunction, hypertrophic cardiomyopathy (especially obstructive), concomitant therapy with beta-blockers or digoxin, edema, or increased intracranial pressure with cranial tumors; do not abruptly withdraw (may cause chest pain); elderly may experience hypotension and constipation more readily.

Pregnancy Risk Factor C

Adverse Reactions

2% to 10%:

Cardiovascular: Peripheral edema (2% to 17%), tachycardia (0.4% to 2.5%), flushing (4% to 7%)

Central nervous system: Headache (11% to 15%)

Gastrointestinal: Gingival hyperplasia

0.5% to 1.5%

<1% (limited to important or life-threatening symptoms): Chest pain, facial edema, flu-like illness, myocardial infarction, hypotension, syncope, angina pectoris, arrhythmia,

premature beats, abdominal pain, diarrhea, vomiting, dry mouth, flatulence, acid, MI, CVA, CHF, regurgitation, gynecomastia, anemia, arthralgia, back pain, leg pain, foot pain, muscle cramps, myalgia, arm pain, knee pain, hip pain, insomnia, depression, anxiety disorders, irritability, nervousness, somnolence, decreased libido, dyspnea, pharyngitis, bronchitis, influenza, sinusitis, epistaxis, respiratory infection, contusion, erythema, urticaria, visual disturbances, impotence, urinary frequency, urinary urgency, dysuria, polyuria, gingival hyperplasia, flushing, palpitations, nausea, constipation, dizziness, paresthesias

Drug Interactions CYP3A3/4 enzyme substrate

Azole antifungals may inhibit calcium channel blocker's metabolism; avoid this combination. Try an antifungal like terbinafine (if appropriate) or monitor closely for altered effect of the calcium channel blocker

Beta-blockers may have increased pharmacokinetic or pharmacodynamic interactions with felodipine

Calcium may reduce the calcium channel blocker's effects, particularly hypotension

Carbamazepine significantly reduces felodipine's bioavailability; avoid this combination

Cyclosporine increases felodipine's serum concentration; avoid the combination or reduce dose of felodipine and monitor blood pressure

Ethanol increases felodipine's absorption; watch for a greater hypotensive effect

Erythromycin decreases felodipine's metabolism; monitor blood pressure

Nafcillin decreases plasma concentration of felodipine; avoid this combination

Rifampin increases the metabolism of the calcium channel blocker; adjust the dose of the calcium channel blocker to maintain efficacy

Alcohol Interactions Avoid use (may increase felodipine's absorption)

Onset 2-5 hours

Duration 16-24 hours

Half-Life 11-16 hours

Education and Monitoring Issues

Patient Education: Take without food. Take as prescribed; do not stop abruptly without consulting prescriber immediately. Swallow whole; do not crush or chew. You may experience headache (if unrelieved, consult prescriber), nausea or vomiting (frequent small meals may help), constipation (increased dietary bulk and fluids may help), depression (should resolve when drug is discontinued). May cause dizziness or drowsiness; use caution when driving or engaging in tasks that require alertness until response to drug is known. Report any chest pain or swelling of hands or feet, respiratory distress, sudden weight gain, or unresolved constipation.

Dietary Considerations: Should be taken without food; the bioavailability of felodipine is influenced by the presence of food and has been shown to increase more than twofold when taken with concentrated grapefruit juice

Manufacturer AstraZeneca

Related Information

Calcium Channel Blocking Agents Comparison *on page 1236*
Enalapril and Felodipine *on page 311*
Pharmaceutical Manufacturers Directory *on page 1020*

♦ **Femara™** *see* Letrozole *on page 512*
♦ **Femcet®** *see* Butalbital Compound *on page 123*
♦ **Femguard®** *see* Sulfabenzamide, Sulfacetamide, and Sulfathiazole *on page 875*
♦ **FemHrt™** *see* Ethinyl Estradiol and Norethindrone *on page 342*
♦ **Femiron® [OTC]** *see* Ferrous Fumarate *on page 359*
♦ **Femizole-7® [OTC]** *see* Clotrimazole *on page 220*
♦ **Femizol-M® [OTC]** *see* Miconazole *on page 600*
♦ **Femogen®** *see* Estrone *on page 334*
♦ **Femogex** *see* Estradiol *on page 327*
♦ **FemPatch® Transdermal** *see* Estradiol *on page 327*
♦ **Femstat®** *see* Butoconazole *on page 124*
♦ **Fenesin™** *see* Guaifenesin *on page 423*
♦ **Fenesin™ DM** *see* Guaifenesin and Dextromethorphan *on page 424*

Fenofibrate (fen oh FYE brate)

Pharmacologic Class Antilipemic Agent (Fibric Acid)

U.S. Brand Names TriCor™

Mechanism of Action Fenofibric acid is believed to increase VLDL catabolism by enhancing the synthesis of lipoprotein lipase; as a result of a decrease in VLDL levels, total plasma triglycerides are reduced by 30% to 60%; modest increase in HDL occurs in some hypertriglyceridemic patients

Use Adjunct to dietary therapy for the treatment of adults with very high elevations of serum triglyceride levels (types IV and V hyperlipidemia) who are at risk of pancreatitis and who do not respond adequately to a determined dietary effort; its efficacy can be enhanced by combination with other hypolipidemic agents that have a different mechanism of action; safety and efficacy may be greater than that of clofibrate

(Continued)

Fenofibrate *(Continued)*

USUAL DOSAGE Adults: Oral: Initial: 67 mg/day, up to 3 capsules (201 mg); requires 6-8 weeks of therapy to determine efficacy; once titrated to 67 mg capsules 3 times/day, the patient may be switched to one 200 mg capsule once daily

Dosing adjustment/comments in renal impairment: Decrease dose or increase dosing interval for patients with renal failure

Dosage Forms CAP: 67 mg, 200 mg

Warnings/Precautions The hypoprothrombinemic effect of anticoagulants is significantly increased with concomitant fenofibrate administration; use with caution in patients with severe renal dysfunction

Pregnancy Risk Factor C

Pregnancy Implications Although teratogenicity and mutagenicity tests in animals have been negative, significant risk has been identified with clofibrate, an agent similar in action to fenofibrate. Use should be avoided, if possible, in pregnant women since the neonatal glucuronide conjugation pathways are immature.

Adverse Reactions

>10%: Gastrointestinal: Nausea, gastric discomfort

1% to 10%:

Dermatologic: Skin reactions

Gastrointestinal: Constipation, diarrhea

<1%: Arthralgia, dizziness, fatigue, headache, insomnia, myalgia, transient increases in LFTs

Drug Interactions

Chlorpropamide: May increase risk of hypoglycemia

Furosemide: Increased blood levels of both in hypoalbuminemia

HMG-CoA reductase inhibitors (atorvastatin, cerivastatin, fluvastatin, lovastatin, pravastatin, simvastatin) may increase the risk of myopathy and rhabdomyolysis. The manufacturer warns against concomitant use. However, combination therapy with statins has been used in some patients with resistant hyperlipidemias (with great caution).

Rifampin: Decreased fenofibrate blood levels

Warfarin: Increased hypoprothrombinemic response; monitor INRs closely when fenofibrate is initiated or discontinued

Half-Life Fenofibrate: 21 hours (30 hours in the elderly, 44-54 hours in hepatic impairment)

Education and Monitoring Issues

Patient Education: Take with food. Do not change dosage without consulting prescriber. Maintain diet and exercise program as prescribed. You may experience mild GI disturbances (eg, gas, diarrhea, constipation, nausea); inform prescriber if these are severe. Report skin rash or irritation, insomnia, unusual muscle pain or tremors, or persistent dizziness.

Monitoring Parameters: Total serum cholesterol and triglyceride concentration and CLDL, LDL, and HDL levels should be measured periodically; if only marginal changes are noted in 6-8 weeks, the drug should be discontinued; serum transaminases should be measured every 3 months; if ALT values increase >100 units/L, therapy should be discontinued. Monitor LFTs prior to initiation, at 6 and 12 weeks after initiation of first dose, then periodically thereafter.

Manufacturer Abbott Laboratories (Pharmaceutical Product Division)

Related Information

Pharmaceutical Manufacturers Directory *on page 1020*

Fenoprofen (fen oh PROE fen)

Pharmacologic Class Nonsteroidal Anti-Inflammatory Agent (NSAID)

U.S. Brand Names Nalfon®

Generic Available Yes

Mechanism of Action Inhibits prostaglandin synthesis by decreasing the activity of the enzyme, cyclo-oxygenase, which results in decreased formation of prostaglandin precursors

Use Symptomatic treatment of acute and chronic rheumatoid arthritis and osteoarthritis; relief of mild to moderate pain

USUAL DOSAGE Adults: Oral:

Rheumatoid arthritis: 300-600 mg 3-4 times/day up to 3.2 g/day

Mild to moderate pain: 200 mg every 4-6 hours as needed

Dosage Forms CAP: 200 mg, 300 mg. **TAB:** 600 mg

Contraindications Known hypersensitivity to fenoprofen or other NSAIDs

Warnings/Precautions Use with caution in patients with congestive heart failure, hypertension, decreased renal or hepatic function, history of GI disease, or those receiving anticoagulants

Pregnancy Risk Factor B; D (if used in 3rd trimester or near delivery)

Adverse Reactions

>10%:

Central nervous system: Dizziness

Dermatologic: Rash

Gastrointestinal: Abdominal cramps, heartburn, indigestion, nausea

1% to 10%:

Central nervous system: Headache, nervousness

Dermatologic: Itching

Endocrine & metabolic: Fluid retention

Gastrointestinal: Vomiting

Otic: Tinnitus

<1%: Acute renal failure, agranulocytosis, allergic rhinitis, anemia, angioedema, arrhythmias, aseptic meningitis, bone marrow suppression, blurred vision, confusion, congestive heart failure, conjunctivitis, cystitis, decreased hearing, drowsiness, dry eyes, epistaxis, erythema multiforme, gastritis, GI ulceration, hallucinations, hemolytic anemia, hepatitis, hot flashes, hypertension, insomnia, leukopenia, mental depression, peripheral neuropathy, polydipsia, polyuria, shortness of breath, Stevens-Johnson syndrome, tachycardia, thrombocytopenia, toxic amblyopia, toxic epidermal necrolysis, urticaria

Drug Interactions

Decreased effect with phenobarbital

Increased effect/toxicity of phenytoin, sulfonamides, sulfonylureas

Increased toxicity with salicylates, oral anticoagulants

Alcohol Interactions Avoid use (may enhance gastric mucosal irritation)

Onset Begins in a few days

Half-Life 2.5-3 hours

Education and Monitoring Issues

Patient Education: Take this medication exactly as directed; do not increase dose without consulting prescriber. Do not crush tablets or break capsules. Take with food or milk to reduce GI distress. Maintain adequate fluid intake (2-3 L/day of fluids unless instructed to restrict fluid intake). Do not use alcohol, aspirin, or aspirin-containing medication, and all other anti-inflammatory medications without consulting prescriber. You may experience drowsiness, dizziness, nervousness, or headache (use caution when driving or engaging in tasks requiring alertness until response to drug is known); anorexia, nausea, vomiting, or heartburn (frequent small meals, frequent mouth care, sucking lozenges, or chewing gum may help); fluid retention (weigh yourself weekly and report unusual (3-5 lb/week) weight gain). GI bleeding, ulceration, or perforation can occur with or without pain; discontinue medication and contact prescriber if persistent abdominal pain or cramping, or blood in stool occurs. Report breathlessness, difficulty breathing, or unusual cough; chest pain, rapid heartbeat, palpitations; unusual bruising/bleeding; blood in urine, stool, mouth, or vomitus; swollen extremities; skin rash or itching; acute fatigue; or changes in hearing or ringing in ears.

Monitoring Parameters: Monitor CBC, liver enzymes; monitor urine output and BUN/serum creatinine in patients receiving diuretics

Reference Range: Therapeutic: 20-65 μg/mL (SI: 82-268 μmol/L)

Related Information

Nonsteroidal Anti-Inflammatory Agents Comparison *on page 1248*

Fentanyl (FEN ta nil)

Pharmacologic Class Analgesic, Narcotic

U.S. Brand Names Actiq®; Duragesic® Transdermal; Fentanyl Oralet®; Sublimaze® Injection

Generic Available No

Mechanism of Action Binds with stereospecific receptors at many sites within the CNS, increases pain threshold, alters pain reception, inhibits ascending pain pathways

Use Sedation, relief of pain, preoperative medication, adjunct to general or regional anesthesia, management of chronic pain (transdermal product)

Fentanyl Oralet® is indicated only for use in hospital settings as an anesthetic premedication in the operating room, or to induce conscious sedation prior to diagnostic or therapeutic procedures in a monitored hospital setting.

Actiq® is indicated only for management of breakthrough cancer pain in patients who are tolerant to and currently receiving opioid therapy for persistent cancer pain. Actiq® must not be used in patients who are intolerant to opioids. Patients are considered opioid tolerant if they are taking at least 60 mg morphine/day, 50 mcg transdermal fentanyl/hour, or an equivalent dose of another opioid for one week or longer.

USUAL DOSAGE Doses should be titrated to appropriate effects; wide range of doses, dependent upon desired degree of analgesia/anesthesia

Children 1-12 years:

Sedation for minor procedures/analgesia:

I.M., I.V.: 1-2 mcg/kg/dose; may repeat at 30- to 60-minute intervals. **Note:** Children 18-36 months of age may require 2-3 mcg/kg/dose

Transmucosal: Fentanyl Oralet® (dosage strength is based on patient weight, see table): 5 mcg/kg if child is not fearful; fearful children and some younger children may require doses of 5-15 mcg/kg (which also carries an increased risk of hypoventilation); drug effect begins within 10 minutes, with sedation beginning shortly thereafter. Should only be used in pediatric patients who are able to follow administration instructions; (should not be used in patients <10 kg or <2 years of age; maximum dose regardless of weight): 400 mcg

(Continued)

Fentanyl *(Continued)*

Continuous sedation/analgesia: Initial I.V. bolus: 1-2 mcg/kg then 1 mcg/kg/hour; titrate upward; usual: 1-3 mcg/kg/hour

Pain control: Transdermal: Not recommended

Children >12 years and Adults:

Sedation for minor procedures/analgesia:

I.M., I.V.: 0.5-1 mcg/kg/dose; higher doses are used for major procedures

Transmucosal: Fentanyl Oralet®: Do not use doses >15 mcg/kg regardless of age or doses >5 mcg/kg in adults; maximum dose regardless of weight: 400 mcg

See table.

Dosage Recommendations for Transmucosal Fentanyl (Oralet®)

Patient Age/Weight	5-10 mcg/kg/dose	10-15 mcg/kg/dose
Children <2 years of age OR <10 kg	CONTRAINDICATED	CONTRAINDICATED
10 kg	100 mcg	100 mcg
15 kg	100 mcg	200 mcg
20 kg	100 or 200 mcg	200 or 300 mcg
25 kg	200 mcg	300 mcg
30 kg	300 mcg	300 or 400 mcg
35 kg	300 mcg	400 mcg
>40 kg	400 mcg	400 mcg
Adults	400 mcg	400 mcg

Preoperative sedation, adjunct to regional anesthesia, postoperative pain: I.M., I.V.: 50-100 mcg/dose

Adjunct to general anesthesia: I.M., I.V.: 2-50 mcg/kg

General anesthesia without additional anesthetic agents: I.V. 50-100 mcg/kg with O_2 and skeletal muscle relaxant

Breakthrough cancer pain: Adults: Transmucosal: Actiq® dosing should be individually titrated to provide adequate analgesia with minimal side effects. It is indicated only for management of breakthrough cancer pain in patients who are tolerant to and currently receiving opioid therapy for persistent cancer pain. An initial starting dose of 200 mcg should be used for the treatment of breakthrough cancer pain. Patients should be monitored closely in order to determine the proper dose. If redosing for the same episode is necessary, the second dose may be started 15 minutes after completion of the first dose. Dosing should be titrated so that the patient's pain can be treated with one single dose. Generally, 1-2 days is required to determine the proper dose of analgesia with limited side effects. Once the dose has been determined, consumption should be limited to 4 units/day or less. Patients needing more than 4 units/day should have the dose of their long-term opioid re-evaluated. If signs of excessive opioid effects occur before a dose is complete, the unit should be removed from the patients mouth immediately, and subsequent doses decreased.

Pain control: Adults: Transdermal: Initial: 25 mcg/hour system; if currently receiving opiates, convert to fentanyl equivalent and administer equianalgesic dosage titrated to minimize the adverse effects and provide analgesia. To convert patients from oral or parenteral opioids to Duragesic®, the previous 24-hour analgesic requirement should be calculated. This analgesic requirement should be converted to the equianalgesic oral morphine dose. See tables.

Corresponding Doses of Oral/Intramuscular Morphine and Duragesic™

P.O. 24-Hour Morphine (mg/d)	I.M. 24-Hour Morphine (mg/d)	Duragesic™ Dose (mcg/h)
45-134	8-22	25
135-224	28-37	50
225-314	38-52	75
315-404	53-67	100
405-494	68-82	125
495-584	83-97	150
585-674	98-112	175
675-764	113-127	200
765-854	128-142	225
855-944	143-157	250
945-1034	158-172	275
1035-1124	173-187	300

Product information, Duragesic™ — Janssen Pharmaceutica, January, 1991.

Equianalgesic Doses of Opioid Agonists

Drug	Equianalgesic Dose (mg)	
	I.M.	P.O.
Codeine	130	200
Hydromorphone	1.5	7.5
Levorphanol	2	4
Meperidine	75	—
Methadone	10	20
Morphine	10	60
Oxycodone	15	30
Oxymorphone	1	10 (PR)

From *N Engl J Med*, 1985, 313:84-95.

The dosage should not be titrated more frequently than every 3 days after the initial dose or every 6 days thereafter. The majority of patients are controlled on every 72-hour administration, however, a small number of patients require every 48-hour administration.

Elderly >65 years: Transmucosal: Actiq®: Dose should be reduced to 2.5-5 mcg/kg; elderly have been found to be twice as sensitive as younger patients to the effects of fentanyl. Patients in this age group generally require smaller doses of Actiq® than younger patients

Dosing adjustment in renal impairment:

Cl_{cr} 10-50 mL/minute: Administer at 75% of normal dose

Cl_{cr} <10 mL/minute: Administer at 50% of normal dose

Dosing adjustment in renal/hepatic impairment: Actiq®: Although fentanyl kinetics may be altered in renal/hepatic disease, Actiq® can be used successfully in the management of breakthrough cancer pain. Doses should be titrated to reach clinical effect with careful monitoring of patients with severe renal/hepatic disease.

Dosage Forms INJ: 0.05 mg/mL (2 mL, 5 mL, 10 mL, 20 mL, 50 mL). **LOZ, oral transmucosal** (raspberry flavored): 100 mcg, 200 mcg, 300 mcg, 400 mcg, 600 mcg, 800 mcg, 1200 mcg, 1600 mcg. **TRANSDERMAL system:** 25 mcg/hour [10 cm²], 50 mcg/hour [20 cm²], 75 mcg/hour [30 cm²], 100 mcg/hour [40 cm²] (all available in 5s)

Contraindications Hypersensitivity to fentanyl or any component; increased intracranial pressure; severe respiratory depression; severe liver or renal insufficiency

Fentanyl Oralet® is contraindicated in unmonitored settings where a risk of unrecognized hypoventilation exists or in treating acute or chronic pain. Fentanyl Oralet® is contraindicated in children <10 kg; for use at home or any setting outside of a hospital; for the treatment of acute or chronic pain; in doses >15 mcg/kg in children and 5 mcg/kg in adults. The maximum dose of Fentanyl Oralet®, regardless of weight, is 400 mcg.

Actiq® is indicated only for management of breakthrough cancer pain in patients who are tolerant to and currently receiving opioid therapy for persistent cancer pain. Actiq® must not be used in patients who are intolerant to opioids. Patients are considered opioid-tolerant if they are taking at least 60 mg morphine/day, 50 mcg transdermal fentanyl/hour, or an equivalent dose of another opioid for ≥1 week.

Warnings/Precautions Fentanyl shares the toxic potentials of opiate agonists, and precautions of opiate agonist therapy should be observed; use with caution in patients with bradycardia; rapid I.V. infusion may result in skeletal muscle and chest wall rigidity → impaired ventilation → respiratory distress → apnea, bronchoconstriction, laryngospasm; inject slowly over 3-5 minutes; nondepolarizing skeletal muscle relaxant may be required. Tolerance of drug dependence may result from extended use.

Fentanyl Oralet® is not indicated for use in unmonitored settings where there is a risk of unrecognized hypoventilation or in treating acute or chronic pain. Patients should be monitored by direct visual observation and by some means of measuring respiratory function such as pulse oximetry until they are recovered. Facilities for the administration of fluids, opioid antagonists, oxygen and resuscitation equipment (including facilities for endotracheal intubation) should be readily available. Safety and efficacy have not been established in children <2 years of age.

Actiq® should be used only for the care of cancer patients and is intended for use by specialists who are knowledgeable in treating cancer pain. Actiq® preparations contain an amount of medication that can be fatal to children. Keep all units out of the reach of children and discard any open units properly. Patients and caregivers should be counseled on the dangers to children including the risk of exposure to partially-consumed units. Safety and efficacy have not been established in children <16 years of age.

Topical patches: Serum fentanyl concentrations may increase approximately one-third for patients with a body temperature of 40°C secondary to a temperature-dependent increase

(Continued)

Fentanyl *(Continued)*

in fentanyl release from the system and increased skin permeability. Patients who experience adverse reactions should be monitored for at least 12 hours after removal of the patch.

The elderly may be particularly susceptible to the CNS depressant and constipating effects of narcotics

Pregnancy Risk Factor B; D (if used for prolonged periods or in high doses at term)

Adverse Reactions

>10%:

Cardiovascular: Hypotension, bradycardia
Central nervous system: CNS depression, drowsiness, sedation
Gastrointestinal: Nausea, vomiting, constipation
Respiratory: Respiratory depression

1% to 10%:

Cardiovascular: Cardiac arrhythmias, orthostatic hypotension
Central nervous system: Confusion
Gastrointestinal: Biliary tract spasm
Ocular: Miosis

<1%: ADH release, bronchospasm, circulatory depression, CNS excitation or delirium, cold/clammy skin, convulsions, dysesthesia, erythema, itching, laryngospasm, paradoxical dizziness, physical and psychological dependence with prolonged use, pruritus, rash, urinary tract spasm, urticaria

Drug Interactions CYP3A3/4 enzyme substrate

Increased toxicity: CNS depressants, phenothiazines, tricyclic antidepressants may potentiate fentanyl's adverse effects

MAO Inhibitors: Not recommended to use Actiq® or Fentanyl Oralet® within 14 days. Severe and unpredictable potentiation by MAO Inhibitors has been reported with opioid analgesics.

Alcohol Interactions Avoid use (may increase central nervous system depression)

Onset Respiratory depressant effect may last longer than analgesic effect

I.M.: 7-15 minutes
I.V.: Almost immediate
Transmucosal: 5-15 minutes with a maximum reduction in activity/apprehension; Peak analgesia: Within 20-30 minutes

Duration Respiratory depressant effect may last longer than analgesic effect.

I.M.: 1-2 hours; I.V.: 0.5-1 hour; Transmucosal: Related to blood level of the drug

Half-Life 2-4 hours; Transmucosal: 6.6 hours (range: 5-15 hours)

Education and Monitoring Issues

Patient Education: Use exactly as directed; do not increase or discontinue without consulting prescriber. While using this medication, do not use alcohol and other prescription or OTC medications (especially sedatives, tranquilizers, antihistamines, or pain medications) without consulting prescriber. Maintain adequate hydration (2-3 L/day of fluids unless instructed to restrict fluid intake). May cause hypotension, dizziness, drowsiness, impaired coordination, or blurred vision (use caution when driving, climbing stairs, or changing position - rising from sitting or lying to standing, or when engaging in tasks requiring alertness until response to drug is known); nausea or vomiting (frequent mouth care, small frequent meals, chewing gum, or sucking lozenges may help); constipation (increased exercise, fluids, or dietary fruit and fiber may help - if constipation remains an unresolved problem, consult prescriber about use of stool softeners). Report acute dizziness, chest pain, slow or rapid heartbeat, acute headache; confusion or changes in mentation; changes in voiding frequency or amount, swelling of extremities, or unusual weight gain; shortness of breath or difficulty breathing; or changes in vision.

Transdermal: Apply to clean, dry skin, immediately after removing from package. Firmly press in place and hold for 20 seconds.

Dietary Considerations: Food: Glucose may cause hyperglycemia; monitor blood glucose concentrations

Monitoring Parameters: Respiratory and cardiovascular status, blood pressure, heart rate

Related Information

Droperidol and Fentanyl *on page 303*
Lipid-Lowering Agents Comparison *on page 1243*
Narcotic Agonists Comparison *on page 1244*

- **Fentanyl Oralet®** *see* Fentanyl *on page 355*
- **Feosol® [OTC]** *see* Ferrous Sulfate *on page 360*
- **Feostat® [OTC]** *see* Ferrous Fumarate *on page 359*
- **Feratab® [OTC]** *see* Ferrous Sulfate *on page 360*
- **Fergon® [OTC]** *see* Ferrous Gluconate *on page 359*
- **Fer-In-Sol** *see* Ferrous Sulfate *on page 360*
- **Fer-Iron® [OTC]** *see* Ferrous Sulfate *on page 360*
- **Fermalac®** *see Lactobacillus acidophilus* and *Lactobacillus bulgaricus on page 505*

- **Ferodan** *see* Ferrous Sulfate *on page 360*
- **Fero-Grad** *see* Ferrous Sulfate *on page 360*
- **Fero-Gradumet® [OTC]** *see* Ferrous Sulfate *on page 360*
- **Ferospace® [OTC]** *see* Ferrous Sulfate *on page 360*
- **Ferralet® [OTC]** *see* Ferrous Gluconate *on page 359*
- **Ferralyn® Lanacaps® [OTC]** *see* Ferrous Sulfate *on page 360*
- **Ferra-TD® [OTC]** *see* Ferrous Sulfate *on page 360*

Ferric Gluconate (FER ik GLOO koe nate)

Pharmacologic Class Iron Salt

U.S. Brand Names Ferrlecit®

Use Repletion of total body iron content in patients with iron deficiency anemia who are undergoing hemodialysis in conjunction with erythropoietin therapy

USUAL DOSAGE Adults:

Test dose (recommended): 2 mL diluted in 50 mL 0.9% sodium chloride over 60 minutes

Repletion of iron in hemodialysis patients: I.V.: 125 mg (10 mL) in 100 mL 0.9% sodium chloride over 1 hour during hemodialysis. Most patients will require a cumulative dose of 1 g elemental iron over approximately 8 sequential dialysis treatments to achieve a favorable response.

Contraindications Hypersensitivity to ferric gluconate, benzyl alcohol, or any component of the formulation; use in any anemia not caused by iron deficiency, heart failure (of any severity)

Pregnancy Risk Factor B

- **Ferrlecit®** *see* Ferric Gluconate *on page 359*
- **Ferro-Sequels® [OTC]** *see* Ferrous Fumarate *on page 359*

Ferrous Fumarate (FER us FYOO ma rate)

Pharmacologic Class Electrolyte Supplement, Oral

U.S. Brand Names Femiron® [OTC]; Feostat® [OTC]; Ferro-Sequels® [OTC]; Fumasorb® [OTC]; Fumerin® [OTC]; Hemocyte® [OTC]; Ircon® [OTC]; Nephro-Fer™ [OTC]; Span-FF® [OTC]

Use Prevention and treatment of iron deficiency anemias

USUAL DOSAGE Oral **(dose expressed in terms of elemental iron):**

Children:

Severe iron deficiency anemia: 4-6 mg Fe/kg/day in 3 divided doses

Mild to moderate iron deficiency anemia: 3 mg Fe/kg/day in 1-2 divided doses

Prophylaxis: 1-2 mg Fe/kg/day

Adults:

Iron deficiency: 60-100 mg twice daily up to 60 mg 2 times/day

Prophylaxis: 60-100 mg/day

To avoid GI upset, start with a single daily dose and increase by 1 tablet/day each week or as tolerated until desired daily dose is achieved

Elderly: 200 mg 3-4 times/day

Contraindications Hemochromatosis, hemolytic anemia, known hypersensitivity to iron salts

Pregnancy Risk Factor A

Ferrous Gluconate (FER us GLOO koe nate)

Pharmacologic Class Electrolyte Supplement, Oral

U.S. Brand Names Fergon® [OTC]; Ferralet® [OTC]; Simron® [OTC]

Generic Available Yes

Mechanism of Action Replaces iron found in hemoglobin, myoglobin, and enzymes; allows the transportation of oxygen via hemoglobin

Use Prevention and treatment of iron deficiency anemias

USUAL DOSAGE Oral **(dose expressed in terms of elemental iron):**

Children:

Severe iron deficiency anemia: 4-6 mg Fe/kg/day in 3 divided doses

Mild to moderate iron deficiency anemia: 3 mg Fe/kg/day in 1-2 divided doses

Prophylaxis: 1-2 mg Fe/kg/day

Adults:

Iron deficiency: 60 mg twice daily up to 60 mg 4 times/day

Prophylaxis: 60 mg/day

Dosage Forms Amount of elemental iron is listed in brackets **CAP, soft gelatin** (Simron®): 86 mg [10 mg]. **ELIX** (Fergon®): 300 mg/5 mL [34 mg/5 mL] with alcohol 7% (480 mL). **TAB:** 300 mg [34 mg], 325 mg [38 mg]; (Fergon®, Ferralet®): 320 mg [37 mg]; Sustained release (Ferralet® Slow Release): 320 mg [37 mg]

Contraindications Hemochromatosis, hemolytic anemia; known hypersensitivity to iron salts

Warnings/Precautions Administration of iron for >6 months should be avoided except in patients with continued bleeding, menorrhagia, or repeated pregnancies; avoid in patients with peptic ulcer, enteritis, or ulcerative colitis. Anemia in the elderly is often caused by

(Continued)

Ferrous Gluconate *(Continued)*

"anemia of chronic disease" or associated with inflammation rather than blood loss. Iron stores are usually normal or increased, with a serum ferritin >50 ng/mL and a decreased total iron binding capacity. Hence, the "anemia of chronic disease" is not secondary to iron deficiency but the inability of the reticuloendothelial system to reclaim available iron stores.

Pregnancy Risk Factor A

Adverse Reactions

>10%: Gastrointestinal: Stomach cramping, constipation, nausea, vomiting, dark stools

1% to 10%:

Gastrointestinal: Heartburn, diarrhea, staining of teeth

Genitourinary: Discoloration of urine

<1%: Contact irritation

Drug Interactions Absorption of oral preparation of iron and tetracyclines is decreased when both of these drugs are given together; concurrent administration of antacids may decrease iron absorption; iron may decrease absorption of penicillamine when given at the same time. Response to iron therapy may be delayed in patients receiving chloramphenicol. Concurrent administration ≥200 mg vitamin C/30 mg elemental iron increases absorption of oral iron; milk may decrease absorption of iron.

Onset Hematologic response: 3-10 days

Education and Monitoring Issues

Patient Education: May color stool black, take between meals for maximum absorption; may take with food if GI upset occurs, do not take with milk or antacids; keep out of reach of children

Reference Range: Therapeutic: Male: 75-175 μg/dL (SI: 13.4-31.3 μmol/L); Female: 65-165 μg/dL (SI: 11.6-29.5 μmol/L); serum iron level >300 μg/dL usually requires treatment of overdose due to severe toxicity

Ferrous Sulfate (FER us SUL fate)

Pharmacologic Class Electrolyte Supplement, Oral

U.S. Brand Names Feosol® [OTC]; Feratab® [OTC]; Fer-Iron® [OTC]; Fero-Gradumet® [OTC]; Ferospace® [OTC]; Ferralyn® Lanacaps® [OTC]; Ferra-TD® [OTC]; Mol-Iron® [OTC]; Slow FE® [OTC]

Generic Available Yes

Mechanism of Action Replaces iron, found in hemoglobin, myoglobin, and other enzymes; allows the transportation of oxygen via hemoglobin

Use Prevention and treatment of iron deficiency anemias

USUAL DOSAGE Oral:

Children **(dose expressed in terms of elemental iron)**:

Severe iron deficiency anemia: 4-6 mg Fe/kg/day in 3 divided doses

Mild to moderate iron deficiency anemia: 3 mg Fe/kg/day in 1-2 divided doses

Prophylaxis: 1-2 mg Fe/kg/day up to a maximum of 15 mg/day

Adults **(dose expressed in terms of ferrous sulfate)**:

Iron deficiency: 300 mg twice daily up to 300 mg 4 times/day or 250 mg (extended release) 1-2 times/day

Prophylaxis: 300 mg/day

Dosage Forms Amount of elemental iron is listed in brackets **CAP:** Exsiccated, timed release (Feosol®): 159 mg [50 mg]; Exsiccated, timed release (Ferralyn® Lanacaps®, Ferra-TD®): 250 mg [50 mg]; (Ferospace®): 250 mg [50 mg]. **DROPS, oral:** (Fer-In-Sol®): 75 mg/0.6 mL [15 mg/0.6 mL] (50 mL); (Fer-Iron®): 125 mg/mL [25 mg/mL] (50 mL). **ELIX** (Feosol®): 220 mg/5 mL [44 mg/5 mL] with alcohol 5% (473 mL, 4000 mL). **SYR** (Fer-In-Sol®): 90 mg/5 mL [18 mg/5 mL] with alcohol 5% (480 mL). **TAB:** 324 mg [65 mg]; Exsiccated (Feosol®) 200 mg [65 mg]; Exsiccated, timed release (Slow FE®): 160 mg [50 mg]; (Feratab®): 300 mg [60 mg]; (Mol-Iron®): 195 mg [39 mg]; Timed release (Fero-Gradumet®): 525 mg [105 mg]

Contraindications Hemochromatosis, hemolytic anemia; known hypersensitivity to iron salts

Warnings/Precautions Administration of iron for >6 months should be avoided except in patients with continued bleeding, menorrhagia, or repeated pregnancies; avoid in patients with peptic ulcer, enteritis, or ulcerative colitis. Anemia in the elderly is often caused by "anemia of chronic disease" or associated with inflammation rather than blood loss. Iron stores are usually normal or increased, with a serum ferritin >50 ng/mL and a decreased total iron binding capacity. Hence, the "anemia of chronic disease" is not secondary to iron deficiency but the inability of the reticuloendothelial system to reclaim available iron stores.

Pregnancy Risk Factor A

Adverse Reactions

>10%: Gastrointestinal: GI irritation, epigastric pain, nausea, dark stool, vomiting, stomach cramping, constipation

1% to 10%:

Gastrointestinal: Heartburn, diarrhea

Genitourinary: Discoloration of urine

Miscellaneous: Liquid preparations may temporarily stain the teeth

<1%: Contact irritation

Drug Interactions

Decreased effect: Absorption of oral preparation of iron and tetracyclines are decreased when both of these drugs are given together; concurrent administration of antacids may decrease iron absorption; iron may decrease absorption of penicillamine when given at the same time; response to iron therapy may be delayed in patients receiving chloramphenicol; milk may decrease absorption of iron

Increased effect: Concurrent administration ≥200 mg vitamin C per 30 mg elemental Fe increases absorption of oral iron

Onset Hematologic response: 3-10 days

Education and Monitoring Issues

Patient Education: May color stool black, take between meals for maximum absorption; may take with food if GI upset occurs, do not take with milk or antacids; keep out of reach of children

Reference Range:

Serum iron:

Male: 75-175 μg/dL (SI: 13.4-31.3 μmol/L)

Female: 65-165 μg/dL (SI: 11.6-29.5 μmol/L)

Total iron binding capacity: 230-430 μg/dL

Transferrin: 204-360 mg/dL

Percent transferrin saturation: 20% to 50%

Related Information

Ferrous Sulfate, Ascorbic Acid, Vitamin B-Complex, and Folic Acid *on page 361*

Ferrous Sulfate, Ascorbic Acid, Vitamin B-Complex, and Folic Acid

(FER us SUL fate, a SKOR bik AS id, VYE ta min bee KOM pleks, & FOE lik AS id)

Pharmacologic Class Vitamin

U.S. Brand Names Iberet-Folic-500®

Dosage Forms TAB, controlled release: Ferrous sulfate: 105 mg, Ascorbic acid: 500 mg, B_1: 6 mg, B_2: 6 mg, B_3: 30 mg, B_5: 10 mg, B_6: 5 mg, B_{12}: 25 mcg, Folic acid: 800 mcg

Pregnancy Risk Factor A

♦ **Fertinex™** *see* Follitropins *on page 391*

♦ **Fertinic®** *see* Ferrous Gluconate *on page 359*

♦ **Feverall™ [OTC]** *see* Acetaminophen *on page 17*

♦ **Feverall™ Sprinkle Caps [OTC]** *see* Acetaminophen *on page 17*

Feverfew

Pharmacologic Class Herbal

Mechanism of Action Active ingredient is parthenolide (~0.2% concentration), a sesquiterpene which is a serotonin antagonist; also, the plant may be an inhibitor of prostaglandin synthesis and platelet aggregation; has spasmolytic effect on cerebral blood vessels; other anti-inflammatory effects, antimicrobial, antifungal

Use Prophylaxis and treatment of migraine headaches; used to treat menstrual complaints and fever

USUAL DOSAGE 125 mg of a preparation standardized to 0.2% parthenolide (250 mcg) once or twice daily

Contraindications Pregnancy, breast-feeding; children <2 years of age; allergies to feverfew and other members of the Asteraceae, daisy, ragweed, chamomile

Warnings/Precautions Use with caution in patients taking medications with serotonergic properties

Adverse Reactions

>10%: Gastrointestinal: Mouth ulcerations

<10%:

Dermatologic: Contact dermatitis

Gastrointestinal: Swelling of tongue, lips, abdominal pain, nausea, vomiting, loss of taste

Post-feverfew syndrome: Nervousness, insomnia, stiff joints, headache

Drug Interactions Use with caution in patients taking aspirin or anticoagulants due to increased potential for bleeding

Fexofenadine (feks oh FEN a deen)

Pharmacologic Class Antihistamine

U.S. Brand Names Allegra®

Mechanism of Action Fexofenadine is an active metabolite of terfenadine and like terfenadine it competes with histamine for H_1-receptor sites on effector cells in the gastrointestinal tract, blood vessels and respiratory tract; it appears that fexofenadine does not cross the blood brain barrier to any appreciable degree, resulting in a reduced potential for sedation

(Continued)

Fexofenadine *(Continued)*

Use Antihistamine indicated for the relief of seasonal allergic rhinitis and chronic idiopathic urticaria

USUAL DOSAGE Oral:

Children 6-11 years: 30 mg twice daily (once daily in children with impaired renal function)

Children ≥12 years and Adults:

Seasonal allergic rhinitis: 60 mg twice daily **or** 180 mg once daily

Chronic idiopathic urticaria: 60 mg twice daily

Dosing adjustment in renal impairment: Recommended initial doses of 60 mg once daily

Dosage Forms CAP: 60 mg. **TAB:** 30 mg, 60 mg, 180 mg

Contraindications Individuals demonstrating hypersensitivity to fexofenadine or any components of its formulation

Warnings/Precautions Safety and effectiveness in pediatric patients <12 years of age has not been established. Fexofenadine is classified in FDA pregnancy category C and no data is yet available evaluating its use in breast-feeding women.

Pregnancy Risk Factor C

Adverse Reactions 1% to 10%:

Central nervous system: Drowsiness (1.3%), fatigue (1.3%)

Endocrine & metabolic: Dysmenorrhea (1.5%)

Gastrointestinal: Nausea (1.5%), dyspepsia (1.3%)

Miscellaneous: Viral infection (2.5%)

Drug Interactions CYP3A3/4 enzyme substrate

Fexofenadine levels have increased with erythromycin (82% higher) and with ketoconazole (135% higher); this has not been associated with any increased incidence of side effects

In two separate studies, fexofenadine 120 mg twice daily (high doses) was coadministered with standard doses of erythromycin or ketoconazole to healthy volunteers and although fexofenadine peak plasma concentrations increased, no differences in adverse events or QT_c intervals were observed. **It remains unknown if a similar interaction occurs with other azole antifungal agents (eg, itraconazole) or other macrolide antibiotics (eg, clarithromycin).**

Onset 1 hour

Duration Antihistaminic effect: At least 12 hours

Half-Life 14.4 hours

Education and Monitoring Issues

Patient Education: Take as directed; do not exceed recommended dose. Store at room temperature in a dry place. Avoid use of other depressants, alcohol, or sleep-inducing medications unless approved by prescriber. You may experience mild drowsiness or dizziness (use caution when driving or engaging in tasks requiring alertness until response to drug is known); or nausea (frequent small meals, frequent mouth care, chewing gum, or sucking hard candy may help). Report persistent sedation or drowsiness, menstrual irregularities, or lack of improvement or worsening of condition.

Monitoring Parameters: Relief of symptoms

Related Information

Fexofenadine and Pseudoephedrine *on page 362*

Fexofenadine and Pseudoephedrine

(feks oh FEN a deen & soo doe e FED rin)

Pharmacologic Class Antihistamine/Decongestant Combination

U.S. Brand Names Allegra-D™

Dosage Forms TAB, extended release: Fexofenadine hydrochloride 60 mg and pseudoephedrine hydrochloride 120 mg

Pregnancy Risk Factor C

- **Fiberall® Powder [OTC]** *see* Psyllium *on page 793*
- **Fiberall® Wafer [OTC]** *see* Psyllium *on page 793*
- **Fibrepur®** *see* Psyllium *on page 793*

Fibrinolysin and Desoxyribonuclease

(fye brin oh LYE sin & des oks i rye boe NOO klee ase)

Pharmacologic Class Enzyme

U.S. Brand Names Elase-Chloromycetin® Topical; Elase® Topical

Dosage Forms OINT, top: (Elase®): Fibrinolysin 1 unit and desoxyribonuclease 666.6 units per g (10 g, 30 g); (Elase-Chloromycetin®): Fibrinolysin 1 unit and desoxyribonuclease 666.6 units per g with chloramphenicol 10 mg per g (10 g, 30 g). **POWDER, dry:** Fibrinolysin 25 units and desoxyribonuclease 15,000 units per 30 g

Pregnancy Risk Factor C

Filgrastim (fil GRA stim)

Pharmacologic Class Colony Stimulating Factor

U.S. Brand Names Neupogen® Injection

Generic Available No

Mechanism of Action Stimulates the production, maturation, and activation of neutrophils, G-CSF activates neutrophils to increase both their migration and cytotoxicity

Use

Patients with nonmyeloid malignancies receiving myelosuppressive anticancer drugs associated with a significant incidence of neutropenia (FDA-approved indication)

Cancer patients receiving bone marrow transplant (BMT) (FDA-approved indication)

Patients undergoing peripheral blood progenitor cell (PBPC) collection

Patients with severe chronic neutropenia (SCN) (FDA-approved indication)

Chronic administration in symptomatic patients with congenital neutropenia, cyclic neutropenia, or idiopathic neutropenic; filgrastim should not be started until the diagnosis of SCN is confirmed, as it may interfere with diagnostic efforts

Safety and efficacy of G-CSF given simultaneously with cytotoxic chemotherapy have not been established; concurrent treatment may increase myelosuppression; G-CSF should be avoided in patients receiving concomitant chemotherapy and radiation therapy

USUAL DOSAGE Children and Adults:

Dosage should be based on actual body weight (even in morbidly obese patients)

Existing clinical data suggest that starting G-CSF between 24 and 72 hours subsequent to chemotherapy may provide optimal neutrophil recover; continue therapy until the occurrence of an absolute neutrophil count of 10,000 µL after the neutrophil nadir

The available data suggest that rounding the dose to the nearest vial size may enhance patient convenience and reduce costs without clinical detriment

Neonates: 5-10 mcg/kg/day once daily for 3-5 days has been administered to neutropenic neonates with sepsis; there was a rapid and significant increase in peripheral neutrophil counts and the neutrophil storage pool

Children and Adults:

Myelosuppressive chemotherapy S.C. or I.V. infusion: 5 mcg/kg/day

Doses may be increased in increments of 5 mcg/kg for each chemotherapy cycle, according to the duration and severity of the absolute neutrophil count (ANC) nadir

Bone marrow transplant patients: 5-10 mcg/kg/day as an I.V. infusion of 4 or 24 hours or as continuous 24-hour S.C. infusion; administer first dose at least 24 hours after cytotoxic chemotherapy and at least 24 hours after bone marrow infusion; if ANC decreases <1000/mm^3 during the 5 mcg/kg/day dose, increase filgrastim to 10 mcg/kg/day and follow the steps in the table

Filgrastim Dose Based on Neutrophil Response

Absolute Neutrophil Count	Filgrastim Dose Adjustment
When ANC >1000/mm^3 for 3 consecutive days	Reduce to 5 mcg/kg/day
If ANC remains >1000/mm^3 for 3 more consecutive days	Discontinue filgrastim
If ANC decreases to <1000/mm^3	Resume at 5 mcg/kg/day

If ANC decreases <1000/mm^3 during the 5 mcg/kg/day dose, increase filgrastim to 10 mcg/kg/day and follow the above steps in the table.

Peripheral blood progenitor cell (PBPC) collection: 10 mcg/kg/day either S.C. or a bolus or continuous I.V. infusion. It is recommended that G-CSF be given for at least 4 days before the first leukapheresis procedure and continued until the last leukapheresis; although the optimal duration of administration and leukapheresis schedule have not been established, administration of G-CSF for 6-7 days with leukaphereses on days 5,6 and 7 was found to be safe and effective; neutrophil counts should be monitored after 4 days of G-CSF, and G-CSF dose-modification should be considered for those patients who develop a white blood cell count >100,000/mm^3

Severe chronic neutropenia: S.C.:

Congenital neutropenia: 6 mcg/kg/dose twice daily

Idiopathic/cyclic neutropenia: 5 mcg/kg single dose daily

Chronic daily administration is required to maintain clinical benefit; adjust dose based on the patients' clinical course as well as ANC; in phase III studies, the target ANC was 1500-10,000/mm^3. Reduce the dose if the ANC is persistently >10,000/mm^3

Premature discontinuation of G-CSF therapy prior to the time of recovery from the expected neutrophil is generally not recommended; a transient increase in neutrophil counts is typically seen 1-2 days after initiation of therapy

Hemodialysis: Supplemental dose is not necessary

Peritoneal dialysis: Supplemental dose is not necessary

Dosage Forms INJ (preservative free): 300 mcg/mL (1 mL, 1.6 mL)

Contraindications Patients with known hypersensitivity to *E. coli*-derived proteins or G-CSF

Warnings/Precautions Complete blood count and platelet count should be obtained prior to chemotherapy. Do not use G-CSF in the period 12-24 hours before to 24 hours after administration of cytotoxic chemotherapy because of the potential sensitivity of rapidly

(Continued)

Filgrastim *(Continued)*

dividing myeloid cells to cytotoxic chemotherapy. Precaution should be exercised in the usage of G-CSF in any malignancy with myeloid characteristics. G-CSF can potentially act as a growth factor for any tumor type, particularly myeloid malignancies. Tumors of nonhematopoietic origin may have surface receptors for G-CSF.

Allergic-type reactions have occurred in patients receiving G-CSF with first or later doses. Reactions tended to occur more frequently with intravenous administration and within 30 minutes of infusion. Most cases resolved rapidly with antihistamines, steroids, bronchodilators, and/or epinephrine. Symptoms recurred in >50% of patients on rechallenge.

Pregnancy Risk Factor C

Adverse Reactions Effects are generally mild and dose related

>10%:
- Central nervous system: Neutropenic fever, fever
- Dermatologic: Alopecia
- Gastrointestinal: Nausea, vomiting, diarrhea, mucositis,
- Splenomegaly: This occurs more commonly in patients with cyclic neutropenia/congenital agranulocytosis who received S.C. injections for a prolonged (>14 days) period of time; ~33% of these patients experience subclinical splenomegaly (detected by MRI or CT scan); ~3% of these patients experience clinical splenomegaly
- Neuromuscular & skeletal: Medullary bone pain (24% incidence): This occurs most commonly in lower back pain, posterior iliac crest, and sternum and is controlled with non-narcotic analgesics

1% to 10%:
- Cardiovascular: Chest pain, fluid retention
- Central nervous system: Headache
- Dermatologic: Skin rash
- Gastrointestinal: Anorexia, stomatitis, constipation
- Hematologic: Leukocytosis
- Local: Pain at injection site
- Neuromuscular & skeletal: Weakness
- Respiratory: Dyspnea, cough, sore throat

<1%: Anaphylactic reaction pericarditis, thrombophlebitis, transient supraventricular arrhythmia

Drug Interactions Drugs which may potentiate the release of neutrophils (eg, lithium) should be used with caution

Onset Rapid elevation in neutrophil counts within the first 24 hours, reaching a plateau in 3-5 days

Duration ANC decreases by 50% within 2 days after discontinuing G-CSF; white counts return to the normal range in 4-7 days

Half-Life 1.8-3.5 hours

Education and Monitoring Issues

Patient Education: Follow directions for proper storage and administration of S.C. medication. Never reuse syringes or needles. You may experience bone pain (request analgesic); nausea or vomiting (small frequent meals may help); hair loss (reversible); or sore mouth (frequent mouth care with soft toothbrush or cotton swab may help). Report unusual fever or chills; unhealed sores; severe bone pain; pain, redness, or swelling at injection site; unusual swelling of extremities or difficulty breathing; or chest pain and palpitations.

Monitoring Parameters: CBC and platelet count should be obtained twice weekly. Leukocytosis (white blood cell counts ≥100,000/mm^3) has been observed in ~2% of patients receiving G-CSF at doses >5 mcg/kg/day. Monitor platelets and hematocrit regularly.

Reference Range: No clinical benefit seen with ANC >10,000/mm^3

Manufacturer Amgen, Inc

Related Information

Pharmaceutical Manufacturers Directory *on page 1020*
Sargramostim *on page 839*

♦ **Filibon® [OTC]** *see* Vitamins, Multiple *on page 981*

Finasteride (fi NAS teer ide)

Pharmacologic Class Antiandrogen

U.S. Brand Names Propecia®; Proscar®

Generic Available No

Mechanism of Action Finasteride is a 4-azo analog of testosterone and is a competitive inhibitor of both tissue and hepatic 5-alpha reductase. This results in inhibition of the conversion of testosterone to dihydrotestosterone and markedly suppresses serum dihydrotestosterone levels; depending on dose and duration, serum testosterone concentrations may or may not increase. Testosterone-dependent processes such as fertility, muscle strength, potency, and libido are not affected by finasteride.

Use Early data indicate that finasteride is useful in the treatment of symptomatic benign prostatic hyperplasia (BPH); male pattern baldness

Unlabeled use: Adjuvant monotherapy after radical prostatectomy in the treatment of prostatic cancer

USUAL DOSAGE Adults: Male:

Benign prostatic hyperplasia: Oral: 5 mg/day as a single dose; clinical responses occur within 12 weeks to 6 months of initiation of therapy; long-term administration is recommended for maximal response

Male pattern baldness: Oral: 1 mg daily

Dosing adjustment in renal impairment: No dosage adjustment is necessary

Dosing adjustment in hepatic impairment: Use with caution in patients with liver function abnormalities because finasteride is metabolized extensively in the liver

Dosage Forms TAB, film coated: 1 mg, 5 mg

Contraindications History of hypersensitivity to drug, pregnancy, lactation, children

Warnings/Precautions A minimum of 6 months of treatment may be necessary to determine whether an individual will respond to finasteride. Use with caution in those patients with liver function abnormalities. Carefully monitor patients with a large residual urinary volume or severely diminished urinary flow for obstructive uropathy. These patients may not be candidates for finasteride therapy.

Pregnancy Risk Factor X

Adverse Reactions 1% to 10%:

Endocrine & metabolic: Decreased libido

Genitourinary: <4% incidence of impotence, decreased volume of ejaculate

Drug Interactions CYP3A3/4 enzyme substrate

Onset Onset of clinical effect: Within 12 weeks to 6 months of ongoing therapy

Duration

After a single oral dose as small as 0.5 mg: 65% depression of plasma dihydrotestosterone levels persists 5-7 days.

After 6 months of treatment with 5 mg/day: Circulating dihydrotestosterone levels are reduced to castrate levels without significant effects on circulating testosterone. Levels return to normal within 14 days of discontinuation of treatment.

Half-Life

Half-life, serum: Parent drug: ~5-17 hours (mean: 1.9 fasting, 4.2 with breakfast)

Half-life: Adults: 6 hours (3-16); Elderly: 8 hours

Education and Monitoring Issues

Patient Education: Results of therapy may take several months. Take as directed, with fluids, 30 minutes before or 2 hours after meals. You may experience decreased libido or impotence during therapy. Report any increase in urinary volume or voiding patterns occurs.

Dietary Considerations: Food: Administration with food may delay the rate and reduce the extent of oral absorption

Monitoring Parameters: Objective and subjective signs of relief of benign prostatic hyperplasia, including improvement in urinary flow, reduction in symptoms of urgency, and relief of difficulty in micturition

Manufacturer Merck & Co

Related Information

Pharmaceutical Manufacturers Directory *on page 1020*

- **Fiorgen PF®** *see* Butalbital Compound *on page 123*
- **Fioricet®** *see* Butalbital Compound *on page 123*
- **Fiorinal®** *see* Butalbital Compound *on page 123*
- **Flagyl ER® Oral** *see* Metronidazole *on page 597*
- **Flagyl® Oral** *see* Metronidazole *on page 597*
- **Flamazine®** *see* Silver Sulfadiazine *on page 852*
- **Flarex®** *see* Fluorometholone *on page 376*
- **Flavorcee® [OTC]** *see* Ascorbic Acid *on page 72*

Flavoxate (fla VOKS ate)

Pharmacologic Class Antispasmodic Agent, Urinary

U.S. Brand Names Urispas®

Generic Available No

Mechanism of Action Synthetic antispasmodic with similar actions to that of propantheline; it exerts a direct relaxant effect on smooth muscles via phosphodiesterase inhibition, providing relief to a variety of smooth muscle spasms; it is especially useful for the treatment of bladder spasticity, whereby it produces an increase in urinary capacity

Use Antispasmodic to provide symptomatic relief of dysuria, nocturia, suprapubic pain, urgency, and incontinence due to detrusor instability and hyper-reflexia in elderly with cystitis, urethritis, urethrocystitis, urethrotrigonitis, and prostatitis

USUAL DOSAGE Children >12 years and Adults: Oral: 100-200 mg 3-4 times/day; reduce the dose when symptoms improve

Dosage Forms TAB, film coated: 100 mg

Contraindications Pyloric or duodenal obstruction, GI hemorrhage, GI obstruction; ileus; achalasia; obstructive uropathies of lower urinary tract (BPH)

(Continued)

Flavoxate *(Continued)*

Warnings/Precautions May cause drowsiness, vertigo, and ocular disturbances; administer cautiously in patients with suspected glaucoma

Pregnancy Risk Factor B

Adverse Reactions

>10%:

Central nervous system: Drowsiness

Gastrointestinal: Xerostomia, dry throat

1% to 10%:

Cardiovascular: Tachycardia, palpitations,

Central nervous system: Nervousness, fatigue, vertigo, headache, hyperpyrexia

Gastrointestinal: Constipation, nausea, vomiting

<1%: Confusion (especially in the elderly), increased intraocular pressure leukopenia, rash

Onset 55-60 minutes

Education and Monitoring Issues

Patient Education: Take exactly as directed, with water, preferably on an empty stomach (1 hour before or 2 hours after meals). Do not use alcohol or OTC medications without consulting prescriber. You may experience mild drowsiness, nervousness, or dizziness (use caution when driving or engaging in tasks requiring alertness until response to drug is known); nausea, vomiting, dry mouth (small frequent meals, frequent oral care, chewing gum, or sucking hard candy may help); decreased ability to perspire (avoid extremes of heat); constipation (increased exercise or dietary fluid and fiber may help). Report vision changes (blurred vision); rapid heartbeat; or unresolved nausea, vomiting, or constipation.

Monitoring Parameters: Monitor I & O closely

Flecainide (fle KAY nide)

Pharmacologic Class Antiarrhythmic Agent, Class I-C

U.S. Brand Names Tambocor™

Generic Available No

Mechanism of Action Class Ic antiarrhythmic; slows conduction in cardiac tissue by altering transport of ions across cell membranes; causes slight prolongation of refractory periods; decreases the rate of rise of the action potential without affecting its duration; increases electrical stimulation threshold of ventricle, HIS-Purkinje system; possesses local anesthetic and moderate negative inotropic effects

Use Prevention and suppression of documented life-threatening ventricular arrhythmias (ie, sustained ventricular tachycardia); controlling symptomatic, disabling supraventricular tachycardias in patients without structural heart disease in whom other agents fail

USUAL DOSAGE Oral:

Children:

Initial: 3 mg/kg/day or 50-100 mg/m^2/day in 3 divided doses

Usual: 3-6 mg/kg/day or 100-150 mg/m^2/day in 3 divided doses; up to 11 mg/kg/day or 200 mg/m^2/day for uncontrolled patients with subtherapeutic levels

Adults:

Life-threatening ventricular arrhythmias:

Initial: 100 mg every 12 hours

Increase by 50-100 mg/day (given in 2 doses/day) every 4 days; maximum: 400 mg/day

Use of higher initial doses and more rapid dosage adjustments have resulted in an increased incidence of proarrhythmic events and congestive heart failure, particularly during the first few days. Do not use a loading dose. Use very cautiously in patients with history of congestive heart failure or myocardial infarction.

Prevention of paroxysmal supraventricular arrhythmias in patients with disabling symptoms but no structural heart disease:

Initial: 50 mg every 12 hours

Increase by 50 mg twice daily at 4-day intervals; maximum: 300 mg/day

Dosing adjustment in severe renal impairment: Cl_{cr} <35 mL/minute: Decrease initial dose to 50 mg every 12 hours; increase doses at intervals >4 days monitoring plasma levels closely

Dialysis: Not dialyzable (0% to 5%) via hemo- or peritoneal dialysis; no supplemental dose necessary

Dosing adjustment/comments in hepatic impairment: Monitoring of plasma levels is recommended because of significantly increased half-life

When transferring from another antiarrhythmic agent, allow for 2-4 half-lives of the agent to pass before initiating flecainide therapy

Dosage Forms TAB: 50 mg, 100 mg, 150 mg

Contraindications Pre-existing second or third degree A-V block; right bundle-branch block associated with left hemiblock (bifascicular block) or trifascicular block; cardiogenic shock, myocardial depression; known hypersensitivity to the drug; concurrent use of ritonavir

Warnings/Precautions Pre-existing sinus node dysfunction, sick-sinus syndrome, history of congestive heart failure or myocardial dysfunction; increases in P-R interval ≥300 MS,

QRS ≥180 MS, QT_c interval increases, and/or new bundle-branch block; patients with pacemakers, renal impairment, and/or hepatic impairment.

The manufacturer and FDA recommend that this drug be reserved for life-threatening ventricular arrhythmias unresponsive to conventional therapy. Its use for symptomatic nonsustained ventricular tachycardia, frequent premature ventricular complexes (PVCs), uniform and multiform PVCs and/or coupled PVCs is no longer recommended. Flecainide can worsen or cause arrhythmias with an associated risk of death. Proarrhythmic effects range from an increased number of PVCs to more severe ventricular tachycardias (eg, tachycardias that are more sustained or more resistant to conversion to sinus rhythm).

Pregnancy Risk Factor C

Adverse Reactions

>10%:

- Central nervous system: Dizziness (19% to 30%)
- Ocular: Visual disturbances (16%)
- Respiratory: Dyspnea (~10%)

1% to 10%:

- Cardiovascular: Palpitations (6%), chest pain (5%), edema (3.5%), tachycardia (1% to 3%), proarrhythmic (4% to 12%), sinus node dysfunction (1.2%)
- Central nervous system: Headache (4% to 10%), fatigue (8%), nervousness (5%) additional symptoms occurring at a frequency between 1% and 3%: fever, malaise, hypoesthesia, paresis, ataxia, vertigo, syncope, somnolence, tinnitus, anxiety, insomnia, depression
- Dermatologic: Rash (1% to 3%)
- Gastrointestinal: Nausea (9%), constipation (1%), abdominal pain (3%), anorexia (1% to 3%), diarrhea (0.7% to 3%)
- Neuromuscular & skeletal: Tremor (5%), weakness (5%), paresthesias (1%)
- Ocular: Diplopia (1% to 3%), blurred vision

<1% (limited to important or life-threatening symptoms): Bradycardia, paradoxical increase in ventricular rate in atrial fibrillation/flutter, heart block, increased P-R, QRS duration, ventricular arrhythmias, congestive heart failure, flushing, A-V block, angina, hypertension, hypotension, amnesia, confusion, decreased libido, depersonalization, euphoria, apathy, nervousness, twitching, neuropathy, weakness, taste disturbance, urticaria, exfoliative dermatitis, pruritus, alopecia, flatulence, xerostomia, blood dyscrasias, possible hepatic dysfunction, paresthesia, eye pain, photophobia, bronchospasm, pneumonitis, swollen lips/tongue/mouth, arthralgia, myalgia, polyuria, urinary retention, leukopenia, granulocytopenia, thrombocytopenia, metallic taste, alters pacing threshold

Case reports: Tardive dyskinesia, corneal deposits

Drug Interactions CYP2D6 enzyme substrate

- Cimetidine may decrease flecainide's metabolism; monitor cardiac status or use an alternative H_2 antagonist
- Quinidine may decrease flecainide's metabolism; monitor cardiac status
- Digoxin's serum concentration may increase slightly
- Amiodarone increases in flecainide plasma levels; consider reducing flecainide dose by 25% to 33% with concurrent use
- Amprenavir and ritonavir may increase cardiotoxicity of flecainide (decrease metabolism)
- Propranolol (and possibly other beta-blockers) increases flecainide blood levels, and propranolol blood levels are increased with concurrent use; monitor for excessive negative inotropic effects
- Urinary alkalinizers (antacids, sodium bicarbonate, acetazolamide) may increase flecainide blood levels

Half-Life 7-22 hours, increased with congestive heart failure or renal dysfunction; End-stage renal disease: 19-26 hours

Education and Monitoring Issues

Patient Education: Take exactly as directed, around-the-clock. Do not discontinue without consulting prescriber. You will require frequent monitoring while taking this medication. You may experience lightheadedness, nervousness, dizziness, visual disturbances (use caution when driving or engaging in tasks requiring alertness until response to drug is known); or nausea, vomiting, or loss of appetite (small frequent meals may help). Report palpitations, chest pain, excessively slow or rapid heartbeat; acute nervousness, headache, or fatigue; unusual weight gain; unusual cough; difficulty breathing; swelling of hands or ankles; or muscle tremor, numbness, or weakness.

Monitoring Parameters: EKG, blood pressure, pulse, periodic serum concentrations, especially in patients with renal or hepatic impairment

Reference Range: Therapeutic: 0.2-1 μg/mL; pediatric patients may respond at the lower end of the recommended therapeutic range

Manufacturer 3M Pharmaceuticals

Related Information

Pharmaceutical Manufacturers Directory *on page 1020*

♦ **Flexaphen®** *see* Chlorzoxazone *on page 192*

♦ **Flexeril®** *see* Cyclobenzaprine *on page 234*

♦ **Flodine®** *see* Folic Acid *on page 390*

♦ **Flolan® Injection** *see* Epoprostenol *on page 319*

- **Flomax®** *see* Tamsulosin *on page 891*
- **Flonase®** *see* Fluticasone *on page 386*
- **Florical® [OTC]** *see* Calcium Carbonate *on page 130*
- **Florinef®** *see* Fludrocortisone Acetate *on page 370*
- **Florinef® Acetate** *see* Fludrocortisone Acetate *on page 370*
- **Florone®** *see* Diflorasone *on page 270*
- **Florone E®** *see* Diflorasone *on page 270*
- **Floropryl® Ophthalmic** *see* Isoflurophate *on page 487*
- **Florvite®** *see* Vitamins, Multiple *on page 981*
- **Flovent®** *see* Fluticasone *on page 386*
- **Floxin®** *see* Ofloxacin *on page 672*

Fluconazole (floo KOE na zole)

Pharmacologic Class Antifungal Agent, Oral; Antifungal Agent, Parenteral

U.S. Brand Names Diflucan®

Generic Available No

Mechanism of Action Interferes with cytochrome P-450 activity, decreasing ergosterol synthesis (principal sterol in fungal cell membrane) and inhibiting cell membrane formation

Use Indications for use in adult patients: Oral or vaginal candidiasis unresponsive to nystatin or clotrimazole; nonlife-threatening *Candida* infections (eg, cystitis, esophagitis); treatment of hepatosplenic candidiasis and other *Candida* infections in persons unable to tolerate amphotericin B; treatment of cryptococcal infections; secondary prophylaxis for cryptococcal meningitis in persons with AIDS; antifungal prophylaxis in allogeneic bone marrow transplant recipients

Oral fluconazole should be used in persons able to tolerate oral medications; parenteral fluconazole should be reserved for patients who are both unable to take oral medications and are unable to tolerate amphotericin B (eg, due to hypersensitivity or renal insufficiency)

USUAL DOSAGE The daily dose of fluconazole is the same for oral and I.V. administration

Neonates: First 2 weeks of life, especially premature neonates: Same dose as older children every 72 hours

Children: See table for once daily dosing

Fluconazole — Once-Daily Dosing (Children)

Indication	Day 1	Daily Therapy	Minimum Duration of Therapy
Oropharyngeal candidiasis	6 mg/kg	3 mg/kg	14 d
Esophageal candidiasis	6 mg/kg	3-12 mg/kg	21 d and for at least 2 wks following resolution of symptoms
Systemic candidiasis	—	6-12 mg/kg	28 d
Cryptococcal meningitis relapse	12 mg/kg 6 mg/kg	6-12 mg/kg 6 mg/kg	10-12 wk after CSF culture becomes negative

Adults: Oral, I.V.: See table for once daily dosing.

Fluconazole — Once-Daily Dosing (Adults)

Indication	Day 1	Daily Therapy	Minimum Duration of Therapy
Oropharyngeal candidiasis	200 mg	100 mg	14 d
Esophageal candidiasis	200 mg	100 mg	21 d and for at least 14 d following resolution of symptoms
Prevention of candidiasis in bone marrow transplant	400 mg	400 mg	3 d before neutropenia, 7 d after neutrophils >1000 cells/mm^3
Candidiasis UTIs, peritonitis	50-200 mg	50-200 mg	
Systemic candidiasis	400 mg	200 mg	28 d
Cryptococcal meningitis			10-12 wk after CSF culture becomes negative
acute	400 mg	200 mg	
relapse	200 mg	200 mg	
Vaginal candidiasis	150 mg	Single dose	

Dosing adjustment/interval in renal impairment:

No adjustment for vaginal candidiasis single-dose therapy

For multiple dosing, administer usual load then adjust daily doses

Cl_{cr} 11-50 mL/minute: Administer 50% of recommended dose or administer every 48 hours

Hemodialysis: One dose after each dialysis

Continuous arteriovenous or venovenous hemodiafiltration (CAVH) effects: Dose as for Cl_{cr} 10-50 mL/minute

Dosage Forms INJ: 2 mg/mL (100 mL, 200 mL). **POWDER for oral susp:** 10 mg/mL (35 mL); 40 mg/mL (35 mL). **TAB:** 50 mg, 100 mg, 150 mg, 200 mg

Contraindications Known hypersensitivity to fluconazole or other azoles; concomitant administration with terfenadine

Warnings/Precautions Should be used with caution in patients with renal and hepatic dysfunction or previous hepatotoxicity from other azole derivatives. Patients who develop abnormal liver function tests during fluconazole therapy should be monitored closely and discontinued if symptoms consistent with liver disease develop. **Should be used with caution in patients receiving cisapride or astemizole.**

Pregnancy Risk Factor C

Adverse Reactions

1% to 10%:

Central nervous system: Headache

Dermatologic: Rash

Gastrointestinal: Nausea, vomiting, abdominal pain, diarrhea

<1%: Dizziness, hypokalemia, increased AST/ALT/alkaline phosphatase, pallor

Drug Interactions CYP2C9 enzyme inducer; CYP2C9, and 2C19 enzyme inhibitor and CYP3A3/4 enzyme inhibitor (weak)

Decreased effect: Rifampin and cimetidine decrease concentrations of fluconazole; fluconazole may decrease the effect of oral contraceptives

Increased effect/toxicity:

Coadministration with terfenadine or cisapride is contraindicated; use with caution with astemizole due to increased risk of significant cardiotoxicity

Hydrochlorothiazide may decrease fluconazole clearance

Fluconazole may also inhibit warfarin, phenytoin, cyclosporine, and theophylline, zidovudine, sulfonylureas, rifabutin, and warfarin clearance

Nephrotoxicity of tacrolimus may be increased

Half-Life 25-30 hours with normal renal function

Education and Monitoring Issues

Patient Education: Take as directed, around-the-clock. Take full course of medication as ordered. Follow good hygiene measures to prevent reinfection. Frequent blood tests may be required. Maintain adequate hydration (2-3 L/day of fluids unless instructed to restrict fluid intake). You may experience headache, dizziness, drowsiness (use caution when driving or engaging in tasks that require alertness until response to drug is known); nausea, vomiting, or diarrhea (small frequent meals, frequent mouth care, sucking lozenges, or chewing gum may help). Report skin rash, redness, or irritation; persistent GI upset; urinary pattern changes; excessively dry eyes or mouth; changes in color of stool or urine.

Monitoring Parameters: Periodic liver function tests (AST, ALT, alkaline phosphatase) and renal function tests, potassium

Manufacturer Pfizer U.S. Pharmaceutical Group

Related Information

Pharmaceutical Manufacturers Directory *on page 1020*

Treatment of Sexually Transmitted Diseases *on page 1210*

Flucytosine (floo SYE toe seen)

Pharmacologic Class Antifungal Agent, Oral

U.S. Brand Names Ancobon®

Generic Available No

Mechanism of Action Penetrates fungal cells and is converted to fluorouracil which competes with uracil interfering with fungal RNA and protein synthesis

Use Adjunctive treatment of susceptible fungal infections (usually *Candida* or *Cryptococcus*); synergy with amphotericin B for certain fungal infections (*Cryptococcus* spp., *Candida* spp.)

USUAL DOSAGE Children and Adults: Oral: 50-150 mg/kg/day in divided doses every 6 hours

Dosing interval in renal impairment: Use lower initial dose:

Cl_{cr} >50 mL/minute: Administer every 12 hours

Cl_{cr} 10-50 mL/minute: Administer every 16 hours

Cl_{cr} <10 mL/minute: Administer every 24 hours

Hemodialysis: Dialyzable (50% to 100%); administer dose posthemodialysis

Peritoneal dialysis: Adults: Administer 0.5-1 g every 24 hours

Continuous arteriovenous or venovenous hemodiafiltration (CAVH) effects: Dose as for Cl_{cr} 10-50 mL/minute

Dosage Forms CAP: 250 mg, 500 mg

Contraindications Hypersensitivity to flucytosine or any component

(Continued)

Flucytosine *(Continued)*

Warnings/Precautions Use with extreme caution in patients with renal impairment, bone marrow suppression, or in patients with AIDS; dosage modification required in patients with impaired renal function

Pregnancy Risk Factor C

Adverse Reactions

1% to 10%:

Dermatologic: Rash

Gastrointestinal: Abdominal pain, diarrhea, loss of appetite, nausea, vomiting

Hematologic: Anemia, leukopenia, thrombocytopenia

Hepatic: Hepatitis, jaundice

<1%: Anaphylaxis, ataxia, bone marrow suppression, cardiac arrest, confusion, dizziness, drowsiness, elevated liver enzymes, hallucinations, headache, hearing loss, hypoglycemia, hypokalemia, paresthesia, parkinsonism, photosensitivity, psychosis, respiratory arrest, temporary growth failure

Drug Interactions Increased effect/toxicity with concurrent amphotericin administration; cytosine may inactivate flucytosine activity

Half-Life 3-8 hours; Anuria: May be as long as 200 hours; End-stage renal disease: 75-200 hours

Education and Monitoring Issues

Patient Education: Take capsules one at a time over a few minutes with food to reduce GI upset. Take full course of medication as ordered. Do not discontinue without consulting prescriber. Practice good hygiene measures to prevent reinfection. Frequent blood tests may be required. You may experience nausea and vomiting (small, frequent meals may help). Report rash, respiratory difficulty, CNS changes (eg, confusion, hallucinations, ataxia, acute headache), yellowing of skin or eyes, and changes in color of stool or urine, unresolved diarrhea or anorexia, or unusual bleeding or fatigue and weakness.

Monitoring Parameters: Serum creatinine, BUN, alkaline phosphatase, AST, ALT, CBC; serum flucytosine concentrations

Reference Range:

Therapeutic: 25-100 μg/mL (SI: 195-775 μmol/L); levels should not exceed 100-120 μg/mL to avoid toxic bone marrow depressive effects

Trough: Draw just prior to dose administration

Peak: Draw 2 hours after an oral dose administration

Fludrocortisone Acetate (floo droe KOR ti sone AS e tate)

Pharmacologic Class Corticosteroid, Oral

U.S. Brand Names Florinef® Acetate

Generic Available No

Mechanism of Action Promotes increased reabsorption of sodium and loss of potassium from renal distal tubules

Use Partial replacement therapy for primary and secondary adrenocortical insufficiency in Addison's disease; treatment of salt-losing adrenogenital syndrome

USUAL DOSAGE Oral:

Infants and Children: 0.05-0.1 mg/day

Adults: 0.1-0.2 mg/day with ranges of 0.1 mg 3 times/week to 0.2 mg/day

Addison's disease: Initial: 0.1 mg/day; if transient hypertension develops, reduce the dose to 0.05 mg/day. Preferred administration with cortisone (10-37.5 mg/day) or hydrocortisone (10-30 mg/day).

Salt-losing adrenogenital syndrome: 0.1-0.2 mg/day

Dosage Forms TAB: 0.1 mg

Contraindications Known hypersensitivity to fludrocortisone; systemic fungal infections

Warnings/Precautions Taper dose gradually when therapy is discontinued; use with caution with Addison's disease, sodium retention and potassium loss

Pregnancy Risk Factor C

Adverse Reactions 1% to 10%:

Cardiovascular: Hypertension, edema, congestive heart failure

Central nervous system: Convulsions, headache, dizziness

Dermatologic: Acne, rash, bruising

Endocrine & metabolic: Hypokalemic alkalosis, suppression of growth, hyperglycemia, HPA suppression

Gastrointestinal: Peptic ulcer

Neuromuscular & skeletal: Muscle weakness

Ocular: Cataracts

Miscellaneous: Diaphoresis

Drug Interactions Decreased effect:

Anticholinesterases effects are antagonized

Decreased corticosteroid effects by rifampin, barbiturates, and hydantoins

Decreased salicylate levels

Half-Life Plasma: 30-35 minutes; Biological: 18-36 hours

Education and Monitoring Issues

Patient Education: Take exactly as directed. Do not take more than prescribed dose and do not discontinue abruptly; consult prescriber. Take with or after meals. Take once-a-day dose with food in the morning. Limit intake of caffeine or stimulants. Maintain adequate nutrition; consult prescriber for possibility of special dietary recommendations. If diabetic, monitor serum glucose closely and notify prescriber of changes; this medication can alter glucose tolerance. Notify prescriber if you are experiencing higher than normal levels of stress; medication may need adjustment. Periodic ophthalmic examinations will be necessary with long-term use. You will be susceptible to infection; avoid crowds or infected persons or persons with contagious diseases. You may experience insomnia or nervousness; use caution when driving or engaging in tasks requiring alertness until response to drug is known. Report weakness, change in menstrual pattern, vision changes, signs of hyperglycemia, signs of infection (eg, fever, chills, mouth sores, perianal itching, vaginal discharge), other persistent side effects, or worsening of condition.

Monitoring Parameters: Monitor blood pressure and signs of edema when patient is on chronic therapy; very potent mineralocorticoid with high glucocorticoid activity; monitor serum electrolytes, serum renin activity, and blood pressure; monitor for evidence of infection

Related Information

Corticosteroids Comparison *on page 1237*

♦ **Flumadine®** *see* Rimantadine *on page 824*

Flumazenil (FLO may ze nil)

Pharmacologic Class Antidote

U.S. Brand Names Romazicon™ Injection

Generic Available No

Flumazenil

Pediatric Dosage Further studies are needed Pediatric dosage for **reversal of conscious sedation:** Intravenously through a freely running intravenous infusion into a large vein to minimize pain at the injection site	
Initial dose	0.01 mg/kg over 15 seconds (maximum dose of 0.2 mg)
Repeat doses	0.005-0.01 mg/kg (maximum dose of 0.2 mg) repeated at 1-minute intervals
Maximum total cumulative dose	1 mg
Pediatric dosage for **management of benzodiazepine overdose:** Intravenously through a freely running intravenous infusion into a large vein to minimize pain at the injection site	
Initial dose	0.01 mg/kg (maximum dose: 0.2 mg)
Repeat doses	0.01 mg/kg (maximum dose of 0.2 mg) repeated at 1-minute intervals
Maximum total cumulative dose	1 mg
In place of repeat bolus doses, follow-up continuous infusions of 0.005-0.01 mg/kg/hour have been used; further studies are needed.	
Adult Dosage Adult dosage for **reversal of conscious sedation:** Intravenously through a freely running intravenous infusion into a large vein to minimize pain at the injection site	
Initial dose	0.2 mg intravenously over 15 seconds
Repeat doses	If desired level of consciousness is not obtained, 0.2 mg may be repeated at 1-minute intervals.
Maximum total cumulative dose	1 mg (usual dose 0.6-1 mg) **In the event of resedation:** Repeat doses may be given at 20-minute intervals with maximum of 1 mg/dose and 3 mg/hour
Adult dosage for **suspected benzodiazepine overdose:** Intravenously through a freely running intravenous infusion into a large vein to minimize pain at the injection site	
Initial dose	0.2 mg intravenously over 30 seconds
Repeat doses	0.5 mg over 30 seconds repeated at 1-minute intervals
Maximum total cumulative dose	3 mg (usual dose 1-3 mg) Patients with a partial response at 3 mg may require additional titration up to a total dose of 5 mg. If a patient has not responded 5 minutes after cumulative dose of 5 mg, the major cause of sedation is not likely due to benzodiazepines. **In the event of resedation:** May repeat doses at 20-minute intervals with maximum of 1 mg/dose and 3 mg/hour

(Continued)

Flumazenil *(Continued)*

Mechanism of Action Antagonizes the effect of benzodiazepines on the GABA/benzodiazepine receptor complex. Flumazenil is benzodiazepine specific and does not antagonize other nonbenzodiazepine GABA agonists (including ethanol, barbiturates, general anesthetics); flumazenil does not reverse the effects of opiates

Use Benzodiazepine antagonist - reverses sedative effects of benzodiazepines used in general anesthesia; for management of benzodiazepine overdose; flumazenil does **not** antagonize the CNS effects of other GABA agonists (such as ethanol, barbiturates, or general anesthetics), **does not** reverse narcotics

USUAL DOSAGE See table.

Resedation: Repeated doses may be given at 20-minute intervals as needed; repeat treatment doses of 1 mg (at a rate of 0.5 mg/minute) should be given at any time and no more than 3 mg should be given in any hour. After intoxication with high doses of benzodiazepines, the duration of a single dose of flumazenil is not expected to exceed 1 hour; if desired, the period of wakefulness may be prolonged with repeated low intravenous doses of flumazenil, or by an infusion of 0.1-0.4 mg/hour. Most patients with benzodiazepine overdose will respond to a cumulative dose of 1-3 mg and doses >3 mg do not reliably produce additional effects. Rarely, patients with a partial response at 3 mg may require additional titration up to a total dose of 5 mg. **If a patient has not responded 5 minutes after receiving a cumulative dose of 5 mg, the major cause of sedation is not likely to be due to benzodiazepines.**

Dosing in renal impairment: Not significantly affected by renal failure (Cl_{cr} <10 mL/minute) or hemodialysis beginning 1 hour after drug administration

Dosing in hepatic impairment: Initial dose of flumazenil used for initial reversal of benzodiazepine effects is not changed; however, subsequent doses in liver disease patients should be reduced in size or frequency

Dosage Forms INJ: 0.1 mg/mL (5 mL, 10 mL)

Contraindications Known hypersensitivity to flumazenil or benzodiazepines; patients given benzodiazepines for control of potentially life-threatening conditions (eg, control of intracranial pressure or status epilepticus); patients who are showing signs of serious cyclic-antidepressant overdosage

Warnings/Precautions

Risk of seizures = high-risk patients:

- Patients on benzodiazepines for long-term sedation
- Tricyclic antidepressant overdose patients
- Concurrent major sedative-hypnotic drug withdrawal
- Recent therapy with repeated doses of parenteral benzodiazepines
- Myoclonic jerking or seizure activity prior to flumazenil administration

Hypoventilation: Does not reverse respiratory depression/hypoventilation or cardiac depression

Resedation: Occurs more frequently in patients where a large single dose or cumulative dose of a benzodiazepine is administered along with a neuromuscular blocking agent and multiple anesthetic agents

Flumazenil should be used with caution in the intensive care unit because of increased risk of unrecognized benzodiazepine dependence in such settings.

Pregnancy Risk Factor C

Adverse Reactions

>10%: Gastrointestinal: Vomiting, nausea

1% to 10%:

- Cardiovascular: Palpitations
- Central nervous system: Headache, anxiety, nervousness, insomnia, abnormal crying, euphoria, depression, agitation, dizziness, emotional lability, ataxia, depersonalization, increased tears, dysphoria, paranoia
- Endocrine & metabolic: Hot flashes
- Gastrointestinal: Xerostomia
- Local: Pain at injection site
- Neuromuscular & skeletal: Tremor, weakness, paresthesia
- Ocular: Abnormal vision, blurred vision
- Respiratory: Dyspnea, hyperventilation
- Miscellaneous: Diaphoresis

<1%: Abnormal hearing, arrhythmia, bradycardia, chest pain, confusion, generalized convulsions, hiccups, hypertension, shivering, somnolence, speech disorder, tachycardia, withdrawal syndrome

Drug Interactions Use with caution in overdosage involving mixed drug overdose; toxic effects may emerge (especially with cyclic antidepressants) with the reversal of the benzodiazepine effect by flumazenil

Onset 1-3 minutes; 80% response within 3 minutes; Peak effect: 6-10 minutes

Duration Resedation occurs usually within 1 hour. Duration is related to dose given and benzodiazepine plasma concentrations. Reversal effects of flumazenil may wear off before effects of benzodiazepine.

Half-Life Alpha: 7-15 minutes; Terminal: 41-79 minutes

Education and Monitoring Issues

Patient Education: Avoid driving or activities requiring alertness for 18-24 hours after drug use. Memory and judgment may be impaired for 24-48 hours. Avoid alcohol or other CNS depressants for 2-3 days after treatment.

Monitoring Parameters: Monitor patients for return of sedation or respiratory depression

Manufacturer Roche Laboratories

Related Information

Pharmaceutical Manufacturers Directory *on page 1020*

Flunisolide (floo NIS oh lide)

Pharmacologic Class Corticosteroid, Oral Inhaler; Corticosteroid, Nasal

U.S. Brand Names AeroBid®-M Oral Aerosol Inhaler; AeroBid® Oral Aerosol Inhaler; Nasalide® Nasal Aerosol; Nasarel™

Generic Available No

Mechanism of Action Decreases inflammation by suppression of migration of polymorphonuclear leukocytes and reversal of increased capillary permeability; does not depress hypothalamus

Use Steroid-dependent asthma; nasal solution is used for seasonal or perennial rhinitis

USUAL DOSAGE

Children >6 years:

Oral inhalation: 2 inhalations twice daily (morning and evening) up to 4 inhalations/day

Nasal: 1 spray each nostril twice daily (morning and evening), not to exceed 4 sprays/day each nostril

Adults:

Oral inhalation: 2 inhalations twice daily (morning and evening) up to 8 inhalations/day maximum

Nasal: 2 sprays each nostril twice daily (morning and evening); maximum dose: 8 sprays/day in each nostril

Dosage Forms INH: Nasal: (Nasalide®, Nasarel™): 25 mcg/actuation [200 sprays] (25 mL); Oral: (AeroBid®): 250 mcg/actuation [100 metered doses] (7 g), (AeroBid-M®) (menthol flavor): 250 mcg/actuation [100 metered doses] (7 g). **SOLN, spray:** 0.025% [200 actuations] (25 mL)

Contraindications Known hypersensitivity to flunisolide, acute status asthmaticus; viral, tuberculosis, fungal or bacterial respiratory infections, or infections of nasal mucosa

Warnings/Precautions Use with caution in patients with hypothyroidism, cirrhosis, hypertension, congestive heart failure, ulcerative colitis, thromboembolic disorders; do not stop medication abruptly if on prolonged therapy; fatalities have occurred due to adrenal insufficiency in asthmatic patients during and after transfer from systemic corticosteroids to aerosol steroids; several months may be required for recovery of this syndrome; during this period, aerosol steroids do **not** provide the systemic steroid needed to treat patients having trauma, surgery or infections. When consumed in excessive quantities, systemic hypercorticism and adrenal suppression may occur; withdrawal and discontinuation of the corticosteroid should be done carefully. Controlled clinical studies have shown that inhaled and intranasal corticosteroids may cause a reduction in growth velocity in pediatric patients. Growth velocity provides a means of comparing the rate of growth among children of the same age.

In studies involving inhaled corticosteroids, the average reduction in growth velocity was approximately 1 cm (about 1/3 of an inch) per year. It appears that the reduction is related to dose and how long the child takes the drug.

FDA's Pulmonary and Allergy Drugs and Metabolic and Endocrine Drugs advisory committees discussed this issue at a July 1998 meeting. They recommended that the agency develop class-wide labeling to inform healthcare providers so they would understand this potential side effect and monitor growth routinely in pediatric patients who are treated with inhaled corticosteroids, intranasal corticosteroids or both.

Long-term effects of this reduction in growth velocity on final adult height are unknown. Likewise, it also has not yet been determined whether patients' growth will "catch up" if treatment in discontinued. Drug manufacturers will continue to monitor these drugs to learn more about long-term effects. Children are prescribed inhaled corticosteroids to treat asthma. Intranasal corticosteroids are generally used to prevent and treat allergy-related nasal symptoms.

Patients are advised not to stop using their inhaled or intranasal corticosteroids without first speaking to their healthcare providers about the benefits of these drugs compared to their risks.

Pregnancy Risk Factor C

Pregnancy Implications

Clinical effects on the fetus: No data on crossing the placenta or effects on the fetus

Breast-feeding/lactation: No data on crossing into breast milk or effects on the infant

Adverse Reactions

>10%:

Cardiovascular: Pounding heartbeat

Central nervous system: Dizziness, headache, nervousness

(Continued)

Flunisolide *(Continued)*

Dermatologic: Itching, rash
Endocrine & metabolic: Adrenal suppression, menstrual problems
Gastrointestinal: GI irritation, anorexia, sore throat, bitter taste
Local: Nasal burning, *Candida* infections of the nose or pharynx, atrophic rhinitis
Respiratory: Sneezing, coughing, upper respiratory tract infection, bronchitis, nasal congestion, nasal dryness
Miscellaneous: Increased susceptibility to infections

1% to 10%:
Central nervous system: Insomnia, psychic changes
Dermatologic: Acne, urticaria
Gastrointestinal: Increase in appetite, xerostomia, dry throat, loss of taste perception
Ocular: Cataracts
Respiratory: Epistaxis
Miscellaneous: Diaphoresis, loss of smell

<1%: Abdominal fullness, bronchospasm, shortness of breath

Drug Interactions Expected interactions similar to other corticosteroids

Half-Life 1.8 hours

Education and Monitoring Issues

Patient Education: Use as directed; do not use nasal preparations for oral inhalation. Do not increase dosage or discontinue abruptly without consulting prescriber. Review use of inhaler or spray with prescriber or follow package insert for directions. Keep oral inhaler clean and unobstructed. Always rinse mouth and throat after use of inhaler to prevent opportunistic infection. If you are also using an inhaled bronchodilator, wait 10 minutes before using this steroid aerosol. You may experience dizziness, anxiety, or blurred vision (rise slowly from sitting or lying position and use caution when driving or engaging in tasks requiring alertness until response to drug is known); or taste disturbance or aftertaste (frequent mouth care and mouth rinses may help). Report pounding heartbeat or chest pain; acute nervousness or inability to sleep; severe sneezing or nosebleed; difficulty breathing, sore throat, hoarseness, or bronchitis; respiratory difficulty or bronchospasms; disturbed menstrual pattern; vision changes; loss of taste or smell perception; or worsening of condition or lack of improvement.

Related Information

Asthma Guidelines *on page 1077*

Fluocinolone (floo oh SIN oh lone)

Pharmacologic Class Corticosteroid, Topical

U.S. Brand Names Derma-Smoothe/FS®; Fluonid®; Flurosyn®; FS Shampoo®; Synalar®; Synalar-HP®; Synemol®

Generic Available Yes

Mechanism of Action A synthetic corticosteroid which differs structurally from triamcinolone acetonide in the presence of an additional fluorine atom in the 6-alpha position on the steroid nucleus. The mechanism of action for all topical corticosteroids is not well defined, however, is believed to be a combination of three important properties: anti-inflammatory activity, immunosuppressive properties, and antiproliferative actions.

Use Relief of susceptible inflammatory dermatosis [low, medium, high potency topical corticosteroid]

USUAL DOSAGE Children and Adults: Topical: Apply a thin layer to affected area 2-4 times/day. Therapy should be discontinued when control is achieved; if no improvement is seen, reassessment of diagnosis may be necessary.

Dosage Forms CRM, top: 0.01% (15 g, 60 g); 0.025% (15 g, 60 g); (Flurosyn®, Synalar®): 0.01% (15 g, 30 g, 60 g, 425 g); (Flurosyn®, Synalar®, Synemol®): 0.025% (15 g, 60 g, 425 g); (Synalar-HP®): 0.2% (12 g). **OINT, top:** 0.025% (15 g, 60 g); (Flurosyn®, Synalar®): 0.025% (15 g, 30 g, 60 g, 425 g). **OIL** (Derma-Smoothe/FS®): 0.01% (120 mL). **SHAMP** (FS Shampoo®): 0.01% (180 mL). **SOLN, top:** 0.01% (20 mL, 60 mL); (Fluonid®, Synalar®): 0.01% (20 mL, 60 mL)

Contraindications Fungal infection, hypersensitivity to fluocinolone or any component, TB of skin, herpes (including varicella)

Warnings/Precautions Adverse systemic effects may occur when used on large areas of the body, denuded areas, for prolonged periods of time, with an occlusive dressing, and/or in infants or small children. Infants and small children may be more susceptible to adrenal axis suppression from topical corticosteroid therapy.

Pregnancy Risk Factor C

Adverse Reactions <1%: Acne, allergic dermatitis, burning, Cushing's syndrome, dry skin, folliculitis, growth retardation, HPA suppression, hypertrichosis, hypopigmentation, irritation, itching, maceration of the skin, secondary infection, skin atrophy

Education and Monitoring Issues

Patient Education: A thin film of cream or ointment is effective; do not overuse; do not use tight-fitting diapers or plastic pants on children being treated in the diaper area; use only as prescribed, and for no longer than the period prescribed; apply sparingly in light film; rub in lightly; avoid contact with eyes; notify prescriber if condition being treated persists or worsens

Fluocinonide (floo oh SIN oh nide)

Pharmacologic Class Corticosteroid, Topical

U.S. Brand Names Fluonex®; Lidex®; Lidex-E®

Generic Available Yes

Mechanism of Action Fluorinated topical corticosteroid considered to be of high potency. The mechanism of action for all topical corticosteroids is not well defined, however, is felt to be a combination of three important properties: anti-inflammatory activity, immunosuppressive properties, and antiproliferative actions.

Use Anti-inflammatory, antipruritic, relief of inflammatory and pruritic manifestations [high potency topical corticosteroid]

USUAL DOSAGE Children and Adults: Topical: Apply thin layer to affected area 2-4 times/day depending on the severity of the condition. Therapy should be discontinued when control is achieved; if no improvement is seen, reassessment of diagnosis may be necessary.

Dosage Forms **CRM:** 0.05% (15 g, 30 g, 60 g, 120 g); Anhydrous, emollient (Lidex®): 0.05% (15 g, 30 g, 60 g, 120 g); Aqueous, emollient (Lidex-E®): 0.05% (15 g, 30 g, 60 g, 120 g). **GEL, top:** 0.05% (15 g, 60 g); (Lidex®): 0.05% (15 g, 30 g, 60 g, 120 g). **OINT, top:** 0.05% (15 g, 30 g, 60 g); (Lidex®): 0.05% (15 g, 30 g, 60 g, 120 g). **SOLN, top:** 0.05% (20 mL, 60 mL); (Lidex®): 0.05% (20 mL, 60 mL)

Contraindications Viral, fungal, or tubercular skin lesions, herpes simplex, known hypersensitivity to fluocinonide

Warnings/Precautions Adverse systemic effects may occur when used on large areas of the body, denuded areas, for prolonged periods of time, with an occlusive dressing, and/or in infants or small children

Pregnancy Risk Factor C

Adverse Reactions <1%: Acne, allergic dermatitis, burning, Cushing's syndrome, dry skin, folliculitis, growth retardation, HPA suppression, hypertrichosis, hypopigmentation, intracranial hypertension, irritation, itching, maceration of the skin, secondary infection, skin atrophy

Education and Monitoring Issues

Patient Education: Do not use tight-fitting diapers or plastic pants on children being treated in the diaper area; use only as prescribed, and for no longer than the period prescribed; apply sparingly in a light film; rub in lightly; notify prescriber if condition being treated persists or worsens; avoid contact with eyes

♦ **Fluoderm** *see* Fluocinolone *on page 374*

♦ **Fluonex®** *see* Fluocinonide *on page 375*

♦ **Fluonid®** *see* Fluocinolone *on page 374*

♦ **Fluonide** *see* Fluocinolone *on page 374*

♦ **Fluoracaine® Ophthalmic** *see* Proparacaine and Fluorescein *on page 783*

Fluorescein Sodium (FLURE e seen SOW dee um)

Pharmacologic Class Diagnostic Agent

U.S. Brand Names AK-Fluor; Fluorescite®; Fluorets®; Fluor-I-Strip®; Fluor-I-Strip-AT®; Fluress®; Ful-Glo®; Funduscein®; Ophthifluor®

Use Demonstrates defects of corneal epithelium; diagnostic aid in ophthalmic angiography

USUAL DOSAGE

Ophthalmic:

Solution: Instill 1-2 drops of 2% solution and allow a few seconds for staining; wash out excess with sterile water or irrigating solution

Strips: Moisten strip with sterile water. Place moistened strip at the fornix into the lower cul-de-sac close to the punctum. For best results, patient should close lid tightly over strip until desired amount of staining is obtained. Patient should blink several times after application.

Removal of foreign bodies, sutures or tonometry (Fluress®): Instill 1 or 2 drops (single instillations) into each eye before operating

Deep ophthalmic anesthesia (Fluress®): Instill 2 drops into each eye every 90 seconds up to 3 doses

Injection: Prior to use, perform intradermal skin test; have epinephrine 1:1000, an antihistamine, and oxygen available

Children: 3.5 mg/lb (7.5 mg/kg) injected rapidly into antecubital vein

Adults: 500-750 mg injected rapidly into antecubital vein

Contraindications Hypersensitivity to fluorescein or any other component of the product; do not use with soft contact lenses, as this will cause them to discolor; pregnancy with parenteral product

Pregnancy Risk Factor C (topical); X (parenteral)

♦ **Fluorescite®** *see* Fluorescein Sodium *on page 375*

♦ **Fluorets®** *see* Fluorescein Sodium *on page 375*

Fluoride (FLOR ide)

Pharmacologic Class Mineral, Oral

U.S. Brand Names ACT® [OTC]; Fluorigard® [OTC]; Fluorinse®; Fluoritab®; Flura®; Flura-Drops®; Flura-Loz®; Gel Kam®; Gel-Tin® [OTC]; Karidium®; Karigel®; Karigel®-N; Listermint® with Fluoride [OTC]; Luride®; Luride® Lozi-Tab®; Luride®-SF Lozi-Tab®; Minute-Gel®; Pediaflor®; Pharmaflur®; Phos-Flur®; Point-Two®; PreviDent®; Stop® [OTC]; Thera-Flur®; Thera-Flur-N®

Use Prevention of dental caries

USUAL DOSAGE Oral:

Recommended daily fluoride supplement (2.2 mg of sodium fluoride is equivalent to 1 mg of fluoride ion): See table.

Fluoride Ion

Fluoride Content of Drinking Water	Daily Dose, Oral (mg)
<0.3 ppm	
Birth - 6 mo	0
6 mo - 3 y	0.25
3-6 y	0.5
6-16 y	1
0.3-0.6 ppm	
Birth - 3 y	0
3-6 y	0.25
6-16 y	0.5
>0.6 ppm	
All ages	0

Adapted from *AAP News*, 1995, 11(2):18.

Dental rinse or gel:

Children 6-12 years: 5-10 mL rinse or apply to teeth and spit daily after brushing

Adults: 10 mL rinse or apply to teeth and spit daily after brushing

Contraindications Hypersensitivity to fluoride, tartrazine, or any component; when fluoride content of drinking water exceeds 0.7 ppm; low sodium or sodium-free diets; do not use 1 mg tablets in children <3 years of age or when drinking water fluoride content is ≥0.3 ppm; do not use 1 mg/5 mL rinse (as supplement) in children <6 years of age

Pregnancy Risk Factor C

♦ **Fluorigard® [OTC]** *see* Fluoride *on page 376*

♦ **Fluori-Methane® Topical Spray** *see* Dichlorodifluoromethane and Trichloromonofluoromethane *on page 263*

♦ **Fluorinse®** *see* Fluoride *on page 376*

♦ **Fluor-I-Strip®** *see* Fluorescein Sodium *on page 375*

♦ **Fluor-I-Strip-AT®** *see* Fluorescein Sodium *on page 375*

♦ **Fluoritab®** *see* Fluoride *on page 376*

Fluorometholone (flure oh METH oh lone)

Pharmacologic Class Corticosteroid, Ophthalmic; Corticosteroid, Topical

U.S. Brand Names Flarex®; Fluor-Op®; FML®; FML® Forte

Use Inflammatory conditions of the eye, including keratitis, iritis, cyclitis, and conjunctivitis

USUAL DOSAGE Children >2 years and Adults: Ophthalmic:

Ointment: May be applied every 4 hours in severe cases; 1-3 times/day in mild to moderate cases

Solution: Instill 1-2 drops into conjunctival sac every hour during day, every 2 hours at night until favorable response is obtained, then use 1 drop every 4 hours; for mild to moderate inflammation, instill 1-2 drops into conjunctival sac 2-4 times/day

Contraindications Herpes simplex, keratitis, fungal diseases of ocular structures, most viral diseases, hypersensitivity to any component

Pregnancy Risk Factor C

Related Information

Sulfacetamide Sodium and Fluorometholone *on page 876*

♦ **Fluor-Op®** *see* Fluorometholone *on page 376*

♦ **Fluoroplex® Topical** *see* Fluorouracil *on page 376*

Fluorouracil (flure oh YOOR a sil)

Pharmacologic Class Antineoplastic Agent, Antimetabolite

U.S. Brand Names Adrucil® Injection; Efudex® Topical; Fluoroplex® Topical

Generic Available Yes: Injection

Mechanism of Action A pyrimidine antimetabolite that interferes with DNA synthesis by blocking the methylation of deoxyuridylic acid; 5-FU rapidly enters the cell and is activated to the nucleotide level; there it inhibits thymidylate synthetase (TS), or is incorporated into RNA (most evident during the GI phase of the cell cycle). The reduced folate cofactor is required for tight binding to occur between the 5-FdUMP and TS.

Use Treatment of carcinoma of stomach, colon, rectum, breast, and pancreas; also used topically for management of multiple actinic keratoses and superficial basal cell carcinomas

USUAL DOSAGE Refer to individual protocols

All dosages are based on the patient's actual weight. However, the estimated lean body mass (dry weight) is used if the patient is obese or if there has been a spurious weight gain due to edema, ascites, or other forms of abnormal fluid retention.

Children and Adults:

Intra-arterial:

250-1000 mg/day

15-30 mg/kg for 4-17 days, then 15 mg/kg I.V. weekly

10 mg/kg day

I.V.: Initial: 400-500 mg/m²/day (12 mg/kg/day; maximum: 800 mg/day) for 4-5 days either as a single daily I.V. push or 4-day CIV

I.V.: Maintenance dose regimens:

200-250 mg/m² (6 mg/kg) every other day for 4 days repeated in 4 weeks

500-600 mg/m² (15 mg/kg) weekly as a CIV or I.V. push

I.V.: Concomitant with leucovorin:

370 mg/m²/day x 5 days

500-1000 mg/m² every 2 weeks

600 mg/m² weekly for 6 weeks

Although the manufacturer recommends no daily dose >800 mg, higher doses of up to 2 g/day are routinely administered by CIV; higher daily doses have been successfully used

Hemodialysis: Administer dose posthemodialysis

Dosing adjustment/comments in hepatic impairment: Bilirubin >5 mg/dL: Omit use

Topical:

Actinic or solar keratosis: Apply twice daily for 2-6 weeks

Superficial basal cell carcinomas: Apply 5% twice daily for at least 3-6 weeks and up to 10-12 weeks

Dosage Forms CRM, top: (Efudex®): 5% (25 g); (Fluoroplex®): 1% (30 g). **INJ** (Adrucil®): 50 mg/mL (10 mL, 20 mL, 50 mL, 100 mL). **SOLN, top:** (Efudex®): 2% (10 mL), 5% (10 mL); (Fluoroplex®): 1% (30 mL)

Contraindications Hypersensitivity to fluorouracil or any component, poor nutritional status, bone marrow depression, or potentially serious infections; pregnancy with topical product

Warnings/Precautions The U.S. Food and Drug Administration (FDA) currently recommends that procedures for proper handling and disposal of antineoplastic agents be considered. Use with caution in patients with impaired kidney or liver function. The drug should be discontinued if intractable vomiting or diarrhea, precipitous falls in leukocyte or platelet counts, stomatitis, hemorrhage, or myocardial ischemia occurs. Use with caution in patients who have had high-dose pelvic radiation or previous use of alkylating agents. Patient should be hospitalized during initial course of therapy.

Pregnancy Risk Factor D (injection); X (topical)

Adverse Reactions Toxicity depends on route and duration of infusion

>10%:

Dermatologic: Dermatitis, pruritic maculopapular rash, alopecia

Irritant chemotherapy

Gastrointestinal (route and schedule dependent): Heartburn, nausea, vomiting, anorexia, stomatitis, esophagitis, anorexia, stomatitis, and diarrhea; bolus dosing produces milder GI problems, while continuous infusion tends to produce severe mucositis and diarrhea; vomiting is moderate, occurring in 30% to 60% of patients, and responds well to phenothiazines and dexamethasone

Emetic potential:

<1000 mg: Moderately low (10% to 30%)

≥1000 mg: Moderate (30% to 60%)

Hematologic: Myelosuppressive: Granulocytopenia occurs around 9-14 days after 5-FU and thrombocytopenia around 7-17 days. The marrow recovers after 22 days. Myelosuppression tends to be more pronounced in patients receiving bolus dosing of 5-FU.

WBC: Moderate

Platelets: Mild to moderate

Onset (days): 7-10

Nadir (days): 14

Recovery (days): 21

1% to 10%:

Dermatologic: Dry skin

Gastrointestinal: GI ulceration

<1%: Chest pain, hypotension, EKG changes similar to ischemic changes, and possibly cardiac enzyme abnormalities. Usually occurs within the first two days of therapy, and

(Continued)

Fluorouracil *(Continued)*

may resolve with nitroglycerin and calcium channel blockers. May be due to coronary vessel vasospasm induced by 5-FU.

Cerebellar ataxia, headache, somnolence, ataxia are seen primarily in intracarotid arterial infusions for head and neck tumors. This is believed to be caused by fluorocitrate, a neurotoxic metabolite of the parent compound.

Pruritic maculopapular rash, alopecia, hyperpigmentation of nailbeds, face, hands, and veins used in infusion; photosensitization with UV light; palmar-plantar syndrome (hand-foot syndrome); coagulopathy, hepatotoxicity, conjunctivitis, tear duct stenosis, excessive lacrimation, visual disturbances, shortness of breath

Drug Interactions

Methotrexate: This interaction is schedule dependent; **5-FU should be given following MTX, not prior to**

If MTX is given first: The cells exposed to MTX before 5-FU have a depleted reduced folate pool which inhibits the binding of the 5dUMP to TS. However, it does not interfere with FUTP incorporation into RNA. Polyglutamines, which accumulate in the presence of MTX may be substituted for the folates and allow binding of FdUMP to TS. MTX given prior to 5-FU may actually activate 5-FU due to MTX inhibition of purine synthesis.

If 5-FU is given first: 5-FU inhibits the TS binding and thus the reduced folate pool is not depleted, thereby negating the effect of MTX

Increased effect: Leucovorin: ↑ the folate pool and in certain tumors, may promote TS inhibition and ↑ 5-FU activity. Must be given before or with the 5-FU to prime the cells; it is not used as a rescue agent in this case.

Increased toxicity:

Allopurinol: Inhibits thymidine phosphorylase (an enzyme that activates 5-FU). The antitumor effect of 5-FU appears to be unaltered, but decreases toxicity

Cimetidine: Results in increased plasma levels of 5-FU due to drug metabolism inhibition and reduction of liver blood flow induced by cimetidine

Duration ~3 weeks

Half-Life Biphasic: Initial: 6-20 minutes; doses of 400-600 mg/m^2 produce drug concentrations above the threshold for cytotoxicity for normal tissue and remain there for 6 hours; two metabolites, FdUMP and FUTP, have prolonged half-lives depending on the type of tissue; the clinical effect of these metabolites has not been determined

Education and Monitoring Issues

Patient Education: Avoid alcohol and all OTC drugs unless approved by your oncologist. Maintain adequate hydration (2-3 L/day of fluids unless instructed to restrict fluid intake) and nutrition (small frequent meals may help). You may experience sensitivity to sunlight (use sunblock, wear protective clothing, or avoid direct sunlight); susceptibility to infection (avoid crowds or infected persons or persons with contagious diseases); nausea, vomiting, diarrhea, or loss of appetite (frequent small meals may help - request medication); weakness, lethargy, dizziness, decreased vision (use caution when driving or engaging in tasks requiring alertness until response to drug is known); headache (request medication). Report signs and symptoms of infection (eg, fever, chills, sore throat, burning urination, vaginal itching or discharge, fatigue, mouth sores); bleeding (eg, black or tarry stools, easy bruising, unusual bleeding); vision changes; unremitting nausea, vomiting, or abdominal pain; CNS changes; respiratory difficulty; chest pain or palpitations; severe skin reactions to topical application; or any other adverse reactions.

Topical: Use as directed; do not overuse. Wash hands thoroughly before and after applying medication. Avoid contact with eyes and mouth. Avoid occlusive dressings; use a porous dressing. May cause local reaction (pain, burning, or swelling); if severe contact prescriber.

Monitoring Parameters: CBC with differential and platelet count, renal function tests, liver function tests

Fluoxetine (floo OKS e teen)

Pharmacologic Class Antidepressant, Selective Serotonin Reuptake Inhibitor

U.S. Brand Names Prozac®

Generic Available No

Mechanism of Action Inhibits CNS neuron serotonin uptake; minimal or no effect on reuptake of norepinephrine or dopamine; does not significantly bind to alpha-adrenergic, histamine or cholinergic receptors; may therefore be useful in patients at risk from sedation, hypotension, and anticholinergic effects of tricyclic antidepressants

Use Treatment of major depression; treatment of binge-eating and vomiting in patients with moderate-to-severe bulimia nervosa; obsessive-compulsive disorder

USUAL DOSAGE Oral:

Children <18 years: Dose and safety not established; preliminary experience in children 6-14 years using initial doses of 20 mg/day have been reported

Adults: 20 mg/day in the morning; may increase after several weeks by 20 mg/day increments; maximum: 80 mg/day; doses >20 mg should be divided into morning and noon doses

Usual dosage range:
20-80 mg/day for depression and OCD
20-60 mg/day for obesity
60-80 mg/day for bulimia nervosa
Note: Lower doses of 5 mg/day have been used for initial treatment

Elderly: Some patients may require an initial dose of 10 mg/day with dosage increases of 10 and 20 mg every several weeks as tolerated; should not be taken at night unless patient experiences sedation

Dosing adjustment in renal impairment:
Single dose studies: Pharmacokinetics of fluoxetine and norfluoxetine were similar among subjects with all levels of impaired renal function, including anephric patients on chronic hemodialysis
Chronic administration: Additional accumulation of fluoxetine or norfluoxetine may occur in patients with severely impaired renal function

Hemodialysis: Not removed by hemodialysis

Dosing adjustment in hepatic impairment: Elimination half-life of fluoxetine is prolonged in patients with hepatic impairment; a lower or less frequent dose of fluoxetine should be used in these patients
Cirrhosis patients: Administer a lower dose or less frequent dosing interval
Compensated cirrhosis without ascites: Administer 50% of normal dose

Dosage Forms CAP: 10 mg, 20 mg, 40 mg. **LIQ** (mint flavor): 20 mg/5 mL (120 mL). **TAB:** 10 mg

Contraindications Hypersensitivity to fluoxetine; patients receiving MAO inhibitors currently or in past 2 weeks

Warnings/Precautions Use with caution in patients with hepatic impairment, history of seizures; MAO inhibitors should be discontinued at least 14 days before initiating fluoxetine therapy; add or initiate other antidepressants with caution for up to 5 weeks after stopping fluoxetine

Pregnancy Risk Factor C

Adverse Reactions Predominant adverse effects are CNS and GI

>10%:
Central nervous system: Headache, nervousness, insomnia, drowsiness
Gastrointestinal: Nausea, diarrhea, xerostomia

1% to 10%:
Central nervous system: Anxiety, dizziness, fatigue, sedation
Dermatologic: Rash, pruritus
Endocrine & metabolic: SIADH, hypoglycemia, hyponatremia (elderly or volume-depleted patients)
Gastrointestinal: Anorexia, dyspepsia, constipation
Neuromuscular & skeletal: Tremor
Miscellaneous: Diaphoresis (excessive)

<1%: Allergies, anaphylactoid reactions, erythema nodosum, extrapyramidal reactions (rare), suicidal ideation, visual disturbances

Drug Interactions CYP2D6 enzyme substrate (minor), CYP2C enzyme substrate (minor), CYP3A3/4 enzyme substrate; CYP2C9 enzyme inducer; CYP1A2, 2C9, 2C19, 2D6, and 3A3/4 enzyme inhibitor

Increased effect with tricyclics (2 times increased plasma level)
Increased/decreased effect of lithium (both increased and decreased levels have been reported)
Increased toxicity of diazepam, trazodone via decreased clearance; increased toxicity with MAO inhibitors (hyperpyrexia, tremors, seizures, delirium, coma)
May displace highly protein bound drugs (warfarin)
Selective serotonin reuptake inhibitors have been reported, rarely, to cause weakness, hyper-reflexia, and incoordination when coadministered with sumatriptan. If concomitant treatment with sumatriptan and an SSRI is clinically warranted, appropriate observation of the patient is advised.

Alcohol Interactions Avoid use. Although alcohol may not cause much central nervous depression here, depressed patients should avoid/limit intake.

Onset >2-4 weeks for therapeutic effects

Half-Life 2-3 days; due to long half-life, resolution of adverse reactions after discontinuation may be slow

Education and Monitoring Issues

Patient Education: Take exactly as directed (do not increase dose or frequency); may take 2-3 weeks to achieve desired results; may cause physical and/or psychological dependence. Take once-a-day dose in the morning to reduce incidence of insomnia. Avoid excessive alcohol, caffeine, and other prescription or OTC medications not approved by prescriber. Maintain adequate hydration (2-3 L/day of fluids unless instructed to restrict fluid intake). You may experience drowsiness, lightheadedness, impaired coordination, dizziness, or blurred vision (use caution when driving or engaging in tasks requiring alertness until response to drug is known); constipation (increased exercise, fluids, or dietary fruit and fiber may help); anorexia (maintain regular dietary intake to avoid excessive weight loss); or postural hypotension (use caution when climbing stairs or changing position from lying or sitting to standing). If

(Continued)

Fluoxetine *(Continued)*

diabetic, monitor serum glucose closely (may cause hypoglycemia). Report persistent CNS effects (nervousness, restlessness, insomnia, anxiety, excitation, headache, sedation); rash or skin irritation; muscle cramping, tremors, or change in gait; respiratory depression or difficulty breathing; or worsening of condition.

Reference Range: Therapeutic levels have not been well established

Therapeutic: Fluoxetine: 100-800 ng/mL (SI: 289-2314 nmol/L); Norfluoxetine: 100-600 ng/mL (SI: 289-1735 nmol/L)

Toxic: Fluoxetine plus norfluoxetine: >2000 ng/mL

Manufacturer Eli Lilly and Co

Related Information

Antidepressant Agents Comparison *on page 1231*

Pharmaceutical Manufacturers Directory *on page 1020*

Fluoxymesterone (floo oks i MES te rone)

Pharmacologic Class Androgen

U.S. Brand Names Halotestin®

Generic Available Yes

Mechanism of Action Synthetic androgenic anabolic hormone responsible for the normal growth and development of male sex hormones and development of male sex organs and maintenance of secondary sex characteristics; synthetic testosterone derivative with significant androgen activity; stimulates RNA polymerase activity resulting in an increase in protein production; increases bone development

Use Replacement of endogenous testicular hormone; in females, used as palliative treatment of breast cancer; stimulation of erythropoiesis, angioneurotic edema, postpartum breast engorgement

USUAL DOSAGE Adults: Oral:

Male:

Hypogonadism: 5-20 mg/day

Delayed puberty: 2.5-20 mg/day for 4-6 months

Female:

Inoperable breast carcinoma: 10-40 mg/day in divided doses for 1-3 months

Breast engorgement: 2.5 mg after delivery, 5-10 mg/day in divided doses for 4-5 days

Dosage Forms TAB: 2 mg, 5 mg, 10 mg

Contraindications Serious cardiac disease, liver or kidney disease, hypersensitivity to fluoxymesterone or any component; pregnancy

Warnings/Precautions May accelerate bone maturation without producing compensatory gain in linear growth in children; in prepubertal children perform radiographic examination of the hand and wrist every 6 months to determine the rate of bone maturation and to assess the effect of treatment on the epiphyseal centers

Pregnancy Risk Factor X

Adverse Reactions

>10%:

Males: Priapism

Females: Menstrual problems (amenorrhea), virilism, breast soreness

Cardiovascular: Edema

Dermatologic: Acne

1% to 10%:

Males: Prostatic carcinoma, hirsutism (increase in pubic hair growth), impotence, testicular atrophy

Cardiovascular: Edema

Gastrointestinal: GI irritation, nausea, vomiting

Genitourinary: Prostatic hypertrophy

Hepatic: Hepatic dysfunction

<1%:

Males: Gynecomastia

Females: Amenorrhea

Cholestatic hepatitis, hepatic necrosis, hypercalcemia, hypersensitivity reactions, leukopenia, polycythemia

Drug Interactions

Decreased effect:

Fluphenazine effectiveness with anticholinergics

Barbiturate levels and decreased fluphenazine effectiveness when given together

Increased toxicity:

Anticoagulants: Fluoxymesterone may suppress clotting factors II, V, VII, and X; therefore, bleeding may occur in patients on anticoagulant therapy

Cyclosporine: May elevate cyclosporine serum levels

Insulin: May enhance hypoglycemic effect of insulin therapy

May decrease blood glucose concentrations and insulin requirements in patients with diabetes

With ethanol, effects of both drugs may increase

EPSEs and other CNS effects may increase when coadministered with lithium

May potentiate the effects of narcotics including respiratory depression

Half-Life 10-100 minutes

Education and Monitoring Issues

Patient Education: Take as directed; do not discontinue without consulting prescriber. Diabetics should monitor serum glucose closely and notify prescriber of changes; this medication can alter glucose tolerance. You may experience acne, growth of body hair, loss of libido, impotence, or menstrual irregularity (usually reversible); nausea or vomiting (small frequent meals, frequent mouth care, sucking lozenges, or chewing gum may help). Report changes in menstrual pattern; deepening of voice or unusual growth of body hair; fluid retention (swelling of ankles, feet, or hands, difficulty breathing, or sudden weight gain); change in color of urine or stool; yellowing of eyes or skin; unusual bruising or bleeding; or other adverse reactions.

Monitoring Parameters: In prepubertal children, perform radiographic examination of the head and wrist every 6 months

Fluphenazine (floo FEN a zeen)

Pharmacologic Class Antipsychotic Agent, Phenothazine, Piperazine

U.S. Brand Names Permitil® Oral; Prolixin Decanoate® Injection; Prolixin Enanthate® Injection; Prolixin® Injection; Prolixin® Oral

Generic Available Yes

Mechanism of Action Blocks postsynaptic mesolimbic dopaminergic D_1 and D_2 receptors in the brain; exhibits a strong alpha-adrenergic blocking and anticholinergic effect, depresses the release of hypothalamic and hypophyseal hormones; believed to depress the reticular activating system thus affecting basal metabolism, body temperature, wakefulness, vasomotor tone, and emesis

Use Management of manifestations of psychotic disorders

USUAL DOSAGE Adults:

Oral: 0.5-10 mg/day in divided doses at 6- to 8-hour intervals; some patients may require up to 40 mg/day

I.M.: 2.5-10 mg/day in divided doses at 6- to 8-hour intervals (parenteral dose is $^1/_3$ to $^1/_2$ the oral dose for the hydrochloride salts)

I.M., S.C. (decanoate): 12.5 mg every 3 weeks

Conversion from hydrochloride to decanoate I.M. 0.5 mL (12.5 mg) decanoate every 3 weeks is approximately equivalent to 10 mg hydrochloride/day

I.M., S.C. (enanthate): 12.5-25 mg every 3 weeks

Hemodialysis: Not dialyzable (0% to 5%)

Dosage Forms

Fluphenazine decanoate: **INJ:** Prolixin Decanoate®: 25 mg/mL (1 mL, 5 mL)

Fluphenazine enanthate: **INJ:** Prolixin Enanthate®: 25 mg/mL (5 mL)

Fluphenazine hydrochloride: **CONC, oral:** (Permitil®): 5 mg/mL with alcohol 1% (118 mL); (Prolixin®): 5 mg/mL with alcohol 14% (120 mL). **ELIX** (Prolixin®): 2.5 mg/5 mL with alcohol 14% (60 mL, 473 mL). **INJ:** (Prolixin®): 2.5 mg/mL (10 mL). **TAB:** (Permitil®): 2.5 mg, 5 mg, 10 mg; (Prolixin®): 1 mg, 2.5 mg, 5 mg, 10 mg

Contraindications Hypersensitivity to fluphenazine or any component, cross-sensitivity with other phenothiazines may exist; avoid use in patients with narrow-angle glaucoma

Warnings/Precautions Safety in children <6 months of age has not been established; use with caution in patients with cardiovascular disease or seizures; benefits of therapy must be weighed against risks of therapy; adverse effects may be of longer duration with Depot® form; watch for hypotension when administering I.M. or I.V.; use with caution in patients with severe liver or renal disease

Pregnancy Risk Factor C

Adverse Reactions

Cardiovascular: Hypotension, tachycardia, fluctuations in blood pressure, hypertension, arrhythmias, edema

Central nervous system: Parkinsonian symptoms, akathisia, dystonias, tardive dyskinesia, dizziness, hyper-reflexia, headache, cerebral edema, drowsiness, lethargy, restlessness, excitement, bizarre dreams, EEG changes, depression, seizures, NMS, altered central temperature regulation

Dermatologic: Increased sensitivity to sun, rash, skin pigmentation, itching, erythema, urticaria, seborrhea, eczema, dermatitis

Endocrine & metabolic: Changes in menstrual cycle, breast pain, amenorrhea, galactorrhea, gynecomastia, changes in libido, elevated prolactin, SIADH

Gastrointestinal: Weight gain, loss of appetite, salivation, xerostomia, constipation, paralytic ileus, laryngeal edema

Genitourinary: Ejaculatory disturbances, impotence, polyuria, bladder paralysis, enuresis

Hematologic: Agranulocytosis, leukopenia, thrombocytopenia, nonthrombocytopenic purpura, eosinophilia, pancytopenia

Hepatic: Cholestatic jaundice, hepatotoxicity

Neuromuscular & skeletal: Trembling of fingers, SLE, facial hemispasm

Ocular: Pigmentary retinopathy, cornea and lens changes, blurred vision, glaucoma

Respiratory: Nasal congestion, asthma

Drug Interactions CYP2D6 enzyme substrate; CYP2D6 enzyme inhibitor CYP1A2, 2D6, and 3A3/4 enzyme substrate; CYP2D6 enzyme inhibitor

Phenothiazines inhibit the ability of bromocriptine to lower serum prolactin concentrations

(Continued)

Fluphenazine *(Continued)*

Benztropine (and other anticholinergics) may inhibit the therapeutic response to fluphenazine and excess anticholinergic effects may occur

Chloroquine may increase fluphenazine concentrations

Cigarette smoking may enhance the hepatic metabolism of fluphenazine. Larger doses may be required compared to a nonsmoker.

Concurrent use of fluphenazine with an antihypertensive may produce additive hypotensive effects

Antihypertensive effects of guanethidine and guanadrel may be inhibited by fluphenazine

Concurrent use with TCA may produce increased toxicity or altered therapeutic response

Fluphenazine may inhibit the antiparkinsonian effect of levodopa; avoid this combination

Fluphenazine plus lithium may rarely produce neurotoxicity

Barbiturates may reduce fluphenazine concentrations

Propranolol may increase fluphenazine concentrations

Sulfadoxine-pyrimethamine may increase fluphenazine concentrations

Fluphenazine and possibly other low potency antipsychotics may reverse the pressor effects of epinephrine

Fluphenazine and CNS depressants (ethanol, narcotics) may produce additive CNS depressant effects

Fluphenazine and trazodone may produce additive hypotensive effects

Fluphenazine used with clonidine has resulted in delirium; monitor

Fluphenazine may inhibit the metabolism of tricyclic antidepressants (desipramine, imipramine, nortriptyline); monitor for altered therapeutic response

Alcohol Interactions Avoid use (may increase central nervous system depression)

Onset

Following I.M. or S.C. administration (derivative dependent):

Decanoate (lasts the longest and requires 24-72 hours for onset of action): Onset of action: 24-72 hours; Peak neuroleptic effect: Within 48-96 hours

Hydrochloride salt (acts quickly and persists briefly): Onset of activity: Within 1 hour

Duration Hydrochloride salt: 6-8 hours

Half-Life Derivative dependent: Enanthate: 84-96 hours; Hydrochloride: 33 hours; Decanoate: 163-232 hours

Education and Monitoring Issues

Patient Education: Use exactly as directed (do not increase dose or frequency); may cause physical and/or psychological dependence. Do not discontinue without consulting prescriber. Dilute with water, milk, orange or grapefruit juice; do not dilute with beverages containing caffeine, tannin, or pactinate (eg, coffee, colas, tea, or apple juice). Do not take within 2 hours of any antacid. Avoid excess alcohol or caffeine and other prescription or OTC medications not approved by prescriber. Avoid skin contact with medication; may cause contact dermatitis (wash immediately with warm, soapy water). Maintain adequate hydration (2-3 L/day of fluids unless instructed to restrict fluid intake). You may experience excess drowsiness, lightheadedness, dizziness, or blurred vision (use caution driving or when engaging in tasks requiring alertness until response to drug is known); dry mouth, upset stomach, nausea, vomiting (small frequent meals, frequent mouth care, chewing gum, or sucking lozenges may help); constipation (increased exercise, fluids, or dietary fruit and fiber may help); postural hypotension (use caution climbing stairs or when changing position from lying or sitting to standing); urinary retention (void before taking medication); ejaculatory dysfunction (reversible); decreased perspiration (avoid strenuous exercise in hot environments); or photosensitivity (use sunscreen, wear protective clothing and eyewear, avoid direct sunlight). Report persistent CNS effects (eg, trembling fingers, altered gait or balance, excessive sedation, seizures, unusual movements, anxiety, abnormal thoughts, confusion, personality changes); chest pain, palpitations, rapid heartbeat, severe dizziness; unresolved urinary retention or changes in urinary pattern; altered menstrual pattern, change in libido, swelling or pain in breasts (male or female); vision changes; skin rash or irritation or yellowing of skin; or worsening of condition.

Reference Range: Therapeutic: 5-20 ng/mL; correlation of serum concentrations and efficacy is controversial; most often dosed to best response

- **Flura®** *see* Fluoride *on page 376*
- **Flura-Drops®** *see* Fluoride *on page 376*
- **Flura-Loz®** *see* Fluoride *on page 376*

Flurandrenolide (flure an DREN oh lide)

Pharmacologic Class Corticosteroid, Topical

U.S. Brand Names Cordran®; Cordran® SP

Generic Available No

Mechanism of Action Decreases inflammation by suppression of migration of polymorphonuclear leukocytes and reversal of increased capillary permeability

Use Inflammation of corticosteroid-responsive dermatoses [medium potency topical corticosteroid]

USUAL DOSAGE Topical:

Children:

Ointment, cream: Apply sparingly 1-2 times/day

Tape: Apply once daily

Adults: Cream, lotion, ointment: Apply sparingly 2-3 times/day

Therapy should be discontinued when control is achieved; if no improvement is seen, reassessment of diagnosis may be necessary.

Dosage Forms CRM, emulsified base (Cordran® SP): 0.025% (30 g, 60 g); 0.05% (15 g, 30 g, 60 g). **LOT** (Cordran®): 0.05% (15 mL, 60 mL). **OINT, top** (Cordran®): 0.025% (30 g, 60 g); 0.05% (15 g, 30 g, 60 g). **TAPE, top** (Cordran®): 4 mcg/cm^2 (7.5 cm x 60 cm, 7.5 cm x 200 cm rolls)

Contraindications Viral, fungal, or tubercular skin lesions, known hypersensitivity to flurandrenolide

Warnings/Precautions Adverse systemic effects may occur when used on large areas of the body, denuded areas, for prolonged periods of time, with an occlusive dressing, and/or in infants or small children

Pregnancy Risk Factor C

Adverse Reactions <1%: Acne, acneiform eruptions, allergic contact dermatitis, burning, Cushing's syndrome, dry skin, folliculitis, growth retardation, HPA suppression, hypertrichosis, hypopigmentation, intracranial hypertension, irritation, itching, maceration of the skin, miliaria, perioral dermatitis, secondary infection, skin atrophy, striae

Education and Monitoring Issues

Patient Education: A thin film of cream or ointment is effective; do not overuse; do not use tight-fitting diapers or plastic pants on children being treated in the diaper area; use only as prescribed, and for no longer than the period prescribed; apply sparingly in light film; rub in lightly; avoid contact with eyes; notify prescriber if condition being treated persists or worsens

Flurazepam (flure AZ e pam)

Pharmacologic Class Benzodiazepine

U.S. Brand Names Dalmane®

Generic Available Yes

Mechanism of Action Depresses all levels of the CNS, including the limbic and reticular formation, probably through the increased action of gamma-aminobutyric acid (GABA), which is a major inhibitory neurotransmitter in the brain

Use Short-term treatment of insomnia

USUAL DOSAGE Oral:

Children:

<15 years: Dose not established

>15 years: 15 mg at bedtime

Adults: 15-30 mg at bedtime

Dosage Forms CAP: 15 mg, 30 mg

Contraindications Hypersensitivity to flurazepam or any component (there may be cross-sensitivity with other benzodiazepines); pregnancy, pre-existing CNS depression, respiratory depression, narrow-angle glaucoma

Warnings/Precautions Use with caution in patients receiving other CNS depressants, patients with low albumin, hepatic dysfunction, and in the elderly; do not use in pregnant women; may cause drug dependency; safety and efficacy have not been established in children <15 years of age

Pregnancy Risk Factor X

Adverse Reactions

Cardiovascular: Palpitations, chest pain

Central nervous system: Drowsiness, ataxia, lightheadedness, memory impairment, depression, headache, hangover, confusion, nervousness, dizziness, falling, apprehension, irritability, euphoria, slurred speech, restlessness, hallucinations, paradoxical reactions, talkativeness

Dermatologic: Rash, pruritus

Gastrointestinal: Xerostomia, constipation, excessive salivation, heartburn, upset stomach, nausea, vomiting, diarrhea, increased or decreased appetite, bitter taste, weight gain or loss, increased salivation

Hematologic: Euphoria, granulocytopenia

Hepatic: Elevated ALT/AST, total bilirubin, alkaline phosphatase, cholestatic jaundice

Neuromuscular & skeletal: Dysarthria, body/joint pain, reflex slowing, weakness

Ocular: Blurred vision, burning eyes, difficulty focusing

Otic: Tinnitus

Respiratory: Apnea, shortness of breath

Miscellaneous: Diaphoresis, drug dependence

Drug Interactions

Carbamazepine, rifampin, rifabutin may enhance the metabolism of flurazepam and decrease its therapeutic effect; consider using an alternative sedative/hypnotic agent

Amprenavir, cimetidine, ciprofloxacin, clarithromycin, clozapine, CNS depressants, diltiazem, disulfiram, digoxin, erythromycin, ethanol, fluconazole, fluoxetine, fluvoxamine,

(Continued)

Flurazepam *(Continued)*

isoniazid, itraconazole, ketoconazole, labetalol, levodopa, loxapine, metoprolol, metronidazole, miconazole, nefazodone, omeprazole, phenytoin, rifabutin, rifampin, ritonavir, troleandomycin, valproic acid, verapamil may increase the serum level and/or toxicity of flurazepam; monitor for altered benzodiazepine response

Alcohol Interactions Avoid use (may increase central nervous system depression)

Onset Onset of hypnotic effect: 15-20 minutes; Peak: 3-6 hours

Duration 7-8 hours

Half-Life 40-114 hours

Education and Monitoring Issues

Patient Education: Use exactly as directed (do not increase dose or frequency or discontinue without consulting prescriber); may cause physical and/or psychological dependence. May take with food to decrease GI upset. While using this medication, do not use alcohol or other prescription or OTC medications (especially, pain medications, sedatives, antihistamines, or hypnotics) without consulting prescriber. Maintain adequate hydration (2-3 L/day of fluids unless instructed to restrict fluid intake). You may experience drowsiness, dizziness, lightheadedness, or blurred vision (use caution when driving or engaging in tasks requiring alertness until response to drug is known); dry mouth, nausea or vomiting (small frequent meals, frequent mouth care, chewing gum, or sucking lozenges may help); difficulty urinating (void before taking medication); or altered libido (resolves when medication is discontinued). Report CNS changes (confusion, depression, increased sedation, excitation, headache, abnormal thinking, insomnia, or nightmares, memory impairment, impaired coordination); muscle pain or weakness; difficulty breathing; persistent dizziness, chest pain, or palpitations; alterations in normal gait; vision changes; ringing in ears; or ineffectiveness of medication.

Dietary Considerations: Grapefruit juice may increase serum levels and/or toxicity

Monitoring Parameters: Respiratory and cardiovascular status

Reference Range: Therapeutic: 0-4 ng/mL (SI: 0-9 nmol/L); Metabolite N-desalkylflurazepam: 20-110 ng/mL (SI: 43-240 nmol/L); Toxic: >0.12 µg/mL

Flurbiprofen (flure BI proe fen)

Pharmacologic Class Nonsteroidal Anti-Inflammatory Agent (NSAID); Ophthalmic Agent

U.S. Brand Names Ansaid® Oral; Ocufen® Ophthalmic

Generic Available No

Mechanism of Action Inhibits prostaglandin synthesis by decreasing the activity of the enzyme, cyclo-oxygenase, which results in decreased formation of prostaglandin precursors

Use Inhibition of intraoperative miosis; acute or long-term treatment of signs and symptoms of rheumatoid arthritis and osteoarthritis; prevention and management of postoperative ocular inflammation and postoperative cystoid macular edema remains to be determined

USUAL DOSAGE

Oral: Rheumatoid arthritis and osteoarthritis: 200-300 mg/day in 2, 3, or 4 divided doses

Ophthalmic: Instill 1 drop every 30 minutes, 2 hours prior to surgery (total of 4 drops to each affected eye)

Dosage Forms SOLN, ophth (Ocufen®): 0.03% (2.5 mL, 5 mL, 10 mL). **TAB** (Ansaid®): 50 mg, 100 mg

Contraindications Dendritic keratitis, hypersensitivity to flurbiprofen or any component

Warnings/Precautions Should be used with caution in patients with a history of herpes simplex, keratitis, and patients who might be affected by inhibition of platelet aggregation; slowing of corneal wound healing patients in whom asthma, rhinitis, or urticaria is precipitated by aspirin or other NSAIDs.

Pregnancy Risk Factor C; D (3rd trimester)

Adverse Reactions

Ophthalmic:

>10%: Ocular: Slowing of corneal wound healing, mild ocular stinging, itching and burning eyes, ocular irritation

1% to 10%: Ocular: Eye redness

Oral:

>10%:

Central nervous system: Dizziness
Dermatologic: Rash
Gastrointestinal: Abdominal cramps, heartburn, indigestion, nausea

1% to 10%:

Central nervous system: Headache, nervousness
Dermatologic: Itching
Endocrine & metabolic: Fluid retention
Gastrointestinal: Vomiting
Otic: Tinnitus

<1%: Acute renal failure, agranulocytosis, allergic rhinitis, anemia, angioedema, arrhythmias, aseptic meningitis, blurred vision, bone marrow suppression, confusion, congestive heart failure, conjunctivitis, cystitis, decreased hearing, drowsiness, dry

eyes, epistaxis, erythema multiforme, gastritis, GI ulceration, hallucinations, hemolytic anemia, hepatitis, hot flashes, hypertension, insomnia, leukopenia, mental depression, peripheral neuropathy, polydipsia, polyuria, shortness of breath, Stevens-Johnson syndrome, tachycardia, thrombocytopenia, toxic amblyopia, toxic epidermal necrolysis, urticaria

Drug Interactions CYP2C9 enzyme substrate; CYP2C9 enzyme inhibitor

Decreased effect: When used concurrently with flurbiprofen, reports acetylcholine chloride and carbachol being ineffective

Alcohol Interactions Avoid use (may enhance gastric mucosal irritation)

Half-Life 5.7 hours

Education and Monitoring Issues

Patient Education:

Oral: Take this medication exactly as directed; do not increase dose without consulting prescriber. Do not crush tablets or break capsules. Take with food or milk to reduce GI distress. Maintain adequate fluid intake (2-3 L/day of fluids unless instructed to restrict fluid intake). Do not use alcohol, aspirin, or aspirin-containing medication, and all other anti-inflammatory medications without consulting prescriber. You may experience drowsiness, dizziness, nervousness, or headache (use caution when driving or engaging in tasks requiring alertness until response to drug is known); anorexia, nausea, vomiting, or heartburn (frequent small meals, frequent mouth care, sucking lozenges, or chewing gum may help); fluid retention (weigh yourself weekly and report unusual (3-5 lb/week) weight gain). GI bleeding, ulceration, or perforation can occur with or without pain; discontinue medication and contact prescriber if persistent abdominal pain or cramping, or blood in stool occurs. Report breathlessness, difficulty breathing, or unusual cough; chest pain, rapid heartbeat, palpitations; unusual bruising/bleeding; blood in urine, stool, mouth, or vomitus; swollen extremities; skin rash or itching; acute fatigue; changes in hearing or ringing in ears.

Ophthalmic: Wash hands before instilling. Sit or lie down to instill. Open eye, look at ceiling, and instill prescribed amount of medication. Close eye and roll eye in all directions, and apply gentle pressure to inner corner of eye. Do not let tip of applicator touch eye or contaminate tip of applicator. Use protective dark eyewear until healed; avoid direct sunlight. Temporary stinging or burning may occur. Report persistent pain, burning, redness, vision disturbances, swelling, itching, or worsening of condition.

Related Information

Nonsteroidal Anti-Inflammatory Agents Comparison *on page 1248*

- **Fluress®** *see* Fluorescein Sodium *on page 375*
- **Fluro-Ethyl® Aerosol** *see* Ethyl Chloride and Dichlorotetrafluoroethane *on page 346*
- **Flurosyn®** *see* Fluocinolone *on page 374*

Flutamide (FLOO ta mide)

Pharmacologic Class Antiandrogen

U.S. Brand Names Eulexin®

Generic Available No

Mechanism of Action Nonsteroidal antiandrogen that inhibits androgen uptake or inhibits binding of androgen in target tissues

Use In combination therapy with LHRH agonist analogues in treatment of metastatic prostatic carcinoma. A study has shown that the addition of flutamide to leuprolide therapy in patients with advanced prostatic cancer increased median actuarial survival time to 34.9 months versus 27.9 months with leuprolide alone. To achieve benefit to combination therapy, both drugs need to be started simultaneously.

USUAL DOSAGE Refer to individual protocols

Adults: Oral:

250 mg 3 times/day

1.5 g/day

Dosage Forms CAP: 125 mg

Contraindications Known hypersensitivity to flutamide; severe hepatic impairment; not indicated in women

Warnings/Precautions The U.S. Food and Drug Administration (FDA) currently recommends that procedures for proper handling and disposal of antineoplastic agents be considered. Animal data (based on using doses higher than recommended for humans) produced testicular interstitial cell adenoma. Do not discontinue therapy without prescriber's advice. May cause hepatic failure, which can be fatal. Serum transaminases should be monitored at baseline and monthly for the first four months of therapy, and periodically thereafter. These should also be repeated at the first sign and symptom of liver dysfunction. Use of flutamide is not recommended in patients with baseline elevation of transaminase levels (> twice the upper limit of normal). Flutamide should be discontinued immediately at any time if the patient develops jaundice or elevation in serum transaminase levels (>2 times upper limit of normal).

Pregnancy Risk Factor D

Pregnancy Implications This drug will cause fetal abnormalities - use barrier contraceptives

(Continued)

Flutamide *(Continued)*

Adverse Reactions

>10%:

Gastrointestinal: Nausea, vomiting, diarrhea

Genitourinary: Impotence

Endocrine & metabolic: Loss of libido, hot flashes

1% to 10%:

Endocrine & metabolic: Gynecomastia

Gastrointestinal: Anorexia

Neuromuscular & skeletal: Numbness in extremities

<1%: Abdominal pain, confusion, drowsiness, edema, flu-like syndrome, hepatic failure, hepatitis hypertension, jaundice, nervousness

Drug Interactions CYP3A3/4 enzyme substrate

Half-Life 5-6 hours

Education and Monitoring Issues

Patient Education: Take as directed; do not discontinue without consulting prescriber. You may experience decreased libido, impotence, swelling of breasts, or decreased appetite (small frequent meals may help). Report chest pain or palpitation; acute abdominal pain; pain, tingling, or numbness of extremities; swelling of extremities or unusual weight gain; difficulty breathing; or other persistent adverse effects.

Monitoring Parameters: Serum transaminase levels should be measured prior to starting treatment and should be repeated monthly for the first 4 months of therapy, and periodically thereafter. LFTs should be checked at the first sign or symptom of liver dysfunction (eg, nausea, vomiting, abdominal pain, fatigue, anorexia, flu-like symptoms, hyperbilirubinuria, jaundice, or right upper quadrant tenderness). Other parameters include tumor reduction, testosterone/estrogen, and phosphatase serum levels.

Manufacturer Schering-Plough Corp

Related Information

Pharmaceutical Manufacturers Directory *on page 1020*

♦ **Flutex®** *see* Triamcinolone *on page 944*

Fluticasone (floo TIK a sone)

Pharmacologic Class Corticosteroid, Oral Inhaler; Corticosteroid, Nasal

U.S. Brand Names Cutivate™; Flonase®; Flovent®

Generic Available No

Mechanism of Action Fluticasone belongs to a new group of corticosteroids which utilizes a fluorocarbothioate ester linkage at the 17 carbon position; extremely potent vasoconstrictive and anti-inflammatory activity; has a weak hypothalamic -pituitary- adrenocortical axis (HPA) inhibitory potency when applied topically, which gives the drug a high therapeutic index. The mechanism of action for all topical corticosteroids is believed to be a combination of three important properties: anti-inflammatory activity, immunosuppressive properties, and antiproliferative actions.

Use

Inhalation: Maintenance treatment of asthma as prophylactic therapy. It is also indicated for patients requiring oral corticosteroid therapy for asthma to assist in total discontinuation or reduction of total oral dose. NOT indicated for the relief of acute bronchospasm.

Intranasal: Management of seasonal and perennial allergic rhinitis in patients ≥12 years of age

Topical: Relief of inflammation and pruritus associated with corticosteroid-responsive dermatoses [medium potency topical corticosteroid]

USUAL DOSAGE

Flovent® Rotadisk can now be used in children ≥4 years; Flovent® is still indicated for use ≥12 years of age

Topical product (Cutivate™) approved for use in pediatric patients ≥3 months of age

Adolescents:

Intranasal: Initial: 1 spray (50 mcg/spray) per nostril once daily. Patients not adequately responding or patients with more severe symptoms may use 2 sprays (200 mcg) per nostril. Depending on response, dosage may be reduced to 100 mcg daily. Total daily dosage should not exceed 4 sprays (200 mcg)/day.

Adults:

Inhalation, Oral:

Recommended Oral Inhalation Doses

Previous Therapy	Recommended Starting Dose	Recommended Highest Dose
Bronchodilator alone	88 mcg twice daily	440 mcg twice daily
Inhaled corticosteroids	88–220 mcg twice daily	440 mcg twice daily
Oral corticosteroids	880 mcg twice daily	880 mcg twice daily

Intranasal: Initial: 2 sprays (50 mcg/spray) per nostril once daily; after the first few days, dosage may be reduced to 1 spray per nostril once daily for maintenance therapy; maximum total daily dose should not exceed 4 sprays (200 mcg)/day

Adults and Children >3 months of age:

Topical: Apply sparingly in a thin film twice daily. Therapy should be discontinued when control is achieved. If no improvement is seen, reassessment of diagnosis may be necessary.

Dosage Forms **SPRAY, aero, oral inh** (Flovent®): 44 mcg/actuation (7.9 g = 60 actuations or 13 g = 120 actuations); 110 mcg/actuation (13 g = 120 actuations); 220 mcg/actuation (13 g = 120 actuations). **SPRAY, intranasal** (Flonase®): 50 mcg/actuation (9 g = 60 actuations, 16 g = 120 actuations). **TOP** (Cutivate™): **CRM:** 0.05% (15 g, 30 g, 60 g); **OINT:** 0.005% (15 g, 60 g)

Contraindications Hypersensitivity to any component, bacterial infections, ophthalmic use

Warnings/Precautions Adverse systemic effects may occur when used on large areas of the body, denuded areas, for prolonged periods of time, with an occlusive dressing, and/or in infants or small children. Controlled clinical studies have shown that inhaled and intranasal corticosteroids may cause a reduction in growth velocity in pediatric patients. Growth velocity provides a means of comparing the rate of growth among children of the same age. Use in pediatric patients longer than 4 weeks has not been established.

In studies involving inhaled corticosteroids, the average reduction in growth velocity was approximately 1 cm (about 1/3 of an inch) per year. It appears that the reduction is related to dose and how long the child takes the drug.

FDA's Pulmonary and Allergy Drugs and Metabolic and Endocrine Drugs advisory committees discussed this issue at a July 1998 meeting. They recommended that the agency develop class-wide labeling to inform healthcare providers so they would understand this potential side effect and monitor growth routinely in pediatric patients who are treated with inhaled corticosteroids, intranasal corticosteroids or both.

Long-term effects of this reduction in growth velocity on final adult height are unknown. Likewise, it also has not yet been determined whether patients' growth will "catch up" if treatment in discontinued. Drug manufacturers will continue to monitor these drugs to learn more about long-term effects. Children are prescribed inhaled corticosteroids to treat asthma. Intranasal corticosteroids are generally used to prevent and treat allergy-related nasal symptoms.

Patients are advised not to stop using their inhaled or intranasal corticosteroids without first speaking to their healthcare providers about the benefits of these drugs compared to their risks

Rare cases of vasculitis (Churg-Strauss syndrome) may occur

Use of topical fluticasone in patients <4 years of age has not been established

Pregnancy Risk Factor C

Adverse Reactions

>10%: Oral inhalation:

Central nervous system: Headache

Respiratory: Respiratory infection, pharyngitis, nasal congestion

1% to 10%: Oral Inhalation:

Central nervous system: Dysphonia

Gastrointestinal: Oral candidiasis

Respiratory: Sinusitis

<1%: Acne, allergic dermatitis, burning, Churg-Strauss syndrome, Cushing's syndrome, dry skin, folliculitis, growth retardation, HPA suppression, hypertrichosis, hypopigmentation, irritation, itching, maceration of the skin, secondary infection, skin atrophy

Half-Life 7.8 hours

Education and Monitoring Issues

Patient Education: Use as directed; do not overuse and use only for length of time prescribed.

Topical: For external use only. Apply thin film of cream to affected area only; rub in lightly. Do not apply occlusive covering unless advised by prescriber. Wash hand thoroughly after use; avoid contact with eyes. Notify prescriber if skin condition persists or worsens.

Nasal spray: Shake gently before use. Use at regular intervals, no more frequently than directed. Report unusual cough or spasm; persistent nasal bleeding, burning, or irritation; or worsening of condition.

Manufacturer GlaxoWellcome

Related Information

Asthma Guidelines *on page 1077*

Pharmaceutical Manufacturers Directory *on page 1020*

♦ **Flutone** *see* Diflorasone *on page 270*

Fluvastatin (FLOO va sta tin)

Pharmacologic Class Antilipemic Agent (HMG-CoA Reductase Inhibitor)

U.S. Brand Names Lescol®

(Continued)

Fluvastatin *(Continued)*

Mechanism of Action Acts by competitively inhibiting 3-hydroxyl-3-methylglutaryl-coenzyme A (HMG-CoA) reductase, the enzyme that catalyzes the reduction of HMG-CoA to mevalonate; this is an early rate-limiting step in cholesterol biosynthesis. HDL is increased while total, LDL and VLDL cholesterols, apolipoprotein B, and plasma triglycerides are decreased.

Use Adjunct to dietary therapy to decrease elevated serum total and LDL cholesterol concentrations in primary hypercholesterolemia; reduction of triglycerides and Apo-B in patients with primary hypercholesterolemia and mixed dyslipidemia

USUAL DOSAGE Adults: Oral:

Initial dose: 20-40 mg at bedtime

Usual dose: 20-80 mg at bedtime

Note: Splitting the 80 mg dose into a twice daily regimen may provide a modest improvement in LDL response; maximum response occurs within 4-6 weeks; decrease dose and monitor effects carefully in patients with hepatic insufficiency

Dosage Forms CAP: 20 mg, 40 mg

Contraindications Pregnancy; myopathy or marked elevations of CPK

Warnings/Precautions Avoid combination of clofibrate and fluvastatin due to possible myopathy; consider temporarily withholding therapy in patients with risk of developing renal failure; avoid prolonged exposure to the sun or other ultraviolet light

Pregnancy Risk Factor X

Pregnancy Implications

Clinical effects on the fetus: Skeletal malformations have occurred in animals following agents with similar structure; avoid use in women of childbearing age; discontinue if pregnancy occurs

Breast-feeding/lactation: Avoid use in nursing mothers

Adverse Reactions

>10%: Respiratory: Upper respiratory infection (16%)

1% to 10%:

Central nervous system: Headache (9%), dizziness (2%), insomnia (2% to 3%), fatigue (2% to 3%)

Dermatologic: Rash (2% to 3%)

Gastrointestinal: Dyspepsia (8%), diarrhea (5%), nausea/vomiting (3%), constipation (2% to 3%), flatulence (2% to 3%), abdominal pain (5%)

Neuromuscular & skeletal: Back pain/myalgia (5% to 6%), arthropathy (2% to 4%)

Miscellaneous: Cold/flu symptoms (2% to 5%)

Drug Interactions CYP2C9 enzyme substrate; CYP2C9 enzyme inhibitor

Cimetidine increases fluvastatin blood levels

Cholestyramine reduces fluvastatin absorption; separate administration times by at least 4 hours

Cholestyramine and colestipol (bile acid sequestrants): Cholesterol-lowering effects are additive

Clofibrate and fenofibrate may increase the risk of myopathy and rhabdomyolysis

Gemfibrozil: Increased risk of myopathy and rhabdomyolysis

Omeprazole increases fluvastatin blood levels

Ranitidine increases fluvastatin blood levels

Rifampin decreases fluvastatin blood levels

Ritonavir increases fluvastatin blood levels

Warfarin: Hypoprothrombinemic response is increased; monitor INR closely when fluvastatin is initiated or discontinued

Half-Life 1.2 hours

Education and Monitoring Issues

Patient Education: Take at bedtime since highest rate of cholesterol synthesis occurs between midnight and 5 AM. Follow diet and exercise regimen as prescribed. Have periodic ophthalmic exam to check for cataract development. Avoid prolonged exposure to the sun and other ultraviolet light. Report unexplained muscle pain or weakness, especially if accompanied by fever or malaise.

Manufacturer Novartis

Related Information

Pharmaceutical Manufacturers Directory *on page 1020*

Fluvoxamine (floo VOKS ah meen)

Pharmacologic Class Antidepressant, Selective Serotonin Reuptake Inhibitor

U.S. Brand Names Luvox®

Mechanism of Action Inhibits CNS neuron serotonin uptake; minimal or no effect on reuptake of norepinephrine or dopamine; does not significantly bind to alpha-adrenergic, histamine or cholinergic receptors

Use Treatment of obsessive-compulsive disorder (OCD); effective in the treatment of major depression; may be useful for the treatment of panic disorder

USUAL DOSAGE

Adults: Initial: 50 mg at bedtime; adjust in 50 mg increments at 4- to 7-day intervals; usual dose range: 100-300 mg/day; divide total daily dose into 2 doses; administer larger portion at bedtime

Elderly or hepatic impairment: Reduce dose, titrate slowly

Dosage Forms TAB: 50 mg, 100 mg

Contraindications Concomitant terfenadine or astemizole; during or within 14 days of MAO inhibitors; hypersensitivity to fluvoxamine or any congeners (eg, fluoxetine)

Warnings/Precautions Use with caution in patients with liver dysfunction, suicidal tendencies, history of seizures, mania, or drug abuse, ECT, cardiovascular disease, and the elderly

Pregnancy Risk Factor C

Adverse Reactions

>10%:

- Central nervous system: Headache, somnolence, insomnia, nervousness, dizziness
- Gastrointestinal: Nausea, diarrhea, xerostomia
- Neuromuscular & skeletal: Weakness

1% to 10%:

- Cardiovascular: Palpitations
- Central nervous system: Somnolence, headache, insomnia, dizziness, nervousness, mania, hypomania, vertigo, abnormal thinking, agitation, anxiety, malaise, amnesia, yawning, hypertonia, CNS stimulation, depression
- Endocrine & metabolic: Decreased libido
- Gastrointestinal: Abdominal pain, vomiting, dyspepsia, constipation, abnormal taste, anorexia, flatulence
- Genitourinary: Delayed ejaculation, impotence, anorgasmia, urinary frequency, urinary retention
- Neuromuscular & skeletal: Tremors
- Ocular: Blurred vision
- Respiratory: Dyspnea
- Miscellaneous: Diaphoresis

<1%: Acne, alopecia, anemia, angina, ataxia, bradycardia, delayed menstruation, dermatitis, dry skin, dysuria, elevated liver transaminases, extrapyramidal reactions, lactation, leukocytosis, nocturia, seizures, thrombocytopenia, urticaria

Drug Interactions CYP1A2 enzyme substrate; CYP1A2, 2C9, 2C19, 2D6, and 3A3/4 enzyme inhibitor

Fluvoxamine may inhibit the metabolism of alprazolam and diazepam resulting in elevated serum levels; monitor for increased sedation and psychomotor impairment

Fluvoxamine may cause hyponatremia; additive hyponatremic effects may be seen with combined use of a loop diuretic (bumetanide, furosemide, torsemide); monitor for hyponatremia

Fluvoxamine inhibits the reuptake of serotonin; combined use with a serotonin agonist (buspirone) may cause serotonin syndrome

Fluvoxamine may inhibit the metabolism of carbamazepine resulting in increased carbamazepine levels and toxicity; monitor for altered CBZ response

Cyproheptadine, a serotonin antagonist may inhibit the effects of serotonin reuptake inhibitors (fluvoxamine); monitor for altered antidepressant response

Fluvoxamine should not be used with nonselective MAOIs (isocarboxazid, phenelzine). Fatal reactions have been reported. Wait two weeks after stopping fluvoxamine before starting an MAOI and two weeks after stopping an MAOI before starting fluvoxamine.

Patients receiving fluvoxamine and lithium may develop neurotoxicity; if combination is used; monitor for neurotoxicity

Fluvoxamine inhibits the reuptake of serotonin; combined use with other drugs which inhibit the reuptake (nefazodone, sibutramine) may cause serotonin syndrome. Monitor patient for altered response with nefazodone; avoid sibutramine combination.

Fluvoxamine combined with tramadol (serotonergic effects) may cause serotonin syndrome; monitor

Fluvoxamine may inhibit the metabolism of trazodone resulting in increased toxicity; monitor

Fluvoxamine inhibits the reuptake of serotonin; combination with tryptophan, a serotonin precursor, may cause agitation and restlessness; this combination is best avoided

Fluvoxamine may alter the hypoprothombinemic response to warfarin; monitor

Fluvoxamine inhibits the metabolism of clozapine; adjust clozapine dosage downward or use an alternative SSRI

Fluvoxamine inhibits the metabolism of tacrine; use alternative SSRI

Fluvoxamine inhibits the metabolism of theophylline; monitor for theophylline toxicity or use alternative SSRI

Fluvoxamine inhibits the metabolism of triazolam; monitor for altered response; consider lowering dose of triazolam by 50%

Fluvoxamine may increase serum concentrations of buspirone

Fluvoxamine may inhibit the metabolism of tacrolimus; monitor for adverse effects; consider an alternative SSRI

Alcohol Interactions Avoid use. Although alcohol may not cause much central nervous depression here, depressed patients should avoid/limit intake.

(Continued)

Fluvoxamine *(Continued)*

Onset >2 weeks for therapeutic effect

Half-Life ~15 hours

Education and Monitoring Issues

Patient Education: Take exactly as directed (do not increase dose or frequency); may take 2-3 weeks to achieve desired results; may cause physical and/or psychological dependence. Take once-a-day dose at bedtime. Avoid excessive alcohol, caffeine, and other prescription or OTC medications not approved by prescriber. Maintain adequate hydration (2-3 L/day of fluids unless instructed to restrict fluid intake). You may experience drowsiness, lightheadedness, impaired coordination, dizziness, or blurred vision (use caution when driving or engaging in tasks requiring alertness until response to drug is known); nausea, vomiting, or anorexia (small frequent meals, frequent mouth care, chewing gum, or sucking lozenges may help); constipation (increased exercise, fluids, or dietary fruit and fiber may help); diarrhea (buttermilk, yogurt, or boiled milk may help); postural hypotension (use caution when climbing stairs or changing position from lying or sitting to standing); or decreased sexual function or libido (reversible). Report persistent CNS effects (nervousness, restlessness, insomnia, anxiety, excitation, headache, sedation, seizures, mania, abnormal thinking); rash or skin irritation; muscle cramping, tremors, or change in gait; chest pain or palpitations; change in urinary pattern; or worsening of condition.

Monitoring Parameters: Signs and symptoms of depression, anxiety, weight gain or loss, nutritional intake, sleep

Manufacturer Solvay Pharmaceuticals

Related Information

Antidepressant Agents Comparison *on page 1231*
Pharmaceutical Manufacturers Directory *on page 1020*

- **FML®** *see* Fluorometholone *on page 376*
- **FML® Forte** *see* Fluorometholone *on page 376*
- **FML® Liquifilm** *see* Fluorometholone *on page 376*
- **FML-S® Ophthalmic Suspension** *see* Sulfacetamide Sodium and Fluorometholone *on page 876*
- **Foille® [OTC]** *see* Benzocaine *on page 98*
- **Foille® Medicated First Aid [OTC]** *see* Benzocaine *on page 98*
- **Folex® PFS™** *see* Methotrexate *on page 582*

Folic Acid (FOE lik AS id)

Pharmacologic Class Vitamin, Water Soluble

U.S. Brand Names Folvite®

Generic Available Yes

Mechanism of Action Folic acid is necessary for formation of a number of coenzymes in many metabolic systems, particularly for purine and pyrimidine synthesis; required for nucleoprotein synthesis and maintenance in erythropoiesis; stimulates WBC and platelet production in folate deficiency anemia

Use Treatment of megaloblastic and macrocytic anemias due to folate deficiency; dietary supplement to prevent neural tube defects

USUAL DOSAGE

Infants: 0.1 mg/day
Children <4 years: Up to 0.3 mg/day
Children >4 years and Adults: 0.4 mg/day
Pregnant and lactating women: 0.8 mg/day
RDA:
Adult male: 0.15-0.2 mg/day
Adult female: 0.15-0.18 mg/day

Dosage Forms INJ: 5 mg/mL (10 mL); 10 mg/mL (10 mL); (Folvite®): 5 mg/mL (10 mL). **TAB:** 0.1 mg, 0.4 mg, 0.8 mg, 1 mg; (Folvite®): 1 mg

Contraindications Pernicious, aplastic, or normocytic anemias

Warnings/Precautions Doses >0.1 mg/day may obscure pernicious anemia with continuing irreversible nerve damage progression. Resistance to treatment may occur with depressed hematopoiesis, alcoholism, deficiencies of other vitamins. Injection contains benzyl alcohol (1.5%) as preservative (use care in administration to neonates).

Pregnancy Risk Factor A; C (if dose exceeds RDA recommendation)

Adverse Reactions <1%: Allergic reaction, bronchospasm, general malaise, pruritus, rash, slight flushing

Drug Interactions Decreased effect: In folate-deficient patients, folic acid therapy may increase phenytoin metabolism. Phenytoin, primidone, para-aminosalicylic acid, and sulfasalazine may decrease serum folate concentrations and cause deficiency. Oral contraceptives may also impair folate metabolism producing depletion, but the effect is unlikely to cause anemia or megaloblastic changes. Concurrent administration of chloramphenicol and folic acid may result in antagonism of the hematopoietic response to folic acid; dihydrofolate reductase inhibitors (eg, methotrexate, trimethoprim) may interfere with folic acid utilization.

Onset Peak effect: Oral: Within 0.5-1 hour

Education and Monitoring Issues

Patient Education: Take as prescribed. Toxicity can occur from elevated doses. Do not self medicate. Increase intake of foods high in folic acid (eg, dried beans, nuts, bran, vegetables, fruits) as recommended by prescriber. Excessive use of alcohol increases requirement for folic acid. May turn urine more intensely yellow. Report skin rash.

Reference Range: Therapeutic: 0.005-0.015 µg/mL

Related Information

Ferrous Sulfate, Ascorbic Acid, Vitamin B-Complex, and Folic Acid *on page 361*
Vitamin B Complex With Vitamin C and Folic Acid *on page 979*

♦ **Follistim™** *see* Follitropins *on page 391*

Follitropins (foe li TRO pins)

Pharmacologic Class Ovulation Stimulator

U.S. Brand Names Fertinex™; Follistim™; Gonal-F®

Mechanism of Action Urofollitropin is a preparation of highly purified follicle-stimulating hormone (FSH) extracted from the urine of postmenopausal women. Follitropin alpha and follitropin beta are human FSH preparations of recombinant DNA origin. Follitropins stimulate ovarian follicular growth in women who do not have primary ovarian failure. FSH is required for normal follicular growth, maturation, and gonadal steroid production.

Use

Urofollitropin (Fertinex™):

Polycystic ovary syndrome: Give sequentially with hCG for the stimulation of follicular recruitment and development and the induction of ovulation in patients with polycystic ovary syndrome and infertility, who have failed to respond or conceive following adequate clomiphene citrate therapy

Follicle stimulation: Stimulate the development of multiple follicles in ovulatory patients undergoing Assisted Reproductive Technologies such as *in vitro* fertilization

Follitropin alpha (Gonal-F™)/follitropin beta (Follistim™):

Ovulation induction: For the induction of ovulation and pregnancy in anovulatory infertile patients in whom the cause of infertility is functional and not caused by primary ovarian failure

Follicle stimulation: To stimulate the development of multiple follicles in ovulatory patients undergoing Assisted Reproductive Technologies such as *in vitro* fertilization

USUAL DOSAGE

Urofollitropin (Fertinex™): Adults: S.C.:

Polycystic ovary syndrome: Initial recommended dose of the first cycle: 75 international units/day; consider dose adjustment after 5-7 days; additional dose adjustments may be considered based on individual patient response. The dose should not be increased more than twice in any cycle or by more than 75 international units per adjustment. To complete follicular development and affect ovulation in the absence of an endogenous LH surge, give 5000 to 10,000 units hCG, 1 day after the last dose of urofollitropin. Withhold hCG if serum estradiol is >2000 pg/mL.

Individualize the initial dose administered in subsequent cycles for each patient based on her response in the preceding cycle. Doses of >300 international units of FSH/day are not routinely recommended. As in the initial cycle, 5000 to 10,000 units of hCG must be given 1 day after the last dose of urofollitropin to complete follicular development and induce ovulation.

Give the lowest dose consistent with the expectation of good results. Over the course of treatment, doses may range between 75 to 300 international units/day depending on individual patient response. Administer urofollitropin until adequate follicular development as indicated by serum estradiol and vaginal ultrasonography. A response is generally evident after 5-7 days.

Encourage the couple to have intercourse daily, beginning on the day prior to the administration of hCG until ovulation becomes apparent from the indices employed for determination of progestational activity. Take care to ensure insemination.

Follicle stimulation: For Assisted Reproductive Technologies, initiate therapy with urofollitropin in the early follicular phase (cycle day 2 or 3) at a dose of 150 international units/day, until sufficient follicular development is attained. In most cases, therapy should not exceed 10 days.

Follitropin alpha (Gonal-F®): Adults: S.C.:

Ovulation induction: Initial recommended dose of the first cycle: 75 international units/day. Consider dose adjustment after 5-7 days; additional dose adjustments of up to 37.5 international units may be considered after 14 days. Further dose increases of the same magnitude can be made, if necessary, every 7 days. To complete follicular development and affect ovulation in the absence of an endogenous LH surge, give 5000 to 10,000 units hCG, 1 day after the last dose of follitropin alpha. Withhold hCG if serum estradiol is >2000 pg/mL.

Individualize the initial dose administered in subsequent cycles for each patient based on her response in the preceding cycle. Doses of >300 international units of FSH/day are not routinely recommended. As in the initial cycle, 5000 to 10,000 units of hCG must be given 1 day after the last dose of urofollitropin to complete follicular development and induce ovulation.

(Continued)

Follitropins *(Continued)*

Give the lowest dose consistent with the expectation of good results. Over the course of treatment, doses may range between 75 to 300 international units/day depending on individual patient response. Administer urofollitropin until adequate follicular development as indicated by serum estradiol and vaginal ultrasonography. A response is generally evident after 5-7 days.

Encourage the couple to have intercourse daily, beginning on the day prior to the administration of hCG until ovulation becomes apparent from the indices employed for determination of progestational activity. Take care to ensure insemination.

Follicle stimulation: Initiate therapy with follitropin alpha in the early follicular phase (cycle day 2 or 3) at a dose of 150 international units/day, until sufficient follicular development is attained. In most cases, therapy should not exceed 10 days.

In patients undergoing Assisted Reproductive Technologies, whose endogenous gonadotropin levels are suppressed, initiate follitropin alpha at a dose of 225 international units/day. Continue treatment until adequate follicular development is indicated as determined by ultrasound in combination with measurement of serum estradiol levels. Consider adjustments to dose after 5 days based on the patient's response; adjust subsequent dosage every 3-5 days by ≤75-150 international units additionally at each adjustment. Doses >450 international units/day are not recommended. Once adequate follicular development is evident, administer hCG (5000-10,000 units) to induce final follicular maturation in preparation for oocyte.

Follitropin beta (Follistim™): Adults: S.C. or I.M.:

Ovulation induction: Stepwise approach: Initiate therapy with 75 international units/day for up to 14 days. Increase by 37.5 international units at weekly intervals until follicular growth or serum estradiol levels indicate an adequate response. The maximum, individualized, daily dose that has been safely used for ovulation induction in patients during clinical trials is 300 international units. Treat the patient until ultrasonic visualizations or serum estradiol determinations indicate preovulatory conditions greater than or equal to normal values followed by 5000 to 10,000 units hCG.

During treatment and during a 2-week post-treatment period, examine patients at least every other day for signs of excessive ovarian stimulation. Discontinue follitropin beta administration if the ovaries become abnormally enlarged or abdominal pain occurs.

Encourage the couple to have intercourse daily, beginning on the day prior to the administration of hCG until ovulation becomes apparent from the indices employed for determination of progestational activity. Take care to ensure insemination.

Follicle stimulation: A starting dose of 150-225 international units of follitropin beta is recommended for at least the first 4 days of treatment. The dose may be adjusted for the individual patient based upon their ovarian response. Daily maintenance doses ranging from 75-300 international units for 6-12 days are usually sufficient, although longer treatment may be necessary. However, maintenance doses of up to 375-600 international units may be necessary according to individual response. The maximum daily dose used in clinical studies is 600 international units. When a sufficient number of follicles of adequate size are present, the final maturation of the follicles is induced by administering hCG at a dose of 5000-10,000 international units. Oocyte retrieval is performed 34-36 hours later. Withhold hCG in cases where the ovaries are abnormally enlarged on the last day of follitropin beta therapy.

Dosage Forms POWDER for inj: Urofollitropin (Fertinex®): 75 international units (1, 10, 100 mL ampuls with diluent), 150 international units (1 mL ampuls with diluent); Follitropin alpha (Gonal-F®): 75 international units (1, 10, 100 mL ampuls with diluent), 150 international units (1 mL ampuls with diluent); Follitropin beta (Follistim®): 75 international units (1, 5 mL vials with diluent)

Contraindications High levels of FSH indicating primary ovarian failure; uncontrolled thyroid or adrenal dysfunction; the presence of any cause of infertility other than anovulation; tumor of the ovary, breast, uterus, hypothalamus, or pituitary gland; abnormal vaginal bleeding of undetermined origin; ovarian cysts or enlargement not due to polycystic ovary syndrome; hypersensitivity to the product or any of its components; pregnancy

Warnings/Precautions These medications should only be used by prescribers who are thoroughly familiar with infertility problems and their management. To minimize risks, use only at the lowest effective dose. Monitor ovarian response with serum estradiol and vaginal ultrasound on a regular basis.

Ovarian enlargement which may be accompanied by abdominal distention or abdominal pain, occurs in ~20% of those treated with urofollitropin and hCG, and generally regresses without treatment within 2-3 weeks. Ovarian hyperstimulation syndrome, characterized by severe ovarian enlargement, abdominal pain/distention, nausea, vomiting, diarrhea, dyspnea, and oliguria, and may be accompanied by ascites, pleural effusion, hypovolemia, electrolyte imbalance, hemoperitoneum, and thromboembolic events is reported in about 6% of patients. If hyperstimulation occurs, stop treatment and hospitalize patient. This syndrome develops rapidly within 24 hours to several days and generally occurs during the 7-10 days immediately following treatment. Hemoconcentration associated with fluid loss into the abdominal cavity has occurred and should be assessed by fluid intake & output, weight, hematocrit, serum & urinary electrolytes, urine specific gravity, BUN and creatinine, and abdominal girth. Determinations should be performed daily or more often if the need arises. Treatment is primarily symptomatic and consists of bed rest, fluid and electrolyte replacement and analgesics. The ascitic, pleural and pericardial fluids should never be removed because of the potential danger of injury.

Serious pulmonary conditions (atelectasis, acute respiratory distress syndrome and exacerbation of asthma) have been reported. Thromboembolic events, both in association with and separate from ovarian hyperstimulation syndrome, have been reported.

Multiple pregnancies have been associated with these medications, including triplet and quintuplet gestations. Advise patient of the potential risk of multiple births before starting the treatment.

Pregnancy Risk Factor X

Adverse Reactions 1% to 10%:

Dermatologic: Dry skin, body rash, hair loss, hives

Endocrine & metabolic: Ovarian hyperstimulation syndrome, adnexal torsion, mild to moderate ovarian enlargement, abdominal pain, ovarian cysts, breast tenderness

Gastrointestinal: Nausea, vomiting, diarrhea, abdominal cramps, bloating

Local: Pain, rash, swelling, or irritation at the site of injection

Respiratory: Atelectasis, acute respiratory distress syndrome, exacerbation of asthma

Miscellaneous: Febrile reactions accompanied by chills, musculoskeletal, joint pains, malaise, headache, and fatigue

Half-Life 24-32 hours

Education and Monitoring Issues

Patient Education: Discontinue immediately if possibility of pregnancy. Prior to therapy, inform patients of the following: Duration of treatment and monitoring required; possible adverse reactions; risk of multiple births.

Monitoring Parameters: Monitor sufficient follicular maturation. This may be directly estimated by sonographic visualization of the ovaries and endometrial lining or measuring serum estradiol levels. The combination of both ultrasonography and measurement of estradiol levels is useful for monitoring for the growth and development of follicles and timing hCG administration.

The clinical evaluation of estrogenic activity (changes in vaginal cytology and changes in appearance and volume of cervical mucus) provides an indirect estimate of the estrogenic effect upon the target organs and, therefore, it should only be used adjunctively with more direct estimates of follicular development (ultrasonography and serum estradiol determinations).

The clinical confirmation of ovulation is obtained by direct and indirect indices of progesterone production. The indices most generally used are: rise in basal body temperature, increase in serum progesterone, and menstruation following the shift in basal body temperature.

♦ **Follutein®** *see* Chorionic Gonadotropin *on page 196*

♦ **Folvite®** *see* Folic Acid *on page 390*

Fomivirsen (foe MI vir sen)

Pharmacologic Class Antiviral Agent, Ophthalmic

U.S. Brand Names Vitravene™

Mechanism of Action Inhibits synthesis of viral protein by binding to mRNA which blocks replication of cytomegalovirus through an antisense mechanism

Use Local treatment of cytomegalovirus (CMV) retinitis in patients with acquired immunodeficiency syndrome who are intolerant or insufficiently responsive to other treatments for CMV retinitis or when other treatments for CMV retinitis are contraindicated

USUAL DOSAGE Adults: Intravitreal injection: Induction: 330 mcg (0.05 mL) every other week for 2 doses, followed by maintenance dose of 330 mcg (0.05 mL) every 4 weeks

If progression occurs during maintenance, a repeat of the induction regimen may be attempted to establish resumed control. Unacceptable inflammation during therapy may be managed by temporary interruption, provided response has been established. Topical corticosteroids have been used to reduce inflammation.

Dosage Forms SOLN, for ocular inj: 6.6 mg/mL (0.25 mL)

Contraindications Hypersensitivity to fomivirsen or any component

Warnings/Precautions For ophthalmic use via intravitreal injection only. Uveitis occurs frequently, particularly during induction dosing. Do not use in patients who have received intravenous or intravitreal cidofovir within 2-4 weeks (risk of exaggerated inflammation is increased). Patients should be monitored for CMV disease in the contralateral eye and/or extraocular disease. Commonly increases intraocular pressure - monitoring is recommended.

Pregnancy Risk Factor C

Pregnancy Implications Studies have not been conducted in pregnant women. Should be used in pregnancy only when potential benefit to the mother outweighs the potential risk to the fetus. Excretion in human milk is unknown. Use during breast-feeding is contraindicated - a decision to discontinue nursing or discontinue the drug is should be made.

(Continued)

Fomivirsen *(Continued)*

Adverse Reactions

5% to 10%:

Central nervous system: Fever, headache
Gastrointestinal: Abdominal pain, diarrhea, nausea, vomiting
Hematologic: Anemia
Neuromuscular & skeletal: Asthenia
Ocular: Uveitis, abnormal vision, anterior chamber inflammation, blurred vision, cataract, conjunctival hemorrhage, decreased visual acuity, loss of color vision, eye pain, increased intraocular pressure, photophobia, retinal detachment, retinal edema, retinal hemorrhage, retinal pigment changes, vitreitis
Respiratory: Pneumonia, sinusitis
Miscellaneous: Systemic CMV, sepsis, infection

2% to 5%:

Cardiovascular: Chest pain
Central nervous system: Confusion, depression, dizziness, neuropathy, pain
Endocrine and metabolic: Dehydration
Gastrointestinal: Abnormal LFTs, pancreatitis, anorexia, weight loss
Hematologic: Thrombocytopenia, lymphoma
Neuromuscular & skeletal: Back pain, cachexia
Ocular: Application site reaction, conjunctival hyperemia, conjunctivitis, corneal edema, decreased peripheral vision, eye irritation, keratic precipitates, optic neuritis, photopsia, retinal vascular disease, visual field defect, vitreous hemorrhage, vitreous opacity
Renal: Kidney failure
Respiratory: Bronchitis, dyspnea, cough
Miscellaneous: Allergic reaction, flu-like syndrome, diaphoresis (increased)

Drug Interactions Drug interactions between fomivirsen and other medications have not been conducted.

Education and Monitoring Issues

Monitoring Parameters: Immediately after injection, light perception and optic nerve head perfusion should be monitored. Anterior chamber paracentesis may be necessary if perfusion is not complete within 7-10 minutes after injection. Subsequent patient evaluation should include monitoring for contralateral CMV infection or extraocular CMV disease, and intraocular pressure prior to each injection.

- **Formula 44E** *see* Guaifenesin and Dextromethorphan *on page 424*
- **Formula Q®** *see* Quinine *on page 804*
- **Formulex®** *see* Dicyclomine *on page 266*
- **Fortaz®** *see* Ceftazidime *on page 161*
- **Fortovase®** *see* Saquinavir *on page 838*
- **Fosamax®** *see* Alendronate *on page 31*

Foscarnet (fos KAR net)

Pharmacologic Class Antiviral Agent

U.S. Brand Names Foscavir® Injection

Generic Available No

Mechanism of Action Pyrophosphate analogue which acts as a noncompetitive inhibitor of many viral RNA and DNA polymerases as well as HIV reverse transcriptase. Similar to ganciclovir, foscarnet is a virostatic agent. Foscarnet does not require activation by thymidine kinase.

Use

Herpesvirus infections suspected to be caused by acyclovir - (HSV, VZV) or ganciclovir - (CMV) resistant strains (this occurs almost exclusively in immunocompromised persons, eg, with advanced AIDS), who have received prolonged treatment for a herpesvirus infection
CMV retinitis in persons with AIDS
Other CMV infections in persons unable to tolerate ganciclovir; may be given in combination with ganciclovir in patients who relapse after monotherapy with either drug

USUAL DOSAGE Adolescents and Adults: I.V.:

CMV retinitis:

Induction treatment: 60 mg/kg/dose every 8 hours **or** 100 mg/kg every 12 hours for 14-21 days
Maintenance therapy: 90-120 mg/kg/day as a single infusion

Acyclovir-resistant HSV induction treatment: 40 mg/kg/dose every 8-12 hours for 14-21 days

Dosage adjustment in renal impairment: Refer to tables

Induction Dosing of Foscarnet in Patients with Abnormal Renal Function

Cl_{cr} (mL/min/kg)	HSV	HSV	CMV
	Equivalent to 40 mg/kg q12h	Equivalent to 40 mg/kg q8h	Equivalent to 60 mg/kg q8h
<0.4	not recommended	not recommended	not recommended
≥0.4-0.5	20 mg/kg every 24 hours	35 mg/kg every 24 hours	50 mg/kg every 24 hours
≥0.5-0.6	25 mg/kg every 24 hours	40 mg/kg every 24 hours	60 mg/kg every 24 hours
≥0.6-0.8	35 mg/kg every 24 hours	25 mg/kg every 12 hours	40 mg/kg every 12 hours
≥0.8-1.0	20 mg/kg every 12 hours	35 mg/kg every 12 hours	50 mg/kg every 12 hours
≥1.0-1.4	30 mg/kg every 12 hours	30 mg/kg every 8 hours	45 mg/kg every 8 hours
1.4	40 mg/kg every 12 hours	40 mg/kg every 8 hours	60 mg/kg every 8 hours

Maintenance Dosing of Foscarnet in Patients with Abnormal Renal Function

Cl_{cr} (mL/min/kg)	CMV	CMV
	Equivalent to 90 mg/kg q24h	Equivalent to 120 mg/kg q24h
<0.4	not recommended	not recommended
≥0.4-0.5	50 mg/kg every 48 hours	65 mg/kg every 48 hours
≥0.5-0.6	60 mg/kg every 48 hours	80 mg/kg every 48 hours
≥0.6-0.8	80 mg/kg every 48 hours	105 mg/kg every 48 hours
≥0.8-1.0	50 mg/kg every 24 hours	65 mg/kg every 24 hours
≥1-1.4	70 mg/kg every 24 hours	90 mg/kg every 24 hours
≥1.4	90 mg/kg every 24 hours	120 mg/kg every 24 hours

Hemodialysis:

Foscarnet is highly removed by hemodialysis (30% in 4 hours HD)

Doses of 50 mg/kg/dose posthemodialysis have been found to produce similar serum concentrations as doses of 90 mg/kg twice daily in patients with normal renal function

Doses of 60-90 mg/kg/dose loading dose (posthemodialysis) followed by 45 mg/kg/dose posthemodialysis (3 times/week) with the monitoring of weekly plasma concentrations to maintain peak plasma concentrations in the range of 400-800 μMolar has been recommended by some clinicians

Continuous arteriovenous or venovenous hemodiafiltration (CAVH) effects: Dose as for Cl_{cr} 10-50 mL/minute

Dosage Forms INJ: 24 mg/mL (250 mL, 500 mL)

Contraindications Hypersensitivity to foscarnet, Cl_{cr} <0.4 mL/minute/kg during therapy

Warnings/Precautions Renal impairment occurs to some degree in the majority of patients treated with foscarnet; renal impairment may occur at any time and is usually reversible within 1 week following dose adjustment or discontinuation of therapy, however, several patients have died with renal failure within 4 weeks of stopping foscarnet; therefore, renal function should be closely monitored. Foscarnet is deposited in teeth and bone of young, growing animals; it has adversely affected tooth enamel development in rats; safety and effectiveness in children have not been studied. Imbalance of serum electrolytes or minerals occurs in 6% to 18% of patients (hypocalcemia, low ionized calcium, hypo- or hyperphosphatemia, hypomagnesemia or hypokalemia).

Patients with a low ionized calcium may experience perioral tingling, numbness, paresthesias, tetany, and seizures. Seizures have been experienced by up to 10% of AIDS patients. Risk factors for seizures include a low baseline absolute neutrophil count (ANC), impaired baseline renal function and low total serum calcium. Some patients who have experienced seizures have died, while others have been able to continue or resume foscarnet treatment after their mineral or electrolyte abnormality has been corrected, their underlying disease state treated, or their dose decreased. Foscarnet has been shown to be mutagenic *in vitro* and in mice at very high doses. Information on the use of foscarnet is lacking in the elderly; dose adjustments and proper monitoring must be performed because of the decreased renal function common in older patients.

Pregnancy Risk Factor C

Adverse Reactions

>10%:

Central nervous system: Fever (65%), headache (26%), seizures (10%)

Gastrointestinal: Nausea (47%), diarrhea (30%), vomiting

Hematologic: Anemia (33%)

Renal: Abnormal renal function/decreased creatinine clearance (27%)

1% to 10%:

Central nervous system: Fatigue, malaise, dizziness, hypoesthesia, depression/confusion/anxiety (≥5%)

Dermatologic: Rash

(Continued)

Foscarnet *(Continued)*

Endocrine & metabolic: Electrolyte imbalance (especially potassium, calcium, magnesium, and phosphorus)
Gastrointestinal: Anorexia
Hematologic: Granulocytopenia, leukopenia (≥5%), thrombocytopenia, thrombosis
Local: Injection site pain
Neuromuscular & skeletal: Paresthesia, involuntary muscle contractions, rigors, neuropathy (peripheral), weakness
Ocular: Vision abnormalities
Respiratory: Coughing, dyspnea (≥5%)
Miscellaneous: Sepsis, diaphoresis (increased)

<1%: Abnormal crying, abnormal gait, arrhythmias, ascites, bradycardia, cardiac failure, cerebral edema, cholecystitis, cholelithiasis, coma, decreased gonadotropins, dyskinesia, gynecomastia, hepatitis, hepatosplenomegaly, hypertonia, hypothermia, leg edema, malignant hyperpyrexia, nystagmus, peripheral edema, speech disorders, substernal chest pain, syncope, vertigo, vocal cord paralysis

Drug Interactions Increased toxicity: Pentamidine increases hypocalcemia; concurrent use with ciprofloxacin increases seizure potential; acute renal failure (reversible) has been reported with cyclosporin due most likely to toxic synergistic effect; other nephrotoxic drugs (amphotericin B, I.V. pentamidine, aminoglycosides, etc) should be avoided, if possible, to minimize additive renal risk with foscarnet

Half-Life ~3 hours

Education and Monitoring Issues

Patient Education: Foscarnet is not a cure for the disease; progression may occur during or following therapy. Regular ophthalmic examinations will be necessary. While on the therapy it is important to maintain adequate nutrition and hydration (2-3 L/day of fluids unless instructed to restrict fluid intake); small frequent meals may help. Do not use alcohol or OTC medications without consulting prescriber. You may experience dizziness or confusion; use caution when driving or engaging in tasks that require alertness until response to drug is known. Report immediately any perioral tingling or numbness in the extremities occurring during or after the infusion. Report decrease in urine output, fluid retention, unresolved diarrhea or vomiting, unusual fever, chills, sore throat, unhealed sores, swollen lymph glands or extreme, or malaise. Barrier contraceptives are recommended to reduce transmission of disease.

Manufacturer AstraZeneca

Related Information

Pharmaceutical Manufacturers Directory *on page 1020*

♦ **Foscavir® Injection** *see* Foscarnet *on page 394*

Fosinopril (foe SIN oh pril)

Pharmacologic Class Angiotensin-Converting Enzyme (ACE) Inhibitors

U.S. Brand Names Monopril®

Generic Available No

Mechanism of Action Competitive inhibitor of angiotensin-converting enzyme (ACE); prevents conversion of angiotensin I to angiotensin II, a potent vasoconstrictor; results in lower levels of angiotensin II which causes an increase in plasma renin activity and a reduction in aldosterone secretion; a CNS mechanism may also be involved in hypotensive effect as angiotensin II increases adrenergic outflow from CNS; vasoactive kallikreins may be decreased in conversion to active hormones by ACE inhibitors, thus reducing blood pressure

Use Treatment of hypertension, either alone or in combination with other antihypertensive agents; congestive heart failure; believed to prolong survival in heart failure

USUAL DOSAGE Adults: Oral:

Hypertension: Initial: 10 mg/day; most patients are maintained on 20-40 mg/day; may need to divide the dose into two if trough effect is inadequate; discontinue the diuretic, if possible 2-3 days before initiation of therapy; resume diuretic therapy carefully, if needed.

Heart failure: Initial: 10 mg/day (5 mg if renal dysfunction present) and increase, as needed, to a maximum of 40 mg once daily over several weeks; usual dose: 20-40 mg/day; if hypotension, orthostasis, or azotemia occur during titration, consider decreasing concomitant diuretic dose, if any

Dosing adjustment/comments in renal impairment: None needed since hepatobiliary elimination compensates adequately diminished renal elimination

Hemodialysis: Moderately dialyzable (20% to 50%)

Dosage Forms TAB: 10 mg, 20 mg

Contraindications Renal impairment, collagen vascular disease, hypersensitivity to fosinopril, any component, or other angiotensin-converting enzyme inhibitors

Warnings/Precautions Use with caution and modify dosage in patients with renal impairment (decrease dosage) (especially renal artery stenosis), severe congestive heart failure or with coadministered diuretic therapy; experience in children is limited. Severe hypotension may occur in patients who are sodium and/or volume depleted; initiate lower doses and monitor closely when starting therapy in these patients.

Pregnancy Risk Factor C (1st trimester); D (2nd and 3rd trimesters)

Adverse Reactions Note: Frequency ranges include data from hypertension and heart failure trials. Higher rates of adverse reactions have generally been noted in patients with congestive heart failure. However, the frequency of adverse effects associated with placebo is also increased in this population.

>10%: Central nervous system: Dizziness (1.6% to 11.9%)

1% to 10%: Cardiovascular: Orthostatic hypotension (1.4% to 1.9%), palpitation (1.4%)

Central nervous system: Dizziness (1% to 2%; up to 12% in CHF patients), headache (3.2%), weakness (1.4%), fatigue (1% to 2%)

Endocrine and metabolic: Hyperkalemia (2.6%)

Gastrointestinal: Diarrhea (2.2%), nausea/vomiting (1.2% to 2.2%)

Hepatic: Increased transaminases

Neuromuscular & skeletal: Musculoskeletal pain (<1% to 3.3%), noncardiac chest pain (<1% to 2.2%)

Renal: Increased serum creatinine, worsening of renal function (in patients with bilateral renal artery stenosis or hypovolemia)

Respiratory: Cough (2.2% to 9.7%)

Miscellaneous: Upper respiratory infection (2.2%)

>1% but ≤ frequency in patients receiving placebo: Sexual dysfunction, fever, flu-like syndrome, dyspnea, rash, headache, insomnia

<1% (limited to important or life-threatening symptoms): Angina, myocardial infarction, cerebrovascular accident, syncope, hypotension, hypertensive crisis, claudication, flushing, edema, vertigo, insomnia, memory disturbance, drowsiness, angioedema, urticaria, rash, photosensitivity, pruritus, gout, decreased libido, pancreatitis, hepatitis, dysphagia, abdominal distension, flatulence, constipation, heartburn, xerostomia, lymphadenopathy, arthralgia, myalgia, memory disturbance, tremor, mood change, confusion, paresthesia, sleep disturbance, vertigo, drowsiness, bronchospasm, pharyngitis, laryngitis, epistaxis. tinnitus, vision, taste disturbance, eye irritation, renal insufficiency, urinary frequency, weight gain, hyperhydrosis, lower extremity edema, shock, sudden death, hypertension, bradycardia, tachycardia, hepatomegaly, TIA, cerebral infarction, numbness, behavioral change, sinus abnormality, tracheobronchitis, pleuritic chest pain, anaphylactoid reaction. In a small number of patients, a symptom complex of cough, bronchospasm, and eosinophilia has been observed with fosinopril.

Case reports: Gynecomastia, scleroderma, eosinophilic vasculitis

Other events reported with ACE inhibitors: Neutropenia, agranulocytosis, eosinophilic pneumonitis, cardiac arrest, pancytopenia, hemolytic anemia, anemia, aplastic anemia, thrombocytopenia, acute renal failure, hepatic failure, jaundice, symptomatic hyponatremia, bullous pemphigus, exfoliative dermatitis, Stevens-Johnson syndrome. In addition, a syndrome which may include fever, myalgia, arthralgia, interstitial nephritis, vasculitis, rash, eosinophilia and positive ANA, and elevated ESR has been reported for other ACE inhibitors.

Drug Interactions

Alpha$_1$ blockers: Hypotensive effect increased

Aspirin and NSAIDs may decrease ACE inhibitor efficacy and/or increase risk of renal effects

Diuretics: Hypovolemia due to diuretics may precipitate acute hypotensive events or acute renal failure

Insulin: Risk of hypoglycemia may be increased

Lithium: Risk of lithium toxicity may be increased; monitor lithium levels, especially the first 4 weeks of therapy

Mercaptopurine: Risk of neutropenia may be increased

Potassium-sparing diuretics (amiloride, spironolactone, triamterene): Increased risk of hyperkalemia

Potassium supplements may increase the risk of hyperkalemia

Trimethoprim (high dose) may increase the risk of hyperkalemia

Alcohol Interactions Avoid use (may increase risk of hypotension or dizziness)

Onset 1 hour

Duration 24 hours

Half-Life Serum (fosinoprilat): 12 hours

Education and Monitoring Issues

Patient Education: Take exactly as directed; do not discontinue without consulting prescriber. Take first dose at bedtime. This drug does not eliminate need for diet or exercise as recommended by prescriber. Do not use potassium supplements or salt substitutes containing potassium without consulting prescriber. May cause dizziness, fainting, lightheadedness (use caution when driving or engaging in tasks that require alertness until response to drug is known); postural hypotension (use caution when rising from lying or sitting position or climbing stairs); nausea, dry cough, diarrhea, or transient loss of appetite (small frequent meals, frequent mouth care, sucking lozenges, or chewing gum may help) - report if these persist; sexual dysfunction (will usually resolve). Report chest pain or palpitations; difficulty breathing or unusual cough; acute headache; or other persistent adverse reactions.

(Continued)

Fosinopril *(Continued)*

Monitoring Parameters: Blood pressure (supervise for at least 2 hours after the initial dose or any increase for significant orthostasis); serum potassium, calcium, creatinine, BUN, WBC

Manufacturer Bristol-Myers Squibb Company (Pharmaceutical Division)

Related Information

Angiotensin-Related Agents Comparison *on page 1226*
Heart Failure Guidelines *on page 1099*
Pharmaceutical Manufacturers Directory *on page 1020*

♦ **Fragmin®** *see* Dalteparin *on page 243*
♦ **Froben®** *see* Flurbiprofen *on page 384*
♦ **Froben-SR®** *see* Flurbiprofen *on page 384*
♦ **FS Shampoo®** *see* Fluocinolone *on page 374*
♦ **Ful-Glo®** *see* Fluorescein Sodium *on page 375*
♦ **Fulvicin® P/G** *see* Griseofulvin *on page 422*
♦ **Fulvicin-U/F®** *see* Griseofulvin *on page 422*
♦ **Fumasorb® [OTC]** *see* Ferrous Fumarate *on page 359*
♦ **Fumerin® [OTC]** *see* Ferrous Fumarate *on page 359*
♦ **Funduscein®** *see* Fluorescein Sodium *on page 375*
♦ **Fungoid® Creme** *see* Miconazole *on page 600*
♦ **Fungoid® Solution** *see* Clotrimazole *on page 220*
♦ **Fungoid® Tincture** *see* Miconazole *on page 600*
♦ **Furacin® Topical** *see* Nitrofurazone *on page 659*
♦ **Furadantin®** *see* Nitrofurantoin *on page 658*
♦ **Furalan®** *see* Nitrofurantoin *on page 658*
♦ **Furamide®** *see* Diloxanide Furoate *on page 278*
♦ **Furan®** *see* Nitrofurantoin *on page 658*
♦ **Furanite®** *see* Nitrofurantoin *on page 658*

Furazolidone (fyoor a ZOE li done)

Pharmacologic Class Antiprotozoal

U.S. Brand Names Furoxone®

Generic Available No

Mechanism of Action Inhibits several vital enzymatic reactions causing antibacterial and antiprotozoal action

Use Treatment of bacterial or protozoal diarrhea and enteritis caused by susceptible organisms *Giardia lamblia* and *Vibrio cholerae*

USUAL DOSAGE Oral:

Children >1 month: 5-8 mg/kg/day in 4 divided doses for 7 days, not to exceed 400 mg/day or 8.8 mg/kg/day

Adults: 100 mg 4 times/day for 7 days

Dosage Forms LIQ: 50 mg/15 mL (60 mL, 473 mL). **TAB:** 100 mg

Contraindications Known hypersensitivity to furazolidone; concurrent use of alcohol; patients <1 month of age because of the possibility of producing hemolytic anemia

Warnings/Precautions Use caution in patients with G-6-PD deficiency when administering large doses for prolonged periods; furazolidone inhibits monoamine oxidase

Pregnancy Risk Factor C

Adverse Reactions

>10%: Genitourinary: Discoloration of urine (dark yellow to brown)

1% to 10%:

Central nervous system: Headache

Gastrointestinal: Abdominal pain, diarrhea, nausea, vomiting

<1%: Agranulocytosis, arthralgia, disulfiram-like reaction after alcohol ingestion, dizziness, drowsiness, fever, hemolysis in patients with G-6-PD deficiency, hypoglycemia, leukopenia, malaise, orthostatic hypotension, rash

Drug Interactions

Increases toxicity of sympathomimetic amines, tricyclic antidepressants, MAO inhibitors, meperidine, anorexiants, dextromethorphan, fluoxetine, paroxetine, sertraline, trazodone

Increased effect/toxicity of levodopa

Disulfiram-like reaction with alcohol

Alcohol Interactions Avoid use (may cause a disulfiram-like reaction; symptoms include headache, nausea, vomiting, chest or abdominal pain)

Education and Monitoring Issues

Patient Education: Take as directed. Avoid alcohol and tyramine-containing foods during and for 4 days following therapy. Do not take any other prescription or OTC medications without consulting prescriber. Your urine may turn dark brown or yellow (normal). If diabetic, use something other than Clinitest® for urine glucose testing. Report acute GI pain, unresolved diarrhea, unresolved nausea or vomiting, fever, dizziness, or unusual joint pain. Consult prescriber if condition is not resolved at the end of therapy.

Dietary Considerations: Food: Marked elevation of blood pressure, hypertensive crisis, or hemorrhagic stroke may occur with foods high in amine content

Monitoring Parameters: CBC

Manufacturer Roberts Pharmaceuticals

Related Information

Pharmaceutical Manufacturers Directory *on page 1020*

Furosemide (fyoor OH se mide)

Pharmacologic Class Diuretic, Loop

U.S. Brand Names Lasix®

Generic Available Yes

Mechanism of Action Inhibits reabsorption of sodium and chloride in the ascending loop of Henle and distal renal tubule, interfering with the chloride-binding cotransport system, thus causing increased excretion of water, sodium, chloride, magnesium, and calcium

Use Management of edema associated with congestive heart failure and hepatic or renal disease; used alone or in combination with antihypertensives in treatment of hypertension

USUAL DOSAGE

Infants and Children:

Oral: 1-2 mg/kg/dose increased in increments of 1 mg/kg/dose with each succeeding dose until a satisfactory effect is achieved to a maximum of 6 mg/kg/dose no more frequently than 6 hours

I.M., I.V.: 1 mg/kg/dose, increasing by each succeeding dose at 1 mg/kg/dose at intervals of 6-12 hours until a satisfactory response up to 6 mg/kg/dose

Adults:

Oral: 20-80 mg/dose initially increased in increments of 20-40 mg/dose at intervals of 6-8 hours; usual maintenance dose interval is twice daily or every day; may be titrated up to 600 mg/day with severe edematous states

I.M., I.V.: 20-40 mg/dose, may be repeated in 1-2 hours as needed and increased by 20 mg/dose until the desired effect has been obtained; usual dosing interval: 6-12 hours; for acute pulmonary edema, the usual dose is 40 mg I.V. over 1-2 minutes; if not adequate, may increase dose to 80 mg

Continuous I.V. infusion: Initial I.V. bolus dose of 0.1 mg/kg followed by continuous I.V. infusion doses of 0.1 mg/kg/hour doubled every 2 hours to a maximum of 0.4 mg/kg/hour if urine output is <1 mL/kg/hour have been found to be effective and result in a lower daily requirement of furosemide than with intermittent dosing. Other studies have used a rate of ≤4 mg/minute as a continuous I.V. infusion.

Elderly: Oral, I.M., I.V.: Initial: 20 mg/day; increase slowly to desired response

Refractory heart failure: Oral, I.V.: Doses up to 8 g/day have been used

Dosing adjustment/comments in renal impairment: Acute renal failure: High doses (up to 1-3 g/day - oral/I.V.) have been used to initiate desired response; avoid use in oliguric states

Dialysis: Not removed by hemo- or peritoneal dialysis; supplemental dose is not necessary

Dosing adjustment/comments in hepatic disease: Diminished natriuretic effect with increased sensitivity to hypokalemia and volume depletion in cirrhosis; monitor effects, particularly with high doses

Dosage Forms INJ: 10 mg/mL (2 mL, 4 mL, 5 mL, 6 mL, 8 mL, 10 mL, 12 mL). **SOLN, oral:** 10 mg/mL (60 mL, 120 mL); 40 mg/5 mL (5 mL, 10 mL, 500 mL). **TAB:** 20 mg, 40 mg, 80 mg

Contraindications Hypersensitivity to furosemide, any component, or other sulfonamides; use with sparfloxacin; anuric patients

Warnings/Precautions Loop diuretics are potent diuretics; close medical supervision and dose evaluation is required to prevent fluid and electrolyte imbalance; use caution with other nephrotoxic or ototoxic drugs

Pregnancy Risk Factor C

Pregnancy Implications

Clinical effects on the fetus: Crosses the placenta. Increased fetal urine production, electrolyte disturbances reported. Generally, use of diuretics during pregnancy is avoided due to risk of decreased placental perfusion.

Breast-feeding/lactation: Crosses into breast milk; may suppress lactation. American Academy of Pediatrics has NO RECOMMENDATION.

Adverse Reactions Incidence of adverse events is not reported.

Cardiovascular: Orthostatic hypotension, necrotizing angiitis, thrombophlebitis, chronic aortitis, acute hypotension, sudden death from cardiac arrest (with I.V. or I.M. administration)

Central nervous system: Paresthesias, vertigo, dizziness, lightheadedness, headache, blurred vision, xanthopsia , fever, restlessness

Dermatologic: Exfoliative dermatitis, erythema multiforme, purpura, photosensitivity, urticaria, rash, pruritus, cutaneous vasculitis

Endocrine & metabolic: Hyperglycemia, hyperuricemia, hypokalemia, hypochloremia, metabolic alkalosis, hypocalcemia, hypomagnesemia, gout

(Continued)

Furosemide *(Continued)*

Gastrointestinal: Nausea, vomiting, anorexia, oral and gastric irritation, cramping, diarrhea, constipation, pancreatitis, intrahepatic cholestatic jaundice, ischemia hepatitis

Genitourinary: Urinary bladder spasm, urinary frequency

Hematological: Aplastic anemia (rare), thrombocytopenia, agranulocytosis (rare), hemolytic anemia, leukopenia, anemia, purpura

Neuromuscular & skeletal: Muscle spasm, weakness

Otic: Hearing impairment (reversible or permanent with rapid I.V. or I.M. administration), tinnitus, reversible deafness (with rapid I.V. or I.M. administration)

Renal: Vasculitis, allergic interstitial nephritis, glycosuria, fall in glomerular filtration rate and renal blood flow (due to overdiuresis), transient rise in BUN

Miscellaneous: Anaphylaxis (rare), exacerbate or activate systemic lupus erythematosus

Drug Interactions

ACE inhibitors: Hypotensive effects and/or renal effects are potentiated by hypovolemia

Antidiabetic agents: Glucose tolerance may be decreased

Antihypertensive agents: Hypotensive effects may be enhanced

Cephaloridine or cephalexin: Nephrotoxicity may occur

Cholestyramine or colestipol may reduce bioavailability of furosemide

Clofibrate: Protein binding may be altered in hypoalbuminemic patients receiving furosemide, potentially increasing toxicity

Digoxin: Furosemide-induced hypokalemia may predispose to digoxin toxicity; monitor potassium

Indomethacin (and other NSAIDs) may reduce natriuretic and hypotensive effects of furosemide

Lithium: Renal clearance may be reduced. Isolated reports of lithium toxicity have occurred; monitor lithium levels.

Metformin may decrease furosemide concentrations

Metformin blood levels may be increased by furosemide

NSAIDs: Risk of renal impairment may increase when used in conjunction with furosemide

Ototoxic drugs (aminoglycosides, cis-platinum): Concomitant use of furosemide may increase risk of ototoxicity, especially in patients with renal dysfunction

Peripheral adrenergic-blocking drugs or ganglionic blockers: Effects may be increased

Phenobarbital or phenytoin may reduce diuretic response to furosemide

Salicylates (high-dose) with furosemide may predispose patients to salicylate toxicity due to reduced renal excretion or alter renal function

Sparfloxacin, gatifloxacin, and moxifloxacin: Risk of hypokalemia and cardiotoxicity may be increased Avoid use

Succinylcholine: Action may be potentiated by furosemide

Sucralfate may limit absorption of furosemide, effects may be significantly decreased; separate oral administration by 2 hours

Thiazides: Synergistic diuretic effects occur

Tubocurarine: The skeletal muscle-relaxing effect may be attenuated by furosemide

Onset

Onset of diuresis: Oral: Within 30-60 minutes; I.M.: 30 minutes; I.V.: Within 5 minutes

Peak effect: Oral: Within 1-2 hours

Duration Oral: 6-8 hours; I.V.: 2 hours

Half-Life Normal renal function: 0.5-1.1 hours; End-stage renal disease: 9 hours

Education and Monitoring Issues

Patient Education: Take as directed, with food or milk early in the day (daily), or if twice daily, take last dose in late afternoon in order to avoid sleep disturbance and achieve maximum therapeutic effect. Keep medication in original container, away from light; do not use discolored medication. Include bananas or orange juice (or other potassium-rich foods) in daily diet; do not take potassium supplements without advice of prescriber. Weigh yourself each day, at the same time, in the same clothes when beginning therapy, and weekly on long-term therapy; report unusual or unanticipated weight gain or loss. You may experience dizziness, blurred vision, or drowsiness; use caution when driving or engaging in tasks that require alertness until response to drug is known. Use caution when rising or changing position. You may experience sensitivity to sunlight; use sunblock or wear protective clothing and sunglasses. Report signs of edema (eg, weight gains, swollen ankles, feet or hands), trembling, numbness or fatigue, any cramping or muscle weakness, palpitations, or unresolved nausea or vomiting.

Monitoring Parameters: Monitor weight and I & O daily; blood pressure, serum electrolytes, renal function; in high doses, monitor hearing

Related Information

Heart Failure Guidelines *on page 1099*

- **Furoside®** *see* Furosemide *on page 399*
- **Furoxone®** *see* Furazolidone *on page 398*
- **G-1®** *see* Butalbital Compound *on page 123*

Gabapentin (GA ba pen tin)

Pharmacologic Class Anticonvulsant, Miscellaneous

U.S. Brand Names Neurontin®

Generic Available No

Mechanism of Action Exact mechanism of action is not known, but does have properties in common with other anticonvulsants; although structurally related to GABA, it does not interact with GABA receptors

Use Adjunct for treatment of drug-refractory partial and secondarily generalized seizures in adults with epilepsy; not effective for absence seizures

USUAL DOSAGE If gabapentin is discontinued or if another anticonvulsant is added to therapy, it should be done slowly over a minimum of 1 week

Children >12 years and Adults: Oral:

- Initial: 300 mg on day 1 (at bedtime to minimize sedation), then 300 mg twice daily on day 2, and then 300 mg 3 times/day on day 3
- Total daily dosage range: 900-1800 mg/day administered in 3 divided doses at 8-hour intervals
- Pain: 300-1800 mg/day given in 3 divided doses has been the most common dosage range

Dosing adjustment in renal impairment:

- Cl_{cr} >60 mL/minute: Administer 1200 mg/day
- Cl_{cr} 30-60 mL/minute: Administer 600 mg/day
- Cl_{cr} 15-30 mL/minute: Administer 300 mg/day
- Cl_{cr} <15 mL/minute: Administer 150 mg/day

Hemodialysis: 200-300 mg after each 4-hour dialysis following a loading dose of 300-400 mg

Dosage Forms CAP: 100 mg, 300 mg, 400 mg

Contraindications Hypersensitivity to the drug or its ingredients

Warnings/Precautions Avoid abrupt withdrawal, may precipitate seizures; may be associated with a slight incidence (0.6%) of status epilepticus and sudden deaths (0.0038 deaths/patient year); use cautiously in patients with severe renal dysfunction; rat studies demonstrated an association with pancreatic adenocarcinoma in male rats; clinical implication unknown

Pregnancy Risk Factor C

Pregnancy Implications

Clinical effects on the fetus: No data on crossing the placenta; 4 reports of normal pregnancy outcomes; 1 report of infant with respiratory distress, pyloric stenosis, inguinal hernia following 1st trimester exposure to gabapentin plus carbamazepine; epilepsy itself, number of medications, genetic factors, or a combination of these probably influence the teratogenicity of anticonvulsant therapy

Breast-feeding/lactation: No data available

Adverse Reactions

>10%: Central nervous system: Somnolence, dizziness, ataxia, fatigue

1% to 10%:

- Cardiovascular: Peripheral edema
- Central nervous system: Nervousness, amnesia, depression, abnormal coordination, dysarthria, abnormal thinking, twitching
- Dermatologic: Pruritus
- Gastrointestinal: Dyspepsia, xerostomia, dry throat, constipation, appetite stimulation (weight gain)
- Genitourinary: Impotence
- Hematologic: Leukopenia
- Neuromuscular & skeletal: Back pain, myalgia, tremor
- Ocular: Diplopia, blurred vision, nystagmus
- Respiratory: Rhinitis, pharyngitis, coughing
- Miscellaneous: Hiccups

Drug Interactions

Gabapentin does not modify plasma concentrations of standard anticonvulsant medications (ie, valproic acid, carbamazepine, phenytoin, or phenobarbital)

Antacids reduce the bioavailability of gabapentin by 20%

Cimetidine may decrease clearance (by 14%) of gabapentin; gabapentin may increase C_{max} of norethindrone by 13%

Alcohol Interactions Avoid use (may increase central nervous system depression)

Half-Life 5-6 hours

Education and Monitoring Issues

Patient Education: Take exactly as directed (do not increase dose or frequency or discontinue without consulting prescriber). While using this medication, do not use alcohol and other prescription or OTC medications (especially pain medications, sedatives, antihistamines, or hypnotics) without consulting prescriber. Maintain adequate hydration (2-3 L/day of fluids unless instructed to restrict fluid intake). You may experience drowsiness, dizziness, or blurred vision (use caution when driving or engaging in tasks requiring alertness until response to drug is known); nausea, vomiting, loss of appetite, or dry mouth (small frequent meals, frequent mouth care, chewing gum, or sucking lozenges may help). Wear identification of epileptic status. Report CNS

(Continued)

Gabapentin *(Continued)*

changes, mentation changes, or changes in cognition; muscle cramping, weakness, tremors, changes in gait; persistent GI symptoms (cramping, constipation, vomiting, anorexia); difficulty breathing; impotence or changes in urinary pattern; worsening of seizure activity, or loss of seizure control.

Dietary Considerations:

Food: Does not change rate or extent of absorption; take without regard to meals

Serum lipids: May see increases in total cholesterol, HDL cholesterol and triglycerides. Hyperlipidemia and hypercholesterolemia have been reported with gabapentin.

Monitoring Parameters: Monitor serum levels of concomitant anticonvulsant therapy; routine monitoring of gabapentin levels is not mandatory

Reference Range: Minimum effective serum concentration may be 2 μg/mL; **routine monitoring of drug levels is not required**

Manufacturer Parke-Davis

Related Information

Anticonvulsants by Seizure Type Comparison *on page 1230*

Epilepsy Guidelines *on page 1091*

Pharmaceutical Manufacturers Directory *on page 1020*

- **Gabitril®** *see* Tiagabine *on page 917*

Gallium Nitrate (GAL ee um NYE trate)

Pharmacologic Class Antidote

U.S. Brand Names Ganite™

Generic Available No

Mechanism of Action Primarily via inhibition of bone resorption with associated reduction in urinary calcium excretion. Gallium has increased the calcium content of newly mineralized bone following short-term treatment *in vitro*, and this effect combined with its ability to inhibit bone resorption has suggested the use of gallium for other disorders associated with increased bone loss.

Use Treatment of clearly symptomatic cancer-related hypercalcemia that has not responded to adequate hydration

USUAL DOSAGE Adults:

I.V. infusion (over 24 hours): 200 mg/m^2 for 5 consecutive days in 1 L of NS or D_5W

Mild hypercalcemia/few symptoms: 100 mg/m^2/day for 5 days in 1 L of NS or D_5W

Dosing adjustment/comments in renal impairment: Cl_{cr} <30 mL/minute: Avoid use

Dosage Forms INJ: 25 mg/mL (20 mL)

Contraindications Should not be used in patients with a serum creatinine >2.5 mg/dL, hypersensitivity to any component

Warnings/Precautions Safety and efficacy in children have not been established. Concurrent use of gallium nitrate with other potentially nephrotoxic drugs may increase the risk for developing severe renal insufficiency in patients with cancer-related hypercalcemia; use with caution in patients with impaired renal function or dehydration

Pregnancy Risk Factor C

Adverse Reactions

>10%:

Endocrine & metabolic: Hypophosphatemia

Gastrointestinal: Nausea, vomiting, diarrhea, metallic taste

Renal: Renal toxicity

1% to 10%: Endocrine & metabolic: Hypocalcemia

<1%: Anemia, hearing impairment, optic neuritis

Drug Interactions Increased toxicity: Nephrotoxic drugs (eg, aminoglycosides, amphotericin B)

Half-Life 25-111 hours

Education and Monitoring Issues

Monitoring Parameters: Serum creatinine, BUN, and calcium

Reference Range: Steady-state gallium serum levels: Generally obtained within 2 days following initiation of continuous I.V. infusions of gallium nitrate

- **Gamimune® N** *see* Immune Globulin, Intravenous *on page 465*
- **Gammagard® S/D** *see* Immune Globulin, Intravenous *on page 465*
- **Gammar®-P I.V.** *see* Immune Globulin, Intravenous *on page 465*
- **Gamulin® Rh** *see* Rh_o(D) Immune Globulin (Intramuscular) *on page 816*

Ganciclovir (gan SYE kloe veer)

Pharmacologic Class Antiviral Agent

U.S. Brand Names Cytovene®; Vitrasert®

Generic Available No

Mechanism of Action Ganciclovir is phosphorylated to a substrate which competitively inhibits the binding of deoxyguanosine triphosphate to DNA polymerase resulting in inhibition of viral DNA synthesis

Use

Parenteral: Treatment of CMV retinitis in immunocompromised individuals, including patients with acquired immunodeficiency syndrome; prophylaxis of CMV infection in transplant patients; may be given in combination with foscarnet in patients who relapse after monotherapy with either drug

Oral: Alternative to the I.V. formulation for maintenance treatment of CMV retinitis in immunocompromised patients, including patients with AIDS, in whom retinitis is stable following appropriate induction therapy and for whom the risk of more rapid progression is balanced by the benefit associated with avoiding daily I.V. infusions.

Implant: Treatment of CMV retinitis

USUAL DOSAGE

CMV retinitis: Slow I.V. infusion (dosing is based on total body weight):

Children >3 months and Adults:

Induction therapy: 5 mg/kg/dose every 12 hours for 14-21 days followed by maintenance therapy

Maintenance therapy: 5 mg/kg/day as a single daily dose for 7 days/week or 6 mg/kg/day for 5 days/week

CMV retinitis: Oral: 1000 mg 3 times/day with food **or** 500 mg 6 times/day with food

Prevention of CMV disease in patients with advanced HIV infection and normal renal function: Oral: 1000 mg 3 times/day with food

Prevention of CMV disease in transplant patients: Same initial and maintenance dose as CMV retinitis except duration of initial course is 7-14 days, duration of maintenance therapy is dependent on clinical condition and degree of immunosuppression

Intravitreal implant: One implant for 5- to 8-month period; following depletion of ganciclovir, as evidenced by progression of retinitis, implant may be removed and replaced

Dosing adjustment in renal impairment:

I.V. (Induction):

Cl_{cr} 50-69 mL/minute: Administer 2.5 mg/kg/dose every 12 hours

Cl_{cr} 25-49 mL/minute: Administer 2.5 mg/kg/dose every 24 hours

Cl_{cr} 10-24 mL/minute: Administer 1.25 mg/kg/dose every 24 hours

Cl_{cr} <10 mL/minute: Administer 1.25 mg/kg/dose 3 times/week following hemodialysis

I.V. (Maintenance):

Cl_{cr} 50-69 mL/minute: Administer 2.5 mg/kg/dose every 24 hours

Cl_{cr} 25-49 mL/minute: Administer 1.25 mg/kg/dose every 24 hours

Cl_{cr} 10-24 mL/minute: Administer 0.625 mg/kg/dose every 24 hours

Cl_{cr} <10 mL/minute: Administer 0.625 mg/kg/dose 3 times/week following hemodialysis

Oral:

Cl_{cr} 50-69 mL/minute: Administer 1500 mg/day or 500 mg 3 times/day

Cl_{cr} 25-49 mL/minute: Administer 1000 mg/day or 500 mg twice daily

Cl_{cr} 10-24 mL/minute: Administer 500 mg/day

Cl_{cr} <10 mL/minute: Administer 500 mg 3 times/week following hemodialysis

Hemodialysis effects: Dialyzable (50%) following hemodialysis; administer dose postdialysis. During peritoneal dialysis, dose as for Cl_{cr} <10 mL/minute. During continuous arteriovenous or venovenous hemofiltration (CAVH/CAVHD), administer 2.5 mg/kg/dose every 24 hours.

Dosage Forms CAP: 250 mg. **IMPLANT, intravitreal:** 4.5 mg released gradually over 5-8 months. **POWDER for inj, lyophilized:** 500 mg (10 mL)

Contraindications Absolute neutrophil count <500/mm³; platelet count <25,000/mm³; known hypersensitivity to ganciclovir or acyclovir

Warnings/Precautions Dosage adjustment or interruption of ganciclovir therapy may be necessary in patients with neutropenia and/or thrombocytopenia and patients with impaired renal function. Use with extreme caution in children since long-term safety has not been determined and due to ganciclovir's potential for long-term carcinogenic and adverse reproductive effects; ganciclovir may adversely affect spermatogenesis and fertility; due to its mutagenic potential, contraceptive precautions for female and male patients need to be followed during and for at least 90 days after therapy with the drug; take care to administer only into veins with good blood flow.

Pregnancy Risk Factor C

Adverse Reactions

>10%:

Central nervous system: Fever (38% to 48%)

Dermatologic: Rash (15% - oral, 10% - I.V.)

Gastrointestinal: Abdominal pain (17% to 19%), diarrhea (40%), nausea (25%), anorexia (15%), vomiting (13%)

Hematologic: Anemia (20% to 25%), leukopenia (30% to 40%)

1% to 10%:

Central nervous system: Confusion, neuropathy (8% to 9%), headache (4%)

Dermatologic: Pruritus (5%)

Hematologic: Thrombocytopenia (6%), neutropenia with ANC <500/mm³ (5% - oral, 14% - I.V.)

Neuromuscular & skeletal: Paresthesia (6% to 10%), weakness (6%)

Miscellaneous: Sepsis (4% - oral, 15% - I.V.)

(Continued)

Ganciclovir *(Continued)*

<1%: Alopecia, arrhythmia, ataxia, azotemia, coma, creatinine increased 2.5%, dizziness, dyspnea, edema, eosinophilia, hemorrhage, hypertension, hyphema, hypotension, increased LFTs, increased serum creatinine, inflammation or pain at injection site, malaise, nervousness, psychosis, retinal detachment, seizures, tremor, urticaria, uveitis (intravitreal implant), visual loss

Drug Interactions

Decreased effect: Didanosine: A decrease in steady-state ganciclovir AUC may occur

Increased toxicity:

Immunosuppressive agents may increase cytotoxicity of ganciclovir

Imipenem/cilastatin may increase seizure potential

Zidovudine: Oral ganciclovir increased the AUC of zidovudine, although zidovudine decreases steady state levels of ganciclovir. Since both drugs have the potential to cause neutropenia and anemia, some patients may not tolerate concomitant therapy with these drugs at full dosage.

Probenecid: The renal clearance of ganciclovir is decreased in the presence of probenecid

Didanosine levels are increased with concurrent ganciclovir

Other nephrotoxic drugs (eg, amphotericin and cyclosporine) may have additive nephrotoxicity with ganciclovir

Half-Life 1.7-5.8 hours; increases with impaired renal function; End-stage renal disease: 3.6 hours

Education and Monitoring Issues

Patient Education: Ganciclovir is not a cure for CMV retinitis. Maintain adequate hydration (2-3 L/day of fluids unless instructed to restrict fluid intake). You will need frequent blood tests and regular ophthalmic exams while taking this drug. You may experience increased susceptibility to infection; avoid crowds or exposure to infectious persons. You may experience photosensitivity; use sunscreen, wear protective clothing and eyewear, and avoid direct sunlight. Report fever, chills, unusual bleeding or bruising, infection, or unhealed sores or white plaques in mouth.

Dietary Considerations: Administer with food

Monitoring Parameters: CBC with differential and platelet count, serum creatinine, ophthalmologic exams

Manufacturer Roche Laboratories

Related Information

Pharmaceutical Manufacturers Directory *on page 1020*

♦ **Ganite™** *see* Gallium Nitrate *on page 402*

♦ **Gantanol®** *see* Sulfamethoxazole *on page 879*

♦ **Garamycin®** *see* Gentamicin *on page 408*

♦ **Garatec** *see* Gentamicin *on page 408*

Garlic

Pharmacologic Class Herbal

Mechanism of Action Garlic bulbs contain alliin, a parent to the substance allicin (after the bulb is ground), which is odoriferous and may have some antioxidant activity; ajoene (a byproduct of allicin) has potent platelet inhibition effects; garlic can also decrease LDL cholesterol levels and increase fibrinolytic activity

Use Herbal medicine used for lowering LDL cholesterol and triglycerides, and raising HDL cholesterol; protection against atherosclerosis, hypertension, antiseptic agent; may lower blood glucose and decrease thrombosis; potential anti-inflammatory and antitumor effects

USUAL DOSAGE Adult dose: 4-12 mg allicin/day

Average daily dose for cardiovascular benefits: 0.25-1 g/kg or 1-4 cloves daily in an 80 kg individual in divided doses

Toxic dose: >5 cloves or >25 mL of extract can cause gastrointestinal symptoms

Warnings/Precautions Cholesterol lowering and hypotensive effects may require months. Use with caution in patients receiving treatment for hyperglycemia or hypertension.

Pregnancy Implications Avoid use

Adverse Reactions

Dermatologic: Skin blistering, eczema, systemic contact dermatitis, immunologic contact urticaria

Gastrointestinal: G.I. upset and changes in intestinal flora (in rare cases) per Commission E

Ocular: Lacrimation

Respiratory: Asthma (upon inhalation of garlic dust)

Miscellaneous: Allergic reactions (in rare cases); change in odor of skin and breath per Commission E

Drug Interactions Iodine uptake may be reduced with garlic ingestion; can exacerbate bleeding in patients taking aspirin or anticoagulant agents; may increase risk of hypoglycemia, may increase response to antihypertensives

♦ **Gastrocrom® Oral** *see* Cromolyn Sodium *on page 231*

♦ **Gastrosed™** *see* Hyoscyamine *on page 456*

Gatifloxacin (ga ti FLOKS a sin)

Pharmacologic Class Antibiotic, Quinolone

U.S. Brand Names Tequin™

Mechanism of Action Gatifloxacin is a DNA gyrase inhibitor, and also inhibits topoisomerase IV. DNA gyrase (topoisomerase II) is an essential bacterial enzyme that maintains the superhelical structure of DNA. DNA gyrase is required for DNA replication and transcription, DNA repair, recombination, and transposition; inhibition is bactericidal.

Use Treatment of the following infections when caused by susceptible bacteria: Acute bacterial exacerbation of chronic bronchitis due to *S. pneumoniae, H. influenzae, H. parainfluenzae, M. catarrhalis*, or *S. aureus*; acute sinusitis due to *S. pneumoniae, H. influenzae*; community acquired pneumonia due to *S. pneumoniae, H. influenzae, H. parainfluenzae, M. catarrhalis, S. aureus, M. pneumoniae, C. pneumoniae*, or *L. pneumophilia*; uncomplicated urinary tract infections (cystitis) due to *E. coli, K. pneumoniae*, or *P. mirabilis*; complicated urinary tract infections due to *E. coli, K. pneumoniae*, or *P. mirabilis*; pyelonephritis due to *E. coli*; uncomplicated urethral and cervical gonorrhea; acute, uncomplicated rectal infections in women due to *N. gonorrhoeae*

USUAL DOSAGE Adult: Oral, I.V.:

Acute bacterial exacerbation of chronic bronchitis; 400 mg every 24 hours for 7-10 days

Acute sinusitis: 400 mg every 24 hours for 10 days

Community acquired pneumonia: 400 mg every 24 hours for 7-14 days

Uncomplicated urinary tract infections (cystitis): 200-400 mg every 24 hours for 3 days

Complicated urinary tract infections: 400 mg every 24 hours for 7-10 days

Acute pyelonephritis: 400 mg every 24 hours for 7-10 days

Uncomplicated urethral gonorrhea in men, cervical or rectal gonorrhea in women: 400 mg single dose

Dosage adjustment in renal impairment: Creatinine clearance <40 mL/minute (or patients on hemodialysis/CAPD) should receive an initial dose of 400 mg, followed by a subsequent dose of 200 mg every 24 hours. Patients receiving single-dose or 3-day therapy for appropriate indications do not require dosage adjustment.

Dosage adjustment in hepatic impairment: No dosage adjustment is required in mild-moderate hepatic disease. No data are available in severe hepatic impairment (Child-Pugh Class C).

Elderly: No dosage adjustment is required based on age, however, assessment of renal function is particularly important in this population.

Dosage Forms INF: 2 mg/mL (100 mL, 200 mL). **INJ:** 10 mg/mL (20 mL, 40 mL). **TAB:** 200 mg, 400 mg

Contraindications Hypersensitivity to gatifloxacin, other quinolone antibiotics, or any component

Warnings/Precautions Use with caution in patients with significant bradycardia or acute myocardial ischemia. May have potential to prolong Q-T interval; should avoid in patients with uncorrected hypokalemia, or concurrent administration of other medications known to prolong the Q-T interval (including class Ia and class III antiarrhythmics, cisapride, erythromycin, antipsychotics, and tricyclic antidepressants). Safety and effectiveness in pediatric patients (<18 years of age) have not been established. Experience in immature animals has resulted in permanent arthropathy. Use with caution in individuals at risk of seizures (CNS disorders or concurrent therapy with medications which may lower seizure threshold). Discontinue in patients who experience significant CNS adverse effects (dizziness, hallucinations, suicidal ideation or actions). Use caution in renal dysfunction (dosage adjustment required) and in severe hepatic insufficiency (no data available). Use caution in patients with diabetes - glucose regulation may be altered.

Severe hypersensitivity reactions, including anaphylaxis, have occurred with quinolone therapy. If an allergic reaction occurs (itching, urticaria, dyspnea or facial edema, loss of consciousness, tingling, cardiovascular collapse) discontinue drug immediately. Prolonged use may result in superinfection; pseudomembranous colitis may occur and should be considered in all patients who present with diarrhea. Tendon inflammation and/or rupture has been reported with other quinolone antibiotics. This has not been reported for gatifloxacin. Discontinue at first sign of tendon inflammation or pain.

Pregnancy Risk Factor C

Pregnancy Implications No adequate or well-controlled studies in pregnant women. Should be used during pregnancy only when the potential benefit justifies the potential risk to the fetus.

Adverse Reactions

3% to 10%:

Central nervous system: Headache (3%), dizziness (3%)

Gastrointestinal: Nausea (8%), diarrhea (4%)

Genitourinary: Vaginitis (6%)

Local: Injection site reactions (5%)

0.1% to 3%: Allergic reaction, chills, fever, back pain, chest pain, palpitation, abdominal pain, constipation, dyspepsia, glossitis, oral candidiasis, stomatitis, mouth ulceration, vomiting, peripheral edema, abnormal dreams, insomnia, paresthesia, tremor, vasodilation, vertigo, dyspnea, pharyngitis, rash, sweating, abnormal vision, taste perversion,

(Continued)

Gatifloxacin *(Continued)*

tinnitus, dysuria, hematuria, elevated serum transaminases, elevated alkaline phosphatase, increased serum bilirubin, increased serum amylase

<0.1% (limited to important or life-threatening symptoms): Abnormal thinking, agitation, alcohol intolerance, anorexia, anxiety, arthralgia, arthritis, asthenia, ataxia, bone pain, bradycardia, breast pain, bronchospasm, cheilitis, colitis, confusion, cyanosis, depersonalization, depression, diabetes mellitus, dry skin, dysphagia, ear pain, ecchymosis, edema, epistaxis, euphoria, eye pain, facial edema, flatulence, gastritis, gastrointestinal hemorrhage, gingivitis, halitosis, hallucination, hematemesis, hostility, hyperesthesia, hyperglycemia, hypertension, hypertonia, hyperventilation, hypoglycemia, leg cramps, lymphadenopathy, maculopapular rash, metrorrhagia, migraine, myalgia, myasthenia, neck pain, nervousness, panic attacks, paranoia, parosmia, pruritus, pseudomembranous colitis, psychosis, ptosis, rectal hemorrhage, seizures, somnolence, stress, tachycardia, taste disturbance, thirst, tongue edema, vesiculobullous rash

Drug Interactions

Gatifloxacin may prolong Q-T interval; avoid use with drugs which prolong Q-T interval (including class Ia and class III antiarrhythmics, erythromycin, cisapride, antipsychotics, and cyclic antidepressants).

Metal cations (magnesium, aluminum, iron, and zinc) bind quinolones in the gastrointestinal tract and inhibit absorption (by up to 98%). Antacids, electrolyte supplements, sucralfate, quinapril, and some didanosine formulations should be avoided. Gatifloxacin should be administered 4 hours before or 8 hours after these agents.

Antineoplastic agents may decrease the absorption of quinolones

Calcium carbonate was not found to alter the absorption of gatifloxacin.

Cimetidine, and other H_2 antagonists may inhibit renal elimination of quinolones

Digoxin levels may be increased in some patients by gatifloxacin; monitor for increased effect/concentrations.

Foscarnet has been associated with an increased risk of seizures with some quinolones

H_2 antagonists and proton pump inhibitors may decrease absorption of some quinolones

Loop diuretics: Serum levels of some quinolones are increased by loop diuretic administration. May diminish renal excretion.

NSAIDs: The CNS stimulating effect of some quinolones may be enhanced, resulting in neuroexcitation and/or seizures. This effect has not been observed with gatifloxacin.

Probenecid: Blocks renal secretion of gatifloxacin, increasing AUC and half-life.

Warfarin: The hypoprothrombinemic effect of warfarin is enhanced by some quinolone antibiotics. No significant effect has been demonstrated for gatifloxacin, however, monitoring of the INR during concurrent therapy is recommended by the manufacturer.

Half-Life 7-14 hours (up to 40 hours in ESRD)

Education and Monitoring Issues

Patient Education: I.V.: Report any pain, itching, burning or signs of irritation at infusion site.

Oral: Take exactly as directed with or without food. Do not take antacids, vitamins, ulcer or hypertensive medication 2 hours before or 4 hours after taking gatifloxacin. Do not miss a dose (take a missed dose as soon as possible, unless it is almost time for next dose). Take entire prescription even if feeling better. Maintain adequate hydration (2-3 L/day of fluid, unless instructed to restrict fluids). Following I.V. or oral administration, you may experience nausea, vomiting, taste perversion (small frequent meals, good mouth care, chewing gum, or sucking hard candy may help); headache, dizziness, insomnia, anxiety (use caution when driving or engaged in tasks requiring alertness until response is known). Report immediately any swelling of mouth, lips, tongue or throat; chest pain or tightness, difficulty breathing, back pain, itching, skin rash, or tingling; tendon pain; confusion, dizziness, abnormal thinking, anxiety, or insomnia. Report changes in voiding pattern, vaginal itching, burning, or discharge; changes in vision or hearing; abnormal bruising or bleeding or blood in urine; or other adverse reactions.

Monitoring Parameters: WBC, signs of infection

Manufacturer Bristol-Myers Squibb Company (Pharmaceutical Division)

Related Information

Community Acquired Pneumonia in Adults *on page 1200*
Pharmaceutical Manufacturers Directory *on page 1020*

- **Gee Gee® [OTC]** *see* Guaifenesin *on page 423*
- **Gel Kam®** *see* Fluoride *on page 376*
- **Gel-Ose** *see* Lactulose *on page 506*
- **Gel-Tin® [OTC]** *see* Fluoride *on page 376*
- **Gelucast®** *see* Zinc Gelatin *on page 993*
- **Gemcor®** *see* Gemfibrozil *on page 406*

Gemfibrozil (jem FI broe zil)

Pharmacologic Class Antilipemic Agent (Fibric Acid)

U.S. Brand Names Gemcor®; Lopid®

Generic Available No

Mechanism of Action The exact mechanism of action of gemfibrozil is unknown, however, several theories exist regarding the VLDL effect; it can inhibit lipolysis and decrease subsequent hepatic fatty acid uptake as well as inhibit hepatic secretion of VLDL; together these actions decrease serum VLDL levels; increases HDL cholesterol; the mechanism behind HDL elevation is currently unknown

Use Treatment of hypertriglyceridemia in types IV and V hyperlipidemia for patients who are at greater risk for pancreatitis and who have not responded to dietary intervention; reduction of coronary heart disease in type IIB patients who have low HDL cholesterol, increased LDL cholesterol, and increased triglycerides

USUAL DOSAGE Adults: Oral: 1200 mg/day in 2 divided doses, 30 minutes before breakfast and dinner

Hemodialysis: Not removed by hemodialysis; supplemental dose is not necessary

Dosage Forms CAP: 300 mg. **TAB, film coated:** 600 mg

Contraindications Renal or hepatic dysfunction, gallbladder disease, hypersensitivity to gemfibrozil or any component

Warnings/Precautions Abnormal elevation of AST, ALT, LDH, bilirubin, and alkaline phosphatase has occurred; if no appreciable triglyceride or cholesterol lowering effect occurs after 3 months, the drug should be discontinued; not useful for type I hyperlipidemia; myositis may be more common in patients with poor renal function

Pregnancy Risk Factor C

Adverse Reactions

>10% Gastrointestinal: dyspepsia (19.6%)

1% to 10%:

Central nervous system: Fatigue (3.8%), vertigo (1.5%), headache (1.2%)

Dermatologic: Eczema (1.95), rash (1.7%)

Gastrointestinal: Abdominal pain (9.8%), diarrhea (7.2%), nausea/vomiting (2.5%), constipation (1.4%)

<1% or case reports with probable causation (limited to important or life-threatening symptoms): Hypoesthesia, paresthesia, taste perversion, cataracts, intracranial hemorrhage, peripheral vascular disease, cholestatic jaundice, dizziness, somnolence, peripheral neuritis, decreased libido, depression, headache, blurred vision, impotence, myopathy, myasthenia, myalgia, arthralgia, synovitis, rhabdomyolysis, increased creatinine phosphokinase, increased bilirubin, increased transaminases, increased alkaline phosphatase, anemia, leukopenia, bone marrow hypoplasia, eosinophilia, angioedema, laryngeal edema, urticaria, exfoliative dermatitis, rash, dermatitis, pruritus, vasculitis, Raynaud's phenomenon, hypokalemia, nephrotoxicity, dermatomyositis/polymyositis

Reports where causal relationship has not been established: Weight loss, extrasystoles, pancreatitis, hepatoma, colitis, confusion, seizures, syncope, retinal edema, decreased fertility (male), renal dysfunction, positive ANA, drug-induced lupus-like syndrome, thrombocytopenia, anaphylaxis, vasculitis, alopecia, photosensitivity

Drug Interactions CYP3A3/4 enzyme substrate

Bexarotene's serum concentration is significantly increased; avoid concurrent use

Chlorpropamide: May increase risk of hypoglycemia

Cyclosporine's blood levels may be reduced; monitor cyclosporine levels and renal function

Furosemide: Increased blood levels of both in hypoalbuminemia

Glyburide (and possibly other sulfonylureas): The hypoglycemic effects may be increased

HMG-CoA reductase inhibitors (atorvastatin, cerivastatin, fluvastatin, lovastatin, pravastatin, simvastatin) may increase the risk of myopathy and rhabdomyolysis. The manufacturer warns against the concurrent use of lovastatin. However, combination therapy with statins has been used in some patients with resistant hyperlipidemias (with great caution).

Rifampin: Decreased gemfibrozil blood levels

Warfarin: Hypoprothrombinemic response increased; monitor INRs closely when gemfibrozil is initiated or discontinued

Alcohol Interactions Avoid use (may decrease triglyceride levels)

Onset May require several days

Half-Life 1.4 hours

Education and Monitoring Issues

Patient Education: You must return to provider for assessment of drug effectiveness. Should be taken 30 minutes before meals. Take with milk or meals if GI upset occurs. You may experience loss of appetite and flatulence (frequent small meals may help), muscle aches (mild, temporary pain relievers may be required), dizziness, faintness, or blurred vision (use caution when driving or engaging in tasks that require alertness until response to drug is known). Report severe stomach pain, nausea, vomiting, chills, sore throat, headache, and any vision changes.

Monitoring Parameters: Serum cholesterol, LFTs

- **Gen** *see* Glyburide *on page 415*
- **Genabid®** *see* Papaverine *on page 702*
- **Genagesic®** *see* Propoxyphene and Acetaminophen *on page 786*
- **Genahist® Oral** *see* Diphenhydramine *on page 282*
- **Genapap® [OTC]** *see* Acetaminophen *on page 17*

- **Genapax®** *see* Gentian Violet *on page 410*
- **Genaspor® [OTC]** *see* Tolnaftate *on page 931*
- **Genatuss® [OTC]** *see* Guaifenesin *on page 423*
- **Genatuss DM® [OTC]** *see* Guaifenesin and Dextromethorphan *on page 424*
- **Gencalc® 600 [OTC]** *see* Calcium Carbonate *on page 130*
- **Gen-K®** *see* Potassium Chloride *on page 751*
- **Gen-Lac** *see* Lactulose *on page 506*
- **Gen-Nifedipine** *see* Nifedipine *on page 653*
- **Genoptic® Ophthalmic** *see* Gentamicin *on page 408*
- **Genoptic® S.O.P. Ophthalmic** *see* Gentamicin *on page 408*
- **Genora® 0.5/35** *see* Ethinyl Estradiol and Norethindrone *on page 342*
- **Genora® 1/35** *see* Ethinyl Estradiol and Norethindrone *on page 342*
- **Genora® 1/50** *see* Mestranol and Norethindrone *on page 570*
- **Genotropin® Injection** *see* Human Growth Hormone *on page 438*
- **Gen-Pindolol** *see* Pindolol *on page 738*
- **Genpril® [OTC]** *see* Ibuprofen *on page 458*
- **Gentacidin® Ophthalmic** *see* Gentamicin *on page 408*
- **Gentafair®** *see* Gentamicin *on page 408*
- **Gentak® Ophthalmic** *see* Gentamicin *on page 408*

Gentamicin (jen ta MYE sin)

Pharmacologic Class Antibiotic, Aminoglycoside; Antibiotic, Ophthalmic; Antibiotic, Topical

U.S. Brand Names Garamycin®; Genoptic® Ophthalmic; Genoptic® S.O.P. Ophthalmic; Gentacidin® Ophthalmic; Gentafair®; Gentak® Ophthalmic; Gentrasul®; G-myticin® Topical; I-Gent®; Jenamicin® Injection; Ocumycin®

Generic Available Yes

Mechanism of Action Interferes with bacterial protein synthesis by binding to 30S and 50S ribosomal subunits resulting in a defective bacterial cell membrane

Use Treatment of susceptible bacterial infections, normally gram-negative organisms including *Pseudomonas, Proteus, Serratia,* and gram-positive *Staphylococcus*; treatment of bone infections, respiratory tract infections, skin and soft tissue infections, as well as abdominal and urinary tract infections, endocarditis, and septicemia; used topically to treat superficial infections of the skin or ophthalmic infections caused by susceptible bacteria; prevention of bacterial endocarditis prior to dental or surgical procedures

USUAL DOSAGE Individualization is critical because of the low therapeutic index

Use of ideal body weight (IBW) for determining the mg/kg/dose appears to be more accurate than dosing on the basis of total body weight (TBW).

In morbid obesity, dosage requirement may best be estimated using a dosing weight of IBW + 0.4 (TBW - IBW)

Initial and periodic peak and trough plasma drug levels should be determined, particularly in critically ill patients with serious infections or in disease states known to significantly alter aminoglycoside pharmacokinetics (eg, cystic fibrosis, burns, or major surgery)

Newborns: Intrathecal: 1 mg every day

Infants >3 months: Intrathecal: 1-2 mg/day

Infants and Children <5 years: I.M., I.V.: 2.5 mg/kg/dose every 8 hours*

Cystic fibrosis: 2.5 mg/kg/dose every 6 hours

Children >5 years: I.M., I.V.: 1.5-2.5 mg/kg/dose every 8 hours*

Prevention of bacterial endocarditis: Dental, oral, upper respiratory procedures, GI/GU procedures: 2 mg/kg with ampicillin (50 mg/kg) 30 minutes prior to procedure

*Some patients may require larger or more frequent doses (eg, every 6 hours) if serum levels document the need (ie, cystic fibrosis or febrile granulocytopenic patients)

Adults: I.M., I.V.:

Severe life-threatening infections: 2-2.5 mg/kg/dose

Urinary tract infections: 1.5 mg/kg/dose

Synergy (for gram-positive infections): 1 mg/kg/dose

Prevention of bacterial endocarditis:

Dental, oral, or upper respiratory procedures: 1.5 mg/kg not to exceed 80 mg with ampicillin (1-2 g) 30 minutes prior to procedure

GI/GU surgery: 1.5 mg/kg not to exceed 80 mg with ampicillin 2 g 30 minutes prior to procedure

Children and Adults:

Intrathecal: 4-8 mg/day

Ophthalmic:

Ointment: Instill ½" (1.25 cm) 2-3 times/day to every 3-4 hours

Solution: Instill 1-2 drops every 2-4 hours, up to 2 drops every hour for severe infections

Topical: Apply 3-4 times/day to affected area

Some clinicians suggest a daily dose of 4-7 mg/kg for all patients with normal renal function. This dose is at least as efficacious with similar, if not less, toxicity than conventional dosing

Dosing interval in renal impairment:

Cl_{cr} ≥60 mL/minute: Administer every 8 hours

Cl_{cr} 40-60 mL/minute: Administer every 12 hours

Cl_{cr} 20-40 mL/minute: Administer every 24 hours

Cl_{cr} <20 mL/minute: Loading dose, then monitor levels

Hemodialysis: Dialyzable; removal by hemodialysis: 30% removal of aminoglycosides occurs during 4 hours of HD; administer dose after dialysis and follow levels

Removal by continuous ambulatory peritoneal dialysis (CAPD):

Administration via CAPD fluid:

Gram-negative infection: 4-8 mg/L (4-8 mcg/mL) of CAPD fluid

Gram-positive infection (ie, synergy): 3-4 mg/L (3-4 mcg/mL) of CAPD fluid

Administration via I.V., I.M. route during CAPD: Dose as for Cl_{cr} <10 mL/minute and follow levels

Removal via continuous arteriovenous or venovenous hemofiltration (CAVH/CAVHD): Dose as for Cl_{cr} 10-40 mL/minute and follow levels

Dosing adjustment/comments in hepatic disease: Monitor plasma concentrations

Dosage Forms CRM, top, (Garamycin®, G-myticin®): 0.1% (15 g). **INF,** in D_5W: 60 mg, 80 mg, 100 mg. **INF,** in NS: 40 mg, 60 mg, 80 mg, 90 mg, 100 mg, 120 mg. **INJ:** 40 mg/mL (1 mL, 1.5 mL, 2 mL); Pediatric: 10 mg/mL (2 mL). **INTRATHECAL** (preservative free) (Garamycin®): 2 mg/mL (2 mL). **OINT:** Ophth: 0.3% [3 mg/g] (3.5 g); (Garamycin®, Genoptic® S.O.P., Gentacidin®, Gentak®): 0.3% [3 mg/g] (3.5 g); Top (Garamycin®, G-myticin®): 0.1% (15 g). **SOLN, ophth:** 0.3% (5 mL, 15 mL); (Garamycin®, Genoptic®, Gentacidin®, Gentak®): 0.3% (1 mL, 5 mL, 15 mL)

Contraindications Hypersensitivity to gentamicin or other aminoglycosides

Warnings/Precautions Not intended for long-term therapy due to toxic hazards associated with extended administration; pre-existing renal insufficiency, vestibular or cochlear impairment, myasthenia gravis, hypocalcemia, conditions which depress neuromuscular transmission

Parenteral aminoglycosides have been associated with significant nephrotoxicity or ototoxicity; the ototoxicity may be directly proportional to the amount of drug given and the duration of treatment; tinnitus or vertigo are indications of vestibular injury and impending hearing loss; renal damage is usually reversible

Pregnancy Risk Factor C

Adverse Reactions

>10%:

Central nervous system: Neurotoxicity (vertigo, ataxia)

Neuromuscular & skeletal: Gait instability

Otic: Ototoxicity (auditory), ototoxicity (vestibular)

Renal: Nephrotoxicity, decreased creatinine clearance

1% to 10%:

Cardiovascular: Edema

Dermatologic: Skin itching, reddening of skin, rash

<1%: Agranulocytosis, anorexia, burning, drowsiness, dyspnea, elevated LFTs, enterocolitis, erythema, granulocytopenia, headache, increased salivation, muscle cramps, nausea, photosensitivity, pseudomotor cerebri, stinging, thrombocytopenia, tremors, vomiting, weakness, weight loss

Drug Interactions Increased toxicity:

Penicillins, cephalosporins, amphotericin B, loop diuretics may increase nephrotoxic potential

Neuromuscular blocking agents may increase neuromuscular blockade

Half-Life 1.5-3 hours; end-stage renal disease: 36-70 hours

Education and Monitoring Issues

Patient Education: Take exactly as directed and when prescribed. Drink adequate amounts of water (2-3 L/day of fluids unless instructed to restrict fluid intake). You may experience headaches, ringing in ears, dizziness, blurred vision (use caution when driving or engaging in tasks requiring alertness until response to drug is known); GI upset, loss of appetite (small frequent meals and frequent mouth care may help); photosensitivity (use sunscreen wear protective clothing and eyewear, avoid direct sunlight). Report severe headache, changes in hearing acuity or ringing in ears, changes in urine pattern, difficulty breathing, rash, fever, unhealed sores, sores in mouth, vaginal drainage, muscle or bone pain, change in gait, or worsening of condition.

Ophthalmic: Wash hands before instilling. Sit or lie down to instill. Open eye, look at ceiling, and instill prescribed amount of solution (Ointment: Pull lower lid down gently, instill thin ribbon of ointment inside lid.) Close eye and roll eye in all directions, and apply gentle pressure to inner corner of eye. Do not let tip of applicator touch eye or contaminate tip of applicator. Temporary stinging or blurred vision may occur. Report persistent pain, burning, vision disturbances, swelling, itching, or worsening of condition.

Topical: Apply thin film of ointment to affected area as often as recommended. May apply porous dressing. Report persistent burning, swelling, itching, worsening of condition, or lack of response to therapy.

(Continued)

Gentamicin *(Continued)*

Dietary Considerations: Calcium, magnesium, potassium: Renal wasting may cause hypocalcemia, hypomagnesemia, and/or hypokalemia

Monitoring Parameters: Urinalysis, urine output, BUN, serum creatinine; hearing should be tested before, during, and after treatment; particularly in those at risk for ototoxicity or who will be receiving prolonged therapy (>2 weeks)

Reference Range:

Timing of serum samples: Draw peak 30 minutes after 30-minute infusion has been completed or 1 hour after I.M. injection; draw trough immediately before next dose

Sample size: 0.5-2 mL blood (red top tube) or 0.1-1 mL serum (separated)

Therapeutic levels:

Peak:

Serious infections: 6-8 μg/mL (12-17 μmol/L)

Life-threatening infections: 8-10 μg/mL (17-21 μmol/L)

Urinary tract infections: 4-6 μg/mL

Synergy against gram-positive organisms: 3-5 μg/mL

Trough:

Serious infections: 0.5-1 μg/mL

Life-threatening infections: 1-2 μg/mL

Obtain drug levels after the third dose unless renal dysfunction/toxicity suspected

Related Information

Antibiotic Treatment of Adults With Infective Endocarditis *on page 1179*
Antimicrobial Drugs of Choice *on page 1182*
Prednisolone and Gentamicin *on page 763*
Prevention of Bacterial Endocarditis *on page 1154*
Treatment of Sexually Transmitted Diseases *on page 1210*

Gentian Violet (JEN shun VYE oh let)

Pharmacologic Class Antibacterial, Topical; Antifungal Agent, Topical

U.S. Brand Names Genapax®

Use Treatment of cutaneous or mucocutaneous infections caused by *Candida albicans* and other superficial skin infections

USUAL DOSAGE

Children and Adults: Topical: Apply 0.5% to 2% locally with cotton to lesion 2-3 times/day for 3 days, do not swallow and avoid contact with eyes

Adults: Intravaginal: Insert one tampon for 3-4 hours once or twice daily for 12 days

Contraindications Known hypersensitivity to gentian violet; ulcerated areas; patients with porphyria

Pregnancy Risk Factor C

- **Gen-Timolol** *see* Timolol *on page 922*
- **Gentrasul®** *see* Gentamicin *on page 408*
- **Gen-Triazolam** *see* Triazolam *on page 948*
- **Gen-XENE®** *see* Clorazepate *on page 218*
- **Geocillin®** *see* Carbenicillin *on page 139*
- **Geopen®** *see* Carbenicillin *on page 139*
- **Geref® Injection** *see* Sermorelin Acetate *on page 846*
- **Geridium®** *see* Phenazopyridine *on page 721*
- **Germinal®** *see* Ergoloid Mesylates *on page 322*
- **GG-Cen® [OTC]** *see* Guaifenesin *on page 423*

Ginger

Pharmacologic Class Herbal

Mechanism of Action Unknown; may increase GI motility and thus block nausea feedback from the GI tract; appears to decrease prostaglandin synthesis; may have cardiotonic activity; may inhibit platelet aggregation

Use In herbal medicine as a digestive aid; for treatment of nausea (antiemetic) and motion sickness; also used as a menstruation promoter in Chinese herbal medicine; headaches, colds and flu; ginger oil is used as a flavoring agent in beverages and mouthwashes; may be useful in some forms of arthritis

USUAL DOSAGE

For preventing motion sickness or digestive aid: 1-4 g/day (250 mg of ginger root powder 4 times/day)

Per Commission E: 2-4 g/day or equivalent preparations

Contraindications Gallstones per Commission E

Warnings/Precautions Use with caution in diabetics, patients on cardiac glycosides, and patients receiving anticoagulants

Pregnancy Risk Factor No administration for morning sickness during pregnancy per Commission E; however, two-peer reviewed revision of the literature does not justify this caution; Commission E made its cautions based on animal studies and *in vitro* mutagenicity studies (2) on 1 compound, gingerol. Indian and Chinese women use large amounts of ginger routinely in their diet during pregnancy with no ill effects on pregnancy or fetus. High doses may be abortifacient.

Drug Interactions May alter response to cardiotonic, hypoglycemia, anticoagulant, antiplatelet agents

Ginkgo Biloba

Pharmacologic Class Herbal

Mechanism of Action Inhibits platelet aggregation; ginkgo biloba leaf extract contain terpenoids and flavonoids which can allegedly inactivate oxygen-free radicals causing vasodilatation and antagonize effects of platelet activating factor (PAF); fruit pulp contains ginkolic acids which are allergens (seeds are not sensitizing)

Use Dilates blood vessels; plant/leaf extract has been used in Europe for intermittent claudication, arterial insufficiency, and cerebral vascular disease (dementia); tinnitus, visual disorders, traumatic brain injury, vertigo of vascular origin

Per Commission E: Demential syndromes including memory deficits, etc (tinnitus, headache); depressive emotional conditions, primary degenerative dementia, vascular dementia, or both

Investigational: Asthma, impotence (male)

USUAL DOSAGE Beneficial effects for cerebral ischemia in the elderly occur after one month of use

Usual dosage: ~40 mg 3 times/day with meals; 60-80 mg twice daily to 3 times/day depending on indication; maximum dose: 360 mg/day

Cerebral ischemia: 120 mg/day in 2-3 divided doses (24% flavonoid-glycoside extract, 6% terpene glycosides)

Contraindications Pregnancy, patients with clotting disorders; hypersensitivity to ginkgo biloba preparations per Commission E

Warnings/Precautions Use with caution following recent surgery or trauma; effects may require 1-2 months

Adverse Reactions

Cardiovascular: Palpitations, bilateral subdural hematomas

Central nervous system: Headache (very seldom per Commission E), dizziness, seizures (in children), restlessness

Dermatologic: Urticaria, cheilitis

Gastrointestinal: Nausea, diarrhea, vomiting, stomatitis, proctitis; very seldom stomach or intestinal upsets (per Commission E)

Ocular: Hyphema

Miscellaneous: Allergic skin reactions (very seldom per Commission E)

Drug Interactions Due to effects on PAF, use with caution in patients receiving anticoagulants or platelet inhibitors

Education and Monitoring Issues

Reference Range: Maximum plasma level of ginkogolide A and ginkogolide B after an 80 mg oral dose was 15 mg/mL and 4 mg/mL respectively; maximum plasma level of bilobalide after a 120 mg oral dose is ~18.8 mg/mL

Ginseng

Pharmacologic Class Herbal

Mechanism of Action The active agent (ginsenosides) may have CNS stimulant and estrogen-like effect, anti-inflammatory, antiplatelet; used as an adaptogen; may lower cholesterol; not effective as an aphrodesiac

Use A popular ingredient in herbal teas; has been advocated for its antistress and adaptogenic effects although these effects have not been scientifically confirmed, there's much "suggestive" scientific literature

USUAL DOSAGE Avoid in long-term use

Herbal tea: Usually about 1.75 g; 0.5-2 g/day

Dried root: 0.6-3 g/day of dried root or equivalent preparations

Ethanolic extract: 0.5-6 mL 1-3 times/day

Root: 1-2 g/day

Extract: (7% ginsenosides) 100-300 mg 3 times/day

Contraindications Estrogen-receptor positive breast cancer

Warnings/Precautions Nervousness may occur during first few days; use with caution in hypertensives, diabetes; avoid long-term use

Pregnancy Implications Not recommended in pregnancy or breast-feeding

Adverse Reactions

Cardiovascular: Tachycardia, hypertension, sinus tachycardia

Central nervous system: Nervousness, agitation, mania, headache, sciatic nerve inflammation

Dermatologic: Stevens Johnson syndrome

Endocrine & metabolic: Hypoglycemia, vaginal bleeding, breast nodules

Drug Interactions May decrease effects of loop diuretics (furosemide); theoretically may increase effect of antiplatelet agents, anticoagulants, hypoglycemics, and hypotensive agents

Glatiramer Acetate (gla TIR a mer AS e tate)

Pharmacologic Class Biological, Miscellaneous

U.S. Brand Names Copaxone®

Mechanism of Action Glatiramer is a mixture of random polymers of four amino acids; L-alanine, L-glutamic acid, L-lysine and L-tyrosine, the resulting mixture is antigenically similar to myelin basic protein, which is an important component of the myelin sheath of nerves; glatiramer is thought to suppress T-lymphocytes specific for a myelin antigen, it is also proposed that glatiramer interferes with the antigen-presenting function of certain immune cells opposing pathogenic T-cell function

Use Relapsing-remitting type multiple sclerosis; studies indicate that it reduces the frequency of attacks and the severity of disability; appears to be most effective for patients with minimal disability

USUAL DOSAGE Adults: S.C.: 20 mg daily

Dosage Forms INJ: 20 mg (2 mL)

Contraindications Previous hypersensitivity to any component of the copolymer formulation

Pregnancy Risk Factor B

Adverse Reactions

>10%:
- Cardiovascular: Chest pain (26%)
- Local: Pain

1% to 10%:
- Cardiovascular: Chest tightness, flushing, tachycardia, vasodilatation
- Central nervous system: Anxiety, depression, dizziness
- Dermatologic: Erythema (4%), urticaria
- Hematologic: Transient eosinophilia
- Local: Injection site reactions (6.5%)
- Neuromuscular & skeletal: Tremor
- Respiratory: Dyspnea
- Miscellaneous: Diaphoresis, unintended pregnancy

Education and Monitoring Issues

Patient Education: It is essential to provide the patient with proper handling and reconstitution instruction, since they will most likely have to self-administer the drug for an extended period

Glimepiride (GLYE me pye ride)

Pharmacologic Class Antidiabetic Agent (Sulfonylurea)

U.S. Brand Names Amaryl®

Mechanism of Action Stimulates insulin release from the pancreatic beta cells; reduces glucose output from the liver; insulin sensitivity is increased at peripheral target sites

Use

Management of noninsulin-dependent diabetes mellitus (type II) as an adjunct to diet and exercise to lower blood glucose

Use in combination with insulin to lower blood glucose in patients whose hyperglycemia cannot be controlled by diet and exercise in conjunction with an oral hypoglycemic agent

USUAL DOSAGE Oral (allow several days between dose titrations):

Adults: Initial: 1-2 mg once daily, administered with breakfast or the first main meal; usual maintenance dose: 1-4 mg once daily; after a dose of 2 mg once daily, increase in increments of 2 mg at 1- to 2-week intervals based upon the patient's blood glucose response to a maximum of 8 mg once daily

Elderly: Initial: 1 mg/day

Combination with insulin therapy (fasting glucose level for instituting combination therapy is in the range of >150 mg/dL in plasma or serum depending on the patient): 8 mg once daily with the first main meal

After starting with low-dose insulin, upward adjustments of insulin can be done approximately weekly as guided by frequent measurements of fasting blood glucose. Once stable, combination-therapy patients should monitor their capillary blood glucose on an ongoing basis, preferably daily.

Dosing adjustment/comments in renal impairment: Cl_{cr} <22 mL/minute: Initial starting dose should be 1 mg and dosage increments should be based on fasting blood glucose levels

Dosing adjustment in hepatic impairment: No data available

Dosage Forms TAB: 1 mg, 2 mg, 4 mg

Contraindications Hypersensitivity to glimepiride or any component, other sulfonamides; diabetic ketoacidosis (with or without coma)

Warnings/Precautions

The administration of oral hypoglycemic drugs (ie, tolbutamide) has been reported to be associated with increased cardiovascular mortality as compared to treatment with diet alone or diet plus insulin

All sulfonylurea drugs are capable of producing severe hypoglycemia. Hypoglycemia is more likely to occur when caloric intake is deficient, after severe or prolonged exercise, when alcohol is ingested, or when more than one glucose-lowering drug is used.

Pregnancy Risk Factor C

Adverse Reactions

1% to 10%: Central nervous system: Headache

<1%: Agranulocytosis, anorexia, aplastic anemia, blood dyscrasias, bone marrow suppression, cholestatic jaundice, constipation, diarrhea, diuretic effect, edema, epigastric fullness, heartburn, hemolytic anemia, hypoglycemia, hyponatremia, nausea, photosensitivity, rash, thrombocytopenia, urticaria, vomiting

Drug Interactions CYP2C9 enzyme substrate

Decreased effects: Cholestyramine, hydantoins, rifampin, thiazide diuretics, urinary alkalines, charcoal

Increased effects: H_2-antagonists, anticoagulants, androgens, beta-blockers, fluconazole, salicylates, gemfibrozil, sulfonamides, tricyclic antidepressants, probenecid, MAO inhibitors, methyldopa, NSAIDs, salicylates, sulfonamides, chloramphenicol, coumarins, probenecid, MAO inhibitors, digitalis glycosides, urinary acidifiers

Increased toxicity: Cimetidine may increase hypoglycemic effects; certain drugs tend to produce hyperglycemia and may lead to loss of control. These drugs include the thiazides and other diuretics, corticosteroids, phenothiazines, thyroid products, estrogens, oral contraceptives, phenytoin, nicotinic acid, sympathomimetics, and isoniazid.

Alcohol Interactions Avoid use (may cause hypoglycemia)

Onset Peak blood glucose reductions: Within 2-3 hours

Duration 24 hours

Half-Life 5-9 hours

Education and Monitoring Issues

Patient Education: This medication is used to control diabetes; it is not a cure. Other components of treatment plan are important: follow prescribed diet, medication, and exercise regimen. Take exactly as directed; 30 minutes before meal(s) at the same time each day. Do not change dose or discontinue without consulting prescriber. Avoid alcohol while taking this medication; could cause severe reaction. Inform prescriber of all other prescription or OTC medications you are taking; do not introduce new medication without consulting prescriber. Do not take other medication within 2 hours of this medication unless so advised by prescriber. If you experience hypoglycemic reaction, contact prescriber immediately. Maintain regular dietary intake and exercise routine and always carry quick source of sugar with you. You may experience side effects during first weeks of therapy (headache, nausea); consult prescriber if these persist. Report severe or persistent side effects, extended vomiting or flu-like symptoms, skin rash, easy bruising or bleeding, or change in color of urine or stool.

Monitoring Parameters: Urine for glucose and ketones; monitor for signs and symptoms of hypoglycemia (fatigue, excessive hunger, profuse sweating, numbness of extremities), fasting blood glucose, hemoglobin A_{1c}, fructosamine

Reference Range: Target range: Adults:

Fasting blood glucose: <120 mg/dL

Glycosylated hemoglobin: <7%

Manufacturer Hoechst-Marion Roussel

Related Information

Hypoglycemic Drugs and Thiazolidinedione Information *on page 1240*

Pharmaceutical Manufacturers Directory *on page 1020*

Glipizide (GLIP i zide)

Pharmacologic Class Antidiabetic Agent (Sulfonylurea)

U.S. Brand Names Glucotrol®; Glucotrol® XL

Generic Available No

Mechanism of Action Stimulates insulin release from the pancreatic beta cells; reduces glucose output from the liver; insulin sensitivity is increased at peripheral target sites

Use Management of noninsulin-dependent diabetes mellitus (type II)

USUAL DOSAGE Oral (allow several days between dose titrations): Give ~30 minutes before a meal to obtain the greatest reduction in postprandial hyperglycemia

Adults: Initial: 5 mg/day; adjust dosage at 2.5-5 mg daily increments as determined by blood glucose response at intervals of several days. Maximum recommended once-daily dose: 15 mg; maximum recommended total daily dose: 40 mg.

Elderly: Initial: 2.5 mg/day; increase by 2.5-5 mg/day at 1- to 2-week intervals

Dosing adjustment/comments in renal impairment: Cl_{cr} <10 mL/minute: Some investigators recommend not using

Dosing adjustment in hepatic impairment: Initial dosage should be 2.5 mg/day

Dosage Forms TAB: 5 mg, 10 mg; Extended release: 5 mg, 10 mg

Contraindications Hypersensitivity to glipizide or any component, other sulfonamides, type I diabetes mellitus

Warnings/Precautions Use with caution in patients with severe hepatic disease; a useful agent since few drug to drug interactions and not dependent upon renal elimination of active drug

Pregnancy Risk Factor C

Pregnancy Implications

Clinical effects on the fetus: Crosses the placenta. Insulin is the drug of choice for the control of diabetes mellitus during pregnancy.

(Continued)

Glipizide *(Continued)*

Breast-feeding/lactation: No data available

Adverse Reactions

>10%:

Central nervous system: Headache

Gastrointestinal: Anorexia, nausea, vomiting, diarrhea, epigastric fullness, constipation, heartburn

1% to 10%: Dermatologic: Rash, urticaria, photosensitivity

<1%: Agranulocytosis, aplastic anemia, blood dyscrasias, bone marrow suppression, cholestatic jaundice, diuretic effect edema, hemolytic anemia, hypoglycemia, hyponatremia, thrombocytopenia

Drug Interactions

Decreased effects: Beta-blockers, cholestyramine, hydantoins, rifampin, thiazide diuretics, urinary alkalines, charcoal

Increased effects: H_2-antagonists, anticoagulants, androgens, fluconazole, salicylates, gemfibrozil, sulfonamides, tricyclic antidepressants, probenecid, MAO inhibitors, methyldopa, digitalis glycosides, urinary acidifiers

Increased toxicity: Cimetidine may increase hypoglycemic effects

Alcohol Interactions Avoid use (may cause hypoglycemia)

Onset Peak blood glucose reductions: Within 1.5-2 hours

Duration 12-24 hours

Half-Life 2-4 hours

Education and Monitoring Issues

Patient Education: This medication is used to control diabetes; it is not a cure. Other components of treatment plan are important: follow prescribed diet, medication, and exercise regimen. Take exactly as directed; 30 minutes before meal(s) at the same time each day. Do not chew or crush extended release tablets. Do not change dose or discontinue without consulting prescriber. Avoid alcohol while taking this medication; could cause severe reaction. Inform prescriber of all other prescription or OTC medications you are taking; do not introduce new medication without consulting prescriber. Do not take other medication within 2 hours of this medication unless so advised by prescriber. If you experience hypoglycemic reaction, contact prescriber immediately. Maintain regular dietary intake and exercise routine and always carry quick source of sugar with you. You may be more sensitive to sunlight (use sunscreen, wear protective clothing and eyewear, avoid direct sunlight). You may experience side effects during first weeks of therapy (headache, nausea); consult prescriber if these persist. Report severe or persistent side effects, extended vomiting, diarrhea, or constipation; flu-like symptoms; skin rash; easy bruising or bleeding; or change in color of urine or stool.

Dietary Considerations:

Food: Food delays absorption by 40%; take glipizide before meals

Glucose: Decreases blood glucose concentration. Hypoglycemia may occur. Educate patients how to detect and treat hypoglycemia. Monitor for signs and symptoms of hypoglycemia. Administer glucose if necessary. Evaluate patient's diet and exercise regimen. May need to decrease or discontinue dose of sulfonylurea.

Sodium: Reports of hyponatremia and SIADH. Those at increased risk include patients on medications or who have medical conditions that predispose them to hyponatremia. Monitor sodium serum concentration and fluid status. May need to restrict water intake.

Monitoring Parameters: Urine for glucose and ketones; monitor for signs and symptoms of hypoglycemia (fatigue, excessive hunger, profuse sweating, numbness of extremities), fasting blood glucose, hemoglobin A_{1c}, fructosamine

Reference Range: Target range: Adults:

Fasting blood glucose: <120 mg/dL

Glycosylated hemoglobin: <7%

Related Information

Hypoglycemic Drugs and Thiazolidinedione Information *on page 1240*

Glucagon (GLOO ka gon)

Pharmacologic Class Antidote; Diagnostic Agent, Gastrointestinal

Generic Available No

Mechanism of Action Stimulates adenylate cyclase to produce increased cyclic AMP, which promotes hepatic glycogenolysis and gluconeogenesis, causing a raise in blood glucose levels

Use Management of hypoglycemia; diagnostic aid in the radiologic examination of GI tract when a hypnotic state is needed; used with some success as a cardiac stimulant in management of severe cases of beta-adrenergic blocking agent overdosage

USUAL DOSAGE

Hypoglycemia or insulin shock therapy: I.M., I.V., S.C.:

Children: 0.025-0.1 mg/kg/dose, not to exceed 1 mg/dose, repeated in 20 minutes as needed

Adults: 0.5-1 mg, may repeat in 20 minutes as needed

If patient fails to respond to glucagon, I.V. dextrose must be given

Diagnostic aid: Adults: I.M., I.V.: 0.25-2 mg 10 minutes prior to procedure

Dosage Forms POWDER for inj, lyophilized: 1 mg [1 unit]; 10 mg [10 units]

Contraindications Hypersensitivity to glucagon or any component

Warnings/Precautions Use with caution in patients with a history of insulinoma and/or pheochromocytoma

Pregnancy Risk Factor B

Adverse Reactions 1% to 10%:

Cardiovascular: Hypotension

Dermatologic: Urticaria

Gastrointestinal: Nausea, vomiting

Respiratory: Respiratory distress

Drug Interactions Increased toxicity: Oral anticoagulant - hypoprothrombinemic effects may be increased possibly with bleeding

Onset Peak effect on blood glucose levels: Parenteral: Within 5-20 minutes

Duration 60-90 minutes

Half-Life Plasma: 3-10 minutes

Education and Monitoring Issues

Patient Education: Identify appropriate support person to administer glucagon if necessary. Follow prescribers instructions for administering glucagon. Review diet, insulin administration, and testing procedures with prescriber or diabetic educator.

Monitoring Parameters: Blood pressure, blood glucose

♦ **Glucophage®** *see* Metformin *on page 574*

Glucosamine

Pharmacologic Class Herbal

Mechanism of Action Glucosamine is an amino sugar which is a key component in the synthesis of proteoglycans, a group of proteins found in cartilage. These proteoglycans are negatively charged, and attract water so they can produce synovial fluid in the joints. The theory is that supplying the body with these precursors will replenish important synovial fluid, and lead to production of new cartilage. Glucosamine also appears to inhibit cartilage-destroying enzymes such as collagenase and phospholipase A2, thus stopping the degenerative processes of osteoarthritis. A third mechanism may be glucosamine's ability to prevent production of damaging superoxide radicals, which may lead to cartilage destruction.

Use Osteoarthritis, rheumatoid arthritis, tendonitis, gout, bursitis

USUAL DOSAGE 500 mg of the sulfate form 3 times/day

Adverse Reactions Gastrointestinal: Very few effects (eg, flatulence, nausea)

Drug Interactions None known

♦ **Glucotrol®** *see* Glipizide *on page 413*

♦ **Glucotrol® XL** *see* Glipizide *on page 413*

♦ **Glukor®** *see* Chorionic Gonadotropin *on page 196*

♦ **Glyate® [OTC]** *see* Guaifenesin *on page 423*

Glyburide (GLYE byoor ide)

Pharmacologic Class Antidiabetic Agent (Sulfonylurea)

U.S. Brand Names Diaβeta®; Glynase™ PresTab™; Micronase®

Generic Available No

Mechanism of Action Stimulates insulin release from the pancreatic beta cells; reduces glucose output from the liver; insulin sensitivity is increased at peripheral target sites

Use Management of noninsulin-dependent diabetes mellitus (type II)

USUAL DOSAGE Oral:

Adults:

Initial: 2.5-5 mg/day, administered with breakfast or the first main meal of the day; in patients who are more sensitive to hypoglycemic drugs, start at 1.25 mg/day

Increase in increments of no more than 2.5 mg/day at weekly intervals based on the patient's blood glucose response

Maintenance: 1.25-20 mg/day given as single or divided doses; maximum: 20 mg/day

Elderly: Initial: 1.25-2.5 mg/day, increase by 1.25-2.5 mg/day every 1-3 weeks

Micronized tablets (Glynase PresTab™): Adults:

Initial: 1.5-3 mg/day, administered with breakfast or the first main meal of the day in patients who are more sensitive to hypoglycemic drugs, start at 0.75 mg/day. Increase in increments of no more than 1.5 mg/day in weekly intervals based on the patient's blood glucose response.

Maintenance: 0.75-12 mg/day given as a single dose or in divided doses. Some patients (especially those receiving >6 mg/day) may have a more satisfactory response with twice-daily dosing.

Dosing adjustment/comments in renal impairment: Cl_{cr} <50 mL/minute: **Not recommended**

Dosing adjustment in hepatic impairment: Use conservative initial and maintenance doses and avoid use in severe disease

(Continued)

Glyburide *(Continued)*

Elderly: Patients are prone to develop renal insufficiency, which may put them at risk of hypoglycemia; dose selection should include an assessment of renal function

Dosage Forms TAB (Diaβeta®, Micronase®): 1.25 mg, 2.5 mg, 5 mg; Micronized (Glynase™ PresTab™): 1.5 mg, 3 mg, 4.5 mg, 6 mg

Contraindications Hypersensitivity to glyburide or any component, or other sulfonamides; type I diabetes mellitus, diabetic ketoacidosis with or without coma

Warnings/Precautions Use with caution in patients with hepatic impairment. Elderly: Rapid and prolonged hypoglycemia (>12 hours) despite hypertonic glucose injections have been reported; age and hepatic and renal impairment are independent risk factors for hypoglycemia; dosage titration should be made at weekly intervals. Use with caution in patients with renal and hepatic impairment, malnourished or debilitated conditions, or adrenal or pituitary insufficiency. The administration of oral hypoglycemic drugs (ie, tolbutamide) has been reported to be associated with increased cardiovascular mortality as compared to treatment with diet alone or diet plus insulin.

Pregnancy Risk Factor C

Pregnancy Implications

Clinical effects on the fetus: Crosses the placenta. Hypoglycemia; ear defects reported; other malformations reported but may have been secondary to poor maternal glucose control/diabetes. Insulin is the drug of choice for the control of diabetes mellitus during pregnancy.

Breast-feeding/lactation: No data available

Adverse Reactions

>10%:

Central nervous system: Headache, dizziness

Gastrointestinal: Nausea, epigastric fullness, heartburn, constipation, diarrhea, anorexia

Ocular: Blurred vision

1% to 10%: Dermatologic: Pruritus, rash, urticaria, photosensitivity reaction

<1%: Agranulocytosis, aplastic anemia, arthralgia, bone marrow suppression, cholestatic jaundice, diuretic effect, hemolytic anemia, hypoglycemia, leukopenia, nocturia, paresthesia, thrombocytopenia

Drug Interactions CYP3A3/4 enzyme substrate

Decreased effect: Thiazides may decrease effectiveness of glyburide

Increased effect: Possible interaction between glyburide and fluoroquinolone antibiotics has been reported resulting in a potentiation of hypoglycemic action of glyburide

Increased toxicity:

Since this agent is highly protein bound, the toxic potential is increased when given concomitantly with other highly protein bound drugs (ie, phenylbutazone, oral anticoagulants, hydantoins, salicylates, NSAIDs, beta-blockers, sulfonamides) - increase hypoglycemic effect

Alcohol increases disulfiram reactions

Phenylbutazone can increase hypoglycemic effects

Certain drugs tend to produce hyperglycemia and may lead to loss of control (ie, thiazides and other diuretics, corticosteroids, phenothiazines, thyroid products, estrogens, oral contraceptives, phenytoin, nicotinic acid, sympathomimetics, calcium channel blocking drugs, and isoniazid)

Possible interactions between glyburide and coumarin derivatives have been reported that may either potentiate or weaken the effects of coumarin derivatives

Alcohol Interactions Avoid use (may cause hypoglycemia)

Onset Oral: Insulin levels in the serum begin to increase within 15-60 minutes after a single dose

Duration Up to 24 hours

Half-Life 5-16 hours; may be prolonged with renal insufficiency or hepatic insufficiency

Education and Monitoring Issues

Patient Education: This medication is used to control diabetes; it is not a cure. Other components of treatment plan are important: follow prescribed diet, medication, and exercise regimen. Take exactly as directed; 30 minutes before meal(s) at the same time each day. Do not change dose or discontinue without consulting prescriber. Avoid alcohol while taking this medication; could cause severe reaction. Inform prescriber of all other prescription or OTC medications you are taking; do not introduce new medication without consulting prescriber. Do not take other medication within 2 hours of this medication unless so advised by prescriber. If you experience hypoglycemic reaction, contact prescriber immediately. Maintain regular dietary intake and exercise routine and always carry quick source of sugar with you. You may be more sensitive to sunlight (use sunscreen, wear protective clothing and eyewear, avoid direct sunlight). You may experience side effects during first weeks of therapy (headache, nausea); consult prescriber if these persist. Report severe or persistent side effects, extended vomiting or flu-like symptoms, skin rash, easy bruising or bleeding, or change in color of urine or stool.

Dietary Considerations:

Food: Food does not affect absorption; glyburide may be taken with food

Glucose: Decreases blood glucose concentration. Hypoglycemia may occur. Educate patients how to detect and treat hypoglycemia. Monitor for signs and symptoms of hypoglycemia. Administer glucose if necessary. Evaluate patient's diet and exercise regimen. May need to decrease or discontinue dose of sulfonylurea.

Sodium: Reports of hyponatremia and SIADH. Those at increased risk include patients on medications or who have medical conditions that predispose them to hyponatremia. Monitor sodium serum concentration and fluid status. May need to restrict water intake.

Monitoring Parameters: Signs and symptoms of hypoglycemia, fasting blood glucose, hemoglobin A_{1c}, fructosamine

Reference Range: Target range: Adults:

Fasting blood glucose: <120 mg/dL

Glycosylated hemoglobin: <7%

Related Information

Hypoglycemic Drugs and Thiazolidinedione Information *on page 1240*

♦ **Glycerol-T®** *see* Theophylline and Guaifenesin *on page 906*

Glycopyrrolate (glye koe PYE roe late)

Pharmacologic Class Anticholinergic Agent

U.S. Brand Names Robinul®; Robinul® Forte

Generic Available Yes

Mechanism of Action Blocks the action of acetylcholine at parasympathetic sites in smooth muscle, secretory glands, and the CNS (minimal CNS penetration)

Use Adjunct in treatment of peptic ulcer disease; inhibit salivation and excessive secretions of the respiratory tract preoperatively; reversal of neuromuscular blockade; control of upper airway secretions

USUAL DOSAGE

Children:

Control of secretions:

Oral: 40-100 mcg/kg/dose 3-4 times/day

I.M., I.V.: 4-10 mcg/kg/dose every 3-4 hours; maximum: 0.2 mg/dose or 0.8 mg/24 hours

Intraoperative: I.V.: 4 mcg/kg not to exceed 0.1 mg; repeat at 2- to 3-minute intervals as needed

Preoperative: I.M.:

<2 years: 4.4-8.8 mcg/kg 30-60 minutes before procedure

>2 years: 4.4 mcg/kg 30-60 minutes before procedure

Children and Adults: Neuromuscular blockade: Reversal: Block adverse muscarinic effects of anticholinesterase agents: I.V.: 0.2 mg for each 1 mg of neostigmine or 5 mg of pyridostigmine administered or 5-15 mcg/kg glycopyrrolate with 25-70 mcg/kg of neostigmine or 0.1-0.3 mg/kg of pyridostigmine (agents usually administered simultaneously but glycopyrrolate may be administered first if bradycardia is present)

Adults:

Intraoperative: I.V.: 0.1 mg repeated as needed at 2- to 3-minute intervals

Preoperative: I.M.: 4.4 mcg/kg 30-60 minutes before procedure

Peptic ulcer:

Oral: 1-2 mg 2-3 times/day

I.M., I.V.: 0.1-0.2 mg 3-4 times/day

Dosage Forms INJ: 0.2 mg/mL (1 mL, 2 mL, 5 mL, 20 mL); Robinul®: 0.2 mg/mL (1 mL, 2 mL, 5 mL, 20 mL). **TAB:** (Robinul®): 1 mg, Robinul® Forte: 2 mg

Contraindications Narrow-angle glaucoma, acute hemorrhage, tachycardia, hypersensitivity to glycopyrrolate or any component; ulcerative colitis, obstructive uropathy, paralytic ileus, obstructive disease of GI tract

Warnings/Precautions Not recommended in children <12 years of age for the management of peptic ulcer; infants, patients with Down syndrome, and children with spastic paralysis or brain damage may be hypersensitive to antimuscarine effects. Use caution in elderly, patients with autonomic neuropathy, hepatic or renal disease, ulcerative colitis may predispose megacolon, hyperthyroidism, CAD, CHF, arrhythmias, tachycardia, BPH, hiatal hernia, with reflux.

Pregnancy Risk Factor B

Adverse Reactions

>10%:

Dermatologic: Dry skin

Gastrointestinal: Constipation, dry throat, xerostomia

Local: Irritation at injection site

Respiratory: Dry nose

Miscellaneous: Diaphoresis (decreased)

1% to 10%:

Dermatologic: Increased sensitivity to light

Endocrine & metabolic: Decreased flow of breast milk

Gastrointestinal: Dysphagia

(Continued)

Glycopyrrolate *(Continued)*

<1%: Ataxia, bloated feeling, blurred vision, confusion, drowsiness, dysuria, fatigue, headache, increased intraocular pain, loss of memory, nausea, orthostatic hypotension, palpitations, rash, tachycardia, ventricular fibrillation, vomiting, weakness

Drug Interactions

Decreased effect: Antacids (decreased absorption)

Increased risk of adverse anticholinergic effects with concomitant administration of phenothiazines, amantadine, antiparkinsonian drugs, glutethimide, meperidine, tricyclic antidepressants, antiarrhythmic agents with anticholinergic activity (eg, disopyramide, quinidine, procainamide), select antihistamines, and other anticholinergic agents; antipsychotic effectiveness of phenothiazines may be decreased; may alter response to beta-adrenergic blockers; GI absorption of the following drugs may be affected: acetaminophen, levodopa, ketoconazole, digoxin, (product specific), riboflavin, and potassium chloride wax-matrix preparations

Onset

Oral: Onset of action: Within 50 minutes; Peak effect: Within 1 hour

I.M.: 20-40 minutes

I.V.: 1 minute

Duration

Vagal effects: 2-3 hours

Inhibition of salivation: Up to 7 hours

Anticholinergic effects (after oral administration): 8-12 hours

Half-Life <10 minutes

Education and Monitoring Issues

Patient Education: Take as directed before meals; do not increase dose and do not discontinue without consulting prescriber. Void before taking medication. You may experience dizziness or blurred vision (use caution when driving or engaging in tasks that require alertness until response to drug is known); dry mouth (sucking on lozenges may help); photosensitivity (wear dark glasses in bright sunlight); or impotence (temporary). Report excessive and persistent anticholinergic effects (blurred vision, headache, flushing, tachycardia, nervousness, constipation, dizziness, insomnia, mental confusion or excitement, dry mouth, altered taste perception, dysphagia, palpitations, bradycardia, urinary hesitancy or retention, impotence, decreased sweating).

- **Glycotuss® [OTC]** *see* Guaifenesin *on page 423*
- **Glycotuss-DM® [OTC]** *see* Guaifenesin and Dextromethorphan *on page 424*
- **Glynase™ PresTab™** *see* Glyburide *on page 415*
- **Gly-Oxide® Oral [OTC]** *see* Carbamide Peroxide *on page 139*
- **Glyset™** *see* Miglitol *on page 605*
- **Glytuss® [OTC]** *see* Guaifenesin *on page 423*
- **G-myticin® Topical** *see* Gentamicin *on page 408*

Golden Seal

Pharmacologic Class Herbal

Mechanism of Action Contains the alkaloids hydrastine (4%) and berberine (6%), which at higher doses can cause vasoconstriction, hypertension, and mucosal irritation; berberine can produce hypotension

Use Gastrointestinal and peripheral vascular activity; also used in sterile eye washes, as a mouthwash, laxative, hemorrhoids, and to stop postpartum hemorrhage. Efficacy not established in clinical studies; has been used to treat mucosal inflammation/gastritis

USUAL DOSAGE

Root: 0.5-1 g 3 times/day

Solid form: Usual dosage: 5-10 grains

Contraindications Pregnancy, breast-feeding

Warnings/Precautions Should not be used in patients with hypertension, glaucoma, diabetes, history of stroke, or heart disease

Adverse Reactions Generally high doses:

Central nervous system: Stimulation/agitation

Gastrointestinal: Nausea, vomiting, diarrhea, mouth and throat irritation

Neuromuscular & skeletal: Extremity numbness

Respiratory: Respiratory failure

Drug Interactions May interfere with vitamin B absorption

Gold Sodium Thiomalate (gold SOW dee um thye oh MAL ate)

Pharmacologic Class Gold Compound

U.S. Brand Names Aurolate®

Generic Available No

Mechanism of Action Unknown, may decrease prostaglandin synthesis or may alter cellular mechanisms by inhibiting sulfhydryl systems

Use Treatment of progressive rheumatoid arthritis

USUAL DOSAGE I.M.:

Children: Initial: Test dose of 10 mg is recommended, followed by 1 mg/kg/week for 20 weeks; maintenance: 1 mg/kg/dose at 2- to 4-week intervals thereafter for as long as therapy is clinically beneficial and toxicity does not develop. Administration for 2-4 months is usually required before clinical improvement is observed.

Adults: 10 mg first week; 25 mg second week; then 25-50 mg/week until 1 g cumulative dose has been given; if improvement occurs without adverse reactions, administer 25-50 mg every 2-3 weeks for 2-20 weeks, then every 3-4 weeks indefinitely

Dosing adjustment in renal impairment:

Cl_{cr} 50-80 mL/minute: Administer 50% of normal dose

Cl_{cr} <50 mL/minute: Avoid use

Dosage Forms INJ: 25 mg/mL (1 mL), 50 mg/mL (1 mL, 2 mL, 10 mL)

Contraindications Hypersensitivity to gold compounds or any component; systemic lupus erythematosus; history of blood dyscrasias; congestive heart failure, exfoliative dermatitis, colitis

Warnings/Precautions Frequent monitoring of patients for signs and symptoms of toxicity will prevent serious adverse reactions; nonsteroidal anti-inflammatory drugs (NSAIDs) and corticosteroids may be discontinued after initiating gold therapy; must not be injected I.V.

Explain the possibility of adverse reactions before initiating therapy; signs of gold toxicity include decrease in hemoglobin, leukopenia, granulocytes and platelets; proteinuria, hematuria, pigmentation, pruritus, stomatitis or persistent diarrhea, rash, metallic taste; advise patient to report any symptoms of toxicity; use with caution in patients with liver or renal disease

Pregnancy Risk Factor C

Adverse Reactions

>10%:

- Dermatologic: Itching, rash
- Gastrointestinal: Stomatitis, gingivitis, glossitis
- Ocular: Conjunctivitis

1% to 10%:

- Dermatologic: Urticaria, alopecia
- Hematologic: Eosinophilia, leukopenia, thrombocytopenia
- Renal: Proteinuria, hematuria

<1%: Agranulocytosis, anemia, angioedema, aplastic anemia, dysphagia, GI hemorrhage, hepatotoxicity, interstitial pneumonitis, metallic taste, peripheral neuropathy, ulcerative enterocolitis

Drug Interactions Decreased effect with penicillamine, acetylcysteine

Onset Delayed; may require up to 3 months

Half-Life Single dose: 3-27 days; usual is approximately 5 days; After third dose: 14-40 days; After eleventh dose: Up to 168 days

Education and Monitoring Issues

Patient Education: Minimize exposure to sunlight; benefits from drug therapy may take as long as 3 months to appear; notify prescriber of pruritus, rash, sore mouth; metallic taste may occur

Monitoring Parameters: Signs and symptoms of gold toxicity, CBC with differential and platelet count, urinalysis

Reference Range: Gold: Normal: 0-0.1 µg/mL (SI: 0-0.0064 µmol/L); Therapeutic: 1-3 µg/mL (SI: 0.06-0.18 µmol/L); Urine: <0.1 µg/24 hour

♦ **GoLYTELY®** *see* Polyethylene Glycol-Electrolyte Solution *on page 747*

Gonadorelin (goe nad oh REL in)

Pharmacologic Class Diagnostic Agent, Gonadotrophic Hormone; Gonadotropin

U.S. Brand Names Factrel®; Lutrepulse®

Mechanism of Action Stimulates the release of luteinizing hormone (LH) from the anterior pituitary gland

Use Evaluation of the functional capacity and response of gonadotrophic hormones; evaluate abnormal gonadotropin regulation as in precocious puberty and delayed puberty. Lutrepulse®: Induction of ovulation in females with hypothalamic amenorrhea.

USUAL DOSAGE

Diagnostic test: Children >12 years and Adults (female): I.V., S.C. hydrochloride salt: 100 mcg administered in women during early phase of menstrual cycle (day 1-7)

Primary hypothalamic amenorrhea: Female adults: Acetate: I.V.: 5 mcg every 90 minutes via Lutrepulse® pump kit at treatment intervals of 21 days (pump will pulsate every 90 minutes for 7 days)

Dosage Forms INJ: As acetate (Lutrepulse®): 0.8 mg, 3.2 mg; As hydrochloride (Factrel®): 100 mcg, 500 mcg

Contraindications Known hypersensitivity to gonadorelin, women with any condition that could be exacerbated by pregnancy; patients who have ovarian cysts or causes of anovulation other than those of hypothalamic origin; any condition that may worsened by reproductive hormones

(Continued)

Gonadorelin *(Continued)*

Warnings/Precautions Hypersensitivity and anaphylactic reactions have occurred following multiple-dose administration; multiple pregnancy is a possibility; use with caution in women in whom pregnancy could worsen pre-existing conditions (eg, pituitary prolactinemia). Multiple pregnancy is a possibility with Lutrepulse®.

Pregnancy Risk Factor B

Adverse Reactions

1% to 10%: Local: Pain at injection site

<1%: Abdominal discomfort, flushing, headache, lightheadedness, nausea, rash

Drug Interactions

Decreased levels/effect: Oral contraceptives, digoxin, phenothiazines, dopamine antagonists

Increased levels/effect: Androgens, estrogens, progestins, glucocorticoids, spironolactone, levodopa

Duration 3-5 hours

Half-Life 4 minutes

Education and Monitoring Issues

Patient Education: If receiving this drug via pulsating pump, check all procedures with prescriber, and use exactly as prescribed. Report any rash, pain, or inflammation at injection site, and any change in respiratory status.

Monitoring Parameters: LH, FSH

♦ **Gonal-F®** *see* Follitropins *on page 391*

♦ **Gonic®** *see* Chorionic Gonadotropin *on page 196*

♦ **Gormel® Creme [OTC]** *see* Urea *on page 962*

Goserelin (GOE se rel in)

Pharmacologic Class Antineoplastic Agent, Miscellaneous; Gonadotropin Releasing Hormone Analog; Luteinizing Hormone-Releasing Hormone Analog

U.S. Brand Names Zoladex® Implant

Generic Available No

Mechanism of Action Goserelin is a synthetic analog of luteinizing-hormone-releasing hormone (LHRH). Following an initial increase in luteinizing hormone (LH) and follicle stimulating hormone (FSH), chronic administration of goserelin results in a sustained suppression of pituitary gonadotropins. Serum testosterone falls to levels comparable to surgical castration. The exact mechanism of this effect is unknown, but may be related to changes in the control of LH or down-regulation of LH receptors.

Use

Prostate carcinoma: Palliative treatment of advanced carcinoma of the prostate. Combination with flutamide for the management of locally confined stage T2b-T4 (stage B2-C) carcinoma of the prostate.

3.6 mg implant **only**:

Endometriosis: Management of endometriosis, including pain relief and reduction of endometriotic lesions for the duration of therapy

Advanced breast cancer: Palliative treatment of advanced breast cancer in pre- and perimenopausal women. Estrogen and progesterone receptor values may help to predict whether goserelin therapy is likely to be beneficial.

Note: The 10.8 mg implant is not indicated in women as the data are insufficient to support reliable suppression of serum estradiol

USUAL DOSAGE

Adults: S.C.:

Monthly implant: 3.6 mg injected into upper abdomen every 28 days; do not try to aspirate with the goserelin syringe; if the needle is in a large vessel, blood will immediately appear in syringe chamber. While a delay of a few days is permissible, attempt to adhere to the 28-day schedule.

3-month implant: 10.8 mg injected into the upper abdominal wall every 12 weeks; do not try to aspirate with the goserelin syringe; if the needle is in a large vessel, blood will immediately appear in syringe chamber. While a delay of a few days is permissible, attempt to adhere to the 12-week schedule.

Prostate carcinoma: Intended for long-term administration

Endometriosis: Recommended duration: 6 months; retreatment is not recommended since safety data is not available. If symptoms recur after a course of therapy, and further treatment is contemplated, consider monitoring bone mineral density. Currently, there are no clinical data on the effect of treatment of benign gynecological conditions with goserelin for periods >6 months.

Dosing adjustment in renal/hepatic impairment: No adjustment is necessary

Dosage Forms INJ, implant: 3.6 mg, 10.8 mg

Contraindications In women who are or may become pregnant, patients who are hypersensitive to the drug

Warnings/Precautions Initially, goserelin, transiently increases serum levels of testosterone. Transient worsening of signs and symptoms, usually manifested by an increase in cancer-related pain which was managed symptomatically, may develop during the first few weeks of treatment. Isolated cases of ureteral obstruction and spinal cord compression have been reported; patient's symptoms may initially worsen temporarily during first few weeks of therapy, cancer-related pain can usually be controlled by analgesics

Pregnancy Risk Factor X

Adverse Reactions General: Worsening of signs and symptoms may occur during the first few weeks of therapy and are usually manifested by an increase in bone pain, increased difficulty in urinating, hot flashes, injection site irritation, and weakness; this will subside, but patients should be aware

>10%:
- Endocrine & metabolic: Gynecomastia, postmenopausal symptoms, sexual dysfunction, loss of libido, hot flashes
- Genitourinary: Impotence, decreased erection

1% to 10%:
- Cardiovascular: Edema
- Central nervous system: Headache, spinal cord compression (possible result of tumor flare), lethargy, dizziness, insomnia
- Dermatologic: Rash
- Gastrointestinal: Nausea and vomiting, anorexia, diarrhea, weight gain
- Genitourinary: Vaginal spotting and breakthrough bleeding, breast tenderness/enlargement
- Local: Pain on injection
- Neuromuscular & skeletal: Bone loss, increased bone pain
- Miscellaneous: Diaphoresis

<1%: Hypo/hypertension, osteoporosis

Half-Life Following a bolus S.C. dose: ~5 hours; prolonged in impaired renal function ~12 hours

Education and Monitoring Issues

Patient Education: This drug must be implanted into your abdomen every 28 days; it is important to maintain appointment schedule. You may experience systemic hot flashes (cool clothes and temperatures may help), headache (analgesic may help), constipation (increased bulk and water in diet or stool softener may help), sexual dysfunction (decreased libido, decreased erection). Symptoms may worsen temporarily during first weeks of therapy. Report unusual nausea or vomiting, any chest pain, respiratory difficulty, unresolved dizziness, or constipation.

Granisetron (gra NI se tron)

Pharmacologic Class Selective 5-HT_3 Receptor Antagonist

U.S. Brand Names Kytril™

Mechanism of Action Selective 5-HT_3-receptor antagonist, blocking serotonin, both peripherally on vagal nerve terminals and centrally in the chemoreceptor trigger zone

Use Prophylaxis and treatment of chemotherapy-related emesis; may be prescribed for patients who are refractory to or have severe adverse reactions to standard antiemetic therapy. Granisetron may be prescribed for young patients (ie, <45 years of age who are more likely to develop extrapyramidal reactions to high-dose metoclopramide) who are to receive highly emetogenic chemotherapeutic agents as listed:

Agents with high emetogenic potential (>90%) (dose/m^2):
- Amifostine
- Azacitidine
- Carmustine ≥200 mg/m^2
- Cisplatin ≥50 mg/m^2
- Cyclophosphamide ≥1 g/m^2
- Cytarabine ≥1500 mg/m^2
- Dacarbazine ≥500 mg/m^2
- Dactinomycin
- Doxorubicin ≥60 mg/m^2
- Lomustine ≥60 mg/m^2
- Mechlorethamine
- Melphalan ≥100 mg/m^2
- Streptozocin
- Thiotepa ≥100 mg/m^2

or two agents classified as having high or moderately high emetogenic potential as listed:

Agents with moderately high emetogenic potential (60% to 90%) (dose/m^2):
- Carboplatin 200-400 mg/m^2
- Carmustine <200 mg/m^2
- Cisplatin <50 mg/m^2
- Cyclophosphamide 600-999 mg/m^2
- Dacarbazine <500 mg/m^2
- Doxorubicin 21-59 mg/m^2
- Hexamethyl melamine
- Ifosfamide ≥5000 mg/m^2
- Lomustine <60 mg/m^2
- Methotrexate ≥250 mg/m^2

(Continued)

Granisetron *(Continued)*

Pentostatin
Procarbazine

Granisetron should not be prescribed for chemotherapeutic agents with a low emetogenic potential (eg, bleomycin, busulfan, cyclophosphamide <1000 mg, etoposide, 5-fluorouracil, vinblastine, vincristine)

USUAL DOSAGE

I.V.: Children and Adults: 10 mcg/kg for 1-3 doses. Doses should be administered as a single IVPB over 5 minutes to 1 hour or by undiluted IV push over 30 seconds, given just prior to chemotherapy (15-60 minutes before); as intervention therapy for breakthrough nausea and vomiting, during the first 24 hours following chemotherapy, 2 or 3 repeat infusions (same dose) have been administered, separated by at least 10 minutes

Oral: Adults: 1 mg twice daily; the first 1 mg dose should be given up to 1 hour before chemotherapy, and the second tablet, 12 hours after the first; alternatively may give a single dose of 2 mg, up to 1 hour before chemotherapy

Note: Granisetron should only be given on the day(s) of chemotherapy

Dosing interval in renal impairment: Creatinine clearance values have no relationship to granisetron clearance

Dosing interval in hepatic impairment: Kinetic studies in patients with hepatic impairment showed that total clearance was approximately halved, however, standard doses were very well tolerated

Dosage Forms INJ: 1 mg/mL. **TAB:** 1 mg (2s), (20s)

Contraindications Previous hypersensitivity to granisetron

Warnings/Precautions Use with caution in patients with liver disease or in pregnant patients

Pregnancy Risk Factor B

Adverse Reactions

>10%: Central nervous system: Headache

1% to 10%:

Cardiovascular: Hyper/hypotension
Central nervous system: Dizziness, insomnia, anxiety
Gastrointestinal: Constipation, abdominal pain, diarrhea
Neuromuscular & skeletal: Weakness

<1%: Agitation, arrhythmias, hot flashes, liver enzyme elevations, somnolence

Drug Interactions CYP3A3/4 enzyme substrate

Onset Commonly controls emesis within 1-3 minutes of administration

Duration Effects generally last no more than a maximum of 24 hours

Half-Life Cancer patient: 10-12 hours; Healthy volunteer: 3-4 hours

Education and Monitoring Issues

Patient Education: This drug will be administered on days when you receive chemotherapy to reduce nausea and vomiting. If outpatient chemotherapy, you may be given oral medication to take after return home; take as directed. You may experience drowsiness; use caution when driving. For persistent acute headache request analgesic from prescriber. Frequent mouth care, chewing gum, or sucking on lozenges may relieve persistent nausea. Report unrelieved headache, fever, diarrhea, or constipation.

Manufacturer SmithKline Beecham Pharmaceuticals

Related Information

Pharmaceutical Manufacturers Directory *on page 1020*

- **Granulex** *see* Trypsin, Balsam Peru, and Castor Oil *on page 959*
- **Grifulvin® V** *see* Griseofulvin *on page 422*
- **Grisactin-500®** *see* Griseofulvin *on page 422*
- **Grisactin® Ultra** *see* Griseofulvin *on page 422*

Griseofulvin (gri see oh FUL vin)

Pharmacologic Class Antifungal Agent, Oral

U.S. Brand Names Fulvicin® P/G; Fulvicin-U/F®; Grifulvin® V; Grisactin-500®; Grisactin® Ultra; Gris-PEG®

Generic Available No

Mechanism of Action Inhibits fungal cell mitosis at metaphase; binds to human keratin making it resistant to fungal invasion

Use Treatment of susceptible tinea infections of the skin, hair, and nails

USUAL DOSAGE Oral:

Children:

Microsize: 10-20 mg/kg/day in single or 2 divided doses
Ultramicrosize: >2 years: 5-10 mg/kg/day in single or 2 divided doses

Adults:

Microsize: 500-1000 mg/day in single or divided doses
Ultramicrosize: 330-375 mg/day in single or divided doses; doses up to 750 mg/day have been used for infections more difficult to eradicate such as tinea unguium

Duration of therapy depends on the site of infection:
- Tinea corporis: 2-4 weeks
- Tinea capitis: 4-6 weeks or longer
- Tinea pedis: 4-8 weeks
- Tinea unguium: 3-6 months or longer

Dosage Forms

Microsize: **CAP** (Grisactin®): 125 mg, 250 mg. **SUSP, oral** (Grifulvin® V): 125 mg/5 mL with alcohol 0.2% (120 mL). **TAB:** (Fulvicin-U/F®, Grifulvin® V): 250 mg; (Fulvicin-U/F®, Grifulvin® V, Grisactin-500®): 500 mg

Ultramicrosize: **TAB:** (Fulvicin® P/G): 165 mg, 330 mg; (Fulvicin® P/G, Grisactin® Ultra, Gris-PEG®): 125 mg, 250 mg; (Grisactin® Ultra): 330 mg

Contraindications Hypersensitivity to griseofulvin or any component; severe liver disease, porphyria (interferes with porphyrin metabolism)

Warnings/Precautions Safe use in children <2 years of age has not been established; during long-term therapy, periodic assessment of hepatic, renal, and hematopoietic functions should be performed; may cause fetal harm when administered to pregnant women; avoid exposure to intense sunlight to prevent photosensitivity reactions; hypersensitivity cross reaction between penicillins and griseofulvin is possible

Pregnancy Risk Factor C

Adverse Reactions

>10%: Dermatologic: Rash, urticaria

1% to 10%:
- Central nervous system: Headache, fatigue, dizziness, insomnia, mental confusion
- Dermatologic: Photosensitivity
- Gastrointestinal: Nausea, vomiting, epigastric distress, diarrhea
- Miscellaneous: Oral thrush

<1%: Angioneurotic edema, GI bleeding, hepatotoxicity, leukopenia, menstrual toxicity, nephrosis, proteinuria

Drug Interactions

Decreased effect:
- Barbiturates may decrease levels of griseofulvin
- Decreased warfarin, cyclosporine, and salicylate activity with griseofulvin
- Griseofulvin decreases oral contraceptive effectiveness

Increased toxicity: With alcohol → tachycardia and flushing

Alcohol Interactions Avoid use (may increase central nervous system depression)

Half-Life 9-22 hours

Education and Monitoring Issues

Patient Education: Take as directed; around-the-clock with food. Take full course of medication; do not discontinue without notifying prescriber. Avoid alcohol while taking this drug (disulfiram reactions). Practice good hygiene measures to prevent reinfection. Frequent blood tests may be required with prolonged therapy. You may experience nausea and vomiting (small, frequent meals may help); confusion, dizziness, drowsiness (use caution when driving or engaging in tasks that require alertness until response to drug is known); nausea, vomiting, or diarrhea (small frequent meals, frequent mouth care, sucking lozenges, or chewing gum may help); increased sensitivity to sun (use sunscreen, wear protective clothing and eyewear, and avoid excessive exposure to direct sunlight). Report skin rash, respiratory difficulty, CNS changes (confusion, dizziness, acute headache), changes in color of stool or urine, white plaques in mouth, or worsening of condition.

Monitoring Parameters: Periodic renal, hepatic, and hematopoietic function tests

♦ **Grisovin®-FP** *see* Griseofulvin *on page 422*

♦ **Gris-PEG®** *see* Griseofulvin *on page 422*

Guaifenesin (gwye FEN e sin)

Pharmacologic Class Expectorant

U.S. Brand Names Anti-Tuss® Expectorant [OTC]; Breonesin® [OTC]; Diabetic Tussin EX® [OTC]; Duratuss-G®; Fenesin™; Gee Gee® [OTC]; Genatuss® [OTC]; GG-Cen® [OTC]; Glyate® [OTC]; Glycotuss® [OTC]; Glytuss® [OTC]; Guaifenex LA®; GuiaCough® Expectorant [OTC]; Guiatuss® [OTC]; Halotussin® [OTC]; Humibid® L.A.; Humibid® Sprinkle; Hytuss® [OTC]; Hytuss-2X® [OTC]; Liquibid®; Malotuss® [OTC]; Medi-Tuss® [OTC]; Monafed®; Muco-Fen-LA®; Mytussin® [OTC]; Naldecon® Senior EX [OTC]; Organidin® NR; Pneumomist®; Respa-GF®; Robitussin® [OTC]; Scot-Tussin® [OTC]; Siltussin® [OTC]; Sinumist®-SR Capsulets®; Touro Ex®; Tusibron® [OTC]; Uni-Tussin® [OTC]

Use Temporary control of cough due to minor throat and bronchial irritation

USUAL DOSAGE Oral:

Children:
- <2 years: 12 mg/kg/day in 6 divided doses
- 2-5 years: 50-100 mg every 4 hours, not to exceed 600 mg/day
- 6-11 years: 100-200 mg every 4 hours, not to exceed 1.2 g/day

Children >12 years and Adults: 200-400 mg every 4 hours to a maximum of 2.4 g/day

Contraindications Hypersensitivity to guaifenesin or any component

Pregnancy Risk Factor C

(Continued)

Guaifenesin *(Continued)*

Related Information

Guaifenesin and Codeine *on page 424*
Guaifenesin and Phenylephrine *on page 425*
Guaifenesin, Pseudoephedrine, and Codeine *on page 425*
Hydrocodone and Guaifenesin *on page 445*
Hydrocodone, Pseudoephedrine, and Guaifenesin *on page 446*
Theophylline and Guaifenesin *on page 906*

Guaifenesin and Codeine (gwye FEN e sin & KOE deen)

Pharmacologic Class Antitussive; Cough Preparation; Expectorant

U.S. Brand Names Brontex® Liquid; Brontex® Tablet; Cheracol®; Guaituss AC®; Guiatussin® With Codeine; Mytussin® AC; Robafen® AC; Robitussin® A-C; Tussi-Organidin® NR

Use Temporary control of cough due to minor throat and bronchial irritation

Dosage Forms LIQ [C-V] (Brontex®): Guaifenesin 75 mg and codeine phosphate 2.5 mg per 5 mL. **SYR** [C-V] (Cheracol®, Guaituss AC®, Guiatussin® with Codeine, Mytussin® AC, Robafen® AC, Robitussin® A-C, Tussi-Organidin® NR): Guaifenesin 100 mg and codeine phosphate 10 mg per 5 mL (60 mL, 120 mL, 480 mL). **TAB** [C-III] (Brontex®): Guaifenesin 300 mg and codeine phosphate 10 mg

Pregnancy Risk Factor C

Guaifenesin and Dextromethorphan

(gwye FEN e sin & deks troe meth OR fan)

Pharmacologic Class Antitussive; Cough Preparation; Expectorant

U.S. Brand Names Benylin® Expectorant [OTC]; Cheracol® D [OTC]; Clear Tussin® 30; Contac® Cough Formula Liquid [OTC]; Diabetic Tussin DM® [OTC]; Extra Action Cough Syrup [OTC]; Fenesin™ DM; Genatuss DM® [OTC]; Glycotuss-DM® [OTC]; Guaifenex DM®; GuiaCough® [OTC]; Guiatuss-DM® [OTC]; Halotussin®-DM [OTC]; Humibid® DM [OTC]; Iobid DM®; Kolephrin® GG/DM [OTC]; Monafed® DM; Muco-Fen-DM®; Mytussin® DM [OTC]; Naldecon® Senior DX [OTC]; Phanatuss® Cough Syrup [OTC]; Phenadex® Senior [OTC]; Queltuss®; Respa®-DM; Rhinosyn-DMX® [OTC]; Robafen DM® [OTC]; Robitussin®-DM [OTC]; Safe Tussin® 30 [OTC]; Scot-Tussin® Senior Clear [OTC]; Siltussin DM® [OTC]; Synacol® CF [OTC]; Syracol-CF® [OTC]; Tolu-Sed® DM [OTC]; Tusibron-DM® [OTC]; Tuss-DM® [OTC]; Tussi-Organidin® DM NR; Uni-tussin® DM [OTC]; Vicks® 44E [OTC]; Vicks® Pediatric Formula 44E [OTC]

Use Temporary control of cough due to minor throat and bronchial irritation

USUAL DOSAGE Oral:

Children: Dextromethorphan: 1-2 mg/kg/24 hours divided 3-4 times/day

Children >12 years and Adults: 5 mL every 4 hours or 10 mL every 6-8 hours not to exceed 40 mL/24 hours

Dosage Forms SYR: (Benylin® Expectorant): Guaifenesin 100 mg and dextromethorphan hydrobromide 5 mg per 5 mL (118 mL, 236 mL); (Cheracol® D, Clear Tussin® 30, Genatuss DM®, Mytussin® DM, Robitussin®-DM, Siltussin DM®, Tolu-Sed® DM, Tussi-Organidin® DM NR): Guaifenesin 100 mg and dextromethorphan hydrobromide 10 mg per 5 mL (5 mL, 10 mL, 120 mL, 240 mL, 360 mL, 480 mL, 3780 mL); (Contac® Cough Formula Liquid): Guaifenesin 67 mg and dextromethorphan hydrobromide 10 mg per 5 mL (120 mL); (Extra Action Cough Syrup, GuiaCough®, Guiatuss DM®, Halotussin® DM, Rhinosyn-DMX®, Tusibron-DM®, Uni-tussin® DM): Guaifenesin 100 mg and dextromethorphan hydrobromide 15 mg per 5 mL (120 mL, 240 mL, 480 mL); (Kolephrin® GG/DM): Guaifenesin 150 mg and dextromethorphan hydrobromide 10 mg per 5 mL (120 mL); (Naldecon® Senior DX): Guaifenesin 200 mg and dextromethorphan hydrobromide 15 mg per 5 mL (118 mL, 480 mL); (Phanatuss®): Guaifenesin 85 mg and dextromethorphan hydrobromide 10 mg per 5 mL; (Vicks® 44E): Guaifenesin 66.7 mg and dextromethorphan hydrobromide 6.7 mg per 5 mL. **TAB:** (Extended release Guaifenex DM®, Iobid DM®, Fenesin™ DM, Humibid® DM, Monafed® DM, Respa®-DM): Guaifenesin 600 mg and dextromethorphan hydrobromide 30 mg; (Glycotuss-dM®): Guaifenesin 100 mg and dextromethorphan hydrobromide 10 mg; (Queltuss®): Guaifenesin 100 mg and dextromethorphan hydrobromide 15 mg; (Syracol-CF®): Guaifenesin 200 mg and dextromethorphan hydrobromide 15 mg; (Tuss-DM®): Guaifenesin 200 mg and dextromethorphan hydrobromide 10 mg

Contraindications Hypersensitivity to guaifenesin, dextromethorphan or any component

Warnings/Precautions Should not be used for persistent or chronic cough such as that occurring with smoking, asthma, chronic bronchitis, or emphysema or for cough associated with excessive phlegm

Pregnancy Risk Factor C

Adverse Reactions 1% to 10%:

Central nervous system: Drowsiness, headache
Dermatologic: Rash
Gastrointestinal: Nausea, vomiting

Guaifenesin and Phenylephrine (gwye FEN e sin & fen il EF rin)

Pharmacologic Class Cold Preparation

U.S. Brand Names Deconsal® Sprinkle®; Endal®; Sinupan®

Dosage Forms CAP, sustained release: (Deconsal® Sprinkle®): Guaifenesin 300 mg and phenylephrine hydrochloride 10 mg; (Sinupan®): Guaifenesin 200 mg and phenylephrine hydrochloride 40 mg. **TAB, timed release** (Endal®): Guaifenesin 300 mg and phenylephrine hydrochloride 20 mg

Guaifenesin, Pseudoephedrine, and Codeine

(gwye FEN e sin, soo doe e FED rin, & KOE deen)

Pharmacologic Class Antitussive/Decongestant/Expectorant

U.S. Brand Names Codafed® Expectorant; Cycofed® Pediatric; Decohistine® Expectorant; Deproist® Expectorant With Codeine; Dihistine® Expectorant; Guiatuss DAC®; Guiatussin® DAC; Halotussin® DAC; Isoclor® Expectorant; Mytussin® DAC; Nucofed®; Nucofed® Pediatric Expectorant; Nucotuss®; Phenhist® Expectorant; Robitussin®-DAC; Ryna-CX®; Tussar® SF Syrup

Dosage Forms LIQ: C-III: (Nucofed®, Nucotuss®): Guaifenesin 200 mg, pseudoephedrine hydrochloride 60 mg, and codeine phosphate 20 mg per 5 mL (480 mL); C-V: (Codafed® Expectorant, Decohistine® Expectorant, Deproist® Expectorant with Codeine, Dihistine® Expectorant, Guiatuss DAC®, Guiatussin® DAC, Halotussin® DAC, Isoclor® Expectorant, Mytussin® DAC, Nucofed® Pediatric Expectorant, Phenhist® Expectorant, Robitussin®-DAC, Ryna-CX®, Tussar® SF): Guaifenesin 100 mg, pseudoephedrine hydrochloride 30 mg, and codeine phosphate 10 mg per 5 mL (120 mL, 480 mL, 4000 mL)

Pregnancy Risk Factor C

♦ **Guaifenex DM®** *see* Guaifenesin and Dextromethorphan *on page 424*

♦ **Guaifenex LA®** *see* Guaifenesin *on page 423*

♦ **Guaituss AC®** *see* Guaifenesin and Codeine *on page 424*

Guanabenz (GWAHN a benz)

Pharmacologic Class Alpha$_1$ Agonist

U.S. Brand Names Wytensin®

Use Management of hypertension

USUAL DOSAGE Adults: Oral: Initial: 4 mg twice daily, increase in increments of 4-8 mg/day every 1-2 weeks to a maximum of 32 mg twice daily

Dosing adjustment in hepatic impairment: Probably necessary

Contraindications Hypersensitivity to guanabenz or any component

Pregnancy Risk Factor C

Guanadrel (GWAHN a drel)

Pharmacologic Class Alpha$_1$ Agonist

U.S. Brand Names Hylorel®

Use Considered a second line agent in the treatment of hypertension, usually with a diuretic

USUAL DOSAGE Oral:

Adults: Initial: 10 mg/day (5 mg twice daily); adjust dosage weekly or monthly until blood pressure is controlled, usual dosage: 20-75 mg/day, given twice daily; for larger dosage, 3-4 times/day dosing may be needed

Elderly: Initial: 5 mg once daily

Dosing interval in renal impairment:

Cl_{cr} 10-50 mL/minute: Administer every 12-24 hours

Cl_{cr} <10 mL/minute: Administer every 24-48 hours

Contraindications Known hypersensitivity to guanadrel, pheochromocytoma, patients taking MAO inhibitors

Pregnancy Risk Factor B

Guanethidine (gwahn ETH i deen)

Pharmacologic Class Alpha$_1$ Agonist

U.S. Brand Names Ismelin®

Use Treatment of moderate to severe hypertension

USUAL DOSAGE Oral:

Children: Initial: 0.2 mg/kg/day, increase by 0.2 mg/kg/day at 7- to 10-day intervals to a maximum of 3 mg/kg/day

Adults:

Ambulatory patients: Initial: 10 mg/day, increase at 5- to 7-day intervals to an average of 25-50 mg/day

Hospitalized patients: Initial: 25-50 mg/day, increase by 25-50 mg/day or every other day to desired therapeutic response

Elderly: Initial: 5 mg once daily

Dosing interval in renal impairment: Cl_{cr} <10 mL/minute: Administer every 24-36 hours

Contraindications Pheochromocytoma, patients taking MAO inhibitors, hypersensitivity to guanethidine or any component

Pregnancy Risk Factor C

Guanfacine (GWAHN fa seen)

Pharmacologic Class Alpha$_1$ Agonist

U.S. Brand Names Tenex®

Use Management of hypertension

USUAL DOSAGE Adults: Oral: 1 mg usually at bedtime, may increase if needed at 3- to 4-week intervals; 1 mg/day is most common dose

Contraindications Hypersensitivity to guanfacine or any component

Pregnancy Risk Factor B

- **GuiaCough® [OTC]** *see* Guaifenesin and Dextromethorphan *on page 424*
- **GuiaCough® Expectorant [OTC]** *see* Guaifenesin *on page 423*
- **Guiatuss® [OTC]** *see* Guaifenesin *on page 423*
- **Guiatuss DAC®** *see* Guaifenesin, Pseudoephedrine, and Codeine *on page 425*
- **Guiatuss-DM® [OTC]** *see* Guaifenesin and Dextromethorphan *on page 424*
- **Guiatussin® DAC** *see* Guaifenesin, Pseudoephedrine, and Codeine *on page 425*
- **Guiatussin® With Codeine** *see* Guaifenesin and Codeine *on page 424*
- **G-well®** *see* Lindane *on page 531*
- **Gynecort® [OTC]** *see* Hydrocortisone *on page 447*
- **Gynecure** *see* Tioconazole *on page 923*
- **Gyne-Lotrimin® [OTC]** *see* Clotrimazole *on page 220*
- **Gynergen®** *see* Ergotamine *on page 323*
- **Gyne-Sulf®** *see* Sulfabenzamide, Sulfacetamide, and Sulfathiazole *on page 875*
- **Gynix®** *see* Clotrimazole *on page 220*
- **Gynodiol® Oral** *see* Estradiol *on page 327*
- **Gynogen L.A.® Injection** *see* Estradiol *on page 327*
- **Gyno-Trosyd** *see* Tioconazole *on page 923*
- **Habitrol™ Patch [OTC]** *see* Nicotine *on page 651*

Haemophilus b Conjugate and Hepatitis b Vaccine

(he MOF i lus bee KON joo gate & hep a TYE tis bee vak SEEN)

Pharmacologic Class Vaccine, Inactivated Virus

U.S. Brand Names Comvax™

Mechanism of Action Hib conjugate vaccines use covalent binding of capsular polysaccharide of *Haemophilus influenzae* type b to OMPC carrier to produce an antigen which is postulated to convert a T-independent antigen into a T-dependent antigen to result in enhanced antibody response and on immunologic memory. Recombinant hepatitis B vaccine is a noninfectious subunit viral vaccine. The vaccine is derived from hepatitis B surface antigen (HB_sAg) produced through recombinant DNA techniques from yeast cells. The portion of the hepatitis B gene which codes for HB_sAg is cloned into yeast which is then cultured to produce hepatitis B vaccine.

Use

Immunization against invasive disease caused by *H. influenzae* type b and against infection caused by all known subtypes of hepatitis B virus in infants 8 weeks to 15 months of age born of HB_sAg-negative mothers

Infants born of HB_sAg-positive mothers or mothers of unknown HB_sAg status should receive hepatitis B immune globulin and hepatitis B vaccine (Recombinant) at birth and should complete the hepatitis B vaccination series given according to a particular schedule

USUAL DOSAGE Infants (>8 weeks of age): I.M.: 0.5 mL at 2, 4, and 12-15 months of age (total of 3 doses)

If the recommended schedule cannot be followed, the interval between the first two doses should be at least 2 months and the interval between the second and third dose should be as close as possible to 8-11 months.

Modified Schedule: Children who receive one dose of hepatitis B vaccine at or shortly after birth may receive Comvax™ on a schedule of 2,4, and 12-15 months of age

Dosage Forms INJ: 7.5 mcg *Haemophilus* b PRP and 5 mcg HB_sAg/0.5 mL

Contraindications Hypersensitivity to any component of the vaccine

Warnings/Precautions If used in persons with malignancies or those receiving immunosuppressive therapy or who are otherwise immunocompromised, the expected immune response may not be obtained.

Patients who develop symptoms suggestive of hypersensitivity after an injection should not receive further injections of the vaccine.

The decision to administer or delay vaccination because of current or recent febrile illness depends on the severity of symptoms and the etiology of the disease. Immunization should be delayed during the course of an acute febrile illness.

Pregnancy Risk Factor C

Adverse Reactions When administered during the same visit that DTP, OPV, IPV, Varicella Virus Vaccine, and M-M-R II vaccines are given, the rates of systemic reactions do not differ from those observed only when any of the vaccines are administered. **All serious adverse reactions must be reported to the U.S. Department of Health and**

Human Services (DHHS) Vaccine Adverse Event Reporting System (VAERS) 1-800-822-7967.

>10%: Central nervous system: Acute febrile reactions

1% to 10%:

- Central nervous system: Fever (up to 102.2°F), irritability, lethargy
- Gastrointestinal: Anorexia, diarrhea
- Local: Irritation at injection site

<1%: Allergic or anaphylactic reactions (difficulty in breathing, hives, itching, swelling of eyes, face, unusual tiredness or weakness), convulsions, fever (>102.2°F), vomiting

Education and Monitoring Issues

Patient Education: May use acetaminophen for postdose fever

Haemophilus b Conjugate Vaccine

(hem OF fi lus bee KON joo gate vak SEEN)

Pharmacologic Class Vaccine, Inactivated Bacteria

U.S. Brand Names ActHIB®; HibTITER®; OmniHIB™; PedvaxHIB™; ProHIBiT®; TriHIBIT®

Generic Available No

Mechanism of Action Stimulates production of anticapsular antibodies and provides active immunity to *Haemophilus influenzae*

Use Routine immunization of children 2 months to 5 years of age against invasive disease caused by *H. influenzae*

Unimmunized children ≥5 years of age with a chronic illness known to be associated with increased risk of *Haemophilus influenzae* type b disease, specifically, persons with anatomic or functional asplenia or sickle cell anemia or those who have undergone splenectomy, should receive Hib vaccine.

Haemophilus b conjugate vaccines are not indicated for prevention of bronchitis or other infections due to *H. influenzae* in adults; adults with specific dysfunction or certain complement deficiencies who are at especially high risk of *H. influenzae* type b infection (HIV-infected adults); patients with Hodgkin's disease (vaccinated at least 2 weeks before the initiation of chemotherapy or 3 months after the end of chemotherapy)

USUAL DOSAGE Children: I.M.: 0.5 mL as a single dose should be administered according to one of the following "brand-specific" schedules; do not inject I.V.

Vaccination Schedule for *Haemophilus* b Conjugate Vaccines

Age at 1st Dose (mo)	HibTITER®		PedvaxHIB®		ProHIBiT®	
	Primary Series	Booster	Primary Series	Booster	Primary Series	Booster
2-6*	3 doses, 2 months apart	15 mo†	2 doses, 2 months apart	12 mo†		
7-11	2 doses, 2 months apart	15 mo†	2 doses, 2 months apart	15 mo†		
12-14	1 dose	15 mo†	1 dose	15 mo†		
15-60	1 dose	—	1 dose	—	1 dose	—

*It is not currently recommended that the various *Haemophilus* b conjugate vaccines be interchanged (ie, the same brand should be used throughout the entire vaccination series). If the health care provider does not know which vaccine was previously used, it is prudent that an infant, 2-6 months of age, be given a primary series of three doses.

†At least 2 months after previous dose.

Dosage Forms INJ: (ActHIB®, HibTITER®, OmniHIB™): Capsular oligosaccharide 10 mcg and diphtheria CRM_{197} protein ~25 mcg per 0.5 mL (0.5 mL, 2.5 mL, 5 mL); (PedvaxHIB™): Purified capsular polysaccharide 15 mcg and *Neisseria meningitidis* OMPC 250 mcg per dose (0.5 mL); (ProHIBiT®): Purified capsular polysaccharide 25 mcg and conjugated diphtheria toxoid protein 18 mcg per dose (0.5 mL, 2.5 mL, 5 mL); (TriHIBit® vaccine) [Tripedia® vaccine used to reconstitute ActHIB®]: 0.5 mL

Contraindications Children with any febrile illness or active infection, known hypersensitivity to *Haemophilus* b polysaccharide vaccine (thimerosal), children who are immunosuppressed or receiving immunosuppressive therapy

Warnings/Precautions Have epinephrine 1:1000 available; children in whom DTP or DT vaccination is deferred: The carrier proteins used in HbOC (but not PRP-OMP) are chemically and immunologically related to toxoids contained in DTP vaccine. Earlier or simultaneous vaccination with diphtheria or tetanus toxoids may be required to elicit an optimal anti-PRP antibody response to HbOC. In contrast, the immunogenicity of PRP-OMP is not affected by vaccination with DTP. In infants in whom DTP or DT vaccination is deferred, PRP-OMP may be advantageous for *Haemophilus influenzae* type b vaccination.

Children with immunologic impairment: Children with chronic illness associated with increased risk of *Haemophilus influenzae* type b disease may have impaired anti-PRP antibody responses to conjugate vaccination. Examples include those with HIV infection, immunoglobulin deficiency, anatomic or functional asplenia, and sickle cell disease, as

(Continued)

Haemophilus b Conjugate Vaccine *(Continued)*

well as recipients of bone marrow transplants and recipients of chemotherapy for malignancy. Some children with immunologic impairment may benefit from more doses of conjugate vaccine than normally indicated.

Pregnancy Risk Factor C

Adverse Reactions When administered during the same visit that DTP vaccine is given, the rates of systemic reactions do not differ from those observed only when DTP vaccine is administered. **All serious adverse reactions must be reported to the U.S. Department of Health and Human Services (DHHS) Vaccine Adverse Event Reporting System (VAERS) 1-800-822-7967.**

25%:
- Cardiovascular: Edema
- Dermatologic: Local erythema
- Local: Increased risk of *Haemophilus* b infections in the week after vaccination
- Miscellaneous: Warmth

>10%: Acute febrile reactions

1% to 10%:
- Central nervous system: Fever (up to 102.2°F), irritability, lethargy
- Gastrointestinal: Anorexia, diarrhea
- Local: Irritation at injection site

<1%: Convulsions, dyspnea, edema of the eyes/face, fever (>102.2°F), itching, unusual fatigue, urticaria, vomiting, weakness

Drug Interactions Decreased effect with immunosuppressive agents, immunoglobulins within 1 month may decrease antibody production

Education and Monitoring Issues

Patient Education: May use acetaminophen for postdose fever

Halazepam (hal AZ e pam)

Pharmacologic Class Benzodiazepine

U.S. Brand Names Paxipam®

Use Management of anxiety disorders; short-term relief of the symptoms of anxiety

USUAL DOSAGE Oral:

Adults: 20-40 mg 3-4 times/day; optimal dosage usually ranges from 80-160 mg/day. If side effects occur with the starting dose, lower the dose.

Elderly ≥70 years or debilitated patients: 20 mg 1-2 times/day and adjust dose accordingly

Dosage Forms TAB: 20 mg, 40 mg

Contraindications Hypersensitivity to halazepam or any component, cross-sensitivity with other benzodiazepines may exist; avoid using in patients with pre-existing CNS depression, severe uncontrolled pain, or angle-closure glaucoma

Pregnancy Risk Factor D

Alcohol Interactions Avoid use (may increase central nervous system depression)

Onset Peak levels in 1-3 hours

Half-Life Parent: 14 hours; metabolite (desmethyldiazepam): 50-100 hours

Halcinonide (hal SIN oh nide)

Pharmacologic Class Corticosteroid, Topical

U.S. Brand Names Halog®; Halog®-E

Generic Available No

Mechanism of Action Decreases inflammation by suppression of migration of polymorphonuclear leukocytes and reversal of increased capillary permeability

Use Inflammation of corticosteroid-responsive dermatoses [high potency topical corticosteroid]

USUAL DOSAGE Children and Adults: Topical: Apply sparingly 1-3 times/day, occlusive dressing may be used for severe or resistant dermatoses; a thin film of cream or ointment is effective; do not overuse. Therapy should be discontinued when control is achieved; if no improvement is seen, reassessment of diagnosis may be necessary.

Dosage Forms CRM (Halog®): 0.025% (15 g, 60 g, 240 g); 0.1% (15 g, 30 g, 60 g, 240 g); Emollient base (Halog®-E): 0.1% (15 g, 30 g, 60 g). **OINT, top** (Halog®): 0.1% (15 g, 30 g, 60 g, 240 g). **SOLN** (Halog®): 0.1% (20 mL, 60 mL)

Contraindications Viral, fungal, or tubercular skin lesions, known hypersensitivity to halcinonide or any component

Warnings/Precautions Adverse systemic effects may occur when used on large areas of the body, denuded areas, for prolonged periods of time, with an occlusive dressing, and/or in infants or small children

Pregnancy Risk Factor C

Adverse Reactions <1%: Acneiform eruptions, allergic contact dermatitis, dry skin, folliculitis, hypertrichosis, hypopigmentation, irritation, itching, local burning, miliaria, perioral dermatitis, secondary infection, skin atrophy, skin maceration, striae

Education and Monitoring Issues

Patient Education: A thin film of cream or ointment is effective; do not overuse; do not use tight-fitting diapers or plastic pants on children being treated in the diaper area; use only as prescribed, and for no longer than the period prescribed; apply sparingly in light film; rub in lightly; avoid contact with eyes; notify prescriber if condition being treated persists or worsens

- ♦ **Halcion®** *see* Triazolam *on page 948*
- ♦ **Haldol®** *see* Haloperidol *on page 430*
- ♦ **Haldol® Decanoate** *see* Haloperidol *on page 430*
- ♦ **Halenol® Childrens [OTC]** *see* Acetaminophen *on page 17*
- ♦ **Halfan®** *see* Halofantrine *on page 429*
- ♦ **Halfprin® 81® [OTC]** *see* Aspirin *on page 72*

Halobetasol (hal oh BAY ta sol)

Pharmacologic Class Corticosteroid, Topical

U.S. Brand Names Ultravate™ Topical

Generic Available No

Mechanism of Action Corticosteroids inhibit the initial manifestations of the inflammatory process (ie, capillary dilation and edema, fibrin deposition, and migration and diapedesis of leukocytes into the inflamed site) as well as later sequelae (angiogenesis, fibroblast proliferation)

Use Relief of inflammatory and pruritic manifestations of corticosteroid-response dermatoses [very high potency topical corticosteroid]

USUAL DOSAGE Children and Adults: Topical: Apply sparingly to skin twice daily, rub in gently and completely; treatment should not exceed 2 consecutive weeks and total dosage should not exceed 50 g/week. Therapy should be discontinued when control is achieved; if no improvement is seen, reassessment of diagnosis may be necessary.

Dosage Forms CRM: 0.05% (15 g, 45 g). **OINT, top:** 0.05% (15 g, 45 g)

Contraindications Hypersensitivity to halobetasol or any component; viral, fungal, or tubercular skin lesions

Warnings/Precautions Not for ophthalmic use; may cause adrenal suppression or insufficiency; application to abraded or inflamed areas or too large of areas of the body may increase the risk of systemic absorption and the risk of adrenal suppression, as may prolonged use or the use of >50 g/week. Topical halobetasol should not be used for the treatment of rosacea or perioral dermatitis.

Pregnancy Risk Factor C

Adverse Reactions <1%: Acneiform eruptions, allergic contact dermatitis, dry skin, folliculitis, hypertrichosis, hypopigmentation, irritation, itching, local burning, miliaria, perioral dermatitis, secondary infection, skin atrophy, skin maceration, striae

Education and Monitoring Issues

Patient Education: A thin film of cream or ointment is effective; do not overuse; do not use tight-fitting diapers or plastic pants on children being treated in the diaper area; use only as prescribed, and for no longer than the period prescribed; apply sparingly in light film; rub in lightly; avoid contact with eyes; notify prescriber if condition being treated persists or worsens

Halofantrine (ha loe FAN trin)

Pharmacologic Class Antimalarial Agent

U.S. Brand Names Halfan®

Mechanism of Action Similar to mefloquine; destruction of asexual blood forms, possible inhibition of proton pump

Use Treatment of mild to moderate acute malaria caused by susceptible strains of *Plasmodium falciparum* and *Plasmodium vivax*

USUAL DOSAGE Oral:

Children <40 kg: 8 mg/kg every 6 hours for 3 doses; repeat in 1 week

Adults: 500 mg every 6 hours for 3 doses; repeat in 1 week

Dosage Forms TAB: 250 mg

Contraindications Family history of congenital Q-T_c prolongation; hypersensitivity to halofantrine

Warnings/Precautions Monitor closely for decreased hematocrit and hemoglobin, patients with chronic liver disease

Pregnancy Risk Factor C

Adverse Reactions

>10%: Dermatologic: Pruritus

1% to 10%:

- Cardiovascular: Edema
- Central nervous system: Malaise, headache
- Gastrointestinal: Nausea, vomiting
- Hematologic: Leukocytosis
- Hepatic: Elevated LFTs
- Local: Tenderness
- Neuromuscular & skeletal: Myalgia
- Respiratory: Cough
- Miscellaneous: Lymphadenopathy

(Continued)

Halofantrine *(Continued)*

<1%: Anaphylactic shock, asthma, hypoglycemia, hypotension, sterile abscesses, tachycardia, urticaria

Drug Interactions CYP2D6 and 3A3/4 enzyme substrate

Increased toxicity (Q-T_c interval prolongation) with other agents that cause Q-T_c interval prolongation, especially mefloquine

Half-Life 23 hours

Education and Monitoring Issues

Patient Education: Take on an empty stomach; avoid high fat meals; notify prescriber of persistent nausea, vomiting, abdominal pain, light stools, dark urine

Monitoring Parameters: CBC, LFTs, parasite counts

♦ **Halog®** *see* Halcinonide *on page 428*

♦ **Halog®-E** *see* Halcinonide *on page 428*

Haloperidol (ha loe PER i dole)

Pharmacologic Class Antipsychotic Agent, Butyrophenone

U.S. Brand Names Haldol®; Haldol® Decanoate

Generic Available Yes

Mechanism of Action Blocks postsynaptic mesolimbic dopaminergic D_1 and D_2 receptors in the brain; exhibits a strong alpha-adrenergic blocking and anticholinergic effect, depresses the release of hypothalamic and hypophyseal hormones; believed to depress the reticular activating system thus affecting basal metabolism, body temperature, wakefulness, vasomotor tone, and emesis

Use Treatment of psychoses, Tourette's disorder, and severe behavioral problems in children; may be used for the emergency sedation of severely agitated or delirious patients; may be effective for infantile autism and has been commonly used to reduce disabling choreiform movements associated with Huntington's disease

USUAL DOSAGE

Children: 3-12 years (15-40 kg): Oral:

Initial: 0.05 mg/kg/day or 0.25-0.5 mg/day given in 2-3 divided doses; increase by 0.25-0.5 mg every 5-7 days; maximum: 0.15 mg/kg/day

Usual maintenance:

Agitation or hyperkinesia: 0.01-0.03 mg/kg/day once daily

Nonpsychotic disorders: 0.05-0.075 mg/kg/day in 2-3 divided doses

Psychotic disorders: 0.05-0.15 mg/kg/day in 2-3 divided doses

Children 6-12 years: I.M. (as lactate): 1-3 mg/dose every 4-8 hours to a maximum of 0.15 mg/kg/day; change over to oral therapy as soon as able

Adults:

Oral: 0.5-5 mg 2-3 times/day; usual maximum: 30 mg/day; some patients may require up to 100 mg/day

I.M. (as lactate): 2-5 mg every 4-8 hours as needed

I.M. (as decanoate): Initial: 10-15 times the daily oral dose administered at 3- to 4-week intervals

Sedation in the Intensive Care Unit:

I.M./IVP/IVPB: May repeat bolus doses after 30 minutes until calm achieved then administer 50% of the maximum dose every 6 hours

Mild agitation: 0.5-2 mg

Moderate agitation: 2-5 mg

Severe agitation: 10-20 mg

Continuous intravenous infusion (100 mg/100 mL D_5W): Rates of 1-40 mg/hour have been used

Elderly (nonpsychotic patients, dementia behavior):

Initial: Oral: 0.25-0.5 mg 1-2 times/day; increase dose at 4- to 7-day intervals by 0.25-0.5 mg/day; increase dosing intervals (twice daily, 3 times/day, etc) as necessary to control response or side effects

Maximum daily dose: 50 mg; gradual increases (titration) may prevent side effects or decrease their severity

Hemodialysis/peritoneal dialysis: Supplemental dose is not necessary

Dosage Forms

Haloperidol lactate: **CONC, oral:** 2 mg/mL (5 mL, 10 mL, 15 mL, 120 mL, 240 mL). **INJ:** 5 mg/mL (1 mL, 2 mL, 2.5 mL, 10 mL)

Haloperidol decanoate: **INJ:** 50 mg/mL (1 mL, 5 mL); 100 mg/mL (1 mL, 5 mL). **TAB:** 0.5 mg, 1 mg, 2 mg, 5 mg, 10 mg, 20 mg

Contraindications Hypersensitivity to haloperidol or any component; narrow-angle glaucoma, bone marrow suppression, CNS depression, severe liver or cardiac disease, subcortical brain damage; circulatory collapse; severe hypotension or hypertension

Warnings/Precautions Safety and efficacy have not been established in children <3 years of age; watch for hypotension when administering I.M. or I.V.; use with caution in patients with cardiovascular disease or seizures; benefits of therapy must be weighed against risks of therapy; decanoate form should never be given I.V.; some tablets contain tartrazine which may cause allergic reactions; use caution with CNS depression and severe liver or cardiac disease

Pregnancy Risk Factor C

Adverse Reactions EKG changes, retinal pigmentation are more common than with chlorpromazine

>10%:

Central nervous system: Restlessness, anxiety, extrapyramidal reactions, dystonic reactions, pseudoparkinsonian signs and symptoms, tardive dyskinesia, neuroleptic malignant syndrome (NMS), seizures, altered central temperature regulation, akathisia

Endocrine & metabolic: Edema of the breasts

Gastrointestinal: Weight gain, constipation

1% to 10%:

Cardiovascular: Hypotension (especially orthostatic), tachycardia, arrhythmias, abnormal T waves with prolonged ventricular repolarization

Central nervous system: Hallucinations, sedation, drowsiness, persistent tardive dyskinesia

Genitourinary: Dysuria

<1%: adynamic ileus, agranulocytosis, alopecia, amenorrhea, blurred vision, cholestatic jaundice, contact dermatitis, decreased visual acuity (may be irreversible), galactorrhea, gynecomastia, heat stroke, hyperpigmentation, laryngospasm, leukopenia (usually inpatients with large doses for prolonged periods), nausea, obstructive jaundice, overflow incontinence, photosensitivity (rare), priapism, pruritus, rash, respiratory depression, retinal pigmentation, sexual dysfunction, tardive dystonia, urinary retention, vomiting, xerostomia (problem for denture user)

Drug Interactions CYP1A2 enzyme substrate, CYP2D6 enzyme substrate (minor); CYP2D6 enzyme inhibitor CYP2C8 and 3A3/4 enzyme substrate; CYP1A2, 2C, and 3A3/4 inducer

Antipsychotics inhibit the ability of bromocriptine to lower serum prolactin concentrations

Benztropine (and other anticholinergics) may inhibit the therapeutic response to haloperidol and excess anticholinergic effects may occur

Chloroquine may increase haloperidol concentrations

Cigarette smoking may enhance the hepatic metabolism of haloperidol. Larger doses may be required compared to a nonsmoker.

Concurrent use of haloperidol with an antihypertensive may produce additive hypotensive effects

Concurrent use with TCA may produce increased toxicity or altered therapeutic response

Haloperidol may inhibit the antiparkinsonian effect of levodopa; avoid this combination

Haloperidol plus lithium may rarely produce neurotoxicity

Barbiturates may reduce haloperidol concentrations

Propranolol may increase haloperidol concentrations

Sulfadoxine-pyrimethamine may increase haloperidol concentrations

Haloperidol and CNS depressants (ethanol, narcotics) may produce additive CNS depressant effects

Haloperidol and trazodone may produce additive hypotensive effects

Carbamazepine appears to stimulate the metabolism of haloperidol. Monitor for reduced efficacy

Fluoxetine and paroxetine may inhibit the metabolism of haloperidol resulting in EPS; monitor for EPS

Haloperidol in combination with indomethacin may result in drowsiness, tiredness, and confusion; monitor for adverse effects

Quinidine appears to increase haloperidol concentrations; monitor for EPS

Alcohol Interactions Avoid use (may increase central nervous system depression)

Onset Onset of sedation: I.V.: Within 1 hour

Duration ~3 weeks for decanoate form

Half-Life 20 hours

Education and Monitoring Issues

Patient Education: Use exactly as directed (do not increase dose or frequency); may cause physical and/or psychological dependence. It may take 2-3 weeks to achieve desired results; do not discontinue without consulting prescriber. Dilute oral concentration with water or juice. Do not take within 2 hours of any antacid. Store away from light. Avoid excess alcohol or caffeine and other prescription or OTC medications not approved by prescriber. Maintain adequate hydration (2-3 L/day of fluids unless instructed to restrict fluid intake). Avoid skin contact with medication; may cause contact dermatitis (wash immediately with warm, soapy water). You may experience excess drowsiness, restlessness, dizziness, or blurred vision (use caution driving or when engaging in tasks requiring alertness until response to drug is known); nausea, vomiting (small frequent meals, frequent mouth care, chewing gum, or sucking lozenges may help); constipation (increased exercise, fluids, or dietary fruit and fiber may help); postural hypotension (use caution climbing stairs or when changing position from lying or sitting to standing); urinary retention (void before taking medication); decreased perspiration (avoid strenuous exercise in hot environments). Report persistent CNS effects (eg, trembling fingers, altered gait or balance, excessive sedation, seizures, unusual movements, anxiety, abnormal thoughts, confusion, personality changes); chest pain, palpitations, rapid heartbeat, severe dizziness; unresolved urinary retention

(Continued)

Haloperidol *(Continued)*

or changes in urinary pattern; vision changes; skin rash or yellowing of skin; difficulty breathing; or worsening of condition.

Monitoring Parameters: Monitor orthostatic blood pressures 3-5 days after initiation of therapy or a dose increase; observe for tremor and abnormal movement or posturing (extrapyramidal symptoms)

Reference Range:

Therapeutic: 5-15 ng/mL (SI: 10-30 nmol/L) (psychotic disorders - less for Tourette's and mania)

Toxic: >42 ng/mL (SI: >84 nmol/L)

Haloprogin (ha loe PROE jin)

Pharmacologic Class Antifungal Agent

U.S. Brand Names Halotex®

Generic Available No

Mechanism of Action Interferes with fungal DNA replication to inhibit yeast cell respiration and disrupt its cell membrane

Use Topical treatment of tinea pedis (athlete's foot), tinea cruris (jock itch), tinea corporis (ringworm), tinea manuum caused by *Trichophyton rubrum*, *Trichophyton tonsurans*, *Trichophyton mentagrophytes*, *Microsporum canis*, or *Epidermophyton floccosum*; topical treatment of *Malassezia furfur*

USUAL DOSAGE Topical: Children and Adults: Apply liberally twice daily for 2-3 weeks; intertriginous areas may require up to 4 weeks of treatment

Dosage Forms CRM: 1% (15 g, 30 g). **SOLN, top:** 1% with alcohol 75% (10 mL, 30 mL)

Contraindications Hypersensitivity to haloprogin or any component

Warnings/Precautions Safety and efficacy have not been established in children

Pregnancy Risk Factor B

Adverse Reactions <1%: Burning sensation, erythema, folliculitis, irritation, pruritus, vesicle formation

Education and Monitoring Issues

Patient Education: Avoid contact with eyes; for external use only; improvement should occur within 4 weeks; discontinue use if sensitization or irritation occur

- **Halotestin®** *see* Fluoxymesterone *on page 380*
- **Halotex®** *see* Haloprogin *on page 432*
- **Halotussin® [OTC]** *see* Guaifenesin *on page 423*
- **Halotussin® DAC** *see* Guaifenesin, Pseudoephedrine, and Codeine *on page 425*
- **Halotussin®-DM [OTC]** *see* Guaifenesin and Dextromethorphan *on page 424*
- **Haltran® [OTC]** *see* Ibuprofen *on page 458*

Hawthorn

Pharmacologic Class Herbal

Mechanism of Action Contains flavonoids, catechin, and epicatechin which may be cardioprotective and have vasodilatory properties; shown to dilate coronary vessels

Use In herbal medicine to treat cardiovascular abnormalities (arrhythmia, angina), increased cardiac output, increased contractility of heart muscle; also used as a sedative

USUAL DOSAGE Daily dose of total flavonoids: 10 mg

Per Commission E: 160-900 mg native water-ethanol extract (ethanol 45% v/v or methanol 70% v/v, drug-extract ratio: 4-7:1, with defined flavonoid or procyanidin content), corresponding to 30-168.7 mg procyanidins, calculated as epicatechin, or 3.5-19.8 mg flavonoids, calculated as hyperoside in accordance with DAB 10 [German pharmacopoeia #10] in 2 or 3 individual doses; duration of administration: 6 weeks minimum

Contraindications Pregnancy and breast-feeding

Pregnancy Implications Do not use

Adverse Reactions

Cardiovascular: Hypotension, bradycardia, hypertension

Central nervous system: Depression, fatigue

Dermatologic: Rash

Gastrointestinal: Nausea

Drug Interactions Antihypertensives (effect enhanced), digoxin; effects with Viagra® unknown

- **H-BIG®** *see* Hepatitis B Immune Globulin *on page 435*
- **Head & Shoulders® Intensive Treatment [OTC]** *see* Selenium Sulfide *on page 845*
- **Healon®** *see* Sodium Hyaluronate *on page 859*
- **Healon® GV** *see* Sodium Hyaluronate *on page 859*
- **Heart Failure Guidelines** *see page 1099*
- **Hectorol®** *see* Doxercalciferol *on page 299*
- ***Helicobacter pylori* Treatment** *see page 1107*
- **Helidac™** *see* Bismuth Subsalicylate, Metronidazole, and Tetracycline *on page 109*
- **Helistat®** *see* Microfibrillar Collagen Hemostat *on page 601*

- **Hemabate™** *see* Carboprost Tromethamine *on page 141*
- **Hemocyte® [OTC]** *see* Ferrous Fumarate *on page 359*
- **Hemotene®** *see* Microfibrillar Collagen Hemostat *on page 601*
- **Hemril-HC® Uniserts®** *see* Hydrocortisone *on page 447*
- **Hepalean** *see* Heparin *on page 433*
- **Hepalean-Lok** *see* Heparin *on page 433*

Heparin (HEP a rin)

Pharmacologic Class Anticoagulant

U.S. Brand Names Hep-Lock®; Liquaemin®

Generic Available Yes

Mechanism of Action Potentiates the action of antithrombin III and thereby inactivates thrombin (as well as activated coagulation factors IX, X, XI, XII, and plasmin) and prevents the conversion of fibrinogen to fibrin; heparin also stimulates release of lipoprotein lipase (lipoprotein lipase hydrolyzes triglycerides to glycerol and free fatty acids)

Use Prophylaxis and treatment of thromboembolic disorders

USUAL DOSAGE

Line flushing: When using daily flushes of heparin to maintain patency of single and double lumen central catheters, 10 units/mL is commonly used for younger infants (eg, <10 kg) while 100 units/mL is used for older infants, children, and adults. Capped PVC catheters and peripheral heparin locks require flushing more frequently (eg, every 6-8 hours). Volume of heparin flush is usually similar to volume of catheter (or slightly greater). Additional flushes should be given when stagnant blood is observed in catheter, after catheter is used for drug or blood administration, and after blood withdrawal from catheter.

Addition of heparin (0.5-1 unit/mL) to peripheral and central TPN has been shown to increase duration of line patency. The final concentration of heparin used for TPN solutions may need to be decreased to 0.5 units/mL in small infants receiving larger amounts of volume in order to avoid approaching therapeutic amounts. Arterial lines are heparinized with a final concentration of 1 unit/mL.

Children:

- Intermittent I.V.: Initial: 50-100 units/kg, then 50-100 units/kg every 4 hours
- I.V. infusion: Initial: 50 units/kg, then 15-25 units/kg/hour; increase dose by 2-4 units/kg/hour every 6-8 hours as required

Adults:

- Prophylaxis (low-dose heparin): S.C.: 5000 units every 8-12 hours
- Intermittent I.V.: Initial: 10,000 units, then 50-70 units/kg (5000-10,000 units) every 4-6 hours
- I.V. infusion: 50 units/kg to start, then 15-25 units/kg/hour as continuous infusion; increase dose by 5 units/kg/hour every 4 hours as required according to PTT results, usual range: 10-30 units/hour
  - Weight-based protocol: 80 units/kg I.V. push followed by continuous infusion of 18 units/kg/hour; see table.

Standard Heparin Solution
(25,000 units/500 mL D_5W)

To Administer a Dose of	Set Infusion Rate at
400 units/h	8 mL/h
500 units/h	10 mL/h
600 units/h	12 mL/h
700 units/h	14 mL/h
800 units/h	16 mL/h
900 units/h	18 mL/h
1000 units/h	20 mL/h
1100 units/h	22 mL/h
1200 units/h	24 mL/h
1300 units/h	26 mL/h
1400 units/h	28 mL/h
1500 units/h	30 mL/h
1600 units/h	32 mL/h
1700 units/h	34 mL/h
1800 units/h	36 mL/h
1900 units/h	38 mL/h
2000 units/h	40 mL/h

(Continued)

Heparin *(Continued)*

Dosage Forms

Heparin sodium: **LOCK flush inj:** Beef lung source: 10 units/mL (1 mL, 2 mL, 2.5 mL, 3 mL, 5 mL, 10 mL, 30 mL), 100 units/mL (1 mL, 2 mL, 2.5 mL, 3 mL, 5 mL, 10 mL, 30 mL); Porcine intestinal mucosa source: 10 units/mL (1 mL, 2 mL, 10 mL, 30 mL), 100 units/mL (1 mL, 2 mL, 10 mL, 30 mL); Porcine intestinal mucosa source (preservative free): 10 units/mL (1 mL), 100 units/mL (1 mL). **MULTIPLE-dose vial inj:** Beef lung source (with preservative): 1000 units/mL (5 mL, 10 mL, 30 mL), 5000 units/mL (10 mL), 10,000 units/mL (4 mL, 5 mL, 10 mL), 20,000 units/mL (2 mL, 5 mL, 10 mL), 40,000 units/mL (5 mL); Porcine intestinal mucosa source (with preservative): 1000 units/mL (10 mL, 30 mL), 5000 units/mL (10 mL), 10,000 units/mL (4 mL), 20,000 units/mL (2 mL, 5 mL). **SINGLE-dose vial inj:** Beef lung source: 1000 units/mL (1 mL), 5000 units/mL (1 mL), 10,000 units/mL (1 mL), 20,000 units/mL (1 mL), 40,000 units/mL (1 mL); Porcine intestinal mucosa: 1000 units/mL (1 mL), 5000 units/mL (1 mL), 10,000 units/mL (1 mL), 20,000 units/mL (1 mL), 40,000 units/mL (1 mL). **UNIT-dose inj:** Porcine intestinal mucosa source (with preservative): 1000 units/dose (1 mL, 2 mL), 2500 units/dose (1 mL), 5000 units/dose (0.5 mL, 1 mL), 7500 units/dose (1 mL), 10,000 units/dose (1 mL), 15,000 units/dose (1 mL), 20,000 units/dose (1 mL). **INF:** Porcine intestinal mucosa source: D_5W: 40 units/mL (500 mL), 50 units/mL (250 mL, 500 mL), 100 units/mL (100 mL, 250 mL), NaCl 0.45%: 2 units/mL (500 mL, 1000 mL), 50 units/mL (250 mL), 100 units/mL (250 mL), NaCl 0.9%: 2 units/mL (500 mL, 1000 mL), 5 units/mL (1000 mL), 50 units/mL (250 mL, 500 mL, 1000 mL)

Heparin calcium: **UNIT-dose inj:** Porcine intestinal mucosa (preservative free): 5000 units/dose (0.2 mL), 12,500 units/dose (0.5 mL), 20,000 units/dose (0.8 mL)

Contraindications Hypersensitivity to heparin or any component; severe thrombocytopenia, subacute bacterial endocarditis, suspected intracranial hemorrhage, uncontrollable bleeding (unless secondary to disseminated intravascular coagulation)

Warnings/Precautions

Use with caution as hemorrhaging may occur; risk factors for hemorrhage include I.M. injections, peptic ulcer disease, increased capillary permeability, menstruation; severe renal, hepatic or biliary disease; use with caution in patients with shock, severe hypotension

Some preparations contain benzyl alcohol as a preservative. In neonates, large amounts of benzyl alcohol (>100 mg/kg/day) have been associated with fatal toxicity (gasping syndrome). The use of preservative-free heparin is, therefore, recommended in neonates. Some preparations contain sulfite which may cause allergic reactions.

Heparin does not possess fibrinolytic activity and, therefore, cannot lyse established thrombi; discontinue heparin if hemorrhage occurs; severe hemorrhage or overdosage may require protamine

Use caution with white clot syndrome (new thrombus associated with thrombocytopenia) and heparin resistance

Use caution in patients >60 years of age (particularly women); may be more sensitive and have more bleeding complications

Pregnancy Risk Factor C

Adverse Reactions As with all anticoagulants, bleeding is the major adverse effect of heparin. Hemorrhage may occur at virtually any site. Risk is dependent on multiple variables, including the intensity of anticoagulation and patient susceptibility. Additional adverse effects are often related to idiosyncratic reactions, and the frequency is difficult to estimate.

Cardiovascular: Chest pain, vasospasm (possibly related to thrombosis), hemorrhagic shock

Central nervous system: Fever, headache, chills

Dermatologic: Unexplained bruising, urticaria, alopecia, dysesthesia pedis, purpura, eczema

Endocrine and Metabolic: Hyperkalemia (supression of aldosterone), rebound hyperlipidemia on discontinuation

Gastrointestinal: Nausea, vomiting, constipation, hematemesis

Genitourinary: Frequent or persistent erection

Hematologic: Hemorrhage, blood in urine, bleeding from gums, epistaxis, adrenal hemorrhage, ovarian hemorrhage, retroperitoneal hemorrhage, thrombocytopenia (see note)

Hepatic: Elevated liver enzymes (AST/ALT) Local: Irritation, ulceration, cutaneous necrosis have been rarely reported with deep S.C. injections, I.M. injection (not recommended) is associated with a high incidence of these effects

Neuromuscular & skeletal: Peripheral neuropathy, osteoporosis (chronic therapy effect)

Respiratory: Hemoptysis, pulmonary hemorrhage, asthma, rhinitis

Ocular: Conjunctivitis (allergic reaction)

Miscellaneous: Allergic reactions, anaphylactoid reactions

Note: Thrombocytopenia has been reported to occur at an incidence between 0% and 30%. It is often of no clinical significance. However, immunologically mediated heparin-induced thrombocytopenia has been estimated to occur in 1% to 2% of patients, and is marked by a progressive fall in platelet counts and, in some cases, thromboembolic complications (skin necrosis, pulmonary embolism, gangrene of the extremities, stroke or myocardial infarction); daily platelet counts for 5-7 days at initiation of therapy may help detect the onset of this complication.

Case reports: Bronchospasm, erythematous plaques

Drug Interactions

Cephalosporins which contain the MTT side chain may increase the risk of hemorrhage

Drugs which affect platelet function (eg, aspirin, NSAIDs, dipyridamole, ticlopidine, clopidogrel) may potentiate the risk of hemorrhage

Nitroglycerin (I.V.) may decrease heparin's anticoagulant effect. This interaction has not been validated in some studies, and may only occur at high nitroglycerin dosages.

Penicillins (parenteral) may prolong bleeding time via inhibition of platelet aggregation, potentially increasing the risk of hemorrhage

Thrombolytic agents increase the risk of hemorrhage

Warfarin: Risk of bleeding may be increased during concurrent therapy. Heparin is commonly continued during the initiation of warfarin therapy to assure anticoagulation and to protect against possible transient hypercoagulability

Other drugs reported to increase heparin's anticoagulant effect include antihistamines, tetracycline, quinine, nicotine, and cardiac glycosides (digoxin)

Onset Onset of anticoagulation: I.V.: Immediate with use; S.C.: Within 20-30 minutes

Half-Life

Mean: 1.5 hours

Range: 1-2 hours; affected by obesity, renal function, hepatic function, malignancy, presence of pulmonary embolism, and infections

Education and Monitoring Issues

Patient Education: This drug can only be administered by injection. You may have a tendency to bleed easily while taking this drug; brush teeth with soft brush, floss with waxed floss, use electric razor, avoid scissors or sharp knives, and potentially harmful activities. May discolor urine or stool. Report CNS changes (fever, confusion), unusual fever, persistent nausea or GI upset, unusual bleeding or bruising (bleeding gums, nosebleed, blood in urine, dark stool), pain in joints or back, swelling or pain at injection site.

Monitoring Parameters: Platelet counts, PTT, hemoglobin, hematocrit, signs of bleeding

For intermittent I.V. injections, PTT is measured 3.5-4 hours after I.V. injection

Note: Continuous I.V. infusion is preferred vs I.V. intermittent injections. For full-dose heparin (ie, nonlow-dose), the dose should be titrated according to PTT results. For anticoagulation, an APTT 1.5-2.5 times normal is usually desired. APTT is usually measured prior to heparin therapy, 6-8 hours after initiation of a continuous infusion (following a loading dose), and 6-8 hours after changes in the infusion rate; increase or decrease infusion by 2-4 units/kg/hour dependent on PTT. See table.

Heparin Infusion Dose Adjustment

APTT	Adjustment
>3x control	↓ Infusion rate 50%
2-3x control	↓ Infusion rate 25%
1.5-2x control	No change
<1.5x control	↑ Rate of infusion 25%; max 2500 units/h

Reference Range: Heparin: 0.3-0.5 unit/mL; APTT: 1.5-2.5 times **the patient's baseline**

Related Information

Anticoagulation Guidelines *on page 1068*

Hepatitis B Immune Globulin (hep a TYE tis bee i MYUN GLOB yoo lin)

Pharmacologic Class Immune Globulin

U.S. Brand Names H-BIG®; Hep-B Gammagee®; HyperHep®

Generic Available No

Mechanism of Action Hepatitis B immune globulin (HBIG) is a nonpyrogenic sterile solution containing 10% to 18% protein of which at least 80% is monomeric immunoglobulin G (IgG). HBIG differs from immune globulin in the amount of anti-HB_s. Immune globulin is prepared from plasma that is not preselected for anti-HB_s content. HBIG is prepared from plasma preselected for high titer anti-HB_s. In the U.S., HBIG has an anti-HB_s high titer >1:100,000 by IRA. There is no evidence that the causative agent of AIDS (HTLV-III/LAV) is transmitted by HBIG.

Use Provide prophylactic passive immunity to hepatitis B infection to those individuals exposed; newborns of mothers known to be hepatitis B surface antigen positive; hepatitis B immune globulin is not indicated for treatment of active hepatitis B infections and is ineffective in the treatment of chronic active hepatitis B infection

USUAL DOSAGE I.M.:

Newborns: Hepatitis B: 0.5 mL as soon after birth as possible (within 12 hours); may repeat at 3 months in order for a higher rate of prevention of the carrier state to be achieved; at this time an active vaccination program with the vaccine may begin

(Continued)

Hepatitis B Immune Globulin *(Continued)*

Adults: Postexposure prophylaxis: 0.06 mL/kg as soon as possible after exposure (ie, within 24 hours of needlestick, ocular, or mucosal exposure or within 14 days of sexual exposure); usual dose: 3-5 mL; repeat at 28-30 days after exposure

Note: HBIG may be administered at the same time (but at a different site) or up to 1 month preceding hepatitis B vaccination without impairing the active immune response

Dosage Forms INJ: (H-BIG®): 4 mL, 5 mL; (HyperHep®): 0.5 mL, 1 mL, 5 mL

Contraindications Hypersensitivity to hepatitis B immune globulin or any component; allergies to gamma globulin or anti-immunoglobulin antibodies; allergies to thimerosal; IgA deficiency; I.M. injections in patients with thrombocytopenia or coagulation disorders

Pregnancy Risk Factor C

Adverse Reactions

1% to 10%:

Central nervous system: Dizziness, malaise

Dermatologic: Urticaria, angioedema, rash, erythema

Local: Pain and tenderness at injection site

Neuromuscular & skeletal: Arthralgia

<1%: Anaphylaxis

Drug Interactions Interferes with immune response of live virus vaccines

Related Information

Postexposure Prophylaxis for Hepatitis B *on page 1160*

Prophylaxis for Patients Exposed to Common Communicable Diseases *on page 1161*

♦ **Hep-B Gammagee®** *see* Hepatitis B Immune Globulin *on page 435*

♦ **Hep-Lock®** *see* Heparin *on page 433*

♦ **Heptalac®** *see* Lactulose *on page 506*

♦ **Herbal/Nutritional Information** *see page 1251*

♦ **Herceptin®** *see* Trastuzumab *on page 939*

♦ **Hespan®** *see* Hetastarch *on page 436*

Hetastarch (HET a starch)

Pharmacologic Class Plasma Volume Expander, Colloid

U.S. Brand Names Hespan®

Generic Available No

Mechanism of Action Produces plasma volume expansion by virtue of its highly colloidal starch structure, similar to albumin

Use Blood volume expander used in treatment of shock or impending shock when blood or blood products are not available; does not have oxygen-carrying capacity and is not a substitute for blood or plasma

USUAL DOSAGE I.V. infusion (requires an infusion pump):

Children: Safety and efficacy have not been established

Adults: 500-1000 mL (up to 1500 mL/day) or 20 mL/kg/day (up to 1500 mL/day); larger volumes (15,000 mL/24 hours) have been used safely in small numbers of patients

Dosing adjustment in renal impairment: Cl_{cr} <10 mL/minute: Initial dose is the same but subsequent doses should be reduced by 20% to 50% of normal

Dosage Forms INF, in sodium chloride 0.9%: 6% (500 mL)

Contraindications Severe bleeding disorders, renal failure with oliguria or anuria, or severe congestive heart failure

Warnings/Precautions Anaphylactoid reactions have occurred; use with caution in patients with thrombocytopenia (may interfere with platelet function); large volume may cause drops in hemoglobin concentrations; use with caution in patients at risk from overexpansion of blood volume, including the very young or aged patients, those with congestive heart failure or pulmonary edema; large volumes may interfere with platelet function and prolong PT and PTT times

Pregnancy Risk Factor C

Adverse Reactions <1%: Bleeding, chills, circulatory overload, fever, headaches, heart failure, hypersensitivity, itching, myalgia, peripheral edema; prolongation of PT, PTT, clotting time, and bleeding time; pruritus, vomiting

Onset Onset of volume expansion: I.V.: Within 30 minutes

Duration 24-36 hours

Education and Monitoring Issues

Patient Education: Report immediately any respiratory difficulty, acute headache, muscle pain, or abdominal cramping.

♦ **Hexa-Betalin** *see* Pyridoxine *on page 796*

Hexachlorophene (heks a KLOR oh feen)

Pharmacologic Class Antibacterial, Topical

U.S. Brand Names pHisoHex®; Septisol®

Use Surgical scrub and as a bacteriostatic skin cleanser; control an outbreak of gram-positive infection when other procedures have been unsuccessful

USUAL DOSAGE Children and Adults: Topical: Apply 5 mL cleanser and water to area to be cleansed; lather and rinse thoroughly under running water

Contraindications Known hypersensitivity to halogenated phenol derivatives or hexachlorophene; use in premature infants; use on burned or denuded skin; occlusive dressing; application to mucous membranes

Pregnancy Risk Factor C

- **Hexadrol®** *see* Dexamethasone *on page 256*
- **Hexaphenyl** *see* Hexachlorophene *on page 436*
- **Hexifoam** *see* Chlorhexidine Gluconate *on page 181*
- **Hexit®** *see* Lindane *on page 531*
- **H-F Antidote** *see* Calcium Gluconate *on page 132*
- **Hibiclens® Topical [OTC]** *see* Chlorhexidine Gluconate *on page 181*
- **Hibidil** *see* Chlorhexidine Gluconate *on page 181*
- **Hibistat® Topical [OTC]** *see* Chlorhexidine Gluconate *on page 181*
- **Hibitane** *see* Chlorhexidine Gluconate *on page 181*
- **HibTITER®** *see Haemophilus* b Conjugate Vaccine *on page 427*
- **Hi-Cor-1.0®** *see* Hydrocortisone *on page 447*
- **Hi-Cor-2.5®** *see* Hydrocortisone *on page 447*
- **Hi Potency Cal** *see* Calcium Carbonate *on page 130*
- **Hip-Rex®** *see* Methenamine *on page 579*
- **Histalet Forte® Tablet** *see* Chlorpheniramine, Pyrilamine, Phenylephrine, and Phenylpropanolamine *on page 187*
- **Histantil** *see* Promethazine *on page 779*
- **Histatab® Plus Tablet [OTC]** *see* Chlorpheniramine and Phenylephrine *on page 186*
- **Hista-Vadrin® Tablet** *see* Chlorpheniramine, Phenylephrine, and Phenylpropanolamine *on page 186*
- **Histerone® Injection** *see* Testosterone *on page 898*
- **Histor-D® Syrup** *see* Chlorpheniramine and Phenylephrine *on page 186*
- **Histor-D® Timecelles®** *see* Chlorpheniramine, Phenylephrine, and Methscopolamine *on page 186*

Histrelin (his TREL in)

Pharmacologic Class Gonadotropin Releasing Hormone Analog; Luteinizing Hormone-Releasing Hormone Analog

U.S. Brand Names Supprelin™ Injection

Generic Available No

Mechanism of Action Histrelin is a synthetic long-acting gonadotropin-releasing hormone analog; with daily administration, it desensitizes the pituitary to endogenous gonadotropin-releasing hormone (ie, suppresses gonadotropin release by causing down regulation of the pituitary); this results in a decrease in gonadal sex steroid production which stops the secondary sexual development

Use Treatment of central idiopathic precocious puberty; treatment of estrogen-associated gynecological disorders such as acute intermittent porphyria, endometriosis, leiomyomata uteri, and premenstrual syndrome

USUAL DOSAGE

Central idiopathic precocious puberty: S.C.: Usual dose is 10 mcg/kg/day given as a single daily dose at the same time each day

Acute intermittent porphyria in women: S.C.: 5 mcg/day

Endometriosis: S.C.: 100 mcg/day

Leiomyomata uteri: S.C.: 20-50 mcg/day or 4 mcg/kg/day

Dosage Forms INJ: 7-day kits of single use: 120 mcg/0.6 mL; 300 mcg/0.6 mL; 600 mcg/0.6 mL

Contraindications Hypersensitivity to histrelin, pregnancy, breast-feeding

Warnings/Precautions The site of injection should be varied daily; the dose should be administered at the same time each day. In precocious puberty, changing the dosage schedule or noncompliance may result in inadequate control of the pubertal process.

Pregnancy Risk Factor X

Adverse Reactions

>10%:

- Cardiovascular: Vasodilation
- Central nervous system: Headache
- Gastrointestinal: Abdominal pain
- Genitourinary: Vaginal bleeding, vaginal dryness
- Local: Skin reaction at injection site

1% to 10%:

- Central nervous system: Mood swings, headache, pain
- Dermatologic: Rashes, urticaria
- Endocrine & metabolic: Breast tenderness, hot flashes
- Gastrointestinal: Nausea, vomiting
- Genitourinary: Increased urinary calcium excretion

(Continued)

Histrelin *(Continued)*

Neuromuscular & skeletal: Joint stiffness

Onset

Precocious puberty: Onset of hormonal responses: Within 3 months of initiation of therapy

Acute intermittent porphyria associated with menses: Amelioration of symptoms: After 1-2 months of therapy

Treatment of endometriosis or leiomyomata uteri: Onset of responses: After 3-6 months of treatment

Education and Monitoring Issues

Patient Education: Use as directed - daily at the same time. Maintain regular follow-up schedule. You may experience headache and GI distress (analgesics may help), vaginal bleeding, pain, irritation (during first weeks of therapy), nausea or anorexia (small frequent meals may help), flushing or redness (cold clothes and cool environment may help). Report irregular or rapid heartbeat, unresolved nausea or vomiting, difficulty breathing, or infection at injection sites.

Monitoring Parameters: Precocious puberty: Prior to initiating therapy: Height and weight, hand and wrist x-rays, total sex steroid levels, beta-hCG level, adrenal steroid level, gonadotropin-releasing hormone stimulation test, pelvic/adrenal/testicular ultrasound/head CT; during therapy monitor 3 months after initiation and then every 6-12 months; serial levels of sex steroids and gonadotropin-releasing hormone testing; physical exam; secondary sexual development; histrelin may be discontinued when the patient reaches the appropriate age for puberty

- **Histussin D® Liquid** *see* Hydrocodone and Pseudoephedrine *on page 446*
- **Hivid®** *see* Zalcitabine *on page 988*
- **HMS Liquifilm®** *see* Medrysone *on page 558*

Homatropine (hoe MA troe peen)

Pharmacologic Class Anticholinergic Agent

U.S. Brand Names AK-Homatropine® Ophthalmic; Isopto® Homatropine Ophthalmic

Use Producing cycloplegia and mydriasis for refraction; treatment of acute inflammatory conditions of the uveal tract

USUAL DOSAGE

Children:

Mydriasis and cycloplegia for refraction: Instill 1 drop of 2% solution immediately before the procedure; repeat at 10-minute intervals as needed

Uveitis: Instill 1 drop of 2% solution 2-3 times/day

Adults:

Mydriasis and cycloplegia for refraction: Instill 1-2 drops of 2% solution or 1 drop of 5% solution before the procedure; repeat at 5- to 10-minute intervals as needed; maximum of 3 doses for refraction

Uveitis: Instill 1-2 drops of 2% or 5% 2-3 times/day up to every 3-4 hours as needed

Contraindications Narrow-angle glaucoma, acute hemorrhage or hypersensitivity to the drug or any component in the formulation

Pregnancy Risk Factor C

- **Honvol®** *see* Diethylstilbestrol *on page 269*
- **Humalog®** *see* Insulin Preparations *on page 472*
- **Humalog® 50/50** *see* Insulin Preparations *on page 472*
- **Humalog® 75/25** *see* Insulin Preparations *on page 472*

Human Growth Hormone (HYU man grothe HOR mone)

Pharmacologic Class Growth Hormone

U.S. Brand Names Genotropin® Injection; Humatrope® Injection; Norditropin® Injection; Nutropin® AQ Injection; Nutropin® Depot™; Nutropin® Injection; Protropin® Injection; Saizen® Injection; Serostim® Injection

Generic Available No

Mechanism of Action Somatropin and somatrem are purified polypeptide hormones of recombinant DNA origin; somatropin contains the identical sequence of amino acids found in human growth hormone while somatrem's amino acid sequence is identical plus an additional amino acid, methionine; human growth hormone stimulates growth of linear bone, skeletal muscle, and organs; stimulates erythropoietin which increases red blood cell mass; exerts both insulin-like and diabetogenic effects

Use

Long-term treatment of growth failure from lack of adequate endogenous growth hormone secretion

Nutropin®: Treatment of children who have growth failure associated with chronic renal insufficiency up until the time of renal transplantation

USUAL DOSAGE Children (individualize dose):

Somatrem (Protropin®): I.M., S.C.: Up to 0.1 mg (0.26 units)/kg/dose 3 times/week

Somatropin (Genotropin®): S.C.: Weekly dosage of 0.16-0.24 mg/kg divided into 6-7 doses

Somatropin (Humatrope®): I.M., S.C.: Up to 0.06 mg (0.16 units)/kg/dose 3 times/week

Somatropin (Nutropin®): S.C.:

Growth hormone inadequacy: Weekly dosage of 0.3 mg/kg (0.78 units/kg) administered daily

Chronic renal insufficiency: Weekly dosage of 0.35 mg/kg (0.91 units/kg) administered daily

Therapy should be discontinued when patient has reached satisfactory adult height, when epiphyses have fused, or when the patient ceases to respond

Growth of 5 cm/year or more is expected, if growth rate does not exceed 2.5 cm in a 6-month period, double the dose for the next 6 months, if there is still no satisfactory response, discontinue therapy

Somatropin (Nutropin® Depot™): S.C.:

Once-monthly injection: 1.5 mg/kg body weight administered on the same day of each month; patients >15 kg will require more than one injection per dose

Twice-monthly injection: 0.75 mg/kg body weight administered twice each month on the same days of each month (eg, days 1 and 15 of each month); patients >30 kg will require more than one injection per dose

Dosage Forms POWDER for inj, lyophilized: (Somatropin: Genotropin®): 1.5 mg ~4.5 units (5 mL), 5.8 mg ~17.4 units (5 mL); (Humatrope®): 5 mg ~15 units; (Norditropin®): 4 mg ~12 units, 8 mg ~24 units; (Nutropin®): 5 mg ~15 units (10 mL), 10 mg ~30 units (10 mL); (Nutropin® AQ): 10 mg ~30 units (2 mL); (Saizen®) (rDNA origin): 5 mg ~15 units; (Serostim®): 5 mg ~15 units (5 mL), 6 mg ~18 units (5 mL); (Somatrem, Protropin®): 5 mg ~15 units (10 mL), 10 mg ~26 units (10 mL)

Contraindications Closed epiphyses, known hypersensitivity to drug, benzyl alcohol (somatrem), or m-Cresol or glycerin (somatropin); progression of any underlying intracranial lesion or actively growing intracranial tumor; acute critical illness due to complications following open heart or abdominal surgery; multiple accidental trauma or respiratory failure; evidence of active malignancy

Warnings/Precautions Use with caution in patients with diabetes; when administering to newborns, reconstitute with sterile water for injection; insulin dose may require adjustment; monitor for evidence of glucose intolerance. Examine patients with a history of an intracranial lesion for progression or recurrence.

Pregnancy Risk Factor C

Adverse Reactions S.C. administration can cause local lipoatrophy or lipodystrophy and may enhance the development of neutralizing antibodies

1% to 10%: Endocrine & metabolic: Hypothyroidism

<1%: Hypoglycemia, itching, pain at injection site, pain in hip/knee, rash, small risk for developing leukemia

Nutropin® Depot™:

>10%:

Central nervous system: Headache (13%)

Local: Injection site reactions occur in almost all patients

1% to 10%:

Central nervous system: Fever (7%)

Gastrointestinal: Nausea (8%), vomiting (5%)

Neuromuscular & skeletal: Arthralgia (4%), lower extremity pain (7%), severe pain during injection (7%)

<1%: Edema

Drug Interactions Decreased effect: Glucocorticoid therapy may inhibit growth-promoting effects.

Education and Monitoring Issues

Monitoring Parameters: Growth curve, periodic thyroid function tests, bone age (annually), periodical urine testing for glucose, somatomedin C levels

- **Humatin®** *see* Paromomycin *on page 704*
- **Humatrope® Injection** *see* Human Growth Hormone *on page 438*
- **Humegon™** *see* Menotropins *on page 562*
- **Humibid® DM [OTC]** *see* Guaifenesin and Dextromethorphan *on page 424*
- **Humibid® L.A.** *see* Guaifenesin *on page 423*
- **Humibid® Sprinkle** *see* Guaifenesin *on page 423*
- **HuMist® Nasal Mist [OTC]** *see* Sodium Chloride *on page 858*
- **Humorsol® Ophthalmic** *see* Demecarium *on page 250*
- **Humulin 10/90, 20/80, 30/70, 40/60, and 50/50** *see* Insulin Preparations *on page 472*
- **Humulin® 50/50** *see* Insulin Preparations *on page 472*
- **Humulin® 70/30** *see* Insulin Preparations *on page 472*
- **Humulin® L** *see* Insulin Preparations *on page 472*
- **Humulin® N** *see* Insulin Preparations *on page 472*
- **Hurricaine®** *see* Benzocaine *on page 98*
- **Hyalase** *see* Hyaluronidase *on page 440*
- **Hyalgan®** *see* Sodium Hyaluronate *on page 859*

Hyaluronidase (hye al yoor ON i dase)

Pharmacologic Class Antidote

U.S. Brand Names Wydase® Injection

Use Increases the dispersion and absorption of other drugs; increases rate of absorption of parenteral fluids given by hypodermoclysis; enhances diffusion of locally irritating or toxic drugs in the management of I.V. extravasation

USUAL DOSAGE

Infants and Children:

Management of I.V. extravasation: Reconstitute the 150 unit vial of lyophilized powder with 1 mL normal saline; take 0.1 mL of this solution and dilute with 0.9 mL normal saline to yield 15 units/mL; using a 25- or 26-gauge needle, five 0.2 mL injections are made subcutaneously or intradermally into the extravasation site at the leading edge, changing the needle after each injection

Hypodermoclysis:

S.C.: 1 mL (150 units) is added to 1000 mL of infusion fluid and 0.5 mL (75 units) in injected into each clysis site at the initiation of the infusion

I.V.: 15 units is added to each 100 mL of I.V. fluid to be administered

Children <3 years: Limit volume of single clysis to 200 mL

Premature Infants: Do not exceed 25 mL/kg/day and not >2 mL/minute

Adults: Absorption and dispersion of drugs: 150 units are added to the vehicle containing the drug

Contraindications Hypersensitivity to hyaluronidase or any component; do not inject in or around infected, inflamed, or cancerous areas

Pregnancy Risk Factor C

- **Hybalamin®** *see* Hydroxocobalamin *on page 451*
- **Hybolin™ Decanoate Injection** *see* Nandrolone *on page 635*
- **Hybolin™ Improved Injection** *see* Nandrolone *on page 635*
- **HycoClear Tuss®** *see* Hydrocodone and Guaifenesin *on page 445*
- **Hycodan®** *see* Hydrocodone and Homatropine *on page 445*
- **Hycomine®** *see* Hydrocodone and Phenylpropanolamine *on page 446*
- **Hycomine® Compound** *see* Hydrocodone, Chlorpheniramine, Phenylephrine, Acetaminophen, and Caffeine *on page 446*
- **Hycomine® Pediatric** *see* Hydrocodone and Phenylpropanolamine *on page 446*
- **Hycort®** *see* Hydrocortisone *on page 447*
- **Hycotuss® Expectorant Liquid** *see* Hydrocodone and Guaifenesin *on page 445*
- **Hydergine®** *see* Ergoloid Mesylates *on page 322*
- **Hydergine® LC** *see* Ergoloid Mesylates *on page 322*
- **Hyderm** *see* Hydrocortisone *on page 447*

Hydralazine (hye DRAL a zeen)

Pharmacologic Class Vasodilator

U.S. Brand Names Apresoline®

Generic Available Yes

Mechanism of Action Direct vasodilation of arterioles (with little effect on veins) with decreased systemic resistance

Use Management of moderate to severe hypertension, congestive heart failure, hypertension secondary to pre-eclampsia/eclampsia; also used to treat primary pulmonary hypertension

USUAL DOSAGE

Children:

Oral: Initial: 0.75-1 mg/kg/day in 2-4 divided doses; increase over 3-4 weeks to maximum of 7.5 mg/kg/day in 2-4 divided doses; maximum daily dose: 200 mg/day

I.M., I.V.: 0.1-0.2 mg/kg/dose (not to exceed 20 mg) every 4-6 hours as needed, up to 1.7-3.5 mg/kg/day in 4-6 divided doses

Adults:

Oral: Hypertension:

Initial dose: 10 mg 4 times/day for first 2-4 days; increase to 25 mg 4 times/day for the balance of the first week

Increase by 10-25 mg/dose gradually to 50 mg 4 times/day; 300 mg/day may be required for some patients

Oral: Congestive heart failure:

Initial dose: 10-25 mg 3 times/day

Target dose: 75 mg 3 times/day

Maximum dose: 100 mg 3 times/day

I.M., I.V.:

Hypertension: Initial: 10-20 mg/dose every 4-6 hours as needed, may increase to 40 mg/dose; change to oral therapy as soon as possible

Pre-eclampsia/eclampsia: 5 mg/dose then 5-10 mg every 20-30 minutes as needed

Elderly: Oral: Initial: 10 mg 2-3 times/day; increase by 10-25 mg/day every 2-5 days

Dosing interval in renal impairment:

Cl_{cr} 10-50 mL/minute: Administer every 8 hours

Cl_{cr} <10 mL/minute: Administer every 8-16 hours in fast acetylators and every 12-24 hours in slow acetylators

Hemodialysis: Supplemental dose is not necessary

Peritoneal dialysis: Supplemental dose is not necessary

Dosage Forms **INJ:** 20 mg/mL (1 mL). **TAB:** 10 mg, 25 mg, 50 mg, 100 mg

Contraindications Hypersensitivity to hydralazine or any component, dissecting aortic aneurysm, mitral valve rheumatic heart disease

Warnings/Precautions Discontinue hydralazine in patients who develop SLE-like syndrome or positive ANA. Use with caution in patients with severe renal disease or cerebral vascular accidents or with known or suspected coronary artery disease; monitor blood pressure closely with I.V. use; some formulations may contain tartrazines or sulfites. Slow acetylators, patients with decreased renal function, and patients receiving >200 mg/day (chronically) are at higher risk for SLE. Titrate dosage to patient's response. Usually administered with diuretic and a beta-blocker to counteract side effects of sodium and water retention and reflex tachycardia.

Pregnancy Risk Factor C

Pregnancy Implications

Clinical effects on the fetus: Crosses the placenta. One report of fetal arrhythmia; transient neonatal thrombocytopenia and fetal distress reported following late 3rd trimester use. A large amount of clinical experience with the use of these drugs for management of hypertension during pregnancy is available. Available evidence suggests safe use during pregnancy and breast-feeding.

Breast-feeding/lactation: Crosses into breast milk in extremely small amounts. American Academy of Pediatrics considers **compatible** with breast-feeding.

Adverse Reactions Incidence of reactions are not reported.

Cardiovascular: Tachycardia, angina pectoris, orthostatic hypotension (rare), dizziness (rare), paradoxical hypertension, peripheral edema, vascular collapse (rare), flushing

Central nervous system: Increased intracranial pressure (I.V., in patient with pre-existing increased intracranial pressure), fever (rare), chills (rare), anxiety•, disorientation•, depression•, coma•

Dermatologic: Rash (rare), urticaria (rash), pruritus (rash)

Gastrointestinal: Anorexia, nausea, vomiting, diarrhea, constipation, adynamic ileus

Genitourinary: Difficulty in micturition, impotence

Hematologic: Hemolytic anemia (rare), eosinophilia (rare), decreased hemoglobin concentration (rare), reduced erythrocyte count (rare), leukopenia (rare), agranulocytosis (rare), thrombocytopenia (rare)

Neuromuscular & skeletal: Rheumatoid arthritis, muscle cramps, weakness, tremors, peripheral neuritis (rare)

Ocular: Lacrimation, conjunctivitis

Respiratory: Nasal congestion, dyspnea

Miscellaneous: Drug-induced lupus-like syndrome (dose-related; fever, arthralgia, splenomegaly, lymphadenopathy, asthenia, myalgia, malaise, pleuritic chest pain, edema, positive ANA, positive LE cells, maculopapular facial rash, positive direct Coombs' test, pericarditis, pericardial tamponade), sweating

•Seen in uremic patients and severe hypertension where rapidly escalating doses may have caused hypotension leading to these effects

Drug Interactions

Beta-blockers (metoprolol, propranolol) serum concentrations and pharmacologic effects may be increased. Monitor cardiovascular status.

Propranolol increases hydralazine's serum concentrations. Acebutolol, atenolol, and nadolol (low hepatic clearance or no first-pass metabolism) are unlikely to be affected

NSAIDs may decrease the hemodynamic effects of hydralazine; avoid use if possible or closely monitor cardiovascular status

Onset Oral: 20-30 minutes; I.V.: 5-20 minutes

Duration Oral: 2-4 hours; I.V.: 2-6 hours

Half-Life Normal renal function: 2-8 hours; End-stage renal disease: 7-16 hours

Education and Monitoring Issues

Patient Education: Take as directed, with meals. Do not use alcohol or OTC medication without consulting prescriber. Weigh daily at the same time, in the same clothes. Report weight gain >5 lb/week, swelling of feet or ankles. May cause dizziness or weakness; change position slowly when rising from sitting or lying position and avoid driving or activities requiring alertness until response to drug is known. You may experience nausea (small frequent meals may help), impotence (reversible), or constipation (fluids, exercise, dietary fiber may help). This medication does not replace other antihypertensive interventions; follow instructions for diet and lifestyle changes. Report flu-like symptoms, difficulty breathing, skin rash, blackened stool, or numbness and tingling of extremities.

Dietary Considerations: Food enhances bioavailability of hydralazine

Monitoring Parameters: Blood pressure (monitor closely with I.V. use), standing and sitting/supine, heart rate, ANA titer

Related Information

Heart Failure Guidelines *on page 1099*

Hydralazine and Hydrochlorothiazide *on page 442*

(Continued)

Hydralazine *(Continued)*

Hydralazine, Hydrochlorothiazide, and Reserpine *on page 442*

Hydralazine and Hydrochlorothiazide

(hye DRAL a zeen & hye droe klor oh THYE a zide)

Pharmacologic Class Antihypertensive Agent, Combination

U.S. Brand Names Apresazide®

Dosage Forms CAP: 25/25: Hydralazine hydrochloride 25 mg and hydrochlorothiazide 25 mg; 50/50: Hydralazine hydrochloride 50 mg and hydrochlorothiazide 50 mg; 100/50: Hydralazine hydrochloride 100 mg and hydrochlorothiazide 50 mg

Pregnancy Risk Factor C

Hydralazine, Hydrochlorothiazide, and Reserpine

(hye DRAL a zeen, hye droe klor oh THYE a zide, & re SER peen)

Pharmacologic Class Antihypertensive Agent, Combination

U.S. Brand Names Hydrap-ES®; Marpres®; Ser-Ap-Es®

Dosage Forms TAB: Hydralazine 25 mg, hydrochlorothiazide 15 mg, and reserpine 0.1 mg

Pregnancy Risk Factor C

- **Hydramyn® Syrup [OTC]** *see* Diphenhydramine *on page 282*
- **Hydrap-ES®** *see* Hydralazine, Hydrochlorothiazide, and Reserpine *on page 442*
- **Hydrea®** *see* Hydroxyurea *on page 453*
- **Hydrocet®** *see* Hydrocodone and Acetaminophen *on page 444*

Hydrochlorothiazide (hye droe klor oh THYE a zide)

Pharmacologic Class Diuretic, Thiazide

U.S. Brand Names Esidrix®; Ezide®; HydroDIURIL®; Hydro-Par®; Microzide™; Oretic®

Generic Available Yes: Tablet

Mechanism of Action Inhibits sodium reabsorption in the distal tubules causing increased excretion of sodium and water as well as potassium and hydrogen ions

Use Management of mild to moderate hypertension; treatment of edema in congestive heart failure and nephrotic syndrome

USUAL DOSAGE Oral (effect of drug may be decreased when used every day):

Children (In pediatric patients, chlorothiazide may be preferred over hydrochlorothiazide as there are more dosage formulations (eg, suspension) available):

<6 months: 2-3 mg/kg/day in 2 divided doses

>6 months: 2 mg/kg/day in 2 divided doses

Adults: 25-100 mg/day in 1-2 doses

Maximum: 200 mg/day

Elderly: 12.5-25 mg once daily

Minimal increase in response and more electrolyte disturbances are seen with doses >50 mg/day

Dosing adjustment/comments in renal impairment: Cl_{cr} 25-50 mL/minute: Not effective

Dosage Forms CAP: 12.5 mg. **SOLN, oral** (mint flavor): 50 mg/5 mL (50 mL). **TAB:** 25 mg, 50 mg, 100 mg

Contraindications Anuria, renal decompensation, hypersensitivity to hydrochlorothiazide or any component, cross-sensitivity with other thiazides and sulfonamide derivatives

Warnings/Precautions Use with caution in renal disease, hepatic disease, gout, lupus erythematosus, diabetes mellitus; some products may contain tartrazine. Hydrochlorothiazide is not effective in patients with a Cl_{cr} 25-50 mL/minute, therefore, it may not be a useful agent in many elderly patients.

Pregnancy Risk Factor B (per manufacturer); D (based on expert analysis)

Adverse Reactions

1% to 10%:

Cardiovascular: Orthostatic hypotension, hypotension

Endocrine & metabolic: Hypokalemia

Dermatologic: Photosensitivity

Gastrointestinal: Anorexia, epigastric distress

<1% (limited to important or life-threatening symptoms): Allergic myocarditis, alopecia, exfoliative dermatitis, toxic epidermal necrolysis, erythema multiforme, Stevens-Johnson syndrome, aplastic anemia, hemolytic anemia, leukopenia, agranulocytosis, thrombocytopenia, hepatic function impairment, renal failure, interstitial nephritis, respiratory distress, allergic reactions (possibly with life-threatening anaphylactic shock), eosinophilic pneumonitis

Drug Interactions

Angiotensin-converting enzyme inhibitors: Increased hypotension if aggressively diuresed with a thiazide diuretic

Beta-blockers increase hyperglycemic effects in type 2 diabetes mellitus

Cyclosporine and thiazides can increase the risk of gout or renal toxicity; avoid concurrent use

Digoxin toxicity can be exacerbated if a thiazide induces hypokalemia or hypomagnesemia

Lithium toxicity can occur by reducing renal excretion of lithium; monitor lithium concentration and adjust as needed

Neuromuscular blocking agents can prolong blockade; monitor serum potassium and neuromuscular status

NSAIDs can decrease the efficacy of thiazides reducing the diuretic and antihypertensive effects

Onset Diuretic effect within 2 hours; Peak effect: 4-6 hours

Duration 6-12 hours

Half-Life 5.6-14.8

Education and Monitoring Issues

Patient Education: This medication does not replace other antihypertensive recommendations (diet and lifestyle changes). Take as directed, with meals, early in the day to avoid nocturia. Avoid alcohol or OTC medication unless approved by prescriber. Include bananas and/or orange juice (or other food high in potassium) in daily diet; do not take potassium supplements unless recommended by prescriber. May cause dizziness or postural hypotension (use caution when rising from sitting or lying position, when driving, climbing stairs, or engaging in tasks that require alertness until response to drug is known); nausea or vomiting (small frequent meals, frequent mouth care, sucking lozenges, or chewing gum may help); impotence (reversible); constipation (increased exercise or dietary fruit, fiber, or fluids will help); photosensitivity (use sunscreen, wear protective clothing and eyewear, avoid direct sunlight). If diabetic, monitor serum glucose closely; this medication may increase serum glucose levels. Report persistent flu-like symptoms, chest pain, palpitations, muscle cramping, difficulty breathing, skin rash or itching, unusual bruising or easy bleeding, or excessive fatigue.

Monitoring Parameters: Assess weight, I & O reports daily to determine fluid loss; blood pressure, serum electrolytes, BUN, creatinine

Related Information

Amiloride and Hydrochlorothiazide *on page 46*
Benazepril and Hydrochlorothiazide *on page 98*
Bisoprolol and Hydrochlorothiazide *on page 110*
Captopril and Hydrochlorothiazide *on page 136*
Enalapril and Hydrochlorothiazide *on page 311*
Heart Failure Guidelines *on page 1099*
Hydralazine and Hydrochlorothiazide *on page 442*
Hydralazine, Hydrochlorothiazide, and Reserpine *on page 442*
Hydrochlorothiazide and Reserpine *on page 443*
Hydrochlorothiazide and Spironolactone *on page 443*
Hydrochlorothiazide and Triamterene *on page 443*
Irbesartan and Hydrochlorothiazide *on page 485*
Lisinopril and Hydrochlorothiazide *on page 534*
Losartan and Hydrochlorothiazide *on page 544*
Methyldopa and Hydrochlorothiazide *on page 587*
Moexipril and Hydrochlorothiazide *on page 614*
Propranolol and Hydrochlorothiazide *on page 788*
Valsartan and Hydrochlorothiazide *on page 969*

Hydrochlorothiazide and Reserpine

(hye droe klor oh THYE a zide & re SER peen)

Pharmacologic Class Antihypertensive Agent, Combination

U.S. Brand Names Hydropres®; Hydro-Serp®; Hydroserpine®

Dosage Forms TAB: 25: Hydrochlorothiazide 25 mg and reserpine 0.125 mg, 50: Hydrochlorothiazide 50 mg and reserpine 0.125 mg

Pregnancy Risk Factor C

Hydrochlorothiazide and Spironolactone

(hye droe klor oh THYE a zide & speer on oh LAK tone)

Pharmacologic Class Antihypertensive Agent, Combination

U.S. Brand Names Aldactazide®

Dosage Forms TAB: 25/25: Hydrochlorothiazide 25 mg and spironolactone 25 mg, 50/50: Hydrochlorothiazide 50 mg and spironolactone 50 mg

Pregnancy Risk Factor C

Hydrochlorothiazide and Triamterene

(hye droe klor oh THYE a zide & trye AM ter een)

Pharmacologic Class Antihypertensive Agent, Combination; Diuretic, Potassium Sparing; Diuretic, Thiazide

U.S. Brand Names Dyazide®; Maxzide®

Use Management of mild to moderate hypertension; treatment of edema in congestive heart failure and nephrotic syndrome

(Continued)

Hydrochlorothiazide and Triamterene *(Continued)*

Dosage Forms CAP (Dyazide®): Hydrochlorothiazide 25 mg and triamterene 37.5 mg. **TAB:** (Maxzide®-25): Hydrochlorothiazide 25 mg and triamterene 37.5 mg; (Maxzide®): Hydrochlorothiazide 50 mg and triamterene 75 mg

Pregnancy Risk Factor C

- **Hydrocil® [OTC]** *see* Psyllium *on page 793*
- **Hydro-Cobex®** *see* Hydroxocobalamin *on page 451*

Hydrocodone and Acetaminophen

(hye droe KOE done & a seet a MIN oh fen)

Pharmacologic Class Analgesic, Combination (Narcotic)

U.S. Brand Names Anexsia®; Anodynos-DHC®; Bancap HC®; Co-Gesic®; Dolacet®; DuoCet™; Duradyne DHC®; Hydrocet®; Hydrogesic®; Hy-Phen®; Lorcet®-HD; Lorcet® Plus; Lortab®; Margesic® H; Medipain 5®; Norcet®; Stagesic®; T-Gesic®; Vicodin®; Vicodin® ES; Vicodin® HP; Zydone®

Generic Available Yes

Mechanism of Action See individual agents

Use Relief of moderate to severe pain; antitussive (hydrocodone)

USUAL DOSAGE Oral (doses should be titrated to appropriate analgesic effect):

Children:

Antitussive (hydrocodone): 0.6 mg/kg/day in 3-4 divided doses

A single dose should not exceed 10 mg in children >12 years, 5 mg in children 2-12 years, and 1.25 mg in children <2 years of age

Analgesic (acetaminophen): Refer to Acetaminophen monograph

Adults: Analgesic: 1-2 tablets or capsules every 4-6 hours or 5-10 mL solution every 4-6 hours as needed for pain

Dosage Forms CAP: (Bancap HC®, Dolacet®, Hydrocet®, Hydrogesic®, Lorcet®-HD, Margesic® H, Medipain 5®, Norcet®, Stagesic®, T-Gesic®, Zydone®): Hydrocodone bitartrate 5 mg and acetaminophen 500 mg. **ELIX** (tropical fruit punch flavor) (Lortab®): Hydrocodone bitartrate 2.5 mg and acetaminophen 167 mg per 5 mL with alcohol 7% (480 mL). **SOLN, oral** (tropical fruit punch flavor) (Lortab®): Hydrocodone bitartrate 2.5 mg and acetaminophen 167 mg per 5 mL with alcohol 7% (480 mL). **TAB:** (Lortab® 2.5/500): Hydrocodone bitartrate 2.5 mg and acetaminophen 500 mg; (Anexsia® 5/500, Anodynos-DHC®, Co-Gesic®, DuoCet™, DHC®; Hy-Phen®, Lortab®® 5/500, Vicodin®): Hydrocodone bitartrate 5 mg and acetaminophen 500 mg; (Lortab® 7.5/500): Hydrocodone bitartrate 7.5 mg and acetaminophen 500 mg; (Anexsia® 7.5/650, Lorcet® Plus): Hydrocodone bitartrate 7.5 mg and acetaminophen 650 mg; (Vicodin® ES): Hydrocodone bitartrate 7.5 mg and acetaminophen 750 mg; (Norco™): Hydrocodone bitartrate 10 mg and acetaminophen 325 mg; (Lortab® 10/500): Hydrocodone bitartrate 10 mg and acetaminophen 500 mg; (Lorcet® 10/650): Hydrocodone bitartrate 10 mg and acetaminophen 650 mg; (Vicodin® HP): Hydrocodone bitartrate 10 mg and acetaminophen 660 mg

Contraindications CNS depression, hypersensitivity to hydrocodone, acetaminophen or any component; severe respiratory depression

Warnings/Precautions Use with caution in patients with hypersensitivity reactions to other phenanthrene derivative opioid agonists (morphine, hydrocodone, hydromorphone, levorphanol, oxycodone, oxymorphone); tablets contain metabisulfite which may cause allergic reactions; tolerance or drug dependence may result from extended use

Pregnancy Risk Factor C

Adverse Reactions

>10%:

Cardiovascular: Hypotension

Central nervous system: Lightheadedness, dizziness, sedation, drowsiness, fatigue

Neuromuscular & skeletal: Weakness

1% to 10%:

Cardiovascular: Bradycardia

Central nervous system: Confusion

Gastrointestinal: Nausea, vomiting

Genitourinary: Decreased urination

Respiratory: Shortness of breath, dyspnea

<1%: Anorexia, biliary tract spasm, diplopia, hallucinations, histamine release, hypertension, miosis, physical and psychological dependence with prolonged use, urinary tract spasm, xerostomia

Drug Interactions

Decreased effect with phenothiazines

Increased effect with dextroamphetamine

Increased toxicity with CNS depressants, TCAs; effect of warfarin may be enhanced

Alcohol Interactions Avoid use or limit to <3 drinks/day (may increase acetaminophen toxicity and cause central nervous system depression)

Onset Onset of narcotic analgesia: Within 10-20 minutes

Duration 3-6 hours

Half-Life Hydrocodone: 3.8 hours

Education and Monitoring Issues

Patient Education: If self-administered, use exactly as directed (do not increase dose or frequency); may cause physical and/or psychological dependence. Take with food or milk. While using this medication, do not use alcohol and other prescription or OTC medications (especially sedatives, tranquilizers, antihistamines, or pain medications) without consulting prescriber. Maintain adequate hydration (2-3 L/day of fluids unless instructed to restrict fluid intake). May cause dizziness, lightheadedness, confusion, or drowsiness (use caution when driving, climbing stairs, or changing position - rising from sitting or lying to standing, or when engaging in tasks requiring alertness until response to drug is known); nausea or vomiting (frequent mouth care, frequent sips of fluids, chewing gum, or sucking lozenges may help). Report chest pain or palpitations; persistent dizziness, shortness of breath, or difficulty breathing; unusual bleeding or bruising; or unusual fatigue and weakness.

Monitoring Parameters: Pain relief, respiratory and mental status, blood pressure

Related Information

Lipid-Lowering Agents Comparison *on page 1243*

Hydrocodone and Aspirin (hye droe KOE done & AS pir in)

Pharmacologic Class Analgesic, Combination (Narcotic)

U.S. Brand Names Alor® 5/500; Azdone®; Damason-P®; Lortab® ASA; Panasal® 5/500

Use Relief of moderate to moderately severe pain

USUAL DOSAGE Adults: Oral: 1-2 tablets every 4-6 hours as needed for pain

Pregnancy Risk Factor D

Related Information

Lipid-Lowering Agents Comparison *on page 1243*

Hydrocodone and Chlorpheniramine

(hye droe KOE done & klor fen IR a meen)

Pharmacologic Class Antihistamine/Antitussive

U.S. Brand Names Tussionex®

Dosage Forms SYR (alcohol free): Hydrocodone polistirex 10 mg and chlorpheniramine polistirex 8 mg per 5 mL (480 mL, 900 mL)

Pregnancy Risk Factor C

Alcohol Interactions Avoid use (may increase central nervous system depression)

Duration Hydrocodone: 4-6 hours

Half-Life Hydrocodone: 3.8 hours

Hydrocodone and Guaifenesin (hye droe KOE done & gwye FEN e sin)

Pharmacologic Class Antitussive/Expectorant

U.S. Brand Names Codiclear® DH; HycoClear Tuss®; Hycotuss® Expectorant Liquid; Kwelcof®

Dosage Forms LIQ: Hydrocodone bitartrate 5 mg and guaifenesin 100 mg per 5 mL (120 mL, 480 mL)

Pregnancy Risk Factor C

Alcohol Interactions Avoid use (may increase central nervous system depression)

Duration Hydrocodone: 4-6 hours

Half-Life Hydrocodone: 3.8 hours

Hydrocodone and Homatropine (hye droe KOE done & hoe MA troe peen)

Pharmacologic Class Antitussive

U.S. Brand Names Hycodan®; Hydromet®; Hydropane®; Hydrotropine®; Oncet®; Tussigon®

Use Symptomatic relief of cough

USUAL DOSAGE Oral (based on hydrocodone component):

Children: 0.6 mg/kg/day in 3-4 divided doses; do not administer more frequently than every 4 hours

A single dose should not exceed 1.25 mg in children <2 years of age, 5 mg in children 2-12 years, and 10 mg in children >12 years

Adults: 5-10 mg every 4-6 hours, a single dose should not exceed 15 mg; do not administer more frequently than every 4 hours

Contraindications Increased intracranial pressure, narrow-angle glaucoma, depressed ventilation, hypersensitivity to hydrocodone, homatropine, or any component

Pregnancy Risk Factor C

Related Information

Lipid-Lowering Agents Comparison *on page 1243*

Hydrocodone and Ibuprofen (hye droe KOE done & eye byoo PROE fen)

Pharmacologic Class Analgesic, Combination (Narcotic)

U.S. Brand Names Vicoprofen®

Use Short-term (generally <10 days) management of moderate to severe acute pain; is not indicated for treatment of such conditions as osteoarthritis or rheumatoid arthritis

(Continued)

Hydrocodone and Ibuprofen *(Continued)*

USUAL DOSAGE Adults: Oral: 1-2 tablets every 4-6 hours as needed for pain; maximum: 5 tablets/day

Contraindications Hypersensitivity to any of the ingredients, aspirin allergy, and 3rd trimester pregnancy

Pregnancy Risk Factor C

Related Information

Lipid-Lowering Agents Comparison *on page 1243*

Hydrocodone and Phenylpropanolamine

(hye droe KOE done & fen il proe pa NOLE a meen)

Pharmacologic Class Antitussive/Decongestant

U.S. Brand Names Codamine®; Codamine® Pediatric; Hycomine®; Hycomine® Pediatric; Hydrocodone PA® Syrup

Dosage Forms SYR: (Codamine®, Hycomine®): Hydrocodone bitartrate 5 mg and phenylpropanolamine hydrochloride 25 mg per 5 mL (480 mL); (Codamine® Pediatric, Hycomine® Pediatric): Hydrocodone bitartrate 2.5 mg and phenylpropanolamine hydrochloride 12.5 mg per 5 mL (480 mL)

Pregnancy Risk Factor C

Alcohol Interactions Avoid use (may increase central nervous system depression)

Duration Hydrocodone: 4-6 hours

Half-Life Hydrocodone: 3.8 hours

Hydrocodone and Pseudoephedrine

(hye droe KOE done & soo doe e FED rin)

Pharmacologic Class Cough and Cold Combination

U.S. Brand Names Detussin® Liquid; Entuss-D® LIquid; Histussin D® Liquid; Tyrodone® Liquid

Dosage Forms LIQ: Hydrocodone bitartrate 5 mg and pseudoephedrine hydrochloride 30 mg per 5 mL; hydrocodone bitartrate 5 mg and pseudoephedrine hydrochloride 60 mg per 5 mL

Alcohol Interactions Avoid use (may increase central nervous system depression)

Hydrocodone, Chlorpheniramine, Phenylephrine, Acetaminophen, and Caffeine

(hye droe KOE done, klor fen IR a meen, fen il EF rin, a seet a MIN oh fen, & KAF een)

Pharmacologic Class Antitussive

U.S. Brand Names Hycomine® Compound

Dosage Forms TAB: Hydrocodone bitartrate 5 mg, chlorpheniramine maleate 2 mg, phenylephrine hydrochloride 10 mg, acetaminophen 250 mg, and caffeine 30 mg

Pregnancy Risk Factor C

Alcohol Interactions Avoid use (may increase central nervous system depression)

Duration Hydrocodone: 4-6 hours

Half-Life Hydrocodone: 3.8 hours

♦ **Hydrocodone PA® Syrup** *see* Hydrocodone and Phenylpropanolamine *on page 446*

Hydrocodone, Phenylephrine, Pyrilamine, Phenindamine, Chlorpheniramine, and Ammonium Chloride

(hye droe KOE done, fen il EF rin, peer IL a meen, fen IN da meen, klor fen IR a meen, & a MOE nee um KLOR ide)

Pharmacologic Class Antihistamine/Decongestant/Antitussive

U.S. Brand Names P-V-Tussin®

Dosage Forms SYR: Hydrocodone bitartrate 2.5 mg, phenylephrine hydrochloride 5 mg, pyrilamine maleate 6 mg, phenindamine tartrate 5 mg, chlorpheniramine maleate 2 mg, and ammonium chloride 50 mg per 5 mL with alcohol 5% (480 mL, 3780 mL)

Alcohol Interactions Avoid use (may increase central nervous system depression)

Hydrocodone, Pseudoephedrine, and Guaifenesin

(hye droe KOE done, soo doe e FED rin, & gwye FEN e sin)

Pharmacologic Class Antitussive/Decongestant/Expectorant

U.S. Brand Names Cophene XP®; Detussin® Expectorant; Pancof XP®; SRC® Expectorant; Tussafin® Expectorant

Dosage Forms LIQ: Hydrocodone bitartrate 2.5 mg, pseudoephedrine hydrochloride 15 mg, and guaifenesin 100 mg per 5 mL (25 mL, 473 mL); Hydrocodone bitartrate 5 mg, pseudoephedrine hydrochloride 60 mg, and guaifenesin 200 mg per 5 mL with alcohol 12.5% (480 mL)

Pregnancy Risk Factor C

Alcohol Interactions Avoid use (may increase central nervous system depression)

Duration Hydrocodone: 4-6 hours

Half-Life Hydrocodone: 3.8 hours

♦ **Hydrocort®** *see* Hydrocortisone *on page 447*

Hydrocortisone (hye droe KOR ti sone)

Pharmacologic Class Corticosteroid, Oral; Corticosteroid, Parenteral; Corticosteroid, Rectal

U.S. Brand Names Acticort 100®; Aeroseb-HC®; A-hydroCort®; Ala-Cort®; Ala-Scalp®; Anucort-HC® Suppository; Anuprep HC® Suppository; Anusol® HC-1 [OTC]; Anusol® HC-2.5% [OTC]; Anusol-HC® Suppository; CaldeCORT®; CaldeCORT® Anti-Itch Spray; Cetacort®; Clocort® Maximum Strength; CortaGel® [OTC]; Cortaid® Maximum Strength [OTC]; Cortaid® With Aloe [OTC]; Cort-Dome®; Cortef®; Cortef® Feminine Itch; Cortenema®; Cortifoam®; Cortizone®-5 [OTC]; Cortizone®-10 [OTC]; Delcort®; Dermacort®; Dermarest Dricort®; DermiCort®; Dermolate® [OTC]; Dermtex® HC With Aloe; Eldecort®; Gynecort® [OTC]; Hemril-HC® Uniserts®; Hi-Cor-1.0®; Hi-Cor-2.5®; Hycort®; Hydrocort®; Hydrocortone® Acetate; Hydrocortone® Phosphate; HydroSKIN®; Hydro-Tex® [OTC]; Hytone®; LactiCare-HC®; Lanacort® [OTC]; Locoid®; Nutracort®; Orabase® HCA; Pandel®; Penecort®; Procort® [OTC]; Proctocort™; Scalpicin®; Solu-Cortef®; S-T Cort®; Synacort®; Tegrin®-HC [OTC]; U-Cort™; Westcort®

Generic Available Yes

Mechanism of Action Decreases inflammation by suppression of migration of polymorphonuclear leukocytes and reversal of increased capillary permeability

Use Management of adrenocortical insufficiency; relief of inflammation of corticosteroid-responsive dermatoses (low and medium potency topical corticosteroid); adjunctive treatment of ulcerative colitis

USUAL DOSAGE Dose should be based on severity of disease and patient response

Acute adrenal insufficiency: I.M., I.V.:
- Infants and young Children: Succinate: 1-2 mg/kg/dose bolus, then 25-150 mg/day in divided doses every 6-8 hours
- Older Children: Succinate: 1-2 mg/kg bolus then 150-250 mg/day in divided doses every 6-8 hours
- Adults: Succinate: 100 mg I.V. bolus, then 300 mg/day in divided doses every 8 hours or as a continuous infusion for 48 hours; once patient is stable change to oral, 50 mg every 8 hours for 6 doses, then taper to 30-50 mg/day in divided doses

Chronic adrenal corticoid insufficiency: Adults: Oral: 20-30 mg/day

Anti-inflammatory or immunosuppressive:
- Infants and Children:
  - Oral: 2.5-10 mg/kg/day **or** 75-300 mg/m²/day every 6-8 hours
  - I.M., I.V.: Succinate: 1-5 mg/kg/day **or** 30-150 mg/m²/day divided every 12-24 hours
- Adolescents and Adults: Oral, I.M., I.V.: Succinate: 15-240 mg every 12 hours

Congenital adrenal hyperplasia: Oral: Initial: 30-36 mg/m²/day with 1/3 of dose every morning and 2/3 every evening or 1/4 every morning and mid-day and 1/2 every evening; maintenance: 20-25 mg/m²/day in divided doses

Physiologic replacement: Children:
- Oral: 0.5-0.75 mg/kg/day **or** 20-25 mg/m²/day every 8 hours
- I.M.: Succinate: 0.25-0.35 mg/kg/day **or** 12-15 mg/m²/day once daily

Shock: I.M., I.V.: Succinate:
- Children: Initial: 50 mg/kg, then repeated in 4 hours and/or every 24 hours as needed
- Adolescents and Adults: 500 mg to 2 g every 2-6 hours

Status asthmaticus: Children and Adults: I.V.: Succinate: 1-2 mg/kg/dose every 6 hours for 24 hours, then maintenance of 0.5-1 mg/kg every 6 hours

Rheumatic diseases:
- Adults: Intralesional, intra-articular, soft tissue injection: Acetate:
  - Large joints: 25 mg (up to 37.5 mg)
  - Small joints: 10-25 mg
- Tendon sheaths: 5-12.5 mg
- Soft tissue infiltration: 25-50 mg (up to 75 mg)
- Bursae: 25-37.5 mg
- Ganglia: 12.5-25 mg

Dermatosis: Children >2 years and Adults: Topical: Apply to affected area 3-4 times/day (Buteprate: Apply once or twice daily). Therapy should be discontinued when control is achieved; if no improvement is seen, reassessment of diagnosis may be necessary.

Ulcerative colitis: Adults: Rectal: 10-100 mg 1-2 times/day for 2-3 weeks

Dosage Forms

Acetate: **AERO, rectal** (Cortifoam®): 10% (20 g). **CRM:** (CaldeCORT®, Gynecort®, Cortaid® with Aloe, Cortef® Feminine Itch, Lanacort®): 0.5% (15 g, 22.5 g, 30 g); (Anusol-HC-1®, CaldeCORT®, Clocort® Maximum Strength, Cortaid® Maximum Strength, Dermarest Dricort®, U-Cort™): 1% (15 g, 21 g, 30 g, 120 g). **OINT, top:** 0.5% (15 g, 30 g); 1% (15 g, 21 g, 30 g). **INJ, susp** 25 mg/mL (5 mL, 10 mL), 50 mg/mL (5 mL, 10 mL). **SUPP, rectal:** 10 mg, 25 mg.

Base: **AERO, top:** (Aeroseb-HC®, CaldeCORT® Anti-Itch Spray, Cortaid®): 0.5% (45 g, 58 g); (Cortaid® Maximum Strength): 1% (45 mL). **CRM:** (Cort-Dome®, Cortizone®-5, DermiCort®, Dermolate®, Dermtex® HC with Aloe, HydroSKIN®, Hydro-Tex®): 0.5% (15 g, 30 g, 120 g, 454 g); (Ala-Cort®, Cort-Dome®, Delcort®, Dermacort®, DermiCort®,

(Continued)

Hydrocortisone *(Continued)*

Eldecort®, Hi-Cor 1.0®, Hycort®, Hytone®, Nutracort®, Penecort®, Synacort®): 1% (15 g, 20 g, 30 g, 60 g, 120 g, 240 g, 454 g); (Anusol-HC-2.5%®, Eldecort®, Hi-Cor-2.5®, Hydrocort®, Hytone®, Synacort®): 2.5% (15 g, 20 g, 30 g, 60 g, 120 g, 240 g, 454 g); Rectal (Proctocort™): 1% (30 g). **GEL:** (CortaGel®): 0.5% (15 g, 30 g); (CortaGel® Extra Strength): 1% (15 g, 30 g). **LOT:** (Cetacort®, DermiCort®, HydroSKIN®, S-T Cort®): 0.5% (60 mL, 120 mL); (Acticort 100®, Cetacort®, Cortizone-10®, Dermacort®, HydroSKIN® Maximum Strength, Hytone®, LactiCare-HC®, Nutracort®): 1% (60 mL, 120 mL); (Ala-Scalp®): 2% (30 mL); (Hytone®, LactiCare-HC®, Nutracort®): 2.5% (60 mL, 120 mL). **OINT, top:** (Cortizone®-5, HydroSKIN®: 0.5% (30 g), Cortizone®-10, Hycort®, HydroSKIN®, Hydro-Tex®, Hytone®, Tegrin®-HC): 1% (15 g, 20 g, 30 g, 60 g, 120 g, 240 g, 454 g); (Hytone®): 2.5% (20 g, 30 g). **SUSP, rectal** (Cortenema®): 100 mg/60 mL (7s). **TAB:** Cortef®: 5 mg, 10 mg, 20 mg; (Hydrocortone®): 10 mg, 20 mg

Butyrate (Locoid®): **CRM:** 0.1% (15 g, 45 g). **OINT, top:** 0.1% (15 g, 45 g). **SOLN, top:** 0.1% (20 mL, 60 mL)

Cypionate: **SUSP, oral** (Cortef®): 10 mg/5 mL (120 mL)

Sodium phosphate: **INJ** (Hydrocortone® Phosphate): 50 mg/mL (2 mL, 10 mL)

Sodium succinate: **INJ** (A-hydroCort®, Solu-Cortef®): 100 mg, 250 mg, 500 mg, 1000 mg

Valerate (Westcort®): **CRM:** 0.2% (15 g, 45 g, 60 g). **OINT, top:** 0.2% (15 g, 45 g, 60 g, 120 g)

Contraindications Serious infections, except septic shock or tuberculous meningitis; known hypersensitivity to hydrocortisone; viral, fungal, or tubercular skin lesions

Warnings/Precautions

Use with caution in patients with hyperthyroidism, cirrhosis, nonspecific ulcerative colitis, hypertension, osteoporosis, thromboembolic tendencies, CHF, convulsive disorders, myasthenia gravis, thrombophlebitis, peptic ulcer, diabetes

Acute adrenal insufficiency may occur with abrupt withdrawal after long-term therapy or with stress; young pediatric patients may be more susceptible to adrenal axis suppression from topical therapy

Because of the risk of adverse effects, systemic corticosteroids should be used cautiously in the elderly, in the smallest possible dose, and for the shortest possible time

Pregnancy Risk Factor C

Adverse Reactions

>10%:

- Central nervous system: Insomnia, nervousness
- Gastrointestinal: Increased appetite, indigestion

1% to 10%:

- Dermatologic: Hirsutism
- Endocrine & metabolic: Diabetes mellitus
- Neuromuscular & skeletal: Arthralgia
- Ocular: Cataracts
- Respiratory: Epistaxis

<1%: Abdominal distention, acne, amenorrhea, bone growth suppression, bruising, Cushing's syndrome, delirium, dermatitis, edema, euphoria, hallucinations, headache, hyperglycemia, hyperpigmentation, hypersensitivity reactions, hypertension, hypokalemia, immunosuppression, mood swings, muscle wasting, pancreatitis, peptic ulcer, seizures, skin atrophy, sodium and water retention, ulcerative esophagitis

Drug Interactions CYP2D6 and 3A3/4 enzyme substrate

Decreased effect:

- Insulin decreases hypoglycemic effect
- Phenytoin, phenobarbital, ephedrine, and rifampin increase metabolism of hydrocortisone and decrease steroid blood level

Increased toxicity:

- Oral anticoagulants change prothrombin time; potassium-depleting diuretics increase risk of hypokalemia
- Cardiac glucosides increase risk of arrhythmias or digitalis toxicity secondary to hypokalemia

Alcohol Interactions Avoid use (may enhance gastric mucosal irritation)

Onset

Hydrocortisone acetate: Slow onset but long duration of action when compared with more soluble preparations.

Hydrocortisone sodium phosphate: A water soluble salt with a rapid onset but short duration of action.

Hydrocortisone sodium succinate: A water soluble salt which is rapidly active.

Half-Life Biologic: 8-12 hours

Education and Monitoring Issues

Patient Education:

Systemic: Take as directed; do not increase doses and do not stop abruptly without consulting prescribed. Dosage of systemic hydrocortisone is usually tapered off gradually. Take oral dose with food to reduce GI upset. Hydrocortisone may cause immunosuppression and mask symptoms of infection; avoid exposure to contagion and notify prescriber of any signs of infection (eg, fever, chills, sore throat, injury) and notify dentist or surgeon (if necessary) that you are taking this medication. You may experience increased appetite, indigestion, or increased nervousness. Report any sudden weight gain (>5 lb/week), swelling of extremities or difficulty breathing, abdominal pain, severe vomiting, black or tarry stools, fatigue, anorexia, weakness, or unusual mood swings.

Topical: Before applying, wash area gently and thoroughly. Apply gel, cream, or ointment in thin film to cleansed area and rub in gently until medication vanishes. Avoid exposing affected area to sunlight; you will be more sensitive and severe sunburn may occur. Consult prescriber if breast-feeding.

Rectal: Insert suppository gently as high as possible with gloved finger while lying down. Avoid injury with long or sharp fingernails. Remain in resting position for 10 minutes after insertion.

Monitoring Parameters: Blood pressure, weight, serum glucose, and electrolytes

Reference Range: Therapeutic: AM: 5-25 µg/dL (SI: 138-690 nmol/L), PM: 2-9 µg/dL (SI: 55-248 nmol/L) depending on test, assay

Related Information

Acetic Acid, Propylene Glycol Diacetate, and Hydrocortisone *on page 20*
Bacitracin, Neomycin, Polymyxin B, and Hydrocortisone *on page 90*
Benzoyl Peroxide and Hydrocortisone *on page 100*
Chloramphenicol, Polymyxin B, and Hydrocortisone *on page 180*
Ciprofloxacin and Hydrocortisone *on page 201*
Clioquinol and Hydrocortisone *on page 209*
Colistin, Neomycin, and Hydrocortisone *on page 227*
Corticosteroids Comparison *on page 1237*
Dibucaine and Hydrocortisone *on page 263*
Iodoquinol and Hydrocortisone *on page 481*
Lidocaine and Hydrocortisone *on page 529*
Neomycin and Hydrocortisone *on page 643*
Neomycin, Polymyxin B, and Hydrocortisone *on page 644*
Oxytetracycline and Hydrocortisone *on page 695*
Polymyxin B and Hydrocortisone *on page 748*
Pramoxine and Hydrocortisone *on page 758*
Urea and Hydrocortisone *on page 963*

- **Hydrocortone® Acetate** *see* Hydrocortisone *on page 447*
- **Hydrocortone® Phosphate** *see* Hydrocortisone *on page 447*
- **Hydro-Crysti-12®** *see* Hydroxocobalamin *on page 451*
- **HydroDIURIL®** *see* Hydrochlorothiazide *on page 442*
- **Hydrogesic®** *see* Hydrocodone and Acetaminophen *on page 444*
- **Hydromet®** *see* Hydrocodone and Homatropine *on page 445*
- **Hydromorph Contin®** *see* Hydromorphone *on page 449*

Hydromorphone (hye droe MOR fone)

Pharmacologic Class Analgesic, Narcotic

U.S. Brand Names Dilaudid®; Dilaudid-5®; Dilaudid-HP®; HydroStat IR®

Generic Available Yes

Mechanism of Action Binds to opiate receptors in the CNS, causing inhibition of ascending pain pathways, altering the perception of and response to pain; causes cough supression by direct central action in the medulla; produces generalized CNS depression

Use Management of moderate to severe pain; antitussive at lower doses

USUAL DOSAGE

Doses should be titrated to appropriate analgesic effects; when changing routes of administration, note that oral doses are less than half as effective as parenteral doses (may be only one-fifth as effective)

Pain: Older Children and Adults:

Oral, I.M., I.V., S.C.: 1-4 mg/dose every 4-6 hours as needed; usual adult dose: 2 mg/dose

Rectal: 3 mg every 6-8 hours

Antitussive: Oral:

Children 6-12 years: 0.5 mg every 3-4 hours as needed

Children >12 years and Adults: 1 mg every 3-4 hours as needed

Dosing adjustment in hepatic impairment: Should be considered

Dosage Forms INJ: (Dilaudid®): 1 mg/mL (1 mL), 2 mg/mL (1 mL, 20 mL), 3 mg/mL (1 mL), 4 mg/mL (1 mL); (Dilaudid-HP®): 10 mg/mL (1 mL, 2 mL, 5 mL). **LIQ:** 5 mg/5 mL (480 mL). **POWDER for inj:** (Dilaudid-HP®): 250 mg. **SUPP, rectal:** 3 mg (6s). **TAB:** 1 mg, 2 mg, 3 mg, 4 mg, 8 mg

Contraindications Hypersensitivity to hydromorphone or any component or other phenanthrene derivative

Warnings/Precautions Tablet and cough syrup contain tartrazine which may cause allergic reactions; hydromorphone shares toxic potential of opiate agonists, and precaution of opiate agonist therapy should be observed; extreme caution should be taken to avoid confusing the highly concentrated injection with the less concentrated injectable

(Continued)

Hydromorphone *(Continued)*

product, injection contains benzyl alcohol; use with caution in patients with hypersensitivity to other phenanthrene opiates, in patients with respiratory disease, or severe liver or renal failure; tolerance or drug dependence may result from extended use

Pregnancy Risk Factor B; D (if used for prolonged periods or in high doses at term)

Adverse Reactions

Percentage unknown: Antidiuretic hormone release, biliary tract spasm, urinary tract spasm, miosis, histamine release, physical and psychological dependence, increased AST, ALT

>10%:

Cardiovascular: Palpitations, hypotension, peripheral vasodilation
Central nervous system: Dizziness, lightheadedness, drowsiness
Gastrointestinal: Anorexia

1% to 10%:

Cardiovascular: Tachycardia, bradycardia, flushing of face
Central nervous system: CNS depression, increased intracranial pressure, fatigue, headache, nervousness, restlessness
Gastrointestinal: Nausea, vomiting, constipation, stomach cramps, xerostomia
Genitourinary: Decreased urination, ureteral spasm
Hepatic: Increased LFTs
Neuromuscular & skeletal: Trembling, weakness
Respiratory: Respiratory depression, dyspnea, shortness of breath

<1%: Hallucinations, mental depression, paralytic ileus, pruritus, rash, urticaria

Drug Interactions Increased toxicity: CNS depressants, phenothiazines, tricyclic antidepressants may potentiate the adverse effects of hydromorphone

Alcohol Interactions Avoid use (may increase central nervous system depression)

Onset Analgesic effect: Within 15-30 minutes; Peak effect: Within 0.5-1.5 hours

Duration 4-5 hours

Half-Life 1-3 hours

Education and Monitoring Issues

Patient Education: If self-administered, use exactly as directed (do not increase dose or frequency); may cause physical and/or psychological dependence. While using this medication, do not use alcohol and other prescription or OTC medications (especially sedatives, tranquilizers, antihistamines, or pain medications) without consulting prescriber. Maintain adequate hydration (2-3 L/day of fluids unless instructed to restrict fluid intake). May cause dizziness, drowsiness, impaired coordination, or blurred vision (use caution when driving, climbing stairs, or changing position - rising from sitting or lying to standing, or when engaging in tasks requiring alertness until response to drug is known); loss of appetite, nausea, or vomiting (frequent mouth care, small frequent meals, chewing gum, or sucking lozenges may help); constipation (increased exercise, fluids, or dietary fruit and fiber may help - if constipation remains an unresolved problem, consult prescriber about use of stool softeners). Report chest pain, slow or rapid heartbeat, acute dizziness, or persistent headache; swelling of extremities or unusual weight gain; changes in urinary elimination; acute headache; back or flank pain or spasms; or other adverse reactions.

Dietary Considerations: Food: Glucose may cause hyperglycemia; monitor blood glucose concentrations

Monitoring Parameters: Pain relief, respiratory and mental status, blood pressure

Related Information

Lipid-Lowering Agents Comparison *on page 1243*
Narcotic Agonists Comparison *on page 1244*

♦ **Hydropane®** *see* Hydrocodone and Homatropine *on page 445*
♦ **Hydro-Par®** *see* Hydrochlorothiazide *on page 442*
♦ **Hydrophed®** *see* Theophylline, Ephedrine, and Hydroxyzine *on page 906*
♦ **Hydropres®** *see* Hydrochlorothiazide and Reserpine *on page 443*

Hydroquinone (HYE droe kwin one)

Pharmacologic Class Depigmenting Agent

U.S. Brand Names Ambi® Skin Tone [OTC]; Eldopaque® [OTC]; Eldopaque Forte®; Eldoquin® [OTC]; Eldoquin® Forte®; Esoterica® Facial [OTC]; Esoterica® Regular [OTC]; Esoterica® Sensitive Skin Formula [OTC]; Esoterica® Sunscreen [OTC]; Melanex®; Melpaque HP®; Melquin HP®; Nuquin HP®; Porcelana® [OTC]; Porcelana® Sunscreen [OTC]; Solaquin® [OTC]; Solaquin Forte®

Use Gradual bleaching of hyperpigmented skin conditions

USUAL DOSAGE Children >12 years and Adults: Topical: Apply thin layer and rub in twice daily

Contraindications Sunburn, depilatory usage, known hypersensitivity to hydroquinone

Pregnancy Risk Factor C

♦ **Hydro-Serp®** *see* Hydrochlorothiazide and Reserpine *on page 443*
♦ **Hydroserpine®** *see* Hydrochlorothiazide and Reserpine *on page 443*
♦ **HydroSKIN®** *see* Hydrocortisone *on page 447*

♦ **Hydrosone** *see* Hydrocortisone *on page 447*
♦ **HydroStat IR®** *see* Hydromorphone *on page 449*
♦ **Hydro-Tex® [OTC]** *see* Hydrocortisone *on page 447*
♦ **Hydrotropine®** *see* Hydrocodone and Homatropine *on page 445*

Hydroxocobalamin (hye droks oh koe BAL a min)

Pharmacologic Class Vitamin, Water Soluble

U.S. Brand Names Alphamin®; Codroxomin®; Hybalamin®; Hydro-Cobex®; Hydro-Crysti-12®; LA-12®

Generic Available No

Mechanism of Action Coenzyme for various metabolic functions, including fat and carbohydrate metabolism and protein synthesis, used in cell replication and hematopoiesis

Use Treatment of pernicious anemia, vitamin B_{12} deficiency, increased B_{12} requirements due to pregnancy, thyrotoxicosis, hemorrhage, malignancy, liver or kidney disease

USUAL DOSAGE Vitamin B_{12} deficiency: I.M.:

Children: 1-5 mg given in single doses of 100 mcg over 2 or more weeks, followed by 30-50 mcg/month

Adults: 30 mcg/day for 5-10 days, followed by 100-200 mcg/month

Dosage Forms INJ: 1000 mcg/mL (10 mL, 30 mL)

Contraindications Hypersensitivity to cyanocobalamin or any component, cobalt; patients with hereditary optic nerve atrophy

Warnings/Precautions Some products contain benzoyl alcohol; avoid use in premature infants; an intradermal test dose should be performed for hypersensitivity; use only if oral supplementation not possible or when treating pernicious anemia

Pregnancy Risk Factor C

Adverse Reactions

1% to 10%:

Dermatologic: Itching

Gastrointestinal: Diarrhea

<1%: Anaphylaxis, peripheral vascular thrombosis, urticaria

Education and Monitoring Issues

Patient Education: Use exactly as directed. Pernicious anemia may require monthly injections for life. Report skin rash; swelling, pain, or redness in extremities; or acute persistent diarrhea.

Hydroxyamphetamine and Tropicamide

(hye droks ee am FET a meen & troe PIK a mide)

Pharmacologic Class Adrenergic Agonist Agent

U.S. Brand Names Paremyd® Ophthalmic

Dosage Forms SOLN, ophth: Hydroxyamphetamine hydrobromide 1% and tropicamide 0.25% (5 mL, 15 mL)

Hydroxychloroquine (hye droks ee KLOR oh kwin)

Pharmacologic Class Aminoquinoline (Antimalarial)

U.S. Brand Names Plaquenil®

Generic Available No

Mechanism of Action Interferes with digestive vacuole function within sensitive malarial parasites by increasing the pH and interfering with lysosomal degradation of hemoglobin; inhibits locomotion of neutrophils and chemotaxis of eosinophils; impairs complement-dependent antigen-antibody reactions

Use Suppresses and treats acute attacks of malaria; treatment of systemic lupus erythematosus and rheumatoid arthritis

USUAL DOSAGE Note: Hydroxychloroquine sulfate 200 mg is equivalent to 155 mg hydroxychloroquine base and 250 mg chloroquine phosphate. Oral:

Children:

Chemoprophylaxis of malaria: 5 mg/kg (base) once weekly; should not exceed the recommended adult dose; begin 2 weeks before exposure; continue for 4-6 weeks after leaving endemic area; if suppressive therapy is not begun prior to the exposure, double the initial dose and give in 2 doses, 6 hours apart

Acute attack: 10 mg/kg (base) initial dose; followed by 5 mg/kg at 6, 24, and 48 hours

JRA or SLE: 3-5 mg/kg/day divided 1-2 times/day; avoid exceeding 7 mg/kg/day

Adults:

Chemoprophylaxis of malaria: 310 mg base weekly on same day each week; begin 2 weeks before exposure; continue for 4-6 weeks after leaving endemic area; if suppressive therapy is not begun prior to the exposure, double the initial dose and give in 2 doses, 6 hours apart

Acute attack: 620 mg first dose day 1; 310 mg in 6 hours day 1; 310 mg in 1 dose day 2; and 310 mg in 1 dose on day 3

Rheumatoid arthritis: 310-465 mg/day to start taken with food or milk; increase dose until optimum response level is reached; usually after 4-12 weeks dose should be reduced by 1/2 and a maintenance dose of 155-310 mg/day given

(Continued)

Hydroxychloroquine *(Continued)*

Lupus erythematosus: 310 mg every day or twice daily for several weeks depending on response; 155-310 mg/day for prolonged maintenance therapy

Dosage Forms TAB: 200 mg [base 155 mg]

Contraindications Retinal or visual field changes attributable to 4-aminoquinolines; hypersensitivity to hydroxychloroquine, 4-aminoquinoline derivatives, or any component

Warnings/Precautions Use with caution in patients with hepatic disease, G-6-PD deficiency, psoriasis, and porphyria; long-term use in children is not recommended; perform baseline and periodic (6 months) ophthalmologic examinations; test periodically for muscle weakness

Pregnancy Risk Factor C

Adverse Reactions

>10%:
- Central nervous system: Headache
- Dermatologic: Itching
- Gastrointestinal: Diarrhea, loss of appetite, nausea, stomach cramps, vomiting
- Ocular: Ciliary muscle dysfunction

1% to 10%:
- Central nervous system: Dizziness, lightheadedness, nervousness, restlessness
- Dermatologic: Bleaching of hair, rash, discoloration of skin (black-blue)
- Ocular: Ocular toxicity, keratopathy, retinopathy

<1%: Agranulocytosis, aplastic anemia, emotional changes, neuromyopathy, neutropenia, ototoxicity, seizures, thrombocytopenia

Drug Interactions

Chloroquine and other 4-aminoquinolones may be decreased due to GI binding with kaolin or magnesium trisilicate

Increased effect: Cimetidine increases levels of chloroquine and probably other 4-aminoquinolones

Onset In rheumatic disease, may require 4-6 weeks to respond (maximum after several months)

Half-Life 32-50 days

Education and Monitoring Issues

Patient Education: It is important to complete full course of therapy which may take up to 6 months for full effect. May be taken with meals to decrease GI upset and bitter aftertaste. Avoid alcohol. You should have regular ophthalmic exams (every 4-6 months) if using this medication over extended periods. You may experience skin discoloration (blue/black), hair bleaching, or skin rash. If you have psoriasis, you may experience exacerbation. You may experience dizziness, headache, nervousness, or lightheadedness (use caution when driving or engaging in tasks requiring alertness until response to drug is known); nausea, vomiting, or loss of appetite (small frequent meals, frequent mouth care, sucking lozenges, or chewing gum may help); or increased sensitivity to sunlight (wear dark glasses and protective clothing, use sunblock, and avoid direct exposure to sunlight). Report vision changes, rash or itching, persistent diarrhea or GI disturbances, change in hearing acuity or ringing in the ears, chest pain or palpitation, CNS changes, unusual fatigue, easy bruising or bleeding, or any other persistent adverse reactions.

Monitoring Parameters: Ophthalmologic exam, CBC

Hydroxyprogesterone Caproate

(hye droks ee proe JES te rone KAP roe ate)

Pharmacologic Class Progestin

U.S. Brand Names Hylutin® Injection; Hyprogest® 250 Injection

Generic Available Yes

Mechanism of Action Natural steroid hormone that induces secretory changes in the endometrium, promotes mammary gland development, relaxes uterine smooth muscle, blocks follicular maturation and ovulation and maintains pregnancy

Use Treatment of amenorrhea, abnormal uterine bleeding, endometriosis, uterine carcinoma

USUAL DOSAGE Adults: Female: I.M.: *Long-acting progestin*

Amenorrhea: 375 mg; if no bleeding, begin cyclic treatment with estradiol valerate

Production of secretory endometrium and desquamation: (Medical D and C): 125-250 mg administered on day 10 of cycle; repeat every 7 days until suppression is no longer desired.

Uterine carcinoma: 1 g one or more times/day (1-7 g/week) for up to 12 weeks

Dosage Forms INJ: 125 mg/mL (10 mL); (Hylutin®, Hyprogest®): 250 mg/mL (5 mL)

Contraindications Thrombophlebitis, thromboembolic disorders, cerebral hemorrhage, liver impairment, carcinoma of the breast, hypersensitivity to hydroxyprogesterone or any component, undiagnosed vaginal bleeding

Warnings/Precautions Use with caution in patients with asthma, seizure disorders, migraine, cardiac or renal impairment, history of mental depression; use of any progestin during the first 4 months of pregnancy is not recommended; observe patients closely for signs and symptoms of thrombotic disorders

Pregnancy Risk Factor D

Adverse Reactions

>10%:

Cardiovascular: Edema

Endocrine & metabolic: Breakthrough bleeding, spotting, changes in menstrual flow, amenorrhea

Gastrointestinal: Anorexia

Local: Pain at injection site

Neuromuscular & skeletal: Weakness

1% to 10%:

Central nervous system: Mental depression, insomnia, fever

Dermatologic: Melasma or chloasma, allergic rash with or without pruritus

Gastrointestinal: Weight gain or loss

Genitourinary: Changes in cervical erosion and secretions, increased breast tenderness

Hepatic: Cholestatic jaundice

Drug Interactions Decreased effect: Rifampin may increase clearance of hydroxyprogesterone

Education and Monitoring Issues

Patient Education: Maintain a regular schedule of injections as prescribed. This drug can only be given deep I.M. injection. If diabetic, monitor serum glucose closely. You may experience some sensitivity to sunlight; wear protective clothing, use sunblock, or avoid sunlight. You may experience dizziness; use caution when driving or engaging in tasks that require alertness until response to drug is known. Report rash, alopecia, radically increased weight gain or swelling, anorexia, muscular weakness, fever, or unresolved nausea or vomiting. Report immediately any swelling or warmth in calves, chest pain or respiratory difficulty, severe headache or acute dizziness, numbness and/or tingling in extremities.

Hydroxyurea (hye droks ee yoor EE a)

Pharmacologic Class Antineoplastic Agent, Antimetabolite

U.S. Brand Names Droxia™; Hydrea®

Generic Available No

Mechanism of Action Hydroxyurea appears to inhibit DNA synthesis, without inhibiting RNA or protein synthesis, by inhibition of ribonucleotide reductase. It may also inhibit incorporation of thymidine into DNA and directly damage DNA. Hydroxyurea is specific for the S phase of the cell cycle, but may also arrest cells in the G_1 phase. Blocking the G_1-S interface, when sensitivity to radiation is at its maximum, may account for the drug's activity as a radiation sensitizer.

Use CML in chronic phase; radiosensitizing agent in the treatment of primary brain tumors, head and neck tumors, uterine cervix and nonsmall cell lung cancer, psoriasis, sickle cell anemia and other hemoglobinopathies; treatment of hematologic conditions such as essential thrombocythemia, polycythemia vera, hypereosinophilia, and hyperleukocytosis due to acute leukemia. Has shown activity against renal cell cancer, melanoma, ovarian cancer, head and neck cancer, and prostate cancer. Management of sickle cell anemia - to reduce the frequency of painful crises and to reduce the need for blood transfusions in adult patients with sickle cell anemia with recurrent moderate to severe painful crises (generally at least 3 during the preceding 12 months). Has been used in combination with didanosine and other antiretrovirals in the treatment of HIV.

USUAL DOSAGE Oral (refer to individual protocols): All dosage should be based on ideal or actual body weight, whichever is less:

Children:

No FDA-approved dosage regimens have been established; dosages of 1500-3000 mg/m^2 as a single dose in combination with other agents every 4-6 weeks have been used in the treatment of pediatric astrocytoma, medulloblastoma, and primitive neuroectodermal tumors

CML: Initial: 10-20 mg/kg/day once daily; adjust dose according to hematologic response

Adults: Dose should always be titrated to patient response and WBC counts; usual oral doses range from 10-30 mg/kg/day or 500-3000 mg/day; if WBC count falls to <2500 cells/mm^3, or the platelet count to <100,000/mm^3, therapy should be stopped for at least 3 days and resumed when values rise toward normal

Solid tumors:

Intermittent therapy: 80 mg/kg as a single dose every third day

Continuous therapy: 20-30 mg/kg/day given as a single dose/day

Concomitant therapy with irradiation: 80 mg/kg as a single dose every third day starting at least 7 days before initiation of irradiation

Resistant chronic myelocytic leukemia: 20-30 mg/kg/day divided daily

HIV: 1000-1500 mg daily in a single dose or divided doses

Sickle cell anemia (moderate/severe disease): Initial: 15 mg/kg/day, increased by 5 mg/kg every 12 weeks if blood counts are in an acceptable range until the maximum tolerated dose of 35 mg/kg/day is achieved or the dose that does not produce toxic effects

(Continued)

Hydroxyurea *(Continued)*

Acceptable range:
Neutrophils ≥2500 cells/mm³
Platelets ≥95,000/mm³
Hemoglobin >5.3 g/dL, and
Reticulocytes ≥95,000/mm³ if the hemoglobin concentration is <9 g/dL
Toxic range:
Neutrophils <2000 cells/mm³
Platelets <80,000/mm³
Hemoglobin <4.5 g/dL
Reticulocytes <80,000/mm³ if the hemoglobin concentration is <9 g/dL
Monitor for toxicity every 2 weeks; if toxicity occurs, stop treatment until the bone marrow recovers; restart at 2.5 mg/kg/day less than the dose at which toxicity occurs; if no toxicity occurs over the next 12 weeks, then the subsequent dose should be increased by 2.5 mg/kg/day; reduced dosage of hydroxyurea alternating with erythropoietin may decrease myelotoxicity and increase levels of fetal hemoglobin in patients who have not been helped by hydroxyurea alone

Dosing adjustment in renal impairment:
Cl_{cr} 10-50 mL/minute: Administer 50% of normal dose
Cl_{cr} <10 mL/minute: Administer 20% of normal dose

Hemodialysis: Supplemental dose is not necessary. Hydroxyurea is a low molecular weight compound with high aqueous solubility that may be freely dialyzable, however, clinical studies confirming this hypothesis have not been performed; peak serum concentrations are reached within 2 hours after oral administration and by 24 hours, the concentration in the serum is zero
CAPD effects: Unknown
CAVH effects: Unknown

Dosage Forms CAP: 500 mg; (Droxia™): 200 mg, 300 mg, 400 mg

Contraindications Severe anemia, severe bone marrow suppression; WBC <2500/mm³ or platelet count <100,000/mm³; hypersensitivity to hydroxyurea

Warnings/Precautions The U.S. Food and Drug Administration (FDA) currently recommends that procedures for proper handling and disposal of antineoplastic agents be considered. Use with caution in patients with renal impairment, in patients who have received prior irradiation therapy, and in the elderly.

Pregnancy Risk Factor D

Adverse Reactions

>10%:
Central nervous system: Drowsiness
Gastrointestinal: Mild to moderate nausea and vomiting may occur, as well as diarrhea, constipation, mucositis, ulceration of the GI tract, anorexia, and stomatitis
Hematologic: Myelosuppression: Dose-limiting toxicity, causes a rapid drop in leukocyte count (seen in 4-5 days in nonhematologic malignancy and more rapidly in leukemia); thrombocytopenia and anemia occur less often; reversal of WBC count occurs rapidly, but the platelet count may take 7-10 days to recover
WBC: Moderate
Platelets: Moderate
Onset (days): 7
Nadir (days): 10
Recovery (days): 21

1% to 10%:
Dermatologic: Dermatologic changes (hyperpigmentation, erythema of the hands and face, maculopapular rash, or dry skin), alopecia
Hepatic: Abnormal LFTs and hepatitis
Renal: Increased creatinine and BUN due to impairment of renal tubular function
Miscellaneous: Carcinogenic potential

<1%: Disorientation, dizziness, dyspnea, dysuria, elevated hepatic enzymes, facial erythema, fever, hallucination, headache, hyperuricemia, neurotoxicity, rarely acute diffuse pulmonary infiltrates, seizures, skin cancer

Drug Interactions
Increased effect: Zidovudine, zalcitabine, didanosine: Synergy
Increased toxicity:
Fluorouracil: The potential for neurotoxicity may increase with concomitant administration
Cytarabine: Modulation of its metabolism and cytotoxicity → reduction of cytarabine dose is recommended

Half-Life 3-4 hours

Education and Monitoring Issues

Patient Education: Take capsules exactly on schedule directed by prescriber (dosage and timing will be specific to purpose of therapy). Contents of capsule may be emptied into a glass of water and taken immediately. You will require frequent monitoring and blood tests while taking this medication to assess effectiveness and monitor adverse reactions. During therapy, do not use alcohol, aspirin-containing products, or OTC medications without consulting prescriber. It is important to maintain adequate nutrition and hydration (2-3 L/day of fluids unless instructed to restrict fluid intake) during therapy; frequent small meals may help. Drowsiness may occur; avoid activities requiring alertness until the effects of the medication are known. You may experience mild nausea or vomiting (frequent small meals, frequent mouth care, sucking lozenges, or chewing gum may help); loss of hair (reversible); mouth sores (frequent mouth care and use of a soft toothbrush or cotton swabs may help). You will be more susceptible to infection (avoid crowds and exposure to infection, and avoid immunizations unless approved by prescriber). Yogurt or buttermilk may help reduce diarrhea. Report extreme fatigue; severe GI upset or diarrhea; bleeding or bruising, fever, chills, sore throat, vaginal discharge; signs of fluid retention (swelling extremities, difficulty breathing, unusual weight gain); yellowing of skin or eyes or change in color of urine or stool. If powder from capsule is spilled, wipe up with damp, disposable towel immediately, and discard the towel in a closed container, such as a plastic bag. Wash hands thoroughly.

Monitoring Parameters: CBC with differential, platelets, hemoglobin, renal function and liver function tests, serum uric acid

Hydroxyzine (hye DROKS i zeen)

Pharmacologic Class Antiemetic; Antihistamine

U.S. Brand Names Anxanil®; Atarax®; Atozine®; Durrax®; Hy-Pam®; Hyzine-50®; Neucalm®; Quiess®; QYS®; Rezine®; Vamate®; Vistacon-50®; Vistaject-25®; Vistaject-50®; Vistaquel®; Vistaril®; Vistazine®

Generic Available Yes

Mechanism of Action Competes with histamine for H_1-receptor sites on effector cells in the gastrointestinal tract, blood vessels, and respiratory tract

Use Treatment of anxiety, as a preoperative sedative, an antipruritic, an antiemetic, and in alcohol withdrawal symptoms

USUAL DOSAGE

Children:
- Oral: 0.6 mg/kg/dose every 6 hours
- I.M.: 0.5-1 mg/kg/dose every 4-6 hours as needed

Adults:
- Antiemetic: I.M.: 25-100 mg/dose every 4-6 hours as needed
- Anxiety: Oral: 25-100 mg 4 times/day; maximum dose: 600 mg/day
- Preoperative sedation:
  - Oral: 50-100 mg
  - I.M.: 25-100 mg
- Management of pruritus: Oral: 25 mg 3-4 times/day

Dosing interval in hepatic impairment: Change dosing interval to every 24 hours in patients with primary biliary cirrhosis

Dosage Forms

Hydroxyzine hydrochloride: **INJ:** 25 mg/mL (1 mL, 2 mL, 10 mL); 50 mg/mL (1 mL, 2 mL, 10 mL). **SYR**: 10 mg/5 mL (120 mL, 480 mL, 4000 mL). **TAB:** 10 mg, 25 mg, 50 mg, 100 mg

Hydroxyzine pamoate: **CAP:** 25 mg, 50 mg, 100 mg. **SUSP, oral**: 25 mg/5 mL (120 mL, 480 mL)

Contraindications Hypersensitivity to hydroxyzine or any component

Warnings/Precautions S.C., intra-arterial and I.V. administration **not** recommended since thrombosis and digital gangrene can occur; extravasation can result in sterile abscess and marked tissue induration; should be used with caution in patients with narrow-angle glaucoma, prostatic hypertrophy, and bladder neck obstruction; should also be used with caution in patients with asthma or COPD

Anticholinergic effects are not well tolerated in the elderly. Hydroxyzine may be useful as a short-term antipruritic, but it is not recommended for use as a sedative or anxiolytic in the elderly.

Pregnancy Risk Factor C

Adverse Reactions

>10%:
- Central nervous system: Slight to moderate drowsiness
- Respiratory: Thickening of bronchial secretions

1% to 10%:
- Central nervous system: Headache, fatigue, nervousness, dizziness
- Gastrointestinal: Appetite increase, weight gain, nausea, diarrhea, abdominal pain, xerostomia
- Neuromuscular & skeletal: Arthralgia
- Respiratory: Pharyngitis

<1%: Angioedema, blurred vision, bronchospasm, depression, edema, epistaxis, hepatitis, hypotension, insomnia, myalgia, palpitations, paradoxical excitement, paresthesia, photosensitivity, rash, sedation, tremor, urinary retention

Drug Interactions CNS depressants, anticholinergics, used in combination with hydroxyzine may result in additive effects

Alcohol Interactions Avoid use (may increase central nervous system depression)

(Continued)

Hydroxyzine *(Continued)*

Onset Within 15-30 minutes

Duration 4-6 hours

Half-Life 3-7 hours

Education and Monitoring Issues

Patient Education: Take this drug as prescribed; do not increase dosage or discontinue without consulting prescriber. Store medication away from light. Maintain adequate hydration (2-3 L/day of fluids unless instructed to restrict fluid intake). Void before taking medication. Do not use alcohol or other CNS depressants or sleeping aids without consulting prescriber. May cause dizziness, drowsiness, or blurred vision (use caution when driving or engaging in tasks requiring alertness until response to drug is known); or nausea, dry mouth, appetite disturbances (small frequent meals, frequent mouth care, or sucking hard candy may help). Report unusual weight gain, unresolved nausea or diarrhea, chest pain or palpitations, muscle or joint pain, excess sedation, sore throat, or difficulty breathing.

Monitoring Parameters: Relief of symptoms, mental status, blood pressure

Related Information

Theophylline, Ephedrine, and Hydroxyzine *on page 906*

- **Hygroton®** *see* Chlorthalidone *on page 191*
- **Hylorel®** *see* Guanadrel *on page 425*
- **Hylutin® Injection** *see* Hydroxyprogesterone Caproate *on page 452*

Hyoscyamine (hye oh SYE a meen)

Pharmacologic Class Anticholinergic Agent

U.S. Brand Names Anaspaz®; A-Spas® S/L; Cystospaz®; Cystospaz-M®; Donnamar®; ED-SPAZ®; Gastrosed™; Levbid®; Levsin®; Levsinex®; Levsin/SL®

Use Treatment of GI tract disorders caused by spasm, adjunctive therapy for peptic ulcers

USUAL DOSAGE

Children: Oral, S.L.: Dose as per table repeated every 4 hours as needed

Hyoscyamine

Weight (kg)	Dose (mcg)	Maximum 24-Hour Dose (mcg)
Children <2 y		
2.3	12.5	75
3.4	16.7	100
5	20.8	125
7	25	150
10	31.3-33.3	200
15	45.8	275
Children 2-10 y		
10	31.3-33.3	Do not exceed 0.75 mg
20	62.5	
40	93.8	
50	125	

Adults:

Oral or S.L.: 0.125-0.25 mg 3-4 times/day before meals or food and at bedtime

Oral: 0.375-0.75 mg (timed release) every 12 hours

I.M., I.V., S.C.: 0.25-0.5 mg every 6 hours

Contraindications Narrow-angle glaucoma, obstructive uropathy, obstructive GI tract disease, myasthenia gravis, known hypersensitivity to belladonna alkaloids

Pregnancy Risk Factor C

Related Information

Hyoscyamine, Atropine, Scopolamine, Kaolin, Pectin, and Opium *on page 457*

Hyoscyamine, Atropine, Scopolamine, and Phenobarbital

(hye oh SYE a meen, A troe peen, skoe POL a meen, & fee noe BAR bi tal)

Pharmacologic Class Anticholinergic Agent; Antispasmodic Agent, Gastrointestinal

U.S. Brand Names Barbidonna®; Barophen®; Donnapine®; Donna-Sed®; Donnatal®; Hyosophen®; Kinesed®; Malatal®; Relaxadon®; Spaslin®; Spasmolin®; Spasmophen®; Spasquid®; Susano®

Generic Available Yes

Mechanism of Action Refer to individual agents

Use Adjunct in treatment of peptic ulcer disease, irritable bowel, spastic colitis, spastic bladder, and renal colic

USUAL DOSAGE Oral:

Children 2-12 years: Kinesed® dose: ½ to 1 tablet 3-4 times/day

Children: Donnatal® elixir: 0.1 mL/kg/dose every 4 hours; maximum dose: 5 mL **or** see table for alternative.

Hyoscyamine, Atropine, Scopolamine, and Phenobarbital

Weight (kg)	Dose (mL)	
	q4h	q6h
4.5	0.5	0.75
10	1	1.5
14	1.5	2
23	2.5	3.8
34	3.8	5
≥45	5	7.5

Adults: 1-2 capsules or tablets 3-4 times/day; or 1 Donnatal® Extentab® in sustained release form every 12 hours; or 5-10 mL elixir 3-4 times/day or every 8 hours

Dosage Forms CAP (Donnatal®, Spasmolin®): Hyoscyamine sulfate 0.1037 mg, atropine sulfate 0.0194 mg, scopolamine hydrobromide 0.0065 mg, and phenobarbital 16.2 mg. **ELIX** (Donnatal®, Hyosophen®, Spasmophen®): Hyoscyamine sulfate 0.1037 mg, atropine sulfate 0.0194 mg, scopolamine hydrobromide 0.0065 mg, and phenobarbital 16.2 mg per 5 mL (120 mL, 480 mL, 4000 mL); **TAB:** (Barbidonna®): Hyoscyamine hydrobromide 0.1286 mg, atropine sulfate 0.025 mg, scopolamine hydrobromide 0.0074 mg, and phenobarbital 16 mg; (Barbidonna® No. 2): Hyoscyamine hydrobromide 0.1286 mg, atropine sulfate 0.025 mg, scopolamine hydrobromide 0.0074 mg, and phenobarbital 32 mg; (Donnatal®, Hyosophen®): Hyoscyamine sulfate 0.1037 mg, atropine sulfate 0.0194 mg, scopolamine hydrobromide 0.0065 mg, and phenobarbital 16.2 mg; Long-acting (Donnatal®): Hyoscyamine sulfate 0.3111 mg, atropine sulfate 0.0582 mg, scopolamine hydrobromide 0.0195 mg, and phenobarbital 48.6 mg; (Spasmophen®): Hyoscyamine sulfate 0.1037 mg, atropine sulfate 0.0194 mg, scopolamine hydrobromide 0.0065 mg, and phenobarbital 15 mg

Contraindications Hypersensitivity to hyoscyamine, atropine, scopolamine, phenobarbital, or any component; narrow-angle glaucoma, tachycardia, GI and GU obstruction, myasthenia gravis

Warnings/Precautions Use with caution in patients with hepatic or renal disease, hyperthyroidism, cardiovascular disease, hypertension, prostatic hypertrophy, autonomic neuropathy in the elderly; abrupt withdrawal may precipitate status epilepticus. Because of the anticholinergic effects of this product, it is not recommended for use in the elderly.

Pregnancy Risk Factor C

Adverse Reactions

>10%:

- Dermatologic: Dry skin
- Gastrointestinal: Constipation, dry throat, xerostomia
- Local: Irritation at injection site
- Respiratory: Dry nose
- Miscellaneous: Diaphoresis (decreased)

1% to 10%:

- Dermatologic: Increased sensitivity to light
- Endocrine & metabolic: Decreased flow of breast milk
- Gastrointestinal: Dysphagia

<1%: Ataxia, bloated feeling, blurred vision, confusion, drowsiness, dysuria, fatigue, headache, increased intraocular pain, loss of memory, nausea, orthostatic hypotension, palpitations, rash, tachycardia, ventricular fibrillation, vomiting

Drug Interactions Increased toxicity: CNS depressants, coumarin anticoagulants, amantadine, antihistamine, phenothiazides, antidiarrheal suspensions, corticosteroids, digitalis, griseofulvin, tetracyclines, anticonvulsants, MAO inhibitors, tricyclic antidepressants

Hyoscyamine, Atropine, Scopolamine, Kaolin, Pectin, and Opium

(hye oh SYE a meen, A troe peen, skoe POL a meen, KAY oh lin, PEK tin, & OH pee um)

Pharmacologic Class Anticholinergic Agent

U.S. Brand Names Donnapectolin-PG®; Kapectolin PG®

Dosage Forms SUSP, oral: Hyoscyamine sulfate 0.1037 mg, atropine sulfate 0.0194 mg, scopolamine hydrobromide 0.0065 mg, kaolin 6 g, pectin 142.8 mg, and powdered opium 24 mg per 30 mL with alcohol 5%

Pregnancy Risk Factor C

♦ **Hyosophen®** *see* Hyoscyamine, Atropine, Scopolamine, and Phenobarbital *on page 456*

♦ **Hy-Pam®** *see* Hydroxyzine *on page 455*

- **Hyperab®** *see* Rabies Immune Globulin (Human) *on page 806*
- **HyperHep®** *see* Hepatitis B Immune Globulin *on page 435*
- **Hyperlipidemia Therapy** *see page 1109*
- **Hypertension Therapy** *see page 1116*
- **Hyper-Tet®** *see* Tetanus Immune Globulin (Human) *on page 900*
- **Hy-Phen®** *see* Hydrocodone and Acetaminophen *on page 444*
- **Hypoglycemic Drugs and Thiazolidinedione Information** *see page 1240*
- **HypRho®-D** *see* Rh_o(D) Immune Globulin (Intramuscular) *on page 816*
- **HypRho®-D Mini-Dose** *see* Rh_o(D) Immune Globulin (Intramuscular) *on page 816*
- **Hyprogest® 250 Injection** *see* Hydroxyprogesterone Caproate *on page 452*
- **Hyrexin-50® Injection** *see* Diphenhydramine *on page 282*
- **Hytakerol®** *see* Dihydrotachysterol *on page 277*
- **Hytone®** *see* Hydrocortisone *on page 447*
- **Hytrin®** *see* Terazosin *on page 895*
- **Hytuss® [OTC]** *see* Guaifenesin *on page 423*
- **Hytuss-2X® [OTC]** *see* Guaifenesin *on page 423*
- **Hyzaar®** *see* Losartan and Hydrochlorothiazide *on page 544*
- **Hyzine-50®** *see* Hydroxyzine *on page 455*
- **Iberet-Folic-500®** *see* Ferrous Sulfate, Ascorbic Acid, Vitamin B-Complex, and Folic Acid *on page 361*
- **Iberet-Folic-500®** *see* Vitamins, Multiple *on page 981*
- **Ibuprin® [OTC]** *see* Ibuprofen *on page 458*

Ibuprofen (eye byoo PROE fen)

Pharmacologic Class Nonsteroidal Anti-Inflammatory Agent (NSAID)

U.S. Brand Names Aches-N-Pain® [OTC]; Advil® [OTC]; Children's Advil® Oral Suspension [OTC]; Children's Motrin® Oral Suspension [OTC]; Excedrin® IB [OTC]; Genpril® [OTC]; Haltran® [OTC]; Ibuprin® [OTC]; Ibuprohm® [OTC]; Ibu-Tab®; Junior Strength Motrin® [OTC]; Medipren® [OTC]; Menadol® [OTC]; Midol® 200 [OTC]; Motrin®; Motrin® IB [OTC]; Nuprin® [OTC]; Pamprin IB® [OTC]; PediaProfen™; Saleto-200® [OTC]; Saleto-400®; Trendar® [OTC]; Uni-Pro® [OTC]

Generic Available Yes: Tablet

Mechanism of Action Inhibits prostaglandin synthesis by decreasing the activity of the enzyme, cyclo-oxygenase, which results in decreased formation of prostaglandin precursors

Use Inflammatory diseases and rheumatoid disorders including juvenile rheumatoid arthritis, mild to moderate pain, fever, dysmenorrhea, gout, ankylosing spondylitis, acute migraine headache

USUAL DOSAGE Oral:

Children:

Antipyretic: 6 months to 12 years: Temperature <102.5°F (39°C): 5 mg/kg/dose; temperature >102.5°F: 10 mg/kg/dose given every 6-8 hours; maximum daily dose: 40 mg/kg/day

Juvenile rheumatoid arthritis: 30-70 mg/kg/24 hours divided every 6-8 hours

<20 kg: Maximum: 400 mg/day

20-30 kg: Maximum: 600 mg/day

30-40 kg: Maximum: 800 mg/day

>40 kg: Adult dosage

Start at lower end of dosing range and titrate upward; maximum: 2.4 g/day

Analgesic: 4-10 mg/kg/dose every 6-8 hours

Adults:

Inflammatory disease: 400-800 mg/dose 3-4 times/day; maximum dose: 3.2 g/day

Analgesia/pain/fever/dysmenorrhea: 200-400 mg/dose every 4-6 hours; maximum daily dose: 1.2 g (unless directed by prescriber)

Dosing adjustment/comments in severe hepatic impairment: Avoid use

Dosage Forms CAPLET: 100 mg. **DROPS, oral** (berry flavor):40 mg/mL (15 mL). **SUSP:** Oral: 100 mg/5 mL [OTC] (60 mL, 120 mL, 480 mL); Drops: 40 mg/mL [OTC], 50 mg/1.25 mL. **TAB:** 100 mg [OTC], 200 mg [OTC], 300 mg, 400 mg, 600 mg, 800 mg; Chewable: 50 mg, 100 mg

Contraindications Hypersensitivity to ibuprofen, any component, aspirin, or other nonsteroidal anti-inflammatory drugs (NSAIDs)

Warnings/Precautions Do not exceed 3200 mg/day; use with caution in patients with congestive heart failure, hypertension, decreased renal or hepatic function, history of GI disease (bleeding or ulcers), or those receiving anticoagulants; safety and efficacy in children <6 months of age have not yet been established; elderly are a high-risk population for adverse effects from nonsteroidal anti-inflammatory agents. As much as 60% of elderly can develop peptic ulceration and/or hemorrhage asymptomatically.

Use lowest effective dose for shortest period possible. Use of NSAIDs can compromise existing renal function especially when Cl_{cr} is <30 mL/minute. CNS adverse effects such as confusion, agitation, and hallucination are generally seen in overdose or high dose situations; but elderly may demonstrate these adverse effects at lower doses than younger adults.

Pregnancy Risk Factor B; D (3rd trimester)

Adverse Reactions

>10%:

Central nervous system: Dizziness, fatigue
Dermatologic: Rash, urticaria
Gastrointestinal: Abdominal cramps, heartburn, indigestion, nausea

1% to 10%:

Central nervous system: Headache, nervousness
Dermatologic: Itching
Endocrine & metabolic: Fluid retention
Gastrointestinal: Dyspepsia, vomiting, abdominal pain, peptic ulcer, GI bleed, GI perforation
Otic: Tinnitus

<1%: Acute renal failure, agranulocytosis, allergic rhinitis, anemia, arrhythmias, aseptic meningitis, blurred vision, bone marrow suppression, confusion, congestive heart failure, conjunctivitis, cystitis, decreased hearing, drowsiness, dry eyes, edema, epistaxis, erythema multiforme, gastritis, GI ulceration, hallucinations, hemolytic anemia, hepatitis, hot flashes, hypertension, inhibition of platelet aggregation, insomnia, leukopenia, mental depression, neutropenia, peripheral neuropathy, polydipsia, polyuria, shortness of breath, Stevens-Johnson syndrome, tachycardia, thrombocytopenia, toxic amblyopia, toxic epidermal necrolysis, vision changes

Drug Interactions CYP2C8 and 2C9 enzyme substrate

Decreased effect: Aspirin may decrease ibuprofen serum concentrations

Increased toxicity: May increase digoxin, methotrexate, and lithium serum concentrations; other nonsteroidal anti-inflammatories may increase adverse gastrointestinal effects

Alcohol Interactions Avoid use (may enhance gastric mucosal irritation)

Onset Onset of analgesia: 30-60 minutes; Onset of anti-inflammatory effect: Up to 7 days; Peak action: 1-2 weeks

Duration 4-6 hours

Half-Life 2-4 hours; End-stage renal disease: Unchanged

Education and Monitoring Issues

Patient Education: If self-administered, use exactly as directed (do not increase dose or frequency); adverse reactions can occur with overuse. Do not take longer than 3 days for fever, or 10 days for pain without consulting medical advisor. Take with food or milk. While using this medication, do not use alcohol, excessive amounts of vitamin C, or salicylate containing foods (curry powder, prunes, raisins, tea, or licorice), other prescription or OTC medications containing aspirin or salicylate, or other NSAIDs without consulting prescriber. Maintain adequate hydration (2-3 L/day of fluids unless instructed to restrict fluid intake). May discolor urine (red/pink). You may experience nausea, vomiting, gastric discomfort (frequent mouth care, small frequent meals, chewing gum, sucking lozenges may help). GI bleeding, ulceration, or perforation can occur with or without pain. Stop taking medication and report ringing in ears; persistent cramping or pain in stomach; unresolved nausea or vomiting; difficulty breathing or shortness of breath; unusual bruising or bleeding (mouth, urine, stool); skin rash; unusual swelling of extremities; chest pain; or palpitations.

Dietary Considerations: Food: May decrease the rate but not the extent of oral absorption; drug may cause GI upset, bleeding, ulceration, perforation; take with food or milk to minimize GI upset

Monitoring Parameters: CBC; occult blood loss and periodic liver function tests; monitor response (pain, range of motion, grip strength, mobility, ADL function), inflammation; observe for weight gain, edema; monitor renal function (urine output, serum BUN and creatinine); observe for bleeding, bruising; evaluate gastrointestinal effects (abdominal pain, bleeding, dyspepsia); mental confusion, disorientation; with long-term therapy, periodic ophthalmic exams

Reference Range: Plasma concentrations >200 μg/mL may be associated with severe toxicity

Related Information

Nonsteroidal Anti-Inflammatory Agents Comparison *on page 1248*

- **Ibuprohm® [OTC]** *see* Ibuprofen *on page 458*
- **Ibu-Tab®** *see* Ibuprofen *on page 458*

Ibutilide (i BYOO ti lide)

Pharmacologic Class Antiarrhythmic Agent, Class III

U.S. Brand Names Corvert®

Mechanism of Action Exact mechanism of action is unknown; prolongs the action potential in cardiac tissue

Use Acute termination of atrial fibrillation or flutter of recent onset; the effectiveness of ibutilide has not been determined in patients with arrhythmias of >90 days in duration

USUAL DOSAGE I.V.: Initial:

<60 kg: 0.01 mg/kg over 10 minutes

(Continued)

Ibutilide *(Continued)*

≥60 kg: 1 mg over 10 minutes

If the arrhythmia does not terminate within 10 minutes after the end of the initial infusion, a second infusion of equal strength may be infused over a 10-minute period

Dosage Forms INJ: 0.1 mg/mL (10 mL)

Contraindications Hypersensitivity to the drug or any component

Warnings/Precautions Potentially fatal arrhythmias (eg, polymorphic ventricular tachycardia) can occur with ibutilide, **usually** in association with torsade de pointes (Q-T prolongation). Studies indicate a 1.7% incidence of arrhythmias in treated patients. The drug should be given in a setting of continuous EKG monitoring and by personnel trained in treating arrhythmias particularly polymorphic ventricular tachycardia. Patients with chronic atrial fibrillation may not be the best candidates for ibutilide since they often revert after conversion and the risks of treatment may not be justified when compared to alternative management. Dosing adjustments in patients with renal or hepatic dysfunction since a maximum of only two 10-minute infusions are indicated and drug distribution is one of the primary mechanisms responsible for termination of the pharmacologic effect; safety and efficacy in children have not been established.

Pregnancy Risk Factor C

Pregnancy Implications

Clinical effects on the fetus: Teratogenic and embryocidal in rats; avoid use in pregnancy

Breast-feeding/lactation: Avoid breast-feeding during therapy

Adverse Reactions

1% to 10%:

Cardiovascular: Sustained polymorphic ventricular tachycardia (ie, torsade de pointes) (1.7% - often requiring cardioversion), nonsustained polymorphic ventricular tachycardia (2.7%), nonsustained monomorphic ventricular tachycardia (4.9%), ventricular extrasystoles (5.1%), nonsustained monomorphic VT (4.9%), tachycardia/supraventricular tachycardia (2.7%), hypotension (2%), bundle branch block (1.9%), A-V block (1.5%), bradycardia (1.2%), Q-T segment prolongation, hypertension (1.2%), palpitations (1%)

Central nervous system: Headache (3.6%)

Gastrointestinal: Nausea (>1%)

<1% (limited to important or life-threatening symptoms): Supraventricular extrasystoles (0.9%), nodal arrhythmia (0.7%), congestive heart failure (0.5%), syncope (0.3% - not > placebo), idioventricular rhythm (0.2%), sustained monomorphic ventricular tachycardia (0.2%), renal failure (0.3%)

Case reports: Erythematous bullous lesions

Drug Interactions

Antiarrhythmics: Class Ia antiarrhythmic drugs (disopyramide, quinidine, and procainamide) and other class III drugs such as amiodarone and sotalol, should not be given concomitantly with ibutilide due to their potential to prolong refractoriness

Other drugs which may prolong Q-T interval: phenothiazines, tricyclic and tetracyclic antidepressants, and cisapride, sparfloxacin, gatifloxacin, moxifloxacin, erythromycin may increase risk of toxicity; avoid concurrent use

Digoxin: Signs of digoxin toxicity may be masked when coadministered with ibutilide

Onset Within 90 minutes after start of infusion (½ of conversions to sinus rhythm occur during infusion)

Half-Life 2-12 hours (average: 6 hours)

Education and Monitoring Issues

Patient Education: This drug is only given I.V. and you will be on continuous cardiac monitoring during and for several hours following administration. You may experience headache or irregular heartbeat during infusion. Report chest pain or respiratory difficulty immediately.

Monitoring Parameters: Observe patient with continuous EKG monitoring for at least 4 hours following infusion or until QT_c has returned to baseline; skilled personnel and proper equipment should be available during administration of ibutilide and subsequent monitoring of the patient

Manufacturer Pharmacia & Upjohn

Related Information

Pharmaceutical Manufacturers Directory *on page 1020*

- **Ideal Body Weight Calculation** *see page 1038*
- **I-Gent®** *see* Gentamicin *on page 408*
- **Iletin II Pork Lente** *see* Insulin Preparations *on page 472*
- **Iletin II Pork NPH** *see* Insulin Preparations *on page 472*
- **Iletin II Pork Regular** *see* Insulin Preparations *on page 472*
- **Iletin Lente** *see* Insulin Preparations *on page 472*
- **Iletin NPH** *see* Insulin Preparations *on page 472*
- **Iletin Regular** *see* Insulin Preparations *on page 472*
- **Iletin Semilente** *see* Insulin Preparations *on page 472*
- **Iletin Ultralente** *see* Insulin Preparations *on page 472*
- **Ilopan®** *see* Dexpanthenol *on page 259*

- **Ilopan-Choline®** *see* Dexpanthenol *on page 259*
- **Ilosone®** *see* Erythromycin *on page 323*
- **Ilozyme®** *see* Pancrelipase *on page 698*
- **Imdur™** *see* Isosorbide Mononitrate *on page 491*
- **I-Methasone®** *see* Dexamethasone *on page 256*

Imipenem and Cilastatin (i mi PEN em & sye la STAT in)

Pharmacologic Class Antibiotic, Carbapenem

U.S. Brand Names Primaxin®

Generic Available No

Mechanism of Action Inhibits bacterial cell wall synthesis by binding to one or more of the penicillin binding proteins (PBPs); which in turn inhibits the final transpeptidation step of peptidoglycan synthesis in bacterial cell walls, thus inhibiting cell wall biosynthesis. Bacteria eventually lyse due to ongoing activity of cell wall autolytic enzymes (autolysins and murein hydrolases) while cell wall assembly is arrested. Cilastatin prevents renal metabolism of imipenem by competitive inhibition of dehydropeptidase along the brush border of the renal tubules.

Use Treatment of respiratory tract, urinary tract, intra-abdominal, gynecologic, bone and joint, skin structure, and polymicrobic infections as well as bacterial septicemia and endocarditis. Antibacterial activity includes resistant gram-negative bacilli (*Pseudomonas aeruginosa* and *Enterobacter* sp), gram-positive bacteria (methicillin-sensitive *Staphylococcus aureus* and *Streptococcus* sp) and anaerobes.

USUAL DOSAGE Dosing based on imipenem component:

Children: I.V.:

3 months to 3 years: 25 mg/kg every 6 hours; maximum: 2 g/day

≥3 years: 15 mg/kg/every 6 hours

Adults: I.V.:

Mild to moderate infection: 250-500 mg every 6-8 hours

Severe infections with only **moderately susceptible** organisms: 1 g every 6-8 hours

Mild to moderate infection **only**: I.M.: 500-750 mg every 12 hours (**Note:** 750 mg is recommended for intra-abdominal and more severe respiratory, dermatologic, or gynecologic infections; total daily I.M. dosages >1500 mg are not recommended; deep I.M. injection should be carefully made into a large muscle mass only)

Dosing adjustment in renal impairment: See table.

Imipenem/Cilastatin

Creatinine Clearance (mL/min/1.73 m²)	Frequency	Dose (mg)
30-70	q8h	500
20-30	q12h	500
5-20	q12h	250

Hemodialysis: Imipenem (**not cilastatin**) is moderately dialyzable (20% to 50%); administer dose postdialysis

Peritoneal dialysis: Dose as for Cl_{cr} <10 mL/minute

Continuous arteriovenous or venovenous hemofiltration (CAVH/CAVHD): Dose as for Cl_{cr} 20-30 mL/minute; monitor for seizure activity; imipenem is well removed by CAVH but cilastatin is not; removes 20 mg of imipenem per liter of filtrate per day

Dosage Forms POWDER for inj: I.M.: Imipenem 500 mg and cilastatin 500 mg, Imipenem 750 mg and cilastatin 750 mg; I.V.: Imipenem 250 mg and cilastatin 250 mg, Imipenem 500 mg and cilastatin 500 mg

Contraindications Hypersensitivity to imipenem/cilastatin or any component

Warnings/Precautions Dosage adjustment required in patients with impaired renal function; safety and efficacy in children <12 years of age have not yet been established; prolonged use may result in superinfection; use with caution in patients with a history of seizures or hypersensitivity to beta-lactams; elderly patients often require lower doses

Pregnancy Risk Factor C

Adverse Reactions

1% to 10%:

Gastrointestinal: Nausea/diarrhea/vomiting (1% to 2%)

Local: Phlebitis (3%)

<1%: Abnormal urinalysis, anemia, emergence of resistant strains of *P. aeruginosa*, eosinophilia, hypotension, increased BUN/creatine, increased LFTs, increased PT, neutropenia (including agranulocytosis), pain at injection site, palpitations, (+) Coombs' test, pseudomembranous colitis, rash, seizures, thrombocytopenia

Drug Interactions Increased toxicity: Beta-lactam antibiotics, probenecid may increase toxic potential

Half-Life Imipenem: 1 hour, extended with renal insufficiency; Cilastatin: 1 hour, extended with renal insufficiency

(Continued)

Imipenem and Cilastatin *(Continued)*

Education and Monitoring Issues

Patient Education: Report warmth, swelling, irritation at infusion or injection site. Maintain adequate hydration (2-3 L/day of fluids unless instructed to restrict fluid intake) and nutrition. Report unresolved nausea or vomiting (small, frequent meals may help). Diabetics must use serum glucose testing rather than Clinitest®. Report feelings of excessive dizziness, palpitations, visual disturbances, and CNS changes. Report chills, or unusual discharge, or foul-smelling urine.

Monitoring Parameters: Periodic renal, hepatic, and hematologic function tests; monitor for signs of anaphylaxis during first dose

Manufacturer Merck & Co

Related Information

Animal and Human Bites Guidelines *on page 1177*
Antimicrobial Drugs of Choice *on page 1182*
Pharmaceutical Manufacturers Directory *on page 1020*

Imipramine (im IP ra meen)

Pharmacologic Class Antidepressant, Tricyclic (Tertiary Amine)

U.S. Brand Names Janimine®; Tofranil®; Tofranil-PM®

Generic Available Yes: Tablet

Mechanism of Action Traditionally believed to increase the synaptic concentration of serotonin and/or norepinephrine in the central nervous system by inhibition of their reuptake by the presynaptic neuronal membrane. However, additional receptor effects have been found including desensitization of adenyl cyclase, down regulation of beta-adrenergic receptors, and down regulation of serotonin receptors.

Use Treatment of various forms of depression, often in conjunction with psychotherapy; enuresis in children; certain types of chronic and neuropathic pain

USUAL DOSAGE Maximum antidepressant effect may not be seen for 2 or more weeks after initiation of therapy.

Children: Oral:
- Depression: 1.5 mg/kg/day with dosage increments of 1 mg/kg every 3-4 days to a maximum dose of 5 mg/kg/day in 1-4 divided doses; monitor carefully especially with doses ≥3.5 mg/kg/day
  - Enuresis: ≥6 years: Initial: 10-25 mg at bedtime, if inadequate response still seen after 1 week of therapy, increase by 25 mg/day; dose should not exceed 2.5 mg/kg/day or 50 mg at bedtime if 6-12 years of age or 75 mg at bedtime if ≥12 years of age
  - Adjunct in the treatment of cancer pain: Initial: 0.2-0.4 mg/kg at bedtime; dose may be increased by 50% every 2-3 days up to 1-3 mg/kg/dose at bedtime

Adolescents: Oral: Initial: 25-50 mg/day; increase gradually; maximum: 100 mg/day in single or divided doses

Adults:
- Oral: Initial: 25 mg 3-4 times/day, increase dose gradually, total dose may be given at bedtime; maximum: 300 mg/day
- I.M.: Initial: Up to 100 mg/day in divided doses; change to oral as soon as possible

Elderly: Initial: 10-25 mg at bedtime; increase by 10-25 mg every 3 days for inpatients and weekly for outpatients if tolerated; average daily dose to achieve a therapeutic concentration: 100 mg/day; range: 50-150 mg/day

Dosage Forms

Imipramine hydrochloride: **INJ** (Tofranil®): 12.5 mg/mL (2 mL). **TAB** (Janimine®, Tofranil®): 10 mg, 25 mg, 50 mg

Imipramine pamoate: **CAP** (Tofranil-PM®): 75 mg, 100 mg, 125 mg, 150 mg

Contraindications Hypersensitivity to imipramine (cross-sensitivity with other tricyclics may occur); patients receiving MAO inhibitors or fluoxetine within past 14 days; narrow-angle glaucoma

Warnings/Precautions Use with caution in patients with cardiovascular disease, conduction disturbances, seizure disorders, urinary retention, hyperthyroidism or those receiving thyroid replacement; do not discontinue abruptly in patients receiving long-term, high-dose therapy; some oral preparations contain tartrazine and injection contains sulfites, both of which can cause allergic reactions

Orthostatic hypotension is a concern with this agent, especially in patients taking other medications that may affect blood pressure; may precipitate arrhythmias in predisposed patients; may aggravate seizures; a less anticholinergic antidepressant may be a better choice

Pregnancy Risk Factor D

Adverse Reactions

Cardiovascular: Orthostatic hypotension, arrhythmias, tachycardia, hypertension, palpitations, myocardial infarction, heart block, EKG changes, CHF, stroke

Central nervous system: Dizziness, drowsiness, headache, agitation, insomnia, nightmares, hypomania, psychosis, fatigue, confusion, hallucinations, disorientation, delusions, anxiety, restlessness, seizures

Endocrine & metabolic: Gynecomastia, breast enlargement, galactorrhea, increase or decrease in libido, increase or decrease in blood sugar, SIADH

Gastrointestinal: Nausea, unpleasant taste, weight gain, xerostomia, constipation, ileus, stomatitis, abdominal cramps, vomiting, anorexia, epigastric disorders, diarrhea, black tongue, weight loss

Genitourinary: Urinary retention, impotence

Neuromuscular & skeletal: Weakness, numbness, tingling, paresthesias, incoordination, ataxia, tremor, peripheral neuropathy, extrapyramidal symptoms

Ocular: Blurred vision, disturbances of accommodation, mydriasis

Otic: Tinnitus

Miscellaneous: Diaphoresis

<1%: Agranulocytosis, alopecia, cholestatic jaundice, eosinophilia, increased liver enzymes, itching, petechiae, photosensitivity, purpura, rash, thrombocytopenia, urticaria

Drug Interactions CYP1A2, 2C9, 2C19, 2D6, and 3A3/4 enzyme substrate

Carbamazepine, phenobarbital, and rifampin may increase the metabolism of imipramine resulting in decreased effect of imipramine

Imipramine inhibits the antihypertensive response to bethanidine, clonidine, debrisoquin, guanadrel, guanethidine, guanabenz, guanfacine; monitor BP; consider alternate antihypertensive agent

Abrupt discontinuation of clonidine may cause hypertensive crisis, imipramine may enhance the response

Use with altretamine may cause orthostatic hypertension

Imipramine may be additive with or may potentiate the action of other CNS depressants (sedatives, hypnotics, or ethanol); with MAO inhibitors, hyperpyrexia, hypertension, tachycardia, confusion, seizures, and **deaths have been reported** (serotonin syndrome), this combination should be avoided; imipramine may increase the prothrombin time in patients stabilized on warfarin

Cimetidine and methylphenidate may decrease the metabolism of imipramine

Additive anticholinergic effects seen with other anticholinergic agents

The SSRIs, to varying degrees, inhibit the metabolism of TCAs and clinical toxicity may result

Use of lithium with a TCA may increase the risk for neurotoxicity

Phenothiazines may increase concentration of some TCAs and TCAs may increase concentration of phenothiazines; monitor for altered clinical response

TCAs may enhance the hypoglycemic effects of tolazamide, chlorpropamide, or insulin; monitor for changes in blood glucose levels

Cholestyramine and colestipol may bind TCAs and reduce their absorption; monitor for altered response

TCAs may enhance the effect of amphetamines; monitor for adverse CV effects

Verapamil and diltiazem appear to decrease the metabolism of imipramine and potentially other TCAs; monitor for increased TCA concentrations. The pressor response to I.V. epinephrine, norepinephrine, and phenylephrine may be enhanced in patients receiving TCAs, this combination is best avoided.

Indinavir, ritonavir may inhibit the metabolism of clomipramine and potentially other TCAs; monitor for altered effects; a decrease in TCA dosage may be required

Quinidine may inhibit the metabolism of TCAs; monitor for altered effect

Combined use of anticholinergics with TCAs may produce additive anticholinergic effects; combined use of beta-agonists with TCAs may predispose patients to cardiac arrhythmias

Alcohol Interactions Avoid use (may increase central nervous system depression)

Onset Peak antidepressant effect: Usually after ≥2 weeks

Half-Life 6-18 hours

Education and Monitoring Issues

Patient Education: Oral: Take exactly as directed (do not increase dose or frequency); may take 2-3 weeks to achieve desired results; may cause physical and/or psychological dependence. Take in the evening. Avoid excessive alcohol, caffeine, and other prescription or OTC medications not approved by prescriber. Maintain adequate hydration (2-3 L/day of fluids unless instructed to restrict fluid intake). You may experience drowsiness, lightheadedness, impaired coordination, dizziness, or blurred vision (use caution when driving or engaging in tasks requiring alertness until response to drug is known); nausea, vomiting, altered taste, dry mouth (small frequent meals, frequent mouth care, chewing gum, or sucking lozenges may help); constipation (increased exercise, fluids, or dietary fruit and fiber may help); diarrhea (buttermilk, yogurt, or boiled milk may help); postural hypotension (use caution when climbing stairs or changing position from lying or sitting to standing); or urinary retention (void before taking medication). Report persistent insomnia; muscle cramping or tremors; chest pain, palpitations, rapid heartbeat, swelling of extremities, or severe dizziness; unresolved urinary retention; rash or skin irritation; yellowing of eyes or skin; pale stools/dark urine; or worsening of condition.

Dietary Considerations: Grapefruit juice may potentially inhibit metabolism of TCAs

Monitoring Parameters: Monitor blood pressure and pulse rate prior to and during initial therapy; EKG, CBC; evaluate mental status

Reference Range: Therapeutic: Imipramine and desipramine: 150-250 ng/mL (SI: 530-890 nmol/L); desipramine: 150-300 ng/mL (SI: 560-1125 nmol/L); Toxic: >500 ng/mL (SI: 446-893 nmol/L); utility of serum level monitoring controversial

(Continued)

Imipramine *(Continued)*

Related Information

Antidepressant Agents Comparison *on page 1231*

Imiquimod (i mi KWI mod)

Pharmacologic Class Topical Skin Product

U.S. Brand Names Aldara™

Use Treatment of external genital and perianal warts/condyloma acuminata in adults

USUAL DOSAGE

Adults: Topical: Apply 3 times/week prior to normal sleeping hours and leave on the skin for 6-10 hours. Following treatment period, remove cream by washing the treated area with mild soap and water. Examples of 3 times/week application schedules are: Monday, Wednesday, Friday; or Tuesday, Thursday, Saturday. Continue imiquimod treatment until there is total clearance of the genital/perianal warts for ≤16 weeks. A rest period of several days may be taken if required by the patient's discomfort or severity of the local skin reaction. Treatment may resume once the reaction subsides.

Nonocclusive dressings such as cotton gauze or cotton underwear may be used in the management of skin reactions. Handwashing before and after cream application is recommended. Imiquimod is packaged in single-use packets that contain sufficient cream to cover a wart area of up to 20 cm^2; avoid use of excessive amounts of cream. Instruct patients to apply imiquimod to external or perianal warts. Apply a thin layer to the wart area and rub in until the cream is no longer visible. Do not occlude the application site.

Contraindications Hypersensitivity to imiquimod

Pregnancy Risk Factor B

♦ **Imitrex®** *see* Sumatriptan Succinate *on page 884*

Immune Globulin, Intramuscular

(i MYUN GLOB yoo lin, IN tra MUS kyoo ler)

Pharmacologic Class Immune Globulin

Generic Available No

Mechanism of Action Provides passive immunity by increasing the antibody titer and antigen-antibody reaction potential

Use Household and sexual contacts of persons with hepatitis A, measles, varicella, and possibly rubella; travelers to high-risk areas outside tourist routes; staff, attendees, and parents of diapered attendees in day-care center outbreaks

For travelers, IG is not an alternative to careful selection of foods and water; immune globulin can interfere with the antibody response to parenterally administered live virus vaccines. Frequent travelers should be tested for hepatitis A antibody, immune hemolytic anemia, and neutropenia (with ITP, I.V. route is usually used).

USUAL DOSAGE I.M.:

Hepatitis A:

Pre-exposure prophylaxis upon travel into endemic areas (hepatitis A vaccine preferred):

0.02 mL/kg for anticipated risk 1-3 months

0.06 mL/kg for anticipated risk >3 months

Repeat approximate dose every 4-6 months if exposure continues

Postexposure prophylaxis: 0.02 mL/kg given within 2 weeks of exposure

Measles:

Prophylaxis: 0.25 mL/kg/dose (maximum dose: 15 mL) given within 6 days of exposure followed by live attenuated measles vaccine in 3 months or at 15 months of age (whichever is later)

For patients with leukemia, lymphoma, immunodeficiency disorders, generalized malignancy, or receiving immunosuppressive therapy: 0.5 mL/kg (maximum dose: 15 mL)

Poliomyelitis: Prophylaxis: 0.3 mL/kg/dose as a single dose

Rubella: Prophylaxis: 0.55 mL/kg/dose within 72 hours of exposure

Varicella:: Prophylaxis: 0.6-1.2 mL/kg (varicella zoster immune globulin preferred) within 72 hours of exposure

IgG deficiency: 1.3 mL/kg, then 0.66 mL/kg in 3-4 weeks

Hepatitis B: Prophylaxis: 0.06 mL/kg/dose (HBIG preferred)

Dosage Forms INJ: I.M.: 165±15 mg (of protein)/mL (2 mL, 10 mL)

Contraindications Thrombocytopenia, hypersensitivity to immune globulin, thimerosal, IgA deficiency

Warnings/Precautions Skin testing should not be performed as local irritation can occur and be misinterpreted as a positive reaction; do not administer I.V.; IG should **not** be used to control outbreaks of measles; epidemiologic and laboratory data indicate current IMIG products do not have a discernible risk of transmitting HIV

Pregnancy Risk Factor C

Adverse Reactions

>10%: Local: Pain, tenderness, muscle stiffness at I.M. site

1% to 10%:

Cardiovascular: Flushing

Central nervous system: Chills
Gastrointestinal: Nausea
<1%: Angioedema, erythema, fever, hypersensitivity reactions, lethargy, myalgia, urticaria, vomiting

Drug Interactions Increased toxicity: Live virus, vaccines (measles, mumps, rubella); do not administer within 3 months after administration of these vaccines

Related Information
Prophylaxis for Patients Exposed to Common Communicable Diseases *on page 1161*

Immune Globulin, Intravenous (i MYUN GLOB yoo lin, IN tra VEE nus)

Pharmacologic Class Immune Globulin

U.S. Brand Names Gamimune® N; Gammagard® S/D; Gammar®-P I.V.; Polygam®; Polygam® S/D; Sandoglobulin®; Venoglobulin®-I; Venoglobulin®-S

Mechanism of Action Replacement therapy for primary and secondary immunodeficiencies; interference with F_c receptors on the cells of the reticuloendothelial system for autoimmune cytopenias and ITP; possible role of contained antiviral-type antibodies

Use Treatment of immunodeficiency sufficiency (hypogammaglobulinemia, agammaglobulinemia, IgG subclass deficiencies, severe combined immunodeficiency syndromes (SCIDS), Wiskott-Aldrich syndrome), idiopathic thrombocytopenic purpura; used in conjunction with appropriate anti-infective therapy *to prevent or modify acute bacterial or viral infections* in patients with iatrogenically-induced or disease-associated immunodepression; *chronic lymphocytic leukemia (CLL) - chronic prophylaxis autoimmune neutropenia, bone marrow transplantation patients, autoimmune hemolytic anemia or neutropenia, refractory dermatomyositis/polymyositis, autoimmune diseases* (myasthenia gravis, SLE, bullous pemphigoid, severe rheumatoid arthritis), Guillain-Barré syndrome; pediatric HIV infection to decrease frequency of serious bacterial infections

USUAL DOSAGE Children and Adults: I.V.:

Dosages should be based on ideal body weight and not actual body weight in morbidly obese patients; approved doses and regimens may vary between brands; check manufacturer guidelines

Primary immunodeficiency disorders: 200-400 mg/kg every 4 weeks or as per monitored serum IgG concentrations

Chronic lymphocytic leukemia (CLL): 400 mg/kg/dose every 3 weeks

Idiopathic thrombocytopenic purpura (ITP): Maintenance dose:
- 400 mg/kg/day for 2-5 consecutive days; or 1000 mg/kg every other day for 3 doses, if needed or
- 1000 mg/kg/day for 2 consecutive days; or up to 2000 mg/kg/day over 2-7 consecutive days

Chronic ITP: 400-2000 mg/kg/dose as needed to maintain appropriate platelet counts

Kawasaki disease:
- 400 mg/kg/day for 4 days within 10 days of onset of fever
- 800 mg/kg/day for 1-2 days within 10 days of onset of fever
- 2 g/kg for one dose only

Acquired immunodeficiency syndrome (patients must be symptomatic):
- 200-250 mg/kg/dose every 2 weeks
- 400-500 mg/kg/dose every month or every 4 weeks

Pediatric HIV: 400 mg/kg every 28 days

Autoimmune hemolytic anemia and neutropenia: 1000 mg/kg/dose for 2-3 days

Autoimmune diseases: 400 mg/kg/day for 4 days

Bone marrow transplant: 500 mg/kg beginning on days 7 and 2 pretransplant, then 500 mg/kg/week for 90 days post-transplant

Adjuvant to severe cytomegalovirus infections: 500 mg/kg/dose every other day for 7 doses

Severe systemic viral and bacterial infections: Children: 500-1000 mg/kg/week

Prevention of gastroenteritis: Infants and Children: Oral: 50 mg/kg/day divided every 6 hours

Guillain-Barré syndrome:
- 400 mg/kg/day for 4 days
- 1000 mg/kg/day for 2 days
- 2000 mg/kg/day for one day

Refractory dermatomyositis: 2 g/kg/dose every month x 3-4 doses

Refractory polymyositis: 1 g/kg/day x 2 days every month x 4 doses

Chronic inflammatory demyelinating polyneuropathy:
- 400 mg/kg/day for 5 doses once each month
- 800 mg/kg/day for 3 doses once each month
- 1000 mg/kg/day for 2 days once each month

Dosing adjustment/comments in renal impairment: Cl_{cr} <10 mL/minute: Avoid use

Dosage Forms INJ: (Gamimune® N): 5% [50 mg/mL] (10 mL, 50 mL, 100 mL, 250 mL); 10% [100 mg/mL] (10 mL, 50 mL, 100 mL, 200 mL). **POWDER for inj, lyophilized:** (Gammar®-P IV): 1 g, 2.5 g, 5 g, 10 g; (Polygam®): 0.5 g, 2.5 g, 5 g, 10 g; (Sandoglobulin®): 1 g, 3 g, 6 g, 12 g; (Venoglobulin®-I): 0.5 g, 2.5 g, 5 g, 10 g; Detergent treated: (Gammagard® S/D): 2.5 g, 5 g, 10 g; (Polygam® S/D): 2.5 g, 5 g, 10 g; (Venoglobulin®-S): 5% [50 mg/mL] (50 mL, 100 mL, 200 mL); 10% [100 mg/mL] (50 mL, 100 mL, 200 mL)

(Continued)

Immune Globulin, Intravenous *(Continued)*

Contraindications Hypersensitivity to immune globulin or any component, IgA deficiency (except with the use of Gammagard®, Polygam®)

Warnings/Precautions Anaphylactic hypersensitivity reactions can occur, especially in IgA-deficient patients; studies indicate that the currently available products have no discernible risk of transmitting HIV or hepatitis B; aseptic meningitis may occur with high doses (≥2 g/kg); renal dysfunction (increased serum creatinine, oliguria, acute renal failure) can rarely occur (usually within 7 days of use)

Pregnancy Risk Factor C

Intravenous Immune Globulin Product Comparison

	Gamimune® N	Gammagard® SD	Gammar®-IV	Polygam®	Sandoglobulin®	Venoglobulin®-I
FDA indication	Primary immunodeficiency, ITP	Primary immunodeficiency, ITP, CLL prophylaxis	Primary immunodeficiency	Primary immunodeficiency, ITP, CLL	Primary immunodeficiency, ITP	Primary immunodeficiency, ITP
Contraindication	IgA deficiency	None (caution with IgA deficiency)	IgA deficiency	None (caution with IgA deficiency)	IgA deficiency	IgA deficiency
IgA content	270 mcg/mL	0.92-1.6 mcg/mL	<20 mcg/mL	0.74±0.33 mcg/mL	720 mcg/mL	20-24 mcg/mL
Adverse reactions (%)	5.2	6	15	6	2.5-6.6	6
Plasma source	>2000 paid donors	4000-5000 paid donors	>8000 paid donors	50,000 voluntary donors	8000-15,000 voluntary donors	6000-9000 paid donors
Half-life	21 d	24 d	21-24 d	21-25 d	21-23 d	29 d
IgG subclass (%)						
IgG_1 (60-70)	60	67 (66.8)[1]	69	67	60.5 (55.3)[1]	62.3[2]
IgG_2 (19-31)	29.4	25 (25.4)	23	25	30.2 (35.7)	32.8
IgG_3 (5-8.4)	6.5	5 (7.4)	6	5	6.6 (6.3)	2.9
IgG_4 (0.7-4)	4.1	3 (0.3)	2	3	2.6 (2.6)	2
Monomers (%)	>95	>95	>98	>95	>92	>98
Gammaglobulin (%)	>98	>90	>98	>90	>96	>98
Storage	Refrigerate	Room temp	Room temp	Room temp	Room temp	Room temp
Recommendations for initial infusion rate	0.01-0.02 mL/kg/min	0.5 mL/kg/h	0.01-0.02 mL/kg/min	0.5 mL/kg/h	0.01-0.03 mL/kg/min	0.01-0.02 mL/kg/min
Maximum infusion rate	0.08 mL/kg/min	4 mL/kg/h	0.06 mL/kg/min	4 mL/kg/h	2.5 mL/min	0.04 mL/kg/min
Maximum concentration for infusion (%)	10	5	5	10	12	10

[1]Skvaril F and Gardi A, "Differences Among Available Immunoglobulin Preparations for Intravenous Use," *Pediatr Infect Dis J*, 1988, 7:543-48.

[2]Roomer J, Morgenthaler JJ, Scherz R, et al, "Characterization of Various Immunoglobulin Preparations for Intravenous Application," *Vox Sang*, 1982, 42:62-73.

Adverse Reactions

1% to 10%:

Cardiovascular: Flushing of the face, tachycardia

Central nervous system: Chills

Gastrointestinal: Nausea

Respiratory: Dyspnea

<1%: Diaphoresis, dizziness, fever, headache, hypersensitivity reactions, hypotension, tightness in the chest

Drug Interactions Increased toxicity: Live virus, vaccines (measles, mumps, rubella); do not administer within 3 months after administration of these vaccines

Onset I.V. provides immediate antibody levels.

Half-Life 21-24 days

Education and Monitoring Issues

Patient Education: This medication can only be administered by infusion. You will be monitored closely during the infusion. If you experience nausea ask for assistance, do not get up alone. Do not have any vaccinations for the next 3 months without consulting prescriber. Immediately report chills; chest pain, tightness, or rapid heartbeat; acute back pain; or difficulty breathing.

- ♦ **Immunization Recommendations** *see page 1138*
- ♦ **Immunizations and Vaccinations** *see page 1139*
- ♦ **Imodium®** *see* Loperamide *on page 538*
- ♦ **Imodium® A-D [OTC]** *see* Loperamide *on page 538*
- ♦ **Imogam®** *see* Rabies Immune Globulin (Human) *on page 806*
- ♦ **Imuran®** *see* Azathioprine *on page 84*
- ♦ **I-Naphline®** *see* Naphazoline *on page 636*
- ♦ **Inapsine®** *see* Droperidol *on page 302*

Indapamide (in DAP a mide)

Pharmacologic Class Diuretic, Thiazide

U.S. Brand Names Lozol®

Generic Available No

Mechanism of Action Diuretic effect is localized at the proximal segment of the distal tubule of the nephron; it does not appear to have significant effect on glomerular filtration rate nor renal blood flow; like other diuretics, it enhances sodium, chloride, and water excretion by interfering with the transport of sodium ions across the renal tubular epithelium

Use Management of mild to moderate hypertension; treatment of edema in congestive heart failure and nephrotic syndrome

USUAL DOSAGE Adults: Oral:

Edema: 2.5-5 mg/day. **Note:** There is little therapeutic benefit to increasing the dose >5 mg/day; there is, however, an increased risk of electrolyte disturbances

Hypertension: 1.25 mg in the morning, may increase to 5 mg/day by increments of 1.25-2.5 mg; consider adding another antihypertensive and decreasing the dose if response is not adequate

Dosage Forms TAB: 1.25 mg, 2.5 mg

Contraindications Anuria, hypersensitivity to indapamide or any component, cross-sensitivity with other thiazides and sulfonamide derivatives

Warnings/Precautions Use with caution in patients with renal or hepatic disease, gout, lupus erythematosus, or diabetes mellitus

Pregnancy Risk Factor B (per manufacturer); D (based on expert analysis)

Adverse Reactions

1% to 10%:

Cardiovascular: Orthostatic hypotension, palpitations, flushing

Central nervous system: Dizziness, lightheadedness, vertigo, headache, weakness, restlessness, drowsiness, fatigue, lethargy, malaise, lassitude, anxiety, agitation, depression, nervousness

Gastrointestinal: Anorexia, gastric irritation, nausea, vomiting, abdominal pain, cramping, bloating, diarrhea, constipation, dry mouth, weight loss

Genitourinary: Nocturia, frequent urination, polyuria

Neuromuscular & skeletal: Muscle cramps, spasm

Ocular: Blurred vision

Respiratory: Rhinorrhea

<1% (limited to important or life-threatening symptoms): Purpura, necrotizing angiitis, vasculitis, cutaneous vasculitis, impotency, reduced libido, hyperglycemia, glycosuria, hyperuricemia

Drug Interactions

Angiotensin-converting enzyme inhibitors: Increased hypotension if aggressively diuresed with a thiazide diuretic

Beta-blockers increase hyperglycemic effects in type 2 diabetes mellitus

Cyclosporine and thiazides can increase the risk of gout or renal toxicity; avoid concurrent use

(Continued)

Indapamide *(Continued)*

Digoxin toxicity can be exacerbated if a thiazide induces hypokalemia or hypomagnesemia

Lithium toxicity can occur by reducing renal excretion of lithium; monitor lithium concentration and adjust as needed

Neuromuscular blocking agents can prolong blockade; monitor serum potassium and neuromuscular status

NSAIDs can decrease the efficacy of thiazides reducing the diuretic and antihypertensive effects

Onset 1-2 hours

Duration Up to 36 hours

Half-Life 14-18 hours

Education and Monitoring Issues

Patient Education: Take as directed, early in the day (last dose late afternoon). Do not exceed recommended dosage. Noninsulin-dependent diabetics should monitor serum glucose closely (medication may decrease effect of oral hypoglycemics). Monitor weight on a regular basis. Report sudden or excessive weight gain, swelling of ankles or hands, or difficulty breathing. You may experience dizziness, weakness, or drowsiness; use caution when changing position (rising from sitting or lying position) and when driving or engaging in tasks that require alertness until response to drug is known. Use may experience sensitivity to sunlight (use sunblock, wear protective clothing or sunglasses), impotence (reversible), dry mouth or thirst (frequent mouth care, chewing gum or sucking on lozenges may help). Report unusual bleeding, palpitations, numbness or tingling or cramping.

Monitoring Parameters: Blood pressure (both standing and sitting/supine), serum electrolytes, renal function, assess weight, I & O reports daily to determine fluid loss

♦ **Inderal®** *see* Propranolol *on page 786*

♦ **Inderal® LA** *see* Propranolol *on page 786*

♦ **Inderide®** *see* Propranolol and Hydrochlorothiazide *on page 788*

Indinavir (in DIN a veer)

Pharmacologic Class Antiretroviral Agent, Protease Inhibitor

U.S. Brand Names Crixivan®

Use Treatment of HIV infection; should always be used as part of a multidrug regimen (at least three antiretroviral agents)

USUAL DOSAGE Adults: Oral: 800 mg every 8 hours; when administered with delavirdine, itraconazole, or ketoconazole, dose should be reduced to 600 mg every 8 hours; when administered with efavirenz, dose should be increased to 1000 mg every 8 hours

Dosage adjustment in hepatic impairment: 600 mg every 8 hours with mild/medium impairment due to cirrhosis

Contraindications Hypersensitivity to the drug or its components

Warnings/Precautions Because indinavir may cause nephrolithiasis the drug should be discontinued if signs and symptoms occur. Indinavir should not be administered concurrently with terfenadine, astemizole, cisapride, triazolam, and midazolam because of competition for metabolism of these drugs through the CYP3A4 system, and potential serious or life-threatening events. Patients with hepatic insufficiency due to cirrhosis should have dose reduction. Fat redistribution can occur with protease inhibitors.

Pregnancy Risk Factor C

Adverse Reactions Protease inhibitors cause dyslipidemia which includes elevated cholesterol and triglycerides and a redistribution of body fat centrally to cause "protease paunch", buffalo hump, facial atrophy, and breast enlargement. These agents also cause hyperglycemia.

1% to 10%:

Central nervous system: Headache (5.6%), insomnia (3.1%)

Gastrointestinal: Mild elevation of indirect bilirubin (10%), abdominal pain (8.7%), nausea (11.7%), diarrhea/vomiting (4% to 5%), taste perversion (2.6%)

Neuromuscular & skeletal: Weakness (3.6%), flank pain (2.6%)

Renal: Kidney stones (2% to 3%)

<1%: Anorexia, decreased hemoglobin, depression, dizziness, increased serum cholesterol, malaise, pancreatitis, somnolence, urticaria, xerostomia

Drug Interactions CYP3A3/4 enzyme substrate; CYP3A3/4 enzyme inhibitor

Decreased effect: Concurrent use of rifampin and rifabutin may decrease the effectiveness of indinavir (dosage increase of indinavir is recommended), dosage decreases of rifampin/rifabutin are recommended; the efficacy of protease inhibitors may be decreased when given with nevirapine or efavirenz.

Increased toxicity: Gastric pH is lowered and absorption may be decreased when didanosine and indinavir are taken <1 hour apart; a reduction of dose is often required when coadministered with ketoconazole; astemizole and cisapride should be avoided with indinavir due to life-threatening cardiotoxicity; benzodiazepines with indinavir may result in prolonged sedation and respiratory depression; ketoconazole, itraconazole, nelfinavir, ritonavir, and delavirdine increased indinavir levels. Indinavir inhibits the metabolism of HMG-CoA reductase inhibitors (atorvastatin, cerivastatin, lovastatin, simvastatin) which increases the risk of rhabdomyolysis. Indinavir increases the AUC of amprenavir.

Drug-Herb interactions: St John's wort (hypericum) appears to induce CYP3A enzymes and has lead to 57% reductions in indinavir AUCs and 81% reductions in trough serum concentrations, which may lead to treatment failures

Manufacturer Merck & Co

Related Information

Antiretroviral Therapy for HIV Infection *on page 1190*
Management of Healthcare Worker Exposures to HIV *on page 1151*
Pharmaceutical Manufacturers Directory *on page 1020*

- **Indocid®** *see* Indomethacin *on page 469*
- **Indocin®** *see* Indomethacin *on page 469*
- **Indocin® I.V.** *see* Indomethacin *on page 469*
- **Indocin® SR** *see* Indomethacin *on page 469*

Indomethacin (in doe METH a sin)

Pharmacologic Class Nonsteroidal Anti-Inflammatory Agent (NSAID)

U.S. Brand Names Indocin®; Indocin® I.V.; Indocin® SR

Generic Available Yes

Mechanism of Action Inhibits prostaglandin synthesis by decreasing the activity of the enzyme, cyclo-oxygenase, which results in decreased formation of prostaglandin precursors

Use Management of inflammatory diseases and rheumatoid disorders; moderate pain; acute gouty arthritis; I.V. form used as alternative to surgery for closure of patent ductus arteriosus in neonates

USUAL DOSAGE

Patent ductus arteriosus: Neonates: I.V.: Initial: 0.2 mg/kg; followed with: 2 doses of 0.1 mg/kg at 12- to 24-hour intervals if age <48 hours at time of first dose; 0.2 mg/kg 2 times if 2-7 days old at time of first dose; or 0.25 mg/kg 2 times if over 7 days at time of first dose; discontinue if significant adverse effects occur. Dose should be withheld if patient has anuria or oliguria.

Analgesia:

Children: Oral: Initial: 1-2 mg/kg/day in 2-4 divided doses; maximum: 4 mg/kg/day; not to exceed 150-200 mg/day

Adults: Oral, rectal: 25-50 mg/dose 2-3 times/day; maximum dose: 200 mg/day; extended release capsule should be given on a 1-2 times/day schedule

Dosage Forms CAP: 25 mg, 50 mg; (Indocin®): 25 mg, 50 mg; Sustained release (Indocin® SR): 75 mg. **POWDER for inj** (Indocin® I.V.): 1 mg. **SUPP, rectal** (Indocin®): 50 mg. **SUSP, oral** (Indocin®): 25 mg/5 mL (5 mL, 10 mL, 237 mL, 500 mL)

Contraindications Hypersensitivity to indomethacin, any component, aspirin, or other nonsteroidal anti-inflammatory drugs (NSAIDs); active GI bleeding, ulcer disease; premature neonates with necrotizing enterocolitis, impaired renal function, active bleeding, thrombocytopenia

Warnings/Precautions Use with caution in patients with cardiac dysfunction, hypertension, renal or hepatic impairment, epilepsy, history of GI bleeding, patients receiving anticoagulants, and for treatment of JRA in children (fatal hepatitis has been reported); may have adverse effects on fetus; may affect platelet and renal function in neonates; elderly are a high-risk population for adverse effects from nonsteroidal anti-inflammatory agents. As much as 60% of elderly can develop peptic ulceration and/or hemorrhage asymptomatically.

Use lowest effective dose for shortest period possible. Use of NSAIDs can compromise existing renal function especially when Cl_{cr} is <30 mL/minute.

CNS adverse effects such as confusion, agitation, and hallucination are generally seen in overdose or high-dose situations; but elderly may demonstrate these adverse effects at lower doses than younger adults.

Pregnancy Risk Factor B; D (if used longer than 48 hours or after 34-week gestation)

Adverse Reactions

>10%:

Central nervous system: Dizziness
Dermatologic: Rash
Gastrointestinal: Nausea, epigastric pain, abdominal pain, anorexia, GI bleeding, ulcers, perforation, abdominal cramps, heartburn, indigestion

1% to 10%:

Central nervous system: Headache, nervousness
Dermatologic: Itching
Endocrine & metabolic: Fluid retention
Gastrointestinal: Vomiting
Otic: Tinnitus

<1%: Agranulocytosis, allergic rhinitis, anemia, angioedema, arrhythmias, aseptic meningitis, blurred vision, bone marrow suppression, confusion, congestive heart failure,

(Continued)

Indomethacin *(Continued)*

conjunctivitis, corneal opacities, cystitis, decreased hearing, depression, dilutional hyponatremia (I.V.), drowsiness, dry eyes, epistaxis, erythema multiforme, fatigue, gastritis, GI ulceration, hallucinations, hemolytic anemia, hepatitis, hot flashes, hyperkalemia, hypersensitivity reactions, hypertension, hypoglycemia (I.V.), inhibition of platelet aggregation, leukopenia, oliguria, peripheral neuropathy, polydipsia, polyuria, renal failure, shortness of breath, somnolence, Stevens-Johnson syndrome, tachycardia, thrombocytopenia, toxic amblyopia, toxic epidermal necrolysis, urticaria

Drug Interactions CYP2C9 enzyme substrate

Decreased effect: May decrease antihypertensive effects of beta-blockers, hydralazine and captopril; indomethacin may decrease antihypertensive and diuretic effects of furosemide and thiazides

Increased toxicity: May increase serum potassium with potassium-sparing diuretics; probenecid may increase indomethacin serum concentrations; other NSAIDs may increase GI adverse effects; may increase nephrotoxicity of cyclosporin

Indomethacin may increase serum concentrations of digoxin, methotrexate, lithium, and aminoglycosides (reported with I.V. use in neonates)

Alcohol Interactions Avoid use (may enhance gastric mucosal irritation)

Onset Within 30 minutes

Duration 4-6 hours

Half-Life 4.5 hours, longer in neonates

Education and Monitoring Issues

Patient Education:

Oral: Take this medication exactly as directed; do not increase dose without consulting prescriber. Do not crush, break, or chew capsules. Take with food or milk to reduce GI distress. Maintain adequate fluid intake (2-3 L/day of fluids unless instructed to restrict fluid intake).

Rectal: Suppositories do not need to be refrigerated. Wash hands before inserting unwrapped suppository high up in rectum. Wearing glove is recommended. (Use caution to avoid damage with long fingernails.)

Do not use alcohol, aspirin, or aspirin-containing medication, and all other anti-inflammatory medications without consulting prescriber. You may experience drowsiness, dizziness, nervousness, or headache (use caution when driving or engaging in tasks requiring alertness until response to drug is known); anorexia, nausea, vomiting, or heartburn (frequent small meals, frequent oral care, sucking lozenges, or chewing gum may help); fluid retention (weigh yourself weekly and report unusual (3-5 lb/week) weight gain). May discolor stool (green). GI bleeding, ulceration, or perforation can occur with or without pain; discontinue medication and contact prescriber if persistent abdominal pain or cramping, or blood in stool occurs. Report breathlessness, difficulty breathing, or unusual cough; chest pain, rapid heartbeat, palpitations; unusual bruising/bleeding; blood in urine, stool, gums, or vomitus; swollen extremities; skin rash, irritation, or itching; acute fatigue; or changes in hearing or ringing in ears.

Dietary Considerations:

Food: May decrease the rate but not the extent of oral absorption. Drug may cause GI upset, bleeding, ulceration, perforation; take with food or milk to minimize GI upset.

Potassium: Hyperkalemia has been reported. The elderly and those with renal insufficiency are at greatest risk. Monitor potassium serum concentration in those at greatest risk. Avoid salt substitutes.

Sodium: Hyponatremia from sodium retention. Suspect secondary to suppression of renal prostaglandin. Monitor serum concentration and fluid status. May need to restrict fluid.

Monitoring Parameters: Monitor response (pain, range of motion, grip strength, mobility, ADL function), inflammation; observe for weight gain, edema; monitor renal function (serum creatinine, BUN); observe for bleeding, bruising; evaluate gastrointestinal effects (abdominal pain, bleeding, dyspepsia); mental confusion, disorientation, CBC, liver function tests

Related Information

Nonsteroidal Anti-Inflammatory Agents Comparison *on page 1248*

- **Infants Feverall™ [OTC]** *see* Acetaminophen *on page 17*
- **Infants' Silapap® [OTC]** *see* Acetaminophen *on page 17*
- **InFed™ Injection** *see* Iron Dextran Complex *on page 485*
- **Inflamase® Forte Ophthalmic** *see* Prednisolone *on page 762*
- **Inflamase® Mild Ophthalmic** *see* Prednisolone *on page 762*

Infliximab (in FLIKS e mab)

Pharmacologic Class Gastrointestinal Agent, Miscellaneous; Monoclonal Antibody

U.S. Brand Names Remicade™

Use Treatment of moderately to severely active Crohn's disease for the reduction of the signs and symptoms in patients who have an inadequate response to conventional therapy or for the treatment of patients with fistulizing Crohn's disease for the reduction in the number of draining enterocutaneous fistula(s). Use with methotrexate in treatment of rheumatoid arthritis patients who have had an inadequate response to methotrexate alone.

USUAL DOSAGE

Moderately to severely active Crohn's disease: Adults: I.V.: 5 mg/kg as a single infusion over a minimum of 2 hours

Fistulizing Crohn's disease: 5 mg/kg as an infusion over a minimum of 2 hours, dose repeated at 2 and 6 weeks after the initial infusion

Rheumatoid arthritis: I.V. infusion (in combination with methotrexate therapy): 3 mg/kg followed by an additional 3 mg/kg at 2 and 6 weeks after the first dose; then repeat every 8 weeks thereafter. Doses have ranged from 3-10 mg/kg intravenous infusion repeated at 4-week intervals or 8-week intervals.

Dosing adjustment in renal impairment: No specific adjustment recommended

Dosing adjustment in hepatic impairment: No specific adjustment recommended

Dosage Forms POWDER for inj: 100 mg

Contraindications Known hypersensitivity to murine proteins or any component

Warnings/Precautions Hypersensitivity reactions, including urticaria, dyspnea, and hypotension have occurred; discontinue the drug if a reaction occurs. Medications for the treatment of hypersensitivity reactions should be available for immediate use. Autoimmune antibodies and a lupus-like syndrome have been reported; if antibodies to double-stranded DNA are confirmed in a patient with lupus-like symptoms, treatment should be discontinued. May affect normal immune responses; effects on development of lymphoma and infection in Crohn's patients are unknown. Treatment may result in the development of human antichimeric antibodies (HACA); presence of these antibodies may predispose patients to infusion reactions. Serious infections, including sepsis and fatal infections, have been reported in patients receiving TNF-blocking agents. Many of the serious infections in patients treated with infliximab have occurred in patients on concomitant immunosuppressive therapy that, in addition to their Crohn's disease or rheumatoid arthritis, could predispose them to infections. Caution should be exercised when considering the use of infliximab in patients with a chronic infection of a history of recurrent infection. Infliximab should not be given to patients with a clinically important, active infection. Patients who develop a new infection while undergoing treatment with infliximab should be monitored closely. If a patient develops a serious infection or sepsis, infliximab should be discontinued.

Pregnancy Risk Factor C

Pregnancy Implications It is not known whether infliximab is secreted in human milk. Because many immunoglobulins are secreted in milk, and the potential for serious adverse reactions exists, a decision should be made whether to discontinue nursing or discontinue the drug, taking into account the importance of the drug to the mother.

Adverse Reactions

>10%:

- Central nervous system: Headache (22.6%), fatigue (10.6%), fever (10.1%)
- Gastrointestinal: Nausea (16.6%), abdominal pain (12.1%)
- Local: Infusion reactions (16%)
- Respiratory: Upper respiratory tract infection (16.1%)
- Miscellaneous: Infections (21%)

1% to 10%:

- Cardiovascular: Chest pain (5.5%)
- Central nervous system: Pain (8.5%), dizziness (8%)
- Dermatologic: Rash (6%), pruritus (5%)
- Gastrointestinal: Vomiting (8.5%)
- Neuromuscular & skeletal: Myalgia (5%), back pain (5%)
- Respiratory: Pharyngitis (8.5%), bronchitis (7%), rhinitis (6%), cough (5%), sinusitis (5%)
- Miscellaneous: Development of antibodies to double-stranded DNA (9%), candidiasis (5%), serious infection (3%)

<1%: Lupus-like syndrome (2 patients); a proportion of patients (12%) with fistulizing disease developed new abscess 8-16 weeks after the last infusion of infliximab

Drug Interactions Specific drug interaction studies have not been conducted

Onset Within 2 weeks

Half-Life 9.5 days

Education and Monitoring Issues

Patient Education: This drug can only be administered by infusion. Report adverse symptoms: headache or unusual fatigue; increased nausea or abdominal pain; cough, runny nose, difficulty breathing; chest pain or persistent dizziness; fatigue, muscle pain or weakness, back pain; fever or chills, mouth sores, vaginal itching or discharge, sore throat, unhealed sores, or frequent infections.

Manufacturer Centocor, Inc

Related Information

Pharmaceutical Manufacturers Directory *on page 1020*

♦ **Infufer®** *see* Iron Dextran Complex *on page 485*

♦ **Infumorph™ Injection** *see* Morphine Sulfate *on page 618*

♦ **Initard 50/50** *see* Insulin Preparations *on page 472*

♦ **Innofem®** *see* Estradiol *on page 327*

♦ **Innovar®** *see* Droperidol and Fentanyl *on page 303*

♦ **Inocor®** *see* Amrinone *on page 62*

♦ **Insta-Char® [OTC]** *see* Charcoal *on page 175*

Insulin Preparations (IN su lin prep a RAY shuns)

Pharmacologic Class Antidiabetic Agent (Insulin); Antidote

U.S. Brand Names Humalog®; Humalog® 50/50; Humalog® 75/25; Humulin® 50/50; Humulin® 70/30; Humulin® L; Humulin® N; Lente® Iletin® I; Lente® Iletin® II; Lente® Insulin; Lente® L; Novolin® 70/30; Novolin® L; Novolin® N; Novolin® R; NPH Iletin® I; NPH-N; Pork NPH Iletin® II; Pork Regular Iletin® II; Regular (Concentrated) Iletin® II U-500; Regular Iletin® I; Regular Insulin; Regular Purified Pork Insulin; Velosulin® BR Human (Buffered); Velosulin® Human

Generic Available Yes

Mechanism of Action The principal hormone required for proper glucose utilization in normal metabolic processes; it is obtained from beef or pork pancreas or a biosynthetic process converting pork insulin to human insulin; insulins are categorized into 3 groups related to promptness, duration, and intensity of action

Use Treatment of insulin-dependent diabetes mellitus, also noninsulin-dependent diabetes mellitus unresponsive to treatment with diet and/or oral hypoglycemics; to assure proper utilization of glucose and reduce glucosuria in nondiabetic patients receiving parenteral nutrition whose glucosuria cannot be adequately controlled with infusion rate adjustments or those who require assistance in achieving optimal caloric intakes; hyperkalemia (use with glucose to shift potassium into cells to lower serum potassium levels)

USUAL DOSAGE Dose requires continuous medical supervision; may administer I.V. (regular), I.M., S.C.

Diabetes mellitus: The number and size of daily doses, time of administration, and diet and exercise require continuous medical supervision. Lispro should be given within 15 minutes of a meal and human regular insulin should be given within 30-60 minutes before a meal. Maintenance doses should be administered subcutaneously and sites should be rotated to prevent lipodystrophy.

Children and Adults: 0.5-1 unit/kg/day in divided doses

Adolescents (growth spurts): 0.8-1.2 units/kg/day in divided doses

Adjust dose to maintain premeal and bedtime blood glucose of 80-140 mg/dL (children <5 years: 100-200 mg/dL)

Hyperkalemia: Administer calcium gluconate and $NaHCO_3$ first then 50% dextrose at 0.5-1 mL/kg and insulin 1 unit for every 4-5 g dextrose given

Diabetic ketoacidosis: Children and Adults: Regular Insulin: I.V. loading dose: 0.1 unit/kg, then maintenance continuous infusion: 0.1 unit/kg/hour (range: 0.05-0.2 units/kg/hour depending upon the rate of decrease of serum glucose - too rapid decrease of serum glucose may lead to cerebral edema).

Optimum rate of decrease (serum glucose): 80-100 mg/dL/hour

Note: Newly diagnosed patients with IDDM presenting in DKA and patients with blood sugars <800 mg/dL may be relatively "sensitive" to insulin and should receive loading and initial maintenance doses approximately $^1/_2$ of those indicated above.

Dosing adjustment in renal impairment (regular): Insulin requirements are reduced due to changes in insulin clearance or metabolism

Cl_{cr} 10-50 mL/minute: Administer at 75% of normal dose

Cl_{cr} <10 mL/minute: Administer at 25% to 50% of normal dose and monitor glucose closely

Hemodialysis: Because of a large molecular weight (6000 daltons), insulin is not significantly removed by either peritoneal or hemodialysis

Supplemental dose is not necessary

Peritoneal dialysis: Supplemental dose is not necessary

Continuous arteriovenous or venovenous hemofiltration effects: Supplemental dose is not necessary

Dosage Forms All insulins are 100 units/mL (10 mL) except where indicated:

RAPID ACTING: **Insulin lispro rDNA origin:** (Humalog®) [*Lilly*] (1.5 mL, 10 mL). **Insulin inj**: (Regular Insulin); Beef and pork: (Regular Iletin® I) [*Lilly*]; Human: rDNA: (Humulin® R) [*Lilly*], (Novolin® R) [*Novo Nordisk*]; Semisynthetic: (Velosulin® Human) [*Novo Nordisk*]; Pork: (Regular Insulin) [*Novo Nordisk*]; Purified pork: (Pork Regular Iletin® II) [*Lilly*], (Regular Purified Pork Insulin) [*Novo Nordisk*], (Regular (Concentrated) Iletin® II U-500) (*Lilly*): 500 units/mL

INTERMEDIATE-ACTING: **Insulin zinc susp** (Lente), Beef and pork: (Lente® Iletin® I) [*Lilly*]; Human, rDNA: (Humulin® L) [*Lilly*], (Novolin® L) [*Novo Nordisk*]; Purified pork: (Lente® Iletin® II) [*Lilly*], (Lente® L) [*Novo Nordisk*]. **Isophane insulin susp** (NPH), Beef and pork: (NPH Iletin® I) [*Lilly*]; Human, rDNA: (Humulin® N) [*Lilly*], (Novolin® N) [*Novo Nordisk*]; Purified pork: (Pork NPH Iletin® II) [*Lilly*], (NPH-N) [*Novo Nordisk*]

LONG-ACTING: **Insulin zinc susp, extended** (Ultralente®), Human, rDNA: Humulin® U [Lilly]

COMBINATIONS: **Isophane insulin susp and insulin inj,** Isophane insulin susp (50%) and insulin inj (50%) human (rDNA): (Humulin® 50/50) [*Lilly*], Isophane insulin susp

(70%) and insulin inj (30%) human (rDNA): (Humulin® 70/30) [*Lilly*], (Novolin® 70/30) [*Novo Nordisk*]

Warnings/Precautions Any change of insulin should be made cautiously; changing manufacturers, type and/or method of manufacture, may result in the need for a change of dosage; human insulin differs from animal-source insulin; regular insulin is the only insulin to be used I.V.; hypoglycemia may result from increased work or exercise without eating

Pregnancy Risk Factor B

Pregnancy Implications

Clinical effects on the fetus: Does not cross the placenta. Insulin is the drug of choice for the control of diabetes mellitus during pregnancy.

Breast-feeding/lactation: The gastrointestinal tract destroys insulin when administered orally and therefore would not be expected to be absorbed intact by the breast-feeding infant.

Adverse Reactions 1% to 10%:

Cardiovascular: Palpitation, tachycardia, pallor

Central nervous system: Fatigue, mental confusion, loss of consciousness, headache, hypothermia

Dermatologic: Urticaria, redness

Endocrine & metabolic: Hypoglycemia

Gastrointestinal: Hunger, nausea, numbness of mouth

Local: Itching, edema, stinging, or warmth at injection site, atrophy or hypertrophy of S.C. fat tissue

Neuromuscular & skeletal: Muscle weakness, paresthesia, tremors

Ocular: Transient presbyopia or blurred vision, blurred vision

Miscellaneous: Diaphoresis, anaphylaxis

Drug Interactions See table.

Drug Interactions With Insulin Injection

Decrease Hypoglycemic Effect of Insulin	Increase Hypoglycemic Effect of Insulin
Contraceptives, oral	Alcohol
Corticosteroids	Alpha-blockers
Dextrothyroxine	Anabolic steroids
Diltiazem	Beta-blockers*
Dobutamine	Clofibrate
Epinephrine	Fenfluramine
Niacin	Guanethidine
Smoking	MAO inhibitors
Thiazide diuretics	Pentamidine
Thyroid hormone	Phenylbutazone
	Salicylates
	Sulfinpyrazone
	Tetracyclines

*Nonselective beta-blockers may delay recovery from hypoglycemic episodes and mask signs/symptoms of hypoglycemia. Cardioselective agents may be alternatives.

Alcohol Interactions Avoid use (may increase hypoglycemia)

Onset

Onset and duration of hypoglycemic effects depend upon preparation administered. See table.

Pharmacokinetics/Pharmacodynamics: Onset and Duration of Hypoglycemic Effects Depend Upon Preparation Administered

	Onset (h)	Peak (h)	Duration (h)
Insulin, regular (Novolin® R)	0.5–1	2-3	5–7
Isophane insulin suspension (NPH) (Novolin® N)	1–1.5	4–12	18–24
Insulin zinc suspension (Lente®)	1–2.5	8–12	18–24
Isophane insulin suspension and regular insulin injection (Novolin® 70/30)	0.5 (0.5)	4-8 (2-12)	24 (24)
Prompt zinc insulin suspension (PZI)	4-8	14-24	36
Extended insulin zinc suspension (Ultralente®)	4-8	16–18	>36

(Continued)

Insulin Preparations *(Continued)*

Onset and duration: Insulin lispro may begin to act in 15-30 minutes. Biosynthetic NPH human insulin shows a more rapid onset and shorter duration of action than corresponding porcine insulins; human insulin and purified porcine regular insulin are similarly efficacious following S.C. administration. The duration of action of highly purified porcine insulins is shorter than that of conventional insulin equivalents. Duration depends on type of preparation and route of administration as well as patient related variables. In general, the larger the dose of insulin, the longer the duration of activity.

Education and Monitoring Issues

Patient Education: This medication is used to control diabetes; it is not a cure. Other components of treatment plan are important: follow prescribed diet, medication, and exercise regimen. Take exactly as directed. Do not change dose or discontinue unless so advised by prescriber. Inform prescriber of all other prescription or OTC medications you are taking; do not introduce new medication without consulting prescriber. If you experience hypoglycemic reaction, contact prescriber immediately. Maintain regular dietary intake and exercise routine and always carry quick source of sugar with you. Report adverse side effects, including chest pain or palpitations; persistent fatigue, confusion, headache; skin rash or redness; numbness of mouth, lips, or tongue; muscle weakness or tremors; changes in vision; difficulty breathing; or nausea, vomiting, or flu-like symptoms.

Dietary Considerations:

Food:

Potassium: Shifts potassium from extracellular to intracellular space. Decreases potassium serum concentration; monitor potassium serum concentration.

Sodium: SIADH; water retention and dilutional hyponatremia may occur. Patients at greatest risk are those with CHF or hepatic cirrhosis. Monitor sodium serum concentration and fluid status.

Monitoring Parameters: Urine sugar and acetone, serum glucose, electrolytes

Reference Range:

Therapeutic, serum insulin (fasting): 5-20 μIU/mL (SI: 35-145 pmol/L)

Glucose, fasting:

Newborns: 60-110 mg/dL

Adults: 60-110 mg/dL

Elderly: 100-180 mg/dL

Related Information

Diabetes Mellitus Treatment *on page 1089*

♦ **Insulin-Toronto (Regular)** *see* Insulin Preparations *on page 472*

♦ **Intal® Nebulizer Solution** *see* Cromolyn Sodium *on page 231*

♦ **Intal® Oral Inhaler** *see* Cromolyn Sodium *on page 231*

Interferon Alfa-2a (in ter FEER on AL fa-too aye)

Pharmacologic Class Biological Response Modulator

U.S. Brand Names Roferon-A®

Generic Available No

Mechanism of Action The exact mechanism of interferon-α's cytotoxic effect is not clear. The antineoplastic effect does not appear to be linked to interferon's antiviral effect. Possible mechanisms by which interferons stimulate existing host defenses against malignancies include induction of gene transcription, inhibition of cell growth, alteration of cellular differentiation, interference with oncogene expression, and augmentation of lymphocyte toxicity. Interferon-α has been shown to increase activation of prenatural killer cells, cytotoxic activity of natural killer cells, macrophage phagocytosis, cytotoxicity of K cells and polymorphonuclear leukocytes, and to alter antibody production.

Use Hairy cell leukemia, AIDS-related Kaposi's sarcoma, chronic myelogenous leukemia (CML), chronic hepatitis C, adjuvant therapy of malignant melanoma

Unlabeled uses: AIDS thrombocytopenia, cutaneous ulcerations of Behçet's disease, brain tumors, metastatic ileal carcinoid tumors, cervical and colorectal cancer, genital warts, idiopathic mixed cryoglobulinemia, hemangioma, hepatitis D, hepatocellular carcinoma, idiopathic hypereosinophilic syndrome, mycosis fungoides, Sézary syndrome, low-grade non-Hodgkin's lymphoma, macular degeneration, multiple myeloma, renal cell carcinoma, basal and squamous cell skin cancer, essential thrombocythemia

USUAL DOSAGE Refer to individual protocols. I.V., I.M., S.C.:

Infants and Children: 1-3 million units/day

Adults:

Hairy cell leukemia: 3 million units/day for 16-24 weeks, then 3 million units 3 times/week for up to 6-24 months

Chronic myelogenous leukemia (CML): 9 million units/day for up to 18 months

Cutaneous T-cell lymphoma: 3-36 million units/day; 65.5 million units/m^2 every month

Melanoma: 3 million units/day for 8-48 weeks

AIDS-related Kaposi's sarcoma: 36 million units/day for 10-12 weeks, then 36 million units 3 times/week for 10-12 weeks

Hepatitis C: 3 million units 3 times/week for 12 months

Genital herpes: 6-18 million units as a single dose or daily for 3 days

Not removed by hemodialysis

Dosage Forms INJ: 3 million units/mL (1 mL); 6 million units/mL (3 mL); 9 million units/mL (0.9 mL, 3 mL); 36 million units/mL (1 mL). **POWDER for inj:** 6 million units/mL when reconstituted

Contraindications Hypersensitivity to alfa-2a interferon or any component; neonates and patients with known hypersensitivity to benzyl alcohol (premixed solutions are preserved with benzyl alcohol)

Warnings/Precautions Use with caution in patients with a history of seizures, brain metastases, multiple sclerosis, cardiac disease, myelosuppression, or hepatic or renal dysfunction. Safety and efficacy in children <18 years of age have not been established. Higher doses in elderly patients or diseases other than hairy cell leukemia may result in increased CNS toxicity. **Due to differences in dosage, patients should not change brands of interferon-α.**

Pregnancy Risk Factor C

Adverse Reactions

>10%:

Central nervous system: Dizziness, fatigue, malaise, fever (usually within 4-6 hours), chills

Dermatologic: Rash

Gastrointestinal: Xerostomia, nausea, vomiting, diarrhea, abdominal cramps, weight loss, metallic taste

Hematologic: Mildly myelosuppressive and well tolerated if used without adjunct antineoplastic agents; thrombocytosis has been reported, leukopenia (mainly neutropenia), anemia, thrombocytopenia, decreased hemoglobin, hematocrit, platelets

Myelosuppressive:

WBC: Mild

Platelets: Mild

Onset (days): 7-10

Nadir (days): 14

Recovery (days): 21

Neuromuscular & skeletal: Rigors, arthralgia

Miscellaneous: Flu-like syndrome, diaphoresis

1% to 10%:

Central nervous system: Headache, delirium, somnolence, neurotoxicity

Dermatologic: Alopecia, dry skin

Gastrointestinal: Anorexia, stomatitis

Hepatic: Hepatotoxicity

Neuromuscular & skeletal: Peripheral neuropathy, leg cramps

Ocular: Blurred vision

Miscellaneous: Diaphoresis

<1%: Usually patient can build up a tolerance to side effects. Arrhythmias, change in taste, chest pain, confusion, coughing, depression, dyspnea, edema, EEG abnormalities, hypotension, hypothyroidism, increased BUN/creatinine, increased hepatic transaminase, increased uric acid level, local sensitivity to injection, myalgia, nasal congestion, neutralizing antibodies, proteinuria, psychiatric effects, sensory neuropathy, SVT, tachycardia, visual disturbances

Drug Interactions

Increased effect:

Cimetidine: May augment the antitumor effects of interferon in melanoma

Theophylline: Clearance has been reported to be decreased in hepatitis patients receiving interferon

Increased toxicity: Vinblastine: Enhances interferon toxicity in several patients; increased incidence of paresthesia has also been noted

Half-Life I.M., I.V.: 2 hours after administration; S.C.: 3 hours

Education and Monitoring Issues

Patient Education: Use as directed; do not change dosage or schedule of administration without consulting prescriber. Maintain adequate hydration (2-3 L/day of fluids unless instructed to restrict fluid intake). You may experience flu-like syndrome (acetaminophen may help); nausea, vomiting, dry mouth, or metallic taste (frequent small meals, frequent mouth care, sucking lozenges, or chewing gum may help); drowsiness, dizziness, agitation, abnormal thinking (use caution when driving or engaging in tasks requiring alertness until response to drug is known). Report unusual bruising or bleeding; persistent abdominal disturbances; unusual fatigue; muscle pain or tremors; chest pain or palpitation; swelling of extremities or unusual weight gain; difficulty breathing; pain, swelling, or redness at injection site; or other unusual symptoms.

Monitoring Parameters: Baseline chest x-ray, EKG, CBC with differential, liver function tests, electrolytes, platelets, weight; patients with pre-existing cardiac abnormalities, or in advanced stages of cancer should have EKGs taken before and during treatment

Manufacturer Roche Laboratories

Related Information

Pharmaceutical Manufacturers Directory *on page 1020*

Interferon Alfa-2b (in ter FEER on AL fa-too bee)

Pharmacologic Class Biological Response Modulator

U.S. Brand Names Intron® A

Generic Available No

Mechanism of Action Alpha interferons are a family of proteins, produced by nucleated cells, that have antiviral, antiproliferative, and immune-regulating activity. There are 16 known subtypes of alpha interferons. Interferons interact with cells through high affinity cell surface receptors. Following activation, multiple effects can be detected including induction of gene transcription. Inhibits cellular growth, alters the state of cellular differentiation, interferes with oncogene expression, alters cell surface antigen expression, increases phagocytic activity of macrophages, and augments cytotoxicity of lymphocytes for target cells

Use Hairy-cell leukemia in patients >18 years, condylomata acuminata, AIDS-related Kaposi's sarcoma in patients >18 years, chronic non-A/non-B/C hepatitis in patients >18 years, chronic hepatitis B in patients >18 years (indications and dosage are specific for a particular brand of interferon)

USUAL DOSAGE Adults (refer to individual protocols):

Hairy cell leukemia: I.M., S.C.: 2 million units/m² 3 times/week for 2 to ≥6 months of therapy

AIDS-related Kaposi's sarcoma: I.M., S.C. (use 50 million international unit vial): 30 million units/m² 3 times/week

Condylomata acuminata: Intralesionally (use 10 million international unit vial): 1 million units/lesion 3 times/week for 4-8 weeks; not to exceed 5 million units per treatment (maximum: 5 lesions at one time)

Chronic hepatitis C (non-A/non-B): I.M., S.C.: 3 million units 3 times/week for approximately a 6-month course

Chronic hepatitis B: I.M., S.C.: 5 million international units/day or 10 million international units 3 times/week for 16 weeks; if severe adverse reactions occur, reduce dosage 50% or temporarily discontinue therapy until adverse reactions abate; when platelet/granulocyte count returns to normal, reinstitute therapy

Hemodialysis: Supplemental dose is not necessary

Peritoneal dialysis: Supplemental dose is not necessary

Dosage Forms INJ (albumin free): 3 million units (0.5 mL); 5 million units (0.5 mL); 10 million units (1 mL); 25 million units. **POWDER for inj, lyophilized:** 18 million units, 50 million units

Contraindications Known hypersensitivity to interferon alfa-2b or any components, patients with pre-existing thyroid disease uncontrolled by medication, coagulation disorders, diabetics prone to DKA, pulmonary disease

Warnings/Precautions Use with caution in patients with seizure disorders, brain metastases, compromised CNS, multiple sclerosis, and patients with pre-existing cardiac disease, severe renal or hepatic impairment, or myelosuppression; safety and efficacy in children <18 years has not been established. Higher doses in the elderly or in malignancies other than hairy cell leukemia may result in severe obtundation. A baseline ocular exam is recommended in patients with diabetes or hypertension.

Pregnancy Risk Factor C

Adverse Reactions

>10%:

- Central nervous system: Dizziness, fatigue, malaise, fever (usually within 4-6 hours), chills
- Dermatologic: Skin rash
- Gastrointestinal: Xerostomia, nausea, vomiting, diarrhea, dizziness, abdominal cramps, weight loss, metallic taste, anorexia
- Hematologic: Mildly myelosuppressive and well tolerated if used without adjunct antineoplastic agents; thrombocytosis has been reported, leukopenia (mainly neutropenia), anemia, thrombocytopenia, decreased hemoglobin, hematocrit, platelets
- Myelosuppressive:
  - WBC: Mild
  - Platelets: Mild
  - Onset (days): 7-10
  - Nadir (days): 14
  - Recovery (days): 21
- Neuromuscular & skeletal: Rigors, arthralgia
- Miscellaneous: Flu-like syndrome, diaphoresis

1% to 10%:

- Central nervous system: Neurotoxicity
- Dermatologic: Dry skin, alopecia
- Gastrointestinal: Stomatitis
- Hepatic: Hepatotoxicity
- Neuromuscular & skeletal: Peripheral neuropathy, leg cramps
- Ocular: Blurred vision
- Miscellaneous: Diaphoresis

<1%: Usually patient can build up a tolerance to side effects. Arrhythmias, cardiotoxicity, change in taste, chest pain, confusion, coughing, delirium, dyspnea, edema, EEG

abnormalities, headache, hypotension, hypothyroidism, increased ALT/AST, increased BUN, increased creatinine, increased hepatic transaminase, increased uric acid level, myalgia, nasal congestion, neutralizing antibodies, partial alopecia, proteinuria, psychiatric effects, rigors, sensitivity to injection, sensory neuropathy, somnolence, SVT, tachycardia, visual disturbances

Drug Interactions

Increased effect: Cimetidine: May augment the antitumor effects of interferon in melanoma

Increased toxicity:

Theophylline: Clearance has been reported to be decreased in hepatitis patients receiving interferon

Vinblastine: Enhances interferon toxicity in several patients; increased incidence of paresthesia has also been noted

Zidovudine: Increased myelosuppression

Half-Life I.M., I.V.: 2 hours; S.C.: 3 hours

Education and Monitoring Issues

Patient Education: Use as directed; do not change dosage or schedule of administration without consulting prescriber. Maintain adequate hydration (2-3 L/day of fluids unless instructed to restrict fluid intake). You may experience flu-like syndrome (acetaminophen may help); nausea, vomiting, dry mouth, or metallic taste (frequent small meals, frequent mouth care, sucking lozenges, or chewing gum may help); drowsiness, dizziness, agitation, abnormal thinking (use caution when driving or engaging in tasks requiring alertness until response to drug is known). Report unusual bruising or bleeding; persistent abdominal disturbances; unusual fatigue; muscle pain or tremors; chest pain or palpitation; swelling of extremities or unusual weight gain; difficulty breathing; pain, swelling, or redness at injection site; or other unusual symptoms.

Monitoring Parameters: Baseline chest x-ray, EKG, CBC with differential, liver function tests, electrolytes, thyroid function tests, platelets, weight; patients with pre-existing cardiac abnormalities, or in advanced stages of cancer should have EKGs taken before and during treatment

Manufacturer Schering-Plough Corp

Related Information

Pharmaceutical Manufacturers Directory *on page 1020*

Interferon Alfa-2b and Ribavirin Combination Pack

(in ter FEER on AL fa-too bee & rye ba VYE rin com bi NAY shun pak)

Pharmacologic Class Antiviral Agent; Biological Response Modulator

U.S. Brand Names Rebetron™

Use The combination therapy of oral ribavirin with interferon alfa-2b, recombinant (Intron® A) injection is indicated for the treatment of chronic hepatitis C in patients with compensated liver disease who have relapsed after alpha interferon therapy.

USUAL DOSAGE The recommended dosage of combination therapy is 3 million int. units of Intron® A injected subcutaneously 3 times/week and 1000-1200 mg of Rebetol® capsules administered orally in a divided daily (morning and evening) dose for 24 weeks; patients weighing 75 kg (165 pounds) or less should receive 1000 mg of Rebetol® daily (2 x 200 mg capsules in the morning and 3 x 200 mg capsules in the evening); while patients weighing more than 75 kg should receive 1200 mg of Rebetol® daily (3 x 200 mg capsules in the morning and 3 x 200 mg capsules in the evening)

Dosage Forms COMBINATION PACKAGE:

For patients ≤75 kg: Each Rebetron™ combination package consists of:

A box containing 6 vials of Intron® A (3 million international units in 0.5 mL per vial) and 6 syringes and alcohol swabs; two boxes containing 35 Rebetrol® capsules each for a total of 70 capsules (5 capsules per blister card)

One 18 million international units multidose vial of Intron® A injection (22.8 million international units/3.8 mL; 3 million international units/0.5 mL) and 6 syringes and alcohol swabs; two boxes containing 35 Rebetrol® capsules each for a total of 70 capsules (5 capsules per blister card)

One 18 million international units Intron® A injection multidose pen (22.5 million international units per 1.5 mL; 3 million international units/0.2 mL) and 6 disposable needles and alcohol swabs; two boxes containing 35 Rebetrol® capsules each for a total of 70 capsules (5 capsules per blister card)

For patients >75 kg: A box containing 6 vials of Intron® A injection (3 million international units in 0.5 mL per vial) and 6 syringes and alcohol swabs; two boxes containing 42 Rebetrol® capsules each for a total of 84 capsules (6 capsules per blister card)

One 18 million international units multidose vial of Intron® A injection (22.5 million international units per 3.8 mL; 3 million international units/0.5 mL) and 6 syringes and alcohol swabs; two boxes containing 42 Rebetrol® capsules each for a total of 84 capsules (6 capsules per blister card)

One 18 million international units Intron® A injection multidose pen (22.5 million international units per 1.5 mL; 3 million international units/0.2 mL) and 6 disposable needles and alcohol swabs; two boxes containing 42 Rebetrol® capsules each for a total of 84 capsules (6 capsules per blister card)

(Continued)

Interferon Alfa-2b and Ribavirin Combination Pack *(Continued)*

For Rebetrol® dose reduction: A box containing 6 vials of Intron® A injection (3 million international units in 0.5 mL per vial) and 6 syringes and alcohol swabs; one box containing 42 Rebetrol® capsules (6 capsules per blister card)

One 18 million international units multidose vial of Intron® A injection (22.8 million international units per 3.8 mL; 3 million international units/0.5 mL) and 6 syringes and alcohol swabs; one box containing 42 Rebetrol® capsules (6 capsules per blister card)

One 18 million international units Introl® A injection multidose pen (22.5 million international units per 1.5 mL; 3 million international units/0.2 mL) and 6 disposable needles and alcohol swabs; one box containing 42 Rebetrol® capsules (6 capsules per blister card)

Pregnancy Risk Factor X

Manufacturer Schering-Plough Corp

Related Information

Pharmaceutical Manufacturers Directory *on page 1020*

Interferon Alfa-n3 (in ter FEER on AL fa-en three)

Pharmacologic Class Biological Response Modulator

U.S. Brand Names Alferon® N

Generic Available No

Mechanism of Action Interferons interact with cells through high affinity cell surface receptors. Following activation, multiple effects can be detected including induction of gene transcription. Inhibits cellular growth, alters the state of cellular differentiation, interferes with oncogene expression, alters cell surface antigen expression, increases phagocytic activity of macrophages, and augments cytotoxicity of lymphocytes for target cells

Use Patients ≥18 years of age: Condylomata acuminata, intralesional treatment of refractory or recurring genital or venereal warts; useful in patients who do not respond or are not candidates for usual treatments; indications and dosage regimens are specific for a particular brand of interferon

USUAL DOSAGE Adults: Inject 250,000 units (0.05 mL) in each wart twice weekly for a maximum of 8 weeks; therapy should not be repeated for at least 3 months after the initial 8-week course of therapy

Dosage Forms INJ: 5 million units (1 mL)

Contraindications Patients with known hypersensitivity to alpha interferon, mouse immunoglobulin, or any component of the product

Warnings/Precautions Use with caution in patients with seizure disorders, brain metastases, compromised CNS function, cardiac disease, severe renal or hepatic impairment, multiple sclerosis; safety and efficacy in children <18 years have not been established.

Pregnancy Risk Factor C

Adverse Reactions

>10%:

- Central nervous system: Fatigue, malaise, fever (usually within 4-6 hours), chills, dizziness
- Dermatologic: Rash
- Gastrointestinal: Xerostomia, nausea, vomiting, diarrhea, abdominal cramps, weight loss, metallic taste, anorexia
- Hematologic: Mildly myelosuppressive and well tolerated if used without adjunct antineoplastic agents; thrombocytosis has been reported, leukopenia (mainly neutropenia), anemia, thrombocytopenia, decreased hemoglobin, hematocrit, platelets
- Myelosuppressive:
  - WBC: Mild
  - Platelets: Mild
  - Onset (days): 7-10
  - Nadir (days): 14
  - Recovery (days): 21
- Neuromuscular & skeletal: Arthralgia, rigors
- Miscellaneous: Flu-like syndrome, diaphoresis

1% to 10%:

- Central nervous system: Headache, delirium, somnolence, neurotoxicity
- Dermatologic: Alopecia, dry skin
- Gastrointestinal: Stomatitis
- Hepatic: Hepatotoxicity
- Neuromuscular & skeletal: Peripheral neuropathy, leg cramps
- Ocular: Blurred vision
- Miscellaneous: Diaphoresis

<1%: Usually patient can build up a tolerance to side effects. Arrhythmias, change in taste, chest pain, confusion, coughing, depression, dyspnea, edema, EEG abnormalities, hypotension, hypothyroidism, increased ALT/AST, increased BUN/creatinine, increased hepatic transaminase, increased uric acid level, myalgia, nasal congestion,

neutralizing antibodies, proteinuria, psychiatric effects, sensitivity to injection, sensory neuropathy, SVT, tachycardia, visual disturbances

Drug Interactions

Increased effect: Cimetidine: May augment the antitumor effects of interferon in melanoma

Increased toxicity:

Vinblastine: Enhances interferon toxicity in several patients; increased incidence of paresthesia has also been noted

Theophylline: Clearance has been reported to be decreased in hepatitis patients receiving interferon

Education and Monitoring Issues

Patient Education: Warts are highly contagious until they completely disappear, abstain from sexual activity or use barrier protection; inform nurse or prescriber if allergy exists to eggs, neomycin, mouse immunoglobulin, or to human interferon alpha; acetaminophen can be used to treat flu-like symptoms

Interferon Beta-1a (in ter FEER on BAY ta-won aye)

Pharmacologic Class Biological Response Modulator

U.S. Brand Names Avonex™

Generic Available No

Mechanism of Action Interferon beta differs from naturally occurring human protein by a single amino acid substitution and the lack of carbohydrate side chains; alters the expression and response to surface antigens and can enhance immune cell activities. Properties of interferon beta that modify biologic responses are mediated by cell surface receptor interactions; mechanism in the treatment of MS is unknown.

Use Treatment of relapsing forms of multiple sclerosis (MS); to slow the accumulation of physical disability and decrease the frequency of clinical exacerbations

USUAL DOSAGE Adults >18 years: I.M.: 30 mcg once weekly

Dosage Forms POWDER for inj, lyophilized: 33 mcg [6.6 million units]

Contraindications History of hypersensitivity to natural or recombinant interferon beta, human albumin, or any other component of the formulation

Warnings/Precautions Interferon beta-1a should be used with caution in patients with a history of depression, seizures, or cardiac disease; because its use has not been evaluated during lactation, its use in breast-feeding mothers may not be safe and should be warned against

Pregnancy Risk Factor C

Adverse Reactions 1% to 10%:

Cardiovascular: CHF (rare), tachycardia, syncope

Central nervous system: Headache, lethargy, depression, emotional lability, anxiety, suicidal ideations, somnolence, agitation, confusion

Dermatologic: Alopecia (rare)

Endocrine & metabolic: Hypocalcemia

Gastrointestinal: Nausea, anorexia, vomiting, diarrhea, chronic weight loss

Hematologic: Leukopenia, thrombocytopenia, anemia (frequent, dose-related, but not usually severe)

Hepatic: Elevated liver enzymes (mild, transient)

Local: Pain/redness at injection site (80%)

Neuromuscular & skeletal: Weakness

Ocular: Retinal toxicity/visual changes

Renal: Elevated BUN and S_{cr}

Miscellaneous: Flu-like syndrome (fever, nausea, malaise, myalgia) occurs in most patients, but is usually controlled by acetaminophen or NSAIDs; dose related abortifacient activity was reported in Rhesus monkeys

Drug Interactions Decreases clearance of zidovudine thus increasing zidovudine toxicity

Half-Life I.M.: 10 hours; S.C.: 8.6 hours

Education and Monitoring Issues

Patient Education: This is not a cure for MS; you will continue to receive regular treatment and follow-up for MS. Use as directed; do not change dosage or schedule of administration without consulting prescriber. Maintain adequate hydration (2-3 L/day of fluids unless instructed to restrict fluid intake). You may experience flu-like syndrome (acetaminophen may help); nausea, vomiting, or loss of appetite (frequent small meals, frequent mouth care, sucking lozenges, or chewing gum may help); drowsiness, dizziness, agitation, or abnormal thinking (use caution when driving or engaging in tasks requiring alertness until response to drug is known). Report unusual bruising or bleeding; persistent abdominal disturbances; unusual fatigue; muscle pain or tremors; chest pain or palpitations, swelling of extremities; visual disturbances; pain, swelling, or redness at injection site; or other unusual symptoms.

Monitoring Parameters: Hemoglobin, liver function, and blood chemistries

Manufacturer Biogen

Related Information

Pharmaceutical Manufacturers Directory *on page 1020*

Interferon Beta-1b (in ter FEER on BAY ta-won bee)

Pharmacologic Class Biological Response Modulator

U.S. Brand Names Betaseron®

Mechanism of Action Interferon beta-1b differs from naturally occurring human protein by a single amino acid substitution and the lack of carbohydrate side chains; alters the expression and response to surface antigens and can enhance immune cell activities. Properties of interferon beta-1b that modify biologic responses are mediated by cell surface receptor interactions; mechanism in the treatment of MS is unknown.

Use Reduces the frequency of clinical exacerbations in ambulatory patients with relapsing-remitting multiple sclerosis (MS)

USUAL DOSAGE S.C.:

Children <18 years: Not recommended

Adults >18 years: 0.25 mg (8 million units) every other day

Dosage Forms POWDER for inj, lyophilized: 0.3 mg [9.6 million units]

Contraindications Hypersensitivity to *E. coli* derived products, natural or recombinant interferon beta, albumin human or any other component of the formulation

Warnings/Precautions The safety and efficacy of interferon beta-1b in chronic progressive MS have not been evaluated; use with caution in women who are breast-feeding; flu-like symptoms complex (ie, myalgia, fever, chills, malaise, sweating) is reported in 53% of patients who receive interferon beta-1b

Pregnancy Risk Factor C

Adverse Reactions Due to the pivotal position of interferon in the immune system, toxicities can affect nearly every organ system: Injection site reactions, injection site necrosis, flu-like symptoms, menstrual disorders, depression (with suicidal ideations), somnolence, palpitations, peripheral vascular disorders, hypertension, blood dyscrasias, dyspnea, laryngitis, cystitis, gastrointestinal complaints, seizures, headache, and liver enzyme elevations

Half-Life I.M., S.C.: 3-6 hours; I.V.: 38 minutes

Education and Monitoring Issues

Patient Education: This is not a cure for MS; you will continue to receive regular treatment and follow-up for MS. Use as directed; do not change dosage or schedule of administration without consulting prescriber. Maintain adequate hydration (2-3 L/day of fluids unless instructed to restrict fluid intake). You may experience flu-like syndrome (acetaminophen may help); nausea, vomiting, or loss of appetite (frequent small meals, frequent mouth care, sucking lozenges, or chewing gum may help); drowsiness, dizziness, agitation, or abnormal thinking (use caution when driving or engaging in tasks requiring alertness until response to drug is known). Report unusual bruising or bleeding; persistent abdominal disturbances; unusual fatigue; muscle pain or tremors; chest pain or palpitations, swelling of extremities; visual disturbances; pain, swelling, or redness at injection site; or other unusual symptoms.

Monitoring Parameters: Hemoglobin, liver function, and blood chemistries

Manufacturer Berlex Laboratories, Inc

Related Information

Pharmaceutical Manufacturers Directory *on page 1020*

- **Intralipid®** *see* Fat Emulsion *on page 351*
- **Intron® A** *see* Interferon Alfa-2b *on page 476*
- **Intropin® Injection** *see* Dopamine *on page 294*
- **Invirase®** *see* Saquinavir *on page 838*
- **Iobid DM®** *see* Guaifenesin and Dextromethorphan *on page 424*
- **Iodex® [OTC]** *see* Povidone-Iodine *on page 756*
- **Iodex-p® [OTC]** *see* Povidone-Iodine *on page 756*

Iodinated Glycerol (EYE oh di nay ted GLI ser ole)

Pharmacologic Class Expectorant

U.S. Brand Names Iophen®; Organidin®; Par Glycerol®; R-Gen®

Use Mucolytic expectorant in adjunctive treatment of bronchitis, bronchial asthma, pulmonary emphysema, cystic fibrosis, or chronic sinusitis

USUAL DOSAGE Oral:

Children: Up to 30 mg 4 times/day

Adults: 60 mg 4 times/day

Contraindications Hypersensitivity to inorganic iodides, iodinated glycerol, or any component; pregnancy, newborns

Pregnancy Risk Factor X

Iodoquinol (eye oh doe KWIN ole)

Pharmacologic Class Amebicide

U.S. Brand Names Yodoxin®

Generic Available No

Mechanism of Action Contact amebicide that works in the lumen of the intestine by an unknown mechanism

Use Treatment of acute and chronic intestinal amebiasis; asymptomatic cyst passers; *Blastocystis hominis* infections; ineffective for amebic hepatitis or hepatic abscess

USUAL DOSAGE Oral:

Children: 30-40 mg/kg/day (maximum: 650 mg/dose) in 3 divided doses for 20 days; not to exceed 1.95 g/day

Adults: 650 mg 3 times/day after meals for 20 days; not to exceed 1.95 g/day

Dosage Forms POWDER: 25 g. **TAB:** 210 mg, 650 mg

Contraindications Known hypersensitivity to iodine or iodoquinol; hepatic damage; pre-existing optic neuropathy

Warnings/Precautions Optic neuritis, optic atrophy, and peripheral neuropathy have occurred following prolonged use; avoid long-term therapy

Pregnancy Risk Factor C

Adverse Reactions

>10%: Gastrointestinal: Diarrhea, nausea, vomiting, stomach pain

1% to 10%:

Central nervous system: Fever, chills, agitation, retrograde amnesia, headache
Dermatologic: Rash, urticaria
Endocrine & metabolic: Thyroid gland enlargement
Neuromuscular & skeletal: Peripheral neuropathy, weakness
Ocular: Optic neuritis, optic atrophy, visual impairment
Miscellaneous: Itching of rectal area

Education and Monitoring Issues

Patient Education: Take as directed; complete full course of therapy. Maintain adequate hydration (2-3 L/day of fluids unless instructed to restrict fluid intake) and nutrition. If GI upset occurs, small frequent meals, frequent mouth care, sucking lozenges, or chewing gum may help. Report unresolved or severe nausea or vomiting, skin rash, fever, or fatigue.

Monitoring Parameters: Ophthalmologic exam

Related Information

Iodoquinol and Hydrocortisone *on page 481*

Iodoquinol and Hydrocortisone

(eye oh doe KWIN ole & hye droe KOR ti sone)

Pharmacologic Class Antifungal Agent, Topical; Corticosteroid, Topical

U.S. Brand Names Vytone® Topical

Dosage Forms CRM: Iodoquinol 1% and hydrocortisone 1% (30 g)

Pregnancy Risk Factor C

- **Iofran ODT®** *see* Ondansetron *on page 676*
- **Ionamin®** *see* Phentermine *on page 726*
- **Iophen®** *see* Iodinated Glycerol *on page 480*
- **Iopidine®** *see* Apraclonidine *on page 70*

Ioxilan (eye OKS ee lan)

Pharmacologic Class Radiopaque Agents

U.S. Brand Names Oxilan®

Mechanism of Action Ioxilan is a nonionic, water soluble, tri-iodinated x-ray contrast agent for intravascular injection. Intravascular injection of a radiopaque diagnostic agent opacifies those vessels in the path of flow of the contrast medium, permitting radiographic visualization of the internal structures of the human body until significant hemodilution occurs.

Use

Intra-arterial: Ioxilan 300 mgI/mL is indicated for cerebral arteriography. Ioxilan 350 mgI/mL is indicated for coronary arteriography and left ventriculography, visceral angiography, aortography, and peripheral arteriography

Intravenous: Both products are indicated for excretory urography and contrast enhanced computed tomographic (CECT) imaging of the head and body

USUAL DOSAGE

Intra-arterial: Coronary arteriography and left ventriculography: For visualization of coronary arteries and left ventricle, ioxilan injection with a concentration of 350 mg iodine/mL is recommended

Usual injection volumes:

Left and right coronary: 2-10 mL (0.7-3.5 g iodine)
Left ventricle: 25-50 mL (8.75-17.5 g iodine)

Total doses should not exceed 250 mL; the injection rate of ioxilan should approximate the flow rate in the vessel injected

Cerebral arteriography: For evaluation of arterial lesions of the brain, a concentration of 300 mg iodine/mL is indicated

Recommended doses: 8-12 mL (2.4-3.6 g iodine)

Total dose should not exceed 150 mL

Dosage Forms SOLN, for inj: 300 mgI/mL, 350 mgI/mL

Contraindications Ioxilan injection is not indicated for intrathecal use

(Continued)

Ioxilan *(Continued)*

Warnings/Precautions Clotting has been reported when blood remains in contact with syringes containing ioxilan; use of plastic syringes in place of glass syringes has been reported to decrease, but not eliminate, the likelihood of *in vitro* clotting. Serious, rarely fatal, thromboembolic events causing myocardial infarction and stroke have been reported during angiographic procedures with both ionic and nonionic contrast media. Therefore, meticulous intravascular administration technique is necessary; caution must be exercised in patients with severely impaired renal function, combined renal and hepatic disease, combined renal and cardiac disease, severe thyrotoxicosis, myelomatosis, or anuria, particularly when large doses are administered.

Intravascularly administered ioxilan is potentially hazardous in patients with multiple myeloma or other paraproteinacious diseases, who are prone to disease-induced renal insufficiency and/or failure. Partial dehydration in the preparation of these patients prior to injection is not recommended since this may predispose the patient to precipitation of the myeloma protein. Reports of thyroid storm following the intravascular use of iodinated radiopaque agents in patients with hyperthyroidism, or with an autonomously functioning thyroid nodule, suggest that this additional risk be evaluated in such patients before use of any contrast agent. Administration of radiopaque materials to patients with known or suspected pheochromocytoma should be performed with extreme caution. Contrast agents may promote sickling in individuals who are homozygous for sickle cell disease when administered intravascularly.

Pregnancy Risk Factor B

Adverse Reactions

1% to 10%:

- Cardiovascular: Angina (1.3%), hypertension (1.1%)
- Central nervous system: Headache (3.6%), fever (1.7%)
- Gastrointestinal: Nausea (1.5%)

<1%: Bradycardia (0.8%), chills (0.6%), diarrhea (0.9%), dizziness (0.8%), hypotension (0.9%), injection site hematomas (0.8%), rash (0.6%), urticaria (0.8%), vomiting (0.9%)

Drug Interactions Increased toxicity: Renal toxicity has been reported in a few patients with liver dysfunction who were given an oral cholecystographic agent followed by intravascular contrast agents such as ioxilan

Education and Monitoring Issues

Patient Education: Patients receiving iodinated intravascular contrast agents should be instructed to:

- Inform prescriber if pregnant
- Inform prescriber if diabetic or have multiple myeloma, pheochromocytoma, homozygous sickle cell disease, or known thyroid disorder
- Inform prescriber if allergic to any drugs or food, or have immune, autoimmune, or immune deficiency disorders; also inform prescriber if previous reactions to injections of dyes used for x-ray procedures
- Inform prescriber about all medications currently being taken, including nonprescription (over-the-counter) drugs, before having this procedure

Monitoring Parameters: Prior to and 24-48 hours after intravascular administration: Thyroid function tests, renal function tests, blood counts, serum electrolytes, and urinalysis should be monitored for and blood pressure, heart rate, electrocardiogram, and temperature should be monitored throughout the procedure

♦ **I-Paracaine®** *see* Proparacaine *on page 782*

Ipecac Syrup (IP e kak SIR up)

Pharmacologic Class Antidote

Generic Available Yes

Mechanism of Action Irritates the gastric mucosa and stimulates the medullary chemoreceptor trigger zone to induce vomiting

Use Treatment of acute oral drug overdosage and in certain poisonings

USUAL DOSAGE Oral:

Children:

- 6-12 months: 5-10 mL followed by 10-20 mL/kg of water; repeat dose one time if vomiting does not occur within 20 minutes
- 1-12 years: 15 mL followed by 10-20 mL/kg of water; repeat dose one time if vomiting does not occur within 20 minutes
- If emesis does not occur within 30 minutes after second dose, ipecac must be removed from stomach by gastric lavage

Adults: 15-30 mL followed by 200-300 mL of water; repeat dose one time if vomiting does not occur within 20 minutes

Dosage Forms SYR: 70 mg/mL (15 mL, 30 mL, 473 mL, 4000 mL)

Contraindications Do not use in unconscious patients when time elapsed since exposure is >1 hour, patients with no gag reflex; following ingestion of strong bases or acids, volatile oils; when seizures are likely

Warnings/Precautions Do not confuse ipecac syrup with ipecac fluid extract, which is 14 times more potent; use with caution in patients with cardiovascular disease and bulimics; may not be effective in antiemetic overdose

Pregnancy Risk Factor C

Adverse Reactions 1% to 10%:

Cardiovascular: Cardiotoxicity
Central nervous system: Lethargy
Gastrointestinal: Protracted vomiting, diarrhea
Neuromuscular & skeletal: Myopathy

Drug Interactions

Decreased effect: Activated charcoal, milk, carbonated beverages
Increased toxicity: Phenothiazines (chlorpromazine has been associated with serious dystonic reactions)

Onset Within 15-30 minutes

Duration 20-25 minutes; can last longer, 60 minutes in some cases

Education and Monitoring Issues

Patient Education: The Poison Control Center should be contacted before administration. Take only as directed; do not take more than recommended or more often than recommended. Follow with 8 oz of water. If vomiting does not occur within 30 minutes, contact the Poison Control Center or emergency services again. Do not administer if vomiting. If vomiting occurs after taking, do not eat or drink until vomiting subsides.

♦ **I-Pentolate®** *see* Cyclopentolate *on page 235*

♦ **I-Phrine® Ophthalmic Solution** *see* Phenylephrine *on page 727*

Ipratropium (i pra TROE pee um)

Pharmacologic Class Anticholinergic Agent

U.S. Brand Names Atrovent®

Generic Available No

Mechanism of Action Blocks the action of acetylcholine at parasympathetic sites in bronchial smooth muscle causing bronchodilation

Use Anticholinergic bronchodilator in bronchospasm associated with COPD, bronchitis, and emphysema

USUAL DOSAGE

Children:

<2 years: Nebulization: 250 mcg 3 times/day
3-14 years: Metered dose inhaler: 1-2 inhalations 3 times/day, up to 6 inhalations/24 hours

Children >12 years and Adults: Nebulization: 500 mcg (1 unit-dose vial) administered 3-4 times/day by oral nebulization, with doses 6-8 hours apart

Children >14 years and Adults: Metered dose inhaler: 2 inhalations 4 times/day every 4-6 hours up to 12 inhalations in 24 hours

Dosage Forms SOLN: Inhalation: 18 mcg/actuation (14 g); Nasal spray: 0.03% (30 mL), 0.06% (15 mL); Nebulizing: 0.02% (2.5 mL)

Contraindications Hypersensitivity to atropine or its derivatives

Warnings/Precautions Not indicated for the initial treatment of acute episodes of bronchospasm; use with caution in patients with narrow-angle glaucoma, prostatic hypertrophy, or bladder neck obstruction; ipratropium has not been specifically studied in the elderly, but it is poorly absorbed from the airways and appears to be safe in this population.

Pregnancy Risk Factor B

Adverse Reactions Note: Ipratropium is poorly absorbed from the lung, so systemic effects are rare

>10%:

Central nervous system: Nervousness, dizziness, fatigue, headache
Gastrointestinal: Nausea, xerostomia, stomach upset
Respiratory: Cough

1% to 10%:

Cardiovascular: Palpitations, hypotension
Central nervous system: Insomnia
Genitourinary: Urinary retention
Neuromuscular & skeletal: Trembling
Ocular: Blurred vision
Respiratory: Nasal congestion

<1%: Rash, stomatitis, urticaria

Drug Interactions

Increased effect with albuterol
Increased toxicity with anticholinergics or drugs with anticholinergic properties, dronabinol

Onset Onset of bronchodilation: 1-3 minutes after administration; Peak effect: Within 1.5-2 hours

Duration Up to 4-6 hours

Education and Monitoring Issues

Patient Education: Use exactly as directed. Do not use more often than recommended. Store solution away from light. Maintain adequate hydration (2-3 L/day of fluids unless instructed to restrict fluid intake). You may experience sensitivity to heat (avoid extremes in temperature); nervousness, dizziness, or fatigue (use caution when driving

(Continued)

Ipratropium *(Continued)*

or engaging in tasks requiring alertness until response to drug is known); dry mouth, unpleasant taste, stomach upset (frequent small meals, frequent mouth care, chewing gum, or sucking hard candy may help); or difficulty urinating (always void before treatment). Report unresolved GI upset, dizziness or fatigue, vision changes, palpitations, persistent inability to void, nervousness, or insomnia.

Related Information

Ipratropium and Albuterol *on page 484*

Ipratropium and Albuterol (i pra TROE pee um & al BYOO ter ole)

Pharmacologic Class Bronchodilator

U.S. Brand Names Combivent®

Dosage Forms AERO: Ipratropium bromide 18 mcg and albuterol sulfate 103 mcg per actuation [200 doses] (14.7 g)

Pregnancy Risk Factor C

Manufacturer Boehringer Ingelheim, Inc

Related Information

Pharmaceutical Manufacturers Directory *on page 1020*

Irbesartan (ir be SAR tan)

Pharmacologic Class Angiotensin II Antagonists

U.S. Brand Names Avapro®

Mechanism of Action Irbesartan is an angiotensin receptor antagonist. Angiotensin II acts as a vasoconstrictor. In addition to causing direct vasoconstriction, angiotensin II also stimulates the release of aldosterone. Once aldosterone is released, sodium as well as water are reabsorbed. The end result is an elevation in blood pressure. Irbesartan binds to the AT1 angiotensin II receptor. This binding prevents angiotensin II from binding to the receptor thereby blocking the vasoconstriction and the aldosterone secreting effects of angiotensin II.

Use Treatment of hypertension alone or in combination with other antihypertensives

USUAL DOSAGE Adults: Oral: 150 mg once daily with or without food; patients may be titrated to 300 mg once daily

Dosage Forms TAB: 75 mg, 150 mg, 300 mg

Contraindications Hypersensitivity to any component

Warnings/Precautions Avoid use or use a much smaller dose in patients who are intravascularly volume-depleted; use caution in patients with unilateral or bilateral renal artery stenosis to avoid a decrease in renal function; AUCs of irbesartan (not the active metabolite) are about 50% greater in patients with Cl_{cr} <30 mL/minute and are doubled in hemodialysis patients

Pregnancy Risk Factor C (1st trimester); D (2nd and 3rd trimesters)

Adverse Reactions

Central nervous system: Fatigue (4%)

Gastrointestinal: Diarrhea (3%), dyspepsia (2%)

Respiratory: Upper respiratory infection (9%), cough (2.8% versus 2.7% in placebo)

>1% but frequency ≤ placebo: Abdominal pain, anxiety, nervousness, chest pain, dizziness, edema, headache, influenza, musculoskeletal pain, pharyngitis, nausea, vomiting, rash, rhinitis, sinus abnormality, tachycardia, urinary tract infection, dizziness, syncope, vertigo

<1% (limited to important or life-threatening symptoms): Hypotension, orthostatic hypotension, fever, chills, facial edema, upper extremity edema, flushing, hypertension, myocardial infarction, angina, arrhythmia, cardiopulmonary arrest, heart failure, hypertensive crisis, pruritus, dermatitis, ecchymosis, erythema, urticaria, sexual dysfunction, decreased libido, gout, constipation, gastroenteritis, flatulence, abdominal distension, muscle cramps, arthritis, muscle aches, chest pain (noncardiac), bursitis, muscle weakness, sleep disturbance, numbness, somnolence, depression, paresthesia, tremor, TIA, cerebrovascular accident, abnormal urination, prostate disorder, epistaxis, bronchitis, congestion, pulmonary congestion, dyspnea, wheezing, vision disturbance, hearing abnormality, ear infection, ear pain, conjunctivitis, increased serum creatinine (0.7% versus 0.9% in placebo). May be associated with worsening of renal function in patients dependent on renin-angiotensin-aldosterone system.

Drug Interactions CYP2C9 enzyme substrate

Inhibitors of CYP2C9 may increase blood levels

Lithium: Risk of toxicity may be increased by irbesartan; monitor lithium levels

Potassium-sparing diuretics (amiloride, potassium, spironolactone, triamterene): Increased risk of hyperkalemia

Potassium supplements may increase the risk of hyperkalemia

Trimethoprim (high dose) may increase the risk of hyperkalemia

Onset Peak levels in 1-2 hours

Duration >24 hours

Half-Life 11-15 hours

Education and Monitoring Issues

Patient Education: Take exactly as directed; do not discontinue without consulting prescriber. Take first dose at bedtime. This drug does not eliminate need for diet or exercise regimen as recommended by prescriber. May cause dizziness, fainting, lightheadedness (use caution when driving or engaging in tasks that require alertness until response to drug is known); nausea, vomiting, or abdominal pain (small frequent meals, frequent mouth care, sucking lozenges, or chewing gum may help); diarrhea (buttermilk, boiled milk, yogurt may help). Report chest pain or palpitations, skin rash, fluid retention (swelling of extremities), difficulty in breathing or unusual cough, or other persistent adverse reactions.

Manufacturer Bristol-Myers Squibb Company (Pharmaceutical Division)

Related Information

Angiotensin-Related Agents Comparison *on page 1226*
Irbesartan and Hydrochlorothiazide *on page 485*
Pharmaceutical Manufacturers Directory *on page 1020*

Irbesartan and Hydrochlorothiazide

(ir be SAR tan & hye droe klor oh THYE a zide)

Pharmacologic Class Antihypertensive Agent, Combination

U.S. Brand Names Avalide®

Dosage Forms TAB: Irbesartan 150 mg and hydrochlorothiazide 12.5 mg; irbesartan 300 mg and hydrochlorothiazide 12.5 mg

Pregnancy Risk Factor C (2nd trimester); D (3rd trimester)

Manufacturer Bristol-Myers Squibb Company (Pharmaceutical Division)

Related Information

Pharmaceutical Manufacturers Directory *on page 1020*

♦ **Ircon® [OTC]** *see* Ferrous Fumarate *on page 359*

Iron Dextran Complex (EYE ern DEKS tran KOM pleks)

Pharmacologic Class Iron Salt

U.S. Brand Names Dexferrum®; InFed™ Injection

Generic Available Yes

Mechanism of Action The released iron, from the plasma, eventually replenishes the depleted iron stores in the bone marrow where it is incorporated into hemoglobin

Use Treatment of microcytic hypochromic anemia resulting from iron deficiency in whom oral administration is infeasible or ineffective

USUAL DOSAGE I.M. (Z-track method should be used for I.M. injection), I.V.:

A 0.5 mL test dose (0.25 mL in infants) should be given prior to starting iron dextran therapy; total dose should be divided into a daily schedule for I.M., total dose may be given as a single continuous infusion

Iron deficiency anemia: Dose (mL) = 0.0476 x wt (kg) x (normal hemoglobin - observed hemoglobin) + (1 mL/5 kg) to maximum of 14 mL for iron stores

Iron replacement therapy for blood loss: Replacement iron (mg) = blood loss (mL) x hematocrit

Maximum daily dose (can administer total dose at one time I.V.):
- Infants <5 kg: 25 mg iron (0.5 mL)
- Children:
  - 5-10 kg: 50 mg iron (1 mL)
  - 10-50 kg: 100 mg iron (2 mL)
- Adults >50 kg: 100 mg iron (2 mL)

Dosage Forms INJ: 50 mg/mL (2 mL, 10 mL)

Contraindications Hypersensitivity to iron dextran, all anemias that are not involved with iron deficiency, hemochromatosis, hemolytic anemia

Warnings/Precautions Use with caution in patients with history of asthma, hepatic impairment, rheumatoid arthritis; not recommended in children <4 months of age; deaths associated with parenteral administration following anaphylactic-type reactions have been reported; use only in patients where the iron deficient state is not amenable to oral iron therapy. A test dose of 0.5 mL I.V. or I.M. should be given to observe for adverse reactions. Anemia in the elderly is often caused by "anemia of chronic disease" or associated with inflammation rather than blood loss. Iron stores are usually normal or increased, with a serum ferritin >50 ng/mL and a decreased total iron binding capacity. I.V. administration of iron dextran is often preferred over I.M. in the elderly secondary to a decreased muscle mass and the need for daily injections.

Pregnancy Risk Factor C

Adverse Reactions

>10%:
- Cardiovascular: Flushing
- Central nervous system: Dizziness, fever, headache, pain
- Gastrointestinal: Nausea, vomiting, metallic taste
- Local: Staining of skin at the site of I.M. injection
- Miscellaneous: Diaphoresis

1% to 10%:
- Cardiovascular: Hypotension (1% to 2%)

(Continued)

Iron Dextran Complex *(Continued)*

Dermatologic: Urticaria (1% to 2%), phlebitis (1% to 2%)
Gastrointestinal: Diarrhea
Genitourinary: Discoloration of urine

<1%: Arthralgia, cardiovascular collapse, chills, leukocytosis, lymphadenopathy, respiratory difficulty

Note: Diaphoresis, urticaria, arthralgia, fever, chills, dizziness, headache, and nausea may be delayed 24-48 hours after I.V. administration or 3-4 days after I.M. administration

Anaphylactoid reactions: Respiratory difficulties and cardiovascular collapse have been reported and occur most frequently within the first several minutes of administration

Drug Interactions Decreased effect with chloramphenicol

Onset Hematologic response: 3-10 days

Education and Monitoring Issues

Patient Education: You will need frequent blood tests while on this therapy. If you have rheumatoid arthritis you may experience increased swelling or joint pain; consult prescriber for medication adjustment. If you experience dizziness or severe headache, use caution when driving or engaging in tasks that require alertness until response to drug is known. Small frequent meals, frequent mouth care, sucking lozenges, or chewing gum may relieve nausea and metallic taste. You may experience increased sweating. Report acute GI problems, fever, difficulty breathing, rapid heartbeat, yellowing of skin or eyes, or swelling of hands and feet.

Monitoring Parameters: Hemoglobin, hematocrit, reticulocyte count, serum ferritin

Reference Range:

Hemoglobin 14.8 mg % (for weight >15 kg), hemoglobin 12.0 mg % (for weight <15 kg)
Serum iron: 40-160 μg/dL
Total iron binding capacity: 230-430 μg/dL
Transferrin: 204-360 mg/dL
Percent transferrin saturation: 20% to 50%

- **Ismelin®** *see* Guanethidine *on page 425*
- **Ismo®** *see* Isosorbide Mononitrate *on page 491*
- **Ismotic®** *see* Isosorbide *on page 490*
- **Isocaine®** *see* Mepivacaine *on page 565*
- **Isocaine® HCl** *see* Mepivacaine *on page 565*
- **Isoclor® Expectorant** *see* Guaifenesin, Pseudoephedrine, and Codeine *on page 425*
- **Isocom®** *see* Acetaminophen, Isometheptene, and Dichloralphenazone *on page 19*
- **Isodine® [OTC]** *see* Povidone-Iodine *on page 756*

Isoetharine (eye soe ETH a reen)

Pharmacologic Class Adrenergic Agonist Agent; Bronchodilator; Sympathomimetic

U.S. Brand Names Arm-a-Med® Isoetharine; Beta-2®; Bronkometer®; Bronkosol®; Dey-Lute® Isoetharine

Generic Available Yes

Mechanism of Action Relaxes bronchial smooth muscle by action on beta$_2$-receptors with very little effect on heart rate

Use Bronchodilator in bronchial asthma and for reversible bronchospasm occurring with bronchitis and emphysema

USUAL DOSAGE Treatments are not usually repeated more than every 4 hours, except in severe cases

Nebulizer: Children: 0.01 mL/kg; minimum dose 0.1 mL; maximum dose: 0.5 mL diluted in 2-3 mL normal saline

Inhalation: Oral: Adults: 1-2 inhalations every 4 hours as needed

Dosage Forms

Isoetharine hydrochloride: **SOLN, inh:** 0.062% (4 mL); 0.08% (3.5 mL); 0.1% (2.5 mL, 5 mL); 0.125% (4 mL); 0.167% (3 mL); 0.17% (3 mL); 0.2% (2.5 mL); 0.25% (2 mL, 3.5 mL); 0.5% (0.5 mL); 1% (0.5 mL, 0.25 mL, 10 mL, 14 mL, 30 mL)

Isoetharine mesylate: **AERO, oral:** 340 mcg/metered spray

Contraindications Known hypersensitivity to isoetharine

Warnings/Precautions Excessive or prolonged use may result in decreased effectiveness

Pregnancy Risk Factor C

Adverse Reactions

1% to 10%:

Cardiovascular: Tachycardia, hypertension, pounding heartbeat
Central nervous system: Dizziness, lightheadedness, headache, nervousness, insomnia
Gastrointestinal: Xerostomia, nausea, vomiting
Neuromuscular & skeletal: Trembling, weakness

<1%: Paradoxical bronchospasm

Drug Interactions
Decreased effect with beta-blockers
Increased toxicity with other sympathomimetics (eg, epinephrine)

Onset Peak effect: Inhaler: Within 5-15 minutes

Duration 1-4 hours

Education and Monitoring Issues

Patient Education: Use as directed. Do not use more often than recommended. Store solution away from light. You may experience nervousness, dizziness, or fatigue (use caution when driving or engaging in tasks requiring alertness until response to drug is known); dry mouth, nausea, or vomiting (frequent small meals and good mouth care may help). Report unresolved/persistent GI upset, rapid heartbeat or palpitations, dizziness or fatigue, trembling, or difficulty breathing.

Monitoring Parameters: Heart rate, blood pressure, respiratory rate

Related Information
Bronchodilators Comparison *on page 1235*

Isoflurophate (eye soe FLURE oh fate)

Pharmacologic Class Cholinergic Agonist

U.S. Brand Names Floropryl® Ophthalmic

Use Treat primary open-angle glaucoma and conditions that obstruct aqueous outflow and to treat accommodative convergent strabismus

USUAL DOSAGE Adults: Ophthalmic:
Glaucoma: Instill 0.25" strip in eye every 8-72 hours
Strabismus: Instill 0.25" strip to each eye every night for 2 weeks then reduce to 0.25" every other night to once weekly for 2 months

Contraindications Active uveal inflammation, angle-closure (narrow-angle) glaucoma, known hypersensitivity to isoflurophate, pregnancy

Pregnancy Risk Factor X

♦ **Isollyl® Improved** *see* Butalbital Compound *on page 123*

Isoniazid (eye soe NYE a zid)

Pharmacologic Class Antitubercular Agent

U.S. Brand Names Laniazid®; Nydrazid®

Generic Available Yes

Mechanism of Action Unknown, but may include the inhibition of myocolic acid synthesis resulting in disruption of the bacterial cell wall

Use Treatment of susceptible tuberculosis infections and prophylactically to those individuals exposed to tuberculosis

USUAL DOSAGE Recommendations often change due to resistant strains and newly developed information; consult *MMWR* for current CDC recommendations: **Oral** (injectable is available for patients who are unable to either take or absorb oral therapy):

Note: A four-drug regimen (isoniazid, rifampin, pyrazinamide, and either streptomycin or ethambutol) is preferred for the initial, empiric treatment of TB. When the drug susceptibility results are available, the regimen should be altered as appropriate.

Infants and Children:
- Prophylaxis: 10 mg/kg/day in 1-2 divided doses (maximum: 300 mg/day) 6 months in patients who do not have HIV infection and 12 months in patients who have HIV infection
- Treatment:
  - Daily therapy: 10-20 mg/kg/day in 1-2 divided doses (maximum: 300 mg/day)
  - Directly observed therapy (DOT): Twice weekly therapy: 20-40 mg/kg (maximum: 900 mg/day); 3 times/week therapy: 20-40 mg/kg (maximum: 900 mg)

Adults:
- Prophylaxis: 300 mg/day for 6 months in patients who do not have HIV infection and 12 months in patients who have HIV infection
- Treatment:
  - Daily therapy: 5 mg/kg/day given daily (usual dose: 300 mg/day); 10 mg/kg/day in 1-2 divided doses in patients with disseminated disease
  - Directly observed therapy (DOT): Twice weekly therapy: 15 mg/kg (maximum: 900 mg); 3 times/week therapy: 15 mg/kg (maximum: 900 mg)

Note: Concomitant administration of 6-50 mg/day pyridoxine is recommended in malnourished patients or those prone to neuropathy (eg, alcoholics, diabetics)

Hemodialysis: Dialyzable (50% to 100%)
Administer dose postdialysis

Peritoneal dialysis effects: Dose for Cl_{cr} <10 mL/minute

Continuous arteriovenous or venovenous hemofiltration (CAVH/CAVHD): Dose for Cl_{cr} <10 mL/minute

Dosing adjustment in hepatic impairment: Dose should be reduced in severe hepatic disease

Dosage Forms INJ: 100 mg/mL (10 mL). **SYR** (orange flavor): 50 mg/5 mL (473 mL). **TAB:** 50 mg, 100 mg, 300 mg

(Continued)

Isoniazid *(Continued)*

Contraindications Acute liver disease; hypersensitivity to isoniazid or any component; previous history of hepatic damage during isoniazid therapy

Warnings/Precautions Use with caution in patients with renal impairment and chronic liver disease. Severe and sometimes fatal hepatitis may occur or develop even after many months of treatment; patients must report any prodromal symptoms of hepatitis, such as fatigue, weakness, malaise, anorexia, nausea, or vomiting. Children with low milk and low meat intake should receive concomitant pyridoxine therapy. Periodic ophthalmic examinations are recommended even when usual symptoms do not occur; pyridoxine (10-50 mg/day) is recommended in individuals likely to develop peripheral neuropathies.

Pregnancy Risk Factor C

Adverse Reactions

>10%:

- Gastrointestinal: Loss of appetite, nausea, vomiting, stomach pain
- Hepatic: Mild increased LFTs (10% to 20%)
- Neuromuscular & skeletal: Weakness, peripheral neuropathy (dose-related incidence, 10% to 20% incidence with 10 mg/kg/day)

1% to 10%:

- Central nervous system: Dizziness, slurred speech, lethargy
- Hepatic: Progressive liver damage (increases with age; 2.3% in patients >50 years of age)
- Neuromuscular & skeletal: Hyper-reflexia

<1%: Arthralgia, blood dyscrasias, blurred vision, fever, loss of vision, mental depression, psychosis, rash, seizures

Drug Interactions CYP2E1 enzyme substrate; CYP2E1 enzyme inducer; and CYP1A2, 2C, 2C9, 2C19, and 3A3/4 enzyme inhibitor

Decreased effect of ketoconazole with isoniazid

Decreased effect/levels of isoniazid with aluminum salts

Increased toxicity/levels of oral anticoagulants, carbamazepine, cycloserine, meperidine, hydantoins, hepatically metabolized benzodiazepines with isoniazid; reaction with disulfiram occurs; enflurane with isoniazid may result in renal failure especially in rapid acetylators

Increased hepatic toxicity with alcohol or with rifampin and isoniazid

Alcohol Interactions Avoid use (increased risk of hepatitis with concurrent use)

Half-Life

Fast acetylators: 30-100 minutes

Slow acetylators: 2-5 hours; half-life may be prolonged in patients with impaired hepatic function or severe renal impairment

Education and Monitoring Issues

Patient Education: Best if taken on an empty stomach (1 hour before or 2 hours after meals). Avoid missing any dose and do not discontinue without notifying prescriber. Avoid alcohol and tyramine-containing foods (eg, fish, preserved meats or sausages, tuna, sauerkraut, aged cheeses, broad beans, liver pate, wine, protein supplements, etc). Increase dietary intake of folate, niacin, magnesium. If diabetic, use serum testing (isoniazid may affect Clinitest® results). You may experience GI distress (taking dose with meals may help). Use caution to prevent injury. You will need to have frequent ophthalmic exams and periodic medical check-ups to evaluate drug effects. Report tingling or numbness in hands or feet, loss of sensation, unusual weakness, fatigue, nausea or vomiting, dark colored urine, change in urinary pattern, yellowing skin or eyes, or change in color of stool.

Monitoring Parameters: Periodic liver function tests; monitoring for prodromal signs of hepatitis

Reference Range: Therapeutic: 1-7 μg/mL (SI: 7-51 μmol/L); Toxic: 20-710 μg/mL (SI: 146-5176 μmol/L)

Manufacturer Hoechst-Marion Roussel

Related Information

Pharmaceutical Manufacturers Directory *on page 1020*
Rifampin and Isoniazid *on page 822*
Rifampin, Isoniazid, and Pyrazinamide *on page 822*
Tuberculosis Test Recommendations and Prophylaxis *on page 1163*
Tuberculosis Treatment Guidelines *on page 1213*

♦ **Isopap®** *see* Acetaminophen, Isometheptene, and Dichloralphenazone *on page 19*
♦ **Isopro®** *see* Isoproterenol *on page 488*

Isoproterenol (eye soe proe TER e nole)

Pharmacologic Class $Beta_1/Beta_2$ Agonist

U.S. Brand Names Aerolone®; Arm-a-Med® Isoproterenol; Dey-Dose® Isoproterenol; Dispos-a-Med® Isoproterenol; Isopro®; Isuprel®; Medihaler-Iso®; Norisodrine®; Vapo-Iso®

Generic Available Yes

Mechanism of Action Stimulates $beta_1$- and $beta_2$-receptors resulting in relaxation of bronchial, GI, and uterine smooth muscle, increased heart rate and contractility, vasodilation of peripheral vasculature

Use Parenterally in ventricular arrhythmias due to A-V nodal block; hemodynamically compromised bradyarrhythmias or atropine-resistant bradyarrhythmias; temporary use in third degree A-V block until pacemaker insertion; low cardiac output; vasoconstrictive shock states; treatment of reversible airway obstruction as in asthma or COPD

USUAL DOSAGE

Children:

Bronchodilation: Inhalation: Metered dose inhaler: 1-2 metered doses up to 5 times/day

Bronchodilation (using 1:200 inhalation solution) 0.01 mL/kg/dose every 4 hours as needed (maximum: 0.05 mL/dose) diluted with NS to 2 mL

Sublingual: 5-10 mg every 3-4 hours, not to exceed 30 mg/day

Cardiac arrhythmias: I.V.: Start 0.1 mcg/kg/minute (usual effective dose 0.2-2 mcg/kg/minute)

Adults:

Bronchodilation: Inhalation: Metered dose inhaler: 1-2 metered doses 4-6 times/day

Bronchodilation: 1-2 inhalations of a 0.25% solution, no more than 2 inhalations at any one time (1-5 minutes between inhalations); no more than 6 inhalations in any hour during a 24-hour period; maintenance therapy: 1-2 inhalations 4-6 times/day. Alternatively: 0.5% solution via hand bulb nebulizer is 5-15 deep inhalations repeated once in 5-10 minutes if necessary; treatments may be repeated up to 5 times/day.

Sublingual: 10-20 mg every 3-4 hours; not to exceed 60 mg/day

Cardiac arrhythmias: I.V.: 5 mcg/minute initially, titrate to patient response (2-20 mcg/minute)

Shock: I.V.: 0.5-5 mcg/minute; adjust according to response

Dosage Forms INH, Aero: 0.2% (1:500) (15 mL, 22.5 mL); 0.25% (1:400) (15 mL). **SOLN for nebulization:** 0.031% (4 mL); 0.062% (4 mL); 0.25% (0.5 mL, 30 mL); 0.5% (0.5 mL, 10 mL, 60 mL); 1% (10 mL). **INJ:** 0.2 mg/mL (1:5000) (1 mL, 5 mL, 10 mL). **TAB, sublingual:** 10 mg, 15 mg

Contraindications Angina, pre-existing cardiac arrhythmias (ventricular); tachycardia or A-V block caused by cardiac glycoside intoxication; allergy to sulfites or isoproterenol or other sympathomimetic amines

Warnings/Precautions Elderly patients, diabetics, renal or cardiovascular disease, hyperthyroidism; excessive or prolonged use may result in decreased effectiveness

Pregnancy Risk Factor C

Adverse Reactions

>10%:

Central nervous system: Insomnia, restlessness

Gastrointestinal: Dry throat, xerostomia, discoloration of saliva (pinkish-red)

1% to 10%:

Cardiovascular: Flushing of the face or skin, ventricular arrhythmias, tachycardias, profound hypotension, hypertension

Central nervous system: Nervousness, anxiety, dizziness, headache, lightheadedness

Gastrointestinal: Vomiting, nausea

Neuromuscular & skeletal: Trembling, tremor, weakness

Miscellaneous: Diaphoresis

<1%: Arrhythmias, chest pain, paradoxical bronchospasm

Drug Interactions

Decreased effect with beta-blockers

Increased pressor effects with sympathomimetics, albuterol, guanethidine, oxytocic agents, TCAs

Arrhythmias with bretylium, theophylline

Onset Onset of bronchodilation: Oral inhalation: Immediately

Duration Oral inhalation: 1 hour; S.C.: Up to 2 hours

Half-Life 2.5-5 minutes

Education and Monitoring Issues

Patient Education:

Sublingual: Do not chew or swallow tables, let them dissolve under the tongue.

Inhalant: Shake canister before use. Administer pressurized inhalation during the second half of inspiration. If more than one dose is necessary, wait at least 1 full minute between inhalations; second inhalation is best delivered after 5-10 minutes. Do not use more often than recommended. Store solution away from light or excess heat or cold.

You may experience nervousness, dizziness, or fatigue (use caution when driving or engaging in tasks requiring alertness until response to drug is known); or dry mouth, nausea, or vomiting (frequent small meals may reduce the incidence of nausea or vomiting). Report chest pain, rapid heartbeat or palpitations, unresolved/persistent GI upset, dizziness, fatigue, trembling, increased anxiety, sleeplessness, or difficulty breathing.

Monitoring Parameters: EKG, heart rate, respiratory rate, arterial blood gas, arterial blood pressure, CVP

Related Information

Bronchodilators Comparison *on page 1235*

Isoproterenol and Phenylephrine *on page 490*

Isoproterenol and Phenylephrine (eye soe proe TER e nole & fen il EF rin)

Pharmacologic Class Adrenergic Agonist Agent

U.S. Brand Names Duo-Medihaler® Aerosol

Dosage Forms AERO: Each actuation releases isoproterenol hydrochloride 0.16 mg and phenylephrine bitartrate 0.24 mg (15 mL, 22.5 mL)

Pregnancy Risk Factor C

- **Isoptin®** *see* Verapamil *on page 975*
- **Isoptin® SR** *see* Verapamil *on page 975*
- **Isopto® Atropine Ophthalmic** *see* Atropine *on page 80*
- **Isopto® Carbachol Ophthalmic** *see* Carbachol *on page 137*
- **Isopto® Carpine Ophthalmic** *see* Pilocarpine *on page 736*
- **Isopto® Cetamide®** *see* Sulfacetamide Sodium *on page 876*
- **Isopto® Cetamide® Ophthalmic** *see* Sulfacetamide Sodium *on page 876*
- **Isopto® Cetapred® Ophthalmic** *see* Sulfacetamide Sodium and Prednisolone *on page 876*
- **Isopto® Eserine** *see* Physostigmine *on page 734*
- **Isopto® Frin Ophthalmic Solution** *see* Phenylephrine *on page 727*
- **Isopto® Homatropine Ophthalmic** *see* Homatropine *on page 438*
- **Isopto® Hyoscine Ophthalmic** *see* Scopolamine *on page 842*
- **Isordil®** *see* Isosorbide Dinitrate *on page 490*

Isosorbide (eye soe SOR bide)

Pharmacologic Class Diuretic, Osmotic

U.S. Brand Names Ismotic®

Generic Available No

Mechanism of Action Elevates osmolarity of glomerular filtrate to hinder the tubular resorption of water and increase excretion of sodium and chloride to result in diuresis; creates an osmotic gradient between plasma and ocular fluids

Use Short-term emergency treatment of acute angle-closure glaucoma and short-term reduction of intraocular pressure prior to and following intraocular surgery; may be used to interrupt an acute glaucoma attack; preferred agent when need to avoid nausea and vomiting

USUAL DOSAGE Adults: Oral: Initial: 1.5 g/kg with a usual range of 1-3 g/kg 2-4 times/day as needed

Dosage Forms SOLN: 45% [450 mg/mL] (220 mL)

Contraindications Severe renal disease, anuria, severe dehydration, acute pulmonary edema, severe cardiac decompensation, known hypersensitivity to isosorbide

Warnings/Precautions Use with caution in patients with impending pulmonary edema and in the elderly due to the elderly's predisposition to dehydration and the fact that they frequently have concomitant diseases which may be aggravated by the use of isosorbide; hypernatremia and dehydration may begin to occur after 72 hours of continuous administration. Maintain fluid/electrolyte balance with multiple doses; monitor urinary output; if urinary output declines, need to review clinical status.

Pregnancy Risk Factor B

Adverse Reactions

1% to 10%:

Central nervous system: Headache, confusion, disorientation

Gastrointestinal: Vomiting

<1%: Abdominal/gastric discomfort (infrequently), anorexia, dizziness, hiccups, hypernatremia, hyperosmolarity, irritability, lethargy, lightheadedness, nausea, rash, syncope, thirst, vertigo

Onset Onset of action: Within 10-30 minutes; Peak action: 1-1.5 hours

Duration 5-6 hours

Half-Life 5-9.5 hours

Education and Monitoring Issues

Monitoring Parameters: Monitor for signs of dehydration, blood pressure, renal output, intraocular pressure reduction

Isosorbide Dinitrate (eye soe SOR bide dye NYE trate)

Pharmacologic Class Vasodilator

U.S. Brand Names Dilatrate®-SR; Isordil®; Sorbitrate®

Generic Available Yes

Mechanism of Action Stimulation of intracellular cyclic-GMP results in vascular smooth muscle relaxation of both arterial and venous vasculature. Increased venous pooling decreases left ventricular pressure (preload) and arterial dilatation decreases arterial resistance (afterload). Therefore, this reduces cardiac oxygen demand by decreasing left ventricular pressure and systemic vascular resistance by dilating arteries. Additionally, coronary artery dilation improves collateral flow to ischemic regions; esophageal smooth muscle is relaxed via the same mechanism.

Use Prevention and treatment of angina pectoris; for congestive heart failure; to relieve pain, dysphagia, and spasm in esophageal spasm with GE reflux

USUAL DOSAGE Adults (elderly should be given lowest recommended daily doses initially and titrate upward): Oral:

Angina: 5-40 mg 4 times/day or 40 mg every 8-12 hours in sustained-release dosage form

Congestive heart failure:

Initial dose: 10 mg 3 times/day

Target dose: 40 mg 3 times/day

Maximum dose: 80 mg 3 times/day

Sublingual: 2.5-10 mg every 4-6 hours

Chew: 5-10 mg every 2-3 hours

Tolerance to nitrate effects develops with chronic exposure

Dose escalation does not overcome this effect. Tolerance can only be overcome by short periods of nitrate absence from the body. Short periods (14 hours) or nitrate withdrawal help minimize tolerance.

Hemodialysis: During hemodialysis, administer dose postdialysis or administer supplemental 10-20 mg dose

Peritoneal dialysis: Supplemental dose is not necessary

See Administration

Dosage Forms CAP, sustained release: 40 mg. **TAB:** Chewable: 5 mg, 10 mg; Oral: 5 mg, 10 mg, 20 mg, 30 mg, 40 mg; Subl: 2.5 mg, 5 mg, 10 mg; Sustained release: 40 mg

Contraindications Severe anemia, closed-angle glaucoma, postural hypotension, cerebral hemorrhage, head trauma, hypersensitivity to isosorbide dinitrate or any component

Warnings/Precautions Use with caution in patients with increased intracranial pressure, hypotension, hypovolemia, glaucoma; sustained release products may be absorbed erratically in patients with GI hypermotility or malabsorption syndrome; do not crush or chew sublingual dosage form; abrupt withdrawal may result in angina; tolerance may develop (adjust dose or change agent). Avoid use with sildenafil.

Pregnancy Risk Factor C

Adverse Reactions Incidence of reactions are not reported.

Cardiovascular: Hypotension (infrequent), postural hypotension, crescendo angina (uncommon), rebound hypertension (uncommon), pallor, cardiovascular collapse, tachycardia, shock, flushing, peripheral edema

Central nervous system: Headache (most common), lightheadedness (related to blood pressure changes), syncope (uncommon), dizziness, restlessness

Gastrointestinal: Nausea, vomiting, bowel incontinence, xerostomia

Genitourinary: Urinary incontinence

Hematologic: Methemoglobinemia (rare, overdose)

Neuromuscular & skeletal: Weakness

Ocular: Blurred vision

Miscellaneous: Cold sweat

The incidence of hypotension and adverse cardiovascular events may be increased when used in combination with sildenafil

Drug Interactions Sildenafil: Significant reduction of systolic and diastolic blood pressure with concurrent use. Do not give sildenafil within 24 hours of a nitrate preparation.

Alcohol Interactions Use with caution (may increase risk of hypotension)

Onset

Sublingual tablet: 2-10 minutes

Chewable tablet: 3 minutes

Oral tablet: 45-60 minutes

Sustained release tablet: 30 minutes

Duration Sublingual tablet: 1-2 hours; Chewable tablet: 0.5-2 hours; Oral tablet: 4-6 hours; Sustained release tablet: 6-12 hours

Half-Life Parent drug: 1-4 hours; Metabolite (5-mononitrate): 4 hours

Education and Monitoring Issues

Patient Education: Take as directed, at the same time each day. Do not chew or swallow sublingual tablets; allow them to dissolve under your tongue. Do not change brands without consulting prescriber. Do not discontinue abruptly. Keep medication in original container, tightly closed. Avoid alcohol; combination may cause severe hypotension. Take medication while sitting down and use caution when changing position (rise from sitting or lying position slowly). May cause dizziness; use caution when driving or engaging in hazardous activities until response to drug is known. If chest pain is unresolved in 15 minutes, seek emergency medical help at once. Report acute headache, rapid heartbeat, unusual restlessness or dizziness, muscular weakness, or blurring vision.

Monitoring Parameters: Monitor for orthostasis

Related Information

Heart Failure Guidelines *on page 1099*

Isosorbide Mononitrate (eye soe SOR bide mon oh NYE trate)

Pharmacologic Class Vasodilator

U.S. Brand Names Imdur™; Ismo®; Monoket®

Generic Available No

(Continued)

Isosorbide Mononitrate *(Continued)*

Mechanism of Action Prevailing mechanism of action for nitroglycerin (and other nitrates) is systemic venodilation, decreasing preload as measured by pulmonary capillary wedge pressure and left ventricular end diastolic volume and pressure; the average reduction in left ventricular end diastolic volume is 25% at rest, with a corresponding increase in ejection fractions of 50% to 60%. This effect improves congestive symptoms in heart failure and improves the myocardial perfusion gradient in patients with coronary artery disease.

Use Long-acting metabolite of the vasodilator isosorbide dinitrate used for the prophylactic treatment of angina pectoris

USUAL DOSAGE Adults: Oral:

Regular tablet: 20 mg twice daily separated by 7 hours; may initiate with 5-10 mg

Asymmetrical dosing regimen of 7 AM and 3 PM or 9 AM and 5 PM to allow for a nitrate-free dosing interval to minimize nitrate tolerance

Extended release tablet (Imdur™): Initial: 30-60 mg once daily; after several days the dosage may be increased to 120 mg/day (given as two 60 mg tablets); daily dose should be taken in the morning upon arising; rarely, 240 mg may be needed

Dosing adjustment in renal impairment: Not necessary for elderly or patients with altered renal or hepatic function

Dosage Forms TAB (Ismo®, Monoket®): 10 mg, 20 mg; Extended release (Imdur™): 30 mg, 60 mg, 120 mg

Contraindications Contraindicated due to potential increases in intracranial pressure in patients with head trauma or cerebral hemorrhage; hypersensitivity or idiosyncrasy to nitrates

Warnings/Precautions Postural hypotension, transient episodes of weakness, dizziness, or syncope may occur even with small doses; alcohol accentuates these effects; tolerance and cross-tolerance to nitrate antianginal and hemodynamic effects may occur during prolonged isosorbide mononitrate therapy; (minimized by using the smallest effective dose, by alternating coronary vasodilators or offering drug-free intervals of as little as 12 hours). Excessive doses may result in severe headache, blurred vision, or dry mouth; increased anginal symptoms may be a result of dosage increases. Avoid use with sildenafil.

Pregnancy Risk Factor C

Adverse Reactions

>10%: Central nervous system: Headache (19% to 38%)

1% to 10%:

Central nervous system: Dizziness (3% to 5%)

Gastrointestinal: Nausea/vomiting (2% to 4%)

<1% (limited to important or life-threatening symptoms): Angina pectoris, arrhythmias, atrial fibrillation, hypotension, palpitations, postural hypotension, premature ventricular contractions, supraventricular tachycardia, syncope, pruritus, rash, abdominal pain, diarrhea, dyspepsia, tenesmus, tooth disorder, vomiting, dysuria, impotence, urinary frequency, asthenia, blurred vision, cold sweat, diplopia, edema, malaise, neck stiffness, rigors, agitation, anxiety, confusion, dyscoordination, hypoesthesia, nightmares, bronchitis, pneumonia, upper respiratory tract infection, arthralgia, methemoglobinemia (rare, overdose)

The incidence of hypotension and adverse cardiovascular events may be increased when used in combination with sildenafil

Drug Interactions Sildenafil: Significant reduction of systolic and diastolic blood pressure with concurrent use. Do not give sildenafil within 24 hours of a nitrate preparation.

Alcohol Interactions Use with caution (may increase risk of hypotension)

Onset Oral: 30-60 minutes

Half-Life Mononitrate: ~4 hours (8 times that of dinitrate)

Education and Monitoring Issues

Patient Education: Take as directed, at the same time each day. Do not chew or crush extended release capsules; swallow with 8 oz of water. Do not change brands without consulting prescriber. Do not discontinue abruptly. Keep medication in original container, tightly closed. Avoid alcohol; combination may cause severe hypotension. Take medication while sitting down and use caution when changing position (rise from sitting or lying position slowly). May cause dizziness; use caution when driving or engaging in hazardous activities until response to drug is known. If chest pain is unresolved in 15 minutes, seek emergency medical help at once. Report acute headache, rapid heartbeat, unusual restlessness or dizziness, muscular weakness, or blurring vision.

Monitoring Parameters: Monitor for orthostasis

Isotretinoin (eye soe TRET i noyn)

Pharmacologic Class Retinoic Acid Derivative

U.S. Brand Names Accutane®

Generic Available No

Mechanism of Action Reduces sebaceous gland size and reduces sebum production; regulates cell proliferation and differentiation

Use Treatment of severe recalcitrant cystic and/or conglobate acne unresponsive to conventional therapy

Investigational: Treatment of children with metastatic neuroblastoma or leukemia that does not respond to conventional therapy

USUAL DOSAGE Oral:

Children: Maintenance therapy for neuroblastoma: 100-250 mg/m²/day in 2 divided doses has been used investigationally

Children and Adults: 0.5-2 mg/kg/day in 2 divided doses (dosages as low as 0.05 mg/kg/day have been reported to be beneficial) for 15-20 weeks or until the total cyst count decreases by 70%, whichever is sooner

Dosing adjustment in hepatic impairment: Dose reductions empirically are recommended in hepatitis disease

Dosage Forms CAP: 10 mg, 20 mg, 40 mg

Contraindications Sensitivity to parabens, vitamin A, or other retinoids; patients who are pregnant or intend to become pregnant during treatment

Warnings/Precautions Use with caution in patients with diabetes mellitus, hypertriglyceridemia; **not to be used in women of childbearing potential** unless woman is capable of complying with effective contraceptive measures; therapy is normally begun on the second or third day of next normal menstrual period; effective contraception must be used for at least 1 month before beginning therapy, during therapy, and for 1 month after discontinuation of therapy. Because of the high likelihood of teratogenic effects (~20%), do not prescribe isotretinoin for women who are or who are likely to become pregnant while using the drug. Isolated reports of depression, psychosis and rarely suicidal thoughts and actions have been reported during isotretinoin usage.

Pregnancy Risk Factor X

Adverse Reactions

>10%:

Dermatologic: Redness, cheilitis, inflammation of lips, dry skin, pruritus, photosensitivity
Endocrine & metabolic: Increased serum concentration of triglycerides
Gastrointestinal: Xerostomia
Local: Burning
Neuromuscular & skeletal: Bone pain, arthralgia, myalgia
Ocular: Itching eyes
Respiratory: Epistaxis, dry nose

1% to 10%:

Cardiovascular: Facial edema, pallor
Central nervous system: Fatigue, headache, mental depression, hypothermia
Dermatologic: Skin peeling on hands or soles of feet, rash, cellulitis
Endocrine & metabolic: Fluid imbalance, acidosis
Gastrointestinal: Stomach upset
Hepatic: Ascites
Neuromuscular & skeletal: Flank pain
Ocular: Dry eyes, photophobia
Miscellaneous: Lymph disorders

<1%: Alopecia, anorexia, bleeding of gums, cataracts, conjunctivitis, corneal opacities, decrease in hemoglobin and hematocrit, hepatitis, hyperuricemia, increase in erythrocyte sedimentation rate, inflammatory bowel syndrome, mood change, nausea, optic neuritis, pruritus, pseudomotor cerebri, vomiting, xerostomia

Drug Interactions

Decreased effect: Increased clearance of carbamazepine

Increased toxicity: Avoid other vitamin A products; may interfere with medications used to treat hypertriglyceridemia

Alcohol Interactions Avoid or limit use (may increase triglyceride levels if taken in excess)

Half-Life Parent drug: 10-20 hours; Metabolite: 11-50 hours

Education and Monitoring Issues

Patient Education: Use exactly as directed; do not take more than recommended. Capsule can be chewed and swallowed, swallowed, or opened with a large needle and contents sprinkled on applesauce or ice cream. Do not take any other vitamin A products, limit vitamin A intake, and increase exercise during therapy. Exacerbations of acne may occur during first weeks of therapy. You may experience headache, loss of night vision, lethargy, or visual disturbances (use caution when driving or engaging in tasks requiring alertness until response to drug is known); photosensitivity (use sunscreen, wear protective clothing and eyewear, avoid direct sunlight); dry mouth or nausea (small frequent meals, sucking hard candy, or chewing gum may may help); dryness, redness, or itching of skin, eye irritation, or increased sensitivity to contact lenses (wear regular glasses). Discontinue therapy and report acute vision changes, rectal bleeding, abdominal cramping, or unresolved diarrhea.

Monitoring Parameters: CBC with differential and platelet count, baseline sedimentation rate, serum triglycerides, liver enzymes

Manufacturer Roche Laboratories

Related Information

Pharmaceutical Manufacturers Directory *on page 1020*

♦ **Isotrex®** *see* Isotretinoin *on page 492*

Isradipine (iz RA di peen)

Pharmacologic Class Calcium Channel Blocker

U.S. Brand Names DynaCirc®

Generic Available No

Mechanism of Action Inhibits calcium ion from entering the "slow channels" or select voltage-sensitive areas of vascular smooth muscle and myocardium during depolarization, producing a relaxation of coronary vascular smooth muscle and coronary vasodilation; increases myocardial oxygen delivery in patients with vasospastic angina

Use Treatment of hypertension, congestive heart failure, migraine prophylaxis

USUAL DOSAGE Adults: 2.5 mg twice daily; antihypertensive response occurs in 2-3 hours; maximal response in 2-4 weeks; increase dose at 2- to 4-week intervals at 2.5-5 mg increments; usual dose range: 5-20 mg/day. **Note:** Most patients show no improvement with doses >10 mg/day except adverse reaction rate increases

Dosage Forms CAP: 2.5 mg, 5 mg

Contraindications Sinus bradycardia; advanced heart block; ventricular tachycardia; cardiogenic shock, hypotension, congestive heart failure; hypersensitivity to isradipine or any component, hypersensitivity to calcium channel blockers and adenosine; atrial fibrillation or flutter associated with accessory conduction pathways; not to be given within a few hours of I.V. beta-blocking agents

Warnings/Precautions Avoid use in hypotension, congestive heart failure, cardiac conduction defects, PVCs, idiopathic hypertrophic subaortic stenosis; may cause platelet inhibition; do not abruptly withdraw (chest pain); may cause hepatic dysfunction or increased angina; increased intracranial pressure with cranial tumors; elderly may have greater hypotensive effect

Pregnancy Risk Factor C

Pregnancy Implications

Clinical effects on the fetus: No data on crossing the placenta

Breast-feeding/lactation: No data on crossing into breast milk. Not recommended due to potential harm to infant.

Adverse Reactions

>10%: Central nervous system: Headache (dose-related 1.9% to 22%)

1% to 10%:

- Cardiovascular: Edema (dose-related 1.2% to 8.7%), palpitations (dose-related 0.8% to 5.1%), flushing (dose-related 0.8% to 5.1%), tachycardia (1% to 3.4%), chest pain (1.7% to 2.7%)
- Central nervous system: Dizziness (1.6% to 8%), fatigue (dose-related 0.4% to 8.5%), flushing (9%)
- Dermatologic: Rash (1.5% to 2%)
- Gastrointestinal: Nausea (1% to 5.1%), abdominal discomfort (0% to 3.3%), vomiting (0% to 1.3%), diarrhea (0% to 3.4%)
- Respiratory: Dyspnea (0.5% to 3.4%)
- Renal: urinary frequency (1.3% to 3.4%)

0.5% to 1% (limited to important or life-threatening symptoms): Pruritus, urticaria, cramps of legs and feet, cough, shortness of breath, hypotension, atrial fibrillation, ventricular fibrillation, myocardial infarction, heart failure, abdominal discomfort, constipation, diarrhea, nocturia, drowsiness, insomnia, lethargy, nervousness, weakness, impotence, decreased libido, depression, syncope, paresthesias,transient ischemic attack, stroke, hyperhidrosis, visual disturbance, dry mouth, gingival hyperplasia (incidence unknown), numbness, throat discomfort, leukopenia, elevated liver function tests

Drug Interactions CYP3A3/4 enzyme substrate

Azole antifungals may inhibit the calcium channel blocker's metabolism; avoid this combination. Try an antifungal like terbinafine (if appropriate) or monitor closely for altered effect of the calcium channel blocker.

Beta-blockers may have increased pharmacokinetic or pharmacodynamic interactions with isradipine

Calcium may reduce the calcium channel blocker's effects, particularly hypotension

Rifampin increases the metabolism of the calcium channel blocker; adjust the dose of the calcium channel blocker to maintain efficacy

Onset Peak serum concentration in 1-2 hours

Duration 8-16 hours

Half-Life 8 hours

Education and Monitoring Issues

Patient Education: Take as prescribed; do not stop abruptly without consulting prescriber immediately. You may experience headache (if unrelieved, consult prescriber), nausea or vomiting (frequent small meals may help), constipation (increased dietary bulk and fluids may help), or depression (should resolve when drug is discontinued). May cause dizziness or drowsiness; use caution when driving or engaging in tasks that require alertness until response to drug is known. Report unrelieved headache, vomiting, constipation, palpitations, swelling of hands or feet, or sudden weight gain.

Manufacturer Novartis

Related Information
Calcium Channel Blocking Agents Comparison *on page 1236*
Pharmaceutical Manufacturers Directory *on page 1020*

♦ **Isuprel®** *see* Isoproterenol *on page 488*

♦ **Isuprel-Neo Mistometer** *see* Isoproterenol and Phenylephrine *on page 490*

Itraconazole (i tra KOE na zole)

Pharmacologic Class Antifungal Agent, Oral; Antifungal Agent, Parenteral

U.S. Brand Names Sporanox®

Generic Available No

Mechanism of Action Interferes with cytochrome P-450 activity, decreasing ergosterol synthesis (principal sterol in fungal cell membrane) and inhibiting cell membrane formation

Use Treatment of susceptible fungal infections in immunocompromised and immunocompetent patients including blastomycosis and histoplasmosis; indicated for aspergillosis, and onychomycosis of the toenail; treatment of onychomycosis of the fingernail without concomitant toenail infection via a pulse-type dosing regimen; has activity against *Aspergillus, Candida, Coccidioides, Cryptococcus, Sporothrix,* tinea unguium

Oral solution (not capsules) is marketed for oral and esophageal candidiasis

Useful in superficial mycoses including dermatophytoses (eg, tinea capitis), pityriasis versicolor, sebopsoriasis, vaginal and chronic mucocutaneous candidiases; systemic mycoses including candidiasis, meningeal and disseminated cryptococcal infections, paracoccidioidomycosis, coccidioidomycoses; miscellaneous mycoses such as sporotrichosis, chromomycosis, leishmaniasis, fungal keratitis, alternariosis, zygomycosis

Intravenous solution is indicated in the treatment of blastomycosis, histoplasmosis (nonmeningeal), and aspergillosis (in patients intolerant or refractory to amphotericin B therapy)

USUAL DOSAGE Oral: Capsule: Absorption is best if taken with food, therefore, it is best to administer itraconazole after meals; Solution: Should be taken on an empty stomach. Absorption of both products is significantly increased when taken with a cola beverage.

Children: Efficacy and safety have not been established; a small number of patients 3-16 years of age have been treated with 100 mg/day for systemic fungal infections with no serious adverse effects reported

Adults:

Oral:

Blastomycosis/histoplasmosis: 200 mg once daily, if no obvious improvement or there is evidence of progressive fungal disease, increase the dose in 100 mg increments to a maximum of 400 mg/day; doses >200 mg/day are given in 2 divided doses; length of therapy varies from 1 day to >6 months depending on the condition and mycological response

Aspergillosis: 200-400 mg/day

Onychomycosis: 200 mg once daily for 12 consecutive weeks

Life-threatening infections: Loading dose: 200 mg 3 times/day (600 mg/day) should be given for the first 3 days of therapy

Oropharyngeal and esophageal candidiasis: Oral solution: 100-200 mg once daily

I.V.: 200 mg twice daily for 4 doses, followed by 200 mg daily

Dosing adjustment in renal impairment: Not necessary; itraconazole injection is not recommended in patients with Cl_{cr} <30 mL/minute

Hemodialysis: Not dialyzable

Dosing adjustment in hepatic impairment: May be necessary, but specific guidelines are not available

Dosage Forms CAP: 100 mg. **INJ kit:** 10 mg/mL - 25 mL ampul, one 50 mL (100 mL capacity) bag 0.9% sodium chloride, one filtered infusion set. **SOLN, oral:** 100 mg/10 mL (150 mL)

Contraindications Known hypersensitivity to other azoles; concurrent administration with astemizole, cisapride, lovastatin, midazolam, simvastatin, or triazolam

Warnings/Precautions Rare cases of serious cardiovascular adverse event, including death, ventricular tachycardia and torsade de pointes have been observed due to increased terfenadine and cisapride concentrations induced by itraconazole. Patients who develop abnormal liver function tests during itraconazole therapy should be monitored and therapy discontinued if symptoms of liver disease develop. Itraconazole injection is not recommended in patients with Cl_{cr} <30 mL/minute.

Pregnancy Risk Factor C

Adverse Reactions Listed incidences are for higher doses appropriate for systemic fungal infections

>10%: Gastrointestinal: Nausea (10.6%)

1% to 10%:

Cardiovascular: Edema (3.5%), hypertension (3.2%)

Central nervous system: Headache (4%), fatigue (2% to 3%), malaise (1.2%), fever (2.5%)

Dermatologic: Rash (8.6%)

Endocrine & metabolic: Decreased libido (1.2%), hypertriglyceridemia

(Continued)

Itraconazole *(Continued)*

Gastrointestinal: Abdominal pain (1.5%), vomiting (5%), diarrhea (3%)
Hepatic: Abnormal LFTs (2.7%), hepatitis

<1%: Adrenal suppression, albuminuria, anorexia, dizziness, gynecomastia, hypokalemia, impotence, pruritus, somnolence

Drug Interactions CYP3A3/4 enzyme substrate; CYP3A3/4 enzyme inhibitor

Decreased effect: Decreased serum levels with carbamazepine, didanosine, isoniazid, phenobarbital, phenytoin, rifabutin, and rifampin. **Should not be administered concomitantly with rifampin**. Absorption requires gastric acidity; therefore, antacids, H_2 antagonists (cimetidine, famotidine, nizatidine, and ranitidine), proton pump inhibitors (omeprazole, lansoprazole, rabeprazole), and sucralfate significantly reduce bioavailability resulting in treatment failures and should not be administered concomitantly; amphotericin B or fluconazole should be used instead

Increased toxicity: Due to inhibition of hepatic CYP3A3/4, itraconazole use is contraindicated with astemizole, cisapride, lovastatin, midazolam, simvastatin, terfenadine, and triazolam due to large substantial increases in the toxicity of these agents, Itraconazole may also increase the levels of amlodipine, benzodiazepines (alprazolam. diazepam, and others), buspirone, busulfan, corticosteroids, cyclosporine, digoxin, HMG-CoA reductase inhibitors (atorvastatin, cerivastatin), oral hypoglycemics (sulfonylureas), phenytoin, protease inhibitors (amprenavir, nelfinavir, ritonavir), tacrolimus, vincristine, vinblastine, and warfarin. Other medications metabolized by CYP3A3/4 should be used with caution.

Half-Life After single 200 mg dose: 21 ±5 hours; 64 hours at steady-state; I.V. steady-state: 35 hours

Education and Monitoring Issues

Patient Education: Take as directed, around-the-clock, with food. Take full course of medication; do not discontinue without notifying prescriber. Practice good hygiene measures to prevent reinfection. If diabetic, test serum glucose regularly (can cause hypoglycemia when given with sulfonylureas). Frequent blood tests may be required with prolonged therapy. You may experience dizziness or drowsiness (use caution when driving or engaging in tasks that require alertness until response to drug is known); nausea, vomiting, or diarrhea (small frequent meals, frequent mouth care, sucking lozenges, or chewing gum may help). Report skin rash or other persistent adverse reactions.

Dietary Considerations:

Capsule: Administer with food; avoid grapefruit juice
Solution: Take without food, if possible

Manufacturer Janssen Pharmaceutical, Inc

Related Information

Pharmaceutical Manufacturers Directory *on page 1020*

♦ **I-Tropine® Ophthalmic** *see* Atropine *on page 80*

Ivermectin (eye ver MEK tin)

Pharmacologic Class Antibiotic, Miscellaneous

U.S. Brand Names Mectizan®; Stromectol®

Generic Available No

Mechanism of Action Ivermectin is a semisynthetic antihelminthic agent; it binds selectively and with strong affinity to glutamate-gated chloride ion channels which occur in invertebrate nerve and muscle cells. This leads to increased permeability of cell membranes to chloride ions then hyperpolarization of the nerve or muscle cell, and death of the parasite.

Use Treatment of the following infections: Strongyloidiasis of the intestinal tract due the nematode parasite *Strongyloides stercoralis*. Onchocerciasis due to the nematode parasite *Onchocerca volvulus*. Ivermectin is only active against the immature form of *Onchocerca volvulus*, and the intestinal forms of *Strongyloides stercoralis*. Ivermectin has been used for other parasitic infections including *Ascaris lumbricoides*, bancroftian filariasis, *Brugia malayi*, scabies, *Enterobius vermicularis*, *Mansonella ozzardi*, *Trichuris trichiura*.

USUAL DOSAGE Oral:

Children ≥5 years: 150 mcg/kg as a single dose; treatment for onchocerciasis may need to be repeated every 3-12 months until the adult worms die

Adults:

Strongyloidiasis: 200 mcg/kg as a single dose; follow-up stool examinations
Onchocerciasis: 150 mcg/kg as a single dose; retreatment may be required every 3-12 months until the adult worms die

Dosage Forms TAB: 6 mg

Contraindications Hypersensitivity to ivermectin or any component

Warnings/Precautions Data have shown that antihelmintic drugs like ivermectin may cause cutaneous and/or systemic reactions (Mazzoti reaction) of varying severity including ophthalmological reactions in patients with onchocerciasis. These reactions are probably due to allergic and inflammatory responses to the death of microfilariae. Patients with hyper-reactive onchodermatitis may be more likely than others to experience severe adverse reactions, especially edema and aggravation of the onchodermatitis. Repeated treatment may be required in immunocompromised patients (eg, HIV); control of extraintestinal strongyloidiasis may necessitate suppressive (once monthly) therapy

Pregnancy Risk Factor C

Adverse Reactions

Percentage unknown: Abdominal pain, blurred vision, diarrhea, dizziness, eosinophilia, headache, hyperthermia, hypotension, increased ALT/AST, insomnia, leukopenia, limbitis, mild conjunctivitis, mild EKG changes, myalgia, nausea, peripheral and facial edema, pruritus, punctate opacity, rash, somnolence, transient tachycardia, tremor, urticaria, vertigo, vomiting, weakness

Mazzotti reaction (with onchocerciasis): Pruritus, edema, rash, fever, lymphadenopathy, ocular damage

Half-Life 16-35 hours

Education and Monitoring Issues

Patient Education: If infected with strongyloidiasis, repeated stool examinations are required to document clearance of the organisms; repeated follow-up and retreatment is usually required in the treatment of onchocerciasis

Monitoring Parameters: Skin and eye microfilarial counts, periodic ophthalmologic exams

Manufacturer Merck & Co

Related Information

Pharmaceutical Manufacturers Directory *on page 1020*

- **IvyBlock®** *see* Bentoquatam *on page 98*
- **Jaa Amp® Trihydrate** *see* Ampicillin *on page 59*
- **Jaa-Prednisone®** *see* Prednisone *on page 763*
- **Jaa Pyral®** *see* Pyrantel Pamoate *on page 793*
- **Janimine®** *see* Imipramine *on page 462*
- **Jenamicin® Injection** *see* Gentamicin *on page 408*
- **Jenest-28™** *see* Ethinyl Estradiol and Norethindrone *on page 342*
- **Junior Strength Motrin® [OTC]** *see* Ibuprofen *on page 458*
- **Junior Strength Panadol® [OTC]** *see* Acetaminophen *on page 17*
- **K-10** *see* Potassium Chloride *on page 751*
- **Kabikinase®** *see* Streptokinase *on page 871*
- **Kadian™** *see* Morphine Sulfate *on page 618*
- **Kalcinate®** *see* Calcium Gluconate *on page 132*
- **Kalium Durules** *see* Potassium Chloride *on page 751*

Kanamycin (kan a MYE sin)

Pharmacologic Class Aminoglycoside (Antibiotic)

U.S. Brand Names Kantrex®

Use

Oral: Preoperative bowel preparation in the prophylaxis of infections and adjunctive treatment of hepatic coma (oral kanamycin is not indicated in the treatment of systemic infections); treatment of susceptible bacterial infection including gram-negative aerobes, gram-positive *Bacillus* as well as some mycobacteria

Parenteral: Rarely used in antibiotic irrigations during surgery

USUAL DOSAGE

Children: Infections: I.M., I.V.: 15 mg/kg/day in divided doses every 8-12 hours

Adults:

Infections: I.M., I.V.: 5-7.5 mg/kg/dose in divided doses every 8-12 hours (<15 mg/kg/day)

Preoperative intestinal antisepsis: Oral: 1 g every 4-6 hours for 36-72 hours

Hepatic coma: Oral: 8-12 g/day in divided doses

Intraperitoneal: After contamination in surgery: 500 mg diluted in 20 mL distilled water; other irrigations: 0.25% solutions

Aerosol: 250 mg 2-4 times/day (250 mg diluted with 3 mL of NS and nebulized)

Dosing adjustment/interval in renal impairment:

Cl_{cr} 50-80 mL/minute: Administer 60% to 90% of dose or administer every 8-12 hours

Cl_{cr} 10-50 mL/minute: Administer 30% to 70% of dose or administer every 12 hours

Cl_{cr} <10 mL/minute: Administer 20% to 30% of dose or administer every 24-48 hours

Hemodialysis: Dialyzable (50% to 100%)

Contraindications Hypersensitivity to kanamycin or any component or other aminoglycosides

Pregnancy Risk Factor D

Related Information

Antimicrobial Drugs of Choice *on page 1182*

Tuberculosis Test Recommendations and Prophylaxis *on page 1163*

Tuberculosis Treatment Guidelines *on page 1213*

- **Kantrex®** *see* Kanamycin *on page 497*
- **Kaochlor®** *see* Potassium Chloride *on page 751*

- **Kaochlor-Eff®** *see* Potassium Bicarbonate, Potassium Chloride, and Potassium Citrate *on page 751*
- **Kaochlor® SF** *see* Potassium Chloride *on page 751*

Kaolin and Pectin With Opium (KAY oh lin & PEK tin with OH pee um)

Pharmacologic Class Antidiarrheal

U.S. Brand Names Parepectolin®

Dosage Forms SUSP, oral: Kaolin 5.5 g, pectin 162 mg, and opium 15 mg per 30 mL [3.7 mL paregoric] (240 mL)

Pregnancy Risk Factor C

- **Kaon** *see* Potassium Gluconate *on page 753*
- **Kaon-Cl®** *see* Potassium Chloride *on page 751*
- **Kaon Cl-10®** *see* Potassium Chloride *on page 751*
- **Kaopectate® II [OTC]** *see* Loperamide *on page 538*
- **Kapectolin PG®** *see* Hyoscyamine, Atropine, Scopolamine, Kaolin, Pectin, and Opium *on page 457*
- **Karidium®** *see* Fluoride *on page 376*
- **Karigel®** *see* Fluoride *on page 376*
- **Karigel®-N** *see* Fluoride *on page 376*
- **Kasof® [OTC]** *see* Docusate *on page 290*

Kava

Pharmacologic Class Herbal

Mechanism of Action Contains alpha-pyrones in root extracts; may possess central dopaminergic antagonistic properties

Use Conditions of nervous anxiety, stress, and restlessness per Commission E; used for sleep inducement and to reduce anxiety

USUAL DOSAGE Per Commission E: Herb and preparations equivalent to 60-120 mg kavalactones

Contraindications Per Commission E: Pregnancy, breast-feeding, endogenous depression. "Extended continuous intake can cause a temporary yellow discoloration of skin, hair and nails. In this case, further application must be discontinued. In rare cases, allergic skin reactions occur. Also, accommodative disturbances (eg, enlargement of the pupils and disturbances of the oculomotor equilibrium) have been described."

Pregnancy Implications Do not use

Adverse Reactions

Central nervous system: Euphoria, depression, somnolence
Dermatologic: Skin discoloration (prolonged use)
Neuromuscular & skeletal: Muscle weakness
Ocular: Eye disturbances

Drug Interactions Coma can occur from concomitant administration of kava and alprazolam; may potentiate alcohol or CNS depressants, barbiturates, psychopharmacological agents

- **Kaybovite-1000®** *see* Cyanocobalamin *on page 233*
- **Kay Ciel®** *see* Potassium Chloride *on page 751*
- **Kayexalate®** *see* Sodium Polystyrene Sulfonate *on page 860*
- **Kaylixir®** *see* Potassium Gluconate *on page 753*
- **K+ Care®** *see* Potassium Chloride *on page 751*
- **K-Dur® 10** *see* Potassium Chloride *on page 751*
- **K-Dur® 20** *see* Potassium Chloride *on page 751*
- **Keflex®** *see* Cephalexin *on page 169*
- **Keflin** *see* Cephalothin *on page 170*
- **Keftab®** *see* Cephalexin *on page 169*
- **Kefurox® Injection** *see* Cefuroxime *on page 165*
- **Kefzol®** *see* Cefazolin *on page 149*
- **Kemadrin®** *see* Procyclidine *on page 775*
- **Kenacort®** *see* Triamcinolone *on page 944*
- **Kenaject-40®** *see* Triamcinolone *on page 944*
- **Kenalog®** *see* Triamcinolone *on page 944*
- **Kenalog-10®** *see* Triamcinolone *on page 944*
- **Kenalog-40®** *see* Triamcinolone *on page 944*
- **Kenalog® H** *see* Triamcinolone *on page 944*
- **Kenalog® in Orabase®** *see* Triamcinolone *on page 944*
- **Kenonel®** *see* Triamcinolone *on page 944*
- **Keppra®** *see* Levetiracetam *on page 517*
- **Keralyt® Gel** *see* Salicylic Acid and Propylene Glycol *on page 836*
- **Kerlone® Oral** *see* Betaxolol *on page 105*
- **Kestrone®** *see* Estrone *on page 334*

Ketoconazole (kee toe KOE na zole)

Pharmacologic Class Antifungal Agent, Oral; Antifungal Agent, Topical

U.S. Brand Names Nizoral®

Generic Available No

Mechanism of Action Alters the permeability of the cell wall by blocking fungal cytochrome P-450; inhibits biosynthesis of triglycerides and phospholipids by fungi; inhibits several fungal enzymes that results in a build-up of toxic concentrations of hydrogen peroxide

Use Treatment of susceptible fungal infections, including candidiasis, oral thrush, blastomycosis, histoplasmosis, paracoccidioidomycosis, coccidioidomycosis, chromomycosis, candiduria, chronic mucocutaneous candidiasis, as well as, certain recalcitrant cutaneous dermatophytoses; used topically for treatment of tinea corporis, tinea cruris, tinea versicolor, and cutaneous candidiasis, seborrheic dermatitis

USUAL DOSAGE

Oral:

Children ≥2 years: 3.3-6.6 mg/kg/day as a single dose for 1-2 weeks for candidiasis, for at least 4 weeks in recalcitrant dermatophyte infections, and for up to 6 months for other systemic mycoses

Adults: 200-400 mg/day as a single daily dose for durations as stated above

Shampoo: Apply twice weekly for 4 weeks with at least 3 days between each shampoo

Topical: Rub gently into the affected area once daily to twice daily

Dosing adjustment in hepatic impairment: Dose reductions should be considered in patients with severe liver disease

Hemodialysis: Not dialyzable (0% to 5%)

Dosage Forms CRM: 2% (15 g, 30 g, 60 g). **SHAMP:** 2% (120 mL). **TAB:** 200 mg

Contraindications Hypersensitivity to ketoconazole or any component; CNS fungal infections (due to poor CNS penetration); coadministration with terfenadine, astemizole, or cisapride is contraindicated due to risk of potentially fatal cardiac arrhythmias

Warnings/Precautions Rare cases of serious cardiovascular adverse event, including death, ventricular tachycardia and torsade de pointes have been observed due to increased terfenadine concentrations induced by ketoconazole. Use with caution in patients with impaired hepatic function; has been associated with hepatotoxicity, including some fatalities; perform periodic liver function tests; high doses of ketoconazole may depress adrenocortical function.

Pregnancy Risk Factor C

Adverse Reactions

Oral:

1% to 10%:

Dermatologic: Pruritus (1.5%)

Gastrointestinal: Nausea/vomiting (3% to 10%), abdominal pain (1.2%)

<1%: Bulging fontanelles, chills, depression, diarrhea, dizziness, fever, gynecomastia, headache, hemolytic anemia, hepatotoxicity, impotence, leukopenia, photophobia, somnolence, thrombocytopenia

Cream: Severe irritation, pruritus, stinging (~5%)

Shampoo: Increases in normal hair loss, irritation (<1%), abnormal hair texture, scalp pustules, mild dryness of skin, itching, oiliness/dryness of hair

Drug Interactions CYP3A3/4 enzyme substrate; CYP1A2, 2C, 2C9, 2C19 (weak), 3A3/4, and 3A5-7 enzyme inhibitor

Decreased effect:

Decreased ketoconazole serum levels with isoniazid and phenytoin; decreased/undetectable serum levels with rifampin - **should not be administered concomitantly with rifampin**; theophylline and oral hypoglycemic serum levels may be decreased

Absorption requires gastric acidity; therefore, antacids, H_2-antagonists (cimetidine and ranitidine), omeprazole, and sucralfate significantly reduce bioavailability resulting in treatment failures; should not be administered concomitantly

Increased toxicity: Due to inhibition of hepatic CYP3A3/4, ketoconazole use is contraindicated with astemizole, cisapride, midazolam, terfenadine, and triazolam due to large substantial increases in the toxicity of these agents. Ketoconazole may also increase the levels of amlodipine, benzodiazepines (alprazolam. diazepam, and others), buspirone, busulfan, corticosteroids, cyclosporine, digoxin, HMG-CoA reductase inhibitors (atorvastatin, cerivastatin, lovastatin, simvastatin), oral hypoglycemics (sulfonylureas), phenytoin, protease inhibitors (amprenavir and indinavir), tacrolimus, vincristine, vinblastine, and warfarin. Other medications metabolized by CYP3A3/4 should be used with caution. A disulfiram-type reaction may occur with concomitant ethanol. Ritonavir increases ketoconazole concentrations.

Alcohol Interactions Avoid use (may cause a disulfiram-like reaction; symptoms include headache, nausea, vomiting, chest or abdominal pain)

Half-Life Biphasic: Initial: 2 hours; Terminal: 8 hours

Education and Monitoring Issues

Patient Education:

Oral: May take with food; at least 2 hours before any antacids. Take full course of medication as directed; some infections may require long periods of therapy. Frequent blood tests may be required with long-term therapy. Practice good hygiene

(Continued)

Ketoconazole *(Continued)*

measures to reduce incidence of reinfection. If diabetic, test serum glucose regularly. You may experience nausea and vomiting (small frequent meals, frequent mouth care, sucking lozenges, or chewing gum may help); headache (mild analgesic may be necessary); or dizziness (use caution when driving). Report unresolved headache, rash or itching, yellowing of eyes or skin, changes in color of urine or stool, chest pain or palpitations, or sense of fullness or ringing in ears.

Topical: Wash and dry area before applying medication thinly. Do not cover with occlusive dressing. Report severe skin irritation or if condition does not improve.

Shampoo: Allow 3 days between shampoos. You may experience some hair loss, scalp irritation, itching, change in hair texture, or scalp pustules. Report severe side effects or if infestation persists.

Monitoring Parameters: Liver function tests

Ketoprofen (kee toe PROE fen)

Pharmacologic Class Nonsteroidal Anti-Inflammatory Agent (NSAID)

U.S. Brand Names Actron® [OTC]; Orudis®; Orudis® KT [OTC]; Oruvail®

Generic Available No

Mechanism of Action Inhibits prostaglandin synthesis by decreasing the activity of the enzyme, cyclo-oxygenase, which results in decreased formation of prostaglandin precursors

Use Acute or long-term treatment of rheumatoid arthritis and osteoarthritis; primary dysmenorrhea; mild to moderate pain

USUAL DOSAGE Oral:

Children 3 months to 14 years: Fever: 0.5-1 mg/kg every 6-8 hours

Children >12 years and Adults:

Rheumatoid arthritis or osteoarthritis: 50-75 mg 3-4 times/day up to a maximum of 300 mg/day

Mild to moderate pain: 25-50 mg every 6-8 hours up to a maximum of 300 mg/day

Dosage Forms CAP: 25 mg, 50 mg, 75 mg; (Orudis®): 25 mg, 50 mg, 75 mg; (Actron®, Orudis® KT [OTC]): 12.5 mg; Extended release (Oruvail®): 100 mg, 150 mg, 200 mg

Contraindications Known hypersensitivity to ketoprofen or other NSAIDs/aspirin

Warnings/Precautions Use with caution in patients with congestive heart failure, hypertension, decreased renal or hepatic function, history of GI disease (bleeding or ulcers), or those receiving anticoagulants; safety and efficacy in children <6 months of age have not yet been established

Pregnancy Risk Factor B; D (3rd trimester)

Adverse Reactions

>10%:

Central nervous system: Dizziness

Dermatologic: Rash

Gastrointestinal: Abdominal cramps, heartburn, indigestion, nausea

1% to 10%:

Central nervous system: Headache, nervousness

Dermatologic: Itching

Endocrine & metabolic: Fluid retention

Gastrointestinal: Vomiting

Otic: Tinnitus

<1%: Acute renal failure, agranulocytosis, allergic rhinitis, anemia, angioedema, arrhythmias, aseptic meningitis, blurred vision, bone marrow suppression, confusion, congestive heart failure, conjunctivitis, cystitis, decreased hearing, drowsiness, dry eyes, epistaxis, erythema multiforme, gastritis, GI ulceration, hallucinations, hemolytic anemia, hepatitis, hot flashes, hypertension, insomnia, leukopenia, mental depression, peripheral neuropathy, polydipsia, polyuria, shortness of breath, Stevens-Johnson syndrome, tachycardia, thrombocytopenia, toxic amblyopia, toxic epidermal necrolysis, urticaria

Drug Interactions CYP2C and 2C9 enzyme inhibitor

Decreased effect of diuretics

Increased effect/toxicity with probenecid, lithium, anticoagulants

Increased toxicity of methotrexate

Alcohol Interactions Avoid use (may enhance gastric mucosal irritation)

Onset Peak levels in 1-2 hours

Half-Life 1-4 hours

Education and Monitoring Issues

Patient Education: Take this medication exactly as directed; do not increase dose without consulting prescriber. Do not crush tablets or break capsules. Take with food or milk to reduce GI distress. Maintain adequate fluid intake (2-3 L/day of fluids unless instructed to restrict fluid intake). Do not use alcohol, aspirin, or aspirin-containing medication, and all other anti-inflammatory medications without consulting prescriber. You may experience drowsiness, dizziness, nervousness, or headache (use caution when driving or engaging in tasks requiring alertness until response to drug is known); anorexia, nausea, vomiting, or heartburn (frequent small meals, frequent mouth care, sucking lozenges, or chewing gum may help); fluid retention (weigh yourself weekly and report unusual (3-5 lb/week) weight gain). GI bleeding, ulceration, or perforation can occur with or without pain; discontinue medication and contact prescriber if persistent abdominal pain or cramping, or blood in stool occurs. Report breathlessness, difficulty breathing, or unusual cough; chest pain, rapid heartbeat, palpitations; unusual bruising/bleeding; blood in urine, stool, mouth, or vomitus; swollen extremities; skin rash or itching; acute fatigue; or changes in hearing or ringing in ears.

Related Information

Nonsteroidal Anti-Inflammatory Agents Comparison *on page 1248*

Ketorolac Tromethamine (KEE toe role ak troe METH a meen)

Pharmacologic Class Nonsteroidal Anti-Inflammatory Agent (NSAID); Ophthalmic Agent

U.S. Brand Names Acular® Ophthalmic; Toradol® Injection; Toradol® Oral

Generic Available No

Mechanism of Action Inhibits prostaglandin synthesis by decreasing the activity of the enzyme, cyclo-oxygenase, which results in decreased formation of prostaglandin precursors

Use Short-term (<5 days) management of pain; first parenteral NSAID for analgesia; 30 mg provides the analgesia comparable to 12 mg of morphine or 100 mg of meperidine

USUAL DOSAGE Note: The use of ketorolac in children <16 years of age is outside of product labeling

Children 2-16 years: Dosing guidelines are not established; **do not exceed adult doses**

Single-dose treatment:

I.M., I.V.: 0.4-1 mg/kg as a single dose; **Note:** Limited information exists. Single I.V. doses of 0.5 mg/kg, 0.75 mg/kg, 0.9 mg/kg and 1 mg/kg have been studied in children 2-16 years of age for postoperative analgesia. One study (Maunuksela, 1992) used a titrating dose starting with 0.2 mg/kg up to a total of 0.5 mg/kg (median dose required: 0.4 mg/kg).

Oral: One study used 1 mg/kg as a single dose for analgesia in 30 children (mean ±SD age: 3 ±2.5 years) undergoing bilateral myringotomy

Multiple-dose treatment: I.M., I.V., Oral: No pediatric studies exist; one report (Buck, 1994) of the clinical experience with ketorolac in 112 children, 6 months to 19 years of age (mean: 9 years), described usual I.V. maintenance doses of 0.5 mg/kg every 6 hours (mean dose: 0.52 mg/kg; range: 0.17-1 mg/kg)

Adults (pain relief usually begins within 10 minutes with parenteral forms):

Oral: 10 mg every 4-6 hours as needed for a maximum of 40 mg/day; on day of transition from I.M. to oral: maximum oral dose: 40 mg (or 120 mg combined oral and I.M.); maximum 5 days administration

I.M.: Initial: 30-60 mg, then 15-30 mg every 6 hours as needed for up to 5 days maximum; maximum dose in the first 24 hours: 150 mg with 120 mg/24 hours for up to 5 days total

I.V.: Initial: 30 mg, then 15-30 mg every 6 hours as needed for up to 5 days **maximum**; maximum daily dose: 120 mg for up to 5 days total

Ophthalmic: Instill 1 drop in eye(s) 4 times/day for up to 7 days

Elderly >65 years: Renal insufficiency or weight <50 kg:

I.M.: 30 mg, then 15 mg every 6 hours

I.V.: 15 mg every 6 hours as needed for up to 5 days total; maximum daily dose: 60 mg

Dosage Forms INJ: 15 mg/mL (1 mL); 30 mg/mL (1 mL, 2 mL). **SOLN, ophth:** 0.5% (5 mL). **TAB:** 10 mg

Contraindications In patients who have developed nasal polyps, angioedema, or bronchospastic reactions to other NSAIDs, active peptic ulcer disease, recent GI bleeding or perforation, patients with advanced renal disease or risk of renal failure, labor and delivery, nursing mothers, patients with hypersensitivity to ketorolac, aspirin, or other NSAIDs, **prophylaxis before major surgery**, suspected or confirmed cerebrovascular bleeding, hemorrhagic diathesis, concurrent ASA or other NSAIDs, epidural or intrathecal administration, concomitant probenecid

Warnings/Precautions Use extra caution and reduce dosages in the elderly because it is cleared renally somewhat slower, and the elderly are also more sensitive to the renal effects of NSAIDs; use with caution in patients with congestive heart failure, hypertension, decreased renal or hepatic function, history of GI disease (bleeding or ulcers), or those receiving anticoagulants

Pregnancy Risk Factor B; D (3rd trimester)

Adverse Reactions

Percentage unknown: Renal impairment, wound bleeding (with I.M.), postoperative hematomas

1% to 10%:

Cardiovascular: Edema

Central nervous system: Drowsiness, dizziness, headache, pain

Gastrointestinal: Nausea, dyspepsia, diarrhea, gastric ulcers, indigestion

Local: Pain at injection site

Miscellaneous: Diaphoresis (increased)

(Continued)

Ketorolac Tromethamine *(Continued)*

<1%: Aphthous stomatitis, change in vision, dyspnea, mental depression, oliguria, peptic ulceration, purpura, rectal bleeding

Drug Interactions

Decreased effect of diuretics

Increased toxicity: Lithium, methotrexate increased drug level; increased effect/toxicity with salicylates, probenecid, anticoagulants

Alcohol Interactions Avoid use (may enhance gastric mucosal irritation)

Onset Analgesic effect: Onset of action: I.M.: Within 10 minutes; Peak effect: Within 75-150 minutes

Duration Analgesic effect: 6-8 hours

Half-Life 2-8 hours; increased 30% to 50% in the elderly

Education and Monitoring Issues

Patient Education: If self-administered, use exactly as directed (do not increase dose or frequency); adverse reactions can occur with overuse. Do not take longer than 5 days without consulting medical advisor. Take with food or milk. While using this medication, do not use alcohol, other prescription or OTC medications including aspirin, aspirin-containing medications, or other NSAIDs without consulting prescriber. Maintain adequate hydration (2-3 L/day of fluids unless instructed to restrict fluid intake). You may experience nausea, vomiting, gastric discomfort (frequent mouth care, small frequent meals, chewing gum, or sucking lozenges may help). GI bleeding, ulceration, or perforation can occur with or without pain. Stop taking medication and report ringing in ears; persistent cramping or pain in stomach; unresolved nausea or vomiting; difficulty breathing or shortness of breath; unusual bruising or bleeding (mouth, urine, stool); skin rash; unusual swelling of extremities; chest pain; or palpitations.

Ophthalmic: Instill drops as often as recommended. Wash hands before instilling. Sit or lie down to instill. Open eye, look at ceiling, and instill prescribed amount of solution. Close eye and roll eye in all directions, and apply gentle pressure to inner corner of eye for 1-2 minutes after instillation. Do not let tip of applicator touch eye or contaminate tip of applicator. Temporary stinging or blurred vision may occur. Report persistent pain, burning, double vision, swelling, itching, worsening of condition. Inform prescriber if you are or intend to be pregnant. Do not breast-feed.

Dietary Considerations:

Potassium: Hyperkalemia has been reported. The elderly and those with renal insufficiency are at greatest risk. Monitor potassium serum concentration in those at greatest risk. Avoid salt substitutes.

Sodium: Hyponatremia from sodium retention. Suspect secondary to suppression of renal prostaglandin. Monitor serum concentration and fluid status. May need to restrict fluid.

Monitoring Parameters: Monitor response (pain, range of motion, grip strength, mobility, ADL function), inflammation; observe for weight gain, edema; monitor renal function (serum creatinine, BUN, urine output); observe for bleeding, bruising; evaluate gastrointestinal effects (abdominal pain, bleeding, dyspepsia); mental confusion, disorientation, CBC, liver function tests

Reference Range: Serum concentration: Therapeutic: 0.3-5 μg/mL; Toxic: >5 μg/mL

Ketotifen (kee toe TYE fen)

Pharmacologic Class Antihistamine, H_1 Blocker, Ophthalmic

U.S. Brand Names Zaditor™

Mechanism of Action Relatively selective, noncompetitive H_1-receptor antagonist and mast cell stabilizer, inhibiting the release of mediators from cells involved in hypersensitivity reactions

Use Temporary prevention of eye itching due to allergic conjunctivitis

USUAL DOSAGE Adults: Ophthalmic: Instill 1 drop into the affected eye (s) every 8-12 hours

Dosage Forms SOLN, ophth: 0.025% (5 mL)

Contraindications Known hypersensitivity to ketotifen or any component of the formulation (the preservative is benzalkonium chloride)

Warnings/Precautions For topical ophthalmic use only. Not to treat contact lens-related irritation. After ketotifen use, soft contact lens wearers should wait at least 10 minutes before putting their lenses in. Do not wear contact lenses if eyes are red. Do not contaminate dropper tip or solution when placing drops in eyes. Safety and efficacy not established for children <3 years of age.

Pregnancy Risk Factor C

Pregnancy Implications Oral treatment administered to pregnant animals have resulted in retarded ossification of the sternebrae, slight increase in postnatal mortality, and a decrease in weight gain in the first 4 days of life. Topical ocular administration has not been studied. Caution should be used when ketotifen is administered to a nursing mother.

Adverse Reactions 1% to 10%:

Ocular: Allergic reactions, burning or stinging, conjunctivitis, discharge, dry eyes, eye pain, eyelid disorder, itching, keratitis, lacrimation disorder, mydriasis, photophobia, rash

Respiratory: Pharyngitis
Miscellaneous: Flu syndrome

Onset Within minutes

Duration 8-12 hours

Education and Monitoring Issues

Patient Education: For topical ophthalmic use only. Not to be used to treat contact lens-related irritation. After ketotifen's use, soft contact lens wearers should wait at least 10 minutes before putting their contact lenses in. Do not wear contact lenses if eyes are red. Do not contaminate dropper tip or solution when placing drops in eyes. Store at room temperature

- **K-Exit** *see* Sodium Polystyrene Sulfonate *on page 860*
- **Key-Pred® Injection** *see* Prednisolone *on page 762*
- **Key-Pred-SP® Injection** *see* Prednisolone *on page 762*
- **K-G®** *see* Potassium Gluconate *on page 753*
- **K-Ide®** *see* Potassium Bicarbonate and Potassium Citrate, Effervescent *on page 751*
- **Kinesed®** *see* Hyoscyamine, Atropine, Scopolamine, and Phenobarbital *on page 456*
- **Klaron® Lotion** *see* Sulfacetamide Sodium *on page 876*
- **Klean-Prep®** *see* Polyethylene Glycol-Electrolyte Solution *on page 747*
- **K-Lease®** *see* Potassium Chloride *on page 751*
- **K-Long** *see* Potassium Chloride *on page 751*
- **Klonopin™** *see* Clonazepam *on page 214*
- **K-Lor™** *see* Potassium Chloride *on page 751*
- **Klor-Con®** *see* Potassium Chloride *on page 751*
- **Klor-Con® 8** *see* Potassium Chloride *on page 751*
- **Klor-Con® 10** *see* Potassium Chloride *on page 751*
- **Klor-Con/25®** *see* Potassium Chloride *on page 751*
- **Klor-Con®/EF** *see* Potassium Bicarbonate and Potassium Citrate, Effervescent *on page 751*
- **Klorvess® Effervescent** *see* Potassium Bicarbonate and Potassium Chloride, Effervescent *on page 751*
- **Klotrix®** *see* Potassium Chloride *on page 751*
- **K-Lyte®** *see* Potassium Bicarbonate and Potassium Citrate, Effervescent *on page 751*
- **K/Lyte/CL®** *see* Potassium Bicarbonate and Potassium Chloride, Effervescent *on page 751*
- **K-Lyte/Cl®** *see* Potassium Chloride *on page 751*
- **K-Med 900** *see* Potassium Chloride *on page 751*
- **K-Norm®** *see* Potassium Chloride *on page 751*
- **Kolephrin® GG/DM [OTC]** *see* Guaifenesin and Dextromethorphan *on page 424*
- **Kolyum®** *see* Potassium Chloride and Potassium Gluconate *on page 753*
- **Konakion®** *see* Phytonadione *on page 735*
- **Konakion® Injection** *see* Phytonadione *on page 735*
- **Kondon's Nasal® [OTC]** *see* Ephedrine *on page 315*
- **Konsyl® [OTC]** *see* Psyllium *on page 793*
- **Konsyl-D® [OTC]** *see* Psyllium *on page 793*
- **K-Phos® Neutral** *see* Potassium Phosphate and Sodium Phosphate *on page 755*
- **K-Phos® Original** *see* Potassium Acid Phosphate *on page 751*
- **K-Tab®** *see* Potassium Chloride *on page 751*
- **Ku-Zyme® HP** *see* Pancrelipase *on page 698*
- **K-Vescent®** *see* Potassium Bicarbonate and Potassium Citrate, Effervescent *on page 751*
- **Kwelcof®** *see* Hydrocodone and Guaifenesin *on page 445*
- **Kwell®** *see* Lindane *on page 531*
- **Kwellada®** *see* Lindane *on page 531*
- **Kytril™** *see* Granisetron *on page 421*
- **LA-12®** *see* Hydroxocobalamin *on page 451*

Labetalol (la BET a lole)

Pharmacologic Class Alpha-/Beta- Blocker; Beta Blocker, Nonselective

U.S. Brand Names Normodyne®; Trandate®

Generic Available No

Mechanism of Action Blocks alpha-, beta$_1$-, and beta$_2$-adrenergic receptor sites; elevated renins are reduced

Use Treatment of mild to severe hypertension with or without other agents; I.V. for hypertensive emergencies

Unlabeled use: Pheochromocytoma, clonidine withdrawal hypertension

USUAL DOSAGE Due to limited documentation of its use, labetalol should be initiated cautiously in pediatric patients with careful dosage adjustment and blood pressure monitoring

(Continued)

Labetalol *(Continued)*

Children:

Oral: Limited information regarding labetalol use in pediatric patients is currently available in literature. Some centers recommend initial oral doses of 4 mg/kg/day in 2 divided doses. Reported oral doses have started at 3 mg/kg/day and 20 mg/kg/day and have increased up to 40 mg/kg/day.

I.V., intermittent bolus doses of 0.3-1 mg/kg/dose have been reported

For treatment of pediatric hypertensive emergencies, initial continuous infusions of 0.4-1 mg/kg/hour with a maximum of 3 mg/kg/hour have been used; administration requires the use of an infusion pump

Adults:

Oral: Initial: 100 mg twice daily, may increase as needed every 2-3 days by 100 mg until desired response is obtained; usual dose: 200-400 mg twice daily; may require up to 2.4 g/day

I.V.: 20 mg (0.25 mg/kg for an 80 kg patient) IVP over 2 minutes, may administer 40-80 mg at 10-minute intervals, up to 300 mg total dose

I.V. infusion: Initial: 2 mg/minute; titrate to response up to 300 mg total dose, if needed; administration requires the use of an infusion pump

I.V. infusion (500 mg/250 mL D_5W) rates:

1 mg/minute: 30 mL/hour
2 mg/minute: 60 mL/hour
3 mg/minute: 90 mL/hour
4 mg/minute: 120 mL/hour
5 mg/minute: 150 mL/hour
6 mg/minute: 180 mL/hour

Dialysis: Not removed by hemo- or peritoneal dialysis; supplemental dose is not necessary

Dosage adjustment in hepatic impairment: Dosage reduction may be necessary

Dosage Forms INJ: 5 mg/mL (20 mL, 40 mL, 60 mL). **TAB:** 100 mg, 200 mg, 300 mg

Contraindications Cardiogenic shock, uncompensated congestive heart failure, bradycardia, pulmonary edema, or heart block

Warnings/Precautions Paradoxical increase in blood pressure has been reported with treatment of pheochromocytoma or clonidine withdrawal syndrome; use with caution in patients with hyper-reactive airway disease, congestive heart failure, diabetes mellitus, hepatic dysfunction; orthostatic hypotension may occur with I.V. administration; patient should remain supine during and for up to 3 hours after I.V. administration; use with caution in impaired hepatic function (discontinue if signs of liver dysfunction occur); may mask the signs and symptoms of hypoglycemia; a lower hemodynamic response rate and higher incidence of toxicity may be observed with administration to elderly patients.

Pregnancy Risk Factor C (per manufacturer); D (2nd or 3rd trimester, based on expert analysis)

Pregnancy Implications

Clinical effects on the fetus: Crosses the placenta. Bradycardia, hypotension, hypoglycemia, intrauterine growth rate (IUGR). IUGR probably related to maternal hypertension. Available evidence suggests safe use during pregnancy and breast-feeding. Monitor breast-fed infant for symptoms of beta-blockade.

Breast-feeding/lactation: Crosses into breast milk. American Academy of Pediatrics considers **compatible** with breast-feeding.

Adverse Reactions

>10%: Central nervous system: Dizziness (1% to 16%)

Gastrointestinal: Nausea (0% to 19%)

1% to 10%:

Cardiovascular: Edema (0% to 2%), hypotension (1% to 5%); with IV use, hypotension may occur in up to 58%

Central nervous system: Fatigue (1% to 10%), paresthesia (1% to 5%), headache (2%), vertigo (2%), weakness (1%)

Dermatologic: Rash (1%), scalp tingling (1% to 5%)

Gastrointestinal: Vomiting (<1% to 3%), dyspepsia (1% to 4%)

Genitourinary: Ejaculatory failure (0% to 5%), impotence (1% to 4%)

Hepatic: Increased transaminases (4%)

Respiratory: Nasal congestion (1% to 6%), dyspnea (2%)

Miscellaneous: Taste disorder (1%), abnormal vision (1%)

<1% (limited to important or life-threatening symptoms): Hypotension, syncope, bradycardia, heart block, fever, diarrhea, drowsiness, increased sweating, systemic lupus erythematosus, positive ANA, dry eyes, antimitochondrial antibodies, hepatic necrosis, hepatitis, cholestatic jaundice, muscle cramps, toxic myopathy, bronchospasm, Peyronie's disease, alopecia (reversible), micturition difficulty, urinary retention, hypersensitivity, urticaria, angioedema, pruritus, anaphylactoid reaction, Raynaud's syndrome, claudication, congestive heart failure, ventricular arrhythmias (I.V.)

Case reports: Fever, toxic myopathy, muscle cramps, systemic lupus erythematosus, diabetes insipidus

Other adverse reactions noted with beta-adrenergic blocking agents include mental depression, catatonia, disorientation, short-term memory loss, emotional lability, clouded sensorium, intensification of pre-existing A-V block, laryngospasm, respiratory distress, agranulocytosis, thrombocytopenic purpura, nonthrombocytopenic purpura, mesenteric artery thrombosis, ischemic colitis

Drug Interactions CYP2D6 substrate/inhibitor

Inhibitors of CYP2D6 including quinidine, paroxetine, and propafenone are likely to increase blood levels of labetalol

Alpha-blockers (prazosin, terazosin): Concurrent use of beta-blockers may increase risk of orthostasis

Cimetidine increases the bioavailability of labetalol

Halothane, isoflurane, enflurane (possibly other inhalational anesthetics): Excessive hypotension may occur

NSAIDs may reduce antihypertensive efficacy of labetalol

Sulfonylureas: Effects may be decreased by beta-blockers

Salicylates may reduce the antihypertensive effects of beta-blockers

NSAIDs (ibuprofen, indomethacin, naproxen, piroxicam) may reduce the antihypertensive effects of beta-blockers

Verapamil or diltiazem may have synergistic or additive pharmacological effects when taken concurrently with beta-blockers; avoid concurrent I.V. use

Alcohol Interactions Limit use (may increase risk of hypotension or dizziness)

Onset

Oral: 20 minutes to 2 hours

I.V.: 2-5 minutes

Peak effect: Oral: 1-4 hours; I.V.: 5-15 minutes

Duration Oral: 8-24 hours (dose-dependent); I.V.: 2-4 hours

Half-Life Normal renal function: 6-8 hours

Education and Monitoring Issues

Patient Education: For I.V. use in emergency situations - patient information is included in general instruction. Oral: Take as directed, with meals. Do not skip dose or discontinue without consulting prescriber. Follow recommended diet and exercise program. Do not use alcohol or OTC medications which may affect blood pressure (eg, cough or cold remedies, diet pills, stay-awake medications) without consulting prescriber. If diabetic, monitor serum glucose closely and notify prescriber of changes; this medication can alter glycemic response. You may experience drowsiness, dizziness, or impaired judgment (use caution when driving or engaging in tasks that require alertness until response to drug is known); postural hypotension (use caution when rising from sitting or lying position or when climbing stairs); dry mouth, nausea, or loss of appetite (frequent mouth care or sucking lozenges may help); or sexual dysfunction (reversible, may resolve with continued use). Report altered CNS status (eg, fatigue, depression, numbness or tingling of fingers, toes, or skin); palpitations or slowed heartbeat; difficulty breathing; edema or cold extremities; or other persistent side effects.

Monitoring Parameters: Blood pressure, standing and sitting/supine, pulse, cardiac monitor and blood pressure monitor required for I.V. administration

Related Information

Beta-Blockers Comparison *on page 1233*

♦ **LaBID®** *see* Theophylline Salts *on page 906*

♦ **LactiCare-HC®** *see* Hydrocortisone *on page 447*

♦ **Lactinex® [OTC]** *see Lactobacillus acidophilus* and *Lactobacillus bulgaricus on page 505*

Lactobacillus acidophilus and *Lactobacillus bulgaricus*

(lak toe ba SIL us as i DOF fil us & lak toe ba SIL us bul GAR i cus)

Pharmacologic Class Antidiarrheal

U.S. Brand Names Bacid® [OTC]; Lactinex® [OTC]; More-Dophilus® [OTC]

Generic Available No

Mechanism of Action Creates an environment unfavorable to potentially pathogenic fungi or bacteria through the production of lactic acid, and favors establishment of an aciduric flora, thereby suppressing the growth of pathogenic microorganisms; helps re-establish normal intestinal flora

Use Treatment of uncomplicated diarrhea particularly that caused by antibiotic therapy; re-establish normal physiologic and bacterial flora of the intestinal tract

USUAL DOSAGE Children >3 years and Adults: Oral:

Capsules: 2 capsules 2-4 times/day

Granules: 1 packet added to or taken with cereal, food, milk, fruit juice, or water, 3-4 times/day

Powder: 1 teaspoonful daily with liquid

Tablet, chewable: 4 tablets 3-4 times/day; may follow each dose with a small amount of milk, fruit juice, or water

Dosage Forms CAP: 50s, 100s. **GRANULES:** 1 g/packet (12 packets/box). **POWDER:** 12 oz. **TAB, chewable:** 50s

Contraindications Allergy to milk or lactose

Warnings/Precautions Discontinue if high fever present; do not use in children <3 years of age

Adverse Reactions 1% to 10%: Gastrointestinal: Intestinal flatus

(Continued)

Lactobacillus acidophilus **and** ***Lactobacillus bulgaricus*** *(Continued)*

Education and Monitoring Issues

Patient Education: Granules may be added to or taken with cereal, food, milk, fruit juice, or water. You may experience increased flatus while taking this medication. Discontinue and notify prescriber if a high fever develops.

- **Lactulax** *see* Lactulose *on page 506*

Lactulose (LAK tyoo lose)

Pharmacologic Class Ammonium Detoxicant; Laxative, Miscellaneous

U.S. Brand Names Cephulac®; Cholac®; Chronulac®; Constilac®; Constulose®; Duphalac®; Enulose®; Evalose®; Heptalac®; Lactulose PSE®

Generic Available Yes

Mechanism of Action The bacterial degradation of lactulose resulting in an acidic pH inhibits the diffusion of NH_3 into the blood by causing the conversion of NH_3 to NH_4+; also enhances the diffusion of NH_3 from the blood into the gut where conversion to NH_4+ occurs; produces an osmotic effect in the colon with resultant distention promoting peristalsis

Use Adjunct in the prevention and treatment of portal-systemic encephalopathy (PSE); treatment of chronic constipation

USUAL DOSAGE Diarrhea may indicate overdosage and responds to dose reduction

Prevention of portal systemic encephalopathy (PSE): Oral:

Infants: 2.5-10 mL/day divided 3-4 times/day; adjust dosage to produce 2-3 stools/day

Older Children: Daily dose of 40-90 mL divided 3-4 times/day; if initial dose causes diarrhea, then reduce it immediately; adjust dosage to produce 2-3 stools/day

Constipation:

Children: 5 g/day (7.5 mL) after breakfast

Adults:

Acute PSE:

Oral: 20-30 g (30-45 mL) every 1-2 hours to induce rapid laxation; adjust dosage daily to produce 2-3 soft stools; doses of 30-45 mL may be given hourly to cause rapid laxation, then reduce to recommended dose; usual daily dose: 60-100 g (90-150 mL) daily

Rectal administration: 200 g (300 mL) diluted with 700 mL of H_20 or NS; administer rectally via rectal balloon catheter and retain 30-60 minutes every 4-6 hours

Constipation: Oral: 15-30 mL/day increased to 60 mL/day if necessary

Dosage Forms SYR: 10 g/15 mL (15 mL, 30 mL, 237 mL, 473 mL, 946 mL, 1890 mL)

Contraindications Patients with galactosemia and require a low galactose diet, hypersensitivity to any component

Warnings/Precautions Use with caution in patients with diabetes mellitus; monitor periodically for electrolyte imbalance when lactulose is used >6 months or in patients predisposed to electrolyte abnormalities (eg, elderly); patients receiving lactulose and an oral anti-infective agent should be monitored for possible inadequate response to lactulose

Pregnancy Risk Factor B

Adverse Reactions

>10%: Gastrointestinal: Flatulence, diarrhea (excessive dose)

1% to 10%: Gastrointestinal: Abdominal discomfort, nausea, vomiting

Drug Interactions Decreased effect: Oral neomycin, laxatives, antacids

Onset 1-4 hours

Education and Monitoring Issues

Patient Education: Not for long-term use. Take as directed, alone, or diluted with water, juice or milk, or take with food. Laxative results may not occur for 24-48 hours; do not take more often than recommended or for a longer time than recommended. Do not use any other laxatives while taking lactulose. Increased fiber, fluids, and exercise may help reduce constipation. Do not use if experiencing abdominal pain, nausea, or vomiting. Diarrhea may indicate overdose. May cause flatulence, belching, or abdominal cramping. Report persistent or severe diarrhea or abdominal cramping.

Monitoring Parameters: Blood pressure, standing/supine; serum potassium, bowel movement patterns, fluid status, serum ammonia

- **Lactulose PSE®** *see* Lactulose *on page 506*
- **Lamictal®** *see* Lamotrigine *on page 507*
- **Lamisil® [OTC]** *see* Terbinafine *on page 896*
- **Lamisil® Dermgel®** *see* Terbinafine *on page 896*

Lamivudine (la MI vyoo deen)

Pharmacologic Class Antiretroviral Agent, Reverse Transcriptase Inhibitor (Non-Nucleoside)

U.S. Brand Names Epivir®; Epivir® HBV

Use Treatment of HIV infection when antiretroviral therapy is warranted; should always be used as part of a multidrug regimen (at least three antiretroviral agents); indicated for the treatment of chronic hepatitis B associated with evidence of hepatitis B viral replication and active liver inflammation

USUAL DOSAGE Oral: Use with at least two other antiretroviral agents when treating HIV

Children 3 months to 12 years: 4 mg/kg twice daily (maximum: 150 mg twice daily)

Adolescents 12-16 years and Adults: 150 mg twice daily

Prevention of HIV following needlesticks: 150 mg twice daily (with zidovudine and a protease inhibitor)

Adults <50 kg: 2 mg/kg twice daily

Treatment of hepatitis B: 100 mg/day

Dosing interval in renal impairment in patients >16 years for HIV:

Cl_{cr} 30-49 mL/minute: Administer 150 mg once daily

Cl_{cr} 15-29 mL/minute: Administer 150 mg first dose, then 100 mg once daily

Cl_{cr} 5-14 mL/minute: Administer 150 mg first dose, then 50 mg once daily

Cl_{cr} <5 mL/minute: Administer 50 mg first dose, then 25 mg once daily

Dosing interval in renal impairment in patients with hepatitis B:

Cl_{cr} 30-49: Administer 100 mg first dose then 50 mg once daily

Cl_{cr} 15-29: Administer 100 mg first dose then 25 mg once daily

Cl_{cr} 5-14: Administer 35 mg first dose then 15 mg once daily

Cl_{cr} <5: Administer 35 mg first dose then 10 mg once daily

Dialysis: No data available

Contraindications Hypersensitivity to lamivudine or any component

Warnings/Precautions A decreased dosage is recommended in patients with renal dysfunction since AUC, C_{max}, and half-life increased with diminishing renal function; use with extreme caution in children with history of pancreatitis or risk factors for development of pancreatitis. Do not use as monotherapy in treatment of HIV.

Pregnancy Risk Factor C

Adverse Reactions

>10%:

- Central nervous system: Headache, insomnia, malaise, fatigue, pain
- Gastrointestinal: Nausea, diarrhea, vomiting
- Neuromuscular & skeletal: Peripheral neuropathy, paresthesia
- Respiratory: Nasal signs and symptoms, cough

1% to 10%:

- Central nervous system: Dizziness, depression, fever, chills
- Dermatologic: Rashes
- Gastrointestinal: Anorexia, abdominal pain, dyspepsia, increased amylase
- Hematologic: Neutropenia, anemia
- Hepatic: Elevated AST/ALT
- Neuromuscular & skeletal: Myalgia, arthralgia

<1%: Hyperbilirubinemia, pancreatitis, thrombocytopenia

Drug Interactions Increased effect: Zidovudine concentrations increase (~39%) with coadministration with lamivudine; trimethoprim/sulfamethoxazole increases lamivudine's AUC and decreases its renal clearance by 44% and 29%, respectively; although the AUC was not significantly affected, absorption of lamivudine was slowed and C_{max} was 40% lower when administered to patients in the fed versus the fasted state

Manufacturer GlaxoWellcome

Related Information

Antiretroviral Therapy for HIV Infection *on page 1190*

Management of Healthcare Worker Exposures to HIV *on page 1151*

Pharmaceutical Manufacturers Directory *on page 1020*

Zidovudine and Lamivudine *on page 992*

Lamotrigine (la MOE tri jeen)

Pharmacologic Class Anticonvulsant, Miscellaneous

U.S. Brand Names Lamictal®

Mechanism of Action A triazine derivative which inhibits release of glutamate (an excitatory amino acid) and inhibits voltage-sensitive sodium channels, which stabilizes neuronal membranes

Use Partial/secondary generalized seizures in adults; childhood epilepsy, including Lennox-Gastaut disorder **(not approved for use in children <2 years of age)**

USUAL DOSAGE Oral:

Children 2-12 years:

With concomitant AEDs including valproic acid therapy: Initial: 0.15 mg/kg/day in 1-2 divided doses for 2 weeks; may increase by 0.3 mg/kg/day in 1-2 divided doses for 2 weeks; may increase by 0.3 mg/kg/day at 1- to 2-week intervals in 1-2 divided doses; see table

With concomitant AEDs without valproic acid therapy: Initial: 0.6 mg/kg/day in 2 divided doses for 2 weeks, then 1-2 mg/kg/day in 2 divided doses for 2 weeks; may increase by 1.2 mg/kg/day (round down to nearest 5 mg) at 1- to 2-week intervals; usual maintenance dose: 5-15 mg/kg/day; maximum: 400 mg/day in 2 divided doses

Adults: Initial: 50-100 mg/day then titrate to daily maintenance dose of 100-400 mg/day in 1-2 divided daily doses

(Continued)

Lamotrigine *(Continued)*

Lamictal® Added to an AED Regimen Containing VPA in Patients 2-12 Years of Age

Weeks 1 and 2	0.15 mg/kg/day in 1 or 2 divided doses, rounded down to the nearest 5 mg; if the initial calculated daily dose is 2.5-5 mg, then 5 mg should be taken on alternate days for the first 2 weeks
Weeks 3 and 4	0.3 mg/kg/day in 1 or 2 divided doses, rounded down to the nearest 5 mg
Usual maintenance dose: 1-5 mg/kg/day (maximum: 200 mg/day in 1-2 divided doses). To achieve usual maintenance dose, subsequent doses should be increased every 1-2 weeks as follows: Calculate 0.3 mg/kg/day, round this amount down to the neares 5 mg, and add this amount to the previously administered daily dose.	

With concomitant valproic acid therapy: Start initial dose at 25 mg/day then titrate to maintenance dose of 50-200 mg/day in 1-2 divided daily doses

Dosage Forms TAB: 25 mg, 100 mg, 150 mg, 200 mg; Chewable: 5 mg, 25 mg

Contraindications History of hypersensitivity to lamotrigine or any component

Warnings/Precautions Lactation, impaired renal, hepatic, or cardiac function; avoid abrupt cessation, taper over at least 2 weeks if possible. Severe and potentially life-threatening skin rashes have been reported; this appears to occur most frequently in pediatric patients. Write/fill prescription carefully; confusion has occurred between Lamictal® (lamotrigine) and Lamisil® (terbinafine)

Pregnancy Risk Factor C

Adverse Reactions

>10%:

Central nervous system: Headache, nausea, dizziness, ataxia, somnolence
Ocular: Diplopia, blurred vision
Respiratory: Rhinitis

1% to 10%:

Cardiovascular: Hot flashes, palpitations
Central nervous system: Depression, anxiety, irritability, confusion, speech disorder, difficulty concentrating, emotional lability, malaise, seizure, incoordination, insomnia
Dermatologic: Hypersensitivity rash, Stevens-Johnson syndrome, angioedema, pruritus, alopecia, acne
Gastrointestinal: Abdominal pain, vomiting, diarrhea, dyspepsia, constipation, psoriasis, xerostomia
Genitourinary: Vaginitis, amenorrhea
Neuromuscular & skeletal: Tremor, arthralgia, joint pain
Ocular: Nystagmus, diplopia
Renal: Hematuria
Respiratory: Cough

Miscellaneous: Flu syndrome, fever

Drug Interactions

Lamotrigine may increase the epoxide metabolite of carbamazepine resulting in toxicity
Carbamazepine, phenytoin, phenobarbital may decrease concentrations of lamotrigine
Valproic acid inhibits the metabolism of lamotrigine
Lamotrigine enhances the metabolism of valproic acid

Alcohol Interactions Avoid use (may increase central nervous system depression)

Half-Life 24 hours; increases to 59 hours with concomitant valproic acid therapy; decreases with concomitant phenytoin or carbamazepine therapy to 15 hours

Education and Monitoring Issues

Patient Education: Take exactly as directed (do not increase dose or frequency or discontinue without consulting prescriber). While using this medication, do not use alcohol and other prescription or OTC medications (especially pain medications, sedatives, antihistamines, or hypnotics) without consulting prescriber. Maintain adequate hydration (2-3 L/day of fluids unless instructed to restrict fluid intake). You may experience drowsiness, dizziness, or blurred vision (use caution when driving or engaging in tasks requiring alertness until response to drug is known); nausea, vomiting, loss of appetite, heartburn, or dry mouth (small frequent meals, frequent mouth care, chewing gum, or sucking lozenges may help). Wear identification of epileptic status and medications. Report CNS changes, mentation changes, or changes in cognition; persistent GI symptoms (cramping, constipation, vomiting, anorexia); skin rash; swelling of face, lips, or tongue; easy bruising or bleeding (mouth, urine, stool); vision changes; worsening of seizure activity, or loss of seizure control.

Dietary Considerations: Food: Has no effect on absorption, take without regard to meals; drug may cause GI upset

Monitoring Parameters: Seizure (frequency and duration); serum levels of concurrent anticonvulsants; hypersensitivity reactions (especially rash)

Reference Range: Therapeutic range: 2-4 μg/mL

Manufacturer GlaxoWellcome

Related Information

Anticonvulsants by Seizure Type Comparison *on page 1230*
Epilepsy Guidelines *on page 1091*

Pharmaceutical Manufacturers Directory *on page 1020*

- **Lamprene®** *see* Clofazimine *on page 210*
- **Lanacane® [OTC]** *see* Benzocaine *on page 98*
- **Lanacort® [OTC]** *see* Hydrocortisone *on page 447*
- **Lanaphilic® Topical [OTC]** *see* Urea *on page 962*
- **Laniazid®** *see* Isoniazid *on page 487*
- **Lanorinal®** *see* Butalbital Compound *on page 123*
- **Lanoxicaps®** *see* Digoxin *on page 272*
- **Lanoxin®** *see* Digoxin *on page 272*

Lansoprazole (lan SOE pra zole)

Pharmacologic Class Proton Pump Inhibitor

U.S. Brand Names Prevacid®

Use Short-term treatment (up to 4 weeks) for healing and symptom relief of active duodenal ulcers (should not be used for maintenance therapy of duodenal ulcers); as part of a multiple drug regimen for *H. pylori* eradication; short-term treatment of symptomatic GERD; up to 8 weeks of treatment for all grades of erosive esophagitis (8 additional weeks can be given for incompletely healed esophageal erosions or for recurrence); and long-term treatment of pathological hypersecretory conditions, including Zollinger-Ellison syndrome

USUAL DOSAGE

Duodenal ulcer: 15 mg once daily for 4 weeks; maintenance therapy: 15 mg once daily

Gastric ulcer: 30 mg once daily for up to 8 weeks

GERD: 15 mg once daily for up to 8 weeks

Erosive esophagitis: 30 mg once daily for up to 8 weeks, continued treatment for an additional 8 weeks may be considered for recurrence or for patients that do not heal after the first 8 weeks of therapy. Maintenance therapy: 15 mg once daily.

Hypersecretory conditions: Initial: 60 mg once daily; adjust dose based upon patient response and to reduce acid secretion to <10 mEq/hour (5 mEq/hour in patients with prior gastric surgery); doses of 90 mg twice daily have been used; administer doses >120 mg/day in divided doses.

Helicobacter pylori-associated antral gastritis: 30 mg twice daily for 2 weeks (in combination with 1 g amoxicillin and 500 mg clarithromycin given twice daily for 14 days). Alternatively, in patients allergic to or intolerant of clarithromycin or in whom resistance to clarithromycin is known or suspected, lansoprazole 30 mg every 8 hours and amoxicillin 1 g every 8 hours may be given for 2 weeks

Dosing adjustment in hepatic impairment: Dose reduction is necessary for severe hepatic impairment

Dosage Forms CAP, delayed release: 15 mg, 30 mg

Contraindications Should not be taken by anyone with a known hypersensitivity to lansoprazole or any of the formulation's components

Warnings/Precautions Liver disease may require dosage reductions

Pregnancy Risk Factor B

Adverse Reactions

1% to 10%:

Central nervous system: Fatigue, dizziness, headache

Gastrointestinal: Abdominal pain, diarrhea, nausea, increased appetite, hypergastrinoma

<1%: Proteinuria, rash, tinnitus

Drug Interactions CYP2C19 enzyme substrate, CYP3A3/4 enzyme substrate (minor)

Decreased effect: Ketoconazole, itraconazole, and other drugs dependent upon acid for absorption; theophylline clearance increased slightly; sucralfate delays and reduces lansoprazole absorption by 30%

Alcohol Interactions Avoid use (may enhance gastric mucosal irritation)

Duration 1 day

Half-Life Healthy patient: 1.5 hours; Elderly: 2.9 hours; Cirrhosis: 7 hours

Education and Monitoring Issues

Patient Education: Take as directed, before eating. Do not crush or chew granules. Patients who may have difficulty swallowing capsules may open the delayed-release capsules and sprinkle the contents on applesauce, pudding, cottage cheese, yogurt, or Ensure. Report unresolved fatigue, diarrhea, or constipation, and appetite changes.

Monitoring Parameters: Patients with Zollinger-Ellison syndrome should be monitored for gastric acid output, which should be maintained at 10 mEq/hour or less during the last hour before the next lansoprazole dose; lab monitoring should include CBC, liver function, renal function, and serum gastrin levels

Manufacturer Tap Pharmaceuticals

Related Information

Helicobacter pylori Treatment *on page 1107*

Pharmaceutical Manufacturers Directory *on page 1020*

- **Lariam®** *see* Mefloquine *on page 559*
- **Larodopa®** *see* Levodopa *on page 520*

♦ **Lasix®** *see* Furosemide *on page 399*

Latanoprost (la TAN oh prost)

Pharmacologic Class Prostaglandin

U.S. Brand Names Xalatan®

Use Reduction of elevated intraocular pressure in patients with open-angle glaucoma and ocular hypertension who are intolerant of the other IOP lowering medications or insufficiently responsive (failed to achieve target IOP determined after multiple measurements over time) to another IOP lowering medication

USUAL DOSAGE Adults: Ophthalmic: 1 drop (1.5 mcg) in the affected eye(s) once daily in the evening; do not exceed the once daily dosage because it has been shown that more frequent administration may decrease the IOP lowering effect

Contraindications Hypersensitivity to any component of product

Pregnancy Risk Factor C

♦ **Laxilose** *see* Lactulose *on page 506*

♦ **LazerSporin-C® Otic** *see* Neomycin, Polymyxin B, and Hydrocortisone *on page 644*

♦ **Le 500 D** *see* Cascara Sagrada *on page 146*

Leflunomide (le FLU no mide)

Pharmacologic Class Antimetabolite; Antirheumatic, Disease Modifying

U.S. Brand Names Arava™

Mechanism of Action Inhibits pyrimidine synthesis, resulting in antiproliferative and anti-inflammatory effects

Use Treatment of active rheumatoid arthritis to reduce signs and symptoms and to retard structural damage as evidenced by x-ray erosions and joint space narrowing

USUAL DOSAGE

Adults: Oral: Initial: 100 mg/day for 3 days, followed by 20 mg/day; dosage may be decreased to 10 mg/day in patients who have difficulty tolerating the 20 mg dose. Due to the long half-life of the active metabolite, plasma levels may require a prolonged period to decline after dosage reduction.

Dosing adjustment in renal impairment: No specific dosage adjustment is recommended. There is no clinical experience in the use of leflunomide in patients with renal impairment. The free fraction of MI is doubled in dialysis patients. Patients should be monitored closely for adverse effects requiring dosage adjustment.

Dosing adjustment in hepatic impairment: No specific dosage adjustment is recommended. Since the liver is involved in metabolic activation and subsequent metabolism/elimination of leflunomide, patients with hepatic impairment should be monitored closely for adverse effects requiring dosage adjustment.

Guidelines for dosage adjustment or discontinuation based on the severity and persistence of ALT elevation secondary to leflunomide have been developed. For ALT elevations >2 times the upper limit of normal, dosage reduction to 10 mg/day may allow continued administration. Cholestyramine 8 g 3 times/day for 1-3 days may be administered to decrease plasma levels. If elevations >2 times but ≤3 times the upper limit of normal persist, liver biopsy is recommended. If elevations >3 times the upper limit of normal persist despite cholestyramine administration and dosage reduction, leflunomide should be discontinued and drug elimination should be enhanced with additional cholestyramine as indicated.

Elderly: Although hepatic function may decline with age, no specific dosage adjustment is recommended. Patients should be monitored closely for adverse effects which may require dosage adjustment.

Dosage Forms TAB: 10 mg, 20 mg, 100 mg

Contraindications Pregnancy/breast-feeding; known hypersensitivity to leflunomide or any component

Warnings/Precautions Hepatic disease (including seropositive hepatitis B or C patients) may increase risk of hepatotoxicity; immunosuppression may increase the risk of lymphoproliferative disorders or other malignancies; women of childbearing potential should not receive leflunomide until pregnancy has been excluded, patients have been counseled concerning fetal risk and reliable contraceptive measures have been confirmed. Caution in renal impairment, immune deficiency, bone marrow dysplasia or severe, uncontrolled infection. Use of live vaccines is not recommended; will increase uric acid excretion.

Pregnancy Risk Factor X

Pregnancy Implications Has been associated with teratogenic and embryolethal effects in animal models at low doses. Leflunomide is contraindicated in pregnant women or women of childbearing potential who are not using reliable contraception. Pregnancy must be excluded prior to initiating treatment. Following treatment, pregnancy should be avoided until the drug elimination procedure is completed (see Additional Information).

Breast-feeding is contraindicated. It is not known whether leflunomide is secreted in human milk; however, there is a potential for serious adverse reactions in nursing infants. A decision should be made whether to discontinue nursing or discontinue the drug, taking into account the importance of the drug to the mother.

Adverse Reactions

>10%:

Gastrointestinal: Diarrhea (17%)

Respiratory: Respiratory tract infection (15%)

1% to 10%:

Cardiovascular: Hypertension (10%), chest pain (2%), palpitation, tachycardia, vasculitis, vasodilation, varicose vein, edema (peripheral)

Central nervous system: Headache (7%), dizziness (4%), pain (2%), fever, malaise, migraine, anxiety, depression, insomnia, sleep disorder

Dermatologic: Alopecia (10%), rash (10%), pruritus (4%), dry skin (2%), eczema (2%), acne, dermatitis, hair discoloration, hematoma, herpes infection, nail disorder, subcutaneous nodule, skin disorder/discoloration, skin ulcer, bruising

Endocrine & metabolic: Hypokalemia (1%), diabetes mellitus, hyperglycemia, hyperlipidemia, hyperthyroidism, menstrual disorder

Gastrointestinal: Nausea (9%), abdominal pain (5%), dyspepsia (5%), weight loss (4%), anorexia (3%), gastroenteritis (3%), stomatitis (3%), vomiting (3%), cholelithiasis, colitis, constipation, esophagitis, flatulence, gastritis, gingivitis, melena, candidiasis (oral), enlarged salivary gland, tooth disorder, xerostomia, taste disturbance

Genitourinary: Urinary tract infection (5%), albuminuria, cystitis, dysuria, hematuria, vaginal candidiasis, prostate disorder, urinary frequency

Hematologic: Anemia

Hepatic: Abnormal LFTs (5%)

Neuromuscular & skeletal: Back pain (5%), joint disorder (4%), weakness (3%), tenosynovitis (3%), synovitis (2%), arthralgia (1%), paresthesia (2%), muscle cramps (1%), neck pain, pelvic pain, increased CPK, arthrosis, bursitis, myalgia, bone necrosis, bone pain, tendon rupture, neuralgia, neuritis

Ocular: Blurred vision, cataract, conjunctivitis, eye disorder

Respiratory: Bronchitis (7%), cough (3%), pharyngitis (3%), pneumonia (2%), rhinitis (2%), sinusitis (2%), asthma, dyspnea, epistaxis, lung disorder

Miscellaneous: Infection (4%), accidental injury (5%), allergic reactions (2%), diaphoresis

<1%: Anaphylaxis, eosinophilia, leukopenia, thrombocytopenia, urticaria

Drug Interactions CYP2C9 enzyme inhibitor

Increased effect: Theoretically, the concomitant use of drugs metabolized by this enzyme, which includes many NSAIDs, may result in increased serum concentrations. Coadministration with methotrexate increases the risk of hepatotoxicity. Leflunomide may also enhance the hepatotoxicity of other drugs. Tolbutamide free fraction may be increased. Rifampin may increase the serum concentrations of the active metabolite of leflunomide. Leflunomide has uricosuric activity and may enhance activity of other uricosuric agents.

Decreased effect: Administration of cholestyramine and activated charcoal enhance the elimination of leflunomide's active metabolite

Half-Life Mean 14-15 days; enterohepatic recycling appears to contribute to the long half-life of this agent, since activated charcoal and cholestyramine substantially reduce plasma half-life

Education and Monitoring Issues

Patient Education: Take as directed; do not increase dose without consulting prescriber. Maintain adequate hydration (2-3 L/day of fluids unless instructed to restrict fluid intake). Store medication away from light. You may experience diarrhea (buttermilk, boiled milk, or yogurt may help); nausea, vomiting, loss of appetite, and flatulence (small frequent meals, frequent mouth care, chewing gum, or sucking lozenges may help); dizziness (use caution when driving or engaging in tasks requiring alertness until response to drug is known). If diabetic, monitor blood sugars closely; this medication may alter glucose levels. Report chest pain, palpitations, rapid heartbeat, or swelling of extremities; persistent gastrointestinal problems; skin rash, redness, irritation, acne, ulcers, or easy bruising; frequency, painful or difficult urination, or genital itching or irritation; depression, acute headache, anxiety, or difficulty sleeping; weakness, muscle tremors, cramping or weakness, back pain, or altered gait; cough, cold symptoms, wheezing, or difficulty breathing; easy bruising/bleeding; blood in vomitus, stool, urine; or other unusual effects related to this medication.

Dietary Considerations: No interactions with food have been noted

Monitoring Parameters: Serum transaminase determinations at baseline and monthly during the initial phase of treatment; if stable, monitoring frequency may be decreased to intervals determined by the individual clinical situation

Manufacturer Hoechst-Marion Roussel

Related Information

Pharmaceutical Manufacturers Directory *on page 1020*

- **Lenoltec No 1, 2, 3, 4** *see* Acetaminophen and Codeine *on page 18*
- **Lens Plus Buffered Saline Solution** *see* Sodium Chloride *on page 858*
- **Lente® Iletin® I** *see* Insulin Preparations *on page 472*
- **Lente® Iletin® II** *see* Insulin Preparations *on page 472*
- **Lente® Insulin** *see* Insulin Preparations *on page 472*
- **Lente® L** *see* Insulin Preparations *on page 472*

♦ **Lescol®** *see* Fluvastatin *on page 387*

Letrozole (LET roe zole)

Pharmacologic Class Antineoplastic Agent, Miscellaneous; Aromatase Inhibitor

U.S. Brand Names Femara™

Mechanism of Action Nonsteroidal, competitive inhibitor of the aromatase enzyme system which binds to the heme group of aromatase, a cytochrome P-450 enzyme which catalyzes conversion of androgens to estrogens (specifically, androstenedione to estrone and testosterone to estradiol). This leads to inhibition of the enzyme and a significant reduction in plasma estrogen levels. Approximately 30% of breast cancers are sensitive to this estrogen deprivation.

Use Treatment of advanced breast cancer in postmenopausal women with disease progression following antiestrogen therapy

USUAL DOSAGE Oral (refer to individual protocols):

Adults: 2.5 mg once daily without regard to meals; continue treatment until tumor progression is evident. Patients treated with letrozole do not require glucocorticoid or mineralocorticoid replacement therapy.

Dosage adjustment in renal impairment: No dosage adjustment is required in patients with renal impairment if Cl_{cr} ≥10 mL/minute

Dosage adjustment in hepatic impairment: No dosage adjustment is recommended for patients with mild-to-moderate hepatic impairment. Patients with severe impairment of liver function have not been studied; dose patients with severe impairment of liver function with caution.

Dosage Forms TAB: 2.5 mg

Contraindications Hypersensitivity to letrozole or any of its excipients

Warnings/Precautions Letrozole was not mutagenic in *in vitro* tests but was observed to be a potential clastogen in *in vitro* assays. Repeated dosing caused sexual inactivity in females and atrophy in the reproductive tract in males and females at doses of 0.6 mg/kg, 0.1 mg/kg, and 0.03 mg/kg in mice, rats, and dogs, respectively (~1 mg/kg, 0.4 mg/kg, and 0.4 mg/kg the maximum recommended human doses, respectively).

Moderate decreases in lymphocyte counts, of uncertain clinical significance, were observed in some patients receiving letrozole 2.5 mg. This depression was transient in ~50% of those affected. Two patients on letrozole developed thrombocytopenia; relationship to the drug was unclear.

Increases in AST, ALT, and GGT ≥5 times the upper limit of normal (ULN) and of bilirubin ≥1.5 times the ULN were most often associated with metastatic disease in the liver.

Pregnancy Risk Factor D

Pregnancy Implications

Clinical effects on the fetus: Letrozole may cause fetal harm when administered to pregnant women. Letrozole is embryotoxic and fetotoxic when administered to rats. There are no studies in pregnant women and letrozole is indicated for postmenopausal women.

Breast-feeding/lactation: It is not known if letrozole is excreted in breast milk; exercise caution when letrozole is administered to nursing women

Adverse Reactions

>10%: Gastrointestinal: Nausea

1% to 10%:

Central nervous system: Headache, somnolence, dizziness
Dermatologic: Hot flashes, rash, pruritus
Gastrointestinal: Vomiting, constipation, diarrhea, abdominal pain, anorexia, dyspepsia
Neuromuscular: Arthralgia
Respiratory: Dyspnea, coughing

<1%: Thromboembolic events, vaginal bleeding

Drug Interactions CYP3A3/4 and 2A6 enzyme substrate; CYP2A6 and 2C19 enzyme inhibitor

Half-Life 2 days

Education and Monitoring Issues

Patient Education: Take as directed, without regard to food. You may experience nausea, vomiting, or loss of appetite (frequent mouth care, frequent small meals, chewing gum, or sucking lozenges may help); musculoskeletal pain or headache (mild analgesics may offer relief); sleepiness, fatigue, or dizziness (use caution when driving, climbing stairs, or engaging in tasks that require alertness until response to drug is known); constipation (increased exercise, or dietary fruit or fluids may help); diarrhea (boiled milk or yogurt may help). Report chest pain, palpitations, or swollen extremities; vaginal bleeding or hot flashes; unusual coughing or difficulty breathing; severe nausea; muscle pain; or skin rash.

Monitoring Parameters: Clinical/radiologic evidence of tumor regression in advanced breast cancer patients. Until the toxicity has been defined in larger patient populations, monitor the following laboratory tests periodically during therapy: complete blood counts, thyroid function tests, serum electrolytes, serum transaminases, and serum creatinine.

Manufacturer Novartis

Related Information

Pharmaceutical Manufacturers Directory *on page 1020*

Leucovorin (loo koe VOR in)

Pharmacologic Class Antidote; Vitamin, Water Soluble

U.S. Brand Names Wellcovorin®

Mechanism of Action Leucovorin is a reduced form of folic acid. Reduced folates function as 1 carbon donors in the synthesis of thymidine and purines for DNA, RNA, and proteins. When given following folic acid antagonists, leucovorin bypasses the inhibition of dihydrofolate reductase induced by the antagonist. This allows for recovery of normal tissues hopefully after irreversible toxicity to tumor tissue has occurred. When given before/with 5-FU, leucovorin provides the folate cofactors that stabilize the binding of 5-dUMP (active nucleotide of 5-FU) and thymidylate synthase; this enhances the activity of 5-FU.

Use Antidote for folic acid antagonists (methotrexate [>100 mg/m^2], trimethoprim, pyrimethamine); treatment of megaloblastic anemias when folate is deficient as in infancy, sprue, pregnancy, and nutritional deficiency when oral folate therapy is not possible; in combination with fluorouracil in the treatment of malignancy

USUAL DOSAGE Children and Adults:

Treatment of folic acid antagonist overdosage (eg, pyrimethamine or trimethoprim): Oral: 2-15 mg/day for 3 days or until blood counts are normal or 5 mg every 3 days; doses of 6 mg/day are needed for patients with platelet counts <100,000/mm^3

Folate-deficient megaloblastic anemia: I.M.: 1 mg/day

Megaloblastic anemia secondary to congenital deficiency of dihydrofolate reductase: I.M.: 3-6 mg/day

Rescue dose (rescue therapy should start within 24 hours of MTX therapy): I.V.: 10 mg/m^2 to start, then 10 mg/m^2 every 6 hours orally for 72 hours until serum MTX concentration is <10^{-8} molar; if serum creatinine (24 hours after methotrexate) is elevated 50% or more above the pre-MTX serum creatinine **or** the serum MTX concentration is >5×10^{-6} molar (see graph), increase dose to 100 mg/m^2/dose (preservative-free) every 3 hours until serum methotrexate level is <1×10^{-8} molar

Investigational: Post I.T. methotrexate: Oral, I.V.: 12 mg/m^2 as a single dose; post high-dose methotrexate: 100-1000 mg/m^2/dose until the serum methotrexate level is less than 1×10^{-7} molar

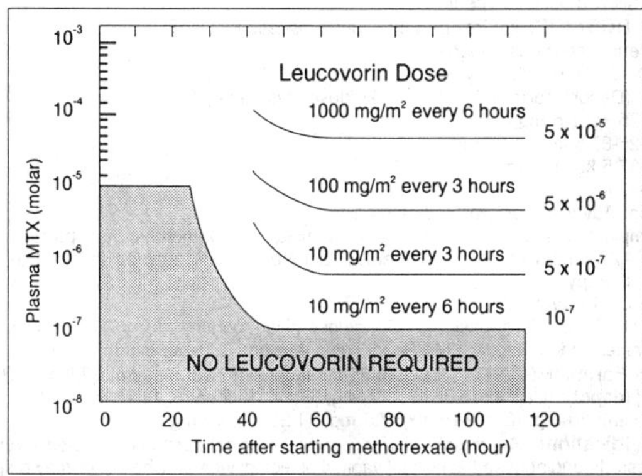

Note: The drug should be given parenterally instead of orally in patients with GI toxicity, nausea, vomiting, and when individual doses are >25 mg

Dosage adjustment in renal/hepatic impairment: No adjustment is necessary. Dosage may be increased and/or prolonged with renal insufficiency to rescue cells from toxicity secondary to delayed elimination of methotrexate.

Dosage Forms INJ: 3 mg/mL (1 mL). **POWDER** For inj: 25 mg, 50 mg, 100 mg, 350 mg; For oral soln: 1 mg/mL (60 mL). **TAB:** 5 mg, 10 mg, 15 mg, 25 mg

Contraindications Pernicious anemia or vitamin B_{12} deficient megaloblastic anemias; should **NOT** be administered Intrathecally/Intraventricularly

Warnings/Precautions Use with caution in patients with a history of hypersensitivity

Pregnancy Risk Factor C

Adverse Reactions <1%: Anaphylactoid reactions, erythema, pruritus, rash, thrombocytosis, urticaria, wheezing

Onset Onset of activity: Oral: Within 30 minutes; I.V.: Within 5 minutes

Half-Life Leucovorin: 15 minutes; Metabolite 5MTHF: 33-35 minutes

(Continued)

Leucovorin *(Continued)*

Education and Monitoring Issues

Patient Education: Take as directed, at evenly spaced intervals around-the-clock. Maintain hydration (2-3 L of water/day while taking for rescue therapy). For folic acid deficiency, eat foods high in folic acid (eg, meat proteins, bran, dried beans, asparagus, green leafy vegetables). Report respiratory difficulty, lethargy, or rash or itching.

Monitoring Parameters: Plasma MTX concentration as a therapeutic guide to high-dose MTX therapy with leucovorin factor rescue

Leucovorin is continued until the plasma MTX level is <1 x 10^{-7} molar

Each dose of leucovorin is increased if the plasma MTX concentration is excessively high (see graph)

With 4- to 6-hour high-dose MTX infusions, plasma drug values in excess of 5 x 10^{-5} and 10^{-6} molar at 24 and 48 hours after starting the infusion, respectively, are often predictive of delayed MTX clearance; see graph.

♦ **Leukeran®** *see* Chlorambucil *on page 177*

♦ **Leukine™** *see* Sargramostim *on page 839*

Leuprolide Acetate (loo PROE lide AS e tate)

Pharmacologic Class Antineoplastic Agent, Miscellaneous; Luteinizing Hormone-Releasing Hormone Analog

U.S. Brand Names Lupron®; Lupron Depot®; Lupron Depot®-3 Month; Lupron Depot®-4 Month; Lupron Depot-Ped®; Viadur®

Generic Available No

Mechanism of Action Continuous daily administration results in suppression of ovarian and testicular steroidogenesis due to decreased levels of LH and FSH with subsequent decrease in testosterone (male) and estrogen (female) levels

Use Palliative treatment of advanced prostate carcinoma (alternative when orchiectomy or estrogen administration are not indicated or are unacceptable to the patient); combination therapy with flutamide for treating metastatic prostatic carcinoma; endometriosis (3.75 mg depot only); central precocious puberty (may be used an agent to treat precocious puberty because of its effect in lowering levels of LH and FSH, testosterone, and estrogen).

Unlabeled use: Treatment of breast, ovarian, and endometrial cancer; leiomyoma uteri; infertility; prostatic hypertrophy

USUAL DOSAGE Requires parenteral administration

Children: Precocious puberty:
- S.C.: 20-45 mcg/kg/day
- I.M. (Depot®) formulation: 0.3 mg/kg/dose given every 28 days
  - ≤25 kg: 7.5 mg
  - >25-37.5 kg: 11.25 mg
  - >37.5 kg: 15 mg

Adults:
- Male: Advanced prostatic carcinoma:
  - Implant (Viadur®): One subcutaneous implant for 12 months; must be removed after 12 months of hormonal therapy; another implant may be inserted to continue therapy
  - S.C.: 1 mg/day **or**
  - I.M., Depot® (suspension): 7.5 mg/dose given monthly (every 28-33 days)
- Female: Endometriosis: I.M., Depot® (suspension): 3.75 mg monthly for up to 6 months

Dosage Forms IMPLANT: (Viadur®): 65 mg leuprolide **INJ:** 5 mg/mL (2.8 mL). **POWDER for inj (depot):** (Depot®): 3.75 mg, 7.5 mg; (Depot-3® Month): 11.25 mg, 22.5 mg; (Depot-4® Month): 30 mg; (Depot-Ped™): 7.5 mg, 11.25 mg, 15 mg

Contraindications Hypersensitivity to leuprolide; spinal cord compression (orchiectomy suggested); undiagnosed abnormal vaginal bleeding; women who are or may be pregnant should not receive Lupron® Depot®

Warnings/Precautions Use with caution in patients hypersensitive to benzyl alcohol; after 6 months use of Depot® leuprolide, vertebral bone density decreased (average 13.5%); long-term safety of leuprolide in children has not been established; urinary tract obstruction may occur upon initiation of therapy. Closely observe patients for weakness, paresthesias, and urinary tract obstruction in first few weeks of therapy. Tumor flare and bone pain may occur at initiation of therapy; transient weakness and paresthesia of lower limbs, hematuria, and urinary tract obstruction in first week of therapy; animal studies have shown dose-related benign pituitary hyperplasia and benign pituitary adenomas after 2 years of use.

Pregnancy Risk Factor X

Adverse Reactions

>10%:
- Central nervous system: Depression, pain
- Endocrine & metabolic: Hot flashes
- Gastrointestinal: Weight gain, nausea, vomiting

1% to 10%:
- Cardiovascular: Cardiac arrhythmias, edema

Central nervous system: Dizziness, lethargy, insomnia, headache
Dermatologic: Rash
Endocrine: Estrogenic effects (gynecomastia, breast tenderness)
Gastrointestinal: Nausea, vomiting, diarrhea, GI bleed
Hematologic: Decreased hemoglobin and hematocrit
Neuromuscular & skeletal: Paresthesia, myalgia
Ocular: Blurred vision

<1%: Myocardial infarction, pulmonary embolism, thrombophlebitis

Onset Serum testosterone levels first increase within 3 days of therapy.

Duration Levels decrease after 2-4 weeks with continued therapy.

Half-Life 3-4.25 hours

Education and Monitoring Issues

Patient Education: Use as directed. Do not discontinue abruptly; consult prescriber. You may experience disease flare (increased bone pain) and urinary retention during early treatment (usually resolves), dizziness, headache, lethargy, or faintness (use caution when driving or engaging in tasks that require alertness until response to drug is known), nausea or vomiting (small frequent meals or analgesics may help), hot flashes - flushing or redness (layered clothing and cool environment may help). Report irregular or rapid heartbeat, unresolved nausea or vomiting, numbness of extremities, breast swelling or pain, difficulty breathing, or infection at injection sites.

Monitoring Parameters: Precocious puberty: GnRH testing (blood LH and FSH levels), testosterone in males and estradiol in females; closely monitor patients with prostatic carcinoma for weakness, paresthesias, and urinary tract obstruction in first few weeks of therapy

Manufacturer Tap Pharmaceuticals

Related Information

Pharmaceutical Manufacturers Directory *on page 1020*

♦ **Leustatin™** *see* Cladribine *on page 204*

Levalbuterol (leve al BYOO ter ole)

Pharmacologic Class Adrenergic Agonist Agent; Beta$_2$ Agonist; Bronchodilator

U.S. Brand Names Xopenex™

Mechanism of Action Relaxes bronchial smooth muscle by action on beta-2 receptors with little effect on heart rate

Use Treatment or prevention of bronchospasm in adults and adolescents ≥12 years of age with reversible obstructive airway disease

USUAL DOSAGE

Pediatric: Safety and efficacy in patients <12 years of age not established

Children >12 years and Adults: Inhalation: 0.63 mg 3 times/day at intervals of 6-8 hours, via nebulization. Dosage may be increased to 1.25 mg 3 times/day with close monitoring for adverse effects. Most patients gain optimal benefit from regular use.

Elderly: Only a small number of patients have been studied. Although greater sensitivity of some elderly patients cannot be ruled out, no overall differences in safety or effectiveness were observed. An initial dose of 0.63 mg should be used in all patients >65 years of age.

Dosage Forms SOLN, inh: 0.63 mg/3 mL, 1.25 mg/3 mL

Contraindications Patients with known hypersensitivity to levalbuterol or any of the formulation's components

Warnings/Precautions May provoke paradoxical bronchospasm (similar to other bronchodilators). Immediate hypersensitivity reactions have occurred, including angioedema, oropharyngeal edema, urticaria, rash, and anaphylaxis. Use with caution in patients with cardiovascular disease, including coronary artery disease, hypertension, and a history of arrhythmias (may increase heart rate, blood pressure, or other symptoms including EKG changes). Do not use doses higher than recommended - fatalities have been associated with excessive use of other sympathomimetics. The need to use bronchodilators more frequently than usual should prompt an evaluation of the need for additional anti-inflammatory medication. Additional anti-inflammatory medication (such as corticosteroids), may be required to control asthma. Use with caution in diabetic patients and in patients with hypokalemia. Use with caution during labor and delivery. Safety and efficacy in patients <12 years of age not established.

Pregnancy Risk Factor C

Pregnancy Implications There are no studies in pregnant women; this drug should be used during pregnancy only if benefit exceeds risk

It is not known whether levalbuterol is excreted in human milk. Because of the tumorigenicity observed in animal studies, a decision should be made whether to discontinue nursing or to discontinue the drug, taking into account the importance of the drug to the mother.

Adverse Reactions Events reported include those ≥2% with incidence higher than placebo.

>10%:

Endocrine and metabolic: Increased serum glucose, decreased serum potassium
Respiratory: Viral infection (6.9% to 12.3%), rhinitis (2.7% to 11.1%)

(Continued)

Levalbuterol *(Continued)*

>2% to <10%:

Cardiovascular: Tachycardia (2.7% to 2.8%)

Central nervous system: Nervousness (2.8% to 9.6%), tremor (0 to 6.8%), anxiety (0 to 2.7%), dizziness (1.4% to 2.7%), migraine (0 to 2.7%), pain (1.4% to 2.8%)

Gastrointestinal: Dyspepsia (1.4% to 2.7%)

Neuromuscular & skeletal: Leg cramps (0 to 2.7%)

Respiratory: Cough (1.4% to 4.1%), nasal edema (1.4% to 2.8%), sinusitis (1.4% to 4.2%)

Miscellaneous: Flu-like syndrome (1.4% to 4.2%), accidental injury (0% to 2.7%)

<2%: Abnormal EKG, anxiety, asthma exacerbation, chest pain, chills, diarrhea, dyspepsia, gastroenteritis, hypertension, hypesthesia (hand), hypotension, insomnia, itching eyes, lymphadenopathy, myalgia, nausea, oropharyngeal dryness, paresthesia, sweating, syncope, vomiting, wheezing

Drug Interactions

Decreased effect:

Beta-blockers (particularly nonselective agents) block the effect of levalbuterol

Digoxin levels may be decreased

Increased effect/toxicity:

May add to effects of medications which deplete potassium (eg, loop or thiazide diuretics)

Cardiac effects may be potentiated in patients receiving MAOIs, tricyclic antidepressants, sympathomimetics (eg, amphetamine, dobutamine), inhaled anesthetics (eg, enflurane)

Onset 10-17 minutes

Duration 5-8 hours

Half-Life 3-4 hours

Education and Monitoring Issues

Patient Education: Use only when necessary or as prescribed; tolerance may develop with overuse. First dose should not be used when you are alone. Avoid OTC medications without consulting prescriber. Maintain adequate hydration (2-3 L/day of fluids unless instructed to restrict fluid intake). Stress or excessive exercising may exacerbate wheezing or bronchospasm (controlled breathing or relaxation techniques may help). If diabetic, you will need to monitor serum glucose levels closely until response is known; notify diabetic advisor if hyperglycemia occurs. You may experience tremor, anxiety, dizziness (use caution when driving or engaging in hazardous activities until response to drug is known); temporarily upset stomach, nausea, or vomiting (frequent small meals, frequent mouth care, chewing gum, or sucking hard candy may help). Paradoxical bronchospasm can occur; stop drug immediately and notify prescriber if any of the following occur: chest pain or tightness, palpitations; severe headache; difficulty breathing; increased nervousness, restlessness, or trembling; muscle cramps or weakness; seizures. Report unusual signs of flu or infection; leg or muscle cramps; unusual cough; persistent GI problems; changes in vision; or other adverse effects.

Use of nebulizer: Wash hands, sit to administer. Shake container, exhale slowly and completely through nose, inhale deeply through mouth while administering aerosol. Hold breath for 2-3 seconds, then exhale slowly. Allow 1 minute between inhalations. Wash mouthpiece with soap and water after each use. Rinse mouth to remove any unpleasant taste.

Monitoring Parameters: Asthma symptoms, FEV_1 and/or peak expiratory flow rate, heart rate, blood pressure, CNS status, arterial blood gases (if condition warrants). In selected patients: Serum, glucose, and potassium

Levamisole (lee VAM i sole)

Pharmacologic Class Immune Modulator

U.S. Brand Names Ergamisol®

Generic Available No

Mechanism of Action Clinically, combined therapy with levamisole and 5-fluorouracil has been effective in treating colon cancer patients, whereas demonstrable activity has been demonstrated. Due to the broad range of pharmacologic activities of levamisole, it has been suggested that the drug may act as a biochemical modulator (of fluorouracil, for example, in colon cancer), an effect entirely independent of immune modulation. Further studies are needed to evaluate the mechanisms of action of the drug in cancer patients.

Use Adjuvant treatment with fluorouracil in Dukes stage C colon cancer

USUAL DOSAGE Adults: Oral: Initial: 50 mg every 8 hours for 3 days, then 50 mg every 8 hours for 3 days every 2 weeks (fluorouracil is always given concomitantly)

Dosing adjustment in hepatic impairment: May be necessary in patients with liver disease, but no specific guidelines are available

Dosage Forms TAB, as base: 50 mg

Contraindications Previous hypersensitivity to the drug

Warnings/Precautions Agranulocytosis can occur asymptomatically and flu-like symptoms can occur without hematologic adverse effects; frequent hematologic monitoring is necessary

Pregnancy Risk Factor C

Adverse Reactions

>10%: Gastrointestinal: Nausea, diarrhea

1% to 10%:

Cardiovascular: Edema

Central nervous system: Fatigue, fever, dizziness, headache, somnolence, depression, nervousness, insomnia

Dermatologic: Dermatitis, alopecia

Gastrointestinal: Stomatitis, vomiting, anorexia, abdominal pain, constipation, taste perversion

Hematologic: Leukopenia

Neuromuscular & skeletal: Rigors, arthralgia, myalgia, paresthesia

Miscellaneous: Infection

<1%: Abnormal tearing, altered sense of smell, anemia, anxiety, blurred vision, chest pain, conjunctivitis, dyspepsia, epistaxis, flatulence, granulocytopenia, pruritus, Stevens-Johnson syndrome, thrombocytopenia, urticaria

Drug Interactions

Increased toxicity/serum levels of phenytoin

Disulfiram-like reaction with alcohol

Half-Life 2-6 hours

Education and Monitoring Issues

Patient Education: Take as directed, at regular intervals around-the-clock. Avoid alcohol (may cause disulfiram-like effect). Avoid all aspirin-containing medications. You may experience GI upset (small frequent meals may help); diarrhea (request medication); sensitivity to sun (use sunblock, wear protective clothing, and avoid direct sun); or dizziness, drowsiness, or impaired judgment (use caution when driving, climbing stairs, or engaging in tasks requiring alertness until response to drug is known). You will be more susceptible to infection; avoid crowds or infected persons. Report chills or fever, confusion, persistent or violent vomiting, persistent diarrhea, or respiratory difficulty.

Monitoring Parameters: CBC with platelet count prior to therapy and weekly prior to treatment; LFTs every 3 months

Manufacturer Janssen Pharmaceutical, Inc

Related Information

Pharmaceutical Manufacturers Directory *on page 1020*

♦ **Levaquin™** *see* Levofloxacin *on page 522*

♦ **Levate®** *see* Amitriptyline *on page 51*

♦ **Levbid®** *see* Hyoscyamine *on page 456*

Levetiracetam (lev e tir AS e tam)

Pharmacologic Class Anticonvulsant, Miscellaneous

U.S. Brand Names Keppra®

Mechanism of Action The precise mechanism by which levetiracetam exerts its antiepileptic effect is unknown and does not appear to derive from any interaction with known mechanisms involved in inhibitory and excitatory neurotransmission

Use Indicated as adjunctive therapy in the treatment of partial onset seizures in adults with epilepsy

USUAL DOSAGE

Adults: Initial: 500 mg twice daily; additional dosing increments may be given (1000 mg/day additional every 2 weeks) to a maximum recommended daily dose of 3000 mg

Dosing adjustment in renal impairment:

Cl_{cr} >80 mL/min: 500-1500 mg every 12 hours

Cl_{cr} 50-80 mL/min: 500-1000 mg every 12 hours

Cl_{cr} 30-50 mL/min: 250-750 mg every 12 hours

Cl_{cr} <30 mL/min: 250-500 mg every 12 hours

End-stage renal disease patients using dialysis: 500-2000 mg every 24 hours

Dosage Forms TAB: 250 mg, 500 mg, 750 mg

Contraindications Should not be administered to patients who have previously exhibited hypersensitivity to levetiracetam or any of the inactive ingredients in the tablets

Warnings/Precautions Associated with the occurrence of central nervous system adverse events; somnolence and fatigue, which were treated by discontinuation, reduction, or hospitalization; coordination difficulty was treated by reduction, and only one patient was hospitalized. Behavioral abnormalities, such as psychosis, hallucinations, psychotic depression and other behavioral symptoms (agitation, hostility, anxiety, apathy, emotional lability, depersonalization, and depression) were treated by reduction of dose and in some cases hospitalization. Levetiracetam should be withdrawn gradually to minimize the potential of increased seizure frequency.

Pregnancy Risk Factor C

Adverse Reactions

>10%:

Central nervous system: Somnolence (14.8% vs 8.4% with placebo)

Neuromuscular & skeletal: Weakness (14.7% vs 9.1% with placebo)

(Continued)

Levetiracetam *(Continued)*

<10%:

Central nervous system: Psychotic symptoms (0.7%), amnesia (2% vs 1% with placebo), ataxia (3% vs 1% with placebo), depression (4% vs 2% with placebo), dizziness (9% vs 4% with placebo), emotional lability (2%), nervousness (4% vs 2% with placebo), vertigo (3% vs 1% with placebo)

Hematologic: Decreased erythrocyte counts (3.2%), decreased leukocytes (2.4-3.2%)

Neuromuscular & skeletal: Ataxia and other coordination difficulties (3.4% vs 1.6% with placebo), pain (7% vs 6% with placebo)

Ophthalmic: Diplopia (2% vs 1% with placebo)

Onset 1 hour

Half-Life 6-8 hours

Education and Monitoring Issues

Patient Education: Take exactly as directed (do not increase dose or frequency or discontinue without consulting prescriber). While using this medication, do not use alcohol and other prescription or OTC medications (especially pain medications, sedatives, antihistamines, or hypnotics) without consulting prescriber. Maintain adequate hydration (2-3 L/day of fluids unless instructed to restrict fluid intake). You may experience drowsiness, dizziness, or blurred vision (use caution when driving or engaging in tasks requiring alertness until response to drug is known); nausea, vomiting, loss of appetite, or dry mouth (small frequent meals, frequent mouth care, chewing gum, or sucking lozenges may help). Wear identification of epileptic status and medications. Report CNS changes, mentation changes, or changes in cognition; muscle cramping, weakness, tremors, changes in gait; persistent GI symptoms (cramping, constipation, vomiting, anorexia); rash or skin irritations; unusual bruising or bleeding (mouth, urine, stool); worsening of seizure activity, or loss of seizure control.

Manufacturer UCB Pharmaceuticals, Inc

Related Information

Epilepsy Guidelines *on page 1091*

Pharmaceutical Manufacturers Directory *on page 1020*

♦ **Levlen®** *see* Ethinyl Estradiol and Levonorgestrel *on page 341*

♦ **Levlite®** *see* Ethinyl Estradiol and Levonorgestrel *on page 341*

Levobetaxolol (lee voe be TAX oh lol)

Pharmacologic Class Beta-Adrenergic Blocker, Ophthalmic

U.S. Brand Names Betaxon®

Mechanism of Action Levobetaxolol is a cardioselective, $beta_1$-adrenergic receptor antagonist. It is the more active enantiomer of betaxolol. Reduces intraocular pressure by reducing the production of aqueous humor.

Use Lowering of intraocular pressure in patients with chronic open-angle glaucoma or ocular hypertension

USUAL DOSAGE Adults: Ophthalmic: Instill 1 drop in affected eye(s) twice daily

Dosage Forms SOLN, ophth: 0.5% (5 mL, 10 mL, 15 mL)

Contraindications Hypersensitivity to levobetaxolol or any component; sinus bradycardia; greater than first degree heart block (without a functional pacemaker); cardiogenic shock; decompensated heart failure

Warnings/Precautions Monitor for bronchospasm, bradycardia, or heart failure since topically-applied beta-blockers can sometimes be absorbed systemically. Use caution in patients with a history of heart failure, heart block (without a functional pacemaker), or pulmonary dysfunction. Use caution in labile diabetic patients. Beta-blockers may mask signs of hypoglycemia and hyperthyroidism. May potentiate muscle weakness in myasthenia.

Pregnancy Risk Factor C

Pregnancy Implications There are no adequate studies in pregnant women. Should be used during pregnancy only if the benefit outweighs the potential risk to the fetus. It is not known if levobetaxolol is excreted in human milk. Exercise caution when administering to breast-feeding women.

Adverse Reactions

>10%: Ocular: Transient discomfort (11%)

2% to 10%: Ocular: Transient blurred vision (2%)

<2%:

Central nervous system: Anxiety, dizziness, vertigo, headache

Cardiovascular: Bradycardia, heart block, hypertension, hypotension, tachycardia

Dermatologic: Alopecia, dermatitis, psoriasis

Endocrine & metabolic: Diabetes, hyperthyroidism, gout, hypercholesterolemia, hyperlipidemia

Gastrointestinal: Constipation, dyspepsia, taste perversion

Genitourinary: Cystitis

Neuromuscular & skeletal: Hypertonia, arthritis, tendonitis

Ocular: Cataracts, vitreous disorders

Otic: Ear pain, otitis media, tinnitus

Respiratory: Bronchitis, dyspnea, pharyngitis, pneumonia, rhinitis, sinusitis

Miscellaneous: Breast abscess, infection

Drug Interactions Increased toxicity (hypotension): systemic beta-blockers, catecholamine-depleting agents (reserpine), adrenergic psychotropic agents

Onset 30 minutes

Duration 12 hours

Half-Life 20 hours

Education and Monitoring Issues

Patient Education: May sting on instillation; do not touch dropper tip to eye; visual acuity may be decreased after administration; apply gentle pressure to the inside corner of the eye during and immediately following instillation to avoid systemic absorption. Stop the medicine if breathing problems occur and contact healthcare provider. Do not use with contact lenses in the eyes. Shake well before using.

Monitoring Parameters: Intraocular pressure

Manufacturer Alcon Laboratories, Inc

Related Information

Pharmaceutical Manufacturers Directory *on page 1020*

Levobunolol (lee voe BYOO noe lole)

Pharmacologic Class Beta Blocker

U.S. Brand Names AKBeta®; Betagan® Liquifilm®

Use To lower intraocular pressure in chronic open-angle glaucoma or ocular hypertension

USUAL DOSAGE Adults: Instill 1 drop in the affected eye(s) 1-2 times/day

Contraindications Known hypersensitivity to levobunolol; bronchial asthma, severe COPD, sinus bradycardia, second or third degree A-V block, cardiac failure, cardiogenic shock

Pregnancy Risk Factor C

Levocabastine (LEE voe kab as teen)

Pharmacologic Class Antihistamine

U.S. Brand Names Livostin®

Mechanism of Action Potent, selective histamine H_1-receptor antagonist for topical ophthalmic use

Use Treatment of allergic conjunctivitis

USUAL DOSAGE Children >12 years and Adults: Instill 1 drop in affected eye(s) 4 times/day for up to 2 weeks

Dosage Forms SUSP, ophth: 0.05% (2.5 mL, 5 mL, 10 mL)

Contraindications Hypersensitivity to any component of product; while soft contact lenses are being worn

Warnings/Precautions Safety and efficacy in children <12 years of age have not been established; not for injection; not for use in patients wearing soft contact lenses during treatment

Pregnancy Risk Factor C

Adverse Reactions

>10%: Local: Transient burning, stinging, discomfort

1% to 10%:

Central nervous system: Headache, somnolence, fatigue

Dermatologic: Rash

Gastrointestinal: Xerostomia

Ocular: Blurred vision, eye pain, somnolence, red eyes, eyelid edema

Respiratory: Dyspnea

Levocarnitine (lee voe KAR ni teen)

Pharmacologic Class Nutritional Supplement

U.S. Brand Names Carnitor® Injection; Carnitor® Oral; VitaCarn® Oral

Mechanism of Action Carnitine is a naturally occurring metabolic compound which functions as a carrier molecule for long-chain fatty acids within the mitochondria, facilitating energy production. Carnitine deficiency is associated with accumulation of excess acyl-CoA esters and disruption of intermediary metabolism. Carnitine supplementation increases carnitine plasma concentrations. The effects on specific metabolic alterations have not been evaluated. ESRD patients on maintenance HD may have low plasma carnitine levels because of reduced intake of meat and dairy products, reduced renal synthesis, and dialytic losses. Certain clinical conditions (malaise, muscle weakness, cardiomyopathy and arrhythmias) in HD patients may be related to carnitine deficiency.

Use

Oral: Primary systemic carnitine deficiency; acute and chronic treatment of patients with an inborn error of metabolism which results in secondary carnitine deficiency

I.V. Acute and chronic treatment of patients with an inborn error of metabolism which results in secondary carnitine deficiency; prevention and treatment of carnitine deficiency in patients with end stage renal disease who are undergoing hemodialysis.

(Continued)

Levocarnitine *(Continued)*

USUAL DOSAGE

Oral:

Infants/Children: Initial: 50 mg/kg/day; titrate to 50-100 mg/kg/day in divided doses with a maximum dose of 3 g/day

Adults: 990 mg (oral tablets) 2-3 times/day or 1-3 g/day (oral solution)

I.V.:

Metabolic disorders: 50 mg/kg as a slow 2- to 3-minute I.V. bolus or by I.V. infusion

Severe metabolic crisis:

A loading dose of 50 mg/kg followed by an equivalent dose over the following 24 hours administered as q3h or q4h (never less than q6h either by infusion or by intravenous injection)

All subsequent daily doses are recommended to be in the range of 50 mg/kg or as therapy may require

The highest dose administered has been 300 mg/kg

It is recommended that a plasma carnitine concentration be obtained prior to beginning parenteral therapy accompanied by weekly and monthly monitoring

ESRD patients on hemodialysis:

Predialysis levocarnitine concentrations below normal (40-50 μmol/L): 10-20 mg/kg dry body weight as a slow 2- to 3-minute bolus after each dialysis session

Dosage adjustments should be guided by predialysis trough levocarnitine concentrations and downward dose adjustments (to 5 mg/kg after dialysis) may be made as early as every 3rd or 4th week of therapy

Dosage Forms INJ: 200 mg/mL (2.5 mL, 5 mL). **SOLN, oral:** 100 mg/mL (118 mL). **TAB:** 330 mg

Contraindications There are no known contraindications to this agent

Warnings/Precautions Caution in patients with seizure disorders or in those at risk of seizures (CNS mass or medications which may lower seizure threshold). Both new-onset seizure activity as well as an increased frequency of seizures has been observed.

Pregnancy Risk Factor B

Pregnancy Implications No adequate or well controlled studies in pregnant women. However, carnitine is a naturally occurring substance in mammalian metabolism. In breast-feeding women, use must be weighed against the potential exposure of the infant to increased carnitine intake. Use caution in breast-feeding women.

Adverse Reactions I.V. therapy in HD patients: >5%:

Central nervous system: Dizziness (10% to 18%), fever (5% to 12%), paresthesia (3% to 12%), depression (5% to 6%)

Cardiovascular: Hypertension (18% to 21%), peripheral edema (3% to 6%)

Endocrine & metabolic: Hypercalcemia (6% to 15%)

Gastrointestinal: Diarrhea (9% to 35%), abdominal pain (5% to 21%), vomiting (9% to 21%), nausea (5% to 12%)

Neuromuscular & skeletal: Weakness (9% to 12%)

Miscellaneous: Allergic reaction (2% to 6%)

Half-Life 17.4 hours

Education and Monitoring Issues

Patient Education: I.V.: Report immediately any dizziness, loss of feeling, acute headache, tremors, or nausea.

Oral: Take exactly as directed; do not alter dose or frequency except as directed by prescriber. Dissolve solution in any liquid and drink with or following meals. You may experience abdominal pain, nausea, or vomiting (small frequent meals, chewing gum, or sucking hard candy); diarrhea (yogurt or buttermilk may help); dizziness (use caution driving or when engaged in hazardous activities until response to medication is known). Report acute headache, chest pain, tremors, or visual changes; muscle or skeletal weakness; skin rash; swelling of extremities; or other adverse effects. Consult prescriber about breast-feeding.

Monitoring Parameters: Plasma concentrations should be obtained prior to beginning parenteral therapy, and should be monitored weekly to monthly. In metabolic disorders: monitor blood chemistry, vital signs, and plasma carnitine levels (maintain between 35-60 μmol/L). In ESRD patients on dialysis: Plasma levels below the normal range should prompt initiation of therapy. Monitor predialysis (trough) plasma carnitine levels.

Reference Range: Normal carnitine levels are 40-50 μmol/L; levels should be maintained on therapy between 35-60 μmol/L

Manufacturer Sigma-Tau Pharmaceuticals, Inc

Related Information

Pharmaceutical Manufacturers Directory *on page 1020*

Levodopa (lee voe DOE pa)

Pharmacologic Class Diagnostic Agent; Dopaminergic Agent (Antiparkinson's)

U.S. Brand Names Dopar®; Larodopa®

Use Treatment of Parkinson's disease; used as a diagnostic agent for growth hormone deficiency

USUAL DOSAGE Oral:

Children (administer as a single dose to evaluate growth hormone deficiency):

0.5 g/m^2 **or**

<30 lbs: 125 mg

30-70 lbs: 250 mg

>70 lbs: 500 mg

Adults: 500-1000 mg/day in divided doses every 6-12 hours; increase by 100-750 mg/day every 3-7 days until response or total dose of 8,000 mg is reached

A significant therapeutic response may not be obtained for 6 months

Contraindications Hypersensitivity to levodopa or any component; narrow-angle glaucoma, MAO inhibitor therapy, melanomas or any undiagnosed skin lesions

Pregnancy Risk Factor C

Levodopa and Carbidopa (lee voe DOE pa & kar bi DOE pa)

Pharmacologic Class Anti-Parkinson's Agent (Dopamine Agonist)

U.S. Brand Names Atamet®; Sinemet®; Sinemet® CR

Generic Available No

Mechanism of Action Parkinson's symptoms are due to a lack of striatal dopamine; levodopa circulates in the plasma to the blood-brain-barrier (BBB), where it crosses, to be converted by striatal enzymes to dopamine; carbidopa inhibits the peripheral plasma breakdown of levodopa by inhibiting its decarboxylation, and thereby increases available levodopa at the BBB

Use Treatment of parkinsonian syndrome; 50-100 mg/day of carbidopa is needed to block the peripheral conversion of levodopa to dopamine. "On-off" can be managed by giving smaller, more frequent doses of Sinemet® or adding a dopamine agonist or selegiline; when adding a new agent, doses of Sinemet® should usually be decreased.

USUAL DOSAGE Oral:

Adults: Initial: 25/100 2-4 times/day, increase as necessary to a maximum of 200/2000 mg/day

Elderly: Initial: 25/100 twice daily, increase as necessary

Conversion from Sinemet® to Sinemet® CR (50/200): (Sinemet® [total daily dose of levodopa] / Sinemet® CR)

300-400 mg / 1 tablet twice daily

500-600 mg / 1½ tablets twice daily or one 3 times/day

700-800 mg / 4 tablets in 3 or more divided doses

900-1000 mg / 5 tablets in 3 or more divided doses

Intervals between doses of Sinemet® CR should be 4-8 hours while awake

Dosage Forms TAB: 10/100: Carbidopa 10 mg and levodopa 100 mg; 25/100: Carbidopa 25 mg and levodopa 100 mg; 25/250: Carbidopa 25 mg and levodopa 250 mg; Sustained release: Carbidopa 25 mg and levodopa 100 mg; carbidopa 50 mg and levodopa 200 mg

Contraindications Narrow-angle glaucoma, MAO inhibitors, hypersensitivity to levodopa, carbidopa, or any component; do not use in patients with malignant melanoma or undiagnosed skin lesions

Warnings/Precautions Use with caution in patients with history of myocardial infarction, arrhythmias, asthma, wide angle glaucoma, peptic ulcer disease; sudden discontinuation of levodopa may cause a worsening of Parkinson's disease; some tablets may contain tartrazine. The elderly may be more sensitive to the CNS effects of levodopa. Protein in the diet should be distributed throughout the day to avoid fluctuations in levodopa absorption.

Pregnancy Risk Factor C

Adverse Reactions

Cardiovascular: Orthostatic hypotension, arrhythmias, chest pain, hypertension, syncope, palpitations, phlebitis

Central nervous system: Dizziness, anxiety, confusion, nightmares, headache, hallucinations, on-off phenomenon, decreased mental acuity, memory impairment, disorientation, delusions, euphoria, agitation, somnolence, insomnia, gait abnormalities, nervousness, ataxia, EPS, falling

Gastrointestinal: Anorexia, nausea, vomiting, constipation, GI bleeding, duodenal ulcer, diarrhea, dyspepsia, taste alterations, sialorrhea, heartburn

Genitourinary: Discoloration of urine, urinary frequency

Hematologic: Hemolytic anemia, agranulocytosis, thrombocytopenia, leukopenia, decreased hemoglobin and hematocrit, abnormalities in AST and ALT, LDH, bilirubin, BUN, Coombs' test

Neuromuscular & skeletal: Choreiform and involuntary movements, paresthesia, bone pain, shoulder pain, muscle cramps, weakness

Ocular: Blepharospasm

Renal: Difficult urination

Respiratory: Dyspnea, cough

Miscellaneous: Hiccups, discoloration of sweat

Drug Interactions

Benzodiazepines may inhibit the antiparkinsonian effects of levodopa; monitor for reduced effect

(Continued)

Levodopa and Carbidopa *(Continued)*

Antipsychotics may inhibit the antiparkinsonian effects of levodopa via dopamine receptor blockade; use antipsychotics with low dopamine blockade (clozapine, olanzapine, quetiapine)

High-protein diets may inhibit levodopa's efficacy; avoid high protein foods

Iron binds levodopa and reduces its bioavailability; separate doses of iron and levodopa

Concurrent use of levodopa with nonselective MAOIs may result in hypertensive reactions via an increased storage and release of dopamine, norepinephrine, or both. Use with carbidopa to minimize reactions if combination is necessary; otherwise avoid combination.

L-methionine, phenytoin, pyridoxine, and spiramycin may inhibit levodopa's antiparkinsonian effects

Tacrine may inhibit the effects of levodopa via enhanced cholinergic activity; monitor

Duration Variable, 6-12 hours; longer with CR dosage forms

Half-Life Carbidopa: 1-2 hours; Levodopa: 1.2-2.3 hours

Education and Monitoring Issues

Patient Education: Take exactly as directed; do not change dosage or discontinue without consulting prescriber. Therapeutic effects may take several weeks or months to achieve and you may need frequent monitoring during first weeks of therapy. Take with meals if GI upset occurs, before meals if dry mouth occurs, after eating if drooling or if nausea occurs. Take at the same time each day. Maintain adequate hydration (2-3 L/day of fluids unless instructed to restrict fluid intake); void before taking medication. Do not use alcohol and prescription or OTC sedatives or CNS depressants without consulting prescriber. Urine or perspiration may appear darker. You may experience drowsiness, dizziness, confusion, or vision changes (use caution when driving, climbing stairs, or engaging in tasks requiring alertness until response to drug is known); orthostatic hypotension (use caution when changing position - rising to standing from sitting or lying); increased susceptibility to heat stroke, decreased perspiration (use caution in hot weather - maintain adequate fluids and reduce exercise activity); constipation (increased exercise, fluids, or dietary fruit and fiber may help); dry skin or nasal passages (consult prescriber for appropriate relief); nausea, vomiting, loss of appetite, or stomach discomfort (small frequent meals, frequent mouth care, chewing gum, or sucking lozenges may help). Report unresolved constipation or vomiting; chest pain or irregular heartbeat; difficulty breathing; acute headache or dizziness; CNS changes (hallucination, loss of memory, nervousness, etc); painful or difficult urination; abdominal pain or blood in stool; increased muscle spasticity or rigidity; skin rash; or significant worsening of condition.

Monitoring Parameters: Blood pressure, standing and sitting/supine; symptoms of parkinsonism, dyskinesias, mental status

Related Information

Parkinson's Disease Dosing *on page 1249*

♦ **Levo-Dromoran** *see* Levorphanol *on page 525*

Levofloxacin (lee voe FLOKS a sin)

Pharmacologic Class Antibiotic, Quinolone

U.S. Brand Names Levaquin™

Mechanism of Action As the S (-) enantiomer of the fluoroquinolone, ofloxacin, levofloxacin, inhibits DNA-gyrase in susceptible organisms thereby inhibits relaxation of supercoiled DNA and promotes breakage of DNA strands. DNA gyrase (topoisomerase II), is an essential bacterial enzyme that maintains the superhelical structure of DNA and is required for DNA replication and transcription, DNA repair, recombination, and transposition.

Use Acute maxillary sinusitis due to *S. pneumoniae*, *H. influenzae*, or *M. catarrhalis*; uncomplicated urinary tract infection due to *E. coli*, *K. pneumoniae*, or *S. saprophyticus*; also for acute bacterial exacerbation of chronic bronchitis and community-acquired pneumonia (including penicillin-resistant pneumococci) due to *S. aureus*, *S. pneumoniae*, *H. influenzae*, *H. parainfluenzae*, or *M. catarrhalis*, *C. pneumoniae*, *L. pneumophila*, or *M. pneumoniae*; may be used for uncomplicated skin and skin structure infection (due to *S. aureus* or *S. pyogenes*) and complicated urinary tract infection due to gram-negative *Enterobacter* sp, including acute pyelonephritis (caused by *E. coli*)

USUAL DOSAGE Adults: Oral, I.V. (infuse I.V. solution over 60 minutes):

Acute bacterial exacerbation of chronic bronchitis: 500 mg every 24 hours for at least 7 days

Community acquired pneumonia: 500 mg every 24 hours for 7-14 days

Acute maxillary sinusitis: 500 mg every 24 hours for 10-14 days

Uncomplicated skin infections: 500 mg every 24 hours for 7-10 days

Uncomplicated urinary tract infections: 250 mg once daily for 3 days

Complicated urinary tract infections include acute pyelonephritis: 250 mg every 24 hours for 10 days

Dosing adjustment in renal impairment:

Cl_{cr} 20-49 mL/minute: Administer 250 mg every 24 hours (initial: 500 mg)

Cl_{cr} 10-19 mL/minute: Administer 250 mg every 48 hours (initial: 500 mg for most infections; 250 mg for renal infections)

Hemodialysis/CAPD: 250 mg every 48 hours (initial: 500 mg)

Dosage Forms INF, in D_5W: 5 mg/mL (50 mL, 100 mL). **INJ:** 25 mg/mL (20 mL). **TAB:** 250 mg, 500 mg

Contraindications Hypersensitivity to levofloxacin, any component, or other quinolones; pregnancy, lactation

Warnings/Precautions Not recommended in children <18 years of age; other quinolones have caused transient arthropathy in children; CNS stimulation may occur (tremor, restlessness, confusion, and very rarely hallucinations or seizures); use with caution in patients with known or suspected CNS disorders or renal dysfunction; prolonged use may result in superinfection; if an allergic reaction (itching, urticaria, dyspnea, pharyngeal or facial edema, loss of consciousness, tingling, cardiovascular collapse) occurs, discontinue the drug immediately; use caution to avoid possible photosensitivity reactions during and for several days following fluoroquinolone therapy; pseudomembranous colitis may occur and should be considered in patients who present with diarrhea

Pregnancy Risk Factor C

Pregnancy Implications

Clinical effects on the fetus: Avoid use in pregnant women unless the benefit justifies the potential risk to the fetus

Breast-feeding/lactation: Quinolones are known to distribute well into breast milk; consequently, use during lactation should be avoided, if possible

Adverse Reactions >1%:

Central nervous system: Dizziness, headache, insomnia

Dermatologic: Rash

Gastrointestinal: Nausea, vomiting, increased transaminases

Hematologic: Leukopenia, thrombocytopenia

Neuromuscular & skeletal: Tremor, arthralgia

Drug Interactions CYP1A2 enzyme inhibitor (minor)

Decreased effect: Decreased absorption with didanosine and antacids containing aluminum, magnesium, and/or calcium (by up to 98% if given at the same time), and with metal cations; phenytoin serum levels may be reduced by quinolones; antineoplastic agents may also decrease serum levels of fluoroquinolones

Increased toxicity/serum levels: Quinolones may cause increased levels of digoxin, caffeine, warfarin, cyclosporine. Cimetidine and probenecid increase quinolone levels; an increased incidence of seizures may occur with foscarnet.

Half-Life 6 hours; prolonged in renal impairment

Education and Monitoring Issues

Patient Education: Oral: Take per recommended schedule, preferably on an empty stomach (1 hour before or 2 hours after meals). Maintain adequate hydration (2-3 L/day of fluids unless instructed to restrict fluid intake). Take complete prescription; do not skip doses. Do not take with antacids. You may experience dizziness, lightheadedness, or confusion; use caution when driving or engaging in tasks that require alertness until response to drug is known. Small frequent meals and frequent mouth care may reduce nausea or vomiting. You may experience photosensitivity; use sunscreen, wear protective clothing and eyewear, and avoid direct sunlight. Report palpitations or chest pain, persistent diarrhea, GI disturbances or abdominal pain, muscle tremor or pain, yellowing of eyes or skin, easy bruising or bleeding, unusual fatigue, fever, chills, signs of infection, or worsening of condition. Report immediately any rash; itching; unusual CNS changes; pain, inflammation, or rupture of tendon; or any facial swelling.

Monitoring Parameters: Evaluation of organ system functions (renal, hepatic, ophthalmologic, and hematopoietic) is recommended periodically during therapy; the possibility of crystalluria should be assessed; WBC and signs of infection

Manufacturer Ortho-McNeil Pharmaceutical

Related Information

Antimicrobial Drugs of Choice *on page 1182*

Community Acquired Pneumonia in Adults *on page 1200*

Pharmaceutical Manufacturers Directory *on page 1020*

Levomethadyl Acetate Hydrochloride

(lee voe METH a dil AS e tate hye droe KLOR ide)

Pharmacologic Class Analgesic, Narcotic

U.S. Brand Names ORLAAM®

Use Management of opiate dependence

USUAL DOSAGE Adults: Oral: 20-40 mg 3 times/week, with ranges of 10 mg to as high as 140 mg 3 times/week; always dilute before administration and mix with diluent prior to dispensing

Dosage Forms SOLN, oral: 10 mg/mL (474 mL)

Warnings/Precautions Not recommended for use outside of the treatment of opiate addiction; shall be dispensed only by treatment programs approved by FDA, DEA, and the designated state authority. Approved treatment programs shall dispense and use levomethadyl in oral form only and according to the treatment requirements stipulated in federal regulations. Failure to abide by these requirements may result in injunction

(Continued)

Levomethadyl Acetate Hydrochloride *(Continued)*

precluding operation of the program, seizure of the drug supply, revocation of the program approval, and possible criminal prosecution.

Adverse Reactions

>10%:

Central nervous system: Malaise

Miscellaneous: Flu syndrome

1% to 10%:

Central nervous system: CNS depression, sedation, chills, abnormal dreams, anxiety, euphoria, headache, insomnia, nervousness, hypesthesia

Endocrine & metabolic: Hot flashes (males 2:1)

Gastrointestinal: Abdominal pain, constipation, diarrhea, xerostomia, nausea, vomiting

Genitourinary: Urinary tract spasm, difficult ejaculation, impotence, decreased sex drive

Neuromuscular & skeletal: Arthralgia, back pain, weakness

Ocular: Miosis, blurred vision

<1%: Myalgia, postural hypotension, tearing

Drug Interactions

Sedative, tranquilizers, propoxyphene, antidepressants, benzodiazepines, alcohol used in combination with ORLAAM® may result in serious overdose

ORLAAM® used in combination with naloxone, naltrexone, pentazocine, nalbuphine, butorphanol, and buprenorphine may result in withdrawal symptoms

Meperidine and propoxyphene may be ineffective in patients taking ORLAAM®

Carbamazepine, phenobarbital, rifampin, phenytoin may enhance the metabolism of ORLAAM® leading to an increase in ORLAAM®'s peak effect and shorten its duration of action

Erythromycin, cimetidine, and ketoconazole may slow the onset, lower the activity, and/or increase the duration of action of ORLAAM® via enzyme inhibitors

Half-Life 2-4 days

Education and Monitoring Issues

Monitoring Parameters: Patient adherence with regimen and avoidance of illicit substances; random drug testing is recommended

Manufacturer Roxane Laboratories, Inc

Related Information

Pharmaceutical Manufacturers Directory *on page 1020*

Levonorgestrel (LEE voe nor jes trel)

Pharmacologic Class Contraceptive

U.S. Brand Names Norplant® Implant; Plan B™

Generic Available No

Mechanism of Action First, ovulation is inhibited in about 50% to 60% of implant users from a negative feedback mechanism on the hypothalamus, leading to reduced secretion of follicle stimulating hormone (FSH) and luteinizing hormone (LH). An insufficient luteal phase has also been demonstrated with levonorgestrel administration and may result from defective gonadotropin stimulation of the ovary or from a direct effect of the drug on progesterone synthesis by the corpora lutea.

Use Prevention of pregnancy. The net cumulative 5-year pregnancy rate for levonorgestrel implant use has been reported to be from 1.5-3.9 pregnancies/100 users. Norplant® is a very efficient, yet reversible, method of contraception. The long duration of action may be particularly advantageous in women who desire an extended period of contraceptive protection without sacrificing the possibility of future fertility.

USUAL DOSAGE Total administration doses (implanted): 216 mg in 6 capsules which should be implanted during the first 7 days of onset of menses subdermally in the upper arm; each Norplant® silastic capsule releases 80 mcg of drug/day for 6-18 months, following which a rate of release of 25-30 mcg/day is maintained for ≤5 years; capsules should be removed by end of 5th year

Emergency contraception: One 0.75 mg tablet as soon as possible within 72 hours of unprotected sex; a second 0.75 mg tablet should be taken 12 hours after the first dose

Dosage Forms CAP, subdermal implantation: 36 mg (6s). **TAB:** 0.75 mg

Contraindications Women with undiagnosed abnormal uterine bleeding, hemorrhagic diathesis, known or suspected pregnancy, active hepatic disease, active thrombophlebitis, thromboembolic disorders, or known or suspected carcinoma of the breast

Warnings/Precautions Patients presenting with lower abdominal pain should be evaluated for follicular atresia and ectopic pregnancy. Plan B™ tablets are not intended to be used for routine contraception.

Pregnancy Risk Factor X

Adverse Reactions

>10%: Hormonal: Prolonged menstrual flow, spotting

1% to 10%:

Central nervous system: Headache, nervousness, dizziness

Dermatologic: Dermatitis, acne

Endocrine & metabolic: Amenorrhea, irregular menstrual cycles, scanty bleeding, breast discharge

Gastrointestinal: Nausea, change in appetite, weight gain
Genitourinary: Vaginitis, leukorrhea
Local: Pain or itching at implant site
Neuromuscular & skeletal: Myalgia
<1%: Infection at implant site, induration, bruising, nerve injury, phlebitis

Drug Interactions Decreased effect: Carbamazepine/phenytoin/rifampin; for women receiving long-term therapy with hepatic enzyme inducers, another method of contraception should be considered

Half-Life 11-45 hours

Education and Monitoring Issues

Patient Education: Do not attempt to remove implants - see prescriber. You may experience photosensitivity (use sunscreen, wear protective clothing and eyewear, avoid direct sunlight); dizziness or sleeplessness (use caution when driving or engaging in hazardous tasks until response to drug is known); skin rash, change in skin color, loss of hair, or unusual menses (breakthrough bleeding, irregularity, excessive bleeding - these should resolve after the first month). Report swelling, pain, or excessive feelings of warmth in calves, sudden acute headache, or visual disturbance, unusual nausea or vomiting, and any loss of feeling in arms or legs, unusual menses (if they persist past first month), and irritation at insertion site.

♦ **Levora®** *see* Ethinyl Estradiol and Levonorgestrel *on page 341*

Levorphanol (lee VOR fa nole)

Pharmacologic Class Analgesic, Narcotic

U.S. Brand Names Levo-Dromoran®

Generic Available No

Mechanism of Action Levorphanol tartrate is a synthetic opioid agonist that is classified as a morphinan derivative. Opioids interact with stereospecific opioid receptors in various parts of the central nervous system and other tissues. Analgesic potency parallels the affinity for these binding sites. These drugs do not alter the threshold or responsiveness to pain, but the perception of pain.

Use Relief of moderate to severe pain; also used parenterally for preoperative sedation and an adjunct to nitrous oxide/oxygen anesthesia; 2 mg levorphanol produces analgesia comparable to that produced by 10 mg of morphine

USUAL DOSAGE Adults:

Oral: 2 mg every 6-24 hours as needed
S.C.: 2 mg, up to 3 mg if necessary, every 6-8 hours

Dosing adjustment in hepatic disease: Reduction is necessary in patients with liver disease

Dosage Forms INJ: 2 mg/mL (1 mL, 10 mL). **TAB:** 2 mg

Contraindications Hypersensitivity to levorphanol or any component

Warnings/Precautions Use with caution in patients with hypersensitivity reactions to other phenanthrene derivative opioid agonists (morphine, hydrocodone, hydromorphone, levorphanol, oxycodone, oxymorphone); respiratory diseases including asthma, emphysema, COPD or severe liver or renal insufficiency; some preparations contain sulfites which may cause allergic reactions; tolerance or dependence may result from extended use; dextromethorphan has equivalent antitussive activity but has much lower toxicity in accidental overdose. Elderly may be particularly susceptible to the CNS depressant and constipating effects of narcotics.

Pregnancy Risk Factor B; D (if used for prolonged periods or in high doses at term)

Adverse Reactions

>10%:

Cardiovascular: Palpitations, hypotension, bradycardia, peripheral vasodilation
Central nervous system: CNS depression, fatigue, drowsiness, dizziness
Dermatologic: Pruritus
Gastrointestinal: Nausea, vomiting
Neuromuscular & skeletal: Weakness

1% to 10%:

Central nervous system: Nervousness, headache, restlessness, anorexia, malaise, confusion
Gastrointestinal: Stomach cramps, xerostomia, constipation
Endocrine & metabolic: Antidiuretic hormone release
Gastrointestinal: Biliary tract spasm
Genitourinary: Decreased urination, urinary tract spasm
Local: Pain at injection site
Ocular: Miosis
Respiratory: Respiratory depression

<1%: Hallucinations, histamine release, increased intracranial pressure, mental depression, paradoxical CNS stimulation, paralytic ileus, physical and psychological dependence rash, urticaria

Drug Interactions Increased toxicity: CNS depressants increase CNS depression

Alcohol Interactions Avoid use (may increase central nervous system depression)

Onset Oral: 10-60 minutes

Duration 4-8 hours

(Continued)

Levorphanol *(Continued)*

Half-Life 12-16 hours

Education and Monitoring Issues

Patient Education: If self-administered, use exactly as directed (do not increase dose or frequency); may cause physical and/or psychological dependence. While using this medication, do not use alcohol and other prescription or OTC medications (especially sedatives, tranquilizers, antihistamines, or pain medications) without consulting prescriber. Maintain adequate hydration (2-3 L/day of fluids unless instructed to restrict fluid intake). May cause hypotension, dizziness, drowsiness, impaired coordination, or blurred vision (use caution when driving, climbing stairs, or changing position - rising from sitting or lying to standing, or when engaging in tasks requiring alertness until response to drug is known); loss of appetite, nausea, or vomiting (frequent mouth care, small frequent meals, chewing gum, or sucking lozenges may help); constipation (increased exercise, fluids, or dietary fruit and fiber may help - if constipation remains an unresolved problem, consult prescriber about use of stool softeners). Report chest pain, slow or rapid heartbeat, acute dizziness, or persistent headache; swelling of extremities or unusual weight gain; changes in urinary elimination; acute headache; back or flank pain or spasms; blurred vision; skin rash; or shortness of breath.

Dietary Considerations: Food: Glucose may cause hyperglycemia; monitor blood glucose concentrations

Monitoring Parameters: Pain relief, respiratory and mental status, blood pressure

Related Information

Lipid-Lowering Agents Comparison *on page 1243*
Narcotic Agonists Comparison *on page 1244*

♦ **Levo-T™** *see* Levothyroxine *on page 526*
♦ **Levothroid®** *see* Levothyroxine *on page 526*

Levothyroxine (lee voe thye ROKS een)

Pharmacologic Class Thyroid Product

U.S. Brand Names Eltroxin®; Levo-T™; Levothroid®; Levoxyl®; Synthroid®

Generic Available Yes

Mechanism of Action Exact mechanism of action is unknown; however, it is believed the thyroid hormone exerts its many metabolic effects through control of DNA transcription and protein synthesis; involved in normal metabolism, growth, and development; promotes gluconeogenesis, increases utilization and mobilization of glycogen stores, and stimulates protein synthesis, increases basal metabolic rate

Use Replacement or supplemental therapy in hypothyroidism; some clinicians suggest levothyroxine is the drug of choice for replacement therapy

USUAL DOSAGE

Children: Congenital hypothyroidism:

Oral:

0-6 months: 8-10 mcg/kg/day **or** 25-50 mcg/day
6-12 months: 6-8 mcg/kg/day **or** 50-75 mcg/day
1-5 years: 5-6 mcg/kg/day **or** 75-100 mcg/day
6-12 years: 4-5 mcg/kg/day **or** 100-150 mcg/day
>12 years: 2-3 mcg/kg/day **or** ≥150 mcg/day

I.M., I.V.: 50% to 75% of the oral dose

Adults:

Oral: Initial: 0.05 mg/day, then increase by increments of 25 mcg/day at intervals of 2-3 weeks; average adult dose: 100-200 mcg/day; maximum dose: 200 mcg/day

I.M., I.V.: 50% of the oral dose

Myxedema coma or stupor: I.V.: 200-500 mcg one time, then 100-300 mcg the next day if necessary

Thyroid suppression therapy: Oral: 2-6 mcg/kg/day for 7-10 days

Dosage Forms POWDER for inj, lyophilized: 200 mcg/vial (6 mL, 10 mL), 500 mcg/vial (6 mL, 10 mL). **TAB:** 25 mcg, 50 mcg, 75 mcg, 88 mcg, 100 mcg, 112 mcg, 125 mcg, 150 mcg, 175 mcg, 200 mcg, 300 mcg

Contraindications Recent myocardial infarction or thyrotoxicosis, uncorrected adrenal insufficiency, hypersensitivity to levothyroxine sodium or any component

Warnings/Precautions Ineffective for weight reduction; high doses may produce serious or even life-threatening toxic effects particularly when used with some anorectic drugs. Use with caution and reduce dosage in patients with angina pectoris or other cardiovascular disease; levothyroxine tablets contain tartrazine dye which may cause allergic reactions in susceptible individuals; use cautiously in elderly since they may be more likely to have compromised cardiovascular functions. Patients with adrenal insufficiency, myxedema, diabetes mellitus and insipidus may have symptoms exaggerated or aggravated; thyroid replacement requires periodic assessment of thyroid status. Chronic hypothyroidism predisposes patients to coronary artery disease.

Pregnancy Risk Factor A

Adverse Reactions <1%: Abdominal cramps, alopecia, ataxia, cardiac arrhythmias, changes in menstrual cycle, chest pain, constipation, diaphoresis, diarrhea, fever, hand tremors, headache, increased appetite, insomnia, myalgia, nervousness, palpitations, shortness of breath, tachycardia, tremor, weight loss

Drug Interactions

Decreased effect:

Phenytoin may decrease levothyroxine levels

Cholestyramine may decrease absorption of levothyroxine

Increased oral hypoglycemic requirements

Increased effect: Increased effects of oral anticoagulants

Increased toxicity: Tricyclic antidepressants may increase toxic potential of both drugs

Onset

Onset of therapeutic effect: Oral: 3-5 days; I.V. Within 6-8 hours

Peak effect: I.V.: Within 24 hours

Half-Life 6-7 days

Education and Monitoring Issues

Patient Education: Thyroid replacement therapy is generally for life. Take as directed, in the morning before breakfast. Do not change brands and do not discontinue without consulting prescriber. Consult prescriber if drastically increasing or decreasing intake of goitrogenic food (eg, asparagus, cabbage, peas, turnip greens, broccoli, spinach, brussels sprouts, lettuce, soybeans). Report chest pain, rapid heart rate, palpitations, heat intolerance, excessive sweating, increased nervousness, agitation, or lethargy.

Monitoring Parameters: Thyroid function test (serum thyroxine, thyrotropin concentrations), resin triiodothyronine uptake (RT_3U), free thyroxine index (FTI), T_4, TSH, heart rate, blood pressure, clinical signs of hypo- and hyperthyroidism; TSH is the most reliable guide for evaluating adequacy of thyroid replacement dosage. TSH may be elevated during the first few months of thyroid replacement despite patients being clinically euthyroid. In cases where T_4 remains low and TSH is within normal limits, an evaluation of "free" (unbound) T_4 is needed to evaluate further increase in dosage

Reference Range: Pediatrics: Cord T_4 and values in the first few weeks are much higher, falling over the first months and years. ≥10 years: ~5.8-11 µg/dL (SI: 75-142 nmol/L). Borderline low: ≤4.5-5.7 µg/dL (SI: 58-73 nmol/L); low: ≤4.4 µg/dL (SI: 57 nmol/L); results <2.5 µg/dL (SI: <32 nmol/L) are strong evidence for hypothyroidism.

Approximate adult normal range: 4-12 µg/dL (SI: 51-154 nmol/L). Borderline high: 11.1-13 µg/dL (SI: 143-167 nmol/L); high: ≥13.1 µg/dL (SI: 169 nmol/L). Normal range is increased in women on birth control pills (5.5-12 µg/dL); normal range in pregnancy: ~5.5-16 µg/dL (SI: ~71-206 nmol/L). TSH: 0.4-10 (for those ≥80 years) mIU/L; T_4: 4-12 µg/dL (SI: 51-154 nmol/L); T_3 (RIA) (total T_3): 80-230 ng/dL (SI: 1.2-3.5 nmol/L); T_4 free (free T_4): 0.7-1.8 ng/dL (SI: 9-23 pmol/L).

- **Levoxyl®** *see* Levothyroxine *on page 526*
- **Levsin®** *see* Hyoscyamine *on page 456*
- **Levsinex®** *see* Hyoscyamine *on page 456*
- **Levsin/SL®** *see* Hyoscyamine *on page 456*
- **Levulan® Kerastick™** *see* Aminolevulinic Acid *on page 47*
- **Lexxel™** *see* Enalapril and Felodipine *on page 311*
- **Librax®** *see* Clidinium and Chlordiazepoxide *on page 208*
- **Libritabs®** *see* Chlordiazepoxide *on page 180*
- **Librium®** *see* Chlordiazepoxide *on page 180*
- **Lice-Enz® Shampoo [OTC]** *see* Pyrethrins *on page 795*
- **Lida-Mantle HC® Topical** *see* Lidocaine and Hydrocortisone *on page 529*
- **Lidemol** *see* Fluocinonide *on page 375*
- **Lidex®** *see* Fluocinonide *on page 375*
- **Lidex-E®** *see* Fluocinonide *on page 375*

Lidocaine (LYE doe kane)

Pharmacologic Class Antiarrhythmic Agent, Class I-B; Local Anesthetic

U.S. Brand Names Anestacon®; Dermaflex® Gel; Dilocaine®; Dr Scholl's® Cracked Heel Relief Cream [OTC]; Duo-Trach®; Lidoderm® Patch; LidoPen® Auto-Injector; Nervocaine®; Octocaine®; Solarcaine® Aloe Extra Burn Relief [OTC]; Xylocaine®; Zilactin-L® [OTC]

Generic Available Yes

Mechanism of Action Class IB antiarrhythmic; suppresses automaticity of conduction tissue, by increasing electrical stimulation threshold of ventricle, HIS-Purkinje system, and spontaneous depolarization of the ventricles during diastole by a direct action on the tissues; blocks both the initiation and conduction of nerve impulses by decreasing the neuronal membrane's permeability to sodium ions, which results in inhibition of depolarization with resultant blockade of conduction

Use Local anesthetic and acute treatment of ventricular arrhythmias from myocardial infarction, cardiac manipulation, digitalis intoxication; topical local anesthetic; drug of choice for ventricular ectopy, ventricular tachycardia, ventricular fibrillation; for pulseless VT or VF preferably administer **after** defibrillation and epinephrine; control of premature ventricular contractions, wide-complex PSVT; relief of pain associated with postherpetic neuralgia

(Continued)

Lidocaine *(Continued)*

USUAL DOSAGE

Topical: Apply to affected area as needed; maximum: 3 mg/kg/dose; do not repeat within 2 hours

Postherpetic neuralgia: Lidoderm® patch: Apply patch to most painful area; up to 3 patches may be applied in a single application; patch may remain in place for up to 12 hours in any 24-hour period

Injectable local anesthetic: Varies with procedure, degree of anesthesia needed, vascularity of tissue, duration of anesthesia required, and physical condition of patient; maximum: 4.5 mg/kg/dose; do not repeat within 2 hours

I.M.: Adults: 300 mg (best in deltoid muscle; only 10% solution)

Children: Endotracheal, intraosseous, I.V.: Loading dose: 1 mg/kg; may repeat in 10-15 minutes for 2 doses; after loading dose, start I.V. continuous infusion 20-50 mcg/kg/minute (300 mcg/kg/minute per American Heart Association)

Use 20 mcg/kg/minute in patients with shock, hepatic disease, mild congestive heart failure (CHF)

Moderate to severe CHF may require 1/2 loading dose and lower infusion rates to avoid toxicity

Adults: Antiarrhythmic:

I.V.: 1-1.5 mg/kg bolus over 2-3 minutes; may repeat doses of 0.5-0.75 mg/kg in 5-10 minutes up to a total of 3 mg/kg; continuous infusion: 1-4 mg/minute

I.V. (2 g/250 mL D_5W) infusion rates (infusion pump should be used for I.V. infusion administration):

1 mg/minute: 7 mL/hour
2 mg/minute: 15 mL/hour
3 mg/minute: 21 mL/hour
4 mg/minute: 30 mL/hour

Ventricular fibrillation (after defibrillation and epinephrine): Initial dose: 1.5 mg/kg, may repeat boluses as above; follow with continuous infusion after return of perfusion

Prevention of ventricular fibrillation: I.V.: Initial bolus: 0.5 mg/kg; repeat every 5-10 minutes to a total dose of 2 mg/kg

Refractory ventricular fibrillation: Repeat 1.5 mg/kg bolus may be given 3-5 minutes after initial dose

Endotracheal: 2-2.5 times the I.V. dose

Decrease dose in patients with CHF, shock, or hepatic disease

Dosing adjustment/comments in hepatic disease: Reduce dose in acute hepatitis and decompensated cirrhosis by 50%

Dialysis: Not dialyzable (0% to 5%) by hemo- or peritoneal dialysis; supplemental dose not necessary

Dosage Forms CRM: 2% (56 g). **INJ:** 0.5% [5 mg/mL] (50 mL); 1% [10 mg/mL] (2 mL, 5 mL, 10 mL, 20 mL, 30 mL, 50 mL); 1.5% [15 mg/mL] (20 mL); 2% [20 mg/mL] (2 mL, 5 mL, 10 mL, 20 mL, 30 mL, 50 mL); 4% [40 mg/mL] (5 mL); 10% [100 mg/mL] (10 mL); 20% [200 mg/mL] (10 mL, 20 mL). **INJ:** I.M. use: 10% [100 mg/mL] (3 mL, 5 mL); Direct I.V.: 1% [10 mg/mL] (5 mL, 10 mL), 20 mg/mL (5 mL); I.V. admixture (preservative free): 4% [40 mg/mL] (25 mL, 30 mL), 10% [100 mg/mL] (10 mL), 20% [200 mg/mL] (5 mL, 10 mL); I.V. infusion, in D_5W: 0.2% [2 mg/mL] (500 mL), 0.4% [4 mg/mL] (250 mL, 500 mL, 1000 mL), 0.8% [8 mg/mL] (250 mL, 500 mL). **GEL, top:** 2% (30 mL), 2.5% (15 mL). **LIQ:** Top: 2.5% (7.5 mL); Viscous: 2% (20 mL, 100 mL). **OINT, top:** 2.5% [OTC], 5% (35 g). **PATCH, transdermal:** 5%. **SOLN, top:** 2% (15 mL, 240 mL), 4% (50 mL)

Contraindications Known hypersensitivity to amide-type local anesthetics; patients with Adams-Stokes syndrome or with severe degree of S-A, A-V, or intraventricular heart block (without a pacemaker)

Warnings/Precautions Avoid use of preparations containing preservatives for spinal or epidural (including caudal) anesthesia. Use extreme caution in patients with hepatic disease, heart failure, marked hypoxia, severe respiratory depression, hypovolemia or shock, incomplete heart block or bradycardia, and atrial fibrillation.

Due to decreases in phase I metabolism and possibly decrease in splanchnic perfusion with age, there may be a decreased clearance or increased half-life in elderly and increased risk for CNS side effects and cardiac effects

Pregnancy Risk Factor B (per manufacturer); C (based on expert analysis)

Adverse Reactions

1% to 10%:

Cardiovascular: Hypotension
Central nervous system: Positional headache
Miscellaneous: Shivering

<1%: Agitation, anxiety, arrhythmias, blurred vision, cardiovascular collapse, coma, diplopia, dyspnea, edema of the skin, euphoria, hallucinations, heart block, itching, lethargy, nausea, paresthesias, rash, respiratory depression or arrest, seizures, slurred speech, vomiting

Drug Interactions CYP3A3/4 enzyme substrate

Increased toxicity:

Concomitant cimetidine or beta-blockers may result in increased serum concentrations of lidocaine with resultant toxicity; procainamide and tocainide may result in additive cardiodepressant action

Effect of succinylcholine may be enhanced

Amprenavir may increase the toxicity of lidocaine

Onset Single bolus dose: 45-90 seconds

Duration 10-20 minutes

Half-Life Biphasic: Increased with CHF, liver disease, shock, severe renal disease; Initial: 7-30 minutes; Terminal: 1.5-2 hours

Education and Monitoring Issues

Patient Education: I.V.: You will be monitored during infusion. Do not get up without assistance. Report dizziness, numbness, double vision, nausea, pain or burning at infusion site, nightmares, hearing strange noises, seeing unusual visions, or difficulty breathing.

Dermatologic: You will experience decreased sensation to pain, heat, or cold in the area and/or decreased muscle strength (depending on area of application) until effects wear off; use necessary caution to reduce incidence of possible injury until full sensation returns. Report irritation, pain, burning at injection site, persistent numbness, tingling, swelling; restlessness, dizziness, acute weakness; blurred vision; ringing in ears; or difficulty breathing.

Oral: Lidocaine can cause numbness of tongue, cheeks, and throat. Do not eat or drink for 1 hour after use. Take small sips of water at first to ensure that you can swallow without difficulty. Your tongue and mouth may be numb; use caution avoid biting yourself. Immediately report swelling of face, lips, or tongue.

Patch: Patch may be cut to appropriate size. Apply patch to most painful area. Up to 3 patches may be applied in a single application. Patch may remain in place for up to 12 hours in any 24-hour period. Remove immediately if burning sensation occurs. Wash hands after application.

Reference Range:

Therapeutic: 1.5-5.0 μg/mL (SI: 6-21 μmol/L)

Potentially toxic: >6 μg/mL (SI: >26 μmol/L)

Toxic: >9 μg/mL (SI: >38 μmol/L)

Related Information

Lidocaine and Hydrocortisone *on page 529*

Lidocaine and Epinephrine (LYE doe kane & ep i NEF rin)

Pharmacologic Class Local Anesthetic

U.S. Brand Names Octocaine® With Epinephrine; Xylocaine® With Epinephrine

Mechanism of Action Lidocaine blocks both the initiation and conduction of nerve impulses via decreased permeability of sodium ions; epinephrine increases the duration of action of lidocaine by causing vasoconstriction (via alpha effects) which slows the vascular absorption of lidocaine

Use Local infiltration anesthesia; AVS for nerve block

USUAL DOSAGE

Children: Use lidocaine concentrations of 0.5% to 1% (or even more diluted) to decrease possibility of toxicity; lidocaine dose should not exceed 7 mg/kg/dose; do not repeat within 2 hours

Adults: Dosage varies with the anesthetic procedure, degree of anesthesia needed, vascularity of tissue, duration of anesthesia required, and physical condition of patient

Dosage Forms INJ, with epinephrine: 1:200,000: Lidocaine hydrochloride 0.5% [5 mg/mL] (50 mL), 1% [10 mg/mL] (30 mL), 1.5% [15 mg/mL] (5 mL, 10 mL, 30 mL), 2% [20 mg/mL] (20 mL); 1:100,000: Lidocaine hydrochloride 1% [10 mg/mL] (20 mL, 50 mL), 2% [20 mg/mL] (1.8 mL, 20 mL, 50 mL); 1:50,000: Lidocaine hydrochloride 2% [20 mg/mL] (1.8 mL)

Contraindications Hypersensitivity to local anesthetics of the amide type, myasthenia gravis, shock, or cardiac conduction disease

Warnings/Precautions Do not use solutions in distal portions of the body (digits, nose, ears, penis); use with caution in endocrine, heart, hepatic, or thyroid disease

Pregnancy Risk Factor B

Adverse Reactions Refer to Lidocaine monograph

Onset Peak: within 5 minutes

Duration ~2 hours

Lidocaine and Hydrocortisone (LYE doe kane & hye droe KOR ti sone)

Pharmacologic Class Anesthetic/Corticosteroid

U.S. Brand Names Lida-Mantle HC® Topical

Dosage Forms CRM: Lidocaine 3% and hydrocortisone 0.5% (15 g, 30 g)

Pregnancy Risk Factor B (lidocaine); C (hydrocortisone)

Lidocaine and Prilocaine (LYE doe kane & PRIL oh kane)

Pharmacologic Class Local Anesthetic

U.S. Brand Names EMLA® Anesthetic Disc; EMLA® Cream

(Continued)

Lidocaine and Prilocaine *(Continued)*

Mechanism of Action Local anesthetic action occurs by stabilization of neuronal membranes and inhibiting the ionic fluxes required for the initiation and conduction of impulses

Use Topical anesthetic for use on normal intact skin for local analgesia, genital mucous membranes for superficial minor surgery, and as pretreatment for infiltration anesthesia; EMLA® is **not** recommended in any clinical situation in which penetration or migration beyond the tympanic membrane into the middle ear is possible

USUAL DOSAGE Although the incidence of systemic adverse effects with EMLA® is very low, caution should be exercised, particularly when applying over large areas and leaving on for >2 hours

Children (intact skin): EMLA® should **not** be used in neonates with a gestation age <37 weeks nor in infants <12 months of age who are receiving treatment with methoglobin-inducing agents

Dosing is based on child's age and weight:

Age & Body Weight Requirements	Maximum Application Area	Maximum Applicaiton Time (h)	Maximum Total Dose of EMLA® (g)
0 up to 3 mo or <5 kg	10 cm²	1	1
3 mo up to 12 mo and >5 kg	20 cm²	4	2
1-6 y and >10 kg	100 cm²	4	10
7-12 y and >20 kg	200 cm²	4	20

Adults (intact skin):

EMLA® cream and EMLA® anesthetic disc: A thick layer of EMLA® cream is applied to intact skin and covered with an occlusive dressing, or alternatively, an EMLA® anesthetic disc is applied to intact skin

Minor dermal procedures (eg, I.V. cannulation or venipuncture): apply 2.5 g of cream (1/2 of the 5 g tube) over 20-25 cm of skin surface area, or 1 anesthetic disc (1 g over 10 cm^2) for at least 1 hour. **Note:** In clinical trials, 2 sites were usually prepared in case there was a technical problem with cannulation or venipuncture at the first site.

EMLA® cream: A thick layer of cream is applied to intact skin and covered with an occlusive dressing

Major dermal procedures (eg, more painful dermatological procedures involving a larger skin area such as split thickness skin graft harvesting): Apply 2 g of cream per 10 cm^2 of skin and allow to remain in contact with the skin for at least 2 hours.

Adult male genital skin (eg, pretreatment prior to local anesthetic infiltration): Apply a thick layer of cream (1 g/10 cm^2) to the skin surface for 15 minutes. Local anesthetic infiltration should be performed immediately after removal of EMLA® cream.

Note: Dermal analgesia can be expected to increase for up to 3 hours under occlusive dressing and persist for 1-2 hours after removal of the cream

Adult females: Genital mucous membranes: Minor procedures (eg, removal of condylomata acuminata, pretreatment for local anesthetic infiltration): Apply 5-10 g (thick layer) of cream for 5-10 minutes

Dosage Forms CRM: Lidocaine 2.5% and prilocaine 2.5% [2 Tegaderm® dressings] (5 g, 30 g). **DISC,** anesthetic: 1

Contraindications

Children <1 month of age

Administration on mucous membranes

Administration on broken or inflamed skin

Children with congenital or idiopathic methemoglobinemia, or in children who are receiving medications associated with drug-induced methemoglobinemia [ie, acetaminophen (overdosage), benzocaine, chloroquine, dapsone, nitrofurantoin, nitroglycerin, nitroprusside, phenazopyridine, phenelzine, phenobarbital, phenytoin, quinine, sulfonamides]

Patients with a known history of sensitivity to local anesthetics of the amide type or to any other component of the product

Warnings/Precautions EMLA® should not be used in patients with congenital or idiopathic methemoglobinemia and in infants <12 months of age who are receiving treatment with methemoglobin-inducing agents. Very young patients or patients with glucose-6-phosphate deficiencies are more susceptible to methemoglobinemia. Patients taking drugs associated with drug-induced methemoglobinemia (sulfonamides, acetaminophen, acetanilide, analine dyes, benzocaine, chloroquine, dapsone, naphthalene, nitrates/nitrites, nitrofurantoin, nitroglycerin, nitroprusside, pamoquine, para-aminosalicylic acid, phenacetin, phenobarbital, phenytoin, primaquine, quinine) are at greater risk for developing methemoglobinemia. Reports of significant methemoglobinemia have occurred in infants and children following excessive applications of EMLA® cream. These cases involved the use of large doses, larger than recommended areas of application, infants <3 months of age who did not have fully mature enzyme systems. Treatment with I.V. methylene blue may be effective if required.

Neonates and infants up to 3 months of age should be monitored for Met-Hb levels before, during, and after application of EMLA®, provided the test results can be obtained quickly.

Use with caution in patients who may be more sensitive to the systemic effects of lidocaine and prilocaine, including acutely ill, debilitated, or elderly patients.

Use with caution in patients with severe hepatic disease, because their inability to metabolize local anesthetics normally puts them at greater risk of developing toxic plasma concentrations of lidocaine and prilocaine.

Pregnancy Risk Factor B

Pregnancy Implications Neither lidocaine nor prilocaine are contraindicated in labor and delivery. Total doses contributed by all formations must be considered if used concomitantly with other products containing lidocaine and/or prilocaine. Lidocaine, and probably prilocaine, are excreted in human milk. Caution should be considered when EMLA® is administered to a nursing mother.

Adverse Reactions

1% to 10%:

Dermatologic: Angioedema, contact dermatitis

Local: Burning, stinging

<1%: Alteration in temperature sensation, blanching, blurred vision, bradycardia, bronchospasm, CNS excitation, confusion, convulsions, dizziness, drowsiness, edema, erythema, euphoria, hypotension, itching, methemoglobinemia in infants, nervousness, rash, respiratory depression, shock, tenderness, tinnitus, tremors, urticaria

Drug Interactions Increased toxicity:

Class I antiarrhythmic drugs (tocainide, mexiletine): Effects are additive and potentially synergistic

Drugs known to induce methemoglobinemia

Onset 1 hour for sufficient dermal analgesia; Peak effect: 2-3 hours

Duration 1-2 hours after removal of the cream

Half-Life

Lidocaine: 65-150 minutes, prolonged with cardiac or hepatic dysfunction

Prilocaine: 10-150 minutes, prolonged in hepatic or renal dysfunction

Education and Monitoring Issues

Patient Education: This drug will block sensation to the applied area. Report irritation, pain, burning at application site.

- **Lidoderm® Patch** *see* Lidocaine *on page 527*
- **LidoPen® Auto-Injector** *see* Lidocaine *on page 527*
- **Limbitrol® DS 10-25** *see* Amitriptyline and Chlordiazepoxide *on page 52*
- **Linctus Codeine Blac** *see* Codeine *on page 223*
- **Linctus With Codeine Phosphate** *see* Codeine *on page 223*

Lindane (LIN dane)

Pharmacologic Class Antiparasitic Agent, Topical; Pediculocide; Scabicidal Agent

U.S. Brand Names G-well®; Kwell®; Scabene®

Generic Available Yes

Mechanism of Action Directly absorbed by parasites and ova through the exoskeleton; stimulates the nervous system resulting in seizures and death of parasitic arthropods

Use Treatment of scabies (*Sarcoptes scabiei*), *Pediculus capitis* (head lice), and *Pediculus pubis* (crab lice); FDA recommends reserving lindane as a second-line agent or with inadequate response to other therapies

USUAL DOSAGE Children and Adults: Topical:

Scabies: Apply a thin layer of lotion or cream and massage it on skin from the neck to the toes (head to toe in infants). For adults, bathe and remove the drug after 8-12 hours; for children, wash off 6-8 hours after application (for infants, wash off 6 hours after application); repeat treatment in 7 days if lice or nits are still present

Pediculosis, capitis and pubis: 15-30 mL of shampoo is applied and lathered for 4-5 minutes; rinse hair thoroughly and comb with a fine tooth comb to remove nits; repeat treatment in 7 days if lice or nits are still present

Dosage Forms CRM: 1% (60 g, 454 g). **LOT:** 1% (60 mL, 473 mL, 4000 mL). **SHAMP:** 1% (60 mL, 473 mL, 4000 mL)

Contraindications Hypersensitivity to lindane or any component; premature neonates; acutely inflamed skin or raw, weeping surfaces

Warnings/Precautions Not considered a drug of first choice; use with caution in infants and small children, and patients with a history of seizures; avoid contact with face, eyes, mucous membranes, and urethral meatus. Because of the potential for systemic absorption and CNS side effects, lindane should be used with caution; consider permethrin or crotamiton agent first.

Pregnancy Risk Factor B

Pregnancy Implications Clinical effects on the fetus: There are no well controlled studies in pregnant women; treat no more than twice during a pregnancy

Adverse Reactions <1%: Aplastic anemia, ataxia, burning and stinging, cardiac arrhythmia, contact dermatitis, dizziness, eczematous eruptions, headache, hematuria,

(Continued)

Lindane *(Continued)*

hepatitis, nausea, pulmonary edema, restlessness, seizures, skin and adipose tissue may act as repositories, vomiting

Drug Interactions Increased toxicity: Oil-based hair dressing may increase toxic potential

Half-Life 17-22 hours

Education and Monitoring Issues

Patient Education: For external use only. Do not apply to face and avoid getting in eyes. Do not apply immediately after hot soapy bath. Apply from neck to toes. Bathe to remove drug after 8-12 hours. Repeat in 7 days if lice or nits are still present. Clothing and bedding must be washed in hot water or dry cleaned to kill nits. Wash combs and brushes with lindane shampoo and thoroughly rinse. May need to treat all members of household and all sexual contacts concurrently. Report if condition persists or infection occurs.

Linezolid (li NE zoh lid)

Pharmacologic Class Antibiotic, Macrolide Combination

U.S. Brand Names Zyvox™

Mechanism of Action Binds to 50S ribosomal subunit near the interface with the 30S subunit resulting in distortion that prevents the 30S initiation complex. Inhibits the initiation of translation. Interacts with the translation component that is involved in binding mRNA during the start of translation.

Use Treatment of various infections causes by susceptible gram-positive organisms including vancomycin-resistant enterococcus faecium and faecalis

USUAL DOSAGE Adults: Oral or I.V.: 600 mg

Dosage Forms

Injection, I.V.: 200 mg, 600 mg (premade minibags)
Suspension, oral, powder for reconstitution: 100 mg/5 mL
Tablet, film-coated: 400 mg, 600 mg

Contraindications Allergy to linezolid or other oxazolidinones

Warnings/Precautions Linezolid has mild monoamine oxidase inhibitor properties and has the potential to have the same interactions as other MAOIs

Adverse Reactions

Cardiovascular: Hypertension
Central nervous system: Headache, insomnia, dizziness, fever
Dermatologic: Pruritus
Endocrine & metabolic: Oral and vaginal *monilia*
Gastrointestinal: Nausea, diarrhea, vomiting, dyspepsia, abdominal pain, constipation
Hepatic: Increased LFTs
Local: Localized pain

- **Lioresal®** *see* Baclofen *on page 90*
- **Lipid-Lowering Agents Comparison** *see page 1243*
- **Lipitor®** *see* Atorvastatin *on page 78*
- **Liposyn®** *see* Fat Emulsion *on page 351*
- **Lipram®** *see* Pancrelipase *on page 698*
- **Liquaemin®** *see* Heparin *on page 433*
- **Liquibid®** *see* Guaifenesin *on page 423*
- **Liqui-Char® [OTC]** *see* Charcoal *on page 175*
- **Liquid Pred®** *see* Prednisone *on page 763*
- **Liquiprin® [OTC]** *see* Acetaminophen *on page 17*

Lisinopril (lyse IN oh pril)

Pharmacologic Class Angiotensin-Converting Enzyme (ACE) Inhibitors

U.S. Brand Names Prinivil®; Zestril®

Generic Available No

Mechanism of Action Competitive inhibitor of angiotensin-converting enzyme (ACE); prevents conversion of angiotensin I to angiotensin II, a potent vasoconstrictor; results in lower levels of angiotensin II which causes an increase in plasma renin activity and a reduction in aldosterone secretion; a CNS mechanism may also be involved in hypotensive effect as angiotensin II increases adrenergic outflow from CNS; vasoactive kallikreins may be decreased in conversion to active hormones by ACE inhibitors, thus reducing blood pressure

Use Treatment of hypertension, either alone or in combination with other antihypertensive agents; adjunctive therapy in treatment of CHF (afterload reduction); treatment of hemodynamically stable patients within 24 hours of acute myocardial infarction, to improve survival

USUAL DOSAGE

Hypertension:

Adults: Initial: 10 mg/day; increase doses 5-10 mg/day at 1- to 2-week intervals; maximum daily dose: 40 mg

Elderly: Initial: 2.5-5 mg/day; increase doses 2.5-5 mg/day at 1- to 2-week intervals; maximum daily dose: 40 mg

Patients taking diuretics should have them discontinued 2-3 days prior to initiating lisinopril if possible; restart diuretic after blood pressure is stable if needed; if diuretic cannot be discontinued prior to therapy, begin with 5 mg with close supervision until stable blood pressure; in patients with hyponatremia (<130 mEq/L), start dose at 2.5 mg/day

Congestive heart failure: Adults: 5 mg initially with diuretics and digitalis; usual maintenance: 5-20 mg/day as a single dose

Acute myocardial infarction (within 24 hours in hemodynamically stable patients): Oral: 5 mg immediately, then 5 mg at 24 hours, 10 mg at 48 hours, and 10 mg every day thereafter for 6 weeks; patients should continue to receive standard treatments such as thrombolytics, aspirin, and beta-blockers

Dosing adjustment in renal impairment:

Cl_{cr} 10-50 mL/minute: Administer 50% to 75% of normal dose

Cl_{cr} <10 mL/minute: Administer 25% to 50% of normal dose

Hemodialysis: Dialyzable (50%)

Dosage Forms TAB: 2.5 mg, 5 mg, 10 mg, 20 mg, 40 mg

Contraindications Hypersensitivity to lisinopril or any component or other ACE inhibitors

Warnings/Precautions Use with caution and modify dosage in patients with renal impairment (decrease dosage) (especially renal artery stenosis), severe congestive heart failure, or with coadministered diuretic therapy; experience in children is limited. Severe hypotension may occur in patients who are sodium and/or volume depleted, initiate lower doses and monitor closely when starting therapy in these patients.

Pregnancy Risk Factor C (1st trimester); D (2nd and 3rd trimesters)

Pregnancy Implications

Clinical effects on the fetus: No data available on crossing the placenta. Cranial defects, hypocalvaria/acalvaria, oligohydramnios, persistent anuria following delivery, hypotension, renal defects, renal dysgenesis/dysplasia, renal failure, pulmonary hypoplasia, limb contractures secondary to oligohydramnios and stillbirth reported. ACE inhibitors should be avoided during pregnancy.

Breast-feeding/lactation: Crosses into breast milk. American Academy of Pediatrics considers **compatible** with breast-feeding.

Adverse Reactions Note: Frequency ranges include data from hypertension and heart failure trials. Higher rates of adverse reactions have generally been noted in patients with congestive heart failure. However, the frequency of adverse effects associated with placebo is also increased in this population.

1% to 10%:

Cardiovascular: Orthostatic effects (1.2%), hypotension (1.2% to 4.4%)

Central nervous system: Headache (4.4% to 5.7%), dizziness (5.4% to 11.8%), fatigue (2.5%), weakness (1.3%)

Dermatologic: Rash (1.3% to 1.7%)

Endocrine and metabolic: Hyperkalemia (2.2% to 4.8%)

Gastrointestinal: Diarrhea (2.7% to 3.7%), nausea (2.0%), vomiting (1.1%), abdominal pain (2.2%)

Genitourinary: Impotence (1%)

Hematologic: Decreased hemoglobin (small)

Neuromuscular & skeletal: Chest pain (3.4%)

Renal: Increased serum creatinine (often transient), increased BUN (2%); deterioration in renal function (in patients with bilateral renal artery stenosis or hypovolemia)

Respiratory: Cough (3.5% to 8.5%), upper respiratory infection (1.5% to 2.1%)

>1% but ≤ frequency in patients receiving placebo: Chest pain, back pain, angina, dyspnea, pruritus

<1% (limited to important or life-threatening symptoms): Angioedema, anaphylactoid reactions, edema, cardiac arrest, myocardial infarction, cerebrovascular accident, pulmonary embolism, arrhythmia, palpitation, TIA, paroxysmal nocturnal dyspnea, orthostatic hypotension, peripheral edema, vasculitis, pancreatitis, hepatitis, jaundice (cholestatic), vomiting, heartburn, gastrointestinal cramps, constipation, flatulence, xerostomia, bone marrow suppression, neutropenia, thrombocytopenia, diabetes mellitus, weight loss, dehydration, volume overload, gout, weight gain, arthritis, arthralgia, stroke, ataxia, memory impairment, tremor, peripheral neuropathy, paresthesia, confusion, insomnia, somnolence, irritability, nervousness, bronchospasm, infiltrates, asthma, pleural effusion, bronchitis, wheezing, epistaxis, laryngitis, sinusitis, pharyngitis, rhinitis, rhinorrhea, urticaria, alopecia, photosensitivity, pemphigus, erythema, flushing, diaphoresis, toxic epidermal necrolysis, Stevens-Johnson syndromes, vision loss, diplopia, blurred vision, tinnitus, photophobia, acute renal failure, oliguria, anuria, azotemia, renal dysfunction, dyspepsia, muscle cramps, paresthesia, decreased libido, vertigo, nasal congestion, increased transaminases, increased bilirubin, hyperkalemia, hyponatremia, gout

Case reports: Hepatitis, systemic lupus erythematosus. In addition, a syndrome which may include fever, myalgia, arthralgia, interstitial nephritis, vasculitis, rash, eosinophilia and positive ANA, and elevated ESR has been reported with ACE inhibitors

Drug Interactions

Allopurinol: Case reports (rare) indicate a possible increased risk of hypersensitivity reactions when combined with lisinopril

(Continued)

Lisinopril *(Continued)*

Alpha$_1$ blockers: Hypotensive effect increased
Aspirin and NSAIDs may decrease ACE inhibitor efficacy and/or increase adverse renal effects
Diuretics: Hypovolemia due to diuretics may precipitate acute hypotensive events or acute renal failure
Insulin: Risk of hypoglycemia may be increased
Lithium: Risk of lithium toxicity may be increased; monitor lithium levels, especially the first 4 weeks of therapy
Mercaptopurine: Risk of neutropenia may be increased
Potassium-sparing diuretics (amiloride, spironolactone, triamterene): Increased risk of hyperkalemia
Potassium supplements may increase the risk of hyperkalemia
Trimethoprim (high dose) may increase the risk of hyperkalemia

Alcohol Interactions Avoid use (may increase risk of hypotension or dizziness)

Onset 1 hour; Peak hypotensive effect: Oral: Within 6 hours

Duration 24 hours

Half-Life 11-12 hours

Education and Monitoring Issues

Patient Education: Take exactly as directed; do not discontinue without consulting prescriber. Take first dose at bedtime. This drug does not eliminate need for diet or exercise regimen as recommended by prescriber. Do not take potassium supplements or salt substitutes containing potassium without consulting prescriber. May cause dizziness, fainting, lightheadedness (use caution when driving or engaging in tasks that require alertness until response to drug is known); postural hypotension (use caution when rising from lying or sitting position or climbing stairs); nausea, vomiting, abdominal pain, dry mouth, or transient loss of appetite (small frequent meals, frequent mouth care, sucking lozenges, or chewing gum may help) - report if these persist. Report chest pain or palpitations; mouth sores; fever or chills; skin rash; numbness, tingling, or pain in muscles; difficulty in breathing or unusual cough; or other persistent adverse reactions.

Monitoring Parameters: Serum calcium levels, BUN, serum creatinine, renal function, WBC, and potassium

Related Information

Angiotensin-Related Agents Comparison *on page 1226*
Heart Failure Guidelines *on page 1099*
Lisinopril and Hydrochlorothiazide *on page 534*

Lisinopril and Hydrochlorothiazide

(lyse IN oh pril & hye droe klor oh THYE a zide)

Pharmacologic Class Antihypertensive Agent, Combination

U.S. Brand Names Prinzide®; Zestoretic®

Dosage Forms TAB: Lisinopril 10 mg and hydrochlorothiazide 12.5 mg, [12.5]-Lisinopril 20 mg and hydrochlorothiazide 12.5 mg, [25]-Lisinopril 20 mg and hydrochlorothiazide 25 mg

Pregnancy Risk Factor C (1st trimester); D (2nd and 3rd trimesters)

Alcohol Interactions Avoid use (may increase risk of hypotension or dizziness)

♦ **Listermint® with Fluoride [OTC]** *see* Fluoride *on page 376*

♦ **Lithane®** *see* Lithium *on page 534*

Lithium (LITH ee um)

Pharmacologic Class Lithium

U.S. Brand Names Eskalith®; Eskalith CR®; Lithane®; Lithobid®; Lithonate®; Lithotabs®

Generic Available Yes

Mechanism of Action Alters cation transport across cell membrane in nerve and muscle cells and influences reuptake of serotonin and/or norepinephrine

Use Management of acute manic episodes, bipolar disorders, and depression

USUAL DOSAGE Oral: Monitor serum concentrations and clinical response (efficacy and toxicity) to determine proper dose

Children 6-12 years: 15-60 mg/kg/day in 3-4 divided doses; dose not to exceed usual adult dosage
Adults: 300-600 mg 3-4 times/day; usual maximum maintenance dose: 2.4 g/day or 450-900 mg of sustained release twice daily
Elderly: Initial dose: 300 mg twice daily; increase weekly in increments of 300 mg/day, monitoring levels; rarely need >900-1200 mg/day

Dosing adjustment in renal impairment:

Cl_{cr} 10-50 mL/minute: Administer 50% to 75% of normal dose
Cl_{cr} <10 mL/minute: Administer 25% to 50% of normal dose

Hemodialysis: Dialyzable (50% to 100%)

Dosage Forms

Lithium carbonate: **CAP:** 150 mg, 300 mg, 600 mg. **TAB:** 300 mg; Controlled release: 450 mg; Slow release: 300 mg

Lithium citrate: **SYR:** 300 mg/5 mL (5 mL, 10 mL, 480 mL)

Contraindications Hypersensitivity to lithium or any component; severe cardiovascular or renal disease

Warnings/Precautions Lithium toxicity is closely related to serum levels and can occur at therapeutic doses; serum lithium determinations are required to monitor therapy. Use with caution in patients with cardiovascular or thyroid disease, severe debilitation, dehydration or sodium depletion, or in patients receiving diuretics. Some elderly patients may be extremely sensitive to the effects of lithium; see dosage and therapeutic levels.

Pregnancy Risk Factor D

Adverse Reactions

Cardiovascular: Cardiac arrhythmias, hypotension, sinus node dysfunction, flattened or inverted T waves (reversible), edema

Central nervous system: Dizziness, vertigo, slurred speech, blackout spells, seizures, sedation, restlessness, confusion, psychomotor retardation, stupor, coma, dystonia, fatigue, lethargy, headache, pseudotumor cerebri

Dermatologic: Dry or thinning of hair, folliculitis, alopecia, exacerbation of psoriasis, rash

Endocrine & metabolic: Euthyroid goiter and/or hypothyroidism, hyperthyroidism, hyperglycemia, diabetes insipidus

Gastrointestinal: Polydipsia, anorexia, nausea, vomiting, diarrhea, xerostomia, metallic taste, weight gain

Genitourinary: Incontinence, polyuria, glycosuria, oliguria, albuminuria

Hematologic: Leukocytosis

Neuromuscular & skeletal: Tremor, muscle hyperirritability, ataxia, choreoathetoid movements, hyperactive deep tendon reflexes

Ocular: Nystagmus, blurred vision

Miscellaneous: Discoloration of fingers and toes

Drug Interactions

Concurrent use of lithium with carbamazepine, diltiazem, fluoxetine, fluvoxamine, haloperidol, methyldopa, phenothiazines, TCAs, and verapamil may increase the risk for neurotoxicity; monitor

NSAIDs decrease renal lithium excretion leading to increased serum lithium concentrations; sulindac and aspirin may be the exceptions; monitor

Combined use of lithium and chlorpromazine may lower serum concentrations of both drugs; monitor

ACE inhibitors may increase the risk of lithium toxicity via sodium depletion; monitor

Lithium and MAOIs should generally be avoided due to use reports of fatal malignant hyperpyrexia

Losartan may reduce the renal clearance of lithium; monitor

Phenytoin may enhance lithium toxicity; monitor

Potassium iodide may enhance the hypothyroid effects of lithium; monitor

Combined use of lithium with sibutramine may increase the risk of serotonin syndrome; this combination is best avoided

Sodium bicarbonate and high sodium intake may reduce serum lithium concentrations via enhanced excretion; monitor

Thiazide diuretics increase serum lithium concentration via sodium depletion

Onset Peak serum concentration: 30 minutes to 2 hours

Half-Life 18-24 hours; can increase to more than 36 hours in the elderly or in patients with renal impairment

Education and Monitoring Issues

Patient Education: Take exactly as directed; do not change dosage without consulting prescriber. Do not crush or chew tablets or capsules. Maintain adequate fluid intake (2-3 L/day of fluids unless instructed to restrict fluid intake) especially in summer. Frequent blood test and monitoring will be necessary. You may experience decreased appetite or altered taste sensation (small frequent meals may help maintain nutrition); or drowsiness or dizziness, especially during early therapy (use caution when driving or engaging in tasks requiring alertness until response to drug is known). Immediately report unresolved diarrhea, abrupt changes in weight, muscular tremors or lack of coordination, fever, or changes in urinary volume.

Monitoring Parameters: Serum lithium every 3-4 days during initial therapy; draw lithium serum concentrations 8-12 hours postdose; renal, hepatic, thyroid, and cardiovascular function; fluid status; serum electrolytes; CBC with differential, urinalysis; monitor for signs of toxicity

Reference Range: Levels should be obtained twice weekly until both patient's clinical status and levels are stable then levels may be obtained every 1-2 months

Timing of serum samples: Draw trough just before next dose

Therapeutic levels:

Acute mania: 0.6-1.2 mEq/L (SI: 0.6-1.2 mmol/L)

Protection against future episodes in most patients with bipolar disorder: 0.8-1 mEq/L (SI: 0.8-1.0 mmol/L); a higher rate of relapse is described in subjects who are maintained at <0.4 mEq/L (SI: 0.4 mmol/L)

Elderly patients can usually be maintained at lower end of therapeutic range (0.6-0.8 mEq/L)

Toxic concentration: >2 mEq/L (SI: >2 mmol/L)

(Continued)

Lithium *(Continued)*

Adverse effect levels:
GI complaints/tremor: 1.5-2 mEq/L
Confusion/somnolence: 2-2.5 mEq/L
Seizures/death: >2.5 mEq/L

- **Lithobid®** *see* Lithium *on page 534*
- **Lithonate®** *see* Lithium *on page 534*
- **Lithotabs®** *see* Lithium *on page 534*
- **Liver Disease** *see page 1046*
- **Livostin®** *see* Levocabastine *on page 519*
- **LKV-Drops® [OTC]** *see* Vitamins, Multiple *on page 981*
- **LoCHOLEST®** *see* Cholestyramine Resin *on page 192*
- **LoCHOLEST® Light** *see* Cholestyramine Resin *on page 192*
- **Locoid®** *see* Hydrocortisone *on page 447*
- **Lodine®** *see* Etodolac *on page 347*
- **Lodine® XL** *see* Etodolac *on page 347*
- **Lodosyn®** *see* Carbidopa *on page 139*

Lodoxamide Tromethamine (loe DOKS a mide troe METH a meen)

Pharmacologic Class Mast Cell Stabilizer
U.S. Brand Names Alomide® Ophthalmic
Use Treatment of vernal keratoconjunctivitis, vernal conjunctivitis, and vernal keratitis
USUAL DOSAGE Children >2 years and Adults: Instill 1-2 drops in eye(s) 4 times/day for up to 3 months
Contraindications Hypersensitivity to any component of product
Pregnancy Risk Factor B

- **Loestrin®** *see* Ethinyl Estradiol and Norethindrone *on page 342*
- **Loestrin 1.5/30** *see* Ethinyl Estradiol and Norethindrone *on page 342*
- **Lofene®** *see* Diphenoxylate and Atropine *on page 283*
- **Logen®** *see* Diphenoxylate and Atropine *on page 283*
- **Lomanate®** *see* Diphenoxylate and Atropine *on page 283*

Lomefloxacin (loe me FLOKS a sin)

Pharmacologic Class Antibiotic, Quinolone
U.S. Brand Names Maxaquin®
Mechanism of Action Inhibits DNA-gyrase in susceptible organisms thereby inhibits relaxation of supercoiled DNA and promotes breakage of DNA strands. DNA gyrase (topoisomerase II), is an essential bacterial enzyme that maintains the superhelical structure of DNA and is required for DNA replication and transcription, DNA repair, recombination, and transposition.
Use Lower respiratory infections, acute bacterial exacerbation of chronic bronchitis, skin infections, sexually transmitted diseases, and urinary tract infections caused by *E. coli*, *K. pneumoniae*, *P. mirabilis*, *P. aeruginosa*; also has gram-positive activity including *S. pneumoniae* and some staphylococci
USUAL DOSAGE
Lower respiratory and urinary tract infections (UTI): Adults: Oral: 400 mg once daily for 10-14 days
Urinary tract infection (UTI) due to susceptible organisms:
Uncomplicated cystitis caused by *Escherichia coli*: Adult female: Oral: 400 mg once daily for 3 successive days
Uncomplicated cystitis caused by *Klebsiella pneumoniae*, *Proteus mirabilis*, or *Staphylococcus saprophyticus*: Adult female: 400 mg once daily for 10 successive days
Complicated UTI caused by *Escherichia coli*, *Klebsiella pneumoniae*, *Proteus mirabilis*, or *Pseudomonas aeruginosa*: Adults: Oral: 400 mg once daily for 14 successive days
Surgical prophylaxis: 400 mg 2-6 hours before surgery
Uncomplicated gonorrhea: 400 mg as a single dose
No dosage adjustment is needed for elderly patients with normal renal function
Dosing adjustment in renal impairment:
Cl_{cr} 11-39 mL/minute: Loading dose: 400 mg; then 200 mg every day
Hemodialysis: Same as above
Dosage Forms TAB: 400 mg
Contraindications Hypersensitivity to lomefloxacin or other members of the quinolone group such as nalidixic acid, oxolinic acid, cinoxacin, norfloxacin, and ciprofloxacin; avoid use in children <18 years of age due to association of other quinolones with transient arthropathies
Warnings/Precautions Use with caution in patients with epilepsy or other CNS diseases which could predispose them to seizures; risk of photosensitivity may be reduced by taking in the evening
Pregnancy Risk Factor C

Adverse Reactions

1% to 10%:

Central nervous system: Headache, dizziness

Dermatologic: Photosensitivity

Gastrointestinal: Nausea

<1%: Abdominal pain, abnormal taste, allergic reaction, angina pectoris, anuria, arrhythmia, back pain, bradycardia, cardiac failure, chest pain, chills, coma, constipation, convulsions, cough, cyanosis, decreased heat tolerance, diaphoresis (increased), discoloration of tongue, dyspnea, dysuria, earache, edema, epistaxis, extrasystoles, facial edema, fatigue, flatulence, flu-like symptoms, flushing, gout, hematuria, hyperkinesia, hypertension, hypoglycemia, hypotension, increased fibrinolysis, leg cramps, malaise, myalgia, myocardial infarction, paresthesias, purpura, rash, syncope, tachycardia, thirst, thrombocytopenia, tremor, urinary disorders, vertigo, vomiting, weakness, xerostomia

Drug Interactions

Decreased effect: Decreased absorption with antacids containing aluminum, magnesium, and/or calcium (by up to 98% if given at the same time), sucralfate, didanosine, divalent and trivalent cations

Increased toxicity/serum levels: Quinolones cause increased levels of caffeine, warfarin, cyclosporine, and theophylline; cimetidine, probenecid increase quinolone levels

Half-Life 5-7.5 hours

Education and Monitoring Issues

Patient Education: Take as directed, preferably on an empty stomach 1 hour before or 2 hours after meals. Complete entire prescription even if feeling better. Maintain adequate hydration (2-3 L/day of fluids unless instructed to restrict fluid intake). You may experience dizziness or drowsiness; use caution when driving or engaging in tasks that require alertness until response to drug is known. You may experience photosensitivity (use sunscreen, wear protective clothing and eyewear, avoid direct sunlight). Report any signs of opportunistic infection (eg, fever, chills, vaginal itching or foul-smelling vaginal discharge, oral thrush, easy bruising). Report immediately any signs of allergic reaction (eg, rash, itching or tingling of skin); joint pain; difficulty breathing; CNS changes (excitability, seizures); pain, inflammation, or rupture of tendon; or abdominal cramping or pain.

Dietary Considerations: May be taken without regard to meals

Manufacturer Unimed

Related Information

Pharmaceutical Manufacturers Directory *on page 1020*

- **Lomodix®** *see* Diphenoxylate and Atropine *on page 283*
- **Lomotil®** *see* Diphenoxylate and Atropine *on page 283*

Lomustine (loe MUS teen)

Pharmacologic Class Antineoplastic Agent, Alkylating Agent

U.S. Brand Names CeeNU®

Generic Available No

Mechanism of Action A nitrosourea alkylating agent, lomustine acts by both alkylation and carbamylation. It appears to alkylate DNA, prevent DNA repair, and alter the structure of RNA and the structure and function of a variety of enzymes and proteins. It appears that carbamylation of DNA polymerase, not DNA structure modifications, are responsible for the inhibition of DNA synthesis. Lomustine is cell-cycle nonspecific, but may be active primarily in late G_1 or early S phase.

Use Treatment of brain tumors and Hodgkin's disease, non-Hodgkin's lymphoma, melanoma, renal carcinoma, lung cancer, colon cancer

USUAL DOSAGE Oral (refer to individual protocols):

Children: 75-150 mg/m^2 as a single dose every 6 weeks; subsequent doses are readjusted after initial treatment according to platelet and leukocyte counts

Adults: 100-130 mg/m^2 as a single dose every 6 weeks; readjust after initial treatment according to platelet and leukocyte counts

With compromised marrow function: Initial dose: 100 mg/m^2 as a single dose every 6 weeks

Repeat courses should only be administered after adequate recovery: WBC >4000 and platelet counts >100,000

Subsequent dosing adjustment based on nadir:

Leukocytes 2000-2900/mm^3, platelets 25,000-74,999/mm^3: Administer 70% of prior dose

Leukocytes <2000/mm^3, platelets <25,000/mm^3: Administer 50% of prior dose

Dosage adjustment in renal impairment:

Cl_{cr} 10-50 mL/minute: Administer 75% of normal dose

Cl_{cr} <10 mL/minute: Administer 50% of normal dose

Hemodialysis: Supplemental dose is not necessary

Peritoneal dialysis: Significant drug removal is unlikely based on physiochemical characteristics

Dosage Forms CAP: 10 mg, 40 mg, 100 mg. **DOSE PACK:** 10 mg (2s), 100 mg (2s), 40 mg (2s)

(Continued)

Lomustine *(Continued)*

Contraindications Hypersensitivity to lomustine or any component

Warnings/Precautions The U.S. Food and Drug Administration (FDA) currently recommends that procedures for proper handling and disposal for antineoplastic agents be considered. Bone marrow suppression, notably thrombocytopenia and leukopenia, may lead to bleeding and overwhelming infections in an already compromised patient; will last for at least 6 weeks after a dose, do not administer courses more frequently than every 6 weeks because the toxicity is cumulative. Use with caution in patients with depressed platelet, leukocyte or erythrocyte counts, liver function abnormalities.

Pregnancy Risk Factor D

Adverse Reactions

>10%:

Gastrointestinal: Nausea and vomiting occur 3-6 hours after oral administration; this is due to a centrally mediated mechanism, not a direct effect on the GI lining; if vomiting occurs, it is not necessary to replace the dose unless it occurs immediately after drug administration

Emetic potential:

<60 mg: Moderately high (60% to 90%)

≥60 mg: High (>90%)

Time course of nausea/vomiting: Onset: 2-6 hours; Duration: 4-6 hours

Hematologic: Myelosuppression: Anemia; effects occur 4-6 weeks after a dose and may persist for 1-2 weeks

WBC: Moderate

Platelets: Severe

Onset (days): 14

Nadir (weeks): 4-5

Recovery (weeks): 6

1% to 10%:

Central nervous system: Neurotoxicity

Dermatologic: Skin rash

Gastrointestinal: Stomatitis, diarrhea

Hematologic: Anemia

<1%: Alopecia, ataxia, disorientation, dysarthria, hepatotoxicity, lethargy, pulmonary fibrosis with cumulative doses >600 mg, renal failure

Drug Interactions CYP2D6 enzyme inhibitor

Decreased effect with phenobarbital, resulting in decreased efficacy of both drugs

Increased toxicity with cimetidine, reported to cause bone marrow suppression or to potentiate the myelosuppressive effects of lomustine

Duration Marrow recovery may require 6 weeks

Half-Life Parent drug: 16-72 hours; Active metabolite: 1.3-2 days

Education and Monitoring Issues

Patient Education: Take with fluids on an empty stomach; do not eat or drink for 2 hours following administration. Do not use alcohol, aspirin, aspirin-containing medications, or OTC medications without consulting prescriber. Maintain adequate fluid intake (2-3 L/day of fluids unless instructed to restrict fluid intake). May cause hair loss (reversible); easy bleeding or bruising (use soft toothbrush or cotton swabs and frequent mouth care, use electric razor, avoid sharp knives or scissors); increased susceptibility to infection (avoid crowds and exposure to infection, and avoid immunizations unless approved by prescriber). Report unusual bleeding or bruising or persistent fever or sore throat; blood in urine, stool, or vomitus; delayed healing of any wounds; skin rash; yellowing of skin or eyes; changes in color of urine of stool.

Monitoring Parameters: CBC with differential and platelet count, hepatic and renal function tests, pulmonary function tests

Manufacturer Bristol-Myers Squibb Company (Pharmaceutical Division)

Related Information

Pharmaceutical Manufacturers Directory *on page 1020*

♦ **Loniten®** *see* Minoxidil *on page 607*

♦ **Lonox®** *see* Diphenoxylate and Atropine *on page 283*

♦ **Lo/Ovral®** *see* Ethinyl Estradiol and Norgestrel *on page 345*

Loperamide (loe PER a mide)

Pharmacologic Class Antidiarrheal

U.S. Brand Names Diar-Aid® [OTC]; Imodium®; Imodium® A-D [OTC]; Kaopectate® II [OTC]; Pepto® Diarrhea Control [OTC]

Generic Available Yes

Mechanism of Action Acts directly on intestinal muscles to inhibit peristalsis and prolongs transit time enhancing fluid and electrolyte movement through intestinal mucosa; reduces fecal volume, increases viscosity, and diminishes fluid and electrolyte loss; demonstrates antisecretory activity; exhibits peripheral action

Use Treatment of acute diarrhea and chronic diarrhea associated with inflammatory bowel disease; chronic functional diarrhea (idiopathic), chronic diarrhea caused by bowel resection or organic lesions; to decrease the volume of ileostomy discharge

Unlabeled use: Treatment of traveler's diarrhea in combination with trimethoprim-sulfamethoxazole (co-trimoxazole) (3 days therapy)

USUAL DOSAGE Oral:

Children:

Acute diarrhea: Initial doses (in first 24 hours):

2-6 years: 1 mg 3 times/day

6-8 years: 2 mg twice daily

8-12 years: 2 mg 3 times/day

Maintenance: After initial dosing, 0.1 mg/kg doses after each loose stool, but not exceeding initial dosage

Chronic diarrhea: 0.08-0.24 mg/kg/day divided 2-3 times/day, maximum: 2 mg/dose

Adults: Initial: 4 mg (2 capsules), followed by 2 mg after each loose stool, up to 16 mg/day (8 capsules)

Dosage Forms CAPLET: 2 mg. **CAP:** 2 mg. **LIQ, oral:** 1 mg/5 mL (60 mL, 90 mL, 120 mL). **TAB:** 2 mg

Contraindications Patients who must avoid constipation, diarrhea resulting from some infections, or in patients with pseudomembranous colitis, hypersensitivity to specific drug or component, bloody diarrhea

Warnings/Precautions Large first-pass metabolism, use with caution in hepatic dysfunction; should not be used if diarrhea accompanied by high fever, blood in stool

Pregnancy Risk Factor B

Adverse Reactions Percentage unknown: Abdominal cramping, abdominal distention, constipation, dizziness, drowsiness, fatigue, nausea, rash, sedation, vomiting, xerostomia

Drug Interactions Increased toxicity: CNS depressants, phenothiazines, tricyclic antidepressants may potentiate the adverse effects

Onset Oral: Within 0.5-1 hour

Half-Life 7-14 hours

Education and Monitoring Issues

Patient Education: Do not take more than 8 capsules or 80 mL in 24 hours. May cause drowsiness. If acute diarrhea lasts longer than 48 hours, consult prescriber. Do not take if diarrhea is bloody.

♦ **Lopid®** *see* Gemfibrozil *on page 406*

♦ **Lopressor®** *see* Metoprolol *on page 595*

♦ **Loprox®** *see* Ciclopirox *on page 197*

♦ **Lorabid™** *see* Loracarbef *on page 539*

Loracarbef (lor a KAR bef)

Pharmacologic Class Antibiotic, Carbacephem

U.S. Brand Names Lorabid™

Generic Available No

Mechanism of Action Inhibits bacterial cell wall synthesis by binding to one or more of the penicillin binding proteins (PBPs); inhibits the final transpeptidation step of peptidoglycan synthesis in bacterial cell walls, thus inhibiting cell wall biosynthesis. It is thought that beta-lactam antibiotics inactivate transpeptidase via acylation of the enzyme with cleavage of the CO-N bond of the beta-lactam ring. Upon exposure to beta-lactam antibiotics, bacteria eventually lyse due to ongoing activity of cell wall autolytic enzymes (autolysins and murein hydrolases) while cell wall assembly is arrested.

Use Infections caused by susceptible organisms involving the respiratory tract, acute otitis media, sinusitis, skin and skin structure, bone and joint, and urinary tract and gynecologic

USUAL DOSAGE Oral:

Children:

Acute otitis media: 15 mg/kg twice daily for 10 days

Pharyngitis and impetigo: 7.5-15 mg/kg twice daily for 10 days

Adults:

Uncomplicated urinary tract infections: 200 mg once daily for 7 days

Skin and soft tissue: 200-400 mg every 12-24 hours

Uncomplicated pyelonephritis: 400 mg every 12 hours for 14 days

Upper/lower respiratory tract infection: 200-400 mg every 12-24 hours for 7-14 days

Dosing comments in renal impairment:

Cl_{cr} 10-49 mL/minute: 50% of usual dose at usual interval or usual dose given half as often

Cl_{cr} <10 mL/minute: Administer usual dose every 3-5 days

Hemodialysis: Doses should be administered after dialysis sessions

Dosage Forms CAP: 200 mg, 400 mg. **SUSP, oral:** 100 mg/5 mL (50 mL, 100 mL), 200 mg/5 mL (50 mL, 100 mL)

Contraindications Patients with a history of hypersensitivity to loracarbef or cephalosporins

Warnings/Precautions Modify dosage in patients with severe renal impairment; prolonged use may result in superinfection; use with caution in patients with a previous history of hypersensitivity to other beta-lactam antibiotics (eg, penicillins, cephalosporins)

Pregnancy Risk Factor B

(Continued)

Loracarbef *(Continued)*

Adverse Reactions

>1%: Gastrointestinal: Diarrhea

<1%: Arthralgia, candidiasis, cholestatic jaundice, eosinophilia, headache, hemolytic anemia, interstitial nephritis, nausea, nephrotoxicity with transient elevations of BUN/creatinine, nervousness, neutropenia, positive Coombs' test, pruritus, pseudomembranous colitis, rash, seizures (with high doses and renal dysfunction), serum sickness, slightly increased AST/ALT, Stevens-Johnson syndrome, thrombocytopenia, urticaria, vomiting

Drug Interactions

Increased effect: Probenecid may decrease cephalosporin elimination

Increased toxicity: Furosemide, aminoglycosides may be a possible additive to nephrotoxicity

Half-Life ~1 hour; prolonged in renal impairment

Education and Monitoring Issues

Patient Education: Take as directed, preferably on an empty stomach (30 minutes before or 2 hours after meals). Take entire prescription even if feeling better. Maintain adequate hydration (2-3 L/day of fluids unless instructed to restrict fluid intake). You may experience nausea, vomiting, or anorexia (small frequent meals, frequent mouth care, sucking lozenges, or chewing gum may help). Report immediately any signs of skin rash, joint or back pain, or difficulty breathing. Report unusual fever, chills, vaginal itching or foul-smelling vaginal discharge, or easy bruising or bleeding.

Manufacturer Eli Lilly and Co

Related Information

Pharmaceutical Manufacturers Directory *on page 1020*

Loratadine (lor AT a deen)

Pharmacologic Class Antihistamine

U.S. Brand Names Claritin®

Mechanism of Action Long-acting tricyclic antihistamine with selective peripheral histamine H_1-receptor antagonistic properties

Use Relief of nasal and non-nasal symptoms of seasonal allergic rhinitis

USUAL DOSAGE Children ≥6 years and Adults: Oral: 10 mg/day on an empty stomach

Dosing interval in hepatic impairment: 10 mg every other day to start

Dosage Forms SYR: 1 mg/mL (480 mL). **TAB:** 10 mg; Rapid-disintegrating: 10 mg (RediTabs®)

Contraindications Patients hypersensitive to loratadine or any of its components

Warnings/Precautions Patients with liver impairment should start with a lower dose (10 mg every other day), since their ability to clear the drug will be reduced; use with caution in lactation, safety in children <12 years of age has not been established

Pregnancy Risk Factor B

Adverse Reactions

>10%:

Central nervous system: Headache, somnolence, fatigue

Gastrointestinal: Xerostomia

1% to 10%:

Cardiovascular: Hypotension, hypertension, palpitations, tachycardia

Central nervous system: Anxiety, depression

Endocrine & metabolic: Breast pain

Neuromuscular & skeletal: Hyperkinesia, arthralgias

Respiratory: Nasal dryness, pharyngitis, dyspnea

Miscellaneous: Diaphoresis

Drug Interactions CYP2D6 and 3A3/4 enzyme substrate

Increased plasma concentrations of loratadine and its active metabolite with ketoconazole; erythromycin increases the AUC of loratadine and its active metabolite; no change in QT_c interval was seen

Protease inhibitors (amprenavir, ritonavir, nelfinavir) may increase the serum levels of loratadine

Increased toxicity: Procarbazine, other antihistamines, alcohol

Onset Within 1-3 hours; Peak effect: 8-12 hours

Duration >24 hours

Half-Life 12-15 hours

Education and Monitoring Issues

Patient Education: Take as directed; do not exceed recommended dose. Avoid use of other depressants, alcohol, or sleep-inducing medications unless approved by prescriber. You may experience drowsiness or dizziness (use caution when driving or engaging in tasks requiring alertness until response to drug is known); or dry mouth or nausea (frequent small meals, frequent mouth care, chewing gum, or sucking hard candy may help). Report persistent dizziness, sedation, or seizures; chest pain, rapid heartbeat, or palpitations; swelling of face, mouth, lips, or tongue; difficulty breathing; changes in urinary pattern; yellowing of skin or eyes, dark urine, or pale stool; or lack of improvement or worsening of condition.

Manufacturer Schering-Plough Corp

Related Information

Loratadine and Pseudoephedrine *on page 541*
Pharmaceutical Manufacturers Directory *on page 1020*

Loratadine and Pseudoephedrine (lor AT a deen & soo doe e FED rin)

Pharmacologic Class Antihistamine/Decongestant Combination

U.S. Brand Names Claritin-D®; Claritin-D® 24-Hour

Dosage Forms TAB: Loratadine 5 mg and pseudoephedrine sulfate 120 mg; Extended release: Loratadine 10 mg and pseudoephedrine sulfate 240 mg

Pregnancy Risk Factor B

Manufacturer Schering-Plough Corp

Related Information

Pharmaceutical Manufacturers Directory *on page 1020*

Lorazepam (lor A ze pam)

Pharmacologic Class Benzodiazepine

U.S. Brand Names Ativan®

Generic Available Yes

Mechanism of Action Depresses all levels of the CNS, including the limbic and reticular formation, probably through the increased action of gamma-aminobutyric acid (GABA), which is a major inhibitory neurotransmitter in the brain

Use Management of anxiety, status epilepticus, preoperative sedation, for desired amnesia, and as an antiemetic adjunct

Unapproved uses: Alcohol detoxification, insomnia, psychogenic catatonia, partial complex seizures

USUAL DOSAGE

Antiemetic:
- Children 2-15 years: I.V.: 0.05 mg/kg (up to 2 mg/dose) prior to chemotherapy
- Adults: Oral, I.V.: 0.5-2 mg every 4-6 hours as needed

Anxiety and sedation:
- Infants and Children: Oral, I.V.: Usual: 0.05 mg/kg/dose (range: 0.02-0.09 mg/kg) every 4-8 hours
- Adults: Oral: 1-10 mg/day in 2-3 divided doses; usual dose: 2-6 mg/day in divided doses

Insomnia: Adults: Oral: 2-4 mg at bedtime

Preoperative: Adults:
- I.M.: 0.05 mg/kg administered 2 hours before surgery; maximum: 4 mg/dose
- I.V.: 0.044 mg/kg 15-20 minutes before surgery; usual maximum: 2 mg/dose

Operative amnesia: Adults: I.V.: Up to 0.05 mg/kg; maximum: 4 mg/dose

Status epilepticus: I.V.:
- Infants and Children: 0.1 mg/kg slow I.V. over 2-5 minutes, do not exceed 4 mg/single dose; may repeat second dose of 0.05 mg/kg slow I.V. in 10-15 minutes if needed
- Adolescents: 0.07 mg/kg slow I.V. over 2-5 minutes; maximum: 4 mg/dose; may repeat in 10-15 minutes
- Adults: 4 mg/dose given slowly over 2-5 minutes; may repeat in 10-15 minutes; usual maximum dose: 8 mg

Dosage Forms INJ: 2 mg/mL (1 mL, 10 mL), 4 mg/mL (1 mL, 10 mL). **SOLN, oral concentrated** (alcohol and dye free): 2 mg/mL (30 mL). **TAB:** 0.5 mg, 1 mg, 2 mg

Contraindications Hypersensitivity to lorazepam or any component; there may be a cross-sensitivity with other benzodiazepines; do not use in a comatose patient, those with pre-existing CNS depression, narrow-angle glaucoma, severe uncontrolled pain, severe hypotension

Warnings/Precautions Use caution in patients with renal or hepatic impairment, organic brain syndrome, myasthenia gravis, or Parkinson's disease. Dilute injection prior to I.V. use with equal volume of compatible diluent (D_5W, 0.9% sodium chloride, sterile water for injection); do **not** inject intra-arterially, arteriospasm and gangrene may occur; injection contains benzyl alcohol 2%, polyethylene glycol and propylene glycol, which may be toxic to newborns in high doses, may reduce effectiveness of ECT; oral doses >0.09 mg/kg produced increased ataxia without increased sedative benefit versus lower doses

Pregnancy Risk Factor D

Pregnancy Implications

Clinical effects on the fetus: Crosses the placenta. Respiratory depression or hypotonia if administered near time of delivery.

Breast-feeding/lactation: Crosses into breast milk and no data on clinical effects on the infant. American Academy of Pediatrics states MAY BE OF CONCERN.

Adverse Reactions

>10%:
- Cardiovascular: Tachycardia, chest pain
- Central nervous system: Drowsiness, confusion, ataxia, amnesia, slurred speech, paradoxical excitement, rage, headache, depression, anxiety, fatigue, lightheadedness, insomnia
- Dermatologic: Rash

(Continued)

Lorazepam *(Continued)*

Endocrine & metabolic: Decreased libido
Gastrointestinal: Xerostomia, constipation, diarrhea, nausea, vomiting, increased or decreased appetite, decreased salivation
Local: Phlebitis, pain with injection
Neuromuscular & skeletal: Dysarthria
Ocular: Blurred vision, diplopia
Miscellaneous: Diaphoresis

1% to 10%:
Cardiovascular: Cardiac arrest, hypotension, bradycardia, cardiovascular collapse, syncope
Central nervous system: Confusion, nervousness, dizziness, akathisia
Neuromuscular & skeletal: Rigidity, tremor, muscle cramps
Dermatologic: Dermatitis
Gastrointestinal: Weight gain or loss
Otic: Tinnitus
Respiratory: Nasal congestion, hyperventilation

<1%: Blood dyscrasias, increased salivation, menstrual irregularities, physical and psychological dependence with prolonged use, reflex slowing

Drug Interactions
Alcohol and other CNS depressants may increase the CNS effects of lorazepam
Oral contraceptives may increase the clearance of lorazepam
Lorazepam may decrease the antiparkinsonian efficacy of levodopa
Scopolamine in combination with parenteral lorazepam may increase the incidence of sedation, hallucinations, and irrational behavior
Theophylline and other CNS stimulants may antagonize the sedative effects of lorazepam
There are rare reports of significant respiratory depression, stupor, and/or hypotension with concomitant use of loxapine and lorazepam. Use caution if concomitant administration of loxapine and CNS drugs is required.

Alcohol Interactions Avoid use (may increase central nervous system depression)

Onset
Onset of hypnosis: I.M.: 20-30 minutes
Sedation, anticonvulsant: I.V.: 5 minutes; oral: 30 minutes to 1 hour

Duration 6-8 hours

Half-Life Adults: 12.9 hours; Elderly: 15.9 hours; End-stage renal disease: 32-70 hours

Education and Monitoring Issues

Patient Education: Oral: Take exactly as directed (do not increase dose or frequency); may cause physical and/or psychological dependence. Do not use excessive alcohol or other prescription or OTC medications (especially pain medications, sedatives, antihistamines, or hypnotics) without consulting prescriber. Maintain adequate hydration (2-3 L/day of fluids unless instructed to restrict fluid intake). You may experience drowsiness, lightheadedness, impaired coordination, dizziness, or blurred vision (use caution when driving or engaging in tasks requiring alertness until response to drug is known); nausea, vomiting, or dry mouth (small frequent meals, frequent mouth care, chewing gum, or sucking lozenges may help); constipation (increased exercise, fluids, or dietary fruit and fiber may help); altered sexual drive or ability (reversible); or photosensitivity (use sunscreen, wear protective clothing and eyewear, avoid direct sunlight). Report persistent CNS effects (eg, confusion, depression, increased sedation, excitation, headache, agitation, insomnia or nightmares, dizziness, fatigue, impaired coordination, changes in personality, or changes in cognition); changes in urinary pattern; chest pain, palpitations, or rapid heartbeat; muscle cramping, weakness, tremors, or rigidity; ringing in ears or visual disturbances; excessive perspiration, or excessive GI symptoms (cramping, constipation, vomiting, anorexia); or worsening of condition.

Monitoring Parameters: Respiratory and cardiovascular status, blood pressure, heart rate, symptoms of anxiety

Reference Range: Therapeutic: 50-240 ng/mL (SI: 156-746 nmol/L)

♦ **Lorcet®-HD** *see* Hydrocodone and Acetaminophen *on page 444*
♦ **Lorcet® Plus** *see* Hydrocodone and Acetaminophen *on page 444*
♦ **Lortab®** *see* Hydrocodone and Acetaminophen *on page 444*
♦ **Lortab® ASA** *see* Hydrocodone and Aspirin *on page 445*

Losartan (loe SAR tan)

Pharmacologic Class Angiotensin II Antagonists

U.S. Brand Names Cozaar®

Mechanism of Action As a selective and competitive, nonpeptide angiotensin II receptor antagonist, losartan blocks the vasoconstrictor and aldosterone-secreting effects of angiotensin II; losartan interacts reversibly at the AT1 and AT2 receptors of many tissues and has slow dissociation kinetics; its affinity for the AT1 receptor is 1000 times greater than the AT2 receptor. Angiotensin II receptor antagonists may induce a more complete inhibition of the renin-angiotensin system than ACE inhibitors, they do not affect the response to bradykinin, and are less likely to be associated with nonrenin-angiotensin effects (eg, cough and angioedema). Losartan increases urinary flow rate and in addition to being natriuretic and kaliuretic, increases excretion of chloride, magnesium, uric acid, calcium, and phosphate.

Use Treatment of hypertension with or without concurrent use of thiazide diuretics; may prolong survival in heart failure; recommended for patients unable to tolerated ACE inhibitors

USUAL DOSAGE

Oral: The usual starting dose is 50 mg once daily; can be administered once or twice daily with total daily doses ranging from 25 mg to 100 mg

Usual initial doses in patients receiving diuretics or those with intravascular volume depletion: 25 mg

Patients not receiving diuretics: 50 mg

Dosing adjustment in renal impairment: None necessary

Dosing adjustment in hepatic impairment or elderly patients: Reduce the initial dose to 25 mg; divide dosage intervals into two

Not removed via hemodialysis

Dosage Forms TAB, film coated 25 mg, 50 mg

Contraindications Hypersensitivity to losartan or any components; pregnancy

Warnings/Precautions Avoid use or use a much smaller dose in patients who are intravascularly volume-depleted; use caution in patients with unilateral or bilateral renal artery stenosis to avoid a decrease in renal function; AUCs of losartan (not the active metabolite) are about 50% greater in patients with Cl_{cr} <30 mL/minute and are doubled in hemodialysis patients

Pregnancy Risk Factor C (1st trimester); D (2nd and 3rd trimesters)

Pregnancy Implications Breast-feeding/lactation: Avoid use in the nursing mother, if possible, since it is postulated that losartan is excreted in breast milk

Adverse Reactions

1% to 10%:

Central nervous system: Dizziness (3.5%), insomnia (1.4%)

Cardiovascular: First dose hypotension (dose-related; 0.5% with 50 mg, 2.2% with 100 mg)

Gastrointestinal: Diarrhea (2.4%), dyspepsia (1.3%), abdominal pain (1.6%), Nausea (1.5%)

Neuromuscular & skeletal: Back pain (1.8%), muscle cramps (1.1%), myalgia (1%), leg pain (1%)

Upper respiratory infection (7.9%), cough (3.4% versus 3.3% in placebo), nasal congestion (2%), sinus disorder (1.2%), sinusitis (1%)

>1% but frequency ≤ placebo: Asthenia, fatigue, edema, abdominal pain, chest pain, nausea, headache, pharyngitis

<1% (limited to important or life-threatening symptoms): Angioedema, anaphylactic reactions, hyponatremia, hepatitis, hyperkalemia, facial edema, fever, orthostatic effects, syncope, angina, A-V block (second degree), CVA, hypotension, myocardial infarction, arrhythmias, palpitations, bradycardia, tachycardia, ventricular arrhythmias, anorexia, constipation, dental pain, xerostomia, flatulence, gastritis, vomiting, anemia, gout, arm pain, hip pain, joint swelling, arthralgia, arthritis, muscle weakness, anxiety, ataxia, confusion, depression, hypesthesia, decreased libido, memory impairment, migraine, nervousness, paresthesia, peripheral neuropathy, sleep disorder, somnolence, tremor, vertigo, dyspnea, bronchitis, pharyngitis, epistaxis, rhinitis, alopecia, dermatitis, dry skin, ecchymosis, erythema, flushing, photosensitivity, pruritus, rash, sweating, urticaria, blurred vision, conjunctivitis, taste perversion, tinnitus, decreased visual acuity, impotence, nocturia, urinary frequency, increased serum creatinine, increased BUN, decreased hemoglobin, decreased hematocrit, increased transaminases, increased bilirubin. May be associated with worsening of renal function in patients dependent on renin-angiotensin-aldosterone system, panic disorder

Case reports: Henoch-Schönlein purpura, anemia, acute psychosis with paranoid delusions, pancreatitis, dysgeusia, ageusia, maculopapular rash

Drug Interactions CYP2C9 substrate and CYP3A3/4 substrate

Inhibitors of CYP2C9 or CYP3A3/4 may increase blood levels

Fluconazole (and possibly other azoles) decreases the plasma level of losartan's active metabolite; monitor for decreased efficacy

Lithium: Risk of toxicity may be increased by losartan; monitor lithium levels

Potassium-sparing diuretics (amiloride, potassium, spironolactone, triamterene): Increased risk of hyperkalemia

Potassium supplements may increase the risk of hyperkalemia

Rifampin may reduce antihypertensive efficacy of losartan

Trimethoprim (high dose) may increase the risk of hyperkalemia

Onset 6 hours

Half-Life Losartan: 1.5-2 hours; Metabolite (E-3174): 6-9 hours

Education and Monitoring Issues

Patient Education: Take exactly as directed; do not discontinue without consulting prescriber. Take first dose at bedtime. This drug does not eliminate need for diet or exercise regimen as recommended by prescriber. May cause dizziness, fainting, lightheadedness (use caution when driving or engaging in tasks that require alertness until response to drug is known); diarrhea (buttermilk, boiled milk, yogurt may help). Report

(Continued)

Losartan *(Continued)*

chest pain or palpitations; unrelenting headache; swelling of extremities, face, or tongue; difficulty in breathing or unusual cough; flu-like symptoms; or other persistent adverse reactions

Monitoring Parameters: Supine blood pressure, electrolytes, serum creatinine, BUN, urinalysis, symptomatic hypotension and tachycardia, CBC

Manufacturer Merck & Co

Related Information

Angiotensin-Related Agents Comparison *on page 1226*
Losartan and Hydrochlorothiazide *on page 544*
Pharmaceutical Manufacturers Directory *on page 1020*

Losartan and Hydrochlorothiazide

(loe SAR tan & hye droe klor oh THYE a zide)

Pharmacologic Class Antihypertensive Agent, Combination

U.S. Brand Names Hyzaar®

Dosage Forms TAB: Losartan potassium 50 mg and hydrochlorothiazide 12.5 mg; Losartan potassium 100 mg and hydrochlorothiazide 25 mg

Pregnancy Risk Factor C (1st trimester); D (2nd and 3rd trimesters)

Manufacturer Merck & Co

Related Information

Pharmaceutical Manufacturers Directory *on page 1020*

- **Losec®** *see* Omeprazole *on page 675*
- **Lotemax®** *see* Loteprednol *on page 544*
- **Lotensin®** *see* Benazepril *on page 97*
- **Lotensin® HCT** *see* Benazepril and Hydrochlorothiazide *on page 98*

Loteprednol (loe te PRED nol)

Pharmacologic Class Corticosteroid, Ophthalmic

U.S. Brand Names Alrex™; Lotemax®

Use

0.2% suspension (Alrex™): Temporary relief of signs and symptoms of seasonal allergic conjunctivitis

0.5% suspension (Lotemax®): Inflammatory conditions (treatment of steroid-responsive inflammatory conditions of the palpebral and bulbar conjunctiva, cornea, and anterior segment of the globe such as allergic conjunctivitis, acne rosacea, superficial punctate keratitis, herpes zoster keratitis, iritis, cyclitis, selected infective conjunctivitis, when the inherent hazard of steroid use is accepted to obtain an advisable diminution in edema and inflammation) and treatment of postoperative inflammation following ocular surgery

USUAL DOSAGE Adults: Ophthalmic:

0.2% suspension (Alrex™): Instill 1 drop into affected eye(s) 4 times/day

0.5% suspension (Lotemax®):

Inflammatory conditions: Apply 1-2 drops into the conjunctival sac of the affected eye(s) 4 times/day. During the initial treatment within the first week, the dosing may be increased up to 1 drop every hour. Advise patients not to discontinue therapy prematurely. If signs and symptoms fail to improve after 2 days, re-evaluate the patient.

Postoperative inflammation: Apply 1-2 drops into the conjunctival sac of the operated eye(s) 4 times/day beginning 24 hours after surgery and continuing throughout the first 2 weeks of the postoperative period

Contraindications Viral diseases of the cornea and conjunctiva; mycobacterial infection of the eye; fungal diseases of ocular structures; hypersensitivity to loteprednol and any ingredients; hypersensitivity to other corticosteroids

Pregnancy Risk Factor C

- **Lotrel®** *see* Amlodipine and Benazepril *on page 54*
- **Lotriderm®** *see* Betamethasone and Clotrimazole *on page 105*
- **Lotrimin®** *see* Clotrimazole *on page 220*
- **Lotrimin® AF Cream [OTC]** *see* Clotrimazole *on page 220*
- **Lotrimin® AF Lotion [OTC]** *see* Clotrimazole *on page 220*
- **Lotrimin® AF Powder [OTC]** *see* Miconazole *on page 600*
- **Lotrimin® AF Solution [OTC]** *see* Clotrimazole *on page 220*
- **Lotrimin® AF Spray Liquid [OTC]** *see* Miconazole *on page 600*
- **Lotrimin® AF Spray Powder [OTC]** *see* Miconazole *on page 600*
- **Lotrisone®** *see* Betamethasone and Clotrimazole *on page 105*
- **Lotronex®** *see* Alosetron *on page 36*

Lovastatin (LOE va sta tin)

Pharmacologic Class Antilipemic Agent (HMG-CoA Reductase Inhibitor)

U.S. Brand Names Mevacor®

Generic Available No

Mechanism of Action Lovastatin acts by competitively inhibiting 3-hydroxyl-3-methylglutaryl-coenzyme A (HMG-CoA) reductase, the enzyme that catalyzes the rate-limiting step in cholesterol biosynthesis

Use Adjunct to dietary therapy to decrease elevated serum total and LDL cholesterol concentrations in primary hypercholesterolemia

USUAL DOSAGE Adults: Oral: Initial: 20 mg with evening meal, then adjust at 4-week intervals; maximum dose: 80 mg/day; before initiation of therapy, patients should be placed on a standard cholesterol-lowering diet for 3-6 months and the diet should be continued during drug therapy

Dosage Forms TAB: 10 mg, 20 mg, 40 mg

Contraindications Pregnancy; active liver disease, hypersensitivity to lovastatin or any component

Warnings/Precautions May elevate aminotransferases; LFTs should be performed before and every 4- 6 weeks during the first 12-15 months of therapy and periodically thereafter; can also cause myalgia and rhabdomyolysis; use with caution in patients who consume large quantities of alcohol or who have a history of liver disease

Pregnancy Risk Factor X

Adverse Reactions

>10%: Neuromuscular and skeletal: Increased CPK (>2x normal) (11%)

1% to 10%:

Central nervous system: Headache (2.1% to 3.2%), dizziness (0.5% to 1.2%)

Dermatologic: Rash (0.8% to 1.3%)

Gastrointestinal: Abdominal pain (2.0% to 2.5%), constipation (2.0% to 3.5%), diarrhea (2.2% to 2.6%), dyspepsia (1.0% to 1.6%), flatulence (3.7% to 4.5%), nausea (1.9% to 2.5%)

Neuromuscular & skeletal: Myalgia (1.8% to 3.0%), weakness (1.2% to 1.7%), muscle cramps (0.6% to 1.1%)

Ocular: Blurred vision (0.8% to 1.3%)

<1% (limited to important or life-threatening symptoms): Chest pain, acid regurgitation, xerostomia, vomiting, leg pain, arthralgia, insomnia, paresthesia, alopecia, pruritus, eye irritation

Additional class-related events or case reports (not necessarily reported with lovastatin therapy): Myopathy, increased CPK (>10x normal), rhabdomyolysis, renal failure (secondary to rhabdomyolysis), alteration in taste, impaired extraocular muscle movement, facial paresis, tremor, memory loss, vertigo, paresthesia, peripheral neuropathy, peripheral nerve palsy, anxiety, depression, psychic disturbance, hypersensitivity reaction, angioedema, anaphylaxis, systemic lupus erythematosus-like syndrome, polymyalgia rheumatica, dermatomyositis, vasculitis, purpura, thrombocytopenia, leukopenia, hemolytic anemia, positive ANA, increased ESR, eosinophilia, arthritis, urticaria, photosensitivity, fever, chills, flushing, malaise, dyspnea, rash, toxic epidermal necrolysis, erythema multiforme, Stevens-Johnson syndrome, pancreatitis, hepatitis, cholestatic jaundice, fatty liver, cirrhosis, fulminant hepatic necrosis, hepatoma, anorexia, vomiting, alopecia, pruritus, nodules, skin discoloration, dryness of skin/mucous membranes, nail changes, gynecomastia, decreased libido, erectile dysfunction, impotence, cataracts, ophthalmoplegia, elevated transaminases, increased alkaline phosphatase, increased GGT, hyperbilirubinemia, thyroid dysfunction

Drug Interactions CYP3A3/4 substrate

Inhibitors of CYP3A3/4 (amprenavir, clarithromycin, cyclosporine, danazol, diltiazem, fluvoxamine, erythromycin, fluconazole, indinavir, itraconazole, ketoconazole, miconazole, nefazodone, nelfinavir, ritonavir, saquinavir, troleandomycin, and verapamil) increase lovastatin blood levels; may increase the risk of lovastatin-induced myopathy and rhabdomyolysis

Cholestyramine reduces absorption of several HMG-CoA reductase inhibitors. Separate administration times by at least 4 hours.

Cholestyramine and colestipol (bile acid sequestrants): Cholesterol-lowering effects are additive

Clofibrate and fenofibrate may increase the risk of myopathy and rhabdomyolysis

Gemfibrozil: Increased risk of myopathy and rhabdomyolysis

Isradipine may decrease lovastatin blood levels

Niacin may increase risk of myopathy and rhabdomyolysis

Warfarin effect (hypoprothrombinemic response) may be increased; monitor INR closely when lovastatin is initiated or discontinued

Onset 3 days of therapy required for LDL cholesterol concentration reductions

Half-Life 1.1-1.7 hours

Education and Monitoring Issues

Patient Education: Take with evening meal (highest rate of cholesterol synthesis occurs from midnight to morning). If sleep disturbances occur, take earlier in the day. Do not change dosage without consulting prescriber. Maintain diet and exercise program as identified by prescriber. Have periodic ophthalmic exams while taking lovastatin (check for cataracts). You may experience mild GI disturbances (eg, gas, diarrhea, constipation); inform prescriber if these are severe or if you experience severe muscle pain, weakness, or tenderness.

(Continued)

Lovastatin *(Continued)*

Dietary Considerations: Grapefruit juice may inhibit metabolism of lovastatin via CYP3A3/4; avoid high dietary intakes of grapefruit juice

Monitoring Parameters: Plasma triglycerides, cholesterol, and liver function tests

Manufacturer Merck & Co

Related Information

Pharmaceutical Manufacturers Directory *on page 1020*

- **Lovenox® Injection** *see* Enoxaparin *on page 312*
- **Low-Ogestrel-21®** *see* Ethinyl Estradiol and Norgestrel *on page 345*
- **Low-Ogestrel-28®** *see* Ethinyl Estradiol and Norgestrel *on page 345*
- **Low-Quel®** *see* Diphenoxylate and Atropine *on page 283*
- **Loxapac®** *see* Loxapine *on page 546*

Loxapine (LOKS a peen)

Pharmacologic Class Antipsychotic Agent, Dibenzoxazepine

U.S. Brand Names Loxitane®; Loxitane® C; Loxitane® I.M.

Generic Available No

Mechanism of Action Unclear, thought to be similar to chlorpromazine

Use Management of psychotic disorders

USUAL DOSAGE Adults:

Oral: 10 mg twice daily, increase dose until psychotic symptoms are controlled; usual dose range: 60-100 mg/day in divided doses 2-4 times/day; dosages >250 mg/day are not recommended

I.M.: 12.5-50 mg every 4-6 hours or longer as needed and change to oral therapy as soon as possible

Dosage Forms

Loxapine hydrochloride: **CONC, oral:** 25 mg/mL (120 mL dropper bottle). **INJ:** 50 mg/mL (1 mL)

Loxapine succinate: **CAP:** 5 mg, 10 mg, 25 mg, 50 mg

Contraindications Hypersensitivity to chlorpromazine or any component, cross-sensitivity with other phenothiazines may exist; avoid use in patients with narrow-angle glaucoma, bone marrow suppression, severe liver or cardiac disease, severe CNS depression, coma

Warnings/Precautions Watch for hypotension when administering I.M.; safety in children <6 months of age has not been established; use with caution in patients with cardiovascular disease or seizures; benefits of therapy must be weighed against risks of therapy; should not be given I.V.

Pregnancy Risk Factor C

Adverse Reactions

Cardiovascular: Orthostatic hypotension, tachycardia, arrhythmias, abnormal T-waves with prolonged ventricular repolarization, hypertension, hypotension, lightheadedness, syncope

Central nervous system: Drowsiness, extrapyramidal reactions (dystonia, akathisia, pseudoparkinsonism, tardive dyskinesia, akinesia), dizziness, faintness, ataxia, insomnia, agitation, tension, seizures, slurred speech, confusion, headache, neuroleptic malignant syndrome (NMS), altered central temperature regulation

Dermatologic: Rash, pruritus, photosensitivity, dermatitis, alopecia, seborrhea

Endocrine & metabolic: Enlargement of breasts, galactorrhea, amenorrhea, gynecomastia, menstrual irregularity

Gastrointestinal: Xerostomia, constipation, nausea, vomiting, nasal congestion, weight gain or loss, adynamic ileus, polydipsia

Genitourinary: Urinary retention, sexual dysfunction

Hematologic: Agranulocytosis, leukopenia, thrombocytopenia

Neuromuscular & skeletal: Weakness

Ocular: Blurred vision

Drug Interactions

Antipsychotics inhibit the ability of bromocriptine to lower serum prolactin concentrations

Benztropine (and other anticholinergics) may inhibit the therapeutic response to loxapine and excess anticholinergic effects may occur

Chloroquine may increase loxapine concentrations

Cigarette smoking may enhance the hepatic metabolism of loxapine. Larger doses may be required compared to a nonsmoker.

Concurrent use of loxapine with an antihypertensive may produce additive hypotensive effects

Concurrent use with TCA may produce increased toxicity or altered therapeutic response

Loxapine may inhibit the antiparkinsonian effect of levodopa

Loxapine plus lithium may rarely produce neurotoxicity

Barbiturates may reduce loxapine concentrations

Propranolol may increase loxapine concentrations

Sulfadoxine-pyrimethamine may increase loxapine concentrations

Loxapine and possibly other low potency antipsychotic may reverse the pressor effects of epinephrine

Loxapine and CNS depressants (ethanol, narcotics) may produce additive CNS depressant effects

Loxapine and trazodone may produce additive hypotensive effects

There are rare reports of significant respiratory depression, stupor, and/or hypotension with the concomitant use of loxapine and lorazepam; use caution if the concomitant administration of loxapine and CNS drugs is required

Alcohol Interactions Avoid use (may increase central nervous system depression)

Onset Onset of neuroleptic effect: Oral: Within 20-30 minutes; Peak effect: 1.5-3 hours

Duration ~12 hours

Half-Life Half-life, biphasic: Initial: 5 hours; Terminal: 12-19 hours

Education and Monitoring Issues

Patient Education: Use exactly as directed (do not increase dose or frequency); may cause physical and/or psychological dependence. It may take 2-3 weeks to achieve desired results; do not discontinue without consulting prescriber. Dilute oral concentration with water or juice. Do not take within 2 hours of any antacid. Avoid excess alcohol or caffeine and other prescription or OTC medications not approved by prescriber. Maintain adequate hydration (2-3 L/day of fluids unless instructed to restrict fluid intake). You may experience excess drowsiness, restlessness, dizziness, or blurred vision (use caution driving or when engaging in tasks requiring alertness until response to drug is known); nausea, vomiting (small frequent meals, frequent mouth care, chewing gum, or sucking lozenges may help); constipation (increased exercise, fluids, or dietary fruit and fiber may help); postural hypotension (use caution climbing stairs or when changing position from lying or sitting to standing); urinary retention (void before taking medication); or decreased perspiration (avoid strenuous exercise in hot environments). Report persistent CNS effects (eg, trembling fingers, altered gait or balance, excessive sedation, seizures, unusual movements, anxiety, abnormal thoughts, confusion, personality changes); chest pain, palpitations, rapid heartbeat, severe dizziness; unresolved urinary retention or changes in urinary pattern; vision changes; skin rash or yellowing of skin; difficulty breathing; or worsening of condition.

- **Loxitane®** *see* Loxapine *on page 546*
- **Loxitane® C** *see* Loxapine *on page 546*
- **Loxitane® I.M.** *see* Loxapine *on page 546*
- **Lozide®** *see* Indapamide *on page 467*
- **Lozol®** *see* Indapamide *on page 467*
- **Luminal®** *see* Phenobarbital *on page 723*
- **Lupron®** *see* Leuprolide Acetate *on page 514*
- **Lupron Depot®** *see* Leuprolide Acetate *on page 514*
- **Lupron Depot®-3 Month** *see* Leuprolide Acetate *on page 514*
- **Lupron Depot®-4 Month** *see* Leuprolide Acetate *on page 514*
- **Lupron Depot-Ped®** *see* Leuprolide Acetate *on page 514*
- **Luride®** *see* Fluoride *on page 376*
- **Luride® Lozi-Tab®** *see* Fluoride *on page 376*
- **Luride®-SF Lozi-Tab®** *see* Fluoride *on page 376*
- **Lutrepulse®** *see* Gonadorelin *on page 419*
- **Luvox®** *see* Fluvoxamine *on page 388*
- **Luxiq™** *see* Betamethasone *on page 103*
- **Lyderm** *see* Fluocinonide *on page 375*

Lyme Disease Vaccine (LIME dee seas vak SEEN)

Pharmacologic Class Vaccine

U.S. Brand Names LYMErix™

Mechanism of Action Lyme disease vaccine is a recombinant, noninfectious lipoprotein (OspA) derived from the outer surface of *Borrelia burgdorfi*, the causative agent of Lyme disease. Vaccination stimulates production of antibodies directed against this organism, including antibodies against the LA-2 epitope, which have bactericidal activity. Since OspA expression is down-regulated after inoculation into the human host, at least part of the vaccine's efficacy may be related to neutralization of bacteria within the midgut of the tick vector, preventing transmission to the human host.

Use Active immunization against Lyme disease in individuals between 15-70 years of age. Individuals most at risk are those who live, work, or travel to *B. burgdorferi*-infected, tick-infested, grassy/wooded areas.

USUAL DOSAGE Adults: I.M.: Vaccination with 3 doses of 30 mcg (0.5 mL), administered at 0, 1, and 12 months, is recommended for optimal protection

Dosage Forms INJ: Vial: 30 mcg/0.5 mL; Prefilled syringe (Tip-Lok™): 30 mcg/0.5 mL

Contraindications Known hypersensitivity to any component of the vaccine. Vaccination should be postponed during acute moderate to severe febrile illness (minor illness is generally not a contraindication). Safety and efficacy in patients <15 years of age have not been established.

Warnings/Precautions Do not administer to patients with treatment-resistant Lyme arthritis. Will not prevent disease in patients with prior infection and offers no protection

(Continued)

Lyme Disease Vaccine *(Continued)*

against other tick-borne diseases. Immunosuppressed patients or those receiving immunosuppressive therapy (vaccine may not be effective) - defer vaccination until 3 months after therapy. Avoid in patients receiving anticoagulant therapy (due to intramuscular injection). The prescriber should take all known precautions for prevention of allergic or other reactions. Administer with caution to patients with known or suspected latex allergy (applies only to the LMErix Tip-Lok™ syringe, vaccine vial does not contain natural rubber). Duration of immunity has not been established.

Pregnancy Risk Factor C

Pregnancy Implications It is not known whether Lyme disease vaccine is excreted in human milk. Because many drugs are excreted in milk, caution should be exercised when the vaccine is given to nursing mothers. Healthcare professionals are encouraged to register pregnant women who receive the vaccine with the SKB vaccination pregnancy registry (1-800-366-8900, ext 5231).

Adverse Reactions (Limited to overall self-reported events occurring within 30 days following a dose)

>10%: Local: Injection site pain (21.9%)

1% to 10%:

- Central nervous system: Headache (5.6%), fatigue (3.9%), fever (2.6%), chills (2%), dizziness (1%)
- Dermatologic: Rash (1.4%)
- Gastrointestinal: Nausea (1.1%)
- Neuromuscular & skeletal: Arthralgia (6.8%), myalgia (4.8%), muscle aches (2.8%), back pain (1.9%), stiffness (1%)
- Respiratory: Upper respiratory tract infection (4.4%), sinusitis (3.2%), pharyngitis (2.5%), rhinitis (2.4%), cough (1.5%), bronchitis (1.1%)
- Miscellaneous: Viral infection (2.8%), flu-like syndrome (2.5%)

Solicited adverse event rates were higher than unsolicited event rates (above). These included local reactions of soreness (93.5%), redness (41.8%), and swelling (29.9%). In addition, general systemic symptoms included fatigue (40.8%), headache (38.6%), arthralgia (25.6%), rash (11.7%), and fever (3.5%)

Patients with a history of Lyme disease were noted to experience a higher frequency of early musculoskeletal reactions. Other differences in the observed rate of adverse reactions were not significantly different between vaccine and placebo recipients.

Drug Interactions No data available

Education and Monitoring Issues

Patient Education: You will require two more injections over the next 12 months; schedule appointments for those injections as directed by prescriber. You may experience headache, mild nausea, chills, fever, or dizziness following injection. These should subside, if not contact prescriber. Report persistent redness, swelling, or pain at injection site; skin rash; persistent flu-like symptoms; or muscle aches of stiffness.

Manufacturer SmithKline Beecham Pharmaceuticals

Related Information

Pharmaceutical Manufacturers Directory *on page 1020*

♦ **LYMErix™** *see* Lyme Disease Vaccine *on page 547*

Lymphocyte Immune Globulin (LIM foe site i MYUN GLOB yoo lin)

Pharmacologic Class Immunosuppressant Agent

U.S. Brand Names Atgam®

Generic Available No

Mechanism of Action May involve elimination of antigen-reactive T-lymphocytes (killer cells) in peripheral blood or alteration of T-cell function

Use Prevention and treatment of acute renal and other solid organ allograft rejection; treatment of moderate to severe aplastic anemia in patients not considered suitable candidates for bone marrow transplantation; prevention of graft-versus-host disease following bone marrow transplantation

USUAL DOSAGE An intradermal skin test is recommended prior to administration of the initial dose of ATG; use 0.1 mL of a 1:1000 dilution of ATG in normal saline. A positive skin reaction consists of a wheal ≥10 mm in diameter. If a positive skin test occurs, the first infusion should be administered in a controlled environment with intensive life support immediately available. A systemic reaction precludes further administration of the drug. The absence of a reaction does **not** preclude the possibility of an immediate sensitivity reaction.

First dose: Premedicate with diphenhydramine 50 mg orally 30 minutes prior to and hydrocortisone 100 mg I.V. 15 minutes prior to infusion and acetaminophen 650 mg 2 hours after start of infusion

Children: I.V.:

- Aplastic anemia protocol: 10-20 mg/kg/day for 8-14 days; then administer every other day for 7 more doses; addition doses may be given every other day for 21 total doses in 28 days
- Renal allograft: 5-25 mg/kg/day

Adults: I.V.:
  Aplastic anemia protocol: 10-20 mg/kg/day for 8-14 days, then administer every other day for 7 more doses
  Renal allograft:
    Rejection prophylaxis: 15 mg/kg/day for 14 days followed by 14 days of alternative day therapy at the same dose; the first dose should be administered within 24 hours before or after transplantation
    Rejection treatment: 10-15 mg/kg/day for 14 days, then administer every other day for 10-14 days up to 21 doses in 28 days

Dosage Forms INJ: 50 mg of equine IgG/mL (5 mL)

Contraindications Known hypersensitivity to ATG, thimerosal, or other equine gamma globulins; severe, unremitting leukopenia and/or thrombocytopenia

Warnings/Precautions Must be administered via central line due to chemical phlebitis; should only be used by prescribers experienced in immunosuppressive therapy or management of solid organ or bone marrow transplant patients; adequate laboratory and supportive medical resources must be readily available in the facility for patient management; rash, dyspnea, hypotension, or anaphylaxis precludes further administration of the drug. Dose must be administered over at least 4 hours; patient may need to be pretreated with an antipyretic, antihistamine, and/or corticosteroid. Intradermal skin testing is recommended prior to first-dose administration.

Pregnancy Risk Factor C

Adverse Reactions
  >10%:
    Central nervous system: Fever, chills
    Dermatologic: Rash
    Hematologic: Leukopenia, thrombocytopenia
    Miscellaneous: Systemic infection
  1% to 10%:
    Cardiovascular: Hypotension, hypertension, tachycardia, edema, chest pain
    Central nervous system: Headache, malaise, pain
    Gastrointestinal: Diarrhea, nausea, stomatitis, GI bleeding
    Respiratory: Dyspnea
    Local: Edema or redness at injection site, thrombophlebitis
    Neuromuscular & skeletal: Myalgia, back pain, arthralgia
    Renal: Abnormal renal function tests
    Miscellaneous: Sensitivity reactions: Anaphylaxis may be indicated by hypotension, respiratory distress; serum sickness, viral infection
  <1%: Acute renal failure, anemia, arthralgia, hemolysis, lymphadenopathy, pruritus, seizures, urticaria, weakness

Half-Life Plasma: 1.5-12 days

Education and Monitoring Issues
  Patient Education: This medication can only be administered by infusion. You will be monitored closely during the infusion. Do not get up alone; ask for assistance if you must get up or change position. Do not have any vaccinations for the next 3 months without consulting prescriber. Immediately report chills; persistent dizziness or nausea; itching or stinging; acute back pain; chest pain or tightness or rapid heartbeat; or difficulty breathing.
  Monitoring Parameters: Lymphocyte profile, CBC with differential and platelet count, vital signs during administration

♦ **Lyphocin®** *see* Vancomycin *on page 970*

Lypressin (lye PRES in)

Pharmacologic Class Antidiuretic Hormone Analog

U.S. Brand Names Diapid® Nasal Spray

Generic Available No

Mechanism of Action Increases cyclic adenosine monophosphate (cAMP) which increases water permeability at the renal tubule resulting in decreased urine volume and increased osmolality; causes peristalsis by directly stimulating the smooth muscle in the GI tract

Use Controls or prevents signs and complications of neurogenic diabetes insipidus

USUAL DOSAGE Children and Adults: Instill 1-2 sprays into one or both nostrils whenever frequency of urination increases or significant thirst develops; usual dosage is 1-2 sprays 4 times/day; range: 1 spray/day at bedtime to 10 sprays each nostril every 3-4 hours

Dosage Forms SPRAY: 0.185 mg/mL (equivalent to 50 USP posterior pituitary units/mL) (8 mL)

Contraindications Known hypersensitivity to lypressin

Warnings/Precautions Use with caution in patients with coronary artery disease

Pregnancy Risk Factor C

Adverse Reactions
  1% to 10%:
    Cardiovascular: Chest tightness
    Central nervous system: Dizziness, headache
  (Continued)

Lypressin *(Continued)*

Endocrine & metabolic: Water intoxication
Gastrointestinal: Abdominal cramping, increased bowel movements
Local: Irritation or burning
Respiratory: Coughing, dyspnea, rhinorrhea, nasal congestion
<1%: Inadvertent inhalation

Drug Interactions Increased effect: Chlorpropamide, clofibrate, carbamazepine → prolongation of antidiuretic effects

Onset Onset of antidiuretic effect: Intranasal spray: Within 0.5-2 hours

Duration 3-8 hours

Half-Life 15-20 minutes

Education and Monitoring Issues

Patient Education: To control nocturia, an additional dose may be given at bedtime. Notify prescriber if drowsiness, fatigue, headache, shortness of breath, abdominal cramps, or severe nasal irritation occurs.

- **Lysatec-rt-PA®** *see* Alteplase *on page 39*
- **Macrobid®** *see* Nitrofurantoin *on page 658*
- **Macrodantin®** *see* Nitrofurantoin *on page 658*

Mafenide (MA fe nide)

Pharmacologic Class Antibiotic, Topical

U.S. Brand Names Sulfamylon® Topical

Use Adjunct in the treatment of second and third degree burns to prevent septicemia caused by susceptible organisms such as *Pseudomonas aeruginosa*; prevention of graft loss of meshed autografts on excised burn wounds

USUAL DOSAGE Children and Adults: Topical: Apply once or twice daily with a sterile gloved hand; apply to a thickness of approximately 16 mm; the burned area should be covered with cream at all times

Contraindications Hypersensitivity to mafenide, sulfites, or any component

Pregnancy Risk Factor C

Magnesium Citrate (mag NEE zhum SIT rate)

Pharmacologic Class Laxative

U.S. Brand Names Evac-Q-Mag® [OTC]

Use Evacuation of bowel prior to certain surgical and diagnostic procedures or overdose situations

USUAL DOSAGE Cathartic: Oral:

Children:
<6 years: 0.5 mL/kg up to a maximum of 200 mL repeated every 4-6 hours until stools are clear
6-12 years: 100-150 mL
Adults ≥12 years: ½ to 1 full bottle (120-300 mL)

Contraindications Renal failure, appendicitis, abdominal pain, intestinal impaction, obstruction or perforation, diabetes mellitus, complications in gastrointestinal tract, patients with colostomy, ileostomy, ulcerative colitis or diverticulitis

Pregnancy Risk Factor B

Magnesium Hydroxide (mag NEE zhum hye DROKS ide)

Pharmacologic Class Antacid; Electrolyte Supplement, Oral; Laxative

U.S. Brand Names Phillips'® Milk of Magnesia [OTC]

Use Short-term treatment of occasional constipation and symptoms of hyperacidity, magnesium replacement therapy

USUAL DOSAGE Oral:

Average daily intakes of dietary magnesium have declined in recent years due to processing of food; the latest estimate of the average American dietary intake was 349 mg/day

Laxative:
<2 years: 0.5 mL/kg/dose
2-5 years: 5-15 mL/day or in divided doses
6-12 years: 15-30 mL/day or in divided doses
≥12 years: 30-60 mL/day or in divided doses

Antacid:
Children: 2.5-5 mL as needed up to 4 times/day
Adults: 5-15 mL up to 4 times/day as needed

Dosing in renal impairment: Patients in severe renal failure should not receive magnesium due to toxicity from accumulation. Patients with a Cl_{cr} <25 mL/minute receiving magnesium should be monitored by serum magnesium levels.

Contraindications Patients with colostomy or an ileostomy, intestinal obstruction, fecal impaction, renal failure, appendicitis, hypersensitivity to any component

Pregnancy Risk Factor B

Magnesium Oxide (mag NEE zhum OKS ide)

Pharmacologic Class Antacid; Electrolyte Supplement, Oral; Laxative

U.S. Brand Names Maox®

Use Short-term treatment of occasional constipation and symptoms of hyperacidity

USUAL DOSAGE Adults: Oral:

Dietary supplement: 20-40 mEq (1-2 tablets) 2-3 times

Antacid: 140 mg 3-4 times/day **or** 400-840 mg/day

Laxative: 2-4 g at bedtime with full glass of water

Dosing in renal impairment: Patients in severe renal failure should not receive magnesium due to toxicity from accumulation. Patients with a Cl_{cr} <25 mL/minute should be monitored by serum magnesium levels.

Note: Oral magnesium is not generally adequate for repletion in patients with serum magnesium concentrations <1.5 mEq/L

Contraindications Patients with colostomy or an ileostomy, appendicitis, ulcerative colitis, diverticulitis, heart block, myocardial damage, serious renal impairment, hepatitis, Addison's disease, hypersensitivity to any component

Pregnancy Risk Factor B

Magnesium Salts (Other) (mag NEE zhum salts OTH er)

Pharmacologic Class Magnesium Salt

U.S. Brand Names Almora® (Gluconate); Magonate® (Gluconate) [OTC]; Magtrate® (Gluconate); Slow-Mag® (Chloride)

Generic Available Yes

Mechanism of Action Magnesium is important as a cofactor in many enzymatic reactions in the body involving protein synthesis and carbohydrate metabolism, (at least 300 enzymatic reactions require magnesium). Actions on lipoprotein lipase have been found to be important in reducing serum cholesterol and on sodium/potassium ATPase in promoting polarization (ie, neuromuscular functioning).

Use Dietary supplement for treatment of magnesium deficiencies

USUAL DOSAGE Oral:

Average daily intakes of dietary magnesium have declined in recent years due to processing of food; the latest estimate of the average American dietary intake was 349 mg/day

Adequate intakes:

- Infants:
  - 0-6 months: 30 mg
  - 7-12 months: 75 mg

Recommended dietary allowance:

- Children:
  - 1-3 years: 80 mg/day
  - 4-8 years: 130 mg/day
- Male:
  - 9-13 years: 240 mg/day
  - 14-18 years: 130 mg/day
  - 19-30 years: 400 mg/day
  - ≥31 years: 420 mg/day
- Female:
  - 9-13 years: 240 mg/day
  - 14-18 years: 360 mg/day
  - 19-30 years: 310 mg/day
  - ≥31 years: 320 mg/day
- Female: Pregnancy:
  - ≤18 years: 400 mg/day
  - 19-30 years: 350 mg/day
  - 31-50 years: 360 mg/day
- Female: Lactation:
  - ≤18 years: 360 mg/day
  - 19-30 years: 310 mg/day
  - 31-50 years: 320 mg/day

Hypomagnesemia: There are no specific dosage recommendations for this product in replacement of magnesium. Extrapolation from dosage recommendations of magnesium sulfate are as follows:

Children: 10-20 mg/kg/dose **elemental** magnesium 4 times/day

Adults: 300 mg **elemental** magnesium 4 times/day

The recommended dietary allowance (RDA) of magnesium is 4.5 mg/kg which is a total daily allowance of 350-400 mg for adult men and 280-300 mg for adult women. During pregnancy the RDA is 300 mg and during lactation the RDA is 355 mg.

Dietary supplement: Oral:

Children: 3-6 mg/kg/day in divided doses 3-4 times/day; maximum: 400 mg/day

Adults: 54-483 mg/day in divided doses; refer to product labeling

(Continued)

Magnesium Salts (Other) *(Continued)*

Dosing in renal impairment: Patients in severe renal failure should not receive magnesium due to toxicity from accumulation. Patients with a Cl_{cr} <25 mL/minute receiving magnesium should be monitored by serum magnesium levels.

Dosage Forms

Gluconate: **LIQ:** 54 mg/5 mL as magnesium. **TAB:** 500 mg (elemental magnesium 27 mg)

Chloride: **TAB, sustained release:** 535 mg (64 mg magnesium)

Amino acids chelate: **TAB:** 500 mg (100 mg magnesium)

Contraindications Patients with heart block, severe renal disease

Warnings/Precautions Use with caution in patients with impaired renal function; hypermagnesemia and toxicity may occur due to decreased renal clearance of absorbed magnesium

Adverse Reactions

1% to 10%: Gastrointestinal: Diarrhea (excessive dose)

<1%: Abdominal cramps, hypermagnesemia, hypotension, muscle weakness, respiratory depression

Drug Interactions

Increased effect of nondepolarizing neuromuscular blockers

Decreased absorption of aminoquinolones, digoxin, nitrofurantoin, penicillamine, and tetracyclines may occur with magnesium salts

Education and Monitoring Issues

Reference Range: Serum magnesium:

Children: 1.5-1.9 mg/dL ~1.2-1.6 mEq/L

Adults: 2.2-2.8 mg/dL ~1.8-2.3 mEq/L

Magnesium Sulfate (mag NEE zhum SUL fate)

Pharmacologic Class Anticonvulsant; Electrolyte Supplement, Oral; Laxative

Generic Available Yes

Mechanism of Action Promotes bowel evacuation by causing osmotic retention of fluid which distends the colon with increased peristaltic activity when taken orally; parenterally, decreases acetylcholine in motor nerve terminals and acts on myocardium by slowing rate of S-A node impulse formation and prolonging conduction time

Use Treatment and prevention of hypomagnesemia and in seizure prevention in severe pre-eclampsia or eclampsia, pediatric acute nephritis; also used as short-term treatment of constipation, postmyocardial infarction, and torsade de pointes

USUAL DOSAGE The recommended dietary allowance (RDA) of magnesium is 4.5 mg/kg which is a total daily allowance of 350-400 mg for adult men and 280-300 mg for adult women. During pregnancy the RDA is 300 mg and during lactation the RDA is 355 mg. Average daily intakes of dietary magnesium have declined in recent years due to processing of food. The latest estimate of the average American dietary intake was 349 mg/day. Dose represented as $MgSO_4$ unless stated otherwise.

Note: Serum magnesium is poor reflection of repletional status as the majority of magnesium is intracellular; serum levels may be transiently normal for a few hours after a dose is given, therefore, aim for consistently high normal serum levels in patients with normal renal function for most efficient repletion

Hypomagnesemia:

Neonates: I.V.: 25-50 mg/kg/dose (0.2-0.4 mEq/kg/dose) every 8-12 hours for 2-3 doses

Children: I.M., I.V.: 25-50 mg/kg/dose (0.2-0.4 mEq/kg/dose) every 4-6 hours for 3-4 doses, maximum single dose: 2000 mg (16 mEq), may repeat if hypomagnesemia persists (higher dosage up to 100 mg/kg/dose $MgSO_4$ I.V. has been used); maintenance: I.V.: 30-60 mg/kg/day (0.25-0.5 mEq/kg/day)

Adults:

Oral: 3 g every 6 hours for 4 doses as needed

I.M., I.V.: 1 g every 6 hours for 4 doses; for severe hypomagnesemia: 8-12 g $MgSO_4$/day in divided doses has been used

Management of seizures and hypertension: Children: I.M., I.V.: 20-100 mg/kg/dose every 4-6 hours as needed; in severe cases doses as high as 200 mg/kg/dose have been used

Eclampsia, pre-eclampsia: Adults:

I.M.: 1-4 g every 4 hours

I.V.: Initial: 4 g, then switch to I.M. or 1-4 g/hour by continuous infusion

Maximum dose should not exceed 30-40 g/day; maximum rate of infusion: 1-2 g/hour

Maintenance electrolyte requirements:

Daily requirements: 0.2-0.5 mEq/kg/24 hours or 3-10 mEq/1000 kcal/24 hours

Maximum: 8-16 mEq/24 hours

Cathartic: Oral:

Children: 0.25 g/kg every 4-6 hours

Adults: 10-15 g in a glass of water

Dosing adjustment/comments in renal impairment: Cl_{cr} <25 mL/minute: Do not administer or monitor serum magnesium levels carefully

Dosage Forms GRANULES: ~40 mEq magnesium/5 g (240 g). **INJ:** 100 mg/mL (20 mL), 125 mg/mL (8 mL), 250 mg/mL (150 mL), 500 mg/mL (2 mL, 5 mL, 10 mL, 30 mL, 50 mL). **SOLN, oral:** 50% [500 mg/mL] (30 mL)

Contraindications Heart block, serious renal impairment, myocardial damage, hepatitis, Addison's disease

Warnings/Precautions Use with caution in patients with impaired renal function (accumulation of magnesium which may lead to magnesium intoxication); use with caution in digitalized patients (may alter cardiac conduction leading to heart block); monitor serum magnesium level, respiratory rate, deep tendon reflex, renal function when $MgSO_4$ is administered parenterally

Pregnancy Risk Factor B

Adverse Reactions 1% to 10%:

Serum magnesium levels >3 mg/dL:
- Central nervous system: Depressed CNS
- Gastrointestinal: Diarrhea
- Neuromuscular & skeletal: Blocked peripheral neuromuscular transmission leading to anticonvulsant effects

Serum magnesium levels >5 mg/dL:
- Cardiovascular: Flushing
- Central nervous system: Somnolence

Serum magnesium levels >12.5 mg/dL:
- Cardiovascular: Complete heart block
- Respiratory: Respiratory paralysis

Drug Interactions

Decreased effect: Nifedipine decreased blood pressure and neuromuscular blockade

Increased toxicity: Aminoglycosides increased neuromuscular blockade; CNS depressants increased CNS depression; neuromuscular antagonists, betamethasone (pulmonary edema), ritodrine increased cardiotoxicity

Onset Oral: Onset of cathartic action: Within 1-2 hours; I.M.: 1 hour; I.V.: Immediate

Duration I.M.: 3-4 hours; I.V.: 30 minutes

Education and Monitoring Issues

Monitoring Parameters: Monitor blood pressure when administering $MgSO_4$ I.V.; serum magnesium levels should be monitored to avoid overdose; monitor for diarrhea; monitor for arrhythmias, hypotension, respiratory and CNS depression during rapid I.V. administration

Reference Range: Serum magnesium:

Children: 1.5-1.9 mg/dL (1.2-1.6 mEq/L)

Adults: 1.5-2.5 mg/dL (1.2-2.0 mEq/L)

Note: Serum magnesium is poor reflection of repletional status as the majority of magnesium is intracellular; serum levels may be transiently normal for a few hours after a dose is given, therefore, aim for consistently high normal serum levels in patients with normal renal function for most efficient repletion

- **Magonate® (Gluconate) [OTC]** *see* Magnesium Salts (Other) *on page 551*
- **Magtrate® (Gluconate)** *see* Magnesium Salts (Other) *on page 551*
- **Malatal®** *see* Hyoscyamine, Atropine, Scopolamine, and Phenobarbital *on page 456*

Malathion (mal a THYE on)

Pharmacologic Class Scabicides/Pediculicides

U.S. Brand Names Ovide™

Generic Available No

Use Treatment of head lice and their ova

USUAL DOSAGE Sprinkle Ovide™ lotion on dry hair and rub gently until the scalp is thoroughly moistened; pay special attention to the back of the head and neck. Allow to dry naturally - use no heat and leave uncovered. After 8-12 hours, the hair should be washed with a nonmedicated shampoo; rinse and use a fine-toothed comb to remove dead lice and eggs. If required, repeat with second application in 7-9 days. Further treatment is generally not necessary. Other family members should be evaluated to determine if infested and if so, receive treatment.

Dosage Forms LOT: 0.5% (59 mL)

Contraindications Known hypersensitivity to malathion

Pregnancy Risk Factor B

Education and Monitoring Issues

Patient Education: Topical use only

- **Mallamint® [OTC]** *see* Calcium Carbonate *on page 130*
- **Mallisol® [OTC]** *see* Povidone-Iodine *on page 756*
- **Malogen Aqueous** *see* Testosterone *on page 898*
- **Malogen in Oil** *see* Testosterone *on page 898*
- **Malogex** *see* Testosterone *on page 898*
- **Malotuss® [OTC]** *see* Guaifenesin *on page 423*
- **Management of Healthcare Worker Exposures to HIV** *see page 1151*

♦ **Mandelamine®** *see* Methenamine *on page 579*
♦ **Mandol®** *see* Cefamandole *on page 148*

Manganese (MAN ga nees)

Pharmacologic Class Trace Element, Parenteral
U.S. Brand Names Chelated Manganese® [OTC]
Generic Available Yes
Mechanism of Action Cofactor in many enzyme systems, stimulates synthesis of cholesterol and fatty acids in liver, and influences mucopolysaccharide synthesis
Use Trace element added to TPN (total parenteral nutrition) solution to prevent manganese deficiency; orally as a dietary supplement
USUAL DOSAGE
Infants: I.V.: 2-10 mcg/kg/day usually administered in TPN solutions
Adults:
Oral: 20-50 mg/day
RDA: 2-5 mg/day
I.V.: 150-800 mcg/day usually administered in TPN solutions
Dosage Forms INJ: As chloride: 0.1 mg/mL (10 mL); As sulfate: 0.1 mg/mL (10 mL, 30 mL). **TAB:** 20 mg, 50 mg
Contraindications High manganese levels; patients with severe liver dysfunction or cholestasis (conjugated bilirubin >2 mg/dL) due to reduced biliary excretion
Pregnancy Risk Factor C
Education and Monitoring Issues
Monitoring Parameters: Periodic manganese plasma level
Reference Range: 4-14 μg/L

Mannitol (MAN i tole)

Pharmacologic Class Diuretic, Osmotic
U.S. Brand Names Osmitrol® Injection; Resectisol® Irrigation Solution
Generic Available Yes
Mechanism of Action Increases the osmotic pressure of glomerular filtrate, which inhibits tubular reabsorption of water and electrolytes and increases urinary output
Use Reduction of increased intracranial pressure associated with cerebral edema; promotion of diuresis in the prevention and/or treatment of oliguria or anuria due to acute renal failure; reduction of increased intraocular pressure; promoting urinary excretion of toxic substances; genitourinary irrigant in transurethral prostatic resection or other transurethral surgical procedures
USUAL DOSAGE I.V.:
Children:
Test dose (to assess adequate renal function): 200 mg/kg over 3-5 minutes to produce a urine flow of at least 1 mL/kg for 1-3 hours
Initial: 0.5-1 g/kg
Maintenance: 0.25-0.5 g/kg given every 4-6 hours
Adults:
Test dose (to assess adequate renal function): 12.5 g (200 mg/kg) over 3-5 minutes to produce a urine flow of at least 30-50 mL of urine per hour over the next 2-3 hours
Initial: 0.5-1 g/kg
Maintenance: 0.25-0.5 g/kg every 4-6 hours; usual adult dose: 20-200 g/24 hours
Intracranial pressure: Cerebral edema: 1.5-2 g/kg/dose I.V. as a 15% to 20% solution over ≥30 minutes; maintain serum osmolality 310-320 mOsm/kg
Preoperative for neurosurgery: 1.5-2 g/kg administered 1-1.5 hours prior to surgery
Transurethral irrigation: Use urogenital solution as required for irrigation
Dosage Forms INJ: 5% [50 mg/mL] (1000 mL), 10% [100 mg/mL] (500 mL, 1000 mL), 15% [150 mg/mL] (150 mL, 500 mL), 20% [200 mg/mL] (150 mL, 250 mL, 500 mL); 25% [250 mg/mL] (50 mL). **SOLN, urogenital:** 0.54% [5.4 mg/mL] (2000 mL)
Contraindications Severe renal disease (anuria), dehydration, or active intracranial bleeding, severe pulmonary edema or congestion, hypersensitivity to any component
Warnings/Precautions Should not be administered until adequacy of renal function and urine flow is established; cardiovascular status should also be evaluated; do not administer electrolyte-free mannitol solutions with blood
Pregnancy Risk Factor C
Adverse Reactions
>10%:
Central nervous system: Headache
Gastrointestinal: Nausea, vomiting
Genitourinary: Polyuria
1% to 10%:
Central nervous system: Dizziness
Dermatologic: Rash
Ocular: Blurred vision
<1%: Allergic reactions chills, circulatory overload, congestive heart failure, convulsions, dehydration and hypovolemia secondary to rapid diuresis, dysuria, fluid and electrolyte

imbalance, headache, pulmonary edema, tissue necrosis, water intoxication, xerostomia

Onset Onset of diuresis: Injection: Within 1-3 hours; Onset of reduction in intracerebral pressure: Within 15 minutes

Duration Duration of reduction in intracerebral pressure: 3-6 hours

Half-Life 1.1-1.6 hours

Education and Monitoring Issues

Patient Education: This medication can only be given by infusion. Report immediately any muscle weakness, numbness, tingling, acute headache, nausea, dizziness, blurred vision, eye pain, difficulty breathing, chest pain, or pain at infusion site.

Monitoring Parameters: Renal function, daily fluid I & O, serum electrolytes, serum and urine osmolality; for treatment of elevated intracranial pressure, maintain serum osmolality 310-320 mOsm/kg

- **Maox®** *see* Magnesium Oxide *on page 551*
- **Mapap® [OTC]** *see* Acetaminophen *on page 17*
- **Maranox® [OTC]** *see* Acetaminophen *on page 17*
- **Marax®** *see* Theophylline, Ephedrine, and Hydroxyzine *on page 906*
- **Marbaxin®** *see* Methocarbamol *on page 581*
- **Marcaine®** *see* Bupivacaine *on page 118*
- **Marcillin®** *see* Ampicillin *on page 59*
- **Margesic®** *see* Butalbital Compound *on page 123*
- **Margesic® H** *see* Hydrocodone and Acetaminophen *on page 444*
- **Marinol®** *see* Dronabinol *on page 302*
- **Marnal®** *see* Butalbital Compound *on page 123*
- **Marpres®** *see* Hydralazine, Hydrochlorothiazide, and Reserpine *on page 442*
- **Marthritic®** *see* Salsalate *on page 837*
- **Marvelon** *see* Ethinyl Estradiol and Desogestrel *on page 341*

Masoprocol (ma SOE pro kole)

Pharmacologic Class Topical Skin Product, Acne

U.S. Brand Names Actinex® Topical

Use Treatment of actinic keratosis

USUAL DOSAGE Adults: Topical: Wash and dry area; gently massage into affected area every morning and evening for 28 days

Contraindications Hypersensitivity to masoprocol or any component

Pregnancy Risk Factor B

- **Massengill® Medicated** *see* Povidone-Iodine *on page 756*
- **Massengill® Medicated Douche w/Cepticin [OTC]** *see* Povidone-Iodine *on page 756*
- **Maternal and Fetal Guidelines** *see page 1219*
- **Matulane®** *see* Procarbazine *on page 771*
- **Mavik®** *see* Trandolapril *on page 936*
- **Maxair™ Autohaler™** *see* Pirbuterol *on page 743*
- **Maxair™ Inhalation Aerosol** *see* Pirbuterol *on page 743*
- **Maxalt®** *see* Rizatriptan *on page 829*
- **Maxalt-MLT™** *see* Rizatriptan *on page 829*
- **Maxaquin®** *see* Lomefloxacin *on page 536*
- **Maxeran®** *see* Metoclopramide *on page 592*
- **Maxidex®** *see* Dexamethasone *on page 256*
- **Maxiflor®** *see* Diflorasone *on page 270*
- **Maximum Strength Anbesol® [OTC]** *see* Benzocaine *on page 98*
- **Maximum Strength Desenex® Antifungal Cream [OTC]** *see* Miconazole *on page 600*
- **Maximum Strength Dex-A-Diet® [OTC]** *see* Phenylpropanolamine *on page 729*
- **Maximum Strength Dexatrim® [OTC]** *see* Phenylpropanolamine *on page 729*
- **Maximum Strength Nytol® [OTC]** *see* Diphenhydramine *on page 282*
- **Maximum Strength Orajel® [OTC]** *see* Benzocaine *on page 98*
- **Maxipime®** *see* Cefepime *on page 151*
- **Maxitrol®** *see* Neomycin, Polymyxin B, and Dexamethasone *on page 644*
- **Maxivate®** *see* Betamethasone *on page 103*
- **Maxolon®** *see* Metoclopramide *on page 592*
- **Maxzide®** *see* Hydrochlorothiazide and Triamterene *on page 443*
- **Mazepine®** *see* Carbamazepine *on page 137*
- **Mebaral** *see* Mephobarbital *on page 565*

Mebendazole (me BEN da zole)

Pharmacologic Class Anthelmintic

U.S. Brand Names Vermox®

(Continued)

Mebendazole *(Continued)*

Generic Available No

Mechanism of Action Selectively and irreversibly blocks glucose uptake and other nutrients in susceptible adult intestine-dwelling helminths

Use Treatment of pinworms (*Enterobius vermicularis*), whipworms (*Trichuris trichiura*), roundworms (*Ascaris lumbricoides*), and hookworms (*Ancylostoma duodenale*)

USUAL DOSAGE Children and Adults: Oral:

Pinworms: 100 mg as a single dose; may need to repeat after 2 weeks; treatment should include family members in close contact with patient

Whipworms, roundworms, hookworms: One tablet twice daily, morning and evening on 3 consecutive days; if patient is not cured within 3-4 weeks, a second course of treatment may be administered

Capillariasis: 200 mg twice daily for 20 days

Dosing adjustment in hepatic impairment: Dosage reduction may be necessary in patients with liver dysfunction

Hemodialysis: Not dialyzable (0% to 5%)

Dosage Forms TAB, chewable: 100 mg

Contraindications Hypersensitivity to mebendazole or any component

Warnings/Precautions Pregnancy and children <2 years of age are relative contraindications since safety has not been established; not effective for hydatid disease

Pregnancy Risk Factor C

Adverse Reactions

1% to 10%: Gastrointestinal: Abdominal pain, diarrhea, nausea, vomiting

<1%: Alopecia (with high doses), angioedema, dizziness, fever, headache, itching, neutropenia (sore throat, unusual fatigue), rash, seizures, unusual weakness

Drug Interactions Decreased effect: Anticonvulsants such as carbamazepine and phenytoin may increase metabolism of mebendazole

Half-Life 2.8-9 hours

Education and Monitoring Issues

Patient Education: Take exactly as directed for full course of medication. Tablets may be chewed, swallowed whole, or crushed and mixed with food. Increase dietary intake of fruit juices. All family members and close friends should also be treated. To reduce possibility of reinfection, wash hands and scrub nails carefully with soap and hot water before handling food, before eating, and before and after toileting. Keep hands out of mouth. Disinfect toilet daily and launder bed lines, undergarments, and nightclothes daily with hot water and soap. Do not go barefoot and do not sit directly on grass or ground. May cause abdominal pain, nausea, or vomiting (frequent small meals, frequent mouth care, sucking lozenges, or chewing gum may help); hair loss (reversible). Report skin rash or itching, unusual fatigue or sore throat, unresolved diarrhea or vomiting, or CNS changes.

Monitoring Parameters: Check for helminth ova in feces within 3-4 weeks following the initial therapy

Manufacturer McNeil Consumer Products Co

Related Information

Pharmaceutical Manufacturers Directory *on page 1020*

♦ **Meclan® Topical** *see* Meclocycline *on page 557*

Meclizine (MEK li zeen)

Pharmacologic Class Antihistamine

U.S. Brand Names Antivert®; Antrizine®; Bonine® [OTC]; Dizmiss® [OTC]; Dramamine® II [OTC]; Meni-D®; Nico-Vert® [OTC]; Ru-Vert-M®; Vergon® [OTC]

Generic Available Yes

Mechanism of Action Has central anticholinergic action by blocking chemoreceptor trigger zone; decreases excitability of the middle ear labyrinth and blocks conduction in the middle ear vestibular-cerebellar pathways

Use Prevention and treatment of symptoms of motion sickness; management of vertigo with diseases affecting the vestibular system

USUAL DOSAGE Children >12 years and Adults: Oral:

Motion sickness: 12.5-25 mg 1 hour before travel, repeat dose every 12-24 hours if needed; doses up to 50 mg may be needed

Vertigo: 25-100 mg/day in divided doses

Dosage Forms CAP: 15 mg, 25 mg, 30 mg. **TAB:** 12.5 mg, 25 mg, 50 mg; Chewable: 25 mg; Film coated: 25 mg

Contraindications Hypersensitivity to meclizine or any component; pregnancy

Warnings/Precautions Use with caution in patients with angle-closure glaucoma, prostatic hypertrophy, pyloric or duodenal obstruction, or bladder neck obstruction; use with caution in hot weather, and during exercise; elderly may be at risk for anticholinergic side effects such as glaucoma, prostatic hypertrophy, constipation, gastrointestinal obstructive disease; if vertigo does not respond in 1-2 weeks, it is advised to discontinue use

Pregnancy Risk Factor B

Pregnancy Implications

Clinical effects on the fetus: No data available on crossing the placenta. Probably no effect on the fetus (insufficient data). Available evidence suggests safe use during pregnancy.

Breast-feeding/lactation: No data available

Adverse Reactions

>10%:

Central nervous system: Slight to moderate drowsiness

Respiratory: Thickening of bronchial secretions

1% to 10%:

Central nervous system: Headache, fatigue, nervousness, dizziness

Gastrointestinal: Appetite increase, weight gain, nausea, diarrhea, abdominal pain, xerostomia

Neuromuscular & skeletal: Arthralgia

Respiratory: Pharyngitis

<1%: Angioedema, blurred vision, bronchospasm, depression, epistaxis, hepatitis, hypotension, myalgia, palpitations, paresthesia, photosensitivity, rash, sedation, tremor, urinary retention

Drug Interactions Increased toxicity: CNS depressants, neuroleptics, anticholinergics

Alcohol Interactions Avoid use (may increase central nervous system depression)

Onset Oral: Within 1 hour

Duration 8-24 hours

Half-Life 6 hours

Education and Monitoring Issues

Patient Education: Take exactly as prescribed; do not increase dose. If taking for motion sickness, take before travel begins. Avoid alcohol, other CNS depressants, sleeping aids without consulting prescriber. You may experience dizziness, drowsiness, or blurred vision (use caution when driving or engaging in tasks that require alertness until response to drug is known); dry mouth (frequent mouth care, sucking lozenges, or chewing gum may help); constipation (increased dietary fluid, fiber, and fruit and exercise may help); heat intolerance (avoid excessive exercise, hot environments, maintain adequate fluid intake). Report CNS change (hallucination, confusion, nervousness); sudden or unusual weight gain; unresolved nausea or diarrhea; chest pain or palpitations; muscle pain; or changes in urinary pattern.

Meclocycline (me kloe SYE kleen)

Pharmacologic Class Antibiotic, Topical; Topical Skin Product, Acne

U.S. Brand Names Meclan® Topical

Use Topical treatment of inflammatory acne vulgaris

USUAL DOSAGE Children >11 years and Adults: Topical: Apply generously to affected areas twice daily

Contraindications Known hypersensitivity to tetracyclines or any component

Pregnancy Risk Factor B

Meclofenamate (me kloe fen AM ate)

Pharmacologic Class Analgesic, Non-narcotic; Nonsteroidal Anti-inflammatory Drug (NSAID)

U.S. Brand Names Meclomen®

Use Treatment of inflammatory disorders

USUAL DOSAGE Children >14 years and Adults: Oral:

Mild to moderate pain: 50 mg every 4-6 hours, not to exceed 400 mg/day

Rheumatoid arthritis/osteoarthritis: 200-400 mg/day in 3-4 equal doses

Contraindications Active GI bleeding, ulcer disease, hypersensitivity to aspirin, meclofenamate, or other NSAIDs

Pregnancy Risk Factor B; D (3rd trimester)

- **Meclomen®** *see* Meclofenamate *on page 557*
- **Mectizan®** *see* Ivermectin *on page 496*
- **Medigesic®** *see* Butalbital Compound *on page 123*
- **Medihaler-Iso®** *see* Isoproterenol *on page 488*
- **Medilium®** *see* Chlordiazepoxide *on page 180*
- **Medimet®** *see* Methyldopa *on page 586*
- **Medipain 5®** *see* Hydrocodone and Acetaminophen *on page 444*
- **Medipren® [OTC]** *see* Ibuprofen *on page 458*
- **Medi-Quick® Topical Ointment [OTC]** *see* Bacitracin, Neomycin, and Polymyxin B *on page 90*
- **Meditran®** *see* Meprobamate *on page 565*
- **Medi-Tuss® [OTC]** *see* Guaifenesin *on page 423*
- **Medralone® Injection** *see* Methylprednisolone *on page 589*
- **Medrol® Oral** *see* Methylprednisolone *on page 589*
- **Medrol Veriderm** *see* Methylprednisolone *on page 589*

Medroxyprogesterone Acetate (me DROKS ee proe JES te rone AS e tate)

Pharmacologic Class Contraceptive; Progestin

U.S. Brand Names Amen®; Curretab®; Cycrin®; Depo-Provera® Injection; Provera®

Generic Available Yes

Mechanism of Action Inhibits secretion of pituitary gonadotropins, which prevents follicular maturation and ovulation, stimulates growth of mammary tissue

Use Endometrial carcinoma or renal carcinoma as well as secondary amenorrhea or abnormal uterine bleeding due to hormonal imbalance; prevention of pregnancy

USUAL DOSAGE

Adolescents and Adults: Oral:

Amenorrhea: 5-10 mg/day for 5-10 days or 2.5 mg/day

Abnormal uterine bleeding: 5-10 mg for 5-10 days starting on day 16 or 21 of cycle

Accompanying cyclic estrogen therapy, postmenopausal: 2.5-10 mg the last 10-13 days of estrogen dosing each month

Adults: I.M.:

Endometrial or renal carcinoma: 400-1000 mg/week

Contraception: 150 mg every 3 months

Dosing adjustment in hepatic impairment: Dose needs to be lowered in patients with alcoholic cirrhosis

Dosage Forms INJ, susp: 100 mg/mL (5 mL), 150 mg/mL (1 mL), 400 mg/mL (1 mL, 2.5 mL, 10 mL). **TAB:** 2.5 mg, 5 mg, 10 mg

Contraindications Pregnancy, thrombophlebitis; hypersensitivity to medroxyprogesterone or any component; cerebral apoplexy, undiagnosed vaginal bleeding, liver dysfunction

Warnings/Precautions Use with caution in patients with depression, diabetes, epilepsy, asthma, migraines, renal or cardiac dysfunction; pretreatment exams should include PAP smear, physical exam of breasts and pelvic areas. May increase serum cholesterol, LDL, decrease HDL and triglycerides; use of any progestin during the first 4 months of pregnancy is not recommended; monitor patient closely for loss of vision, sudden onset of proptosis, diplopia, migraine, and signs and symptoms of thromboembolic disorders.

Pregnancy Risk Factor X

Adverse Reactions

>10%:

Cardiovascular: Edema

Endocrine & metabolic: Breakthrough bleeding, spotting, changes in menstrual flow, amenorrhea

Gastrointestinal: Anorexia

Local: Pain at injection site

Neuromuscular & skeletal: Weakness

1% to 10%:

Cardiovascular: Embolism, central thrombosis

Central nervous system: Mental depression, fever, insomnia

Dermatologic: Melasma or chloasma, allergic rash with or without pruritus

Endocrine & metabolic: Changes in cervical erosion and secretions, increased breast tenderness

Gastrointestinal: Weight gain or loss

Hepatic: Cholestatic jaundice

Local: Thrombophlebitis

Drug Interactions Decreased effect: Aminoglutethimide may decrease effects by increasing hepatic metabolism

Half-Life 30 days

Education and Monitoring Issues

Patient Education: Follow dosage schedule and do not take more than prescribed. You may experience sensitivity to sunlight (use sunblock, wear protective clothing and eyewear, and avoid extensive exposure to direct sunlight); dizziness, anxiety, depression (use caution when driving or engaging in tasks that require alertness until response to drug is known); changes in appetite (maintain adequate hydration and diet - 2-3 L/day of fluids unless instructed to restrict fluid intake); decreased libido or increased body hair (reversible when drug is discontinued); hot flashes (cool clothes and environment may help). May cause discoloration of stool (green). Report swelling of face, lips, or mouth; absence or altered menses; abdominal pain; vaginal itching, irritation, or discharge; heat, warmth, redness, or swelling of extremities; or sudden onset change in vision.

Monitoring Parameters: Monitor closely for loss of vision, sudden onset of proptosis, diplopia, migraine, and signs and symptoms of thromboembolic disorders; must have pregnancy test prior to beginning therapy

Related Information

Estrogens and Medroxyprogesterone *on page 330*

Medrysone (ME dri sone)

Pharmacologic Class Corticosteroid, Ophthalmic

U.S. Brand Names HMS Liquifilm®

Use Treatment of allergic conjunctivitis, vernal conjunctivitis, episcleritis, ophthalmic epinephrine sensitivity reaction

USUAL DOSAGE Children and Adults: Ophthalmic: Instill 1 drop in conjunctival sac 2-4 times/day up to every 4 hours; may use every 1-2 hours during first 1-2 days

Contraindications Fungal, viral, or untreated pus-forming bacterial ocular infections; not for use in iritis and uveitis

Pregnancy Risk Factor C

Mefloquine (ME floe kwin)

Pharmacologic Class Antimalarial Agent

U.S. Brand Names Lariam®

Generic Available No

Mechanism of Action Mefloquine is a quinoline-methanol compound structurally similar to quinine; mefloquine's effectiveness in the treatment and prophylaxis of malaria is due to the destruction of the asexual blood forms of the malarial pathogens that affect humans, *Plasmodium falciparum, P. vivax, P. malariae, P. ovale*

Use Treatment of acute malarial infections and prevention of malaria

USUAL DOSAGE Oral:

Children: Malaria prophylaxis:
- 15-19 kg: 1/4 tablet
- 20-30 kg: 1/2 tablet
- 31-45 kg: 3/4 tablet
- >45 kg: 1 tablet
- Administer weekly starting 1 week before travel, continuing weekly during travel and for 4 weeks after leaving endemic area

Adults:
- Treatment of mild to moderate malaria infection: 5 tablets (1250 mg) as a single dose with at least 8 oz of water
- Malaria prophylaxis: 1 tablet (250 mg) weekly starting 1 week before travel, continuing weekly during travel and for 4 weeks after leaving endemic area

Dosage Forms TAB: 250 mg

Contraindications Hypersensitivity to any component

Warnings/Precautions Caution is warranted with lactation; discontinue if unexplained neuropsychiatric disturbances occur, caution in epilepsy patients or in patients with significant cardiac disease. If mefloquine is to be used for a prolonged period, periodic evaluations including liver function tests and ophthalmic examinations should be performed. In cases of life-threatening, serious, or overwhelming malaria infections due to *Plasmodium falciparum*, patients should be treated with intravenous antimalarial drug. Mefloquine may be given orally to complete the course. Caution should be exercised with regard to driving, piloting airplanes, and operating machines since dizziness, disturbed sense of balance; neuropsychiatric reactions have been reported with mefloquine. In patients with epilepsy, mefloquine may increase the risk of convulsions. Administration of mefloquine with quinine or quinidine may produce electrocardiographic change; when administered with halofantrine, life-threatening prolongation of Q-T interval may occur.

Pregnancy Risk Factor C

Adverse Reactions

1% to 10%:
- Central nervous system: Difficulty concentrating, headache, insomnia, lightheadedness, vertigo, dizziness, fever, myalgia
- Dermal: Skin rash
- Gastrointestinal: Vomiting (3%), diarrhea, stomach pain, nausea, loss of appetite
- Ocular: Visual disturbances
- Otic: Tinnitus

<1%: Anxiety, bradycardia, confusion, dizziness, extrasystoles, hair loss, hallucinations, mental depression, psychosis, seizures, syncope,

Drug Interactions

Decreased effect of valproic acid

Increased toxicity of beta-blockers; chloroquine, quinine, and quinidine (hold treatment until at least 12 hours after these later drugs); when administered concurrently with halofantrine, life-threatening prolongation of Q-T interval may occur

Half-Life 21-22 days

Education and Monitoring Issues

Patient Education: Take on schedule as directed, with a full 8 oz glass of water. Ophthalmic exams will be necessary when used long-term. When taking for prophylaxis, begin 1 week before traveling to endemic areas, continue during travel period, and for 4 weeks following return. You may experience GI distress (frequent small meals may help). You may experience dizziness, changes in mentation, insomnia, headache, visual disturbances (use caution when driving or engaging in tasks that require alertness until response to drug is known).

Monitoring Parameters: LFTS; ocular examination

♦ **Mefoxin®** *see* Cefoxitin *on page 158*

♦ **Mega-B® [OTC]** *see* Vitamins, Multiple *on page 981*

♦ **Mega-Cal** *see* Calcium Carbonate *on page 130*

♦ **Megace®** *see* Megestrol Acetate *on page 560*

♦ **Megacillin® Susp** *see* Penicillin G Benzathine, Parenteral *on page 710*

Megestrol Acetate (me JES trole AS e tate)

Pharmacologic Class Antineoplastic Agent, Miscellaneous; Progestin

U.S. Brand Names Megace®

Generic Available Yes

Mechanism of Action Exact mechanism of megestrol as an antineoplastic agent is unknown. The drug is a synthetic progestogen; pituitary inhibition as a consequence of an antiluteinizing effect has been postulated.

Use Palliative treatment of breast and endometrial carcinomas, appetite stimulation, and promotion of weight gain in cachexia

USUAL DOSAGE Adults: Oral (refer to individual protocols):

Female:

Breast carcinoma: 40 mg 4 times/day

Endometrial: 40-320 mg/day in divided doses; use for 2 months to determine efficacy; maximum doses used have been up to 800 mg/day

Uterine bleeding: 40 mg 2-4 times/day

Male/Female: HIV-related cachexia: Initial dose: 800 mg/day; daily doses of 400 and 800 mg/day were found to be clinically effective

Dosing adjustment in renal impairment: No data available; however, the urinary excretion of megestrol acetate administered in doses of 4-90 mg ranged from 56% to 78% within 10 days

Hemodialysis: Megestrol acetate has not been tested for dialyzability; however, due to its low solubility, it is postulated that dialysis would not be an effective means of treating an overdose

Dosage Forms SUSP, oral: 40 mg/mL with alcohol 0.06% (236.6 mL). **TAB:** 20 mg, 40 mg

Contraindications Hypersensitivity to megestrol or any component; pregnancy

Warnings/Precautions The U.S. Food and Drug Administration (FDA) currently recommends that procedures for proper handling and disposal of antineoplastic agents be considered. Use during the first few months of pregnancy is not recommended. Use with caution in patients with a history of thrombophlebitis. Elderly females may have vaginal bleeding or discharge and need to be forewarned of this side effect and inconvenience.

Pregnancy Risk Factor X

Adverse Reactions

>10%:

Cardiovascular: Edema

Endocrine & metabolic: Breakthrough bleeding and amenorrhea, spotting, changes in menstrual flow

Neuromuscular & skeletal: Weakness

1% to 10%:

Central nervous system: Insomnia, depression, fever, headache

Dermatologic: Allergic rash with or without pruritus, melasma or chloasma, rash, and rarely alopecia

Endocrine & metabolic: Changes in cervical erosion and secretions, increased breast tenderness, changes in vaginal bleeding pattern, edema, fluid retention, hyperglycemia

Gastrointestinal: Weight gain (not attributed to edema or fluid retention), nausea, vomiting, stomach cramps

Hepatic: Cholestatic jaundice, hepatotoxicity

Hematologic: Myelosuppressive:

WBC: None

Platelets: None

Local: Thrombophlebitis

Neuromuscular & skeletal: Carpal tunnel syndrome

Respiratory: Hyperpnea

Onset At least 2 months of continuous therapy is necessary.

Half-Life 15-20 hours

Education and Monitoring Issues

Patient Education: Follow dosage schedule and do not take more than prescribed. You may experience sensitivity to sunlight (use sunblock, wear protective clothing, and avoid extended exposure to direct sunlight); dizziness, anxiety, depression (use caution when driving or engaging in tasks that require alertness until response to drug is known); change in appetite (maintain adequate hydration and diet - 2-3 L/day of fluids unless instructed to restrict fluid intake); decreased libido or increased body hair (reversible when drug is discontinued); hot flashes (cool clothes and environment may help). Report swelling of face, lips, or mouth; absence or altered menses; abdominal pain; vaginal itching, irritation, or discharge; heat, warmth, redness, or swelling of extremities; or sudden onset change in vision.

Monitoring Parameters: Monitor for tumor response; observe for signs of thromboembolic phenomena; monitor for thromboembolism

♦ **Melanex®** *see* Hydroquinone *on page 450*

Melatonin (mel ah TOE nin)

Pharmacologic Class Hormone

Mechanism of Action Melatonin is a hormone responsible for regulating the body's circadian rhythm and sleep patterns. Its release is prompted by darkness and inhibited by light. Secretion appears to peak during childhood, and declines gradually through adolescence and adulthood. Melatonin receptors have been found in blood cells, the brain, gut, and ovaries. This substance may also have a role in regulating cardiovascular and reproductive function through its antioxidant properties.

Use Sleep disorders (eg, jet lag, insomnia, neurologic problems, shift work); aging; cancer; immune system support

USUAL DOSAGE Sleep disturbances: 0.3-5 mg/day

Contraindications Patients with immune disorders

Pregnancy Implications Do not use if thinking about becoming pregnant, during pregnancy, or lactation

Adverse Reactions Central nervous system: Reduced alertness, headache, irritability, increased fatigue, drowsiness, sedation

Drug Interactions Medications commonly used as sedatives or hyphotics, or those that induce sedation, drowsiness (eg, benzodiazepines, narcotics); CNS depressants (prescription, supplements such as 5-HTP); other herbs known to cause sedation include kava kava, valerian

♦ **Mellaril®** *see* Thioridazine *on page 912*
♦ **Mellaril-S®** *see* Thioridazine *on page 912*
♦ **Melpaque HP®** *see* Hydroquinone *on page 450*

Melphalan (MEL fa lan)

Pharmacologic Class Antineoplastic Agent, Alkylating Agent

U.S. Brand Names Alkeran®

Generic Available No

Mechanism of Action Alkylating agent which is a derivative of mechlorethamine that inhibits DNA and RNA synthesis via formation of carbonium ions; cross-links strands of DNA

Use Palliative treatment of multiple myeloma and nonresectable epithelial ovarian carcinoma; neuroblastoma, rhabdomyosarcoma, breast cancer

USUAL DOSAGE

Oral (refer to individual protocols); dose should always be adjusted to patient response and weekly blood counts:

Children: 4-20 mg/m^2/day for 1-21 days

Adults:

Multiple myeloma: 6 mg/day initially adjusted as indicated **or** 0.15 mg/kg/day for 7 days **or** 0.25 mg/kg/day for 4 days; repeat at 4- to 6-week intervals

Ovarian carcinoma: 0.2 mg/kg/day for 5 days, repeat every 4-5 weeks

Intravenous (refer to individual protocols):

Children:

Pediatric rhabdomyosarcoma: 10-35 mg/m^2/dose every 21-28 days

High-dose melphalan with bone marrow transplantation for neuroblastoma: 70-100 mg/m^2/day on day 7 and 6 before BMT **or** 140-220 mg/m^2 single dose before BMT **or** 50 mg/m^2/day for 4 days **or** 70 mg/m^2/day for 3 days

Adults:

Multiple myeloma: 16 mg/m^2 administered at 2-week intervals for 4 doses, then repeat monthly as per protocol for multiple myeloma

Dosing adjustment in renal impairment:

Cl_{cr} 10-50 mL/minute: Administer at 75% of normal dose

Cl_{cr} <10 mL/minute: Administer at 50% of normal dose

or

BUN >30 mg/dL: Reduce dose by 50%

Serum creatinine >1.5 mg/dL: Reduce dose by 50%

Hemodialysis: Unknown

CAPD effects: Unknown

CAVH effects: Unknown

Dosage Forms POWDER for inj: 50 mg. **TAB:** 2 mg

Contraindications Hypersensitivity to melphalan or any component; severe bone marrow suppression; patients whose disease was resistant to prior therapy

Warnings/Precautions The U.S. Food and Drug Administration (FDA) currently recommends that procedures for proper handling and disposal for antineoplastic agents be considered. Is potentially mutagenic, carcinogenic, and teratogenic; produces amenorrhea. Reduce dosage or discontinue therapy if leukocyte count <3000/mm^3 or platelet count <100,000/mm^3; use with caution in patients with bone marrow suppression, impaired renal function, or who have received prior chemotherapy or irradiation; will cause amenorrhea. Toxicity to immunosuppressives is increased in elderly. Start with lowest recommended adult doses. Signs of infection, such as fever and WBC rise, may not occur. Lethargy and confusion may be more prominent signs of infection.

Pregnancy Risk Factor D

(Continued)

Melphalan *(Continued)*

Adverse Reactions

>10%:

Hematologic: Myelosuppressive: Leukopenia and thrombocytopenia are the most common effects of melphalan. Irreversible bone marrow failure has been reported.

WBC: Moderate
Platelets: Moderate
Onset (days): 7
Nadir (days): 8-10 and 27-32
Recovery (days): 42-50

Second malignancies: Reported are melphalan more frequently

1% to 10%:

Cardiovascular: Vasculitis
Dermatologic: Vesiculation of skin, alopecia, pruritus, rash
Endocrine & metabolic: SIADH, sterility and amenorrhea
Gastrointestinal: Nausea and vomiting are mild; stomatitis and diarrhea are infrequent
Genitourinary: Bladder irritation, hemorrhagic cystitis
Hematologic: Anemia, agranulocytosis, hemolytic anemia
Respiratory: Pulmonary fibrosis, interstitial pneumonitis
Miscellaneous: Hypersensitivity

Drug Interactions

Decreased effect: Cimetidine and other H_2-antagonists: The reduction in gastric pH has been reported to decrease bioavailability of melphalan by 30%

Increased toxicity: Cyclosporine: Increased incidence of nephrotoxicity

Half-Life 1.5 hours

Education and Monitoring Issues

Patient Education: Infusion: Report promptly any pain, irritation, or redness at infusion site. Oral: Preferable to take on an empty stomach, 1 hour prior to or 2 hours after meals. Do not take alcohol, aspirin, aspirin-containing medications, or OTC medications without consulting prescriber. Inform prescriber of all prescription medication you are taking. Maintain adequate fluid intake (2-3 L/day of fluids unless instructed to restrict fluid intake). May cause hair loss (reversible); easy bleeding or bruising (use soft toothbrush or cotton swabs and frequent mouth care, use electric razor, avoid sharp knives or scissors); increased susceptibility to infection (avoid crowds or exposure to infection - do not have any vaccinations unless approved by prescriber). Report unusual bleeding or bruising or persistent fever or sore throat; blood in urine, stool, or vomitus; delayed healing of any wounds; skin rash; yellowing of skin or eyes; changes in color of urine or black stool; pain or burning on urination; respiratory difficulty; or other severe adverse reactions.

Monitoring Parameters: CBC with differential and platelet count, serum electrolytes, serum uric acid

Manufacturer GlaxoWellcome

Related Information

Pharmaceutical Manufacturers Directory *on page 1020*

♦ **Melquin HP®** *see* Hydroquinone *on page 450*
♦ **Menadol® [OTC]** *see* Ibuprofen *on page 458*
♦ **Menest®** *see* Estrogens, Esterified *on page 333*
♦ **Meni-D®** *see* Meclizine *on page 556*

Menotropins (men oh TROE pins)

Pharmacologic Class Gonadotropin; Ovulation Stimulator

U.S. Brand Names Humegon™; Pergonal®; Repronex™

Generic Available No

Mechanism of Action Actions occur as a result of both follicle stimulating hormone (FSH) effects and luteinizing hormone (LH) effects; menotropins stimulate the development and maturation of the ovarian follicle (FSH), cause ovulation (LH), and stimulate the development of the corpus luteum (LH); in males it stimulates spermatogenesis (LH)

Use Sequentially with hCG to induce ovulation and pregnancy in the infertile woman with functional anovulation or in patients who have previously received pituitary suppression; used with hCG in men to stimulate spermatogenesis in those with primary hypogonadotropic hypogonadism

USUAL DOSAGE Adults: I.M.:

Male: Following pretreatment with hCG, 1 ampul 3 times/week and hCG 2000 units twice weekly until sperm is detected in the ejaculate (4-6 months) then may be increased to 2 ampuls of menotropins (150 units FSH/150 units LH) 3 times/week

Female: 1 ampul/day (75 units of FSH and LH) for 9-12 days followed by 10,000 units hCG 1 day after the last dose; repeated at least twice at same level before increasing dosage to 2 ampuls (150 units FSH/150 units LH)

Repronex™: I.M., S.C.:

Infertile patients with oligo-anovulation: Initial: 150 int. units daily for the first 5 days of treatment. Adjustments should not be made more frequently than once every 2 days and should not exceed 75-150 int. units per adjustment. Maximum daily dose should not exceed 450 int. units and dosing beyond 12 days is not recommended. If patient's response to Repronex™ is appropriate, hCG 5000-10,000 units should be given one day following the last dose of Repronex™.

Assisted reproductive technologies: Initial (in patients who have received GnRH agonist or antagonist pituitary suppression): 225 int. units; adjustments in dose should not be made more frequently than once every 2 days and should not exceed more than 75-50 int. units per adjustment. The maximum daily doses of Repronex™ given should not exceed 450 int. units and dosing beyond 12 days is not recommended. Once adequate follicular development is evident, hCG (5000-10,000 units) should be administered to induce final follicular maturation in preparation for oocyte retrieval.

Dosage Forms INJ: Follicle stimulating hormone activity 75 units and luteinizing hormone activity 75 units per 2 mL ampul, Follicle stimulating hormone activity 150 units and luteinizing hormone activity 150 units per 2 mL ampul

Contraindications Primary ovarian failure, overt thyroid and adrenal dysfunction, abnormal bleeding, pregnancy, men with normal urinary gonadotropin concentrations, elevated gonadotropin levels indicating primary testicular failure

Warnings/Precautions Advise patient of frequency and potential hazards of multiple pregnancy; to minimize the hazard of abnormal ovarian enlargement, use the lowest possible dose

Pregnancy Risk Factor X

Adverse Reactions

Male:

>10%: Endocrine & metabolic: Gynecomastia

1% to 10%: Erythrocytosis (shortness of breath, dizziness, anorexia, syncope, epistaxis)

Female:

>10%:

Endocrine & metabolic: Ovarian enlargement

Gastrointestinal: Abdominal distention

Local: Pain/rash at injection site

1% to 10%: Ovarian hyperstimulation syndrome

<1%: Febrile reactions, pain, thromboembolism,

Education and Monitoring Issues

Patient Education: Self injection: Follow prescriber's recommended schedule for injections. Multiple ovulations resulting in multiple pregnancies have been reported. Male infertility and/or breast enlargement may occur. Report pain at injection site; enlarged breasts (male); difficulty breathing; nosebleeds; acute abdominal discomfort; or fever, pain, redness, or swelling of calves.

♦ **Mentax®** *see* Butenafine *on page 124*

♦ **Mepergan®** *see* Meperidine and Promethazine *on page 564*

Meperidine (me PER i deen)

Pharmacologic Class Analgesic, Narcotic

U.S. Brand Names Demerol®

Generic Available Yes

Mechanism of Action Binds to opiate receptors in the CNS, causing inhibition of ascending pain pathways, altering the perception of and response to pain; produces generalized CNS depression

Use Management of moderate to severe pain; adjunct to anesthesia and preoperative sedation

USUAL DOSAGE Doses should be titrated to appropriate analgesic effect; when changing route of administration, note that oral doses are about half as effective as parenteral dose

Children: Oral, I.M., I.V., S.C.: 1-1.5 mg/kg/dose every 3-4 hours as needed; 1-2 mg/kg as a single dose preoperative medication may be used; maximum 100 mg/dose

Adults: Oral, I.M., I.V.: S.C.: 50-150 mg/dose every 3-4 hours as needed

Elderly:

Oral: 50 mg every 4 hours

I.M.: 25 mg every 4 hours

Dosing adjustment in renal impairment:

Cl_{cr} 10-50 mL/minute: Administer at 75% of normal dose

Cl_{cr} <10 mL/minute: Administer at 50% of normal dose

Dosing adjustment/comments in hepatic disease: Increased narcotic effect in cirrhosis; reduction in dose more important for oral than I.V. route

Dosage Forms INJ: Multiple-dose vials: 50 mg/mL (30 mL), 100 mg/mL (20 mL); Single-dose: 10 mg/mL (5 mL, 10 mL, 30 mL), 25 mg/dose (0.5 mL, 1 mL), 50 mg/dose (1 mL), 75 mg/dose (1 mL, 1.5 mL), 100 mg/dose (1 mL). **SYR:** 50 mg/5 mL (500 mL). **TAB:** 50 mg, 100 mg

Contraindications Hypersensitivity to meperidine or any component; patients receiving MAO inhibitors presently or in the past 14 days

Warnings/Precautions Use with caution in patients with pulmonary, hepatic, renal disorders, or increased intracranial pressure; use with caution in patients with renal failure or seizure disorders or those receiving high-dose meperidine; normeperidine (an active metabolite and CNS stimulant) may accumulate and precipitate twitches, tremors, or

(Continued)

Meperidine *(Continued)*

seizures; some preparations contain sulfites which may cause allergic reaction; not recommended as a drug of first choice for the treatment of chronic pain in the elderly due to the accumulation of normeperidine; for acute pain, its use should be limited to 1-2 doses; tolerance or drug dependence may result from extended use

Pregnancy Risk Factor B; D (if used for prolonged periods or in high doses at term)

Adverse Reactions

>10%:
- Cardiovascular: Hypotension
- Central nervous system: Fatigue, drowsiness, dizziness
- Gastrointestinal: Nausea, vomiting, constipation
- Neuromuscular & skeletal: Weakness
- Miscellaneous: Histamine release

1% to 10%:
- Central nervous system: Nervousness, headache, restlessness, malaise, confusion
- Gastrointestinal: Anorexia, stomach cramps, xerostomia, biliary spasm
- Genitourinary: Ureteral spasms, decreased urination
- Local: Pain at injection site
- Respiratory: Dyspnea, shortness of breath

<1%: Hallucinations, increased intracranial pressure, mental depression, paradoxical CNS stimulation, paralytic ileus, physical and psychological dependence, rash, urticaria

Drug Interactions CYP2D6 enzyme substrate

Decreased effect: Phenytoin may decrease the analgesic effects

Increased toxicity: May aggravate the adverse effects of isoniazid; MAO inhibitors, fluoxetine, and other serotonin uptake inhibitors greatly potentiate the effects of meperidine; acute opioid overdosage symptoms can be seen, including severe toxic reactions; CNS depressants, tricyclic antidepressants, phenothiazines may potentiate the effects of meperidine; ritonavir increases the formation of normeperidine, potentially increasing the risk of CNS toxicity

Alcohol Interactions Avoid use (may increase central nervous system depression)

Onset

Oral, S.C., I.M.: Onset of analgesic effect: Within 10-15 minutes; Peak effect: Within 1 hour

I.V.: Onset of effects: Within 5 minutes

Duration 2-4 hours

Half-Life

Parent drug: Terminal phase: Adults: 2.5-4 hours; Adults with liver disease: 7-11 hours

Normeperidine (active metabolite): 15-30 hours; is dependent on renal function and can accumulate with high doses or in patients with decreased renal function

Education and Monitoring Issues

Patient Education: If self-administered, use exactly as directed (do not increase dose or frequency); may cause physical and/or psychological dependence. While using this medication, do not use alcohol and other prescription or OTC medications (especially sedatives, tranquilizers, antihistamines, or pain medications) without consulting prescriber. Maintain adequate hydration (2-3 L/day of fluids unless instructed to restrict fluid intake). May cause hypotension, dizziness, drowsiness, impaired coordination, or blurred vision (use caution when driving, climbing stairs, or changing position - rising from sitting or lying to standing, or when engaging in tasks requiring alertness until response to drug is known); loss of appetite, nausea, or vomiting (frequent mouth care, small frequent meals, chewing gum, or sucking lozenges may help); constipation (increased exercise, fluids, or dietary fruit and fiber may help - if constipation remains an unresolved problem, consult prescriber about use of stool softeners). Report chest pain, slow or rapid heartbeat, acute dizziness or persistent headache; changes in mental status; swelling of extremities or unusual weight gain; changes in urinary elimination; acute headache; back or flank pain or muscle spasms; blurred vision; skin rash; or shortness of breath.

Dietary Considerations: Food: Glucose may cause hyperglycemia; monitor blood glucose concentrations

Monitoring Parameters: Pain relief, respiratory and mental status, blood pressure; observe patient for excessive sedation, CNS depression, seizures, respiratory depression

Reference Range: Therapeutic: 70-500 ng/mL (SI: 283-2020 nmol/L); Toxic: >1000 ng/mL (SI: >4043 nmol/L)

Related Information

Lipid-Lowering Agents Comparison *on page 1243*
Meperidine and Promethazine *on page 564*
Narcotic Agonists Comparison *on page 1244*

Meperidine and Promethazine (me PER i deen & proe METH a zeen)

Pharmacologic Class Analgesic, Combination (Narcotic)

U.S. Brand Names Mepergan®

Dosage Forms CAP: Meperidine hydrochloride 50 mg and promethazine hydrochloride 25 mg. **INJ:** Meperidine hydrochloride 25 mg and promethazine hydrochloride 25 per mL (2 mL, 10 mL)

Pregnancy Risk Factor B; D (if used for prolonged periods or in high doses at term)

Alcohol Interactions Avoid use (may increase central nervous system depression)

Mephobarbital (me foe BAR bi tal)

Pharmacologic Class Barbiturate

U.S. Brand Names Mebaral®

Use Sedative; treatment of grand mal and petit mal epilepsy

USUAL DOSAGE Oral:

Epilepsy:

Children: 6-12 mg/kg/day in 2-4 divided doses

Adults: 200-600 mg/day in 2-4 divided doses

Sedation:

Children:

<5 years: 16-32 mg 3-4 times/day

>5 years: 32-64 mg 3-4 times/day

Adults: 32-100 mg 3-4 times/day

Dosing adjustment in renal or hepatic impairment: Use with caution and reduce dosages

Contraindications Hypersensitivity to mephobarbital, other barbiturates, or any component; pre-existing CNS depression; respiratory depression; severe uncontrolled pain; history of porphyria

Pregnancy Risk Factor D

♦ **Mephyton® Oral** *see* Phytonadione *on page 735*

Mepivacaine (me PIV a kane)

Pharmacologic Class Local Anesthetic

U.S. Brand Names Carbocaine®; Isocaine® HCl; Polocaine®

Generic Available Yes

Mechanism of Action Mepivacaine is an amino amide local anesthetic similar to lidocaine; like all local anesthetics, mepivacaine acts by preventing the generation and conduction of nerve impulses

Use Local anesthesia by nerve block; infiltration in dental procedures; **not** for use in spinal anesthesia

USUAL DOSAGE Children and Adults: Injectable local anesthetic: Varies with procedure, degree of anesthesia needed, vascularity of tissue, duration of anesthesia required, and physical condition of patient

Dosage Forms INJ: 1% [10 mg/mL] (30 mL, 50 mL); 1.5% [15 mg/mL] (30 mL); 2% [20 mg/mL] (20 mL, 50 mL); 3% [30 mg/mL] (1.8 mL)

Contraindications Hypersensitivity to mepivacaine or any component or other amide anesthetics, allergy to sodium bisulfate

Warnings/Precautions Use with caution in patients with cardiac disease, renal disease, and hyperthyroidism; convulsions due to systemic toxicity leading to cardiac arrest have been reported presumably due to intravascular injection

Pregnancy Risk Factor C

Adverse Reactions <1%: Anaphylactoid reactions, anxiety, blurred vision, bradycardia, cardiovascular collapse, chills, confusion, disorientation, drowsiness, edema, hypotension, myocardial depression, nausea, respiratory arrest, restlessness, seizures, shivering, tinnitus, transient stinging or burning at injection site, tremors, unconsciousness, urticaria, vomiting

Onset Epidural: Within 7-15 minutes

Duration 2-2.5 hours; similar onset and duration is seen following infiltration

Half-Life 1.9 hours

Education and Monitoring Issues

Patient Education: You will experience decreased sensation to pain, heat, or cold in the area and/or decreased muscle strength (depending on area of application) until effects wear off; use necessary caution to reduce incidence of possible injury until full sensation returns. Report irritation, pain, burning at injection site; chest pain or palpitations; or difficulty breathing.

Oral: This will cause numbness of your mouth. Do not eat or drink for 1 hour after use. Take small sips of water at first to ensure that you can swallow without difficulty. Your tongue and/or mouth may be numb - use caution to avoid biting yourself. Report irritation, pain, burning at injection site; chest pain or palpitations; or difficulty breathing.

Meprobamate (me proe BA mate)

Pharmacologic Class Antianxiety Agent, Miscellaneous

U.S. Brand Names Equanil®; Miltown®; Neuramate®

Generic Available Yes

(Continued)

Meprobamate *(Continued)*

Mechanism of Action Precise mechanism is not yet clear, but many effects have been ascribed to its central depressant actions

Use Management of anxiety disorders; insomnia; preprocedure sedation and relaxation

Unlabeled use: Demonstrated value for muscle contraction, headache, premenstrual tension, external sphincter spasticity, muscle rigidity, opisthotonos-associated with tetanus

USUAL DOSAGE Oral:

Children 6-12 years: 100-200 mg 2-3 times/day
Sustained release: 200 mg twice daily

Adults: 400 mg 3-4 times/day, up to 2400 mg/day
Sustained release: 400-800 mg twice daily

Dosing interval in renal impairment:

Cl_{cr} 10-50 mL/minute: Administer every 9-12 hours
Cl_{cr} <10 mL/minute: Administer every 12-18 hours

Hemodialysis: Moderately dialyzable (20% to 50%)

Dosing adjustment in hepatic impairment: Probably necessary in patients with liver disease

Dosage Forms CAP, sustained release: 200 mg, 400 mg. **TAB:** 200 mg, 400 mg, 600 mg

Contraindications Acute intermittent porphyria; hypersensitivity to meprobamate or any component; do not use in patients with pre-existing CNS depression, narrow-angle glaucoma, or severe uncontrolled pain

Warnings/Precautions Physical and psychological dependence and abuse may occur; not recommended in children <6 years of age; allergic reaction may occur in patients with history of dermatological condition (usually by fourth dose); use with caution in patients with renal or hepatic impairment, or with a history of seizures

Pregnancy Risk Factor D

Adverse Reactions

Cardiovascular: Syncope, peripheral edema, palpitations, tachycardia, arrhythmia
Central nervous system: Drowsiness, ataxia, dizziness, paradoxical excitement, confusion, slurred speech, headache, euphoria, chills, vertigo, paresthesia, overstimulation
Dermatologic: Rashes, purpura, dermatitis, Stevens-Johnson syndrome, petechiae, ecchymosis
Gastrointestinal: Diarrhea, vomiting, nausea
Hematologic: Leukopenia, eosinophilia, agranulocytosis, aplastic anemia
Neuromuscular & skeletal: Weakness
Ocular: Blurred vision, impairment of accommodation
Renal: Renal failure
Respiratory: Wheezing, dyspnea, bronchospasm, angioneurotic edema

Drug Interactions Increased toxicity: CNS depressants (ethanol) may increase CNS depression

Alcohol Interactions Avoid use (may increase central nervous system depression)

Onset Onset of sedation: Oral: Within 1 hour

Half-Life 10 hours

Education and Monitoring Issues

Patient Education: Take exactly as directed (do not increase dose or frequency); may cause physical and/or psychological dependence. Do not chew or crush extended release capsule. Do not use excessive alcohol or other prescription or OTC medications (especially pain medications, sedatives, antihistamines, or hypnotics) without consulting prescriber. Maintain adequate hydration (2-3 L/day of fluids unless instructed to restrict fluid intake). You may experience drowsiness, lightheadedness, impaired coordination, dizziness, or blurred vision (use caution when driving or engaging in tasks requiring alertness until response to drug is known); nausea, vomiting, or dry mouth (small frequent meals, frequent mouth care, chewing gum, or sucking lozenges may help); or diarrhea (boiled milk, yogurt, or buttermilk may help). Report persistent CNS effects, skin rash or irritation, changes in urinary pattern, wheezing or respiratory difficulty, or worsening of condition.

Monitoring Parameters: Mental status

Reference Range: Therapeutic: 6-12 μg/mL (SI: 28-55 μmol/L); Toxic: >60 μg/mL (SI: >275 μmol/L)

Related Information

Aspirin and Meprobamate *on page 76*

♦ **Mepron™** *see* Atovaquone *on page 79*

Mequinol and Tretinoin (ME kwi nol & TRET i noyn)

Pharmacologic Class Retinoic Acid Derivative; Vitamin A Derivative; Vitamin, Topical

U.S. Brand Names Solagé™ Topical Solution

Mechanism of Action Solar lentigines are localized, pigmented, macular lesions of the skin on areas of the body chronically exposed to the sun. Mequinol is a substrate for the enzyme tyrosinase and acts as a competitive inhibitor of the formation of melanin precursors. The mechanisms of depigmentation for both drugs is unknown.

Use Treatment of solar lentigines; the efficacy of using Solagé™ daily for >24 weeks has not been established. The local cutaneous safety of Solagé™ in non-Caucasians has not been adequately established.

USUAL DOSAGE Adults: Topical: Apply twice daily to solar lentigines using the applicator tip while avoiding application to the surrounding skin. Separate application by at least 8 hours or as directed by prescriber.

Dosage Forms LIQ, top: Mequinol 2% and tretinoin 0.01% (30 mL)

Contraindications Pregnancy, women of childbearing potential, hypersensitivity to mequinol, tretinoin, or any component

Warnings/Precautions Discontinue if hypersensitivity is noted. Use extreme caution in eczematous skin conditions. Safety and efficacy have not been established in moderately or heavily pigmented skin. Not to be taken with photosensitizing drugs (eg, thiazides, tetracyclines, fluoroquinolones, phenothiazines, sulfonamides). Avoid sun (including sun lamps) or use protective clothing. Do not use in sunburned patients until they have fully recovered. Use extreme caution in patients who have significant exposure to the sun through their occupation. Use caution in patient with history or family history of vitiligo. For external use only. Weather extremes (wind, cold) may be irritating to users of Solagé™. Do not use in pediatric patients. No bathing or showering for at least 6 hours after application. Effects of chronic use (>52 weeks) are unknown.

Pregnancy Risk Factor X

Pregnancy Implications May cause fetal harm when administered to a pregnant woman. It is unknown if mequinol or tretinoin are excreted in breast milk. Use caution in breast-feeding.

Adverse Reactions

>10%: Dermatologic: Erythema (49%), burning, stinging or tingling (26%), desquamation (14%), pruritus (12%),

1% to 10%: Dermatologic: Skin irritation (5%), hypopigmentation (5%), halo hypopigmentation (7%), rash (3%), dry skin (3%), crusting (3%), vesicular bullae rash (2%), contact allergic reaction (1%)

Drug Interactions

Topical products with skin drying effects (eg, those containing alcohol, astringents, spices, or lime; medicated soaps or shampoos; permanent wave solutions; hair depilatories or waxes; and others) may increase skin irritation. Avoid concurrent use.

Photosensitizing drugs (eg, thiazides, tetracyclines, fluoroquinolones, phenothiazines, sulfonamides) can further increase sun sensitivity. Avoid concurrent use.

Education and Monitoring Issues

Patient Education: No bathing or showering for at least 6 hours after application. Avoid eyes, mouth, paranasal creases, and mucous membranes when applying. Application of larger amounts or more frequently will not result in more rapid or better results. Follow application directions closely. Wait 30 minutes after use before applying cosmetics. Avoid sun exposure (including sun lamps) or use protective clothing. Some reappearance of freckles may occur after discontinuation. After application, short-term stinging, burning, or irritation may occur.

Manufacturer Bristol-Myers Squibb Company (Pharmaceutical Division)

Related Information

Pharmaceutical Manufacturers Directory *on page 1020*

♦ **Meridia®** *see* Sibutramine *on page 849*

♦ **Meronem®** *see* Meropenem *on page 567*

Meropenem (mer oh PEN em)

Pharmacologic Class Antibiotic, Carbapenem

U.S. Brand Names Meronem®; Merrem® I.V.

Generic Available No

Mechanism of Action Inhibits bacterial cell wall synthesis by binding to several of the penicillin-binding proteins, which in turn inhibit the final transpeptidation step of peptidoglycan synthesis in bacterial cell walls, thus inhibiting cell wall biosynthesis; bacteria eventually lyse due to ongoing activity of cell wall autolytic enzymes (autolysins and murein hydrolases) while cell wall assembly is arrested

Use Intra-abdominal infections (complicated appendicitis and peritonitis) caused by viridans group streptococci, *E. coli*, *K. pneumoniae*, *P. aeruginosa*, *B. fragilis*, *B. thetaiotaomicron*, and *Peptostreptococcus* sp; also indicated for bacterial meningitis in pediatric patients >3 months of age caused by *S. pneumoniae*, *H. influenzae*, and *N. meningitidis*; meropenem has also been used to treat soft tissue infections, febrile neutropenia, and urinary tract infections

USUAL DOSAGE I.V.:

Neonates:

Preterm: 20 mg/kg/dose every 12 hours (may be increased to 40 mg/kg/dose if treating a highly resistant organism such as *Pseudomonas aeruginosa*)

Full-term (<3 months of age): 20 mg/kg/dose every 8 hours (may be increased to 40 mg/kg/dose if treating a highly resistant organism such as *Pseudomonas aeruginosa*)

Children >3 months (<50 kg):

Intra-abdominal infections: 20 mg/kg every 8 hours (maximum dose: 1 g every 8 hours)

(Continued)

Meropenem *(Continued)*

Meningitis: 40 mg/kg every 8 hours (maximum dose: 2 g every 8 hours)
Children >50 kg:
Intra-abdominal infections: 1 g every 8 hours
Meningitis: 2 g every 8 hours
Adults: 1 g every 8 hours
Dosing adjustment in renal impairment: Adults:
Cl_{cr} 26-50 mL/minute: Administer 1 g every 12 hours
Cl_{cr} 10-25 mL/minute: Administer 500 mg every 12 hours
Cl_{cr} <10 mL/minute: Administer 500 mg every 24 hours
Dialysis: Meropenem and its metabolites are readily dialyzable
Continuous arteriovenous or venovenous hemodiafiltration (CAVH) effects: Dose as Cl_{cr} 10-50 mL/minute

Dosage Forms INF: 500 mg (100 mL), 1 g (100 mL); ADD-vantage®: 500 mg (15 mL), 1 g (15 mL). **INJ:** 25 mg/mL (20 mL), 33.3 mg/mL (30 mL)

Contraindications Patients with known hypersensitivity to meropenem, any component, or other carbapenems (eg, imipenem); patients who have experienced anaphylactic reactions to other beta-lactams

Warnings/Precautions Pseudomembranous colitis and hypersensitivity reactions have occurred and often require immediate drug discontinuation; thrombocytopenia has been reported in patients with significant renal dysfunction; seizures have occurred in patients with underlying neurologic disorders (less frequent than with Primaxin®); safety and efficacy have not been established for children <3 months of age; superinfection possible with long courses of therapy

Pregnancy Risk Factor B

Pregnancy Implications Although no teratogenic or infant harm has been found in studies, excretion in breast milk is not known and this drug should be used during pregnancy and lactation only if clearly indicated

Adverse Reactions
1% to 10%:
Central nervous system: Headache (2.8%)
Dermatologic: Rash, pruritus (1% to 2%)
Gastrointestinal: Diarrhea (5%), nausea/vomiting (4%), constipation (1.2%)
Local: Pain at injection site (3%), phlebitis, thrombophlebitis (1%)
Respiratory: Apnea (1.2%)
<1%: Agitation, anemia, anorexia, cholestatic jaundice, confusion, depression, dysuria, edema, fever, flatulence, glossitis, hallucinations, heart failure (MI and arrhythmias), hepatic failure, hypertension, hypotension, hypo- and hypercytosis, bleeding events (epistaxis, melena, etc), ileus, increased creatinine/BUN, increased LFTs, insomnia, oral moniliasis, paresthesia, RBCs in urine, renal failure, seizures, tachycardia, urticaria, whole body pain

Drug Interactions Increased effect: Probenecid competes with meropenem for active tubular secretion and inhibits the renal excretion of meropenem (half-life increased by 38%)

Half-Life ~1 hour

Education and Monitoring Issues
Patient Education: Report pain at infusion/injection site, rash, or respiratory difficulty. You may experience gastric distress, diarrhea, mouth sores, respiratory difficulty, or headache (consult prescriber for appropriate medication).
Monitoring Parameters: Monitor for signs of anaphylaxis during first dose

Manufacturer AstraZeneca

Related Information
Antimicrobial Drugs of Choice *on page 1182*
Pharmaceutical Manufacturers Directory *on page 1020*

♦ **Merrem** *see* Meropenem *on page 567*
♦ **Merrem® I.V.** *see* Meropenem *on page 567*

Mesalamine (me SAL a meen)

Pharmacologic Class 5-Aminosalicylic Acid Derivative

U.S. Brand Names Asacol® Oral; Pentasa® Oral; Rowasa® Rectal

Generic Available No

Mechanism of Action Mesalamine (5-aminosalicylic acid) is the active component of sulfasalazine; the specific mechanism of action of mesalamine is unknown; however, it is thought that it modulates local chemical mediators of the inflammatory response, especially leukotrienes; action appears topical rather than systemic

Use
Oral: Remission and treatment of mildly to moderately active ulcerative colitis
Rectal: Treatment of active mild to moderate distal ulcerative colitis, proctosigmoiditis, or proctitis

USUAL DOSAGE Adults (usual course of therapy is 3-6 weeks):
Oral:
Capsule: 1 g 4 times/day

Tablet: 800 mg 3 times/day

Retention enema: 60 mL (4 g) at bedtime, retained overnight, approximately 8 hours

Rectal suppository: Insert 1 suppository in rectum twice daily

Some patients may require rectal and oral therapy concurrently

Dosage Forms CAP, controlled release (Pentasa®): 250 mg. **SUPP, rectal** (Rowasa®): 500 mg. **SUSP, rectal** (Rowasa®): 4 g/60 mL (7s). **TAB, enteric coated** (Asacol®): 400 mg

Contraindications Known hypersensitivity to mesalamine, sulfasalazine, sulfites, or salicylates

Warnings/Precautions Pericarditis should be considered in patients with chest pain; pancreatitis should be considered in any patient with new abdominal complaints. Elderly may have difficulty administering and retaining rectal suppositories. Given renal function decline with aging, monitor serum creatinine often during therapy. Use caution in patients with impaired hepatic function.

Pregnancy Risk Factor B

Adverse Reactions

>10%:

Central nervous system: Headache, malaise

Gastrointestinal: Abdominal pain, cramps, flatulence, gas

1% to 10%: Dermatologic: Alopecia, rash

<1%: Acute intolerance syndrome (bloody diarrhea, severe abdominal cramps, severe headache), anal irritation, pericarditis, fatal myocarditis, hypersensitivity pneumonitis, allergic reactions, pancreatitis, nephrotic syndrome, interstitial nephritis, hepatitis, aplastic anemia, pancytopenia, leukopenia, agranulocytosis or anemia, elevated transaminases, LDH, alkaline, phosphatase, bilirubin, jaundice, cholestatic jaundice, liver necrosis/failure, Kawasaki-like syndrome

Drug Interactions Decreased effect: Decreased digoxin bioavailability

Half-Life 5-ASA: 0.5-1.5 hours; Acetyl 5-ASA: 5-10 hours

Education and Monitoring Issues

Patient Education: Take as directed. Oral: Do not chew or break tablets. Enemas: Shake well before using, retain for 8 hours or as long as possible. Suppository: After removing foil wrapper, insert high in rectum without excessive handling (warmth will melt suppository). You may experience flatulence, headache, or hair loss (reversible). Report abdominal pain, unresolved diarrhea, severe headache, or chest pain.

♦ **Mesasal** *see* Mesalamine *on page 568*

♦ **M-Eslon®** *see* Morphine Sulfate *on page 618*

Mesoridazine (mez oh RID a zeen)

Pharmacologic Class Antipsychotic Agent, Phenothazine, Piperidine

U.S. Brand Names Serentil®

Generic Available No

Mechanism of Action Blockade of postsynaptic CNS dopamine receptors

Use Symptomatic management of psychotic disorders, including schizophrenia, behavioral problems, alcoholism as well as reducing anxiety and tension occurring in neurosis

USUAL DOSAGE Concentrate may be diluted just prior to administration with distilled water, acidified tap water, orange or grape juice; do not prepare and store bulk dilutions

Adults:

Oral: 25-50 mg 3 times/day; maximum: 100-400 mg/day

I.M.: Initial: 25 mg, repeat in 30-60 minutes as needed; optimal dosage range: 25-200 mg/day

Hemodialysis: Not dialyzable (0% to 5%)

Dosage Forms INJ: 25 mg/mL (1 mL). **LIQ, oral:** 25 mg/mL (118 mL). **TAB:** 10 mg, 25 mg, 50 mg, 100 mg

Contraindications Hypersensitivity to mesoridazine or any component, cross-sensitivity with other phenothiazines may exist

Warnings/Precautions Safety in children <6 months of age has not been established; use with caution in patients with cardiovascular disease or seizures; benefits of therapy must be weighed against risks of therapy; doses >1 g/day frequently cause pigmentary retinopathy; some products contain sulfites and/or tartrazine; use with caution in patients with narrow-angle glaucoma, bone marrow suppression, severe liver disease

Pregnancy Risk Factor C

Adverse Reactions

Cardiovascular: Hypotension, orthostatic hypotension, tachycardia, Q-T prolongation, syncope, edema

Central nervous system: Pseudoparkinsonism, akathisia, dystonias, tardive dyskinesia, dizziness, drowsiness, restlessness, ataxia, slurred speech, neuroleptic malignant syndrome (NMS), impairment of temperature regulation, lowering of seizure threshold

Dermatologic: Increased sensitivity to sun, rash, itching, angioneurotic edema, dermatitis, discoloration of skin (blue-gray)

Endocrine & metabolic: Changes in menstrual cycle, changes in libido, gynecomastia, lactation, galactorrhea

Gastrointestinal: Constipation, xerostomia, weight gain, nausea, vomiting, stomach pain

(Continued)

Mesoridazine *(Continued)*

Genitourinary: Difficulty in urination, ejaculatory disturbances, impotence, enuresis, incontinence, priapism, urinary retention

Hematologic: Agranulocytosis, leukopenia, eosinophilia, thrombocytopenia, anemia, aplastic anemia

Hepatic: Cholestatic jaundice, hepatotoxicity

Neuromuscular & skeletal: Weakness, tremor, rigidity

Ocular: Pigmentary retinopathy, photophobia, blurred vision, cornea and lens changes

Respiratory: Nasal congestion

Miscellaneous: Diaphoresis (decreased)

Drug Interactions

Phenothiazines inhibit the ability of bromocriptine to lower serum prolactin concentrations

Benztropine (and other anticholinergics) may inhibit the therapeutic response to mesoridazine and excess anticholinergic effects may occur

Chloroquine may increase mesoridazine concentrations

Cigarette smoking may enhance the hepatic metabolism of mesoridazine. Larger doses may be required compared to a nonsmoker.

Concurrent use of mesoridazine with an antihypertensive may produce additive hypotensive effects

Antihypertensive effects of guanethidine and guanadrel may be inhibited by mesoridazine

Concurrent use with TCA may produce increased toxicity or altered therapeutic response

Mesoridazine may inhibit the antiparkinsonian effect of levodopa; avoid this combination

Mesoridazine plus lithium may rarely produce neurotoxicity

Barbiturates may reduce mesoridazine concentrations

Propranolol may increase mesoridazine concentrations

Sulfadoxine-pyrimethamine may increase mesoridazine concentrations

Mesoridazine and possibly other low potency antipsychotics may reverse the pressor effects of epinephrine

Mesoridazine and CNS depressants (ethanol, narcotics) may produce additive CNS depressant effects

Mesoridazine and trazodone may produce additive hypotensive effects

Alcohol Interactions Avoid use (may increase central nervous system depression)

Duration 4-6 hours

Half-Life Time to steady-state serum: 4-7 days

Education and Monitoring Issues

Patient Education: Use exactly as directed (do not increase dose or frequency); may cause physical and/or psychological dependence. It may take 2-3 weeks to achieve desired results; do not discontinue without consulting prescriber. Dilute oral concentration with water, orange or grape juice. Do not take within 2 hours of any antacid. Avoid excess alcohol or caffeine and other prescription or OTC medications not approved by prescriber. Maintain adequate hydration (2-3 L/day of fluids unless instructed to restrict fluid intake). Avoid skin contact with medication; may cause contact dermatitis (wash immediately with warm, soapy water). You may experience excess drowsiness, restlessness, dizziness, or blurred vision (use caution driving or when engaging in tasks requiring alertness until response to drug is known); dry mouth, nausea, vomiting (small frequent meals, frequent mouth care, chewing gum, or sucking lozenges may help); constipation (increased exercise, fluids, or dietary fruit and fiber may help); postural hypotension (use caution climbing stairs or when changing position from lying or sitting to standing); urinary retention (void before taking medication); photosensitivity (use sunscreen, wear protective clothing and eyewear, avoid direct sunlight); decreased perspiration (avoid strenuous exercise in hot environments); or changes in menstrual cycle, libido, ejaculation (will resolve when medication is discontinued). Report persistent CNS effects (eg, trembling fingers, altered gait or balance, excessive sedation, seizures, unusual movements, anxiety, abnormal thoughts, confusion, personality changes); chest pain, palpitations, rapid heartbeat, severe dizziness; unresolved urinary retention or changes in urinary pattern; menstrual pattern, change in libido, swelling or pain in breasts (male or female); vision changes; skin rash or yellowing of skin; difficulty breathing; or worsening of condition.

♦ **Mestatin®** *see* Nystatin *on page 670*

♦ **Mestinon®** *see* Pyridostigmine *on page 795*

♦ **Mestinon® Time-Span®** *see* Pyridostigmine *on page 795*

Mestranol and Norethindrone (MES tra nole & nor eth IN drone)

Pharmacologic Class Contraceptive, Oral

U.S. Brand Names Genora® 1/50; Nelova™ 1/50M; Norethin™ 1/50M; Norinyl® 1+50; Ortho-Novum™ 1/50

Generic Available Yes

Mechanism of Action Combination oral contraceptives inhibit ovulation via a negative feedback mechanism on the hypothalamus, which alters the normal pattern of gonadotropin secretion of a follicle-stimulating hormone (FSH) and luteinizing hormone by the anterior pituitary. The follicular phase FSH and midcycle surge of gonadotropins are inhibited. In addition, oral contraceptives produce alterations in the genital tract, including changes in the cervical mucus, rendering it unfavorable for sperm penetration even if ovulation occurs. Changes in the endometrium may also occur, producing an unfavorable environment for nidation. Oral contraceptive drugs may alter the tubal transport of the ova through the fallopian tubes. Progestational agents may also alter sperm fertility.

Use Prevention of pregnancy; treatment of hypermenorrhea, endometriosis, female hypogonadism [monophasic oral contraceptive]

USUAL DOSAGE Adults: Female: Oral:

Contraception: 1 tablet daily, beginning on day 5 of menstrual cycle (first day of menstrual flow is day 1). With 20-tablet and 21-tablet packages, new dosing cycle begins 7 days after last tablet taken. With 28-tablet packages, dosage is 1 tablet daily without interruption; extra tablets are placebos or contain iron. If next menstrual period does not begin on schedule, rule out pregnancy before starting new dosing cycle. If menstrual period begins, start new dosing cycle 7 days after last tablet was taken. If all doses have been taken on schedule and one menstrual period is missed, continue dosing cycle. If two consecutive menstrual periods are missed, pregnancy test is required before new dosing cycle is started.

One dose missed: Take as soon as remembered or take 2 tablets next day

Two doses missed: Take 2 tablets as soon as remembered or 2 tablets next 2 days

Three doses missed: Begin new compact of tablets starting on day 1 of next cycle

Dosage Forms TAB: Mestranol 0.05 mg and norethindrone 1 mg (21s and 28s)

Contraindications Known or suspected breast cancer, undiagnosed abnormal vaginal bleeding, carcinoma of the breast, estrogen-dependent tumor, pregnancy

Warnings/Precautions Use with caution in patients with a history of thromboembolism, stroke, myocardial infarction, liver tumor, hypertension, cardiac, renal or hepatic insufficiency; use of any progestin during the first 4 months of pregnancy is not recommended; risk of cardiovascular side effects increases in those women who smoke cigarettes and in women >35 years of age

Pregnancy Risk Factor X

Adverse Reactions

>10%:

Cardiovascular: Peripheral edema

Central nervous system: Headache

Endocrine: Enlargement of breasts, breast tenderness, increased libido

Gastrointestinal: Nausea, anorexia, bloating

1% to 10%: Gastrointestinal: Vomiting, diarrhea

<1%: Alterations in frequency and flow of menses, amenorrhea, anxiety, breast tumors, chloasma, cholestatic jaundice, decreased glucose tolerance, depression, dizziness, edema, GI distress, hypertension, increased susceptibility to *Candida* infection, increased triglycerides and LDL, intolerance to contact lenses, melasma, myocardial infarction, rash, stroke, thromboembolism

See tables.

Achieving Proper Hormonal Balance in an Oral Contraceptive

Estrogen		Progestin	
Excess	**Deficiency**	**Excess**	**Deficiency**
Nausea, bloating	Early or midcycle breakthrough bleeding	Increased appetite	Late breakthrough bleeding
Cervical mucorrhea, polyposis	Increased spotting	Weight gain	Amenorrhea
Melasma	Hypomenorrhea	Tiredness, fatigue	Hypermenorrhea
Migraine headache		Hypomenorrhea	
Breast fullness or tenderness		Acne, oily scalp*	
Edema		Hair loss, hirsutism*	
Hypertension		Depression	
		Monilial vaginitis	
		Breast regression	

*Result of androgenic activity of progestins.

Pharmacological Effects of Progestins Used in Oral Contraceptives

	Progestin	Estrogen	Antiestrogen	Androgen
Norgestrel/levonorgestrel	+++	0	++	+++
Ethynodiol diacetate	++	+*	+*	+
Norethindrone acetate	+	+	+++	+
Norethindrone	+	+*	+*	+
Norethynodrel	+	+++	0	0

*Has estrogenic effect at low doses; may have antiestrogenic effect at higher doses.

+++ = pronounced effect

++ = moderate effect

+ = slight effect

0 = no effect

(Continued)

Mestranol and Norethindrone *(Continued)*

Drug Interactions

Decreased effect:

Tetracyclines, penicillins, griseofulvin, rifampin, acetaminophen, barbiturates, hydantoins may increase contraceptive failures

Decreases acetaminophen, estrogen levels, and anticoagulants

Increased toxicity: Increases benzodiazepines, caffeine, metoprolol, theophyllines, and tricyclic antidepressants

Education and Monitoring Issues

Patient Education: Take exactly as directed; use additional method of birth control during first week of administration of first cycle; photosensitivity may occur

Women should inform their prescribers if signs or symptoms of any of the following occur thromboembolic or thrombotic disorders including sudden severe headache or vomiting, disturbance of vision or speech, loss of vision, numbness or weakness in an extremity, sharp or crushing chest pain, calf pain, shortness of breath, severe abdominal pain or mass, mental depression or unusual bleeding

Women should be advised that if they miss one daily dose, they should take the tablet as soon as remembered. If 2 daily doses are missed, 2 tablets should be taken daily for 2 days and the regular schedule resumed. If 3 or more daily doses are missed, therapy should be discontinued. Therapy with a new cycle can be resumed in 7 or 8 days. When any doses are missed, alternative contraceptive methods should be used for the next 2 days or until 2 days into the new cycle.

Women should discontinue taking the medication if they suspect they are pregnant or become pregnant

- ♦ **Metadate ER®** *see* Methylphenidate *on page 588*
- ♦ **Metahydrin®** *see* Trichlormethiazide *on page 949*
- ♦ **Metamucil® [OTC]** *see* Psyllium *on page 793*
- ♦ **Metamucil® Instant Mix [OTC]** *see* Psyllium *on page 793*
- ♦ **Metandren®** *see* Methyltestosterone *on page 591*
- ♦ **Metaprel® Syrup** *see* Metaproterenol *on page 572*

Metaproterenol (met a proe TER e nol)

Pharmacologic Class Beta$_2$ Agonist

U.S. Brand Names Alupent®; Arm-a-Med® Metaproterenol; Dey-Dose® Metaproterenol; Metaprel® Syrup; Prometa®

Generic Available Yes (except inhaler)

Mechanism of Action Relaxes bronchial smooth muscle by action on beta$_2$-receptors with very little effect on heart rate

Use Bronchodilator in reversible airway obstruction due to asthma or COPD; because of its delayed onset of action (1 hour) and prolonged effect (4 or more hours), this may not be the drug of choice for assessing response to a bronchodilator

USUAL DOSAGE

Oral:

Children:

<2 years: 0.4 mg/kg/dose given 3-4 times/day; in infants, the dose can be given every 8-12 hours

2-6 years: 1-2.6 mg/kg/day divided every 6 hours

6-9 years: 10 mg/dose 3-4 times/day

Children >9 years and Adults: 20 mg 3-4 times/day

Elderly: Initial: 10 mg 3-4 times/day, increasing as necessary up to 20 mg 3-4 times/day

Inhalation: Children >12 years and Adults: 2-3 inhalations every 3-4 hours, up to 12 inhalations in 24 hours

Nebulizer:

Infants and Children: 0.01-0.02 mL/kg of 5% solution; minimum dose: 0.1 mL; maximum dose: 0.3 mL diluted in 2-3 mL normal saline every 4-6 hours (may be given more frequently according to need)

Adolescents and Adults: 5-20 breaths of full strength 5% metaproterenol **or** 0.2 to 0.3 mL 5% metaproterenol in 2.5-3 mL normal saline until nebulized every 4-6 hours (can be given more frequently according to need)

Dosage Forms AERO, oral: 0.65 mg/dose (5 mL, 10 mL). **SOLN for inh** (preservative free): 0.4% [4 mg/mL] (2.5 mL), 0.6 [6 mg/mL] (2.5 mL), 5% [50 mg/mL] (10 mL, 30 mL). **SYR:** 10 mg/5 mL (480 mL). **TAB:** 10 mg, 20 mg

Contraindications Hypersensitivity to metaproterenol or any components, pre-existing cardiac arrhythmias associated with tachycardia

Warnings/Precautions Use with caution in patients with hypertension, CHF, hyperthyroidism, CAD, diabetes, or sensitivity to sympathomimetics; excessive prolonged use may result in decreased efficacy or increased toxicity and death; use caution in patients with pre-existing cardiac arrhythmias associated with tachycardia. Metaproterenol has more beta$_1$ activity than other sympathomimetics such as albuterol and, therefore, may no longer be the beta agonist of first choice. All patients should utilize a spacer device when using a metered dose inhaler. Oral use should be avoided due to the increased incidence of adverse effects.

Pregnancy Risk Factor C

Pregnancy Implications

Clinical effects on the fetus: No data on crossing the placenta. Reported association with polydactyly in 1 study; may be secondary to severe maternal disease or chance.

Breast-feeding/lactation: No data on crossing into breast milk or clinical effects on the infant

Adverse Reactions

>10%:

- Central nervous system: Nervousness
- Neuromuscular & skeletal: Tremor

1% to 10%:

- Cardiovascular: Tachycardia, palpitations, hypertension
- Central nervous system: Headache, dizziness
- Gastrointestinal: Nausea, vomiting, bad taste
- Neuromuscular & skeletal: Trembling, muscle cramps, weakness
- Respiratory: Coughing
- Miscellaneous: Diaphoresis (increased)

<1%: Paradoxical bronchospasm

Drug Interactions

Decreased effect: Beta-blockers

Increased toxicity: Sympathomimetics, TCAs, MAO inhibitors

Onset

Oral: Onset of bronchodilation: Within 15 minutes; Peak effect: Within 1 hour

Inhalation: Onset of bronchodilation: Within 60 seconds

Duration Oral or inhalation: ~1-5 hours, regardless of route administered

Education and Monitoring Issues

Patient Education: Use exactly as directed. Do not use more often than recommended. Maintain adequate hydration (2-3 L/day of fluids unless instructed to restrict fluid intake). You may experience nervousness, dizziness, or fatigue (use caution when driving or engaging in tasks requiring alertness until response to drug is known); dry mouth, unpleasant aftertaste, stomach upset (frequent small meals, frequent mouth care, chewing gum, or sucking hard candy may help); or increased perspiration. Report unresolved GI upset; dizziness or fatigue; vision changes; chest pain, rapid heartbeat, or palpitations; nervousness or insomnia; muscle cramping or tremor; or unusual cough.

Monitoring Parameters: Assess lung sounds, pulse, and blood pressure before administration and during peak of medication; observe patient for wheezing after administration, if this occurs, call prescriber; monitor heart rate, respiratory rate, blood pressure, and arterial or capillary blood gases if applicable

Related Information

Bronchodilators Comparison *on page 1235*

♦ **Metastron** *see* Strontium-89 *on page 874*

Metaxalone (me TAKS a lone)

Pharmacologic Class Skeletal Muscle Relaxant

U.S. Brand Names Skelaxin®

Generic Available No

Mechanism of Action Does not have a direct effect on skeletal muscle; most of its therapeutic effect comes from actions on the central nervous system

Use Relief of discomfort associated with acute, painful musculoskeletal conditions

USUAL DOSAGE Children >12 years and Adults: Oral: 800 mg 3-4 times/day

Dosage Forms TAB: 400 mg

Contraindications Impaired hepatic or renal function, known hypersensitivity to metaxalone, history of drug-induced hemolytic anemias or other anemias

Warnings/Precautions Use with caution in patients with impaired hepatic function

Pregnancy Risk Factor C

Adverse Reactions

>10%:

- Gastrointestinal: Nausea, vomiting, stomach cramps
- Central nervous system: Paradoxical stimulation, headache, drowsiness, dizziness

<1%: Allergic dermatitis, anaphylaxis, hemolytic anemia, hepatotoxicity, leukopenia

Drug Interactions Increased effect of alcohol, CNS depressants

Onset ~1 hour

Duration 4-6 hours

Half-Life 2-3 hours

Education and Monitoring Issues

Patient Education: Avoid alcohol and other CNS depressants; may cause drowsiness, impairment of judgment, or coordination; notify prescriber of dark urine, pale stools, yellowing of eyes, severe nausea, vomiting, or abdominal pain

Metformin (met FOR min)

Pharmacologic Class Antidiabetic Agent (Biguanide)

U.S. Brand Names Glucophage®

Mechanism of Action Decreases hepatic glucose production, decreasing intestinal absorption of glucose and improves insulin sensitivity (increases peripheral glucose uptake and utilization)

Use Management of noninsulin-dependent diabetes mellitus (type II) as monotherapy when hyperglycemia cannot be managed on diet alone. May be used concomitantly with a sulfonylurea when diet and metformin or sulfonylurea alone do not result in adequate glycemic control.

Investigational: Data suggests that some patients with NIDDM with secondary failure to sulfonylurea therapy may obtain significant improvement in metabolic control when metformin in combination with insulin and a sulfonylurea is used in lieu of insulin alone

USUAL DOSAGE Oral (allow 1-2 weeks between dose titrations): Generally, clinically significant responses are not seen at doses <1500 mg daily; however, a lower recommended starting dose and gradual increased dosage is recommended to minimize gastrointestinal symptoms

Adults:

500 mg tablets: Initial: 500 mg twice daily (give with the morning and evening meals). Dosage increases should be made in increments of 1 tablet every week, given in divided doses, up to a maximum of 2500 mg/day. Doses of up to 2000 mg/day may be given twice daily. If a dose of 2500 mg/day is required, it may be better tolerated 3 times/day (with meals).

850 mg tablets: Initial: 850 mg once daily (give with the morning meal). Dosage increases should be made in increments of 1 tablet every **other** week, given in divided doses, up to a maximum of 2550 mg/day. Usual maintenance dose: 850 mg twice daily (with the morning and evening meals). Some patients may be given 850 mg 3 times/day (with meals).

Elderly: The initial and maintenance dosing should be conservative, due to the potential for decreased renal function. Generally, elderly patients should not be titrated to the maximum dose of metformin.

Transfer from other antidiabetic agents: No transition period is generally necessary except when transferring from chlorpropamide. When transferring from chlorpropamide, care should be exercised during the first 2 weeks because of the prolonged retention of chlorpropamide in the body, leading to overlapping drug effects and possible hypoglycemia.

Concomitant metformin and oral sulfonylurea therapy: If patients have not responded to 4 weeks of the maximum dose of metformin monotherapy, consideration to a gradual addition of an oral sulfonylurea while continuing metformin at the maximum dose, even if prior primary or secondary failure to a sulfonylurea has occurred.

Dosing adjustment/comments in renal impairment: The plasma and blood half-life of metformin is prolonged and the renal clearance is decreased in proportion to the decrease in creatinine clearance. Metformin is contraindicated in the presence of renal dysfunction defined as a serum creatinine >1.5 mg/dL in males or >1.4 mg/dL in females or an abnormal creatinine clearance.

Dosing adjustment in hepatic impairment: No studies have been conducted, however, metformin should be avoided because the presence of liver disease is a risk factor for the development of lactic acidosis during metformin therapy.

Dosage Forms TAB: 500 mg, 625 mg, 750 mg, 850 mg, 1000 mg

Contraindications Hypersensitivity to metformin or any component; renal disease or renal dysfunction (serum creatinine ≥1.5 mg/dL in males or ≥1.4 mg/dL in females or abnormal clearance); clinical situations predisposing to hypoxemia, including conditions such as cardiovascular collapse, respiratory failure, acute myocardial infarction, acute congestive heart failure, and septicemia; acute or chronic metabolic acidosis with or without coma (including diabetic ketoacidosis); should be temporarily discontinued for 48 hours in patients undergoing radiologic studies involving the intravascular administration of iodinated contrast materials (potential for acute alteration in renal function).

Warnings/Precautions Administration of oral antidiabetic drugs has been reported to be associated with increased cardiovascular mortality as compared to treatment with diet alone or diet plus insulin.

Lactic acidosis is a rare, but potentially severe consequence of therapy with metformin. Withhold therapy in hypoxemia, dehydration or sepsis. The risk of lactic acidosis is increased in any patient with CHF requiring pharmacologic management. This risk is particularly high during acute or unstable congestive heart failure (see Contraindications) because of the risk of hypoperfusion and hypoxemia.

Metformin is substantially excreted by the kidney. The risk of accumulation and lactic acidosis increases with the degree of impairment of renal function. Patients with renal function below the limit of normal for their age should not receive metformin. In elderly patients, renal function should be monitored regularly. should not be used in any patient 80 years of age or older unless measurement of creatinine clearance verifies normal renal function. Use of concomitant medications that may affect renal function (ie, affect tubular secretion) may also affect metformin disposition. Therapy should be suspended for any surgical procedures - resume only after normal intake resumed and normal renal function is verified. Avoid use in patients with impaired liver function. Patient must be instructed to avoid excessive acute or chronic ethanol use.

Lactic acidosis should be suspected in any diabetic patient receiving metformin who has evidence of acidosis when evidence of ketoacidosis is lacking.

Pregnancy Risk Factor B

Adverse Reactions

>10%: Gastrointestinal: Anorexia, nausea, vomiting, diarrhea, epigastric fullness, constipation, heartburn

1% to 10%:

Dermatologic: Rash, urticaria, photosensitivity

Miscellaneous: Decreased vitamin B_{12} levels

<1%: Agranulocytosis, aplastic anemia, blood dyscrasias, bone marrow suppression, hemolytic anemia, thrombocytopenia

Drug Interactions

Decreased effect: Drugs which tend to produce hyperglycemia (eg, diuretics, corticosteroids, phenothiazines, thyroid products, estrogens, oral contraceptives, phenytoin, nicotinic acid, sympathomimetics, calcium channel blocking drugs, isoniazid) may lead to a loss of glycemic control

Increased effect: Furosemide increased the metformin plasma and blood C_{max} without altering metformin renal clearance in a single dose study

Increased toxicity:

Cationic drugs (eg, amiloride, digoxin, morphine, procainamide, quinidine, quinine, ranitidine, triamterene, trimethoprim, and vancomycin) which are eliminated by renal tubular secretion could have the potential for interaction with metformin by competing for common renal tubular transport systems

Cimetidine increases (by 60%) peak metformin plasma and whole blood concentrations

Alcohol Interactions Alcohol intake may increase risk of lactic acidosis. Avoid concurrent use.

Onset Within days, maximum effects up to 2 weeks

Half-Life 6.2 hours; prolonged in renal impairment

Education and Monitoring Issues

Patient Education: This medication is used to control diabetes; it is not a cure. Other components of treatment plan are important: follow prescribed diet, medication, and exercise regimen. Take exactly as directed; with meal(s) at the same time each day. Do not change dose or discontinue without consulting prescriber. Avoid alcohol while taking this medication; could cause severe reaction. Inform prescriber of all other prescription or OTC medications you are taking; do not introduce new medication without consulting prescriber. Do not take other medication within 2 hours of this medication unless so advised by prescriber. You may experience side effects during first weeks of therapy (headache, nausea); consult prescriber if these persist. Report severe or persistent side effects, extended vomiting or flu-like symptoms, skin rash, easy bruising or bleeding, or change in color of urine or stool.

Dietary Considerations:

Food: Food decreases the extent and slightly delays the absorption. Drug may cause GI upset; take with food to decrease GI upset.

Glucose: Decreases blood glucose concentration. Hypoglycemia does not usually occur unless a patient is predisposed. Monitor blood glucose concentration. Exercise caution with administration in patients predisposed to hypoglycemia (eg, cases of reduced caloric intake, strenuous exercise without repletion of calories, alcohol ingestion or when metformin is combined with another oral antidiabetic agent).

Vitamin B_{12}: Decreases absorption of Vitamin B_{12}; monitor for signs and symptoms of vitamin B_{12} deficiency

Folic acid: Decreases absorption of folic acid; monitor for signs and symptoms of folic acid deficiency

Monitoring Parameters: Urine for glucose and ketones, fasting blood glucose, hemoglobin A_{1c}, and fructosamine. Initial and periodic monitoring of hematologic parameters (eg, hemoglobin/hematocrit and red blood cell indices) and renal function should be performed, at least annually. While megaloblastic anemia has been rarely seen with metformin, if suspected, vitamin B_{12} deficiency should be excluded.

Reference Range: Target range: Adults:

Fasting blood glucose: <120 mg/dL

Glycosylated hemoglobin: <7%

Manufacturer Bristol-Myers Squibb Company (Pharmaceutical Division)

Related Information

Hypoglycemic Drugs and Thiazolidinedione Information *on page 1240*

Pharmaceutical Manufacturers Directory *on page 1020*

Methacholine (meth a KOLE leen)

Pharmacologic Class Diagnostic Agent

U.S. Brand Names Provocholine®

Generic Available No

(Continued)

Methacholine *(Continued)*

Mechanism of Action Methacholine chloride is a cholinergic (parasympathomimetic) synthetic analogue of acetylcholine. The drug stimulates muscarinic, postganglionic parasympathetic receptors, which results in smooth muscle contraction of the airways and increased tracheobronchial secretions.

Use Diagnosis of bronchial airway hyperactivity in subjects who do not have clinically apparent asthma

USUAL DOSAGE Before inhalation challenge, perform baseline pulmonary function tests; the patient must have an FEV_1 of at least 70% of the predicted value. The following is a suggested schedule for administration of methacholine challenge. Calculate cumulative units by multiplying number of breaths by concentration given. Total cumulative units is the sum of cumulative units for each concentration given. See table.

Methacholine

Vial	Serial Concentration (mg/mL)	No. of Breaths	Cumulative Units per Concentration	Total Cumulative Units
E	0.025	5	0.125	0.125
D	0.25	5	1.25	1.375
C	2.5	5	12.5	13.88
B	10	5	50	63.88
A	25	5	125	188.88

Determine FEV_1 within 5 minutes of challenge, a postive challenge is a 20% reduction in FEV_1

Dosage Forms POWDER for reconstitution, inhalation: 100 mg/5 mL

Contraindications Concomitant use of beta-blockers; hypersensitivity to the drug; because of the potential for severe bronchoconstriction, methacholine challenge should not be performed on any patient with clinically apparent asthma, wheezing, or very low baseline pulmonary function tests (forced expiratory volume in one second less than 70% of predicted value).

Warnings/Precautions Methacholine is a bronchoconstrictor for diagnostic purposes only. Perform inhalation challenge under the supervision of a prescriber trained in and thoroughly familiar with all aspects of the technique, all contraindications, warnings, and precautions of methacholine challenge and the management of respiratory distress. Have emergency equipment and medication immediately available to treat acute respiratory distress. Administer only by inhalation; severe bronchoconstriction and reduction in respiratory function can result. Patients with severe hyper-reactivity of the airways can experience bronchoconstriction at a dosage as low as 0.025 mg/mL (0.125 cumulative units). If severe bronchoconstriction occurs, reverse immediately by administration of a rapid-acting inhaled bronchodilator (beta-agonist).

Pregnancy Risk Factor C

Adverse Reactions <1%: Complete heart block, cough, dyspnea, headache, hypotension, itching, lightheadedness, substernal pain, syncope, tightness of the chest, throat irritation, wheezing

Onset Rapid

Duration 15-75 minutes

Methadone (METH a done)

Pharmacologic Class Analgesic, Narcotic

U.S. Brand Names Dolophine®

Generic Available Yes

Mechanism of Action Binds to opiate receptors in the CNS, causing inhibition of ascending pain pathways, altering the perception of and response to pain; produces generalized CNS depression

Use Management of severe pain, used in narcotic detoxification maintenance programs

USUAL DOSAGE Doses should be titrated to appropriate effects

Children: Analgesia:

- Oral, I.M., S.C.: 0.7 mg/kg/24 hours divided every 4-6 hours as needed or 0.1-0.2 mg/kg every 4-12 hours as needed; maximum: 10 mg/dose
- I.V.: 0.1 mg/kg every 4 hours initially for 2-3 doses, then every 6-12 hours as needed; maximum: 10 mg/dose

Adults:

- Analgesia: Oral, I.M., S.C.: 2.5-10 mg every 3-8 hours as needed, up to 5-20 mg every 6-8 hours
- Detoxification: Oral: 15-40 mg/day; should not exceed 21 days and may not be repeated earlier than 4 weeks after completion of preceding course
- Maintenance of opiate dependence: Oral: 20-120 mg/day

Dosing adjustment in renal impairment: Cl_{cr} <10 mL/minute: Administer at 50% to 75% of normal dose

Dosing adjustment/comments in hepatic disease: Avoid in severe liver disease

Important note: Methadone accumulates with repeated doses and dosage may need to be adjusted downward after 3-5 days to prevent toxic effects. Some patients may benefit from every 8- to 12-hour dosing interval (pain control).

Dosage Forms INJ: 10 mg/mL (1 mL, 10 mL, 20 mL). **SOLN:** Oral: 5 mg/5 mL (5 mL, 500 mL), 10 mg/5 mL (500 mL); Oral, concentrate: 10 mg/mL (30 mL). **TAB:** 5 mg, 10 mg; Dispersible: 40 mg

Contraindications Hypersensitivity to methadone or any component

Warnings/Precautions Tablets are to be used only for oral administration and **must not** be used for injection; use with caution in patients with respiratory diseases including asthma, emphysema, or COPD and in patients with severe liver disease; because methadone's effects on respiration last much longer than its analgesic effects, the dose must be titrated slowly; because of its long half-life and risk of accumulation, it is not considered a drug of first choice in the elderly, who may be particularly susceptible to its CNS depressant and constipating effects; tolerance or drug dependence may result from extended use

Pregnancy Risk Factor B; D (if used for prolonged periods or in high doses at term)

Adverse Reactions

Cardiovascular: Bradycardia, peripheral vasodilation, cardiac arrest, syncope, faintness

Central nervous system: Euphoria, dysphoria, headache, insomnia, agitation, disorientation, drowsiness, dizziness, lightheadedness, sedation

Dermatologic: Pruritus, urticaria, rash

Endocrine & metabolic: Decreased libido

Gastrointestinal: Nausea, vomiting, constipation, anorexia, stomach cramps, xerostomia, biliary tract spasm

Genitourinary: Urinary retention or hesitancy, antidiuretic effect, impotence

Neuromuscular & skeletal: Weakness

Ocular: Miosis, visual disturbances

Respiratory: Respiratory depression, respiratory arrest

Miscellaneous: Physical and psychological dependence

Drug Interactions CYP1A2, 2D6, and 3A3/4 enzyme substrate; CYP2D6 inhibitor

Decreased effect: Phenytoin, pentazocine, ritonavir and rifampin may increase the metabolism of methadone and may precipitate withdrawal

Increased toxicity: CNS depressants, phenothiazines, tricyclic antidepressants, MAO inhibitors may potentiate the adverse effects of methadone

Alcohol Interactions Avoid use (may increase central nervous system depression)

Onset

Oral: Onset of analgesia: Within 0.5-1 hour

Parenteral: Onset of analgesia: Within 10-20 minutes; Peak effect: Within 1-2 hours

Duration Oral: 6-8 hours, increases to 22-48 hours with repeated doses

Half-Life 15-29 hours, may be prolonged with alkaline pH

Education and Monitoring Issues

Patient Education: If self-administered, use exactly as directed (do not increase dose or frequency); may cause physical and/or psychological dependence. While using this medication, do not use alcohol and other prescription or OTC medications (especially sedatives, tranquilizers, antihistamines, or pain medications) without consulting prescriber. Maintain adequate hydration (2-3 L/day of fluids unless instructed to restrict fluid intake). May cause hypotension, dizziness, drowsiness, impaired coordination, or blurred vision (use caution when driving, climbing stairs, or changing position - rising from sitting or lying to standing, or when engaging in tasks requiring alertness until response to drug is known); loss of appetite, nausea, or vomiting (frequent mouth care, small frequent meals, chewing gum, or sucking lozenges may help); constipation (increased exercise, fluids, or dietary fruit and fiber may help - if constipation remains an unresolved problem, consult prescriber about use of stool softeners). Report chest pain, slow or rapid heartbeat, acute dizziness or persistent headache; changes in mental status; swelling of extremities or unusual weight gain; changes in urinary elimination; acute headache; back or flank pain or muscle spasms; blurred vision; skin rash; or shortness of breath.

Dietary Considerations: Food: Glucose may cause hyperglycemia; monitor blood glucose concentrations

Monitoring Parameters: Pain relief, respiratory and mental status, blood pressure

Reference Range: Therapeutic: 100-400 ng/mL (SI: 0.32-1.29 μmol/L); Toxic: >2 μg/mL (SI: >6.46 μmol/L)

Related Information

Lipid-Lowering Agents Comparison *on page 1243*
Narcotic Agonists Comparison *on page 1244*

♦ **Methadose®** *see* Methadone *on page 576*

Methamphetamine (meth am FET a meen)

Pharmacologic Class Amphetamine

U.S. Brand Names Desoxyn®; Desoxyn Gradumet®

Generic Available No

(Continued)

Methamphetamine *(Continued)*

Use Treatment of narcolepsy, exogenous obesity, abnormal behavioral syndrome in children (minimal brain dysfunction)

USUAL DOSAGE

Attention deficit disorder: Children >6 years: 2.5-5 mg 1-2 times/day, may increase by 5 mg increments weekly until optimum response is achieved, usually 20-25 mg/day

Exogenous obesity: Children >12 years and Adults: 5 mg, 30 minutes before each meal; long-acting formulation: 10-15 mg in morning; treatment duration should not exceed a few weeks; see "Obesity Treatment Guidelines for Adults" in Appendix

Dosage Forms TAB: 5 mg; Extended release (Gradumet®): 5 mg, 10 mg, 15 mg

Contraindications Known hypersensitivity to methamphetamine

Warnings/Precautions Cardiovascular disease, nephritis, angina pectoris, hypertension, glaucoma, patients with a history of drug abuse, known hypersensitivity to amphetamine

Pregnancy Risk Factor C

Adverse Reactions

Cardiovascular: Hypertension, tachycardia, palpitations

Central nervous system: Restlessness, headache, exacerbation of motor and phonic tics and Tourette's syndrome, dizziness, psychosis, dysphoria, overstimulation, euphoria, insomnia

Dermatologic: Rash, urticaria

Endocrine & metabolic: Change in libido

Gastrointestinal: Diarrhea, nausea, vomiting, stomach cramps, constipation, anorexia, weight loss, xerostomia, unpleasant taste

Genitourinary: Impotence

Neuromuscular & skeletal: Tremor

Miscellaneous: Suppression of growth in children, tolerance and withdrawal with prolonged use

Drug Interactions CYP2D6 enzyme substrate

Insulin and oral hypoglycemic requirements in diabetes may be lessened with the use of methamphetamine and the concomitant diet

Methamphetamine may decrease hypotensive effects of guanethidine

Methamphetamine is contraindicated with MAOIs

Antipsychotics may antagonize the CNS stimulant effect of methamphetamine

Concurrent use of methamphetamine and TCAs and indirect-acting sympathomimetic amines should be dosed carefully

Duration 12-24 hours

Half-Life 4-5 hours

Education and Monitoring Issues

Patient Education: Take during day to avoid insomnia; do not discontinue abruptly, may cause physical and psychological dependence with prolonged use; do not crush or chew extended release tablet

Monitoring Parameters: Heart rate, respiratory rate, blood pressure, and CNS activity

Methazolamide (meth a ZOE la mide)

Pharmacologic Class Carbonic Anhydrase Inhibitor; Diuretic, Carbonic Anhydrase Inhibitor; Ophthalmic Agent, Antiglaucoma

U.S. Brand Names Neptazane®

Generic Available No

Mechanism of Action Noncompetitive inhibition of the enzyme carbonic anhydrase; thought that carbonic anhydrase is located at the luminal border of cells of the proximal tubule. When the enzyme is inhibited, there is an increase in urine volume and a change to an alkaline pH with a subsequent decrease in the excretion of titratable acid and ammonia.

Use Adjunctive treatment of open-angle or secondary glaucoma; short-term therapy of narrow-angle glaucoma when delay of surgery is desired

USUAL DOSAGE Adults: Oral: 50-100 mg 2-3 times/day

Dosage Forms TAB: 25 mg, 50 mg

Contraindications Marked kidney or liver dysfunction, severe pulmonary obstruction, hypersensitivity to methazolamide or any component

Warnings/Precautions Sulfonamide-type reactions, melena, anorexia, nausea, vomiting, constipation, hematuria, glycosuria, urinary frequency, renal colic, renal calculi, crystalluria, polyuria, hepatic insufficiency, various CNS effects, transient myopia, bone marrow suppression, thrombocytopenia/purpura, hemolytic anemia, leukopenia, pancytopenia, agranulocytosis, urticaria, pruritus, rash, Stevens-Johnson syndrome, weight loss, fever, acidosis; use with caution in patients with respiratory acidosis and diabetes mellitus; impairment of mental alertness and/or physical coordination. Malaise and complaints of tiredness and myalgia are signs of excessive dosing and acidosis in the elderly.

Pregnancy Risk Factor C

Adverse Reactions

>10%:

Central nervous system: Malaise

Gastrointestinal: Metallic taste, anorexia

Genitourinary: Polyuria
Neuromuscular & skeletal: Weakness
1% to 10%:
Central nervous system: Mental depression, drowsiness, dizziness
Genitourinary: Crystalluria
<1%: Black tarry stools, bone marrow suppression, constipation, dysuria, fatigue, fever, GI irritation, headache, hyperchloremic metabolic acidosis, hyperglycemia, hypersensitivity, hypokalemia, loss of smell, myopia, paresthesia, rash, seizures, Stevens-Johnson syndrome, sulfonamide rash, tinnitus, trembling, unsteadiness, xerostomia

Drug Interactions
Increased toxicity:
May induce hypokalemia which would sensitize a patient to digitalis toxicity
May increase the potential for salicylate toxicity
Hypokalemia may be compounded with concurrent diuretic use or steroids
Primidone absorption may be delayed
Decreased effect: Increased lithium excretion and altered excretion of other drugs by alkalinization of the urine, such as amphetamines, quinidine, procainamide, methenamine, phenobarbital, salicylates

Onset Slow in comparison with acetazolamide (2-4 hours); Peak effect: 6-8 hours

Duration 10-18 hours

Half-Life ~14 hours

Education and Monitoring Issues
Patient Education: Take with food; swallow whole, do not chew or crush. You may experience gastrointestinal upset and loss of appetite; frequent small meals are advised to reduce these effects and the metallic taste that sometimes occurs with this medication. Maintain adequate fluid intake (2-3 L/day unless instructed to restrict fluid intake). If diabetic, monitor blood sugars closely (may cause elevated blood sugars). You may experience lightheadedness, depression, dizziness, or weakness for a few days; use caution when driving or engaging in tasks that require alertness until response to drug is known. Report excessive tiredness; loss of appetite; cramping, pain, or weakness in muscles; acute GI symptoms; changes in CNS (depression, drowsiness); difficulty or pain on urination; visual changes; or skin rash.

Methenamine (meth EN a meen)

Pharmacologic Class Antibiotic, Miscellaneous

U.S. Brand Names Hiprex®; Mandelamine®; Urex®

Generic Available Yes

Mechanism of Action Methenamine is hydrolyzed to formaldehyde and ammonia in acidic urine; formaldehyde has nonspecific bactericidal action

Use Prophylaxis or suppression of recurrent urinary tract infections; urinary tract discomfort secondary to hypermotility

USUAL DOSAGE Oral:
Children:
<6 years: 0.25 g/30 lb 4 times/day
6-12 years:
Hippurate: 25-50 mg/kg/day divided every 12 hours or 0.5-1 g twice daily
Mandelate: 50-75 mg/kg/day divided every 6 hours or 0.5 g 4 times/day
Children >12 years and Adults:
Hippurate: 1 g twice daily
Mandelate: 1 g 4 times/day after meals and at bedtime
Dosing adjustment/comments in renal impairment: Cl_{cr} <50 mL/minute: Avoid use

Dosage Forms SUSP, oral: 0.5 g/5 mL (480 mL). **TAB:** As hippurate (Hiprex®, Urex®): 1 g (Hiprex® contains tartrazine dye); As mandelate, enteric coated: 500 mg, 1 g

Contraindications Severe dehydration, renal insufficiency, hepatic insufficiency in patients receiving hippurate salt, hypersensitivity to methenamine or any component; patients receiving sulfonamides

Warnings/Precautions Use with caution in patients with hepatic disease, gout, and the elderly; doses of 8 g/day for 3-4 weeks may cause bladder irritation, some products may contain tartrazine; methenamine should not be used to treat infections outside of the lower urinary tract. Use care to maintain an acid pH of the urine, especially when treating infections due to urea splitting organisms (eg, *Proteus* and strains of *Pseudomonas*); reversible increases in LFTs have occurred during therapy especially in patients with hepatic dysfunction.

Pregnancy Risk Factor C

Adverse Reactions
1% to 10%:
Dermatologic: Rash (3.5%)
Gastrointestinal: Nausea, dyspepsia (3.5%)
Genitourinary: Dysuria (3.5%)
<1%: Bladder irritation, crystalluria (especially with large doses), increased AST/ALT (reversible, rare)

(Continued)

Methenamine *(Continued)*

Drug Interactions

Decreased effect: Sodium bicarbonate and acetazolamide will decrease effect secondary to alkalinization of urine

Increased toxicity: Sulfonamides (may precipitate)

Half-Life 3-6 hours

Education and Monitoring Issues

Patient Education: Take per recommended schedule, at regular intervals around-the-clock. Complete full course of therapy; do not skip doses. Maintain adequate hydration (2-3 L/day of fluids unless instructed to restrict fluid intake). Avoid excessive citrus fruits, milk, or alkalizing medications. You may experience nausea or vomiting or GI upset (small frequent meals, frequent mouth care, sucking lozenges, or chewing gum may help). Report pain on urination or blood in urine, skin rash, other persistent adverse effects, or if condition does not improve.

Monitoring Parameters: Urinalysis, periodic liver function tests in patients

♦ **Methergine®** *see* Methylergonovine *on page 588*

Methicillin (meth i SIL in)

Pharmacologic Class Antibiotic, Penicillin

U.S. Brand Names Staphcillin®

Use Treatment of susceptible bacterial infections such as osteomyelitis, septicemia, endocarditis, and CNS infections due to penicillinase-producing strains of *Staphylococcus*; other antistaphylococcal penicillins are usually preferred

USUAL DOSAGE I.M., I.V.:

Infants:

>7 days and >2000 g: 100 mg/kg/day in divided doses every 6 hours (for meningitis: 200 mg/kg/day)

>7 days and <2000 g: 75 mg/kg/day in divided doses every 8 hours (for meningitis: 150 mg/kg/day)

<7 days and >2000 g: Same as above

<7 days and <2000 g: 50 mg/kg/day in divided doses every 12 hours (for meningitis: 100 mg/kg/day)

Children: 100-300 mg/kg/day in divided doses every 4-6 hours

Adults: 4-12 g/day in divided doses every 4-6 hours

Dosing interval in renal impairment:

Cl_{cr} 10-50 mL/minute: Administer every 6-8 hours

Cl_{cr} <10 mL/minute: Administer every 8-12 hours

Hemodialysis: Not dialyzable (0% to 5%)

Contraindications Known hypersensitivity to methicillin or any penicillin

Pregnancy Risk Factor B

Methimazole (meth IM a zole)

Pharmacologic Class Antithyroid Agent

U.S. Brand Names Tapazole®

Generic Available No

Mechanism of Action Inhibits the synthesis of thyroid hormones by blocking the oxidation of iodine in the thyroid gland, blocking iodine's ability to combine with tyrosine to form thyroxine and triiodothyronine (T_3), does not inactivate circulating T_4 and T_3

Use Palliative treatment of hyperthyroidism, return the hyperthyroid patient to a normal metabolic state prior to thyroidectomy, and to control thyrotoxic crisis that may accompany thyroidectomy. The use of antithyroid thioamides is as effective in elderly as they are in younger adults; however, the expense, potential adverse effects, and inconvenience (compliance, monitoring) make them undesirable. The use of radioiodine due to ease of administration and less concern for long-term side effects and reproduction problems (some older males) makes it a more appropriate therapy.

USUAL DOSAGE Oral: Administer in 3 equally divided doses at approximately 8-hour intervals

Children: Initial: 0.4 mg/kg/day in 3 divided doses; maintenance: 0.2 mg/kg/day in 3 divided doses up to 30 mg/24 hours maximum

Alternatively: Initial: 0.5-0.7 mg/kg/day **or** 15-20 mg/m²/day in 3 divided doses

Maintenance: $^1/_3$ to $^2/_3$ of the initial dose beginning when the patient is euthyroid

Maximum: 30 mg/24 hours

Adults: Initial: 15 mg/day for mild hyperthyroidism; 30-40 mg/day in moderately severe hyperthyroidism; 60 mg/day in severe hyperthyroidism; maintenance: 5-15 mg/day

Adjust dosage as required to achieve and maintain serum T_3, T_4, and TSH levels in the normal range. An elevated T_3 may be the sole indicator of inadequate treatment. An elevated TSH indicates excessive antithyroid treatment.

Dosing adjustment in renal impairment: Adjustment is not necessary

Dosage Forms TAB: 5 mg, 10 mg

Contraindications Hypersensitivity to methimazole or any component, nursing mothers (per manufacturer; however, expert analysis and the American Academy of Pediatrics state this drug may be used with caution in nursing mothers)

Warnings/Precautions Use with extreme caution in patients receiving other drugs known to cause myelosuppression particularly agranulocytosis, patients >40 years of age; avoid doses >40 mg/day (↑ myelosuppression); may cause acneiform eruptions or worsen the condition of the thyroid

Pregnancy Risk Factor D

Adverse Reactions

>10%:

Central nervous system: Fever

Hematologic: Leukopenia

1% to 10%:

Central nervous system: Dizziness

Gastrointestinal: Nausea, vomiting, stomach pain, abnormal taste

Hematologic: Agranulocytosis

Miscellaneous: SLE-like syndrome

<1%: Alopecia, aplastic anemia, arthralgia, cholestatic jaundice, constipation, drowsiness, edema, goiter, headache, nephrotic syndrome, paresthesia, pruritus, rash, swollen salivary glands, thrombocytopenia, urticaria, vertigo, weight gain

Drug Interactions Increased toxicity: Iodinated glycerol, lithium, potassium iodide; anticoagulant activity increased

Onset Onset of antithyroid effect: Oral: Within 30-40 minutes

Duration 2-4 hours

Half-Life 4-13 hours

Education and Monitoring Issues

Patient Education: Take as directed, at the same time each day around-the-clock; do not miss doses or make up missed doses. This drug will need to be taken for an extended period of time to achieve appropriate results. You may experience nausea or vomiting (small frequent meals may help), dizziness or drowsiness (use caution when driving or engaging in tasks that require alertness until response to drug is known). Report rash, fever, unusual bleeding or bruising, unresolved headache, yellowing of eyes or skin, or changes in color of urine or feces, unresolved malaise.

Monitoring Parameters: Monitor for signs of hypothyroidism, hyperthyroidism, T_4, T_3; CBC with differential, liver function (baseline and as needed), serum thyroxine, free thyroxine index

Methocarbamol (meth oh KAR ba mole)

Pharmacologic Class Skeletal Muscle Relaxant

U.S. Brand Names Delaxin®; Marbaxin®; Robaxin®; Robomol®

Generic Available Yes

Mechanism of Action Causes skeletal muscle relaxation by reducing the transmission of impulses from the spinal cord to skeletal muscle

Use Treatment of muscle spasm associated with acute painful musculoskeletal conditions, supportive therapy in tetanus

USUAL DOSAGE

Children: Recommended **only** for use in tetanus I.V.: 15 mg/kg/dose or 500 mg/m²/dose, may repeat every 6 hours if needed; maximum dose: 1.8 g/m²/day for 3 days only

Adults: Muscle spasm:

Oral: 1.5 g 4 times/day for 2-3 days, then decrease to 4-4.5 g/day in 3-6 divided doses

I.M., I.V.: 1 g every 8 hours if oral not possible

Dosing adjustment/comments in renal impairment: Do not administer parenteral formulation to patients with renal dysfunction

Dosage Forms INJ: 100 mg/mL in polyethylene glycol 50% (10 mL). **TAB:** 500 mg, 750 mg

Contraindications Renal impairment, hypersensitivity to methocarbamol or any component

Warnings/Precautions Rate of injection should not exceed 3 mL/minute; solution is hypertonic; avoid extravasation; use with caution in patients with a history of seizures

Pregnancy Risk Factor C

Adverse Reactions

>10%: Central nervous system: Drowsiness, dizziness, lightheadedness

1% to 10%:

Cardiovascular: Flushing of face, bradycardia

Dermatologic: Allergic dermatitis

Gastrointestinal: Nausea, vomiting

Ocular: Nystagmus

Respiratory: Nasal congestion

<1%: Allergic manifestations, blurred vision, convulsions, leukopenia, pain at injection site, renal impairment, syncope, thrombophlebitis

Drug Interactions Increased effect/toxicity with CNS depressants

Alcohol Interactions Avoid use (may increase central nervous system depression)

Onset Onset of muscle relaxation: Oral: Within 30 minutes

Half-Life 1-2 hours

(Continued)

Methocarbamol *(Continued)*

Education and Monitoring Issues

Patient Education: Take exactly as directed. Do not increase dose or discontinue without consulting prescriber. Do not use alcohol, prescriptive or OTC antidepressants, sedatives, or pain medications without consulting prescriber. You may experience drowsiness, dizziness, lightheadedness (avoid driving or engaging in tasks requiring alertness until response to drug is known); or nausea or vomiting (small, frequent meals, frequent mouth care, or sucking hard candy may help). Report excessive drowsiness or mental agitation, chest pain, skin rash, swelling of mouth/face, difficulty speaking, or vision disturbances.

Related Information

Methocarbamol and Aspirin *on page 582*

Methocarbamol and Aspirin (meth oh KAR ba mole & AS pir in)

Pharmacologic Class Skeletal Muscle Relaxant

U.S. Brand Names Robaxisal®

Dosage Forms TAB: Methocarbamol 400 mg and aspirin 325 mg

Pregnancy Risk Factor C; D (if full-dose aspirin in 3rd trimester)

Alcohol Interactions Avoid use (may increase central nervous system depression and enhance gastric mucosal irritation)

Methotrexate (meth oh TREKS ate)

Pharmacologic Class Antimetabolite; Antineoplastic Agent, Antimetabolite; Antirheumatic, Disease Modifying

U.S. Brand Names Folex® PFS™; Rheumatrex®

Generic Available Yes

Mechanism of Action An antimetabolite that inhibits DNA synthesis and cell reproduction in malignant cells

Folates must be in the reduced form (FH_4) to be active

Folates are activated by dihydrofolate reductase (DHFR)

DHFR is inhibited by MTX (by binding irreversibly), causing an increase in the intracellular dihydrofolate pool (the inactive cofactor) and inhibition of both purine and thymidylate synthesis (TS)

MTX enters the cell through an energy-dependent and temperature-dependent process which is mediated by an intramembrane protein; this carrier mechanism is also used by naturally occurring reduced folates, including folinic acid (leucovorin), making this a competitive process

At high drug concentrations (>20 μM), MTX enters the cell by a second mechanism which is not shared by reduced folates; the process may be passive diffusion or a specific, saturable process, and provides a rationale for high-dose MTX

A small fraction of MTX is converted intracellularly to polyglutamates, which leads to a prolonged inhibition of DHFR

The MOA in the treatment of rheumatoid arthritis is unknown, but may affect immune function

In psoriasis, methotrexate is thought to target rapidly proliferating epithelial cells in the skin

Use Treatment of trophoblastic neoplasms; leukemias; psoriasis; rheumatoid arthritis; breast, head and neck, and lung carcinomas; osteosarcoma; sarcomas; carcinoma of gastric, esophagus, testes; lymphomas

USUAL DOSAGE Refer to individual protocols. May be administered orally, I.M., intra-arterially, intrathecally, or I.V.

Leucovorin may be administered concomitantly or within 24 hours of methotrexate - refer to Leucovorin *on page 513* for details

Methotrexate Dosing Schedules

Dose	Route	Frequency
Conventional		
15-20 mg/m²	P.O.	Twice weekly
30-50 mg/m²	P.O., I.V.	Weekly
15 mg/day for 5 days	P.O., I.M.	Every 2-3 weeks
Intermediate		
50-150 mg/m²	I.V. push	Every 2-3 weeks
240 mg/m²*	I.V. infusion	Every 4-7 days
0.5-1 g/m²*	I.V. infusion	Every 2-3 weeks
High		
1-12 g/m²*	I.V. infusion	Every 1-3 weeks

*Followed with leucovorin rescue - refer to Leucovorin monograph for details.

Children:

Dermatomyositis: Oral: 15-20 mg/m²/week as a single dose once weekly or 0.3-1 mg/kg/dose once weekly

Juvenile rheumatoid arthritis: Oral, I.M.: 5-15 mg/m²/week as a single dose **or** as 3 divided doses given 12 hours apart

Antineoplastic dosage range:

Oral, I.M.: 7.5-30 mg/m²/week **or** every 2 weeks

I.V.: 10-18,000 mg/m² bolus dosing **or** continuous infusion over 6-42 hours

Pediatric solid tumors (high-dose): I.V.:

<12 years: 12 g/m² (dosage range: 12-18 g)

≥12 years: 8 g/m² (maximum: 18 g)

Acute lymphocytic leukemia (intermediate-dose): I.V.: Loading: 100 mg/m² over 1 hour, followed by a 35-hour infusion of 900 mg/m²/day

Meningeal leukemia: I.T.: 10-15 mg/m² (maximum dose: 15 mg) **or**

≤3 months: 3 mg/dose

4-11 months: 6 mg/dose

1 year: 8 mg/dose

2 years: 10 mg/dose

≥3 years: 12 mg/dose

I.T. doses are prepared with preservative-free MTX only. Hydrocortisone may be added to the I.T. preparation; total volume should range from 3-6 mL. Doses should be repeated at 2- to 5-day intervals until CSF counts return to normal followed by a dose once weekly for 2 weeks then monthly thereafter.

Adults: I.V.: Range is wide from 30-40 mg/m²/week to 100-12,000 mg/m² with leucovorin rescue

Doses **not** requiring leucovorin rescue range from 30-40 mg/m² I.V. or I.M. repeated weekly, or oral regimens of 10 mg/m² twice weekly

High-dose MTX is considered to be >100 mg/m² and can be as high as 1500-7500 mg/m². These doses **require** leucovorin rescue. Patients receiving doses ≥1000 mg/m² should have their urine alkalinized with bicarbonate or Bicitra® prior to and following MTX therapy.

Trophoblastic neoplasms: Oral, I.M.: 15-30 mg/day for 5 days; repeat in 7 days for 3-5 courses

Head and neck cancer: Oral, I.M., I.V.: 25-50 mg/m² once weekly

Rheumatoid arthritis: Oral: 7.5 mg once weekly **OR** 2.5 mg every 12 hours for 3 doses/week; not to exceed 20 mg/week

Psoriasis: Oral: 2.5-5 mg/dose every 12 hours for 3 doses given weekly **or** Oral, I.M.: 10-25 mg/dose given once weekly

Ectopic pregnancy: I.M./I.V.: 50 mg/m² single-dose without leucovorin rescue

Elderly: Rheumatoid arthritis/psoriasis: Oral: Initial: 5 mg once weekly; if nausea occurs, split dose to 2.5 mg every 12 hours for the day of administration; dose may be increased to 7.5 mg/week based on response, not to exceed 20 mg/week

Dosing adjustment in renal impairment:

Cl_{cr} 61-80 mL/minute: Reduce dose to 75% of usual dose

Cl_{cr} 51-60 mL/minute: Reduce dose to 70% of usual dose

Cl_{cr} 10-50 mL/minute: Reduce dose to 30% to 50% of usual dose

Cl_{cr} <10 mL/minute: Avoid use

Hemodialysis: Not dialyzable (0% to 5%); supplemental dose is not necessary

Peritoneal dialysis: Supplemental dose is not necessary

Dosage adjustment in hepatic impairment:

Bilirubin 3.1-5 mg/dL OR AST >180 units: Administer 75% of usual dose

Bilirubin >5 mg/dL: Do not use

Dosage Forms INJ: 2.5 mg/mL (2 mL), 25 mg/mL (2 mL, 4 mL, 8 mL, 10 mL); Preservative free: 25 mg (2 mL, 4 mL, 8 mL, 10 mL). **POWDER, for inj:** 20 mg, 25 mg, 50 mg, 100 mg, 250 mg, 1 g. **TAB:** 2.5 mg; Dose pack: 2.5 mg (4 cards with 2, 3, 4, 5, or 6 tabs each)

Contraindications Hypersensitivity to methotrexate or any component; severe renal or hepatic impairment; pre-existing profound bone marrow suppression in patients with psoriasis or rheumatoid arthritis, alcoholic liver disease, AIDS, pre-existing blood dyscrasias

Warnings/Precautions The U.S. Food and Drug Administration (FDA) currently recommends that procedures for proper handling and disposal of antineoplastic agents be considered

Bone and soft tissue necrosis may occur following radiation treatment. Painful plaque erosions may occur with psoriasis treatment.

May cause photosensitivity-type reaction. Reduce dosage in patients with renal or hepatic impairment. Methotrexate penetrates slowly into 3rd space fluids, such as pleural effusions or ascites, and exits slowly from these compartments (slower than from plasma). Drain ascites and pleural effusions prior to treatment. Use with caution in patients with peptic ulcer disease, ulcerative colitis, pre-existing bone marrow suppression. Monitor closely for pulmonary disease; use with caution in the elderly.

Because of the possibility of severe toxic reactions, fully inform patient of the risks involved. Do not use in women of childbearing age unless benefit outweighs risks; may

(Continued)

Methotrexate *(Continued)*

cause hepatotoxicity, fibrosis, and cirrhosis, along with marked bone marrow depression. Death from intestinal perforation may occur.

Patients should receive 1-2 L of I.V. fluid prior to initiation of high-dose methotrexate. Patients should receive sodium bicarbonate to alkalinize their urine during and after high-dose methotrexate (urine SG <1.010 and pH >7 should be maintained for at least 24 hours after infusion).

Toxicity to methotrexate or any immunosuppressive is increased in elderly; must monitor carefully. For rheumatoid arthritis and psoriasis, immunosuppressive therapy should only be used when disease is active and less toxic, traditional therapy is ineffective. Recommended doses should be reduced when initiating therapy in elderly due to possible decreased metabolism, reduced renal function, and presence of interacting diseases and drugs.

Pregnancy Risk Factor D

Adverse Reactions

>10%:

- Central nervous system (with I.T. administration only):
  - Arachnoiditis: Acute reaction manifested as severe headache, nuchal rigidity, vomiting, and fever; may be alleviated by reducing the dose
  - Subacute toxicity: 10% of patients treated with 12-15 mg/m^2 of I.T. MTX may develop this in the second or third week of therapy; consists of motor paralysis of extremities, cranial nerve palsy, seizures, or coma. This has also been seen in pediatric cases receiving very high-dose I.V. MTX (when enough MTX can get across into the CSF).
  - Demyelinating encephalopathy: Seen months or years after receiving MTX; usually in association with cranial irradiation or other systemic chemotherapy
- Dermatologic: Reddening of skin
- Endocrine & metabolic: Hyperuricemia, defective oogenesis or spermatogenesis
- Gastrointestinal: Ulcerative stomatitis, glossitis, gingivitis, nausea, vomiting, diarrhea, anorexia, intestinal perforation, mucositis (dose-dependent; appears in 3-7 days after therapy, resolving within 2 weeks)
  - Emetic potential:
  - <100 mg: Moderately low (10% to 30%)
  - ≥100 mg or <250 mg: Moderate (30% to 60%)
  - ≥250 mg: Moderately high (60% to 90%)
- Hematologic: Leukopenia, thrombocytopenia
- Renal: Renal failure, azotemia, nephropathy
- Respiratory: Pharyngitis

1% to 10%:

- Cardiovascular: Vasculitis
- Central nervous system: Dizziness, malaise, encephalopathy, seizures, fever, chills
- Dermatitis: Alopecia, rash, photosensitivity, depigmentation or hyperpigmentation of skin
- Endocrine & metabolic: Diabetes
- Genitourinary: Cystitis
- Hematologic: Hemorrhage
- Myelosuppressive: This is the primary dose-limiting factor (along with mucositis) of MTX; occurs about 5-7 days after MTX therapy, and should resolve within 2 weeks
  - WBC: Mild
  - Platelets: Moderate
  - Onset (days): 7
  - Nadir (days): 10
  - Recovery (days): 21
- Hepatic: Cirrhosis and portal fibrosis have been associated with chronic MTX therapy; acute elevation of liver enzymes are common after high-dose MTX, and usually resolve within 10 days
- Neuromuscular & skeletal: Arthralgia
- Ocular: Blurred vision
- Renal: Renal dysfunction: Manifested by an abrupt rise in serum creatinine and BUN and a fall in urine output; more common with high-dose MTX, and may be due to precipitation of the drug. The best treatment is prevention: Aggressively hydrate with 3 L/m^2/day starting 12 hours before therapy and continue for 24-36 hours; alkalinize the urine by adding 50 mEq of bicarbonate to each liter of fluid; keep urine flow >100 mL/hour and urine pH >7.
- Respiratory: Pneumonitis: Associated with fever, cough, and interstitial pulmonary infiltrates; treatment is to withhold MTX during the acute reaction
- Miscellaneous: Anaphylaxis, decreased resistance to infection

Drug Interactions

Decreased effect:

- Corticosteroids: Reported to decrease uptake of MTX into leukemia cells. Administration of these drugs should be separated by 12 hours. Dexamethasone has been reported to not affect methotrexate influx into cells.
- Decreases phenytoin, 5-FU

Increased toxicity:

Live virus vaccines → vaccinia infections

Vincristine: Inhibits MTX efflux from the cell, leading to increased and prolonged MTX levels in the cell; the dose of VCR needed to produce this effect is not achieved clinically

Organic acids: Salicylates, sulfonamides, probenecid, and high doses of penicillins compete with MTX for transport and reduce renal tubular secretion. Salicylates and sulfonamides may also displace MTX from plasma proteins, increase MTX levels.

Ara-C: Increased formation of the ara-C nucleotide can occur when MTX precedes ara-C, thus promoting the action of ara-C

Cyclosporine: CSA and MTX interfere with each other's renal elimination, which may result in increased toxicity

Nonsteroidal anti-inflammatory drugs (NSAIDs): Should not be used during moderate or high-dose methotrexate due to increased and prolonged methotrexate levels; may increase toxicity

Patients receiving concomitant therapy with methotrexate and other potential hepatotoxins (eg, azathioprine, retinoids, sulfasalazine) should be closely monitored for possible increased risk of hepatotoxicity.

Alcohol Interactions Avoid use

Onset Antirheumatic effects may require several weeks

Half-Life 8-12 hours with high doses and 3-10 hours with low doses

Education and Monitoring Issues

Patient Education: Avoid alcohol to prevent serious side effects. Avoid intake of extra dietary folic acid, maintain adequate hydration (2-3 L/day of fluids unless instructed to restrict fluid intake) and adequate nutrition (frequent small meals may help). You may experience nausea and vomiting (small frequent meals may help or request antiemetic from prescriber); drowsiness (avoid driving or engaging in tasks that require alertness until response to drug is known), tingling, numbness, blurred vision; mouth sores (frequent oral care is necessary); loss of hair; permanent sterility; skin rash; photosensitivity (use sunscreen, wear protective clothing and eyewear, avoid direct sunlight). You will be more susceptible to infection (avoid crowds and exposure to infection, and avoid immunizations unless approved by prescriber). Report black or tarry stools, fever, chills, unusual bleeding or bruising, shortness of breath or difficulty breathing, yellowing of skin or eyes, dark or bloody urine, or acute joint pain or other side effects you may experience.

Monitoring Parameters: For prolonged use (especially rheumatoid arthritis, psoriasis) a baseline liver biopsy, repeated at each 1-1.5 g cumulative dose interval, should be performed; WBC and platelet counts every 4 weeks; CBC and creatinine, LFTs every 3-4 months; chest x-ray

Reference Range: Refer to chart in Leucovorin Calcium monograph. Therapeutic levels: Variable; Toxic concentration: Variable; therapeutic range is dependent upon therapeutic approach.

High-dose regimens produce drug levels between 10^{-6}Molar and 10^{-7}Molar 24-72 hours after drug infusion

10^{-6} Molar unit = 1 microMolar unit

Toxic: Low-dose therapy: >9.1 ng/mL; high-dose therapy: >454 ng/mL

Methoxsalen (meth OKS a len)

Pharmacologic Class Psoralen

U.S. Brand Names 8-MOP®; Oxsoralen® Topical; Oxsoralen-Ultra® Oral

Generic Available No

Mechanism of Action Bonds covalently to pyrimidine bases in DNA, inhibits the synthesis of DNA, and suppresses cell division. The augmented sunburn reaction involves excitation of the methoxsalen molecule by radiation in the long-wave ultraviolet light (UVA), resulting in transference of energy to the methoxsalen molecule producing an excited state ("triplet electronic state"). The molecule, in this "triplet state", then reacts with cutaneous DNA.

Use

Oral: Symptomatic control of severe, recalcitrant disabling psoriasis, not responsive to other therapy when to diagnosis has been supported by biopsy. Administer only in conjunction with a schedule of controlled doses of long wave ultraviolet (UV) radiation; also used with long wave ultraviolet (UV) radiation for repigmentation of idiopathic vitiligo.

Topical: Repigmenting agent in vitiligo, used in conjunction with controlled doses of UVA or sunlight

USUAL DOSAGE

Psoriasis: Adults: Oral: 10-70 mg 1½-2 hours before exposure to ultraviolet light, 2-3 times at least 48 hours apart; dosage is based upon patient's body weight and skin type

Vitiligo: Children >12 years and Adults:

Oral: 20 mg 2-4 hours before exposure to UVA light or sunlight; limit exposure to 15-40 minutes based on skin basic color and exposure

Topical: Apply lotion 1-2 hours before exposure to UVA light, no more than once weekly

(Continued)

Methoxsalen *(Continued)*

Dosage Forms CAP: 10 mg. **LOT:** 1% (30 mL). **SOLN:** 20 mcg/mL

Contraindications Diseases associated with photosensitivity, cataract, invasive squamous cell cancer, known hypersensitivity to methoxsalen (psoralens), and children <12 years of age

Warnings/Precautions Family history of sunlight allergy or chronic infections; lotion should only be applied under direct supervision of a prescriber and should not be dispensed to the patient; for use only if inadequate response to other forms of therapy, serious burns may occur from UVA or sunlight even through glass if dose and or exposure schedule is not maintained; some products may contain tartrazine; use caution in patients with hepatic or cardiac disease

Pregnancy Risk Factor C

Adverse Reactions

>10%:

Dermatologic: Itching

Gastrointestinal: Nausea

1% to 10%:

Cardiovascular: Severe edema, hypotension

Central nervous system: Nervousness, vertigo, depression

Dermatologic: Painful blistering, burning, and peeling of skin; pruritus, freckling, hypopigmentation, rash, cheilitis, erythema

Neuromuscular & skeletal: Loss of muscle coordination

Drug Interactions Increased toxicity: Concomitant therapy with other photosensitizing agents such as anthralin, coal tar, griseofulvin, phenothiazines, nalidixic acid, sulfanilamides, tetracyclines, thiazides

Onset Peak: 2-4 hours

Education and Monitoring Issues

Patient Education: This medication is used in conjunction with specific ultraviolet treatment. Follow prescriber's directions exactly for oral medication. Can be taken with food or milk to reduce nausea. Consult prescriber for specific dietary instructions. Avoid use of any other skin treatments unless approved by prescriber. Control exposure to direct sunlight as per prescriber's instructions. If sunlight cannot be avoided, use sunblock (consult prescriber for specific SPF level), wear protective clothing and wraparound protective eyewear. Consult prescriber immediately if burning, blistering, or skin irritation occur.

Manufacturer ICN Pharmaceuticals, Inc

Related Information

Pharmaceutical Manufacturers Directory *on page 1020*

Methyldopa (meth il DOE pa)

Pharmacologic Class False Neurotransmitter

U.S. Brand Names Aldomet®

Generic Available Yes

Mechanism of Action Stimulation of central alpha-adrenergic receptors by a false transmitter that results in a decreased sympathetic outflow to the heart, kidneys, and peripheral vasculature

Use Management of moderate to severe hypertension

USUAL DOSAGE

Children:

Oral: Initial: 10 mg/kg/day in 2-4 divided doses; increase every 2 days as needed to maximum dose of 65 mg/kg/day; do not exceed 3 g/day

I.V.: 5-10 mg/kg/dose every 6-8 hours up to a total dose of 65 mg/kg/24 hours or 3 g/24 hours

Adults:

Oral: Initial: 250 mg 2-3 times/day; increase every 2 days as needed; usual dose 1-1.5 g/day in 2-4 divided doses; maximum dose: 3 g/day

I.V.: 250-500 mg every 6-8 hours; maximum dose: 1 g every 6 hours

Dosing interval in renal impairment:

Cl_{cr} >50 mL/minute: Administer every 8 hours

Cl_{cr} 10-50 mL/minute: Administer every 8-12 hours

Cl_{cr} <10 mL/minute: Administer every 12-24 hours

Hemodialysis: Slightly dialyzable (5% to 20%)

Dosage Forms INJ, as methyldopate hydrochloride: 50 mg/mL (5 mL, 10 mL). **SUSP, oral:** 250 mg/5 mL (5 mL, 473 mL). **TAB:** 125 mg, 250 mg, 500 mg

Contraindications Hypersensitivity to methyldopa or any component; (oral suspension contains benzoic acid and sodium bisulfite; injection contains sodium bisulfite); liver disease, pheochromocytoma, coadministration with MAO inhibitors

Warnings/Precautions May rarely produce hemolytic anemia and liver disorders; positive Coombs' test occurs in 10% to 20% of patients (perform periodic CBCs); sedation usually transient may occur during initial therapy or whenever the dose is increased. Use with caution in patients with previous liver disease or dysfunction, the active metabolites of methyldopa accumulate in uremia. Patients with impaired renal function may respond to smaller doses. Elderly patients may experience syncope (avoid by giving smaller doses). Tolerance may occur usually between the second and third month of therapy. Adding a diuretic or increasing the dosage of methyldopa frequently restores blood pressure control. Because of its CNS effects, methyldopa is not considered a drug of first choice in the elderly.

Pregnancy Risk Factor B (oral); C (I.V.)

Pregnancy Implications

Clinical effects on the fetus: Crosses the placenta. Hypotension reported. A large amount of clinical experience with the use of these drugs for the management of hypertension during pregnancy is available. Available evidence suggests safe use during pregnancy and breast-feeding.

Breast-feeding/lactation: Crosses into breast milk at extremely low levels. American Academy of Pediatrics considers **compatible** with breast-feeding.

Adverse Reactions

>10%: Cardiovascular: Peripheral edema

1% to 10%:

Central nervous system: Drug fever, mental depression, anxiety, nightmares, drowsiness, headache

Gastrointestinal: Dry mouth

<1% (limited to important or life-threatening symptoms): Orthostatic hypotension, bradycardia (sinus), sodium retention, sexual dysfunction, gynecomastia, hyperprolactinemia, thrombocytopenia, hemolytic anemia, positive Coombs' test, leukopenia, transient leukopenia or granulocytopenia, cholestasis or hepatitis and heptocellular injury, increased liver enzymes, jaundice, cirrhosis, dyspnea, SLE-like syndrome

Drug Interactions

Iron supplements can interact and cause a significant **increase** in blood pressure

Barbiturates and TCAs may reduce response to methyldopa

Beta-blockers, MAO inhibitors, phenothiazines, and sympathomimetics: Hypertension, sometimes severe, may occur

Lithium: Methyldopa may increase lithium toxicity; monitor lithium levels

Tolbutamide, haloperidol, anesthetics, and levodopa effects/toxicity are increased with methyldopa

Onset Peak hypotensive effect: Oral, parenteral: Within 3-6 hours

Duration 12-24 hours

Half-Life 75-80 minutes; End-stage renal disease: 6-16 hours

Education and Monitoring Issues

Patient Education: Take as directed. Do not skip dose or discontinue without consulting prescriber. Follow recommended diet and exercise program. Do not use OTC medications which may affect blood pressure (eg, cough or cold remedies, diet pills, stay-awake medications) without consulting prescriber. This medication may cause altered color of urine (normal); drowsiness, dizziness, or impaired judgment (use caution when driving or engaging in tasks that require alertness until response to drug is known); postural hypotension (use caution when rising from sitting or lying position or when climbing stairs); or dry mouth or nausea (frequent mouth care or sucking lozenges may help). Report altered CNS status (eg, nightmares, depression, anxiety, increased nervousness); sudden weight gain (weigh yourself in the same clothes at the same time of day once a week); unusual or persistent swelling of ankles, feet, or extremities; palpitations or rapid heartbeat; persistent weakness, fatigue, or unusual bleeding; or other persistent side effects.

Monitoring Parameters: Blood pressure, standing and sitting/lying down, CBC, liver enzymes, Coombs' test (direct); blood pressure monitor required during I.V. administration

Related Information

Chlorothiazide and Methyldopa *on page 185*
Methyldopa and Hydrochlorothiazide *on page 587*

Methyldopa and Hydrochlorothiazide

(meth il DOE pa & hye droe klor oh THYE a zide)

Pharmacologic Class Antihypertensive Agent, Combination

U.S. Brand Names Aldoril®

Dosage Forms TAB: 15: Methyldopa 250 mg and hydrochlorothiazide 15 mg; 25: Methyldopa 250 mg and hydrochlorothiazide 25 mg; D30: Methyldopa 500 mg and hydrochlorothiazide 30 mg; D50: Methyldopa 500 mg and hydrochlorothiazide 50 mg

Pregnancy Risk Factor C

Methylene Blue (METH i leen bloo)

Pharmacologic Class Antidote

U.S. Brand Names Urolene Blue®

Use Antidote for cyanide poisoning and drug-induced methemoglobinemia, indicator dye, chronic urolithiasis.

Unlabeled use: Has been used topically (0.1% solutions) in conjunction with polychromatic light to photoinactivate viruses such as herpes simplex; has been used alone or in combination with vitamin C for the management of chronic urolithiasis

(Continued)

Methylene Blue *(Continued)*

USUAL DOSAGE

Children: NADPH-methemoglobin reductase deficiency: Oral: 1-1.5 mg/kg/day (maximum: 300 mg/day) given with 5-8 mg/kg/day of ascorbic acid

Children and Adults: Methemoglobinemia: I.V.: 1-2 mg/kg or 25-50 mg/m^2 over several minutes; may be repeated in 1 hour if necessary

Adults: Genitourinary antiseptic: Oral: 65-130 mg 3 times/day with a full glass of water (maximum: 390 mg/day)

Contraindications Renal insufficiency, hypersensitivity to methylene blue or any component, intraspinal injection

Pregnancy Risk Factor C (D if injected intra-amniotically)

Methylergonovine (meth il er goe NOE veen)

Pharmacologic Class Ergot Derivative

U.S. Brand Names Methergine®

Generic Available No

Mechanism of Action Similar smooth muscle actions as seen with ergotamine; however, it affects primarily uterine smooth muscles producing sustained contractions and thereby shortens the third stage of labor

Use Prevention and treatment of postpartum and postabortion hemorrhage caused by uterine atony or subinvolution

USUAL DOSAGE Adults:

Oral: 0.2 mg 3-4 times/day for 2-7 days

I.M.: 0.2 mg after delivery of anterior shoulder, after delivery of placenta, or during puerperium; may be repeated as required at intervals of 2-4 hours

I.V.: Same dose as I.M., but should not be routinely administered I.V. because of possibility of inducing sudden hypertension and cerebrovascular accident

Dosage Forms INJ: 0.2 mg/mL (1 mL). **TAB:** 0.2 mg

Contraindications Induction of labor, threatened spontaneous abortion, hypertension, toxemia, hypersensitivity to methylergonovine or any component, pregnancy

Warnings/Precautions Use caution in patients with sepsis, obliterative vascular disease, hepatic, or renal involvement, hypertension; administer with extreme caution if using I.V.

Pregnancy Risk Factor C

Adverse Reactions

>10%: Cardiovascular: Hypertension

1% to 10%: Gastrointestinal: Nausea, vomiting

<1%: Diaphoresis, diarrhea, dizziness, dyspnea, foul taste, hallucinations, headache, hematuria, leg cramps, nasal congestion, palpitations, seizures, temporary chest pain, thrombophlebitis, tinnitus, water intoxication

Drug Interactions Augmented effects may occur with concurrent use of methylergonovine and vasoconstrictors or ergot alkaloids

Onset Onset of oxytocic effect: Oral: 5-10 minutes; I.M.: 2-5 minutes; I.V.: Immediately

Duration Oral: ~3 hours; I.M.: ~3 hours; I.V.: 45 minutes

Half-Life Biphasic: Initial: 1-5 minutes; Terminal: 30 minutes to 2 hours

Education and Monitoring Issues

Patient Education: This drug will generally not be needed for more than a week. You may experience nausea and vomiting (small frequent meals may help), dizziness, headache, or ringing in the ears (will reverse when drug is discontinued). Report any respiratory difficulty, acute headache, or numb cold extremities, or severe abdominal cramping.

♦ **Methylone®** *see* Methylprednisolone *on page 589*

Methylphenidate (meth il FEN i date)

Pharmacologic Class Stimulant

U.S. Brand Names Metadate ER®; Ritalin®; Ritalin-SR®

Generic Available Yes

Mechanism of Action Blocks the reuptake mechanism of dopaminergic neurons; appears to stimulate the cerebral cortex and subcortical structures similar to amphetamines

Use Treatment of attention deficit disorder and symptomatic management of narcolepsy; many unlabeled uses

USUAL DOSAGE Oral: (Discontinue periodically to re-evaluate or if no improvement occurs within 1 month)

Children ≥6 years: Attention deficit disorder: Initial: 0.3 mg/kg/dose or 2.5-5 mg/dose given before breakfast and lunch; increase by 0.1 mg/kg/dose or by 5-10 mg/day at weekly intervals; usual dose: 0.5-1 mg/kg/day; maximum dose: 2 mg/kg/day or 60 mg/day

Adults:

Narcolepsy: 10 mg 2-3 times/day, up to 60 mg/day

Depression: Initial: 2.5 mg every morning before 9 AM; dosage may be increased by 2.5-5 mg every 2-3 days as tolerated to a maximum of 20 mg/day; may be divided (ie,

7 AM and 12 noon), but should not be given after noon; do not use sustained release product

Dosage Forms TAB: 5 mg, 10 mg, 20 mg; Sustained release: 20 mg; Extended release: 10 mg, 20 mg

Contraindications Hypersensitivity to methylphenidate or any components; glaucoma, motor tics, Tourette's syndrome, patients with marked agitation, tension, and anxiety

Warnings/Precautions Use with caution in patients with hypertension, dementia (may worsen agitation or confusion) seizures; has high potential for abuse. Treatment should include "drug holidays" or periodic discontinuation in order to assess the patient's requirements and to decrease tolerance and limit suppression of linear growth and weight; it is often useful in treating elderly patients who are discouraged, withdrawn, apathetic, or disinterested in their activities. In particular, it is useful in patients who are starting a rehabilitation program but have resigned themselves to fail; these patients may not have a major depressive disorder; will not improve memory or cognitive function.

Pregnancy Risk Factor C

Adverse Reactions

Cardiovascular: Tachycardia, bradycardia, angina, hypertension, hypotension, palpitations, cardiac arrhythmias

Central nervous system: Nervousness, insomnia, headache, dyskinesia, toxic psychosis, Tourette's syndrome, NMS, dizziness, drowsiness

Dermatologic: Rash

Endocrine & metabolic: Growth retardation

Gastrointestinal: Nausea, vomiting, anorexia, nausea, abdominal pain, weight loss

Hematologic: Thrombocytopenia, anemia, leukopenia

Ocular: Blurred vision

Miscellaneous: Hypersensitivity reactions

Drug Interactions

Methylphenidate may antagonize the adrenergic blockade of guanethidine and guanadrel and inhibit the antihypertensive effect; use alternative antihypertensive

Methylphenidate may cause hypertensive effects when used in combination with MAOIs; it is best to avoid this combination

NMS has been reported in a patient receiving methylphenidate and venlafaxine

Onset Immediate release tablet: Peak cerebral stimulation effect: Within 2 hours; Sustained release tablet: Peak effect: Within 4-7 hours

Duration Immediate release tablet: 3-6 hours; Sustained release tablet: 8 hours

Half-Life 2-4 hours

Education and Monitoring Issues

Patient Education: Take exactly as directed; do not change dosage or discontinue without consulting prescriber. Response may take some time. Do not crush or chew sustained release tables. Avoid alcohol, caffeine, or other stimulants. Maintain adequate fluid intake (2-3 L/day of fluids unless instructed to restrict fluid intake). You may experience decreased appetite or weight loss (small frequent meals may help maintain adequate nutrition); restlessness, impaired judgment, or dizziness, especially during early therapy (use caution when driving or engaging in tasks requiring alertness until response to drug is known); Report unresolved rapid heartbeat; excessive agitation, nervousness, insomnia, tremors, or dizziness; blackened stool; skin rash or irritation; or altered gait or movement.

Methylprednisolone (meth il pred NIS oh lone)

Pharmacologic Class Corticosteroid, Parenteral

U.S. Brand Names Adlone® Injection; A-methaPred® Injection; depMedalone® Injection; Depoject® Injection; Depo-Medrol® Injection; Depopred® Injection; D-Med® Injection; Duralone® Injection; Medralone® Injection; Medrol® Oral; Methylone®; M-Prednisol® Injection; Solu-Medrol® Injection

Generic Available Yes

Mechanism of Action In a tissue-specific manner, corticosteroids regulate gene expression subsequent to binding specific intracellular receptors and translocation into the nucleus. Corticosteroids exert a wide array of physiologic effects including modulation of carbohydrate, protein, and lipid metabolism and maintenance of fluid and electrolyte homeostasis. Moreover cardiovascular, immunologic, musculoskeletal, endocrine, and neurologic physiology are influenced by corticosteroids. Decreases inflammation by suppression of migration of polymorphonuclear leukocytes and reversal of increased capillary permeability.

Use Primarily as an anti-inflammatory or immunosuppressant agent in the treatment of a variety of diseases including those of hematologic, allergic, inflammatory, neoplastic, and autoimmune origin. Prevention and treatment of graft-versus-host disease following allogeneic bone marrow transplantation.

USUAL DOSAGE Dosing should be based on the lesser of ideal body weight or actual body weight

Only sodium succinate may be given I.V.; methylprednisolone sodium succinate is highly soluble and has a rapid effect by I.M. and I.V. routes. Methylprednisolone acetate has a low solubility and has a sustained I.M. effect.

(Continued)

Methylprednisolone *(Continued)*

Children:

Anti-inflammatory or immunosuppressive: Oral, I.M., I.V. (sodium succinate): 0.5-1.7 mg/kg/day **or** 5-25 mg/m^2/day in divided doses every 6-12 hours; "Pulse" therapy: 15-30 mg/kg/dose over ≥30 minutes given once daily for 3 days

Status asthmaticus: I.V. (sodium succinate): Loading dose: 2 mg/kg/dose, then 0.5-1 mg/kg/dose every 6 hours for up to 5 days

Acute spinal cord injury: I.V. (sodium succinate): 30 mg/kg over 15 minutes, followed in 45 minutes by a continuous infusion of 5.4 mg/kg/hour for 23 hours

Lupus nephritis: I.V. (sodium succinate): 30 mg/kg over ≥30 minutes every other day for 6 doses

High-dose therapy for acute spinal cord injury: I.V. bolus: 30 mg/kg over 15 minutes, followed 45 minutes later by an infusion of 5.4 mg/kg/hour for 23 hours

Adults:

Anti-inflammatory or immunosuppressive: Oral: 2-60 mg/day in 1-4 divided doses to start, followed by gradual reduction in dosage to the lowest possible level consistent with maintaining an adequate clinical response

I.M. (sodium succinate): 10-80 mg/day once daily

I.M. (acetate): 10-80 mg every 1-2 weeks

I.V. (sodium succinate): 10-40 mg over a period of several minutes and repeated I.V. or I.M. at intervals depending on clinical response; when high dosages are needed, administer 30 mg/kg over a period of ≥30 minutes and may be repeated every 4-6 hours for 48 hours

Status asthmaticus: I.V. (sodium succinate): Loading dose: 2 mg/kg/dose, then 0.5-1 mg/kg/dose every 6 hours for up to 5 days

High-dose therapy for acute spinal cord injury: I.V. bolus: 30 mg/kg over 15 minutes, followed 45 minutes later by an infusion of 5.4 mg/kg/hour for 23 hours

Lupus nephritis: High-dose "pulse" therapy: I.V. (sodium succinate): 1 g/day for 3 days

Aplastic anemia: I.V. (sodium succinate): 1 mg/kg/day or 40 mg/day (whichever dose is higher), for 4 days. After 4 days, change to oral and continue until day 10 or until symptoms of serum sickness resolve, then rapidly reduce over approximately 2 weeks.

Hemodialysis: Slightly dialyzable (5% to 20%); administer dose posthemodialysis

Intra-articular (acetate): Administer every 1-5 weeks

Large joints: 20-80 mg

Small joints: 4-10 mg

Intralesional (acetate): 20-60 mg every 1-5 weeks

Dosage Forms INJ: As acetate: 20 mg/mL (5 mL, 10 mL), 40 mg/mL (1 mL, 5 mL, 10 mL), 80 mg/mL (1 mL, 5 mL); As sodium succinate: 40 mg (1 mL, 3 mL), 125 mg (2 mL, 5 mL), 500 mg (1 mL, 4 mL, 8 mL, 20 mL), 1000 mg (1 mL, 8 mL, 50 mL), 2000 mg (30.6 mL). **TAB:** 2 mg, 4 mg, 8 mg, 16 mg, 24 mg, 32 mg; Dose pack: 4 mg (21s)

Contraindications Serious infections, except septic shock or tuberculous meningitis; known hypersensitivity to methylprednisolone; viral, fungal, or tubercular skin lesions; administration of live virus vaccines. Methylprednisolone formulations containing benzyl alcohol preservative are contraindicated in infants.

Warnings/Precautions Use with caution in patients with hyperthyroidism, cirrhosis, nonspecific ulcerative colitis, hypertension, osteoporosis, thromboembolic tendencies, CHF, convulsive disorders, myasthenia gravis, thrombophlebitis, peptic ulcer, diabetes; because of the risk of adverse effects, systemic corticosteroids should be used cautiously in the elderly, in the smallest possible dose, and for the shortest possible time

Acute adrenal insufficiency may occur with abrupt withdrawal after long-term therapy or with stress; young pediatric patients may be more susceptible to adrenal axis suppression from topical therapy

Pregnancy Risk Factor C (not assigned per manufacturer; however, similar agents like prednisolone are classified as "C")

Adverse Reactions

>10%:

Central nervous system: Insomnia, nervousness

Gastrointestinal: Increased appetite, indigestion

1% to 10%:

Dermatologic: Hirsutism

Endocrine & metabolic: Diabetes mellitus, adrenal suppression, hyperlipidemia

Hematologic: Transient leukocytosis

Neuromuscular & skeletal: Arthralgia

Ocular: Cataracts, glaucoma

Miscellaneous: Infections

<1%: Abdominal distention, acne, alkalosis, amenorrhea, arrhythmias, avascular necrosis, bruising, Cushing's syndrome, delirium, edema, euphoria, fractures, glucose intolerance, growth suppression, hallucinations, headache, hyperglycemia, hyperpigmentation, hypersensitivity reactions, hypertension, hypokalemia, intractable hiccups,

mood swings, muscle weakness, nausea, osteoporosis, pancreatitis, peptic ulcer, pituitary-adrenal axis suppression, pseudotumor cerebri, psychoses, secondary malignancy, seizures, skin atrophy, sodium and water retention, ulcerative esophagitis, vertigo, vomiting

Drug Interactions CYP3A enzyme inducer

Decreased effect:

Phenytoin, phenobarbital, rifampin increase clearance of methylprednisolone

Potassium depleting diuretics enhance potassium depletion

Increased toxicity:

Skin test antigens, immunizations decrease response and increase potential infections

Methylprednisolone may increase circulating glucose levels and may need adjustments of insulin or oral hypoglycemics

Onset Methylprednisolone sodium succinate is highly soluble and has a rapid effect by I.M. and I.V. routes. Methylprednisolone acetate has a low solubility and has a sustained I.M. effect.

Duration

Peak effect: Oral: 1-2 hours; I.M.: 4-8 days; Intra-articular: 1 week

Duration: Oral: 30-36 hours; I.M.: 1-4 weeks; Intra-articular: 1-5 weeks

Half-Life 3-3.5 hours

Education and Monitoring Issues

Patient Education: Maintain adequate nutritional intake; consult prescriber for possibility of special dietary instructions. If diabetic, monitor serum glucose closely and notify prescriber of any changes; this medication can increase blood glucose levels. Inform prescriber if you are experiencing unusual stress; dosage may need to be adjusted. You will be susceptible to infection; avoid crowds or infected persons or persons with contagious diseases. You may experience insomnia or nervousness; use caution when driving or engaging in tasks requiring alertness until response to drug is known. Report increased pain, swelling, or redness in area being treated; excessive or sudden weight gain; swelling of extremities; difficulty breathing; muscle pain or weakness; change in menstrual pattern; vision changes; signs of hyperglycemia; signs of infection (eg, fever, chills, mouth sores, perianal itching, vaginal discharge); blackened stool; other persistent side effects; or worsening of condition.

Intra-articular: Refrain from excessive use of joint following therapy, even if pain is gone.

Monitoring Parameters: Blood pressure, blood glucose, electrolytes

Related Information

Corticosteroids Comparison *on page 1237*

Methyltestosterone (meth il tes TOS te rone)

Pharmacologic Class Androgen

U.S. Brand Names Android®; Metandren®; Oreton® Methyl; Testred®; Virilon®

Generic Available Yes

Mechanism of Action Stimulates receptors in organs and tissues to promote growth and development of male sex organs and maintains secondary sex characteristics in androgen-deficient males

Use

Male: Hypogonadism; delayed puberty; impotence and climacteric symptoms

Female: Palliative treatment of metastatic breast cancer; postpartum breast pain and/or engorgement

USUAL DOSAGE Adults (buccal absorption produces twice the androgenic activity of oral tablets):

Male:

- Hypogonadism, male climacteric and impotence: Oral: 10-40 mg/day
- Androgen deficiency:
  - Oral: 10-50 mg/day
  - Buccal: 5-25 mg/day
- Postpubertal cryptorchidism: Oral: 30 mg/day

Female:

- Breast pain/engorgement:
  - Oral: 80 mg/day for 3-5 days
  - Buccal: 40 mg/day for 3-5 days
- Breast cancer:
  - Oral: 50-200 mg/day
  - Buccal: 25-100 mg/day

Dosage Forms CAP: 10 mg. **TAB:** 10 mg, 25 mg; Buccal: 5 mg, 10 mg

Contraindications Hypersensitivity to methyltestosterone or any component, known or suspected carcinoma of the breast or the prostate, pregnancy

Warnings/Precautions Use with extreme caution in patients with liver or kidney disease or serious heart disease; may accelerate bone maturation without producing compensatory gain in linear growth

Pregnancy Risk Factor X

(Continued)

Methyltestosterone *(Continued)*

Adverse Reactions

>10%:

Cardiovascular: Edema

Males: Virilism, priapism

Females: Virilism, menstrual problems (amenorrhea), breast soreness

Dermatologic: Acne

1% to 10%:

Males: Prostatic hypertrophy, prostatic carcinoma, impotence, testicular

Females: Hirsutism (increase in pubic hair growth) atrophy

Gastrointestinal: GI irritation, nausea, vomiting

Hepatic: Hepatic dysfunction

<1%: Amenorrhea, cholestatic hepatitis, gynecomastia, hepatic necrosis, hypercalcemia, hypersensitivity reactions, leukopenia, polycythemia

Drug Interactions Decreased effect: Oral anticoagulant effect or decrease insulin requirements

Education and Monitoring Issues

Patient Education: Take as directed; do not discontinue without consulting prescriber. Diabetics should monitor serum glucose closely and notify prescriber of changes; this medication can alter blood glucose levels. You may experience acne, growth of body hair, loss of libido, impotence, or menstrual irregularity (usually reversible); nausea or vomiting (small frequent meals, frequent mouth care, sucking lozenges, or chewing gum may help). Report changes in menstrual pattern; deepening of voice or unusual growth of body hair; fluid retention (swelling of ankles, feet, or hands, difficulty breathing, or sudden weight gain); change in color of urine or stool; yellowing of eyes or skin; unusual bruising or bleeding; or other adverse reactions.

Related Information

Estrogens and Methyltestosterone *on page 330*

Methysergide (meth i SER jide)

Pharmacologic Class Ergot Derivative

U.S. Brand Names Sansert®

Use Prophylaxis of vascular headache

USUAL DOSAGE Adults: Oral: 4-8 mg/day with meals; if no improvement is noted after 3 weeks, drug is unlikely to be beneficial; must not be given continuously for longer than 6 months, and a drug-free interval of 3-4 weeks must follow each 6-month course

Dosage Forms TAB: 2 mg

Contraindications Peripheral vascular disease, severe arteriosclerosis, pulmonary disease, severe hypertension, phlebitis, serious infections, pregnancy

Pregnancy Risk Factor X

Half-Life ~10 hours

Education and Monitoring Issues

Patient Education: This drug is meant to prevent migraine headaches, not treat acute attacks. Take as directed; do not take more than recommended and do not discontinue without consulting prescriber (must be discontinued slowly). You may experience weight gain (monitor dietary intake and exercise) or dizziness or vertigo (use caution when driving or engaging in tasks that require alertness until response to drug is known). Small frequent meals may reduce nausea or vomiting. Diarrhea will lessen with use. Report cold, numb, tingling, or painful extremities or leg cramps, chest pain, difficulty breathing or shortness of breath, or pain on urination.

- **Meticorten®** *see* Prednisone *on page 763*
- **Metimyd** *see* Sulfacetamide Sodium and Prednisolone *on page 876*
- **Metimyd® Ophthalmic** *see* Sulfacetamide Sodium and Prednisolone *on page 876*

Metipranolol (met i PRAN oh lol)

Pharmacologic Class Beta Blocker

U.S. Brand Names OptiPranolol® Ophthalmic

Use Agent for lowering intraocular pressure in patients with chronic open-angle glaucoma

USUAL DOSAGE Ophthalmic: Adults: Instill 1 drop in the affected eye(s) twice daily

Contraindications Bronchial asthma, sinus bradycardia, second and third degree A-V block, cardiac failure, cardiogenic shock, hypersensitivity to betaxolol or any component, pregnancy

Pregnancy Risk Factor C

Metoclopramide (met oh kloe PRA mide)

Pharmacologic Class Gastrointestinal Agent, Prokinetic

U.S. Brand Names Clopra®; Maxolon®; Octamide®; Reglan®

Generic Available Yes

Mechanism of Action Blocks dopamine receptors in chemoreceptor trigger zone of the CNS; enhances the response to acetylcholine of tissue in upper GI tract causing enhanced motility and accelerated gastric emptying without stimulating gastric, biliary, or pancreatic secretions

Use Symptomatic treatment of diabetic gastric stasis, gastroesophageal reflux; prevention of nausea associated with chemotherapy or postsurgery and facilitates intubation of the small intestine

USUAL DOSAGE

Children:

Gastroesophageal reflux: Oral: 0.1-0.2 mg/kg/dose up to 4 times/day; efficacy of continuing metoclopramide beyond 12 weeks in reflux has not been determined; total daily dose should not exceed 0.5 mg/kg/day

Gastrointestinal hypomotility (gastroparesis): Oral, I.M., I.V.: 0.1 mg/kg/dose up to 4 times/day, not to exceed 0.5 mg/kg/day

Antiemetic (chemotherapy-induced emesis): I.V.: 1-2 mg/kg 30 minutes before chemotherapy and every 2-4 hours

Facilitate intubation of GI tract for radiographic examination: I.V.:

<6 years: 0.1 mg/kg

6-14 years: 2.5-5 mg

Adults:

Gastroesophageal reflux: Oral: 10-15 mg/dose up to 4 times/day 30 minutes before meals or food and at bedtime; single doses of 20 mg are occasionally needed for provoking situations; efficacy of continuing metoclopramide beyond 12 weeks in reflux has not been determined

Gastrointestinal hypomotility (gastroparesis):

Oral: 10 mg 30 minutes before each meal and at bedtime for 2-8 weeks

I.V. (for severe symptoms): 10 mg over 1-2 minutes; 10 days of I.V. therapy may be necessary for best response

Antiemetic (chemotherapy-induced emesis): I.V.: 1-2 mg/kg 30 minutes before chemotherapy and every 2-4 hours to every 4-6 hours (and usually given with diphenhydramine 25-50 mg I.V./oral)

Postoperative nausea and vomiting: I.M.: 10 mg near end of surgery; 20 mg doses may be used

Facilitate intubation: I.V.: 10 mg

Elderly:

Gastroesophageal reflux: Oral: 5 mg 4 times/day (30 minutes before meals and at bedtime); increase dose to 10 mg 4 times/day if no response at lower dose

Gastrointestinal hypomotility:

Oral: Initial: 5 mg 30 minutes before meals and at bedtime for 2-8 weeks; increase if necessary to 10 mg doses

I.V.: Initiate at 5 mg over 1-2 minutes; increase to 10 mg if necessary

Postoperative nausea and vomiting: I.M.: 5 mg near end of surgery; may repeat dose if necessary

Dosing adjustment in renal impairment:

Cl_{cr} 10-40 mL/minute: Administer at 50% of normal dose

Cl_{cr} <10 mL/minute: Administer at 25% of normal dose

Hemodialysis: Not dialyzable (0% to 5%); supplemental dose is not necessary

Dosage Forms INJ: 5 mg/mL (2 mL, 10 mL, 30 mL, 50 mL, 100 mL). **SOLN, oral, concentrated:** 10 mg/mL (10 mL, 30 mL). **SYR** (sugar free): 5 mg/5 mL (10 mL, 480 mL). **TAB:** 5 mg, 10 mg

Contraindications Hypersensitivity to metoclopramide or any component; GI obstruction, perforation or hemorrhage, pheochromocytoma, history of seizure disorder

Warnings/Precautions Use with caution in patients with Parkinson's disease and in patients with a history of mental illness; dosage and/or frequency of administration should be modified in response to degree of renal impairment; extrapyramidal reactions, depression; may exacerbate seizures in seizure patients; to prevent extrapyramidal reactions, patients may be pretreated with diphenhydramine; elderly are more likely to develop dystonic reactions than younger adults; use lowest recommended doses initially

Pregnancy Risk Factor B

Pregnancy Implications

Clinical effects on the fetus: Crosses the placenta. Available evidence suggests safe use during pregnancy and breast-feeding.

Breast-feeding/lactation: Crosses into breast milk

Clinical effects on the infant: Increased milk production; 2 reports of mild intestinal discomfort; American Academy of Pediatrics states MAY BE OF CONCERN

Adverse Reactions

>10%:

Central nervous system: Restlessness, drowsiness

Gastrointestinal: Diarrhea

Neuromuscular & skeletal: Weakness

1% to 10%:

Central nervous system: Insomnia, depression

Dermatologic: Rash

Endocrine & metabolic: Breast tenderness, prolactin stimulation

Gastrointestinal: Nausea, xerostomia

(Continued)

Metoclopramide *(Continued)*

<1%: Agitation, anxiety, constipation, extrapyramidal reactions*, fatigue, hypertension or hypotension, methemoglobinemia, tachycardia, tardive dyskinesia

***Note:** A recent study suggests the incidence of extrapyramidal reactions due to metoclopramide may be as high as 34% and the incidence appears more often in the elderly

Drug Interactions CYP1A2 and 2D6 enzyme substrate

Anticholinergic agents antagonize metoclopramide's actions

Cyclosporine levels may be increased by metoclopramide

Digoxin: Absorption of some digoxin formulations (lower bioavailability tablets) may be reduced

Levodopa: The absorption of levodopa may be altered by metoclopramide; levodopa may blunt the efficacy of metoclopramide

Opiate analgesics may increase CNS depression

Succinylcholine: Neuromuscular blockade may be prolonged by metoclopramide

Alcohol Interactions Avoid use (may increase central nervous system depression)

Onset Oral: Within 0.5-1 hour; I.V.: Within 1-3 minutes

Duration Duration of therapeutic effect: 1-2 hours, regardless of route administered

Half-Life Normal renal function: 4-7 hours (may be dose-dependent)

Education and Monitoring Issues

Patient Education: Take this drug as prescribed, 30 minutes prior to eating. Do not increase dosage. Do not use alcohol or other CNS depressant or sleeping aids without consulting prescriber. May cause dizziness, drowsiness, or blurred vision; use caution when driving or engaging in tasks that require alertness until response to drug is known. May cause restlessness, anxiety, depression, or insomnia (will reverse when medication is discontinued). Report any CNS changes, involuntary movements, unresolved diarrhea. If diabetic, monitor serum glucose regularly.

Monitoring Parameters: Periodic renal function test; monitor for dystonic reactions; monitor for signs of hypoglycemia in patients using insulin and those being treated for gastroparesis; monitor for agitation and irritable confusion

Metolazone (me TOLE a zone)

Pharmacologic Class Diuretic, Thiazide

U.S. Brand Names Mykrox®; Zaroxolyn®

Generic Available No

Mechanism of Action Inhibits sodium reabsorption in the distal tubules causing increased excretion of sodium and water, as well as, potassium and hydrogen ions

Use Management of mild to moderate hypertension; treatment of edema in congestive heart failure and nephrotic syndrome, impaired renal function

USUAL DOSAGE Adults: Oral:

Edema: 5-20 mg/dose every 24 hours

Hypertension: 2.5-5 mg/dose every 24 hours

Hypertension (Mykrox®): 0.5 mg/day; if response is not adequate, increase dose to maximum of 1 mg/day

Dialysis: Not dialyzable (0% to 5%) via hemo- or peritoneal dialysis; supplemental dose is not necessary

Dosage Forms TAB: (Zaroxolyn®) (slow acting): 2.5 mg, 5 mg, 10 mg; (Mykrox®) (rapidly acting): 0.5 mg

Contraindications Hypersensitivity to metolazone or any component, other thiazides, and sulfonamide derivatives; patients with hepatic coma, anuria

Warnings/Precautions Use with caution in renal disease, hepatic disease, gout, lupus erythematosus, diabetes mellitus; some products may contain tartrazine. **Mykrox® is not bioequivalent to Zaroxolyn® and should not be interchanged for one another.**

Pregnancy Risk Factor B (per manufacturer); D (based on expert analysis)

Adverse Reactions

>10%: Central nervousness: Dizziness

1% to 10%:

Cardiovascular: Orthostatic hypotension, palpitations, chest pain, cold extremities (rapidly acting), edema (rapidly acting), venous thrombosis (slow acting), syncope (slow acting)

Central nervous system: Headache, fatigue, lethargy, malaise, lassitude, anxiety, depression, nervousness, "weird" feeling (rapidly acting), chills (slow acting)

Endocrine & metabolic: Hypokalemia, impotence, reduced libido, excessive volume depletion (slow acting), hemoconcentration (slow acting), acute gouty attach (slow acting), weakness

Dermatologic: Rash, pruritus, dry skin (rapidly acting)

Gastrointestinal: Nausea, vomiting, abdominal pain, cramping, bloating, diarrhea or constipation, dry mouth

Genitourinary: Nocturia

Neuromuscular & skeletal: Muscle cramps, spasm

Ocular: Eye itching (rapidly acting)

Otic: Tinnitus (rapidly acting)

Respiratory: Cough (rapidly acting), epistaxis (rapidly acting), sinus congestion (rapidly acting), sore throat (rapidly acting),

<1% (limited to important or life-threatening symptoms): Purpura, hyperglycemia, glycosuria, leukopenia, agranulocytosis, aplastic anemia, hepatitis, pancreatitis, gout

Drug Interactions

Angiotensin-converting enzyme inhibitors: Increased hypotension if aggressively diuresed with a thiazide-type diuretic

Beta-blockers increase hyperglycemic effects in type 2 diabetes mellitus

Cyclosporine and thiazide-type compounds can increase the risk of gout or renal toxicity; avoid concurrent use

Digoxin toxicity can be exacerbated if a diuretic induces hypokalemia or hypomagnesemia

Lithium toxicity can occur due to a reduced renal excretion of lithium; monitor lithium concentration and adjust as needed

Neuromuscular blocking agents effects may be prolonged; monitor serum potassium and neuromuscular status

NSAIDs can decrease the efficacy of thiazide-type diuretics

Onset Onset of diuresis: Within 60 minutes

Duration 12-24 hours

Half-Life 6-20 hours, renal function dependent

Education and Monitoring Issues

Patient Education: Take exactly as directed - with meals. May take early in day to avoid nocturia. Include bananas, orange juice, or other potassium-rich foods in daily diet but do not take dietary potassium supplements without advice or consultation of prescriber. Do not use alcohol or OTC medication without consulting prescriber. Weigh weekly at the same time, in the same clothes. Report weight gain >5 lb/week. May cause dizziness or weakness (change position slowly when rising from sitting or lying, avoid driving or tasks requiring alertness until response to drug is known). You may experience nausea or loss of appetite (small frequent meals may help), impotence (reversible), constipation (fluids, exercise, dietary fiber may help), photosensitivity (use sunscreen, wear protective clothing and eyewear, avoid direct sunlight). This medication does not replace other antihypertensive interventions; follow instructions for diet and lifestyle changes. Report flu-like symptoms, headache, joint soreness or weakness, difficulty breathing, skin rash, excessive fatigue, swelling of extremities, or difficulty breathing.

Monitoring Parameters: Serum electrolytes (potassium, sodium, chloride, bicarbonate), renal function, blood pressure (standing, sitting/supine)

Related Information

Heart Failure Guidelines *on page 1099*

Metoprolol (me toe PROE lole)

Pharmacologic Class Beta Blocker, Beta$_1$ Selective

U.S. Brand Names Lopressor®; Toprol XL®

Generic Available No

Mechanism of Action Selective inhibitor of beta$_1$-adrenergic receptors; competitively blocks beta$_1$-receptors, with little or no effect on beta$_2$-receptors at doses <100 mg; does not exhibit any membrane stabilizing or intrinsic sympathomimetic activity

Use Treatment of hypertension and angina pectoris; prevention of myocardial infarction, atrial fibrillation, flutter, symptomatic treatment of hypertrophic subaortic stenosis

Unlabeled use: Treatment of ventricular arrhythmias, atrial ectopy, migraine prophylaxis, essential tremor, aggressive behavior, adjunct for class II/III congestive heart failure

USUAL DOSAGE

Children: Oral: 1-5 mg/kg/24 hours divided twice daily; allow 3 days between dose adjustments

Adults:

Oral: 100-450 mg/day in 2-3 divided doses, begin with 50 mg twice daily and increase doses at weekly intervals to desired effect

Extended release: Same daily dose administered as a single dose

I.V.: 5 mg every 2 minutes for 3 doses in early treatment of myocardial infarction; thereafter administer 50 mg orally every 6 hours 15 minutes after last I.V. dose and continue for 48 hours; then administer a maintenance dose of 100 mg twice daily

Elderly: Oral: Initial: 25 mg/day; usual range: 25-300 mg/day

Hemodialysis: Administer dose posthemodialysis or administer 50 mg supplemental dose; supplemental dose is not necessary following peritoneal dialysis

Dosing adjustment/comments in hepatic disease: Reduced dose probably necessary

Dosage Forms

Metoprolol succinate: **TAB, sustained release:** 50 mg, 100 mg, 200 mg

Metoprolol tartrate: **INJ:** 1 mg/mL (5 mL). **TAB:** 50 mg, 100 mg

Contraindications Hypersensitivity to beta-blocking agents, uncompensated congestive heart failure; cardiogenic shock; bradycardia (heart rate <45 bpm) or heart block; sinus node dysfunction; A-V conduction abnormalities, systolic blood pressure <100 mm Hg; diabetes mellitus. Although metoprolol primarily blocks beta$_1$-receptors, high doses can result in beta$_2$-receptor blockage; therefore, use with caution in elderly with bronchospastic lung disease.

(Continued)

Metoprolol *(Continued)*

Warnings/Precautions Use with caution in patients with inadequate myocardial function; those undergoing anesthesia, patients with CHF, myasthenia gravis, impaired hepatic or renal function, severe peripheral vascular disease, bronchospastic disease, diabetes mellitus or hyperthyroidism. Abrupt withdrawal of the drug should be avoided (may result in an exaggerated cardiac beta-adrenergic response, tachycardia, hypertension, ischemia, angina, myocardial infarction, and sudden death), drug should be discontinued over 1-2 weeks; do not use in pregnant or nursing women; may potentiate hypoglycemia in a diabetic patient and mask signs and symptoms; sweating will continue.

Pregnancy Risk Factor C (per manufacturer); D (2nd and 3rd trimester, based on expert analysis)

Pregnancy Implications

Clinical effects on the fetus: Crosses the placenta. None; mild IUGR probably secondary to maternal hypertension. Available evidence suggests safe use during pregnancy and breast-feeding. Monitor breast-fed infant for symptoms of beta-blockade.

Breast-feeding/lactation: Crosses into breast milk. American Academy of Pediatrics considers **compatible** with breast-feeding.

Adverse Reactions

>10%:

Central nervous system: Drowsiness, insomnia

Endocrine & metabolic: Decreased sexual ability

1% to 10%:

Cardiovascular: Bradycardia, palpitations, edema, congestive heart failure, reduced peripheral circulation

Central nervous system: Mental depression

Gastrointestinal: Diarrhea or constipation, nausea, vomiting, stomach discomfort

Respiratory: Bronchospasm

Miscellaneous: Cold extremities

<1% (limited to important or life-threatening symptoms): Chest pain, arrhythmias, orthostatic hypotension, nervousness, headache, depression, hallucinations, confusion (especially in the elderly), thrombocytopenia, leukopenia, shortness of breath, hepatitis, hepatic dysfunction, jaundice

Drug Interactions CYP2D6 enzyme substrate

Alpha-blockers (prazosin, terazosin): Concurrent use of beta-blockers may increase risk of orthostasis

Clonidine: Hypertensive crisis after or during withdrawal of either agent

Drugs which slow A-V conduction (digoxin): effects may be additive with beta-blockers

Fluoxetine may inhibit the metabolism of metoprolol resulting in cardiac toxicity

Glucagon: Metoprolol may blunt the hyperglycemic action of glucagon

Hydralazine may enhance the bioavailability of metoprolol

Insulin and oral hypoglycemics: Metoprolol may mask tachycardia from hypoglycemia

Metoprolol reduces antipyrine's clearance by 18%

NSAIDs (ibuprofen, indomethacin, naproxen, piroxicam) may reduce the antihypertensive effects of beta-blockers

Oral contraceptives may increase the AUC and C_{max} of metoprolol

Salicylates may reduce the antihypertensive effects of beta-blockers

Sulfonylureas: Beta-blockers may alter response to hypoglycemic agents

Verapamil or diltiazem may have synergistic or additive pharmacological effects when taken concurrently with beta-blockers; avoid concurrent I.V. use

Alcohol Interactions Limit use (may increase risk of hypotension or dizziness)

Onset Peak antihypertensive effect: Oral: Within 1.5-4 hours

Duration 10-20 hours

Half-Life 3-4 hours; End-stage renal disease: 2.5-4.5 hours

Education and Monitoring Issues

Patient Education: I.V. use in emergency situations - patient information is included in general instructions.

Oral: Take exactly as directed. Do not increase, decrease, or adjust dosage without consulting prescriber. Take pulse daily, prior to medication and follow prescriber's instruction about holding medication. Do not take with antacids. Do not use alcohol or OTC medications (eg, cold remedies) without consulting prescriber. If diabetic, monitor serum sugars closely (may alter glucose tolerance or mask signs of hypoglycemia). May cause fatigue, dizziness, or postural hypotension; use caution when changing position from lying or sitting to standing, when driving, or when climbing stairs until response to medication is known. May cause alteration in sexual performance (reversible). Report unresolved swelling of extremities, difficulty breathing or new cough, unresolved fatigue, unusual weight gain, unresolved constipation, or unusual muscle weakness.

Monitoring Parameters: Blood pressure, apical and radial pulses, fluid I & O, daily weight, respirations, mental status, and circulation in extremities before and during therapy

Related Information

Beta-Blockers Comparison *on page 1233*

♦ **Metreton® Ophthalmic** *see* Prednisolone *on page 762*
♦ **MetroGel® Topical** *see* Metronidazole *on page 597*
♦ **MetroGel®-Vaginal** *see* Metronidazole *on page 597*
♦ **Metro I.V.® Injection** *see* Metronidazole *on page 597*

Metronidazole (me troe NI da zole)

Pharmacologic Class Amebicide; Antibiotic, Topical; Antibiotic, Miscellaneous; Antiprotozoal

U.S. Brand Names Flagyl ER® Oral; Flagyl® Oral; MetroGel® Topical; MetroGel®-Vaginal; Metro I.V.® Injection; Noritate® Cream; Protostat® Oral

Generic Available Yes

Mechanism of Action Reduced to a product which interacts with DNA to cause a loss of helical DNA structure and strand breakage resulting in inhibition of protein synthesis and cell death in susceptible organisms

Use Treatment of susceptible anaerobic bacterial and protozoal infections in the following conditions: amebiasis, symptomatic and asymptomatic trichomoniasis; skin and skin structure infections; CNS infections; intra-abdominal infections; systemic anaerobic infections; topically for the treatment of acne rosacea; treatment of antibiotic-associated pseudomembranous colitis (AAPC), bacterial vaginosis; used in combination with other agents (eg, tetracycline, bismuth subsalicylate, and an H_2-antagonist) to treat duodenal ulcer disease due to *Helicobacter pylori*; also used in Crohn's disease and hepatic encephalopathy

USUAL DOSAGE

Neonates: Anaerobic infections: Oral, I.V.:
- 0-4 weeks: <1200 g: 7.5 mg/kg/dose every 48 hours
- Postnatal age <7 days:
  - 1200-2000 g: 7.5 mg/kg/day every 24 hours
  - >2000 g: 15 mg/kg/day in divided doses every 12 hours
- Postnatal age >7 days:
  - 1200-2000 g: 15 mg/kg/day in divided doses every 12 hours
  - >2000 g: 30 mg/kg/day in divided doses every 12 hours

Infants and Children:
- Amebiasis: Oral: 35-50 mg/kg/day in divided doses every 8 hours for 10 days
- Trichomoniasis: Oral: 15-30 mg/kg/day in divided doses every 8 hours for 7 days
- Anaerobic infections:
  - Oral: 15-35 mg/kg/day in divided doses every 8 hours
  - I.V.: 30 mg/kg/day in divided doses every 6 hours
- *Clostridium difficile* (antibiotic-associated colitis): Oral: 20 mg/kg/day divided every 6 hours
  - Maximum dose: 2 g/day

Adults:
- Amebiasis: Oral: 500-750 mg every 8 hours for 5-10 days
- Trichomoniasis: Oral: 250 mg every 8 hours for 7 days or 2 g as a single dose
- Anaerobic infections: Oral, I.V.: 500 mg every 6-8 hours, not to exceed 4 g/day
- Antibiotic-associated pseudomembranous colitis: Oral: 250-500 mg 3-4 times/day for 10-14 days
- *H. pylori*: 1 capsule with meals and at bedtime for 14 days in combination with other agents (eg, tetracycline, bismuth subsalicylate, and H_2-antagonist)
- Vaginosis: 1 applicatorful (~37.5 mg metronidazole) intravaginally once or twice daily for 5 days; apply once in morning and evening if using twice daily, if daily, use at bedtime

Elderly: Use lower end of dosing recommendations for adults, do not administer as a single dose

Topical (acne rosacea therapy): Apply and rub a thin film twice daily, morning and evening, to entire affected areas after washing. Significant therapeutic results should be noticed within 3 weeks. Clinical studies have demonstrated continuing improvement through 9 weeks of therapy.

Dosing adjustment in renal impairment: Cl_{cr} <10 mL/minute: Administer every 12 hours

Hemodialysis: Extensively removed by hemodialysis and peritoneal dialysis (50% to 100%); administer dose posthemodialysis

Peritoneal dialysis: Dose as for Cl_{cr} <10 mL/minute

Continuous arteriovenous or venovenous hemofiltration (CAVH/CAVHD): Administer usual dose

Dosing adjustment/comments in hepatic disease: Unchanged in mild liver disease; reduce dosage in severe liver disease

Dosage Forms CAP: 375 mg. **GEL:** Top: 0.75% [7.5 mg/mL] (30 g); Vag: 0.75% (5 g applicator delivering 37.5 mg; 70 g tube). **INJ,** ready-to-use: 5 mg/mL (100 mL). **POWDER for inj:** 500 mg. **TAB:** 250 mg, 500 mg; Extended release: 750 mg

Contraindications Hypersensitivity to metronidazole or any component, 1st trimester of pregnancy since found to be carcinogenic in rats

Warnings/Precautions Use with caution in patients with liver impairment due to potential accumulation, blood dyscrasias; history of seizures, congestive heart failure, or other sodium retaining states; reduce dosage in patients with severe liver impairment, CNS

(Continued)

Metronidazole *(Continued)*

disease, and severe renal failure (Cl_{cr} <10 mL/minute); if *H. pylori* is not eradicated in patients being treated with metronidazole in a regimen, it should be assumed that metronidazole-resistance has occurred and it should not again be used; seizures and neuropathies have been reported especially with increased doses and chronic treatment; if this occurs, discontinue therapy

Pregnancy Risk Factor B (may be contraindicated in 1st trimester)

Adverse Reactions

>10%:

Central nervous system: Dizziness, headache

Gastrointestinal (12%): Nausea, diarrhea, loss of appetite, vomiting

<1%: Ataxia, change in taste sensation, dark urine, disulfiram-type reaction with alcohol, furry tongue, hypersensitivity, leukopenia, metallic taste, neuropathy, pancreatitis, seizures, thrombophlebitis, vaginal candidiasis, xerostomia

Drug Interactions CYP2C9 enzyme substrate; CYP2C9, 3A3/4, and 3A5-7 enzyme inhibitor

Decreased effect: Phenytoin, phenobarbital may decrease metronidazole half-life

Increased toxicity: Alcohol results in disulfiram-like reactions; metronidazole increases P-T prolongation with warfarin and increases lithium levels/toxicity; cimetidine may increase metronidazole levels

Alcohol Interactions Metronidazole inhibits alcohol's usual metabolism. Avoid all alcohol or any alcohol containing drugs (may cause a disulfiram-like reaction; symptoms include headache, nausea, vomiting, chest or abdominal pain).

Half-Life 6-8 hours, increases with hepatic impairment; End-stage renal disease: 21 hours

Education and Monitoring Issues

Patient Education: Take exactly as directed, with meals. Avoid alcohol during and for 24 hours after last dose. With alcohol your may experience severe flushing, headache, nausea, vomiting, or chest and abdominal pain. May discolor urine (brown/black/dark) (normal). You may experience "metallic" taste disturbance or nausea or vomiting (small frequent meals, frequent mouth care, chewing gum, or sucking lozenges may help). Refrain from intercourse or use a barrier contraceptive if being treated for trichomoniasis. Report unresolved or severe fatigue; weakness; fever or chills; mouth or vaginal sores; numbness, tingling, or swelling of extremities; difficulty breathing; or lack of improvement or worsening of condition.

Topical: Wash hands and area before applying and medication thinly. Wash hands after applying. Avoid contact with eyes. Do not cover with occlusive dressing. Report severe skin irritation or if condition does not improve.

Dietary Considerations: Food: Peak antibiotic serum concentration lowered and delayed, but total drug absorbed not affected. Take on an empty stomach. Drug may cause GI upset; if GI upset occurs, take with food.

Related Information

Antimicrobial Drugs of Choice *on page 1182*
Bismuth Subsalicylate, Metronidazole, and Tetracycline *on page 109*
Community Acquired Pneumonia in Adults *on page 1200*
Helicobacter pylori Treatment *on page 1107*
Treatment of Sexually Transmitted Diseases *on page 1210*

♦ **Mevacor®** *see* Lovastatin *on page 544*
♦ **Meval®** *see* Diazepam *on page 261*

Mexiletine (MEKS i le teen)

Pharmacologic Class Antiarrhythmic Agent, Class I-B

U.S. Brand Names Mexitil®

Generic Available No

Mechanism of Action Class IB antiarrhythmic, structurally related to lidocaine, which inhibits inward sodium current, decreases rate of rise of phase 0, increases effective refractory period/action potential duration ratio

Use Management of serious ventricular arrhythmias; use with lesser arrhythmias is generally not recommended

Unlabeled use: Diabetic neuropathy, reduction of ventricular tachycardia and other arrhythmias in the acute phase of myocardial infarction (mortality may not be reduced)

USUAL DOSAGE Adults: Oral: Initial: 200 mg every 8 hours (may load with 400 mg if necessary); adjust dose every 2-3 days; usual dose: 200-300 mg every 8 hours; maximum dose: 1.2 g/day (some patients respond to every 12-hour dosing); patients with hepatic impairment or CHF may require dose reduction; when switching from another antiarrhythmic, initiate a 200 mg dose 6-12 hours after stopping former agents, 3-6 hours after stopping procainamide

Dosage Forms CAP: 150 mg, 200 mg, 250 mg

Contraindications Cardiogenic shock, second or third degree heart block, hypersensitivity to mexiletine or any component

Warnings/Precautions Exercise extreme caution in patients with pre-existing sinus node dysfunction; mexiletine can worsen CHF, bradycardias, and other arrhythmias; mexiletine, like other antiarrhythmic agents, is proarrhythmic; CAST study indicates a trend toward increased mortality with antiarrhythmics in the face of cardiac disease (myocardial infarction); elevation of AST/ALT; hepatic necrosis reported; leukopenia, agranulocytopenia, and thrombocytopenia; seizures; alterations in urinary pH may change urinary excretion; electrolyte disturbances (hypokalemia, hyperkalemia, etc) after drug response

Pregnancy Risk Factor C

Adverse Reactions

>10%:

Central nervous system: Lightheadedness (10.5% to 25%), dizziness (20% to 25%), nervousness (5% to 10%), incoordination (10.2%)

Gastrointestinal: GI distress (41%), nausea/vomiting (40%)

Neuromuscular & skeletal: Trembling, unsteady gait, tremor (12.6%), ataxia (10% to 20%)

1% to 10%:

Cardiovascular: Chest pain (2.5% to 7.5%), premature ventricular contractions (1% to 2%), palpitations (4% to 8%), angina (1.7%), proarrhythmic (10% to 15% in patients with malignant arrhythmias)

Central nervous system: Confusion, headache, insomnia (5% to 7%), depression (2.4%)

Dermatologic: Rash (3.8% to 4.2%)

Gastrointestinal: Constipation or diarrhea (4% to 5%), xerostomia (2.8%), abdominal pain (1.2%)

Neuromuscular & skeletal: Weakness (5%), numbness of fingers or toes (2% to 4%), paresthesias (2.4%), arthralgias (1.4%)

Ocular: Blurred vision (5% to 7%), nystagmus (6%)

Otic: Tinnitus (2% to 2.5%)

Respiratory: Shortness of breath(3%)

<1% (limited to important or life-threatening symptoms): Leukopenia, agranulocytosis, thrombocytopenia, positive antinuclear antibody, SLE syndrome, increased LFTs, diplopia, syncope, edema, hot flashes, hypertension, short-term memory loss, psychological changes, psychosis, convulsion, diaphoresis, urinary hesitancy, urinary retention, malaise, impotence, decreased libido, pharyngitis, dysphagia, esophageal ulceration, upper GI bleeding, increased transaminases, hepatitis, hepatic necrosis, exfoliative dermatitis, Stevens-Johnson syndrome, congestive heart failure (patients with pre-existing ventricular dysfunction), diaphoresis, salivary changes, alopecia, pancreatitis (rare), myelofibrosis (patients with pre-existing myeloid abnormalities), hypotension, sinus arrest, A-V block, conduction disturbances, cardiogenic shock, torsade de pointes, hallucinations, seizures, peptic ulcer, drug-induced lupus-like syndrome

Case reports: Pulmonary fibrosis, urticaria

Drug Interactions CYP2D6 enzyme substrate; CYP1A2 enzyme inhibitor

Decreased plasma levels: Phenobarbital, phenytoin, rifampin, and other hepatic enzyme inducers, cimetidine and drugs which make the urine acidic

Increased effect: Allopurinol

Increased toxicity/levels of caffeine and theophylline

Half-Life 10-14 hours (average: 14.4 hours elderly, 12 hours in younger adults); increase in half-life with hepatic or heart failure

Education and Monitoring Issues

Patient Education: Take exactly as directed, with food or antacids, around-the-clock. Do not take additional doses or discontinue without consulting prescriber. Do not change diet without consulting prescriber. You will need regular cardiac checkups and blood tests while taking this medication. You may experience drowsiness or dizziness, numbness, or visual changes (use caution when driving or engaging in tasks requiring alertness until response to drug is known); nausea, vomiting, or heartburn (small frequent meals, frequent mouth care, chewing gum, or sucking lozenges may help); or headaches or sleep disturbances (usually temporary, if persistent consult prescriber). Report chest pain, palpitation, or erratic heartbeat; increased weight or swelling of hands or feet; chills, fever, or persistent sore throat; numbness, weakness, trembling, or unsteady gait; blurred vision or ringing in ears; or difficulty breathing.

Reference Range: Therapeutic range: 0.5-2 µg/mL; potentially toxic: >2 µg/mL

♦ **Mexitil®** *see* Mexiletine *on page 598*

♦ **Mezlin®** *see* Mezlocillin *on page 599*

Mezlocillin (mez loe SIL in)

Pharmacologic Class Antibiotic, Penicillin

U.S. Brand Names Mezlin®

Generic Available No

Mechanism of Action Inhibits bacterial cell wall synthesis by binding to one or more of the penicillin binding proteins (PBPs); which in turn inhibits the final transpeptidation step of peptidoglycan synthesis in bacterial cell walls, thus inhibiting cell wall biosynthesis. Bacteria eventually lyse due to ongoing activity of cell wall autolytic enzymes (autolysins and murein hydrolases) while cell wall assembly is arrested.

Use Treatment of infections caused by susceptible gram-negative aerobic bacilli (*Klebsiella, Proteus, Escherichia coli, Enterobacter, Pseudomonas aeruginosa, Serratia*) involving the

(Continued)

Mezlocillin *(Continued)*

skin and skin structure, bone and joint, respiratory tract, urinary tract, gastrointestinal tract, as well as, septicemia

USUAL DOSAGE I.M., I.V.:

Infants:

≤7 days, ≤2000 g: 75 mg/kg every 12 hours
≤7 days, >2000 g: Same as above
>7 days, ≤2000 g: 75 mg/kg every 8 hours
>7 days, >2000 g: 75 mg/kg every 6 hours

Children: 300 mg/kg/day divided every 4-6 hours; maximum: 24 g/day

Adults: Usual: 3-4 g every 4-6 hours

Uncomplicated urinary tract infection: 1.5-2 g every 6 hours
Serious infections: 200-300 mg/kg/day in 4-6 divided doses

Dosing interval in renal impairment:

Cl_{cr} 10-30 mL/minute: Administer every 6-8 hours
Cl_{cr} <10 mL/minute: Administer every 8 hours

Hemodialysis: Moderately dialyzable (20% to 50%)

Dosing adjustment in hepatic impairment: Reduce dose by 50%

Dosage Forms POWDER for inj: 1 g, 2 g, 3 g, 4 g, 20 g

Contraindications Hypersensitivity to mezlocillin, any component, or penicillins

Warnings/Precautions If bleeding occurs during therapy, mezlocillin should be discontinued; dosage modification required in patients with impaired renal function; use with caution in patients with renal impairment or biliary obstruction, or history of allergy to cephalosporins

Pregnancy Risk Factor B

Adverse Reactions

1% to 10%: Gastrointestinal: Nausea, diarrhea

<1%: Agranulocytosis, dizziness, elevated BUN/serum creatinine, elevated liver enzymes, eosinophilia, exfoliative dermatitis, fever, headache, hematuria, hemolytic anemia, hepatotoxicity, hypernatremia, hypokalemia, interstitial nephritis, leukopenia, neutropenia, positive Coombs' [direct], prolonged bleeding time, rash, seizures, serum sickness-like reactions, thrombocytopenia, vomiting

Drug Interactions Aminoglycosides (synergy), probenecid (decreased clearance), vecuronium (increased duration of neuromuscular blockade), heparin (increased risk of bleeding); possible decrease in effectiveness of oral contraceptives; bacteriostatic action of tetracycline may impair bactericidal effects of the penicillins

Half-Life Dose dependent: 50-70 minutes, increased in renal impairment

Education and Monitoring Issues

Patient Education: This medication can only be administered by infusion or injection. Maintain adequate hydration (2-3 L/day of fluids unless instructed to restrict fluid intake). Small frequent meals, frequent mouth care, and adequate fluids may reduce incidence of nausea or vomiting. If diabetic, drug may cause false tests with Clinitest® urine glucose monitoring; use of glucose oxidase methods (Clinistix®) or serum glucose monitoring is preferable. This drug may interfere with oral contraceptives; an alternate form of birth control should be used. Report difficulty breathing, acute diarrhea, systemic rash, fever, white plaques in mouth, or mouth sores.

Monitoring Parameters: Observe for signs and symptoms of anaphylaxis during first dose

Related Information

Antimicrobial Drugs of Choice *on page 1182*
Community Acquired Pneumonia in Adults *on page 1200*

- **Miacalcin® Injection** *see* Calcitonin *on page 128*
- **Miacalcin® Nasal Spray** *see* Calcitonin *on page 128*
- **Micanol® Cream** *see* Anthralin *on page 66*
- **Micardis®** *see* Telmisartan *on page 892*
- **Micatin® Topical [OTC]** *see* Miconazole *on page 600*

Miconazole (mi KON a zole)

Pharmacologic Class Antifungal Agent, Parenteral; Antifungal Agent, Topical; Antifungal Agent, Vaginal

U.S. Brand Names Absorbine® Antifungal Foot Powder [OTC]; Breezee® Mist Antifungal [OTC]; Femizol-M® [OTC]; Fungoid® Creme; Fungoid® Tincture; Lotrimin® AF Powder [OTC]; Lotrimin® AF Spray Liquid [OTC]; Lotrimin® AF Spray Powder [OTC]; Maximum Strength Desenex® Antifungal Cream [OTC]; Micatin® Topical [OTC]; Monistat-Derm™ Topical; Monistat i.v.™ Injection; Monistat™ Vaginal; M-Zole® 7 Dual Pack [OTC]; Ony-Clear® Spray; Prescription Strength Desenex® [OTC]; Zeasorb-AF® Powder [OTC]

Generic Available No

Mechanism of Action Inhibits biosynthesis of ergosterol, damaging the fungal cell wall membrane, which increases permeability causing leaking of nutrients

Use

I.V.: Treatment of severe systemic fungal infections and fungal meningitis that are refractory to standard treatment

Topical: Treatment of vulvovaginal candidiasis and a variety of skin and mucous membrane fungal infections

USUAL DOSAGE

Children:

<1 year: 15-30 mg/kg/day

1-12 years:

I.V.: 20-40 mg/kg/day divided every 8 hours (do not exceed 15 mg/kg/dose)

Topical: Apply twice daily for up to 1 month

Adults:

Topical: Apply twice daily for up to 1 month

I.T.: 20 mg every 1-2 days

I.V.: Initial: 200 mg, then 0.6-3.6 g/day divided every 8 hours for up to 20 weeks

Bladder candidal infections: 200 mg diluted solution instilled in the bladder

Vaginal: Insert contents of 1 applicator of vaginal cream (100 mg) or 100 mg suppository at bedtime for 7 days, or 200 mg suppository at bedtime for 3 days

Hemodialysis: Not dialyzable (0% to 5%)

Dosage Forms CRM: Top: 2% (15 g, 30 g, 56.7 g, 85 g); Vag: 2% (45 g is equivalent to 7 doses). **DUAL PACK:** Vag supp and external vulvar crm 2%. **INJ:** 1% [10 mg/mL] (20 mL). **LOT:** 2% (30 mL, 60 mL). **POWDER, top:** 2% (45 g, 90 g, 113 g). **SPRAY, top:** 2% (105 mL). **SUPP, vag:** 100 mg (7s); 200 mg (3s). **TINCTURE:** 2% with alcohol (7.39 mL, 29.57 mL)

Contraindications Hypersensitivity to miconazole, fluconazole, ketoconazole, polyoxyl 35 castor oil, or any component; concomitant administration with cisapride

Warnings/Precautions Administer I.V. with caution to patients with hepatic insufficiency; the safety of miconazole in patients <1 year of age has not been established; cardiorespiratory and anaphylaxis have occurred with excessively rapid administration

Pregnancy Risk Factor C

Adverse Reactions

>10%:

Central nervous system: Fever, chills (10%)

Dermatologic: Rash, itching, pruritus (21%)

Gastrointestinal: Anorexia, diarrhea, nausea (18%), vomiting (7%)

Local: Pain at injection site

1% to 10%: Dermatologic: Rash (9%)

<1%: Anemia, drowsiness, flushing of face or skin, thrombocytopenia

Drug Interactions CYP3A3/4 enzyme substrate; CYP2C enzyme inhibitor, CYP3A3/4 enzyme inhibitor (moderate), and CYP3A5-7 enzyme inhibitor

Warfarin (increased anticoagulant effect), oral sulfonylureas, amphotericin B (decreased antifungal effect of both agents), phenytoin (levels may be increased)

Increased risk of significant cardiotoxicity with concurrent administration of cisapride - concomitant administration is contraindicated (see interactions associated with ketoconazole)

Half-Life I.V.: Multiphasic: Initial: 40 minutes; Secondary: 126 minutes; Terminal phase: 24 hours

Education and Monitoring Issues

Patient Education: Take full course of therapy as directed; do not discontinue without consulting prescriber. Some infections may require long periods of therapy. Practice good hygiene measures to prevent reinfection.

Topical: Wash and dry area before applying medication; apply thinly. Do not get in or near eyes.

Vaginal: Insert high in vagina. Refrain from intercourse during treatment.

If you are diabetic you should test serum glucose regularly at the same time of day. You may experience nausea and vomiting (small, frequent meals may help) or headache, dizziness (use caution when driving). Report unresolved headache, rash, burning, itching, anorexia, unusual fatigue, diarrhea, nausea, or vomiting.

Related Information

Treatment of Sexually Transmitted Diseases *on page 1210*

♦ **MICRhoGAM™** *see* Rh_o(D) Immune Globulin (Intramuscular) *on page 816*

Microfibrillar Collagen Hemostat

(mye kro FI bri lar KOL la jen HEE moe stat)

Pharmacologic Class Hemostatic Agent

U.S. Brand Names Avitene®; Helistat®; Hemotene®

Use Adjunct to hemostasis when control of bleeding by ligature is ineffective or impractical

USUAL DOSAGE Apply dry directly to source of bleeding

Contraindications Closure of skin incisions, contaminated wounds

Pregnancy Risk Factor C

♦ **Micro-K** *see* Potassium Chloride *on page 751*

♦ **Micro-K® 10** *see* Potassium Chloride *on page 751*

♦ **Micro-K® Extencaps®** *see* Potassium Chloride *on page 751*
♦ **Micro-K® LS®** *see* Potassium Chloride *on page 751*
♦ **Micronase®** *see* Glyburide *on page 415*
♦ **Microsulfon®** *see* Sulfadiazine *on page 877*
♦ **Microzide™** *see* Hydrochlorothiazide *on page 442*
♦ **Midamor®** *see* Amiloride *on page 45*

Midazolam (MID aye zoe lam)

Pharmacologic Class Benzodiazepine

U.S. Brand Names Versed®

Generic Available No

Mechanism of Action Depresses all levels of the CNS, including the limbic and reticular formation, probably through the increased action of gamma-aminobutyric acid (GABA), which is a major inhibitory neurotransmitter in the brain

Use Preoperative sedation and provides conscious sedation prior to diagnostic or radiographic procedures

Unlabeled use: Anxiety, status epilepticus

USUAL DOSAGE The dose of midazolam needs to be individualized based on the patient's age, underlying diseases, and concurrent medications. Decrease dose (by ~30%) if narcotics or other CNS depressants are administered concomitantly. **Personnel and equipment needed for standard respiratory resuscitation should be immediately available during midazolam administration.**

Neonates: Conscious sedation during mechanical ventilation: I.V. continuous infusion: 0.15-1 mcg/kg/minute. Use smallest dose possible; use lower doses (up to 0.5 mcg/kg/minute) for preterm neonates

Infants <2 months and Children: Status epilepticus refractory to standard therapy: I.V.: Loading dose: 0.15 mg/kg followed by a continuous infusion of 1 mcg/kg/minute; titrate dose upward very 5 minutes until clinical seizure activity is controlled; mean infusion rate required in 24 children was 2.3 mcg/kg/minute with a range of 1-18 mcg/kg/minute

Children:

- Preoperative sedation:
  - Oral: Single dose preprocedure: 0.25-0.5 mg/kg, up to a maximum of 20 mg, depending on the status of the patient and desired effect; patients between 6 months and younger than 6 years, or less cooperative patients may require as much as 0.1 mg/kg as a single dose
  - I.M.: 0.07-0.08 mg/kg 30-60 minutes presurgery
  - I.V.: 0.035 mg/kg/dose, repeat over several minutes as required to achieve the desired sedative effect up to a total dose of 0.1-0.2 mg/kg
- Conscious sedation during mechanical ventilation: I.V.: Loading dose: 0.05-0.2 mg/kg then follow with initial continuous infusion: 1-2 mcg/kg/minute; titrate to the desired effect; usual range: 0.4-6 mcg/kg/minute
- Conscious sedation for procedures:
  - Oral, Intranasal: 0.2-0.4 mg/kg (maximum: 15 mg) 30-45 minutes before the procedure
  - I.V.: 0.05 mg/kg 3 minutes before procedure

Adolescents >12 years: I.V.: 0.5 mg every 3-4 minutes until effect achieved

Adults:

- Preoperative sedation: I.M.: 0.07-0.08 mg/kg 30-60 minutes presurgery; usual dose: 5 mg
- Conscious sedation: I.V.: Initial: 0.5-2 mg slow I.V. over at least 2 minutes; slowly titrate to effect by repeating doses every 2-3 minutes if needed; usual total dose: 2.5-5 mg; use decreased doses in elderly
  - Healthy Adults <60 years: Some patients respond to doses as low as 1 mg; no more than 2.5 mg should be administered over a period of 2 minutes. Additional doses of midazolam may be administered after a 2-minute waiting period and evaluation of sedation after each dose increment. A total dose >5 mg is generally not needed. If narcotics or other CNS depressants are administered concomitantly, the midazolam dose should be reduced by 30%.

Elderly: I.V.: Conscious sedation: Initial: 0.5 mg slow I.V.; give no more than 1.5 mg in a 2-minute period; if additional titration is needed, give no more than 1 mg over 2 minutes, waiting another 2 or more minutes to evaluate sedative effect; a total dose of >3.5 mg is rarely necessary

Sedation in mechanically intubated patients: I.V. continuous infusion: 100 mg in 250 mL D_5W or NS, (if patient is fluid-restricted, may concentrate up to a maximum of 0.5 mg/mL); initial dose: 0.01-0.05 mg/kg (~0.5-4 mg for a typical adult) initially and either repeated at 10-15 minute intervals until adequate sedation is achieved or continuous infusion rates of 0.02-0.1 mg/kg/hour (1-7 mg/hour) and titrate to reach desired level of sedation

Hemodialysis: Supplemental dose is not necessary

Peritoneal dialysis: Significant drug removal is unlikely based on physiochemical characteristics

Dosage Forms INJ: 1 mg/mL (2 mL, 5 mL, 10 mL), 5 mg/mL (1 mL, 2 mL, 5 mL, 10 mL). **SYR:** 2 mg/mL (118 mL)

Contraindications Hypersensitivity to midazolam or any component (cross-sensitivity with other benzodiazepines may occur); uncontrolled pain; existing CNS depression; shock; narrow-angle glaucoma; concurrent use of amprenavir, nelfinavir or ritonavir

Warnings/Precautions Use with caution in patients with congestive heart failure, renal impairment, pulmonary disease, hepatic dysfunction, the elderly, and those receiving concomitant narcotics; midazolam may cause respiratory depression/arrest; deaths and hypoxic encephalopathy have resulted when these were not promptly recognized and treated appropriately. Serious respiratory reactions have occurred after midazolam syrup, most often when used in combination with other CNS depressants. It should only be used in hospital or ambulatory care settings that are equipped with the capabilities to monitor cardiac and respiratory function.

Pregnancy Risk Factor D

Adverse Reactions

>10%: Respiratory: Decreased tidal volume and/or respiratory rate decrease, apnea

1% to 10%:

- Central nervous system: Drowsiness, oversedation, headache
- Gastrointestinal: Nausea, vomiting
- Local: Pain and local reactions at injection site (severity less than diazepam)
- Respiratory: Coughing
- Miscellaneous: Physical and psychological dependence with prolonged use, hiccups

<1% (limited to important or life-threatening symptoms): PVC, bradycardia, tachycardia, bigeminy, acid taste, excessive salivation, amnesia, euphoria, hallucinations, confusion, emergence delirium, agitation, rash, wheezing, laryngospasm, bronchospasm, dyspnea, hyperventilation

Drug Interactions CYP3A3/4 enzyme substrate

Decreased effect: Theophylline may antagonize the sedative effects of midazolam

Increased toxicity: CNS depressants, may increase sedation and respiratory depression; doses of anesthetic agents should be reduced when used in conjunction with midazolam; cimetidine may increase midazolam serum concentrations

Protease inhibitors (amprenavir, nelfinavir, ritonavir) may increase the toxicity of midazolam - concurrent use should be avoided

If narcotics or other CNS depressants are administered concomitantly, the midazolam dose should be reduced by 30%, if <65 years of age or by at least 50%, if >65 years of age.

Alcohol Interactions Avoid use (may increase central nervous system depression)

Onset

I.M.: Within 15 minutes; Peak effect: 0.5-1 hour

I.V.: Within 1-5 minutes

Duration I.M.: 2 hours mean, up to 6 hours

Half-Life 1-4 hours, increased with cirrhosis, CHF, obesity, elderly

Education and Monitoring Issues

Patient Education: Avoid use of alcohol or prescription or OTC sedatives or hypnotics for a minimum of 24 hours after administration. Avoid driving or engaging in any tasks that require alertness for 24 hours following administration. You may experience some loss of memory following administration.

Monitoring Parameters: Respiratory and cardiovascular status, blood pressure, blood pressure monitor required during I.V. administration

Manufacturer Roche Laboratories

Related Information

Pharmaceutical Manufacturers Directory *on page 1020*

♦ **Midchlor®** *see* Acetaminophen, Isometheptene, and Dichloralphenazone *on page 19*

Midodrine (MI doe dreen)

Pharmacologic Class Alpha$_1$ Agonist

U.S. Brand Names ProAmatine®

Mechanism of Action Midodrine forms an active metabolite, desglymidodrine, that is an alpha$_1$-agonist. This agent increases arteriolar and venous tone resulting in a rise in standing, sitting, and supine systolic and diastolic blood pressure in patients with orthostatic hypotension.

Use Treatment of symptomatic orthostatic hypotension

Investigational: Management of urinary incontinence

USUAL DOSAGE Adults: Oral: 10 mg 3 times/day during daytime hours (every 3-4 hours) when patient is upright (maximum: 40 mg/day)

Dosing adjustment in renal impairment: 2.5 mg 3 times/day, gradually increasing as tolerated

Dosage Forms TAB: 2.5 mg, 5 mg

Contraindications Severe organic heart disease, urinary retention, pheochromocytoma, thyrotoxicosis, persistent and significant supine hypertension; hypersensitivity to midodrine or any component; concurrent use of fludrocortisone

(Continued)

Midodrine *(Continued)*

Causes of Orthostatic Hypotension

Causes
Primary Autonomic Causes
Pure autonomic failure (Bradbury-Eglleston syndrome, idiopathic orthostatic hypotension)
Autonomic failure with multiple system atrophy (Shy-Drager syndrome)
Familial dysautonomia (Riley-Day syndrome)
Dopamine beta-hydroxylase deficiency
Secondary Autonomic Causes
Chronic alcoholism
Parkinson's disease
Diabetes mellitus
Porphyria
Amyloidosis
Various carcinomas
Vitamin B_1 or B_{12} deficiency
Nonautonomic Causes
Hypovolemia (such as associated with hemorrhage, burns, or hemodialysis) and dehydration
Diminished homeostatic regulation (such as associated with aging, pregnancy, fever, or prolonged best rest)
Medications (eg, antihypertensives, insulin, tricyclic antidepressants)

Warnings/Precautions Only indicated for patients for whom orthostatic hypotension significantly impairs their daily life. Use is not recommended with supine hypertension and caution should be exercised in patients with diabetes, visual problems, urinary retention (reduce initial dose) or hepatic dysfunction; monitor renal and hepatic function prior to and periodically during therapy; safety and efficacy has not been established in children; discontinue and re-evaluate therapy if signs of bradycardia occur.

Pregnancy Risk Factor C

Pregnancy Implications Clinical effects on the fetus: No studies are available; use during pregnancy and lactation should be avoided unless the potential benefit outweighs the risk to the fetus

Adverse Reactions

>10%:
- Dermatologic: Piloerection (13%), pruritus (12%)
- Genitourinary: Urinary urgency, retention, or polyuria, dysuria (up to 13%)
- Neuromuscular & skeletal: Paresthesia (18.3%)

1% to 10%:
- Cardiovascular: Supine hypertension, (7%) facial flushing
- Central nervous system: Confusion, anxiety, dizziness, chills (5%)
- Dermatologic: Rash, dry skin (2%)
- Gastrointestinal: Xerostomia, nausea, abdominal pain
- Neuromuscular & skeletal: Pain (5%)

<1%: Flatulence, flushing, headache, insomnia, leg cramps, visual changes

Drug Interactions Increased effect: Concomitant fludrocortisone results in hypernatremia or an increase in intraocular pressure and glaucoma; bradycardia may be accentuated with concomitant administration of cardiac glycosides, psychotherapeutics, and beta-blockers; alpha-agonists may increase the pressure effects and alpha-antagonists may negate the effects of midodrine

Onset Within 1 hour

Duration May last for 2-3 hours

Half-Life ~3-4 hours (active drug); 25 minutes (prodrug)

Education and Monitoring Issues

Patient Education: This drug may relieve positional hypotension; effects must be evaluated regularly. Take prescribed amount 3 times daily (shortly before rising in the morning, at midday, and in late afternoon); do not take after 6 PM or within 4 hours of bedtime or when lying down for any length of time. Follow recommended diet and exercise program. Do not use OTC medications which may affect blood pressure (eg, cough or cold remedies, diet pills, stay-awake medications) without consulting prescriber. You may experience urinary urgency or retention (void before taking or consult prescriber if difficulty persists); or dizziness, drowsiness, or headache (use caution when driving or engaging in tasks that require alertness until response to drug is known). Report skin rash, severe gastric upset or pain, muscle weakness or pain, or other persistent side effects.

Monitoring Parameters: Blood pressure, renal and hepatic parameters

♦ **Midol® 200 [OTC]** *see* Ibuprofen *on page 458*

♦ **Midol Douche** *see* Acetic Acid *on page 19*

♦ **Midrin®** *see* Acetaminophen, Isometheptene, and Dichloralphenazone *on page 19*

Miglitol (MIG li tol)

Pharmacologic Class Antidiabetic Agent (Miscellaneous)

U.S. Brand Names Glyset™

Mechanism of Action In contrast to sulfonylureas, miglitol does not enhance insulin secretion; the antihyperglycemic action of miglitol results from a reversible inhibition of membrane-bound intestinal alpha-glucosidases which hydrolyze oligosaccharides and disaccharides to glucose and other monosaccharides in the brush border of the small intestine; in diabetic patients, this enzyme inhibition results in delayed glucose absorption and lowering of postprandial hyperglycemia

Use

Noninsulin-dependent diabetes mellitus (NIDDM)

Monotherapy adjunct to diet to improve glycemic control in patients with NIDDM whose hyperglycemia cannot be managed with diet alone

Combination therapy with a sulfonylurea when diet plus either miglitol or a sulfonylurea alone do not result in adequate glycemic control. The effect of miglitol to enhance glycemic control is additive to that of sulfonylureas when used in combination.

USUAL DOSAGE Adults: Oral: 25 mg 3 times/day with the first bite of food at each meal; the dose may be increased to 50 mg 3 times/day after 4-8 weeks; maximum recommended dose: 100 mg 3 times/day

Dosing adjustment in renal impairment: Miglitol is primarily excreted by the kidneys; there is little information of miglitol in patients with a Cl_{cr} <25 mL/minute

Dosing adjustment in hepatic impairment: No adjustment necessary

Dosage Forms TAB: 25 mg, 50 mg, 100 mg

Contraindications Diabetic ketoacidosis, inflammatory bowel disease, colonic ulceration, partial intestinal obstruction, patients predisposed to intestinal obstruction, chronic intestinal diseases associated with marked disorders of digestion or absorption or with conditions that may deteriorate as a result of increased gas formation in the intestine; hypersensitivity to drug or any of its components

Warnings/Precautions GI symptoms are the most common reactions. The incidence of abdominal pain and diarrhea tend to diminish considerably with continued treatment. Long-term clinical trials in diabetic patients with significant renal dysfunction (serum creatinine >2 mg/dL) have not been conducted. Treatment of these patients is not recommended. Because of its mechanism of action, miglitol administered alone should not cause hypoglycemia in the fasting of postprandial state. In combination with a sulfonylurea will cause a further lowering of blood glucose and may increase the hypoglycemic potential of the sulfonylurea.

Pregnancy Risk Factor B

Adverse Reactions

>10%: Gastrointestinal: Flatulence (41.5%), diarrhea (28.7%), abdominal pain (11.7%)

1% to 10%: Dermatologic: Rash

Drug Interactions Decreased effect:

Miglitol may decrease the absorption and bioavailability of digoxin, propranolol, ranitidine

Digestive enzymes (amylase, pancreatin, charcoal) may reduce the effect of miglitol and should **not** be taken concomitantly

Half-Life ~2 hours

Education and Monitoring Issues

Patient Education: Take this medication exactly as directed, with the first bite of each main meal. Do not change dosage or discontinue without first consulting prescriber. Do not take other medications with or within 2 hours of this medication unless so advised by prescriber. It is important to follow dietary and lifestyle recommendations of prescriber. You will be instructed in signs of hypo-/hyperglycemia by prescriber or diabetic educator. If combining miglitol with other diabetic medication (eg, sulfonylureas, insulin), keep source of glucose (sugar) on hand in case hypoglycemia occurs. You may experience mild side effects during first weeks of therapy (eg, bloating, flatulence, diarrhea, abdominal discomfort); these should diminish over time. Report severe or persistent side effects, fever, extended vomiting or flu, or change in color of urine or stool.

Monitoring Parameters: Monitor therapeutic response by periodic blood glucose tests; measurement of glycosylated hemoglobin is recommended for the monitoring of long-term glycemic control

Reference Range: Target range: Adults:

Fasting blood glucose: <120 mg/dL

Glycosylated hemoglobin: <7%

Manufacturer Pharmacia & Upjohn

Related Information

Hypoglycemic Drugs and Thiazolidinedione Information *on page 1240*

Pharmaceutical Manufacturers Directory *on page 1020*

♦ **Migranal® Nasal Spray** *see* Dihydroergotamine *on page 277*

♦ **Migratine®** *see* Acetaminophen, Isometheptene, and Dichloralphenazone *on page 19*

♦ **Miles Nervine® Caplets [OTC]** *see* Diphenhydramine *on page 282*

♦ **Milliequivalent and Millimole Calculations & Conversions** *see page 1039*

♦ **Milophene®** *see* Clomiphene *on page 212*

Milrinone (MIL ri none)

Pharmacologic Class Phosphodiesterase Enzyme Inhibitor

U.S. Brand Names Primacor®

Mechanism of Action Phosphodiesterase inhibitor resulting in vasodilation

Use Short-term I.V. therapy of congestive heart failure; used for calcium antagonist intoxication

USUAL DOSAGE Adults: I.V.: Loading dose: 50 mcg/kg administered over 10 minutes followed by a maintenance dose titrated according to the hemodynamic and clinical response, see table.

Maintenance Dosage	Dose Rate (mcg/kg/min)	Total Dose (mg/kg/24 h)
Minimum	0.375	0.59
Standard	0.500	0.77
Maximum	0.750	1.13

Dosing adjustment in renal impairment:

Cl_{cr} 50 mL/minute/1.73 m^2: Administer 0.43 mcg/kg/minute
Cl_{cr} 40 mL/minute/1.73 m^2: Administer 0.38 mcg/kg/minute
Cl_{cr} 30 mL/minute/1.73 m^2: Administer 0.33 mcg/kg/minute
Cl_{cr} 20 mL/minute/1.73 m^2: Administer 0.28 mcg/kg/minute
Cl_{cr} 10 mL/minute/1.73 m^2: Administer 0.23 mcg/kg/minute
Cl_{cr} 5 mL/minute/1.73 m^2: Administer 0.2 mcg/kg/minute

Dosage Forms INJ: 1 mg/mL (5 mL, 10 mL, 20 mL)

Contraindications Hypersensitivity to drug or amrinone

Warnings/Precautions Severe obstructive aortic or pulmonic valvular disease, history of ventricular arrhythmias; atrial fibrillation, flutter; renal dysfunction. Life-threatening arrhythmias were infrequent and have been associated with pre-existing arrhythmias, metabolic abnormalities, abnormal digoxin levels, and catheter insertion

Pregnancy Risk Factor C

Adverse Reactions

1% to 10%:
- Cardiovascular: Arrhythmias, hypotension
- Central nervous system: Headache

<1% (limited to important or life-threatening symptoms): Ventricular fibrillation, chest pain, hypokalemia, thrombocytopenia

Drug Interactions When furosemide is admixed with milrinone, a precipitate immediately forms

Half-Life I.V.: 136 minutes in patients with CHF; patients with severe CHF have a more prolonged half-life, with values ranging from 1.7-2.7 hours. Patients with CHF have a reduction in the systemic clearance of milrinone, resulting in a prolonged elimination half-life. Alternatively, one study reported that 1 month of therapy with milrinone did not change the pharmacokinetic parameters for patients with CHF despite improvement in cardiac function.

Education and Monitoring Issues

Patient Education: This drug can only be given intravenously. If you experience increased voiding call for assistance. Report pain at infusion site, numbness or tingling of extremities, or difficulty breathing.

Monitoring Parameters: Cardiac monitor and blood pressure monitor required; serum potassium

Therapeutic: Patients should be monitored for improvement in the clinical signs and symptoms of congestive heart failure

Toxic: Patients should be monitored for ventricular arrhythmias and exacerbation of anginal symptoms; during I.V. therapy with milrinone, blood pressure and heart rate should be monitored

Manufacturer Sanofi Winthrop Pharmaceuticals

Related Information

Pharmaceutical Manufacturers Directory *on page 1020*

♦ **Miltown®** *see* Meprobamate *on page 565*
♦ **Minestrin** *see* Ethinyl Estradiol and Norethindrone *on page 342*
♦ **Minidyne® [OTC]** *see* Povidone-Iodine *on page 756*
♦ **Mini-Gamulin® Rh** *see* Rh_o(D) Immune Globulin (Intramuscular) *on page 816*
♦ **Minims® Pilocarpine** *see* Pilocarpine *on page 736*
♦ **Minipress®** *see* Prazosin *on page 760*
♦ **Minitran®** *see* Nitroglycerin *on page 659*
♦ **Minitran® Patch** *see* Nitroglycerin *on page 659*
♦ **Minizide®** *see* Prazosin and Polythiazide *on page 761*
♦ **Minocin® IV Injection** *see* Minocycline *on page 607*

♦ **Minocin® Oral** *see* Minocycline *on page 607*

Minocycline (mi noe SYE kleen)

Pharmacologic Class Antibiotic, Tetracycline Derivative

U.S. Brand Names Dynacin® Oral; Minocin® IV Injection; Minocin® Oral

Generic Available Yes

Mechanism of Action Inhibits bacterial protein synthesis by binding with the 30S and possibly the 50S ribosomal subunit(s) of susceptible bacteria; cell wall synthesis is not affected

Use Treatment of susceptible bacterial infections of both gram-negative and gram-positive organisms; acne, meningococcal carrier state

USUAL DOSAGE

Children >8 years: Oral, I.V.: Initial: 4 mg/kg followed by 2 mg/kg/dose every 12 hours

Adults:

Infection: Oral, I.V.: 200 mg stat, 100 mg every 12 hours not to exceed 400 mg/24 hours

Acne: Oral: 50 mg 1-3 times/day

Hemodialysis: Not dialyzable (0% to 5%)

Dosage Forms CAP: 50 mg, 100 mg; (Dynacin®): 50 mg, 100 mg; Pellet-filled (Minocin®): 50 mg, 100 mg. **INJ** (Minocin® IV): 100 mg. **SUSP, oral** (Minocin®): 50 mg/5 mL (60 mL)

Contraindications Hypersensitivity to minocycline, other tetracyclines, or any component; children <8 years of age

Warnings/Precautions Should be avoided in renal insufficiency, children ≤8 years of age, pregnant and nursing women; photosensitivity reactions can occur with minocycline

Pregnancy Risk Factor D

Adverse Reactions

>10%: Miscellaneous: Discoloration of teeth in children

1% to 10%:

Dermatologic: Photosensitivity

Gastrointestinal: Nausea, diarrhea

<1%: Abdominal cramps, acute renal failure, anaphylaxis, anorexia, azotemia, bulging fontanels in infants, dermatologic effects, diabetes insipidus syndrome, esophagitis, exfoliative dermatitis, increased intracranial pressure, paresthesia, pericarditis, pigmentation of nails, pruritus, rash, superinfections, vomiting

Drug Interactions

Decreased effect with antacids (aluminum, calcium, zinc, or magnesium), bismuth salts, sodium bicarbonate, barbiturates, carbamazepine, hydantoins; decreased effect of oral contraceptives

Increased effect of warfarin

Drug-Herb interactions: Berberine is a chemical extracted from **goldenseal** (*Hydrastis canadensis*), **barberry** (*Berberis vulgaris*), and **Oregon grape** (*Berberis aquifolium*), which has been shown to have antibacterial activity. One double-blind study found that giving berberine concurrently with tetracycline reduced the efficacy of tetracycline in the treatment of cholera. Berberine may decrease absorption of tetracycline. Another double-blind trial did not find that berberine interfered with tetracycline in cholera patients. Until more studies are completed, berberine-containing herbs should not be taken concomitantly with tetracyclines.

Half-Life 15 hours

Education and Monitoring Issues

Patient Education: Take as directed, at regular intervals around-the-clock. May be taken with food or milk. Complete full course of therapy; do not discontinue even if condition is resolved. You may experience sensitivity to sun; avoid sun, use sunblock, or wear protective clothing. Frequent small meals may help reduce nausea, vomiting or diarrhea. If diabetic, drug may cause false tests with Clinitest® urine glucose monitoring; use of glucose oxidase methods (Clinistix®) or serum glucose monitoring is preferable. Report any burning or stinging at infusion site. Report rash or itching, respiratory difficulty, yellowing of skin or eyes, change in color of urine or stool, fever or chills, unusual bruising or bleeding, or unresolved diarrhea.

Related Information

Antimicrobial Drugs of Choice *on page 1182*

Community Acquired Pneumonia in Adults *on page 1200*

♦ **Min-Ovral** *see* Ethinyl Estradiol and Levonorgestrel *on page 341*

Minoxidil (mi NOKS i dil)

Pharmacologic Class Topical Skin Product; Vasodilator

U.S. Brand Names Loniten®; Rogaine® Extra Strength for Men [OTC]; Rogaine® for Men [OTC]; Rogaine® for Women [OTC]

Generic Available Yes: Tablet

Mechanism of Action Produces vasodilation by directly relaxing arteriolar smooth muscle, with little effect on veins; effects may be mediated by cyclic AMP; stimulation of hair growth is secondary to vasodilation, increased cutaneous blood flow and stimulation of resting hair follicles

(Continued)

Minoxidil *(Continued)*

Use Management of severe hypertension (usually in combination with a diuretic and beta-blocker); treatment of male pattern baldness (alopecia androgenetica)

USUAL DOSAGE

Children <12 years: Hypertension: Oral: Initial: 0.1-0.2 mg/kg once daily; maximum: 5 mg/day; increase gradually every 3 days; usual dosage: 0.25-1 mg/kg/day in 1-2 divided doses; maximum: 50 mg/day

Children >12 years and Adults:

Hypertension: Oral: Initial: 5 mg once daily, increase gradually every 3 days; usual dose: 10-40 mg/day in 1-2 divided doses; maximum: 100 mg/day

Alopecia: Topical: Apply twice daily; 4 months of therapy may be necessary for hair growth

Elderly: Initial: 2.5 mg once daily; increase gradually

Note: Dosage adjustment is needed when added to concomitant therapy

Dialysis: Supplemental dose is not necessary via hemo- or peritoneal dialysis

Dosage Forms SOLN, top: 2% [20 mg/metered dose] (60 mL); 5% [50 mg/metered dose] (60 mL). **TAB:** 2.5 mg, 10 mg

Contraindications Pheochromocytoma, hypersensitivity to minoxidil or any component

Warnings/Precautions Note: Minoxidil can cause pericardial effusion, occasionally progressing to tamponade and it can exacerbate angina pectoris; use with caution in patients with pulmonary hypertension, significant renal failure, or congestive heart failure; use with caution in patients with coronary artery disease or recent myocardial infarction; renal failure or dialysis patients may require smaller doses; usually used with a beta-blocker (to treat minoxidil-induced tachycardia) and a diuretic (for treatment of water retention/edema); may take 1-6 months for hypertrichosis to totally reverse after minoxidil therapy is discontinued.

Pregnancy Risk Factor C

Adverse Reactions

Oral: Incidence of reactions not always reported.

Cardiovascular: Peripheral edema (7%), sodium and water retention, congestive heart failure, tachycardia, angina pectoris, pericardial effusion with or without tamponade, pericarditis, EKG changes (T-wave changes, 60%), rebound hypertension (in children after a gradual withdrawal)

Central nervous system: Headache (rare), fatigue

Dermatologic: Hypertrichosis (common, 80%), transient pruritus, changes in pigmentation (rare), serosanguineous bullae (rare), rash (rare), Stevens-Johnson syndrome

Endocrine & metabolic: Breast tenderness (rare, <1%), gynecomastia (rare), polymenorrhea (rare)

Gastrointestinal: Weight gain, nausea (rare), vomiting

Hematologic: Intermittent claudication (rare), thrombocytopenia (rare), decreased hematocrit (hemodilution), decreased hemoglobin (hemodilution), decreased erythrocyte count (hemodilution), leukopenia (rare)

Hepatic: Increased alkaline phosphatase

Renal: Transient increase in serum BUN and creatinine

Respiratory: Pulmonary edema

Topical: Incidence of adverse events is not always reported.

Cardiovascular: Increased left ventricular end-diastolic volume, increased cardiac output, increased left ventricular mass, dizziness, tachycardia, edema, transient chest pain, palpitation, increase or decrease in blood pressure, increase or decrease in pulse rate (1.5%, placebo 1.6%)

Central nervous system: Headache, dizziness, weakness, taste alterations, faintness, lightheadedness (3.4%, placebo 3.5%), vertigo (1.2%, placebo 1.2%), anxiety (rare), mental depression (rare), fatigue (rare 0.4%, placebo 1%)

Dermatologic: Local irritation, dryness, erythema, allergic contact dermatitis (7.4%, placebo 5.4%), pruritus, scaling/flaking, eczema, seborrhea, papular rash, folliculitis, local erythema, flushing, exacerbation of hair loss, alopecia, hypertrichosis, increased hair growth outside the area of application (face, beard, eyebrows, ear, arm)

Endocrine & metabolic: Menstrual changes, breast symptoms (0.5%, placebo 0.5%)

Gastrointestinal: Diarrhea, nausea, vomiting (4.3%, placebo 6.6%), weight gain (1.2%, placebo 1.3%)

Genitourinary: Urinary tract infections (rare), renal calculi (rare), urethritis (rare), prostatitis (rare), epididymitis (rare), impotence (rare)

Hematologic: Lymphadenopathy, thrombocytopenia, anemia (0.3%, placebo 0.6%)

Neuromuscular & skeletal: Fractures, back pain, retrosternal chest pain of muscular origin, tendonitis (2.6%, placebo 2.2%)

Ocular: Conjunctivitis, visual disturbances, decreased visual acuity

Respiratory: Bronchitis, upper respiratory infections, sinusitis (7.2%, placebo 8.6%)

Drug Interactions

Guanethidine can cause severe orthostasis; avoid concurrent use - discontinue 1-3 weeks prior to initiating minoxidil

Antihypertensives: Effects may be additive

Onset Oral: Within 30 minutes

Duration Up to 2-5 days

Half-Life 3.5-4.2 hours

Education and Monitoring Issues

Patient Education: Topical product must be used every day. Hair growth usually takes 4 months. Notify prescriber if any of the following occur: Heart rate ≥20 beats per minute over normal; rapid weight gain >5 lb (2 kg); unusual swelling of extremities, face, or abdomen; breathing difficulty, especially when lying down; rise slowly from prolonged lying or sitting; new or aggravated angina symptoms (chest, arm, or shoulder pain); severe indigestion; dizziness, lightheadedness, or fainting; nausea or vomiting may occur. Do not make up for missed doses.

Monitoring Parameters: Blood pressure, standing and sitting/supine; fluid and electrolyte balance and body weight should be monitored

- **Minoxigaine®** *see* Minoxidil *on page 607*
- **Mintezol®** *see* Thiabendazole *on page 910*
- **Minute-Gel®** *see* Fluoride *on page 376*
- **Miochol** *see* Acetylcholine *on page 20*
- **Miochol-E®** *see* Acetylcholine *on page 20*
- **Miostat** *see* Carbachol *on page 137*
- **Miostat® Intraocular** *see* Carbachol *on page 137*
- **Mirapex®** *see* Pramipexole *on page 757*
- **Mireze®** *see* Nedocromil Sodium *on page 639*

Mirtazapine (mir TAZ a peen)

Pharmacologic Class Antidepressant, Alpha-2 Antagonist

U.S. Brand Names Remeron®

Mechanism of Action Mirtazapine is a tetracyclic antidepressant that works by its central presynaptic $alpha_2$-adrenergic antagonist effects, which results in increased release of norepinephrine and serotonin. It is also a potent antagonist of 5-HT_2 and 5-HT_3 serotonin receptors and H_1 histamine receptors and a moderate peripheral $alpha_1$-adrenergic and muscarinic antagonist; it does not inhibit the reuptake of norepinephrine or serotonin.

Use Treatment of depression

USUAL DOSAGE Adults: Oral: Initial: 15 mg nightly, titrate up to 15-45 mg/day with dose increases made no more frequently than every 1-2 weeks

Dosage Forms TAB: 15 mg, 30 mg

Contraindications Patients with a known hypersensitivity to mirtazapine, use during or within 14 days of monoamine oxidase inhibitor therapy

Warnings/Precautions Hepatic or renal dysfunction, predisposition to conditions that could be exacerbated by hypotension, history of mania or hypomania, seizure disorders, immunocompromized patients, the elderly, or during pregnancy or nursing

Pregnancy Risk Factor C

Adverse Reactions

>10%:

Central nervous system: Somnolence

Endocrine & metabolic: Increased cholesterol

Gastrointestinal: Constipation, xerostomia, increased appetite, weight gain

1% to 10%:

Cardiovascular: Hypertension, vasodilatation, peripheral edema, edema

Central nervous system: Dizziness, abnormal dreams, abnormal thoughts, confusion, malaise

Endocrine & metabolic: Increased triglycerides

Gastrointestinal: Vomiting, anorexia

Genitourinary: Urinary frequency

Neuromuscular & skeletal: Myalgia, back pain, arthralgias, tremor, weakness

Respiratory: Dyspnea

Miscellaneous: Flu-like symptoms, thirst

<1%: Agranulocytosis, dehydration, liver function test increases, lymphadenopathy, neutropenia, orthostatic hypotension, seizures (1 case reported), weight loss

Drug Interactions CYP1A2, 2C9, 2D6, and 3A3/4 enzyme substrate

Impairment of cognitive and motor skills are additive with those produced by alcohol, benzodiazepines, and other CNS depressants

Possibly serious or fatal reactions can occur when given with or when given within 14 days of a monoamine oxidase inhibitor

Alcohol Interactions Avoid use (may increase central nervous system depression)

Onset Therapeutic effects general >2 weeks

Half-Life 20-40 hours

Education and Monitoring Issues

Patient Education: Take exactly as directed (do not increase dose or frequency); may take 2-3 weeks to achieve desired results; may cause physical and/or psychological dependence. Take once-a-day dose at bedtime. Avoid excessive alcohol, caffeine, and other prescription or OTC medications not approved by prescriber. Maintain adequate

(Continued)

Mirtazapine *(Continued)*

hydration (2-3 L/day of fluids unless instructed to restrict fluid intake). You may experience drowsiness, dizziness, or lightheadedness (use caution when driving or engaging in tasks requiring alertness until response to drug is known); nausea, vomiting, anorexia, or dry mouth (small frequent meals, frequent mouth care, chewing gum, or sucking lozenges may help); or orthostatic hypotension (use caution when climbing stairs or changing position from lying or sitting to standing). Report persistent insomnia, agitation, or confusion; muscle cramping, tremors, weakness, or change in gait; breathlessness or difficulty breathing; chest pain, palpitations, or rapid heartbeat; change in urinary pattern; vision changes or eye pain; yellowing of eyes or skin; pale stools/dark urine; or worsening of condition.

Monitoring Parameters: Patients should be monitored for signs of agranulocytosis or severe neutropenia such as sore throat, stomatitis or other signs of infection or a low WBC; monitor for improvement in clinical signs and symptoms of depression, improvement may be observed within 1-4 weeks after initiating therapy

Manufacturer Organon, Inc

Related Information

Antidepressant Agents Comparison *on page 1231*
Pharmaceutical Manufacturers Directory *on page 1020*

Misoprostol (mye soe PROST ole)

Pharmacologic Class Prostaglandin

U.S. Brand Names Cytotec®

Generic Available No

Mechanism of Action Misoprostol is a synthetic prostaglandin E_1 analog that replaces the protective prostaglandins consumed with prostaglandin-inhibiting therapies eg, nonsteroidal anti-inflammatory drugs

Use Prevention of NSAID-induced gastric ulcers

USUAL DOSAGE Adults: Oral: 200 mcg 4 times/day with food; if not tolerated, may decrease dose to 100 mcg 4 times/day with food or 200 mcg twice daily with food

Dosage Forms TAB: 100 mcg, 200 mcg

Contraindications Pregnancy; hypersensitivity to misoprostol or any component

Warnings/Precautions Safety and efficacy have not been established in children <18 years of age; use with caution in patients with renal impairment and the elderly; not to be used in pregnant women or women of childbearing potential unless woman is capable of complying with effective contraceptive measures; therapy is normally begun on the second or third day of next normal menstrual period

Pregnancy Risk Factor X

Adverse Reactions

>10%: Gastrointestinal: Diarrhea, abdominal pain

1% to 10%:

Central nervous system: Headache

Gastrointestinal: Constipation, flatulence

<1%: Nausea, uterine stimulation, vaginal bleeding, vomiting

Half-Life Parent and metabolite combined: 1.5 hours

Education and Monitoring Issues

Patient Education: Take as directed; continue taking your NSAIDs while taking this medication. Take with meals or after meals to prevent nausea, diarrhea, and flatulence. Avoid using antacids. You may experience increased menstrual pain, or cramping; request analgesics. Report abnormal menstrual periods, spotting (may occur even in postmenstrual women), or severe menstrual bleeding.

Manufacturer Searle

Related Information

Pharmaceutical Manufacturers Directory *on page 1020*

♦ **Mitran® Oral** *see* Chlordiazepoxide *on page 180*

♦ **Mivacron®** *see* Mivacurium *on page 610*

Mivacurium (mye va KYOO ree um)

Pharmacologic Class Skeletal Muscle Relaxant

U.S. Brand Names Mivacron®

Generic Available No

Mechanism of Action Mivacurium is a short-acting, nondepolarizing, neuromuscular-blocking agent. Like other nondepolarizing drugs, mivacurium antagonizes acetylcholine by competitively binding to cholinergic sites on motor endplates in skeletal muscle. This inhibits contractile activity in skeletal muscle leading to muscle paralysis. This effect is reversible with cholinesterase inhibitors such as edrophonium, neostigmine, and physostigmine.

Use Short-acting nondepolarizing neuromuscular blocking agent; an adjunct to general anesthesia; facilitates endotracheal intubation; provides skeletal muscle relaxation during surgery or mechanical ventilation; does not relieve pain or produce sedation

USUAL DOSAGE Dose to effect; doses will vary due to interpatient variability; use ideal body weight for obese patients

Children 2-12 years (duration of action is shorter and dosage requirements are higher): 0.2 mg/kg I.V. followed by average infusion rate of 14 mcg/kg/minute (range: 5-31 mcg/kg/minute) upon evidence of spontaneous recovery from initial dose

Adults: Initial: I.V.: 0.15-0.25 mg/kg bolus followed by maintenance doses of 0.1 mg/kg at approximately 15-minute intervals; for prolonged neuromuscular block, initial infusion of 9-10 mcg/kg/minute is used upon evidence of spontaneous recovery from initial dose, usual infusion rate of 6-7 mcg/kg/minute (1-15 mcg/kg/minute) under balanced anesthesia; initial dose after succinylcholine for intubation (balanced anesthesia): Adults: 0.1 mg/kg

Pretreatment/priming: 10% of intubating dose given 3-5 minutes before initial dose

Dosing adjustment in renal impairment: 0.15 mg/kg I.V. bolus; duration of action of blockade: 1.5 times longer in ESRD, may decrease infusion rates by as much as 50%, dependent on degree of renal impairment

Dosing adjustment in hepatic impairment: 0.15 mg/kg I.V. bolus; duration of blockade: 3 times longer in ESLD, may decrease rate of infusion by as much as 50% in ESLD, dependent on the degree of impairment

Dosage Forms **INF,** in D_5W: 0.5 mg/mL (50 mL). **INJ:** 2 mg/mL (5 mL, 10 mL)

Contraindications Hypersensitivity to mivacurium chloride or other benzylisoquinolinium agents; use of multidose vials in patients with allergy to benzyl alcohol

Pregnancy Risk Factor C

Adverse Reactions

>10%: Cardiovascular: Flushing of face

1% to 10%: Cardiovascular: Hypotension

<1%: Bradycardia, bronchospasm, cutaneous erythema, dizziness, endogenous histamine release, hypoxemia, injection site reaction, muscle spasms, rash, tachycardia, wheezing

Drug Interactions See table.

Potential Drug Interactions

Potentiation	Antagonism
Anesthetics	Calcium
Desflurane, sevoflurane, enflurane and	Carbamazepine
isoflurane > halothane > nitrous	Phenytoin
oxide-narcotics	Steroids (chronic administration)
Antibiotics	Theophylline
Aminoglycosides, polymyxins,	Anticholinesterases*
clindamycin, vancomycin	Neostigmine, pyridostigmine,
Magnesium sulfate	edrophonium, echothiophate
Antiarrhythmics	ophthalmic solution
Quinidine, procainamide, bretylium, and	Caffeine
possibly lidocaine	Azathioprine
Diuretics	
Furosemide, mannitol	
Amphotericin B (secondary to hypokalemia)	
Local anesthetics	
Dantrolene (directly depresses skeletal muscle)	
Beta agonists	
Beta blockers	
Calcium channel blockers	
Ketamine	
Lithium	
Succinylcholine (when administered prior to nondepolarizing NMB agent)	
Cyclosporine	

*Can prolong the effects of acetylcholine

Onset 2-3 minutes

Duration 15-30 minutes

Manufacturer GlaxoWellcome

Related Information

Pharmaceutical Manufacturers Directory *on page 1020*

♦ **Mixtard 15/85, 30/70, 50/50** *see* Insulin Preparations *on page 472*

♦ **Mixtard 30/70** *see* Insulin Preparations *on page 472*

♦ **Moban®** *see* Molindone *on page 614*

♦ **Mobenol®** *see* Tolbutamide *on page 928*

Modafinil (moe DAF i nil)

Pharmacologic Class Central Nervous System Stimulant, Nonamphetamine

U.S. Brand Names Provigil®

Mechanism of Action The exact mechanism of action is unclear, it does not appear to alter the release of dopamine or norepinephrine, it may exert its stimulant effects by decreasing GABA-mediated neurotransmission, although this theory has not yet been fully evaluated; several studies also suggest that an intact central alpha-adrenergic system is required for modafinil's activity; the drug increases high-frequency alpha waves while decreasing both delta and theta wave activity, and these effects are consistent with generalized increases in mental alertness

Use Improve wakefulness in patients with excessive daytime sleepiness associated with narcolepsy

Investigational use: ADHA; treatment of fatigue in MS and other disorders

USUAL DOSAGE

Narcolepsy: Initial: 200 mg as a single daily dose in the morning

Doses of 400 mg/day, given as a single dose, have been well tolerated, but there is no consistent evidence that this dose confers additional benefit

Dosing adjustment in elderly: Elimination of modafinil and its metabolites may be reduced as a consequence of aging and as a result, lower doses should be considered.

Dosing adjustment in renal impairment: Inadequate data to determine safety and efficacy in severe renal impairment

Dosing adjustment in hepatic impairment: Dose should be reduced to one-half of that recommended for patients with normal liver function

Dosage Forms TAB: 100 mg, 200 mg

Contraindications Hypersensitivity to modafinil or any component

Warnings/Precautions History of angina, ischemic EKG changes, left ventricular hypertrophy, or clinically significant mitral valve prolapse in association with CNS stimulant use; caution should be exercised when modafinil is given to patients with a history of psychosis, recent history of myocardial infarction, and because it has not yet been adequately studied in patients with hypertension, periodic monitoring of hypertensive patients receiving modafinil may be appropriate; caution is warranted when operating machinery or driving, although functional impairment has not been demonstrated with modafinil, all CNS-active agents may alter judgment, thinking and/or motor skills. Efficacy of oral contraceptives may be reduced, therefore, use of alternative contraception should be considered.

Pregnancy Risk Factor C

Pregnancy Implications Currently, there are no studies in humans evaluating its teratogenicity. Embryotoxicity of modafinil has been observed in animal models at dosages above those employed therapeutically. As a result, it should be used cautiously during pregnancy and should be used only when the potential risk of drug therapy is outweighed by the drug's benefits. It remains unknown if modafinil is secreted into human milk and, therefore, should be used cautiously in nursing women.

Adverse Reactions Limited to reports that were equal to or greater than placebo-related events:

<10%:

Cardiovascular: Chest pain (2%), hypertension (2%), hypotension (2%), vasodilation (1%), arrhythmia (1%), syncope (1%)

Central nervous system: Headache (50%, compared to 40% with placebo), nervousness (8%), dizziness (5%), depression (4%), anxiety (4%), cataplexy (3%), insomnia (3%), chills (2%), fever (1%), confusion (1%), amnesia (1%), emotional lability (1%), ataxia (1%)

Dermatologic: Dry skin (1%)

Endocrine & metabolic: Hyperglycemia (1%), albuminuria (1%)

Gastrointestinal: Diarrhea (8%), nausea (13%, compared to 4% with placebo), xerostomia (5%), anorexia (5%), vomiting (1%), mouth ulceration (1%), gingivitis (1%)

Genitourinary: Abnormal urine (1%), urinary retention (1%), ejaculatory disturbance (1%)

Hematologic: Eosinophilia (1%)

Hepatic: Abnormal LFTs (3%)

Neuromuscular & skeletal: Paresthesias (3%), dyskinesia (2%), neck pain (2%), hypertonia (2%), neck rigidity (1%), joint disorder (1%), tremor (1%)

Ocular: Amblyopia (2%), abnormal vision (2%)

Respiratory: Pharyngitis (6%), rhinitis (11%, compared to 8% with placebo), lung disorder (4%), dyspnea (2%), asthma (1%), epistaxis (1%)

Drug Interactions Modafinil may interact with drugs that inhibit, induce, or are metabolized by cytochrome P-450 isoenzymes; specifically modafinil is a 3A4 isoenzyme substrate and induces CYP1A2, CYP2B6, and CYP3A4 isoenzymes, as a result modafinil may decrease serum concentrations of 3A4 metabolized drugs such as oral contraceptives, cyclosporine, and to a lesser degree, theophylline; agents that induce CYP3A4, including phenobarbital, carbamazepine, and rifampin may result in decreased modafinil levels; there is evidence to suggest that modafinil may induce its own metabolism.

Increased effects: As a result of its inhibition of CYP2C19 isoenzymes, serum concentrations of drugs metabolized by this enzyme can be increased, these agents include diazepam, mephenytoin, phenytoin, and propranolol and due to modafinil's potential inhibition of the CYP2C9 isoenzyme, warfarin and phenytoin levels may be increased; in populations deficient in the CYP2D6 isoenzyme, where CYP2C19 acts as a secondary metabolic pathway, concentrations of tricyclic antidepressants and selective serotonin reuptake inhibitors may be increased during coadministration

Onset Peak zone: 2-4 hours

Half-Life 15 hours

Education and Monitoring Issues

Patient Education: Take exactly as prescribed; do not exceed recommended dosage without consulting prescriber. Maintain healthy sleep hygiene. Do not share medication with anyone else. Void before taking medication. You may experience headache, nervousness, confusion, or dizziness (use caution when driving or engaging in tasks requiring alertness until response to drug is known); diarrhea (yogurt or buttermilk may help); or dry mouth or sore mouth, loss of appetite, or vomiting (small frequent meals, frequent mouth care, chewing gum, or sucking lozenges may help). Diabetics should monitor glucose levels closely. Report chest pain or palpitations; difficulty breathing; excessive insomnia, CNS agitation, depression, or memory disturbances; vision changes; changes in urinary pattern or ejaculation disturbances; or persistent joint pain or stiffness.

- **Modane® Bulk [OTC]** *see* Psyllium *on page 793*
- **Modane® Soft [OTC]** *see* Docusate *on page 290*
- **Modecate®** *see* Fluphenazine *on page 381*
- **Modecate® Enantha** *see* Fluphenazine *on page 381*
- **Modicon™** *see* Ethinyl Estradiol and Norethindrone *on page 342*
- **Moduret®** *see* Amiloride and Hydrochlorothiazide *on page 46*
- **Moduretic®** *see* Amiloride and Hydrochlorothiazide *on page 46*

Moexipril (mo EKS i pril)

Pharmacologic Class Angiotensin-Converting Enzyme (ACE) Inhibitors

U.S. Brand Names Univasc®

Mechanism of Action Competitive inhibitor of angiotensin-converting enzyme (ACE); prevents conversion of angiotensin I to angiotensin II, a potent vasoconstrictor; results in lower levels of angiotensin II which causes an increase in plasma renin activity and a reduction in aldosterone secretion

Use Treatment of hypertension, alone or in combination with thiazide diuretics in a once daily dosing regimen

USUAL DOSAGE Adults: Oral: Initial: 7.5 mg once daily (in patients **not** receiving diuretics), one hour prior to a meal **or** 3.75 mg once daily (when combined with thiazide diuretics); maintenance dose: 7.5-30 mg/day in 1 or 2 divided doses one hour before meals

Dosing adjustment in renal impairment: Cl_{cr} ≤40 mL/minute: Patients may be cautiously placed on 3.75 mg once daily, then upwardly titrated to a maximum of 15 mg/day

Dosage Forms TAB: 7.5 mg, 15 mg

Contraindications Hypersensitivity to moexipril, moexiprilat, or component; hypersensitivity or allergic reactions or angioedema related to an ACE inhibitor

Warnings/Precautions Do not administer in pregnancy; use with caution and modify dosage in patients with renal impairment especially renal artery stenosis, severe congestive heart failure, or with coadministered diuretic therapy; experience in children is limited. Severe hypotension may occur in patients who are sodium and/or volume depleted; initiate lower doses and monitor closely when starting therapy in these patients; ACE inhibitors may be preferred agents in elderly patients with congestive heart failure and diabetes mellitus (diabetic proteinuria is reduced, minimal CNS effects, and enhanced insulin sensitivity), however due to decreased renal function, tolerance must be carefully monitored; if possible, discontinue the diuretic 2-3 days prior to initiating moexipril in patients receiving them to reduce the risk of symptomatic hypotension.

Pregnancy Risk Factor C (1st trimester); D (2nd and 3rd trimesters)

Adverse Reactions

1% to 10%:

Cardiovascular: Hypotension, peripheral edema

Central nervous system: Headache, dizziness, fatigue

Dermatologic: Rash, alopecia, flushing, rash

Endocrine & metabolic: Hyperkalemia

Gastrointestinal: Diarrhea, nausea, heartburn

Genitourinary: Polyuria

Neuromuscular & skeletal: Myalgia

Renal: Reversible increases in creatinine or BUN

Respiratory: Cough, pharyngitis, upper respiratory infection, sinusitis

<1% (limited to important or life-threatening symptoms): Chest pain, myocardial infarction, palpitations, arrhythmias, syncope, cerebrovascular accident, orthostatic hypotension,

(Continued)

Moexipril *(Continued)*

hypercholesterolemia, anemia, elevated LFTs, hepatitis, oliguria, proteinuria, bronchospasm, dyspnea, eosinophilic pneumonitis

Drug Interactions

Allopurinol: Potential for allergic reactions increased with moexipril

$Alpha_1$ blockers: Hypotensive effect increased

Aspirin and NSAIDs may decrease ACE inhibitor efficacy and/or increase potential to alter renal function

Diuretics: Hypovolemia due to diuretics may precipitate acute hypotensive events or acute renal failure

Insulin: Risk of hypoglycemia may be increased

Lithium: Risk of lithium toxicity may be increased; monitor lithium levels, especially the first 4 weeks of therapy

Mercaptopurine: Risk of neutropenia may be increased

Potassium-sparing diuretics (amiloride, potassium, spironolactone, triamterene): Increased risk of hyperkalemia

Potassium supplements may increase the risk of hyperkalemia

Probenecid: Blood levels of moexipril are increased (may occur with other ACE inhibitors)

Trimethoprim (high dose) may increase the risk of hyperkalemia

Alcohol Interactions Avoid use (may increase risk of hypotension or dizziness)

Onset Peak concentrations in 1-2 hours

Duration >24 hours

Half-Life Moexipril: 1 hour; Moexiprilat: 2-10 hours

Education and Monitoring Issues

Patient Education: Take exactly as directed; do not discontinue without consulting prescriber. Take first dose at bedtime. This drug does not eliminate need for diet or exercise regimen as recommended by prescriber. Do not take potassium supplements or salt substitutes containing potassium without consulting prescriber. May cause dizziness, fainting, lightheadedness (use caution when driving or engaging in tasks that require alertness until response to drug is known); postural hypotension (use caution when rising from lying or sitting position or climbing stairs); nausea, vomiting, abdominal pain, dry mouth, or transient loss of appetite (small frequent meals, frequent mouth care, sucking lozenges, or chewing gum may help) - report if these persist. Report chest pain or palpitations; difficulty in breathing or unusual cough; or other persistent adverse reactions.

Monitoring Parameters: Blood pressure, heart rate, electrolytes, CBC, symptoms of hypotension

Manufacturer Schwarz Pharma

Related Information

Angiotensin-Related Agents Comparison *on page 1226*

Moexipril and Hydrochlorothiazide *on page 614*

Pharmaceutical Manufacturers Directory *on page 1020*

Moexipril and Hydrochlorothiazide

(mo EKS i pril & hye droe klor oh THYE a zide)

Pharmacologic Class Antihypertensive Agent, Combination

U.S. Brand Names Uniretic™

Dosage Forms TAB: Moexipril hydrochloride 7.5 mg and hydrochlorothiazide 12.5 mg, moexipril hydrochloride 15 mg and hydrochlorothiazide 25 mg

Pregnancy Risk Factor C (1st trimester); D (2nd and 3rd trimesters)

Alcohol Interactions Avoid use (may increase risk of hypotension or dizziness)

Manufacturer Schwarz Pharma

Related Information

Pharmaceutical Manufacturers Directory *on page 1020*

Molindone (moe LIN done)

Pharmacologic Class Antipsychotic Agent, Dihydoindoline

U.S. Brand Names Moban®

Generic Available No

Mechanism of Action Mechanism of action mimics that of chlorpromazine; however, it produces more extrapyramidal effects and less sedation than chlorpromazine

Use Management of psychotic disorder

USUAL DOSAGE Oral:

Children:

3-5 years: 1-2.5 mg/day divided into 4 doses

5-12 years: 0.5-1 mg/kg/day in 4 divided doses

Adults: 50-75 mg/day increase at 3- to 4-day intervals up to 225 mg/day

Dosage Forms CONC, oral: 20 mg/mL (120 mL). **TAB:** 5 mg, 10 mg, 25 mg, 50 mg, 100 mg

Contraindications Narrow-angle glaucoma, hypersensitivity to molindone or any component

Warnings/Precautions Use with caution in patients with cardiovascular disease or seizures, CNS depression, or hepatic impairment

Pregnancy Risk Factor C

Adverse Reactions

Cardiovascular: Orthostatic hypotension, tachycardia, arrhythmias

Central nervous system: Extrapyramidal reactions (akathisia, pseudoparkinsonism, dystonia, tardive dyskinesia), mental depression, altered central temperature regulation, sedation, drowsiness, restlessness, anxiety, hyperactivity, euphoria, seizures, neuroleptic malignant syndrome (NMS)

Dermatologic: Pruritus, rash, photosensitivity

Endocrine & metabolic: Change in menstrual periods, edema of breasts, amenorrhea, galactorrhea, gynecomastia

Gastrointestinal: Constipation, xerostomia, nausea, salivation, weight gain, weight loss

Genitourinary: Urinary retention, priapism

Hematologic: Leukopenia, leukocytosis

Ocular: Blurred vision, retinal pigmentation

Miscellaneous: Diaphoresis (decreased)

Drug Interactions CYP2D6 enzyme substrate

Antipsychotics inhibit the ability of bromocriptine to lower serum prolactin concentrations

Benztropine (and other anticholinergics) may inhibit the therapeutic response to molindone and excess anticholinergic effects may occur

Chloroquine may increase molindone concentrations

Cigarette smoking may enhance the hepatic metabolism of molindone. Larger doses may be required compared to a nonsmoker.

Concurrent use of molindone with an antihypertensive may produce additive hypotensive effects

Antihypertensive effects of guanethidine and guanadrel may be inhibited by molindone

Concurrent use with TCA may produce increased toxicity or altered therapeutic response

Molindone may inhibit the antiparkinsonian effect of levodopa; avoid this combination

Molindone plus lithium may rarely produce neurotoxicity

Barbiturates may reduce molindone concentrations

Propranolol may increase molindone concentrations

Sulfadoxine-pyrimethamine may increase molindone concentrations

Molindone and possibly other low potency antipsychotics may reverse the pressor effects of epinephrine

Molindone and CNS depressants (ethanol, narcotics) may produce additive CNS depressant effects

Molindone and trazodone may produce additive hypotensive effects

Alcohol Interactions Avoid use (may increase central nervous system depression)

Half-Life 1.5 hours

Education and Monitoring Issues

Patient Education: Use exactly as directed (do not increase dose or frequency); may cause physical and/or psychological dependence. It may take 2-3 weeks to achieve desired results; do not discontinue without consulting prescriber. Avoid excess alcohol or caffeine and other prescription or OTC medications not approved by prescriber. Maintain adequate hydration (2-3 L/day of fluids unless instructed to restrict fluid intake). You may experience excess drowsiness, restlessness, dizziness, or blurred vision (use caution driving or when engaging in tasks requiring alertness until response to drug is known); constipation (increased exercise, fluids, or dietary fruit and fiber may help); postural hypotension (use caution climbing stairs or when changing position from lying or sitting to standing); or decreased perspiration (avoid strenuous exercise in hot environments). Report persistent CNS effects (eg, trembling fingers, altered gait or balance, excessive sedation, seizures, unusual movements, anxiety, abnormal thoughts, confusion, personality changes); chest pain, palpitations, rapid heartbeat, severe dizziness; unresolved urinary retention or changes in urinary pattern; changes in menstrual pattern or breast tenderness; vision changes; skin rash or yellowing of skin; difficulty breathing; or worsening of condition.

Monitoring Parameters: Monitor blood pressure and pulse rate prior to and during initial therapy evaluate mental status; monitor weight

- **Mol-Iron® [OTC]** *see* Ferrous Sulfate *on page 360*
- **Mollifene® Ear Wax Removing Formula [OTC]** *see* Carbamide Peroxide *on page 139*

Mometasone Furoate (moe MET a sone FYOOR oh ate)

Pharmacologic Class Corticosteroid, Topical

U.S. Brand Names Elocon® Topical; Nasonex®

Generic Available No

Mechanism of Action May depress the formation, release, and activity of endogenous chemical mediators of inflammation (kinins, histamine, liposomal enzymes, prostaglandins). Leukocytes and macrophages may have to be present for the initiation of responses mediated by the above substances. Inhibits the margination and subsequent cell migration to the area of injury, and also reverses the dilatation and increased vessel permeability in the area resulting in decreased access of cells to the sites of injury.

(Continued)

Mometasone Furoate *(Continued)*

Use Relief of the inflammatory and pruritic manifestations of corticosteroid-responsive dermatoses (medium potency topical corticosteroid); treatment of nasal symptoms of seasonal and perennial rhinitis in adults and children ≥3 years of age

USUAL DOSAGE

Nasal spray:

Children 3-12 years of age: Nasal spray: 1 spray in each nostril daily

Children ≥12 years and Adults: 2 sprays in each nostril daily

Topical: Adults: Apply sparingly to area once daily, do not use occlusive dressings. Therapy should be discontinued when control is achieved; if no improvement is seen, reassessment of diagnosis may be necessary.

Dosage Forms CRM: 0.1% (15 g, 45 g). **LOT:** 0.1% (30 mL, 60 mL). **OINT, top:** 0.1% (15 g, 45 g). **SPRAY,** nasal: 50 mcg/spray (17 g)

Contraindications Hypersensitivity to mometasone or any component; fungal, viral, or tubercular skin lesions, herpes simplex or zoster

Warnings/Precautions Adverse systemic effects may occur when used on large areas of the body, denuded areas, for prolonged periods of time, with an occlusive dressing, and/or in infants or small children

Pregnancy Risk Factor C

Adverse Reactions <1%: Acne, allergic dermatitis, burning, Cushing's syndrome, dryness, folliculitis, growth retardation, HPA suppression, hypertrichosis, hypopigmentation, irritation, itching, maceration of the skin, miliaria, secondary infection skin atrophy, striae

Education and Monitoring Issues

Patient Education: Before applying, gently wash area to reduce risk of infection; apply a thin film to cleansed area and rub in gently and thoroughly until medication vanishes; avoid exposure to sunlight, severe sunburn may occur

Manufacturer Schering-Plough Corp

Related Information

Pharmaceutical Manufacturers Directory *on page 1020*

- **Monafed®** *see* Guaifenesin *on page 423*
- **Monafed® DM** *see* Guaifenesin and Dextromethorphan *on page 424*
- **Monazole-7®** *see* Miconazole *on page 600*
- **Monistat-Derm™ Topical** *see* Miconazole *on page 600*
- **Monistat i.v.™ Injection** *see* Miconazole *on page 600*
- **Monistat™ Vaginal** *see* Miconazole *on page 600*
- **Monitan®** *see* Acebutolol *on page 16*
- **Monocid®** *see* Cefonicid *on page 154*
- **Mono-Gesic®** *see* Salsalate *on page 837*
- **Monoket®** *see* Isosorbide Mononitrate *on page 491*
- **Monopril®** *see* Fosinopril *on page 396*

Montelukast (mon te LOO kast)

Pharmacologic Class Leukotriene Receptor Antagonist

U.S. Brand Names Singulair®

Mechanism of Action Selective leukotriene receptor antagonist that inhibits the cysteinyl leukotriene receptor. Cysteinyl leukotrienes and leukotriene receptor occupation have been correlated with the pathophysiology of asthma, including airway edema, smooth muscle contraction, and altered cellular activity associated with the inflammatory process, which contribute to the signs and symptoms of asthma.

Use Prophylaxis and chronic treatment of asthma in adults and children ≥2 years of age

USUAL DOSAGE Oral:

Children:

<2 years: Safety and efficacy have not been established

2-5 years: Chew one 4 mg chewable tablet/day, taken in the evening

6 to 14 years: Chew one 5 mg chewable tablet/day, taken in the evening

Children ≥15 years and Adults: 10 mg/day, taken in the evening

Dosing adjustment in hepatic impairment: Mild moderate: No adjustment necessary

Dosage Forms TAB: 10 mg; Chewable, cherry: 4 mg, 5 mg

Contraindications Hypersensitivity to any component

Warnings/Precautions Montelukast is not indicated for use in the reversal of bronchospasm in acute asthma attacks, including status asthmaticus. Should not be used as monotherapy for the treatment and management of exercise-induced bronchospasm. Advise patients to have appropriate rescue medication available. Appropriate clinical monitoring and caution are recommended when systemic corticosteroid reduction is considered in patients receiving montelukast. Inform phenylketonuric patients that the chewable tablet contains phenylalanine 0.842 mg/5 mg chewable tablet.

In rare cases, patients on therapy with montelukast may present with systemic eosinophilia, sometimes presenting with clinical features of vasculitis consistent with Churg-

Strauss syndrome, a condition which is often treated with systemic corticosteroid therapy. See Adverse Reactions.

Pregnancy Risk Factor B

Adverse Reactions

>10%: Central nervous system: Headache

1% to 10%:

Central nervous system: Dizziness, fatigue, fever

Dermatologic: Rash

Gastrointestinal: Dyspepsia, dental pain, gastroenteritis, diarrhea, nausea, abdominal pain

Neuromuscular & skeletal: Weakness

Respiratory: Cough, nasal congestion, laryngitis, pharyngitis

Miscellaneous: Flu-like symptoms, trauma

In rare cases, patients on therapy with montelukast may present with systemic eosinophilia, sometimes presenting with clinical features of vasculitis consistent with Churg-Strauss syndrome, a condition which is often treated with systemic corticosteroid therapy. Prescribers should be alert to eosinophilia, vasculitic rash, worsening pulmonary symptoms, cardiac complications, and/or neuropathy presenting in their patients. A casual association between montelukast and these underlying conditions has not been established.

Drug Interactions CYP2A6, and 2C9, 3A3/4, enzyme substrate

Decreased effect: Phenobarbital, rifampin induce hepatic metabolism and decrease the AUC of montelukast

Onset Time to peak: 2-4 hours

Duration >24 hours

Half-Life 3-6 hours

Education and Monitoring Issues

Patient Education: This medication is not for an acute asthmatic attack; in acute attack, follow instructions of prescriber. Do not stop other asthma medication unless advised by prescriber. Take every evening on a continuous basis; do not discontinue even if feeling better (this medication may help reduce incidence of acute attacks). You may experience mild headache (mild analgesic may help); fatigue or dizziness (use caution when driving). Report skin rash or itching, abdominal pain or persistent GI upset, unusual cough or congestion, or worsening of asthmatic condition.

Manufacturer Merck & Co

Related Information

Pharmaceutical Manufacturers Directory *on page 1020*

♦ **8-MOP®** *see* Methoxsalen *on page 585*

♦ **More-Dophilus® [OTC]** *see Lactobacillus acidophilus* and *Lactobacillus bulgaricus on page 505*

Moricizine (mor I siz een)

Pharmacologic Class Antiarrhythmic Agent, Class I

U.S. Brand Names Ethmozine®

Generic Available No

Mechanism of Action Class I antiarrhythmic agent; reduces the fast inward current carried by sodium ions, shortens Phase I and Phase II repolarization, resulting in decreased action potential duration and effective refractory period

Use Treatment of ventricular tachycardia and life-threatening ventricular arrhythmias

Unlabeled use: PVCs, complete and nonsustained ventricular tachycardia

USUAL DOSAGE Adults: Oral: 200-300 mg every 8 hours, adjust dosage at 150 mg/day at 3-day intervals. See table for dosage recommendations of transferring from other antiarrhythmic agents to Ethmozine®.

Moricizine

Transferred From	Start Ethmozine®
Encainide, propafenone, tocainide, or mexiletine	8-12 hours after last dose
Flecainide	12-24 hours after last dose
Procainamide	3-6 hours after last dose
Quinidine, disopyramide	6-12 hours after last dose

Dosing interval in renal or hepatic impairment: Start at 600 mg/day or less

Dosage Forms TAB: 200 mg, 250 mg, 300 mg

Contraindications Pre-existing second or third degree A-V block and in patients with right bundle-branch block when associated with left hemiblock, unless pacemaker is present; cardiogenic shock; known hypersensitivity to the drug

(Continued)

Moricizine *(Continued)*

Warnings/Precautions Considering the known proarrhythmic properties and lack of evidence of improved survival for any antiarrhythmic drug in patients without life-threatening arrhythmias, it is prudent to reserve the use for patients with life-threatening ventricular arrhythmias; CAST II trial demonstrated a trend towards decreased survival for patients treated with moricizine; proarrhythmic effects occur as with other antiarrhythmic agents; hypokalemia, hyperkalemia, hypomagnesemia may effect response to class I agents; use with caution in patients with sick-sinus syndrome, hepatic, and renal impairment

Pregnancy Risk Factor B

Adverse Reactions

>10%: Central nervous system: Dizziness

1% to 10%:

Cardiovascular: Proarrhythmia, palpitations, cardiac death, EKG abnormalities, congestive heart failure

Central nervous system: Headache, fatigue, insomnia

Endocrine & metabolic: Decreased libido

Gastrointestinal: Nausea, diarrhea, ileus

Ocular: Blurred vision, periorbital edema

Respiratory: Dyspnea

<1% (limited to important or life-threatening symptoms): Ventricular tachycardia, cardiac chest pain, hypotension or hypertension, syncope, supraventricular arrhythmias, myocardial infarction, apnea

Drug Interactions CYP1A2 inducer

Cimetidine increases moricizine levels by 50%

Digoxin may result in additive prolongation of the PR interval when combined with moricizine (but not rate of second- and third-degree A-V block)

Diltiazem increases moricizine levels resulting in an increased incidence of side effects. Moricizine decreases diltiazem plasma levels and decreases its half-life.

Drugs which may prolong Q-T interval (including cisapride, erythromycin, phenothiazines, cyclic antidepressants, and some quinolones) are contraindicated with type Ia antiarrhythmics. Moricizine has some type Ia activity, and caution should be used.

Theophylline levels are decreased by 50% with moricizine due to increased clearance

Half-Life Normal patient: 3-4 hours; Cardiac disease patient: 6-13 hours

Education and Monitoring Issues

Patient Education: Take exactly as directed; do not take additional doses or discontinue without consulting prescriber. You will need regular cardiac checkups and blood tests while taking this medication. You may experience dizziness or visual changes (use caution when driving or engaging in tasks requiring alertness until response to drug is known); nausea or vomiting (small frequent meals, frequent mouth care, chewing gum, or sucking lozenges may help); or headaches, sleep disturbances, or decreased libido (usually temporary, if persistent consult prescriber). Report chest pain, palpitation, or erratic heartbeat; increased weight or swelling of hands or feet; blurred vision or facial swelling; acute diarrhea; changes in bowel or bladder patterns; or difficulty breathing.

Manufacturer Roberts Pharmaceuticals

Related Information

Pharmaceutical Manufacturers Directory *on page 1020*

♦ **Morphine-HP®** *see* Morphine Sulfate *on page 618*

Morphine Sulfate (MOR feen SUL fate)

Pharmacologic Class Analgesic, Narcotic

U.S. Brand Names Astramorph™ PF Injection; Duramorph® Injection; Infumorph™ Injection; Kadian™; MS Contin® Oral; MSIR® Oral; MS/L®; MS/S®; OMS® Oral; Oramorph SR™ Oral; RMS® Rectal; Roxanol™ Oral; Roxanol Rescudose®; Roxanol SR™ Oral

Generic Available Yes

Mechanism of Action Binds to opiate receptors in the CNS, causing inhibition of ascending pain pathways, altering the perception of and response to pain; produces generalized CNS depression

Use Relief of moderate to severe acute and chronic pain; pain of myocardial infarction; relieves dyspnea of acute left ventricular failure and pulmonary edema; preanesthetic medication

USUAL DOSAGE Doses should be titrated to appropriate effect; when changing routes of administration in chronically treated patients, please note that oral doses are approximately one-half as effective as parenteral dose

Infants and Children:

Oral: Tablet and solution (prompt release): 0.2-0.5 mg/kg/dose every 4-6 hours as needed; tablet (controlled release): 0.3-0.6 mg/kg/dose every 12 hours

I.M., I.V., S.C.: 0.1-0.2 mg/kg/dose every 2-4 hours as needed; usual maximum: 15 mg/dose; may initiate at 0.05 mg/kg/dose

I.V., S.C. continuous infusion: Sickle cell or cancer pain: 0.025-2 mg/kg/hour; postoperative pain: 0.01-0.04 mg/kg/hour

Sedation/analgesia for procedures: I.V.: 0.05-0.1 mg/kg 5 minutes before the procedure
Adolescents >12 years: Sedation/analgesia for procedures: I.V.: 3-4 mg and repeat in 5 minutes if necessary
Adults:
Oral: Prompt release: 10-30 mg every 4 hours as needed; controlled release: 15-30 mg every 8-12 hours
I.M., I.V., S.C.: 2.5-20 mg/dose every 2-6 hours as needed; usual: 10 mg/dose every 4 hours as needed
I.V., S.C. continuous infusion: 0.8-10 mg/hour; may increase depending on pain relief/ adverse effects; usual range: up to 80 mg/hour
Epidural: Initial: 5 mg in lumbar region; if inadequate pain relief within 1 hour, administer 1-2 mg, maximum dose: 10 mg/24 hours
Intrathecal ($^1/_{10}$ of epidural dose): 0.2-1 mg/dose; repeat doses **not** recommended
Rectal: 10-20 mg every 4 hours

Dosing adjustment in renal impairment:
Cl_{cr} 10-50 mL/minute: Administer at 75% of normal dose
Cl_{cr} <10 mL/minute: Administer at 50% of normal dose

Dosing adjustment/comments in hepatic disease: Unchanged in mild liver disease; substantial extrahepatic metabolism may occur; excessive sedation may occur in cirrhosis

Dosage Forms CAP (MSIR®): 15 mg, 30 mg; Sustained release (Kadian™): 20 mg, 50 mg, 100 mg. **INJ:** 0.5 mg/mL (10 mL), 1 mg/mL (10 mL, 30 mL, 60 mL), 2 mg/mL (1 mL, 2 mL, 60 mL), 3 mg/mL (50 mL), 4 mg/mL (1 mL, 2 mL), 5 mg/mL (1 mL, 30 mL), 8 mg/mL (1 mL, 2 mL), 10 mg/mL (1 mL, 2 mL, 10 mL), 15 mg/mL (1 mL, 2 mL, 20 mL), 25 mg/mL (4 mL, 10 mL, 20 mL, 40 mL), 50 mg/mL (10 mL, 20 mL, 40 mL); Preservative free (Astramorph™ PF, Duramorph®): 0.5 mg/mL (2 mL, 10 mL), 1 mg/mL (2 mL, 10 mL), 10 mg/mL (20 mL), 25 mg/mL (20 mL). **I.V. via PCA pump:** 1 mg/mL (10 mL, 30 mL, 60 mL), 5 mg/mL (30 mL). **I.V. infusion preparation:** 25 mg/mL (4 mL, 10 mL, 20 mL). **SOLN, oral:** 10 mg/5 mL (5 mL, 10 mL, 100 mL, 120 mL, 500 mL), 20 mg/5 mL (5 mL, 100 mL, 120 mL, 500 mL); (MSIR®): 10 mg/5 mL (5 mL, 120 mL, 500 mL), 20 mg/5 mL (5 mL 120 mL, 500 mL), 20 mg/mL (30 mL, 120 mL); (MS/L®): 100 mg/5 mL (120 mL) 20 mg/5 mL; (OMS®): 20 mg/mL (30 mL, 120 mL); (Roxanol™): 10 mg/2.5 mL (2.5 mL), 20 mg/mL (1 mL, 1.5 mL, 30 mL, 120 mL, 240 mL). **SUPP, rectal:** 5 mg, 10 mg, 20 mg, 30 mg; (MS/S®, RMS®, Roxanol™): 5 mg, 10 mg, 20 mg, 30 mg. **TAB:** 15 mg, 30 mg; (MSIR®): 15 mg, 30 mg; Controlled release: (MS Contin®): 15 mg, 30 mg, 60 mg, 100 mg, 200 mg; (Roxanol™ SR): 30 mg; Soluble: 10 mg, 15 mg, 30 mg; Sustained release (Oramorph SR™): 30 mg, 60 mg, 100 mg

Contraindications Known hypersensitivity to morphine sulfate; increased intracranial pressure; severe respiratory depression

Warnings/Precautions Some preparations contain sulfites which may cause allergic reactions; infants <3 months of age are more susceptible to respiratory depression, use with caution and generally in reduced doses in this age group; use with caution in patients with impaired respiratory function or severe hepatic dysfunction and in patients with hypersensitivity reactions to other phenanthrene derivative opioid agonists (codeine, hydrocodone, hydromorphone, levorphanol, oxycodone, oxymorphone). Morphine shares the toxic potential of opiate agonists and usual precautions of opiate agonist therapy should be observed; may cause hypotension in patients with acute myocardial infarction. Tolerance or drug dependence may result from extended use.

Elderly may be particularly susceptible to the CNS depressant and constipating effects of narcotics

Pregnancy Risk Factor B; D (if used for prolonged periods or in high doses at term)

Adverse Reactions

Percentage unknown: Flushing, CNS depression, drowsiness, sedation, increased intracranial pressure, antidiuretic hormone release, physical and psychological dependence, diaphoresis

>10%:
Cardiovascular: Palpitations, hypotension, bradycardia
Central nervous system: Dizziness
Gastrointestinal: Nausea, vomiting, constipation, xerostomia
Local: Pain at injection site
Neuromuscular & skeletal: Weakness
Miscellaneous: Histamine release

1% to 10%:
Central nervous system: Restlessness, headache, false feeling of well being, confusion
Gastrointestinal: Anorexia, GI irritation, paralytic ileus
Genitourinary: Decreased urination
Neuromuscular & skeletal: Trembling
Ocular: Vision problems
Respiratory: Respiratory depression, shortness of breath

<1%: Biliary tract spasm, hallucinations, increased intracranial pressure, increased liver function tests, insomnia, mental depression, miosis, muscle rigidity, paradoxical CNS stimulation, peripheral vasodilation, pruritus, urinary tract spasm

Drug Interactions CYP2D6 enzyme substrate

(Continued)

Morphine Sulfate *(Continued)*

Decreased effect: Phenothiazines may antagonize the analgesic effect of morphine and other opiate agonists

Increased toxicity: CNS depressants, tricyclic antidepressants may potentiate the effects of morphine and other opiate agonists; dextroamphetamine may enhance the analgesic effect of morphine and other opiate agonists

Alcohol Interactions Avoid use (may increase central nervous system depression)

Onset Oral: 1 hour; I.V.: 5-10 minutes

Duration 3-5 hours (up to 12 hours for extended release)

Half-Life 2-4 hours

Education and Monitoring Issues

Patient Education: If self-administered, use exactly as directed (do not increase dose or frequency); may cause physical and/or psychological dependence. While using this medication, do not use alcohol and other prescription or OTC medications (especially sedatives, tranquilizers, antihistamines, or pain medications) without consulting prescriber. Maintain adequate hydration (2-3 L/day of fluids unless instructed to restrict fluid intake). May cause hypotension, dizziness, drowsiness, impaired coordination, or blurred vision (use caution when driving, climbing stairs, or changing position - rising from sitting or lying to standing, or when engaging in tasks requiring alertness until response to drug is known); loss of appetite, nausea, or vomiting (frequent mouth care, small frequent meals, chewing gum, or sucking lozenges may help); constipation (increased exercise, fluids, or dietary fruit and fiber may help - if constipation remains an unresolved problem, consult prescriber about use of stool softeners). Report chest pain, slow or rapid heartbeat, acute dizziness, or persistent headache; changes in mental status; swelling of extremities or unusual weight gain; changes in urinary elimination or pain on urination; acute headache; back or flank pain or muscle spasms; blurred vision; skin rash; or shortness of breath.

Dietary Considerations:

Food:

Glucose may cause hyperglycemia; monitor blood glucose concentrations

Administration of oral morphine solution with food may increase bioavailability (ie, a report of 34% increase in morphine AUC when morphine oral solution followed a high-fat meal). Morphine may cause GI upset. Be consistent when taking morphine with or without meals. Take with food if GI upset.

Monitoring Parameters: Pain relief, respiratory and mental status, blood pressure

Reference Range: Therapeutic: Surgical anesthesia: 65-80 ng/mL (SI: 227-280 nmol/L); Toxic: 200-5000 ng/mL (SI: 700-17,500 nmol/L)

Related Information

Lipid-Lowering Agents Comparison *on page 1243*
Narcotic Agonists Comparison *on page 1244*

♦ **Motofen®** *see* Difenoxin and Atropine *on page 270*
♦ **Motrin®** *see* Ibuprofen *on page 458*
♦ **Motrin® IB [OTC]** *see* Ibuprofen *on page 458*

Moxifloxacin (mox i FLOKS a sin)

Pharmacologic Class Antibiotic, Quinolone

U.S. Brand Names Avelox™

Mechanism of Action Moxifloxacin is a DNA gyrase inhibitor, and also inhibits topoisomerase IV. DNA gyrase (topoisomerase II) is an essential bacterial enzyme that maintains the superhelical structure of DNA. DNA gyrase is required for DNA replication and transcription, DNA repair, recombination, and transposition; inhibition is bactericidal.

Use Treatment of mild to moderate community-acquired pneumonia, acute bacterial exacerbation of chronic bronchitis, and acute bacterial sinusitis

USUAL DOSAGE Adult: Oral:

Community acquired pneumonia or acute bacterial sinusitis: 400 mg every 24 hours for 10 days

Chronic bronchitis, acute bacterial exacerbation: 400 mg every 24 hours for 5 days

Dosage adjustment in renal impairment: No dosage adjustment is required.

Dosage adjustment in hepatic impairment: No dosage adjustment is required in mild hepatic insufficiency (Child-Pugh Class A). Not recommended in patients with moderate to severe hepatic insufficiency.

Elderly: No dosage adjustments are required based on age.

Dosage Forms TAB: 400 mg

Contraindications Hypersensitivity to moxifloxacin, other quinolone antibiotics, or any component

Warnings/Precautions Use with caution in patients with significant bradycardia or acute myocardial ischemia. Moxifloxacin causes a dose-dependent Q-T prolongation. Coadministration of moxifloxacin with other drugs that also prolong the Q-T interval or induce bradycardia (eg, beta-blockers, amiodarone) should be avoided. Careful consideration should be given in the use of moxifloxacin in patients with cardiovascular disease, particularly in those with conduction abnormalities. Safety and effectiveness in pediatric patients (<18 years of age) have not been established. Experience in immature animals has resulted in permanent arthropathy. Use with caution in individuals at risk of seizures (CNS disorders or concurrent therapy with medications which may lower seizure threshold). Discontinue in patients who experience significant CNS adverse effects (dizziness, hallucinations, suicidal ideation or actions). Not recommended in patients with moderate to severe hepatic insufficiency. Use with caution in diabetes; glucose regulation may be altered.

Severe hypersensitivity reactions, including anaphylaxis, have occurred with quinolone therapy. If an allergic reaction occurs (itching, urticaria, dyspnea or facial edema, loss of consciousness, tingling, cardiovascular collapse) discontinue drug immediately. Prolonged use may result in superinfection; pseudomembranous colitis may occur and should be considered in all patients who present with diarrhea. Tendon inflammation and/or rupture has been reported with other quinolone antibiotics. This has not been reported for moxifloxacin. Discontinue at first sign of tendon inflammation or pain.

Pregnancy Risk Factor C

Pregnancy Implications No adequate or well-controlled studies in pregnant women. Should be used during pregnancy only when the potential benefit justifies the potential risk to the fetus. Moxifloxacin may be excreted in human breast milk. Breast-feeding is not recommended.

Adverse Reactions

1% to 10%:

Central nervous system: Dizziness (3%), headache (2%)

Gastrointestinal: Nausea (8%), diarrhea (6%), abdominal pain (2%), vomiting (2%), dyspepsia (1%), taste perversion (1%)

Hepatic: Abnormal liver function test (1%)

<1% (limited to important or life-threatening symptoms): Asthenia, moniliasis, pain, malaise, allergic reaction, leg pain, back pain, fever, chills, chest pain, palpitation, vasodilation, tachycardia, hypertension, peripheral edema, hypotension, insomnia, nervousness, anxiety, confusion, hallucinations, depersonalization, hypertonia, incoordination, somnolence, tremor, vertigo, paresthesia, dry mouth, constipation, anorexia, stomatitis, gastritis, glossitis, cholestatic jaundice, GGTP increased, decreased prothrombin time, increased prothrombin time, thrombocytopenia, eosinophilia, leukopenia, increased amylase, hyperglycemia, hyperlipidemia, increased LDH, arthralgia, myalgia, asthma, dyspnea, increased cough, pneumonia, pharyngitis, rhinitis, sinusitis, rash, pruritus, sweating, urticaria, dry skin, tinnitus, amblyopia, vaginitis, cystitis, abnormal renal function, Q-T prolongation (see Warnings)

Drug Interactions

Drugs which prolong Q-T interval (including Class Ia and Class III antiarrhythmics, erythromycin, cisapride, antipsychotics, and cyclic antidepressants) are contraindicated with moxifloxacin.

Metal cations (magnesium, aluminum, iron, and zinc) bind quinolones in the gastrointestinal tract and inhibit absorption (by up to 98%). Antacids, electrolyte supplements, sucralfate, quinapril, and some didanosine formulations should be avoided. Moxifloxacin should be administered 4 hours before or 8 hours after these agents.

Antineoplastic agents may decrease the absorption of quinolones.

Cimetidine, and other H_2 antagonists may inhibit renal elimination of quinolones.

Digoxin levels may be increased in some patients by quinolones; monitor for increased effect/concentrations.

Foscarnet has been associated with an increased risk of seizures with some quinolones.

Loop diuretics: Serum levels of some quinolones are increased by loop diuretic administration. May diminish renal excretion.

NSAIDs: The CNS stimulating effect of some quinolones may be enhanced, resulting in neuroexcitation and/or seizures. This effect has not been observed with moxifloxacin.

Probenecid: Blocks renal secretion of quinolones, increasing concentrations.

Warfarin: The hypoprothrombinemic effect of warfarin is enhanced by some quinolone antibiotics. No significant effect has been demonstrated for moxifloxacin, however, monitoring of the INR during concurrent therapy is recommended by the manufacturer.

Half-Life 12 hours

Education and Monitoring Issues

Patient Education: I.V.: Report any pain, itching, burning or signs of irritation at infusion site.

Oral: Take exactly as directed with or without food. Do not take antacids, vitamins, ulcer or hypertensive medication 4 hours before or 8 hours after taking moxifloxacin. Do not miss a dose (take a missed dose as soon as possible, unless it is almost time for next dose). Take entire prescription even if feeling better. Maintain adequate hydration (2-3 L/day of fluid, unless instructed to restrict fluids). Following I.V. or oral administration, you may experience nausea, vomiting, taste perversion (small frequent meals, good mouth care, chewing gum, or sucking hard candy may help); headache, dizziness, insomnia, anxiety (use caution when driving or engaged in tasks requiring alertness until response is known). Report immediately any swelling of mouth, lips, tongue or throat; chest pain or tightness, difficulty breathing, back pain, itching, skin rash, or tingling; tendon pain; confusion, dizziness, abnormal thinking, anxiety, or insomnia. Report changes in voiding pattern, vaginal itching, burning, or

(Continued)

Moxifloxacin *(Continued)*

discharge; changes in vision or hearing; abnormal bruising or bleeding or blood in urine; or other adverse reactions.

Monitoring Parameters: WBC, signs of infection

Manufacturer Bayer Corp (Biological and Pharmaceutical Division)

Related Information

Community Acquired Pneumonia in Adults *on page 1200*

Pharmaceutical Manufacturers Directory *on page 1020*

- **M-Prednisol® Injection** *see* Methylprednisolone *on page 589*
- **MS Contin® Oral** *see* Morphine Sulfate *on page 618*
- **MSD® Enteric Coated ASA** *see* Aspirin *on page 72*
- **MS-IR®** *see* Morphine Sulfate *on page 618*
- **MSIR® Oral** *see* Morphine Sulfate *on page 618*
- **MS/L®** *see* Morphine Sulfate *on page 618*
- **MS/S®** *see* Morphine Sulfate *on page 618*
- **MST Continus** *see* Morphine Sulfate *on page 618*
- **Mucinum Herbal** *see* Senna *on page 845*
- **Muco-Fen-DM®** *see* Guaifenesin and Dextromethorphan *on page 424*
- **Muco-Fen-LA®** *see* Guaifenesin *on page 423*
- **Mucomyst®** *see* Acetylcysteine *on page 20*
- **Mucosil™** *see* Acetylcysteine *on page 20*
- **Multipax®** *see* Hydroxyzine *on page 455*
- **Multitest CMI®** *see* Skin Test Antigens, Multiple *on page 855*
- **Multi Vit® Drops [OTC]** *see* Vitamins, Multiple *on page 981*

Mupirocin (myoo PEER oh sin)

Pharmacologic Class Antibiotic, Topical

U.S. Brand Names Bactroban®; Bactroban® Nasal

Use Topical treatment of impetigo due to *Staphylococcus aureus*, beta-hemolytic *Streptococcus*, and *S. pyogenes*

USUAL DOSAGE

Topical: Children and Adults: Apply small amount to affected area 2-5 times/day for 5-14 days

Nasal: In adults (12 years of age and older), approximately one-half of the ointment from the single-use tube should be applied into one nostril and the other half into the other nostril twice daily for 5 days

Contraindications Known hypersensitivity to mupirocin or polyethylene glycol

Pregnancy Risk Factor B

- **Murine®** *see* Carbamide Peroxide *on page 139*
- **Murine® Ear Drops [OTC]** *see* Carbamide Peroxide *on page 139*
- **Muro 128® Ophthalmic [OTC]** *see* Sodium Chloride *on page 858*
- **Murocoll-2® Ophthalmic** *see* Phenylephrine and Scopolamine *on page 729*

Muromonab-CD3 (myoo roe MOE nab-see dee three)

Pharmacologic Class Immunosuppressant Agent

U.S. Brand Names Orthoclone® OKT3

Generic Available No

Mechanism of Action Reverses graft rejection by binding to T cells and interfering with their function by binding T-cell receptor-associated CD3 glycoprotein

Use Treatment of acute allograft rejection in renal transplant patients; treatment of acute hepatic, kidney, and pancreas rejection episodes resistant to conventional treatment. Acute graft-versus-host disease following bone marrow transplantation resistant to conventional treatment.

USUAL DOSAGE I.V. (refer to individual protocols):

Children <30 kg: 2.5 mg/day once daily for 7-14 days

Children >30 kg: 5 mg/day once daily for 7-14 days

OR

Children <12 years: 0.1 mg/kg/day once daily for 10-14 days

Children ≥12 years and Adults: 5 mg/day once daily for 10-14 days

Hemodialysis: Molecular size of OKT3 is 150,000 daltons; not dialyzed by most standard dialyzers; however, may be dialyzed by high flux dialysis; OKT3 will be removed by plasmapheresis; administer following dialysis treatments

Peritoneal dialysis: Significant drug removal is unlikely based on physiochemical characteristics

Dosage Forms INJ: 5 mg/5 mL

Contraindications Hypersensitivity to OKT3 or any murine product; patients in fluid overload or those with >3% weight gain within 1 week prior to start of mouse antibody titers >1:1000

Warnings/Precautions It is imperative, especially prior to the first few doses, that there be no clinical evidence of volume overload, uncontrolled hypertension, or uncompensated heart failure, including a clear chest x-ray and weight restriction of ≤3% above the patient's minimum weight during the week prior to injection.

May result in an increased susceptibility to infection; dosage of concomitant immunosuppressants should be reduced during OKT3 therapy; cyclosporine should be decreased to 50% usual maintenance dose and maintenance therapy resumed about 4 days before stopping OKT3.

Severe pulmonary edema has occurred in patients with fluid overload.

First dose effect (flu-like symptoms, anaphylactic-type reaction): may occur within 30 minutes to 6 hours up to 24 hours after the first dose and may be minimized by using the recommended regimens. See table.

Suggested Prevention/Treatment of Muromonab-CD3 First-Dose Effects

Adverse Reaction	Effective Prevention or Palliation	Supportive Treatment
Severe pulmonary edema	Clear chest x-ray within 24 hours preinjection; weight restriction to ≤3% gain over 7 days preinjection	Prompt intubation and oxygenation 24 hours close observation
Fever, chills	15 mg/kg methylprednisolone sodium succinate 1 hour preinjection; fever reduction to <37.8°C (100°F) 1 hour preinjection; acetaminophen (1 g orally) and diphenhydramine (50 mg orally) 1 hour preinjection	Cooling blanket Acetaminophen prn
Respiratory effects	100 mg hydrocortisone sodium succinate 30 minutes postinjection	Additional 100 mg hydrocortisone sodium succinate prn for wheezing; if respiratory distress, give epinephrine 1:1000 (0.3 mL S.C.)

Cardiopulmonary resuscitation may be needed. If the patient's temperature is >37.8°C, reduce before administering OKT3

Pregnancy Risk Factor C

Adverse Reactions

>10%:

"First-dose" (cytokine release) effects: Onset: 1-3 hours after the dose; duration: 12-16 hours. Severity is mild to life-threatening. Signs and symptoms include fever, chilling, dyspnea, wheezing, chest pain, chest tightness, nausea, vomiting, and diarrhea. Hypervolemic pulmonary edema, nephrotoxicity, meningitis, and encephalopathy are possible. Reactions tend to decrease with repeated doses.

Cardiovascular: Tachycardia (including ventricular)
Central nervous system: Dizziness, faintness
Gastrointestinal: Diarrhea, nausea, vomiting
Hematologic: Transient lymphopenia
Neuromuscular & skeletal: Trembling
Respiratory: Shortness of breath

1% to 10%:

Central nervous system: Headache
Neuromuscular & skeletal: Stiff neck
Ocular: Photophobia
Respiratory: Pulmonary edema

<1%: Arthralgia, aseptic meningitis, chest pain, chest tightness, confusion, coma, dyspnea, fatigue, hallucinations, hypertension, hypotension, increased BUN and creatinine, pruritus, pyrexia, rash, seizures, tremor, wheezing. Sensitivity reactions: Anaphylactic-type reactions, flu-like symptoms (ie, fever, chills), infection, pancytopenia, secondary lymphoproliferative disorder or lymphoma, thrombosis of major vessels in renal allograft.

Drug Interactions Decreased effect: Immunosuppressive drugs; it is recommended to decrease dose of azathioprine to 1 mg/kg and decrease dose of cyclosporine by 50% until 4 days prior to stopping OKT3

Half-Life Time to steady-state: Trough level: 3-14 days; pretreatment levels are restored within 7 days after treatment is terminated.

Education and Monitoring Issues

Patient Education: There may be a severe reaction to the first infusion of this medication. You may experience high fever, chills, difficulty breathing, or congestion. You will be closely monitored and comfort measures provided. Effects are substantially reduced with subsequent infusions. During the period of therapy and for some time after the regimen of infusions you will be susceptible to infection. People may wear masks and gloves while caring for you to protect you as much as possible from infection (avoid

(Continued)

Muromonab-CD3 *(Continued)*

crowds and people with infections or contagious diseases). You may experience dizziness, faintness, or trembling (use caution until response to medication is known); nausea or vomiting (frequent small meals, frequent mouth care); sensitivity to direct sunlight (wear dark glasses, and protective clothing, use sunscreen, or avoid exposure to direct sunlight). Report chest pain or tightness; symptoms of respiratory infection, wheezing, or difficulty breathing; vision change; or muscular trembling.

Monitoring Parameters: Chest x-ray, weight gain, CBC with differential, temperature, vital signs (blood pressure, temperature, pulse, respiration); immunologic monitoring of T cells, serum levels of OKT3

Reference Range:

OKT3 serum concentrations:

Serum level monitoring should be performed in conjunction with lymphocyte subset determinations; Trough concentration sampling best correlates with clinical outcome. Serial monitoring may provide a better early indicator of inadequate dosing during induction or rejection.

Mean serum trough levels rise during the first 3 days, then average 0.9 mcg/mL on days 3-14

Circulating levels ≥0.8 mcg/mL block the function of cytotoxic T cells *in vitro* and *in vivo*

Several recent analysis have suggested appropriate dosage adjustments of OKT3 induction course are better determined with OKT3 serum levels versus lymphocyte subset determination; however, no prospective controlled trials have been performed to validate the equivalency of these tests in predicting clinical outcome.

Lymphocyte subset monitoring: CD3+ cells: Trough sample measurement is preferable and reagent utilized defines reference range.

OKT3-FITC: <10-50 cells/mm^3 or <3% to 5%

CD3(IgG1)-FITC: similar to OKT3-FITC

Leu-4a: Higher number of CD3+ cells appears acceptable

Dosage adjustments should be made in conjunction with clinical response and based upon trends over several consecutive days

Manufacturer Ortho Biotech, Inc

Related Information

Pharmaceutical Manufacturers Directory *on page 1020*

- **Muroptic-5® [OTC]** *see* Sodium Chloride *on page 858*
- **Muro's Opcon®** *see* Naphazoline *on page 636*
- **Muse® Pellet** *see* Alprostadil *on page 38*
- **M.V.I.®** *see* Vitamins, Multiple *on page 981*
- **M.V.I.®-12** *see* Vitamins, Multiple *on page 981*
- **M.V.I.® Concentrate** *see* Vitamins, Multiple *on page 981*
- **M.V.I.® Pediatric** *see* Vitamins, Multiple *on page 981*
- **Myambutol®** *see* Ethambutol *on page 339*
- **Mycelex®** *see* Clotrimazole *on page 220*
- **Mycelex®-7** *see* Clotrimazole *on page 220*
- **Mycelex®-G** *see* Clotrimazole *on page 220*
- **Mycifradin** *see* Neomycin *on page 642*
- **Mycifradin® Sulfate Oral** *see* Neomycin *on page 642*
- **Mycifradin® Sulfate Topical** *see* Neomycin *on page 642*
- **Mycinettes® [OTC]** *see* Benzocaine *on page 98*
- **Mycitracin® Topical [OTC]** *see* Bacitracin, Neomycin, and Polymyxin B *on page 90*
- **Myclo-Derm** *see* Clotrimazole *on page 220*
- **Myclo-Gyne** *see* Clotrimazole *on page 220*
- **Mycobutin®** *see* Rifabutin *on page 819*
- **Mycogen II Topical** *see* Nystatin and Triamcinolone *on page 670*
- **Mycolog®-II Topical** *see* Nystatin and Triamcinolone *on page 670*
- **Myconel® Topical** *see* Nystatin and Triamcinolone *on page 670*

Mycophenolate (mye koe FEN oh late)

Pharmacologic Class Immunosuppressant Agent

U.S. Brand Names CellCept®

Mechanism of Action Inhibition of purine synthesis of human lymphocytes and proliferation of human lymphocytes

Use Immunosuppressant used with corticosteroids and cyclosporine to prevent organ rejection in patients receiving allogenic renal and cardiac transplants; treatment of rejection in liver transplant patients unable to tolerate tacrolimus or cyclosporine due to neurotoxicity; mild rejection in heart transplant patients; treatment of moderate-severe psoriasis

Intravenous formulation is an alternative dosage form to oral capsules and tablets

Mycophenolate Adverse Reactions Reported in >10%

Adverse Reaction	MM 2 g/day	MM 3 g/day
Body as a Whole		
Pain	33	31.2
Abdominal pain	12.1-24.7	11.9-27.6
Fever	20.4	23.3
Headache	20.1	16.1
Infection	12.7-18.2	15.6-20.9
Sepsis	17.6-20.8	17.5-19.7
Asthenia	13.7	16.1
Chest pain	13.4	13.3
Back pain	11.6	12.1
Hypertension	17.6-32.4	16.9-28.2
Central Nervous System		
Tremor	11	11.8
Insomnia	8.9	11.8
Dizziness	5.7	11.2
Dermatologic		
Acne	10.1	9.7
Rash	7.7	6.4
Gastrointestinal		
Diarrhea	16.4-31	18.8-36.1
Constipation	21.9	18.5
Nausea	19.9	23.6
Dyspepsia	17.6	13.6
Vomiting	12.5	13.6
Nausea & vomiting	10.4	9.7
Oral monoliasis	10.1	12.1
Hemic/Lymphatic		
Anemia	25.6	25.8
Leukopenia	11.5-23.2	16.3-34.5
Thrombocytopenia	10.1	8.2
Hypochromic anemia	7.4	11.5
Leukocytosis	7.1	10.9
Metabolic/Nutritional		
Peripheral edema	28.6	27
Hypercholesterolemia	12.8	8.5
Hypophosphatemia	12.5	15.8
Edema	12.2	11.8
Hypokalemia	10.1	10
Hyperkalemia	8.9	10.3
Hyperglycemia	8.6	12.4
Respiratory		
Infection	15.8-21	13.1-23.9
Dyspnea	15.5	17.3
Cough increase	15.5	13.3
Pharyngitis	9.5	11.2
Bronchitis	8.5	11.9
Pneumonia	3.6	10.6
Urogenital		
UTI	37.2-45.5	37-44.4
Hematuria	14	12.1
Kidney tubular necrosis	6.3	10
Urinary tract disorder	6.7	10.6

USUAL DOSAGE

Oral:

Children: 600 mg/m^2/dose twice daily; **Note:** Limited information regarding mycophenolate use in pediatric patients is currently available in the literature: 32 pediatric patients (14 underwent living donor and 18 receiving cadaveric donor renal transplants) received mycophenolate 8-30 mg/kg/dose orally twice daily with cyclosporine, prednisone, and Atgam® induction; however, pharmacokinetic studies suggest that doses of mycophenolate adjusted to body surface area resulted in AUCs which better approximated those of adults versus doses adjusted for body weight which resulted in lower AUCs in pediatric patients

(Continued)

Mycophenolate *(Continued)*

Adults: 1 g twice daily within 72 hours of transplant (although 3 g daily has been given in some clinical trials, there was decreased tolerability and no efficacy advantage)

Dosing adjustment in renal impairment: Doses >2 g/day are not recommended in these patients because of the possibility for enhanced immunosuppression as well as toxicities

Dosing adjustment in severe chronic renal impairment: Cl_{cr} <25 mL/minute/1.73 m^2: Doses of >1 g administered twice daily should be avoided; patients should also be carefully observed; no dose adjustments are needed in renal transplant patients experiencing delayed graft function postoperatively

Hemodialysis: Not removed; supplemental dose is not necessary

Peritoneal dialysis: Supplemental dose is not necessary

Dosing adjustment for neutropenia: ANC <1.3 x 10^3/µL: Dosing should be interrupted or the dose reduced, appropriate diagnostic tests performed and patients managed appropriately

Dosage Forms CAP: 250 mg. **POWDER for inj:** 500 mg. **TAB, film coated:** 500 mg

Contraindications Hypersensitivity to mycophenolate mofetil, mycophenolic acid or any ingredient; intravenous is contraindicated in patients who are allergic to polysorbate 80

Warnings/Precautions Increased risk for infection and development of lymphoproliferative disorders. Patients should be monitored appropriately and given supportive treatment should these conditions occur. Increased toxicity in patients with renal impairment. Should be used with caution in patients with active peptic ulcer disease.

Because mycophenolate mofetil has demonstrated teratogenic effects in rats and rabbits, tablets should not be crushed and capsules should not be opened or crushed. Avoid inhalation or direct contact with skin or mucous membranes of the powder contained in the capsules. Caution should be exercised in the handling and preparation of solutions of intravenous mycophenolate. Avoid skin contact with the solution. If such contact occurs, wash thoroughly with soap and water, rinse eyes with plain water.

Pregnancy Risk Factor C

Adverse Reactions 1% to 10%: Thrombophlebitis and thrombosis (4%) with intravenous administration

See table on previous page

Drug Interactions

Decreased effect: Antacids decrease C_{max} and AUC, **do not administer together**; cholestyramine decreases AUC, **do not administer together**

Increased toxicity: Acyclovir and ganciclovir levels may increase due to competition for tubular secretion of these drugs; probenecid may increase mycophenolate levels due to inhibition of tubular secretion; salicylates: high doses may increase free fraction of mycophenolic acid

Half-Life 18 hours; Serum concentrations: Correlation of toxicity or efficacy is still being developed, however, one study indicated that 12-hour AUCs >40 mcg/mL/hour were correlated with efficacy and decreased episodes of rejection.

Education and Monitoring Issues

Patient Education: Take as directed, preferably 1 hour before or 2 hours after meals. Do not take within 1 hour before or 2 hours after antacids or cholestyramine medications. Do not alter dose and do not discontinue without consulting prescriber. Maintain adequate hydration (2-3 L/day of fluids unless instructed to restrict fluid intake) during entire course of therapy. You will be susceptible to infection (avoid crowds and people with infections or contagious diseases). If you are diabetic, monitor glucose levels closely (may alter glucose levels). You may experience dizziness or trembling (use caution until response to medication is known); nausea or vomiting (frequent small meals, frequent mouth care may help); diarrhea (boiled milk, yogurt, or buttermilk may help); sores or white plaques in mouth (frequent rinsing of mouth and frequent mouth care may help); or muscle or back pain (mild analgesics may be recommended). Report chest pain; acute headache or dizziness; symptoms of respiratory infection, cough, or difficulty breathing; unresolved gastrointestinal effects; fatigue, chills, fever unhealed sores, white plaques in mouth; irritation in genital area or unusual discharge; unusual bruising or bleeding; or other unusual effects related to this medication.

Manufacturer Roche Laboratories

Related Information

Pharmaceutical Manufacturers Directory *on page 1020*

- ♦ **Mycostatin®** *see* Nystatin *on page 670*
- ♦ **Myco-Triacet® II** *see* Nystatin and Triamcinolone *on page 670*
- ♦ **Mydfrin® Ophthalmic Solution** *see* Phenylephrine *on page 727*
- ♦ **Mydriacyl®** *see* Tropicamide *on page 958*
- ♦ **Mykrox®** *see* Metolazone *on page 594*
- ♦ **Mylanta AR® [OTC]** *see* Famotidine *on page 350*
- ♦ **Mylanta® Gelcaps®** *see* Calcium Carbonate and Magnesium Carbonate *on page 131*
- ♦ **Myleran®** *see* Busulfan *on page 122*
- ♦ **Myotonachol™** *see* Bethanechol *on page 106*
- ♦ **Myphetane DC®** *see* Brompheniramine, Phenylpropanolamine, and Codeine *on page 114*

- ♦ **Mysoline®** *see* Primidone *on page 766*
- ♦ **Mytrex® F Topical** *see* Nystatin and Triamcinolone *on page 670*
- ♦ **Mytussin® [OTC]** *see* Guaifenesin *on page 423*
- ♦ **Mytussin® AC** *see* Guaifenesin and Codeine *on page 424*
- ♦ **Mytussin® DAC** *see* Guaifenesin, Pseudoephedrine, and Codeine *on page 425*
- ♦ **Mytussin® DM [OTC]** *see* Guaifenesin and Dextromethorphan *on page 424*
- ♦ **M-Zole® 7 Dual Pack [OTC]** *see* Miconazole *on page 600*

Nabumetone (na BYOO me tone)

Pharmacologic Class Nonsteroidal Anti-Inflammatory Agent (NSAID)

U.S. Brand Names Relafen®

Generic Available No

Mechanism of Action Nabumetone is a nonacidic, nonsteroidal anti-inflammatory drug that is rapidly metabolized after absorption to a major active metabolite, 6-methoxy-2-naphthylacetic acid. As found with previous nonsteroidal anti-inflammatory drugs, nabumetone's active metabolite inhibits the cyclo-oxygenase enzyme which is indirectly responsible for the production of inflammation and pain during arthritis by way of enhancing the production of endoperoxides and prostaglandins E_2 and I_2 (prostacyclin). The active metabolite of nabumetone is felt to be the compound primarily responsible for therapeutic effect. Comparatively, the parent drug is a poor inhibitor of prostaglandin synthesis.

Use Management of osteoarthritis and rheumatoid arthritis

Unlabeled use: Sunburn, mild to moderate pain

USUAL DOSAGE Adults: Oral: 1000 mg/day; an additional 500-1000 mg may be needed in some patients to obtain more symptomatic relief; may be administered once or twice daily

Dosing adjustment in renal impairment: None necessary; however, adverse effects due to accumulation of inactive metabolites of nabumetone that are renally excreted have not been studied and should be considered

Dosage Forms TAB: 500 mg, 750 mg

Contraindications Hypersensitivity to nabumetone; should not be administered to patients with active peptic ulceration and those with severe hepatic impairment or in patients in whom nabumetone, aspirin, or other NSAIDs have induced asthma, urticaria, or other allergic-type reactions; fatal asthmatic reactions have occurred following NSAID administration

Warnings/Precautions Elderly patients may sometimes require lower doses; patients with impaired renal function may need a dose reduction; use with caution in patients with severe hepatic impairment

Pregnancy Risk Factor C; D (3rd trimester)

Adverse Reactions

>10%:

Central nervous system: Dizziness
Dermatologic: Rash
Gastrointestinal: Abdominal cramps, heartburn, indigestion, nausea

1% to 10%:

Central nervous system: Headache, nervousness
Dermatologic: Itching
Endocrine & metabolic: Fluid retention
Gastrointestinal: Vomiting
Otic: Tinnitus

<1%: Acute renal failure, agranulocytosis, allergic rhinitis, anemia, angioedema, arrhythmia, aseptic meningitis, bone marrow suppression, blurred vision, confusion, congestive heart failure, conjunctivitis, cystitis, decreased hearing, drowsiness, dry eyes, epistaxis, erythema multiforme, gastritis, GI ulceration, hallucinations, hemolytic anemia, hepatitis, hot flashes, hypertension, insomnia, leukopenia, mental depression, peripheral neuropathy, polydipsia, polyuria, Stevens-Johnson syndrome, tachycardia, thrombocytopenia, toxic amblyopia, toxic epidermal necrolysis, urticaria

Alcohol Interactions Avoid use (may enhance gastric mucosal irritation)

Onset May require several days to maximum effect

Half-Life Major metabolite: 24 hours

Education and Monitoring Issues

Patient Education: Take this medication exactly as directed; do not increase dose without consulting prescriber. Do not crush tablets or break capsules. Take with food or milk to reduce GI distress. Maintain adequate fluid intake (2-3 L/day of fluids unless instructed to restrict fluid intake). Do not use alcohol, aspirin, or aspirin-containing medication, and all other anti-inflammatory medications without consulting prescriber. You may experience drowsiness, dizziness, nervousness, or headache (use caution when driving or engaging in tasks requiring alertness until response to drug is known); anorexia, nausea, vomiting, or heartburn (frequent small meals, frequent oral care, sucking lozenges, or chewing gum may help); fluid retention (weigh yourself weekly and report unusual (3-5 lb/week) weight gain). GI bleeding, ulceration, or perforation can occur with or without pain; discontinue medication and contact prescriber if persistent

(Continued)

Nabumetone *(Continued)*

abdominal pain or cramping, or blood in stool occurs. Report breathlessness, difficulty breathing, or unusual cough; chest pain, rapid heartbeat, palpitations; unusual bruising/bleeding; blood in urine, stool, mouth, or vomitus; swollen extremities; skin rash or itching; acute fatigue; or changes in hearing or ringing in ears.

Dietary Considerations: Food: Increases the rate but not the extent of oral absorption. Take without regard to meals OR take with food or milk to minimize GI upset.

Manufacturer SmithKline Beecham Pharmaceuticals

Related Information

Nonsteroidal Anti-Inflammatory Agents Comparison *on page 1248*
Pharmaceutical Manufacturers Directory *on page 1020*

Nadolol (nay DOE lole)

Pharmacologic Class Beta Blocker, Nonselective

U.S. Brand Names Corgard®

Generic Available No

Mechanism of Action Competitively blocks response to $beta_1$- and $beta_2$-adrenergic stimulation; does not exhibit any membrane stabilizing or intrinsic sympathomimetic activity

Use Treatment of hypertension and angina pectoris; prevention of myocardial infarction; prophylaxis of migraine headaches

USUAL DOSAGE Oral:

Adults: Initial: 40 mg/day, increase dosage gradually by 40-80 mg increments at 3- to 7-day intervals until optimum clinical response is obtained with profound slowing of heart rate; doses up to 160-240 mg/day in angina and 240-320 mg/day in hypertension may be necessary

Elderly: Initial: 20 mg/day; increase doses by 20 mg increments at 3- to 7-day intervals; usual dosage range: 20-240 mg/day

Dosing adjustment in renal impairment:

Cl_{cr} 31-40 mL/minute: Administer every 24-36 hours or administer 50% of normal dose
Cl_{cr} 10-30 mL/minute: Administer every 24-48 hours or administer 50% of normal dose
Cl_{cr} <10 mL/minute: Administer every 40-60 hours or administer 25% of normal dose

Hemodialysis: Moderately dialyzable (20% to 50%); administer dose postdialysis or administer 40 mg supplemental dose

Peritoneal dialysis: Supplemental dose is not necessary

Dosing adjustment/comments in hepatic disease: Reduced dose probably necessary

Dosage Forms TAB: 20 mg, 40 mg, 80 mg, 120 mg, 160 mg

Contraindications Uncompensated congestive heart failure, cardiogenic shock, bradycardia or heart block, hypersensitivity to any component, bronchial asthma, bronchospasms, diabetes mellitus

Warnings/Precautions Increase dosing interval in patients with renal dysfunction; abrupt withdrawal of beta-blockers may result in an exaggerated cardiac beta-adrenergic responsiveness; symptomatology has included reports of tachycardia, hypertension, ischemia, angina, myocardial infarction, and sudden death; it is recommended that patients be tapered gradually off of beta-blockers over a period of 1-2 weeks rather than via abrupt discontinuation; use with caution in patients with bronchial asthma, bronchospasms, CHF, or diabetes mellitus

Pregnancy Risk Factor C

Pregnancy Implications

Clinical effects on the fetus: No data available on crossing the placenta. Bradycardia, hypotension, hypoglycemia, respiratory depression, hypothermia, IUGR reported. IUGR probably related to maternal hypertension. Alternative beta-blockers are preferred for use during pregnancy due to limited data. Monitor breast-fed infant for symptoms of beta-blockade.

Breast-feeding/lactation: Crosses into breast milk. American Academy of Pediatrics considers **compatible** with breast-feeding.

Adverse Reactions

>5%:

Central nervous system: Nightmares
Neuromuscular & skeletal: Paresthesia of toes and fingers

1% to 5%:

Cardiovascular: Bradycardia, reduced peripheral circulation, congestive heart failure, chest pain, orthostatic hypotension, Raynaud's syndrome, edema
Central nervous system: Mental depression, dizziness, drowsiness, vivid dreams, insomnia, lethargy, fatigue (2%), confusion, headache
Dermatologic: Itching, rash
Endocrine & metabolic: Decreased sexual ability
Gastrointestinal: Constipation, vomiting, stomach discomfort, diarrhea, nausea
Genitourinary: Impotence
Hematologic: Thrombocytopenia
Neuromuscular & skeletal: Weakness
Ocular: Dry eyes
Respiratory: Dyspnea, wheezing, nasal congestion

Miscellaneous: Cold extremities

Drug Interactions

Albuterol (and other $beta_2$ agonists): Effects may be blunted by nonspecific beta-blockers

Alpha-blockers (prazosin, terazosin): Concurrent use of beta-blockers may increase risk of orthostasis

Clonidine: Hypertensive crisis after or during withdrawal of either agent

Drugs which slow A-V conduction (digoxin): Effects may be additive with beta-blockers

Epinephrine (including local anesthetics with epinephrine): Propranolol may cause hypertension

Glucagon: Nadolol may blunt the hyperglycemic action of glucagon

Insulin and oral hypoglycemics: Nadolol may mask symptoms of hypoglycemia.

Nadolol increases antipyrine's half-life

NSAIDs (ibuprofen, indomethacin, naproxen, piroxicam) may reduce the antihypertensive effects of beta-blockers

Salicylates may reduce the antihypertensive effects of beta-blockers

Sulfonylureas: Beta-blockers may alter response to hypoglycemic agents

Verapamil or diltiazem may have synergistic or additive pharmacological effects when taken concurrently with beta-blockers

Alcohol Interactions Limit use (may increase risk of hypotension or dizziness)

Duration 24 hours

Half-Life 10-24 hours; increased half-life with decreased renal function; End-stage renal disease: 45 hours

Education and Monitoring Issues

Patient Education: Check pulse daily prior to taking medication. If pulse is <50, hold medication and consult prescriber. Do not adjust dosage without consulting prescriber. May cause dizziness, fatigue, blurred vision; change position slowly (lying/sitting to standing) and use caution when driving or engaging in tasks that require alertness until response to drug is known. Exercise and increasing bulk or fiber in diet may help resolve constipation. If diabetic, monitor serum glucose closely (the drug may mask symptoms of hypoglycemia). Report swelling in feet or legs, difficulty breathing or persistent cough, unresolved fatigue, unusual weight gain >5 lb/week, or unresolved constipation.

Related Information

Beta-Blockers Comparison *on page 1233*

♦ **Nadopen-V®** *see* Penicillin V Potassium *on page 713*

♦ **Nadostine®** *see* Nystatin *on page 670*

Nafarelin (NAF a re lin)

Pharmacologic Class Hormone, Posterior Pituitary; Luteinizing Hormone-Releasing Hormone Analog

U.S. Brand Names Synarel®

Generic Available No

Mechanism of Action Potent synthetic decapeptide analogue of gonadotropin-releasing hormone (GnRH; LHRH) which is approximately 200 times more potent than GnRH in terms of pituitary release of luteinizing hormone (LH) and follicle-stimulating hormone (FSH). Effects on the pituitary gland and sex hormones are dependent upon its length of administration. After acute administration, an initial stimulation of the release of LH and FSH from the pituitary is observed; an increase in androgens and estrogens subsequently follows. Continued administration of nafarelin, however, suppresses gonadotrope responsiveness to endogenous GnRH resulting in reduced secretion of LH and FSH and, secondarily, decreased ovarian and testicular steroid production.

Use Treatment of endometriosis, including pain and reduction of lesions; treatment of central precocious puberty (gonadotropin-dependent precocious puberty) in children of both sexes

USUAL DOSAGE

Endometriosis: Adults: Female: 1 spray (200 mcg) in 1 nostril each morning and the other nostril each evening starting on days 2-4 of menstrual cycle for 6 months

Central precocious puberty: Children: Males/Females: 2 sprays (400 mcg) into each nostril in the morning 2 sprays (400 mcg) into each nostril in the evening. If inadequate suppression, may increase dose to 3 sprays (600 mcg) into alternating nostrils 3 times/day.

Dosage Forms SOLN, nasal: 2 mg/mL (10 mL)

Contraindications Hypersensitivity to GnRH, GnRH-agonist analogs or any components of this product; undiagnosed abnormal vaginal bleeding; pregnancy; lactation

Warnings/Precautions Use with caution in patients with risk factors for decreased bone mineral content, nafarelin therapy may pose an additional risk; hypersensitivity reactions occur in 0.2% of the patients; safety and efficacy in children have not been established

Pregnancy Risk Factor X

Adverse Reactions

>10%:

Central nervous system: Headache, emotional lability

Dermatologic: Acne

(Continued)

Nafarelin *(Continued)*

Endocrine & metabolic: Hot flashes, decreased libido, decreased breast size
Genitourinary: Vaginal dryness
Neuromuscular & skeletal: Myalgia
Respiratory: Nasal irritation

1% to 10%:
Cardiovascular: Edema, chest pain
Central nervous system: Insomnia
Dermatologic: Urticaria, rash, pruritus, seborrhea
Respiratory: Shortness of breath

<1%: Increased libido, weight loss

Education and Monitoring Issues

Patient Education: You will begin this treatment between days 2-4 of your regular menstrual cycle. Use as directed - daily at the same time (arising and bedtime), and rotate nostrils. Maintain regular follow-up schedule. You may experience hot flashes, flushing or redness (layered clothing and cool environment may help), decreased or increased libido, emotional lability, weight gain, decreased breast size, or hirsutism. Report any breakthrough bleeding or continuing menstruation or musculoskeletal pain. Do not use a nasal decongestant within 30 minutes after nafarelin.

Manufacturer Searle

Related Information

Pharmaceutical Manufacturers Directory *on page 1020*

♦ **Nafazair®** *see* Naphazoline *on page 636*
♦ **Nafcil™ Injection** *see* Nafcillin *on page 630*

Nafcillin (naf SIL in)

Pharmacologic Class Antibiotic, Penicillin

U.S. Brand Names Nafcil™ Injection; Nallpen® Injection; Unipen® Injection; Unipen® Oral

Generic Available Yes

Mechanism of Action Interferes with bacterial cell wall synthesis during active multiplication, causing cell wall death and resultant bactericidal activity against susceptible bacteria

Use Treatment of infections such as osteomyelitis, septicemia, endocarditis, and CNS infections caused by susceptible strains of staphylococci species

USUAL DOSAGE

Neonates:
<2000 g, <7 days: 50 mg/kg/day divided every 12 hours
<2000 g, >7 days: 75 mg/kg/day divided every 8 hours
>2000 g, <7 days: 50 mg/kg/day divided every 8 hours
>2000 g, >7 days: 75 mg/kg/day divided every 6 hours

Children:
Oral: 25-50 mg/kg/day in 4 divided doses
I.M.: 25 mg/kg twice daily
I.V.:
Mild to moderate infections: 50-100 mg/kg/day in divided doses every 6 hours
Severe infections: 100-200 mg/kg/day in divided doses every 4-6 hours
Maximum dose: 12 g/day

Adults:
Oral: 250-500 mg (up to 1 g) every 4-6 hours
I.M.: 500 mg every 4-6 hours
I.V.: 500-2000 mg every 4-6 hours

Dosing adjustment in renal impairment: Not necessary

Dialysis: Not dialyzable (0% to 5%) via hemodialysis; supplemental dosage not necessary with hemo- or peritoneal dialysis or continuous arteriovenous or venovenous hemofiltration (CAVH/CAVHD)

Dosage Forms CAP: 250 mg. **POWDER for inj:** 500 mg, 1 g, 2 g, 4 g, 10 g. **SOLN:** 250 mg/5 mL (100 mL). **TAB:** 500 mg

Contraindications Hypersensitivity to nafcillin or any component or penicillins

Warnings/Precautions Extravasation of I.V. infusions should be avoided; modification of dosage is necessary in patients with both severe renal and hepatic impairment; elimination rate will be slow in neonates; use with caution in patients with cephalosporin hypersensitivity

Pregnancy Risk Factor B

Adverse Reactions Percentage unknown: Acute interstitial nephritis, diarrhea, fever, hypersensitivity reactions, nausea, neutropenia, oxacillin (less likely to cause phlebitis) is often preferred in pediatric patients, pain, rash, thrombophlebitis

Drug Interactions

Decreased effect: Efficacy of oral contraceptives may be reduced; warfarin/anticoagulants
Increased effect: Disulfiram, probenecid may increase penicillin levels

Half-Life 0.5-1.5 hours, with normal hepatic function; End-stage renal disease: 1.2 hours

Education and Monitoring Issues

Patient Education: Oral: Take at regular intervals around-the-clock, preferably on and empty stomach with full glass of water. Take complete course of treatment as prescribed. You may experience nausea or vomiting; small frequent meals and good mouth care may help. If diabetic, drug may cause false tests with Clinitest® urine glucose monitoring; use of glucose oxidase methods (Clinistix®) or serum glucose monitoring is preferable. This drug may interfere with oral contraceptives; an alternate form of birth control should be used. Report persistent fever, sore throat, sores in mouth, diarrhea, unusual bleeding or bruising. Report difficulty breathing or skin rash. Notify prescriber if condition does not respond to treatment.

Monitoring Parameters: Periodic CBC, urinalysis, BUN, serum creatinine, AST and ALT; observe for signs and symptoms of anaphylaxis during first dose

Related Information

Antibiotic Treatment of Adults With Infective Endocarditis *on page 1179*

Community Acquired Pneumonia in Adults *on page 1200*

Naftifine (NAF ti feen)

Pharmacologic Class Antifungal Agent

U.S. Brand Names Naftin®

Use Topical treatment of tinea cruris (jock itch), tinea corporis (ringworm), and tinea pedis (athlete's foot)

USUAL DOSAGE Adults: Topical: Apply cream once daily and gel twice daily (morning and evening) for up to 4 weeks

Contraindications Hypersensitivity to any component

Pregnancy Risk Factor B

♦ **Naftin®** *see* Naftifine *on page 631*

Nalbuphine (NAL byoo feen)

Pharmacologic Class Analgesic, Narcotic

U.S. Brand Names Nubain®

Generic Available Yes

Mechanism of Action Binds to opiate receptors in the CNS, causing inhibition of ascending pain pathways, altering the perception of and response to pain; produces generalized CNS depression

Use Relief of moderate to severe pain; preoperative analgesia, postoperative and surgical anesthesia, and obstetrical analgesia during labor and delivery

USUAL DOSAGE I.M., I.V., S.C.:

Children 10 months to 14 years: Premedication: 0.2 mg/kg; maximum: 20 mg/dose

Adults: 10 mg/70 kg every 3-6 hours; maximum single dose: 20 mg; maximum daily dose: 160 mg

Dosing adjustment/comments in hepatic impairment: Use with caution and reduce dose

Dosage Forms INJ: 10 mg/mL (1 mL, 10 mL), 20 mg/mL (1 mL, 10 mL)

Contraindications Hypersensitivity to nalbuphine or any component, including sulfites

Warnings/Precautions Use with caution in patients with recent myocardial infarction, biliary tract surgery, or sulfite sensitivity; may produce respiratory depression; use with caution in women delivering premature infants; use with caution in patients with a history of drug dependence, head trauma or increased intracranial pressure, decreased hepatic or renal function, or pregnancy; tolerance or drug dependence may result from extended use

Pregnancy Risk Factor B; D (if used for prolonged periods or in high doses at term)

Adverse Reactions

>10%:

Central nervous system: Drowsiness, CNS depression, narcotic withdrawal

Miscellaneous: Histamine release

1% to 10%:

Cardiovascular: Hypotension, flushing

Central nervous system: Dizziness, headache

Dermatologic: Urticaria, rash

Gastrointestinal: Nausea, vomiting, anorexia, xerostomia

Local: Pain at injection site

Neuromuscular & skeletal: Weakness

Respiratory: Pulmonary edema

<1%: Biliary spasm, blurred vision, confusion, decreased urination, hallucinations, hypertension, insomnia, GI irritation, mental depression, nervousness, nightmares, paradoxical CNS stimulation, respiratory depression, restlessness, shortness of breath, tachycardia, toxic megacolon, ureteral spasm

Drug Interactions Increased toxicity: Barbiturate anesthetics may increase CNS depression

Alcohol Interactions Avoid use (may increase central nervous system depression)

Onset Peak effect: I.M.: 30 minutes; I.V.: 1-3 minutes

Half-Life 3.5-5 hours

Education and Monitoring Issues

Patient Education: If self-administered, use exactly as directed (do not increase dose or frequency); may cause physical and/or psychological dependence. While using this

(Continued)

Nalbuphine *(Continued)*

medication, do not use alcohol and other prescription or OTC medications (especially sedatives, tranquilizers, antihistamines, or pain medications) without consulting prescriber. Maintain adequate hydration (2-3 L/day of fluids unless instructed to restrict fluid intake). May cause hypotension, dizziness, drowsiness, impaired coordination, or blurred vision (use caution when driving, climbing stairs, or changing position - rising from sitting or lying to standing, or when engaging in tasks requiring alertness until response to drug is known); loss of appetite, nausea, or vomiting (frequent mouth care, small frequent meals, chewing gum, or sucking lozenges may help); constipation (increased exercise, fluids, or dietary fruit and fiber may help - if constipation remains an unresolved problem, consult prescriber about use of stool softeners). Report chest pain, slow or rapid heartbeat, acute dizziness or persistent headache; changes in mental status; swelling of extremities or unusual weight gain; changes in urinary elimination or pain on urination; acute headache; back or flank pain or muscle spasms; blurred vision; skin rash; or shortness of breath.

Monitoring Parameters: Relief of pain, respiratory and mental status, blood pressure

Related Information

Lipid-Lowering Agents Comparison *on page 1243*
Narcotic Agonists Comparison *on page 1244*

- **Naldecon®** *see* Chlorpheniramine, Phenyltoloxamine, Phenylpropanolamine, and Phenylephrine *on page 187*
- **Naldecon® Senior DX [OTC]** *see* Guaifenesin and Dextromethorphan *on page 424*
- **Naldecon® Senior EX [OTC]** *see* Guaifenesin *on page 423*
- **Naldelate®** *see* Chlorpheniramine, Phenyltoloxamine, Phenylpropanolamine, and Phenylephrine *on page 187*
- **Nalfon®** *see* Fenoprofen *on page 354*
- **Nalgest®** *see* Chlorpheniramine, Phenyltoloxamine, Phenylpropanolamine, and Phenylephrine *on page 187*
- **Nallpen® Injection** *see* Nafcillin *on page 630*

Nalmefene (NAL me feen)

Pharmacologic Class Antidote

U.S. Brand Names Revex®

Mechanism of Action As a 6-methylene analog of naltrexone, nalmefene acts as a competitive antagonist at opioid receptor sites, preventing or reversing the respiratory depression, sedation, and hypotension induced by opiates; no pharmacologic activity of its own (eg, opioid agonist activity) has been demonstrated

Use Complete or partial reversal of opioid drug effects, including respiratory depression induced by natural or synthetic opioids; reversal of postoperative opioid depression; management of known or suspected opioid overdose (if opioid dependence is suspected, nalmefene should only be used in opioid overdose if the likelihood of overdose is high based on history or the clinical presentation of respiratory depression with concurrent pupillary constriction is present)

USUAL DOSAGE

Reversal of postoperative opioid depression: Blue labeled product (100 mcg/mL): Titrate to reverse the undesired effects of opioids; initial dose for nonopioid dependent patients: 0.25 mcg/kg followed by 0.25 mcg/kg incremental doses at 2- to 5-minute intervals; after a total dose of >1 mcg/kg, further therapeutic response is unlikely

Management of known/suspected opioid overdose: Green labeled product (1000 mcg/mL): Initial dose: 0.5 mg/70 kg; may repeat with 1 mg/70 kg in 2-5 minutes; further increase beyond a total dose of 1.5 mg/70 kg will not likely result in improved response and may result in cardiovascular stress and precipitated withdrawal syndrome. (If opioid dependency is suspected, administer a challenge dose of 0.1 mg/70 kg; if no withdrawal symptoms are observed in 2 minutes, the recommended doses can be administered.)

Dosing adjustment in renal or hepatic impairment: Not necessary with single uses, however, slow administration (over 60 seconds) of incremental doses is recommended to minimize hypertension and dizziness

Dosage Forms INJ: 100 mcg/mL [blue label] (1 mL); 1000 mcg/mL [green label] (2 mL)

Contraindications Hypersensitivity to nalmefene, naltrexone, or components

Warnings/Precautions May induce symptoms of acute withdrawal in opioid-dependent patients; recurrence of respiratory depression is possible if the opioid involved is long-acting; observe patients until there is no reasonable risk of recurrent respiratory depression; dosage may need to be decreased in renal and hepatic impairment; safety and efficacy have not been established in children; avoid abrupt reversal of opioid effects in patients of high cardiovascular risk or who have received potentially cardiotoxic drugs; animal studies indicate nalmefene may not completely reverse buprenorphine-induced respiratory depression

Pregnancy Risk Factor B

Pregnancy Implications Limited information available; do not use in pregnant or lactating women if possible

Adverse Reactions
>10%: Gastrointestinal: Nausea
1% to 10%:
Cardiovascular: Tachycardia, hypertension, hypotension, vasodilation
Central nervous system: Fever, dizziness, headache, chills
Gastrointestinal: Vomiting
Miscellaneous: Postoperative pain
<1%: Agitation, arrhythmia, bradycardia, confusion, depression, diarrhea, myoclonus, nervousness, pharyngitis, pruritus, somnolence, tremor, urinary retention, xerostomia

Drug Interactions Increased effect: Potential increased risk of seizures exists with use of flumazenil and nalmefene coadministration

Onset I.M., S.C.: 5-15 minutes

Half-Life 10.8 hours

Education and Monitoring Issues
Patient Education: This drug can only be administered I.V. You may experience drowsiness, dizziness, or blurred vision for several days; use caution when driving or engaging in tasks requiring alertness until response to drug is known. Small frequent meals and good mouth care may reduce any nausea or vomiting. Report yellowing of eyes or skin, unusual bleeding, dark or tarry stools, acute headache, or palpitations.

Manufacturer Baxter Pharmaceutical Products, Inc

Related Information
Pharmaceutical Manufacturers Directory *on page 1020*

Naloxone (nal OKS one)

Pharmacologic Class Antidote

U.S. Brand Names Narcan® Injection

Generic Available Yes

Mechanism of Action Competes and displaces narcotics at narcotic receptor sites

Use Reverses CNS and respiratory depression in suspected narcotic overdose; neonatal opiate depression; coma of unknown etiology
Investigational: Shock, PCP and alcohol ingestion

USUAL DOSAGE I.M., I.V. (preferred), intratracheal, S.C.:
Postanesthesia narcotic reversal: Infants and Children: 0.01 mg/kg; may repeat every 2-3 minutes as needed based on response
Opiate intoxication:
Birth (including premature infants) to 5 years or <20 kg: 0.1 mg/kg; repeat every 2-3 minutes if needed; may need to repeat doses every 20-60 minutes
>5 years or ≥20 kg: 2 mg/dose; if no response, repeat every 2-3 minutes; may need to repeat doses every 20-60 minutes
Continuous infusion: I.V.: Children and Adults: If continuous infusion is required, calculate dosage/hour based on effective intermittent dose used and duration of adequate response seen, titrate dose 0.04-0.16 mg/kg/hour for 2-5 days in children, up to 0.8 mg/kg/hour in adults; alternatively, continuous infusion utilizes $^2/_3$ of the initial naloxone bolus on an hourly basis; add 10 times this dose to each liter of D_5W and infuse at a rate of 100 mL/hour; $^1/_2$ of the initial bolus dose should be readministered 15 minutes after initiation of the continuous infusion to prevent a drop in naloxone levels; increase infusion rate as needed to assure adequate ventilation
Narcotic overdose: Adults: I.V.: 0.4-2 mg every 2-3 minutes as needed; may need to repeat doses every 20-60 minutes, if no response is observed after 10 mg, question the diagnosis. **Note:** Use 0.1-0.2 mg increments in patients who are opioid dependent and in postoperative patients to avoid large cardiovascular changes.

Dosage Forms INJ: 0.4 mg/mL (1 mL, 2 mL, 10 mL); 1 mg/mL (2 mL, 10 mL); Neonatal: 0.02 mg/mL (2 mL)

Contraindications Hypersensitivity to naloxone or any component

Warnings/Precautions Use with caution in patients with cardiovascular disease; excessive dosages should be avoided after use of opiates in surgery, because naloxone may cause an increase in blood pressure and reversal of anesthesia; may precipitate withdrawal symptoms in patients addicted to opiates, including pain, hypertension, sweating, agitation, irritability, shrill cry, failure to feed

Pregnancy Risk Factor B

Adverse Reactions
Cardiovascular: Hypertension, hypotension, tachycardia, ventricular arrhythmias, cardiac arrest
Central nervous system: Irritability, anxiety, narcotic withdrawal, restlessness, seizures
Gastrointestinal: Nausea, vomiting, diarrhea
Neuromuscular & skeletal: Tremulousness
Respiratory: Dyspnea, pulmonary edema, runny nose, sneezing
Miscellaneous: Diaphoresis

Drug Interactions Decreased effect of narcotic analgesics

Onset Endotracheal, I.M., S.C.: Within 2-5 minutes; I.V.: Within 2 minutes

Duration 20-60 minutes; since shorter than that of most opioids, repeated doses are usually needed
(Continued)

Naloxone *(Continued)*

Half-Life 1-1.5 hours

Education and Monitoring Issues

Patient Education: If patient is responsive, instructions are individualized. This drug can only be administered I.V. Report difficulty breathing, palpitations, or tremors.

Monitoring Parameters: Respiratory rate, heart rate, blood pressure

Related Information

Lipid-Lowering Agents Comparison *on page 1243*

Narcotic Agonists Comparison *on page 1244*

♦ **Nalspan®** *see* Chlorpheniramine, Phenyltoloxamine, Phenylpropanolamine, and Phenylephrine *on page 187*

Naltrexone (nal TREKS one)

Pharmacologic Class Antidote

U.S. Brand Names ReVia®

Generic Available No

Mechanism of Action Naltrexone is a cyclopropyl derivative of oxymorphone similar in structure to naloxone and nalorphine (a morphine derivative); it acts as a competitive antagonist at opioid receptor sites

Use Adjunct to the maintenance of an opioid-free state in detoxified individual; alcoholism

USUAL DOSAGE Do not give until patient is opioid-free for 7-10 days as required by urine analysis; Adults: Oral:

25 mg; if no withdrawal signs within 1 hour give another 25 mg; maintenance regimen is flexible, variable and individualized (50 mg/day to 100-150 mg 3 times/week)

Adjunct in the management of alcoholism: A flexible approach to dosing is recommended by the manufacturer; the following are acceptable regimens:

- 50 mg once daily
- 50 mg once daily on weekdays and 100 mg on Saturdays
- 100 mg every other day
- 150 mg every third day

Dosage Forms TAB: 50 mg

Contraindications Acute hepatitis, liver failure, known hypersensitivity to naltrexone

Warnings/Precautions Dose-related hepatocellular injury is possible; the margin of separation between the apparent safe and hepatotoxic doses appear to be only fivefold or less

Pregnancy Risk Factor C

Adverse Reactions

>10%:

Central nervous system: Insomnia, nervousness, headache, low energy

Gastrointestinal: Abdominal cramping, nausea, vomiting

Neuromuscular & skeletal: Arthralgia

1% to 10%:

Central nervous system: Increased energy, feeling down, irritability, dizziness, anxiety, somnolence

Dermatologic: Rash

Endocrine & metabolic: Polydipsia

Gastrointestinal: Diarrhea, constipation

Genitourinary: Delayed ejaculation, impotency

<1%: Bad dreams, blurred vision, confusion, depression, disorientation, edema, fatigue, hallucinations, increased blood pressure, itching rhinorrhea, narcotic withdrawal, nasal congestion, nightmares, palpitations, paranoia, restlessness, sneezing, suicide attempts, tachycardia

Drug Interactions

Naltrexone decreases effects of opioid-containing products

Lethargy and somnolence have been reported with the combination of naltrexone and thioridazine

Alcohol Interactions Avoid use (may increase central nervous system depression)

Duration 50 mg: 24 hours; 100 mg: 48 hours; 150 mg: 72 hours

Half-Life 4 hours; active metabolite, 6-β-naltrexol: 13 hours

Education and Monitoring Issues

Patient Education: This medication will help you achieve abstinence from opiates if taken as directed. Do not increase or change dose. Do not use opiates or any medications not approved by your prescriber during naltrexone therapy. You may experience drowsiness, dizziness, or blurred vision (use caution when driving or engaging in tasks requiring alertness until response to drug is known); nausea or vomiting (small frequent meals, frequent mouth care, chewing gum, or sucking lozenges may help); decreased sexual function (reversible when drug is discontinued). Report yellowing of skin or eyes, change in color of stool or urine, increased perspiration or chills, acute headache, palpitations, or unusual joint pain.

Manufacturer DuPont Merck Pharmaceutical

Related Information

Pharmaceutical Manufacturers Directory *on page 1020*

Nandrolone (NAN droe lone)

Pharmacologic Class Androgen

U.S. Brand Names Anabolin® Injection; Androlone®-D Injection; Androlone® Injection; Deca-Durabolin® Injection; Durabolin® Injection; Hybolin™ Decanoate Injection; Hybolin™ Improved Injection; Neo-Durabolic Injection

Generic Available Yes

Mechanism of Action Promotes tissue-building processes, increases production of erythropoietin, causes protein anabolism; increases hemoglobin and red blood cell volume

Use Control of metastatic breast cancer; management of anemia of renal insufficiency

USUAL DOSAGE Deep I.M. (into gluteal muscle):

Children 2-13 years: (decanoate): 25-50 mg every 3-4 weeks
Adults:
  Male:
    Breast cancer (phenpropionate): 50-100 mg/week
    Anemia of renal insufficiency (decanoate): 100-200 mg/week
  Female: 50-100 mg/week
    Breast cancer (phenpropionate): 50-100 mg/week
    Anemia of renal insufficiency (decanoate): 50-100 mg/week

Dosage Forms

Nandrolone phenpropionate: **INJ in oil:** 25 mg/mL (5 mL), 50 mg/mL (2 mL)
Nandrolone decanoate: **INJ**: In oil: 50 mg/mL (1 mL, 2 mL), 100 mg/mL (1 mL, 2 mL), 200 mg/mL (1 mL); Repository: 50 mg/mL (2 mL), 100 mg/mL (2 mL), 200 mg/mL (2 mL)

Contraindications Carcinoma of breast or prostate, nephrosis, pregnancy and infants, hypersensitivity to any component

Warnings/Precautions Monitor diabetic patients carefully; anabolic steroids may cause peliosis hepatis, liver cell tumors, and blood lipid changes with increased risk of arteriosclerosis; use with caution in elderly patients, they may be at greater risk for prostatic hypertrophy; use with caution in patients with cardiac, renal, or hepatic disease or epilepsy

Pregnancy Risk Factor X

Adverse Reactions

Male:

Postpubertal:
  >10%:
    Dermatologic: Acne
    Endocrine & metabolic: Gynecomastia
    Genitourinary: Bladder irritability, priapism
  1% to 10%:
    Central nervous system: Insomnia, chills
    Endocrine & metabolic: Decreased libido, hepatic dysfunction
    Gastrointestinal: Nausea, diarrhea
    Genitourinary: Prostatic hypertrophy (elderly)
    Hematologic: Iron deficiency anemia, suppression of clotting factors
  <1%: Hepatic necrosis, hepatocellular carcinoma
Prepubertal:
  >10%:
    Dermatologic: Acne
    Endocrine & metabolic: Virilism
  1% to 10%:
    Central nervous system: Chills, insomnia
    Dermatologic: Hyperpigmentation
    Gastrointestinal: Diarrhea, nausea
    Hematologic: Iron deficiency anemia, suppression of clotting
  <1%: Hepatocellular carcinoma, necrosis

Female:

  >10%: Endocrine & metabolic: Virilism
  1% to 10%:
    Central nervous system: Chills, insomnia
    Endocrine & metabolic: Hypercalcemia
    Gastrointestinal: Nausea, diarrhea
    Hematologic: Iron deficiency anemia, suppression of clotting factors
    Hepatic: Hepatic dysfunction
  <1%: Hepatic necrosis, hepatocellular carcinoma

Drug Interactions Increased toxicity: Oral anticoagulants, insulin, oral hypoglycemic agents, adrenal steroids, ACTH

Onset 3-6 months

Duration 30 days

Education and Monitoring Issues

Patient Education: This drug can only be given I.M. Diabetics should monitor serum glucose closely and notify prescriber of changes; this medication can alter glycemic response. You may experience acne, growth of body hair, loss of libido, impotence, or menstrual irregularity (usually reversible); nausea or vomiting (small frequent meals,

(Continued)

Nandrolone *(Continued)*

frequent mouth care, sucking lozenges, or chewing gum may help); diarrhea (buttermilk, boiled milk, yogurt may help). Report changes in menstrual pattern; enlarged or painful breasts; deepening of voice or unusual growth of body hair; fluid retention (swelling of ankles, feet, or hands, difficulty breathing, or sudden weight gain); unresolved changes in CNS (nervousness, chills, insomnia); change in color of urine or stool; yellowing of eyes or skin; unusual bruising or bleeding; or other adverse reactions.

Naphazoline (naf AZ oh leen)

Pharmacologic Class Adrenergic Agonist Agent

U.S. Brand Names AK-Con®; Albalon® Liquifilm®; Allerest® Eye Drops [OTC]; Clear Eyes® [OTC]; Comfort® [OTC]; Degest® 2 [OTC]; Estivin® II [OTC]; I-Naphline®; Muro's Opcon®; Nafazair®; Naphcon® [OTC]; Naphcon Forte®; Opcon®; Privine®; VasoClear® [OTC]; Vasocon Regular®

Use Topical ocular vasoconstrictor; will temporarily relieve congestion, itching, and minor irritation, and to control hyperemia in patients with superficial corneal vascularity; treatment of nasal congestion; adjunct for sinusitis

USUAL DOSAGE

Nasal:

Children:

<6 years: Intranasal: Not recommended (especially infants) due to CNS depression

6-12 years: 1 spray of 0.05% into each nostril every 6 hours if necessary; therapy should not exceed 3-5 days

Children >12 years and Adults: 0.05%, instill 1-2 drops or sprays every 6 hours if needed; therapy should not exceed 3-5 days

Ophthalmic:

Children <6 years: Not recommended for use due to CNS depression (especially in infants)

Children >6 years and Adults: Instill 1-2 drops into conjunctival sac of affected eye(s) every 3-4 hours; therapy generally should not exceed 3-4 days

Contraindications Hypersensitivity to naphazoline or any component, narrow-angle glaucoma, prior to peripheral iridectomy (in patients susceptible to angle block)

Pregnancy Risk Factor C

- **Naphcon® [OTC]** *see* Naphazoline *on page 636*
- **Naphcon Forte®** *see* Naphazoline *on page 636*
- **Naprelan®** *see* Naproxen *on page 636*
- **Naprosyn®** *see* Naproxen *on page 636*

Naproxen (na PROKS en)

Pharmacologic Class Nonsteroidal Anti-Inflammatory Agent (NSAID)

U.S. Brand Names Aleve® [OTC]; Anaprox®; Naprelan®; Naprosyn®

Generic Available No

Mechanism of Action Inhibits prostaglandin synthesis by decreasing the activity of the enzyme, cyclo-oxygenase, which results in decreased formation of prostaglandin precursors

Use Management of inflammatory disease and rheumatoid disorders (including juvenile rheumatoid arthritis); acute gout; mild to moderate pain; dysmenorrhea; fever, migraine headache

USUAL DOSAGE Oral:

Children >2 years:

Fever: 2.5-10 mg/kg/dose; maximum: 10 mg/kg/day

Juvenile arthritis: 10 mg/kg/day in 2 divided doses

Adults:

Rheumatoid arthritis, osteoarthritis, and ankylosing spondylitis: 500-1000 mg/day in 2 divided doses; may increase to 1.5 g/day of naproxen base for limited time period

Mild to moderate pain or dysmenorrhea: Initial: 500 mg, then 250 mg every 6-8 hours; maximum: 1250 mg/day naproxen base

Dosing adjustment in hepatic impairment: Reduce dose to 50%

Dosage Forms SUSP, oral: 125 mg/5 mL (15 mL, 30 mL, 480 mL). **TAB:** (Aleve®): 200 mg; (Naprosyn®): 250 mg, 375 mg, 500 mg; Controlled release (Naprelan®): 375 mg, 500 mg; As sodium: 220 mg (200 mg base), (Anaprox®): 220 mg (200 mg base), 275 mg (250 mg base), 550 mg (500 mg base)

Contraindications Hypersensitivity to naproxen, aspirin, or other nonsteroidal anti-inflammatory drugs (NSAIDs)

Warnings/Precautions Use with caution in patients with GI disease (bleeding or ulcers), cardiovascular disease (CHF, hypertension), renal or hepatic impairment, and patients receiving anticoagulants; perform ophthalmologic evaluation for those who develop eye complaints during therapy (blurred vision, diminished vision, changes in color vision, retinal changes); NSAIDs may mask signs/symptoms of infections; photosensitivity reported; elderly are at especially high-risk for adverse effects

Pregnancy Risk Factor B; D (if used in 3rd trimester or near delivery)

Adverse Reactions

>10%:

Central nervous system: Dizziness

Dermatologic: Pruritus, rash

Gastrointestinal: Abdominal discomfort, nausea, heartburn, constipation, GI bleeding, ulcers, perforation, indigestion

1% to 10%:

Central nervous system: Headache, nervousness

Dermatologic: Itching

Endocrine & metabolic: Fluid retention

Gastrointestinal: Vomiting

Otic: Tinnitus

<1%: Acute renal failure, agranulocytosis, allergic rhinitis, anemia, angioedema, arrhythmias, aseptic meningitis, blurred vision, bone marrow suppression, confusion, congestive heart failure, conjunctivitis, cystitis, decreased hearing, drowsiness, dry eyes, edema, epistaxis, erythema multiforme, fatigue, gastritis, GI ulceration, hallucinations, hemolytic anemia, hepatitis, hot flashes, hypertension, inhibits platelet aggregation, insomnia, leukopenia, mental depression, peripheral neuropathy, polydipsia, polyuria, prolongs bleeding time, renal dysfunction, shortness of breath, Stevens-Johnson syndrome, tachycardia, thrombocytopenia, toxic amblyopia, toxic epidermal necrolysis, urticaria

Drug Interactions CYP2C8, 2C9, and 2C18 enzyme substrate

Decreased effect of furosemide

Increased toxicity:

Naproxen could displace other highly protein bound drugs, such as oral anticoagulants, hydantoins, salicylates, sulfonamides, and sulfonylureas

Naproxen and warfarin may cause a slight increase in free warfarin

Naproxen and probenecid may cause increased plasma half-life of naproxen

Naproxen and methotrexate may significantly increase and prolong blood methotrexate concentration, which may be severe or fatal

Alcohol Interactions Avoid use (may enhance gastric mucosal irritation; may cause excessive impairment in cognition/motor function)

Onset Analgesia: 1 hour; Anti-inflammatory: Within 2 weeks

Duration Analgesia: Up to 7 hours; Anti-inflammatory: Peak: 2-4 weeks

Half-Life Normal renal function: 12-15 hours; End-stage renal disease: Unchanged

Education and Monitoring Issues

Patient Education: Take this medication exactly as directed; do not increase dose without consulting prescriber. Do not crush tablets or break capsules. Take with food or milk to reduce GI distress. Maintain adequate fluid intake (2-3 L/day of fluids unless instructed to restrict fluid intake). Do not use alcohol, aspirin, or aspirin-containing medication, and all other anti-inflammatory medications without consulting prescriber. You may experience drowsiness, dizziness, lightheadedness, or headache (use caution when driving or engaging in tasks requiring alertness until response to drug is known); anorexia, nausea, vomiting, or heartburn (frequent small meals, frequent mouth care, sucking lozenges, or chewing gum may help); fluid retention (weigh yourself weekly and report unusual (3-5 lb/week) weight gain). GI bleeding, ulceration, or perforation can occur with or without pain; discontinue medication and contact prescriber if persistent abdominal pain or cramping, or blood in stool occurs. Report breathlessness, difficulty breathing, or unusual cough; chest pain, rapid heartbeat, palpitations; unusual bruising/bleeding; blood in urine, stool, mouth, or vomitus; swollen extremities; skin rash or itching; acute fatigue; or changes in eyesight (double vision, color changes, blurred vision), hearing, or ringing in ears.

Dietary Considerations: Food: Food may decrease the rate but not the extent of oral absorption. Drug may cause GI upset, bleeding, ulceration, perforation; take with food or milk to minimize GI upset.

Monitoring Parameters: Occult blood loss, periodic liver function test, CBC, BUN, serum creatinine

Related Information

Nonsteroidal Anti-Inflammatory Agents Comparison *on page 1248*

♦ **Naqua®** *see* Trichlormethiazide *on page 949*

Naratriptan (NAR a trip tan)

Pharmacologic Class Serotonin 5-HT_{1D} Receptor Agonist

U.S. Brand Names Amerge®

Mechanism of Action The therapeutic effect for migraine is due to serotonin agonist activity

Use Treatment of acute migraine headache with or without aura

USUAL DOSAGE

Adults: Oral: 1-2.5 mg at the onset of headache; it is recommended to use the lowest possible dose to minimize adverse effects. If headache returns or does not fully resolve, the dose may be repeated after 4 hours; do not exceed 5 mg in 24 hours.

Elderly: Not recommended for use in the elderly

(Continued)

Naratriptan *(Continued)*

Dosing in renal impairment:

Cl_{cr}: 18-39 mL/minute: Initial: 1 mg; do not exceed 2.5 mg in 24 hours

Cl_{cr}: <15 mL/minute: Do not use

Dosing in hepatic impairment: Contraindicated in patients with severe liver failure; maximum dose: 2.5 mg in 24 hours for patients with mild or moderate liver failure; recommended starting dose: 1 mg

Dosage Forms TAB: 1 mg, 2.5 mg

Contraindications Hypersensitivity to naratriptan or any component; cerebrovascular, peripheral vascular disease (ischemic bowel disease), ischemic heart disease (angina pectoris, history of myocardial infarction, or proven silent ischemia); or in patients with symptoms consistent with ischemic heart disease, coronary artery vasospasm, or Prinzmetal's variant angina; uncontrolled hypertension or patients who have received within 24 hours another 5-HT agonist (sumatriptan, zolmitriptan) or ergotamine-containing product; patients with known risk factors associated with coronary artery disease; patients with severe hepatic or renal disease (Cl_{cr} <15 mL/minute); do not administer naratriptan to patients with hemiplegic or basilar migraine

Warnings/Precautions Use only if there is a clear diagnosis of migraine. Patients who are at risk of CAD but have had a satisfactory cardiovascular evaluation may receive naratriptan but with extreme caution (ie, in a prescriber's office where there are adequate precautions in place to protect the patient). Blood pressure may increase with the administration of naratriptan. Monitor closely, especially with the first administration of the drug. If the patient does not respond to the first dose, re-evaluate the diagnosis of migraine before trying a second dose.

Pregnancy Risk Factor C

Adverse Reactions

1% to 10%:

Central nervous system: Dizziness, drowsiness, malaise/fatigue

Gastrointestinal: Nausea, vomiting

Neuromuscular & skeletal: Paresthesias

Miscellaneous: Pain or pressure in throat or neck

<1% (limited to important or life-threatening symptoms): allergic reaction, atrial flutter/fibrillation), abnormal bilirubin tests, abnormal liver function tests, bradycardia, convulsions, coronary artery vasospasm, EKG changes (PR prolongation, QT_c prolongation, premature ventricular contractions, eye hemorrhage, glycosuria, hallucinations, heart murmurs, hypercholesterolemia, hyperglycemia, hyperlipidemia, hypertension, hypotension, hypothyroidism, ketonuria, myocardial infarction, palpitations, panic, transient myocardial ischemia, ventricular fibrillation, ventricular tachycardia

Drug Interactions

Decreased effect: Smoking increases the clearance of naratriptan

Increased effect/toxicity: Ergot-containing drugs (dihydroergotamine or methysergide) may cause vasospastic reactions when taken with naratriptan. Avoid concomitant use with ergots; separate dose of naratriptan and ergots by at least 24 hours. Oral contraceptives taken with naratriptan reduced the clearance of naratriptan +30% which may contribute to adverse effects. Selective serotonin reuptake inhibitors (SSRIs) (eg, fluoxetine, fluvoxamine, paroxetine, sertraline) may cause lack of coordination, hyperreflexia, or weakness and should be avoided when taking naratriptan.

Alcohol Interactions Avoid use (may cause or worsen headaches)

Onset 30 minutes

Education and Monitoring Issues

Patient Education: This drug is to be used to reduce your migraine, not to prevent or reduce the number of attacks. If headache returns or is not fully resolved, the dose may be repeated after 4 hours. If you have no relief with first dose, do not take a second dose without consulting prescriber. **Do not exceed 5 mg in 24 hours. Do not take within 24 hours of any other migraine medication without first consulting prescriber.** You may experience some dizziness, fatigue, or drowsiness; use caution when driving or engaging in tasks that require alertness until response to drug is known. Frequent mouth care and sucking on lozenges may relieve dry mouth. Report immediately any chest pain, heart throbbing, tightness in throat, skin rash or hives, hallucinations, anxiety, or panic.

Manufacturer GlaxoWellcome

Related Information

Pharmaceutical Manufacturers Directory *on page 1020*

- **Narcan® Injection** *see* Naloxone *on page 633*
- **Narcotic Agonists Comparison** *see page 1244*
- **Nardil®** *see* Phenelzine *on page 722*
- **Naropin™** *see* Ropivacaine *on page 833*
- **Nasacort®** *see* Triamcinolone *on page 944*
- **Nasacort® AQ** *see* Triamcinolone *on page 944*
- **NāSal™ [OTC]** *see* Sodium Chloride *on page 858*
- **Nasalcrom® Nasal Solution** *see* Cromolyn Sodium *on page 231*

♦ **Nasalide® Nasal Aerosol** *see* Flunisolide *on page 373*
♦ **Nasal Moist® [OTC]** *see* Sodium Chloride *on page 858*
♦ **Nasarel™** *see* Flunisolide *on page 373*
♦ **Nascobal®** *see* Cyanocobalamin *on page 233*
♦ **Nasonex®** *see* Mometasone Furoate *on page 615*
♦ **Natabec® [OTC]** *see* Vitamins, Multiple *on page 981*
♦ **Natabec® FA [OTC]** *see* Vitamins, Multiple *on page 981*
♦ **Natabec® Rx** *see* Vitamins, Multiple *on page 981*
♦ **Natacyn® Ophthalmic** *see* Natamycin *on page 639*
♦ **Natalins® [OTC]** *see* Vitamins, Multiple *on page 981*
♦ **Natalins® Rx** *see* Vitamins, Multiple *on page 981*

Natamycin (na ta MYE sin)

Pharmacologic Class Antifungal Agent, Ophthalmic

U.S. Brand Names Natacyn® Ophthalmic

Use Treatment of blepharitis, conjunctivitis, and keratitis caused by susceptible fungi (*Aspergillus, Candida*), *Cephalosporium, Curvularia, Fusarium, Penicillium, Microsporum, Epidermophyton, Blastomyces dermatitidis, Coccidioides immitis, Cryptococcus neoformans, Histoplasma capsulatum, Sporothrix schenckii,* and *Trichomonas vaginalis*

USUAL DOSAGE Adults: Ophthalmic: Instill 1 drop in conjunctival sac every 1-2 hours, after 3-4 days reduce to one drop 6-8 times/day; usual course of therapy is 2-3 weeks.

Contraindications Known hypersensitivity to natamycin or any component

Pregnancy Risk Factor C

♦ **Natisedine** *see* Quinidine *on page 802*
♦ **Natulan** *see* Procarbazine *on page 771*
♦ **Navane®** *see* Thiothixene *on page 914*
♦ **Naxen®** *see* Naproxen *on page 636*
♦ **Nebcin® Injection** *see* Tobramycin *on page 924*
♦ **NebuPent™ Inhalation** *see* Pentamidine *on page 714*

Nedocromil Sodium (ne doe KROE mil SOW dee um)

Pharmacologic Class Mast Cell Stabilizer

U.S. Brand Names Alocril™; Tilade® Inhalation Aerosol

Mechanism of Action Inhibits the activation of and mediator release from a variety of inflammatory cell types associated with asthma including eosinophils, neutrophils, macrophages, mast cells, monocytes, and platelets; it inhibits the release of histamine, leukotrienes, and slow-reacting substance of anaphylaxis; it inhibits the development of early and late bronchoconstriction responses to inhaled antigen

Use

Aerosol: Maintenance therapy in patients with mild to moderate bronchial asthma

Ophthalmic: Treatment of itching associated with allergic conjunctivitis

USUAL DOSAGE Children ≥6 years and Adults: Inhalation: 2 inhalations 4 times/day; may reduce dosage to 2-3 times/day once desired clinical response to initial dose is observed

Dosage Forms AERO: 1.75 mg/activation (16.2 g). **SOLN, ophth:** 2% (5 mL)

Contraindications Hypersensitivity to nedocromil or other ingredients in the preparation

Warnings/Precautions If systemic or inhaled steroid therapy is at all reduced, monitor patients carefully; nedocromil is **not** a bronchodilator and, therefore, should not be used for reversal of acute bronchospasm

Pregnancy Risk Factor B

Adverse Reactions

Aerosol: 1% to 10%:
- Cardiovascular: Chest pain
- Central nervous system: Dizziness, dysphonia, headache, fatigue
- Dermatologic: Rash
- Gastrointestinal: Nausea, vomiting, dyspepsia, diarrhea, abdominal pain, xerostomia, unpleasant taste
- Hepatic: Increased ALT
- Neuromuscular & skeletal: Arthritis, tremor
- Respiratory: Cough, pharyngitis, rhinitis, bronchitis, upper respiratory infection, bronchospasm, increased sputum production

Ophthalmic solution:
- >10:
  - Central nervous system: Headache (40%)
  - Gastrointestinal: Unpleasant taste
  - Ocular: Burning, irritation, stinging
  - Respiratory: Nasal congestion
- 1% to 10%:
  - Ocular: Conjunctivitis, eye redness, photophobia
  - Respiratory: Asthma, rhinitis

Duration 2 hours

(Continued)

Nedocromil Sodium *(Continued)*

Half-Life 1.5-2 hours

Education and Monitoring Issues

Patient Education: Do not use during acute bronchospasm. Use exactly as directed; do not use more often than instructed or discontinue without consulting prescriber. You may experience drowsiness, dizziness, fatigue, especially during early therapy (use caution when driving or engaging in tasks requiring alertness until response to drug is known); dry mouth, nausea, or vomiting (small frequent meals, frequent mouth care, chewing gum, or sucking lozenges may help). Report persistent runny nose, cough, cold symptoms; unresolved gastrointestinal effects; skin rash; joint pain or tremor; or if breathing difficulty persists or worsens.

Manufacturer Rhone-Poulenc Rorer Pharmaceuticals, Inc

Related Information

Pharmaceutical Manufacturers Directory *on page 1020*

♦ **N.E.E.® 1/35** *see* Ethinyl Estradiol and Norethindrone *on page 342*

Nefazodone (nef AY zoe done)

Pharmacologic Class Antidepressant, Serotonin Reuptake Inhibitor/Antagonist

U.S. Brand Names Serzone®

Mechanism of Action Inhibits serotonin (5-HT) reuptake and is a potent antagonist at type 2 serotonin (5-HT) receptors; minimal affinity for cholinergic, histaminic, or alpha$_1$-adrenergic receptors

Use Treatment of depression

USUAL DOSAGE Oral: Adults: 200 mg/day, administered in two divided doses initially, with a range of 300-600 mg/day in two divided doses thereafter

Dosage Forms TAB: 50 mg, 100 mg, 150 mg, 200 mg, 250 mg

Contraindications Hypersensitivity to nefazodone or any component; concomitant use of any MAO inhibitors, pimozide, terfenadine, astemizole, or cisapride

Warnings/Precautions Safety and efficacy in children <18 years of age have not been established; monitor closely and use with extreme caution in patients with cardiac disease, cerebrovascular disease or seizures; very sedating and can be dehydrating; therapeutic effects may take up to 4 weeks to occur; therapy is normally maintained for several months and optimum response is reached to prevent recurrence of depression, discontinue therapy and re-evaluate if priapism occurs

Pregnancy Risk Factor C

Adverse Reactions

>10%:

- Central nervous system: Headache, drowsiness, insomnia, agitation, dizziness
- Gastrointestinal: Xerostomia, nausea, constipation
- Neuromuscular & skeletal: Weakness

1% to 10%:

- Cardiovascular: Postural hypotension
- Central nervous system: Lightheadedness, confusion, memory impairment, abnormal dreams, decreased concentration, ataxia
- Dermatologic: Pruritus, rash
- Gastrointestinal: Vomiting, dyspepsia, diarrhea, increased appetite, thirst, taste perversion
- Neuromuscular & skeletal: Arthralgia, paresthesia, tremor
- Ocular: Blurred vision, abnormal vision, visual field defect
- Respiratory: Cough
- Otic: Tinnitus
- Miscellaneous: Flu syndrome

Drug Interactions CYP3A3/4 enzyme substrate; CYP3A3/4 enzyme inhibitor

Statins (especially lovastatin and simvastatin) have been associated with myositis and rhabdomyolysis when used in combination with nefazodone

Nefazodone likely increases cisapride serum concentrations via CYP3A4 inhibition; this combination may lead to cardiac arrhythmias and should be avoided

Pimozide serum concentration may be elevated; concurrent use is contraindicated

Combined use of nefazodone with an SSRI may produce serotonin syndrome

Nefazodone inhibits the metabolism of triazolam (decrease dose by 75%) and alprazolam (decrease dose by 50%)

Alcohol Interactions Avoid use (may increase central nervous system depression)

Onset Therapeutic effects take at least 2 weeks to appear

Half-Life 2-4 hours (parent compound), active metabolites persist longer

Education and Monitoring Issues

Patient Education: Take exactly as directed (do not increase dose or frequency); may take 2-3 weeks to achieve desired results; may cause physical and/or psychological dependence. Avoid excessive alcohol, caffeine, and other prescription or OTC medications not approved by prescriber. Maintain adequate hydration (2-3 L/day of fluids unless instructed to restrict fluid intake). You may experience drowsiness, dizziness, or lightheadedness (use caution when driving or engaging in tasks requiring alertness until response to drug is known); nausea or vomiting (small frequent meals, frequent mouth care, chewing gum, or sucking lozenges may help); or orthostatic hypotension (use caution when climbing stairs or changing position from lying or sitting to standing). Report persistent insomnia or excessive daytime sedation; muscle cramping, tremors, weakness, or change in gait; chest pain, palpitations, or rapid heartbeat; vision changes or eye pain; difficulty breathing or breathlessness; abdominal pain or blood in stool; or worsening of condition.

Reference Range: Therapeutic plasma levels have not yet been defined

Related Information

Antidepressant Agents Comparison *on page 1231*

Nelfinavir (nel FIN a veer)

Pharmacologic Class Antiretroviral Agent, Protease Inhibitor

U.S. Brand Names Viracept®

Use In combination with other antiretroviral therapy in the treatment of HIV infection

USUAL DOSAGE Oral:

Children 2-13 years: 20-30 mg/kg 3 times/day with a meal or light snack; if tablets are unable to be taken, use oral powder in small amount of water, milk, formula, or dietary supplements; do not use acidic food/juice or store for >6 hours

Adults: 750 mg 3 times/day with meals or 1250 mg twice daily with meals in combination with other antiretroviral therapies

Dosing adjustment in renal impairment: No adjustment needed

Dosing adjustment in hepatic impairment: Use caution when administering to patients with hepatic impairment since eliminated predominantly by the liver

Contraindications Hypersensitivity to nelfinavir or product components; phenylketonuria; concurrent therapy with terfenadine, astemizole, cisapride, triazolam, or midazolam

Warnings/Precautions Avoid use of powder in phenylketonurics since contains phenylalanine; use extreme caution when administered to patients with hepatic insufficiency since nelfinavir is metabolized in the liver and excreted predominantly in the feces; avoid use, if possible, with terfenadine, astemizole, cisapride, triazolam, or midazolam. Concurrent use with some anticonvulsants may significantly limit nelfinavir's effectiveness. Also, avoid concurrent use of amiodarone, quinidine, and ergot alkaloids. Redistribution of fate can occur with protease inhibitors.

Pregnancy Risk Factor B

Adverse Reactions Protease inhibitors cause dyslipidemia which includes elevated cholesterol and triglycerides and a redistribution of body fat centrally to cause "protease paunch", buffalo hump, facial atrophy, and breast enlargement. These agents also cause hyperglycemia.

>10%: Gastrointestinal: Diarrhea (19%)

1% to 10%:

Central nervous system: Decreased concentration

Dermatologic: Rash

Gastrointestinal: Nausea, flatulence, abdominal pain

Neuromuscular & skeletal: Weakness

<1%: Allergy, anemia, anorexia, anxiety, arthralgia, arthritis, back pain, cramps, depression, dermatitis, diaphoresis, dizziness, dyspepsia, dyspnea, emotional lability, epigastric pain, fever, GI bleeding, headache, hepatitis, hyperkinesia, hyperlipemia, hyperuricemia, hypoglycemia, increased LFTs, insomnia, jaundice, kidney calculus, leukopenia, malaise, metabolic acidosis, migraine, mouth ulceration, myalgia, myasthenia, myopathy, pancreatitis, paresthesia, pharyngitis, pruritus, redistribution of body fat, rhinitis, seizures, sexual dysfunction, sinusitis, sleep disorder, somnolence, suicide ideation, thrombocytopenia, urticaria, vomiting

Drug Interactions CYP3A3/4 enzyme substrate; CYP3A3/4 enzyme inducer; CYP3A3/4 enzyme inhibitor

Increased effect:

Nelfinavir inhibits the metabolism of cisapride and astemizole and should, therefore, not be administered concurrently due to risk of life-threatening cardiac arrhythmias.

A 20% increase in rifabutin plasma AUC has been observed when coadministered with nelfinavir (decrease rifabutin's dose by 50%).

An increase in midazolam and triazolam serum levels may occur resulting in significant oversedation when administered with nelfinavir. These drugs should not be administered together. Use caution with other benzodiazepines.

Amiodarone, quinidine, and ergot alkaloids: Serum levels/toxicity may be increased by nelfinavir - avoid concurrent use.

Indinavir and ritonavir may increase nelfinavir plasma concentrations resulting in potential increases in side effects (the safety of these combinations have not been established).

Nelfinavir increases indinavir concentrations

Decreased effect:

Rifampin decreases nelfinavir's plasma AUC by ~82%; the two drugs should not be administered together.

Ethinyl estradiol concentrations are decreased by nelfinavir.

(Continued)

Nelfinavir *(Continued)*

Oral contraceptives: Serum levels of the hormones in oral contraceptives may decrease significantly with administration of nelfinavir. Patients should use alternative methods of contraceptives during nelfinavir therapy.

Norethindrone concentrations are decreased by nelfinavir.

Phenobarbital, phenytoin, and carbamazepine may decrease serum levels and consequently effectiveness of nelfinavir.

Nelfinavir's effectiveness may be decreased with concomitant nevirapine

Manufacturer Agouron Pharmaceuticals

Related Information

Antiretroviral Therapy for HIV Infection *on page 1190*
Management of Healthcare Worker Exposures to HIV *on page 1151*
Pharmaceutical Manufacturers Directory *on page 1020*

♦ **Nelova™ 0.5/35E** *see* Ethinyl Estradiol and Norethindrone *on page 342*
♦ **Nelova™ 1/50M** *see* Mestranol and Norethindrone *on page 570*
♦ **Nelova™ 10/11** *see* Ethinyl Estradiol and Norethindrone *on page 342*
♦ **Neo Cal** *see* Calcium Carbonate *on page 130*
♦ **Neo-Calglucon® [OTC]** *see* Calcium Glubionate *on page 131*
♦ **Neo-Codema®** *see* Hydrochlorothiazide *on page 442*
♦ **Neo-Cortef** *see* Neomycin and Hydrocortisone *on page 643*
♦ **NeoDecadron®** *see* Neomycin and Dexamethasone *on page 643*
♦ **NeoDecadron® Ophthalmic** *see* Neomycin and Dexamethasone *on page 643*
♦ **NeoDecadron® Topical** *see* Neomycin and Dexamethasone *on page 643*
♦ **Neo-Dexameth® Ophthalmic** *see* Neomycin and Dexamethasone *on page 643*
♦ **Neo-Durabolic Injection** *see* Nandrolone *on page 635*
♦ **Neo-Estrone®** *see* Estrogens, Esterified *on page 333*
♦ **Neo-Estrone®** *see* Estrone *on page 334*
♦ **Neofed® [OTC]** *see* Pseudoephedrine *on page 792*
♦ **Neo-Fer** *see* Ferrous Fumarate *on page 359*
♦ **Neo-fradin® Oral** *see* Neomycin *on page 642*
♦ **Neomixin® Topical [OTC]** *see* Bacitracin, Neomycin, and Polymyxin B *on page 90*

Neomycin (nee oh MYE sin)

Pharmacologic Class Ammonium Detoxicant; Antibiotic, Aminoglycoside; Antibiotic, Topical

U.S. Brand Names Mycifradin® Sulfate Oral; Mycifradin® Sulfate Topical; Neo-fradin® Oral; Neo-Tabs® Oral

Generic Available Yes

Mechanism of Action Interferes with bacterial protein synthesis by binding to 30S ribosomal subunits

Use Orally to prepare GI tract for surgery; topically to treat minor skin infections; treat diarrhea caused by *E. coli*; adjunct in the treatment of hepatic encephalopathy

USUAL DOSAGE

Children: Oral:

Preoperative intestinal antisepsis: 90 mg/kg/day divided every 4 hours for 2 days; or 25 mg/kg at 1 PM, 2 PM, and 11 PM on the day preceding surgery as an adjunct to mechanical cleansing of the intestine and in combination with erythromycin base

Hepatic coma: 50-100 mg/kg/day in divided doses every 6-8 hours or 2.5-7 g/m^2/day divided every 4-6 hours for 5-6 days not to exceed 12 g/day

Children and Adults: Topical: Apply ointment 1-4 times/day; topical solutions containing 0.1% to 1% neomycin have been used for irrigation

Adults: Oral:

Preoperative intestinal antisepsis: 1 g each hour for 4 doses then 1 g every 4 hours for 5 doses; or 1 g at 1 PM, 2 PM, and 11 PM on day preceding surgery as an adjunct to mechanical cleansing of the bowel and oral erythromycin; or 6 g/day divided every 4 hours for 2-3 days

Hepatic coma: 500-2000 mg every 6-8 hours or 4-12 g/day divided every 4-6 hours for 5-6 days

Chronic hepatic insufficiency: 4 g/day for an indefinite period

Hemodialysis: Dialyzable (50% to 100%)

Dosage Forms CRM: 0.5% (15 g). **INJ:** 500 mg. **OINT, top:** 0.5% (15 g, 30 g, 120 g). **SOLN, oral:** 125 mg/5 mL (480 mL). **TAB:** 500 mg [base 300 mg]

Contraindications Hypersensitivity to neomycin or any component, or other aminoglycosides; patients with intestinal obstruction

Warnings/Precautions Use with caution in patients with renal impairment, pre-existing hearing impairment, neuromuscular disorders; neomycin is more toxic than other aminoglycosides when given parenterally; **do not administer parenterally**; topical neomycin is a contact sensitizer with sensitivity occurring in 5% to 15% of patients treated with the drug; symptoms include itching, reddening, edema, and failure to heal; **do not use as peritoneal lavage** due to significant systemic adsorption of the drug

Pregnancy Risk Factor C

Adverse Reactions

1% to 10%:

Dermatologic: Dermatitis, rash, urticaria, erythema

Local: Burning

Ocular: Contact conjunctivitis

<1%: Diarrhea, nausea, nephrotoxicity, neuromuscular blockade, ototoxicity, vomiting

Drug Interactions

Decreased effect: May decrease GI absorption of digoxin and methotrexate

Increased effect: Synergistic effects with penicillins

Increased toxicity:

Oral neomycin may potentiate the effects of oral anticoagulants

Increased adverse effects with other neurotoxic, ototoxic, or nephrotoxic drugs

Half-Life 3 hours (age and renal function dependent)

Education and Monitoring Issues

Patient Education:

Oral: Take as directed. Maintain adequate hydration (2-3 L/day of fluids unless instructed to restrict fluid intake). You may experience nausea or vomiting (small frequent meals, frequent mouth care, sucking lozenges, or chewing gum may help); constipation (exercise, increased fluid or fiber in diet may help, or consult prescriber); or diarrhea (buttermilk, boiled milk, or yogurt may help). Report immediately any change in hearing,; ringing or sense of fullness in ears; persistent diarrhea; changes in voiding patterns; or numbness, tingling, or pain in any extremity.

Topical: Apply a thin film of cream or ointment; do not overuse. Report rash, itching, redness, or failure of condition to improve.

Monitoring Parameters: Renal function tests, audiometry in symptomatic patients

Related Information

Bacitracin, Neomycin, and Polymyxin B *on page 90*
Bacitracin, Neomycin, Polymyxin B, and Hydrocortisone *on page 90*
Colistin, Neomycin, and Hydrocortisone *on page 227*
Neomycin and Dexamethasone *on page 643*
Neomycin and Hydrocortisone *on page 643*
Neomycin and Polymyxin B *on page 643*
Neomycin, Polymyxin B, and Dexamethasone *on page 644*
Neomycin, Polymyxin B, and Hydrocortisone *on page 644*
Neomycin, Polymyxin B, and Prednisolone *on page 644*

Neomycin and Dexamethasone (nee oh MYE sin & deks a METH a sone)

Pharmacologic Class Antibiotic/Corticosteroid, Ophthalmic; Antibiotic/Corticosteroid, Topical

U.S. Brand Names NeoDecadron® Ophthalmic; NeoDecadron® Topical; Neo-Dexameth® Ophthalmic

Dosage Forms CRM: Neomycin sulfate 0.5% [5 mg/g] and dexamethasone 0.1% [1 mg/g] (15 g, 30 g). **OINT, ophth:** Neomycin sulfate 0.35% [3.5 mg/g] and dexamethasone 0.05% [0.5 mg/g] (3.5 g). **SOLN, ophth:** Neomycin sulfate 0.35% [3.5 mg/mL] and dexamethasone 0.1% [1 mg/mL] (5 mL)

Pregnancy Risk Factor C

Neomycin and Hydrocortisone (nee oh MYE sin & hye droe KOR ti sone)

Pharmacologic Class Antibiotic/Corticosteroid, Ophthalmic; Antibiotic/Corticosteroid, Topical

U.S. Brand Names Neo-Cortef®

Dosage Forms CRM: Neomycin sulfate 0.5% and hydrocortisone 1% (20 g). **OINT, top:** Neomycin sulfate 0.5% and hydrocortisone 0.5% (20 g), neomycin sulfate 0.5% and hydrocortisone 1% (20 g). **SOLN, ophth:** Neomycin sulfate 0.5% and hydrocortisone 0.5% (5 mL)

Pregnancy Risk Factor C

Neomycin and Polymyxin B (nee oh MYE sin & pol i MIKS in bee)

Pharmacologic Class Antibiotic, Topical

U.S. Brand Names Neosporin® Cream [OTC]; Neosporin® G.U. Irrigant

Use Short-term as a continuous irrigant or rinse in the urinary bladder to prevent bacteriuria and gram-negative rod septicemia associated with the use of indwelling catheters; to help prevent infection in minor cuts, scrapes, and burns

USUAL DOSAGE Children and Adults:

Bladder irrigation: **Not for injection**; add 1 mL irrigant to 1 liter isotonic saline solution and connect container to the inflow of lumen of 3-way catheter. Continuous irrigant or rinse in the urinary bladder for up to a maximum of 10 days with administration rate adjusted to patient's urine output; usually no more than 1 L of irrigant is used per day.

Topical: Apply cream 1-4 times/day to affected area

Dosage Forms CRM: Neomycin sulfate 3.5 mg and polymyxin B sulfate 10,000 units per g (0.94 g, 15 g). **SOLN, irrigant:** Neomycin sulfate 40 mg and polymyxin B sulfate 200,000 units per mL (1 mL, 20 mL)

(Continued)

Neomycin and Polymyxin B *(Continued)*

Pregnancy Risk Factor C; D (G.U. irrigant)

Neomycin, Polymyxin B, and Dexamethasone

(nee oh MYE sin, pol i MIKS in bee, & deks a METH a sone)

Pharmacologic Class Antibiotic/Corticosteroid, Ophthalmic

U.S. Brand Names AK-Trol®; Dexacidin®; Dexasporin®; Maxitrol®

Use Steroid-responsive inflammatory ocular conditions in which a corticosteroid is indicated and where bacterial infection or a risk of bacterial infection exists

USUAL DOSAGE Children and Adults: Ophthalmic:

Ointment: Place a small amount (~½") in the affected eye 3-4 times/day or apply at bedtime as an adjunct with drops

Solution: Instill 1-2 drops into affected eye(s) every 3-4 hours; in severe disease, drops may be used hourly and tapered to discontinuation

Pregnancy Risk Factor C

Neomycin, Polymyxin B, and Gramicidin

(nee oh MYE sin, pol i MIKS in bee, & gram i SYE din)

Pharmacologic Class Antibiotic, Ophthalmic

U.S. Brand Names AK-Spore® Ophthalmic Solution; Neosporin® Ophthalmic Solution; Ocutricin® Ophthalmic Solution

Use Treatment of superficial ocular infection

USUAL DOSAGE Children and Adults: Ophthalmic: Instill 1-2 drops 4-6 times/day or more frequently as required for severe infections

Contraindications Hypersensitivity to neomycin, polymyxin B, gramicidin or any component

Pregnancy Risk Factor C

Neomycin, Polymyxin B, and Hydrocortisone

(nee oh MYE sin, pol i MIKS in bee, & hye droe KOR ti sone)

Pharmacologic Class Antibiotic/Corticosteroid, Ophthalmic; Antibiotic/Corticosteroid, Otic; Antibiotic/Corticosteroid, Topical

U.S. Brand Names AK-Spore H.C.® Ophthalmic Suspension; AK-Spore H.C.® Otic; Antibi-Otic® Otic; Bacticort® Otic; Cortatrigen® Otic; Cortisporin® Ophthalmic Suspension; Cortisporin® Otic; Cortisporin® Topical Cream; Drotic® Otic; Ear-Eze® Otic; LazerSporin-C® Otic; Octicair® Otic; Otic-Care® Otic; OtiTricin® Otic; Otocort® Otic; Otomycin-HPN® Otic; Otosporin® Otic; PediOtic® Otic; UAD® Otic

Use Steroid-responsive inflammatory condition for which a corticosteroid is indicated and where bacterial infection or a risk of bacterial infection exists

USUAL DOSAGE Duration of use should be limited to 10 days unless otherwise directed by the prescriber

Otic solution is used **only** for swimmer's ear (infections of external auditory canal)

Otic:

Children: Instill 3 drops into affected ear 3-4 times/day

Adults: Instill 4 drops 3-4 times/day; otic suspension is the preferred otic preparation

Children and Adults:

Ophthalmic: Drops: Instill 1-2 drops 2-4 times/day, or more frequently as required for severe infections; in acute infections, instill 1-2 drops every 15-30 minutes gradually reducing the frequency of administration as the infection is controlled

Topical: Apply a thin layer 1-4 times/day

Dosage Forms CRM, top: Neomycin sulfate 5 mg, polymyxin B sulfate 10,000 units, and hydrocortisone 10 mg per mL (7.5 g). **SOLN, otic:** Neomycin sulfate 5 mg, polymyxin B sulfate 10,000 units, and hydrocortisone 10 mg per mL (10 mL). **SUSP:** Ophth: Neomycin sulfate 5 mg, polymyxin B sulfate 10,000 units, and hydrocortisone 10 mg per mL (7.5 mL); Otic: Neomycin sulfate 5 mg, polymyxin B sulfate 10,000 units, and hydrocortisone 10 mg per mL (10 mL)

Pregnancy Risk Factor C

Neomycin, Polymyxin B, and Prednisolone

(nee oh MYE sin, pol i MIKS in bee, & pred NIS oh lone)

Pharmacologic Class Antibiotic/Corticosteroid, Ophthalmic

U.S. Brand Names Poly-Pred® Ophthalmic Suspension

Use Steroid-responsive inflammatory ocular condition in which bacterial infection or a risk of bacterial ocular infection exists

USUAL DOSAGE Children and Adults: Ophthalmic: Instill 1-2 drops every 3-4 hours; acute infections may require every 30-minute instillation initially with frequency of administration reduced as the infection is brought under control. To treat the lids: Instill 1-2 drops every 3-4 hours, close the eye and rub the excess on the lids and lid margins.

Pregnancy Risk Factor C

♦ **Neopap® [OTC]** *see* Acetaminophen *on page 17*

♦ **Neo-Pause** *see* Estradiol and Testosterone *on page 329*

- **Neoral® Oral** *see* Cyclosporine *on page 237*
- **Neosar® Injection** *see* Cyclophosphamide *on page 235*
- **Neosporin®** *see* Neomycin and Polymyxin B *on page 643*
- **Neosporin®** *see* Neomycin, Polymyxin B, and Gramicidin *on page 644*
- **Neosporin® Cream [OTC]** *see* Neomycin and Polymyxin B *on page 643*
- **Neosporin® G.U. Irrigant** *see* Neomycin and Polymyxin B *on page 643*
- **Neosporin® Ophthalmic Ointment** *see* Bacitracin, Neomycin, and Polymyxin B *on page 90*
- **Neosporin® Ophthalmic Solution** *see* Neomycin, Polymyxin B, and Gramicidin *on page 644*
- **Neosporin® Topical Ointment [OTC]** *see* Bacitracin, Neomycin, and Polymyxin B *on page 90*

Neostigmine (nee oh STIG meen)

Pharmacologic Class Acetylcholinesterase Inhibitor (Peripheral)

U.S. Brand Names Prostigmin®

Generic Available No

Mechanism of Action Inhibits destruction of acetylcholine by acetylcholinesterase which facilitates transmission of impulses across myoneural junction

Use Diagnosis and treatment of myasthenia gravis and prevent and treat postoperative bladder distention and urinary retention; reversal of the effects of nondepolarizing neuromuscular blocking agents after surgery

USUAL DOSAGE

Myasthenia gravis: Diagnosis: I.M.:
- Children: 0.04 mg/kg as a single dose
- Adults: 0.02 mg/kg as a single dose

Myasthenia gravis: Treatment:
- Children:
  - Oral: 2 mg/kg/day divided every 3-4 hours
  - I.M., I.V., S.C.: 0.01-0.04 mg/kg every 2-4 hours
- Adults:
  - Oral: 15 mg/dose every 3-4 hours up to 375 mg/day maximum
  - I.M., I.V., S.C.: 0.5-2.5 mg every 1-3 hours up to 10 mg/24 hours maximum

Reversal of nondepolarizing neuromuscular blockade after surgery in conjunction with atropine: I.V.:
- Infants: 0.025-0.1 mg/kg/dose
- Children: 0.025-0.08 mg/kg/dose
- Adults: 0.5-2.5 mg; total dose not to exceed 5 mg

Bladder atony: Adults: I.M., S.C.:
- Prevention: 0.25 mg every 4-6 hours for 2-3 days
- Treatment: 0.5-1 mg every 3 hours for 5 doses after bladder has emptied

Dosing adjustment in renal impairment:
- Cl_{cr} 10-50 mL/minute: Administer 50% of normal dose
- Cl_{cr} <10 mL/minute: Administer 25% of normal dose

Dosage Forms INJ, as methylsulfate: 0.25 mg/mL (1 mL), 0.5 mg/mL (1 mL, 10 mL), 1 mg/mL (10 mL). **TAB,** as bromide: 15 mg

Contraindications Hypersensitivity to neostigmine, bromides or any component; GI or GU obstruction

Warnings/Precautions Does **not** antagonize and may prolong the phase I block of depolarizing muscle relaxants (eg, succinylcholine); use with caution in patients with epilepsy, asthma, bradycardia, hyperthyroidism, cardiac arrhythmias, or peptic ulcer; adequate facilities should be available for cardiopulmonary resuscitation when testing and adjusting dose for myasthenia gravis; have atropine and epinephrine ready to treat hypersensitivity reactions; overdosage may result in cholinergic crisis, this must be distinguished from myasthenic crisis; anticholinesterase insensitivity can develop for brief or prolonged periods

Pregnancy Risk Factor C

Adverse Reactions

>10%:
- Gastrointestinal: Hyperperistalsis, nausea, vomiting, salivation, diarrhea, stomach cramps
- Miscellaneous: Diaphoresis (increased)

1% to 10%:
- Genitourinary: Urge to urinate
- Ocular: Small pupils, lacrimation
- Respiratory: Increased bronchial secretions

<1%: Agitation, A-V block, bradyarrhythmias, bradycardia, bronchoconstriction, diplopia, drowsiness, dysphoria, fasciculations, headache, hyper-reactive cholinergic responses, hypersensitivity, hypotension, laryngospasm, miosis, muscle spasms, respiratory paralysis, restlessness, seizures, thrombophlebitis, tremor, weakness

Drug Interactions

Decreased effect: Antagonizes effects of nondepolarizing muscle relaxants (eg, pancuronium, tubocurarine); atropine antagonizes the muscarinic effects of neostigmine

(Continued)

Neostigmine *(Continued)*

Increased effect: Neuromuscular blocking agents effects are increased

Onset I.M.: Within 20-30 minutes; I.V.: Within 1-20 minutes

Duration I.M.: 2.5-4 hours; I.V.: 1-2 hours

Half-Life Normal renal function: 0.5-2.1 hours; End-stage renal disease: Prolonged

Education and Monitoring Issues

Patient Education: Take this drug exactly as prescribed. You may experience visual difficulty (eg, blurring and dark adaptation - use caution at night) or urinary frequency. Promptly report any muscle weakness, respiratory difficulty, severe or unresolved diarrhea, persistent abdominal cramping or vomiting, sweating, or tearing.

- **Neostrata® HQ** *see* Hydroquinone *on page 450*
- **Neo-Synephrine® Nasal Solution [OTC]** *see* Phenylephrine *on page 727*
- **Neo-Synephrine® Ophthalmic Solution** *see* Phenylephrine *on page 727*
- **Neo-Tabs® Oral** *see* Neomycin *on page 642*
- **Neotopic** *see* Bacitracin, Neomycin, and Polymyxin B *on page 90*
- **Neotricin HC® Ophthalmic Ointment** *see* Bacitracin, Neomycin, Polymyxin B, and Hydrocortisone *on page 90*
- **NeoVadrin® [OTC]** *see* Vitamins, Multiple *on page 981*
- **Neo-Zol** *see* Clotrimazole *on page 220*
- **Nephro-Calci® [OTC]** *see* Calcium Carbonate *on page 130*
- **Nephrocaps®** *see* Vitamin B Complex With Vitamin C and Folic Acid *on page 979*
- **Nephro-Fer™ [OTC]** *see* Ferrous Fumarate *on page 359*
- **Nephronex®** *see* Nitrofurantoin *on page 658*
- **Nephrox Suspension [OTC]** *see* Aluminum Hydroxide *on page 41*
- **Neptazane®** *see* Methazolamide *on page 578*
- **Nervocaine®** *see* Lidocaine *on page 527*
- **Nesacaine®** *see* Chloroprocaine *on page 182*
- **Nesacaine®-MPF** *see* Chloroprocaine *on page 182*
- **Nestrex®** *see* Pyridoxine *on page 796*

Netilmicin (ne til MYE sin)

Pharmacologic Class Aminoglycoside (Antibiotic)

U.S. Brand Names Netromycin®

Use Short-term treatment of serious or life-threatening infections including septicemia, peritonitis, intra-abdominal abscess, lower respiratory tract infections, urinary tract infections; skin, bone, and joint infections caused by susceptible organisms; active against *Pseudomonas aeruginosa, E. coli, Proteus, Klebsiella, Serratia, Enterobacter, Citrobacter,* and other gram-negative bacilli

USUAL DOSAGE Individualization is critical because of the low therapeutic index. Use of ideal body weight (IBW) for determining the mg/kg/dose appears to be more accurate than dosing on the basis of total body weight (TBW). In morbid obesity, dosage requirement may best be estimated using a dosing weight of IBW + 0.4 (TBW - IBW). Peak and trough plasma drug levels should be determined, particularly in critically ill patients with serious infections or in disease states known to significantly alter aminoglycoside pharmacokinetics (eg, cystic fibrosis, burns, or major surgery).

I.M., I.V.:

Neonates <6 weeks: 2-3.25 mg/kg/dose every 12 hours

Children 6 weeks to 12 years: 1-2.5 mg/kg/dose every 8 hours

Children >12 years and Adults: 1.5-2 mg/kg/dose every 8-12 hours

Some clinicians suggest a daily dose of 4-7 mg/kg for all patients with normal renal function. This dose is at least as efficacious with similar, if not less, toxicity than conventional dosing

Dosing adjustment in renal impairment: Initial dose:

All patients should receive a loading dose of at least 2 mg/kg (subsequent dosing should be base on serum concentrations)

Cl_{cr} ≥60 mL/minute: Administer every 8 hours

Cl_{cr} 40-60 mL/minute: Administer every 12 hours

Cl_{cr} 20-40 mL/minute: Administer every 24 hours

Continuous arteriovenous or venovenous hemodiafiltration (CAVH) effects: Dose as for Cl_{cr} 10-40 mL/minute and follow levels

Contraindications Known hypersensitivity to netilmicin (aminoglycosides, bisulfites)

Pregnancy Risk Factor D

- **Netromycin®** *see* Netilmicin *on page 646*
- **Neucalm®** *see* Hydroxyzine *on page 455*
- **Neumega®** *see* Oprelvekin *on page 679*
- **Neupogen® Injection** *see* Filgrastim *on page 363*
- **Neuramate®** *see* Meprobamate *on page 565*
- **Neurontin®** *see* Gabapentin *on page 401*

- **Neut® Injection** *see* Sodium Bicarbonate *on page 856*
- **Neutra-Phos®** *see* Potassium Phosphate and Sodium Phosphate *on page 755*
- **Neutra-Phos®-K** *see* Potassium Phosphate *on page 754*
- **Neutrexin® Injection** *see* Trimetrexate Glucuronate *on page 954*

Nevirapine (ne VYE ra peen)

Pharmacologic Class Antiretroviral Agent, Reverse Transcriptase Inhibitor (Non-Nucleoside)

U.S. Brand Names Viramune®

Use In combination therapy with other antiretroviral agents for the treatment of HIV-1 in adults

USUAL DOSAGE Adults: Oral:

Initial: 200 mg once daily for 14 days

Maintenance: 200 mg twice daily (in combination with an additional antiretroviral agent)

Contraindications Previous hypersensitivity to nevirapine or its components; concurrent use with oral contraceptives and protease inhibitors (indinavir, nelfinavir, ritonavir, saquinavir)

Warnings/Precautions Consider alteration of antiretroviral therapies if disease progression occurs while patients are receiving nevirapine. Resistant HIV virus emerges rapidly and uniformly when nevirapine is administered as monotherapy. Therefore, always administer in combination with at least 1 additional antiretroviral agent. Severe skin reactions (eg, Stevens-Johnson syndrome) have occurred, usually within 6 weeks. Therapy should be discontinued if any rash which develops does not resolve; mild to moderate alterations in LFTs are not uncommon, however, severe hepatotoxic reactions may occur rarely, and if abnormalities reoccur after temporarily discontinuing therapy, treatment should be permanently halted. Safety and efficacy have not been established in children.

Pregnancy Risk Factor C

Adverse Reactions

>10%:

Central nervous system: Headache (11%), fever (8% to 11%)

Dermatologic: Rash (15% to 20%)

Gastrointestinal: Diarrhea (15% to 20%)

Hematologic: Neutropenia (10% to 11%)

1% to 10%:

Gastrointestinal: Ulcerative stomatitis (4%), nausea, abdominal pain (2%)

Hematologic: Anemia

Hepatic: Hepatitis, increased LFTs (2% to 4%)

Neuromuscular & skeletal: Peripheral neuropathy, paresthesia (2%), myalgia

<1%: Hepatic necrosis, hepatotoxicity, Stevens-Johnson syndrome, thrombocytopenia

Drug Interactions CYP3A3/4 enzyme substrate; CYP3A3/4 enzyme inducer; CYP3A3/4 enzyme inhibitor

Decreased effect: Rifampin and rifabutin may decrease nevirapine trough concentrations due to induction of CYP3A; since nevirapine may decrease concentrations of protease inhibitors, they should not be administered concomitantly or doses should be increased; nevirapine may decrease the effectiveness of oral contraceptives - suggest alternate method of birth control; decreased effect of ketoconazole; nevirapine may decrease plasma concentrations of methadone

Increased effect/toxicity with cimetidine, macrolides, ketoconazole; other drugs metabolized by CYP3A3/4 should be used with caution

Manufacturer Roxane Laboratories, Inc

Related Information

Antiretroviral Therapy for HIV Infection *on page 1190*

Pharmaceutical Manufacturers Directory *on page 1020*

- **New Decongestant®** *see* Chlorpheniramine, Phenyltoloxamine, Phenylpropanolamine, and Phenylephrine *on page 187*
- **New Drugs Introduced or Approved by the FDA in 1999** *see page 1007*
- **NF Cough Syrup with Codeine** *see* Guaifenesin, Pseudoephedrine, and Codeine *on page 425*
- **N.G.T.® Topical** *see* Nystatin and Triamcinolone *on page 670*

Niacin (NYE a sin)

Pharmacologic Class Antilipemic Agent; Vitamin, Water Soluble

U.S. Brand Names Niaspan®; Nicobid® [OTC]; Nicolar® [OTC]; Nicotinex [OTC]; Slo-Niacin® [OTC]

Generic Available Yes

Mechanism of Action Component of two coenzymes which is necessary for tissue respiration, lipid metabolism, and glycogenolysis; inhibits the synthesis of very low density lipoproteins

Use Adjunctive treatment of hyperlipidemias; peripheral vascular disease and circulatory disorders; treatment of pellagra; dietary supplement

(Continued)

Niacin *(Continued)*

USUAL DOSAGE Administer I.M., I.V., or S.C. only if oral route is unavailable and use only for vitamin deficiencies (not for hyperlipidemia)

Children: Oral:
- Pellagra: 50-100 mg/dose 3 times/day
- Recommended daily allowances:
  - 0-0.5 years: 5 mg/day
  - 0.5-1 year: 6 mg/day
  - 1-3 years: 9 mg/day
  - 4-6 years: 12 mg/day
  - 7-10 years: 13 mg/day

Children and Adolescents: Oral: Recommended daily allowances:
- Male:
  - 11-14 years: 17 mg/day
  - 15-18 years: 20 mg/day
  - 19-24 years: 19 mg/day
- Female: 11-24 years: 15 mg/day

Adults: Oral:
- Recommended daily allowances:
  - Male: 25-50 years: 19 mg/day; >51 years: 15 mg/day
  - Female: 25-50 years: 15 mg/day; >51 years: 13 mg/day
- Hyperlipidemia: 1.5-6 g/day in 3 divided doses with or after meals
  - Extended release: 375-2000 mg/day at bedtime in a titrated schedule
- Pellagra: 50-100 mg 3-4 times/day, maximum: 500 mg/day
- Niacin deficiency: 10-20 mg/day, maximum: 100 mg/day

Dosage Forms CAP, timed release: 125 mg, 250 mg, 300 mg, 400 mg, 500 mg. **ELIX:** 50 mg/5 mL (473 mL, 4000 mL). **INJ:** 100 mg/mL (30 mL). **TAB:** 25 mg, 50 mg, 100 mg, 250 mg, 500 mg; Timed release: 150 mg, 250 mg, 500 mg, 750 mg; Extended release: 500 mg, 750 mg, 1000 mg

Contraindications Liver disease, peptic ulcer, severe hypotension, arterial hemorrhaging, hypersensitivity to niacin

Warnings/Precautions Monitor liver function tests, blood glucose; may elevate uric acid levels; use with caution in patients predisposed to gout; large doses should be administered with caution to patients with gallbladder disease, jaundice, liver disease, or diabetes; some products may contain tartrazine

Pregnancy Risk Factor A; C (if used in doses greater than RDA suggested doses)

Adverse Reactions

1% to 10%:
- Cardiovascular: Generalized flushing
- Central nervous system: Headache
- Gastrointestinal: Bloating, flatulence, nausea
- Hepatic: Abnormalities of hepatic function tests, jaundice
- Neuromuscular & skeletal: Paresthesia in extremities
- Miscellaneous: Increased sebaceous gland activity, sensation of warmth

<1% (limited to important or life-threatening symptoms): Tachycardia, syncope, vasovagal attacks, dizziness, rash, liver damage (dose-related incidence), blurred vision, wheezing

Drug Interactions
- Oral hypoglycemics: Effect may be decreased by niacin
- Sulfinpyrazone and probenecid; niacin may inhibit uricosuric effects
- Aspirin decreases adverse effect of flushing
- Lovastatin (and possibly other HMG CoA reductase inhibitors): Increased risk of toxicity (myopathy)
- Adrenergic blocking agents → additive vasodilating effect and postural hypotension

Education and Monitoring Issues

Patient Education: Take this medication with food. Do not crush sustained release capsule. May experience transient cutaneous flushing and sensation of warmth, especially of face and upper body. Itching or tingling, and headache may occur, these adverse effects may be decreased by increasing the dose slowly or by taking aspirin or a NSAID 30 minutes to 1 hour prior to taking niacin. May cause GI upset, take with food. If dizziness occurs, avoid sudden changes in posture. Report any persistent nausea, vomiting, abdominal pain, dark urine, or pale stools to the prescriber.

Monitoring Parameters: Blood glucose, liver function tests (with large doses or prolonged therapy), serum cholesterol

Niacinamide (nye a SIN a mide)

Pharmacologic Class Vitamin, Water Soluble

Generic Available Yes

Mechanism of Action Used by the body as a source of niacin; is a component of two coenzymes which is necessary for tissue respiration, lipid metabolism, and glycogenolysis; inhibits the synthesis of very low density lipoproteins; does not have hypolipidemia or vasodilating effects

Use Prophylaxis and treatment of pellagra

USUAL DOSAGE Oral:

Children: Pellagra: 100-300 mg/day in divided doses

Adults: 50 mg 3-10 times/day

Pellagra: 300-500 mg/day

Recommended daily allowance: 13-19 mg/day

Dosage Forms TAB: 50 mg, 100 mg, 125 mg, 250 mg, 500 mg

Contraindications Liver disease, peptic ulcer, known hypersensitivity to niacin

Warnings/Precautions Large doses should be administered with caution to patients with gallbladder disease or diabetes; monitor blood glucose; may elevate uric acid levels; use with caution in patients predisposed to gout; some products may contain tartrazine

Pregnancy Risk Factor A; C (if used in doses greater than RDA suggested doses)

Adverse Reactions Percentage unknown: Tachycardia, rash, bloating, flatulence, nausea, paresthesia in extremities, blurred vision, wheezing, increased sebaceous gland activity

Drug Interactions

Oral hypoglycemics: Effect may be decreased by niacin

Sulfinpyrazone and probenecid; niacin may inhibit uricosuric effects

Aspirin decreases adverse effect of flushing

Lovastatin (and possibly other HMG CoA reductase inhibitors): Increased risk of toxicity (myopathy)

Adrenergic blocking agents → additive vasodilating effect and postural hypotension

♦ **Niaspan®** *see* Niacin *on page 647*

Nicardipine (nye KAR de peen)

Pharmacologic Class Calcium Channel Blocker

U.S. Brand Names Cardene®; Cardene® SR; Cardene® I.V.

Generic Available No

Mechanism of Action Inhibits calcium ion from entering the "slow channels" or select voltage-sensitive areas of vascular smooth muscle and myocardium during depolarization, producing a relaxation of coronary vascular smooth muscle and coronary vasodilation; increases myocardial oxygen delivery in patients with vasospastic angina

Use Chronic stable angina (immediate-release product only); management of essential hypertension (immediate and sustained release; parenteral only for short time that oral treatment is not feasible), migraine prophylaxis

Unlabeled use: Congestive heart failure

USUAL DOSAGE Adults:

Oral:

Immediate release: Initial: 20 mg 3 times/day; usual: 20-40 mg 3 times/day (allow 3 days between dose increases)

Sustained release: Initial: 30 mg twice daily, titrate up to 60 mg twice daily

I.V. (dilute to 0.1 mg/mL): Initial: 5 mg/hour increased by 2.5 mg/hour every 15 minutes to a maximum of 15 mg/hour

Dosing adjustment in renal impairment: Titrate dose beginning with 20 mg 3 times/day (immediate release) or 30 mg twice daily (sustained release)

Dosing adjustment in hepatic impairment: Starting dose: 20 mg twice daily (immediate release) with titration

Equivalent Oral vs I.V. Infusion Doses

Oral Dose	Equivalent I.V. Infusion
20 mg q8h	0.5 mg/h
30 mg q8h	1.2 mg/h
40 mg q8h	2.2 mg/h

Dosage Forms CAP: 20 mg, 30 mg; Sustained release: 30 mg, 45 mg, 60 mg. **INJ:** 2.5 mg/mL (10 mL)

Contraindications Contraindicated in severe hypotension or second and third degree heart block, sinus bradycardia, advanced heart block, ventricular tachycardia, cardiogenic shock, atrial fibrillation or flutter associated with accessory conduction pathways, CHF; hypersensitivity to nicardipine or any component, calcium channel blockers, and adenosine; not to be given within a few hours of I.V. beta-blocking agents

Warnings/Precautions Use with caution in titrating dosages for impaired renal or hepatic function patients; may increase frequency, severity, and duration of angina during initiation of therapy; do not abruptly withdraw (chest pain); may have a greater hypotensive effect in the elderly

Pregnancy Risk Factor C

Pregnancy Implications

Clinical effects on the fetus: Crosses the placenta; may exhibit tocolytic effect

Breast-feeding/lactation: No data available

(Continued)

Nicardipine *(Continued)*

Adverse Reactions

1% to 10%:

Cardiovascular: Flushing (6% to 10%), palpitations (3.3% to 4%), tachycardia (1% to 3.4%), peripheral edema (dose-related 7% to 8%), increased angina (dose-related 5.6%)

Central nervous system: Headache (6.4% to 8%), dizziness (4% to 7%), somnolence (4.2% to 6%), paresthesia (1%)

Dermatologic: Rash (1.2%)

Gastrointestinal: Nausea (1.9% to 2.2%), dry mouth (1.4%)

Neuromuscular & skeletal: Weakness (4.2% to 6%), myalgia (1%)

<1% (limited to important or life-threatening symptoms): Abnormal EKG, insomnia, malaise, abnormal dreams, vomiting, constipation, nocturia, tremor, nervousness, malaise, dyspnea, gingival hyperplasia, syncope, sustained tachycardia

Case report: Parotitis

Drug Interactions CYP3A3/4 enzyme substrate

Azole antifungals may inhibit the calcium channel blocker's metabolism; avoid this combination. Try an antifungal like terbinafine (if appropriate) or monitor closely for altered effect of the calcium channel blocker.

Calcium may reduce the calcium channel blocker's effects, particularly hypotension

Cyclosporine's serum concentrations are increased by nicardipine; avoid this combination. Use another calcium channel blocker or monitor cyclosporine trough levels and renal function closely.

Nafcillin decreases plasma concentration of nicardipine; avoid this combination

Protease inhibitors (amprenavir, ritonavir, nelfinavir) may increase the serum levels of nicardipine

Rifampin increases the metabolism of the calcium channel blocker; adjust the dose of the calcium channel blocker to maintain efficacy

Alcohol Interactions Avoid use

Onset Oral: 1-2 hours; I.V.: 10 minutes

Duration 2-6 hours

Half-Life 2-4 hours

Education and Monitoring Issues

Patient Education: Take as directed; do not alter dosage regimen or increase, decrease, or discontinue without consulting prescriber. Do not crush or chew tablets or capsules. Take with nonfatty food. Avoid caffeine and alcohol. Consult prescriber before increasing exercise routine (decreased angina does not mean it is safe to increase exercise). Change position slowly to prevent orthostatic events. May cause dizziness or fatigue; use caution when driving or engaging in tasks that require alertness until response to drug is known. Frequent small meals, frequent mouth care, sucking lozenges, or chewing gum may reduce nausea. Report swelling, difficulty breathing or new cough, unresolved fatigue, unusual weight gain, or unresolved dizziness.

Related Information

Calcium Channel Blocking Agents Comparison *on page 1236*

♦ **N'ice® Vitamin C Drops [OTC]** *see* Ascorbic Acid *on page 72*

♦ **Niclocide®** *see* Niclosamide *on page 650*

Niclosamide (ni KLOE sa mide)

Pharmacologic Class Anthelmintic

U.S. Brand Names Niclocide®

Generic Available No

Mechanism of Action Inhibits the synthesis of ATP through inhibition of oxidative phosphorylation in the mitochondria of cestodes

Use Treatment of intestinal beef and fish tapeworm infections and dwarf tapeworm infections

USUAL DOSAGE Oral:

Beef and fish tapeworm:

Children:

11-34 kg: 1 g (2 tablets) as a single dose

>34 kg: 1.5 g (3 tablets) as a single dose

Adults: 2 g (4 tablets) in a single dose

May require a second course of treatment 7 days later

Dwarf tapeworm:

Children:

11-34 g: 1 g (2 tablets) chewed thoroughly in a single dose the first day, then 500 mg/day (1 tablet) for next 6 days

>34 g: 1.5 g (3 tablets) in a single dose the first day, then 1 g/day for 6 days

Adults: 2 g (4 tablets) in a single daily dose for 7 days

Dosage Forms TAB, chewable (vanilla flavor): 500 mg

Contraindications Known hypersensitivity to niclosamide

Warnings/Precautions Affects cestodes of the intestine only; it is without effect in cysticercosis

Pregnancy Risk Factor B

Adverse Reactions

1% to 10%:

Central nervous system: Drowsiness, dizziness, headache

Gastrointestinal: Nausea, vomiting, loss of appetite, diarrhea

<1%: Alopecia, backache, bad taste in mouth, constipation, diaphoresis, edema in the arm, fever, oral irritation, palpitations, pruritus ani, rash, rectal bleeding, weakness

Education and Monitoring Issues

Patient Education: Chew tablets thoroughly; tablets can be pulverized and mixed with water to form a paste for administration to children; can be taken with food; a mild laxative can be used for constipation

Monitoring Parameters: Stool cultures

♦ **Nicobid® [OTC]** *see* Niacin *on page 647*

♦ **Nicoderm® Patch [OTC]** *see* Nicotine *on page 651*

♦ **Nicolar® [OTC]** *see* Niacin *on page 647*

♦ **Nicorette®** *see* Nicotine *on page 651*

♦ **Nicorette® DS Gum [OTC]** *see* Nicotine *on page 651*

♦ **Nicorette® Gum [OTC]** *see* Nicotine *on page 651*

♦ **Nicorette® Plus** *see* Nicotine *on page 651*

Nicotine (nik oh TEEN)

Pharmacologic Class Smoking Cessation Aid

U.S. Brand Names Habitrol™ Patch [OTC]; Nicoderm® Patch [OTC]; Nicorette® DS Gum [OTC]; Nicorette® Gum [OTC]; Nicotrol® NS Nasal Spray; Nicotrol® Patch; ProStep® Patch

Generic Available No

Mechanism of Action Nicotine is one of two naturally-occurring alkaloids which exhibit their primary effects via autonomic ganglia stimulation. The other alkaloid is lobeline which has many actions similar to those of nicotine but is less potent. Nicotine is a potent ganglionic and central nervous system stimulant, the actions of which are mediated via nicotine-specific receptors. Biphasic actions are observed depending upon the dose administered. The main effect of nicotine in small doses is stimulation of all autonomic ganglia; with larger doses, initial stimulation is followed by blockade of transmission. Biphasic effects are also evident in the adrenal medulla; discharge of catecholamines occurs with small doses, whereas prevention of catecholamines release is seen with higher doses as a response to splanchnic nerve stimulation. Stimulation of the central nervous system (CNS) is characterized by tremors and respiratory excitation. However, convulsions may occur with higher doses, along with respiratory failure secondary to both central paralysis and peripheral blockade to respiratory muscles.

Use Treatment aid to smoking cessation while participating in a behavioral modification program under medical supervision

USUAL DOSAGE Patients should be advised to completely stop smoking upon initiation of therapy

Gum: Chew 1 piece of gum when urge to smoke, up to 30 pieces/day; most patients require 10-12 pieces of gum/day

Transdermal patch: Apply new patch every 24 hours to nonhairy, clean, dry skin on the upper body or upper outer arm; each patch should be applied to a different site

24-hour patches (some 24-hour duration patches may be worn for 16 hours/day and then removed at bedtime):

Initial starting dose: 21 mg/day for 4-8 weeks for most patients

First weaning dose: 14 mg/day for 2-4 weeks

Second weaning dose: 7 mg/day for 2-4 weeks

Initial starting dose for patients <100 pounds, smoke <10 cigarettes/day, have a history of cardiovascular disease: 14 mg/day for 4-8 weeks followed by 7 mg/day for 2-4 weeks

In patients who are receiving >600 mg/day of cimetidine: Decrease to the next lower patch size

16-hour patches:

One patch worn for 16 hours daily (remove at bedtime) for 6 weeks, then discontinue; these patches are not intended for lighter smokers

Benefits of use of nicotine transdermal patches beyond 3 months have not been demonstrated

Spray: 1-2 sprays/hour; do not exceed more than 5 doses (10 sprays) per hour; each dose (2 sprays) contains 1 mg of nicotine. **Warning:** A dose of 40 mg can cause fatalities.

Inhaler: Patients may self-titrate doses; most patients use between 6 and 16 cartridges daily during the first 3 months of therapy and then gradually reduce their daily dose over the ensuing 6-12 weeks; no tapering strategy has been shown to be superior to any other; the best clinical effects are seen with frequent continuous inhaler puffing (20 minutes). The recommended duration of treatment is 3 months and some patients may require up to 6 months of therapy.

(Continued)

Nicotine *(Continued)*

Dosage Forms INH: Each inhaler cartridge delivers 4 mg of nicotine. **PATCH, transdermal:** (Habitrol™): 21 mg/day; 14 mg/day; 7 mg/day (30 systems/box); (Nicoderm®): 21 mg/day; 14 mg/day; 7 mg/day (14 systems/box); (Nicotrol® [OTC]): 15 mg/day (gradually released over 16 hours); (ProStep®): 22 mg/day; 11 mg/day (7 systems/box). **PIECES, chewing gum,** as polacrilex: 2 mg/square [OTC] (96 pieces/box); 4 mg/square (96 pieces/box). **SPRAY, nasal:** 0.5 mg/actuation [10 mg/mL (200 actuations)] (10 mL)

Contraindications Nonsmokers, patients with a history of hypersensitivity or allergy to nicotine or any components used in the transdermal system, pregnant or nursing women, patients who are smoking during the postmyocardial infarction period, patients with life-threatening arrhythmias, or severe or worsening angina pectoris, active temporomandibular joint disease (gum)

Warnings/Precautions Use with caution in oropharyngeal inflammation and in patients with history of esophagitis, peptic ulcer, coronary artery disease, vasospastic disease, angina, hypertension, hyperthyroidism, diabetes, and hepatic dysfunction; nicotine is known to be one of the most toxic of all poisons; while the gum is being used to help the patient overcome a health hazard, it also must be considered a hazardous drug vehicle. Nicotine nasal spray: Fatal dose: 40 mg

Pregnancy Risk Factor D (transdermal); X (chewing gum)

Adverse Reactions

Chewing gum:

>10%:

- Cardiovascular: Tachycardia
- Central nervous system: Headache (mild)
- Gastrointestinal: Nausea, vomiting, indigestion, excessive salivation, belching, increased appetite
- Miscellaneous: Mouth or throat soreness, jaw muscle ache, hiccups

1% to 10%:

- Central nervous system: Insomnia, dizziness, nervousness
- Endocrine & metabolic: Dysmenorrhea
- Gastrointestinal: GI distress, eructation
- Neuromuscular & skeletal: Muscle pain
- Respiratory: Hoarseness
- Miscellaneous: Hiccups

<1% (limited to important or life-threatening symptoms): Atrial fibrillation, erythema, itching, hypersensitivity reactions,

Transdermal systems:

>10%:

- Central nervous system: Insomnia, abnormal dreams
- Dermatologic: Pruritus, erythema
- Local: Application site reaction
- Respiratory: Rhinitis, cough, pharyngitis, sinusitis

1% to 10%:

- Cardiovascular: Chest pain
- Central nervous system: Dysphoria, anxiety, difficulty concentrating, dizziness, somnolence
- Dermatologic: Rash
- Gastrointestinal: Diarrhea, dyspepsia, nausea, xerostomia, constipation, anorexia, abdominal pain
- Neuromuscular & skeletal: Arthralgia, myalgia

<1% (limited to important or life-threatening symptoms): Atrial fibrillation, nervousness, tremor, taste perversion, thirst, itching, hypersensitivity reactions

Drug Interactions CYP2B6 and 2A6 enzyme substrate; CYP1A2 enzyme inducer

Adenosine: Nicotine increases the hemodynamic and A-V blocking effects of adenosine; monitor

Cimetidine increases nicotine concentrations; therefore, may decrease amount of gum or patches needed

Bupropion: Monitor for treatment-emergent hypertension in patients treated with the combination of nicotine patch and bupropion

Onset Intranasal nicotine may more closely approximate the time course of plasma nicotine levels observed after cigarette smoking than other dosage forms.

Duration Transdermal: 24 hours

Half-Life 4 hours

Education and Monitoring Issues

Patient Education: Use exactly as directed; do not use more often than prescribed. Stop smoking completely during therapy.

Gum: Chew slowly for 30 minutes. Discard chewed gum away from access by children.

Transdermal patch: Follow directions in package for dosing schedule and use. Do not cut patches. Apply to clean, dry skin in different site each day. Do not touch eyes; wash hands after application. You may experience dizziness or lightheadedness; use caution driving or when engaging in tasks requiring alertness until response to drug is known. For nausea, vomiting or GI upset, small frequent meals, chewing gum, frequent oral care may help. Report persistent vomiting, diarrhea, chills, sweating, chest pain or palpitations, or burning or redness at application site.

Spray: Follow directions in package. Blow nose gently before use. Use 1-2 sprays/hour; do not exceed 5 doses (10 sprays) per hour. Excessive use can result in severe (even life-threatening) reactions. You may experience temporary stinging or burning after spray.

Related Information

Nicotine Products Comparison *on page 1247*

- **Nicotine Products Comparison** *see page 1247*
- **Nicotinex [OTC]** *see* Niacin *on page 647*
- **Nicotrol® NS Nasal Spray** *see* Nicotine *on page 651*
- **Nicotrol® Patch** *see* Nicotine *on page 651*
- **Nico-Vert® [OTC]** *see* Meclizine *on page 556*

Nifedipine (nye FED i peen)

Pharmacologic Class Calcium Channel Blocker

U.S. Brand Names Adalat®; Adalat® CC; Procardia®; Procardia XL®

Generic Available Yes: Capsule

Mechanism of Action Inhibits calcium ion from entering the "slow channels" or select voltage-sensitive areas of vascular smooth muscle and myocardium during depolarization, producing a relaxation of coronary vascular smooth muscle and coronary vasodilation; increases myocardial oxygen delivery in patients with vasospastic angina

Use Angina, hypertrophic cardiomyopathy, hypertension (sustained release only), pulmonary hypertension; Raynaud's disease, migraine headaches.

USUAL DOSAGE Oral:

Children: Hypertrophic cardiomyopathy: 0.6-0.9 mg/kg/24 hours in 3-4 divided doses

Adolescents and Adults: (**Note:** When switching from immediate release to sustained release formulations, total daily dose will start the same)

Initial: 10 mg 3 times/day as capsules or 30 mg once daily as sustained release

Usual dose: 10-30 mg 3 times/day as capsules or 30-60 mg once daily as sustained release

Maximum dose: 120-180 mg/day

Increase sustained release at 7- to 14-day intervals

Hemodialysis: Supplemental dose is not necessary

Peritoneal dialysis effects: Supplemental dose is not necessary

Dosing adjustment in hepatic impairment: Reduce oral dose by 50% to 60% in patients with cirrhosis

Dosage Forms CAP, liquid-filled (Adalat®): 10 mg; (Procardia®): 10 mg, 20 mg. **TAB:** Extended release (Adalat® CC): 30 mg, 60 mg, 90 mg; Sustained release (Procardia XL®): 30 mg, 60 mg, 90 mg

Contraindications Known hypersensitivity to nifedipine or any other calcium channel blocker and adenosine; sick-sinus syndrome, 2nd or 3rd degree A-V block, hypotension (<90 mm Hg systolic); advanced aortic stenosis; acute myocardial infarction

Warnings/Precautions The routine use of short-acting nifedipine capsules in hypertensive emergencies and pseudoemergencies is not recommended. **The FDA has concluded that the use of sublingual short-acting nifedipine in hypertensive emergencies is neither safe or effective and SHOULD BE ABANDONED!** Serious adverse events (cerebrovascular ischemia, syncope, heart block, stroke, sinus arrest, severe hypotension, acute myocardial infarction, EKG changes, and fetal distress) have been reported in relation to the administration of short-acting nifedipine in hypertensive emergencies.

Increased angina may be seen upon starting or increasing doses; may increase frequency, duration, and severity of angina during initiation of therapy; use with caution in patients with congestive heart failure or aortic stenosis (especially with concomitant beta-adrenergic blocker); severe left ventricular dysfunction, hepatic or renal impairment, hypertrophic cardiomyopathy (especially obstructive), concomitant therapy with beta-blockers or digoxin, edema

Mild and transient elevations in liver function enzymes may be apparent within 8 weeks of therapy initiation.

Therapeutic potential of sustained-release formulation (elementary osmotic pump, gastrointestinal therapeutic system [GITS]) may be decreased in patients with certain GI disorders that accelerate intestinal transit time (eg, short bowel syndrome, inflammatory bowel disease, severe diarrhea).

Note: Elderly patients may experience a greater hypotensive response and the use of the immediate release formulation in patients >71 years of age has been associated with a nearly fourfold increased risk for all-cause mortality when compared to beta blockers, ACE inhibitors, or other classes of calcium channel blockers

Pregnancy Risk Factor C

Pregnancy Implications

Clinical effects on the fetus: Use in pregnancy only when clearly needed and when the benefits outweigh the potential hazard to the fetus. No data on crossing the placenta.

(Continued)

Nifedipine *(Continued)*

Hypotension, IUGR reported. IUGR probably related to maternal hypertension. May exhibit tocolytic effects. Available evidence suggests safe use during pregnancy and breast-feeding.

Breast-feeding/lactation: Crosses into breast milk. American Academy of Pediatrics considers **compatible** with breast-feeding.

Adverse Reactions

>10%:

Cardiovascular: Flushing (10% to 25%), peripheral edema (dose-related 7% to 10%; up to 50%)

Central nervous system: Dizziness/lightheadedness/giddiness (10% to 27%), headache (10% to 23%)

Gastrointestinal: Nausea/heartburn (10% to 11%)

Neuromuscular & skeletal: Weakness (10% to 12%)

1% to 10%:

Cardiovascular: Palpitations (≤2% to 7%), transient hypotension (dose-related 5%), CHF (2%)

Central nervous system: Nervousness/mood changes (≤2% to 7%), shakiness (≤2%), jitteriness (≤2%), sleep disturbances (≤2%), difficulties in balance (≤2%), fever (≤2%), chills (≤2%)

Gastrointestinal: Diarrhea (≤2%), constipation (≤2%), cramps (≤2%), flatulence (≤2%), gingival hyperplasia (≤10%)

Neuromuscular & skeletal: Muscle cramps/tremor (≤2% to 8%), weakness (10%), inflammation (≤2%), joint stiffness (≤2%)

Respiratory: Dyspnea/cough/wheezing (6%), nasal congestion/sore throat (≤2% to 6%), chest congestion (≤2%), shortness of breath (≤2%)

Ocular: Blurred vision (≤2%)

Dermatologic: Dermatitis (≤2%), pruritus (≤2%), urticaria (≤2%)

Endocrine and metabolic: Sexual difficulties (≤2%)

Miscellaneous: Sweating (≤2%)

<1% (limited to important or life-threatening symptoms): Syncope, erythromelalgia, thrombocytopenia, anemia, leukopenia, purpura, allergic hepatitis, angioedema, gingival hyperplasia, depression, paranoid syndrome, transient blindness, tinnitus, nocturia, polyuria, arthritis with positive ANA, exfoliative dermatitis, gynecomastia, myalgia, memory dysfunction, fever, bezoars (sustained-release preparations), reflux, myoclonus, angina, ischemia, myoclonus

Case reports: Phototoxicity, EPS, aplastic anemia, agranulocytosis, purpura, Stevens-Johnson syndrome, cerebral ischemia, parotitis, dysgeusia, dysosmia, nocturnal enuresis, erythema multiforme, myocardial infarction, cerebral ischemia

Drug Interactions CYP3A3/4 and 3A5-7 enzyme substrate

Azole antifungals may inhibit the calcium channel blocker's metabolism; avoid this combination. Try an antifungal like terbinafine (if appropriate) or monitor closely for altered effect of the calcium channel blocker.

Beta-blockers may have increased pharmacokinetic or pharmacodynamic interactions with nifedipine

Calcium may reduce the calcium channel blocker's effects, particularly hypotension

Cimetidine reduced diltiazem's metabolism; consider an alternative H_2 antagonist

Cisapride increases nifedipine's effects; monitor blood pressure

Ethanol increased nifedipine's AUC by 53%; watch for a greater hypotensive effect

Nafcillin decreases plasma concentration of nifedipine; avoid this combination

Phenobarbital reduces the plasma concentration of nifedipine. May require much higher dose of nifedipine.

Protease inhibitors (amprenavir, ritonavir, nelfinavir) may increase the serum levels of nifedipine

Quinidine's serum concentration is reduced and nifedipine's is increased; adjust doses as needed

Rifampin increases the metabolism of the calcium channel blocker; adjust the dose of the calcium channel blocker to maintain efficacy

Tacrolimus's serum concentrations are increased by verapamil; avoid the combination. Use another calcium channel blocker or monitor tacrolimus trough levels and renal function closely.

Vincristine's half-life is increased by nifedipine; monitor closely for vincristine dose adjustment

Alcohol Interactions Avoid use (may increase nifedipine levels)

Onset Oral: Within 20 minutes

Half-Life Adults, normal: 2-5 hours; Adults with cirrhosis: 7 hours

Education and Monitoring Issues

Patient Education: Take as directed; do not alter dosage regimen or increase, decrease, or discontinue without consulting prescriber. Do not crush or chew tablets or capsules. Consult prescriber before increasing exercise routine (decreased angina does not mean it is safe to increase exercise). Change position slowly to prevent orthostatic events. May cause dizziness or fatigue; use caution when driving or engaging in tasks that require alertness until response to drug is known. Maintain good oral care and inspect gums for swelling or redness. May cause frequent urination at night. Report irregular heartbeat, swelling, difficulty breathing or new cough, unresolved fatigue, unusual weight gain, unresolved dizziness or constipation, and swollen or bleeding gums.

Dietary Considerations: Grapefruit juice increases the bioavailability of nifedipine; monitor for altered nifedipine effects

Monitoring Parameters: Heart rate, blood pressure, signs and symptoms of CHF, peripheral edema

Related Information

Calcium Channel Blocking Agents Comparison *on page 1236*

- **Niferex®-PN** *see* Vitamins, Multiple *on page 981*
- **Nilandron™** *see* Nilutamide *on page 655*
- **Nilstat®** *see* Nystatin *on page 670*

Nilutamide (ni LU ta mide)

Pharmacologic Class Antineoplastic Agent, Miscellaneous

U.S. Brand Names Nilandron™

Mechanism of Action Acts as an antiandrogen by inhibiting androgen uptake and/or inhibiting nuclear binding of androgen in target tissues; it specifically blocks the action of androgens by interacting with cytosolic androgen receptor F sites in the target tissues

Use In combination with surgical castration in treatment of metastatic prostatic carcinoma (Stage D_2); for maximum benefit, nilutamide treatment must begin on the same day as or on the day after surgical castration

USUAL DOSAGE Refer to individual protocol. Oral:

100 mg every 8 hours, daily
150 mg twice daily
300 mg daily for 30 days, then 150 mg/day

Dosage Forms TAB: 50 mg

Contraindications Severe hepatic impairment; severe respiratory insufficiency; hypersensitivity to nilutamide or any component of this preparation

Warnings/Precautions The U.S. Food and Drug Administration (FDA) currently recommends that procedures for proper handling and disposal of antineoplastic agents be considered.

Interstitial pneumonitis has been reported in 2% of patients exposed to nilutamide. Patients typically experienced progressive exertional dyspnea, and possibly cough, chest pain and fever. X-rays showed interstitial or alveolo-interstitial changes. The suggestive signs of pneumonitis most often occurred within the first 3 months of nilutamide treatment.

Hepatitis or marked increases in liver enzymes leading to drug discontinuation occurred in 1% of nilutamide patients. There has been a report of elevated hepatic enzymes followed by death in a 65 year old patient treated with nilutamide.

Foreign postmarketing surveillance has revealed isolated cases of aplastic anemia in which a causal relationship with nilutamide could not be ascertained.

13% to 57% of patients receiving nilutamide reported a delay in adaptation to the dark, ranging from seconds to a few minutes. This effect sometimes does not abate as drug treatment is continued. Caution patients who experience this effect about driving at night or through tunnels. This effect can be alleviated by wearing tinted glasses.

Pregnancy Risk Factor C

Adverse Reactions

>10%:

Central nervous system: Pain, headache, insomnia
Gastrointestinal: Nausea, constipation, anorexia
Genitourinary: Impotence, testicular atrophy, gynecomastia
Endocrine & metabolic: Loss of libido, hot flashes
Neuromuscular & skeletal: Weakness
Ocular: Impaired adaption to dark

1% to 10%:

Cardiovascular: Hypertension
Central nervous system: Flu syndrome, fever, dizziness, depression, hypesthesia
Dermatologic: Alopecia, dry skin, rash
Gastrointestinal: Dyspepsia, vomiting, abdominal pain
Genitourinary: Urinary tract infection, hematuria, urinary tract disorder, nocturia
Ocular: Chromatopsia, impaired adaption to light, abnormal vision
Respiratory: Dyspnea, upper respiratory infection, pneumonia
Miscellaneous: Diaphoresis

Half-Life 38-59 hours

Education and Monitoring Issues

Patient Education: Take as prescribed; do not change dosing schedule or stop taking without consulting prescriber. Avoid alcohol while taking this medication; may cause severe reaction. Periodic laboratory tests are necessary while taking this medication. You may experience dizziness, confusion, or blurred vision (avoid driving or engaging

(Continued)

Nilutamide *(Continued)*

in tasks that require alertness until response to drug is known); loss of light accommodation (avoid night driving and use caution in poorly lighted or changing light situations); impotence; or loss of libido (discuss with prescriber). Report any decreased respiratory function (eg, dyspnea, increased cough); yellowing of skin or eyes; change in color of urine or stool; unusual bruising or bleeding; chest pain; difficulty or painful voiding.

Dietary Considerations: Food: Can be taken without regard to food

Monitoring Parameters:

Perform routine chest x-rays before treatment, and tell patients to report immediately any dyspnea or aggravation of pre-existing dyspnea. At the onset of dyspnea or worsening of pre-existing dyspnea any time during therapy, interrupt nilutamide until it can be determined if respiratory symptoms are drug-related. Obtain a chest x-ray, and if there are findings suggestive of interstitial pneumonitis, discontinue treatment with nilutamide. The pneumonitis is almost always reversible when treatment is discontinued. If the chest x-ray appears normal, perform pulmonary function tests.

Measure serum hepatic enzyme levels at baseline and at regular intervals (3 months); if transaminases increase over 2-3 times the upper limit of normal, discontinue treatment. Perform appropriate laboratory testing at the first symptom/sign of liver injury (eg, jaundice, dark urine, fatigue, abdominal pain or unexplained GI symptoms) and nilutamide treatment must be discontinued immediately if transaminases exceed 3 times the upper limit of normal.

Manufacturer Hoechst-Marion Roussel

Related Information

Pharmaceutical Manufacturers Directory *on page 1020*

Nimodipine (nye MOE di peen)

Pharmacologic Class Calcium Channel Blocker

U.S. Brand Names Nimotop®

Generic Available No

Mechanism of Action Nimodipine shares the pharmacology of other calcium channel blockers; animal studies indicate that nimodipine has a greater effect on cerebral arterials than other arterials; this increased specificity may be due to the drug's increased lipophilicity and cerebral distribution as compared to nifedipine; inhibits calcium ion from entering the "slow channels" or select voltage sensitive areas of vascular smooth muscle and myocardium during depolarization

Use Improvement of neurological deficits due to spasm following subarachnoid hemorrhage from ruptured congenital intracranial aneurysms in patients who are in good neurological condition postictus

USUAL DOSAGE Adults: Oral: 60 mg every 4 hours for 21 days, start therapy within 96 hours after subarachnoid hemorrhage

Dialysis: Not removed by hemo- or peritoneal dialysis; supplemental dose is not necessary

Dosing adjustment in hepatic impairment: Reduce dosage to 30 mg every 4 hours in patients with liver failure

Dosage Forms CAP, liquid-filled: 30 mg

Contraindications Hypersensitivity to nimodipine or any component

Warnings/Precautions Use with caution and titrate dosages for patients with impaired renal or hepatic function; use caution when treating patients with congestive heart failure, sick-sinus syndrome, PVCs, severe left ventricular dysfunction, hypertrophic cardiomyopathy (especially obstructive, IHSS), concomitant therapy with beta-blockers or digoxin, edema, or increased intracranial pressure with cranial tumors; do not abruptly withdraw (may cause chest pain); elderly may experience hypotension and constipation more readily

Pregnancy Risk Factor C

Pregnancy Implications

Clinical effects on the fetus: Use in pregnancy only when clearly needed and when the benefits outweigh the potential hazard to the fetus. Teratogenic and embryotoxic effects have been demonstrated in small animals. No well controlled studies have been conducted in pregnant women.

Breast milk/lactation: Appears in breast milk at levels higher than maternal plasma levels; no recommendations are currently available on breast-feeding

Adverse Reactions

1% to 10%:

Cardiovascular: Reductions in systemic blood pressure (1.2% to 8.1%)
Central nervous system: Headache (1.2% to 4.1%)
Dermatologic: Rash (0.6% to 2.4%)
Gastrointestinal: Diarrhea (1.7% to 4.2%), abdominal discomfort (2%)

<1% (limited to important or life-threatening symptoms): Edema (0.3% to 1.2%), EKG abnormalities (0.6% to 1.4%), tachycardia (0% to 1.4%), bradycardia (0.6% to 1%), depression (0% to 1.4%), acne (0% to 1.4%), nausea (0.6% to 1.4%), hemorrhage, hepatitis, muscle cramps/pain (0.2% to 1.4%), dyspnea (0% to 1.4%), itching, GI hemorrhage, thrombocytopenia, anemia, palpitations, vomiting, flushing, diaphoresis,

wheezing, lightheadedness, dizziness, rebound vasospasm, jaundice, hypertension, hematoma, neurological deterioration, congestive heart failure, hyponatremia, disseminated intravascular coagulation, deep vein thrombosis

Case report: DIC

Drug Interactions CYP3A3/4 enzyme substrate

Increased toxicity/effect/levels:

Nimodipine and cimetidine may increase bioavailability of nimodipine as with other calcium blockers

Nimodipine and omeprazole may increase bioavailability of nimodipine

Nimodipine, propranolol, and other beta-blockers may have minimal increase of depressant effects on A-V conduction

Protease inhibitors (amprenavir, ritonavir, nelfinavir) may increase the serum levels of nimodipine

Half-Life 3 hours, increases with reduced renal function

Education and Monitoring Issues

Patient Education: Take as prescribed, for the length of time prescribed; do not discontinue without consulting prescriber. You may experience headache (if unrelieved, consult prescriber), nausea or vomiting (frequent small meals may help), constipation (increased dietary bulk and fluids may help). Promptly report any chest pain or swelling of hands or feet, respiratory distress, sudden weight gain, or unresolved constipation.

Manufacturer Bayer Corp (Biological and Pharmaceutical Division)

Related Information

Pharmaceutical Manufacturers Directory *on page 1020*

♦ **Nimotop®** *see* Nimodipine *on page 656*

♦ **Nipride** *see* Nitroprusside *on page 661*

Nisoldipine (NYE sole di peen)

Pharmacologic Class Calcium Channel Blocker

U.S. Brand Names Sular®

Mechanism of Action As a dihydropyridine calcium channel blocker, structurally similar to nifedipine, nisoldipine impedes the movement of calcium ions into vascular smooth muscle and cardiac muscle. Dihydropyridines are potent vasodilators and are not as likely to suppress cardiac contractility and slow cardiac conduction as other calcium antagonists such as verapamil and diltiazem; nisoldipine is 5-10 times as potent a vasodilator as nifedipine.

Use Management of hypertension, may be used alone or in combination with other antihypertensive agents

USUAL DOSAGE Adults: Oral: Initial: 20 mg once daily, then increase by 10 mg/week (or longer intervals) to attain adequate control of blood pressure; doses >60 mg once daily are not recommended. A starting dose not exceeding 10 mg/day is recommended for the elderly and those with hepatic impairment.

Dosage Forms TAB, extended release: 10 mg, 20 mg, 30 mg, 40 mg

Contraindications Hypersensitivity to nisoldipine or any component or other dihydropyridine calcium channel blocker

Warnings/Precautions Increased angina and/or myocardial infarction in patients with coronary artery disease

Pregnancy Risk Factor C

Adverse Reactions

>10%:

Cardiovascular: Peripheral edema (dose-related 7% to 29%)

Central nervous system: Headache (22%)

1% to 10%:

Cardiovascular: Chest pain (2%), palpitations (3%), vasodilation (4%)

Central nervous system: Dizziness (3% to 10%)

Dermatologic: Rash (2%)

Gastrointestinal: Nausea (2%)

Respiratory: Pharyngitis (5%), sinusitis (3%), dyspnea (3%), cough (5%)

<1%: Chills, facial edema, fever, flu syndrome, malaise, atria fibrillation, CVA, congestive heart failure, first-degree A-V block, hypertension, angina, pulmonary edema, jugular venous distention, migraine, myocardial infarction, postural hypertension, ventricular extrasystoles, supraventricular tachycardia, syncope, systolic ejection murmur, T-wave abnormalities on EKG (flattening, inversion, nonspecific changes), venous insufficiency, abnormal liver function tests, anorexia, colitis, diarrhea, dry mouth, dyspepsia, dysphagia, flatulence, gastritis, gastrointestinal hemorrhage, gingival hyperplasia, glossitis, hepatomegaly, increased appetite, melena, mouth ulceration, diabetes mellitus, thyroiditis, anemia, ecchymoses, leukopenia, petechiae, gout, hypokalemia, increased serum creatine kinase, increased nonprotein nitrogen, weight gain, weight loss, arthralgia, arthritis, leg cramps, myalgia, myasthenia, myositis, tenosynovitis, abnormal dreams, abnormal thinking and confusion, amnesia, anxiety, ataxia, cerebral ischemia, decreased libido, depression, hypesthesia, hypertonia, insomnia, nervousness, paresthesia, somnolence, tremor, vertigo, asthma, dyspnea, end inspiratory wheeze and fine rales, epistaxis, gynecomastia, increased cough, laryngitis, pharyngitis, pleural effusions, rhinitis, sinusitis, acne, alopecia, dry skin, exfoliative dermatitis, fungal dermatitis,

(Continued)

Nisoldipine *(Continued)*

herpes simplex, herpes zoster, maculopapular rash, pruritus, pustular rash, skin discoloration, skin ulcer, sweating, urticaria, abnormal vision, amblyopia, blepharitis, conjunctivitis, ear pain, glaucoma, itchy eyes, keratoconjunctivitis, otitis media, retinal detachment, tinnitus, watery eyes, taste disturbance, temporary unilateral loss of vision, vitreous floater, watery eyes, dysuria, hematuria, impotence, nocturia, urinary frequency, increased BUN and serum creatinine, vaginal hemorrhage, vaginitis

Case report: Cholestatic jaundice

Drug Interactions CYP3A3/4 enzyme substrate

Azole antifungals may inhibit the calcium channel blocker's metabolism; avoid this combination. Try an antifungal like terbinafine (if appropriate) or monitor closely for altered effect of the calcium channel blocker.

Beta-blockers may have increased pharmacokinetic or pharmacodynamic interactions with nisoldipine

Calcium may reduce the calcium channel blocker's effects, particularly hypotension

Cimetidine reduced diltiazem's metabolism; consider an alternative H_2 antagonist

Phenytoin decreases nisoldipine to undetectable levels; avoid use of any CYP3A4 inducer with nisoldipine

Rifampin increases the metabolism of the calcium channel blocker; adjust the dose of the calcium channel blocker to maintain efficacy

Tacrolimus's serum concentrations are increased by nifedipine; avoid the combination. Use another calcium channel blocker or monitor tacrolimus trough levels and renal function closely.

Duration >24 hours

Half-Life 7-12 hours

Education and Monitoring Issues

Patient Education: Take as prescribed - swallow whole (do not crush or break). May be taken with food but avoid grapefruit products and high fat foods. Do not stop abruptly without consulting prescriber. You may experience headache (if unrelieved, consult prescriber), nausea or vomiting (frequent small meals may help), constipation (increased dietary bulk and fluids may help), depression (should resolve when drug is discontinued). May cause dizziness or drowsiness; use caution when driving or engaging in tasks that require alertness until response to drug is known. Promptly report any chest pain or swelling of hands or feet, respiratory distress, sudden weight gain, or unresolved constipation.

Dietary Considerations: Grapefruit juice increases the bioavailability of nisoldipine; monitor for altered nisoldipine effects

Manufacturer AstraZeneca

Related Information

Calcium Channel Blocking Agents Comparison *on page 1236*
Pharmaceutical Manufacturers Directory *on page 1020*

- **Nitrek® Patch** *see* Nitroglycerin *on page 659*
- **Nitro-Bid®** *see* Nitroglycerin *on page 659*
- **Nitro-Bid® I.V. Injection** *see* Nitroglycerin *on page 659*
- **Nitro-Bid® Ointment** *see* Nitroglycerin *on page 659*
- **Nitrodisc® Patch** *see* Nitroglycerin *on page 659*
- **Nitro-Dur®** *see* Nitroglycerin *on page 659*
- **Nitro-Dur® Patch** *see* Nitroglycerin *on page 659*

Nitrofurantoin (nye troe fyoor AN toyn)

Pharmacologic Class Antibiotic, Miscellaneous

U.S. Brand Names Furadantin®; Furalan®; Furan®; Furanite®; Macrobid®; Macrodantin®

Generic Available Yes: Tablet and suspension

Mechanism of Action Inhibits several bacterial enzyme systems including acetyl coenzyme A interfering with metabolism and possibly cell wall synthesis

Use Prevention and treatment of urinary tract infections caused by susceptible gram-negative and some gram-positive organisms; *Pseudomonas*, *Serratia*, and most species of *Proteus* are generally resistant to nitrofurantoin

USUAL DOSAGE Oral:

Children >1 month: 5-7 mg/kg/day in divided doses every 6 hours; maximum: 400 mg/day

Chronic therapy: 1-2 mg/kg/day in divided doses every 12-24 hours; maximum dose: 100 mg/day

Adults: 50-100 mg/dose every 6 hours

Macrocrystal/monohydrate: 100 mg twice daily

Prophylaxis or chronic therapy: 50-100 mg/dose at bedtime

Dosing adjustment in renal impairment: Cl_{cr} <50 mL/minute: Avoid use

Avoid use in hemo and peritoneal dialysis and continuous arteriovenous or venovenous hemofiltration (CAVH/CAVHD)

Dosage Forms CAP: 50 mg, 100 mg; Macrocrystal: 25 mg, 50 mg, 100 mg; Macrocrystal/monohydrate: 100 mg. **SUSP, oral:** 25 mg/5 mL (470 mL)

Contraindications Hypersensitivity to nitrofurantoin or any component; renal impairment; infants <1 month (due to the possibility of hemolytic anemia)

Warnings/Precautions Use with caution in patients with G-6-PD deficiency, patients with anemia, vitamin B deficiency, diabetes mellitus or electrolyte abnormalities; therapeutic concentrations of nitrofurantoin are not attained in urine of patients with Cl_{cr} <40 mL/minute (elderly); use with caution if prolonged therapy is anticipated due to possible pulmonary toxicity; acute, subacute, or chronic (usually after 6 months of therapy) pulmonary reactions have been observed in patients treated with nitrofurantoin; if these occur, discontinue therapy; monitor closely for malaise, dyspnea, cough, fever, radiologic evidence of diffuse interstitial pneumonitis or fibrosis

Pregnancy Risk Factor B

Adverse Reactions Percentage unknown: Arthralgia, *C. difficile*-colitis, chest pains, chills, cough, diarrhea, dizziness, drowsiness, dyspnea, exfoliative dermatitis, fatigue, fever, headache, hemolytic anemia, hepatitis, hypersensitivity, increased LFTs, itching, loss of appetite/vomiting/nausea (most common), lupus-like syndrome, numbness, paresthesia, rash, sore throat, stomach upset, weakness

Drug Interactions

Decreased effect: Antacids, especially magnesium salts, decrease absorption of nitrofurantoin; nitrofurantoin may antagonize effects of norfloxacin

Increased toxicity: Probenecid (decreases renal excretion of nitrofurantoin); anticholinergic drugs increase absorption of nitrofurantoin

Alcohol Interactions Avoid use

Half-Life 20-60 minutes; prolonged with renal impairment

Education and Monitoring Issues

Patient Education: Take per recommended schedule, at regular intervals around-the-clock. Complete full course of therapy; do not skip doses. Maintain adequate hydration (2-3 L/day of fluids unless instructed to restrict fluid intake). Diabetics should consult prescriber if using Clinitest® for glucose testing. Nitrofurantoin may discolor urine dark yellow or brown (normal). You may experience nausea or vomiting or GI upset (small frequent meals, frequent mouth care, sucking lozenges, or chewing gum may help); fatigue, drowsiness, blurred vision (use caution when driving or engaging in tasks that require alertness until response to drug is known). Report chest pains or palpitations; pain on urination or blood in urine; skin rash; muscle weakness, pain, or tremors; excessive fatigue or weakness; other persistent adverse effects; or if condition does not improve.

Monitoring Parameters: Signs of pulmonary reaction, signs of numbness or tingling of the extremities, periodic liver function tests

Related Information

Antimicrobial Drugs of Choice *on page 1182*

Nitrofurazone (nye troe FYOOR a zone)

Pharmacologic Class Antibiotic, Topical

U.S. Brand Names Furacin® Topical

Use Antibacterial agent in second and third degree burns and skin grafting

USUAL DOSAGE Children and Adults: Topical: Apply once daily or every few days to lesion or place on gauze

Contraindications Hypersensitivity to nitrofurazone or any component

Pregnancy Risk Factor C

♦ **Nitrogard** *see* Nitroglycerin *on page 659*

♦ **Nitrogard® Buccal** *see* Nitroglycerin *on page 659*

Nitroglycerin (nye troe GLI ser in)

Pharmacologic Class Vasodilator

U.S. Brand Names Deponit® Patch; Minitran® Patch; Nitrek® Patch; Nitro-Bid® I.V. Injection; Nitro-Bid® Ointment; Nitrodisc® Patch; Nitro-Dur® Patch; Nitrogard® Buccal; Nitroglyn® Oral; Nitrolingual® Translingual Spray; Nitrol® Ointment; Nitrong® Oral Tablet; Nitrostat® Sublingual; Nitro-Time® Capsules; Transdermal-NTG® Patch; Transderm-Nitro® Patch; Tridil® Injection

Generic Available Yes

Mechanism of Action Reduces cardiac oxygen demand by decreasing left ventricular pressure and systemic vascular resistance; dilates coronary arteries and improves collateral flow to ischemic regions

Use Treatment and prevention of angina pectoris; I.V. for congestive heart failure (especially when associated with acute myocardial infarction); pulmonary hypertension; hypertensive emergencies (especially those associated with coronary complications); control of blood pressure in perioperative hypertension (especially during cardiovascular surgery); controlled hypotension during surgical procedures

USUAL DOSAGE Note: Hemodynamic and antianginal tolerance often develop within 24-48 hours of continuous nitrate administration

Children: Pulmonary hypertension: Continuous infusion: Start 0.25-0.5 mcg/kg/minute and titrate by 1 mcg/kg/minute at 20- to 60-minute intervals to desired effect; usual dose: 1-3 mcg/kg/minute; maximum: 5 mcg/kg/minute

(Continued)

Nitroglycerin *(Continued)*

Adults:

Buccal: Initial: 1 mg every 3-5 hours while awake (3 times/day); titrate dosage upward if angina occurs with tablet in place

Oral: 2.5-9 mg 2-4 times/day (up to 26 mg 4 times/day)

I.V.: 5 mcg/minute, increase by 5 mcg/minute every 3-5 minutes to 20 mcg/minute; if no response at 20 mcg/minute increase by 10 mcg/minute every 3-5 minutes, up to 200 mcg/minute

Ointment: ½" upon rising and ½" 6 hours later; the dose may be doubled and even doubled again as needed

Patch, transdermal: Initial: 0.2-0.4 mg/hour, titrate to doses of 0.4-0.8 mg/hour; tolerance is minimized by using a patch-on period of 12-14 hours and patch-off period of 10-12 hours

Sublingual: 0.2-0.6 mg every 5 minutes for maximum of 3 doses in 15 minutes; may also use prophylactically 5-10 minutes prior to activities which may provoke an attack

Translingual: 1-2 sprays into mouth under tongue every 3-5 minutes for maximum of 3 doses in 15 minutes, may also be used 5-10 minutes prior to activities which may provoke an attack prophylactically

Hemodialysis: Supplemental dose is not necessary

Peritoneal dialysis: Supplemental dose is not necessary

May need to use nitrate-free interval (10-12 hours/day) to avoid tolerance development; gradually decrease dose in patients receiving NTG for prolonged period to avoid withdrawal reaction

Dosage Forms CAP, sustained release: 2.5 mg, 6.5 mg, 9 mg, 13 mg. **INJ:** 0.5 mg/mL (10 mL); 0.8 mg/mL (10 mL); 5 mg/mL (1 mL, 5 mL, 10 mL, 20 mL); 10 mg/mL (5 mL, 10 mL). **INJ, solution** in D_5W: 25 mg (250 mL), 50 mg (250 mL, 500 mL), 100 mg (250 mL), 200 mg (500 mL). **OINT, top** (Nitrol®): 2% [20 mg/g] (30 g, 60 g). **PATCH, transdermal, top:** Systems designed to deliver 0.1 mg/hr, 0.2 mg/hr, 0.4 mg/hr, 0.6 mg/hr, 2.5, 5, 7.5, 10, or 15 mg NTG over 24 hours. **SPRAY, translingual:** 0.4 mg/metered spray (5.7, 12 g). **TAB:** Buccal, controlled release: 1 mg, 2 mg, 3 mg; Sublingual (Nitrostat®): 0.3 mg, 0.4 mg, 0.6 mg; Sustained release: 2.6 mg, 6.5 mg, 9 mg

Contraindications Hypersensitivity to nitroglycerin or any component; pericardial tamponade, restrictive cardiomyopathy, or constrictive pericarditis; allergy to adhesive (transdermal), uncorrected hypovolemia (I.V.); transdermal NTG is not effective for immediate relief of angina

Warnings/Precautions Do not use extended release preparations in patients with GI hypermotility or malabsorptive syndrome; use with caution in patients with hepatic impairment, CHF, or acute myocardial infarction; available preparations of I.V. nitroglycerin differ in concentration or volume; pay attention to dilution and dosage; I.V. preparations contain alcohol and/or propylene glycol; avoid loss of nitroglycerin in standard PVC tubing; dosing instructions must be followed with care when the appropriate infusion sets are used

Hypotension may occur, use with caution in patients who are volume-depleted, are hypotensive, have inadequate circulation; nitrate therapy may aggravate angina caused by hypertrophic cardiomyopathy

Pregnancy Risk Factor C

Adverse Reactions

Spray or patch:

>10%: Central nervous system: Headache (patch 63%, spray 50%)

1% to 10%:

Cardiovascular: Hypotension (patch 4%), increased angina (patch 2%)

Central nervous system: Lightheadedness (patch 6%), syncope (patch 4%)

<1% (limited to important or life-threatening symptoms): Allergic reactions, application site irritation (patch), rash, dizziness, weakness, restlessness, pallor, perspiration, collapse, exfoliative dermatitis, vertigo, palpitations, methemoglobinemia (rare, overdose)

Topical, sublingual, intravenous: Incidence of reactions are not reported:

Cardiovascular: Hypotension (infrequent), postural hypotension, crescendo angina (uncommon), rebound hypertension (uncommon), pallor, cardiovascular collapse, tachycardia, shock, flushing, peripheral edema

Central nervous system: Headache (most common), lightheadedness (related to blood pressure changes), syncope (uncommon), dizziness, restlessness

Gastrointestinal: Nausea, vomiting, bowel incontinence, xerostomia

Genitourinary: Urinary incontinence

Hematologic: Methemoglobinemia (rare, overdose)

Neuromuscular & skeletal: Weakness

Ocular: Blurred vision

Miscellaneous: Cold sweat

The incidence of hypotension and adverse cardiovascular events may be increased when used in combination with sildenafil

Drug Interactions

Alteplase (tissue plasminogen activator) has a lesser effect when used with I.V. nitroglycerin; avoid concurrent use

Ergot alkaloids may cause an increase in blood pressure and decrease in antianginal effects; avoid concurrent use

Ethanol can cause hypotension when nitrates are taken 1 hour or more after ethanol ingestion

Heparin's effect may be reduced by I.V. nitroglycerin. May affect only a minority of patients

Sildenafil potentiates the hypotensive effects of nitrates; concurrent use is contraindicated

Alcohol Interactions Avoid use around dose (may cause hypotension)

Onset

Sublingual tablet: 1-3 minutes
Translingual spray: 2 minutes
Buccal tablet: 2-5 minutes
Sustained release: 20-45 minutes
Topical: 15-60 minutes
Transdermal: 40-60 minutes
I.V. drip: Immediate

Duration

Sublingual tablet: 30-60 minutes
Translingual spray: 30-60 minutes
Buccal tablet: 2 hours
Sustained release: 4-8 hours
Topical: 2-12 hours
Transdermal: 18-24 hours
I.V. drip: 3-5 minutes

Half-Life 1-4 minutes

Education and Monitoring Issues

Patient Education:

Oral: Take as directed. Do not chew or swallow sublingual tablets; allow to dissolve under tongue. Do not chew or crush extended release capsules; swallow with 8 oz of water.

Spray: Spray directly on mucous membranes; do not inhale.

Topical: Spread prescribed amount thinly on applicator; rotate application sites.

Transdermal: Place on hair-free area of skin, rotate sites.

Do not change brands without consulting prescriber. Do not discontinue abruptly. Keep medication in original container, tightly closed. Take medication while sitting down and use caution when changing position (rise from sitting or lying position slowly). May cause dizziness; use caution when driving or engaging in hazardous activities until response to drug is known. If chest pain is unresolved in 15 minutes, seek emergency medical help at once. Report acute headache, rapid heartbeat, unusual restlessness or dizziness, muscular weakness, or blurring vision.

Monitoring Parameters: Blood pressure, heart rate, PCWP

- **Nitroglyn® Oral** *see* Nitroglycerin *on page 659*
- **Nitroject** *see* Nitroglycerin *on page 659*
- **Nitrol** *see* Nitroglycerin *on page 659*
- **Nitrolingual®** *see* Nitroglycerin *on page 659*
- **Nitrolingual® Translingual Spray** *see* Nitroglycerin *on page 659*
- **Nitrol® Ointment** *see* Nitroglycerin *on page 659*
- **Nitrong®** *see* Nitroglycerin *on page 659*
- **Nitrong® Oral Tablet** *see* Nitroglycerin *on page 659*
- **Nitropress®** *see* Nitroprusside *on page 661*

Nitroprusside (nye troe PRUS ide)

Pharmacologic Class Vasodilator

U.S. Brand Names Nitropress®

Generic Available Yes

Mechanism of Action Causes peripheral vasodilation by direct action on venous and arteriolar smooth muscle, thus reducing peripheral resistance; will increase cardiac output by decreasing afterload; reduces aortal and left ventricular impedance

Use Management of hypertensive crises; congestive heart failure; used for controlled hypotension to reduce bleeding during surgery

USUAL DOSAGE Administration requires the use of an infusion pump. Average dose: 5 mcg/kg/minute

Children: Pulmonary hypertension: I.V.: Initial: 1 mcg/kg/minute by continuous I.V. infusion; increase in increments of 1 mcg/kg/minute at intervals of 20-60 minutes; titrating to the desired response; usual dose: 3 mcg/kg/minute, rarely need >4 mcg/kg/minute; maximum: 5 mcg/kg/minute.

Adults: I.V. Initial: 0.3-0.5 mcg/kg/minute; increase in increments of 0.5 mcg/kg/minute, titrating to the desired hemodynamic effect or the appearance of headache or nausea; usual dose: 3 mcg/kg/minute; rarely need >4 mcg/kg/minute; maximum: 10 mcg/kg/minute. When >500 mcg/kg is administered by prolonged infusion of faster than 2 mcg/kg/minute, cyanide is generated faster than an unaided patient can handle.

(Continued)

Nitroprusside *(Continued)*

Dosage Forms INJ: 10 mg/mL (5 mL); 25 mg/mL (2 mL)

Contraindications Hypersensitivity to nitroprusside or components; decreased cerebral perfusion; arteriovenous shunt or coarctation of the aorta (ie, compensatory hypertension)

Warnings/Precautions Use with caution in patients with increased intracranial pressure (head trauma, cerebral hemorrhage); severe renal impairment, hepatic failure, hypothyroidism; use only as an infusion with 5% dextrose in water; continuously monitor patient's blood pressure; excessive amounts of nitroprusside can cause cyanide toxicity (usually in patients with decreased liver function) or thiocyanate toxicity (usually in patients with decreased renal function, or in patients with normal renal function but prolonged nitroprusside use)

Pregnancy Risk Factor C

Adverse Reactions 1% to 10%:

Cardiovascular: Excessive hypotensive response, palpitations, substernal distress
Central nervous system: Disorientation, psychosis, headache, restlessness
Endocrine & metabolic: Thyroid suppression
Gastrointestinal: Nausea, vomiting
Neuromuscular & skeletal: Weakness, muscle spasm
Otic: Tinnitus
Respiratory: Hypoxia
Miscellaneous: Sweating, thiocyanate toxicity

Drug Interactions None noted

Onset Onset of hypotensive effect: <2 minutes

Duration Within 1-10 minutes following discontinuation of therapy, effects cease

Half-Life Parent drug: <10 minutes; Thiocyanate: 2.7-7 days

Education and Monitoring Issues

Patient Education: Patient condition should indicate extent of education and instruction needed. This drug can only be given I.V. You will be monitored at all times during infusion. Promptly report any chest pain or pain/burning at site of infusion.

Monitoring Parameters: Blood pressure, heart rate; monitor for cyanide and thiocyanate toxicity; monitor acid-base status as acidosis can be the earliest sign of cyanide toxicity; monitor thiocyanate levels if requiring prolonged infusion (>3 days) or dose ≥4 mcg/kg/minute or patient has renal dysfunction; monitor cyanide blood levels in patients with decreased hepatic function; cardiac monitor and blood pressure monitor required

Reference Range: Monitor thiocyanate levels if requiring prolonged infusion (>4 days) or ≥4 µg/kg/minute; not to exceed 100 µg/mL (or 10 mg/dL) plasma thiocyanate

Thiocyanate:
- Therapeutic: 6-29 µg/mL
- Toxic: 35-100 µg/mL
- Fatal: >200 µg/mL

Cyanide: Normal <0.2 µg/mL; normal (smoker): <0.4 µg/mL
- Toxic: >2 µg/mL
- Potentially lethal: >3 µg/mL

♦ **Nitrostat®** *see* Nitroglycerin *on page 659*
♦ **Nitrostat® Sublingual** *see* Nitroglycerin *on page 659*
♦ **Nitro-Time® Capsules** *see* Nitroglycerin *on page 659*
♦ **Nix®** *see* Permethrin *on page 719*
♦ **Nix™ Creme Rinse** *see* Permethrin *on page 719*

Nizatidine (ni ZA ti deen)

Pharmacologic Class Histamine H_2 Antagonist

U.S. Brand Names Axid® AR [OTC]; Axid®

Generic Available No

Mechanism of Action Nizatidine is an H_2-receptor antagonist. In healthy volunteers, nizatidine has been effective in suppressing gastric acid secretion induced by pentagastrin infusion or food. Nizatidine reduces gastric acid secretion by 29.4% to 78.4%. This compares with a 60.3% reduction by cimetidine. Nizatidine 100 mg is reported to provide equivalent acid suppression as cimetidine 300 mg.

Use Treatment and maintenance of duodenal ulcer; treatment of gastroesophageal reflux disease (GERD); OTC tablet used for the prevention of meal-induced heartburn, acid indigestion, and sour stomach

USUAL DOSAGE Adults: Oral:

Active duodenal ulcer:
- Treatment: 300 mg at bedtime or 150 mg twice daily
- Maintenance: 150 mg/day

Meal-induced heartburn, acid indigestion, and sour stomach:
- 75 mg tablet [OTC] twice daily, 30 to 60 minutes prior to consuming food or beverages

Dosing adjustment in renal impairment:
- Cl_{cr} 50-80 mL/minute: Administer 75% of normal dose
- Cl_{cr} 10-50 mL/minute: Administer 50% of normal dose or 150 mg/day for active treatment and 150 mg every other day for maintenance treatment

Cl_{cr} <10 mL/minute: Administer 25% of normal dose or 150 mg every other day for treatment and 150 mg every 3 days for maintenance treatment

Dosage Forms CAP: 150 mg, 300 mg. **TAB** [OTC]: 75 mg

Contraindications Hypersensitivity to nizatidine or any component of the preparation; hypersensitivity to other H_2-antagonists since a cross-sensitivity has been observed with this class of drugs

Warnings/Precautions Use with caution in children <12 years of age; use with caution in patients with liver and renal impairment; dosage modification required in patients with renal impairment

Pregnancy Risk Factor C

Adverse Reactions

1% to 10%:

Central nervous system: Dizziness, headache

Gastrointestinal: Constipation, diarrhea

<1%: Abdominal discomfort, acne, agranulocytosis, allergic reaction, anorexia, belching, bradycardia, bronchospasm, drowsiness, dry skin, fatigue, fever, flatulence, hypertension, increased AST/ALT, increased BUN/creatinine, insomnia, neutropenia, palpitations, paresthesia, proteinuria, pruritus, seizures, tachycardia, thrombocytopenia, urticaria, weakness

Alcohol Interactions Avoid use (may enhance gastric mucosal irritation)

Half-Life Normal renal function: 1-2 hours; End-stage renal disease: 3.5-11 hours

Education and Monitoring Issues

Patient Education: Take as directed; do not increase dose. It may take several days before you notice relief. If antacids approved by prescriber, take 1 hour between antacid and nizatidine. Avoid OTC medications, especially cold or cough medication and aspirin or anything containing aspirin. Follow diet as prescriber recommends. May cause drowsiness; use caution when driving or engaging in tasks that require alertness until response to drug is known. Report fever, sore throat, tarry stools, changes in CNS, or muscle or joint pain.

Manufacturer Eli Lilly and Co

Related Information

Pharmaceutical Manufacturers Directory *on page 1020*

- **Nizoral®** *see* Ketoconazole *on page 499*
- **Nobesine®** *see* Diethylpropion *on page 268*
- **Nolamine®** *see* Chlorpheniramine, Phenindamine, and Phenylpropanolamine *on page 186*
- **Nolvadex®** *see* Tamoxifen *on page 890*
- **Nonsteroidal Anti-Inflammatory Agents Comparison** *see page 1248*
- **Norcet®** *see* Hydrocodone and Acetaminophen *on page 444*
- **Nordette®** *see* Ethinyl Estradiol and Levonorgestrel *on page 341*
- **Norditropin® Injection** *see* Human Growth Hormone *on page 438*
- **Nordryl® Injection** *see* Diphenhydramine *on page 282*
- **Nordryl® Oral** *see* Diphenhydramine *on page 282*
- **Norethin™ 1/35E** *see* Ethinyl Estradiol and Norethindrone *on page 342*
- **Norethin™ 1/50M** *see* Mestranol and Norethindrone *on page 570*
- **Norflex™** *see* Orphenadrine *on page 681*

Norfloxacin (nor FLOKS a sin)

Pharmacologic Class Antibiotic, Quinolone

U.S. Brand Names Chibroxin™ Ophthalmic; Noroxin® Oral

Generic Available No

Mechanism of Action Norfloxacin is a DNA gyrase inhibitor. DNA gyrase is an essential bacterial enzyme that maintains the superhelical structure of DNA. DNA gyrase is required for DNA replication and transcription, DNA repair, recombination, and transposition; bactericidal

Use Uncomplicated urinary tract infections and cystitis caused by susceptible gram-negative and gram-positive bacteria; sexually transmitted disease (eg, uncomplicated urethral and cervical gonorrhea) caused by *N. gonorrhoeae*; prostatitis due to *E. coli*; ophthalmic solution for conjunctivitis

USUAL DOSAGE

Ophthalmic: Children >1 year and Adults: Instill 1-2 drops in affected eye(s) 4 times/day for up to 7 days

Oral: Adults:

Urinary tract infections: 400 mg twice daily for 3-21 days depending on severity of infection or organism sensitivity; maximum: 800 mg/day

Uncomplicated gonorrhea: 800 mg as a single dose (CDC recommends as an alternative regimen to ciprofloxacin or ofloxacin)

Prostatitis: 400 mg every 12 hours for 4 weeks

Dosing interval in renal impairment:

Cl_{cr} 10-30 mL/minute: Administer every 24 hours

Cl_{cr} <10 mL/minute: Do not use

(Continued)

Norfloxacin *(Continued)*

Dosage Forms SOLN, ophth: 0.3% [3 mg/mL] (5 mL). **TAB:** 400 mg

Contraindications Known hypersensitivity to quinolones

Warnings/Precautions Not recommended in children <18 years of age; other quinolones have caused transient arthropathy in children; CNS stimulation may occur which may lead to tremor, restlessness, confusion, and very rarely to hallucinations or convulsive seizures; use with caution in patients with known or suspected CNS disorders; has rarely caused ruptured tendons (discontinue immediately with signs of inflammation or tendon pain)

Pregnancy Risk Factor C

Adverse Reactions

1% to 10%:

Central nervous system: Headache (2.7%), dizziness (1.8%), fatigue

Gastrointestinal: Nausea (2.8%)

<1%: Abdominal pain, acute renal failure, anorexia, back pain, bitter taste, constipation, depression, diarrhea, dyspepsia, erythema, fever, flatulence, GI bleeding, heartburn, hyperhidrosis, increased liver enzymes, increased serum creatinine/BUN, insomnia, loose stools, pruritus, rash, ruptured tendons, somnolence, vomiting, weakness, xerostomia

Drug Interactions CYP1A2 and 3A3/4 enzyme inhibitor

Decreased effect: Decreased absorption with antacids containing aluminum, magnesium, and/or calcium (by up to 98% if given at the same time); decreased serum levels of fluoroquinolones by antineoplastics; nitrofurantoin may antagonize effects of norfloxacin; phenytoin serum levels may be decreased by fluoroquinolones

Increased toxicity/serum levels: Quinolones cause increased levels or toxicity of digoxin, caffeine, warfarin, cyclosporine, and possibly theophylline. Cimetidine and probenecid increase quinolone levels.

Half-Life 4.8 hours (can be higher with reduced glomerular filtration rates)

Education and Monitoring Issues

Patient Education:

Oral: Take per recommended schedule, preferably on an empty stomach (1 hour before or 2 hours after meals). Maintain adequate hydration (2-3 L/day of fluids unless instructed to restrict fluid intake). Take complete prescription; do not skip doses. Do not take with antacids. You may experience dizziness, lightheadedness; use caution when driving or engaging in tasks that require alertness until response to drug is known. Small frequent meals and frequent mouth care may reduce nausea or vomiting. You may experience photosensitivity; use sunscreen, wear protective clothing and eyewear, and avoid direct sunlight. Report persistent diarrhea or GI disturbances; excessive sleepiness or agitation; tremors; rash; pain, inflammation, or rupture of tendon; or changes in vision.

Ophthalmic: Tilt head back and instill 1-2 drops in affected eye 4 times a day for length of time prescribed. Do not allow tip of applicator to touch eye or any contaminated surface.

♦ **Norgesic®** *see* Orphenadrine, Aspirin, and Caffeine *on page 681*

♦ **Norgesic® Forte** *see* Orphenadrine, Aspirin, and Caffeine *on page 681*

Norgestrel (nor JES trel)

Pharmacologic Class Contraceptive, Progestin Only

U.S. Brand Names Ovrette®

Generic Available No

Mechanism of Action Inhibits secretion of pituitary gonadotropin (LH) which prevents follicular maturation and ovulation

Use Prevention of pregnancy; **progestin only products have higher risk of failure in contraceptive use**

USUAL DOSAGE Administer daily, starting the first day of menstruation, take 1 tablet at the same time each day, every day of the year. If one dose is missed, take as soon as remembered, then next tablet at regular time; if two doses are missed, take 1 tablet and discard the other, then take daily at usual time; if three doses are missed, use an additional form of birth control until menses or pregnancy is ruled out.

Ovrette®: One dose (20 yellow pills which are equivalent to 0.75 mg levonorgestrel) within 72 hours after unprotected intercourse, and a second dose 12 hours after the first dose

Note: Use of progestin-only ECPs reduces the risk of pregnancy by about 88%. This does not mean that 12% of women will become pregnant. Rather, if 100 women have unprotected intercourse once during the second or third week of their menstrual cycle, about 8 will become pregnant. If those same women had used progestin-only ECPs, only one would have become pregnant (an 88% reduction). Therapy is more effective the earlier it is initiated with the 72-hour window.

Dosage Forms TAB: 0.075 mg

Contraindications Known hypersensitivity to norgestrel; thromboembolic disorders, severe hepatic disease, breast cancer, undiagnosed vaginal bleeding, pregnancy

Warnings/Precautions Discontinue if sudden loss of vision or if diplopia or proptosis occur; use with caution in patients with a history of mental depression; use of any progestin during the first 4 months of pregnancy is not recommended

Pregnancy Risk Factor X

Adverse Reactions

>10%:

Cardiovascular: Edema

Endocrine & metabolic: Breakthrough bleeding, spotting, changes in menstrual flow, amenorrhea

Gastrointestinal: Anorexia

Neuromuscular & skeletal: Weakness

1% to 10%:

Cardiovascular: Embolism, central thrombosis

Central nervous system: Mental depression, fever, insomnia

Dermatologic: Melasma or chloasma, allergic rash with or without pruritus

Endocrine & metabolic: Changes in cervical erosion and secretions, increased breast tenderness

Gastrointestinal: Weight gain or loss

Hepatic: Cholestatic jaundice

Local: Thrombophlebitis

Drug Interactions Decreased effect: Aminoglutethimide may decrease effects by increasing hepatic metabolism

Half-Life ~20 hours

Education and Monitoring Issues

Patient Education: Take this medicine only as directed; do not take more of it and do not take it for a longer period of time; if you suspect you may have become pregnant, stop taking this medicine; report any loss of vision or vision changes immediately; avoid excessive exposure to sunlight

- ♦ **Norinyl® 1+35** *see* Ethinyl Estradiol and Norethindrone *on page 342*
- ♦ **Norinyl® 1+50** *see* Mestranol and Norethindrone *on page 570*
- ♦ **Norinyl® 1/80** *see* Mestranol and Norethindrone *on page 570*
- ♦ **Norinyl® 2** *see* Mestranol and Norethindrone *on page 570*
- ♦ **Norisodrine®** *see* Isoproterenol *on page 488*
- ♦ **Noritate® Cream** *see* Metronidazole *on page 597*
- ♦ **Normodyne®** *see* Labetalol *on page 503*
- ♦ **Noroxin® Oral** *see* Norfloxacin *on page 663*
- ♦ **Norpace®** *see* Disopyramide *on page 287*
- ♦ **Norplant® Implant** *see* Levonorgestrel *on page 524*
- ♦ **Norpramin®** *see* Desipramine *on page 252*
- ♦ **Nor-tet® Oral** *see* Tetracycline *on page 903*

Nortriptyline (nor TRIP ti leen)

Pharmacologic Class Antidepressant, Tricyclic (Secondary Amine)

U.S. Brand Names Aventyl® Hydrochloride; Pamelor®

Generic Available No

Mechanism of Action Traditionally believed to increase the synaptic concentration of serotonin and/or norepinephrine in the central nervous system by inhibition of their reuptake by the presynaptic neuronal membrane. However, additional receptor effects have been found including desensitization of adenyl cyclase, down regulation of beta-adrenergic receptors, and down regulation of serotonin receptors.

Use Treatment of various forms of depression, often in conjunction with psychotherapy. Maximum antidepressant effect may not be seen for 2 or more weeks after initiation of therapy; has also demonstrated effectiveness for chronic pain.

USUAL DOSAGE Oral:

Nocturnal enuresis:

Children:

6-7 years (20-25 kg): 10 mg/day

8-11 years (25-35 kg): 10-20 mg/day

>11 years (35-54 kg): 25-35 mg/day

Depression:

Adolescents: 30-50 mg/day in divided doses

Adults: 25 mg 3-4 times/day up to 150 mg/day

Elderly:

Initial: 10-25 mg at bedtime

Dosage can be increased by 25 mg every 3 days for inpatients and weekly for outpatients if tolerated

Usual maintenance dose: 75 mg as a single bedtime dose, however, lower or higher doses may be required to stay within the therapeutic window

Dosing adjustment in hepatic impairment: Lower doses and slower titration dependent on individualization of dosage is recommended

(Continued)

Nortriptyline *(Continued)*

Dosage Forms CAP: 10 mg, 25 mg, 50 mg, 75 mg. **SOLN:** 10 mg/5 mL (473 mL)

Contraindications Narrow-angle glaucoma, avoid use during pregnancy and lactation, hypersensitivity to tricyclic antidepressants

Warnings/Precautions Use with caution in patients with cardiac conduction disturbances, history of hyperthyroid; should not be abruptly discontinued in patients receiving high doses for prolonged periods; use with caution with renal or hepatic impairment

Pregnancy Risk Factor D

Adverse Reactions

Cardiovascular: Postural hypotension, arrhythmias, hypertension, heart block, tachycardia, palpitations, myocardial infarction

Central nervous system: Confusion, delirium, hallucinations, restlessness, insomnia, disorientation, delusions, anxiety, agitation, panic, nightmares, hypomania, exacerbation of psychosis, incoordination, ataxia, extrapyramidal symptoms, seizures

Dermatologic: Alopecia, photosensitivity, rash, petechiae, urticaria, itching

Endocrine & metabolic: Sexual dysfunction, gynecomastia, breast enlargement, galactorrhea, increase or decrease in libido, increase in blood sugar, SIADH

Gastrointestinal: Xerostomia, constipation, vomiting, anorexia, diarrhea, abdominal cramps, black tongue, nausea, unpleasant taste, weight gain or loss

Genitourinary: Urinary retention, delayed micturition, impotence, testicular edema

Hematologic: Rarely agranulocytosis, eosinophilia, purpura, thrombocytopenia

Hepatic: Increased liver enzymes, cholestatic jaundice

Neuromuscular & skeletal: Tremor, numbness, tingling, paresthesias, peripheral neuropathy

Ocular: Blurred vision, eye pain, disturbances in accommodation, mydriasis

Otic: Tinnitus

Miscellaneous: Diaphoresis (excessive), allergic reactions

Drug Interactions CYP1A2 and 2D6 enzyme substrate

Carbamazepine, phenobarbital, and rifampin may increase the metabolism of nortriptyline resulting in decreased effect of nortriptyline

Nortriptyline inhibits the antihypertensive response to bethanidine, clonidine, debrisoquin, guanadrel, guanethidine, guanabenz, guanfacine; monitor BP; consider alternate antihypertensive agent

Abrupt discontinuation of clonidine may cause hypertensive crisis, nortriptyline may enhance the response

Use with altretamine may cause orthostatic hypertension

Nortriptyline may be additive with or may potentiate the action of other CNS depressants (sedatives, hypnotics, or ethanol); with MAO inhibitors, hyperpyrexia, hypertension, tachycardia, confusion, seizures, and **deaths have been reported** (serotonin syndrome), this combination should be avoided

Nortriptyline may increase the prothrombin time in patients stabilized on warfarin

Cimetidine and methylphenidate may decrease the metabolism of nortriptyline

Additive anticholinergic effects seen with other anticholinergic agents

The SSRIs, to varying degrees, inhibit the metabolism of TCAs and clinical toxicity may result

Use of lithium with a TCA may increase the risk for neurotoxicity

Phenothiazines may increase concentration of some TCAs and TCAs may increase concentration of phenothiazines; monitor for altered clinical response

TCAs may enhance the hypoglycemic effects of tolazamide, chlorpropamide, or insulin; monitor for changes in blood glucose levels

Cholestyramine and colestipol may bind TCAs and reduce their absorption; monitor for altered response

TCAs may enhance the effect of amphetamines; monitor for adverse CV effects

Verapamil and diltiazem appear to decrease the metabolism of imipramine and potentially other TCAs; monitor for increased TCA concentrations. The pressor response to I.V. epinephrine, norepinephrine, and phenylephrine may be enhanced in patients receiving TCAs, this combination is best avoided.

Indinavir, ritonavir may inhibit the metabolism of clomipramine and potentially other TCAs; monitor for altered effects; a decrease in TCA dosage may be required

Quinidine may inhibit the metabolism of TCAs; monitor for altered effect

Combined use of anticholinergics with TCAs may produce additive anticholinergic effects; combined use of beta-agonists with TCAs may predispose patients to cardiac arrhythmias

Alcohol Interactions Avoid use (may increase central nervous system depression)

Onset 1-3 weeks before therapeutic effects are seen

Half-Life 28-31 hours

Education and Monitoring Issues

Patient Education: Oral: Take exactly as directed (do not increase dose or frequency); may take 2-3 weeks to achieve desired results; may cause physical and/or psychological dependence. Take once-a-day dose at bedtime. Avoid excessive alcohol, caffeine, and other prescription or OTC medications not approved by prescriber. Maintain adequate hydration (2-3 L/day of fluids unless instructed to restrict fluid intake). You may experience drowsiness, lightheadedness, impaired coordination, dizziness, or blurred vision (use caution when driving or engaging in tasks requiring alertness until response to drug is known); nausea, vomiting, altered taste, dry mouth (small frequent meals, frequent mouth care, chewing gum, sucking lozenges may help); constipation (increased exercise, fluids, or dietary fruit and fiber may help); diarrhea (buttermilk, yogurt, or boiled milk may help); increased appetite (monitor dietary intake to avoid excess weight gain); postural hypotension (use caution when climbing stairs or changing position from lying or sitting to standing); urinary retention (void before taking medication); or sexual dysfunction (reversible). Report persistent CNS effects (eg, insomnia, nervousness, restlessness, hallucinations, daytime sedation, impaired cognitive function); muscle cramping or tremors; chest pain, palpitations, rapid heartbeat, swelling of extremities, or severe dizziness; blurred vision or eye pain; yellowing of eyes or skin; pale stools/dark urine; or worsening of condition.

Dietary Considerations: Grapefruit juice may potentially inhibit the metabolism of TCAs

Monitoring Parameters: Monitor blood pressure and pulse rate prior to and during initial therapy; evaluate mental status; monitor weight

Reference Range:

Plasma levels do not always correlate with clinical effectiveness
Therapeutic: 50-150 ng/mL (SI: 190-570 nmol/L)
Toxic: >500 ng/mL (SI: >1900 nmol/L)

Related Information

Antidepressant Agents Comparison *on page 1231*

- **Norvasc®** *see* Amlodipine *on page 53*
- **Norvir®** *see* Ritonavir *on page 827*
- **Norzine®** *see* Thiethylperazine *on page 912*
- **Nostril® Nasal Solution [OTC]** *see* Phenylephrine *on page 727*
- **Novacet® Topical** *see* Sulfur and Sulfacetamide Sodium *on page 883*
- **Novahistine® Decongestant** *see* Phenylephrine *on page 727*
- **Novamilor** *see* Amiloride and Hydrochlorothiazide *on page 46*
- **Novamoxin®** *see* Amoxicillin *on page 56*
- **Novasen** *see* Aspirin *on page 72*
- **Novo** *see* Clonidine *on page 216*
- **Novo** *see* Dipyridamole *on page 285*
- **Novo-Alprazol** *see* Alprazolam *on page 37*
- **Novo-Atenol** *see* Atenolol *on page 76*
- **Novo-AZT** *see* Zidovudine *on page 991*
- **Novo-Butamide** *see* Tolbutamide *on page 928*
- **Novocain** *see* Procaine *on page 771*
- **Novocain® Injection** *see* Procaine *on page 771*
- **Novo-Captopril** *see* Captopril *on page 134*
- **Novo-Carbamaz** *see* Carbamazepine *on page 137*
- **Novo-Chlorhydrate** *see* Chloral Hydrate *on page 176*
- **Novo-Cimetine** *see* Cimetidine *on page 198*
- **Novo-Clopate** *see* Clorazepate *on page 218*
- **Novo-Cloxin** *see* Cloxacillin *on page 220*
- **Novo-Cromolyn** *see* Cromolyn Sodium *on page 231*
- **Novo-Cycloprine** *see* Cyclobenzaprine *on page 234*
- **Novo-Difenac®** *see* Diclofenac *on page 263*
- **Novo-Difenac®-SR** *see* Diclofenac *on page 263*
- **Novo-Diflunisal** *see* Diflunisal *on page 271*
- **Novo-Digoxin** *see* Digoxin *on page 272*
- **Novo-Diltazem** *see* Diltiazem *on page 278*
- **Novo-Dipam** *see* Diazepam *on page 261*
- **Novo-Doparil** *see* Methyldopa and Hydrochlorothiazide *on page 587*
- **Novo-Doxepin** *see* Doxepin *on page 298*
- **Novo-Doxylin** *see* Doxycycline *on page 300*
- **Novo E** *see* Vitamin E *on page 980*
- **Novo-Famotidine** *see* Famotidine *on page 350*
- **Novo-Ferrogluc** *see* Ferrous Gluconate *on page 359*
- **Novo-Ferrosulfate** *see* Ferrous Sulfate *on page 360*
- **Novo-Fibrate** *see* Clofibrate *on page 211*
- **Novo-Flupam** *see* Flurazepam *on page 383*
- **Novo-Flurazine** *see* Trifluoperazine *on page 950*
- **Novo-Flurprofen** *see* Flurbiprofen *on page 384*
- **Novo-Flutamide** *see* Flutamide *on page 385*
- **Novo-Folacid** *see* Folic Acid *on page 390*
- **Novo-Fumar** *see* Ferrous Fumarate *on page 359*

- ♦ **Novo-Furan** *see* Nitrofurantoin *on page 658*
- ♦ **Novo-Gesic-C8** *see* Acetaminophen and Codeine *on page 18*
- ♦ **Novo-Gesic-C15** *see* Acetaminophen and Codeine *on page 18*
- ♦ **Novo-Gesic-C30** *see* Acetaminophen and Codeine *on page 18*
- ♦ **Novo-Hexidyl** *see* Trihexyphenidyl *on page 952*
- ♦ **Novo-Hydrazide** *see* Hydrochlorothiazide *on page 442*
- ♦ **Novo-Hydrocort** *see* Hydrocortisone *on page 447*
- ♦ **Novo-Hylazin** *see* Hydralazine *on page 440*
- ♦ **Novo-Ipramide** *see* Ipratropium *on page 483*
- ♦ **Novo-Keto-EC** *see* Ketoprofen *on page 500*
- ♦ **Novolente-K** *see* Potassium Chloride *on page 751*
- ♦ **Novo-Lexin** *see* Cephalexin *on page 169*
- ♦ **Novolin® 10/90, 20/80, 30/70, 40/60, 50/50** *see* Insulin Preparations *on page 472*
- ♦ **Novolin® 70/30** *see* Insulin Preparations *on page 472*
- ♦ **Novolin® L** *see* Insulin Preparations *on page 472*
- ♦ **Novolin® Lente** *see* Insulin Preparations *on page 472*
- ♦ **Novolin® N** *see* Insulin Preparations *on page 472*
- ♦ **Novolin® NPH** *see* Insulin Preparations *on page 472*
- ♦ **Novolin® R** *see* Insulin Preparations *on page 472*
- ♦ **Novolin® Toronto** *see* Insulin Preparations *on page 472*
- ♦ **Novolin® Ultralente** *see* Insulin Preparations *on page 472*
- ♦ **Novo-Lorazepam** *see* Lorazepam *on page 541*
- ♦ **Novo-Medopa®** *see* Methyldopa *on page 586*
- ♦ **Novo-Medrone** *see* Medroxyprogesterone Acetate *on page 558*
- ♦ **Novo-Mepro** *see* Meprobamate *on page 565*
- ♦ **Novo-Metformin** *see* Metformin *on page 574*
- ♦ **Novo-Methacin** *see* Indomethacin *on page 469*
- ♦ **Novo-Metoprolol** *see* Metoprolol *on page 595*
- ♦ **Novo-Mucilax** *see* Psyllium *on page 793*
- ♦ **Novo-Naprox** *see* Naproxen *on page 636*
- ♦ **Novo-Nidazol** *see* Metronidazole *on page 597*
- ♦ **Novo-Nifedin** *see* Nifedipine *on page 653*
- ♦ **Novo-Oxazepam** *see* Oxazepam *on page 686*
- ♦ **Novo-Pen-VK®** *see* Penicillin V Potassium *on page 713*
- ♦ **Novo-Peridol** *see* Haloperidol *on page 430*
- ♦ **Novo-Pindol** *see* Pindolol *on page 738*
- ♦ **Novo-Piroxicam** *see* Piroxicam *on page 744*
- ♦ **Novo-Poxide** *see* Chlordiazepoxide *on page 180*
- ♦ **Novo-Pramine** *see* Imipramine *on page 462*
- ♦ **Novo-Prazin** *see* Prazosin *on page 760*
- ♦ **Novo-Prednisolone** *see* Prednisolone *on page 762*
- ♦ **Novo-Profen®** *see* Ibuprofen *on page 458*
- ♦ **Novo-Propamide** *see* Chlorpropamide *on page 189*
- ♦ **Novo-Propoxyn** *see* Propoxyphene *on page 784*
- ♦ **Novo-Propoxyn Compound (contains caffeine)** *see* Propoxyphene and Aspirin *on page 786*
- ♦ **Novo-Purol** *see* Allopurinol *on page 34*
- ♦ **Novo-Ranidine** *see* Ranitidine Hydrochloride *on page 809*
- ♦ **Novo-Reserpine** *see* Reserpine *on page 814*
- ♦ **Novo-Ridazine** *see* Thioridazine *on page 912*
- ♦ **Novo-Rythro Encap** *see* Erythromycin *on page 323*
- ♦ **Novo-Salmol** *see* Albuterol *on page 27*
- ♦ **Novo-Selegiline** *see* Selegiline *on page 843*
- ♦ **Novo-Semide** *see* Furosemide *on page 399*
- ♦ **Novo-Soxazole** *see* Sulfisoxazole *on page 881*
- ♦ **Novo-Spiroton** *see* Spironolactone *on page 867*
- ♦ **Novo-Spirozine** *see* Hydrochlorothiazide and Spironolactone *on page 443*
- ♦ **Novo-Sucralate** *see* Sucralfate *on page 874*
- ♦ **Novo-Sundac** *see* Sulindac *on page 883*
- ♦ **Novo-Tamoxifen** *see* Tamoxifen *on page 890*
- ♦ **Novo-Tetra** *see* Tetracycline *on page 903*
- ♦ **Novo-Thalidone** *see* Chlorthalidone *on page 191*
- ♦ **Novo-Timol** *see* Timolol *on page 922*
- ♦ **Novo-Tolmetin** *see* Tolmetin *on page 930*
- ♦ **Novo-Triamzide** *see* Hydrochlorothiazide and Triamterene *on page 443*

- **Novo-Trimel** *see* Co-Trimoxazole *on page 230*
- **Novo-Triolam** *see* Triazolam *on page 948*
- **Novo-Tripramine** *see* Trimipramine *on page 955*
- **Novo-Tryptin** *see* Amitriptyline *on page 51*
- **Novo-Veramil** *see* Verapamil *on page 975*
- **Novo-Zolamide®** *see* Acetazolamide *on page 19*
- **NP-27® [OTC]** *see* Tolnaftate *on page 931*
- **NPH Iletin® I** *see* Insulin Preparations *on page 472*
- **NPH-N** *see* Insulin Preparations *on page 472*
- **Nu-Alprax** *see* Alprazolam *on page 37*
- **Nu-Amilzide** *see* Amiloride and Hydrochlorothiazide *on page 46*
- **Nu-Amoxi** *see* Amoxicillin *on page 56*
- **Nu-Ampi Tri** *see* Ampicillin *on page 59*
- **Nu-Atenol** *see* Atenolol *on page 76*
- **Nubain®** *see* Nalbuphine *on page 631*
- **Nu-Ca** *see* Captopril *on page 134*
- **Nu-Carbamazepine** *see* Carbamazepine *on page 137*
- **Nu-Cephalex** *see* Cephalexin *on page 169*
- **Nu-Cimet** *see* Cimetidine *on page 198*
- **Nu-Cloxi** *see* Cloxacillin *on page 220*
- **Nucofed®** *see* Guaifenesin, Pseudoephedrine, and Codeine *on page 425*
- **Nucofed® Pediatric Expectorant** *see* Guaifenesin, Pseudoephedrine, and Codeine *on page 425*
- **Nu-Cotrimox** *see* Co-Trimoxazole *on page 230*
- **Nucotuss®** *see* Guaifenesin, Pseudoephedrine, and Codeine *on page 425*
- **Nu-Diclo** *see* Diclofenac *on page 263*
- **Nu-Diflunisal** *see* Diflunisal *on page 271*
- **Nu-Diltiaz** *see* Diltiazem *on page 278*
- **Nu-Doxycycline** *see* Doxycycline *on page 300*
- **Nu-Famotidine** *see* Famotidine *on page 350*
- **Nu-Flurprofen** *see* Flurbiprofen *on page 384*
- **Nu-Gemfibrozil** *see* Gemfibrozil *on page 406*
- **Nu-Hydral** *see* Hydralazine *on page 440*
- **Nu-Ibuprofen** *see* Ibuprofen *on page 458*
- **Nu-Indo** *see* Indomethacin *on page 469*
- **Nu-Ketoprofen** *see* Ketoprofen *on page 500*
- **Nu-Ketoprofen-E** *see* Ketoprofen *on page 500*
- **Nu-Loraz** *see* Lorazepam *on page 541*
- **NuLytely®** *see* Polyethylene Glycol-Electrolyte Solution *on page 747*
- **Nu-Medopa** *see* Methyldopa *on page 586*
- **Numorphan®** *see* Oxymorphone *on page 694*
- **Numzitdent® [OTC]** *see* Benzocaine *on page 98*
- **Numzit Teething® [OTC]** *see* Benzocaine *on page 98*
- **Nu-Naprox** *see* Naproxen *on page 636*
- **Nu-Nifedin** *see* Nifedipine *on page 653*
- **Nu-Pen-VK** *see* Penicillin V Potassium *on page 713*
- **Nu-Pindol** *see* Pindolol *on page 738*
- **Nu-Pirox** *see* Piroxicam *on page 744*
- **Nu-Prazo** *see* Prazosin *on page 760*
- **Nuprin® [OTC]** *see* Ibuprofen *on page 458*
- **Nu-Prochlor** *see* Prochlorperazine *on page 773*
- **Nu-Propranolol** *see* Propranolol *on page 786*
- **Nuquin HP®** *see* Hydroquinone *on page 450*
- **Nu-Ranit** *see* Ranitidine Hydrochloride *on page 809*
- **Nu-Tetra** *see* Tetracycline *on page 903*
- **Nu-Timolol** *see* Timolol *on page 922*
- **Nutracort®** *see* Hydrocortisone *on page 447*
- **Nutraplus® Topical [OTC]** *see* Urea *on page 962*
- **Nu-Triazide** *see* Hydrochlorothiazide and Triamterene *on page 443*
- **Nu-Triazo** *see* Triazolam *on page 948*
- **Nutrilipid®** *see* Fat Emulsion *on page 351*
- **Nu-Trimipramine** *see* Trimipramine *on page 955*
- **Nutropin® AQ Injection** *see* Human Growth Hormone *on page 438*
- **Nutropin® Depot™** *see* Human Growth Hormone *on page 438*
- **Nutropin® Injection** *see* Human Growth Hormone *on page 438*

- **Nu-Verap** *see* Verapamil *on page 975*
- **Nyaderm** *see* Nystatin *on page 670*
- **Nydrazid®** *see* Isoniazid *on page 487*

Nystatin (nye STAT in)

Pharmacologic Class Antifungal Agent, Oral Nonabsorbed; Antifungal Agent, Topical; Antifungal Agent, Vaginal

U.S. Brand Names Mycostatin®; Nilstat®; Nystat-Rx®; Nystex®; O-V Staticin®

Use Treatment of susceptible cutaneous, mucocutaneous, and oral cavity fungal infections normally caused by the *Candida* species

USUAL DOSAGE

Oral candidiasis:

Suspension (swish and swallow orally):

Premature infants: 100,000 units 4 times/day

Infants: 200,000 units 4 times/day or 100,000 units to each side of mouth 4 times/day

Children and Adults: 400,000-600,000 units 4 times/day

Troche: Children and Adults: 200,000-400,000 units 4-5 times/day

Powder for compounding: Children and Adults: $^1/_8$ teaspoon (500,000 units) to equal approximately $^1/_2$ cup of water; give 4 times/day

Mucocutaneous infections: Children and Adults: Topical: Apply 2-3 times/day to affected areas; very moist topical lesions are treated best with powder

Intestinal infections: Adults: Oral tablets: 500,000-1,000,000 units every 8 hours

Vaginal infections: Adults: Vaginal tablets: Insert 1 tablet/day at bedtime for 2 weeks

Contraindications Hypersensitivity to nystatin or any component

Pregnancy Risk Factor B/C (oral)

Related Information

Nystatin and Triamcinolone *on page 670*

Nystatin and Triamcinolone (nye STAT in & trye am SIN oh lone)

Pharmacologic Class Antifungal Agent, Topical; Corticosteroid, Topical

U.S. Brand Names Mycogen II Topical; Mycolog®-II Topical; Myconel® Topical; Myco-Triacet® II; Mytrex® F Topical; N.G.T.® Topical; Tri-Statin® II Topical

Use Treatment of cutaneous candidiasis

USUAL DOSAGE Children and Adults: Topical: Apply sparingly 2-4 times/day

Dosage Forms CRM: Nystatin 100,000 units and triamcinolone acetonide 0.1% (1.5 g, 15 g, 30 g, 60 g, 120 g). **OINT, top:** Nystatin 100,000 units and triamcinolone acetonide 0.1% (15 g, 30 g, 60 g, 120 g)

Pregnancy Risk Factor C

- **Nystat-Rx®** *see* Nystatin *on page 670*
- **Nystex®** *see* Nystatin *on page 670*
- **Nytol® Extra Strength** *see* Diphenhydramine *on page 282*
- **Nytol® Oral [OTC]** *see* Diphenhydramine *on page 282*
- **Occlucort®** *see* Betamethasone *on page 103*
- **Ocean Nasal Mist [OTC]** *see* Sodium Chloride *on page 858*
- **OCL®** *see* Polyethylene Glycol-Electrolyte Solution *on page 747*
- **Octamide®** *see* Metoclopramide *on page 592*
- **Octicair® Otic** *see* Neomycin, Polymyxin B, and Hydrocortisone *on page 644*
- **Octocaine®** *see* Lidocaine *on page 527*
- **Octocaine** *see* Lidocaine and Epinephrine *on page 529*
- **Octocaine® With Epinephrine** *see* Lidocaine and Epinephrine *on page 529*
- **Octostim®** *see* Desmopressin Acetate *on page 254*

Octreotide Acetate (ok TREE oh tide AS e tate)

Pharmacologic Class Antidiarrheal; Antisecretory Agent; Somatostatin Analog

U.S. Brand Names Sandostatin®; Sandostatin LAR® Depot

Generic Available No

Mechanism of Action Mimics natural somatostatin by inhibiting serotonin release, and the secretion of gastrin, VIP, insulin, glucagon, secretin, motilin, and pancreatic polypeptide

Use Control of symptoms in patients with metastatic carcinoid and vasoactive intestinal peptide-secreting tumors (VIPomas); pancreatic tumors, gastrinoma, secretory diarrhea, acromegaly

Unlabeled use: AIDS-associated secretory diarrhea, control of bleeding of esophageal varices, breast cancer, cryptosporidiosis, Cushing's syndrome, insulinomas, small bowel fistulas, postgastrectomy dumping syndrome, chemotherapy-induced diarrhea, graft-versus-host disease (GVHD) induced diarrhea, Zollinger-Ellison syndrome

USUAL DOSAGE Adults: S.C.: Initial: 50 mcg 1-2 times/day and titrate dose based on patient tolerance and response

Carcinoid: 100-600 mcg/day in 2-4 divided doses

VIPomas: 200-300 mcg/day in 2-4 divided doses

Diarrhea: Initial: I.V.: 50-100 mcg every 8 hours; increase by 100 mcg/dose at 48-hour intervals; maximum dose: 500 mcg every 8 hours

Esophageal varices bleeding: I.V. bolus: 25-50 mcg followed by continuous I.V. infusion of 25-50 mcg/hour

Acromegaly, carcinoid tumors, and VIPomas (depot injection): Patients must be stabilized on subcutaneous octreotide for at least 2 weeks before switching to the long-acting depot: Upon switch: 20 mg I.M. intragluteally every 4 weeks for 2-3 months, then the dose may be modified based upon response

Dosage adjustment for acromegaly: After 3 months of depot injections the dosage may be continued or modified as follows:

GH ≤2.5 ng/mL, IGF-1 is normal, symptoms are controlled: Maintain octreotide LAR® at 20 mg I.M. every 4 weeks

GH >2.5 ng/mL, IGF-1 is elevated, or symptoms: Increase octreotide LAR® to 10 mg I.M. every 4 weeks

GH ≤1 ng/mL, IGF-1 is normal, symptoms controlled: Reduce octreotide LAR® to 10 mg I.M. every 4 weeks

Dosages >40 mg are not recommended

Dosage adjustment for carcinoid tumors and VIPomas: After 2 months of depot injections the dosage may be continued or modified as follows:

Increase to 30 mg I.M. every 4 weeks if symptoms are inadequately controlled

Decrease to 10 mg I.M. every 4 weeks, for a trial period, if initially responsive to 20 mg dose

Dosage >30 mg is not recommended

Dosage Forms INJ: 0.05 mg/mL (1 mL); 0.1 mg/mL (1 mL); 0.2 mg/mL (5 mL); 0.5 mg/mL (1 mL); 1 mg/mL (5 mL); Suspension, depot: 10 mg (5 mL); 20 mg (5 mL); 30 mg (5 mL)

Contraindications Known hypersensitivity to octreotide or any component

Warnings/Precautions Dosage adjustment may be required to maintain symptomatic control; insulin requirements may be reduced as well as sulfonylurea requirements; monitor patients for cholelithiasis, hyper- or hypoglycemia; use with caution in patients with renal impairment

Pregnancy Risk Factor B

Adverse Reactions

1% to 10%:

Cardiovascular: Flushing, edema

Central nervous system: Fatigue, headache, dizziness, vertigo, anorexia, depression

Endocrine & metabolic: Hypoglycemia or hyperglycemia (1%), hypothyroidism, galactorrhea

Gastrointestinal: Nausea, vomiting, diarrhea, constipation, abdominal pain, cramping, discomfort, fat malabsorption, loose stools, flatulence

Hepatic: Jaundice, hepatitis, increase LFTs, cholelithiasis has occurred, presumably by altering fat absorption and decreasing the motility of the gallbladder

Local: Pain at injection site (dose-related)

Neuromuscular & skeletal: Weakness

<1%: Alopecia, anxiety, Bell's palsy, burning eyes, chest pain, fever, hyperesthesia, hypertensive reaction, leg cramps, muscle cramping, rash, rhinorrhea, shortness of breath, throat discomfort, thrombophlebitis, wheal/erythema

Drug Interactions CYP2D6 (high dose) and 3A enzyme inhibitor

Decreased effect: Cyclosporine (case report of a transplant rejection due to reduction of serum cyclosporine levels)

Duration 6-12 hours (S.C.)

Half-Life 60-110 minutes

Education and Monitoring Issues

Patient Education: Schedule injections between meals to decrease GI effects. May affect dietary fat and vitamin B_{12}. Consult prescriber about appropriate diet. Diabetic patients should monitor serum glucose closely (this drug may increase the effects of insulin or sulfonylureas); report abnormal glucose levels so appropriate adjustment can be made. You may experience skin flushing; nausea or vomiting (small frequent meals, frequent mouth care, sucking lozenges, or chewing gum may help); dizziness, fatigue, or drowsiness (use caution when driving or engaging in tasks that require alertness until response to drug is known). Report weight gain, swelling of extremities, or respiratory difficulty; acute or persistent GI distress (eg, diarrhea, vomiting, constipation, abdominal pain); muscle weakness or tremors or loss of motor function; chest pain or palpitations; blurred vision; pain, redness, or swelling at injection site; or emotional depression.

Reference Range: Vasoactive intestinal peptide: <75 ng/L; levels vary considerably between laboratories

Manufacturer Novartis

Related Information

Pharmaceutical Manufacturers Directory *on page 1020*

♦ **Ocu-Carpine® Ophthalmic** *see* Pilocarpine *on page 736*

♦ **Ocu-Dex®** *see* Dexamethasone *on page 256*

♦ **Ocufen® Ophthalmic** *see* Flurbiprofen *on page 384*

♦ **Ocuflox®** *see* Ofloxacin *on page 672*

Ofloxacin (oh FLOKS a sin)

Pharmacologic Class Antibiotic, Ophthalmic; Antibiotic, Otic; Antibiotic, Quinolone

U.S. Brand Names Floxin®; Ocuflox™ Ophthalmic

Generic Available No

Mechanism of Action Ofloxacin is a DNA gyrase inhibitor. DNA gyrase is an essential bacterial enzyme that maintains the superhelical structure of DNA. DNA gyrase is required for DNA replication and transcription, DNA repair, recombination, and transposition; bactericidal

Use

Quinolone antibiotic for skin and skin structure, lower respiratory and urinary tract infections and sexually transmitted diseases. Active against many gram-positive and gram-negative aerobic bacteria.

Ophthalmic: Treatment of superficial ocular infections involving the conjunctiva or cornea due to strains of susceptible organisms

USUAL DOSAGE

Children >1 year and Adults: Ophthalmic: Instill 1-2 drops in affected eye(s) every 2-4 hours for the first 2 days, then use 4 times/day for an additional 5 days

Children >1 year and 12 years: Otic: Place five (5) drops in affected ear(s) twice daily for 10 days

Children >12 years: Otic: Place ten (10) drops in affected ear(s) twice daily for 10 days

Adults: I.V., Oral:

- Lower respiratory tract infection: 400 mg every 12 hours for 10 days
- Gonorrhea: 400 mg as a single dose
- Cervicitis due to *C. trachomatis* and/or *N. gonorrhoeae*: 300 mg every 12 hours for 7 days
- Skin/skin structure: 400 mg every 12 hours for 10 days
- Urinary tract infection: 200-400 mg every 12 hours for 3-10 days
- Prostatitis: 300 mg every 12 hours for 6 weeks

Dosing adjustment/interval in renal impairment: Adults: I.V., Oral:

- Cl_{cr} 10-50 mL/minute: Administer 200-400 mg every 24 hours
- Cl_{cr} <10 mL/minute: Administer 100-200 mg every 24 hours

Continuous arteriovenous or venovenous hemodiafiltration (CAVH) effects: Administer 300 mg every 24 hours

Dosage Forms INJ: 200 mg (50 mL); 400 mg (10 mL, 20 mL, 100 mL). **SOLN:** Ophth: 0.3% (5 mL); Otic: 0.3% (5 mL). **TAB:** 200 mg, 300 mg, 400 mg

Contraindications Hypersensitivity to ofloxacin or other members of the quinolone group such as nalidixic acid, oxolinic acid, cinoxacin, norfloxacin, and ciprofloxacin

Warnings/Precautions Use with caution in patients with epilepsy or other CNS diseases which could predispose seizures; use with caution in patients with renal impairment; failure to respond to an ophthalmic antibiotic after 2-3 days may indicate the presence of resistant organisms, or another causative agent; use caution with systemic preparation in children <18 years of age due to association of other quinolones with transient arthropathy; has rarely caused ruptured tendons (discontinue immediately with signs of inflammation or tendon pain)

Pregnancy Risk Factor C

Adverse Reactions

1% to 10%:

- Cardiovascular: Chest pain (1% to 3%)
- Central nervous system: Headache (1% to 9%), insomnia (3% to 7%), dizziness (1% to 5%), fatigue (1% to 3%), somnolence (1% to 3%), sleep disorders, nervousness (1% to 3%), pyrexia (1% to 3%), pain
- Dermatologic: Rash/pruritus (1% to 3%)
- Gastrointestinal: Diarrhea (1% to 4%), vomiting (1% to 3%), GI distress, cramps, abdominal cramps (1% to 3%), flatulence (1% to 3%), abnormal taste (1% to 3%), xerostomia (1% to 3%), decreased appetite, nausea (3% to 10%)
- Genitourinary: Vaginitis (1% to 3%), external genital pruritus in women
- Local: Pain at injection site
- Ocular: Superinfection (ophthalmic), photophobia, lacrimation, dry eyes, stinging, visual disturbances (1% to 3%)

Miscellaneous: Trunk pain

<1%: Anxiety, chills, cognitive change, cough, decreased hearing acuity, depression, dream abnormality, edema, euphoria, extremity pain, hallucinations, hepatitis, hypertension, malaise, palpitations, paresthesia, photophobia, photosensitivity, ruptured tendons, syncope, thirst, tinnitus, Tourette's syndrome, vasculitis, vasodilation, vertigo, weakness, weight loss

Drug Interactions

Decreased effect: Decreased oral absorption with antacids containing aluminum, magnesium, and/or calcium, sucralfate, didanosine, iron, vitamins with minerals, mineral supplements (by up to 98% if given at the same time); fluoroquinolones may be decreased by antineoplastic agents

Increased toxicity/serum levels: Quinolones cause increased caffeine, warfarin, cyclosporine, procainamide, and possibly theophylline levels. Cimetidine and probenecid increase quinolone levels.

Half-Life 5-7.5 hours; prolonged in renal impairment

Education and Monitoring Issues

Patient Education:

Oral: Take per recommended schedule; complete full course of therapy and do not skip doses. Take on an empty stomach (1 hour before or 2 hours after meals, dairy products, antacids, or other medication). Maintain adequate hydration (2-3 L/day of fluids unless instructed to restrict fluid intake).

Oral/I.V.: You may experience dizziness, lightheadedness (use caution when driving or engaging in tasks that require alertness until response to drug is known); nausea, vomiting, or taste perversion (small frequent meals, frequent mouth care, sucking lozenges, or chewing gum may help); photosensitivity (use sunscreen, wear protective clothing and eyewear, avoid direct sunlight). Report GI disturbances, CNS changes (excessive sleepiness, agitation, or tremors), skin rash, changes in vision, difficulty breathing, signs of opportunistic infection (sore throat, chills, fever, burning, itching on urination, vaginal discharge, white plaques in mouth), or worsening of condition.

Ophthalmic: Tilt head back, instill 1-2 drops in affected eye as frequently as prescribed. Do not allow tip of applicator to touch eye or any contaminated surface. You may experience some stinging or burning or a bad taste in you mouth after instillation. Report persistent pain, burning, swelling, or visual disturbances.

Related Information

Antimicrobial Drugs of Choice *on page 1182*
Treatment of Sexually Transmitted Diseases *on page 1210*
Tuberculosis Treatment Guidelines *on page 1213*

♦ **Ogen® Oral** *see* Estropipate *on page 335*
♦ **Ogen® Vaginal** *see* Estropipate *on page 335*

Olanzapine (oh LAN za peen)

Pharmacologic Class Antipsychotic Agent, Thienobenzodiaepine

U.S. Brand Names Zyprexa™

Mechanism of Action Olanzapine is a thienobenzodiazepine neuroleptic; thought to work by antagonizing dopamine and serotonin activities. It is a selective monoaminergic antagonist with high affinity binding to serotonin 5-HT_{2A} and 5-HT_{2C}, dopamine D_{1-4}, muscarinic M_{1-5}, histamine H_1 and alpha$_1$-adrenergic receptor sites.

Use Treatment of the manifestations of psychotic disorders; treatment of acute mania associated with bipolar disorder

USUAL DOSAGE Adults >18 years: Oral: Usual starting dose: 5-10 mg once daily; increase to 10 mg once daily within 5-7 days, thereafter adjust by 5 mg/day at 1-week intervals, up to a maximum of 20 mg/day

Acute mania associated with bipolar disorder: Initial: 10-15 mg once daily

Dosage Forms TAB: 2.5 mg, 5 mg, 7.5 mg, 10 mg, 15 mg

Warnings/Precautions Use with caution in patients with cardiovascular disease, cerebrovascular disease, hypovolemia, dehydration, seizure disorders, Alzheimer's disease, hepatic impairment, prostatic hypertrophy, narrow-angle glaucoma, history of paralytic ileus or a history of breast cancer, the elderly, and in pregnancy or with nursing patients

Pregnancy Risk Factor C

Adverse Reactions

>10%: Central nervous system: Headache, somnolence, insomnia, agitation, nervousness, hostility, dizziness

1% to 10%:

Cardiovascular: Postural hypotension, tachycardia, hypotension, peripheral edema

Central nervous system: Dystonic reactions, parkinsonian events, amnesia, euphoria, stuttering, akathisia, anxiety, personality changes, fever

Dermatologic: Rash

Gastrointestinal: Xerostomia, constipation, abdominal pain, weight gain, increased appetite

Genitourinary: Premenstrual syndrome

Neuromuscular & skeletal: Arthralgia, neck rigidity, twitching, hypertonia, tremor

Ocular: Amblyopia

(Continued)

Olanzapine *(Continued)*

Respiratory: Rhinitis, cough, pharyngitis

<1%: Neuroleptic malignant syndrome, priapism, seizures, tardive dyskinesia

Drug Interactions CYP1A2 enzyme substrate, CYP2C19 enzyme substrate (minor), and CYP2D6 enzyme substrate (minor)

Reduction of effects may be seen with cytochrome P-450 enzyme inducers such as rifampin, omeprazole, carbamazepine, cigarette smoking

Effects may be potentiated with $CYP1A_2$ inhibitors such as fluvoxamine

Increased sedation with alcohol or other CNS depressants, increased risk of hypotension and orthostatic hypotension with antihypertensives

Olanzapine may antagonize the effects of levodopa and dopamine agonists

Activated charcoal decreased the C_{max} and AUC of olanzapine by 60%

Alcohol Interactions Avoid use (may increase central nervous system depression)

Half-Life 21-54 hours (mean 30 hours)

Education and Monitoring Issues

Patient Education: Use exactly as directed (do not increase dose or frequency); may cause physical and/or psychological dependence. It may take 2-3 weeks to achieve desired results; do not discontinue without consulting prescriber. Avoid excess alcohol or caffeine and other prescription or OTC medications not approved by prescriber. Maintain adequate hydration (2-3 L/day of fluids unless instructed to restrict fluid intake). You may experience excess drowsiness, restlessness, dizziness, or blurred vision (use caution driving or when engaging in tasks requiring alertness until response to drug is known); or constipation (increased exercise, fluids, or dietary fruit and fiber may help). Report persistent CNS effects (eg, trembling fingers, altered gait or balance, excessive sedation, seizures, unusual movements, anxiety, abnormal thoughts, confusion, personality changes); unresolved constipation or gastrointestinal effects; vision changes; difficulty breathing; unusual cough or flu-like symptoms; or worsening of condition.

Manufacturer Eli Lilly and Co

Related Information

Pharmaceutical Manufacturers Directory *on page 1020*

Olopatadine (oh LOP ah tah deen)

Pharmacologic Class Antihistamine

U.S. Brand Names Patanol®

Generic Available No

Use Allergic conjunctivitis

USUAL DOSAGE Adults: Ophthalmic: 1 drop in affected eye(s) every 6-8 hours (twice daily)

Dosage Forms SOLN, ophthalmic: 0.1% (5 mL)

Olsalazine (ole SAL a zeen)

Pharmacologic Class 5-Aminosalicylic Acid Derivative

U.S. Brand Names Dipentum®

Generic Available No

Mechanism of Action The mechanism of action appears to be topical rather than systemic

Use Maintenance of remission of ulcerative colitis in patients intolerant to sulfasalazine

USUAL DOSAGE Adults: Oral: 1 g/day in 2 divided doses

Dosage Forms CAP: 250 mg

Contraindications Hypersensitivity to salicylates

Warnings/Precautions Diarrhea is a common adverse effect of olsalazine; use with caution in patients with hypersensitivity to salicylates, sulfasalazine, or mesalamine

Pregnancy Risk Factor C

Adverse Reactions

>10%: Gastrointestinal: Diarrhea, cramps, abdominal pain

1% to 10%:

Central nervous system: Headache, fatigue, depression

Dermatologic: Rash, itching

Gastrointestinal: Nausea, dyspepsia, bloating, anorexia

Neuromuscular & skeletal: Arthralgia

<1%: Bloody diarrhea, blood dyscrasias, fever, hepatitis

Education and Monitoring Issues

Patient Education: Take as directed, with meals, in evenly divided doses. You may experience flu-like symptoms or muscle pain (a mild analgesic may help); diarrhea (boiled milk or yogurt may help); or nausea or loss of appetite (small frequent meals, frequent mouth care, sucking lozenges, or chewing gum may help). Report persistent diarrhea or abdominal cramping, skin rash or itching, or other adverse reactions.

Manufacturer Pharmacia & Upjohn

Related Information

Pharmaceutical Manufacturers Directory *on page 1020*

Omapatrilat (o ma PAT ri lat)

Pharmacologic Class Vasopeptidase Inhibitor

Mechanism of Action Inhibits both neutral endopeptidase and angiotensin-converting enzyme. These inhibitions increase natriuretic and vasodilatory peptides including atrial natriuretic peptide (ANP), brain natriuretic peptide (BNP) of myocardial cell origin, and C-type natriuretic peptide (CNP) of endothelial cell origin. The half-life of other vasodilator peptides are also increased including bradykinin and adrenomedullin. Vasopeptide inhibitors reduce vasoconstriction and enhance vasodilation.

ANA is found in cardiac atria, BNP is found in ventricular myocardium, and CNP is found in kidney, lung, heart, and vascular endothelium. ANP is released in response to atrial distension; BNP is released in response to ventricular volume and pressure overload; CNP is released in response to endothelium stress. ANP and BNP have multiple effects including improved ventricular relaxation, increased vasodilation, natriuresis, and glomerular filtration rate. They also lower blood pressure, urine osmolality, renin secretion, cardiac preload and afterload, and potassium excretion. CNP reduces cardiac filling pressure, output and venous return, and is a coronary vasodilator.

Use Potential uses: Hypertension, heart failure

Note: Omapatrilat, in animal studies, has demonstrated an antihypertensive effect regardless of the renin state of the animal. It has also increased cardiac output, decreased left ventricular end-diastolic and peak systolic pressures, and decreased peripheral vascular resistance in other animal studies.

In human pilot studies, omapatrilat has reduced blood pressure effectively in patients with mild to moderate hypertension in a dosage range of 5-75 mg once daily. The magnitude of the antihypertensive affect appears to be dose-dependent. The blood pressure response was similar, regardless of baseline renin level and race/ethnicity. The average blood pressure changes ranged as follows: with 5 mg/day, the mean systolic blood pressure decrease was 9-11 mg Hg, the mean diastolic blood pressure decrease was 6-9 mm Hg. With 40 mg/day the mean systolic blood pressure decrease was 16-17 mm Hg and the mean diastolic blood pressure decrease was 11-12 mm Hg.

Omeprazole (oh ME pray zol)

Pharmacologic Class Proton Pump Inhibitor

U.S. Brand Names Prilosec™

Generic Available No

Mechanism of Action Suppresses gastric acid secretion by inhibiting the parietal cell H+/K+ ATP pump

Use Short-term (4-8 weeks) treatment of severe erosive esophagitis (grade 2 or above), diagnosed by endoscopy and short-term treatment of symptomatic gastroesophageal reflux disease (GERD) poorly responsive to customary medical treatment; treatment of heartburn and other symptoms associated with GERD; pathological hypersecretory conditions; peptic ulcer disease; gastric ulcer therapy; maintenance of healing of erosive esophagitis; approved for combination use in the eradication of *H. pylori* in patients with active duodenal ulcer.

Unlabeled use: Healing NSAID-induced ulcers

USUAL DOSAGE Adults: Oral:

Active duodenal ulcer: 20 mg/day for 4-8 weeks

GERD or erosive esophagitis: 20 mg/day for 4-8 weeks

Pathological hypersecretory conditions: 60 mg once daily to start; doses up to 120 mg 3 times/day have been administered; administer daily doses >80 mg in divided doses

Helicobacter pylori: Combination therapy with bismuth subsalicylate, tetracycline, and clarithromycin; or with clarithromycin alone. Adult dose: Oral: 20 mg twice daily

Gastric ulcers: 40 mg/day for 4-8 weeks

Dosage Forms CAP, delayed release: 10 mg, 20 mg, 40 mg

Contraindications Known hypersensitivity to omeprazole

Warnings/Precautions In long-term (2-year) studies in rats, omeprazole produced a dose-related increase in gastric carcinoid tumors. While available endoscopic evaluations and histologic examinations of biopsy specimens from human stomachs have not detected a risk from short-term exposure to omeprazole, further human data on the effect of sustained hypochlorhydria and hypergastrinemia are needed to rule out the possibility of an increased risk for the development of tumors in humans receiving long-term therapy. Bioavailability may be increased in the elderly.

Pregnancy Risk Factor C

Pregnancy Implications

Clinical effects on the fetus: Crosses the placenta

Breast-feeding/lactation: No data available. American Academy of Pediatrics makes NO RECOMMENDATION.

Adverse Reactions

1% to 10%:

- Central nervous system: Headache (6.9%), dizziness (1.5%)
- Dermatologic: Rash (1.5%)
- Gastrointestinal: Diarrhea (3%), abdominal pain (2.4%), nausea (2.2%), vomiting (1.5%), constipation (1.1%), taste perversion (<1% to 15%)

(Continued)

Omeprazole *(Continued)*

Neuromuscular & skeletal: Weakness (1.1%), back pain (1.1%)

Respiratory: Upper respiratory infection (1.9%), cough (1.1%)

<1%: Abdominal swelling, abnormal dreams, aggression, agranulocytosis, alopecia, anemia, angina, angioedema, anorexia, anxiety, apathy, benign gastric polyps, bradycardia, confusion, depression, dry mouth, dry skin, elevated serum creatinine, elevated serum transaminases, epistaxis, erythema multiforme, esophageal candidiasis, fatigue, fecal discoloration, fever, flatulence, gastroduodenal carcinoids, glycosuria, gynecomastia, hallucinations, hematuria, hemifacial dysesthesia, hemolytic anemia, hepatic encephalopathy, hepatic failure, hepatic necrosis, hypertension, hypoglycemia, hyponatremia, increased serum alkaline phosphatase, increased sweating, insomnia, interstitial nephritis, irritable colon, jaundice, joint pain, leg pain, leukocytosis, liver disease (hepatocellular, cholestatic, mixed), malaise, microscopic pyuria, mucosal atrophy (tongue), muscle cramps, muscle weakness, myalgia, nervousness, neutropenia, pain, palpitation, pancreatitis, pancytopenia, paresthesia, peripheral edema, pharyngeal pain, proteinuria, pruritus, psychic disturbance, skin inflammation, somnolence, Stevens-Johnson syndrome, tachycardia, testicular pain, thrombocytopenia, tinnitus, toxic epidermal necrolysis, tremor, urinary frequency, urinary tract infection, urticaria, vertigo, weight gain

Drug Interactions CYP2C8, 2C9, 2C18, 2C19, and 3A3/4 enzyme substrate; CYP1A2 enzyme inducer; CYP2C19, 2C8, 2C9, and 2C19 enzyme inhibitor, CYP3A3/4 enzyme inhibitor (weak)

Decreased effect: Decreased ketoconazole; decreased itraconazole

Increased toxicity: Diazepam may increase half-life; increased digoxin, increased phenytoin, increased warfarin

Alcohol Interactions Avoid use (may enhance gastric mucosal irritation)

Onset Onset of antisecretory action: Oral: Within 1 hour; Peak effect: 2 hours

Duration 72 hours

Half-Life 30-90 minutes

Education and Monitoring Issues

Patient Education: Take as directed, before eating. Do not crush or chew capsules. You may experience anorexia; small frequent meals may help to maintain adequate nutrition. Report changes in urination or pain on urination, unresolved severe diarrhea, testicular pain, or changes in respiratory status.

Manufacturer AstraZeneca

Related Information

Helicobacter pylori Treatment *on page 1107*

Pharmaceutical Manufacturers Directory *on page 1020*

♦ **Omnicef®** *see* Cefdinir *on page 150*

♦ **OmniHIB™** *see Haemophilus* b Conjugate Vaccine *on page 427*

♦ **Omnipen®** *see* Ampicillin *on page 59*

♦ **Omnipen®-N** *see* Ampicillin *on page 59*

♦ **OMS® Oral** *see* Morphine Sulfate *on page 618*

♦ **Oncet®** *see* Hydrocodone and Homatropine *on page 445*

Ondansetron (on DAN se tron)

Pharmacologic Class Selective 5-HT_3 Receptor Antagonist

U.S. Brand Names Iofran ODT®; Zofran®

Generic Available No

Mechanism of Action Selective 5-HT_3-receptor antagonist, blocking serotonin, both peripherally on vagal nerve terminals and centrally in the chemoreceptor trigger zone

Use Prevention of nausea and vomiting associated with highly emetogenic cancer chemotherapy; may be prescribed for patients who are refractory to or have severe adverse reactions to standard antiemetic therapy. Ondansetron may be prescribed for young patients (ie, <45 years of age who are more likely to develop extrapyramidal reactions to high-dose metoclopramide) who are to receive highly emetogenic chemotherapeutic agents as listed:

Ondansetron should not be prescribed for chemotherapeutic agents with a low emetogenic potential (eg, bleomycin, busulfan, cyclophosphamide <1000 mg, etoposide, 5-fluorouracil, vinblastine, vincristine)

USUAL DOSAGE

Chemotherapy-induced emesis: Oral:

Children 4-11 years: 4 mg 30 minutes before chemotherapy; repeat 4 and 8 hours after initial dose, then 4 mg every 8 hours for 1-2 days after chemotherapy completed

Children >11 years and Adults: 8 mg every 8 hours for 2 doses beginning 30 minutes before chemotherapy, then 8 mg every 12 hours for 1-2 days after chemotherapy completed

Total body irradiation: Adults: 8 mg 1-2 hours before each fraction of radiotherapy administered each day

Single high-dose fraction radiotherapy to abdomen: 8 mg 1-2 hours before irradiation, then 8 mg every 8 hours after first dose for 1-2 days after completion of radiotherapy

Daily fractionated radiotherapy to abdomen: 8 mg 1-2 hours before irradiation, then 8 mg every 8 hours after first dose for each day of radiotherapy

Prophylaxis with moderate-emetogenic chemotherapy (not FDA-approved): 8 mg twice daily has been shown to be as effective as doses given 3 times/day

I.V.: Administer either three 0.15 mg/kg doses or a single 32 mg dose; with the 3-dose regimen, the initial dose is given 30 minutes prior to chemotherapy with subsequent doses administered 4 and 8 hours after the first dose. With the single-dose regimen 32 mg is infused over 15 minutes beginning 30 minutes before the start of emetogenic chemotherapy. Dosage should be calculated based on weight:

Children: Pediatric dosing should follow the manufacturer's guidelines for 0.15 mg/kg/dose administered 30 minutes prior to chemotherapy, 4 and 8 hours after the first dose. While not as yet FDA-approved, literature supports the day's total dose administered as a single dose 30 minutes prior to chemotherapy.

Adults:

>80 kg: 12 mg IVPB

45-80 kg: 8 mg IVPB

<45 kg: 0.15 mg/kg/dose IVPB

Postoperative emesis: I.V.:

Children >2 years: 0.1 mg/kg I.V. slow push; if over 40 kg weight, administer 4 mg IVP over 2-5 minutes (no faster than 30 seconds); give I.V. as s single dose immediately before induction of anesthesia or shortly following procedure if vomiting occurs

Adults (infuse in not less than 30 seconds, preferably over 2-5 minutes, as undiluted drug): 4 mg as a single dose immediately before induction of anesthesia; or shortly following procedure if vomiting occurs

Dosing in hepatic impairment: Maximum daily dose: 8 mg in cirrhotic patients with severe liver disease

Dosage Forms **INJ:** 2 mg/mL (2 mL, 20 mL); 32 mg (single-dose vials). **SOLN:** 4 mg/5 mL. **TAB:** 4 mg, 8 mg, 24 mg; Orally disintegrating: 4 mg, 8 mg

Contraindications Hypersensitivity to ondansetron or any component

Warnings/Precautions **Ondansetron should be used on a scheduled basis, not as an "as needed" (PRN) basis,** since data supports the use of this drug in the prevention of nausea and vomiting and not in the rescue of nausea and vomiting. Ondansetron should only be used in the first 24-48 hours of receiving chemotherapy. Data does not support any increased efficacy of ondansetron in delayed nausea and vomiting.

Pregnancy Risk Factor B

Pregnancy Implications

Clinical effects on the fetus: No data available on crossing the placenta; no effects on the fetus from 2 case reports

Breast-feeding/lactation: No data available. American Academy of Pediatrics has NO RECOMMENDATION.

Adverse Reactions

>10%:

Central nervous system: Headache, fever

Gastrointestinal: Constipation, diarrhea

1% to 10%:

Central nervous system: Dizziness

Gastrointestinal: Abdominal cramps, xerostomia

Hepatic: AST/ALT elevations (5%)

Neuromuscular & skeletal: Weakness

<1%: Angina, bronchospasm, hypokalemia, lightheadedness, rash, seizures, shortness of breath, tachycardia, transient elevations in serum levels of aminotransferases and bilirubin, wheezing

Drug Interactions CYP1A2, 2D6, 2E1, and 3A3/4 enzyme substrate

Decreased effect: Metabolized by the hepatic cytochrome P-450 enzymes; therefore, the drug's clearance and half-life may be changed with concomitant use of cytochrome P-450 inducers (eg, barbiturates, carbamazepine, rifampin, phenytoin, and phenylbutazone)

Increased toxicity: Inhibitors (eg, cimetidine, allopurinol, and disulfiram)

Onset Within 30 minutes

Half-Life 4 hours

Education and Monitoring Issues

Patient Education: This drug may cause drowsiness; use caution when driving or engaging in tasks that require alertness until response to drug is known. You may experience constipation and headache (request appropriate treatment from prescriber). Do not change position rapidly (rise slowly). Good mouth care and sucking on lozenges may help relieve nausea. Report persistent headache, excessive drowsiness, fever, numbness or tingling, or severe changes in elimination patterns (constipation or diarrhea), chest pain, or palpitations.

Dietary Considerations:

Food: Increases the extent of absorption. The C_{max} and T_{max} does not change much; take without regard to meals

Potassium: Hypokalemia; monitor potassium serum concentration

Manufacturer GlaxoWellcome

(Continued)

Ondansetron *(Continued)*

Related Information

Pharmaceutical Manufacturers Directory *on page 1020*

- **Ony-Clear® Spray** *see* Miconazole *on page 600*
- **Onyvul®** *see* Urea *on page 962*
- **Opcon®** *see* Naphazoline *on page 636*
- **Operand® [OTC]** *see* Povidone-Iodine *on page 756*
- **Ophthetic®** *see* Proparacaine *on page 782*
- **Ophthifluor®** *see* Fluorescein Sodium *on page 375*
- **Ophtho-Bunolol** *see* Levobunolol *on page 519*
- **Ophthocort** *see* Chloramphenicol, Polymyxin B, and Hydrocortisone *on page 180*
- **Ophtho-Sulf** *see* Sulfacetamide Sodium *on page 876*

Opium Tincture (OH pee um TING chur)

Pharmacologic Class Analgesic, Narcotic; Antidiarrheal

Generic Available No

Mechanism of Action Contains many narcotic alkaloids including morphine; its mechanism for gastric motility inhibition is primarily due to this morphine content; it results in a decrease in digestive secretions, an increase in GI muscle tone, and therefore a reduction in GI propulsion

Use Treatment of diarrhea or relief of pain

USUAL DOSAGE Oral:

Children:

Diarrhea: 0.005-0.01 mL/kg/dose every 3-4 hours for a maximum of 6 doses/24 hours

Analgesia: 0.01-0.02 mL/kg/dose every 3-4 hours

Adults:

Diarrhea: 0.3-1 mL/dose every 2-6 hours to maximum of 6 mL/24 hours

Analgesia: 0.6-1.5 mL/dose every 3-4 hours

Dosage Forms LIQ: 10% [0.6 mL equivalent to morphine 6 mg]

Contraindications Increased intracranial pressure, severe respiratory depression, severe liver or renal insufficiency, known hypersensitivity to morphine sulfate

Warnings/Precautions Opium shares the toxic potential of opiate agonists, and usual precautions of opiate agonist therapy should be observed; some preparations contain sulfites which may cause allergic reactions; infants <3 months of age are more susceptible to respiratory depression, use with caution and generally in reduced doses in this age group; this is **not** paregoric, dose accordingly

Pregnancy Risk Factor B; D (if used for prolonged periods or in high doses at term)

Adverse Reactions

>10%:

Cardiovascular: Palpitations, hypotension, bradycardia

Central nervous system: Drowsiness, dizziness

Neuromuscular & skeletal: Weakness

1% to 10%:

Central nervous system: Restlessness, headache, malaise

Genitourinary: Decreased urination

Miscellaneous: Histamine release

<1%: Anorexia, biliary tract spasm, CNS depression, constipation, increased intracranial pressure, insomnia, mental depression, miosis, nausea, peripheral vasodilation, physical and psychological dependence, respiratory depression, stomach cramps, urinary tract spasm, vomiting

Drug Interactions

Decreased effect: Phenothiazines may antagonize the analgesic effect of opiate agonists

Increased toxicity: CNS depressants, MAO inhibitors, tricyclic antidepressants may potentiate the effects of opiate agonists; dextroamphetamine may enhance the analgesic effect of opiate agonists

Alcohol Interactions Avoid use (may increase central nervous system depression)

Duration 4-5 hours

Education and Monitoring Issues

Patient Education: If self-administered, use exactly as directed (do not increase dose or frequency); may cause physical and/or psychological dependence. While using this medication, do not use alcohol and other prescription or OTC medications (especially sedatives, tranquilizers, antihistamines, or pain medications) without consulting prescriber. Maintain adequate hydration (2-3 L/day of fluids unless instructed to restrict fluid intake). May cause hypotension, dizziness, drowsiness, impaired coordination, or blurred vision (use caution when driving, climbing stairs, or changing position - rising from sitting or lying to standing, or when engaging in tasks requiring alertness until response to drug is known); dry mouth (frequent mouth care, small frequent meals, chewing gum, or sucking lozenges may help). Report slow or rapid heartbeat, acute dizziness, or persistent headache; changes in mental status; swelling of extremities or unusual weight gain; changes in urinary elimination or pain on urination; acute headache; trembling or muscle spasms; blurred vision; skin rash; or shortness of breath.

Monitoring Parameters: Observe patient for excessive sedation, respiratory depression, implement safety measures, assist with ambulation

Oprelvekin (oh PREL ve kin)

Pharmacologic Class Platelet Growth Factor

U.S. Brand Names Neumega®

Generic Available No

Mechanism of Action Oprelvekin stimulates multiple stages of megakaryocytopoiesis and thrombopoiesis, resulting in proliferation of megakaryocyte progenitors and megakaryocyte maturation

Use Prevention of severe thrombocytopenia and the reduction of the need for platelet transfusions following myelosuppressive chemotherapy in patients with nonmyeloid malignancies who are at high risk of severe thrombocytopenia.

USUAL DOSAGE S.C.:

Children: 75-100 mcg/kg once daily for 10-21 days (until postnadir platelet count ≥50,000 cells/μL)

Adults: 50 mcg/kg once daily for 10-21 days (until postnadir platelet count ≥50,000 cells/μL)

Dosage Forms POWDER for inj, lyophilized: 5 mg

Contraindications Hypersensitivity to oprelvekin, or any component

Warnings/Precautions Oprelvekin should be used cautiously in patients with conditions where expansion of plasma volume should be avoided (eg, left ventricular dysfunction, congestive heart failure, hypertension); cardiac arrhythmias or conduction defects, respiratory disease; history of thromboembolic problems; hepatic or renal dysfunction; not indicated following myeloablative chemotherapy

Pregnancy Risk Factor C

Adverse Reactions

>10%:

- Cardiovascular: Tachycardia (19% to 30%), palpitations (14% to 24%), atrial arrhythmias (12%), peripheral edema (60% to 75%)
- Central nervous system: Headache (41%), dizziness (38%), insomnia (33%), fatigue (30%), fever (36%)
- Dermatologic: Rash (25%)
- Endocrine & metabolic: Fluid retention
- Gastrointestinal: Nausea (50% to 77%), vomiting, anorexia
- Hematologic: Anemia (100%), probably a dilutional phenomena; appears within 3 days of initiation of therapy, resolves in about 2 weeks after cessation of oprelvekin
- Neuromuscular & skeletal: Arthralgia, myalgias
- Respiratory: Dyspnea (48%), pleural effusions (10%)

1% to 10%:

- Cardiovascular: Syncope (6% to 13%)
- Gastrointestinal: Weight gain (5%)

Half-Life 5-8 hours

Education and Monitoring Issues

Patient Education: Report any swelling in the arms or legs (peripheral edema), shortness of breath (congestive failure, anemia), irregular heartbeat, headaches

Monitoring Parameters: Monitor fluid balance during therapy, appropriate medical management is advised. If a diuretic is used, carefully monitor fluid and electrolyte balance. Obtain a CBC prior to chemotherapy and at regular intervals during therapy. Monitor platelet counts during the time of the expected nadir and until adequate recovery has occurred (postnadir counts ≥50,000 cells/μL).

Manufacturer Genetics Institute

Related Information

Pharmaceutical Manufacturers Directory *on page 1020*

- **Opticrom®** *see* Cromolyn Sodium *on page 231*
- **Opticyl®** *see* Tropicamide *on page 958*
- **Optimine®** *see* Azatadine *on page 84*
- **Optimyxin Plus** *see* Neomycin, Polymyxin B, and Gramicidin *on page 644*
- **OptiPranolol® Ophthalmic** *see* Metipranolol *on page 592*
- **Orabase®-B [OTC]** *see* Benzocaine *on page 98*
- **Orabase® HCA** *see* Hydrocortisone *on page 447*
- **Orabase®-O [OTC]** *see* Benzocaine *on page 98*
- **Oracit®** *see* Sodium Citrate and Citric Acid *on page 859*
- **Oracort** *see* Triamcinolone *on page 944*
- **Oradexon** *see* Dexamethasone *on page 256*
- **Orafen** *see* Ketoprofen *on page 500*
- **Orajel® Brace-Aid Oral Anesthetic [OTC]** *see* Benzocaine *on page 98*
- **Orajel® Maximum Strength [OTC]** *see* Benzocaine *on page 98*
- **Orajel® Mouth-Aid [OTC]** *see* Benzocaine *on page 98*
- **Orajel® Perioseptic® [OTC]** *see* Carbamide Peroxide *on page 139*

- **Oramorph SR™ Oral** *see* Morphine Sulfate *on page 618*
- **Orap™** *see* Pimozide *on page 737*
- **Orasept® [OTC]** *see* Benzocaine *on page 98*
- **Orasol® [OTC]** *see* Benzocaine *on page 98*
- **Orasone®** *see* Prednisone *on page 763*
- **Oratect™ [OTC]** *see* Benzocaine *on page 98*
- **Orazinc® [OTC]** *see* Zinc Supplements *on page 993*
- **Orbenin®** *see* Cloxacillin *on page 220*
- **Ordrine AT® Extended Release Capsule** *see* Caramiphen and Phenylpropanolamine *on page 137*
- **Oretic®** *see* Hydrochlorothiazide *on page 442*
- **Oreton® Methyl** *see* Methyltestosterone *on page 591*
- **Orfenace** *see* Orphenadrine *on page 681*
- **Organex** *see* Vitamin E *on page 980*
- **Organidin®** *see* Iodinated Glycerol *on page 480*
- **Organidin® NR** *see* Guaifenesin *on page 423*
- **Orgaran®** *see* Danaparoid *on page 244*
- **Orinase® Diagnostic Injection** *see* Tolbutamide *on page 928*
- **Orinase® Oral** *see* Tolbutamide *on page 928*
- **ORLAAM®** *see* Levomethadyl Acetate Hydrochloride *on page 523*

Orlistat (OR li stat)

Pharmacologic Class Lipase Inhibitor

U.S. Brand Names Xenical®

Mechanism of Action A reversible inhibitor of gastric and pancreatic lipases thus inhibiting absorption of dietary fats by 30% (at doses of 120 mg 3 times/day)

Use Management of obesity, including weight loss and weight management when used in conjunction with a reduced-calorie diet; reduce the risk of weight regain after prior weight loss; indicated for obese patients with an initial body mass index (BMI) ≥30 kg/m^2 or ≥27 kg/m^2 in the presence of other risk factors; see "Guidelines for Treatment of Obesity" in Appendix

USUAL DOSAGE 120 mg 3 times daily with each main meal containing fat (during or up to 1 hour after the meal); omit dose if meal is occasionally missed or contains no fat

Dosage Forms CAP: 120 mg

Contraindications Chronic malabsorption syndrome or cholestasis; hypersensitivity to orlistat or any component

Warnings/Precautions Patients should be advised to adhere to dietary guidelines; gastrointestinal adverse events may increase if taken with a diet high in fat (>30% total daily calories from fat). The daily intake of fat should be distributed over three main meals. If taken with any one meal very high in fat, the possibility of gastrointestinal effects increases. Patients should be counseled to take a multivitamin supplement that contains fat-soluble vitamins to ensure adequate nutrition because orlistat has been shown to reduce the absorption of some fat-soluble vitamins and beta-carotene. The supplement should be taken once daily at least 2 hours before or after the administration of orlistat (ie, bedtime). Some patients may develop increased levels of urinary oxalate following treatment; caution should be exercised when prescribing it to patients with a history of hyperoxaluria or calcium oxalate nephrolithiasis. As with any weight-loss agent, the potential exists for misuse in appropriate patient populations (eg, patients with anorexia nervosa or bulimia). Write and fill prescriptions carefully; confusion has occurred between Xenical® and Xeloda®.

Pregnancy Risk Factor B

Pregnancy Implications There are no adequate and well-controlled studies of orlistat in pregnant women. Because animal reproductive studies are not always predictive of human response, orlistat is not recommended for use during pregnancy. Teratogenicity studies were conducted in rats and rabbits at doses up to 800 mg/kg/day. Neither study showed embryotoxicity or teratogenicity. This dose is 23 and 47 times the daily human dose calculated on a body surface area basis for rats and rabbits, respectively. It is not know if orlistat is secreted in human milk. Therefore, it should not be taken by nursing women.

Adverse Reactions Anxiety, arthritis, back pain, depression, dizziness, dry skin, ear/nose/throat symptoms, fatty/oily stool (20%), fecal incontinence (12%), fecal urgency (30%), flatus with discharge (40%), headache, increased defecation (11%), influenza, joint disorder, myalgia, oily evacuation (14.3%), oily spotting (33.%), otitis, pain of lower extremities, rash, respiratory tract infection, sleep disorder, tendonitis

Most symptoms last <1 week; increased GI effects when taken with a high fat meal

Drug Interactions

Decreased effect: Vitamin A, D, K, and beta carotene absorption may be decreased when taken with orlistat

Additive lipid lowering effects with selected statin lipid lowering agents

Education and Monitoring Issues

Patient Education: Take this medication exactly as ordered; do not alter prescribed dose without consulting prescriber. Maintain prescribed diet (high fat meals may result in GI distress), exercise regimen, and vitamin supplements as prescribed. You may experience dizziness or lightheadedness (use caution when driving or engaging in tasks requiring alertness until response to drug is known) or increased flatus and fecal urgency (this may lessen with continued use). Report persistent back, muscle, or joint pain; signs of respiratory tract infection or flu-like symptoms; skin rash or irritation; or other reactions.

Monitoring Parameters: Changes in coagulation parameters

Manufacturer Roche Laboratories

Related Information

Pharmaceutical Manufacturers Directory *on page 1020*

- **Ormazine** *see* Chlorpromazine *on page 187*
- **Ornidyl®** *see* Eflornithine *on page 308*
- **Oro-Clense** *see* Chlorhexidine Gluconate *on page 181*

Orphenadrine (or FEN a dreen)

Pharmacologic Class Anti-Parkinson's Agent (Anticholinergic); Skeletal Muscle Relaxant

U.S. Brand Names Norflex™

Generic Available Yes

Mechanism of Action Indirect skeletal muscle relaxant thought to work by central atropine-like effects; has some euphorigenic and analgesic properties

Use Treatment of muscle spasm associated with acute painful musculoskeletal conditions; supportive therapy in tetanus

USUAL DOSAGE Adults:

Oral: 100 mg twice daily

I.M., I.V.: 60 mg every 12 hours

Dosage Forms INJ: 30 mg/mL (2 mL, 10 mL). **TAB:** 100 mg; Sustained release: 100 mg

Contraindications Glaucoma, GI obstruction, cardiospasm, myasthenia gravis, hypersensitivity to orphenadrine or any component

Warnings/Precautions Use with caution in patients with CHF or cardiac arrhythmias; some products contain sulfites

Pregnancy Risk Factor C

Adverse Reactions

>10%:

Central nervous system: Drowsiness, dizziness

Ocular: Blurred vision

1% to 10%:

Cardiovascular: Flushing of face, tachycardia, syncope

Dermatologic: Rash

Gastrointestinal: Nausea, vomiting, constipation

Genitourinary: Decreased urination

Neuromuscular & skeletal: Weakness

Ocular: Nystagmus, increased intraocular pressure

Respiratory: Nasal congestion

<1%: Aplastic anemia, hallucinations

Drug Interactions CYP2B6, 2D6, and 3A3/4 enzyme substrate; CYP2B6 enzyme inhibitor

Alcohol Interactions Avoid use (may increase central nervous system depression)

Onset Peak effect: Oral: Within 2-4 hours

Duration 4-6 hours

Half-Life 14-16 hours

Education and Monitoring Issues

Patient Education: Take exactly as directed. Do not increase dose or discontinue without consulting prescriber. Do not chew or crush sustained release tablets. Do not use alcohol, prescriptive or OTC antidepressants, sedatives, or pain medications without consulting prescriber. You may experience drowsiness, dizziness, lightheadedness (avoid driving or engaging in tasks requiring alertness until response to drug is known); nausea or vomiting (small, frequent meals, frequent mouth care, or sucking hard candy may help); constipation (increased dietary fluids and fibers or increased exercise may help); or decreased urination (void before taking medication). Report excessive drowsiness or mental agitation, chest pain, skin rash, swelling of mouth/face, difficulty speaking, or vision disturbances.

Related Information

Orphenadrine, Aspirin, and Caffeine *on page 681*

Orphenadrine, Aspirin, and Caffeine

(or FEN a dreen, AS pir in, & KAF een)

Pharmacologic Class Skeletal Muscle Relaxant

U.S. Brand Names Norgesic®; Norgesic® Forte

(Continued)

Orphenadrine, Aspirin, and Caffeine *(Continued)*

Dosage Forms TAB: Orphenadrine citrate 25 mg, aspirin 385 mg, and caffeine 30 mg; (Norgesic® Forte): Orphenadrine citrate 50 mg, aspirin 770 mg, and caffeine 60 mg

Pregnancy Risk Factor D

Alcohol Interactions Avoid use (may increase central nervous system depression and enhance gastric mucosal irritation)

- **Ortho 0.5/35** *see* Ethinyl Estradiol and Norethindrone *on page 342*
- **Ortho 1/35** *see* Ethinyl Estradiol and Norethindrone *on page 342*
- **Ortho 7/7/7** *see* Ethinyl Estradiol and Norethindrone *on page 342*
- **Ortho 10/11** *see* Ethinyl Estradiol and Norethindrone *on page 342*
- **Ortho-Cept®** *see* Ethinyl Estradiol and Desogestrel *on page 341*
- **Orthoclone® OKT3** *see* Muromonab-CD3 *on page 622*
- **Ortho-Cyclen®:** *see* Ethinyl Estradiol and Norgestimate *on page 344*
- **Ortho® Dienestrol Vaginal** *see* Dienestrol *on page 268*
- **Ortho-Est® Oral** *see* Estropipate *on page 335*
- **Ortho-Novum 0.5 mg** *see* Mestranol and Norethindrone *on page 570*
- **Ortho-Novum® 1/35** *see* Ethinyl Estradiol and Norethindrone *on page 342*
- **Ortho-Novum™ 1/50** *see* Mestranol and Norethindrone *on page 570*
- **Ortho-Novum 1/80** *see* Mestranol and Norethindrone *on page 570*
- **Ortho-Novum 2 mg** *see* Mestranol and Norethindrone *on page 570*
- **Ortho-Novum® 7/7/7** *see* Ethinyl Estradiol and Norethindrone *on page 342*
- **Ortho-Novum® 10/11** *see* Ethinyl Estradiol and Norethindrone *on page 342*
- **Ortho-Prefest®** *see* Ethinyl Estradiol and Norgestimate *on page 344*
- **Ortho Tri-Cyclen®** *see* Ethinyl Estradiol and Norgestimate *on page 344*
- **Or-Tyl® Injection** *see* Dicyclomine *on page 266*
- **Orudis®** *see* Ketoprofen *on page 500*
- **Orudis® KT [OTC]** *see* Ketoprofen *on page 500*
- **Oruvail®** *see* Ketoprofen *on page 500*
- **Os-Cal® 500 [OTC]** *see* Calcium Carbonate *on page 130*

Oseltamivir (o sel TAM e veer)

Pharmacologic Class Neuraminidase Inhibitor

U.S. Brand Names Tamiflu™

Mechanism of Action Oseltamivir, a prodrug, is hydrolyzed to the active form, oseltamivir carboxylate. It is thought to inhibit influenza virus neuraminidase, with the possibility of alteration of virus particle aggregation and release. In clinical studies of the influenza virus, 1.3% of post-treatment isolates had decreased neuraminidase susceptibility to oseltamivir carboxylate.

Use Indicated for the treatment of uncomplicated acute illness due to influenza infection in adults who have been symptomatic for no more than 2 days

Investigational use: Prophylaxis against influenza A/B infection

USUAL DOSAGE

Adults: Oral: 75 mg twice daily initiated within 2 days of onset of symptoms; duration of treatment: 5 days

Prophylaxis (investigational use): 75 mg once daily for duration of exposure period (6 weeks has been used in clinical trials)

Dosage adjustment in renal impairment:

Cl_{cr} 10-30 mL/minute: Reduce dose to 75 mg once daily for 5 days

Cl_{cr} <10 mL/minute: Has not been studied

Dosage adjustment in hepatic impairment: Has not been evaluated

Elderly: No adjustments required

Dosage Forms CAP: 75 mg (blister package 10)

Contraindications Hypersensitivity to any components of the product

Warnings/Precautions Dosage adjustment is required for creatinine clearance between 10-30 mL/minute, only for Influenza A or B infections; has not been evaluated in prevention of these infections; this medicine is not a substitute for the flu shot. Safe and efficacious use in children (<18 years) has not been established. Also consider primary or concomitant bacterial infections.

Pregnancy Risk Factor C

Pregnancy Implications There are insufficient human data to determine the risk to a pregnant woman or developing fetus. Studies evaluating the effects on embryo-fetal development in rats and rabbits showed a dose-dependent increase in the rates of minor skeleton abnormalities in exposed offspring. The rate of each abnormality remained within the background rate of occurrence in the species studied. Oseltamivir and its metabolite are excreted in the breast milk of lactating rats. It is unknown if they appear in human milk.

Adverse Reactions

1% to 10%:

Central nervous system: Insomnia (1.1%), vertigo (1%)

Gastrointestinal: Nausea (10%), vomiting (9%)

<1%: Anemia, humerus fracture, peritonsillar abscess, pneumonia, pseudomembranous colitis, pyrexia, unstable angina

Drug Interactions Cimetidine and amoxicillin have no effect on plasma concentrations. Probenecid increases oseltamivir carboxylate serum concentration by twofold. Dosage adjustments are not required.

Half-Life 6-10 hours

Education and Monitoring Issues

Patient Education: This is not a substitute for the flu shot. Must be taken within 2 days of flu symptoms (eg, fever, cough, headache, fatigue, muscular weakness, and sore throat). Take as directed, do not increase dose or frequency, and do not miss a dose. You may experience nausea or vomiting (small frequent meals, good mouth care, chewing gum, or sucking hard candy may help). Report significant adverse effects to your healthcare provider.

Dietary Considerations: Take with or without food; take with food to improve tolerance

Manufacturer Roche Laboratories

Related Information

Pharmaceutical Manufacturers Directory *on page 1020*

- **Osmitrol®** *see* Mannitol *on page 554*
- **Osmitrol® Injection** *see* Mannitol *on page 554*
- **Osteocalcin® Injection** *see* Calcitonin *on page 128*
- **Osteoporosis Management - Quick Reference** *see page 1127*
- **Ostoforte®** *see* Ergocalciferol *on page 321*
- **Otic-Care® Otic** *see* Neomycin, Polymyxin B, and Hydrocortisone *on page 644*
- **Otic Domeboro®** *see* Aluminum Acetate and Acetic Acid *on page 41*
- **OtiTricin® Otic** *see* Neomycin, Polymyxin B, and Hydrocortisone *on page 644*
- **Otobiotic® Otic** *see* Polymyxin B and Hydrocortisone *on page 748*
- **Otocalm® Ear** *see* Antipyrine and Benzocaine *on page 67*
- **Otocort® Otic** *see* Neomycin, Polymyxin B, and Hydrocortisone *on page 644*
- **Otomycin-HPN® Otic** *see* Neomycin, Polymyxin B, and Hydrocortisone *on page 644*
- **Otosporin® Otic** *see* Neomycin, Polymyxin B, and Hydrocortisone *on page 644*
- **Ovcon® 35** *see* Ethinyl Estradiol and Norethindrone *on page 342*
- **Ovcon® 50** *see* Ethinyl Estradiol and Norethindrone *on page 342*
- **Ovide™** *see* Malathion *on page 553*
- **Ovral®** *see* Ethinyl Estradiol and Norgestrel *on page 345*
- **Ovrette®** *see* Norgestrel *on page 664*
- **O-V Staticin®** *see* Nystatin *on page 670*

Oxacillin (oks a SIL in)

Pharmacologic Class Antibiotic, Penicillin

U.S. Brand Names Bactocill®; Prostaphlin®

Generic Available Yes

Mechanism of Action Inhibits bacterial cell wall synthesis by binding to one or more of the penicillin binding proteins (PBPs); which in turn inhibits the final transpeptidation step of peptidoglycan synthesis in bacterial cell walls, thus inhibiting cell wall biosynthesis. Bacteria eventually lyse due to ongoing activity of cell wall autolytic enzymes (autolysins and murein hydrolases) while cell wall assembly is arrested.

Use Treatment of infections such as osteomyelitis, septicemia, endocarditis, and CNS infections caused by susceptible strains of *Staphylococcus*

USUAL DOSAGE

Neonates: I.M., I.V.:
- Postnatal age <7 days:
  - <2000 g: 25 mg/kg/dose every 12 hours
  - >2000 g: 25 mg/kg/dose every 8 hours
- Postnatal age >7 days:
  - <1200 g: 25 mg/kg/dose every 12 hours
  - 1200-2000 g: 30 mg/kg/dose every 8 hours
  - >2000 g: 37.5 mg/kg/dose every 6 hours

Infants and Children:
- Oral: 50-100 mg/kg/day divided every 6 hours
- I.M., I.V.: 150-200 mg/kg/day in divided doses every 6 hours; maximum dose: 12 g/day

Adults:
- Oral: 500-1000 mg every 4-6 hours for at least 5 days
- I.M., I.V.: 250 mg to 2 g/dose every 4-6 hours

Dosing adjustment in renal impairment: Cl_{cr} <10 mL/minute: Use lower range of the usual dosage

Hemodialysis: Not dialyzable (0% to 5%)

Dosage Forms CAP: 250 mg, 500 mg. **POWDER:** For injection: 250 mg, 500 mg, 1 g, 2 g, 4 g, 10 g; For oral solution: 250 mg/5 mL (100 mL)

Contraindications Hypersensitivity to oxacillin or other penicillins or any component

(Continued)

Oxacillin *(Continued)*

Warnings/Precautions Elimination rate will be slow in neonates; modify dosage in patients with renal impairment and in the elderly; use with caution in patients with cephalosporin hypersensitivity

Pregnancy Risk Factor B

Adverse Reactions

1% to 10%: Gastrointestinal: Nausea, diarrhea

<1%: Acute interstitial nephritis, agranulocytosis, eosinophilia, fever, hematuria, hepatotoxicity, increased AST, leukopenia, neutropenia, rash, serum sickness-like reactions, thrombocytopenia, vomiting

Drug Interactions

Decreased effect: Efficacy of oral contraceptives may be reduced; effects of penicillins may be impaired by tetracycline

Increased effect: Disulfiram, probenecid may increase penicillin levels, increased effect of anticoagulants are possible with large I.V. doses

Half-Life Absorption: Oral: 35% to 67%; Adults: 23-60 minutes (prolonged with reduced renal function and in neonates)

Education and Monitoring Issues

Patient Education: Take at regular intervals around-the-clock, preferably on an empty stomach with a full glass of water. Take complete course of treatment as prescribed. You may experience nausea or vomiting; small frequent meals and good mouth care may help. If diabetic, drug may cause false tests with Clinitest® urine glucose monitoring; use of glucose oxidase methods (Clinistix®) or serum glucose monitoring is preferable. This drug may interfere with oral contraceptives; an alternate form of birth control should be used. Report persistent fever, sore throat, sores in mouth, diarrhea, unusual bleeding or bruising, difficulty breathing, or skin rash. Notify prescriber if condition does not respond to treatment.

Monitoring Parameters: Observe for signs and symptoms of anaphylaxis during first dose

Related Information

Antibiotic Treatment of Adults With Infective Endocarditis *on page 1179*
Community Acquired Pneumonia in Adults *on page 1200*

Oxamniquine (oks AM ni kwin)

Pharmacologic Class Anthelmintic

U.S. Brand Names Vansil™

Generic Available No

Mechanism of Action Not fully elucidated; causes worms to dislodge from their usual site of residence (mesenteric veins to the liver) by paralysis and contraction of musculature and subsequently phagocytized

Use Treatment of all stages of *Schistosoma mansoni* infection

USUAL DOSAGE Oral:

Children <30 kg: 20 mg/kg in 2 divided doses of 10 mg/kg at 2- to 8-hour intervals

Adults: 12-15 mg/kg as a single dose

Dosage Forms CAP: 250 mg

Warnings/Precautions Rare epileptiform convulsions have been observed within the first few hours of administration, especially in patients with a history of CNS pathology

Pregnancy Risk Factor C

Adverse Reactions

>10%: Central nervous system: Dizziness, drowsiness, headache

<10%:

Central nervous system: Insomnia, malaise, hallucinations, behavior changes
Gastrointestinal: GI effects, orange/red discoloration of urine
Hepatic: Elevated LFTs
Dermatologic: Rash, urticaria, pruritus
Renal: Proteinuria

Drug Interactions May be synergistic with praziquantel

Half-Life 1-2.5 hours

Education and Monitoring Issues

Patient Education: Take with food

Manufacturer Pfizer U.S. Pharmaceutical Group

Related Information

Pharmaceutical Manufacturers Directory *on page 1020*

♦ **Oxandrin®** *see* Oxandrolone *on page 684*

Oxandrolone (oks AN droe lone)

Pharmacologic Class Androgen

U.S. Brand Names Oxandrin®

Mechanism of Action Synthetic testosterone derivative with similar androgenic and anabolic actions

Use Adjunctive therapy to promote weight gain after weight loss following extensive surgery, chronic infections, or severe trauma, and in some patients who, without definite pathophysiologic reasons, fail to gain or to maintain normal weight

USUAL DOSAGE

Children: Total daily dose: ≤0.1 mg/kg **or** ≤0.045 mg/lb

Adults: 2.5 mg 2-4 times/day; however, since the response of individuals to anabolic steroids varies, a daily dose of as little as 2.5 mg or as much as 20 mg may be required to achieve the desired response. A course of therapy of 2-4 weeks is usually adequate. This may be repeated intermittently as needed.

Dosing adjustment in renal impairment: Caution is recommended because of the propensity of oxandrolone to cause edema and water retention

Dosing adjustment in hepatic impairment: Caution is advised but there are not specific guidelines for dosage reduction

Dosage Forms TAB: 2.5 mg

Contraindications Nephrosis, carcinoma of breast or prostate, pregnancy, hypersensitivity to oxandrolone or any component

Warnings/Precautions May stunt bone growth in children; anabolic steroids may cause peliosis hepatis, liver cell tumors, and blood lipid changes with increased risk of arteriosclerosis; monitor diabetic patients carefully; use with caution in elderly patients, they may be at greater risk for prostatic hypertrophy; use with caution in patients with cardiac, renal, or hepatic disease or epilepsy

Pregnancy Risk Factor X

Adverse Reactions

Male:

Postpubertal:

- >10%:
  - Dermatologic: Acne
  - Endocrine & metabolic: Gynecomastia
  - Genitourinary: Bladder irritability, priapism
- 1% to 10%:
  - Central nervous system: Insomnia, chills
  - Endocrine & metabolic: Decreased libido, hepatic dysfunction
  - Gastrointestinal: Nausea, diarrhea
  - Genitourinary: Prostatic hypertrophy (elderly)
  - Hematologic: Iron deficiency anemia, suppression of clotting factors
- <1%: Hepatic necrosis, hepatocellular carcinoma

Prepubertal:

- >10%:
  - Dermatologic: Acne
  - Endocrine & metabolic: Virilism
- 1% to 10%:
  - Central nervous system: Chills, insomnia,
  - Dermatologic: Hyperpigmentation
  - Gastrointestinal: Diarrhea, nausea
  - Hematologic: Iron deficiency anemia, suppression of clotting factors
- <1%: Hepatic necrosis, hepatocellular carcinoma

Female:

- >10%: Endocrine & metabolic: Virilism
- 1% to 10%:
  - Central nervous system: Chills, insomnia
  - Endocrine & metabolic: Hypercalcemia
  - Gastrointestinal: Nausea, diarrhea
  - Hematologic: Iron deficiency anemia, suppression of clotting factors
  - Hepatic: Hepatic dysfunction
- <1%: Hepatic necrosis, hepatocellular carcinoma

Drug Interactions Increased toxicity: ACTH, adrenal steroids may increase risk of edema and acne; stanozolol enhances the hypoprothrombinemic effects of oral anticoagulants; enhances the hypoglycemic effects of insulin and sulfonylureas (oral hypoglycemics)

Onset 1 month

Education and Monitoring Issues

Patient Education: High protein, high caloric diet is suggested, restrict salt intake; glucose tolerance may be altered in diabetics

Oxaprozin (oks a PROE zin)

Pharmacologic Class Nonsteroidal Anti-Inflammatory Agent (NSAID)

U.S. Brand Names Daypro™

Mechanism of Action Inhibits prostaglandin synthesis by decreasing the activity of the enzyme, cyclo-oxygenase, which results in decreased formation of prostaglandin precursors

Use Acute and long-term use in the management of signs and symptoms of osteoarthritis and rheumatoid arthritis

USUAL DOSAGE Adults: Oral (individualize dosage to lowest effective dose to minimize adverse effects):

(Continued)

Oxaprozin *(Continued)*

Osteoarthritis: 600-1200 mg once daily
Rheumatoid arthritis: 1200 mg once daily
Maximum dose: 1800 mg/day or 26 mg/kg (whichever is lower) in divided doses

Dosage Forms TAB: 600 mg

Contraindications Aspirin allergy, 3rd trimester pregnancy or allergy to oxaprozin, history of GI disease, renal or hepatic dysfunction, bleeding disorders, cardiac failure, elderly, debilitated, nursing mothers

Pregnancy Risk Factor C; D (3rd trimester)

Adverse Reactions

1% to 10%:

Central nervous system: CNS inhibition, disturbance of sleep
Dermatologic: Rash
Gastrointestinal: Nausea, dyspepsia, abdominal pain, anorexia, flatulence, vomiting
Genitourinary: Dysuria or frequency

<1%: Acute interstitial nephritis, acute renal failure, agranulocytosis, anaphylaxis, anemia, blurred vision, change in blood pressure, conjunctivitis, decreased menstrual flow, ecchymosis, edema, erythema multiforme, exfoliative dermatitis, hematuria, leukopenia, LFT abnormalities, malaise, nephrotic syndrome, pancreatitis, pancytopenia, peptic ulcer and/or GI bleed, photosensitivity, pruritus, rectal bleeding, renal insufficiency, serum sickness, Stevens-Johnson syndrome, stomatitis, symptoms of upper respiratory infection, thrombocytopenia, urticaria, weakness, weight gain, weight loss

Drug Interactions Increased toxicity: Aspirin, oral anticoagulants, diuretics

Alcohol Interactions Avoid use (may enhance gastric mucosal irritation)

Onset Steady-state 4-7 days

Duration Absorption: Almost completely; Protein binding: >99%; Half-life: 40-50 hours; Time to peak: 2-4 hours

Half-Life 40-50 hours

Education and Monitoring Issues

Patient Education: Take this medication exactly as directed; do not increase dose without consulting prescriber. Do not crush tablets or break capsules. Take with food or milk to reduce GI distress. Maintain adequate fluid intake (2-3 L/day of fluids unless instructed to restrict fluid intake). Do not use alcohol, aspirin, or aspirin-containing medication, and all other anti-inflammatory medications without consulting prescriber. You may experience drowsiness, dizziness, or nervousness (use caution when driving or engaging in tasks requiring alertness until response to drug is known); anorexia, nausea, vomiting, or heartburn (frequent small meals, frequent mouth care, sucking lozenges, or chewing gum may help). GI bleeding, ulceration, or perforation can occur with or without pain; discontinue medication and contact prescriber if persistent abdominal pain or cramping, or blood in stool occurs. Report vaginal bleeding; breathlessness, difficulty breathing, or unusual cough; chest pain, rapid heartbeat, palpitations; unusual bruising/bleeding; blood in urine, stool, mouth, or vomitus; swollen extremities; skin rash or itching; acute fatigue; or swelling of face, lips, tongue, or throat.

Monitoring Parameters: Monitor blood, hepatic, renal, and ocular function

Manufacturer Searle

Related Information

Nonsteroidal Anti-Inflammatory Agents Comparison *on page 1248*
Pharmaceutical Manufacturers Directory *on page 1020*

Oxazepam (oks A ze pam)

Pharmacologic Class Benzodiazepine

Generic Available Yes

Mechanism of Action Benzodiazepine anxiolytic sedative that produces CNS depression at the subcortical level, except at high doses, whereby it works at the cortical level

Use Treatment of anxiety and management of alcohol withdrawal; may also be used as an anticonvulsant in management of simple partial seizures

USUAL DOSAGE Oral:

Children: 1 mg/kg/day has been administered
Adults:

Anxiety: 10-30 mg 3-4 times/day
Alcohol withdrawal: 15-30 mg 3-4 times/day
Hypnotic: 15-30 mg

Hemodialysis: Not dialyzable (0% to 5%)

Dosage Forms CAP: 10 mg, 15 mg, 30 mg

Contraindications Hypersensitivity to oxazepam or any component, cross-sensitivity with other benzodiazepines may exist

Warnings/Precautions Avoid using in patients with pre-existing CNS depression, severe uncontrolled pain, or narrow-angle glaucoma; use with caution in patients using other CNS depressants and in the elderly

Pregnancy Risk Factor D

Adverse Reactions

Cardiovascular: Syncope (rare), edema

Central nervous system: Drowsiness, ataxia, dizziness, vertigo, memory impairment, headache, paradoxical reactions (excitement, stimulation of effect), lethargy, amnesia, euphoria
Dermatologic: Rash
Endocrine & metabolic: Decreased libido, menstrual irregularities
Genitourinary: Incontinence
Hematologic: Leukopenia, blood dyscrasias
Hepatic: Jaundice
Neuromuscular & skeletal: Dysarthria, tremor, reflex slowing
Ocular: Blurred vision, diplopia
Miscellaneous: Drug dependence

Drug Interactions
Alcohol and other CNS depressants may increase the CNS effects of oxazepam
Oral contraceptives may increase the clearance of oxazepam
Oxazepam may decrease the antiparkinsonian efficacy of levodopa
Theophylline and other CNS stimulants may antagonize the sedative effects of oxazepam
Phenytoin may increase the clearance of oxazepam

Alcohol Interactions Avoid use (may increase central nervous system depression)

Onset Peak serum concentration: 1-2 hours

Half-Life 2.8-5.7 hours

Education and Monitoring Issues

Patient Education: Take exactly as directed (do not increase dose or frequency); may take 2-3 weeks to achieve desired results; may cause physical and/or psychological dependence. Do not use excessive alcohol or other prescription or OTC medications (especially pain medications, sedatives, antihistamines, or hypnotics) without consulting prescriber. Maintain adequate hydration (2-3 L/day of fluids unless instructed to restrict fluid intake). You may experience drowsiness, lightheadedness, impaired coordination, dizziness, or blurred vision (use caution when driving or engaging in tasks requiring alertness until response to drug is known); nausea, vomiting, or dry mouth (small frequent meals, frequent mouth care, chewing gum, or sucking lozenges may help); constipation (increased exercise, fluids, or dietary fruit and fiber may help); altered sexual drive or ability (reversible); or photosensitivity (use sunscreen, wear protective clothing and eyewear, avoid direct sunlight). Report persistent CNS effects (eg, confusion, depression, increased sedation, excitation, headache, agitation, insomnia or nightmares, dizziness, fatigue, impaired coordination, changes in personality, or changes in cognition); changes in urinary pattern; muscle cramping, weakness, tremors, or rigidity; ringing in ears or visual disturbances; chest pain, palpitations, or rapid heartbeat; excessive perspiration, excessive GI symptoms (cramping, constipation, vomiting, anorexia); or worsening of condition.

Monitoring Parameters: Respiratory and cardiovascular status

Reference Range: Therapeutic: 0.2-1.4 µg/mL (SI: 0.7-4.9 µmol/L)

Oxcarbazepine (ox car BAZ e peen)

Pharmacologic Class Anticonvulsant, Miscellaneous

U.S. Brand Names Trileptal®

Mechanism of Action Pharmacological activity results from both oxcarbazepine and its monohydroxy metabolite (MHD). Precise mechanism of anticonvulsant effect has not been defined. Oxcarbazepine and MHD block voltage sensitive sodium channels, stabilizing hyperexcited neuronal membranes, inhibiting repetitive firing, and decreasing the propagation of synaptic impulses. These actions are believed to prevent the spread of seizures. Oxcarbazepine and MHD also increase potassium conductance and modulate the activity of high-voltage activated calcium channels.

Use Monotherapy or adjunctive therapy in the treatment of partial seizures in adults with epilepsy and as adjunctive therapy in the treatment of partial seizures in children ages 4-16 with epilepsy

USUAL DOSAGE

Children:

Adjunctive therapy: 8-10 mg/kg/day, not to exceed 600 mg/day, given in two divided daily doses. Maintenance dose should be achieved over 2 weeks, and is dependent upon patient weight, according to the following chart:

Adjunctive Maintenance Doses in Children

Weight	Maintenance Dose (given in two divided doses)
20-29 kg	900 mg/day
29.1-39 kg	1200 mg/day
>39 kg	1800 mg/day.

Adults:

Adjunctive therapy: Initial: 300 mg twice daily; dose may be increased by as much as 600 mg/day at weekly intervals; recommended daily dose: 1200 mg/day in 2 divided doses

(Continued)

Oxcarbazepine *(Continued)*

Conversion to monotherapy: Oxcarbazepine 600 mg/day in twice daily divided doses while simultaneously initiating the reduction of the dose of the concomitant antiepileptic drug. The concomitant dosage should be withdrawn over 3-6 weeks, while the maximum dose of oxcarbazepine should be reached in about 2-4 weeks. Recommended daily dose: 2400 mg/day.

Initiation of monotherapy: Oxcarbazepine should be initiated at a dose of 600 mg/day in twice daily divided doses; doses may be titrated upward by 300 mg/day every third day to a final dose of 1200 mg/day given in 2 daily divided doses

Dosing adjustment in renal impairment: Therapy should be initiated at one-half the usual starting dose (300 mg/day) and increased slowly to achieve the desired clinical response

Dosage Forms TAB: 150 mg, 300 mg, 600 mg

Contraindications Hypersensitivity to oxcarbazepine or any of its components

Warnings/Precautions Clinically significant hyponatremia (sodium <125 mmol/L) can develop during oxcarbazepine use. As with all antiepileptic drugs, oxcarbazepine should be withdrawn gradually to minimize the potential of increased seizure frequency. Use of oxcarbazepine has been associated with CNS related adverse events, most significant of these were cognitive symptoms including psychomotor slowing, difficulty with concentration, and speech or language problems, somnolence or fatigue, and coordination abnormalities, including ataxia and gait disturbances.

Pregnancy Risk Factor C

Pregnancy Implications Although many epidemiological studies of congenital anomalies in infants born to women treated with various anticonvulsants during pregnancy have been reported, none of these investigations includes enough women treated with oxcarbazepine to assess possible teratogenic effects of this drug. The frequencies of malformations were not significantly increased among the offspring of pregnant mice treated with 20-46 times the usual human dose of oxcarbazepine. This treatment produced plasma levels in the mice that were at least 6-16 times greater than those that are usually seen in human anticonvulsant therapy. Oxcarbazepine and its active metabolite (MHD) are excreted in human breast milk. A milk-to-plasma concentration ratio of 0.5 was found for both. Because of the potential for serious adverse reactions to oxcarbazepine in nursing infants, a decision should be made whether to discontinue nursing or to discontinue the drug in nursing women.

Adverse Reactions

Monotherapy:

>10%

Central nervous system: Headache (13% to 31%), dizziness (22% to 28%), somnolence (19%), fatigue (21%)

Gastrointestinal: Nausea (16% to 22%), vomiting (7% to 15%)

Ocular: Abnormal vision (4% to 14%), diplopia (12%)

1% to 10%

Central nervous system: Anxiety (7%), ataxia (5% to 7%), confusion (7%), nervousness (5% to 7%), insomnia (6%), tremor (4% to 6%), amnesia (4% to 5%), exacerbation of seizures (5%), emotional lability (3%), hypoesthesia (3%), fever (3%), vertigo (3%), abnormal coordination (2% to 4%), speech disorder (2%)

Cardiovascular: Edema (2%), chest pain (2%)

Dermatologic: Rash (4%), purpura (2%)

Endocrine and metabolic: Hyponatremia (5%), hot flashes (2%),

Gastrointestinal: Diarrhea (7%), dyspepsia (5%), anorexia (5%), abdominal pain (5%), constipation (5%), taste perversion (5%), xerostomia (3%), rectal hemorrhage (2%)

Genitourinary: Urinary tract infection (5%), urinary frequency (2%), vaginitis (2%)

Hematologic: Lymphadenopathy (2%)

Miscellaneous: Viral infection (7%), infection (2%), allergy (2%), thirst (2%), toothache (2%)

Neuromuscular and skeletal: Back pain (4%)

Respiratory: Upper respiratory infection (7% to 10%), coughing (5%), epistaxis (4%), sinusitis (4%), bronchitis (3%), pharyngitis (3%)

Ocular: Nystagmus (2%)

Otic: Earache (2%), ear infection (2%)

Adjunctive therapy (600-2400 mg/day): Frequencies noted in patients receiving other anticonvulsants

>10%:

Central nervous system: Headache (26% to 32%), dizziness (26% to 49%), somnolence (20% to 36%), ataxia (9% to 31%), fatigue (12% to 15%), vertigo (6% to 15%)

Gastrointestinal: Nausea (15% to 29%), vomiting (13% to 36%), abdominal pain (10% to 13%)

Neuromuscular & skeletal: Abnormal gait (5% to 17%)

Ocular: Diplopia (14% to 40%), nystagmus (7% to 26%), visual abnormalities (6% to 14%)

1% to 10%:

Central nervous system: Tremor (3% to 16%), nervousness (2% to 4%), insomnia (2% to 4%), agitation (1% to 2%), incoordination (1% to 3%), confusion (1% to 2%), EEG abnormalities (0% to 2%), abnormal thinking (0% to 4%)

Cardiovascular: Leg edema (1% to 2%), hypotension (0% to 2%)

Dermatologic: Acne (1% to 2%)

Endocrine & metabolic: Hyponatremia (1% to 3%), weight gain (1% to 2%)

Gastrointestinal: Diarrhea (5% to 7%), dyspepsia (5% to 6%), constipation (2% to 6%), gastritis (1% to 2%)

Neuromuscular & skeletal: Weakness (3% to 6%), muscle weakness (1% to 2%), sprains and strains (0% to 2%)

Miscellaneous: Speech disorder (1% to 3%), cranial injury (0% to 2%)

Ocular: Abnormal accommodation (0% to 2%)

Respiratory: Rhinitis (2% to 5%)

Pediatrics:

>10%:

Central nervous system: Headache (31%), somnolence (31%), dizziness (28%), ataxia (13%), fatigue (13%)

Gastrointestinal: Vomiting (33%), nausea (19%)

Ocular: Diplopia (17%), visual abnormalities (13%)

1% to 10%:

Central nervous system: Emotional lability (8%), tremor (6%), speech disorder (3%), impaired concentration (2%), convulsions (2%), vertigo (2%)

Dermatologic: Bruising (4%)

Gastrointestinal: Constipation (4%), dyspepsia (2%)

Miscellaneous: Allergic reaction (2%), increased sweating (3%)

Neuromuscular and skeletal: Abnormal gait (8%), weakness (2%), involuntary muscle contractions (2%)

Ocular: Nystagmus (9%)

Respiratory: Rhinitis (10%), pneumonia (2%)

<1% (all populations): Fever, malaise, chest pain, rigors, weight loss, bradycardia, cardiac failure, cerebral hemorrhage, hypertension, postural hypotension, palpitation, syncope, tachycardia, appetite (increased), cholelithiasis, colitis, duodenal ulcer, dysphagia, enteritis, eructation, esophagitis, flatulence, gastric ulcer, bleeding gums, gingival hyperplasia, hematemesis, rectal hemorrhage, hemorrhoids, hiccups, xerostomia, biliary pain, sialoadenitis, stomatitis, ulcerative stomatitis, leukopenia, thrombocytopenia, increased GGT, hyperglycemia, hypocalcemia, hypoglycemia, hypokalemia, elevation of transaminases, hypertonia, aggressiveness, anxiety, aphasia, aura, aggravated convulsions, delirium, delusion, decreased consciousness, dysphonia, dystonia, euphoria, extrapyramidal symptoms, hemiplegia, hyperkinesia, hyper-reflexia, hypoesthesia, hypokinesis, hyporeflexia, hypotonia, hysteria, decreased libido, manic reaction, migraine, nervousness, involuntary muscle contractions, nervousness, neuralgia, occulogyric crisis, panic disorder, paralysis, paranoid reaction, personality disorder, psychoses, ptosis, stupor, tetany, asthma, dyspnea, epistaxis, laryngismus, pleurisy, acne, alopecia, angioedema, bruising, contact dermatitis, eczema, rash (facial), flushing, folliculitis, heat rash, hot flashes, photosensitivity, pruritus, psoriasis, purpura, erythematous rash, maculopapular rash, vitiligo, abnormal accommodation, cataracts, conjunctival hemorrhage, ocular edema, hemianopia, mydriasis, otitis externa, photophobia, scotoma, taste perversion, tinnitus, xerophthalmia, dysuria, hematuria, intermenstrual bleeding, leukorrhea, menorrhagia, urinary frequency, renal pain, urinary tract pain, polyuria, priapism, renal calculi, systemic lupus erythematosus.

Rare, severe dermatologic adverse reactions have been reported in postmarketing reports, including Stevens-Johnson syndrome, erythema multiforme, and toxic epidermal necrolysis.

A rare, multiorgan hypersensitivity disorder characterized by rash, fever, lymphadenopathy, abnormal liver function tests, eosinophilia and arthralgia has been described.

Drug Interactions CYP2C19 enzyme inhibitor; CYP3A3/4 inducer

Oxcarbazepine can inhibit CYP2C19 and induce CYP3A4/5 with potentially important effects on plasma concentrations of others drugs. In addition, several anticonvulsants that are cytochrome P-450 inducers can decrease plasma concentrations of oxcarbazepine and its active metabolite (MHD)

Decreased effect: Oxcarbazepine and MHD induce CYPA3A isozymes (CYP3A4 and CYP3A5) responsible for the metabolism of dihydropyridine calcium antagonists and oral contraceptives, resulting in a lower plasma concentration of these drugs. Oxcarbazepine with oral contraceptives has been shown to decrease plasma concentrations of the two hormonal components, ethinyl estradiol (48% and 52%) and levonorgestrel (32% and 52%). Oxcarbazepine may decrease the effectiveness of these contraceptive products. Oxcarbazepine has been shown to lower the AUC of felodipine by 28% and verapamil produced a decrease of 20% of plasma levels of oxcarbazepine metabolite MHD.

Alcohol Interactions Avoid use (may increase central nervous system depression)

Half-Life 2 hours; Metabolite: 9 hours

(Continued)

Oxcarbazepine *(Continued)*

Education and Monitoring Issues

Patient Education: Take exactly as directed (do not increase dose or frequency or discontinue without consulting prescriber). While using the medication do not use alcohol and other prescription or OTC medications (especially medications to relieve pain, induce sleep, reduce anxiety, treat or prevent cold, coughs, or allergies) unless approved by prescriber. Maintain adequate hydration (2-3 L/day of fluid, unless instructed to restrict fluids). You may experience drowsiness, dizziness, or blurred vision (use caution when driving or engaging in tasks requiring alertness until response to drug is known); nausea or vomiting (small frequent meals, good mouth care, chewing gum, or sucking hard candy may help, or contact prescriber); Report CNS changes, mentation changes, changes in cognition or memory, acute fatigue or weakness, or insomnia; muscle cramping, weakness, or pain; rash or skin irritations; unusual bruising or bleeding (mouth, urine, stool); swelling of extremities; or other adverse response.

Manufacturer Novartis

Related Information

Anticonvulsants by Seizure Type Comparison *on page 1230*
Epilepsy Guidelines *on page 1091*
Pharmaceutical Manufacturers Directory *on page 1020*

Oxiconazole (oks i KON a zole)

Pharmacologic Class Antifungal Agent

U.S. Brand Names Oxistat®

Use Treatment of tinea pedis (athlete's foot), tinea cruris (jock itch), and tinea corporis (ringworm)

USUAL DOSAGE Children and Adults: Topical: Apply once to twice daily to affected areas for 2 weeks (tinea corporis/tinea cruris) to 1 month (tinea pedis)

Contraindications Hypersensitivity to this agent; not for ophthalmic use

Pregnancy Risk Factor B

♦ **Oxilan®** *see* loxilan *on page 481*
♦ **Oxistat®** *see* Oxiconazole *on page 690*
♦ **Oxpam®** *see* Oxazepam *on page 686*
♦ **Oxsoralen® Topical** *see* Methoxsalen *on page 585*
♦ **Oxsoralen-Ultra® Oral** *see* Methoxsalen *on page 585*

Oxybutynin (oks i BYOO ti nin)

Pharmacologic Class Antispasmodic Agent, Urinary

U.S. Brand Names Ditropan®; Ditropan XL®

Generic Available Yes

Mechanism of Action Direct antispasmodic effect on smooth muscle, also inhibits the action of acetylcholine on smooth muscle (exhibits $^1/_5$ the anticholinergic activity of atropine, but is 4-10 times the antispasmodic activity); does not block effects at skeletal muscle or at autonomic ganglia; increases bladder capacity, decreases uninhibited contractions, and delays desire to void; therefore, decreases urgency and frequency

Use Antispasmodic for neurogenic bladder (urgency, frequency, urge incontinence) and uninhibited bladder

USUAL DOSAGE Oral:

Children:
- 1-5 years: 0.2 mg/kg/dose 2-4 times/day
- >5 years: 5 mg twice daily, up to 5 mg 4 times/day maximum

Adults: 5 mg 2-3 times/day up to 5 mg 4 times/day maximum
- Extended release: Initial: 5 mg once daily, may increase in 5-10 mg increments; maximum: 30 mg daily

Elderly: 2.5-5 mg twice daily; increase by 2.5 mg increments every 1-2 days

Note: Should be discontinued periodically to determine whether the patient can manage without the drug and to minimize resistance to the drug

Dosage Forms SYR: 5 mg/5 mL (473 mL). **TAB:** 5 mg; Extended release: 5 mg, 10 mg, 15 mg

Contraindications Glaucoma, myasthenia gravis, partial or complete GI obstruction, GU obstruction, ulcerative colitis, hypersensitivity to drug or specific component, intestinal atony, megacolon, toxic megacolon

Warnings/Precautions Use with caution in patients with urinary tract obstruction, angle-closure glaucoma, hyperthyroidism, reflux esophagitis, heart disease, hepatic or renal disease, prostatic hypertrophy, autonomic neuropathy, ulcerative colitis (may cause ileus and toxic megacolon), hypertension, hiatal hernia. Caution should be used in elderly due to anticholinergic activity (eg, confusion, constipation, blurred vision, and tachycardia).

Pregnancy Risk Factor B

Adverse Reactions

>10%:
- Central nervous system: Drowsiness
- Gastrointestinal: Xerostomia, constipation

Miscellaneous: Diaphoresis (decreased)

1% to 10%:

Cardiovascular: Tachycardia, palpitations

Central nervous system: Dizziness, insomnia, fever, headache

Dermatologic: Rash

Endocrine & metabolic: Decreased flow of breast milk, decreased sexual ability, hot flashes

Gastrointestinal: Nausea, vomiting

Genitourinary: Urinary hesitancy or retention

Neuromuscular & skeletal: Weakness

Ocular: Blurred vision, mydriatic effect

<1%: Allergic reaction, increased intraocular pressure

Drug Interactions Increased toxicity:

Additive sedation with CNS depressants and alcohol

Additive anticholinergic effects with antihistamines and anticholinergic agents

Alcohol Interactions Avoid use (may increase central nervous system depression)

Onset Oral: 30-60 minutes; Peak effect: 3-6 hours

Duration 6-10 hours

Half-Life 1-2.3 hours

Education and Monitoring Issues

Patient Education: Take prescribed dose preferably on an empty stomach (1 hour before or 2 hours after meals). You may experience dizziness, lightheadedness, or drowsiness (use caution when driving or engaging in tasks requiring alertness until response to drug is known); dry mouth or changes in appetite (small frequent meals, frequent mouth care, sucking lozenges, or chewing gum may help); constipation (frequent exercise or increased dietary fiber, fruit, and fluid or stool softener may help); decreased sexual ability (reversible with discontinuance of drug); decreased sweating (use caution in hot weather, avoid extreme exercise or activity). Report rapid heartbeat, palpitations, or chest pain; difficulty voiding; or vision changes. Swallow extended-release tablets whole, do not chew or crush.

Monitoring Parameters: Incontinence episodes, postvoid residual (PVR)

- **Oxycocet** *see* Oxycodone and Acetaminophen *on page 692*
- **Oxycodan** *see* Oxycodone and Aspirin *on page 692*

Oxycodone (oks i KOE done)

Pharmacologic Class Analgesic, Narcotic

U.S. Brand Names Endocodone®; OxyContin®; OxyIR™; Percolone®; Roxicodone™

Generic Available No

Mechanism of Action Binds to opiate receptors in the CNS, causing inhibition of ascending pain pathways, altering the perception of and response to pain; produces generalized CNS depression

Use Management of moderate to severe pain, normally used in combination with non-narcotic analgesics

USUAL DOSAGE Oral:

Immediate release:

Children:

6-12 years: 1.25 mg every 6 hours as needed

>12 years: 2.5 mg every 6 hours as needed

Adults: 5 mg every 6 hours as needed

Controlled release: Adults: 10 mg every 12 hours around-the-clock

Dosing adjustment in hepatic impairment: Reduce dosage in patients with severe liver disease

Dosage Forms CAP, immediate release (OxyIR™): 5 mg. **LIQ, oral:** 5 mg/5 mL (500 mL). **SOLN, oral concentrate:** 20 mg/mL (30 mL). **TAB:** 5 mg; Endocone®: 5 mg; Roxicodone™: 10 mg, 30 mg; Percolone®: 5 mg; Controlled release (OxyContin®): 10 mg, 20 mg, 40 mg, 80 mg

Contraindications Hypersensitivity to oxycodone or any component

Warnings/Precautions Use with caution in patients with hypersensitivity reactions to other phenanthrene derivative opioid agonists (morphine, hydrocodone, hydromorphone, levorphanol, oxycodone, oxymorphone); respiratory diseases including asthma, emphysema, COPD, or severe liver or renal insufficiency; some preparations contain sulfites which may cause allergic reactions; dextromethorphan has equivalent antitussive activity but has much lower toxicity in accidental overdose; tolerance or drug dependence may result from extended use

Pregnancy Risk Factor B; D (if used for prolonged periods or in high doses at term)

Adverse Reactions

>10%:

Cardiovascular: Hypotension

Central nervous system: Fatigue, drowsiness, dizziness

Gastrointestinal: Nausea, vomiting

Neuromuscular & skeletal: Weakness

(Continued)

Oxycodone *(Continued)*

1% to 10%:

Central nervous system: Nervousness, headache, restlessness, malaise, confusion
Gastrointestinal: Anorexia, stomach cramps, xerostomia, constipation, biliary spasm
Genitourinary: Ureteral spasms, decreased urination
Local: Pain at injection site
Respiratory: Dyspnea, shortness of breath

<1%: Hallucinations, histamine release, increased intracranial pressure, mental depression, paradoxical CNS stimulation, paralytic ileus, physical and psychological dependence, skin rash, urticaria

Drug Interactions CYP2D6 enzyme substrate

Decreased effect: Phenothiazines may antagonize the analgesic effect of opiate agonists

Increased toxicity: CNS depressants, monoamine oxidase inhibitors, general anesthetics, and tricyclic antidepressants may potentiate the effects of opiate agonists; dextroamphetamine may enhance the analgesic effect of opiate agonists

Alcohol Interactions Avoid use (may increase central nervous system depression)

Onset Oral: Within 10-15 minutes

Duration 4-5 hours; up to 12 hours for controlled release

Education and Monitoring Issues

Patient Education: If self-administered, use exactly as directed (do not increase dose or frequency); may cause physical and/or psychological dependence. While using this medication, do not use alcohol and other prescription or OTC medications (especially sedatives, tranquilizers, antihistamines, or pain medications) without consulting prescriber. Maintain adequate hydration (2-3 L/day of fluids unless instructed to restrict fluid intake). May cause hypotension, dizziness, drowsiness, impaired coordination, or blurred vision (use caution when driving, climbing stairs, or changing position - rising from sitting or lying to standing, or when engaging in tasks requiring alertness until response to drug is known); nausea, vomiting or dry mouth (frequent mouth care, small frequent meals, chewing gum, or sucking lozenges may help); constipation (increased exercise, fluids, or dietary fruit and fiber may help - if constipation remains an unresolved problem, consult prescriber about use of stool softeners). Report persistent dizziness or headache; excessive fatigue or sedation; changes in mental status; changes in urinary elimination or pain on urination; weakness or trembling; blurred vision; or shortness of breath.

Monitoring Parameters: Pain relief, respiratory and mental status, blood pressure

Reference Range: Blood level of 5 mg/L associated with fatality

Related Information

Narcotic Agonists Comparison *on page 1244*

Oxycodone and Acetaminophen (oks i KOE done & a seet a MIN oh fen)

Pharmacologic Class Analgesic, Combination (Narcotic)

U.S. Brand Names Endocet®; Percocet® 2.5/325; Percocet® 5/325; Percocet® 7.5/500; Percocet® 10/650; Roxicet® 5/500; Roxilox™; Tylox®

Use Management of moderate to severe pain

USUAL DOSAGE Oral (doses should be titrated to appropriate analgesic effects):

Children: Oxycodone: 0.05-0.15 mg/kg/dose to 5 mg/dose (maximum) every 4-6 hours as needed

Adults: 1-2 tablets every 4-6 hours as needed for pain
Maximum daily dose of acetaminophen: 4 g/day

Dosing adjustment in hepatic impairment: Dose should be reduced in patients with severe liver disease

Dosage Forms CAPLET: Oxycodone hydrochloride 5 mg and acetaminophen 500 mg. **CAP:** Oxycodone hydrochloride 5 mg and acetaminophen 500 mg. **SOLN, oral:** Oxycodone hydrochloride 5 mg and acetaminophen 325 mg per 5 mL (5 mL, 500 mL). **TAB:** Oxycodone hydrochloride 2.5 mg and acetaminophen 325 mg; Oxycodone hydrochloride 5 mg and acetaminophen 325 mg; Oxycodone hydrochloride 7.5 mg and acetaminophen 500 mg; Oxycodone hydrochloride 10 mg and acetaminophen 650 mg

Pregnancy Risk Factor C

Alcohol Interactions Avoid use (may increase central nervous system depression)

Related Information

Lipid-Lowering Agents Comparison *on page 1243*

Oxycodone and Aspirin (oks i KOE done & AS pir in)

Pharmacologic Class Analgesic, Combination (Narcotic)

U.S. Brand Names Codoxy®; Percodan®; Percodan®-Demi; Roxiprin®

Use Relief of moderate to moderately severe pain

USUAL DOSAGE Oral (based on oxycodone combined salts):

Children: 0.05-0.15 mg/kg/dose every 4-6 hours as needed; maximum: 5 mg/dose (1 tablet Percodan® or 2 tablets Percodan®-Demi/dose)

Adults: Percodan®: 1 tablet every 6 hours as needed for pain or Percodan®-Demi: 1-2 tablets every 6 hours as needed for pain

Dosing adjustment in hepatic impairment: Dose should be reduced in patients with severe liver disease

Dosage Forms TAB: (Percodan®): Oxycodone hydrochloride 4.5 mg, oxycodone terephthalate 0.38 mg, and aspirin 325 mg; (Percodan®-Demi): Oxycodone hydrochloride 2.25 mg, oxycodone terephthalate 0.19 mg, and aspirin 325 mg

Pregnancy Risk Factor D

Alcohol Interactions Avoid use (may increase central nervous system depression and enhance gastric mucosal irritation)

Related Information

Lipid-Lowering Agents Comparison *on page 1243*

♦ **OxyContin®** *see* Oxycodone *on page 691*

♦ **OxyIR™** *see* Oxycodone *on page 691*

Oxymetholone (oks i METH oh lone)

Pharmacologic Class Anabolic Steroid

U.S. Brand Names Anadrol®

Generic Available No

Mechanism of Action Stimulates receptors in organs and tissues to promote growth and development of male sex organs and maintains secondary sex characteristics in androgen-deficient males

Use Anemias caused by the administration of myelotoxic drugs

USUAL DOSAGE Adults: Erythropoietic effects: Oral: 1-5 mg/kg/day in one daily dose; usual effective dose: 1-2 mg/kg/day; give for a minimum trial of 3-6 months because response may be delayed

Dosing adjustment in hepatic impairment:

Mild to moderate hepatic impairment: Oxymetholone should be used with caution in patients with liver dysfunction because of it's hepatotoxic potential

Severe hepatic impairment: Oxymetholone should **not** be used

Dosage Forms TAB: 50 mg

Contraindications Carcinoma of breast or prostate, nephrosis, pregnancy, hypersensitivity to any component

Warnings/Precautions Anabolic steroids may cause peliosis hepatis, liver cell tumors, and blood lipid changes with increased risk of arteriosclerosis; monitor diabetic patients carefully; use with caution in elderly patients, they may be at greater risk for prostatic hypertrophy; use with caution in patients with cardiac, renal, or hepatic disease or epilepsy

Pregnancy Risk Factor X

Adverse Reactions

Male:

Postpubertal:

- >10%:
  - Dermatologic: Acne
  - Endocrine & metabolic: Gynecomastia
  - Genitourinary: Bladder irritability, priapism
- 1% to 10%:
  - Central nervous system: Insomnia, chills
  - Endocrine & metabolic: Decreased libido
  - Gastrointestinal: Nausea, diarrhea
  - Genitourinary: Prostatic hypertrophy (elderly)
  - Hematologic: Iron deficiency anemia, suppression of clotting factors
- Hepatic: Hepatic dysfunction
- <1%: Hepatic necrosis, hepatocellular carcinoma

Prepubertal:

- >10%:
  - Dermatologic: Acne
  - Endocrine & metabolic: Virilism
- 1% to 10%:
  - Central nervous system: Chills, insomnia
  - Dermatologic: Hyperpigmentation
  - Gastrointestinal: Diarrhea, nausea
  - Hematologic: Iron deficiency anemia, suppression of clotting factors
- <1%: Hepatic necrosis, hepatocellular carcinoma

Female:

- >10%: Endocrine & metabolic: Virilism
- 1% to 10%:
  - Central nervous system: Chills, insomnia
  - Endocrine & metabolic: Hypercalcemia
  - Gastrointestinal: Nausea, diarrhea
  - Hematologic: Iron deficiency anemia, suppression of clotting factors
  - Hepatic: Hepatic dysfunction
- <1%: Hepatic necrosis, hepatocellular carcinoma

(Continued)

Oxymetholone *(Continued)*

Drug Interactions Increased toxicity: Increased oral anticoagulants, insulin requirements may be decreased

Half-Life 9 hours

Education and Monitoring Issues

Patient Education: Take as directed; do not exceed recommended dosage. If diabetic, monitor serum glucose closely and notify prescriber of changes; this medication can alter glucose tolerance. You may experience acne, growth of body hair or baldness, deepening of voice, loss of libido, impotence, swelling of breasts, menstrual irregularity, or priapism (most are reversible); drowsiness, dizziness, or blurred vision (use caution driving or engaging in tasks that require alertness until response to drug is known); or nausea or vomiting (small frequent meals and good mouth care may help). Report persistent GI distress or diarrhea; change in color of urine or stool; yellowing of eyes or skin; swelling of ankles, feet, or hands; unusual bruising or bleeding; or other adverse reactions.

Monitoring Parameters: Liver function tests

Oxymorphone (oks i MOR fone)

Pharmacologic Class Analgesic, Narcotic

U.S. Brand Names Numorphan®

Generic Available No

Mechanism of Action Oxymorphone hydrochloride (Numorphan®) is a potent narcotic analgesic with uses similar to those of morphine. The drug is a semisynthetic derivative of morphine (phenanthrene derivative) and is closely related to hydromorphone chemically (Dilaudid®).

Use Management of moderate to severe pain and preoperatively as a sedative and a supplement to anesthesia

USUAL DOSAGE Adults:

I.M., S.C.: 0.5 mg initially, 1-1.5 mg every 4-6 hours as needed
I.V.: 0.5 mg initially
Rectal: 5 mg every 4-6 hours

Dosage Forms INJ: 1 mg (1 mL); 1.5 mg/mL (1 mL, 10 mL). **SUPP, rectal:** 5 mg

Contraindications Hypersensitivity to oxymorphone or any component, increased intracranial pressure; severe respiratory depression

Warnings/Precautions Some preparations contain sulfites which may cause allergic reactions; infants <3 months of age are more susceptible to respiratory depression, use with caution and generally in reduced doses in this age group; use with caution in patients with impaired respiratory function or severe hepatic dysfunction and in patients with hypersensitivity reactions to other phenanthrene derivative opioid agonists (codeine, hydrocodone, hydromorphone, levorphanol, oxycodone, oxymorphone); tolerance or drug dependence may result from extended use

Pregnancy Risk Factor B; D (if used for prolonged periods or in high doses at term)

Adverse Reactions

>10%:
- Cardiovascular: Hypotension
- Central nervous system: Fatigue, drowsiness, dizziness
- Gastrointestinal: Nausea, vomiting, constipation
- Neuromuscular & skeletal: Weakness
- Miscellaneous: Histamine release

1% to 10%:
- Central nervous system: Nervousness, headache, restlessness, malaise, confusion
- Gastrointestinal: Anorexia, stomach cramps, xerostomia, biliary spasm
- Genitourinary: Decreased urination, ureteral spasms
- Local: Pain at injection site
- Respiratory: Dyspnea, shortness of breath

<1%: Hallucinations, histamine release, increased intracranial pressure, mental depression, paradoxical CNS stimulation, paralytic ileus, physical and psychological dependence, rash, urticaria

Drug Interactions

Decreased effect with phenothiazines
Increased effect/toxicity with CNS depressants, TCAs, dextroamphetamine

Alcohol Interactions Avoid use (may increase central nervous system depression)

Onset Onset of analgesia: I.V., I.M., S.C.: Within 5-10 minutes; Rectal: Within 15-30 minutes

Duration Duration of analgesia: Parenteral, rectal: 3-4 hours

Half-Life 1-2 hours

Education and Monitoring Issues

Patient Education: If self-administered, use exactly as directed (do not increase dose or frequency or discontinue without consulting prescriber); may cause physical and/or psychological dependence. While using this medication, do not use alcohol and other prescription or OTC medications (especially sedatives, tranquilizers, antihistamines, or pain medications) without consulting prescriber. Maintain adequate hydration (2-3 L/day of fluids unless instructed to restrict fluid intake). May cause hypotension, dizziness, drowsiness, impaired coordination, or blurred vision (use caution when driving, climbing stairs, or changing position - rising from sitting or lying to standing, or when engaging in tasks requiring alertness until response to drug is known); nausea, vomiting or dry mouth (frequent mouth care, small frequent meals, chewing gum, or sucking lozenges may help); constipation (increased exercise, fluids, or dietary fruit and fiber may help - if constipation remains an unresolved problem, consult prescriber about use of stool softeners). Report persistent dizziness or headache; excessive fatigue or sedation; changes in mental status; changes in urinary elimination or pain on urination; weakness or trembling; blurred vision; or shortness of breath.

Monitoring Parameters: Respiratory rate, heart rate, blood pressure, CNS activity

Related Information

Lipid-Lowering Agents Comparison *on page 1243*
Narcotic Agonists Comparison *on page 1244*

Oxytetracycline (oks i tet ra SYE kleen)

Pharmacologic Class Tetracycline Derivative

U.S. Brand Names Terramycin® I.M. Injection; Terramycin® Oral; Uri-Tet® Oral

Use Treatment of susceptible bacterial infections; both gram-positive and gram-negative, as well as, *Rickettsia* and *Mycoplasma* organisms

USUAL DOSAGE

Oral:

Children >8 years: 40-50 mg/kg/day in divided doses every 6 hours (maximum: 2 g/24 hours)

Adults: 250-500 mg/dose every 6-12 hours depending on severity of the infection

I.M.:

Children >8 years: 15-25 mg/kg/day (maximum: 250 mg/dose) in divided doses every 8-12 hours

Adults: 250 mg every 24 hours or 300 mg/day divided every 8-12 hours

Syphilis: 30-40 g in divided doses over 10-15 days

Gonorrhea: 1.5 g, then 500 mg every 6 hours for total of 9 g

Uncomplicated chlamydial infections: 500 mg every 6 hours for 7 days

Severe acne: 1 g/day then decrease to 125-500 mg/day

Dosing interval in renal impairment:

Cl_{cr} <10 mL/minute: Administer every 24 hours or avoid use if possible

Dosing adjustment/comments in hepatic impairment: Avoid use in patients with severe liver disease

Contraindications Hypersensitivity to tetracycline or any component

Pregnancy Risk Factor D

Related Information

Oxytetracycline and Hydrocortisone *on page 695*
Oxytetracycline and Polymyxin B *on page 695*

Oxytetracycline and Hydrocortisone

(oks i tet ra SYE kleen & hye droe KOR ti sone)

Pharmacologic Class Antibiotic/Corticosteroid, Ophthalmic

U.S. Brand Names Terra-Cortril® Ophthalmic Suspension

Dosage Forms SUSP, ophth: Oxytetracycline hydrochloride 0.5% and hydrocortisone 0.5% (5 mL)

Pregnancy Risk Factor C

Oxytetracycline and Polymyxin B

(oks i tet ra SYE kleen & pol i MIKS in bee)

Pharmacologic Class Antibiotic, Ophthalmic

U.S. Brand Names Terak® Ophthalmic Ointment; Terramycin® Ophthalmic Ointment; Terramycin® w/Polymyxin B Ophthalmic Ointment

Dosage Forms OINT, ophth/otic: Oxytetracycline hydrochloride 5 mg and polymyxin B 10,000 units per g (3.5 g). **TAB, vag:** Oxytetracycline hydrochloride 100 mg and polymyxin B 100,000 units (10s)

Pregnancy Risk Factor D

Oxytocin (oks i TOE sin)

Pharmacologic Class Oxytocic Agent

U.S. Brand Names Pitocin® Injection

Generic Available Yes

Mechanism of Action Produces the rhythmic uterine contractions characteristic to delivery and stimulates breast milk flow during nursing

Use Induces labor at term; controls postpartum bleeding; nasal preparation used to promote milk letdown in lactating females

USUAL DOSAGE I.V. administration requires the use of an infusion pump

(Continued)

Oxytocin *(Continued)*

Adults:

Induction of labor: I.V.: 0.001-0.002 units/minute; increase by 0.001-0.002 units every 15-30 minutes until contraction pattern has been established; maximum dose should not exceed 20 milliunits/minute

Postpartum bleeding:

I.M.: Total dose of 10 units after delivery

I.V.: 10-40 units by I.V. infusion in 1000 mL of intravenous fluid at a rate sufficient to control uterine atony

Promotion of milk letdown: Intranasal: 1 spray or 3 drops in one or both nostrils 2-3 minutes before breast-feeding

Dosage Forms INJ: 10 units/mL (1 mL, 10 mL). **SOLN, nasal:** 40 units/mL (2 mL, 5 mL)

Contraindications Hypersensitivity to oxytocin or any component; significant cephalopelvic disproportion, unfavorable fetal positions, fetal distress, hypertonic or hyperactive uterus, contraindicated vaginal delivery, prolapse, total placenta previa, and vasa previa

Warnings/Precautions To be used for medical rather than elective induction of labor; may produce antidiuretic effect (ie, water intoxication and excess uterine contractions); high doses or hypersensitivity to oxytocin may cause uterine hypertonicity, spasm, tetanic contraction, or rupture of the uterus; severe water intoxication with convulsions, coma, and death is associated with a slow oxytocin infusion over 24 hours

Pregnancy Risk Factor X

Adverse Reactions

Fetal: <1%: Arrhythmias, bradycardia, brain damage, death, hypoxia, intracranial hemorrhage, neonatal jaundice

Maternal: <1%: Anaphylactic reactions, arrhythmias, cardiac arrhythmias, coma, death, fatal afibrinogenemia, hypotension, increased blood loss, increased uterine motility, nausea, pelvic hematoma, postpartum hemorrhage, premature ventricular contractions, seizures, SIADH with hyponatremia, tachycardia, vomiting

Drug Interactions Sympathomimetic pressor effects may be increased by oxytocin resulting in postpartum hypertension

Onset Onset of uterine contractions: I.V.: Within 1 minute

Duration <30 minutes

Half-Life 1-5 minutes

Education and Monitoring Issues

Patient Education:

I.V., I.M.: Generally used in emergency situations. Drug teaching should be incorporated in other situational teaching.

Intranasal spray: While sitting up, hold bottle upright and squeeze into nostril.

Monitoring Parameters: Fluid intake and output during administration; fetal monitoring

- **Oyst-Cal 500 [OTC]** *see* Calcium Carbonate *on page 130*
- **Oystercal® 500** *see* Calcium Carbonate *on page 130*
- **Pacerone®** *see* Amiodarone *on page 48*
- **Palafer®** *see* Ferrous Fumarate *on page 359*
- **Palgic-D® [OTC]** *see* Carbinoxamine and Pseudoephedrine *on page 140*

Palivizumab (pah li VIZ u mab)

Pharmacologic Class Monoclonal Antibody

U.S. Brand Names Synagis®

Mechanism of Action Exhibits neutralizing and fusion-inhibitory activity against RSV; these activities inhibit RSV replication in laboratory and clinical studies

Use Prevention of serious lower respiratory tract disease caused by respiratory syncytial virus (RSV) in pediatric patients at high risk of RSV disease; safety and efficacy were established in infants with bronchopulmonary dysplasia (BPD) and infants with a history of prematurity (≤35 weeks gestational age)

USUAL DOSAGE Children: I.M.: 15 mg/kg of body weight, monthly throughout RSV season (First dose administered prior to commencement of RSV season)

Dosage Forms INJ, lyophilized: 100 mg

Contraindications Patients with a history of severe prior reaction to palivizumab or other components of the product

Warnings/Precautions Anaphylactoid reactions have not been observed following palivizumab administration; however, can occur after administration of proteins. Safety and efficacy of palivizumab have not been demonstrated in the treatment of established RSV disease.

Pregnancy Risk Factor C

Pregnancy Implications Animal reproduction studies have not been conducted; it is not known whether palivizumab can cause fetal harm when administered to a pregnant woman or could affect reproductive capacity

Adverse Reactions The incidence of adverse events was similar between the palivizumab and placebo groups

>1%:

Central nervous system: Nervousness

Dermatologic: Fungal dermatitis, eczema, seborrhea
Gastrointestinal: Diarrhea, vomiting, gastroenteritis
Hematologic: Anemia
Hepatic: ALT increase, abnormal LFTs
Local: Injection site reaction
Ocular: Conjunctivitis
Respiratory: Cough, wheezing, bronchiolitis, pneumonia, bronchitis, asthma, croup, dyspnea, sinusitis, apnea
Miscellaneous: Oral moniliasis, failure to thrive, viral infection, flu syndrome

Drug Interactions No formal drug interaction studies have been conducted

Manufacturer Medimmune, Inc

Related Information

Pharmaceutical Manufacturers Directory *on page 1020*

♦ **Palmitate-A® 5000 [OTC]** *see* Vitamin A *on page 978*

♦ **Pamelor®** *see* Nortriptyline *on page 665*

♦ **Pamergan** *see* Meperidine and Promethazine *on page 564*

Pamidronate (pa mi DROE nate)

Pharmacologic Class Antidote; Bisphosphonate Derivative

U.S. Brand Names Aredia™

Generic Available No

Mechanism of Action A biphosphonate which inhibits bone resorption via actions on osteoclasts or on osteoclast precursors. Does not appear to produce any significant effects on renal tubular calcium handling and is poorly absorbed following oral administration (high oral doses have been reported effective); therefore, I.V. therapy is preferred.

Use Treatment of hypercalcemia associated with malignancy; treatment of osteolytic bone lesions associated with multiple myeloma or metastatic breast cancer; moderate to severe Paget's disease of bone

USUAL DOSAGE Drug must be properly diluted before administration and slowly infused intravenously (over at least 1 hour). Adults: I.V.:

Hypercalcemia of malignancy:

Moderate cancer-related hypercalcemia (corrected serum calcium: 12-13 mg/dL): 60-90 mg given as a slow infusion over 2-24 hours

Severe cancer-related hypercalcemia (corrected serum calcium: >13.5 mg/dL): 90 mg as a slow infusion over 2-24 hours

A period of 7 days should elapse before the second course; repeat infusions every 2-3 weeks have been suggested, however, could be administered every 2-3 months according to the degree and of severity of hypercalcemia and/or the type of malignancy

Note: Dose recommendations for hypercalcemia are somewhat arbitrary. Some investigators have suggested a lack of a dose-response relationship. Courses of pamidronate for hypercalcemia may be repeated at varying intervals, depending on the duration of normocalcemia (median 2-3 weeks), but the manufacturer recommends a minimum interval between courses of 7 days. Oral etidronate at a dose of 20 mg/kg/day has been used to maintain the calcium lowering effect following I.V. bisphosphonates, although it is of limited effectiveness.

Osteolytic bone lesions with multiple myeloma: 90 mg in 500 mL D_5W, 0.45% NaCl or 0.9% NaCl administered over 4 hours on a monthly basis

Osteolytic bone lesions with metastatic breast cancer: 90 mg in 250 mL D_5W, 0.45% NaCl or 0.9% NaCl administered over 2 hours, repeated every 3-4 weeks

Paget's disease: 30 mg in 500 mL 0.45% NaCl, 0.9% NaCl or D_5W administered over 4 hours for 3 consecutive days

Dosing adjustment in renal impairment: Adjustment is not necessary

Dosage Forms POWDER for inj, lyophilized: 30 mg, 60 mg, 90 mg

Contraindications Previous hypersensitivity to pamidronate or other biphosphonates

Warnings/Precautions Use caution in patients with renal impairment as nephropathy was seen in animal studies. However, in contrast to reports of renal failure with other biphosphonates, impairment of renal function has not been reported with pamidronate in studies to date. However, further experience is needed to assess the nephrotoxic potential with higher doses and prolonged administration. Use caution in patients who are pregnant or in the breast-feeding period; leukopenia has been observed with oral pamidronate and monitoring of white blood cell counts is suggested. Vein irritation and thrombophlebitis may occur with infusions. Has not been studied exclusively in the elderly; monitor serum electrolytes periodically since elderly are often receiving diuretics which can result in decreases in serum calcium, potassium, and magnesium.

Pregnancy Risk Factor C

Adverse Reactions

1% to 10%:

Central nervous system: Malaise, fever, convulsions
Endocrine & metabolic: Hypomagnesemia, hypocalcemia, hypokalemia, fluid overload, hypophosphatemia
Gastrointestinal: GI symptoms, nausea, diarrhea, constipation, anorexia

(Continued)

Pamidronate *(Continued)*

Hepatic: Abnormal hepatic function
Neuromuscular & skeletal: Bone pain
Respiratory: Dyspnea

<1%: Abnormal taste, angioedema, hypersensitivity reactions, increased risk of fractures, leukopenia, nephrotoxicity, occult blood in stools, pain, skin rash

Onset Onset of effect: 24-48 hours; Maximum effect: 5-7 days

Half-Life Distribution half-life: 1.6 hours; Urinary (elimination) half-life: 2.5 hours; Bone half-life: 300 days

Education and Monitoring Issues

Patient Education: This medication can only be administered I.V. Avoid foods high in calcium or vitamins with minerals during infusion or for 2-3 hours after completion. You may experience nausea or vomiting (small frequent meals and good mouth care may help); or recurrent bone pain (consult prescriber for analgesic). Report unusual muscle twitching or spasms, severe diarrhea/constipation, or acute bone pain.

Monitoring Parameters: Serum electrolytes, monitor for hypocalcemia for at least 2 weeks after therapy; serum calcium, phosphate, magnesium, potassium, serum creatinine, CBC with differential

Reference Range: Calcium (total): Adults: 9.0-11.0 mg/dL (SI: 2.05-2.54 mmol/L), may slightly decrease with aging; Phosphorus: 2.5-4.5 mg/dL (SI: 0.81-1.45 mmol/L)

Manufacturer Novartis

Related Information

Pharmaceutical Manufacturers Directory *on page 1020*

- **Pamprin IB® [OTC]** *see* Ibuprofen *on page 458*
- **Panadol® [OTC]** *see* Acetaminophen *on page 17*
- **Panasal® 5/500** *see* Hydrocodone and Aspirin *on page 445*
- **Pancof XP®** *see* Hydrocodone, Pseudoephedrine, and Guaifenesin *on page 446*
- **Pancrease®** *see* Pancrelipase *on page 698*
- **Pancrease® MT 4** *see* Pancrelipase *on page 698*
- **Pancrease® MT 10** *see* Pancrelipase *on page 698*
- **Pancrease® MT 16** *see* Pancrelipase *on page 698*
- **Pancrease® MT 20** *see* Pancrelipase *on page 698*

Pancrelipase (pan kre LI pase)

Pharmacologic Class Enzyme, Gastrointestinal

U.S. Brand Names Cotazym®; Cotazym-S®; Creon® 10; Creon® 20; Ilozyme®; Ku-Zyme® HP; Lipram®; Pancrease®; Pancrease® MT 4; Pancrease® MT 10; Pancrease® MT 16; Pancrease® MT 20; Protilase®; Ultrase® MT12; Ultrase® MT20; Viokase®; Zymase®

Generic Available No

Mechanism of Action Replaces endogenous pancreatic enzymes to assist in digestion of protein, starch and fats

Use Replacement therapy in symptomatic treatment of malabsorption syndrome caused by pancreatic insufficiency

USUAL DOSAGE Oral:

Powder: Actual dose depends on the digestive requirements of the patient
Children <1 year: Start with $^1/_8$ teaspoonful with feedings
Adults: 0.7 g with meals

Enteric coated microspheres and microtablets: The following dosage recommendations are only an approximation for initial dosages. The actual dosage will depend on the digestive requirements of the individual patient.
Children:
<1 year: 2000 units of lipase with meals
1-6 years: 4000-8000 units of lipase with meals and 4000 units with snacks
7-12 years: 4000-12,000 units of lipase with meals and snacks
Adults: 4000-16,000 units of lipase with meals and with snacks or 1-3 tablets/capsules before or with meals and snacks; in severe deficiencies, dose may be increased to 8 tablets/capsules

Occluded feeding tubes: One tablet of Viokase® crushed with one 325 mg tablet of sodium bicarbonate (to activate the Viokase®) in 5 mL of water can be instilled into the nasogastric tube and clamped for 5 minutes; then, flushed with 50 mL of tap water

Dosage Forms

CAP: (Cotazym®): Lipase 8000 units, protease 30,000 units, amylase 30,000 units; (Ku-Zyme® HP): Lipase 8000 units, protease 30,000 units, amylase 30,000 units; (Lipram-PN16®): Lipase 16,000 units, protease 48,000 units, amylase 48,000 units; (Lipram-CR20®): Lipase 20,000 units, protease 75,000 units, amylase 66,400 units; (Lipram-UL12®): Lipase 12,000 units, protease 39,000 units, amylase 39,000 units; (Lipram-PN10®): Lipase 10,000 units, protease 30,000 units, amylase 30,000 units; (Lipram-UL18®): Lipase 18,000 units, protease 58,500 units, amylase 58,500 units; (Lipram-UL20®): Lipase 20,000 units, protease 65,000 units, amylase 65,000 units; (Ultrase® MT12): Lipase 12,000 units, protease 39,000 units, amylase 39,000 units; (Ultrase® MT20): Lipase 20,000 units, protease 65,000 units, amylase 65,000 units;

Enteric coated microspheres (Pancrease®): Lipase 4000 units, protease 25,000 units, amylase 20,000 units; Enteric coated microtablets: (Pancrease® MT 4): Lipase 4500 units, protease 12,000 units, amylase 12,000 units; (Pancrease® MT 10): Lipase 10,000 units, protease 30,000 units, amylase 30,000 units; (Pancrease® MT 16): Lipase 16,000 units, protease 48,000 units, amylase 48,000 units; (Pancrease® MT 20): Lipase 20,000 units, protease 44,000 units, amylase 56,000 units; Enteric coated spheres: (Cotazym-S®): Lipase 5000 units, protease 20,000 units, amylase 20,000 units; (Pancrelipase, Protilase®): Lipase 4000 units, protease 25,000 units, amylase 20,000 units; (Zymase®): Lipase 12,000 units, protease 24,000 units, amylase 24,000 units; Delayed release: (Creon® 10): Lipase 10,000 units, protease 37,500 units, amylase 33,200 units; (Creon® 20): Lipase 20,000 units, protease 75,000 units, amylase 66,400 units. **POWDER** (Viokase®): Lipase 16,800 units, protease 70,000 units, amylase 70,000 units per 0.7 g. **TAB:** (Ilozyme®): Lipase 11,000 units, protease 30,000 units, amylase 30,000 units; (Viokase®): Lipase 8000 units, protease 30,000 units, amylase 30,000 units

Contraindications Hypersensitivity to pancrelipase or any component, pork protein

Warnings/Precautions Pancrelipase is inactivated by acids; use microencapsulated products whenever possible, since these products permit better dissolution of enzymes in the duodenum and protect the enzyme preparations from acid degradation in the stomach

Pregnancy Risk Factor C

Adverse Reactions

1% to 10%: High doses:

- Endocrine & metabolic: Hyperuricemia
- Gastrointestinal: Nausea, cramps, constipation, diarrhea
- Genitourinary: Hyperuricosuria
- Ocular: Lacrimation
- Respiratory: Sneezing, bronchospasm

<1%: Bronchospasm, irritation of the mouth, rash, shortness of breath

Drug Interactions

Decreased effect: Calcium carbonate, magnesium hydroxide

Increased effect: H_2-antagonists (eg, ranitidine, cimetidine)

Education and Monitoring Issues

Patient Education: Take before or with meals. Avoid taking with alkaline food. Do not chew, crush, or dissolve delayed release capsules; swallow whole. Do not inhale powder when preparing. You may experience some gastric discomfort. Report unusual joint pain or swelling, respiratory difficulty, or persistent GI upset.

Pancuronium (pan kyoo ROE nee um)

Pharmacologic Class Skeletal Muscle Relaxant

U.S. Brand Names Pavulon®

Generic Available Yes

Mechanism of Action Prevents depolarization of muscle membrane and subsequent muscle contraction by acting as a competitive antagonist to acetylcholine at the alpha subunits of the nicotinic cholinergic receptors on the motor endplates in skeletal muscle, also interferes with the mobilization of acetylcholine presynaptically; the neuromuscular blockade can be pharmacologically reversed with an anticholinesterase agent (neostigmine, edrophonium, pyridostigmine)

Use Drug of choice for neuromuscular blockade except in patients with renal failure, hepatic failure, or cardiovascular instability, or in situations not suited for pancuronium's long duration of action

Adjunct to general anesthesia to facilitate endotracheal intubation and to relax skeletal muscles during surgery; to facilitate mechanical ventilation in ICU patients; does not relieve pain or produce sedation

USUAL DOSAGE Administer I.V.; dose to effect; doses will vary due to interpatient variability; use ideal body weight for obese patients

Surgery:

Neonates <1 month:

Test dose: 0.02 mg/kg to measure responsiveness

Initial: 0.03 mg/kg/dose repeated twice at 5- to 10-minute intervals as needed; maintenance: 0.03-0.09 mg/kg/dose every 30 minutes to 4 hours as needed

Infants >1 month, Children, and Adults: Initial: 0.06-0.1 mg/kg or 0.05 mg/kg after initial dose of succinylcholine for intubation; maintenance dose: 0.01 mg/kg 60-100 minutes after initial dose and then 0.01 mg/kg every 25-60 minutes

Pretreatment/priming: 10% of intubating dose given 3-5 minutes before initial dose

ICU: 0.05-0.1 mg/kg bolus followed by 0.8-1.7 mcg/kg/minute once initial recovery from bolus observed or 0.1-0.2 mg/kg every 1-3 hours

Dosing adjustment in renal impairment: Elimination half-life is doubled, plasma clearance is reduced and rate of recovery is sometimes much slower

Cl_{cr} 10-50 mL/minute: Administer 50% of normal dose

Cl_{cr} <10 mL/minute: Do not use

Dosing adjustment/comments in hepatic/biliary tract disease: Elimination half-life is doubled, plasma clearance is reduced, recovery time is prolonged, volume of distribution is increased (50%) and results in a slower onset, higher total initial dosage and prolongation of neuromuscular blockade

(Continued)

Pancuronium *(Continued)*

Dosage Forms INJ: 1 mg/mL (10 mL); 2 mg/mL (2 mL, 5 mL)

Contraindications Hypersensitivity to pancuronium, bromide, or any component

Warnings/Precautions Ventilation must be supported during neuromuscular blockade; use with caution in patients with renal and/or hepatic impairment (adjust dose appropriately); certain clinical conditions may result in potentiation or antagonism of neuromuscular blockade, see table.

Clinical Conditions Affecting Neuromuscular Blockade

Potentiation	Antagonism
Electrolyte abnormalities	Alkalosis
Severe hyponatremia	Hypercalcemia
Severe hypocalcemia	Demyelinating lesions
Severe hypokalemia	Peripheral neuropathies
Hypermagnesemia	Diabetes mellitus
Neuromuscular diseases	
Acidosis	
Acute intermittent porphyria	
Renal failure	
Hepatic failure	

Increased sensitivity in patients with myasthenia gravis, Eaton-Lambert syndrome; resistance in burn patients (>30% of body) for period of 5-70 days postinjury; resistance in patients with muscle trauma, denervation, immobilization, infection

Pregnancy Risk Factor C

Potential Drug Interactions

Potentiation	Antagonism
Anesthetics	Calcium
Desflurane, sevoflurane, enflurane and	Carbamazepine
isoflurane > halothane > nitrous	Phenytoin
oxide-narcotics	Steroids (chronic administration)
Antibiotics	Theophylline
Aminoglycosides, polymyxins, clindamycin, vancomycin	Anticholinesterases*
Magnesium sulfate	Neostigmine, pyridostigmine,
Antiarrhythmics	edrophonium, echothiophate
Quinidine, procainamide, bretylium, and	ophthalmic solution
possibly lidocaine	Caffeine
Diuretics	Azathioprine
Furosemide, mannitol	
Amphotericin B (secondary to hypokalemia)	
Local anesthetics	
Dantrolene (directly depresses skeletal muscle)	
Beta agonists	
Beta blockers	
Calcium channel blockers	
Ketamine	
Lithium	
Succinylcholine (when administered prior to nondepolarizing NMB agent)	
Cyclosporine	

*Can prolong the effects of acetylcholine

Adverse Reactions

1% to 10%:

Cardiovascular: Elevation in pulse rate, elevated blood pressure, tachycardia, hypertension

Dermatologic: Rash, itching

Gastrointestinal: Excessive salivation

<1%: Bronchospasm, burning sensation along the vein, circulatory collapse, edema, erythema, hypersensitivity reaction, profound muscle weakness, skin flushing, wheezing

Causes of prolonged neuromuscular blockade:
Excessive drug administration
Cumulative drug effect, decreased metabolism/excretion (hepatic and/or renal impairment)
Accumulation of active metabolites
Electrolyte imbalance (hypokalemia, hypocalcemia, hypermagnesemia, hypernatremia)
Hypothermia
Drug interactions
Increased sensitivity to muscle relaxants (eg, neuromuscular disorders such as myasthenia gravis or polymyositis)

In the ICU setting, reports of prolonged paralysis and generalized myopathy following discontinuation of agent (may be minimized by appropriately monitoring degree of blockade)

Drug Interactions See table on previous page

Onset 2-3 minutes

Duration 40-60 minutes

Half-Life 110 minutes

Education and Monitoring Issues

Monitoring Parameters: Degree of muscle relaxation (via peripheral nerve stimulator and presence of spontaneous movement); vital signs (heart rate, blood pressure, respiratory rate); renal function and liver function

- **Pandel®** *see* Hydrocortisone *on page 447*
- **Panmycin® Oral** *see* Tetracycline *on page 903*
- **Panretin®** *see* Alitretinoin *on page 33*
- **Panthoderm® [OTC]** *see* Dexpanthenol *on page 259*

Pantoprazole (pan TOE pra zole)

Pharmacologic Class Proton Pump Inhibitor

U.S. Brand Names Protonix®

Mechanism of Action Suppresses gastric acid secretin by inhibiting the parietal cell H+/K+ ATP pump

Use Short-term treatment of erosive esophagitis associated with GERD

Investigational use: Hypersecretory disorders, peptic ulcer disease, active ulcer bleeding with parenterally-administered pantoprazole

USUAL DOSAGE Adults: Oral: 40 mg every day for up to 8 weeks; an additional 8 weeks may be used in patients who have not healed after an 8-week course

Dosage adjustment in renal impairment: Not required; pantoprazole is not removed by hemodialysis

Dosage adjustment in hepatic impairment: Dosage adjustment is not required for mild to moderate impairment. Specific guidelines are not available for patients with severe hepatic impairment.

Elderly: Dosage adjustment not required

Dosage Forms TAB: 40 mg

Contraindications Hypersensitivity to pantoprazole or any component

Warnings/Precautions Symptomatic response does not preclude gastric malignancy; not indicated for maintenance therapy; safety and efficacy for use beyond 16 weeks have not been established; safety and efficacy in pediatric patients have not been established

Pregnancy Risk Factor B

Pregnancy Implications No adequate and well-controlled studies have been done in pregnant women. Use in pregnancy only if clearly needed. Pantoprazole and its metabolites are excreted in the milk of rats. It is unknown if pantoprazole is excreted in human milk. Do not use in women who are breast-feeding.

Adverse Reactions

1% to 10%:
Cardiovascular: Chest pain
Central nervous system: Pain, migraine, anxiety, dizziness
Endocrine & metabolic: Hyperglycemia (1%), hyperlipidemia
Gastrointestinal: Diarrhea (4%), constipation, dyspepsia, gastroenteritis, nausea, rectal disorder, vomiting
Genitourinary: Urinary frequency, urinary tract infection
Hepatic: Liver function test abnormality increased SGPT
Neuromuscular & skeletal: Weakness, back pain, neck pain, arthralgia, hypertonia
Respiratory: Bronchitis, increased cough, dyspnea, pharyngitis, rhinitis, sinusitis, upper respiratory tract infection
Miscellaneous: Flu syndrome, infection

<1%: Rash, allergic reaction, fever, generalized edema, neoplasm, angina pectoris, arrhythmia, congestive heart failure, ECG abnormality, hemorrhage, hypertension, hypotension, myocardial ischemia, palpitation, retinal vascular disorder, syncope, tachycardia, thrombosis, vasodilation, anorexia, aphthous stomatitis, colitis, dry mouth, duodenitis, dysphagia, gastrointestinal carcinoma, gastrointestinal hemorrhage, gastrointestinal moniliasis, gingivitis, glossitis, halitosis, increased appetite, mouth ulceration, oral moniliasis, rectal hemorrhage, stomach ulcer, stomatitis, tongue discoloration,

(Continued)

Pantoprazole *(Continued)*

diabetes mellitus, glycosuria, goiter,cholecystitis, cholelithiasis, cholestatic jaundice, hepatitis, increased alkaline phosphatase, increased transaminases, ecchymosis, eosinophilia, anemia, leukocytosis, leukopenia, thrombocytopenia, dehydration, gout, arthritis, bone pain, bursitis, leg cramps, neck rigidity, myalgia, tenosynovitis, confusion, convulsion, depression, dysarthria, hallucinations, hyperkinesia, decreased libido, nervousness, neuralgia, neuritis, paresthesia, decrease reflexes, somnolence, tremor, vertigo, asthma, epistaxis, laryngitis, pneumonia, voice alteration, acne, alopecia, contact dermatitis, dry skin, eczema, fungal dermatitis, herpes simplex, herpes zoster, lichenoid dermatitis, maculopapular rash, pain, pruritus, skin ulcer, sweating, urticaria, abnormal vision, amblyopia, cataract, deafness, diplopia, ear pain, extraocular palsy, glaucoma, otitis externa, taste perversion, tinnitus, albuminuria, balanitis, breast pain, cystitis, dysmenorrhea, dysuria, epididymitis, hematuria, impotence, kidney calculus, kidney pain, nocturia, pyelonephritis, scrotal edema, urethritis, impaired urination, vaginitis, anaphylaxis, angioedema, anterior ischemic optic neuropathy, erythema multiforme, Stevens-Johnson syndrome, toxic epidermal necrolysis, pancreatitis, hypokinesia, speech disorder, increased salivation, vertigo, increased creatinine, hypercholesterolemia, hyperuricemia

Drug Interactions CYP2C19 and 3A4 enzyme substrate

Drugs (eg, itraconazole, ketoconazole, and other azole antifungals, ampicillin esters, iron salts) where absorption is determined by an acidic gastric pH, may have decreased absorption when used concurrently. Monitor for change in effectiveness.

Alcohol Interactions Avoid use (may enhance gastric mucosal irritation)

Onset 2-5 hours

Half-Life 1 hour

Education and Monitoring Issues

Patient Education: Take as directed. Do not chew or crush tablet. May cause dizziness (avoid driving or engaging in tasks that require alertness until response to drug is known); nausea or vomiting (small frequent meals, good mouth care, chewing gum, or sucking lozenges may help); diarrhea (yogurt or boiled milk may offer relief). Report severe headache or anxiety; persistent GI effects; neck, back, or joint pain; unusual cough; or signs of upper respiratory infection.

Dietary Considerations: Take with or without food

Manufacturer Wyeth-Ayerst Laboratories

Related Information

Pharmaceutical Manufacturers Directory *on page 1020*

Papaverine (pa PAV er een)

Pharmacologic Class Vasodilator

U.S. Brand Names Genabid®; Pavabid®; Pavatine®

Generic Available Yes

Mechanism of Action Smooth muscle spasmolytic producing a generalized smooth muscle relaxation including: vasodilatation, gastrointestinal sphincter relaxation, bronchiolar muscle relaxation, and potentially a depressed myocardium (with large doses); muscle relaxation may occur due to inhibition or cyclic nucleotide phosphodiesterase, increasing cyclic AMP; muscle relaxation is unrelated to nerve innervation; papaverine increases cerebral blood flow in normal subjects; oxygen uptake is unaltered

Use Oral: Relief of peripheral and cerebral ischemia associated with arterial spasm and myocardial ischemia complicated by arrhythmias

Investigational: Parenteral: Various vascular spasms associated with muscle spasms as in myocardial infarction, angina, peripheral and pulmonary embolism, peripheral vascular disease, angiospastic states, and visceral spasm (ureteral, biliary, and GI colic); testing for impotence

USUAL DOSAGE Adults: Oral, sustained release: 150-300 mg every 12 hours; in difficult cases: 150 mg every 8 hours

Dosage Forms CAP, sustained release 150 mg

Contraindications Hypersensitivity to papaverine or its components

Warnings/Precautions Use with caution in patients with glaucoma; administer I.V. cautiously since apnea and arrhythmias may result; may, in large doses, depress A-V and intraventricular cardiac conduction leading to serious arrhythmias (eg, premature beats, paroxysmal tachycardia); chronic hepatitis noted with jaundice, eosinophilia, and abnormal LFTs

Pregnancy Risk Factor C

Adverse Reactions <1%: Abdominal distress, anorexia, chronic hepatitis, constipation, diarrhea, drowsiness, flushing of the face, headache, hepatic hypersensitivity, lethargy, mild hypertension, nausea, sedation, tachycardias, vertigo

Drug Interactions CYP2D6 enzyme substrate

Decreased effect: Papaverine decreases the effects of levodopa

Increased toxicity: Additive effects with CNS depressants

Onset Oral: Rapid

Half-Life 0.5-1.5 hours

Education and Monitoring Issues

Patient Education: Oral: Take as directed; do not alter dosage without consulting prescriber. Do not chew, crush, or dissolve extended release tablets. Avoid alcohol while taking this medication. May cause dizziness, confusion, or blurred vision (avoid driving or engaging in tasks that require alertness until response to drug is known). Increased fiber in diet, exercise, and adequate hydration (2-3 L/day of fluids unless instructed to restrict fluid intake) may help if you experience constipation. Report rapid heartbeat or palpitations, CNS depression, persistent sedation or lethargy, or acute headache.

- **Papulex** *see* Niacinamide *on page 648*
- **Paraflex®** *see* Chlorzoxazone *on page 192*
- **Parafon Forte™ DSC** *see* Chlorzoxazone *on page 192*
- **Par Decon®** *see* Chlorpheniramine, Phenyltoloxamine, Phenylpropanolamine, and Phenylephrine *on page 187*

Paregoric (par e GOR ik)

Pharmacologic Class Analgesic, Narcotic

Generic Available Yes

Mechanism of Action Increases smooth muscle tone in GI tract, decreases motility and peristalsis, diminishes digestive secretions

Use Treatment of diarrhea or relief of pain; neonatal opiate withdrawal

USUAL DOSAGE Oral:

Neonatal opiate withdrawal: Instill 3-6 drops every 3-6 hours as needed, or initially 0.2 mL every 3 hours; increase dosage by approximately 0.05 mL every 3 hours until withdrawal symptoms are controlled; it is rare to exceed 0.7 mL/dose. Stabilize withdrawal symptoms for 3-5 days, then gradually decrease dosage over a 2- to 4-week period.

Children: 0.25-0.5 mL/kg 1-4 times/day

Adults: 5-10 mL 1-4 times/day

Dosage Forms LIQ: 2 mg morphine equivalent/5 mL [equivalent to 20 mg opium powder] (5 mL, 60 mL, 473 mL, 4000 mL)

Contraindications Hypersensitivity to opium or any component; diarrhea caused by poisoning until the toxic material has been removed

Warnings/Precautions Use with caution in patients with respiratory, hepatic or renal dysfunction, severe prostatic hypertrophy, or history of narcotic abuse; opium shares the toxic potential of opiate agonists, and usual precautions of opiate agonist therapy should be observed; some preparations contain sulfites which may cause allergic reactions; infants <3 months of age are more susceptible to respiratory depression, use with caution and generally in reduced doses in this age group; tolerance or drug dependence may result from extended use

Pregnancy Risk Factor B; D (when used long-term or in high doses)

Adverse Reactions

>10%:

Cardiovascular: Hypotension

Central nervous system: Drowsiness, dizziness

Gastrointestinal: Constipation

Neuromuscular & skeletal: Weakness

1% to 10%:

Central nervous system: Restlessness, headache, malaise

Genitourinary: Ureteral spasms, decreased urination

Miscellaneous: Histamine release

<1%: Anorexia, biliary tract spasm, CNS depression, increased intracranial pressure, increased liver function tests, insomnia, mental depression, miosis, nausea, peripheral vasodilation, physical and psychological dependence, respiratory depression, stomach cramps, urinary tract spasm, vomiting

Drug Interactions Increased effect/toxicity with CNS depressants (eg, alcohol, narcotics, benzodiazepines, TCAs, MAO inhibitors, phenothiazine)

Alcohol Interactions Avoid use (may increase central nervous system depression)

Education and Monitoring Issues

Patient Education: Take exactly as directed; do not increase dosage. May cause dependence with prolonged or excessive use. Avoid alcohol and all other prescription and OTC that may cause sedation (sleeping medications, some cough/cold remedies, antihistamines, etc). You may experience drowsiness, dizziness, or impaired judgment (use caution when driving or engaging in tasks that require alertness until response to drug is known) or postural hypotension (use caution when rising from sitting or lying position or when climbing stairs). You may experience nausea or loss of appetite (frequent small meals may help) or constipation (a laxative may be necessary). Report unresolved nausea, vomiting, respiratory difficulty (shortness of breath or decreased respirations), chest pain, or palpitations.

- **Paremyd® Ophthalmic** *see* Hydroxyamphetamine and Tropicamide *on page 451*
- **Parepectolin®** *see* Kaolin and Pectin With Opium *on page 498*
- **Par Glycerol®** *see* Iodinated Glycerol *on page 480*

Paricalcitol (par eh CAL ci tol)

Pharmacologic Class Vitamin D Analog

U.S. Brand Names Zemplar™

Mechanism of Action Synthetic vitamin D analog which has been shown to reduce PTH serum concentrations

Use Prevention and treatment of secondary hyperparathyroidism associated with chronic renal failure. Has been evaluated only in hemodialysis patients.

USUAL DOSAGE Adults: I.V.: 0.04-0.1 mcg/kg (2.8-7 mcg) given as a bolus dose no more frequently than every other day at any time during dialysis; doses as high as 0.24 mcg/kg (16.8 mcg) have been administered safely; usually start with 0.04 mcg/kg 3 times/week by I.V. bolus, increased by 0.04 mcg/kg every 2 weeks; the dose of paricalcitol should be adjusted based on serum PTH levels

Serum PTH Levels

PTH Level	Paricalcitol Dose
Same or increasing	Increase
Decreased by <30%	Increase
Decreased by <30% and <60%	Maintain
Decreased by >60%	Decrease
1.5-3 times upper limit of normal	Maintain

Dosage Forms INJ: 5 mcg/mL (1 mL, 2 mL, 5 mL)

Contraindications Should not be given to patients with evidence of vitamin D toxicity, hypercalcemia, or hypersensitivity to any of the ingredients of this product

Warnings/Precautions The most frequently reported adverse reactions with paricalcitol include nausea, vomiting, and edema. Chronic administration can place patients at risk of hypercalcemia, elevated calcium-phosphorus product and metastatic calcification; it should not be used in patients with evidence of hypercalcemia or vitamin D toxicity.

Pregnancy Risk Factor C

Adverse Reactions The three most frequently reported events in clinical studies were nausea, vomiting, and edema, which are commonly seen in hemodialysis patients.

>10%: Gastrointestinal: Nausea (13%)

1% to 10%:

- Cardiovascular: Palpitations, peripheral edema (7%)
- Central nervous system: Chills, malaise, fever, lightheadedness (5%)
- Gastrointestinal: Vomiting (8%), GI bleeding (5%), xerostomia (3%)
- Respiratory: Pneumonia (5%)
- Miscellaneous: Flu-like symptoms, sepsis

Drug Interactions Phosphate or vitamin D-related compounds should not be taken concurrently; digitalis toxicity is potentiated by hypercalcemia

Education and Monitoring Issues

Patient Education: Take as directed; do not increase dosage without consulting prescriber. Adhere to diet as recommended (do not take any other phosphate or vitamin D related compounds while taking paricalcitol). You may experience nausea or vomiting (small frequent meals, frequent mouth care, chewing gum, or sucking lozenges may help); swelling of extremities (elevate feet when sitting); lightheadedness or dizziness (use caution when driving or engaging in tasks requiring alertness until response to drug is known). Report persistent fever, gastric disturbances, abdominal pain or blood in stool, chest pain or palpitations, or signs of respiratory infection or flu.

Monitoring Parameters: Serum calcium and phosphorus should be monitored closely (eg, twice weekly) during dose titration; monitor for signs and symptoms of vitamin D intoxication; serum PTH; in trials, a mean PTH level reduction of 30% was achieved within 6 weeks

Manufacturer Abbott Laboratories (Pharmaceutical Product Division)

Related Information

Pharmaceutical Manufacturers Directory *on page 1020*

♦ **Parkinson's Disease Dosing** *see page 1249*

♦ **Parkinson's Disease Management** *see page 1130*

♦ **Parlodel®** *see* Bromocriptine *on page 113*

♦ **Parnate®** *see* Tranylcypromine *on page 938*

Paromomycin (par oh moe MYE sin)

Pharmacologic Class Amebicide

U.S. Brand Names Humatin®

Generic Available No

Mechanism of Action Acts directly on ameba; has antibacterial activity against normal and pathogenic organisms in the GI tract; interferes with bacterial protein synthesis by binding to 30S ribosomal subunits

Use Treatment of acute and chronic intestinal amebiasis; preoperatively to suppress intestinal flora; tapeworm infestations; treatment of *Cryptosporidium*

USUAL DOSAGE Oral:

Intestinal amebiasis: Children and Adults: 25-35 mg/kg/day in 3 divided doses for 5-10 days

Dientamoeba fragilis: Children and Adults: 25-30 mg/kg/day in 3 divided doses for 7 days

Cryptosporidium: Adults with AIDS: 1.5-2.25 g/day in 3-6 divided doses for 10-14 days (occasionally courses of up to 4-8 weeks may be needed)

Tapeworm (fish, dog, bovine, porcine):

Children: 11 mg/kg every 15 minutes for 4 doses

Adults: 1 g every 15 minutes for 4 doses

Hepatic coma: Adults: 4 g/day in 2-4 divided doses for 5-6 days

Dwarf tapeworm: Children and Adults: 45 mg/kg/dose every day for 5-7 days

Dosage Forms CAP: 250 mg

Contraindications Intestinal obstruction, renal failure, known hypersensitivity to paromomycin or components

Warnings/Precautions Use with caution in patients with impaired renal function or possible or proven ulcerative bowel lesions

Pregnancy Risk Factor C

Adverse Reactions

1% to 10%: Gastrointestinal: Diarrhea, abdominal cramps, nausea, vomiting, heartburn

<1%: Eosinophilia, exanthema, headache, ototoxicity, pruritus, rash, secondary enterocolitis, steatorrhea, vertigo

Drug Interactions

Decreased effect of digoxin, vitamin A, and methotrexate

Increased effect of oral anticoagulants, neuromuscular blockers, and polypeptide antibiotics

Education and Monitoring Issues

Patient Education: Take full course of therapy; do not skip doses; notify prescriber if ringing in ears, hearing loss, or dizziness occurs

Paroxetine (pa ROKS e teen)

Pharmacologic Class Antidepressant, Selective Serotonin Reuptake Inhibitor

U.S. Brand Names Paxil™; Paxil® CR™

Mechanism of Action Paroxetine is a selective serotonin reuptake inhibitor, chemically unrelated to tricyclic, tetracyclic, or other antidepressants; presumably, the inhibition of serotonin reuptake from brain synapse stimulated serotonin activity in the brain

Use Treatment of depression; treatment of panic disorder and obsessive-compulsive disorder; social anxiety disorder

USUAL DOSAGE Adults: Oral:

Depression and social anxiety disorder: 20 mg once daily (maximum: 50 mg/day), preferably in the morning; in elderly, debilitated, or patients with hepatic or renal impairment, start with 10 mg/day (maximum: 40 mg/day); adjust doses at 7-day intervals

Paxil® CR™: Initial: 25 mg once daily; may be increased in 12.5 mg increments at intervals of at least 1 week (range: 26-62.5 mg)

Panic disorder and obsessive compulsive disorder: Recommended average daily dose: 40 mg, this dosage should be given after an adequate trial on 20 mg/day and then titrating upward

Social anxiety disorder: 20 mg/day

Dosage Forms SUSP, oral: 10 mg/5 mL. **TAB:** 10 mg, 20 mg, 30 mg, 40 mg; Controlled release (Paxil® CR™): 12.5 mg, 25 mg

Contraindications Do not use within 14 days of MAO inhibitors

Warnings/Precautions Use cautiously in patients with a history of seizures, mania, renal disease, cardiac disease, suicidal patients, children, or during breast-feeding in lactating women

Pregnancy Risk Factor C

Adverse Reactions

>10%:

Central nervous system: Headache, somnolence, dizziness, insomnia

Gastrointestinal: Nausea, xerostomia, constipation, diarrhea

Genitourinary: Ejaculatory disturbances

Neuromuscular & skeletal: Weakness

Miscellaneous: Diaphoresis

1% to 10%:

Cardiovascular: Palpitations, vasodilation, postural hypotension

Central nervous system: Nervousness, anxiety, yawning, abnormal dreams

Dermatologic: Rash

Endocrine & metabolic: Decreased libido, delayed ejaculation

Gastrointestinal: Anorexia, flatulence, vomiting, dyspepsia, taste perversion

Genitourinary: Urinary frequency, impotence

Neuromuscular & skeletal: Tremor, paresthesia, myopathy, myalgia

(Continued)

Paroxetine *(Continued)*

<1%: Acne, akinesia, alopecia, amenorrhea, anemia, arthritis, asthma, bradycardia, bruxism, colitis, ear pain, eye pain, EPS, hypotension, leukopenia, mania, migraine, thirst

Drug Interactions CYP2D6 enzyme substrate (minor); CYP2D6 and 1A2 enzyme inhibitor (high dose) (weak), and CYP3A3/4 enzyme inhibitor (weak)

Paroxetine inhibits the metabolism of tricyclic antidepressants (amitriptyline, desipramine, imipramine, nortriptyline) resulting is elevated serum levels. If combination is warranted, a low dose of TCA (10-25 mg/day) should be utilized.

Paroxetine may cause hyponatremia. Additive hyponatremic effects may be seen with combined use of a loop diuretic (bumetanide, furosemide, torsemide); monitor for hyponatremia

Paroxetine inhibits the reuptake of serotonin. Combined use with a serotonin agonist (buspirone) may cause serotonin syndrome

Paroxetine inhibits the metabolism of dextromethorphan; visual hallucinations occurred in a patient receiving this combination; monitor for serotonin syndrome

Paroxetine may inhibit the metabolism of haloperidol and cause extrapyramidal symptoms (EPS); monitor patients for EPS if combination is utilized

Paroxetine should not be used with nonselective MAOIs (isocarboxazid, phenelzine). Fatal reactions have been reported. Wait two weeks after stopping paroxetine before starting an MAOI and two weeks after stopping an MAOI before starting paroxetine.

Paroxetine inhibits the reuptake of serotonin; combined use with other drugs which inhibit the reuptake (nefazodone, sibutramine) may cause serotonin syndrome. Monitor patient for altered response with nefazodone; avoid sibutramine combination.

Paroxetine has been reported to cause mania or hypertension when combined with selegiline; this combination is best avoided

Paroxetine combined with tramadol (serotonergic effects) may cause serotonin syndrome; monitor

Paroxetine may alter the hypoprothombinemic response to warfarin; monitor

Cimetidine may reduce the first-pass metabolism of paroxetine resulting in elevated paroxetine serum concentrations; consider an alternative H_2 antagonist

Alcohol Interactions Avoid use. Although alcohol may not cause central nervous system depression here, depressed patients should avoid/limit intake.

Onset Steady-state: ~10 days; therapeutic effects: >2 weeks

Half-Life 21 hours

Education and Monitoring Issues

Patient Education: Take exactly as directed (do not increase dose or frequency); may take 2-3 weeks to achieve desired results; may cause physical and/or psychological dependence. Take in the morning to reduce the incidence of insomnia. Avoid excessive alcohol, caffeine, and other prescription or OTC medications not approved by prescriber. Maintain adequate hydration (2-3 L/day of fluids unless instructed to restrict fluid intake). You may experience drowsiness, dizziness, or lightheadedness (use caution when driving or engaging in tasks requiring alertness until response to drug is known); nausea, vomiting, anorexia, or dry mouth (small frequent meals, frequent mouth care, chewing gum, or sucking lozenges may help); or orthostatic hypotension (use caution when climbing stairs or changing position from lying or sitting to standing). Report persistent insomnia or excessive daytime sedation; muscle cramping, tremors, weakness, or change in gait; chest pain, palpitations, or rapid heartbeat; vision changes or eye pain; difficulty breathing or breathlessness; abdominal pain or blood in stool; or worsening of condition.

Manufacturer SmithKline Beecham Pharmaceuticals

Related Information

Antidepressant Agents Comparison *on page 1231*
Pharmaceutical Manufacturers Directory *on page 1020*

- **Parvolex** *see* Acetylcysteine *on page 20*
- **Patanol®** *see* Olopatadine *on page 674*
- **Pathocil®** *see* Dicloxacillin *on page 265*
- **Patient Education for Management of Common Side Effects** *see page 1002*
- **Pavabid®** *see* Papaverine *on page 702*
- **Pavatine®** *see* Papaverine *on page 702*
- **Paveral Stanley Syrup With Codeine Phosphate** *see* Codeine *on page 223*
- **Pavulon®** *see* Pancuronium *on page 699*
- **Paxil™** *see* Paroxetine *on page 705*
- **Paxil® CR™** *see* Paroxetine *on page 705*
- **Paxipam®** *see* Halazepam *on page 428*
- **PCE®** *see* Erythromycin *on page 323*
- **PediaCare® Oral** *see* Pseudoephedrine *on page 792*
- **Pediacof®** *see* Chlorpheniramine, Phenylephrine, and Codeine *on page 186*
- **Pediaflor®** *see* Fluoride *on page 376*
- **Pediapred® Oral** *see* Prednisolone *on page 762*

- **PediaProfen™** *see* Ibuprofen *on page 458*
- **Pediatric Triban®** *see* Trimethobenzamide *on page 953*
- **Pediatrix** *see* Acetaminophen *on page 17*
- **Pediazole®** *see* Erythromycin and Sulfisoxazole *on page 325*
- **Pedi-Cort V® Creme** *see* Clioquinol and Hydrocortisone *on page 209*
- **PediOtic® Otic** *see* Neomycin, Polymyxin B, and Hydrocortisone *on page 644*
- **Pedituss®** *see* Chlorpheniramine, Phenylephrine, and Codeine *on page 186*
- **PedvaxHIB™** *see Haemophilus* b Conjugate Vaccine *on page 427*

Pegademase Bovine (peg A de mase BOE vine)

Pharmacologic Class Enzyme

U.S. Brand Names Adagen™

Generic Available No

Mechanism of Action Adenosine deaminase is an enzyme that catalyzes the deamination of both adenosine and deoxyadenosine. Hereditary lack of adenosine deaminase activity results in severe combined immunodeficiency disease, a fatal disorder of infancy characterized by profound defects of both cellular and humoral immunity. It is estimated that 25% of patients with the autosomal recessive form of severe combined immunodeficiency lack adenosine deaminase.

Use Enzyme replacement therapy for adenosine deaminase (ADA) deficiency in patients with severe combined immunodeficiency disease (SCID) who can not benefit from bone marrow transplant; not a cure for SCID, unlike bone marrow transplants, injections must be used the rest of the child's life, therefore is not really an alternative

USUAL DOSAGE Children: I.M.: Dose given every 7 days, 10 units/kg the first dose, 15 units/kg the second dose, and 20 units/kg the third dose; maintenance dose: 20 units/kg/week is recommended depending on patient's ADA level; maximum single dose: 30 units/kg

Dosage Forms INJ: 250 units/mL (1.5 mL)

Contraindications Hypersensitivity to pegademase bovine; not to be used as preparatory or support therapy for bone marrow transplantation

Warnings/Precautions Use with caution in patients with thrombocytopenia

Pregnancy Risk Factor C

Adverse Reactions <1%: Headache, pain at injection site

Drug Interactions Decreased effect: Vidarabine

Half-Life 48-72 hours

Education and Monitoring Issues

Patient Education: Not a cure for SCID; unlike bone marrow transplants, injections must be used the rest of the child's life; frequent blood tests are necessary to monitor effect and adjust the dose as needed

- **Peglyte®** *see* Polyethylene Glycol-Electrolyte Solution *on page 747*

Pemirolast (pe MIR oh last)

Pharmacologic Class Mast Cell Stabilizer; Ophthalmic Agent, Miscellaneous

U.S. Brand Names Alamast™

Mechanism of Action Mast cell stabilizer that inhibits the *in vivo* type I immediate hypersensitivity reaction; in addition, inhibits chemotaxis of eosinophils into the ocular tissue and blocks their release of mediators; also reported to prevent calcium influx into mast cells following antigen stimulation

Use Prevent itching of the eye due to allergic conjunctivitis

USUAL DOSAGE Children >3 years and Adults: 1-2 drops instilled in affected eye(s) 4 times/day

Dosage Forms SOLN, ophth: 0.1% (10 mL)

Contraindications Hypersensitivity to pemirolast or any component

Warnings/Precautions Safety and efficacy in children <3 years of age have not been established; not for injection or oral use; ophthalmic use only; not indicated to treat contact lens irritation; do not wear contact lens if eye is red. In nonred eyes, soft contact lenses should not be applied for 10 minutes after the instillation of pemirolast potassium to avoid absorption of lauralkonium chloride (a preservative in Alamast™).

Pregnancy Risk Factor C

Pregnancy Implications There are no adequate and well-controlled studies in pregnant women. Should only be used during pregnancy if the benefit outweighs the risk to the fetus. It is not known if pemirolast potassium is excreted in human milk; caution should be used if administered to a breast-feeding woman.

Adverse Reactions

>10%:

Central nervous system: Headache (10% to 25%)

Respiratory: Rhinitis (10% to 25%)

Miscellaneous: Cold/flu symptoms (10% to 25%)

<5%:

Central nervous system: Fever

Endocrine & metabolic: Dysmenorrhea

(Continued)

Pemirolast *(Continued)*

Ocular: Burning eyes, dry eyes, foreign body sensation, ocular discomfort
Neuromuscular & skeletal: Back pain
Respiratory: Bronchitis, cough, sinusitis, sneezing/nasal congestion

Drug Interactions None reported

Onset Within a few days; Peak effect: 4 weeks

Half-Life 4-5 hours

Education and Monitoring Issues

Patient Education: Decreased itching may occur within a few days; however, longer treatment (up to 4 weeks) is frequently required. Do not use to treat contact lens irritation; do not wear contact lenses if eyes are red. Soft contact lens wearers using pemirolast in nonred eyes should wait at least 10 minutes after application before inserting contact lenses to avoid absorption of the preservative, lauralkonium chloride. In order to prevent contamination, do not allow the dropper tip to touch the eyelid or surrounding areas. When not in use, keep bottle tightly closed.

Dietary Considerations: None reported

Pemoline (PEM oh leen)

Pharmacologic Class Stimulant

U.S. Brand Names Cylert®

Use Treatment of attention deficit/hyperactivity disorder (ADHD); narcolepsy

USUAL DOSAGE Children ≥6 years: Oral: Initial: 37.5 mg given once daily in the morning, increase by 18.75 mg/day at weekly intervals; usual effective dose range: 56.25-75 mg/day; maximum: 112.5 mg/day; dosage range: 0.5-3 mg/kg/24 hours; significant benefit may not be evident until third or fourth week of administration

Dosing adjustment/comments in renal impairment: Cl_{cr} <50 mL/minute: Avoid use

Contraindications Liver disease; hypersensitivity to pemoline or any component; children <6 years of age; Tourette's syndrome, psychoses

Pregnancy Risk Factor B

Penciclovir (pen SYE kloe veer)

Pharmacologic Class Antiviral Agent

U.S. Brand Names Denavir™

Use Topical treatment of herpes simplex labialis (cold sores); potentially used for Epstein-Barr virus infections

USUAL DOSAGE Apply cream at the first sign or symptom of cold sore (eg, tingling, swelling); apply every 2 hours during waking hours for 4 days

Contraindications Previous and significant adverse reactions to famciclovir; hypersensitivity to the product or any of its components

Pregnancy Risk Factor B

- **Pending Drugs or Drugs in Clinical Trials** *see page 1006*
- **Penecort®** *see* Hydrocortisone *on page 447*
- **Penetrex™** *see* Enoxacin *on page 312*
- **Penglobe** *see* Bacampicillin *on page 89*

Penicillamine (pen i SIL a meen)

Pharmacologic Class Chelating Agent

U.S. Brand Names Cuprimine®; Depen®

Generic Available No

Mechanism of Action Chelates with lead, copper, mercury and other heavy metals to form stable, soluble complexes that are excreted in urine; depresses circulating IgM rheumatoid factor, depresses T-cell but not B-cell activity; combines with cystine to form a compound which is more soluble, thus cystine calculi are prevented

Use Treatment of Wilson's disease, cystinuria, adjunct in the treatment of rheumatoid arthritis; lead, mercury, copper, and possibly gold poisoning. (**Note:** Oral DMSA is preferable for lead or mercury poisoning); primary biliary cirrhosis; as adjunctive therapy following initial treatment with calcium EDTA or BAL

USUAL DOSAGE Oral:

Rheumatoid arthritis:

Children: Initial: 3 mg/kg/day (≤250 mg/day) for 3 months, then 6 mg/kg/day (≤500 mg/day) in divided doses twice daily for 3 months to a maximum of 10 mg/kg/day in 3-4 divided doses

Adults: 125-250 mg/day, may increase dose at 1- to 3-month intervals up to 1-1.5 g/day

Wilson's disease (doses titrated to maintain urinary copper excretion >1 mg/day):

Infants <6 months: 250 mg/dose once daily

Children <12 years: 250 mg/dose 2-3 times/day

Adults: 250 mg 4 times/day

Cystinuria:

Children: 30 mg/kg/day in 4 divided doses

Adults: 1-4 g/day in divided doses every 6 hours

Lead poisoning (continue until blood lead level is <60 μg/dL): Children and Adults: 25-35 mg/kg/d, administered in 3-4 divided doses; initiating treatment at 25% of this dose and gradually increasing to the full dose over 2-3 weeks may minimize adverse reactions

Primary biliary cirrhosis: 250 mg/day to start, increase by 250 mg every 2 weeks up to a maintenance dose of 1 g/day, usually given 250 mg 4 times/day

Arsenic poisoning: Children: 100 mg/kg/day in divided doses every 6 hours for 5 days; maximum: 1 g/day

Dosing adjustment/comments in renal impairment: Cl_{cr} <50 mL/minute: Avoid use

Dosage Forms CAP: 125 mg, 250 mg. **TAB:** 250 mg

Contraindications Hypersensitivity to penicillamine or components; renal insufficiency; patients with previous penicillamine-related aplastic anemia or agranulocytosis; concomitant administration with other hematopoietic-depressant drugs (eg, gold, immunosuppressants, antimalarials, phenylbutazone)

Warnings/Precautions Cross-sensitivity with penicillin is possible; therefore, should be used cautiously in patients with a history of penicillin allergy. Patients on penicillamine for Wilson's disease or cystinuria should receive pyridoxine supplementation 25 mg/day; once instituted for Wilson's disease or cystinuria, continue treatment on a daily basis; interruptions of even a few days have been followed by hypersensitivity with reinstitution of therapy. Penicillamine has been associated with fatalities due to agranulocytosis, aplastic anemia, thrombocytopenia, Goodpasture's syndrome, and myasthenia gravis; patients should be warned to report promptly any symptoms suggesting toxicity; approximately 33% of patients will experience an allergic reaction; since toxicity may be dose related, it is recommended not to exceed 750 mg/day in elderly.

Pregnancy Risk Factor D

Adverse Reactions

>10%:

- Dermatologic: Rash, urticaria, itching (44% to 50%)
- Gastrointestinal: Hypogeusia (25% to 33%)
- Neuromuscular & skeletal: Arthralgia

1% to 10%:

- Cardiovascular: Edema of the face, feet, or lower legs
- Central nervous system: Fever, chills
- Gastrointestinal: Weight gain, sore throat
- Genitourinary: Bloody or cloudy urine
- Hematologic: Aplastic or hemolytic anemia, leukopenia (2%), thrombocytopenia (4%)
- Miscellaneous: White spots on lips or mouth, positive ANA

<1%: Allergic reactions, anorexia, cholestatic jaundice, coughing, fatigue, hepatitis, increased friability of the skin, iron deficiency, lymphadenopathy, myasthenia gravis syndrome, nausea, nephrotic syndrome, optic neuritis, pancreatitis, pemphigus, SLE-like syndrome, spitting of blood, tinnitus, toxic epidermal necrolysis, vomiting, weakness, wheezing

Drug Interactions

Decreased effect with iron and zinc salts, antacids (magnesium, calcium, aluminum) and food

Decreased effect/levels of digoxin

Increased effect of gold, antimalarials, immunosuppressants, phenylbutazone (hematologic, renal toxicity)

Half-Life 1.7-3.2 hours

Education and Monitoring Issues

Patient Education: Take this medication exactly as directed; do not increase dose without consulting prescriber. Capsules may be opened and contents mixed in 15-30 mL of chilled fruit juice or puree; do not take with milk or milk products. Avoid alcohol or excess intake of vitamin A. It is preferable to take penicillamine on an empty stomach (1 hour before or 2 hours after meals). Maintain adequate hydration (2-3 L/day of fluids unless instructed to restrict fluid intake).

Wilson's disease: Avoid chocolate, shellfish, nuts, mushrooms, liver, broccoli, molasses.

Lead poisoning: Decrease dietary calcium.

Cystinuria: Take with large amounts of water.

You may experience anorexia, nausea, vomiting (frequent small meals, frequent mouth care, sucking lozenges, or chewing gum may help). Report persistent fever or chills, unhealed sores, white spots or sores in mouth or vaginal area, extreme fatigue, or signs of infection; breathlessness, difficulty breathing, or unusual cough; unusual bruising/bleeding; blood in urine, stool, mouth, or vomitus; swollen face or extremities; skin rash or itching; muscle pain or cramping; or pain on urination.

Monitoring Parameters: Urinalysis, CBC with differential, platelet count, liver function tests; weekly measurements of urinary and blood concentration of the intoxicating metal is indicated (3 months has been tolerated)

CBC: WBC <3500/mm^3, neutrophils <2000/mm^3 or monocytes >500/mm^3 indicate need to stop therapy immediately; quantitative 24-hour urine protein at 1- to 2-week intervals initially (first 2-3 months); urinalysis, LFTs occasionally; platelet counts <100,000/mm^3 indicate need to stop therapy until numbers of platelets increase

Penicillin G Benzathine and Procaine Combined

(pen i SIL in jee BENZ a theen & PROE kane KOM bined)

Pharmacologic Class Penicillin

U.S. Brand Names Bicillin® C-R; Bicillin® C-R 900/300

Generic Available No

Mechanism of Action Inhibits bacterial cell wall synthesis by binding to one or more of the penicillin binding proteins (PBPs); which in turn inhibits the final transpeptidation step of peptidoglycan synthesis in bacterial cell walls, thus inhibiting cell wall biosynthesis. Bacteria eventually lyse due to ongoing activity of cell wall autolytic enzymes (autolysins and murein hydrolases) while cell wall assembly is arrested.

Use May be used in specific situations in the treatment of streptococcal infections

USUAL DOSAGE I.M.:

Children:

<30 lb: 600,000 units in a single dose

30-60 lb: 900,000 units to 1.2 million units in a single dose

Children >60 lb and Adults: 2.4 million units in a single dose

Dosage Forms INJ: 300,000 units [150,000 units each of penicillin g benzathine and penicillin g procaine] (10 mL); 600,000 units [300,000 units each penicillin g benzathine and penicillin g procaine] (1 mL); 1,200,000 units [600,000 units each penicillin g benzathine and penicillin g procaine] (2 mL); 2,400,000 units [1,200,000 units each penicillin g benzathine and penicillin g procaine] (4 mL). **INJ:** Penicillin g benzathine 900,000 units and penicillin g procaine 300,000 units per dose (2 mL)

Contraindications Known hypersensitivity to penicillin or any component

Warnings/Precautions Use with caution in patients with impaired renal function, impaired cardiac function or seizure disorder

Pregnancy Risk Factor B

Drug Interactions Probenecid, tetracyclines, methotrexate, aminoglycosides

Education and Monitoring Issues

Monitoring Parameters: Observe for signs and symptoms for anaphylaxis during first dose

Penicillin G Benzathine, Parenteral

(pen i SIL in jee BENZ a theen, pa REN ter al)

Pharmacologic Class Antibiotic, Penicillin

U.S. Brand Names Bicillin® L-A; Permapen®

Generic Available No

Mechanism of Action Interferes with bacterial cell wall synthesis during active multiplication, causing cell wall death and resultant bactericidal activity against susceptible bacteria

Use Active against some gram-positive organisms, few gram-negative organisms such as *Neisseria gonorrhoeae*, and some anaerobes and spirochetes; used in the treatment of syphilis; used only for the treatment of mild to moderately severe infections caused by organisms susceptible to low concentrations of penicillin G or for prophylaxis of infections caused by these organisms

USUAL DOSAGE I.M.: Administer undiluted injection; higher doses result in more sustained rather than higher levels. Use a penicillin G benzathine-penicillin G procaine combination to achieve early peak levels in acute infections.

Infants and Children:

Group A streptococcal upper respiratory infection: 25,000-50,000 units/kg as a single dose; maximum: 1.2 million units

Prophylaxis of recurrent rheumatic fever: 25,000-50,000 units/kg every 3-4 weeks; maximum: 1.2 million units/dose

Early syphilis: 50,000 units/kg as a single injection; maximum: 2.4 million units

Syphilis of more than 1-year duration: 50,000 units/kg every week for 3 doses; maximum: 2.4 million units/dose

Adults:

Group A streptococcal upper respiratory infection: 1.2 million units as a single dose

Prophylaxis of recurrent rheumatic fever: 1.2 million units every 3-4 weeks or 600,000 units twice monthly

Early syphilis: 2.4 million units as a single dose in 2 injection sites

Syphilis of more than 1-year duration: 2.4 million units in 2 injection sites once weekly for 3 doses

Not indicated as single drug therapy for neurosyphilis, but may be given 1 time/week for 3 weeks following I.V. treatment (refer to Penicillin G monograph for dosing)

Dosage Forms INJ: 300,000 units/mL (10 mL); 600,000 units/mL (1 mL, 2 mL, 4 mL)

Contraindications Known hypersensitivity to penicillin or any component

Warnings/Precautions Use with caution in patients with impaired renal function, seizure disorder, or history of hypersensitivity to other beta-lactams; CDC and AAP do not currently recommend the use of penicillin G benzathine to treat congenital syphilis or neurosyphilis due to reported treatment failures and lack of published clinical data on its efficacy

Pregnancy Risk Factor B

Adverse Reactions

1% to 10%: Local: Pain

<1%: Acute interstitial nephritis, anaphylaxis, confusion, convulsions, drowsiness, electrolyte imbalance, fever, hemolytic anemia, hypersensitivity reactions, Jarisch-Herxheimer reaction, myoclonus, positive Coombs' reaction, rash, thrombophlebitis

Drug Interactions

Decreased effect: Tetracyclines may decrease penicillin effectiveness; decreased oral contraceptive effect is possible

Increased effect:

Probenecid may increase penicillin levels

Aminoglycosides → synergistic efficacy; heparin and parenteral penicillins may result in increased bleeding

Education and Monitoring Issues

Patient Education: Take as directed, for full course of therapy. Maintain adequate hydration (2-3 L/day of fluids unless instructed to restrict fluid intake). If begin treated for sexually transmitted disease, partner will also need to be treated. Small frequent meals, frequent mouth care, sucking lozenges, or chewing gum may reduce nausea or dry mouth. Important to maintain good oral and vaginal hygiene to reduce incidence of opportunistic infection. If diabetic, drug may cause false tests with Clinitest® urine glucose monitoring; use of glucose oxidase methods (Clinistix®) or serum glucose monitoring is preferable. This drug may interfere with oral contraceptives; an alternate form of birth control should be used. Report persistent diarrhea, fever, chills, unhealed sores, bloody urine or stool, muscle pain, mouth sores, or difficulty breathing.

Monitoring Parameters: Observe for signs and symptoms of anaphylaxis during first dose

Related Information

Treatment of Sexually Transmitted Diseases *on page 1210*

Penicillin G, Parenteral, Aqueous

(pen i SIL in jee, pa REN ter al, AYE kwee us)

Pharmacologic Class Antibiotic, Penicillin

U.S. Brand Names Pfizerpen®

Generic Available No

Mechanism of Action Interferes with bacterial cell wall synthesis during active multiplication, causing cell wall death and resultant bactericidal activity against susceptible bacteria

Use Active against some gram-positive organisms, generally not *Staphylococcus aureus*; some gram-negative organisms such as *Neisseria gonorrhoeae*, and some anaerobes and spirochetes

USUAL DOSAGE I.M., I.V.:

Infants:

>7 days, >2000 g: 100,000 units/kg/day in divided doses every 6 hours

>7 days, <2000 g: 75,000 units/kg/day in divided doses every 8 hours

<7 days, >2000 g: 50,000 units/kg/day in divided doses every 8 hours

<7 days, <2000 g: 50,000 units/kg/day in divided doses every 12 hours

Infants and Children (sodium salt is preferred in children): 100,000-250,000 units/kg/day in divided doses every 4 hours

Severe infections: Up to 400,000 units/kg/day in divided doses every 4 hours; maximum dose: 24 million units/day

Adults: 2-24 million units/day in divided doses every 4 hours depending on sensitivity of the organism and severity of the infection

Congenital syphilis:

Newborns: 50,000 units/kg/day I.V. every 8-12 hours for 10-14 days

Infants: 50,000 units/kg every 4-6 hours for 10-14 days

Disseminated gonococcal infections or gonococcus ophthalmia (if organism proven sensitive): 100,000 units/kg/day in 2 equal doses (4 equal doses/day for infants >1 week)

Gonococcal meningitis: 150,000 units/kg in 2 equal doses (4 doses/day for infants >1 week)

Dosing interval in renal impairment:

Cl_{cr} 30-50 mL/minute: Administer every 6 hours

Cl_{cr} 10-30 mL/minute: Administer every 8 hours

Cl_{cr} <10 mL/minute: Administer every 12 hours

Hemodialysis: Moderately dialyzable (20% to 50%)

Continuous arteriovenous or venovenous hemodiafiltration (CAVH) effects: Dose as for Cl_{cr} 10-50 mL/minute

Dosage Forms INJ: As sodium: 5 million units; Frozen premixed, as potassium: 1 million units, 2 million units, 3 million units. **POWDER,** as potassium: 1 million units, 5 million units, 10 million units, 20 million units

Contraindications Known hypersensitivity to penicillin or any component

Warnings/Precautions Avoid intra-arterial administration or injection into or near major peripheral nerves or blood vessels since such injections may cause severe and/or permanent neurovascular damage; use with caution in patients with renal impairment (dosage reduction required), pre-existing seizure disorders, or with a history of hypersensitivity to cephalosporins

(Continued)

Penicillin G, Parenteral, Aqueous *(Continued)*

Pregnancy Risk Factor B

Adverse Reactions <1%: Acute interstitial nephritis, anaphylaxis confusion, convulsions, drowsiness, electrolyte imbalance, fever, hemolytic anemia, hypersensitivity reactions, Jarisch-Herxheimer reaction, myoclonus, positive Coombs' reaction, rash, thrombophlebitis

Drug Interactions

Decreased effect: Tetracyclines may decrease penicillin effectiveness; decreased oral contraceptive effect is possible

Increased effect:

Probenecid may increase penicillin levels

Aminoglycosides may result in synergistic efficacy; heparin and parenteral penicillins may result in increased bleeding

Half-Life Normal renal function: 20-50 minutes; End-stage renal disease: 3.3-5.1 hours

Education and Monitoring Issues

Patient Education: This medication will be administered I.V. or I.M. Maintain adequate hydration (2-3 L/day of fluids unless instructed to restrict fluid intake). If being treated for sexually transmitted disease, partner will also need to be treated. Small frequent meals, frequent mouth care, sucking lozenges, or chewing gum may reduce nausea or dry mouth. Important to maintain good oral and vaginal hygiene to reduce incidence of opportunistic infection. If diabetic, drug may cause false tests with Clinitest® urine glucose monitoring; use of glucose oxidase methods (Clinistix®) or serum glucose monitoring is preferable. This drug may interfere with oral contraceptives; an alternate form of birth control should be used. Report persistent diarrhea, fever, chills, unhealed sores, bloody urine or stool, muscle pain, mouth sores, or difficulty breathing.

Monitoring Parameters: Observe for signs and symptoms of anaphylaxis during first dose

Related Information

Antibiotic Treatment of Adults With Infective Endocarditis *on page 1179*
Antimicrobial Drugs of Choice *on page 1182*
Treatment of Sexually Transmitted Diseases *on page 1210*

Penicillin G Procaine (pen i SIL in jee PROE kane)

Pharmacologic Class Antibiotic, Penicillin

U.S. Brand Names Crysticillin® A.S.; Wycillin®

Generic Available Yes

Mechanism of Action Inhibits bacterial cell wall synthesis by binding to one or more of the penicillin binding proteins (PBPs); which in turn inhibits the final transpeptidation step of peptidoglycan synthesis in bacterial cell walls, thus inhibiting cell wall biosynthesis. Bacteria eventually lyse due to ongoing activity of cell wall autolytic enzymes (autolysins and murein hydrolases) while cell wall assembly is arrested.

Use Moderately severe infections due to *Treponema pallidum* and other penicillin G-sensitive microorganisms that are susceptible to low but prolonged serum penicillin concentrations

USUAL DOSAGE I.M.:

Children: 25,000-50,000 units/kg/day in divided doses 1-2 times/day; not to exceed 4.8 million units/24 hours

Congenital syphilis: 50,000 units/kg/day for 10-14 days

Adults: 0.6-4.8 million units/day in divided doses every 12-24 hours

Endocarditis caused by susceptible viridans *Streptococcus* (when used in conjunction with an aminoglycoside): 1.2 million units every 6 hours for 2-4 weeks

Neurosyphilis: I.M.: 2-4 million units/day with 500 mg probenecid by mouth 4 times/day for 10-14 days; **penicillin G aqueous I.V. is the preferred agent**

Hemodialysis: Moderately dialyzable (20% to 50%)

Dosage Forms INJ, suspension: 300,000 units/mL (10 mL); 500,000 units/mL (1.2 mL); 600,000 units/mL (1 mL, 2 mL, 4 mL)

Contraindications Known hypersensitivity to penicillin or any component; also contraindicated in patients hypersensitive to procaine

Warnings/Precautions May need to modify dosage in patients with severe renal impairment, seizure disorders, or history of hypersensitivity to cephalosporins; avoid I.V., intravascular, or intra-arterial administration of penicillin G procaine since severe and/or permanent neurovascular damage may occur

Pregnancy Risk Factor B

Adverse Reactions

>10%: Local: Pain at injection site

<1%: CNS stimulation, conduction disturbances, confusion, drowsiness, hemolytic anemia, hypersensitivity reactions, interstitial nephritis, Jarisch-Herxheimer reaction, myocardial depression, myoclonus, positive Coombs' reaction, pseudoanaphylactic reactions, seizures, sterile abscess at injection site, vasodilation

Drug Interactions

Decreased effect: Tetracyclines may decrease penicillin effectiveness; decreased oral contraceptive effect is possible

Increased effect:

Probenecid may increase penicillin levels

Aminoglycosides may result in synergistic efficacy; heparin and parenteral penicillins may result in increased bleeding

Education and Monitoring Issues

Patient Education: Take as directed, for full course of therapy. Maintain adequate hydration (2-3 L/day of fluids unless instructed to restrict fluid intake). If being treated for sexually transmitted disease, partner will also need to be treated. Small frequent meals, frequent mouth care, sucking lozenges, or chewing gum may reduce nausea or dry mouth. Important to maintain good oral and vaginal hygiene to reduce incidence of opportunistic infection. If diabetic, drug may cause false tests with Clinitest® urine glucose monitoring; use of glucose oxidase methods (Clinistix®) or serum glucose monitoring is preferable. This drug may interfere with oral contraceptives; an alternate form of birth control should be used. Report persistent diarrhea, fever, chills, unhealed sores, bloody urine or stool, muscle pain, mouth sores, or difficulty breathing.

Monitoring Parameters: Periodic renal and hematologic function tests with prolonged therapy; fever, mental status, WBC count

Related Information

Treatment of Sexually Transmitted Diseases *on page 1210*

Penicillin V Potassium (pen i SIL in vee poe TASS ee um)

Pharmacologic Class Antibiotic, Penicillin

U.S. Brand Names Beepen-VK®; Betapen®-VK; Pen.Vee® K; Robicillin® VK; V-Cillin K®; Veetids®

Generic Available Yes

Mechanism of Action Inhibits bacterial cell wall synthesis by binding to one or more of the penicillin binding proteins (PBPs); which in turn inhibits the final transpeptidation step of peptidoglycan synthesis in bacterial cell walls, thus inhibiting cell wall biosynthesis. Bacteria eventually lyse due to ongoing activity of cell wall autolytic enzymes (autolysins and murein hydrolases) while cell wall assembly is arrested.

Use Treatment of infections caused by susceptible organisms involving the respiratory tract, otitis media, sinusitis, skin, and urinary tract; prophylaxis in rheumatic fever

USUAL DOSAGE Oral:

Systemic infections:

Children <12 years: 25-50 mg/kg/day in divided doses every 6-8 hours; maximum dose: 3 g/day

Children ≥12 years and Adults: 125-500 mg every 6-8 hours

Prophylaxis of pneumococcal infections:

Children <5 years: 125 mg twice daily

Children ≥5 years and Adults: 250 mg twice daily

Prophylaxis of recurrent rheumatic fever:

Children <5 years: 125 mg twice daily

Children ≥5 years and Adults: 250 mg twice daily

Dosing interval in renal impairment: Cl_{cr} <10 mL/minute: Administer 250 mg every 6 hours

Dosage Forms 250 mg = 400,000 units **POWDER for oral soln:** 125 mg/5 mL (3 mL, 100 mL, 150 mL, 200 mL); 250 mg/5 mL (100 mL, 150 mL, 200 mL). **TAB:** 125 mg, 250 mg, 500 mg

Contraindications Known hypersensitivity to penicillin or any component

Warnings/Precautions Use with caution in patients with severe renal impairment (modify dosage), history of seizures, or hypersensitivity to cephalosporins

Pregnancy Risk Factor B

Adverse Reactions

>10%: Gastrointestinal: Mild diarrhea, vomiting, nausea, oral candidiasis

<1%: Acute interstitial nephritis, anaphylaxis, convulsions, fever, hemolytic anemia, hypersensitivity reactions, positive Coombs' reaction

Drug Interactions

Decreased effect: Tetracyclines may decrease penicillin effectiveness; decreased oral contraceptive effect is possible

Increased effect:

Probenecid may increase penicillin levels

Aminoglycosides may result in synergistic efficacy; heparin and parenteral penicillins may result in increased bleeding

Half-Life 0.5 hours; prolonged in patients with renal impairment

Education and Monitoring Issues

Patient Education: Take at regular intervals around-the-clock, preferably on an empty stomach (1 hour before or 2 hours after meals) with 8 oz of water. Take entire prescription; do not skip doses or discontinue without consulting prescriber. Small frequent meals, frequent mouth care, sucking lozenges, or chewing gum may reduce nausea or dry mouth. Important to maintain good oral and vaginal hygiene to reduce incidence of opportunistic infection. If diabetic, drug may cause false tests with Clinitest® urine glucose monitoring; use of glucose oxidase methods (Clinistix®) or serum glucose monitoring is preferable. This drug may interfere with oral contraceptives; an alternate

(Continued)

Penicillin V Potassium *(Continued)*

form of birth control should be used. Report persistent diarrhea, fever, chills, unhealed sores, bloody urine or stool, muscle pain, mouth sores, and difficulty breathing.

Dietary Considerations: Food: Decreases drug absorption rate; decreases drug serum concentration. Take on an empty stomach 1 hour before or 2 hours after meals.

Monitoring Parameters: Periodic renal and hematologic function tests during prolonged therapy; monitor for signs of anaphylaxis during first dose

Related Information

Animal and Human Bites Guidelines *on page 1177*
Antimicrobial Drugs of Choice *on page 1182*

♦ **Penlac™** *see* Ciclopirox *on page 197*
♦ **Pentacarinat® Injection** *see* Pentamidine *on page 714*
♦ **Pentam-300® Injection** *see* Pentamidine *on page 714*

Pentamidine (pen TAM i deen)

Pharmacologic Class Antibiotic, Miscellaneous

U.S. Brand Names NebuPent™ Inhalation; Pentacarinat® Injection; Pentam-300® Injection

Generic Available No

Mechanism of Action Interferes with RNA/DNA, phospholipids and protein synthesis, through inhibition of oxidative phosphorylation and/or interference with incorporation of nucleotides and nucleic acids into RNA and DNA, in protozoa

Use Treatment and prevention of pneumonia caused by *Pneumocystis carinii*; treatment of trypanosomiasis and visceral leishmaniasis

USUAL DOSAGE

Children:

Treatment: I.M., I.V. (I.V. preferred): 4 mg/kg/day once daily for 10-14 days

Prevention:

I.M., I.V.: 4 mg/kg monthly or every 2 weeks

Inhalation (aerosolized pentamidine in children ≥5 years): 300 mg/dose given every 3-4 weeks via Respirgard® II inhaler (8 mg/kg dose has also been used in children <5 years)

Treatment of trypanosomiasis: I.V.: 4 mg/kg/day once daily for 10 days

Adults:

Treatment: I.M., I.V. (I.V. preferred): 4 mg/kg/day once daily for 14-21 days

Prevention: Inhalation: 300 mg every 4 weeks via Respirgard® II nebulizer

Dialysis: Not removed by hemo or peritoneal dialysis or continuous arteriovenous or venovenous hemofiltration (CAVH/CAVHD); supplemental dosage is not necessary

Dosing adjustment in renal impairment: Adults: I.V.:

Cl_{cr} 10-50 mL/minute: Administer 4 mg/kg every 24-36 hours

Cl_{cr} <10 mL/minute: Administer 4 mg/kg every 48 hours

Dosage Forms INH: 300 mg. **POWDER for inj, lyophilized:** 300 mg

Contraindications Hypersensitivity to pentamidine isethionate or any component (inhalation and injection)

Warnings/Precautions Use with caution in patients with diabetes mellitus, renal or hepatic dysfunction; hypertension or hypotension; leukopenia, thrombocytopenia, asthma, hypo/hyperglycemia

Pregnancy Risk Factor C

Adverse Reactions Injection (I); Aerosol (A)

>10%:

Cardiovascular: Chest pain (A - 10% to 23%)

Central nervous system: Fatigue (A - 50% to 70%); dizziness (A - 31% to 47%)

Dermatologic: Rash (31% to 47%)

Endocrine & metabolic: Hyperkalemia

Gastrointestinal: Anorexia (A - 50% to 70%), nausea (A - 10% to 23%)

Local: Local reactions at injection site

Renal: Increased creatinine (I - 23%)

Respiratory: Wheezing (A - 10% to 23%), dyspnea (A - 50% to 70%), coughing (A - 31% to 47%), pharyngitis (10% to 23%)

1% to 10%:

Cardiovascular: Hypotension (I - 4%)

Central nervous system: Confusion/hallucinations (1% to 2%), headache (A - 1% to 5%)

Dermatologic: Rash (I - 3.3%)

Endocrine & metabolic: Hypoglycemia <25 mg/dL (I - 2.4%)

Gastrointestinal: Nausea/anorexia (I - 6%), diarrhea (A - 1% to 5%), vomiting

Hematologic: Severe leukopenia (I - 2.8%), thrombocytopenia <20,000/mm^3 (I - 1.7%), anemia (A - 1% to 5%)

Hepatic: Increased LFTs (I - 8.7%)

<1%: Arrhythmias, dizziness (I), extrapulmonary pneumocystosis, fatigue (I), fever, granulocytopenia, hyperglycemia or hypoglycemia, hypocalcemia, hypotension <60 mm Hg systolic (I - 0.9%), irritation of the airway, Jarisch-Herxheimer-like reaction, leukopenia,

megaloblastic anemia, mild renal or hepatic injury, pancreatitis, pneumothorax, renal insufficiency, tachycardia

Drug Interactions CYP2C19 enzyme substrate

Half-Life 6.4-9.4 hours; may be prolonged in patients with severe renal impairment

Education and Monitoring Issues

Patient Education: I.V. or I.M. preparations must be given every day. For inhalant use as directed. Prepare solution and nebulizer as directed. Protect medication from light. You will be required to have frequent laboratory tests and blood pressure monitoring while taking this drug. PCP pneumonia may still occur despite pentamidine use. Maintain adequate hydration (2-3 L/day of fluids unless instructed to restrict fluid intake). Frequent mouth care or sucking on lozenges may relieve the metallic taste. Diabetics should check glucose levels frequently. You may experience dizziness or weakness with posture changes; rise or change position slowly. Report unusual confusion or hallucinations, chest pain, unusual bleeding, or rash.

Monitoring Parameters: Liver function tests, renal function tests, blood glucose, serum potassium and calcium, EKG, blood pressure

- **Pentamycetin®** *see* Chloramphenicol *on page 178*
- **Pentasa® Oral** *see* Mesalamine *on page 568*

Pentazocine (pen TAZ oh seen)

Pharmacologic Class Analgesic, Narcotic

U.S. Brand Names Talwin®; Talwin® NX

Use Relief of moderate to severe pain; has also been used as a sedative prior to surgery and as a supplement to surgical anesthesia

USUAL DOSAGE

Children: I.M., S.C.:

5-8 years: 15 mg

8-14 years: 30 mg

Children >12 years and Adults: Oral: 50 mg every 3-4 hours; may increase to 100 mg/dose if needed, but should not exceed 600 mg/day

Adults:

I.M., S.C.: 30-60 mg every 3-4 hours, not to exceed total daily dose of 360 mg

I.V.: 30 mg every 3-4 hours

Dosing adjustment in renal impairment:

Cl_{cr} 10-50 mL/minute: Administer 75% of normal dose

Cl_{cr} <10 mL/minute: Administer 50% of normal dose

Dosing adjustment in hepatic impairment: Reduce dose or avoid use in patients with liver disease

Contraindications Hypersensitivity to pentazocine or any component, increased intracranial pressure (unless the patient is mechanically ventilated)

Pregnancy Risk Factor B; D (if used for prolonged periods or in high doses at term)

Related Information

Lipid-Lowering Agents Comparison *on page 1243*

Narcotic Agonists Comparison *on page 1244*

Pentoxifylline (pen toks I fi leen)

Pharmacologic Class Blood Viscosity Reducer Agent

U.S. Brand Names Trental®

Generic Available No

Mechanism of Action Mechanism of action remains unclear; is thought to reduce blood viscosity and improve blood flow by altering the rheology of red blood cells

Use Symptomatic management of peripheral vascular disease, mainly intermittent claudication

Unapproved use: AIDS patients with increased TNF, CVA, cerebrovascular diseases, diabetic atherosclerosis, diabetic neuropathy, gangrene, hemodialysis shunt thrombosis, vascular impotence, cerebral malaria, septic shock, sickle cell syndromes, and vasculitis

USUAL DOSAGE Adults: Oral: 400 mg 3 times/day with meals; may reduce to 400 mg twice daily if GI or CNS side effects occur

Dosage Forms TAB, controlled release: 400 mg

Contraindications Hypersensitivity to pentoxifylline or any component and other xanthine derivatives; patients with recent cerebral and/or retinal hemorrhage

Warnings/Precautions Use with caution in patients with renal impairment

Pregnancy Risk Factor C

Adverse Reactions

1% to 10%:

Central nervous system: Dizziness, headache

Gastrointestinal: Dyspepsia, nausea, vomiting

<1%: Angina, agitation, blurred vision, earache mild hypotension

Drug Interactions

Increased effect/toxic potential with cimetidine (increased levels) and other H_2-antagonists, warfarin; increased effect of antihypertensives

(Continued)

Pentoxifylline *(Continued)*

Increased toxicity with theophylline

Half-Life Parent drug: 24-48 minutes; Metabolites: 60-96 minutes

Education and Monitoring Issues

Patient Education: Take as prescribed for full length of prescription. This may relieve pain of claudication, but additional therapy may be recommended. You may experience dizziness (use caution when driving); GI upset (small frequent meals may help). Report chest pain, persistent headache, nausea or vomiting.

♦ **Pen.Vee® K** *see* Penicillin V Potassium *on page 713*
♦ **Pepcid®** *see* Famotidine *on page 350*
♦ **Pepcid® AC Acid Controller [OTC]** *see* Famotidine *on page 350*
♦ **Pepcid RPD™** *see* Famotidine *on page 350*

Peppermint

Pharmacologic Class Herb

Mechanism of Action Peppermint oil has an antispasmodic action on the ileum. Peppermint oil may block calcium exciting stimuli, with the antispasmodic properties being characteristic of calcium channel blockers. Reports suggest that enteric-coated peppermint oil is effective in relieving symptoms of IBS.

Use

Carminative, spasmolytic (Schulz, 1996)
Irritable bowel syndrome (Liu, 1997)

USUAL DOSAGE Oral:

One tablet (enteric coated), 2-3 times/day, containing 0.2 mL oil per tablet

Note: The oil should contain:

- ≥4.5% w/v and ≤10% w/w of esters calculated as menthyl acetate
- ≥44% w/v of free alcohols calculated as menthol
- ≥15% w/v and ≤32% w/v ketones calculated as menthone

Infants and Children ≤6 years of age: Infuse 1 teaspoonful of dried leaf per cup of boiling water; cool before using; give 1-2 teaspoonfuls 1-3 times/day

Contraindications Due to pharmacological activity, do not use in individuals presenting with biliary tract obstruction, cholecystitis, gallstones, hiatal hernia, or severe liver damage (Pittler, 1998). Calcium channel blocking activity has been observed in animal models (Beesley, 1996); use with caution in individuals receiving other calcium channel blockers.

Warnings/Precautions Use all herbal supplements with extreme caution in children <2 years of age and in pregnancy or lactation. Some herbs are contraindicated in pregnancy or lactation; make sure to observe warnings. Use with caution in individuals on medication and with pre-existing medical conditions. Always review for potential herb-drug interactions (HDIs) and other warnings. Large and prolonged doses may increase the potential for adverse effects. Herbs may cause transient adverse effects such as nausea, vomiting, and GI distress due to a variety of chemical constituents. Caution should be used in individuals having known allergies to plants.

Drug Interactions Calcium channel blocking agents

♦ **Pepto-Bismol® [OTC]** *see* Bismuth *on page 108*
♦ **Pepto® Diarrhea Control [OTC]** *see* Loperamide *on page 538*
♦ **Peptol®** *see* Cimetidine *on page 198*
♦ **Percocet® 2.5/325** *see* Oxycodone and Acetaminophen *on page 692*
♦ **Percocet® 5/325** *see* Oxycodone and Acetaminophen *on page 692*
♦ **Percocet® 7.5/500** *see* Oxycodone and Acetaminophen *on page 692*
♦ **Percocet® 10/650** *see* Oxycodone and Acetaminophen *on page 692*
♦ **Percocet®-Demi** *see* Oxycodone and Acetaminophen *on page 692*
♦ **Percodan®** *see* Oxycodone and Aspirin *on page 692*
♦ **Percodan®-Demi** *see* Oxycodone and Aspirin *on page 692*
♦ **Percolone®** *see* Oxycodone *on page 691*
♦ **Perdiem® Plain [OTC]** *see* Psyllium *on page 793*

Pergolide (PER go lide)

Pharmacologic Class Anti-Parkinson's Agent (Dopamine Agonist); Ergot Derivative

U.S. Brand Names Permax®

Generic Available No

Mechanism of Action Pergolide is a semisynthetic ergot alkaloid similar to bromocriptine but stated to be more potent and longer-acting; it is a centrally-active dopamine agonist stimulating both D_1 and D_2 receptors

Use Adjunctive treatment to levodopa/carbidopa in the management of Parkinson's Disease

USUAL DOSAGE When adding pergolide to levodopa/carbidopa, the dose of the latter can usually and should be decreased. Patients no longer responsive to bromocriptine may benefit by being switched to pergolide.

Adults: Oral: Start with 0.05 mg/day for 2 days, then increase dosage by 0.1 or 0.15 mg/day every 3 days over next 12 days, increase dose by 0.25 mg/day every 3 days until optimal therapeutic dose is achieved, up to 5 mg/day maximum; usual dosage range: 2-3 mg/day in 3 divided doses

Dosage Forms TAB: 0.05 mg, 0.25 mg, 1 mg

Contraindications Known hypersensitivity to pergolide mesylate or other ergot derivatives

Warnings/Precautions Symptomatic hypotension occurs in 10% of patients; use with caution in patients with a history of cardiac arrhythmias, hallucinations, or mental illness

Pregnancy Risk Factor B

Adverse Reactions

>10%:

Central nervous system: Dizziness, somnolence, confusion, hallucinations, dystonia
Gastrointestinal: Nausea, constipation
Neuromuscular & skeletal: Dyskinesia
Respiratory: Rhinitis

1% to 10%:

Cardiovascular: Myocardial infarction, postural hypotension, syncope, arrhythmias, peripheral edema, vasodilation, palpitations, chest pain, hypertension
Central nervous system: Chills, insomnia, anxiety, psychosis, EPS, incoordination
Dermatologic: Rash
Gastrointestinal: Diarrhea, abdominal pain, xerostomia, anorexia, weight gain, dyspepsia, taste perversion
Hematologic: Anemia
Neuromuscular & skeletal: Weakness, myalgia, tremor, NMS (with rapid dose reduction), pain
Ocular: Abnormal vision, diplopia
Respiratory: Dyspnea, epistaxis
Miscellaneous: Flu syndrome, hiccups

Drug Interactions

Use caution with other highly plasma protein bound drugs

Dopamine antagonists (ie, antipsychotics, metoclopramide) may diminish the effects of pergolide; these combinations should generally be avoided

Half-Life 27 hours

Education and Monitoring Issues

Patient Education: Take exactly as directed (may be prescribed in conjunction with levodopa/carbidopa); do not change dosage or discontinue without consulting prescriber. Therapeutic effects may take several weeks or months to achieve and you may need frequent monitoring during first weeks of therapy. Take with meals if GI upset occurs, before meals if dry mouth occurs, after eating if drooling or if nausea occurs. Take at the same time each day. Maintain adequate hydration (2-3 L/day of fluids unless instructed to restrict fluid intake); void before taking medication. Do not use alcohol and prescription or OTC sedatives or CNS depressants without consulting prescriber. You may experience drowsiness, dizziness, confusion, or vision changes (use caution when driving, climbing stairs, or engaging in tasks requiring alertness until response to drug is known); orthostatic hypotension (use caution when changing position - rising to standing from sitting or lying); constipation (increased exercise, fluids, or dietary fruit and fiber may help); runny nose or flu-like symptoms (consult prescriber for appropriate relief); nausea, vomiting, loss of appetite, or stomach discomfort (small frequent meals, frequent mouth care, chewing gum, or sucking lozenges may help); photosensitivity (use sunscreen, wear protective clothing and eyewear, avoid direct sunlight). Report unresolved constipation or vomiting; chest pain, palpitations, irregular heartbeat; ringing in ears; CNS changes (hallucination, loss of memory, seizures, acute headache, nervousness, etc); painful or difficult urination; increased muscle spasticity, rigidity, or involuntary movements; skin rash; or significant worsening of condition.

Monitoring Parameters: Blood pressure (both sitting/supine and standing), symptoms of parkinsonism, dyskinesias, mental status

Related Information

Parkinson's Disease Dosing *on page 1249*

- **Pergonal®** *see* Menotropins *on page 562*
- **Periactin®** *see* Cyproheptadine *on page 240*
- **Peridex® Oral Rinse** *see* Chlorhexidine Gluconate *on page 181*
- **Peridol** *see* Haloperidol *on page 430*

Perindopril Erbumine (per IN doe pril er BYOO meen)

Pharmacologic Class Angiotensin-Converting Enzyme (ACE) Inhibitors

U.S. Brand Names Aceon®

Mechanism of Action Competitive inhibitor of angiotensin-converting enzyme (ACE); prevents conversion of angiotensin I to angiotensin II, a potent vasoconstrictor; results in lower levels of angiotensin II which, in turn, causes an increase in plasma renin activity and a reduction in aldosterone secretion

Use Treatment of stage I or II hypertension and congestive heart failure treatment of left ventricular dysfunction after myocardial infarction

USUAL DOSAGE Adults: Oral:

Congestive heart failure: 4 mg once daily

(Continued)

Perindopril Erbumine *(Continued)*

Hypertension: Initial: 4 mg/day but may be titrated to response; usual range: 4-8 mg/day, maximum: 16 mg/day

Dosing adjustment in renal impairment:

Cl_{cr} >60 mL/minute: Administer 4 mg/day

Cl_{cr} 30-60 mL/minute: Administer 2 mg/day

Cl_{cr} 15-29 mL/minute: Administer 2 mg every other day

Cl_{cr} <15 mL/minute: Administer 2 mg on the day of dialysis

Hemodialysis: Perindopril and its metabolites are dialyzable

Dosing adjustment in hepatic impairment: None needed

Dosing adjustment in elderly patients: Due to greater bioavailability and lower renal clearance of the drug in elderly subjects, dose reduction of 50% is recommended

Dosage Forms TAB: 2 mg, 4 mg, 8 mg

Contraindications Hypersensitivity to perindopril or any component; angioedema related to previous treatment with an ACE inhibitor; bilateral renal artery stenosis; primary hyperaldosteronism; pregnancy (2nd and 3rd trimesters)

Warnings/Precautions Anaphylactic reactions can occur. Angioedema can occur at any time during treatment (especially following first dose). Careful blood pressure monitoring with first dose (hypotension can occur especially in volume depleted patients). Dosage adjustment needed in renal impairment. Use with caution in hypovolemia; collagen vascular diseases; valvular stenosis (particularly aortic stenosis); hyperkalemia; or before, during, or immediately after anesthesia. Avoid rapid dosage escalation, which may lead to renal insufficiency. Neutropenia/agranulocytosis with myeloid hyperplasia can rarely occur. If patient has renal impairment then a baseline WBC with differential and serum creatinine should be evaluated and monitored closely during the first 3 months of therapy. Hypersensitivity reactions may be seen during hemodialysis with high-flux dialysis membranes (eg, AN69). Use with caution in unilateral renal artery stenosis and pre-existing renal insufficiency.

Pregnancy Risk Factor C (1st trimester); D (2nd and 3rd trimesters)

Pregnancy Implications When used in pregnancy during the 2nd and 3rd trimesters, ACE inhibitors can cause injury and even death to the developing fetus. Perindopril erbumine should be discontinued as soon as possible when pregnancy is detected. Small amounts enter breast milk, any effect this has on the infant is unknown.

Adverse Reactions

>10% Central nervous system: Headache (23%)

1% to 10%:

Cardiovascular: Edema (3.9%), chest pain (2.4%)

Central nervous system: Dizziness (8.2%), sleep disorders (2.5%), depression (2%), fever (1.5%), weakness (7.9%), nervousness (1%)

Dermatologic: Rash (2.3%)

Endocrine and metabolic: Hyperkalemia (1.4%), increased triglycerides (1.3%)

Gastrointestinal: Nausea (2.3%), diarrhea (4.3%), vomiting (1.5%), dyspepsia (1.9%), abdominal pain (2.7%), flatulence (1%)

Genitourinary: Sexual dysfunction (male: 1.4%)

Hepatic: Increased ALT (1.7%)

Neuromuscular & skeletal: Back pain (5.8%), upper extremity pain (2.8%), lower extremity pain (4.7%), paresthesia (2.3%), joint pain (1.1%), myalgia (1.1%), arthritis (1%)

Renal: Proteinuria (1.5%)

Respiratory: Cough (incidence is higher in women, 3:1) (12%), sinusitis (5.2%), rhinitis (4.8%), pharyngitis (3.3%)

Otic: Tinnitus (1.5%)

Miscellaneous: Viral infection (3.4%)

Note: Some reactions occurred at an incidence >1% but ≤ placebo:

<1% (limited to important or life-threatening symptoms): Angioedema (0.1%), anaphylaxis, facial edema, malaise, pain, chills, orthostatic hypotension, constipation, xerostomia, increased appetite, gastroenteritis, bronchitis, rhinorrhea, dyspnea, sneezing, epistaxis, pulmonary fibrosis (<0.1%), vaginitis, nephrolithiasis, urinary frequency, urinary retention, flank pain, hypotension, ventricular extrasystole, myocardial infarction, vasodilation, syncope, conduction abnormalities, gout, hematoma, bruising, arthralgia, migraine, amnesia, vertigo, cerebrovascular accident (0.2%), anxiety, psychosocial disorder, sweating, pruritus, dry skin, erythema, purpura (0.1%), conjunctivitis, earache, hypokalemia, decreased uric acid, increased alkaline phosphatase, increased serum creatinine, increased AST, hematuria, and hyperglycemia.

Additional adverse effects associated with with ACE inhibitors include agranulocytosis (especially in patients with renal impairment or collagen vascular disease), neutropenia, decreases in creatinine clearance in some elderly hypertensive patients or those with chronic renal failure, and worsening of renal function in patients with bilateral renal artery stenosis or hypovolemic patients (diuretic therapy). In addition, a syndrome which may include fever, myalgia, arthralgia, interstitial nephritis, vasculitis, rash, eosinophilia and positive ANA, and elevated ESR has been reported with ACE inhibitors.

Drug Interactions

$Alpha_1$ blockers: Hypotensive effect increased.

Aspirin and NSAIDs may decrease ACE inhibitor efficacy and/or increase risk of renal effects.

Diuretics: Hypovolemia due to diuretics may precipitate acute hypotensive events or acute renal failure.

Insulin: Risk of hypoglycemia may be increased.

Lithium: Risk of lithium toxicity may be increased; monitor lithium levels, especially the first 4 weeks of therapy.

Mercaptopurine: Risk of neutropenia may be increased.

Potassium-sparing diuretics (amiloride, spironolactone, triamterene): Increased risk of hyperkalemia.

Potassium supplements may increase the risk of hyperkalemia.

Trimethoprim (high dose) may increase the risk of hyperkalemia.

Alcohol Interactions Avoid use (may increase risk of hypotension and dizziness)

Onset Peak concentrations: 1-2 hours

Half-Life Parent drug: 1.5-3 hours; Metabolite: 25-30 hours

Education and Monitoring Issues

Patient Education: This medication does not replace the need to follow exercise and diet recommendations for hypertension. Take as directed; do not miss doses, alter dosage, or discontinue without consulting prescriber. Consult prescriber for appropriate diet. Change position slowly when rising from sitting or lying. May cause transient drowsiness; avoid driving or engaging in tasks that require alertness until response to drug is known. Small frequent meals may help reduce any nausea, vomiting, or epigastric pain. You may experience persistent cough; contact prescriber. Report unusual weight gain or swelling of ankles and hands; persistent fatigue; dry cough; difficulty breathing; palpitations; or swelling of face, eyes, or lips.

Dietary Considerations: Perindopril active metabolite concentrations may be lowered if taken with food

Monitoring Parameters: Serum creatinine, electrolytes, and WBC with differential initially and repeated at 2-week intervals for at least 90 days; urinalysis for protein

Manufacturer Solvay Pharmaceuticals

Related Information

Angiotensin-Related Agents Comparison *on page 1226*
Pharmaceutical Manufacturers Directory *on page 1020*

♦ **PerioChip®** *see* Chlorhexidine Gluconate *on page 181*
♦ **PerioGard®** *see* Chlorhexidine Gluconate *on page 181*
♦ **Periostat®** *see* Doxycycline *on page 300*
♦ **Permapen®** *see* Penicillin G Benzathine, Parenteral *on page 710*
♦ **Permax®** *see* Pergolide *on page 716*

Permethrin (per METH rin)

Pharmacologic Class Antiparasitic Agent, Topical; Scabicidal Agent

U.S. Brand Names Acticin® Cream; Elimite™ Cream; Nix™ Creme Rinse

Use Single application treatment of infestation with *Pediculus humanus capitis* (head louse) and its nits or *Sarcoptes scabiei* (scabies); indicated for prophylactic use during epidemics of lice

USUAL DOSAGE Topical: Children >2 months and Adults:

Head lice: After hair has been washed with shampoo, rinsed with water, and towel dried, apply a sufficient volume of topical liquid to saturate the hair and scalp. Leave on hair for 10 minutes before rinsing off with water; remove remaining nits; may repeat in 1 week if lice or nits still present.

Scabies: Apply cream from head to toe; leave on for 8-14 hours before washing off with water; for infants, also apply on the hairline, neck, scalp, temple, and forehead; may reapply in 1 week if live mites appear

Permethrin 5% cream was shown to be safe and effective when applied to an infant <1 month of age with neonatal scabies; time of application was limited to 6 hours before rinsing with soap and water

Contraindications Known hypersensitivity to pyrethyroid, pyrethrin, or chrysanthemums

Pregnancy Risk Factor B

♦ **Permitil® Oral** *see* Fluphenazine *on page 381*

Perphenazine (per FEN a zeen)

Pharmacologic Class Antipsychotic Agent, Phenothazine, Piperazine

U.S. Brand Names Trilafon®

Generic Available Yes

Mechanism of Action Blocks postsynaptic mesolimbic dopaminergic receptors in the brain; exhibits a strong alpha-adrenergic blocking effect and depresses the release of hypothalamic and hypophyseal hormones

Use Management of manifestations of psychotic disorders, depressive neurosis, alcohol withdrawal, nausea and vomiting, nonpsychotic symptoms associated with dementia in elderly, Tourette's syndrome, Huntington's chorea, spasmodic torticollis and Reye's syndrome

(Continued)

Perphenazine *(Continued)*

USUAL DOSAGE

Children:

Psychoses: Oral:

1-6 years: 4-6 mg/day in divided doses

6-12 years: 6 mg/day in divided doses

>12 years: 4-16 mg 2-4 times/day

I.M.: 5 mg every 6 hours

Nausea/vomiting: I.M.: 5 mg every 6 hours

Adults:

Psychoses:

Oral: 4-16 mg 2-4 times/day not to exceed 64 mg/day

I.M.: 5 mg every 6 hours up to 15 mg/day in ambulatory patients and 30 mg/day in hospitalized patients

Nausea/vomiting:

Oral: 8-16 mg/day in divided doses up to 24 mg/day

I.M.: 5-10 mg every 6 hours as necessary up to 15 mg/day in ambulatory patients and 30 mg/day in hospitalized patients

I.V. (severe): 1 mg at 1- to 2-minute intervals up to a total of 5 mg

Hemodialysis: Not dialyzable (0% to 5%)

Dosing adjustment in hepatic impairment: Dosage reductions should be considered in patients with liver disease although no specific guidelines are available

Dosage Forms CONC, oral: 16 mg/5 mL (118 mL). **INJ:** 5 mg/mL (1 mL). **TAB:** 2 mg, 4 mg, 8 mg, 16 mg

Contraindications Hypersensitivity to perphenazine or any component, cross-sensitivity with other phenothiazines may exist; avoid use in patients with narrow-angle glaucoma, bone marrow suppression, severe liver or cardiac disease; subcortical brain damage; circulatory collapse; severe hypotension or hypertension

Warnings/Precautions Safety in children <6 months of age has not been established; use with caution in patients with cardiovascular disease or seizures, bone marrow suppression, severe liver or cardiac disease

Pregnancy Risk Factor C

Adverse Reactions

Cardiovascular: Hypotension, orthostatic hypotension, hypertension, tachycardia, bradycardia, dizziness, cardiac arrest

Central nervous system: Extrapyramidal signs (pseudoparkinsonism, akathisia, dystonias, tardive dyskinesia), dizziness, cerebral edema, seizures, headache, drowsiness, paradoxical excitement, restlessness, hyperactivity, insomnia, neuroleptic malignant syndrome (NMS), impairment of temperature regulation

Dermatologic: Increased sensitivity to sun, rash, discoloration of skin (blue-gray)

Endocrine & metabolic: Hypoglycemia, hyperglycemia, galactorrhea, lactation, breast enlargement, gynecomastia, menstrual irregularity, amenorrhea, SIADH, changes in libido

Gastrointestinal: Constipation, weight gain, vomiting, stomach pain, nausea, xerostomia, salivation, diarrhea, anorexia, ileus

Genitourinary: Difficulty in urination, ejaculatory disturbances, incontinence, polyuria, ejaculating dysfunction, priapism

Hematologic: Agranulocytosis, leukopenia, eosinophilia, hemolytic anemia, thrombocytopenic purpura, pancytopenia

Hepatic: Cholestatic jaundice, hepatotoxicity

Neuromuscular & skeletal: Tremor

Ocular: Pigmentary retinopathy, blurred vision, cornea and lens changes

Respiratory: Nasal congestion

Miscellaneous: Diaphoresis

Drug Interactions CYP2D6 enzyme substrate; CYP2D6 enzyme inhibitor

Phenothiazines inhibit the ability of bromocriptine to lower serum prolactin concentrations

Benztropine (and other anticholinergics) may inhibit the therapeutic response to perphenazine and excess anticholinergic effects may occur

Chloroquine may increase perphenazine concentrations

Cigarette smoking may enhance the hepatic metabolism of perphenazine. Larger doses may be required compared to a nonsmoker.

Concurrent use of perphenazine with an antihypertensive may produce additive hypotensive effects

Concurrent use with TCA may produce increased toxicity or altered therapeutic response

Perphenazine may inhibit the antiparkinsonian effect of levodopa; avoid this combination

Perphenazine plus lithium may rarely produce neurotoxicity

Barbiturates may reduce perphenazine concentrations

Propranolol may increase perphenazine concentrations

Sulfadoxine-pyrimethamine may increase perphenazine concentrations

Perphenazine and possibly other low potency antipsychotics may reverse the pressor effects of epinephrine

Perphenazine and CNS depressants (ethanol, narcotics) may produce additive CNS depressant effects

Perphenazine and trazodone may produce additive hypotensive effects

Alcohol Interactions Avoid use (may increase central nervous system depression)

Half-Life 9 hours

Education and Monitoring Issues

Patient Education: Use exactly as directed (do not increase dose or frequency); may cause physical and/or psychological dependence. It may take 2-3 weeks to achieve desired results; do not discontinue without consulting prescriber. Dilute oral concentration with milk, water, or citrus; do not dilute with liquids containing coffee, tea, or apple juice. Do not take within 2 hours of any antacid. Avoid excess alcohol or caffeine and other prescription or OTC medications not approved by prescriber. Maintain adequate hydration (2-3 L/day of fluids unless instructed to restrict fluid intake). Avoid skin contact with medication; may cause contact dermatitis (wash immediately with warm, soapy water). You may experience excess drowsiness, restlessness, dizziness, or blurred vision (use caution driving or when engaging in tasks requiring alertness until response to drug is known); dry mouth, nausea, vomiting (small frequent meals, frequent mouth care, chewing gum, or sucking lozenges may help); constipation (increased exercise, fluids, or dietary fruit and fiber may help); postural hypotension (use caution climbing stairs or when changing position from lying or sitting to standing); urinary retention (void before taking medication); or photosensitivity (use sunscreen, wear protective clothing and eyewear, avoid direct sunlight); or decreased perspiration (avoid strenuous exercise in hot environments). Report persistent CNS effects (eg, trembling fingers, altered gait or balance, excessive sedation, seizures, unusual movements, anxiety, abnormal thoughts, confusion, personality changes); chest pain, palpitations, rapid heartbeat, severe dizziness; unresolved urinary retention or changes in urinary pattern; menstrual pattern, change in libido, or ejaculatory difficulty; vision changes; skin rash or yellowing of skin; difficulty breathing; or worsening of condition.

Reference Range: 2-6 nmol/L

Related Information

Amitriptyline and Perphenazine *on page 52*

- **Persantine®** *see* Dipyridamole *on page 285*
- **Pfizerpen®** *see* Penicillin G, Parenteral, Aqueous *on page 711*
- **Phanatuss® Cough Syrup [OTC]** *see* Guaifenesin and Dextromethorphan *on page 424*
- **Pharmacal** *see* Calcium Carbonate *on page 130*
- **Pharmaceutical Manufacturers Directory** *see page 1020*
- **Pharmaflur®** *see* Fluoride *on page 376*
- **Pharmalose** *see* Lactulose *on page 506*
- **Pharmitussin DM** *see* Guaifenesin and Dextromethorphan *on page 424*
- **Phenadex® Senior [OTC]** *see* Guaifenesin and Dextromethorphan *on page 424*
- **Phenahist-TR®** *see* Chlorpheniramine, Phenylephrine, Phenylpropanolamine, and Belladonna Alkaloids *on page 187*
- **Phenameth® DM** *see* Promethazine and Dextromethorphan *on page 780*
- **Phenaphen® With Codeine** *see* Acetaminophen and Codeine *on page 18*
- **Phenazine®** *see* Promethazine *on page 779*
- **Phenazo** *see* Phenazopyridine *on page 721*
- **Phenazodine®** *see* Phenazopyridine *on page 721*

Phenazopyridine (fen az oh PEER i deen)

Pharmacologic Class Analgesic, Urinary

U.S. Brand Names Azo-Standard® [OTC]; Baridium® [OTC]; Geridium®; Phenazodine®; Prodium™ [OTC]; Pyridiate®; Pyridium®; Urodine®; Urogesic®

Generic Available Yes

Mechanism of Action An azo dye which exerts local anesthetic or analgesic action on urinary tract mucosa through an unknown mechanism

Use Symptomatic relief of urinary burning, itching, frequency and urgency in association with urinary tract infection or following urologic procedures

USUAL DOSAGE Oral:

Children: 12 mg/kg/day in 3 divided doses administered after meals for 2 days

Adults: 100-200 mg 3 times/day after meals for 2 days when used concomitantly with an antibacterial agent

Dosing interval in renal impairment:

Cl_{cr} 50-80 mL/minute: Administer every 8-16 hours

Cl_{cr} <50 mL/minute: Avoid use

Dosage Forms TAB: (Azo-Standard®, Prodium™): 95 mg; (Baridium®, Geridium®, Pyridiate®, Pyridium®, Urodine®, Urogesic®): 100 mg; (Geridium®, Phenazodine®, Pyridium®, Urodine®): 200 mg

Contraindications Hypersensitivity to phenazopyridine or any component; kidney or liver disease

Warnings/Precautions Does not treat infection, acts only as an analgesic; drug should be discontinued if skin or sclera develop a yellow color; use with caution in patients with renal

(Continued)

Phenazopyridine *(Continued)*

impairment. Use of this agent in the elderly is limited since accumulation of phenazopyridine can occur in patients with renal insufficiency. It should not be used in patients with a Cl_{cr} <50 mL/minute.

Pregnancy Risk Factor B

Adverse Reactions

1% to 10%:

Central nervous system: Headache, dizziness

Gastrointestinal: Stomach cramps

<1%: Acute renal failure, hemolytic anemia, hepatitis, methemoglobinemia, rash, skin pigmentation, vertigo

Education and Monitoring Issues

Patient Education: Take prescribed dose after meals. May discolor urine (orange/yellow) or feces (orange/red); this is normal but will stain fabric. Report persistent headache, dizziness, or stomach cramping.

Related Information

Sulfamethoxazole and Phenazopyridine *on page 879*

Sulfisoxazole and Phenazopyridine *on page 882*

♦ **Phenchlor® S.H.A.** *see* Chlorpheniramine, Phenylephrine, Phenylpropanolamine, and Belladonna Alkaloids *on page 187*

♦ **Phendry® Oral [OTC]** *see* Diphenhydramine *on page 282*

Phenelzine (FEN el zeen)

Pharmacologic Class Antidepressant, Monoamine Oxidase Inhibitor

U.S. Brand Names Nardil®

Generic Available No

Mechanism of Action Thought to act by increasing endogenous concentrations of epinephrine, norepinephrine, dopamine and serotonin through inhibition of the enzyme (monoamine oxidase) responsible for the breakdown of these neurotransmitters

Use Symptomatic treatment of atypical, nonendogenous or neurotic depression. The MAO inhibitors are usually reserved for patients who do not tolerate or respond to the traditional "cyclic" or "second generation" antidepressants. The brain activity of monoamine oxidase increases with age and even more so in patients with Alzheimer's disease. Therefore, the MAO inhibitors may have an increased role in patients with Alzheimer's disease who are depressed. Phenelzine is less stimulating than tranylcypromine.

USUAL DOSAGE Oral:

Adults: 15 mg 3 times/day; may increase to 60-90 mg/day during early phase of treatment, then reduce to dose for maintenance therapy slowly after maximum benefit is obtained; takes 2-4 weeks for a significant response to occur

Elderly: Initial: 7.5 mg/day; increase by 7.5-15 mg/day every 3-4 days as tolerated; usual therapeutic dose: 15-60 mg/day in 3-4 divided doses

Dosage Forms TAB: 15 mg

Contraindications Pheochromocytoma, hepatic or renal disease, cerebrovascular defect, cardiovascular disease, hypersensitivity to phenelzine or any component, do not use within 5 weeks of fluoxetine or 2 weeks of sertraline or paroxetine discontinuance

Warnings/Precautions Safety in children <16 years of age has not been established; use with caution in patients who are hyperactive, hyperexcitable, or who have glaucoma; avoid use of meperidine within 2 weeks of phenelzine use. Hypertensive crisis may occur with tyramine.

The MAO inhibitors are effective and generally well tolerated by older patients. It is the potential interactions with tyramine or tryptophan-containing foods and other drugs, and their effects on blood pressure that have limited their use.

Pregnancy Risk Factor C

Adverse Reactions

Cardiovascular: Orthostatic hypotension, edema

Central nervous system: Dizziness, headache, drowsiness, sleep disturbances, fatigue, hyper-reflexia, twitching, ataxia, mania

Dermatologic: Rash, pruritus

Endocrine & metabolic: Decreased sexual ability (anorgasmia, ejaculatory disturbances, impotence), hypernatremia, hypermetabolic syndrome

Gastrointestinal: Xerostomia, constipation, weight gain

Genitourinary: Urinary retention

Hematologic: Leukopenia

Hepatic: Hepatitis

Neuromuscular & skeletal: Weakness, tremor, myoclonus

Ocular: Blurred vision, glaucoma

Miscellaneous: Diaphoresis

Drug Interactions

In general, the combined use of phenelzine with TCAs, venlafaxine, trazodone, and SSRIs should be avoided due to the potential for severe adverse reactions (serotonin syndrome, death)

MAOIs may inhibit the metabolism of barbiturates and prolong their effect

MAOIs in combination with dexfenfluramine, sibutramine, meperidine, fenfluramine, and dextromethorphan may cause serotonin syndrome; these combinations are best avoided

MAOIs in combination with amphetamines, other stimulants (methylphenidate), metaraminol, and decongestants (pseudoephedrine) may result in severe hypertensive reaction; these combinations are best avoided

Foods (eg, cheese) and beverages (eg, ethanol) containing tyramine, should be avoided in patients receiving an MAOI; hypertensive crisis may result

MAOIs inhibit the antihypertensive response to guanadrel or guanethidine; use an alternative antihypertensive agent

MAOIs in combination with levodopa and reserpine may result in hypertensive reactions; monitor

MAOIs in combination with lithium have resulted in malignant hyperpyrexia; this combination is best avoided

MAOIs may increase the pressor response of norepinephrine; monitor

MAOIs may prolong the muscle relaxation produced by succinylcholine via decreased plasma pseudocholinesterase

Tramadol may increase the risk of seizures and serotonin syndrome in patients receiving an MAOI

MAOIs may produce hypoglycemia in patients with diabetes; monitor

MAOIs may produce delirium in patients receiving disulfiram; monitor

Alcohol Interactions Avoid use (alcoholic beverages containing tyramine and tyramine-containing foods may induce a severe hypertensive response)

Onset Within 2-4 weeks

Duration May continue to have a therapeutic effect and interactions 2 weeks after discontinuing therapy

Education and Monitoring Issues

Patient Education: Take exactly as directed (do not increase dose or frequency); may take 2-3 weeks to achieve desired results; may cause physical and/or psychological dependence. Avoid excessive alcohol, caffeine, and other prescription or OTC medications not approved by prescriber. Avoid tyramine-containing foods (eg, pickles, aged cheese, wine). Maintain adequate hydration (2-3 L/day of fluids unless instructed to restrict fluid intake). You may experience postural hypotension (use caution when climbing stairs or changing position from lying or sitting to standing); drowsiness, lightheadedness, dizziness (use caution when driving or engaging in tasks requiring alertness until response to drug is known); anorexia, dry mouth (small frequent meals, frequent mouth care, chewing gum, or sucking lozenges may help); constipation (increased exercise, fluids, or dietary fruit and fiber may help); or diarrhea (buttermilk, yogurt, or boiled milk may help). Diabetic patients should monitor serum glucose closely (Nardil® may effect glucose levels). Report persistent insomnia; chest pain, palpitations, irregular or rapid heartbeat, or swelling of extremities; muscle cramping, tremors, or altered gait; blurred vision or eye pain; yellowing of eyes or skin; pale stools/dark urine; or worsening of condition.

Dietary Considerations: Food: Avoid tyramine-containing foods

Monitoring Parameters: Blood pressure, heart rate, diet, weight, mood (if depressive symptoms)

Manufacturer Parke-Davis

Related Information

Antidepressant Agents Comparison *on page 1231*

Pharmaceutical Manufacturers Directory *on page 1020*

♦ **Phenerbel-S®** *see* Belladonna, Phenobarbital, and Ergotamine Tartrate *on page 96*

♦ **Phenergan®** *see* Promethazine *on page 779*

♦ **Phenergan® VC Syrup** *see* Promethazine and Phenylephrine *on page 780*

♦ **Phenergan® VC With Codeine** *see* Promethazine, Phenylephrine, and Codeine *on page 780*

♦ **Phenergan® With Codeine** *see* Promethazine and Codeine *on page 780*

♦ **Phenergan® With Dextromethorphan** *see* Promethazine and Dextromethorphan *on page 780*

♦ **Phenhist® Expectorant** *see* Guaifenesin, Pseudoephedrine, and Codeine *on page 425*

Pheniramine, Phenylpropanolamine, and Pyrilamine

(fen EER a meen, fen il proe pa NOLE a meen, & peer IL a meen)

Pharmacologic Class Antihistamine/Decongestant Combination

U.S. Brand Names Triaminic® Oral Infant Drops

Dosage Forms DROPS: Pheniramine maleate 10 mg, phenylpropanolamine hydrochloride 20 mg, and pyrilamine maleate 10 mg per mL (15 mL)

Pregnancy Risk Factor C

Phenobarbital (fee noe BAR bi tal)

Pharmacologic Class Anticonvulsant, Barbiturate; Barbiturate

U.S. Brand Names Barbita®; Luminal®; Solfoton®

(Continued)

Phenobarbital *(Continued)*

Generic Available Yes

Mechanism of Action Interferes with transmission of impulses from the thalamus to the cortex of the brain resulting in an imbalance in central inhibitory and facilitatory mechanisms

Use Management of generalized tonic-clonic (grand mal) and partial seizures; neonatal seizures; febrile seizures in children; sedation; may also be used for prevention and treatment of neonatal hyperbilirubinemia and lowering of bilirubin in chronic cholestasis

USUAL DOSAGE

Children:

Sedation: Oral: 2 mg/kg 3 times/day

Hypnotic: I.M., I.V., S.C.: 3-5 mg/kg at bedtime

Preoperative sedation: Oral, I.M., I.V.: 1-3 mg/kg 1-1.5 hours before procedure

Anticonvulsant: Status epilepticus: **Loading dose:** I.V.:

Infants and Children: 10-20 mg/kg in a single or divided dose; in select patients may administer additional 5 mg/kg/dose every 15-30 minutes until seizure is controlled or a total dose of 40 mg/kg is reached

Adults: 300-800 mg initially followed by 120-240 mg/dose at 20-minute intervals until seizures are controlled or a total dose of 1-2 g

Anticonvulsant maintenance dose: Oral, I.V.:

Infants: 5-8 mg/kg/day in 1-2 divided doses

Children:

1-5 years: 6-8 mg/kg/day in 1-2 divided doses

5-12 years: 4-6 mg/kg/day in 1-2 divided doses

Children >12 years and Adults: 1-3 mg/kg/day in divided doses or 50-100 mg 2-3 times/day

Adults:

Sedation: Oral, I.M.: 30-120 mg/day in 2-3 divided doses

Hypnotic: Oral, I.M., I.V., S.C.: 100-320 mg at bedtime

Preoperative sedation: I.M.: 100-200 mg 1-1.5 hours before procedure

Dosing interval in renal impairment: Cl_{cr} <10 mL/minute: Administer every 12-16 hours

Hemodialysis: Moderately dialyzable (20% to 50%)

Dosing adjustment/comments in hepatic disease: Increased side effects may occur in severe liver disease; monitor plasma levels and adjust dose accordingly

Dosage Forms CAP: 16 mg. **ELIX:** 15 mg/5 mL (5 mL, 10 mL, 20 mL); 20 mg/5 mL (3.75 mL, 5 mL, 7.5 mL, 120 mL, 473 mL, 946 mL, 4000 mL). **INJ:** 30 mg/mL (1 mL); 60 mg/mL (1 mL); 65 mg/mL (1 mL); 130 mg/mL (1 mL). **POWDER for inj:** 120 mg. **TAB:** 8 mg, 15 mg, 16 mg, 30 mg, 32 mg, 60 mg, 65 mg, 100 mg

Contraindications Hypersensitivity to phenobarbital or any component; pre-existing CNS depression, severe uncontrolled pain, porphyria, severe respiratory disease with dyspnea or obstruction

Warnings/Precautions Use with caution in patients with hypovolemic shock, congestive heart failure, hepatic impairment, respiratory dysfunction or depression, previous addiction to the sedative/hypnotic group, chronic or acute pain, renal dysfunction, and the elderly, due to its long half-life and risk of dependence, phenobarbital is not recommended as a sedative in the elderly; tolerance or psychological and physical dependence may occur with prolonged use. **Abrupt withdrawal in patients with epilepsy may precipitate status epilepticus.**

Pregnancy Risk Factor D

Pregnancy Implications

Clinical effects on the fetus: Crosses the placenta. Cardiac defect reported; hemorrhagic disease of newborn due to fetal vitamin K depletion may occur; may induce maternal folic acid deficiency; withdrawal symptoms observed in infant following delivery. Epilepsy itself, number of medications, genetic factors, or a combination of these probably influence the teratogenicity of anticonvulsant therapy. Benefit:risk ratio usually favors continued use during pregnancy and breast-feeding.

Breast-feeding/Lactation: Crosses into breast milk

Clinical effects on the infant: Sedation; withdrawal with abrupt weaning reported. American Academy of Pediatrics recommends USE WITH CAUTION.

Adverse Reactions

Cardiovascular: Bradycardia, hypotension, syncope

Central nervous system: Drowsiness, lethargy, CNS excitation or depression, impaired judgment, "hangover" effect, confusion, somnolence, agitation, hyperkinesia, ataxia, nervousness, headache, insomnia, nightmares, hallucinations, anxiety, dizziness

Dermatologic: Rash, exfoliative dermatitis, Stevens-Johnson syndrome

Gastrointestinal: Nausea, vomiting, constipation

Hematologic: Agranulocytosis, thrombocytopenia, megaloblastic anemia

Local: Pain at injection site, thrombophlebitis with I.V. use

Renal: Oliguria

Respiratory: Laryngospasm, respiratory depression, apnea (especially with rapid I.V. use), hypoventilation, apnea

Miscellaneous: Gangrene with inadvertent intra-arterial injection

Drug Interactions CYP1A2, 2B6, 2C, 2C8, 3A3/4, and 3A5-7 inducer

Barbiturates are enzyme inducers. Patients should be monitored when these drugs are started or stopped for a decreased or increased therapeutic effect respectively.

Decreased effect: Phenobarbital may reduce the efficacy of beta-blockers, chloramphenicol, cimetidine, clozapine, corticosteroids, cyclosporine, disopyramide, doxycycline, ethosuximide, furosemide, griseofulvin, haloperidol, lamotrigine, methadone, nifedipine, oral contraceptives, phenothiazine, phenytoin, propafenone, psychotropics, quinidine, tacrolimus, TCAs, theophylline, warfarin, and verapamil

Increased toxicity when combined with other CNS depressants, benzodiazepines, valproic acid, chloramphenicol, or antidepressants; respiratory and CNS depression may be additive

MAOIs may prolong the effect of phenobarbital

Barbiturates stimulate the metabolism of beta-blockers and decrease their serum concentrations; consider a renally-eliminated beta-blocker (atenolol, nadolol)

Barbiturates may enhance the hepatotoxic potential of acetaminophen via an increased formation of toxic metabolites

Barbiturates may increase chloramphenicol metabolism and chloramphenicol may inhibit the metabolism of barbiturates

Barbiturates may increase the metabolism of corticosteroids, cyclosporine, disopyramide, griseofulvin, nifedipine, oral contraceptives, phenytoin, propafenone, quinidine, verapamil; dosage adjustments may be useful

Barbiturates may enhance the metabolism of methadone resulting in methadone withdrawal

Felbamate may increase phenobarbital concentrations leading to toxicity

Phenobarbital may reduce the diuretic response to furosemide; monitor

Concurrent use of phenobarbital with meperidine may result in increased CNS depression

Concurrent use of phenobarbital with primidone may result in elevated phenobarbital serum concentrations

Valproic acid inhibits the metabolism of phenobarbital resulting in elevated serum phenobarbital concentrations

Alcohol Interactions Avoid use (may increase central nervous system depression)

Onset Oral: 20-60 minutes

Duration Oral: 6-10 hours

Half-Life Adults: 53-140 hours

Education and Monitoring Issues

Patient Education: I.V./I.M.: Patient instructions and information are determined by patient condition and therapeutic purpose. If self-administered, use exactly as directed (do not increase dose or frequency); may cause physical and/or psychological dependence. While using this medication, do not use alcohol and other prescription or OTC medications (especially pain medications, sedatives, antihistamines, or hypnotics) without consulting prescriber. Maintain adequate hydration (2-3 L/day of fluids unless instructed to restrict fluid intake). You may experience drowsiness, dizziness, or blurred vision (use caution when driving or engaging in tasks requiring alertness until response to drug is known); nausea, vomiting, or loss of appetite (small frequent meals, frequent mouth care, chewing gum, or sucking lozenges may help); constipation (increased exercise, fluids, or dietary fruit and fiber may help). Report skin rash or irritation; CNS changes (confusion, depression, increased sedation, excitation, headache, insomnia, or nightmares); difficulty breathing or shortness of breath; changes in urinary pattern or menstrual pattern; muscle weakness or tremors; or difficulty swallowing or feeling of tightness in throat.

Dietary Considerations:

Food:

Protein-deficient diets: Increases duration of action of barbiturates. Should not restrict or delete protein from diet unless discussed with prescriber. Be consistent with protein intake during therapy with barbiturates.

Fresh fruits containing vitamin C: Displaces drug from binding sites, resulting in increased urinary excretion of barbiturate. Educate patients regarding the potential for a decreased anticonvulsant effect of barbiturates with consumption of foods high in vitamin C.

Vitamin D: Loss in vitamin D due to malabsorption; increase intake of foods rich in vitamin D. Supplementation of vitamin D may be necessary.

Monitoring Parameters: Phenobarbital serum concentrations, mental status, CBC, LFTs, seizure activity

Reference Range:

Therapeutic:

Infants and children: 15-30 μg/mL (SI: 65-129 μmol/L)

Adults: 20-40 μg/mL (SI: 86-172 μmol/L)

Toxic: >40 μg/mL (SI: >172 μmol/L)

Toxic concentration: Slowness, ataxia, nystagmus: 35-80 μg/mL (SI: 150-344 μmol/L)

Coma with reflexes: 65-117 μg/mL (SI: 279-502 μmol/L)

Coma without reflexes: >100 μg/mL (SI: >430 μmol/L)

Related Information

Anticonvulsants by Seizure Type Comparison *on page 1230*

Belladonna, Phenobarbital, and Ergotamine Tartrate *on page 96*

Epilepsy Guidelines *on page 1091*

(Continued)

Phenobarbital *(Continued)*

Theophylline, Ephedrine, and Phenobarbital *on page 906*

♦ **Phenoxine® [OTC]** *see* Phenylpropanolamine *on page 729*

Phentermine (FEN ter meen)

Pharmacologic Class Anorexiant

U.S. Brand Names Adipex-P®; Fastin®; Ionamin®; Zantryl®

Generic Available Yes

Mechanism of Action Phentermine is structurally similar to dextroamphetamine and is comparable to dextroamphetamine as an appetite suppressant, but is generally associated with a lower incidence and severity of CNS side effects. Phentermine, like other anorexiants, stimulates the hypothalamus to result in decreased appetite; anorexiant effects are most likely mediated via norepinephrine and dopamine metabolism. However, other CNS effects or metabolic effects may be involved.

Use Short-term adjunct in exogenous obesity in patients with an initial body mass index (BMI) ≥30 kg/m^2 or a BMI ≥27 kg/m^2 when other risk factors are present (eg, hypertension, diabetes, hyperlipidemia); see "Guidelines for Treatment of Obesity" in Appendix

USUAL DOSAGE Oral:

Children 3-15 years: 5-15 mg/day for 4 weeks

Adults: 8 mg 3 times/day 30 minutes before meals or food or 15-37.5 mg/day before breakfast or 10-14 hours before retiring

Dosage Forms CAP: 15 mg, 18.75 mg, 30 mg, 37.5 mg; Resin complex: 15 mg, 30 mg. **TAB:** 8 mg, 37.5 mg

Contraindications Known hypersensitivity to phentermine

Warnings/Precautions Do not use in children ≤16 years of age. Use with caution in patients with diabetes mellitus, cardiovascular disease, nephritis, angina pectoris, hypertension, glaucoma, patients with a history of drug abuse. **Primary pulmonary hypertension (PPH),** a rare and frequently fatal pulmonary disease, has been reported to occur in patients receiving a combination of phentermine and fenfluramine or dexfenfluramine. The possibility of an association between PPH and the use of phentermine alone cannot be ruled out.

Pregnancy Risk Factor C

Adverse Reactions

Cardiovascular: Hypertension, palpitations, tachycardia, primary pulmonary hypertension and/or regurgitant cardiac valvular disease

Central nervous system: Euphoria, insomnia, overstimulation, dizziness, dysphoria, headache, restlessness, psychosis

Dermatologic: Urticaria

Gastrointestinal: Nausea, constipation, xerostomia, unpleasant taste, diarrhea

Endocrine & metabolic: Changes in libido, impotence

Hematologic: Blood dyscrasias

Neuromuscular & skeletal: Tremor

Ocular: Blurred vision

Drug Interactions

Phentermine may decrease the hypotensive effect of guanethidine and other antihypertensives

Hypoglycemic agents may need to be adjusted when phentermine is used in a diabetic receiving a special diet

Half-Life 20 hours

Education and Monitoring Issues

Patient Education: Take during day to avoid insomnia; do not discontinue abruptly, may cause physical and psychological dependence with prolonged use

Monitoring Parameters: CNS

Phentolamine (fen TOLE a meen)

Pharmacologic Class Alpha$_1$ Blockers

U.S. Brand Names Regitine®

Generic Available No

Mechanism of Action Competitively blocks alpha-adrenergic receptors to produce brief antagonism of circulating epinephrine and norepinephrine to reduce hypertension caused by alpha effects of these catecholamines; also has a positive inotropic and chronotropic effect on the heart

Use Diagnosis of pheochromocytoma and treatment of hypertension associated with pheochromocytoma or other caused by excess sympathomimetic amines; as treatment of dermal necrosis after extravasation of drugs with alpha-adrenergic effects (norepinephrine, dopamine, epinephrine, dobutamine)

USUAL DOSAGE

Treatment of alpha-adrenergic drug extravasation: S.C.:

Children: 0.1-0.2 mg/kg diluted in 10 mL 0.9% sodium chloride infiltrated into area of extravasation within 12 hours

Adults: Infiltrate area with small amount of solution made by diluting 5-10 mg in 10 mL 0.9% sodium chloride within 12 hours of extravasation

If dose is effective, normal skin color should return to the blanched area within 1 hour

Diagnosis of pheochromocytoma: I.M., I.V.:

Children: 0.05-0.1 mg/kg/dose, maximum single dose: 5 mg

Adults: 5 mg

Surgery for pheochromocytoma: Hypertension: I.M., I.V.:

Children: 0.05-0.1 mg/kg/dose given 1-2 hours before procedure; repeat as needed every 2-4 hours until hypertension is controlled; maximum single dose: 5 mg

Adults: 5 mg given 1-2 hours before procedure and repeated as needed every 2-4 hours

Hypertensive crisis: Adults: 5-20 mg

Dosage Forms INJ: 5 mg/mL (1 mL)

Contraindications Hypersensitivity to phentolamine or any component; renal impairment; coronary or cerebral arteriosclerosis

Warnings/Precautions Myocardial infarction, cerebrovascular spasm and cerebrovascular occlusion have occurred following administration; use with caution in patients with gastritis or peptic ulcer, tachycardia, or a history of cardiac arrhythmias

Pregnancy Risk Factor C

Adverse Reactions

>10%:

Cardiovascular: Hypotension, tachycardia, arrhythmias, reflex tachycardia, anginal pain, orthostatic hypotension

Gastrointestinal: Nausea, vomiting, diarrhea, exacerbation of peptic ulcer, abdominal pain

Respiratory: Nasal congestion

1% to 10%:

Cardiovascular: Flushing of face, syncope

Central nervous system: Dizziness

Neuromuscular & skeletal: Weakness

Respiratory: Nasal congestion

<1%: Myocardial infarction, severe headache

Drug Interactions

Epinephrine, ephedrine: Effects may be decreased

Ethanol: Increased toxicity (disulfiram reaction)

Onset I.M.: Within 15-20 minutes; I.V.: Immediate

Duration I.M.: 30-45 minutes; I.V.: 15-30 minutes

Half-Life 19 minutes

Education and Monitoring Issues

Patient Education: Immediately report pain at infusion site. Report any dizziness, feelings of faintness, or palpitations. Do not change position rapidly; rise slowly or ask for assistance.

Monitoring Parameters: Blood pressure, heart rate

♦ **Phenyldrine® [OTC]** *see* Phenylpropanolamine *on page 729*

Phenylephrine (fen il EF rin)

Pharmacologic Class Alpha/Beta Agonist; Ophthalmic Agent, Antiglaucoma; Ophthalmic Agent, Mydriatic

U.S. Brand Names AK-Dilate® Ophthalmic Solution; AK-Nefrin® Ophthalmic Solution; Alconefrin® Nasal Solution [OTC]; Doktors® Nasal Solution [OTC]; I-Phrine® Ophthalmic Solution; Isopto® Frin Ophthalmic Solution; Mydfrin® Ophthalmic Solution; Neo-Synephrine® Nasal Solution [OTC]; Neo-Synephrine® Ophthalmic Solution; Nostril® Nasal Solution [OTC]; Prefrin™ Ophthalmic Solution; Relief® Ophthalmic Solution; Rhinall® Nasal Solution [OTC]; Sinarest® Nasal Solution [OTC]; St. Joseph® Measured Dose Nasal Solution [OTC]; Vicks® Sinex® Nasal Solution [OTC]

Generic Available Yes

Mechanism of Action Potent, direct-acting alpha-adrenergic stimulator with weak beta-adrenergic activity; causes vasoconstriction of the arterioles of the nasal mucosa and conjunctiva; activates the dilator muscle of the pupil to cause contraction; produces vasoconstriction of arterioles in the body; produces systemic arterial vasoconstriction

Use Treatment of hypotension, vascular failure in shock; as a vasoconstrictor in regional analgesia; symptomatic relief of nasal and nasopharyngeal mucosal congestion; as a mydriatic in ophthalmic procedures and treatment of wide-angle glaucoma; supraventricular tachycardia

USUAL DOSAGE

Ophthalmic procedures:

Infants <1 year: Instill 1 drop of 2.5% 15-30 minutes before procedures

Children and Adults: Instill 1 drop of 2.5% or 10% solution, may repeat in 10-60 minutes as needed

Nasal decongestant: (therapy should not exceed 5 continuous days)

Children:

2-6 years: Instill 1 drop every 2-4 hours of 0.125% solution as needed

6-12 years: Instill 1-2 sprays or instill 1-2 drops every 4 hours of 0.25% solution as needed

(Continued)

Phenylephrine *(Continued)*

Children >12 years and Adults: Instill 1-2 sprays or instill 1-2 drops every 4 hours of 0.25% to 0.5% solution as needed; 1% solution may be used in adult in cases of extreme nasal congestion; do not use nasal solutions more than 3 days

Hypotension/shock:

Children:

I.M., S.C.: 0.1 mg/kg/dose every 1-2 hours as needed (maximum: 5 mg)

I.V. bolus: 5-20 mcg/kg/dose every 10-15 minutes as needed

I.V. infusion: 0.1-0.5 mcg/kg/minute

Adults:

I.M., S.C.: 2-5 mg/dose every 1-2 hours as needed (initial dose should not exceed 5 mg)

I.V. bolus: 0.1-0.5 mg/dose every 10-15 minutes as needed (initial dose should not exceed 0.5 mg)

I.V. infusion: 10 mg in 250 mL D_5W or NS (1:25,000 dilution) (40 mcg/mL); start at 100-180 mcg/minute (2-5 mL/minute; 50-90 drops/minute) initially; when blood pressure is stabilized, maintenance rate: 40-60 mcg/minute (20-30 drops/minute)

Paroxysmal supraventricular tachycardia: I.V.:

Children: 5-10 mcg/kg/dose over 20-30 seconds

Adults: 0.25-0.5 mg/dose over 20-30 seconds

Dosage Forms INJ (Neo-Synephrine®): 1% [10 mg/mL] (1 mL). **NASAL:** Soln: Drops: (Neo-Synephrine®): 0.125% (15 mL); (Alconefrin® 12): 0.16% (30 mL); (Alconefrin® 25, Neo-Synephrine®, Children's Nostril®, Rhinall®): 0.25% (15 mL, 30 mL, 40 mL); (Alconefrin®, Neo-Synephrine®): 0.5% (15 mL, 30 mL). **SPRAY:** (Alconefrin® 25, Neo-Synephrine®, Rhinall®): 0.25% (15 mL, 30 mL, 40 mL); (Neo-Synephrine®, Nostril®, Sinex®): 0.5% (15 mL, 30 mL); (Neo-Synephrine®): 1% (15 mL). **SOLN, ophth:** (AK-Nefrin®, Prefrin™ Liquifilm®, Relief®): 0.12% (0.3 mL, 15 mL, 20 mL); (AK-Dilate®, Mydfrin®, Neo-Synephrine®, Phenoptic®): 2.5% (2 mL, 3 mL, 5 mL, 15 mL); (AK-Dilate®, Neo-Synephrine®, Neo-Synephrine® Viscous): 10% (1 mL, 2 mL, 5 mL, 15 mL)

Contraindications Pheochromocytoma, severe hypertension, bradycardia, ventricular tachyarrhythmias; hypersensitivity to phenylephrine or any component; narrow-angle glaucoma (ophthalmic preparation), acute pancreatitis, hepatitis, peripheral or mesenteric vascular thrombosis, myocardial disease, severe coronary disease

Warnings/Precautions Injection may contain sulfites which may cause allergic reaction in some patients; do not use if solution turns brown or contains a precipitate; use with extreme caution in elderly patients, patients with hyperthyroidism, bradycardia, partial heart block, myocardial disease, or severe arteriosclerosis; infuse into large veins to help prevent extravasation which may cause severe necrosis; the 10% ophthalmic solution has caused increased blood pressure in elderly patients and its use should, therefore, be avoided

Pregnancy Risk Factor C

Adverse Reactions Incidence of adverse events is not reported.

Cardiovascular: Reflex bradycardia, excitability, restlessness, arrhythmias (rare), precordial pain or discomfort, pallor, hypertension, severe peripheral and visceral vasoconstriction

Central nervous system: Headache, anxiety, weakness, dizziness, tremor, paresthesia

Endocrine and metabolic: Metabolic acidosis

Local: Extravasation which may lead to necrosis and sloughing of surrounding tissue, blanching of skin

Neuromuscular & skeletal: Pilomotor response

Renal: Decreased renal perfusion, reduced urine output, reduced urine output

Respiratory: Respiratory distress

Drug Interactions

Beta-blockers (nonselective ones) may increase hypertensive effect; avoid concurrent use

Cocaine may cause malignant arrhythmias; avoid concurrent use

Guanethidine can increase the pressor response; be aware of the patient's drug regimen

Methyldopa can increase the pressor response; be aware of patient's drug regimen

Phenytoin administration during a dopamine infusion may result in hypotension and possibly cardiac arrest; use cautiously

Reserpine increases the pressor response; be aware of patient's drug regimen

TCAs increase the pressor response; be aware of patient's drug regimen

MAO inhibitors potentiate hypertension and hypertensive crisis; avoid concurrent use

Onset I.M., S.C.: Within 10-15 minutes; I.V.: Immediate

Duration I.M.: 30 minutes to 2 hours; I.V.: 15-30 minutes; S.C.: 1 hour

Half-Life 2.5 hours

Education and Monitoring Issues

Patient Education:

Nasal decongestant: Do not use for more than 5 days in a row. Clear nose as much as possible before use. Tilt head back and instill recommended dose of drops or spray. Do not blow nose for 5-10 minutes. You may experience transient stinging or burning.

Ophthalmic: Open eye, look at ceiling, and instill prescribed amount of solution. Close eye and roll eye in all directions, and apply gentle pressure to inner corner of eye for

1-2 minutes after instillation. Do not let tip of applicator touch eye or contaminate tip of applicator. Temporary stinging or blurred vision may occur. Report persistent pain, burning, double vision, severe headache, or if condition worsens.

Monitoring Parameters: Blood pressure, heart rate, arterial blood gases, central venous pressure

Related Information

Chlorpheniramine and Phenylephrine *on page 186*
Chlorpheniramine, Ephedrine, Phenylephrine, and Carbetapentane *on page 186*
Chlorpheniramine, Phenylephrine, and Codeine *on page 186*
Chlorpheniramine, Phenylephrine, and Methscopolamine *on page 186*
Chlorpheniramine, Phenylephrine, and Phenylpropanolamine *on page 186*
Chlorpheniramine, Phenylephrine, and Phenyltoloxamine *on page 186*
Chlorpheniramine, Phenylephrine, Phenylpropanolamine, and Belladonna Alkaloids *on page 187*
Chlorpheniramine, Phenyltoloxamine, Phenylpropanolamine, and Phenylephrine *on page 187*
Chlorpheniramine, Pyrilamine, and Phenylephrine *on page 187*
Chlorpheniramine, Pyrilamine, Phenylephrine, and Phenylpropanolamine *on page 187*
Cyclopentolate and Phenylephrine *on page 235*
Guaifenesin and Phenylephrine *on page 425*
Hydrocodone, Chlorpheniramine, Phenylephrine, Acetaminophen, and Caffeine *on page 446*
Hydrocodone, Phenylephrine, Pyrilamine, Phenindamine, Chlorpheniramine, and Ammonium Chloride *on page 446*
Isoproterenol and Phenylephrine *on page 490*
Phenylephrine and Scopolamine *on page 729*
Promethazine and Phenylephrine *on page 780*
Promethazine, Phenylephrine, and Codeine *on page 780*
Sulfacetamide Sodium and Phenylephrine *on page 876*

Phenylephrine and Scopolamine (fen il EF rin & skoe POL a meen)

Pharmacologic Class Anticholinergic/Adrenergic Agonist

U.S. Brand Names Murocoll-2® Ophthalmic

Dosage Forms SOLN, ophth: Phenylephrine hydrochloride 10% and scopolamine hydrobromide 0.3% (7.5 mL)

Pregnancy Risk Factor C

Phenylpropanolamine (fen il proe pa NOLE a meen)

Pharmacologic Class Alpha/Beta Agonist

U.S. Brand Names Acutrim® 16 Hours [OTC]; Acutrim® II, Maximum Strength [OTC]; Acutrim® Late Day [OTC]; Control® [OTC]; Dexatrim® Pre-Meal [OTC]; Maximum Strength Dex-A-Diet® [OTC]; Maximum Strength Dexatrim® [OTC]; Phenoxine® [OTC]; Phenyldrine® [OTC]; Prolamine® [OTC]; Propagest® [OTC]; Rhindecon®; Unitrol® [OTC]

Generic Available Yes

Mechanism of Action Releases tissue stores of epinephrine and thereby produces an alpha- and beta-adrenergic stimulation; this causes vasoconstriction and nasal mucosa blanching; also appears to depress central appetite centers

Use Anorexiant; nasal decongestant

USUAL DOSAGE Oral:

Children: Decongestant:
- 2-6 years: 6.25 mg every 4 hours
- 6-12 years: 12.5 mg every 4 hours not to exceed 75 mg/day

Adults:
- Decongestant: 25 mg every 4 hours or 50 mg every 8 hours, not to exceed 150 mg/day
- Anorexic: 25 mg 3 times/day 30 minutes before meals or 75 mg (timed release) once daily in the morning; see "Obesity Treatment Guidelines for Adults" in Appendix
- Precision release: 75 mg after breakfast

Dosage Forms CAP: 37.5 mg; Timed release: 25 mg, 75 mg. **TAB:** 25 mg, 50 mg; Precision release: 75 mg, Timed release: 75 mg

Contraindications Known hypersensitivity to drug

Warnings/Precautions Use with caution in patients with high blood pressure, tachyarrhythmias, pheochromocytoma, bradycardia, cardiac disease, arteriosclerosis; do not use for more than 3 weeks for weight loss

Pregnancy Risk Factor C

Adverse Reactions

>10%: Cardiovascular: Hypertension, palpitations

1% to 10%:
- Central nervous system: Insomnia, restlessness, dizziness
- Gastrointestinal: Xerostomia, nausea

<1%: Angina, anxiety, arrhythmias, bradycardia, dysuria, nervousness, restlessness, severe headache, tightness in chest

Drug Interactions

Decreased effect of antihypertensives

(Continued)

Phenylpropanolamine *(Continued)*

Increased effect/toxicity with MAO inhibitors (hypertensive crisis), beta-blockers (increased pressor effects)

Duration Up to 24 hours (timed release)

Half-Life 4.6-6.6 hours

Education and Monitoring Issues

Patient Education: Nasal decongestant: Do not use for longer than recommended (4-5 days in a row). Anorexiant: Do not use for longer than 3 weeks. With timed release form, take early in day; do not chew or crush. Do not use more often, or in greater dose than prescribed. You may experience dizziness or blurred vision (use caution when driving or engaging in tasks requiring alertness until response to drug is known). With nasal use you may experience burning or stinging (this will resolve). Report rapid heartbeat, chest pain, palpitations; persistent vomiting; excessive nervousness, trembling, or insomnia; difficult or painful urination; unresolved burning or stinging (eyes or nose); or acute headache.

Monitoring Parameters: Blood pressure, heart rate

Related Information

Brompheniramine, Phenylpropanolamine, and Codeine *on page 114*
Caramiphen and Phenylpropanolamine *on page 137*
Chlorpheniramine, Phenindamine, and Phenylpropanolamine *on page 186*
Chlorpheniramine, Phenylephrine, and Phenylpropanolamine *on page 186*
Chlorpheniramine, Phenylephrine, Phenylpropanolamine, and Belladonna Alkaloids *on page 187*
Chlorpheniramine, Phenyltoloxamine, Phenylpropanolamine, and Phenylephrine *on page 187*
Chlorpheniramine, Pyrilamine, Phenylephrine, and Phenylpropanolamine *on page 187*
Clemastine and Phenylpropanolamine *on page 207*
Hydrocodone and Phenylpropanolamine *on page 446*
Pheniramine, Phenylpropanolamine, and Pyrilamine *on page 723*
Phenyltoloxamine, Phenylpropanolamine, and Acetaminophen *on page 730*
Phenyltoloxamine, Phenylpropanolamine, Pyrilamine, and Pheniramine *on page 730*

Phenyltoloxamine, Phenylpropanolamine, and Acetaminophen

(fen il tol OKS a meen, fen il proe pa NOLE a meen, & a seet a MIN oh fen)

Pharmacologic Class Antihistamine/Decongestant/Analgesic

U.S. Brand Names Sinubid®

Dosage Forms TAB: Phenyltoloxamine citrate 22 mg, phenylpropanolamine hydrochloride 25 mg, and acetaminophen 325 mg

Pregnancy Risk Factor C

Phenyltoloxamine, Phenylpropanolamine, Pyrilamine, and Pheniramine

(fen il tol OKS a meen, fen il proe pa NOLE a meen, peer IL a meen, & fen IR a meen)

Pharmacologic Class Cold Preparation

U.S. Brand Names Poly-Histine-D® Capsule

Dosage Forms CAP: Phenyltoloxamine citrate 16 mg, phenylpropanolamine hydrochloride 50 mg, pyrilamine maleate 16 mg, and pheniramine maleate 16 mg

Phenytoin (FEN i toyn)

Pharmacologic Class Antiarrhythmic Agent, Class I-B; Anticonvulsant, Hydantoin

U.S. Brand Names Dilantin®; Diphenylan Sodium®

Generic Available Yes

Mechanism of Action Stabilizes neuronal membranes and decreases seizure activity by increasing efflux or decreasing influx of sodium ions across cell membranes in the motor cortex during generation of nerve impulses; prolongs effective refractory period and suppresses ventricular pacemaker automaticity, shortens action potential in the heart

Use Management of generalized tonic-clonic (grand mal), simple partial and complex partial seizures; prevention of seizures following head trauma/neurosurgery; ventricular arrhythmias, including those associated with digitalis intoxication, prolonged Q-T interval and surgical repair of congenital heart diseases in children; also used for epidermolysis bullosa

USUAL DOSAGE

Status epilepticus: I.V.:

Infants and Children: Loading dose: 15-20 mg/kg in a single or divided dose; maintenance dose: Initial: 5 mg/kg/day in 2 divided doses, usual doses:

6 months to 3 years: 8-10 mg/kg/day
4-6 years: 7.5-9 mg/kg/day
7-9 years: 7-8 mg/kg/day
10-16 years: 6-7 mg/kg/day, some patients may require every 8 hours dosing

Adults: Loading dose: 15-20 mg/kg in a single or divided dose, followed by 100-150 mg/dose at 30-minute intervals up to a maximum of 1500 mg/24 hours; maintenance dose: 300 mg/day or 5-6 mg/kg/day in 3 divided doses or 1-2 divided doses using extended release

Anticonvulsant: Children and Adults: Oral:

Loading dose: 15-20 mg/kg; based on phenytoin serum concentrations and recent dosing history; administer oral loading dose in 3 divided doses given every 2-4 hours to decrease GI adverse effects and to ensure complete oral absorption; maintenance dose: same as I.V.

Dosing adjustment/comments in renal impairment or hepatic disease: Safe in usual doses in mild liver disease; clearance may be substantially reduced in cirrhosis and plasma level monitoring with dose adjustment advisable. Free phenytoin levels should be monitored closely.

Dosage Forms CAP: Extended release: 30 mg, 100 mg; Prompt release: 100 mg. **INJ:** 50 mg/mL (2 mL, 5 mL). **SUSP, oral:** 30 mg/5 mL (5 mL, 240 mL), 125 mg/5 mL (5 mL, 240 mL). **TAB, chewable:** 50 mg

Contraindications Hypersensitivity to phenytoin, other hydantoins, or any component; heart block, sinus bradycardia

Warnings/Precautions May increase frequency of petit mal seizures; I.V. form may cause hypotension, skin necrosis at I.V. site; avoid I.V. administration in small veins; use with caution in patients with porphyria; discontinue if rash or lymphadenopathy occurs; use with caution in patients with hepatic dysfunction, sinus bradycardia, S-A block, A-V block, or hepatic impairment; elderly may have reduced hepatic clearance and low albumin levels, which will increase the free fraction of phenytoin in the serum and, therefore, the pharmacologic response

Pregnancy Risk Factor D

Pregnancy Implications

Clinical effects on the fetus: Crosses the placenta. Cardiac defects and multiple other malformations reported; characteristic pattern of malformations called "fetal hydantoin syndrome"; hemorrhagic disease of newborn due to fetal vitamin K depletion, maternal folic acid deficiency may occur. Epilepsy itself, number of medications, genetic factors, or a combination of these probably influence the teratogenicity of anticonvulsant therapy. Benefit:risk ratio usually favors continued use during pregnancy and breast-feeding.

Breast-feeding/lactation: Crosses into breast milk

Clinical effects on the infant: Methemoglobinemia, drowsiness and decreased sucking reported in 1 case. American Academy of Pediatrics considers **compatible** with breast-feeding.

Adverse Reactions I.V. effects: Hypotension, bradycardia, cardiac arrhythmias, cardiovascular collapse (especially with rapid I.V. use), venous irritation and pain, thrombophlebitis

Effects not related to plasma phenytoin concentrations: Hypertrichosis, gingival hypertrophy, thickening of facial features, carbohydrate intolerance, folic acid deficiency, peripheral neuropathy, vitamin D deficiency, osteomalacia, systemic lupus erythematosus

Dose-related effects: Nystagmus, blurred vision, diplopia, ataxia, slurred speech, dizziness, drowsiness, lethargy, coma, rash, fever, nausea, vomiting, gum tenderness, confusion, mood changes, folic acid depletion, osteomalacia, hyperglycemia

Related to elevated concentrations:

>20 mcg/mL: Far lateral nystagmus

>30 mcg/mL: 45° lateral gaze nystagmus and ataxia

>40 mcg/mL: Decreased mentation

>100 mcg/mL: Death

Cardiovascular: Hypotension, bradycardia, cardiac arrhythmias, cardiovascular collapse

Central nervous system: Psychiatric changes, slurred speech, dizziness, drowsiness, headache, insomnia

Dermatologic: Rash

Gastrointestinal: Constipation, nausea, vomiting, gingival hyperplasia, enlargement of lips

Hematologic: Leukopenia, thrombocytopenia, agranulocytosis

Hepatic: Hepatitis

Local: Thrombophlebitis

Neuromuscular & skeletal: Tremor, peripheral neuropathy, paresthesia

Ocular: Diplopia, nystagmus, blurred vision

Rarely seen effects: SLE-like syndrome, lymphadenopathy, hepatitis, Stevens-Johnson syndrome, blood dyscrasias, dyskinesias, pseudolymphoma, lymphoma, venous irritation and pain, coarsening of the facial features, hypertrichosis

Drug Interactions CYP2C9 and 2C19 enzyme substrate; CYP1A2, 2B6, 2C, 3A3/4, and 3A5-7 enzyme inducer

Decreased effect: Phenytoin with rifampin, cisplatin, vinblastine, bleomycin, folic acid, theophylline, and continuous NG feedings

Amiodarone or disulfiram decreases metabolism of phenytoin

(Continued)

Phenytoin *(Continued)*

Carbamazepine, cisplatin, diazoxide, ethanol (chronic), folic acid, phenobarbital, pyridoxine, and rifampin may enhance the metabolism of phenytoin resulting in decreased serum concentrations

Concurrent use of acetazolamide and phenytoin may result in an increased risk of osteomalacia

Concurrent use of I.V. phenytoin with dopamine may result in an increased risk of hypotension

Concurrent use of phenytoin and lithium has resulted in lithium intoxication

Isoniazid, chloramphenicol, or fluconazole may increase phenytoin serum concentrations

Phenytoin enhances the conversion of primidone to phenobarbital resulting in elevated phenobarbital serum concentrations

Phenytoin may decrease the effect of oral contraceptives, itraconazole, mebendazole, methadone, oral midazolam, valproic acid, cyclosporine, theophylline, doxycycline, quinidine, mexiletine, disopyramide

Phenytoin may enhance the hepatotoxic potential of acetaminophen

Phenytoin may increase the effect of dopamine (enhanced hypotension), warfarin (enhanced anticoagulation), increase the rate of conversion of primidone to phenobarbital resulting in increased phenobarbital serum concentrations

Phenytoin may increase the metabolism of alprazolam, amiodarone, bromfenac, carbamazepine, clozapine, cyclosporine, diazepam, disopyramide, doxycycline, felbamate, furosemide, itraconazole, lamotrigine, mebendazole, meperidine, methadone, metyrapone, mexiletine, midazolam, oral contraceptives, quetiapine, quinidine, tacrolimus, teniposide, theophylline, thyroid hormones, triazolam, and valproic acid resulting in decreased levels/effect

Phenytoin may inhibit the anti-Parkinson effect of levodopa

Phenytoin transiently increased the hypothrombinemia response to warfarin initially; this is followed by an inhibition of the hypoprothombinemic response

Sucralfate may reduce the GI absorption of phenytoin

Ticlopidine increases serum phenytoin concentrations to increase toxicity of phenytoin

Amiodarone, chloramphenicol, cimetidine, ciprofloxacin, disulfiram, enoxacin, norfloxacin, felbamate, fluconazole, fluoxetine, influenza vaccine, isoniazid, metronidazole, nifedipine, omeprazole, phenylbutazone, phenobarbital, sulfamethizole, sulfamethoxazole, sulfaphenazole, and trimethoprim inhibit the metabolism of phenytoin resulting in increased serum phenytoin concentrations/effects; monitor

Valproic acid may increase, decrease, or have no effect on phenytoin serum concentrations

Valproic acid and sulfisoxazole may displace phenytoin from binding sites

Vigabatrin and theophylline may reduce phenytoin serum concentrations

Alcohol Interactions Avoid use (may increase central nervous system depression)

Acute use: Inhibits metabolism of phenytoin

Chronic use: Stimulates metabolism of phenytoin

Onset I.V.: within 30 minutes to 1 hour; onset of fosphenytoin may be more rapid due to more rapid infusion

Half-Life Oral: 22 hours (range: 7-42 hours); I.V.: 10-15 hours

Education and Monitoring Issues

Patient Education: Take this drug as directed, with food. Do not change brands or discontinue without consulting prescriber. Follow good oral hygiene practices and have frequent dental checkups. If diabetic, monitor your serum glucose regularly as directed by prescriber; insulin dosage may need to be adjusted. You may experience dizziness, confusion, or vision changes; use caution when driving or engaging in tasks requiring alertness until response to drug is known. If GI upset occurs, frequent small meals may help. May discolor urine (red/pink). Report rash; unresolved nausea or vomiting; slurring speech or coordination difficulties; swollen glands; swollen, sore, or bleeding gums; yellowish color to skin or eyes; unusual bleeding and/or bruising; erection problems; difficulty breathing; or palpitations. Do not crush or open extended-release capsules.

Dietary Considerations:

Food:

Folic acid: Low erythrocyte and CSF folate concentrations. Phenytoin may decrease mucosal uptake of folic acid; to avoid folic acid deficiency and megaloblastic anemia, some clinicians recommend giving patients on anticonvulsants prophylactic doses of folic acid and cyanocobalamin.

Calcium: Hypocalcemia has been reported in patients taking prolonged high-dose therapy with an anticonvulsant. Phenytoin may decrease calcium absorption. Monitor calcium serum concentration and for bone disorders (eg, rickets, osteomalacia). Some clinicians have given an additional 4,000 Units/week of vitamin D (especially in those receiving poor nutrition and getting no sun exposure) to prevent hypocalcemia.

Vitamin D: Phenytoin interferes with vitamin D metabolism and osteomalacia may result; may need to supplement with vitamin D

Glucose: Hyperglycemia and glycosuria may occur in patients receiving high-dose therapy. Monitor blood glucose concentration, especially in patients with impaired renal function.

Tube feedings: Tube feedings decrease phenytoin bioavailability; to avoid decreased serum levels with continuous NG feeds, hold feedings for 2 hours prior to and 2 hours after phenytoin administration, if possible. There is a variety of opinions on how to administer phenytoin with enteral feedings. BE CONSISTENT throughout therapy.

Monitoring Parameters: Blood pressure, vital signs (with I.V. use), plasma phenytoin level, CBC, liver function tests

Reference Range: Timing of serum samples: Because it is slowly absorbed, peak blood levels may occur 4-8 hours after ingestion of an oral dose. The serum half-life varies with the dosage and the drug follows Michaelis-Menten kinetics. The average adult half-life is about 24 hours. Steady-state concentrations are reached in 5-10 days.

Neonates: 8-15 μg/mL total phenytoin; 1-2 μg/mL free phenytoin

Children and Adults: Toxicity is measured clinically, and some patients require levels outside the suggested therapeutic range
- Toxic: 30-50 μg/mL;
- **Lethal**: >100 μg/mL

Therapeutic range:
- Total phenytoin: 10-20 μg/mL (children and adults), 8-15 μg/mL (neonates)
- Concentrations of 5-10 μg/mL may be therapeutic for some patients but concentrations <5 μg/mL are not likely to be effective
- 50% of patients show decreased frequency of seizures at concentrations >10 μg/mL
- 86% of patients show decreased frequency of seizures at concentrations >15 μg/mL
- Add another anticonvulsant if satisfactory therapeutic response is not achieved with a phenytoin concentration of 20 μg/mL

Free phenytoin: 1-2.5 μg/mL

Toxic: <30-50 μg/mL (SI: <120-200 μmol/L)

Lethal: >100 μg/mL (SI: >400 μmol/L)

When to draw levels: This is dependent on the disease state being treated and the clinical condition of the patient

Key points:
- Slow absorption minimizes fluctuations between peak and trough concentrations, timing of sampling not crucial
- Trough concentrations are generally recommended for routine monitoring. Daily levels are not necessary and may result in incorrect dosage adjustments. If it is determined essential to monitor free phenytoin concentrations, concomitant monitoring of total phenytoin concentrations is not necessary and expensive.

After a loading dose: Draw level within 48-96 hours

Rapid achievement: Draw within 2-3 days of therapy initiation to ensure that the patient's metabolism is not remarkably different from that which would be predicted by average literature-derived pharmacokinetic parameters; early levels should be used cautiously in design of new dosing regimens

Second concentration: Draw within 6-7 days with subsequent doses of phenytoin adjusted accordingly

Adjustment of Serum Concentration in Patients With Low Serum Albumin

Measured Total Phenytoin Concentration (mcg/mL)	Patient's Serum Albumin (g/dL)			
	3.5	3	2.5	2
	Adjusted Total Phenytoin Concentration (mcg/mL)*			
5	6	7	8	10
10	13	14	17	20
15	19	21	25	30

*Adjusted concentration = measured total concentration ÷ [(0.2 x albumin) + 0.1].

Adjustment of Serum Concentration in Patients With Renal Failure (Cl_{cr} ≤10 mL/min)

Measured Total Phenytoin Concentration (mcg/mL)	Patient's Serum Albumin (g/dL)				
	4	3.5	3	2.5	2
	Adjusted Total Phenytoin Concentration (mcg/mL)*				
5	10	11	13	14	17
10	20	22	25	29	33
15	30	33	38	43	50

*Adjusted concentration = measured total concentration ÷ [(0.1 x albumin) + 0.1].

In stable patients requiring long-term therapy, generally monitor levels at 3- to 12-month intervals

Phenytoin *(Continued)*

If plasma concentrations have not changed over a 3- to 5-day period, monitoring interval may be increased to once weekly in the acute clinical setting

Related Information

Anticonvulsants by Seizure Type Comparison *on page 1230*
Epilepsy Guidelines *on page 1091*

- **Pherazine® VC w/ Codeine** *see* Promethazine, Phenylephrine, and Codeine *on page 780*
- **Pherazine® w/DM** *see* Promethazine and Dextromethorphan *on page 780*
- **Pherazine® With Codeine** *see* Promethazine and Codeine *on page 780*
- **Phillips'® Magnesia Tablets** *see* Magnesium Hydroxide *on page 550*
- **Phillips'® Milk of Magnesia** *see* Magnesium Hydroxide *on page 550*
- **pHisoHex®** *see* Hexachlorophene *on page 436*
- **Phos-Ex® 125** *see* Calcium Acetate *on page 130*
- **Phos-Flur®** *see* Fluoride *on page 376*
- **PhosLo®** *see* Calcium Acetate *on page 130*
- **Phospholine Iodide** *see* Echothiophate Iodide *on page 305*
- **Phospholine Iodide® Ophthalmic** *see* Echothiophate Iodide *on page 305*
- **Photofrin®** *see* Porfimer *on page 749*
- **Phrenilin®** *see* Butalbital Compound *on page 123*
- **Phrenilin® Forte** *see* Butalbital Compound *on page 123*
- **Phyllocontin®** *see* Theophylline Salts *on page 906*

Physostigmine (fye zoe STIG meen)

Pharmacologic Class Acetylcholinesterase Inhibitor (Peripheral); Ophthalmic Agent, Antiglaucoma

U.S. Brand Names Antilirium®; Isopto® Eserine

Generic Available Yes: Ophthalmic

Mechanism of Action Inhibits destruction of acetylcholine by acetylcholinesterase which facilitates transmission of impulses across myoneural junction and prolongs the central and peripheral effects of acetylcholine

Use Reverse toxic CNS effects caused by anticholinergic drugs; used as miotic in treatment of glaucoma

USUAL DOSAGE

Children: Anticholinergic drug overdose: Reserve for life-threatening situations only: I.V.: 0.01-0.03 mg/kg/dose, (maximum: 0.5 mg/minute); may repeat after 5-10 minutes to a maximum total dose of 2 mg or until response occurs or adverse cholinergic effects occur

Adults: Anticholinergic drug overdose:

I.M., I.V., S.C.: 0.5-2 mg to start, repeat every 20 minutes until response occurs or adverse effect occurs

Repeat 1-4 mg every 30-60 minutes as life-threatening signs (arrhythmias, seizures, deep coma) recur; maximum I.V. rate: 1 mg/minute

Ophthalmic:

Ointment: Instill a small quantity to lower fornix up to 3 times/day
Solution: Instill 1-2 drops into eye(s) up to 4 times/day

Dosage Forms INJ as salicylate: 1 mg/mL (2 mL). **OINT, ophth** as sulfate: 0.25% (3.5 g, 3.7 g)

Contraindications Hypersensitivity to physostigmine or any component; GI or GU obstruction; physostigmine therapy of drug intoxications should be used with extreme caution in patients with asthma, gangrene, severe cardiovascular disease, or mechanical obstruction of the GI tract or urogenital tract. In these patients, physostigmine should be used only to treat life-threatening conditions.

Warnings/Precautions Use with caution in patients with epilepsy, asthma, diabetes, gangrene, cardiovascular disease, bradycardia. Discontinue if excessive salivation or emesis, frequent urination or diarrhea occur. Reduce dosage if excessive sweating or nausea occurs. Administer I.V. slowly or at a controlled rate not faster than 1 mg/minute. Due to the possibility of hypersensitivity or overdose/cholinergic crisis, atropine should be readily available; ointment may delay corneal healing, may cause loss of dark adaptation; not intended as a first-line agent for anticholinergic toxicity or Parkinson's disease.

Pregnancy Risk Factor C

Adverse Reactions

Ophthalmic:

>10%:

Ocular: Lacrimation, marked miosis, blurred vision, eye pain
Miscellaneous: Diaphoresis

1% to 10%:

Central nervous system: Headache, browache
Dermatologic: Burning, redness

Systemic:

>10%:

Gastrointestinal: Nausea, salivation, diarrhea, stomach pains

Ocular: Lacrimation

Miscellaneous: Diaphoresis

1% to 10%:

Cardiovascular: Palpitations, bradycardia

Central nervous system: Restlessness, nervousness, hallucinations, seizures

Genitourinary: Frequent urge to urinate

Neuromuscular & skeletal: Muscle twitching

Ocular: Miosis

Respiratory: Dyspnea, bronchospasm, respiratory paralysis, pulmonary edema

Drug Interactions Increased toxicity: Bethanechol, methacholine, succinylcholine may increase neuromuscular blockade with systemic administration

Onset Ophthalmic instillation: Within 2 minutes; Parenteral: Within 5 minutes

Duration Ophthalmic: 12-48 hours; Parenteral: 0.5-5 hours

Half-Life 15-40 minutes

Education and Monitoring Issues

Patient Education: Systemic: Maintain adequate hydration (2-3 L/day of fluids unless instructed to restrict fluid intake). May cause dizziness, drowsiness, or hypotension (rise slowly from sitting or lying position and use caution when driving or climbing stairs); vomiting or loss of appetite (frequent small meals, frequent mouth care, chewing gum, or sucking lozenges may help); or diarrhea (boiled milk, yogurt, or buttermilk may help). Report persistent abdominal discomfort; significantly increased salivation, sweating, tearing, or urination; flushed skin; chest pain or palpitations; acute headache; unresolved diarrhea; excessive fatigue, insomnia, dizziness, or depression; increased muscle, joint, or body pain; vision changes or blurred vision; or shortness of breath or wheezing.

Ophthalmic: For ophthalmic use only. Wash hands before using. Tilt head back and look upward. Put drops of suspension or apply thin ribbon of ointment inside lower eyelid. Close eye and roll eyeball in all directions. Do not blink for ½ minute. Apply gentle pressure to inner corner of eye for 30 seconds. Do not use any other eye preparation for at least 10 minutes. Do not touch tip of applicator to eye or contaminate tip of applicator. Do not share medication with anyone else. Wear sunglasses when in sunlight; you may be more sensitive to bright light. Inform prescriber if condition worsens or fails to improve or if you experience eye pain, vision disturbances, or other adverse eye response; excess sweating; urinary frequency; severe headache; or skin rash, redness, or burning.

Phytonadione (fye toe na DYE one)

Pharmacologic Class Vitamin, Fat Soluble

U.S. Brand Names AquaMEPHYTON® Injection; Konakion® Injection; Mephyton® Oral

Generic Available No

Mechanism of Action Promotes liver synthesis of clotting factors (II, VII, IX, X); however, the exact mechanism as to this stimulation is unknown. Menadiol is a water soluble form of vitamin K; phytonadione has a more rapid and prolonged effect than menadione; menadiol sodium diphosphate (K_4) is half as potent as menadione (K_3).

Use Prevention and treatment of hypoprothrombinemia caused by drug-induced or anticoagulant-induced vitamin K deficiency, hemorrhagic disease of the newborn; phytonadione is more effective and is preferred to other vitamin K preparations in the presence of impending hemorrhage; oral absorption depends on the presence of bile salts

USUAL DOSAGE I.V. route should be restricted for emergency use only

Minimum daily requirement: Not well established

Infants: 1-5 mcg/kg/day

Adults: 0.03 mcg/kg/day

Hemorrhagic disease of the newborn:

Prophylaxis: I.M.: 0.5-1 mg within 1 hour of birth

Treatment: I.M., S.C.: 1-2 mg/dose/day

Oral anticoagulant overdose:

Infants: I.M., S.C.: 1-2 mg/dose every 4-8 hours

Children and Adults: Oral, I.M., I.V., S.C.: 2.5-10 mg/dose; rarely up to 25-50 mg has been used; may repeat in 6-8 hours if given by I.M., I.V., S.C. route; may repeat 12-48 hours after oral route

Vitamin K deficiency: Due to drugs, malabsorption or decreased synthesis of vitamin K

Infants and Children:

Oral: 2.5-5 mg/24 hours

I.M., I.V.: 1-2 mg/dose as a single dose

Adults:

Oral: 5-25 mg/24 hours

I.M., I.V.: 10 mg

Dosage Forms INJ: Aqueous colloidal: 2 mg/mL (0.5 mL); 10 mg/mL (1 mL, 2.5 mL, 5 mL); Aqueous (I.M. only): 2 mg/mL (0.5 mL); 10 mg/mL (1 mL). **TAB:** 5 mg

Contraindications Hypersensitivity to phytonadione or any component

(Continued)

Phytonadione *(Continued)*

Warnings/Precautions Severe reactions resembling anaphylaxis or hypersensitivity have occurred rarely during or immediately after I.V. administration (even with proper dilution and rate of administration); restrict I.V. administration for emergency use only; ineffective in hereditary hypoprothrombinemia, hypoprothrombinemia caused by severe liver disease; severe hemolytic anemia has been reported rarely in neonates following large doses (10-20 mg) of phytonadione

Pregnancy Risk Factor C

Adverse Reactions <1%: Abnormal taste, anaphylaxis, cyanosis, diaphoresis, dizziness (rarely), dyspnea, GI upset (oral), hemolysis in neonates and in patients with G-6-PD deficiency, hypersensitivity reactions, pain, rarely hypotension, tenderness at injection site, transient flushing reaction

Drug Interactions Decreased effect: Warfarin sodium, dicumarol, anisindione effects antagonized by phytonadione; mineral oil may decrease GI absorption of vitamin K

Onset Onset of increased coagulation factors: Oral: Within 6-12 hours; Parenteral: Within 1-2 hours; prothrombin may become normal after 12-14 hours

Education and Monitoring Issues

Patient Education: Oral: Take only as directed; do not take more or more often than prescribed. Avoid excessive or increased intake of vitamin K containing food (eg, green leafy vegetables, dairy products, meats) unless recommended by prescriber. Avoid alcohol and any OTC or prescribed medications containing aspirin that are not approved by prescriber. Report bleeding gums; blood in urine, stool, or vomitus; unusual bruising of bleeding; or abdominal cramping.

Monitoring Parameters: PT

- **Pilagan® Ophthalmic** *see* Pilocarpine *on page 736*
- **Pilocar® Ophthalmic** *see* Pilocarpine *on page 736*

Pilocarpine (pye loe KAR peen)

Pharmacologic Class Cholinergic Agonist; Ophthalmic Agent, Antiglaucoma; Ophthalmic Agent, Miotic

U.S. Brand Names Adsorbocarpine® Ophthalmic; Isopto® Carpine Ophthalmic; Ocu-Carpine® Ophthalmic; Ocusert Pilo-20® Ophthalmic; Ocusert Pilo-40® Ophthalmic; Pilagan® Ophthalmic; Pilocar® Ophthalmic; Pilopine HS® Ophthalmic; Piloptic® Ophthalmic; Pilostat® Ophthalmic; Salagen® Oral

Use

Ophthalmic: Management of chronic simple glaucoma, chronic and acute angle-closure glaucoma; counter effects of cycloplegics

Oral: Symptomatic treatment of xerostomia caused by salivary gland hypofunction resulting from radiotherapy for cancer of the head and neck

USUAL DOSAGE Adults:

Ophthalmic:

Nitrate solution: Shake well before using; instill 1-2 drops 2-4 times/day

Hydrochloride solution:

Instill 1-2 drops up to 6 times/day; adjust the concentration and frequency as required to control elevated intraocular pressure

To counteract the mydriatic effects of sympathomimetic agents: Instill 1 drop of a 1% solution in the affected eye

Gel: Instill 0.5" ribbon into lower conjunctival sac once daily at bedtime

Ocular systems: Systems are labeled in terms of mean rate of release of pilocarpine over 7 days; begin with 20 mcg/hour at night and adjust based on response

Oral: 5 mg 3 times/day, titration up to 10 mg 3 times/day may be considered for patients who have not responded adequately

Contraindications Acute inflammatory disease of anterior chamber, hypersensitivity to pilocarpine or any component

Pregnancy Risk Factor C

Related Information

Pilocarpine and Epinephrine *on page 736*

Pilocarpine and Epinephrine (pye loe KAR peen & ep i NEF rin)

Pharmacologic Class Ophthalmic Agent, Antiglaucoma; Ophthalmic Agent, Miotic

U.S. Brand Names E-Pilo-x® Ophthalmic; P_xE_x® Ophthalmic

Dosage Forms SOLN, ophth: Epinephrine bitartrate 1% and pilocarpine hydrochloride 1%, 2%, 3%, 4%, 6% (15 mL)

Pregnancy Risk Factor C

- **Pilopine HS® Ophthalmic** *see* Pilocarpine *on page 736*
- **Piloptic® Ophthalmic** *see* Pilocarpine *on page 736*
- **Pilostat® Ophthalmic** *see* Pilocarpine *on page 736*
- **Pima®** *see* Potassium Iodide *on page 754*

Pimozide (PI moe zide)

Pharmacologic Class Antipsychotic Agent, Diphenylbutylperidine

U.S. Brand Names Orap™

Generic Available No

Mechanism of Action A potent centrally-acting dopamine-receptor antagonist resulting in its characteristic neuroleptic effects

Use Suppression of severe motor and phonic tics in patients with Tourette's disorder

USUAL DOSAGE Children >12 years and Adults: Oral: Initial: 1-2 mg/day, then increase dosage as needed every other day; range is usually 7-16 mg/day, maximum dose: 20 mg/day or 0.3 mg/kg/day should not be exceeded

Dosing adjustment in hepatic impairment: Reduction of dose is necessary in patients with liver disease

Dosage Forms TAB: 2 mg

Contraindications Simple tics other than Tourette's, history of cardiac dysrhythmias, known hypersensitivity to pimozide; use in patients receiving nefazodone, zileuton, macrolide antibiotics such as clarithromycin, erythromycin, azithromycin, troleandomycin and dirithromycin, azole antifungal agents such as itraconazole and ketoconazole, and/or protease inhibitors such as ritonavir, saquinavir, indinavir, nelfinavir, other inhibitors of CYP3A4

Warnings/Precautions Sudden, unexpected deaths have been known to occur in patients taking high doses (>10 mg) of pimozide. One possible explanation is prolongation of Q-T intervals predisposing the patients to arrhythmias. May alter cardiac conduction - life-threatening arrhythmias have occurred with therapeutic doses of phenothiazines. May cause hypotension, use with caution in patients with autonomic instability. Moderately sedating, use with caution in disorders where CNS depression is a feature. Use with caution in Parkinson's disease. Caution in patients with hemodynamic instability; bone marrow suppression; predisposition to seizures; subcortical brain damage; severe cardiac, hepatic, renal, or respiratory disease. Esophageal dysmotility and aspiration have been associated with antipsychotic use - use with caution in patients at risk of pneumonia (ie, Alzheimer's disease). Caution in breast cancer or other prolactin-dependent tumors (may elevate prolactin levels). May alter temperature regulation or mask toxicity of other drugs due to antiemetic effects. May cause orthostatic hypotension - use with caution in patients at risk of this effect or those who would tolerate transient hypotensive episodes (cerebrovascular disease, cardiovascular disease, or other medications which may predispose).

May cause anticholinergic effects (confusion, agitation, constipation, dry mouth, blurred vision, urinary retention); therefore, use with caution in patients with decreased gastrointestinal motility, urinary retention, BPH, xerostomia, or visual problems. Conditions which also may be exacerbated by cholinergic blockade include narrow-angle glaucoma (screening is recommended) and worsening of myasthenia gravis. Relative to neuroleptics, pimozide has a moderate potency of cholinergic blockade.

May cause extrapyramidal reactions, including pseudoparkinsonism, acute dystonic reactions, akathisia, and tardive dyskinesia (risk of these reactions is high relative to other neuroleptics). May be associated with neuroleptic malignant syndrome (NMS) or pigmentary retinopathy.

Avoid concurrent grapefruit juice, macrolide antibiotics, azole antifungal agents, protease inhibitors, nefazodone, and zileuton due to their potential inhibition of pimozide metabolism, leading to the accumulation of active compound and the increased chance of serious arrhythmias

Pregnancy Risk Factor C

Adverse Reactions

Cardiovascular: Swelling of face, tachycardia, orthostatic hypotension, chest pain, hypertension, palpitations, ventricular arrhythmias, Q-T prolongation

Central nervous system: Extrapyramidal signs (akathisia, akinesia, dystonia, pseudoparkinsonism, tardive dyskinesia), drowsiness, NMS, headache, dizziness, excitement

Dermatologic: Rash

Endocrine & metabolic: Edema of breasts, decreased libido

Gastrointestinal: Constipation, xerostomia, weight gain or loss, nausea, salivation, vomiting, anorexia

Genitourinary: Impotence

Hematologic: Blood dyscrasias

Hepatic: Jaundice

Neuromuscular & skeletal: Weakness, tremor

Ocular: Visual disturbance, decreased accommodation, blurred vision

Miscellaneous: Diaphoresis

Drug Interactions CYP1A2 enzyme substrate (minor); CYP3A3/4 enzyme substrate

Antipsychotics inhibit the ability of bromocriptine to lower serum prolactin concentrations

Benztropine (and other anticholinergics) may inhibit the therapeutic response to pimozide and excess anticholinergic effects may occur

Chloroquine may increase pimozide concentrations

(Continued)

Pimozide *(Continued)*

Cigarette smoking may enhance the hepatic metabolism of pimozide. Larger doses may be required compared to a nonsmoker
Concurrent use of pimozide with an antihypertensive may produce additive hypotensive effects
Antihypertensive effects of guanethidine and guanadrel may be inhibited by pimozide
Concurrent use with TCA may produce increased toxicity or altered therapeutic response
Fluoxetine concurrent use caused bradycardia (case report)
Pimozide may inhibit the antiparkinsonian effect of levodopa; avoid this combination
Pimozide plus lithium may rarely produce neurotoxicity
Barbiturates may reduce pimozide concentrations
Propranolol may increase pimozide concentrations
Protease inhibitors (amprenavir, ritonavir, nelfinavir) may increase the serum levels of pimozide
Sulfadoxine-pyrimethamine may increase pimozide concentrations
Pimozide and possibly other low potency antipsychotics may reverse the pressor effects of epinephrine
Pimozide and CNS depressants (ethanol, narcotics) may produce additive CNS depressant effects
Pimozide and trazodone may produce additive hypotensive effects
Carbamazepine may stimulate the metabolism of pimozide; monitor for reduced efficacy
Macrolide antibiotics (clarithromycin, erythromycin, dirithromycin, azithromycin, and troleandomycin), azole antifungals, protease inhibitors, nefazodone, and zileuton inhibit metabolism of pimozide and may predispose to life-threatening arrhythmias

Alcohol Interactions Avoid use (may increase central nervous system depression)

Half-Life 50 hours

Education and Monitoring Issues

Patient Education: Use exactly as directed (do not increase dose or frequency); may cause physical and/or psychological dependence. It may take 2-3 weeks to achieve desired results; do not discontinue without consulting prescriber. Avoid excess alcohol or caffeine and other prescription or OTC medications not approved by prescriber. Maintain adequate hydration (2-3 L/day of fluids unless instructed to restrict fluid intake). You may experience excess drowsiness, restlessness, dizziness, or blurred vision (use caution driving or when engaging in tasks requiring alertness until response to drug is known); or constipation, dry mouth, anorexia (increased exercise, fluids, or dietary fruit and fiber may help). Report persistent CNS effects (eg, trembling fingers, altered gait or balance, excessive sedation, seizures, unusual muscle or facial movements, anxiety, abnormal thoughts, confusion, personality changes); unresolved constipation or gastrointestinal effects; breast swelling (male and female) or decreased sexual ability; vision changes; difficulty breathing; unusual cough or flu-like symptoms; or worsening of condition.

Dietary Considerations: Grapefruit juice may potentially inhibit the metabolism of pimozide leading to the accumulation of active compound and the increased chance of serious arrhythmias; avoid concurrent use

Pindolol (PIN doe lole)

Pharmacologic Class Beta Blocker (with Intrinsic Sympathomimetic Activity)

U.S. Brand Names Visken®

Use Management of hypertension

Unlabeled use: Ventricular arrhythmias/tachycardia, antipsychotic-induced akathisia, situational anxiety; aggressive behavior associated with dementia

USUAL DOSAGE

Adults: Initial: 5 mg twice daily, increase as necessary by 10 mg/day every 3-4 weeks; maximum daily dose: 60 mg

Elderly: Initial: 5 mg once daily, increase as necessary by 5 mg/day every 3-4 weeks

Dosing adjustment in renal and hepatic impairment: Reduction is necessary in severely impaired

Contraindications Uncompensated congestive heart failure, cardiogenic shock, bradycardia or heart block, asthma, COPD; hypersensitivity to any component

Pregnancy Risk Factor B (per manufacturer); D (2nd and 3rd trimester, based on expert analysis)

Related Information

Beta-Blockers Comparison *on page 1233*

♦ **Pink Bismuth® [OTC]** *see* Bismuth *on page 108*
♦ **Pin-Rid® [OTC]** *see* Pyrantel Pamoate *on page 793*
♦ **Pin-X® [OTC]** *see* Pyrantel Pamoate *on page 793*

Pioglitazone (pye oh GLI ta zone)

Pharmacologic Class Antidiabetic Agent (Thiazolidinedione)

U.S. Brand Names Actos™

Mechanism of Action Thiazolidinedione antidiabetic agent that lowers blood glucose by improving target cell response to insulin, without increasing pancreatic insulin secretion. It has a mechanism of action that is dependent on the presence of insulin for activity. Pioglitazone is a potent and selective agonist for peroxisome proliferator-activated receptor-gamma (PPARgamma). Activation of nuclear PPARgamma receptors influences the production of a number of gene products involved in glucose and lipid metabolism.

Use

Type 2 diabetes, monotherapy: Adjunct to diet and exercise, to improve glycemic control

Type 2 diabetes, combination therapy with sulfonylurea, metformin, or insulin: When diet, exercise, and a single agent alone does not result in adequate glycemic control

USUAL DOSAGE Adults: Oral:

Monotherapy: Initial: 15-30 mg once daily; if response is inadequate, the dosage may be increased in increments up to 45 mg once daily; maximum recommended dose: 45 mg once daily

Combination therapy:

With sulfonylureas: Initial: 15-30 mg once daily; dose of sulfonylurea should be reduced if the patient reports hypoglycemia

With metformin: Initial: 15-30 mg once daily; it is unlikely that the dose of metformin will need to be reduced due to hypoglycemia

With insulin: Initial: 15-30 mg once daily; dose of insulin should be reduced by 10% to 25% if the patient reports hypoglycemia or if the plasma glucose falls to below 100 mg/dL. Doses greater than 30 mg/day have not been evaluated in combination regimens.

A 1-week washout period is recommended in patients with normal liver enzymes who are changed from troglitazone to pioglitazone therapy.

Dosage adjustment in renal impairment: No dosage adjustment is required.

Dosage adjustment in hepatic impairment: Clearance is significantly lower in hepatic impairment. Therapy should not be initiated if the patient exhibits active liver disease or increased transaminases (>2.5 times the upper limit of normal) at baseline.

Elderly patients: No dosage adjustment is recommended in elderly patients.

Dosage Forms TAB: 15 mg, 30 mg, 45 mg

Contraindications Hypersensitivity to pioglitazone or any component of the formulation. Active liver disease (transaminases >2.5 times the upper limit of normal at baseline).

Warnings/Precautions Should not be used in diabetic ketoacidosis. Mechanism requires the presence of insulin, therefore use in type 1 diabetes is not recommended. May potentiate hypoglycemia when used in combination with sulfonylureas or insulin. Use with caution in premenopausal, anovulatory women - may result in a resumption of ovulation, increasing the risk of pregnancy. Use with caution in patients with anemia (may reduce hemoglobin and hematocrit). Use with caution in patients with heart failure or edema - may increase plasma volume and/or increase cardiac hypertrophy. In general, use should be avoided in patients with NYHA class III or IV heart failure. Use with caution in patients with elevated transaminases (AST or ALT) - see Contraindications and Monitoring Parameters. Idiosyncratic hepatotoxicity has been reported with another thiazolidinedione agent (troglitazone) - monitoring should include periodic determinations of liver function.

Pregnancy Risk Factor C

Pregnancy Implications Treatment during mid-late gestation was associated with delayed partuition, embryotoxicity and postnatal growth retardation in animal models. In animal studies, pioglitazone has been found to be excreted in milk. It is not known whether pioglitazone is excreted in human milk. Should not be administered to a nursing woman.

Adverse Reactions

>10%:

Endocrine & metabolic: Decreased serum triglycerides, increased HDL cholesterol

Gastrointestinal: Weight gain

Respiratory: Upper respiratory tract infection (13.2%)

1% to 10%:

Cardiovascular: Edema (4.8%)

Central nervous system: Headache (9.1%), fatigue (3.6%)

Endocrine & metabolic: Aggravation of diabetes mellitus (5.1%), hypoglycemia (range 2% to 15% when used in combination with sulfonylureas or insulin)

Hematologic; Anemia (1%)

Neuromuscular & skeletal: Myalgia (5.4%)

Respiratory: Sinusitis (6.3%), pharyngitis (5.1%)

<1%: Elevated CPK, elevated transaminases

In combination trials with sulfonylureas or insulin, the incidence of edema was as high as 15%.

Drug Interactions CYP2C8 and CYP3A4 substrate

Decreased effect: Effects of oral contraceptives may be decreased, based on data from a related compound. This has not been specifically evaluated for pioglitazone.

Increased effect/toxicity: Ketoconazole (*in vitro*) inhibits metabolism of pioglitazone. Other inhibitors of CYP3A4, including itraconazole, are likely to decrease pioglitazone metabolism. Patients receiving inhibitors of CYP3A4 should have their glycemic control evaluated more frequently.

Alcohol Interactions Avoid use (may cause hypoglycemia)

Onset Delayed, may require several weeks to reach maximum effect

Half-Life 16-24 hours

(Continued)

Pioglitazone *(Continued)*

Education and Monitoring Issues

Patient Education: Use exactly as directed (do not increase dose or frequency or discontinue without consulting prescriber). May be taken without regard to meals; avoid alcohol while taking this medication. If dose is missed, take as soon as possible. If dose is missed completely one day, do not double dose the next day. Follow dietary, exercise, and glucose monitoring instructions of prescriber (more frequent monitoring may be advised in periods of stress, trauma, surgery, increased exercise, etc). Report respiratory infection, unusual weight gain, aggravation of hyper- or hypoglycemic condition, unusual swelling of extremities, fatigue, yellowing of skin or eyes, dark urine, pale stool, nausea/vomiting, or muscle pain.

Dietary Considerations: Peak concentrations are delayed when administered with food, but the extent of absorption is not affected. Pioglitazone may be taken without regard to meals. Management of type 2 diabetes should include diet control.

Monitoring Parameters: Hemoglobin A_{1c}, liver enzymes (prior to initiation and every 2 months for the first year of treatment, then periodically). If the ALT is increased to >2.5 times the upper limit of normal, liver function testing should be performed more frequently until the levels return to normal or pretreatment values. Patients with an elevation in ALT >3 times the upper limit of normal should be rechecked as soon as possible. If the ALT levels remain >3 times the upper limit of normal, therapy with rosiglitazone should be discontinued.

Manufacturer Takeda Pharmaceuticals America, Inc

Related Information

Hypoglycemic Drugs and Thiazolidinedione Information *on page 1240*
Pharmaceutical Manufacturers Directory *on page 1020*

Piperacillin (pi PER a sil in)

Pharmacologic Class Antibiotic, Penicillin

U.S. Brand Names Pipracil®

Generic Available No

Mechanism of Action Inhibits bacterial cell wall synthesis by binding to one or more of the penicillin binding proteins (PBPs); which in turn inhibits the final transpeptidation step of peptidoglycan synthesis in bacterial cell walls, thus inhibiting cell wall biosynthesis. Bacteria eventually lyse due to ongoing activity of cell wall autolytic enzymes (autolysins and murein hydrolases) while cell wall assembly is arrested.

Use Treatment of susceptible infections such as septicemia, acute and chronic respiratory tract infections, skin and soft tissue infections, and urinary tract infections due to susceptible strains of *Pseudomonas, Proteus,* and *Escherichia coli* and *Enterobacter,* active against some streptococci and some anaerobic bacteria

USUAL DOSAGE

Neonates: 100 mg/kg every 12 hours

Infants and Children: I.M., I.V.: 200-300 mg/kg/day in divided doses every 4-6 hours

Higher doses have been used in cystic fibrosis: 350-500 mg/kg/day in divided doses every 4-6 hours

Adults: I.M., I.V.:

Moderate infections (urinary tract infections): 2-3 g/dose every 6-12 hours; maximum: 2 g I.M./site

Serious infections: 3-4 g/dose every 4-6 hours; maximum: 24 g/24 hours

Uncomplicated gonorrhea: 2 g I.M. in a single dose accompanied by 1 g probenecid 30 minutes prior to injection

Dosing adjustment in renal impairment: Adults: I.V.:

Cl_{cr} 20-40 mL/minute: Administer 3-4 g every 8 hours

Cl_{cr} <20 mL/minute: Administer 3-4 g every 12 hours

Moderately dialyzable (20% to 50%)

Continuous arteriovenous or venovenous hemodiafiltration (CAVH) effects: Dose as for Cl_{cr} 10-50 mL/minute

Dosage Forms POWDER for inj: 2 g, 3 g, 4 g, 40 g

Contraindications Hypersensitivity to piperacillin or any component or penicillins

Warnings/Precautions Dosage modification required in patients with impaired renal function; history of seizure activity; use with caution in patients with a history of beta-lactam allergy

Pregnancy Risk Factor B

Adverse Reactions Percentage unknown: Abnormal platelet aggregation and prolonged PT (high doses), acute interstitial nephritis, anaphylaxis, confusion, convulsions, drowsiness, electrolyte imbalance, fever, hemolytic anemia, hypersensitivity reactions, Jarisch-Herxheimer reaction, myoclonus, positive Coombs' reaction, rash, thrombophlebitis

Drug Interactions

Decreased effect: Tetracyclines may decrease penicillin effectiveness; aminoglycosides → physical inactivation of aminoglycosides in the presence of high concentrations of piperacillin and potential toxicity in patients with mild to moderate renal dysfunction; decreased efficacy of oral contraceptives is possible

Increased effect:

Probenecid may increase penicillin levels

Neuromuscular blockers may increase duration of blockade
Aminoglycosides → synergistic efficacy
Heparin with high-dose parenteral penicillins may result in increased risk of bleeding

Half-Life Dose-dependent; prolonged with moderately severe renal or hepatic impairment: 36-80 minutes

Education and Monitoring Issues

Patient Education: This medication will be administered I.V. or I.M. Maintain adequate hydration (2-3 L/day of fluids unless instructed to restrict fluid intake). If being treated for sexually transmitted disease, partner will also need to be treated. Small frequent meals, frequent mouth care, sucking lozenges, or chewing gum may reduce nausea or dry mouth. Important to maintain good oral and vaginal hygiene to reduce incidence of opportunistic infection. Diabetics should use serum glucose testing while on this medication. If diabetic, drug may cause false tests with Clinitest® urine glucose monitoring; use of glucose oxidase methods (Clinistix®) or serum glucose monitoring is preferable. This drug may interfere with oral contraceptives; an alternate form of birth control should be used. Report persistent diarrhea, fever, chills, unhealed sores, bloody urine or stool, muscle pain, mouth sores, or difficulty breathing.

Monitoring Parameters: Observe for signs and symptoms for anaphylaxis during first dose

Manufacturer Lederle Laboratories

Related Information

Antimicrobial Drugs of Choice *on page 1182*
Community Acquired Pneumonia in Adults *on page 1200*
Pharmaceutical Manufacturers Directory *on page 1020*

Piperacillin and Tazobactam Sodium

(pi PER a sil in & ta zoe BAK tam SOW dee um)

Pharmacologic Class Antibiotic, Penicillin

U.S. Brand Names Zosyn™

Mechanism of Action Inhibits bacterial cell wall synthesis by binding to one or more of the penicillin binding proteins (PBPs); which in turn inhibits the final transpeptidation step of peptidoglycan synthesis in bacterial cell walls, thus inhibiting cell wall biosynthesis. Bacteria eventually lyse due to ongoing activity of cell wall autolytic enzymes (autolysins and murein hydrolases) while cell wall assembly is arrested. Tazobactam inhibits many beta-lactamases, including staphylococcal penicillinase and Richmond and Sykes types II, III, IV, and V, including extended spectrum enzymes; it has only limited activity against class I beta-lactamases other than class Ic types.

Use Treatment of infections of lower respiratory tract, urinary tract, skin and skin structures, gynecologic, bone and joint infections, and septicemia caused by susceptible organisms. Tazobactam expands activity of piperacillin to include beta-lactamase producing strains of *S. aureus*, *H. influenzae*, *Bacteroides*, and other gram-negative bacteria.

USUAL DOSAGE

Children <12 years: Not recommended due to lack of data

Children >12 years and Adults:

Severe infections: I.V.: Piperacillin/tazobactam 4/0.5 g every 8 hours or 3/0.375 g every 6 hours

Moderate infections: I.M.: Piperacillin/tazobactam 2/0.25 g every 6-8 hours; treatment should be continued for ≥7-10 days depending on severity of disease (Note: I.M. route not FDA-approved)

Dosing interval in renal impairment:

Cl_{cr} 20-40 mL/minute: Administer 2/0.25 g every 6 hours

Cl_{cr} <20 mL/minute: Administer 2/0.25 g every 8 hours

Hemodialysis: Administer 2/0.25 g every 8 hours with an additional dose of 0.75 g after each dialysis

Continuous arteriovenous or venovenous hemodiafiltration (CAVH) effects: Dose as for Cl_{cr} 10-50 mL/minute

Dosage Forms INJ: Piperacillin sodium 2 g and tazobactam sodium 0.25 g; piperacillin sodium 3 g and tazobactam sodium 0.375 g; Piperacillin sodium 4 g and tazobactam sodium 0.5 g (vials at an 8:1 ratio of piperacillin sodium/tazobactam sodium)

Contraindications Hypersensitivity to penicillins, beta-lactamase inhibitors, or any component

Warnings/Precautions Due to sodium load and to the adverse effects of high serum concentrations of penicillins, dosage modification is required in patients with impaired or underdeveloped renal function; use with caution in patients with seizures or in patients with history of beta-lactam allergy; safety and efficacy have not been established in children <12 years of age

Pregnancy Risk Factor B

Pregnancy Implications Breast-feeding/lactation: Use by the breast-feeding mother may result in diarrhea, candidiasis, or allergic response in the infant

Adverse Reactions

>10%: Gastrointestinal: Diarrhea (11.3%)

1% to 10%:

Cardiovascular: Hypertension (1.6%)

(Continued)

Piperacillin and Tazobactam Sodium *(Continued)*

Central nervous system: Insomnia (6.7%), headache (7% to 8%), agitation (2%), fever (2.4%), dizziness (1.4%)

Dermatologic: Rash (4%), pruritus (3%)

Gastrointestinal: Constipation (7% to 8%), nausea (6.9%), vomiting/dyspepsia (3.3%)

Respiratory: Rhinitis/dyspnea (~1%)

Miscellaneous: Serum sickness-like reaction

<1%: Bronchospasm, confusion, edema, hypotension, pseudomembranous colitis

Several laboratory abnormalities have rarely been associated with piperacillin/tazobactam including reversible eosinophilia, and neutropenia (associated most often with prolonged therapy), positive direct Coombs' test, prolonged PT and PTT, transient elevations of LFT, increases in creatinine

Drug Interactions

Decreased effect: Tetracyclines may decrease penicillin effectiveness; aminoglycosides → physical inactivation of aminoglycosides in the presence of high concentrations of piperacillin and potential toxicity in patients with mild to moderate renal dysfunction; decreased efficacy of oral contraceptives is possible

Increased effect:

Probenecid may increase penicillin levels

Neuromuscular blockers may increase duration of blockade

Aminoglycosides → synergistic efficacy

Heparin with high-dose parenteral penicillins may result in increased risk of bleeding

Half-Life Piperacillin: 1 hour; Piperacillin (desethyl) metabolite: 1-1.5 hours; Tazobactam: 0.7-0.9 hour

Education and Monitoring Issues

Patient Education: This medication will be administered I.V. or I.M. Maintain adequate hydration (2-3 L/day of fluids unless instructed to restrict fluid intake). Small frequent meals, frequent mouth care, sucking lozenges, or chewing gum may reduce nausea or dry mouth. Important to maintain good oral and vaginal hygiene to reduce incidence of opportunistic infection. Diabetics should use serum glucose testing while receiving this medication. If diabetic, drug may cause false tests with Clinitest® urine glucose monitoring; use of glucose oxidase methods (Clinistix®) or serum glucose monitoring is preferable. This drug may interfere with oral contraceptives; an alternate form of birth control should be used. Report persistent diarrhea, fever, chills, unhealed sores, bloody urine or stool, muscle pain, mouth sores, or difficulty breathing, or skin rash.

Monitoring Parameters: LFTs, creatinine, BUN, CBC with differential, serum electrolytes, urinalysis, PT, PTT; monitor for signs of anaphylaxis during first dose

Manufacturer Lederle Laboratories

Related Information

Antimicrobial Drugs of Choice *on page 1182*

Community Acquired Pneumonia in Adults *on page 1200*

Pharmaceutical Manufacturers Directory *on page 1020*

Piperazine (PI per a zeen)

Pharmacologic Class Anthelmintic

U.S. Brand Names Vermizine®

Generic Available Yes

Mechanism of Action Causes muscle paralysis of the roundworm by blocking the effects of acetylcholine at the neuromuscular junction

Use Treatment of pinworm and roundworm infections (used as an alternative to first-line agents, mebendazole, or pyrantel pamoate)

USUAL DOSAGE Oral:

Pinworms: Children and Adults: 65 mg/kg/day (not to exceed 2.5 g/day) as a single daily dose for 7 days; in severe infections, repeat course after a 1-week interval

Roundworms:

Children: 75 mg/kg/day as a single daily dose for 2 days; maximum: 3.5 g/day

Adults: 3.5 g/day for 2 days (in severe infections, repeat course, after a 1-week interval)

Dosage Forms SYR: 500 mg/5 mL (473 mL, 4000 mL). **TAB:** 250 mg

Contraindications Seizure disorders, liver or kidney impairment, hypersensitivity to piperazine or any component

Warnings/Precautions Use with caution in patients with anemia or malnutrition; avoid prolonged use especially in children

Pregnancy Risk Factor B

Adverse Reactions <1%: Bronchospasms, diarrhea, dizziness, EEG changes, headache, hemolytic anemia, hypersensitivity reactions, nausea, seizures, vertigo, visual impairment, vomiting, weakness

Drug Interactions Pyrantel pamoate (antagonistic mode of action)

Education and Monitoring Issues

Patient Education: Take on empty stomach; if severe or persistent headache, loss of balance or coordination, dizziness, vomiting, diarrhea, or rash occurs, contact prescriber. If used for pinworm infections, all members of the family should be treated.

Monitoring Parameters: Stool exam for worms and ova

Pipobroman (pi poe BROE man)

Pharmacologic Class Antineoplastic Agent

U.S. Brand Names Vercyte®

Generic Available No

Mechanism of Action Although its exact mechanism of action is not known, pipobroman appears to work as a polyfunctional alkylating agent, forming covalent cross-links with DNA, misreading of the DNA code and inhibition of DNA, RNA, and protein synthesis

Use Treat polycythemia vera; chronic myelocytic leukemia (in patients refractory to busulfan)

USUAL DOSAGE Children >15 years and Adults (refer to individual protocols): Oral:

Polycythemia: 1 mg/kg/day for 30 days; may increase to 1.5-3 mg/kg until hematocrit reduced to 50% to 55%; maintenance: 0.1-0.2 mg/kg/day

Myelocytic leukemia: 1.5-2.5 mg/kg/day until WBC drops to 10,000/mm^3 then start maintenance 7-175 mg/day; stop if WBC falls to <3000/mm^3 or platelets fall to <150,000/mm^3

Dosage Forms TAB: 25 mg

Contraindications Hypersensitivity to pipobroman or any component; pre-existing bone marrow suppression; pregnancy

Warnings/Precautions The U.S. Food and Drug Administration (FDA) currently recommends that procedures for proper handling and disposal of antineoplastic agents be considered. Avoid I.M. injection of medications if platelet count is <100,000/mm^3. Avoid rectal administration of medications if platelet count is <100,000/mm^3 or absolute neutrophil count is <1000/mm^3.

Pregnancy Risk Factor D

Adverse Reactions

>10%: Hematologic: Leukopenia, myelosuppression, thrombocytopenia

1% to 10%:

Dermatologic: Rash

Gastrointestinal: Abdominal cramps, diarrhea, nausea, vomiting

Hematologic: Anemia

Education and Monitoring Issues

Patient Education: Notify prescriber if nausea, vomiting, diarrhea, or rash become severe or if unusual bleeding or bruising, sore throat, or fatigue occur; contraceptives are recommended during therapy

Monitoring Parameters: CBC, liver and renal function tests

♦ **Pipracil®** *see* Piperacillin *on page 740*

Pirbuterol (peer BYOO ter ole)

Pharmacologic Class $Beta_2$ Agonist

U.S. Brand Names Maxair™ Autohaler™; Maxair™ Inhalation Aerosol

Generic Available No

Mechanism of Action Pirbuterol is a $beta_2$-adrenergic agonist with a similar structure to albuterol, specifically a pyridine ring has been substituted for the benzene ring in albuterol. The increased $beta_2$ selectivity of pirbuterol results from the substitution of a tertiary butyl group on the nitrogen of the side chain, which additionally imparts resistance of pirbuterol to degradation by monoamine oxidase and provides a lengthened duration of action in comparison to the less selective previous beta-agonist agents.

Use Prevention and treatment of reversible bronchospasm including asthma

USUAL DOSAGE Children >12 years and Adults: 2 inhalations every 4-6 hours for prevention; two inhalations at an interval of at least 1-3 minutes, followed by a third inhalation in treatment of bronchospasm, not to exceed 12 inhalations/day

Dosage Forms AERO, oral: 0.2 mg per actuation [25.6 g] (300 inhalations); Autohaler™: 0.2 mg per actuation [2.8 g] (80 inhalations), [14 g] (400 inhalations)

Contraindications Hypersensitivity to pirbuterol or albuterol

Warnings/Precautions Excessive use may result in tolerance; some adverse reactions may occur more frequently in children 2-5 years of age; use with caution in patients with hyperthyroidism, diabetes mellitus; cardiovascular disorders including coronary insufficiency or hypertension or sensitivity to sympathomimetic amines

Pregnancy Risk Factor C

Adverse Reactions

>10%:

Central nervous system: Nervousness, restlessness

Neuromuscular & skeletal: Trembling

1% to 10%:

Central nervous system: Headache, dizziness

Gastrointestinal: Taste changes, vomiting, nausea

<1%: Anorexia, arrhythmias, bruising, chest pain, hypertension, insomnia, numbness in hands, paradoxical bronchospasm, weakness

Drug Interactions

Decreased effect with beta-blockers

(Continued)

Pirbuterol *(Continued)*

Increased toxicity with other beta agonists, MAO inhibitors, TCAs

Onset Peak therapeutic effect: Inhalation: 0.5-1 hour

Half-Life 2-3 hours

Education and Monitoring Issues

Patient Education: Use exactly as directed. Do not use more often than recommended. Maintain adequate hydration (2-3 L/day of fluids unless instructed to restrict fluid intake). You may experience nervousness, dizziness, or fatigue (use caution when driving or engaging in tasks requiring alertness until response to drug is known); or dry mouth, stomach upset (frequent small meals, frequent mouth care, chewing gum, or sucking hard candy may help). Report unresolved GI upset; dizziness or fatigue; vision changes; chest pain, rapid heartbeat, or palpitations; nervousness or insomnia; muscle cramping or tremor; or unusual cough.

Monitoring Parameters: Respiratory rate, heart rate, and blood pressure

Manufacturer 3M Pharmaceuticals

Related Information

Bronchodilators Comparison *on page 1235*
Pharmaceutical Manufacturers Directory *on page 1020*

Piroxicam (peer OKS i kam)

Pharmacologic Class Nonsteroidal Anti-Inflammatory Agent (NSAID)

U.S. Brand Names Feldene®

Generic Available No

Mechanism of Action Inhibits prostaglandin synthesis, acts on the hypothalamus heat-regulating center to reduce fever, blocks prostaglandin synthetase action which prevents formation of the platelet-aggregating substance thromboxane A_2; decreases pain receptor sensitivity. Other proposed mechanisms of action for salicylate anti-inflammatory action are lysosomal stabilization, kinin and leukotriene production, alteration of chemotactic factors, and inhibition of neutrophil activation. This latter mechanism may be the most significant pharmacologic action to reduce inflammation.

Use Management of inflammatory disorders; symptomatic treatment of acute and chronic rheumatoid arthritis, osteoarthritis, and ankylosing spondylitis; also used to treat sunburn

USUAL DOSAGE Oral:

Children: 0.2-0.3 mg/kg/day once daily; maximum dose: 15 mg/day

Adults: 10-20 mg/day once daily; although associated with increase in GI adverse effects, doses >20 mg/day have been used (ie, 30-40 mg/day)

Dosing adjustment in hepatic impairment: Reduction of dosage is necessary

Dosage Forms CAP: 10 mg, 20 mg

Contraindications Hypersensitivity to piroxicam, any component, aspirin or other nonsteroidal anti-inflammatory drugs (NSAIDs); active GI bleeding

Warnings/Precautions Use with caution in patients with impaired cardiac function, hypertension, impaired renal function, GI disease (bleeding or ulcers) and patients receiving anticoagulants; elderly have increased risk for adverse reactions to NSAIDs

Pregnancy Risk Factor B; D (3rd trimester)

Adverse Reactions

>10%:

Central nervous system: Dizziness
Dermatologic: Rash
Gastrointestinal: Abdominal cramps, heartburn, indigestion, nausea

1% to 10%:

Central nervous system: Headache, nervousness
Dermatologic: Itching
Endocrine & metabolic: Fluid retention
Gastrointestinal: Vomiting
Otic: Tinnitus

<1%: Acute renal failure, agranulocytosis, allergic rhinitis, anemia, angioedema, arrhythmias, aseptic meningitis, blurred vision, bone marrow suppression, confusion, congestive heart failure, conjunctivitis, cystitis, decreased hearing, drowsiness, dry eyes, epistaxis, erythema multiforme, gastritis, GI ulceration, hallucinations, hemolytic anemia, hepatitis, hot flashes, hypertension, insomnia, leukopenia, mental depression, peripheral neuropathy, polydipsia, polyuria, shortness of breath, Stevens-Johnson syndrome, tachycardia, thrombocytopenia, toxic amblyopia, toxic epidermal necrolysis, urticaria

Drug Interactions CYP2C9 and 2C18 enzyme substrate

Decreased effect of diuretics, beta-blockers; decreased effect with aspirin, antacids, cholestyramine

Increased effect/toxicity of lithium, warfarin, methotrexate (controversial)

Alcohol Interactions Avoid use (may enhance gastric mucosal irritation)

Onset Onset of analgesia: Oral: Within 1 hour; Peak effect: 3-5 hours

Half-Life 45-50 hours

Education and Monitoring Issues

Patient Education: Take this medication exactly as directed; do not increase dose without consulting prescriber. Do not crush tablets or break capsules. Take with food or milk to reduce GI distress. Maintain adequate fluid intake (2-3 L/day of fluids unless instructed to restrict fluid intake). Do not use alcohol, aspirin, or aspirin-containing medication, and all other anti-inflammatory medications without consulting prescriber. You may experience drowsiness, dizziness, or nervousness (use caution when driving or engaging in tasks requiring alertness until response to drug is known); anorexia, nausea, vomiting, flatulence, or heartburn (frequent small meals, frequent mouth care, sucking lozenges, or chewing gum may help); fluid retention (weigh yourself weekly and report unusual (3-5 lb/week) weight gain). GI bleeding, ulceration, or perforation can occur with or without pain; discontinue medication and contact prescriber if persistent abdominal pain or cramping, or blood in stool occurs. Report unusual swelling of extremities or unusual weight gain; breathlessness, difficulty breathing, or unusual cough; chest pain, rapid heartbeat, palpitations; unusual bruising/bleeding; blood in urine, stool, mouth, or vomitus; unusual fatigue; changes in urinary pattern (polyuria or anuria); skin rash or itching; or change in hearing or ringing in ears.

Monitoring Parameters: Occult blood loss, hemoglobin, hematocrit, and periodic renal and hepatic function tests; periodic ophthalmologic exams with chronic use

Related Information

Nonsteroidal Anti-Inflammatory Agents Comparison *on page 1248*

- **Pitocin® Injection** *see* Oxytocin *on page 695*
- **Pitressin® Injection** *see* Vasopressin *on page 972*
- **Pitrex** *see* Tolnaftate *on page 931*
- **Placidyl®** *see* Ethchlorvynol *on page 340*
- **Plan B™** *see* Levonorgestrel *on page 524*
- **Plaquenil®** *see* Hydroxychloroquine *on page 451*
- **Plasbumin®** *see* Albumin *on page 27*
- **Plavix®** *see* Clopidogrel *on page 217*
- **Plendil®** *see* Felodipine *on page 352*
- **Pletal®** *see* Cilostazol *on page 197*
- **PMS-** *see* Oxazepam *on page 686*
- **PMS-Amantadine** *see* Amantadine *on page 42*
- **PMS-Baclofen** *see* Baclofen *on page 90*
- **PMS-Benztropine** *see* Benztropine *on page 100*
- **PMS-Bethanechol Chloride** *see* Bethanechol *on page 106*
- **PMS-Chloral Hydrate** *see* Chloral Hydrate *on page 176*
- **PMS-Cholestyramine** *see* Cholestyramine Resin *on page 192*
- **PMS-Clonazepam** *see* Clonazepam *on page 214*
- **PMS-Cyproheptadine** *see* Cyproheptadine *on page 240*
- **PMS-Desipramine** *see* Desipramine *on page 252*
- **PMS-Diazepam** *see* Diazepam *on page 261*
- **PMS-Dicitrate** *see* Sodium Citrate and Citric Acid *on page 859*
- **PMS-Docusate Calcium** *see* Docusate *on page 290*
- **PMS-Dopazide** *see* Methyldopa and Hydrochlorothiazide *on page 587*
- **PMS-Erythromycin** *see* Erythromycin *on page 323*
- **PMS-Flupam** *see* Flurazepam *on page 383*
- **PMS-Hydromorphone** *see* Hydromorphone *on page 449*
- **PMS-Imipramine** *see* Imipramine *on page 462*
- **PMS-Isoniazid** *see* Isoniazid *on page 487*
- **PMS-Ketoprofen** *see* Ketoprofen *on page 500*
- **PMS-Levazine** *see* Amitriptyline and Perphenazine *on page 52*
- **PMS-Levothyroxine Sodium** *see* Levothyroxine *on page 526*
- **PMS-Lidocaine Viscous** *see* Lidocaine *on page 527*
- **PMS-Lindane** *see* Lindane *on page 531*
- **PMS-Loperamine** *see* Loperamide *on page 538*
- **PMS-Lorazepam** *see* Lorazepam *on page 541*
- **PMS-Methylphenidate** *see* Methylphenidate *on page 588*
- **PMS-Nystatin** *see* Nystatin *on page 670*
- **PMS-Opium & Beladonna** *see* Belladonna and Opium *on page 96*
- **PMS-Perphenazine** *see* Perphenazine *on page 719*
- **PMS-Prochlorperazine** *see* Prochlorperazine *on page 773*
- **PMS-Procyclidine** *see* Procyclidine *on page 775*
- **PMS-Progesterone** *see* Progesterone *on page 775*
- **PMS-Pseudoephedrine** *see* Pseudoephedrine *on page 792*
- **PMS-Pyrazinamide** *see* Pyrazinamide *on page 794*
- **PMS-Sodium Cromoglycate** *see* Cromolyn Sodium *on page 231*

- **PMS-Sulfasa** *see* Sulfasalazine *on page 880*
- **PMS-Thiorid** *see* Thioridazine *on page 912*
- **PMS-Trihexyphenidyl** *see* Trihexyphenidyl *on page 952*
- **Pneumomist®** *see* Guaifenesin *on page 423*
- **Pneumopent** *see* Pentamidine *on page 714*
- **Pod-Ben-25®** *see* Podophyllum Resin *on page 746*
- **Podocon-25™** *see* Podophyllum Resin *on page 746*
- **Podofilm®** *see* Podophyllum Resin *on page 746*
- **Podofin®** *see* Podophyllum Resin *on page 746*

Podophyllin and Salicylic Acid (po DOF fil in & sal i SIL ik AS id)

Pharmacologic Class Keratolytic Agent

U.S. Brand Names Verrex-C&M®

Dosage Forms SOLN, top: Podophyllum 10% and salicylic acid 30% with penederm 0.5% (7.5 mL)

Podophyllum Resin (po DOF fil um REZ in)

Pharmacologic Class Keratolytic Agent

U.S. Brand Names Pod-Ben-25®; Podocon-25™; Podofin®

Use Topical treatment of benign growths including external genital and perianal warts, papillomas, fibroids; compound benzoin tincture generally is used as the medium for topical application

USUAL DOSAGE Topical:

Children and Adults: 10% to 25% solution in compound benzoin tincture; apply drug to dry surface, use 1 drop at a time allowing drying between drops until area is covered; total volume should be limited to <0.5 mL per treatment session

Condylomata acuminatum: 25% solution is applied daily; use a 10% solution when applied to or near mucous membranes

Verrucae: 25% solution is applied 3-5 times/day directly to the wart

Contraindications Not to be used on birthmarks, moles, or warts with hair growth; cervical, urethral, oral warts; not to be used by diabetic patient or patient with poor circulation; pregnant women

Pregnancy Risk Factor X

- **Point-Two®** *see* Fluoride *on page 376*
- **Poladex®** *see* Dexchlorpheniramine *on page 259*
- **Polaramine®** *see* Dexchlorpheniramine *on page 259*
- **Polocaine®** *see* Mepivacaine *on page 565*
- **Polycillin®** *see* Ampicillin *on page 59*
- **Polycillin-N®** *see* Ampicillin *on page 59*
- **Polycitra®** *see* Sodium Citrate and Potassium Citrate Mixture *on page 859*
- **Polycitra®-K** *see* Potassium Citrate and Citric Acid *on page 753*
- **Polydine® [OTC]** *see* Povidone-Iodine *on page 756*

Polyestradiol (pol i es tra DYE ole)

Pharmacologic Class Estrogen Derivative

Generic Available No

Mechanism of Action Estrogens exert their primary effects on the interphase DNA-protein complex (chromatin) by binding to a receptor (usually located in the cytoplasm of a target cell) and initiating translocation of the hormone-receptor complex to the nucleus

Use Palliative treatment of advanced, inoperable carcinoma of the prostate

USUAL DOSAGE Adults: Deep I.M.: 40 mg every 2-4 weeks or less frequently; maximum dose: 80 mg

Dosage Forms POWDER for inj: 40 mg

Contraindications Known or suspected estrogen-dependent neoplasm, carcinoma of the breast, active thromboembolic disorders, hypersensitivity to estrogens or any component, pregnancy

Warnings/Precautions Use with caution in patients with migraine, diabetes, cardiac, or renal impairment

Pregnancy Risk Factor X

Adverse Reactions

>10%:

Cardiovascular: Peripheral edema

Endocrine & metabolic: Enlargement of breasts (female and male), breast tenderness

Gastrointestinal: Nausea, anorexia, bloating

1% to 10%:

Central nervous system: Headache

Endocrine & metabolic: Increased libido (female), decrease libido (male)

Gastrointestinal: Vomiting, diarrhea

<1%: Alterations in frequency and flow of menses, amenorrhea, anxiety, breast tumors, chloasma, cholestatic jaundice, decreased glucose tolerance, depression, dizziness,

edema, GI distress, hypertension, increased susceptibility to *Candida* infection, increased triglycerides and LDL, intolerance to contact lenses, melasma, myocardial infarction, nausea, rash, stroke, thromboembolism

Polyethylene Glycol-Electrolyte Solution

(pol i ETH i leen GLY kol-ee LEK troe lite soe LOO shun)

Pharmacologic Class Cathartic; Laxative, Bowel Evacuant

U.S. Brand Names Colovage®; Colyte®; GoLYTELY®; NuLytely®; OCL®

Use Bowel cleansing prior to GI examination or following toxic ingestion

USUAL DOSAGE The recommended dose for adults is 4 L of solution prior to gastrointestinal examination, as ingestion of this dose produces a satisfactory preparation in >95% of patients. Ideally the patient should fast for approximately 3-4 hours prior to administration, but in no case should solid food be given for at least 2 hours before the solution is given. The solution is usually administered orally, but may be given via nasogastric tube to patients who are unwilling or unable to drink the solution.

Children: Oral: 25-40 mL/kg/hour for 4-10 hours

Adults:

- Oral: At a rate of 240 mL (8 oz) every 10 minutes, until 4 liters are consumed or the rectal effluent is clear; rapid drinking of each portion is preferred to drinking small amounts continuously
- Nasogastric tube: At a rate of 20-30 mL/minute (1.2-1.8 L/hour); the first bowel movement should occur approximately 1 hour after the start of administration

Contraindications Gastrointestinal obstruction, gastric retention, bowel perforation, toxic colitis, megacolon

Pregnancy Risk Factor C

- ♦ **Polygam®** *see* Immune Globulin, Intravenous *on page 465*
- ♦ **Polygam® S/D** *see* Immune Globulin, Intravenous *on page 465*
- ♦ **Poly-Histine CS®** *see* Brompheniramine, Phenylpropanolamine, and Codeine *on page 114*
- ♦ **Poly-Histine-D® Capsule** *see* Phenyltoloxamine, Phenylpropanolamine, Pyrilamine, and Pheniramine *on page 730*
- ♦ **Polymox®** *see* Amoxicillin *on page 56*

Polymyxin B (pol i MIKS in bee)

Pharmacologic Class Antibiotic, Irrigation; Antibiotic, Miscellaneous

Generic Available Yes

Mechanism of Action Binds to phospholipids, alters permeability, and damages the bacterial cytoplasmic membrane permitting leakage of intracellular constituents

Use

- Topical: Wound irrigation and bladder irrigation against *Pseudomonas aeruginosa*; used occasionally for gut decontamination
- Parenteral use of polymyxin B has mainly been replaced by less toxic antibiotics; it is reserved for life-threatening infections caused by organisms resistant to the preferred drugs (eg, pseudomonal meningitis - intrathecal administration)

USUAL DOSAGE

Otic: 1-2 drops, 3-4 times/day; should be used sparingly to avoid accumulation of excess debris

Infants <2 years:

- I.M.: Up to 40,000 units/kg/day divided every 6 hours (not routinely recommended due to pain at injection sites)
- I.V.: Up to 40,000 units/kg/day by continuous I.V. infusion
- Intrathecal: 20,000 units/day for 3-4 days, then 25,000 units every other day for at least 2 weeks after CSF cultures are negative and CSF (glucose) has returned to within normal limits

Children ≥2 years and Adults:

- I.M.: 25,000-30,000 units/kg/day divided every 4-6 hours (not routinely recommended due to pain at injection sites)
- I.V.: 15,000-25,000 units/kg/day divided every 12 hours or by continuous infusion
- Intrathecal: 50,000 units/day for 3-4 days, then every other day for at least 2 weeks after CSF cultures are negative and CSF (glucose) has returned to within normal limits
- Total daily dose should not exceed 2,000,000 units/day
- Bladder irrigation: Continuous irrigant or rinse in the urinary bladder for up to 10 days using 20 mg (equal to 200,000 units) added to 1 L of normal saline; usually no more than 1 L of irrigant is used per day unless urine flow rate is high; administration rate is adjusted to patient's urine output
- Topical irrigation or topical solution: 500,000 units/L of normal saline; topical irrigation should not exceed 2 million units/day in adults
- Gut sterilization: Oral: 15,000-25,000 units/kg/day in divided doses every 6 hours
- *Clostridium difficile* enteritis: Oral: 25,000 units every 6 hours for 10 days
- Ophthalmic: A concentration of 0.1% to 0.25% is administered as 1-3 drops every hour, then increasing the interval as response indicates to 1-2 drops 4-6 times/day

(Continued)

Polymyxin B *(Continued)*

Dosing adjustment/interval in renal impairment:

Cl_{cr} 20-50 mL/minute: Administer 75% to 100% of normal dose every 12 hours
Cl_{cr} 5-20 mL/minute: Administer 50% of normal dose every 12 hours
Cl_{cr} <5 mL/minute: Administer 15% of normal dose every 12 hours

Dosage Forms INJ: 500,000 units (20 mL). **SOLN, otic:** 10,000 units of polymyxin B per mL in combination with hydrocortisone 0.5% solution (eg, Otobiotic®). **SUSP, otic:** 10,000 units of polymixin B per mL in combination with hydrocortisone 1% and neomycin sulfate 0.5% (eg, PediOtic®); also available in a variety of other combination products for ophthalmic and otic use

Contraindications Concurrent use of neuromuscular blockers

Warnings/Precautions Use with caution in patients with impaired renal function, (modify dosage); polymyxin B-induced nephrotoxicity may be manifested by albuminuria, cellular casts, and azotemia. Discontinue therapy with decreasing urinary output and increasing BUN; neurotoxic reactions are usually associated with high serum levels, often in patients with renal dysfunction. Avoid concurrent or sequential use of other nephrotoxic and neurotoxic drugs (eg, aminoglycosides). The drug's neurotoxicity can result in respiratory paralysis from neuromuscular blockade, especially when the drug is given soon after anesthesia or muscle relaxants. Polymyxin B sulfate is most toxic when given parenterally; avoid parenteral use whenever possible.

Pregnancy Risk Factor B

Adverse Reactions <1%: Anaphylactoid reaction, drug fever, facial flushing, hypocalcemia, hypochloremia, hypokalemia, hyponatremia, meningeal irritation with intrathecal administration, nephrotoxicity, neuromuscular blockade, neurotoxicity (irritability, drowsiness, ataxia, perioral paresthesia, numbness of the extremities, and blurring of vision), pain at injection site, respiratory arrest, urticarial rash, weakness

Drug Interactions Polymyxin may increase/prolong effect of neuromuscular blocking agents; aminoglycosides may increase polymyxin's risk of respiratory paralysis and renal dysfunction

Half-Life 4.5-6 hours, increased with reduced renal function

Education and Monitoring Issues

Patient Education: Wound irrigation / bladder irrigation / gut sterilization / or I.V.: Immediately report numbness or tingling of mouth, tongue, or extremities; constant blurring of vision; increased nervousness or irritability; excessive drowsiness; or difficulty breathing.

Ophthalmic: tilt head back, place medication into eyes (as frequently as prescribed), close eyes, apply light pressure over inside corner of the eye for 1 minute. Do not touch medicine dropper to eye or contaminate tip of dropper. You may experience some stinging or burning or temporary blurring of vision - use caution driving or when engaging in hazardous tasks until vision clears. Report any adverse effects including respiratory difficulty or unusual numbness or tingling of mouth or tongue, increased nervousness or irritability, or excessive drowsiness.

Monitoring Parameters: Neurologic symptoms and signs of superinfection; renal function (decreasing urine output and increasing BUN may require discontinuance of therapy)

Reference Range: Serum concentrations >5 μg/mL are toxic in adults

Related Information

Bacitracin and Polymyxin B *on page 90*
Bacitracin, Neomycin, and Polymyxin B *on page 90*
Bacitracin, Neomycin, Polymyxin B, and Hydrocortisone *on page 90*
Chloramphenicol, Polymyxin B, and Hydrocortisone *on page 180*
Neomycin and Polymyxin B *on page 643*
Neomycin, Polymyxin B, and Dexamethasone *on page 644*
Neomycin, Polymyxin B, and Hydrocortisone *on page 644*
Neomycin, Polymyxin B, and Prednisolone *on page 644*
Oxytetracycline and Polymyxin B *on page 695*
Polymyxin B and Hydrocortisone *on page 748*
Trimethoprim and Polymyxin B *on page 954*

Polymyxin B and Hydrocortisone

(pol i MIKS in bee & hye droe KOR ti sone)

Pharmacologic Class Antibiotic/Corticosteroid, Otic

U.S. Brand Names Otobiotic® Otic

Dosage Forms SOLN, otic: Polymyxin B sulfate 10,000 units and hydrocortisone 0.5% [5 mg/mL] per mL (10 mL, 15 mL)

Pregnancy Risk Factor C

- **Poly-Pred® Ophthalmic Suspension** *see* Neomycin, Polymyxin B, and Prednisolone *on page 644*
- **Polysporin® Ophthalmic** *see* Bacitracin and Polymyxin B *on page 90*
- **Polysporin® Topical** *see* Bacitracin and Polymyxin B *on page 90*
- **Polytopic** *see* Bacitracin and Polymyxin B *on page 90*
- **Polytrim** *see* Trimethoprim and Polymyxin B *on page 954*

- **Polytrim® Ophthalmic** *see* Trimethoprim and Polymyxin B *on page 954*
- **Poly-Vi-Flor®** *see* Vitamins, Multiple *on page 981*
- **Poly-Vi-Sol® [OTC]** *see* Vitamins, Multiple *on page 981*
- **Pontocaine®** *see* Tetracaine *on page 902*
- **Pontocaine® With Dextrose Injection** *see* Tetracaine and Dextrose *on page 903*
- **Porcelana® [OTC]** *see* Hydroquinone *on page 450*
- **Porcelana® Sunscreen [OTC]** *see* Hydroquinone *on page 450*

Porfimer (POR fi mer)

Pharmacologic Class Antineoplastic Agent, Miscellaneous

U.S. Brand Names Photofrin®

Mechanism of Action Porfimer's cytotoxic activity is dependent on light and oxygen. Following administration, the drug is selectively retained in neoplastic tissues. Exposure of the drug to laser light at wavelengths >630 nm results in the production of oxygen free-radicals. Release of thromboxane A_2, leading to vascular occlusion and ischemic necrosis, may also occur.

Use Esophageal cancer: Photodynamic therapy (PDT) with porfimer for palliation of patients with completely obstructing esophageal cancer, or of patients with partially obstructing esophageal cancer who cannot be satisfactorily treated with Nd:YAG laser therapy

USUAL DOSAGE I.V. (refer to individual protocols):

Children: Safety and efficacy have not been established

Adults: I.V.: 2 mg/kg over 3-5 minutes

Bladder: 15 joules/cm^2

Esophageal: 90-600 joules/cm^2

Gastric: >90 joules/cm^2

Lung: 150-1575 joules/cm^2

Rectal: 50-200 joules/cm^2

Photodynamic therapy (PDT) is a two-stage process requiring administration of both drug and light. The first stage of PDT is the I.V. injection of porfimer. Illumination with laser light 40-50 hours following the injection with porfimer constitutes the second stage of therapy. A second laser light application may be given 90-120 hours after injection, preceded by gentle debridement of residual tumor.

Patients may receive a second course of PDT a minimum of 30 days after the initial therapy; up to three courses of PDT (each separated by a minimum of 30 days) can be given. Before each course of treatment, evaluate patients for the presence of a tracheoesophageal or bronchoesophageal fistula.

Dosage Forms POWDER for inj: 75 mg

Contraindications Hypersensitivity to porfimer or any component; patients with porphyria, patients with broncho- or tracheoesophageal fistulas or tumors eroding the tracheal/bronchial tree, or a major blood vessel

Warnings/Precautions The U.S. Food and Drug Administration (FDA) currently recommends that procedures for proper handling and disposal of antineoplastic agents be considered. If the esophageal tumor is eroding into the trachea or bronchial tree, the likelihood of tracheoesophageal or bronchoesophageal fistula resulting from treatment is sufficiently high that PDT is not recommended. All patients who receive porfimer sodium will be photosensitive and must observe precautions to avoid exposure of skin and eyes to direct sunlight or bright indoor light for 30 days. The photosensitivity is due to residual drug which will be present in all parts of the skin. Exposure of the skin to ambient indoor light is, however, beneficial because the remaining drug will be inactivated gradually and safely through a photobleaching reaction. Patients should not stay in a darkened room during this period and should be encouraged to expose their skin to ambient indoor light. Ocular discomfort has been reported; for 30 days, when outdoors, patients should wear dark sunglasses which have an average white light transmittance of <4%.

Pregnancy Risk Factor C

Adverse Reactions

>10%:

Cardiovascular: Atrial fibrillation, chest pain

Central nervous system: Fever, pain, insomnia

Dermatologic: Photosensitivity reaction

Gastrointestinal: Abdominal pain, constipation, dysphagia, nausea, vomiting

Hematologic: Anemia

Neuromuscular & skeletal: Back pain

Respiratory: Dyspnea, pharyngitis, pleural effusion, pneumonia, respiratory insufficiency

1% to 10%:

Cardiovascular: Hypertension, hypotension, edema, cardiac failure, tachycardia, chest pain (substernal)

Central nervous system: Anxiety, confusion

Endocrine & metabolic: Dehydration

Gastrointestinal: Diarrhea, dyspepsia, eructation, esophageal edema, esophageal tumor bleeding, esophageal stricture, esophagitis, hematemesis, melena, weight loss, anorexia

(Continued)

Porfimer *(Continued)*

Genitourinary: Urinary tract infection
Neuromuscular & skeletal: Weakness
Respiratory: Coughing, tracheoesophageal fistula
Miscellaneous: Moniliasis, surgical complication

Drug Interactions

Decreased effect: Compounds that quench active oxygen species or scavenge radicals (eg, dimethyl sulfoxide, beta-carotene, ethanol, mannitol) would be expected to decrease PDT activity; allopurinol, calcium channel blockers and some prostaglandin synthesis inhibitors could interfere with porfimer; drugs that decrease clotting, vasoconstriction or platelet aggregation could decrease the efficacy of PDT; glucocorticoid hormones may decrease the efficacy of the treatment

Increased toxicity: Concomitant administration of other photosensitizing agents (eg, tetracyclines, sulfonamides, phenothiazines, sulfonylureas, thiazide diuretics, griseofulvin) could increase the photosensitivity reaction

Half-Life 250 hours

Education and Monitoring Issues

Patient Education: This medication can only be administered I.V. and will be followed by laser light therapy. Avoid any exposure to sunlight or bright indoor light for 30 days following therapy (cover skin with protective clothing and wear dark sunglasses with light transmittance <4% when outdoors - severe blistering, burning, and skin/eye damage can result). After 30 days, test small area of skin (not face) for remaining sensitivity. Retest sensitivity if traveling to a different geographic area with greater sunshine. Exposure to indoor normal light is beneficial since it will help dissipate photosensitivity gradually. Maintain adequate hydration (2-3 L/day of fluids unless instructed to restrict fluid intake); maintain good oral hygiene (use soft toothbrush or cotton applicators several times a day and rinse mouth frequently). Small frequent meals, frequent mouth care, sucking lozenges, or chewing gum may reduce nausea or vomiting. Can cause constipation; increase bulk in diet. Consult prescriber if constipation persists. Report rapid heart rate, chest pain or palpitations, difficulty breathing or air hunger, persistent fever or chills, foul-smelling urine or burning on urination, swelling of extremities, increased anxiety, confusion, or hallucination.

Manufacturer Sanofi Winthrop Pharmaceuticals

Related Information

Pharmaceutical Manufacturers Directory *on page 1020*

- **Pork NPH Iletin® II** *see* Insulin Preparations *on page 472*
- **Pork Regular Iletin® II** *see* Insulin Preparations *on page 472*
- **Postexposure Prophylaxis for Hepatitis B** *see page 1160*
- **Potasalan®** *see* Potassium Chloride *on page 751*

Potassium Acetate (poe TASS ee um AS e tate)

Pharmacologic Class Electrolyte Supplement, Oral

Use Potassium deficiency; to avoid chloride when high concentration of potassium is needed, source of bicarbonate

USUAL DOSAGE I.V. doses should be incorporated into the patient's maintenance I.V. fluids, intermittent I.V. potassium administration should be reserved for severe depletion situations and requires EKG monitoring; doses listed as mEq of potassium

Treatment of hypokalemia: I.V.:
Children: 2-5 mEq/kg/day
Adults: 40-100 mEq/day

I.V. intermittent infusion (must be diluted prior to administration):
Children: 0.5-1 mEq/kg/dose (maximum: 30 mEq/dose) to infuse at 0.3-0.5 mEq/kg/hour (maximum: 1 mEq/kg/hour)
Adults: 5-10 mEq/dose (maximum: 40 mEq/dose) to infuse over 2-3 hours (maximum: 40 mEq over 1 hour)

Note: Continuous cardiac monitor recommended for rates >0.5 mEq/hour

Potassium Dosage/Rate of Infusion Guidelines

Serum Potassium	Maximum Infusion Rate	Maximum Concentration	Maximum 24-Hour Dose
>2.5 mEq/L	10 mEq/h	40 mEq/L	200 mEq
<2.5 mEq/L	40 mEq/h	80 mEq/L	400 mEq

Contraindications Severe renal impairment, hyperkalemia

Pregnancy Risk Factor C

Related Information

Potassium Acetate, Potassium Bicarbonate, and Potassium Citrate *on page 751*

Potassium Acetate, Potassium Bicarbonate, and Potassium Citrate

(poe TASS ee um AS e tate, poe TASS ee um bye KAR bun ate, & poe TASS ee um SIT rate)

Pharmacologic Class Electrolyte Supplement, Oral

U.S. Brand Names Tri-K®

Dosage Forms SOLN, oral: 45 mEq/15 mL from potassium acetate 1500 mg, potassium bicarbonate 1500 mg, and potassium citrate 1500 mg per 15 mL

Pregnancy Risk Factor C

Potassium Acid Phosphate (poe TASS ee um AS id FOS fate)

Pharmacologic Class Urinary Acidifying Agent

U.S. Brand Names K-Phos® Original

Use Acidifies urine and lowers urinary calcium concentration; reduces odor and rash caused by ammoniacal urine; increases the antibacterial activity of methenamine

USUAL DOSAGE Adults: Oral: 1000 mg dissolved in 6-8 oz of water 4 times/day with meals and at bedtime; for best results, soak tablets in water for 2-5 minutes, then stir and swallow

Contraindications Severe renal impairment, hyperkalemia, hyperphosphatemia, and infected magnesium ammonium phosphate stones

Pregnancy Risk Factor C

Potassium Bicarbonate and Potassium Chloride, Effervescent

(poe TASS ee um bye KAR bun ate & poe TASS ee um KLOR ide, ef er VES ent)

Pharmacologic Class Electrolyte Supplement, Oral

U.S. Brand Names Klorvess® Effervescent; K/Lyte/CL®

Dosage Forms GRANULES for oral soln, effervescent (Klorvess®): 20 mEq per packet. **TAB for oral soln, effervescent,** (Klorvess®): 20 mEq per packet, K/Lyte/Cl®: 25 mEq, 50 mEq per packet

Pregnancy Risk Factor C

Education and Monitoring Issues

Patient Education: Take as directed; do not take more than directed. Dissolve granules, powder, or tablets in 4-6 ounces of water or juice and stir before drinking. Do not take on an empty stomach; take with or after meals. Consult prescriber about increasing dietary potassium intake (eg, salt substitutes, orange juice, bananas, etc). Report tingling of hands or feet, unresolved nausea or vomiting, chest pain, palpitations, persistent abdominal pain, muscle cramping or weakness, tarry stools, easy bruising, or unusual bleeding.

Potassium Bicarbonate and Potassium Citrate, Effervescent

(poe TASS ee um bye KAR bun ate & poe TASS ee um SIT rate, ef er VES ent)

Pharmacologic Class Electrolyte Supplement, Oral

U.S. Brand Names Effer-K™; K-Ide®; Klor-Con®/EF; K-Lyte®; K-Vescent®

Use Treatment or prevention of hypokalemia

USUAL DOSAGE Oral:

Children: 1-4 mEq/kg/24 hours in divided doses as required to maintain normal serum potassium

Adults:

Prevention: 16-24 mEq/day in 2-4 divided doses

Treatment: 40-100 mEq/day in 2-4 divided doses

Contraindications Severe renal impairment, hyperkalemia

Pregnancy Risk Factor C

Potassium Bicarbonate, Potassium Chloride, and Potassium Citrate

(poe TASS ee um bye KAR bun ate, poe TASS ee um KLOR ide, & poe TASS ee um SIT rate)

Pharmacologic Class Electrolyte Supplement, Oral

U.S. Brand Names Kaochlor-Eff®

Dosage Forms TAB for oral soln: 20 mEq from potassium bicarbonate 1 g, potassium chloride 600 mg, and potassium citrate 220 mg

Pregnancy Risk Factor C

Related Information

Potassium Chloride and Potassium Gluconate *on page 753*

Potassium Chloride (poe TASS ee um KLOR ide)

Pharmacologic Class Electrolyte Supplement, Oral

U.S. Brand Names Cena-K®; Gen-K®; K+ 10®; Kaochlor®; Kaochlor® SF; Kaon-Cl®; Kaon Cl-10®; Kay Ciel®; K+ Care®; K-Dur® 10; K-Dur® 20; K-Lease®; K-Lor™; Klor-Con®; Klor-

(Continued)

Potassium Chloride *(Continued)*

Con® 8; Klor-Con® 10; Klor-Con/25®; Klotrix®; K-Lyte/Cl®; K-Norm®; K-Tab®; Micro-K® 10; Micro-K® Extencaps®; Micro-K® LS®; Potasalan®; Rum-K®; Slow-K®; Ten-K®

Generic Available Yes

Mechanism of Action Potassium is the major cation of intracellular fluid and is essential for the conduction of nerve impulses in heart, brain, and skeletal muscle; contraction of cardiac, skeletal and smooth muscles; maintenance of normal renal function, acid-base balance, carbohydrate metabolism, and gastric secretion

Use Treatment or prevention of hypokalemia

USUAL DOSAGE I.V. doses should be incorporated into the patient's maintenance I.V. fluids; intermittent I.V. potassium administration should be reserved for severe depletion situations in patients undergoing EKG monitoring.

Normal daily requirements: Oral, I.V.:
- Premature infants: 2-6 mEq/kg/24 hours
- Term infants 0-24 hours: 0-2 mEq/kg/24 hours
- Infants >24 hours: 1-2 mEq/kg/24 hours
- Children: 2-3 mEq/kg/day
- Adults: 40-80 mEq/day

Prevention during diuretic therapy: Oral:
- Children: 1-2 mEq/kg/day in 1-2 divided doses
- Adults: 20-40 mEq/day in 1-2 divided doses

Treatment of hypokalemia: Children:
- Oral: 1-2 mEq/kg initially, then as needed based on frequently obtained lab values. If deficits are severe or ongoing losses are great, I.V. route should be considered.
- I.V.: 1 mEq/kg over 1-2 hours initially, then repeated as needed based on frequently obtained lab values; severe depletion or ongoing losses may require >200% of normal limit needs
- I.V. intermittent infusion: Dose should not exceed 1 mEq/kg/hour, or 40 mEq/hour; if it exceeds 0.5 mEq/kg/hour, prescriber should be at bedside and patient should have continuous EKG monitoring; usual pediatric maximum: 3 mEq/kg/day or 40 mEq/m^2/day

Treatment of hypokalemia: Adults:
- I.V. intermittent infusion: 5-10 mEq/hour (continuous cardiac monitor recommended for rates >5 mEq/hour), not to exceed 40 mEq/hour; usual adult maximum per 24 hours: 400 mEq/day. See table.

Potassium Dosage/Rate of Infusion Guidelines

Serum Potassium	Maximum Infusion Rate	Maximum Concentration	Maximum 24-Hour Dose
>2.5 mEq/L	10 mEq/h	40 mEq/L	200 mEq
<2.5 mEq/L	40 mEq/h	80 mEq/L	400 mEq

Potassium >2.5 mEq/L:
- Oral: 60-80 mEq/day plus additional amounts if needed
- I.V.: 10 mEq over 1 hour with additional doses if needed

Potassium <2.5 mEq/L:
- Oral: Up to 40-60 mEq initial dose, followed by further doses based on lab values
- I.V.: Up to 40 mEq over 1 hour, with doses based on frequent lab monitoring; deficits at a plasma level of 2 mEq/L may be as high as 400-800 mEq of potassium

Dosage Forms CAP, controlled release (microcapsulated): 600 mg [8 mEq]; 750 mg [10 mEq]; (Micro-K® Extencaps®): 600 mg [8 mEq]; (K-Lease®, K-Norm®, Micro-K® 10): 750 mg [10 mEq]. **LIQ:** 10% [20 mEq/15 mL] (480 mL, 4000 mL); 20% [40 mEq/15 mL] (480 mL, 4000 mL); (Cena-K®, Kaochlor®, Kaochlor® SF, Kay Ciel®, Potasalan®): 10% [20 mEq/15 mL] (480 mL, 4000 mL); (Rum-K®): 15% [30 mEq/15 mL] (480 mL, 4000 mL); (Cena-K®, Kaon-Cl® 20%): 20% [40 mEq/15 mL]. **CRYSTALS for oral suspension, extended release** (Micro-K® LS®): 20 mEq per packet. **POWDER:** 20 mEq per packet (30s, 100s); (K+ Care®, K-Lor™): 15 mEq per packet (30s, 100s); (Gen-K®, Kay Ciel®, K+ Care®, K-Lor®, Klor-Con®): 20 mEq per packet (30s, 100s); (K+ Care®, Klor-Con/25®): 25 mEq per packet (30s, 100s); (K-Lyte/Cl®): 25 mEq per dose (30s). **INF, concentrate:** 0.1 mEq/mL, 0.2 mEq/mL, 0.3 mEq/mL, 0.4 mEq/mL. **INJ, concentrate:** 1.5 mEq/mL, 2 mEq/mL, 3 mEq/mL. **TAB, controlled release (microencapsulated):** (K-Dur® 10, Ten-K®): 750 mg [10 mEq]; (K-Dur® 20): 1500 mg [20 mEq]; **TAB, controlled release (wax matrix):** 600 mg [8 mEq]; 750 mg [10 mEq]; (Kaon-Cl®): 500 mg [6.7 mEq]; (Klor-Con® 8, Slow-K®): 600 mg [8 mEq]; (K+ 10®, Kaon-Cl-10®, Klor-Con® 10, Klotrix®, K-Tab®): 750 mg [10 mEq]

Contraindications Severe renal impairment, untreated Addison's disease, heat cramps, hyperkalemia, severe tissue trauma; solid oral dosage forms are contraindicated in patients in whom there is a structural, pathological, and/or pharmacologic cause for delay or arrest in passage through the GI tract; an oral liquid potassium preparation should be used in patients with esophageal compression or delayed gastric emptying time

Warnings/Precautions Use with caution in patients with cardiac disease, severe renal impairment, hyperkalemia

Pregnancy Risk Factor A

Adverse Reactions

>10%: Gastrointestinal: Diarrhea, nausea, stomach pain, flatulence, vomiting (oral)

1% to 10%:

- Cardiovascular: Bradycardia
- Endocrine & metabolic: Hyperkalemia
- Local: Local tissue necrosis with extravasation, pain at the site of injection
- Neuromuscular & skeletal: Weakness
- Respiratory: Dyspnea

<1%: Abdominal pain, alkalosis, arrhythmias, chest pain, heart block, hypotension, mental confusion, paralysis, paresthesias, phlebitis, throat pain

Drug Interactions Increased effect/levels with potassium-sparing diuretics, salt substitutes, ACE inhibitors

Education and Monitoring Issues

Patient Education: Sustained release and wax matrix tablets should be swallowed whole, do not crush or chew; effervescent tablets must be dissolved in water before use; take with food; liquid and granules can be diluted or dissolved in water or juice

Monitoring Parameters: Serum potassium, glucose, chloride, pH, urine output (if indicated), cardiac monitor (if intermittent infusion or potassium infusion rates >0.25 mEq/kg/hour)

Potassium Chloride and Potassium Gluconate

(poe TASS ee um KLOR ide & poe TASS ee um GLOO coe nate)

Pharmacologic Class Electrolyte Supplement, Oral

U.S. Brand Names Kolyum®

Dosage Forms SOLN, oral: Potassium 20 mEq/15 mL

Pregnancy Risk Factor A

Potassium Citrate and Citric Acid

(poe TASS ee um SIT rate & SI trik AS id)

Pharmacologic Class Alkalinizing Agent

U.S. Brand Names Polycitra®-K

Dosage Forms CRYSTALS for reconstitution: Potassium citrate 3300 mg and citric acid 1002 mg per pk. **SOLN, oral:** Potassium citrate 1100 mg and citric acid 334 mg per 5 mL

Pregnancy Risk Factor C

Education and Monitoring Issues

Patient Education: Take as directed; do not take more than directed. Dilute crystals or solution in 4-6 ounces of juice or water; stir and drink. Swallow tablet whole with full glass of water or juice and stir before sipping slowly, with or after meals (do not take on an empty stomach). Take any antacids 2 hours before or after potassium. Consult prescriber about advisability of increasing dietary potassium. Report tingling of hands or feet; unresolved nausea or vomiting; chest pain or palpitations; persistent abdominal pain; feelings of weakness, dizziness, listlessness, confusion, acute muscle weakness or cramping; blood in stool or tarry stools; or easy bruising or unusual bleeding.

Potassium Citrate and Potassium Gluconate

(poe TASS ee um SIT rate & poe TASS ee um GLOO coe nate)

Pharmacologic Class Electrolyte Supplement, Oral

U.S. Brand Names Twin-K®

Dosage Forms SOLN, oral: 20 mEq/5 mL from potassium citrate 170 mg and potassium gluconate 170 mg per 5 mL

Pregnancy Risk Factor C

Potassium Gluconate (poe TASS ee um GLOO coe nate)

Pharmacologic Class Electrolyte Supplement, Oral

U.S. Brand Names Kaon®; Kaylixir®; K-G®

Use Treatment or prevention of hypokalemia

USUAL DOSAGE Oral (doses listed as mEq of potassium):

Normal daily requirement:

- Children: 2-3 mEq/kg/day
- Adults: 40-80 mEq/day

Prevention of hypokalemia during diuretic therapy:

- Children: 1-2 mEq/kg/day in 1-2 divided doses
- Adults: 16-24 mEq/day in 1-2 divided doses

Treatment of hypokalemia:

- Children: 2-5 mEq/kg/day in 2-4 divided doses
- Adults: 40-100 mEq/day in 2-4 divided doses

Contraindications Severe renal impairment, untreated Addison's disease, heat cramps, hyperkalemia, severe tissue trauma; solid oral dosage forms are contraindicated in patients in whom there is a structural, pathological, and/or pharmacologic cause for delay

(Continued)

Potassium Gluconate *(Continued)*

or arrest in passage through the GI tract; an oral liquid potassium preparation should be used in patients with esophageal compression or delayed gastric emptying time

Pregnancy Risk Factor A

Related Information

Potassium Chloride and Potassium Gluconate *on page 753*

Potassium Citrate and Potassium Gluconate *on page 753*

Potassium Iodide (poe TASS ee um EYE oh dide)

Pharmacologic Class Antithyroid Agent; Cough Preparation; Expectorant

U.S. Brand Names Pima®; SSKI®; Thyro-Block®

Use Facilitate bronchial drainage and cough; reduce thyroid vascularity prior to thyroidectomy and management of thyrotoxic crisis; block thyroidal uptake of radioactive isotopes of iodine in a radiation emergency

USUAL DOSAGE Oral:

Adults: RDA: 130 mcg

Expectorant:

- Children: 60-250 mg every 6-8 hours; maximum single dose: 500 mg
- Adults: 300-650 mg 2-3 times/day

Preoperative thyroidectomy: Children and Adults: 50-250 mg (1-5 drops SSKI®) 3 times/day **or** 0.1-0.3 mL (3-5 drops) of strong iodine (Lugol's solution) 3 times/day; administer for 10 days before surgery

Thyrotoxic crisis:

- Infants <1 year: 150-250 mg (3-5 drops SSKI®) 3 times/day
- Children and Adults: 300-500 mg (6-10 drops SSKI®) 3 times/day or 1 mL strong iodine (Lugol's solution) 3 times/day

Sporotrichosis:

- Initial:
  - Preschool: 50 mg/dose 3 times/day
  - Children: 250 mg/dose 3 times/day
  - Adults: 500 mg/dose 3 times/day
- Oral increase 50 mg/dose daily
- Maximum dose:
  - Preschool: 500 mg/dose 3 times/day
  - Children and Adults: 1-2 g/dose 3 times/day
  - Continue treatment for 4-6 weeks after lesions have completely healed

Contraindications Known hypersensitivity to iodine; hyperkalemia, pulmonary tuberculosis, pulmonary edema, bronchitis, impaired renal function

Pregnancy Risk Factor D

Potassium Phosphate (poe TASS ee um FOS fate)

Pharmacologic Class Electrolyte Supplement, Oral

U.S. Brand Names Neutra-Phos®-K

Generic Available Yes

Use Treatment and prevention of hypophosphatemia or hypokalemia

USUAL DOSAGE I.V. doses should be incorporated into the patient's maintenance I.V. fluids; intermittent I.V. infusion should be reserved for severe depletion situations in patients undergoing continuous EKG monitoring. It is difficult to determine total body phosphorus deficit; the following dosages are empiric guidelines:

Normal requirements elemental phosphorus: Oral:

- 0-6 months: 240 mg
- 6-12 months: 360 mg
- 1-10 years: 800 mg
- >10 years: 1200 mg
- Pregnancy lactation: Additional 400 mg/day
- Adults: 800 mg

Treatment: It is difficult to provide concrete guidelines for the treatment of severe hypophosphatemia because the extent of total body deficits and response to therapy are difficult to predict. Aggressive doses of phosphate may result in a transient serum elevation followed by redistribution into intracellular compartments or bone tissue. It is recommended that repletion of severe hypophosphatemia (<1 mg/dL in adults) be done I.V. because large doses of oral phosphate may cause diarrhea and intestinal absorption may be unreliable

Pediatric I.V. phosphate repletion:

Children: 0.25-0.5 mmol/kg **administer over 4-6 hours and repeat if symptomatic hypophosphatemia persists**; to assess the need for further phosphate administration, obtain serum inorganic phosphate after administration of the first dose and base further doses on serum levels and clinical status

Adult I.V. phosphate repletion:

Initial dose: 0.08 mmol/kg if recent uncomplicated hypophosphatemia

Initial dose: 0.16 mmol/kg if prolonged hypophosphatemia with presumed total body deficits; increase dose by 25% to 50% if patient symptomatic with severe hypophosphatemia

Do not exceed 0.24 mmol/kg/day; administer over 6 hours by I.V. infusion

With orders for I.V. phosphate, there is considerable confusion associated with the use of millimoles (mmol) versus milliequivalents (mEq) to express the phosphate requirement. Because inorganic phosphate exists as monobasic and dibasic anions, with the mixture of valences dependent on pH, ordering by mEq amounts is unreliable and may lead to large dosing errors. In addition, I.V. phosphate is available in the sodium and potassium salt; therefore, the content of these cations must be considered when ordering phosphate. The most reliable method of ordering I.V. phosphate is by millimoles, then specifying the potassium or sodium salt. For example, an order for 15 mmol of phosphate as potassium phosphate in one liter of normal saline The dosing of phosphate should be 0.2-0.3 mmol/kg with a usual daily requirement of 30-60 mmol/day or 15 mmol of phosphate per liter of TPN or 15 mmol phosphate per 1000 calories of dextrose. Would also provide 22 mEq of potassium.

Maintenance:

I.V. solutions:

Children: 0.5-1.5 mmol/kg/24 hours I.V. or 2-3 mmol/kg/24 hours orally in divided doses

Adults: 15-30 mmol/24 hours I.V. or 50-150 mmol/24 hours orally in divided doses

Oral:

Children <4 years: 1 capsule (250 mg phosphorus/8 mmol) 4 times/day; dilute as instructed

Children >4 years and Adults: 1-2 capsules (250-500 mg phosphorus/8-16 mmol) 4 times/day; dilute as instructed

Dosage Forms CAP: Neutra-Phos®-K: Phosphorus 250 mg [8 mmol] and potassium 556 mg [14.25 mEq] per capsule. **INJ:** Potassium phosphate monobasic anhydrous 224 mg and potassium phosphate dibasic anhydrous 236 mg per mL, [phosphorus 3 mmol and potassium 4.4 mEq per mL] (15 mL). **POWDER:** Neutra-Phos®-K: Phosphorus 250 mg [8 mmol] and potassium 556 mg [14.25 mEq] per packet

Contraindications Hyperphosphatemia, hyperkalemia, hypocalcemia, hypomagnesemia, renal failure

Warnings/Precautions Use with caution in patients with renal insufficiency, cardiac disease, metabolic alkalosis; admixture of phosphate and calcium in I.V. fluids can result in calcium phosphate precipitation

Pregnancy Risk Factor C

Adverse Reactions

>10%: Gastrointestinal: Diarrhea, nausea, stomach pain, flatulence, vomiting

1% to 10%:

Cardiovascular: Bradycardia

Endocrine & metabolic: Hyperkalemia

Neuromuscular & skeletal: Weakness

Respiratory: Dyspnea

<1%: Abdominal pain, acute renal failure, alkalosis, chest pain, hypocalcemia tetany (with large doses of phosphate), mental confusion, paralysis, paresthesias, phlebitis, throat pain

Drug Interactions

Decreased effect/levels with aluminum and magnesium-containing antacids or sucralfate which can act as phosphate binders

Increased effect/levels with potassium-sparing diuretics, salt substitutes, or ACE-inhibitors; increased effect of digitalis

Education and Monitoring Issues

Patient Education: Do not swallow the capsule; empty contents of capsule into 75 mL (2.5 oz) of water before taking; take with food to reduce the risk of diarrhea

Monitoring Parameters: Serum potassium, calcium, phosphate, sodium, cardiac monitor (when intermittent infusion or high-dose I.V. replacement needed)

Potassium Phosphate and Sodium Phosphate

(poe TASS ee um FOS fate & SOW dee um FOS fate)

Pharmacologic Class Electrolyte Supplement, Oral

U.S. Brand Names K-Phos® Neutral; Neutra-Phos®; Uro-KP-Neutral®

Generic Available Yes

Use Treatment of conditions associated with excessive renal phosphate loss or inadequate GI absorption of phosphate; to acidify the urine to lower calcium concentrations; to increase the antibacterial activity of methenamine; reduce odor and rash caused by ammonia in urine

USUAL DOSAGE All dosage forms to be mixed in 6-8 oz of water prior to administration

Children: 2-3 mmol phosphate/kg/24 hours given 4 times/day **or** 1 capsule 4 times/day

Adults: 1-2 capsules (250-500 mg phosphorus/8-16 mmol) 4 times/day after meals and at bedtime

Dosage Forms CAP (Neutra-Phos®): Phosphorus 8 mmol, potassium 14.25 mEq. **POWDER, conc:** Phosphate 8 mmol, sodium 7.125 mEq, and potassium 7.125 mEq per

(Continued)

Potassium Phosphate and Sodium Phosphate *(Continued)*

75 mL when reconstituted. **TAB:** Phosphate 8 mmol, sodium 13 mEq, and potassium 1.1 mEq (114 mg of phosphorus)

Contraindications Addison's disease, hyperkalemia, hyperphosphatemia, infected urolithiasis or struvite stone formation, patients with severely impaired renal function

Warnings/Precautions Use with caution in patients with renal disease, hyperkalemia, cardiac disease and metabolic alkalosis

Pregnancy Risk Factor C

Adverse Reactions

>10%: Gastrointestinal: Diarrhea, nausea, stomach pain, flatulence, vomiting

1% to 10%:

- Cardiovascular: Bradycardia
- Endocrine & metabolic: Hyperkalemia
- Neuromuscular & skeletal: Weakness
- Respiratory: Dyspnea

<1%: Acute renal failure, alkalosis, arrhythmia, arthralgia, bone pain, chest pain, decreased urine output, edema, mental confusion, pain/weakness of extremities, paralysis, paresthesias, phlebitis, shortness of breath, tetany (with large doses of phosphate), thirst, throat pain, weight gain

Drug Interactions

Decreased effect/levels with aluminum and magnesium-containing antacids or sucralfate which can act as phosphate binders

Increased effect/levels with potassium-sparing diuretics or ACE inhibitors; salicylates

Education and Monitoring Issues

Patient Education: Do not swallow, open capsule and dissolve in 6-8 oz of water; powder packets are to be mixed in 6-8 oz of water; tablets should be crushed and mixed in 6-8 oz of water

Monitoring Parameters: Serum potassium, sodium, calcium, phosphate, EKG

Povidone-Iodine (POE vi done-EYE oh dyne)

Pharmacologic Class Antibacterial, Topical

U.S. Brand Names ACU-dyne® [OTC]; Aerodine® [OTC]; Betadine® [OTC]; Betagan® [OTC]; Biodine [OTC]; Efodine® [OTC]; Iodex® [OTC]; Iodex-p® [OTC]; Isodine® [OTC]; Mallisol® [OTC]; Massengill® Medicated Douche w/Cepticin [OTC]; Minidyne® [OTC]; Operand® [OTC]; Polydine® [OTC]; Summer's Eve® Medicated Douche [OTC]; Yeast-Gard® Medicated Douche

Generic Available Yes

Mechanism of Action Povidone-iodine is known to be a powerful broad spectrum germicidal agent effective against a wide range of bacteria, viruses, fungi, protozoa, and spores.

Use External antiseptic with broad microbicidal spectrum against bacteria, fungi, viruses, protozoa, and yeasts

USUAL DOSAGE

Shampoo: Apply 2 teaspoons to hair and scalp, lather and rinse; repeat application 2 times/week until improvement is noted, then shampoo weekly

Topical: Apply as needed for treatment and prevention of susceptible microbial infections

Dosage Forms AERO: 5% (88.7 mL, 90 mL). **ANTISEPTIC gauze pads:** 10% (3" x 9"). **CLEANSER:** Skin: 7.5% (30 mL, 118 mL); Skin, foam: 7.5% (170 g); Top: 60 mL, 240 mL. **CONCENTRATE, whirlpool:** 3,840 mL. **CRM:** 5% (14 g). **DOUCHE** (10%): 0.5 oz/packet (6 packets/box), 240 mL. **FOAM, topical** (10%): 250 g. **GEL:** Lubricating: 5% (5 g); Vag (10%): 18 g, 90 g. **LIQUID:** 473 mL. **MOUTHWASH** (0.5%): 177 mL. **OINTMENT, topical:** 10% (0.94 g, 3.8 g, 28 g, 30 g, 454 g); 1 g, 1.2 g, 2.7 g packets. **PERINEAL wash concentrate:** 1% (240 mL); 10% (236 mL). **SCRUB, surgical:** 7.5% (15 mL, 473 mL, 946 mL). **SHAMP:** 7.5% (118 mL). **SOLN:** Ophthalmic sterile prep: 5% (50 mL); Prep: 30 mL, 60 mL, 240 mL, 473 mL, 1000 mL, 4000 mL; Swab aid: 1%; Swabsticks: 4"; Top: 10% (15 mL, 30 mL, 120 mL, 237 mL, 473 mL, 480 mL, 1000 mL, 4000 mL). **SUPP, vag:** 10%

Contraindications Hypersensitivity to iodine

Warnings/Precautions Highly toxic if ingested; sodium thiosulfate is the most effective chemical antidote; avoid contact with eyes

Pregnancy Risk Factor D

Adverse Reactions

1% to 10%:

- Dermatologic: Rash, pruritus
- Local: Local edema

<1%: Metabolic acidosis, renal impairment, systemic absorption in extensive burns causing iododerma

Education and Monitoring Issues

Patient Education: Do not swallow; avoid contact with eyes

♦ **Pr** *see* Lorazepam *on page 541*

♦ **Pramet® FA** *see* Vitamins, Multiple *on page 981*

♦ **Pramilet® FA** *see* Vitamins, Multiple *on page 981*

Pramipexole (pra mi PEX ole)

Pharmacologic Class Anti-Parkinson's Agent (Dopamine Agonist)

U.S. Brand Names Mirapex®

Mechanism of Action Pramipexole is a nonergot dopamine agonist with specificity for the D_2 dopamine receptor, but has also been shown to bind to D_3 and D_4 receptors. By binding to these receptors, it is thought that pramipexole can stimulate dopamine activity on the nerves of the striatum and substantia nigra.

Use Treatment of the signs and symptoms of idiopathic Parkinson's Disease; has been evaluated for use in the treatment of depression with positive results

USUAL DOSAGE Adults: Oral: Initial: 0.375 mg/day given in 3 divided doses, increase gradually by 0.125 mg/dose every 5-7 days; range: 1.5-4.5 mg/day

Dosage Forms TAB: 0.125 mg, 0.25 mg, 0.5 mg, 1 mg, 1.25 mg, 1.5 mg

Contraindications Patients with known hypersensitivity to pramipexole or any of the product's ingredients

Warnings/Precautions Caution should be taken in patients with renal insufficiency and in patients with pre-existing dyskinesias. May cause orthostatic hypotension; Parkinson's disease patients appear to have an impaired capacity to respond to a postural challenge. Use with caution in patients at risk of hypotension (such as those receiving antihypertensive drugs) or where transient hypotensive episodes would be poorly tolerated (cardiovascular disease or cerebrovascular disease). Parkinson's patients being treated with dopaminergic agonists ordinarily require careful monitoring for signs and symptoms of postural hypotension, especially during dose escalation, and should be informed of this risk. May cause hallucinations, particularly in older patients. Pathologic degenerative changes were observed in the retinas of albino rats during studies with this agent, but were not observed in the retinas of pigmented rats or in other species. The significance of these data for humans remains uncertain.

Although not reported for pramipexole, other dopaminergic agents have been associated with a syndrome resembling neuroleptic malignant syndrome on withdrawal or significant dosage reduction after long-term use. Dopaminergic agents from the ergot class have also been associated with fibrotic complications, such as retroperitoneum, lungs, and pleura.

Pramipexole has been associated with somnolence, particularly at higher dosages (> 1.5 mg/day). In addition, patients have been reported to fall asleep during activities of daily living, including driving, while taking this medication. Whether these patients exhibited somnolence prior to these events is not clear. Patients should be advised of this issue and factors which may increase risk (sleep disorders, other sedating medications, or concomitant medications which increase pramipexole concentrations) and instructed to report daytime somnolence or sleepiness to the prescriber. Patients should use caution in performing activities which require alertness (driving or operating machinery), and to avoid other medications which may cause CNS depression, including ethanol.

Pregnancy Risk Factor C

Adverse Reactions

>10%:
- Cardiovascular: Postural hypotension
- Central nervous system: Asthenia, dizziness, somnolence, insomnia, hallucinations, abnormal dreams
- Gastrointestinal: Nausea, constipation
- Neuromuscular & skeletal: Weakness, dyskinesia, EPS

1% to 10%:
- Cardiovascular: Edema, postural hypotension, syncope, tachycardia, chest pain
- Central nervous system: Malaise, confusion, amnesia, dystonias, akathisia, thinking abnormalities, myoclonus, hyperesthesia, gait abnormalities, hypertonia, paranoia
- Endocrine & metabolic: Decreased libido
- Gastrointestinal: Anorexia, weight loss, xerostomia
- Genitourinary: Urinary frequency (up to 6%), impotence
- Neuromuscular & skeletal: Muscle twitching, leg cramps, arthritis, bursitis
- Ocular: Vision abnormalities (3%)
- Respiratory: Dyspnea, rhinitis

<1%: Elevated liver transaminase levels

Drug Interactions

Cimetidine in combination with pramipexole produced a 50% increase in AUC and a 40% increase in half-life

Drugs secreted by the cationic transport system (diltiazem, triamterene, verapamil, quinidine, quinine, ranitidine) decrease the clearance of pramipexole by ~20%

Dopamine antagonists (antipsychotics, metoclopramide) may decrease the efficiency of pramipexole

Alcohol Interactions Avoid use (may increase central nervous system depression)

Half-Life ~8 hours (12-14 hours in the elderly)

Education and Monitoring Issues

Patient Education: Do not take other medications, including over-the-counter products without consulting prescriber (especially important are other medicines that could make you sleepy such as sleeping pills, tranquilizers, some cold and allergy medicines,

(Continued)

Pramipexole *(Continued)*

narcotic pain killers, or medicines that relax muscles). Avoid alcohol as this may increase the potential for drowsiness or sedation.

Dietary Considerations: Food intake does not affect the extent of drug absorption, although the time to maximal plasma concentration is delayed by 60 minutes when taken with a meal

Monitoring Parameters: Monitor for improvement in symptoms of Parkinson's disease (eg, mentation, behavior, daily living activities, motor examinations), blood pressure, body weight changes, and heart rate

Manufacturer Pharmacia & Upjohn

Related Information

Parkinson's Disease Dosing *on page 1249*

Pharmaceutical Manufacturers Directory *on page 1020*

- **Pramosone®** *see* Pramoxine and Hydrocortisone *on page 758*
- **Pramox HC** *see* Pramoxine and Hydrocortisone *on page 758*

Pramoxine and Hydrocortisone (pra MOKS een & hye droe KOR ti sone)

Pharmacologic Class Anesthetic/Corticosteroid

U.S. Brand Names Enzone®; Pramosone®; Proctofoam®-HC; Zone-A Forte®

Dosage Forms CRM, top: Pramoxine hydrochloride 1% and hydrocortisone acetate 0.5% (30 g), pramoxine hydrochloride 1% and hydrocortisone acetate 1%. **FOAM, rectal:** Pramoxine hydrochloride 1% and hydrocortisone acetate 1% (10 g). **LOT, top:** Pramoxine hydrochloride 1% and hydrocortisone 0.25%, pramoxine hydrochloride 1% and hydrocortisone 2.5%, pramoxine hydrochloride 2.5% and hydrocortisone 1% (37.5 mL, 120 mL, 240 mL)

Pregnancy Risk Factor C

- **Prandase** *see* Acarbose *on page 14*
- **Prandin™** *see* Repaglinide *on page 812*
- **Pravachol®** *see* Pravastatin *on page 758*

Pravastatin (PRA va stat in)

Pharmacologic Class Antilipemic Agent (HMG-CoA Reductase Inhibitor)

U.S. Brand Names Pravachol®

Generic Available No

Mechanism of Action Pravastatin is a competitive inhibitor of 3-hydroxy-3-methylglutaryl coenzyme A (HMG-CoA) reductase, which is the rate-limiting enzyme involved in *de novo* cholesterol synthesis.

Use

"Primary prevention" in hypercholesterolemic patients without clinically-evident coronary heart disease to reduce the risk of myocardial infarction, reduce the risk of undergoing myocardial revascularization procedures, reduce the risk of cardiovascular mortality with no increase in death from noncardiovascular causes

"Secondary prevention" in hypercholesterolemic patients with clinically-evident coronary artery disease, including prior myocardial infarction, to slow the progression of coronary atherosclerosis, and reduce the risk of acute coronary events

"Secondary prevention" in patients with previous myocardial infarction, and normal cholesterol levels; to reduce the risk of recurrent myocardial infarction; reduce the risk of undergoing myocardial revascularization procedures; and reduce the risk of stroke or transient ischemic attack (TIA)

Adjunct to diet to reduce elevated total cholesterol, LDL cholesterol, apolipoprotein B (apo-B) and triglyceride levels in patients with primary hypercholesterolemia and mixed dyslipidemia (Fredrickson types IIa and IIb); Fredrickson type IV, type III (who do not respond adequately to diet)

USUAL DOSAGE Adults: Oral: 10, 20, or 40 mg once daily

Dosing adjustment in significant renal/hepatic impairment: Start at 10 mg/day

Dosage Forms TAB: 10 mg, 20 mg, 40 mg

Contraindications Previous hypersensitivity, active liver disease, or persistent, unexplained liver function enzyme elevations; specifically contraindicated in pregnant or lactating females

Warnings/Precautions May elevate aminotransferases; LFTs should be performed before and every 4-6 weeks during the first 12-15 months of therapy and periodically thereafter; can also cause myalgia and rhabdomyolysis; use with caution in patients who consume large quantities of alcohol or who have a history of liver disease

Pregnancy Risk Factor X

Adverse Reactions

1% to 10%:

Central nervous system: Headache (1.7% to 6.2%), fatigue (3.8%), dizziness (1% to 3.3%)

Cardiovascular: Chest pain (3.7%)

Dermatologic: Rash (4%)

Gastrointestinal: Nausea/vomiting (7.3%), diarrhea (6.2%), heartburn (2.9%)

Hepatic: Increased transaminases (>3x normal on two occasions - 1.3%)
Neuromuscular & skeletal: Myalgia (2.4%)
Respiratory: Cough (2.6%)
Miscellaneous: Influenza (2.4%)

<1%: Weakness, neuropathy, myopathy

Case reports: Lichenoid eruption, porphyria cutanea tarda

Additional class-related events or case reports (not necessarily reported with pravastatin therapy): Myopathy, increased CPK (>10x normal), rhabdomyolysis, renal failure (secondary to rhabdomyolysis), alteration in taste, impaired extraocular muscle movement, facial paresis, tremor, memory loss, vertigo, paresthesia, peripheral neuropathy, peripheral nerve palsy, anxiety, depression, psychic disturbance, hypersensitivity reaction, angioedema, anaphylaxis, systemic lupus erythematosus-like syndrome, polymyalgia rheumatica, dermatomyositis, vasculitis, purpura, thrombocytopenia, leukopenia, hemolytic anemia, positive ANA, increased ESR, eosinophilia, arthritis, urticaria, photosensitivity, fever, chills, flushing, malaise, dyspnea, rash, toxic epidermal necrolysis, erythema multiforme, Stevens-Johnson syndrome, pancreatitis, hepatitis, cholestatic jaundice, fatty liver, cirrhosis, fulminant hepatic necrosis, hepatoma, anorexia, vomiting, alopecia, pruritus, nodules, skin discoloration, dryness of skin/mucous membranes, nail changes, gynecomastia, decreased libido, erectile dysfunction, impotence, cataracts, ophthalmoplegia, elevated transaminases, increased alkaline phosphatase, increased GGT, hyperbilirubinemia, thyroid dysfunction

Drug Interactions CYP3A3/4 enzyme substrate

Cholestyramine reduces pravastatin absorption; separate administration times by at least 4 hours

Cholestyramine and colestipol (bile acid sequestrants): Cholesterol-lowering effects are additive

Clofibrate and fenofibrate may increase the risk of myopathy and rhabdomyolysis

Colestipol reduces pravastatin absorption

Gemfibrozil: Increased risk of myopathy and rhabdomyolysis

Niacin may increase the risk of myopathy and rhabdomyolysis

Onset Several days

Half-Life ~77 hours for parent and metabolites

Education and Monitoring Issues

Patient Education: Take at bedtime since highest rate of cholesterol synthesis occurs between midnight and 5 AM. Do not change dosage without consulting prescriber. Maintain diet and exercise program as prescribed. Have periodic ophthalmic exam while taking pravastatin (check for cataracts). You may experience mild GI disturbances (gas, diarrhea, constipation); inform prescriber if these are severe, or if you experience severe muscle pain or tenderness accompanied with malaise, blurred vision, or chest pain.

Monitoring Parameters: Creatine phosphokinase due to possibility of myopathy

Manufacturer Bristol-Myers Squibb Company (Pharmaceutical Division)

Related Information

Pharmaceutical Manufacturers Directory *on page 1020*

Praziquantel (pray zi KWON tel)

Pharmacologic Class Anthelmintic

U.S. Brand Names Biltricide®

Generic Available No

Mechanism of Action Increases the cell permeability to calcium in schistosomes, causing strong contractions and paralysis of worm musculature leading to detachment of suckers from the blood vessel walls and to dislodgment

Use All stages of schistosomiasis caused by all *Schistosoma* species pathogenic to humans; clonorchiasis and opisthorchiasis

Unlabeled use: Cysticercosis, flukes, and many intestinal tapeworms

USUAL DOSAGE Children >4 years and Adults: Oral:

Schistosomiasis: 20 mg/kg/dose 2-3 times/day for 1 day at 4- to 6-hour intervals

Flukes: 25 mg/kg/dose every 8 hours for 1-2 days

Cysticercosis: 50 mg/kg/day divided every 8 hours for 14 days

Tapeworms: 10-20 mg/kg as a single dose (25 mg/kg for *Hymenolepis nana*)

Clonorchiasis/opisthorchiasis: 3 doses of 25 mg/kg as a 1-day treatment

Dosage Forms TAB, tri-scored: 600 mg

Contraindications Ocular cysticercosis, known hypersensitivity to praziquantel

Warnings/Precautions Use caution in patients with severe hepatic disease; patients with cerebral cysticercosis require hospitalization

Pregnancy Risk Factor B

Adverse Reactions

1% to 10%:

Central nervous system: Dizziness, drowsiness, headache, malaise
Gastrointestinal: Abdominal pain, loss of appetite, nausea, vomiting
Miscellaneous: Diaphoresis

<1%: CSF reaction syndrome in patients being treated for neurocysticercosis, diarrhea, fever, itching, rash, urticaria

(Continued)

Praziquantel *(Continued)*

Drug Interactions Hydantoins may decrease praziquantel levels causing treatment failures

Half-Life Parent drug: 0.8-1.5 hours; Metabolites: 4.5 hours

Education and Monitoring Issues

Patient Education: Take exactly as directed for full course of medication. Tablets may be chewed, swallowed whole, or crushed and mixed with food. Increase dietary intake of fruit juices. All family members and close friends should also be treated. To reduce possibility of reinfection, wash hands and scrub nails carefully with soap and hot water before handling food, before eating, and before and after toileting. Keep hands out of mouth. Disinfect toilet daily and launder bed lines, undergarments, and nightclothes daily with hot water and soap. Do not go barefoot and do not sit directly on grass or ground. May cause dizziness, fainting, lightheadedness (use caution when driving or engaging in tasks that require alertness until response to drug is known); abdominal pain, nausea, or vomiting (frequent small meals, frequent mouth care, sucking lozenges, or chewing gum may help). Report unusual fatigue, persistent dizziness, CNS changes, change in color of urine or stool, or easy bruising or unusual bleeding.

Manufacturer Bayer Corp (Biological and Pharmaceutical Division)

Related Information

Pharmaceutical Manufacturers Directory *on page 1020*

Prazosin (PRA zoe sin)

Pharmacologic Class Alpha$_1$ Blockers

U.S. Brand Names Minipress®

Generic Available Yes

Mechanism of Action Competitively inhibits postsynaptic alpha-adrenergic receptors which results in vasodilation of veins and arterioles and a decrease in total peripheral resistance and blood pressure

Use Treatment of hypertension, severe refractory congestive heart failure (in conjunction with diuretics and cardiac glycosides); may reduce mortality in stable postmyocardial patients with left ventricular dysfunction (ejection fraction ≤40%)

Unlabeled use: Symptoms of benign prostatic hypertrophy, Raynaud's vasospasm

USUAL DOSAGE Oral:

Children: Initial: 5 mcg/kg/dose (to assess hypotensive effects); usual dosing interval: every 6 hours; increase dosage gradually up to maximum of 25 mcg/kg/dose every 6 hours

Adults:

- CHF, hypertension: Initial: 1 mg/dose 2-3 times/day; usual maintenance dose: 3-15 mg/day in divided doses 2-4 times/day; maximum daily dose: 20 mg
- Hypertensive urgency: 10-20 mg once, may repeat in 30 minutes
- Raynaud's: 0.5-3 mg twice daily
- Benign prostatic hypertrophy: 2 mg twice daily

Dosage Forms CAP: 1 mg, 2 mg, 5 mg

Contraindications Hypersensitivity to prazosin or any component

Warnings/Precautions Marked orthostatic hypotension, syncope, and loss of consciousness may occur with first dose ("first dose phenomenon") occurs more often in patients receiving beta-blockers, diuretics, low sodium diets, or larger first doses (ie, >1 mg/dose in adults); avoid rapid increase in dose; use with caution in patients with renal impairment

Pregnancy Risk Factor C

Adverse Reactions

>10%: Central nervous system: Dizziness (10.3%)

1% to 10%:

- Cardiovascular: Palpitations (5.3%), edema, orthostatic hypotension, syncope (1%)
- Central nervous system: Headache (7.8%), drowsiness (7.6%), weakness (6.5%), vertigo, depression, nervousness
- Dermatologic: Rash (1% to 4%)
- Endocrine & metabolic: Decreased energy (6.9%)
- Gastrointestinal: Nausea (4.9%), vomiting, diarrhea, constipation
- Genitourinary: Urinary frequency (1% to 5%)
- Ocular: Blurred vision, reddened sclera, xerostomia
- Respiratory: Dyspnea, epistaxis, nasal congestion

<1% (limited to important or life-threatening symptoms): Paresthesia, hallucinations, tachycardia, pruritus, alopecia, lichen planus, incontinence, impotence, priapism, abdominal discomfort, liver function abnormalities, pancreatitis, tinnitus, pigmentary mottling and serous retinopathy, cataracts (both development and disappearance have been reported), worsening of narcolepsy, angina, bradycardia, myocardial infarction

Case reports: Leukopenia, cataplexy, enuresis, systemic lupus erythematosus

Drug Interactions

Decreased effect (antihypertensive) with NSAIDs (eg, indomethacin); clonidine's antihypertensive effect may be decreased

Increased effect (hypotensive) with diuretics and antihypertensive medications (especially beta-blockers); verapamil may increase serum prazosin levels and sensitivity to postural hypotension

Alcohol Interactions Use with caution (may increase risk of hypotension or dizziness)

Onset Onset of hypotensive effect: Within 2 hours; Maximum decrease: 2-4 hours

Duration 10-24 hours

Half-Life 2-4 hours; increased with congestive heart failure

Education and Monitoring Issues

Patient Education: Take as directed (first dose at bedtime). Do not skip dose or discontinue without consulting prescriber. Follow recommended diet and exercise program. Do not use alcohol or OTC medications which may affect blood pressure (eg, cough or cold remedies, diet pills, stay-awake medications) without consulting prescriber. You may experience drowsiness, dizziness, or impaired judgment (use caution when driving or engaging in tasks that require alertness until response to drug is known); postural hypotension (use caution when rising from sitting or lying position or when climbing stairs); dry mouth or nausea (frequent mouth care or sucking lozenges may help); or urinary incontinence (void before taking medication). Report altered CNS status (eg, fatigue, lethargy, confusion, nervousness); sudden weight gain (weigh yourself in the same clothes at the same time of day once a week); unusual or persistent swelling of ankles, feet, or extremities; palpitations or rapid heartbeat; difficulty breathing; or other persistent side effects.

Monitoring Parameters: Blood pressure, standing and sitting/supine

Related Information

Prazosin and Polythiazide *on page 761*

Prazosin and Polythiazide (PRA zoe sin & pol i THYE a zide)

Pharmacologic Class Antihypertensive Agent, Combination

U.S. Brand Names Minizide®

Dosage Forms CAP: 1: Prazosin 1 mg and polythiazide 0.5 mg; 2: Prazosin 2 mg and polythiazide 0.5 mg; 5: Prazosin 5 mg and polythiazide 0.5 mg

Pregnancy Risk Factor C

- **Precose®** *see* Acarbose *on page 14*
- **Predair®** *see* Prednisolone *on page 762*
- **Predaject®** *see* Prednisolone *on page 762*
- **Predalone T.B.A.®** *see* Prednisolone *on page 762*
- **Predcor®** *see* Prednisolone *on page 762*
- **Predcor-TBA®** *see* Prednisolone *on page 762*
- **Pred Forte® Ophthalmic** *see* Prednisolone *on page 762*
- **Pred-G® Ophthalmic** *see* Prednisolone and Gentamicin *on page 763*
- **Pred Mild® Ophthalmic** *see* Prednisolone *on page 762*

Prednicarbate (PRED ni kar bate)

Pharmacologic Class Corticosteroid, Topical

U.S. Brand Names Dermatop®

Mechanism of Action Topical corticosteroids have anti-inflammatory, antipruritic, vasoconstrictive, and antiproliferative actions

Use Relief of the inflammatory and pruritic manifestations of corticosteroid-responsive dermatoses (medium potency topical corticosteroid)

USUAL DOSAGE Adults: Topical: Apply a thin film to affected area twice daily. Therapy should be discontinued when control is achieved; if no improvement is seen, reassessment of diagnosis may be necessary.

Dosage Forms CRM: 0.1% (15 g, 60 g)

Contraindications Hypersensitivity to prednicarbate or any component; fungal, viral, or tubercular skin lesions, herpes simplex or zoster

Warnings/Precautions Systemic absorption of topical corticosteroids has produced reversible HPA axis suppression. This is more likely to occur when the preparation is used on large surface or denuded areas for prolonged periods of time or with an occlusive dressing.

Pregnancy Risk Factor C

Adverse Reactions

1% to 10%: Dermatologic: Skin atrophy, shininess, thinness, mild telangiectasia

<1%: Acneiform eruptions, allergic contact dermatitis and rash, burning, edema, folliculitis, hypopigmentation, miliaria, paresthesia, perioral dermatitis, pruritus, secondary infection, striae, urticaria

Education and Monitoring Issues

Patient Education: Use only as prescribed and for no longer than the period prescribed; apply sparingly in a thin film and rub in lightly; avoid contact with eyes; do not apply to the face, underarms, or groin areas; notify prescriber if condition persists or worsens

Monitoring Parameters: Relief of symptoms

- **Prednicen-M®** *see* Prednisone *on page 763*

Prednisolone (pred NIS oh lone)

Pharmacologic Class Corticosteroid, Ophthalmic; Corticosteroid, Parenteral

U.S. Brand Names AK-Pred® Ophthalmic; Articulose-50® Injection; Delta-Cortef® Oral; Econopred® Ophthalmic; Econopred® Plus Ophthalmic; Inflamase® Forte Ophthalmic; Inflamase® Mild Ophthalmic; Key-Pred® Injection; Key-Pred-SP® Injection; Metreton® Ophthalmic; Pediapred® Oral; Predair®; Predaject®; Predalone T.B.A.®; Predcor®; Predcor-TBA®; Pred Forte® Ophthalmic; Pred Mild® Ophthalmic; Prednisol® TBA Injection; Prelone® Oral

Generic Available Yes

Mechanism of Action Decreases inflammation by suppression of migration of polymorphonuclear leukocytes and reversal of increased capillary permeability; suppresses the immune system by reducing activity and volume of the lymphatic system

Use Treatment of palpebral and bulbar conjunctivitis; corneal injury from chemical, radiation, thermal burns, or foreign body penetration; endocrine disorders, rheumatic disorders, collagen diseases, dermatologic diseases, allergic states, ophthalmic diseases, respiratory diseases, hematologic disorders, neoplastic diseases, edematous states, and gastrointestinal diseases; useful in patients with inability to activate prednisone (liver disease)

USUAL DOSAGE Dose depends upon condition being treated and response of patient; dosage for infants and children should be based on severity of the disease and response of the patient rather than on strict adherence to dosage indicated by age, weight, or body surface area. Consider alternate day therapy for long-term therapy. Discontinuation of long-term therapy requires gradual withdrawal by tapering the dose.

Children:
- Acute asthma:
  - Oral: 1-2 mg/kg/day in divided doses 1-2 times/day for 3-5 days
  - I.V. (sodium phosphate salt): 2-4 mg/kg/day divided 3-4 times/day
- Anti-inflammatory or immunosuppressive dose: Oral, I.V., I.M. (sodium phosphate salt): 0.1-2 mg/kg/day in divided doses 1-4 times/day
- Nephrotic syndrome: Oral:
  - Initial (first 3 episodes): 2 mg/kg/day **or** 60 mg/m²/day (maximum: 80 mg/day) in divided doses 3-4 times/day until urine is protein free for 3 consecutive days (maximum: 28 days); followed by 1-1.5 mg/kg/dose **or** 40 mg/m²/dose given every other day for 4 weeks
  - Maintenance (long-term maintenance dose for frequent relapses): 0.5-1 mg/kg/dose given every other day for 3-6 months

Adults:
- Oral, I.V., I.M. (sodium phosphate salt): 5-60 mg/day
- Multiple sclerosis (sodium phosphate): Oral: 200 mg/day for 1 week followed by 80 mg every other day for 1 month
- Rheumatoid arthritis: Oral: Initial: 5-7.5 mg/day; adjust dose as necessary

Elderly: Use lowest effective dose

Dosing adjustment in hyperthyroidism: Prednisolone dose may need to be increased to achieve adequate therapeutic effects

Hemodialysis: Slightly dialyzable (5% to 20%); administer dose posthemodialysis

Peritoneal dialysis: Supplemental dose is not necessary

Intra-articular, intralesional, soft-tissue administration:
- Tebutate salt: 4-40 mg/dose
- Sodium phosphate salt: 2-30 mg/dose

Ophthalmic suspension/solution: Children and Adults: Instill 1-2 drops into conjunctival sac every hour during day, every 2 hours at night until favorable response is obtained, then use 1 drop every 4 hours

Dosage Forms INJ: As acetate (for I.M., intralesional, intra-articular, or soft tissue administration only): 25 mg/mL (10 mL, 30 mL), 50 mg/mL (30 mL); As sodium phosphate (for I.M., I.V., intra-articular, intralesional, or soft tissue administration): 20 mg/mL (2 mL, 5 mL, 10 mL); As tebutate (for intra-articular, intralesional, soft tissue administration only): 20 mg/mL (1 mL, 5 mL, 10 mL). **LIQ, oral,** as sodium phosphate: 5 mg/5 mL (120 mL). **SOLN, ophth,** as sodium phosphate: 0.125% (5 mL, 10 mL, 15 mL), 1% (5 mL, 10 mL, 15 mL). **SUSP ophth,** as acetate: 0.12% (5 mL, 10 mL), 0.125% (5 mL, 10 mL, 15 mL), 1% (1 mL, 5 mL, 10 mL, 15 mL). **SYR:** 15 mg/5 mL (240 mL). **TAB:** 5 mg

Contraindications Acute superficial herpes simplex keratitis; systemic fungal infections; varicella; hypersensitivity to prednisolone or any component

Warnings/Precautions Use with caution in patients with hyperthyroidism, cirrhosis, nonspecific ulcerative colitis, hypertension, osteoporosis, thromboembolic tendencies, CHF, convulsive disorders, myasthenia gravis, thrombophlebitis, peptic ulcer, diabetes; acute adrenal insufficiency may occur with abrupt withdrawal after long-term therapy or with stress; young pediatric patients may be more susceptible to adrenal axis suppression from topical therapy. Because of the risk of adverse effects, systemic corticosteroids should be used cautiously in the elderly, in the smallest possible dose, and for the shortest possible time.

Pregnancy Risk Factor C

Adverse Reactions

>10%:
- Central nervous system: Insomnia, nervousness

Gastrointestinal: Increased appetite, indigestion

1% to 10%:

Dermatologic: Hirsutism

Endocrine & metabolic: Diabetes mellitus

Neuromuscular & skeletal: Arthralgia

Ocular: Cataracts, glaucoma

Respiratory: Epistaxis

<1%: Abdominal distention, acne, alkalosis, amenorrhea, bruising, Cushing's syndrome, delirium, edema, euphoria, fractures, glucose intolerance, growth suppression, hallucinations, headache, hyperglycemia, hyperpigmentation, hypersensitivity reactions, hypertension, hypokalemia, mood swings, muscle wasting, muscle weakness, nausea, osteoporosis, pancreatitis, peptic ulcer, pituitary-adrenal axis suppression, pseudotumor cerebri, psychoses, seizures, skin atrophy, sodium and water retention, ulcerative esophagitis, vertigo, vomiting

Drug Interactions CYP3A enzyme substrate; inducer of cytochrome P-450 enzymes

Decreased effect:

Barbiturates, phenytoin, rifampin decrease corticosteroid effectiveness

Decreases salicylates

Decreases vaccines

Decreases toxoids effectiveness

Alcohol Interactions Avoid use (may enhance gastric mucosal irritation)

Duration 18-36 hours

Half-Life I.V.: 3.6 hours Biological: 18-36 hours; End-stage renal disease: 3-5 hours

Education and Monitoring Issues

Patient Education: Take exactly as directed; do not increase dose or discontinue abruptly without consulting prescriber. Take oral medication with or after meals. Limit intake of caffeine or stimulants. Prescriber may recommend increased dietary vitamins, minerals, or iron. Diabetics should monitor glucose levels closely (antidiabetic medication may need to be adjusted). Inform prescriber if you are experiencing greater than normal levels of stress (medication may need adjustment). Some forms of this medication may cause GI upset (oral medication may be taken with meals to reduce GI upset; small frequent meals and frequent mouth care may reduce GI upset). You may be more susceptible to infection (avoid crowds and persons with contagious or infective conditions). Report promptly excessive nervousness or sleep disturbances; any signs of infection (sore throat, unhealed injuries); excessive growth of body hair or loss of skin color; changes in vision; excessive or sudden weight gain (>3 lb/week); swelling of face or extremities; difficulty breathing; muscle weakness; change in color of stools (black or tarry) or persistent abdominal pain; or worsening of condition or failure to improve.

Ophthalmic: For ophthalmic use only. Wash hands before using. Tilt head back and look upward. Put drops of suspension or apply thin ribbon of ointment inside lower eyelid. Close eye and roll eyeball in all directions. Do not blink for 1/2 minute. Apply gentle pressure to inner corner of eye for 30 seconds. Do not use any other eye preparation for at least 10 minutes. Do not touch tip of applicator to eye or contaminate tip of applicator. Do not share medication with anyone else. Wear sunglasses when in sunlight; you may be more sensitive to bright light. Inform prescriber if condition worsens or fails to improve or if you experience eye pain, disturbances of vision, or other adverse eye response.

Monitoring Parameters: Blood pressure, blood glucose, electrolytes

Related Information

Chloramphenicol and Prednisolone *on page 180*

Corticosteroids Comparison *on page 1237*

Neomycin, Polymyxin B, and Prednisolone *on page 644*

Prednisolone and Gentamicin *on page 763*

Sulfacetamide Sodium and Prednisolone *on page 876*

Prednisolone and Gentamicin (pred NIS oh lone & jen ta MYE sin)

Pharmacologic Class Antibiotic/Corticosteroid, Ophthalmic

U.S. Brand Names Pred-G® Ophthalmic

Dosage Forms **OINT, ophth:** Prednisolone acetate 0.6% and gentamicin sulfate 0.3% (3.5 g). **SUSP, ophth:** Prednisolone acetate 1% and gentamicin sulfate 0.3% (2 mL, 5 mL, 10 mL)

Pregnancy Risk Factor C

♦ **Prednisol® TBA Injection** *see* Prednisolone *on page 762*

Prednisone (PRED ni sone)

Pharmacologic Class Corticosteroid, Oral

U.S. Brand Names Deltasone®; Liquid Pred®; Meticorten®; Orasone®; Prednicen-M®; Sterapred®

Generic Available Yes

Mechanism of Action Decreases inflammation by suppression of migration of polymorphonuclear leukocytes and reversal of increased capillary permeability; suppresses the immune system by reducing activity and volume of the lymphatic system; suppresses adrenal function at high doses. Antitumor effects may be related to inhibition of glucose

(Continued)

Prednisone *(Continued)*

transport, phosphorylation, or induction of cell death in immature lymphocytes. Antiemetic effects are thought to occur due to blockade of cerebral innervation of the emetic center via inhibition of prostaglandin synthesis.

Use Treatment of a variety of diseases including adrenocortical insufficiency, hypercalcemia, rheumatic, and collagen disorders; dermatologic, ocular, respiratory, gastrointestinal, and neoplastic diseases; organ transplantation and a variety of diseases including those of hematologic, allergic, inflammatory, and autoimmune in origin; not available in injectable form, prednisolone must be used

Investigational: Prevention of postherpetic neuralgia and relief of acute pain in the early stages

USUAL DOSAGE Oral: Dose depends upon condition being treated and response of patient; dosage for infants and children should be based on severity of the disease and response of the patient rather than on strict adherence to dosage indicated by age, weight, or body surface area. Consider alternate day therapy for long-term therapy. Discontinuation of long-term therapy requires gradual withdrawal by tapering the dose.

Children:
- Anti-inflammatory or immunosuppressive dose: 0.05-2 mg/kg/day divided 1-4 times/day
- Acute asthma: 1-2 mg/kg/day in divided doses 1-2 times/day for 3-5 days
  - Alternatively (for 3- to 5-day "burst"):
  - <1 year: 10 mg every 12 hours
  - 1-4 years: 20 mg every 12 hours
  - 5-13 years: 30 mg every 12 hours
  - >13 years: 40 mg every 12 hours
- Asthma long-term therapy (alternative dosing by age):
  - <1 year: 10 mg every other day
  - 1-4 years: 20 mg every other day
  - 5-13 years: 30 mg every other day
  - >13 years: 40 mg every other day
- Nephrotic syndrome: Initial (first 3 episodes): 2 mg/kg/day **or** 60 mg/m^2/day (maximum: 80 mg/day) in divided doses 3-4 times/day until urine is protein free for 3 consecutive days (maximum: 28 days); followed by 1-1.5 mg/kg/dose **or** 40 mg/m^2/dose given every other day for 4 weeks
- Maintenance dose (long-term maintenance dose for frequent relapses): 0.5-1 mg/kg/dose given every other day for 3-6 months

Children and Adults: Physiologic replacement: 4-5 mg/m^2/day

Adults: 5-60 mg/day in divided doses 1-4 times/day

Elderly: Use the lowest effective dose

Dosing adjustment in hepatic impairment: Prednisone is inactive and must be metabolized by the liver to prednisolone. This conversion may be impaired in patients with liver disease, however, prednisolone levels are observed to be higher in patients with severe liver failure than in normal patients. Therefore, compensation for the inadequate conversion of prednisone to prednisolone occurs.

Dosing adjustment in hyperthyroidism: Prednisone dose may need to be increased to achieve adequate therapeutic effects

Hemodialysis: Supplemental dose is not necessary

Peritoneal dialysis: Supplemental dose is not necessary

Dosage Forms SOLN, oral: Concentrate (30% alcohol): 5 mg/mL (30 mL); Nonconcentrate (5% alcohol) 5 mg/mL (5 mL, 500 mL). **SYR:** 5 mg/5 mL (120 mL, 240 mL). **TAB:** 1 mg, 2.5 mg, 5 mg, 10 mg, 20 mg, 50 mg

Contraindications Serious infections, except septic shock or tuberculous meningitis; systemic fungal infections; hypersensitivity to prednisone or any component; varicella

Warnings/Precautions Withdraw therapy with gradual tapering of dose, may retard bone growth; use with caution in patients with hypothyroidism, cirrhosis, hypertension, congestive heart failure, ulcerative colitis, thromboembolic disorders, and patients at increased risk for peptic ulcer disease. Because of the risk of adverse effects, systemic corticosteroids should be used cautiously in the elderly, in the smallest possible dose, and for the shortest possible time.

Pregnancy Risk Factor B

Pregnancy Implications

Clinical effects on the fetus: Crosses the placenta. Immunosuppression reported in 1 infant exposed to high-dose prednisone plus azathioprine throughout gestation. One report of congenital cataracts. Available evidence suggests safe use during pregnancy.

Breast-feeding/lactation: Crosses into breast milk. No data on clinical effects on the infant. American Academy of Pediatrics considers **compatible** with breast-feeding.

Adverse Reactions

>10%:
- Central nervous system: Insomnia, nervousness
- Gastrointestinal: Increased appetite, indigestion

1% to 10%:
- Dermatologic: Hirsutism
- Endocrine & metabolic: Diabetes mellitus
- Ocular: Cataracts, glaucoma

Neuromuscular & skeletal: Arthralgia
Respiratory: Epistaxis

<1%: Abdominal distention, acne, alkalosis, amenorrhea, bruising, Cushing's syndrome, delirium, edema, euphoria, fractures, glucose intolerance, growth suppression, hallucinations, headache, hyperglycemia, hyperpigmentation, hypersensitivity reactions, hypertension, hypokalemia, mood swings, muscle wasting, muscle weakness, osteoporosis, pancreatitis, peptic ulcer, pituitary-adrenal axis suppression, pseudotumor cerebri, psychoses, seizures, skin atrophy, sodium and water retention, ulcerative esophagitis, vertigo, vomiting

Drug Interactions CYP3A3/4 enzyme substrate

Decreased effect:

Barbiturates, phenytoin, rifampin decrease corticosteroid effectiveness
Decreases salicylates
Decreases vaccines
Decreases toxoids effectiveness

Alcohol Interactions Avoid use (may enhance gastric mucosal irritation)

Duration 18-36 hours

Half-Life Normal renal function: 2.5-3.5 hours

Education and Monitoring Issues

Patient Education: Take exactly as directed. Do not take more than prescribed dose and do not discontinue abruptly; consult prescriber. Take with or after meals. Take once-a-day dose with food in the morning. Limit intake of caffeine or stimulants. Maintain adequate nutrition; consult prescriber for possibility of special dietary recommendations. If diabetic, monitor serum glucose closely and notify prescriber of changes; this medication can affect blood glucose readings. Notify prescriber if you are experiencing higher than normal levels of stress; medication may need adjustment. Periodic ophthalmic examinations will be necessary with long-term use. You will be susceptible to infection; avoid crowds or infected persons or persons with contagious diseases. You may experience insomnia or nervousness; use caution when driving or engaging in tasks requiring alertness until response to drug is known. Report weakness, change in menstrual pattern, vision changes, signs of hyperglycemia, signs of infection (eg, fever, chills, mouth sores, perianal itching, vaginal discharge), other persistent side effects, or worsening of condition.

Monitoring Parameters: Blood pressure, blood glucose, electrolytes

Related Information

Anticonvulsants by Seizure Type Comparison *on page 1230*
Corticosteroids Comparison *on page 1237*

- **Prefrin® Liquifilm®** *see* Phenylephrine *on page 727*
- **Prefrin™ Ophthalmic Solution** *see* Phenylephrine *on page 727*
- **Pregnyl®** *see* Chorionic Gonadotropin *on page 196*
- **Prelone® Oral** *see* Prednisolone *on page 762*
- **Premarin®** *see* Estrogens, Conjugated *on page 331*
- **Premarin® With Methyltestosterone** *see* Estrogens and Methyltestosterone *on page 330*
- **Premphase™** *see* Estrogens and Medroxyprogesterone *on page 330*
- **Prempro™** *see* Estrogens and Medroxyprogesterone *on page 330*
- **Prenavite® [OTC]** *see* Vitamins, Multiple *on page 981*
- **Pre-Par®** *see* Ritodrine *on page 826*
- **Pre-Pen®** *see* Benzylpenicilloyl-polylysine *on page 101*
- **Prepidil® Vaginal Gel** *see* Dinoprostone *on page 281*
- **Prepulsid®** *see* Cisapride *on page 201*
- **Prescription Strength Desenex® [OTC]** *see* Miconazole *on page 600*
- **Pressyn®** *see* Vasopressin *on page 972*
- **Pretz® [OTC]** *see* Sodium Chloride *on page 858*
- **Pretz-D® [OTC]** *see* Ephedrine *on page 315*
- **Prevacid®** *see* Lansoprazole *on page 509*
- **Prevalite®** *see* Cholestyramine Resin *on page 192*
- **Preven™** *see* Ethinyl Estradiol and Levonorgestrel *on page 341*
- **Prevention of Bacterial Endocarditis** *see page 1154*
- **Prevention of Wound Infection & Sepsis in Surgical Patients** *see page 1158*
- **Prevex HC** *see* Hydrocortisone *on page 447*
- **PreviDent®** *see* Fluoride *on page 376*
- **Priftin®** *see* Rifapentine *on page 822*
- **Prilosec™** *see* Omeprazole *on page 675*
- **Primacor®** *see* Milrinone *on page 606*

Primaquine Phosphate (PRIM a kween FOS fate)

Pharmacologic Class Aminoquinoline (Antimalarial)

Generic Available No

(Continued)

Primaquine Phosphate *(Continued)*

Mechanism of Action Eliminates the primary tissue exoerythrocytic forms of *P. falciparum*; disrupts mitochondria and binds to DNA

Use Provides radical cure of *P. vivax* or *P. ovale* malaria after a clinical attack has been confirmed by blood smear or serologic titer and postexposure prophylaxis

USUAL DOSAGE Oral:

Children: 0.3 mg base/kg/day once daily for 14 days (not to exceed 15 mg/day) or 0.9 mg base/kg once weekly for 8 weeks not to exceed 45 mg base/week

Adults: 15 mg/day (base) once daily for 14 days or 45 mg base once weekly for 8 weeks

CDC treatment recommendations: Begin therapy during last 2 weeks of, or following a course of, suppression with chloroquine or a comparable drug

Dosage Forms TAB: 26.3 mg [15 mg base]

Contraindications Acutely ill patients who have a tendency to develop granulocytopenia (rheumatoid arthritis, SLE); patients receiving other drugs capable of depressing the bone marrow (eg, quinacrine and primaquine)

Warnings/Precautions Use with caution in patients with G-6-PD deficiency, NADH methemoglobin reductase deficiency, acutely ill patients who have a tendency to develop granulocytopenia; patients receiving other drugs capable of depressing the bone marrow; do not exceed recommended dosage

Pregnancy Risk Factor C

Adverse Reactions

>10%:

Gastrointestinal: Abdominal pain, nausea, vomiting

Hematologic: Hemolytic anemia in G-6-PD deficiency

1% to 10%: Hematologic: Methemoglobinemia in NADH-methemoglobin reductase-deficient individuals

<1%: Agranulocytosis, arrhythmias, headache, interference with visual accommodation, leukocytosis, leukopenia, pruritus

Drug Interactions Quinacrine may potentiate the toxicity of antimalarial compounds which are structurally related to primaquine

Half-Life 3.7-9.6 hours

Education and Monitoring Issues

Patient Education: It is important to complete full course of therapy for full effect. May be taken with meals to decrease GI upset and bitter aftertaste. Avoid alcohol. You should have regular ophthalmic exams (every 4-6 months) if using this medication over extended periods. You may experience nausea, vomiting, or loss of appetite (small frequent meals, frequent mouth care, sucking lozenges, or chewing gum may help). Report persistent GI disturbance, chest pain or palpitation, unusual fatigue, easy bruising or bleeding, visual or hearing disturbances, changes in urine (darkening, tinged with red, decreased volume), or any other persistent adverse reactions.

Monitoring Parameters: Periodic CBC, visual color check of urine, glucose, electrolytes; if hemolysis suspected - CBC, haptoglobin, peripheral smear, urinalysis dipstick for occult blood

♦ **Primaxin®** *see* Imipenem and Cilastatin *on page 461*

Primidone (PRI mi done)

Pharmacologic Class Anticonvulsant, Miscellaneous; Barbiturate

U.S. Brand Names Mysoline®

Generic Available Yes: Tablet

Mechanism of Action Decreases neuron excitability, raises seizure threshold similar to phenobarbital; primidone has two active metabolites, phenobarbital and phenylethylmalonamide (PEMA); PEMA may enhance the activity of phenobarbital

Use Management of grand mal, complex partial, and focal seizures

Unlabeled use: Benign familial tremor (essential tremor)

USUAL DOSAGE Oral:

Children <8 years: Initial: 50-125 mg/day given at bedtime; increase by 50-125 mg/day increments every 3-7 days; usual dose: 10-25 mg/kg/day in divided doses 3-4 times/day

Children >8 years and Adults: Initial: 125-250 mg/day at bedtime; increase by 125-250 mg/day every 3-7 days; usual dose: 750-1500 mg/day in divided doses 3-4 times/day with maximum dosage of 2 g/day

Dosing interval in renal impairment:

Cl_{cr} 50-80 mL/minute: Administer every 8 hours

Cl_{cr} 10-50 mL/minute: Administer every 8-12 hours

Cl_{cr} <10 mL/minute: Administer every 12-24 hours

Hemodialysis: Moderately dialyzable (20% to 50%); administer dose postdialysis or administer supplemental 30% dose

Dosage Forms SUSP, oral: 250 mg/5 mL (240 mL). **TAB:** 50 mg, 250 mg

Contraindications Hypersensitivity to primidone, phenobarbital, or any component; porphyria

Warnings/Precautions Use with caution in patients with renal or hepatic impairment, pulmonary insufficiency; abrupt withdrawal may precipitate status epilepticus

Pregnancy Risk Factor D

Pregnancy Implications

Clinical effects on the fetus: Crosses the placenta. Dysmorphic facial features; hemorrhagic disease of newborn due to fetal vitamin K depletion, maternal folic acid deficiency may occur. Epilepsy itself, number of medications, genetic factors, or a combination of these probably influence the teratogenicity of anticonvulsant therapy. Benefit:risk ratio usually favors continued use during pregnancy and breast-feeding.

Breast-feeding/lactation: Crosses into breast milk

Clinical effects on the infant: Sedation; feeding problems reported. American Academy of Pediatrics recommends USE WITH CAUTION.

Adverse Reactions

Central nervous system: Drowsiness, vertigo, ataxia, lethargy, behavior change, fatigue, hyperirritability

Dermatologic: Rash

Gastrointestinal: Nausea, vomiting, anorexia

Genitourinary: Impotence

Hematologic: Agranulocytopenia, agranulocytosis, anemia

Ocular: Diplopia, nystagmus

Drug Interactions CYP1A2, 2B6, 2C, 2C8, 3A3/4, and 3A5-7 enzyme inducer

Barbiturates are enzyme inducers. Patients should be monitored when these drugs are started or stopped for a decreased or increased therapeutic effect respectively.

Primidone may reduce the efficacy of beta-blockers, chloramphenicol, cimetidine, clozapine, corticosteroids, cyclosporine, disopyramide, doxycycline, ethosuximide, furosemide, griseofulvin, haloperidol, lamotrigine, methadone, nifedipine, oral contraceptives, phenothiazine, phenytoin, propafenone, quinidine, tacrolimus, TCAs, theophylline, **warfarin**, and verapamil

Increased toxicity when combined with other CNS depressants, benzodiazepine, valproic acid, chloramphenicol, or antidepressants; respiratory and CNS depression may be additive

MAOIs may prolong the effect of primidone

Barbiturates inhibit the hypoprothombinemic response to warfarin

Alcohol Interactions Avoid use (may increase central nervous system depression)

Half-Life Age dependent: Primidone: 10-12 hours; PEMA: 16 hours; Phenobarbital: 52-118 hours

Education and Monitoring Issues

Patient Education: Take exactly as directed (do not increase dose or frequency or discontinue without consulting prescriber); may cause physical and/or psychological dependence. While using this medication, do not use alcohol and other prescription or OTC medications (especially pain medications, sedatives, antihistamines, or hypnotics) without consulting prescriber. Maintain adequate hydration (2-3 L/day of fluids unless instructed to restrict fluid intake). You may experience drowsiness, dizziness, or blurred vision (use caution when driving or engaging in tasks requiring alertness until response to drug is known); nausea, vomiting, or loss of appetite (small frequent meals, frequent mouth care, chewing gum, or sucking lozenges may help); impotence (reversible). Wear identification of epileptic status and medications. Report behavioral or CNS changes (confusion, depression, increased sedation, excitation, headache, insomnia, or lethargy); muscle weakness, or tremors; unusual bruising or bleeding (mouth, urine, stool); worsening of seizure activity, or loss of seizure control.

Dietary Considerations:

Food:

Folic acid: Low erythrocyte and CSF folate concentrations. Megaloblastic anemia has been reported. To avoid folic acid deficiency and megaloblastic anemia, some clinicians recommend giving patients on anticonvulsants prophylactic doses of folic acid and cyanocobalamin.

Protein-deficient diets: Increases duration of action of primidone. Should not restrict or delete protein from diet unless discussed with prescriber. Be consistent with protein intake during primidone therapy.

Fresh fruits containing vitamin C: Displaces drug from binding sites, resulting in increased urinary excretion of primidone. Educate patients regarding the potential for decreased primidone effect with consumption of foods high in vitamin C.

Monitoring Parameters: Serum primidone and phenobarbital concentration, CBC, neurological status. Due to CNS effects, monitor closely when initiating drug in elderly. Monitor CBC at 6-month intervals to compare with baseline obtained at start of therapy. Since elderly metabolize phenobarbital at a slower rate than younger adults, it is suggested to measure both primidone and phenobarbital levels together.

Reference Range: Therapeutic: Children <5 years: 7-10 μg/mL (SI: 32-46 μmol/L); Adults: 5-12 μg/mL (SI: 23-55 μmol/L); toxic effects rarely present with levels <10 μg/mL (SI: 46 μmol/L) if phenobarbital concentrations are low. Dosage of primidone is adjusted with reference mostly to the phenobarbital level; Toxic: >15 μg/mL (SI: >69 μmol/L)

Related Information

Epilepsy Guidelines *on page 1091*

♦ **Principen®** *see* Ampicillin *on page 59*

- **Prinivil®** *see* Lisinopril *on page 532*
- **Prinzide®** *see* Lisinopril and Hydrochlorothiazide *on page 534*
- **Prioderm** *see* Malathion *on page 553*
- **Priscoline®** *see* Tolazoline *on page 927*
- **Privine®** *see* Naphazoline *on page 636*
- **ProAmatine®** *see* Midodrine *on page 603*
- **Pro-Amox®** *see* Amoxicillin *on page 56*
- **Proavil** *see* Amitriptyline and Perphenazine *on page 52*
- **Probalan®** *see* Probenecid *on page 768*
- **Pro-Banthine®** *see* Propantheline *on page 782*

Probenecid (proe BEN e sid)

Pharmacologic Class Uricosuric Agent

U.S. Brand Names Benemid®; Probalan®

Generic Available Yes

Mechanism of Action Competitively inhibits the reabsorption of uric acid at the proximal convoluted tubule, thereby promoting its excretion and reducing serum uric acid levels; increases plasma levels of weak organic acids (penicillins, cephalosporins, or other beta-lactam antibiotics) by competitively inhibiting their renal tubular secretion

Use Prevention of gouty arthritis; hyperuricemia; prolongation of beta-lactam effect (ie, serum levels)

USUAL DOSAGE Oral:

Children:

<2 years: Not recommended

2-14 years: Prolong penicillin serum levels: 25 mg/kg starting dose, then 40 mg/kg/day given 4 times/day

Gonorrhea: <45 kg: 25 mg/kg x 1 (maximum: 1 g/dose) 30 minutes before penicillin, ampicillin or amoxicillin

Adults:

Hyperuricemia with gout: 250 mg twice daily for one week; increase to 250-500 mg/day; may increase by 500 mg/month, if needed, to maximum of 2-3 g/day (dosages may be increased by 500 mg every 6 months if serum urate concentrations are controlled)

Prolong penicillin serum levels: 500 mg 4 times/day

Gonorrhea: 1 g 30 minutes before penicillin, ampicillin, procaine, or amoxicillin

Pelvic inflammatory disease: Cefoxitin 2 g I.M. plus probenecid 1 g orally as a single dose

Neurosyphilis: Aqueous procaine penicillin 2.4 units/day I.M. plus probenecid 500 mg 4 times/day for 10-14 days

Dosing adjustment in renal impairment: Cl_{cr} <50 mL/minute: Avoid use

Dosage Forms TAB: 500 mg

Contraindications Hypersensitivity to probenecid or any component; high-dose aspirin therapy; moderate to severe renal impairment; children <2 years of age

Warnings/Precautions Use with caution in patients with peptic ulcer; use extreme caution in the use of probenecid with penicillin in patients with renal insufficiency; probenecid may not be effective in patients with a creatinine clearance <30 to 50 mL/minute; may cause exacerbation of acute gouty attack

Pregnancy Risk Factor B

Adverse Reactions

>10%:

Central nervous system: Headache

Gastrointestinal: Anorexia, nausea, vomiting

Neuromuscular & skeletal: Gouty arthritis (acute)

1% to 10%:

Cardiovascular: Flushing of face

Central nervous system: Dizziness

Dermatologic: Rash, itching

Gastrointestinal: Sore gums

Genitourinary: Painful urination

Renal: Renal calculi

<1%: Anaphylaxis, aplastic anemia, hemolytic anemia, hepatic necrosis, leukopenia, nephrotic syndrome, urate nephropathy

Drug Interactions

Decreased effect:

Salicylates (high dose) may decrease uricosuria

Nitrofurantoin may decrease efficacy

Increased toxicity:

Increases methotrexate toxic potential; combination with diflunisal has resulted in 40% decrease in its clearance and as much as a 65% increase in plasma concentrations due to inhibition of diflunisal metabolism

Probenecid decreases clearance of beta-lactams such as penicillins and cephalosporins; increases levels/toxicity of acyclovir, thiopental, clofibrate, dyphylline, pantothenic acid, benzodiazepines, rifampin, sulfonamide, dapsone, sulfonylureas, quinolones, and zidovudine

Avoid concomitant use with ketorolac (and other NSAIDs) since its half-life is increased twofold and levels and toxicity are significantly increased

Allopurinol readministration may be beneficial by increasing the uric acid lowering effect

Pharmacologic effects of penicillamine may be attenuated

Onset Effect on penicillin levels reached in about 2 hours

Half-Life Normal renal function: 6-12 hours and is dose dependent

Education and Monitoring Issues

Patient Education: Take as directed; do not discontinue without consulting prescriber. May take 6-12 months to reduce gouty attacks (attacks may increase in frequency and severity for first few months of therapy). Take with food or antacids or alkaline ash foods (milk, nuts, beets, spinach, turnip greens). Maintain adequate hydration (2-3 L/day of fluids unless instructed to restrict fluid intake). Avoid aspirin, or aspirin-containing substances. Diabetics should use serum glucose monitoring. If you experience severe headache, contact prescriber for medication. You may experience dizziness or lightheadedness (use caution when driving, changing position, or engaging in tasks requiring alertness until response to drug is known); nausea, vomiting, indigestion, or loss of appetite (small frequent meals, frequent mouth care, chewing gum, or sucking lozenges may help). Report skin rash or itching, persistent headache, blood in urine or painful urination, excessive tiredness or easy bruising or bleeding, or sore gums.

Dietary Considerations: Food: Drug may cause GI upset; take with food if GI upset. Drink plenty of fluids.

Monitoring Parameters: Uric acid, renal function, CBC

Related Information

Colchicine and Probenecid *on page 225*

Treatment of Sexually Transmitted Diseases *on page 1210*

Procainamide (proe kane A mide)

Pharmacologic Class Antiarrhythmic Agent, Class I-A

U.S. Brand Names Procanbid™; Promine®; Pronestyl®; Rhythmin®

Generic Available Yes

Mechanism of Action Decreases myocardial excitability and conduction velocity and may depress myocardial contractility, by increasing the electrical stimulation threshold of ventricle, HIS-Purkinje system and through direct cardiac effects

Use Treatment of ventricular tachycardia, premature ventricular contractions, paroxysmal atrial tachycardia, and atrial fibrillation; to prevent recurrence of ventricular tachycardia, paroxysmal supraventricular tachycardia, atrial fibrillation or flutter

USUAL DOSAGE Must be titrated to patient's response

Children:

Oral: 15-50 mg/kg/24 hours divided every 3-6 hours

I.M.: 50 mg/kg/24 hours divided into doses of $^1/_8$ to $^1/_4$ every 3-6 hours in divided doses until oral therapy is possible

I.V. (infusion requires use of an infusion pump):

Load: 3-6 mg/kg/dose over 5 minutes not to exceed 100 mg/dose; may repeat every 5-10 minutes to maximum of 15 mg/kg/load

Maintenance as continuous I.V. infusion: 20-80 mcg/kg/minute; maximum: 2 g/24 hours

Adults:

Oral: 250-500 mg/dose every 3-6 hours or 500 mg to 1 g every 6 hours sustained release; usual dose: 50 mg/kg/24 hours; maximum: 4 g/24 hours (**Note:** Twice daily dosing approved for Procanbid™)

I.M.: 0.5-1 g every 4-8 hours until oral therapy is possible

I.V. (infusion requires use of an infusion pump): Loading dose: 15-18 mg/kg administered as slow infusion over 25-30 minutes or 100-200 mg/dose repeated every 5 minutes as needed to a total dose of 1 g; maintenance dose: 1-6 mg/minute by continuous infusion

Infusion rate: 2 g/250 mL D_5W/NS (I.V. infusion requires use of an infusion pump):

1 mg/minute: 7 mL/hour
2 mg/minute: 15 mL/hour
3 mg/minute: 21 mL/hour
4 mg/minute: 30 mL/hour
5 mg/minute: 38 mL/hour
6 mg/minute: 45 mL/hour

Refractory ventricular fibrillation: 30 mg/minute, up to a total of 17 mg/kg; I.V. maintenance infusion: 1-4 mg/minute; monitor levels and do not exceed 3 mg/minute for >24 hours in adults with renal failure

ACLS guidelines: I.V.: Infuse 20 mg/minute until arrhythmia is controlled, hypotension occurs, QRS complex widens by 50% of its original width, or total of 17 mg/kg is given

Dosing interval in renal impairment:

Cl_{cr} 10-50 mL/minute: Administer every 6-12 hours

(Continued)

Procainamide *(Continued)*

Cl_{cr} <10 mL/minute: Administer every 8-24 hours

Dialysis:

Procainamide: Moderately hemodialyzable (20% to 50%): 200 mg supplemental dose posthemodialysis is recommended

N-acetylprocainamide: Not dialyzable (0% to 5%)

Procainamide/N-acetylprocainamide: Not peritoneal dialyzable (0% to 5%)

Procainamide/N-acetylprocainamide: Replace by blood level during continuous arterio-venous or venovenous hemofiltration (CAVH/CAVHD)

Dosing adjustment in hepatic impairment: Reduce dose 50%

Dosage Forms CAP: 250 mg, 375 mg, 500 mg. **INJ:** 100 mg/mL (10 mL), 500 mg/mL (2 mL). **TAB:** 250 mg, 375 mg, 500 mg; Sustained release: 250 mg, 500 mg, 750 mg, 1000 mg; (Procanbid™): 500 mg, 1000 mg

Contraindications Complete heart block; second or third degree heart block without pacemaker; "torsade de pointes"; hypersensitivity to the drug or procaine, or related drugs; SLE; concurrent use of sparfloxacin. Due to results of the CAST study, procainamide and other antiarrhythmic drugs with potentially proarrhythmic effects should be reserved only for documented ventricular arrhythmias which are life-threatening.

Warnings/Precautions Use with caution in patients with marked A-V conduction disturbances, myasthenia gravis, bundle-branch block, or severe cardiac glycoside intoxication, ventricular arrhythmias with organic heart disease or coronary occlusion, CHF supraventricular tachyarrhythmias unless adequate measures are taken to prevent marked increases in ventricular rates; concurrent therapy with other class IA drugs may accumulate in patients with renal or hepatic dysfunction; some tablets contain tartrazine; injection may contain bisulfite (allergens). Long-term administration leads to the development of a positive antinuclear antibody (ANA) test in 50% of patients which may result in a lupus erythematosus-like syndrome (in 20% to 30% of patients); discontinue procainamide with SLE symptoms and choose an alternative agent; elderly have reduced clearance and frequent drug interactions. Potentially fatal blood dyscrasias have occurred with therapeutic doses; close monitoring is recommended during the first 3 months of therapy.

Pregnancy Risk Factor C

Adverse Reactions

>1%:

Dermatologic: Rash

Gastrointestinal: Diarrhea (3% to 4%), nausea, vomiting, taste disorder, GI complaints (3% to 4%)

<1% (limited to important or life-threatening symptoms): New or worsened arrhythmias (proarrhythmic effect), tachycardia, Q-T prolongation (excessive), hypotension, second-degree heart block, torsade de pointes, ventricular arrhythmias, depressed myocardial contractility, paradoxical increase in ventricular rate in atrial fibrillation/flutter, dizziness, lightheadedness, confusion, hallucinations, mental depression, disorientation, fever, drug fever, rash, urticaria, pruritus, angioneurotic edema, flushing, maculopapular rash, hemolytic anemia, agranulocytosis, neutropenia, thrombocytopenia (0.5%), positive Coombs' test, bone marrow suppression, hypoplastic anemia,leukopenia, pancytopenia, aplastic anemia,elevated transaminases, increased alkaline phosphatase, hyperbilirubinemia, hepatic failure,granulomatous hepatitis, intrahepatic cholestasis, arthralgia, myalgia (<0.5%), worsening of myasthenia gravis, neuromuscular blockade, weakness, peripheral/polyneuropathy, myopathy, pleural effusion, SLE-like syndrome (increased incidence with long-term therapy: arthralgia, pleural pain, abdominal pain, arthralgia, pleural effusion, pericarditis, fever, chills, myalgia, rash); positive ANA

Case reports: Pancreatitis, pseudo-obstruction, tremor, mania, myocarditis, vasculitis, psychosis, cerebellar ataxia, demyelinating polyradiculoneuropathy, respiratory failure due to myopathy, pulmonary embolism, myopathy

Drug Interactions

Amiodarone increases procainamide and NAPA blood levels; consider reducing procainamide dosage by 25% with concurrent use

Cimetidine increases procainamide and NAPA blood concentrations; monitor blood levels closely or use an alternative H_2 antagonist

Cisapride and procainamide may increase the risk of malignant arrhythmia; concurrent use is contraindicated

Neuromuscular blocking agents: Procainamide may potentiate neuromuscular blockade

Ofloxacin may increase procainamide levels due to an inhibition of renal secretion; monitor levels for procainamide closely

Drugs which may prolong the Q-T interval include amiodarone, amitriptyline, bepridil, disopyramide, erythromycin, haloperidol, imipramine, pimozide, quinidine, sotalol, and thioridazine. Effects/toxicity may be increased; use with caution

Sparfloxacin, gatifloxacin, and moxifloxacin may result in additional prolongation of the Q-T interval; concurrent use is contraindicated

Trimethoprim increases procainamide and NAPA blood levels; closely monitor levels

Alcohol Interactions Avoid use (acute alcohol intake reduces procainamide serum concentrations)

Onset I.M. 10-30 minutes

Half-Life

Procainamide: (Dependent upon hepatic acetylator, phenotype, cardiac function, and renal function): Adults: 2.5-4.7 hours; Anephric: 11 hours

NAPA: (Dependent upon renal function): Adults: 6-8 hours; Anephric: 42 hours

Education and Monitoring Issues

Patient Education: Oral: Take exactly as directed; do not take additional doses or discontinue without consulting prescriber. You will need regular cardiac checkups and blood tests while taking this medication. You may experience dizziness, lightheadedness, or visual changes (use caution when driving or engaging in tasks requiring alertness until response to drug is known); loss of appetite (small frequent meals, frequent mouth care, chewing gum, or sucking lozenges may help); headaches (prescriber may recommend mild analgesic); or diarrhea (exercise, yogurt, or boiled milk may help - if persistent consult prescriber). Report chest pain, palpitation, or erratic heartbeat; increased weight or swelling of hands or feet; acute diarrhea; or unusual fatigue and tiredness.

Monitoring Parameters: EKG, blood pressure, CBC with differential, platelet count; cardiac monitor and blood pressure monitor required during I.V. administration

Reference Range:

Timing of serum samples: Draw trough just before next oral dose; draw 6-12 hours after I.V. infusion has started; half-life is 2.5-5 hours

Therapeutic levels: Procainamide: 4-10 μg/mL; NAPA 15-25 μg/mL; Combined: 10-30 μg/mL

Toxic concentration: Procainamide: >10-12 μg/mL

Procaine (PROE kane)

Pharmacologic Class Local Anesthetic

U.S. Brand Names Novocain® Injection

Generic Available Yes

Mechanism of Action Blocks both the initiation and conduction of nerve impulses by decreasing the neuronal membrane's permeability to sodium ions, which results in inhibition of depolarization with resultant blockade of conduction

Use Produces spinal anesthesia and epidural and peripheral nerve block by injection and infiltration methods

USUAL DOSAGE Dose varies with procedure, desired depth, and duration of anesthesia, desired muscle relaxation, vascularity of tissues, physical condition, and age of patient

Dosage Forms INJ: 1% [10 mg/mL] (2 mL, 6 mL, 30 mL, 100 mL); 2% [20 mg/mL] (30 mL, 100 mL); 10% (2 mL)

Contraindications Known hypersensitivity to procaine, PABA, parabens, or other ester local anesthetics

Warnings/Precautions Patients with cardiac diseases, hyperthyroidism, or other endocrine diseases may be more susceptible to toxic effects of local anesthetics; some preparations contain metabisulfite

Pregnancy Risk Factor C

Adverse Reactions

1% to 10%: Local: Burning sensation at site of injection, tissue irritation, pain at injection site

<1%: Anaphylactoid reaction, aseptic meningitis resulting in paralysis can occur, chills, CNS stimulation followed by CNS depression, discoloration of skin, miosis, nausea, tinnitus, vomiting

Drug Interactions

Decreased effect of sulfonamides with the PABA metabolite of procaine, chloroprocaine, and tetracaine

Decreased/increased effect of vasopressors, ergot alkaloids, and MAO inhibitors on blood pressure when using anesthetic solutions with a vasoconstrictor

Onset Onset of effect: Injection: Within 2-5 minutes

Duration 0.5-1.5 hours (dependent upon patient, type of block, concentration, and method of anesthesia)

Half-Life 7.7 minutes

Education and Monitoring Issues

Patient Education: The purpose of this medication is to reduce pain sensation. Report local burning or pain at injection site.

- **Pro-Cal-Sof® [OTC]** *see* Docusate *on page 290*
- **Procanbid™** *see* Procainamide *on page 769*

Procarbazine (proe KAR ba zeen)

Pharmacologic Class Antineoplastic Agent, Alkylating Agent

U.S. Brand Names Matulane®

Generic Available No

Mechanism of Action Mechanism of action is not clear, methylating of nucleic acids; inhibits DNA, RNA, and protein synthesis; may damage DNA directly and suppresses mitosis; metabolic activation required by host

(Continued)

Procarbazine *(Continued)*

Use Treatment of Hodgkin's disease, non-Hodgkin's lymphoma, brain tumor, bronchogenic carcinoma

USUAL DOSAGE Refer to individual protocols. Dose based on patient's ideal weight if the patient is obese or has abnormal fluid retention. Oral:

Children:

BMT aplastic anemia conditioning regimen: 12.5 mg/kg/dose every other day for 4 doses

Hodgkin's disease: MOPP/IC-MOPP regimens: 100 mg/m^2/day for 14 days and repeated every 4 weeks

Neuroblastoma and medulloblastoma: Doses as high as 100-200 mg/m^2/day once daily have been used

Adults: Initial: 2-4 mg/kg/day in single or divided doses for 7 days then increase dose to 4-6 mg/kg/day until response is obtained or leukocyte count decreased <4000/mm^3 or the platelet count decreased <100,000/mm^3; maintenance: 1-2 mg/kg/day

Commonly used doses in combination chemotherapy regimens are in the range of 60-100 mg/m^2/day for 10-14 days. Doses are commonly rounded to the nearest 50 mg. Alternating daily doses may be utilized to achieve an "average" (eg, 150 mg alternating with 200 mg in a 1.7 m^2 patient).

In MOPP, 100 mg/m^2/day on days 1-14 of a 28-day cycle

Dosing in renal/hepatic impairment: Use with caution, may result in increased toxicity

Dosage Forms CAP: 50 mg

Contraindications Hypersensitivity to procarbazine or any component, or pre-existing bone marrow aplasia, alcohol ingestion

Warnings/Precautions The U.S. Food and Drug Administration (FDA) currently recommends that procedures for proper handling and disposal of antineoplastic agents be considered; use with caution in patients with pre-existing renal or hepatic impairment; modify dosage in patients with renal or hepatic impairment, or marrow disorders; reduce dosage with serum creatinine >2 mg/dL or total bilirubin >3 mg/dL; procarbazine possesses MAO inhibitor activity. Procarbazine is a carcinogen which may cause acute leukemia; procarbazine may cause infertility.

Pregnancy Risk Factor D

Adverse Reactions

>10%:

Central nervous system: Mental depression, manic reactions, hallucinations, dizziness, headache, nervousness, insomnia, nightmares, ataxia, disorientation, confusion, seizure, CNS stimulation

Gastrointestinal: Severe nausea and vomiting occur frequently and may be dose-limiting; anorexia, abdominal pain, stomatitis, dysphagia, diarrhea, and constipation; use a nonphenothiazine antiemetic, when possible

Emetic potential: Moderately high (60% to 90%)

Time course of nausea/vomiting: Onset: 24-27 hours; Duration: variable

Hematologic: Thrombocytopenia, hemolytic anemia

Myelosuppressive: May be dose-limiting toxicity; procarbazine should be discontinued if leukocyte count is <4000/mm^3 or platelet count <100,000/mm^3

WBC: Moderate

Platelets: Moderate

Onset (days): 14

Nadir (days): 21

Recovery (days): 28

Neuromuscular & skeletal: Weakness, paresthesia, neuropathies, decreased reflexes, foot drop, tremors

Ocular: Nystagmus

Respiratory: Pleural effusion, cough

1% to 10%:

Dermatologic: Hyperpigmentation

Hepatic: Hepatotoxicity

Neuromuscular & skeletal: Peripheral neuropathy

<1%: Allergic reactions, alopecia, arthralgia, cessation of menses, dermatitis, diplopia, disulfiram-like reaction, flu-like syndrome, hoarseness, hypersensitivity rash, hypertensive crisis, irritability, jaundice, myalgia, orthostatic hypotension, photophobia, pneumonitis, pruritus, secondary malignancy, somnolence

Drug Interactions Increased toxicity:

Procarbazine exhibits weak monoamine oxidase (MAO) inhibitor activity; foods containing high amounts of tyramine should, therefore, be avoided (ie, beer, yogurt, yeast, wine, cheese, pickled herring, chicken liver, and bananas). When a MAO inhibitor is given with food high in tyramine, a hypertensive crisis, intracranial bleeding, and headache have been reported.

Sympathomimetic amines (epinephrine and amphetamines) and antidepressants (tricyclics) should be used cautiously with procarbazine.

Barbiturates, narcotics, phenothiazines, and other CNS depressants can cause somnolence, ataxia, and other symptoms of CNS depression

Alcohol has caused a disulfiram-like reaction with procarbazine; may result in headache, respiratory difficulties, nausea, vomiting, sweating, thirst, hypotension, and flushing

Alcohol Interactions Avoid use, including alcohol-containing products and foods with high tyramine content

Half-Life 1 hour

Education and Monitoring Issues

Patient Education: Take as directed. Maintain adequate hydration (2-3 L/day of fluids unless instructed to restrict fluid intake). Avoid aspirin and aspirin-containing substances. Avoid alcohol; may cause acute disulfiram reaction - flushing, headache, acute vomiting, chest and/or abdominal pain. Avoid tyramine-containing foods (aged cheese, chocolate, pickles, aged meat, wine, etc) and consumption of large amounts of caffeine-containing beverages. Continue to avoid these foods and liquids for 14 days following therapy. You may experience mental depression, nervousness, insomnia, nightmares, dizziness, confusion, or lethargy (use caution when driving or engaging in tasks that require alertness until response to drug is known); photosensitivity (use sunscreen, wear protective clothing and eyewear, avoid direct sunlight). You may experience rash or hair loss (reversible), loss of libido, increased sensitivity to infection (avoid crowds and infected persons). Report persistent fever, chills, sore throat; unusual bleeding; blood in urine, stool (black stool), or vomitus; unresolved depression; mania; hallucinations; nightmares; disorientation; seizures; chest pain or palpitations; or difficulty breathing.

Dietary Considerations: Food: Avoid foods with high tyramine content

Monitoring Parameters: CBC with differential, platelet and reticulocyte count, urinalysis, liver function test, renal function test.

♦ **Procardia®** *see* Nifedipine *on page 653*

♦ **Procardia XL®** *see* Nifedipine *on page 653*

♦ **ProChlorax** *see* Clidinium and Chlordiazepoxide *on page 208*

Prochlorperazine (proe klor PER a zeen)

Pharmacologic Class Antipsychotic Agent, Phenothazine, Piperazine

U.S. Brand Names Compazine®

Generic Available Yes: Injection and tablet

Mechanism of Action Blocks postsynaptic mesolimbic dopaminergic D_1 and D_2 receptors in the brain, including the medullary chemoreceptor trigger zone; exhibits a strong alpha-adrenergic and anticholinergic blocking effect and depresses the release of hypothalamic and hypophyseal hormones; believed to depress the reticular activating system, thus affecting basal metabolism, body temperature, wakefulness, vasomotor tone and emesis

Use Management of nausea and vomiting; acute and chronic psychosis

USUAL DOSAGE

Antiemetic: Children:

Oral, rectal:

>10 kg: 0.4 mg/kg/24 hours in 3-4 divided doses; **or**

9-14 kg: 2.5 mg every 12-24 hours as needed; maximum: 7.5 mg/day

14-18 kg: 2.5 mg every 8-12 hours as needed; maximum: 10 mg/day

18-39 kg: 2.5 mg every 8 hours or 5 mg every 12 hours as needed; maximum: 15 mg/day

I.M.: 0.1-0.15 mg/kg/dose; usual: 0.13 mg/kg/dose; change to oral as soon as possible

I.V.: Not recommended in children <10 kg or <2 years

Antiemetic: Adults:

Oral: 5-10 mg 3-4 times/day; usual maximum: 40 mg/day

I.M.: 5-10 mg every 3-4 hours; usual maximum: 40 mg/day

I.V.: 2.5-10 mg; maximum 10 mg/dose or 40 mg/day; may repeat dose every 3-4 hours as needed

Rectal: 25 mg twice daily

Antipsychotic:

Children 2-12 years:

Oral, rectal: 2.5 mg 2-3 times/day; increase dosage as needed to maximum daily dose of 20 mg for 2-5 years and 25 mg for 6-12 years

I.M.: 0.13 mg/kg/dose; change to oral as soon as possible

Adults:

Oral: 5-10 mg 3-4 times/day; doses up to 150 mg/day may be required in some patients for treatment of severe disturbances

I.M.: 10-20 mg every 4-6 hours may be required in some patients for treatment of severe disturbances; change to oral as soon as possible

Dementia behavior (nonpsychotic): Elderly: Initial: 2.5-5 mg 1-2 times/day; increase dose at 4- to 7-day intervals by 2.5-5 mg/day; increase dosing intervals (twice daily, 3 times/day, etc) as necessary to control response or side effects; maximum daily dose should probably not exceed 75 mg in elderly; gradual increases (titration) may prevent some side effects or decrease their severity

Hemodialysis: Not dialyzable (0% to 5%)

Dosage Forms

SUPP, rectal: 2.5 mg, 5 mg, 25 mg (12/box)

Prochlorperazine edisylate: **INJ:** 5 mg/mL (2 mL, 10 mL); **SYR:** 5 mg/5 mL (120 mL)

(Continued)

Prochlorperazine *(Continued)*

Prochlorperazine maleate: **CAP, sustained action:** 10 mg, 15 mg, 30 mg. **TAB:** 5 mg, 10 mg, 25 mg

Contraindications Hypersensitivity to prochlorperazine or any component; cross-sensitivity with other phenothiazines may exist; avoid use in patients with narrow-angle glaucoma; bone marrow suppression; severe liver or cardiac disease

Warnings/Precautions Injection contains sulfites which may cause allergic reactions; may impair ability to perform hazardous tasks requiring mental alertness or physical coordination; some products contain tartrazine dye, avoid use in sensitive individuals

Tardive dyskinesia: Prevalence rate may be 40% in elderly; development of the syndrome and the irreversible nature are proportional to duration and total cumulative dose over time. May be reversible if diagnosed early in therapy.

High incidence of extrapyramidal reactions, especially in children or the elderly, so reserve use in children <5 years of age to those who are unresponsive to other antiemetics; incidence of extrapyramidal reactions is increased with acute illnesses such as chicken pox, measles, CNS infections, gastroenteritis, and dehydration

Drug-induced **Parkinson's syndrome** occurs often. **Akathisia** is the most common extrapyramidal reaction in elderly.

Increased confusion, memory loss, psychotic behavior, and agitation frequently occur as a consequence of anticholinergic effects

Lowers seizure threshold, use cautiously in patients with seizure history

Orthostatic hypotension is due to alpha-receptor blockade, the elderly are at greater risk for orthostatic hypotension

Antipsychotic associated sedation in nonpsychotic patients is extremely unpleasant due to feelings of depersonalization, derealization, and dysphoria

Life-threatening arrhythmias have occurred at therapeutic doses of antipsychotics

Pregnancy Risk Factor C

Pregnancy Implications

Clinical effects on the fetus: Crosses the placenta. Isolated reports of congenital anomalies, however some included exposures to other drugs. Available evidence with use of occasional low doses suggests safe use during pregnancy.

Breast-feeding/lactation: No data available. American Academy of Pediatrics considers **compatible** with breast-feeding.

Adverse Reactions

Cardiovascular: Hypotension, orthostatic hypotension, hypertension, tachycardia, bradycardia, dizziness, cardiac arrest

Central nervous system: Extrapyramidal signs (pseudoparkinsonism, akathisia, dystonias, tardive dyskinesia), dizziness, cerebral edema, seizures, headache, drowsiness, paradoxical excitement, restlessness, hyperactivity, insomnia, neuroleptic malignant syndrome (NMS), impairment of temperature regulation

Dermatologic: Increased sensitivity to sun, rash, discoloration of skin (blue-gray)

Endocrine & metabolic: Hypoglycemia, hyperglycemia, galactorrhea, lactation, breast enlargement, gynecomastia, menstrual irregularity, amenorrhea, SIADH, changes in libido

Gastrointestinal: Constipation, weight gain, vomiting, stomach pain, nausea, xerostomia, salivation, diarrhea, anorexia, ileus

Genitourinary: Difficulty in urination, ejaculatory disturbances, incontinence, polyuria, ejaculating dysfunction, priapism

Hematologic: Agranulocytosis, leukopenia, eosinophilia, hemolytic anemia, thrombocytopenic purpura, pancytopenia

Hepatic: Cholestatic jaundice, hepatotoxicity

Neuromuscular & skeletal: Tremor

Ocular: Pigmentary retinopathy, blurred vision, cornea and lens changes

Respiratory: Nasal congestion

Miscellaneous: Diaphoresis

Drug Interactions

Phenothiazines inhibit the ability of bromocriptine to lower serum prolactin concentrations

Benztropine (and other anticholinergics) may inhibit the therapeutic response to prochlorperazine and excess anticholinergic effects may occur

Chloroquine may increase prochlorperazine concentrations

Cigarette smoking may enhance the hepatic metabolism of prochlorperazine. Larger doses may be required compared to a nonsmoker.

Concurrent use of prochlorperazine with an antihypertensive may produce additive hypotensive effects

Antihypertensive effects of guanethidine and guanadrel may be inhibited by prochlorperazine

Concurrent use with TCA may produce increased toxicity or altered therapeutic response

Prochlorperazine may inhibit the antiparkinsonian effect of levodopa; avoid this combination

Prochlorperazine plus lithium may rarely produce neurotoxicity

Barbiturates may reduce prochlorperazine concentrations

Propranolol may increase prochlorperazine concentrations

Sulfadoxine-pyrimethamine may increase prochlorperazine concentrations

prochlorperazine and possibly other low potency antipsychotics may reverse the pressor effects of epinephrine

Prochlorperazine and CNS depressants (ethanol, narcotics) may produce additive CNS depressant effects

Prochlorperazine and trazodone may produce additive hypotensive effects

Use with cisapride may increase the risk of malignant arrhythmias, concurrent use is contraindicated

Alcohol Interactions Avoid use (may increase central nervous system depression)

Onset Oral: Within 30-40 minutes; I.M.: Within 10-20 minutes; Rectal: Within 60 minutes

Duration Persists longest with I.M. and oral extended-release doses (12 hours); shortest following rectal and immediate release oral administration (3-4 hours)

Half-Life 23 hours

Education and Monitoring Issues

Patient Education: Take exact amount as prescribed. Do not change brand names. Do not crush or chew tablets or capsules. Do not discontinue without consulting prescriber. Avoid alcohol or other sedatives or sleep-inducing drugs. Avoid skin contact with drug; wash immediately with warm soapy water. You may experience appetite changes; small frequent meals may help. Maintain adequate fluid intake (2-3 L/day of fluids unless instructed to restrict fluid intake). May cause dizziness, tremors, or visual disturbance (especially during early therapy); use caution when driving or engaging in tasks that require alertness until response to drug is known. Do not change position rapidly (rise slowly). May cause photosensitivity reaction; use sunscreen, wear protective clothing and eyewear, and avoid direct sunlight. Report immediately any changes in gait or muscular tremors. Report unresolved changes in voiding or elimination (constipation or diarrhea), acute dizziness or unresolved sedation, any vision changes, palpitations, yellowing of skin or eyes, and changes in color of urine or stool (pink or red brown urine is expected).

- **Procort® [OTC]** *see* Hydrocortisone *on page 447*
- **Procrit®** *see* Epoetin Alfa *on page 316*
- **Proctocort™** *see* Hydrocortisone *on page 447*
- **Proctofoam®-HC** *see* Pramoxine and Hydrocortisone *on page 758*
- **Procyclid** *see* Procyclidine *on page 775*

Procyclidine (proe SYE kli deen)

Pharmacologic Class Anticholinergic Agent; Anti-Parkinson's Agent (Anticholinergic)

U.S. Brand Names Kemadrin®

Use Relieves symptoms of parkinsonian syndrome and drug-induced extrapyramidal symptoms

USUAL DOSAGE Adults: Oral: 2.5 mg 3 times/day after meals; if tolerated, gradually increase dose, maximum of 20 mg/day if necessary

Dosing adjustment in hepatic impairment: Decrease dose to a twice daily dosing regimen

Contraindications Angle-closure glaucoma; safe use in children not established

Pregnancy Risk Factor C

- **Procytox®** *see* Cyclophosphamide *on page 235*
- **Prodiem® Plain** *see* Psyllium *on page 793*
- **Prodium™ [OTC]** *see* Phenazopyridine *on page 721*
- **Profasi® HP** *see* Chorionic Gonadotropin *on page 196*
- **Profenal®** *see* Suprofen *on page 885*
- **Progestasert®** *see* Progesterone *on page 775*

Progesterone (proe JES ter one)

Pharmacologic Class Progestin

U.S. Brand Names Progestasert®; Prometrium®

Generic Available Yes

Mechanism of Action Natural steroid hormone that induces secretory changes in the endometrium, promotes mammary gland development, relaxes uterine smooth muscle, blocks follicular maturation and ovulation, and maintains pregnancy

Use Intrauterine contraception in women who have had at least 1 child, are in a stable, mutually monogamous relationship, and have no history of pelvic inflammatory disease; amenorrhea; functional uterine bleeding; replacement therapy

Oral: Prevention of endometrial hyperplasia in nonhysterectomized postmenopausal women who are receiving conjugated estrogen tablets; secondary amenorrhea

Intravaginal gel: Part of assisted reproductive technology for infertile women with progesterone deficiency; secondary amenorrhea (8% gel is used in those who fail to respond to 4%)

USUAL DOSAGE Adults:

Amenorrhea: I.M.: 5-10 mg/day for 6-8 consecutive days

Functional uterine bleeding: I.M.: 5-10 mg/day for 6 doses

(Continued)

Progesterone *(Continued)*

Contraception: Female: Intrauterine device: Insert a single system into the uterine cavity; contraceptive effectiveness is retained for 1 year and system must be replaced 1 year after insertion

Replacement therapy: Gel: Administer 90 mg once daily in women who require progesterone supplementation

Oral:

Prevention of endometrial hyperplasia (in postmenopausal women with a uterus who are receiving daily conjugated estrogen tablets): 200 mg as a single daily dose every evening for 12 days sequentially per 28 day cycle.

Amenorrhea: 400 mg every evening for 10 days.

Intravaginal gel:

Partial or complete ovarian failure (assisted reproductive technology): 90 mg (8% gel) intravaginally once daily; if pregnancy is achieved, may continue up to 10-12 weeks

Secondary amenorrhea: 45 mg (4% gel) intravaginally every other day for up to 6 doses; women who fail to respond may be increased to 90 mg (8% gel) every other day for up to 6 doses

Dosage Forms CAP: 100 mg. **INJ, in oil:** 50 mg/mL (10 mL). **INTRAUTERINE system, reservoir:** 38 mg in silicone fluid

Contraindications Hypersensitivity to progesterone or any component; pregnancy; thrombophlebitis; undiagnosed vaginal bleeding; carcinoma of the breast; cerebral apoplexy; severe liver dysfunction; capsules contain peanut oil and are contraindicated in patients with allergy to peanuts

Warnings/Precautions Use with caution in patients with impaired liver function, depression, diabetes, and epilepsy. Use of any progestin during the first 4 months of pregnancy is not recommended. Monitor closely for loss of vision, proptosis, diplopia, migraine, and signs or symptoms of embolic disorders. Not a progestin of choice in the elderly for hormonal cycling. Capsules may cause some degree of fluid retention, use with caution in conditions which may be aggravated by this factor, including CHF, renal dysfunction, epilepsy, migraine, or asthma. Patients should be warned that progesterone may cause transient dizziness or drowsiness during initial therapy.

Pregnancy Risk Factor X; B (oral capsules per manufacturer)

Gel: None established for Crinone™

Adverse Reactions

Intrauterine device:

>10%:

Cardiovascular: Edema

Endocrine & metabolic: Breakthrough bleeding, spotting, changes in menstrual flow, amenorrhea

Gastrointestinal: Anorexia

Neuromuscular & skeletal: Weakness

1% to 10%:

Cardiovascular: Embolism, central thrombosis

Central nervous system: Mental depression, fever, insomnia

Dermatologic: Melasma or chloasma, allergic rash with or without pruritus

Endocrine: Changes in cervical erosion and secretions, increased breast tenderness

Gastrointestinal: Weight gain or loss

Hepatic: Cholestatic jaundice

Injection (I.M.):

>10% Local: Pain at injection site

1% to 10%: Local: Thrombophlebitis

Oral capsules:

>10%:

Central nervous system: Dizziness (16%)

Endocrine & metabolic: Breast pain (11%)

5% to 10%:

Central nervous system: Headache (10%), fatigue (7%), emotional lability (6%), irritability (5%)

Gastrointestinal: Abdominal pain (10%), abdominal distention (6%)

Neuromuscular & skeletal: Musculoskeletal pain (6%)

Respiratory: Upper respiratory tract infection (5%)

Miscellaneous: Viral infection (7%)

<5% (limited to important or life-threatening symptoms): Dry mouth, accidental injury, chest pain, fever, hypertension, confusion, somnolence, speech disorder, constipation, dyspepsia, gastroenteritis, hemorrhagic rectum, hiatus hernia, vomiting, earache, palpitation, edema, arthritis, leg cramps, hypertonia, muscle disorder, myalgia, angina pectoris, anxiety, impaired concentration, insomnia, personality disorder, leukorrhea, uterine fibroid, vaginal dryness, fungal vaginitis, vaginitis, abscess, herpes simplex, bronchitis, nasal congestion, pharyngitis, pneumonitis, sinusitis, acne, verruca, urinary tract infection, abnormal vision, lymphadenopathy

Other report adverse effects (incidence unspecified): Hepatitis, elevated transaminases, breakthrough bleeding, change in menstrual flow, amenorrhea, weight change, cervical changes, cholestatic jaundice, anaphylactoid reactions, anaphylaxis, rash, pruritus, melasma, chloasma, pyrexia, insomnia, increased sweating, weakness, tooth disorder, anorexia, increased appetite, nervousness, breast enlargement

Systemic:

>10%:

Cardiovascular: Swelling of face

Central nervous system: Headache, mood changes, nervousness

Endocrine & metabolic: Amenorrhea, irregular menstrual cycles, menorrhagia, spotting, ovarian enlargement, ovarian cyst formation

Gastrointestinal: Abdominal pain

1% to 10%:

Cardiovascular: Hot flashes

Central nervous system: Dizziness, mental depression, insomnia

Dermatologic: Dermatitis, acne, melasma, loss or gain of body, facial, or scalp hair

Endocrine & metabolic: Hyperglycemia, galactorrhea, breast pain, libido decrease

Gastrointestinal: Nausea, change in appetite, weight gain

Genitourinary: Vaginitis, leukorrhea

Neuromuscular & skeletal: Myalgia

<1% (limited to important or life-threatening symptoms): Aggressive reactions, allergic reaction, asthma, forgetfulness, hot flashes, migraine, thromboembolism, tremor

Drug Interactions CYP3A3/4 enzyme substrate; CYP3A3/4 enzyme inducer

Decreased effect: Aminoglutethimide may decrease effect by increasing hepatic metabolism

Increase effect: Ketoconazole may increase the bioavailability of progesterone. Progesterone may increase concentrations of estrogenic compounds during concurrent therapy with conjugated estrogens.

Duration 24 hours

Half-Life 5 minutes

Education and Monitoring Issues

Patient Education: This drug can only be given I.M. on a daily basis for a specific number of days (or inserted vaginally to remain for 1 year as a contraceptive). It is important that you you have an annual physical assessment, Pap smear, and vision assessment while taking this medication. You may experience increased facial hair or loss of head hair (reversible); photosensitivity (use sunscreen, wear protective clothing and eyewear, avoid direct sunlight); loss of appetite (small frequent meals will help); constipation (increased fluids, exercise, dietary fiber, or stool softeners may help). Diabetics should use accurate serum glucose testing to identify any changes in glucose tolerance. Report immediately pain or muscle soreness; swelling, heat, or redness in calves; shortness of breath; sudden loss of vision; unresolved leg or foot swelling; change in menstrual pattern (unusual bleeding, amenorrhea, breakthrough spotting); breast tenderness that does not go away; acute abdominal cramping; signs of vaginal infection (drainage, pain, itching); or changes in CNS (eg, blurred vision, confusion, acute anxiety, or unresolved depression).

Dietary Considerations: Food increases oral bioavailability

Monitoring Parameters: Before starting therapy, a physical exam including the breasts and pelvis are recommended, also a PAP smear; signs or symptoms of depression, glucose in diabetics

- **Progesterone Oil** *see* Progesterone *on page 775*
- **Prograf®** *see* Tacrolimus *on page 887*
- **ProHIBiT®** *see Haemophilus* b Conjugate Vaccine *on page 427*
- **Pro-Indo®** *see* Indomethacin *on page 469*
- **Prolamine® [OTC]** *see* Phenylpropanolamine *on page 729*
- **Proleukin®** *see* Aldesleukin *on page 29*
- **Prolixin Decanoate® Injection** *see* Fluphenazine *on page 381*
- **Prolixin Enanthate® Injection** *see* Fluphenazine *on page 381*
- **Prolixin® Injection** *see* Fluphenazine *on page 381*
- **Prolixin® Oral** *see* Fluphenazine *on page 381*
- **Proloprim®** *see* Trimethoprim *on page 953*

Promazine (PROE ma zeen)

Pharmacologic Class Phenothiazine Derivative

U.S. Brand Names Sparine®

Generic Available Injection only

Mechanism of Action Blocks postsynaptic mesolimbic dopaminergic D_1 and D_2 receptors in the brain; exhibits a strong alpha-adrenergic blocking and anticholinergic effect, depresses the release of hypothalamic and hypophyseal hormones; believed to depress the reticular activating system thus affecting basal metabolism, body temperature, wakefulness, vasomotor tone, and emesis

Use Management of manifestations of psychotic disorders; depressive neurosis; alcohol withdrawal; nausea and vomiting; nonpsychotic symptoms associated with dementia in elderly, Tourette's syndrome; Huntington's chorea; spasmodic torticollis and Reye's syndrome

(Continued)

Promazine *(Continued)*

USUAL DOSAGE Oral, I.M.:

Children >12 years: Antipsychotic: 10-25 mg every 4-6 hours

Adults:

Psychosis: 10-200 mg every 4-6 hours not to exceed 1000 mg/day

Antiemetic: 25-50 mg every 4-6 hours as needed

Hemodialysis: Not dialyzable (0% to 5%)

Dosage Forms INJ: 25 mg/mL (10 mL); 50 mg/mL (1 mL, 2 mL, 10 mL). **TAB:** 25 mg, 50 mg, 100 mg

Contraindications Hypersensitivity to promazine or any component; severe CNS depression, cross-sensitivity to other phenothiazines may exist; avoid use in patients with narrow-angle glaucoma, blood dyscrasias, severe liver or cardiac disease; subcortical brain damage; circulatory collapse; severe hypotension or hypertension

Warnings/Precautions

Tardive dyskinesia: Prevalence rate may be 40% in elderly; development of the syndrome and the irreversible nature are proportional to duration and total cumulative dose over time. May be reversible if diagnosed early in therapy.

Extrapyramidal reactions are more common in elderly with up to 50% developing these reactions after 60 years of age. These reactions may be more common in dementia patients.

Drug-induced **Parkinson's syndrome** occurs often. **Akathisia** is the most common extrapyramidal reaction in elderly.

Increased confusion, memory loss, psychotic behavior, and agitation frequently occur as a consequence of anticholinergic effects

Orthostatic hypotension is due to alpha-receptor blockade, the elderly are at greater risk for orthostatic hypotension

Antipsychotic associated sedation in nonpsychotic patients is extremely unpleasant due to feelings of depersonalization, derealization, and dysphoria

Life-threatening arrhythmias have occurred at therapeutic doses of antipsychotics; use with caution in patients with narrow-angle glaucoma, severe liver disease or severe cardiac disease

Pregnancy Risk Factor C

Adverse Reactions

Cardiovascular: Postural hypotension, tachycardia, dizziness, nonspecific Q-T changes

Central nervous system: Drowsiness, dystonias, akathisia, pseudoparkinsonism, tardive dyskinesia, neuroleptic malignant syndrome, seizures

Dermatologic: Photosensitivity, dermatitis, skin pigmentation (slate gray)

Endocrine & metabolic: Lactation, breast engorgement, false-positive pregnancy test, amenorrhea, gynecomastia, hyper- or hypoglycemia

Gastrointestinal: Xerostomia, constipation, nausea

Genitourinary: Urinary retention, ejaculatory disorder, impotence

Hematologic: Agranulocytosis, eosinophilia, leukopenia, hemolytic anemia, aplastic anemia, thrombocytopenic purpura

Hepatic: Jaundice

Ocular: Blurred vision, corneal and lenticular changes, epithelial keratopathy, pigmentary retinopathy

Drug Interactions

Phenothiazines inhibit the ability of bromocriptine to lower serum prolactin concentrations

Benztropine (and other anticholinergics) may inhibit the therapeutic response to promazine and excess anticholinergic effects may occur

Chloroquine may increase promazine concentrations

Cigarette smoking may enhance the hepatic metabolism of promazine. Larger doses may be required compared to a nonsmoker.

Concurrent use of promazine with an antihypertensive may produce additive hypotensive effects

Antihypertensive effects of guanethidine and guanadrel may be inhibited by promazine

Concurrent use with TCA may produce increased toxicity or altered therapeutic response

Promazine may inhibit the antiparkinsonian effect of levodopa; avoid this combination

Promazine plus lithium may rarely produce neurotoxicity

Barbiturates may reduce promazine concentrations

Propranolol may increase promazine concentrations

Sulfadoxine-pyrimethamine may increase promazine concentrations

Promazine and possibly other low potency antipsychotics may reverse the pressor effects of epinephrine

Promazine and CNS depressants (ethanol, narcotics) may produce additive CNS depressant effects

Promazine and trazodone may produce additive hypotensive effects

Alcohol Interactions Avoid use (may increase central nervous system depression)

Half-Life The specific pharmacokinetics of promazine are poorly established but probably resemble those of other phenothiazines. Most phenothiazines have long half-lives in the range of 24 hours or more.

Education and Monitoring Issues

Patient Education: May cause drowsiness, impair judgment and coordination; may cause photosensitivity; avoid excessive sunlight; notify prescriber of involuntary movements or feelings of restlessness

♦ **Prometa®** *see* Metaproterenol *on page 572*

Promethazine (proe METH a zeen)

Pharmacologic Class Antiemetic

U.S. Brand Names Anergan®; Phenazine®; Phenergan®; Prorex®

Generic Available Yes

Mechanism of Action Blocks postsynaptic mesolimbic dopaminergic receptors in the brain; exhibits a strong alpha-adrenergic blocking effect and depresses the release of hypothalamic and hypophyseal hormones; competes with histamine for the H_1-receptor; reduces stimuli to the brainstem reticular system

Use Symptomatic treatment of various allergic conditions, antiemetic, motion sickness, and as a sedative

USUAL DOSAGE

Children:

- Antihistamine: Oral, rectal: 0.1 mg/kg/dose every 6 hours during the day and 0.5 mg/kg/dose at bedtime as needed
- Antiemetic: Oral, I.M., I.V., rectal: 0.25-1 mg/kg 4-6 times/day as needed
- Motion sickness: Oral, rectal: 0.5 mg/kg/dose 30 minutes to 1 hour before departure, then every 12 hours as needed
- Sedation: Oral, I.M., I.V., rectal: 0.5-1 mg/kg/dose every 6 hours as needed

Adults:

- Antihistamine (including allergic reactions to blood or plasma):
  - Oral, rectal: 12.5 mg 3 times/day and 25 mg at bedtime
  - I.M., I.V.: 25 mg, may repeat in 2 hours when necessary; switch to oral route as soon as feasible
- Antiemetic: Oral, I.M., I.V., rectal: 12.5-25 mg every 4 hours as needed
- Motion sickness: Oral, rectal: 25 mg 30-60 minutes before departure, then every 12 hours as needed
- Sedation: Oral, I.M., I.V., rectal: 25-50 mg/dose

Hemodialysis: Not dialyzable (0% to 5%)

Dosage Forms INJ: 25 mg/mL (1 mL, 10 mL); 50 mg/mL (1 mL, 10 mL). **SUPP, rectal:** 12.5 mg, 25 mg, 50 mg. **SYR:** 6.25 mg/5 mL (5 mL, 120 mL, 240 mL, 480 mL, 4000 mL); 25 mg/5 mL (120 mL, 480 mL, 4000 mL). **TAB:** 12.5 mg, 25 mg, 50 mg

Contraindications Hypersensitivity to promethazine or any component; narrow-angle glaucoma

Warnings/Precautions Do not administer S.C. or intra-arterially, necrotic lesions may occur; injection may contain sulfites which may cause allergic reactions in some patients; use with caution in patients with cardiovascular disease, impaired liver function, asthma, sleep apnea, seizures. Rapid I.V. administration may produce a transient fall in blood pressure, rate of administration should not exceed 25 mg/minute; slow I.V. administration may produce a slightly elevated blood pressure. Because promethazine is a phenothiazine (and can, therefore, cause side effects such as extrapyramidal symptoms), it is not considered an antihistamine of choice in the elderly.

Pregnancy Risk Factor C

Pregnancy Implications

Clinical effects on the fetus: Crosses the placenta. Possible respiratory depression if drug is administered near time of delivery; behavioral changes, EEG alterations, impaired platelet aggregation reported with use during labor. Available evidence with use of occasional low doses suggests safe use during pregnancy.

Breast-feeding/lactation: No data available. American Academy of Pediatrics makes NO RECOMMENDATION.

Adverse Reactions

Cardiovascular: Postural hypotension, tachycardia, dizziness, nonspecific Q-T changes

Central nervous system: Drowsiness, dystonias, akathisia, pseudoparkinsonism, tardive dyskinesia, neuroleptic malignant syndrome, seizures

Dermatologic: Photosensitivity, dermatitis, skin pigmentation (slate gray)

Endocrine & metabolic: Lactation, breast engorgement, false-positive pregnancy test, amenorrhea, gynecomastia, hyper- or hypoglycemia

Gastrointestinal: Xerostomia, constipation, nausea

Genitourinary: Urinary retention, ejaculatory disorder, impotence

Hematologic: Agranulocytosis, eosinophilia, leukopenia, hemolytic anemia, aplastic anemia, thrombocytopenic purpura

Hepatic: Jaundice

Ocular: Blurred vision, corneal and lenticular changes, epithelial keratopathy, pigmentary retinopathy

Drug Interactions CYP2D6 enzyme substrate

Phenothiazines inhibit the ability of bromocriptine to lower serum prolactin concentrations

Benztropine (and other anticholinergics) may inhibit the therapeutic response to promethazine and excess anticholinergic effects may occur

(Continued)

Promethazine *(Continued)*

Chloroquine may increase promethazine concentrations

Cigarette smoking may enhance the hepatic metabolism of promethazine. Larger doses may be required compared to a nonsmoker.

Concurrent use of promethazine with an antihypertensive may produce additive hypotensive effects

Antihypertensive effects of guanethidine and guanadrel may be inhibited by promethazine

Concurrent use with TCA may produce increased toxicity or altered therapeutic response

Promethazine may inhibit the antiparkinsonian effect of levodopa; avoid this combination

Promethazine plus lithium may rarely produce neurotoxicity

Barbiturates may reduce promethazine concentrations

Propranolol may increase promethazine concentrations

Sulfadoxine-pyrimethamine may increase promethazine concentrations

Promethazine and possibly other low potency antipsychotics may reverse the pressor effects of epinephrine

Promethazine and CNS depressants (ethanol, narcotics) may produce additive CNS depressant effects

Promethazine and trazodone may produce additive hypotensive effects

Use with cisapride may increase the risk of malignant arrhythmias; concurrent use is contraindicated

Alcohol Interactions Avoid use (may increase central nervous system depression)

Onset I.V.: Within 20 minutes (3-5 minutes with I.V. injection)

Duration 2-6 hours

Education and Monitoring Issues

Patient Education: Take this drug as prescribed; do not increase dosage. Do not use alcohol or other CNS depressants or sleeping aids without consulting prescriber. May cause dizziness, drowsiness, or blurred vision (use caution when driving or engaging in tasks requiring alertness until response to drug is known); nausea, dry mouth, appetite disturbances (small frequent meals, frequent mouth care, chewing gum, or sucking lozenges may help). Report unusual weight gain, unresolved nausea or diarrhea, chest pain or palpitations, excess sedation or stimulation, or sore throat or difficulty breathing.

Related Information

Meperidine and Promethazine *on page 564*
Promethazine and Codeine *on page 780*
Promethazine and Dextromethorphan *on page 780*
Promethazine and Phenylephrine *on page 780*
Promethazine, Phenylephrine, and Codeine *on page 780*

Promethazine and Codeine (proe METH a zeen & KOE deen)

Pharmacologic Class Antihistamine/Antitussive

U.S. Brand Names Phenergan® With Codeine; Pherazine® With Codeine; Prothazine-DC®

Dosage Forms SYR: Promethazine hydrochloride 6.25 mg and codeine phosphate 10 mg per 5 mL (120 mL, 180 mL, 473 mL)

Pregnancy Risk Factor C

Alcohol Interactions Avoid use (may increase central nervous system depression)

Promethazine and Dextromethorphan

(proe METH a zeen & deks troe meth OR fan)

Pharmacologic Class Antihistamine/Antitussive

U.S. Brand Names Phenameth® DM; Phenergan® With Dextromethorphan; Pherazine® w/ DM

Dosage Forms SYR: Promethazine hydrochloride 6.25 mg and dextromethorphan hydrobromide 15 mg per 5 mL with alcohol 7% (120 mL, 480 mL, 4000 mL)

Pregnancy Risk Factor C

Alcohol Interactions Avoid use (may increase central nervous system depression)

Promethazine and Phenylephrine (proe METH a zeen & fen il EF rin)

Pharmacologic Class Antihistamine/Decongestant Combination

U.S. Brand Names Phenergan® VC Syrup; Promethazine VC Plain Syrup; Promethazine VC Syrup; Prometh VC Plain Liquid

Dosage Forms LIQ: Promethazine hydrochloride 6.25 mg and phenylephrine hydrochloride 5 mg per 5 mL (120 mL, 240 mL, 473 mL)

Pregnancy Risk Factor C

Alcohol Interactions Avoid use (may increase central nervous system depression)

Promethazine, Phenylephrine, and Codeine

(proe METH a zeen, fen il EF rin, & KOE deen)

Pharmacologic Class Antihistamine/Decongestant/Antitussive

U.S. Brand Names Phenergan® VC With Codeine; Pherazine® VC w/ Codeine; Promethist® With Codeine; Prometh® VC With Codeine

Dosage Forms LIQ: Promethazine hydrochloride 6.25 mg, phenylephrine hydrochloride 5 mg, and codeine phosphate 10 mg per 5 mL with alcohol 7% (120 mL, 240 mL, 480 mL, 4000 mL)

Pregnancy Risk Factor C

Alcohol Interactions Avoid use (may increase central nervous system depression)

- **Promethazine VC Plain Syrup** *see* Promethazine and Phenylephrine *on page 780*
- **Promethazine VC Syrup** *see* Promethazine and Phenylephrine *on page 780*
- **Promethist® With Codeine** *see* Promethazine, Phenylephrine, and Codeine *on page 780*
- **Prometh VC Plain Liquid** *see* Promethazine and Phenylephrine *on page 780*
- **Prometh® VC With Codeine** *see* Promethazine, Phenylephrine, and Codeine *on page 780*
- **Prometrium®** *see* Progesterone *on page 775*
- **Promine®** *see* Procainamide *on page 769*
- **Pronestyl®** *see* Procainamide *on page 769*
- **Pronto® Shampoo [OTC]** *see* Pyrethrins *on page 795*
- **Propacet®** *see* Propoxyphene and Acetaminophen *on page 786*
- **Propaderm®** *see* Beclomethasone *on page 94*

Propafenone (proe pa FEEN one)

Pharmacologic Class Antiarrhythmic Agent, Class I-C

U.S. Brand Names Rythmol®

Generic Available No

Mechanism of Action Propafenone is a 1C antiarrhythmic agent which possesses local anesthetic properties, blocks the fast inward sodium current, and slows the rate of increase of the action potential. prolongs conduction and refractoriness in all areas of the myocardium, with a slightly more pronounced effect on intraventricular conduction; it prolongs effective refractory period, reduces spontaneous automaticity and exhibits some beta-blockade activity.

Use Life-threatening ventricular arrhythmias

Unlabeled use: Supraventricular tachycardias, including those patients with Wolff-Parkinson-White syndrome

USUAL DOSAGE Adults: Oral: 150 mg every 8 hours, increase at 3- to 4-day intervals up to 300 mg every 8 hours. **Note:** Patients who exhibit significant widening of QRS complex or second or third degree A-V block may need dose reduction.

Dosing adjustment in hepatic impairment: Reduction is necessary

Dosage Forms TAB: 150 mg, 225 mg, 300 mg

Contraindications Hypersensitivity to propafenone or any component; uncontrolled congestive heart failure; bronchospastic disorders; cardiogenic shock, conduction disorders (A-V block, sick-sinus syndrome); bradycardia; concurrent use of amprenavir or ritonavir

Warnings/Precautions Until evidence to the contrary, propafenone should be considered acceptable only for the treatment of life-threatening arrhythmias; propafenone may cause new or worsened arrhythmias, worsen CHF, decrease A-V conduction and alter pacemaker thresholds; use with caution in patients with recent myocardial infarction, congestive heart failure, hepatic or renal dysfunction; elderly may be at greater risk for toxicity

Pregnancy Risk Factor C

Adverse Reactions

1% to 10%:

Central nervous system: Dizziness (4% to 15%), fatigue (2% to 6%), headache (2% to 5%), weakness (1% to 2%), ataxia (0% to 2%), insomnia (0% to 2%), anxiety (1% to 2%), drowsiness (1%)

Cardiovascular: New or worsened arrhythmias (proarrhythmic effect) (2% to 10%), angina (2% to 5%), congestive heart failure (1% to 4%), ventricular tachycardia (1% to 3%), palpitations (1% to 3%), A-V block (first-degree) (1% to 3%), syncope (1% to 2%), increased QRS interval (1% to 2%), chest pain (1% to 2%), PVCs (1% to 2%), bradycardia (1% to 2%), edema (0% to 1%), bundle branch block (0% to 1%), atrial fibrillation (1%), hypotension (0% to 1%), intraventricular conduction delay (0% to 1%)

Dermatologic: Rash (1% to 3%)

Gastrointestinal: Nausea/vomiting (2% to 11%), unusual taste (3% to 23%), constipation (2% to 7%), dyspepsia (1% to 3%), diarrhea (1% to 3%), xerostomia (1% to 2%), anorexia (1% to 2%), abdominal pain (1% to 2%), flatulence (0% to 1%)

Neuromuscular & skeletal: Tremor (0% to 1%), arthralgia (0% to 1%)

Ocular: Blurred vision (1% to 6%)

Respiratory: Dyspnea (2% to 5%)

Miscellaneous: Diaphoresis (1%)

<1% (limited to important or life-threatening symptoms): Agranulocytosis, leukopenia, thrombocytopenia, purpura, granulocytopenia, anemia, increased bleeding time, hepatitis (0.03%), increased serum transaminases (0.2%), prolonged PR interval, sinus node dysfunction, cholestasis (0.1%), gastroenteritis, positive ANA titers (0.7%), lupus

(Continued)

Propafenone *(Continued)*

erythematosus, A-V block (second or third degree), A-V dissociation, cardiac arrest, flushing, sinus arrest, flushing, abnormal speech, abnormal dreams, abnormal vision, apnea, coma, confusion, depression, memory loss, paresthesia, numbness, psychosis, seizures (0.3%), tinnitus, abnormal smell sensation, vertigo, alopecia, eye irritation, SIADH, hyponatremia, impotence, hyperglycemia, kidney failure, muscle cramps, muscle weakness, nephrotic syndrome, pain, pruritus, congestive heart failure, renal failure, nephrotic syndrome

Case reports: Peripheral neuropathy, mania, amnesia

Drug Interactions CYP2D6 substrate/inhibitor, CYP1A2 substrate

Inhibitors of CYP2D6 or CYP1A2 may increase blood levels of propafenone

Amprenavir and ritonavir may increase propafenone levels; concurrent use is contraindicated

Cimetidine increases propafenone blood levels

Digoxin blood levels are increased; monitor for toxicity

Enzyme inducers (phenobarbital, phenytoin, rifabutin, rifampin) may decrease propafenone blood levels

Metoprolol blood levels are increased

Propranolol blood levels are increased

Quinidine increases propafenone blood levels

Theophylline blood levels may be increased

Warfarin blood levels are increased; response may be increased. Monitor INR closely.

Half-Life After a single dose (100-300 mg): 2-8 hours; half-life after chronic dosing ranges from 10-32 hours

Education and Monitoring Issues

Patient Education: Take exactly as directed; do not take additional doses or discontinue without consulting prescriber. You will need regular cardiac checkups and blood tests while taking this medication. You may experience dizziness, drowsiness, or visual changes (use caution when driving or engaging in tasks requiring alertness until response to drug is known); abnormal taste, nausea or vomiting, or loss of appetite (small frequent meals, frequent mouth care, chewing gum, or sucking lozenges may help); headaches (prescriber may recommend mild analgesic); or diarrhea (exercise, yogurt, or boiled milk may help - if persistent consult prescriber). Report chest pain, palpitation, or erratic heartbeat; difficulty breathing, increased weight or swelling of hands or feet; acute persistent diarrhea or constipation; or changes in vision.

Monitoring Parameters: EKG, blood pressure, pulse (particularly at initiation of therapy)

Manufacturer Knoll Pharmaceutical Company

Related Information

Pharmaceutical Manufacturers Directory *on page 1020*

♦ **Propagest® [OTC]** *see* Phenylpropanolamine *on page 729*

♦ **Propanthel** *see* Propantheline *on page 782*

Propantheline (proe PAN the leen)

Pharmacologic Class Anticholinergic Agent

U.S. Brand Names Pro-Banthine®

Use Adjunctive treatment of peptic ulcer, irritable bowel syndrome, pancreatitis, ureteral and urinary bladder spasm; reduce duodenal motility during diagnostic radiologic procedures

USUAL DOSAGE Oral:

Antisecretory:

Children: 1-2 mg/kg/day in 3-4 divided doses

Adults: 15 mg 3 times/day before meals or food and 30 mg at bedtime

Elderly: 7.5 mg 3 times/day before meals and at bedtime

Antispasmodic:

Children: 2-3 mg/kg/day in divided doses every 4-6 hours and at bedtime

Adults: 15 mg 3 times/day before meals or food and 30 mg at bedtime

Dosage Forms TAB, as bromide: 7.5 mg, 15 mg

Contraindications Narrow-angle glaucoma, known hypersensitivity to propantheline; ulcerative colitis; toxic megacolon; obstructive disease of the GI or urinary tract

Pregnancy Risk Factor C

Onset Oral: Within 30-45 minutes

Duration 4-6 hours

Proparacaine (proe PAR a kane)

Pharmacologic Class Local Anesthetic

U.S. Brand Names AK-Taine®; Alcaine®; I-Paracaine®; Ophthetic®

Use Anesthesia for tonometry, gonioscopy; suture removal from cornea; removal of corneal foreign body; cataract extraction, glaucoma surgery; short operative procedure involving the cornea and conjunctiva

USUAL DOSAGE Children and Adults:

Ophthalmic surgery: Instill 1 drop of 0.5% solution in eye every 5-10 minutes for 5-7 doses

Tonometry, gonioscopy, suture removal: Instill 1-2 drops of 0.5% solution in eye just prior to procedure

Contraindications Known hypersensitivity to proparacaine

Pregnancy Risk Factor C

Proparacaine and Fluorescein (proe PAR a kane & FLURE e seen)

Pharmacologic Class Diagnostic Agent; Local Anesthetic

U.S. Brand Names Fluoracaine® Ophthalmic

Use Anesthesia for tonometry, gonioscopy; suture removal from cornea; removal of corneal foreign body; cataract extraction, glaucoma surgery

USUAL DOSAGE

Ophthalmic surgery: Children and Adults: Instill 1 drop in each eye every 5-10 minutes for 5-7 doses

Tonometry, gonioscopy, suture removal: Adults: Instill 1-2 drops in each eye just prior to procedure

Contraindications Known hypersensitivity to proparacaine or fluorescein or any component or ester-type local anesthetics

Pregnancy Risk Factor C

♦ **Propecia®** *see* Finasteride *on page 364*

♦ **Prophylaxis for Patients Exposed to Common Communicable Diseases** *see page 1161*

♦ **Propine® Ophthalmic** *see* Dipivefrin *on page 285*

♦ **Pro-Piroxicam®** *see* Piroxicam *on page 744*

Propofol (PROE po fole)

Pharmacologic Class General Anesthetic

U.S. Brand Names Diprivan®

Generic Available No

Mechanism of Action Propofol is a hindered phenolic compound with intravenous general anesthetic properties. The drug is unrelated to any of the currently used barbiturate, opioid, benzodiazepine, arylcyclohexylamine, or imidazole intravenous anesthetic agents.

Use Induction or maintenance of anesthesia for inpatient or outpatient surgery; may be used (for patients >18 years of age who are intubated and mechanically ventilated) as an alternative to benzodiazepines for the treatment of agitation in the intensive care unit; pain should be treated with analgesic agents, propofol must be titrated separately from the analgesic agent; has demonstrated antiemetic properties in the postoperative setting

USUAL DOSAGE Dosage must be individualized based on total body weight and titrated to the desired clinical effect; however, as a general guideline:

No pediatric dose has been established; however, induction for children 1-12 years 2-2.8 mg/kg has been used

Induction: I.V.:

- Adults ≤55 years, and/or ASA I or II patients: 2-2.5 mg/kg of body weight (approximately 40 mg every 10 seconds until onset of induction)
- Elderly, debilitated, hypovolemic, and/or ASA III or IV patients: 1-1.5 mg/kg of body weight (approximately 20 mg every 10 seconds until onset of induction)

Maintenance: I.V. infusion:

- Adults ≤55 years, and/or ASA I or II patients: 0.1-0.2 mg/kg of body weight/minute (6-12 mg/kg of body weight/hour)
- Elderly, debilitated, hypovolemic, and/or ASA III or IV patients: 0.05-0.1 mg/kg of body weight/minute (3-6 mg/kg of body weight/hour)

I.V. intermittent: 25-50 mg increments, as needed

ICU sedation: Rapid bolus injection should be avoided. Bolus injection can result in hypotension, oxyhemoglobin desaturation, apnea, airway obstruction, and oxygen desaturation. The preferred route of administration is slow infusion. Doses are based on individual need and titrated to response.

- Recommended starting dose: 5 mcg/kg/minute (0.3-0.6 mg/kg/hour) over 5-10 minutes may be used until the desired level of sedation is achieved; infusion rate should be increased by increments of 5-10 mcg/kg/minute (0.3-0.6 mg/kg/hour) until the desired level of sedation is achieved; most adult patients require maintenance rates of 5-50 mcg/kg/minute (0.3-3 mg/kg/hour) or higher
- Adjustments in dose can occur at 3- to 5-minute intervals. An 80% reduction in dose should be considered in elderly, debilitated, and ASA II or IV patients. Once sedation is established, the dose should be decreased for the maintenance infusion period and adjusted to response.

Dosage Forms INJ: 10 mg/mL (20 mL, 50 mL, 100 mL)

Contraindications

Absolute contraindications:

- Patients with a hypersensitivity to propofol
- Patients with a hypersensitivity to propofol's emulsion which contains soybean oil, egg phosphatide, and glycerol or any of the components
- Patients who are not intubated or mechanically ventilated

(Continued)

Propofol *(Continued)*

Patients who are pregnant or nursing: Propofol is not recommended for obstetrics, including cesarian section deliveries. Propofol crosses the placenta and, therefore, may be associated with neonatal depression.

Relative contraindications:

Pediatric Intensive Care Unit patients: Safety and efficacy of propofol is not established

Patients with severe cardiac disease (ejection fraction <50%) or respiratory disease - propofol may have more profound adverse cardiovascular responses

Patients with a history of epilepsy or seizures

Patients with increased intracranial pressure or impaired cerebral circulation - substantial decreases in mean arterial pressure and subsequent decreases in cerebral perfusion pressure may occur

Patients with hyperlipidemia as evidenced by increased serum triglyceride levels or serum turbidity

Patients who are hypotensive, hypovolemic, or hemodynamically unstable

Warnings/Precautions Use slower rate of induction in the elderly; transient local pain may occur during I.V. injection; perioperative myoclonia has occurred; do not administer with blood or blood products through the same I.V. catheter; not for obstetrics, including cesarean section deliveries. Safety and effectiveness has not been established in children. Abrupt discontinuation prior to weaning or daily wake up assessments should be avoided. Abrupt discontinuation can result in rapid awakening, anxiety, agitation, and resistance to mechanical ventilation; not for use in neurosurgical anesthesia.

Pregnancy Risk Factor B

Adverse Reactions

>10%:

Cardiovascular: Hypotension, intravenous propofol produces a dose-related degree of hypotension and decrease in systemic vascular resistance which is not associated with a significant increase in heart rate or decrease in cardiac output

Local: Pain at injection site occurs at an incidence of 28.5% when administered into smaller veins of hand versus 6% when administered into antecubital veins

Respiratory: Apnea (incidence occurs in 50% to 84% of patients and may be dependent on premedication, speed of administration, dose and presence of hyperventilation and hyperoxia)

1% to 10%:

Anaphylaxis: Several cases of anaphylactic reactions have been reported with propofol

Central nervous system: Dizziness, fever, headache; although propofol has demonstrated anticonvulsant activity, several cases of propofol-induced seizures with opisthotonos have occurred

Gastrointestinal: Nausea, vomiting, abdominal cramps

Respiratory: Cough, apnea

Neuromuscular & skeletal: Twitching

Miscellaneous: Hiccups

Drug Interactions

Increased toxicity:

Neuromuscular blockers:

Atracurium: Anaphylactoid reactions (including bronchospasm) have been reported in patients who have received concomitant atracurium and propofol

Vecuronium: Propofol may potentiate the neuromuscular blockade of vecuronium

Central nervous system depressants: Additive CNS depression and respiratory depression may necessitate dosage reduction when used with: Anesthetics, benzodiazepines, opiates, ethanol, narcotics, phenothiazines

Decreased effect: Theophylline: May antagonize the effect of propofol, requiring dosage increases

Onset Rapid, 30 seconds

Duration 3-10 minutes

Half-Life Initial: 40 minutes; Terminal: 1-3 days

Education and Monitoring Issues

Monitoring Parameters: Cardiac monitor, blood pressure monitor, and ventilator required; serum triglyceride levels should be obtained prior to initiation of therapy (ICU setting) and every 3-7 days, thereafter

Vital signs: Blood pressure, heart rate, cardiac output, pulmonary capillary wedge pressure should be monitored

Manufacturer AstraZeneca

Related Information

Pharmaceutical Manufacturers Directory *on page 1020*

Propoxyphene (proe POKS i feen)

Pharmacologic Class Analgesic, Narcotic

U.S. Brand Names Darvon®; Darvon-N®; Dolene®

Generic Available Yes: Capsule

Mechanism of Action Binds to opiate receptors in the CNS, causing inhibition of ascending pain pathways, altering the perception of and response to pain; produces generalized CNS depression

Use Management of mild to moderate pain

USUAL DOSAGE Oral:

Children: Doses for children are not well established; doses of the hydrochloride of 2-3 mg/kg/d divided every 6 hours have been used

Adults:

Hydrochloride: 65 mg every 3-4 hours as needed for pain; maximum: 390 mg/day

Napsylate: 100 mg every 4 hours as needed for pain; maximum: 600 mg/day

Dosing comments in renal impairment: Cl_{cr} <10 mL/minute: Avoid use

Hemodialysis: Not dialyzable (0% to 5%)

Dosing adjustment in hepatic impairment: Reduced doses should be used

Dosage Forms CAP, as hydrochloride: 65 mg. **TAB,** as napsylate: 100 mg

Contraindications Hypersensitivity to propoxyphene or any component

Warnings/Precautions Administer with caution in patients dependent on opiates, substitution may result in acute opiate withdrawal symptoms, use with caution in patients with severe renal or hepatic dysfunction; when given in excessive doses, either alone or in combination with other CNS depressants or propoxyphene products, propoxyphene is a major cause of drug-related deaths; **do not exceed recommended dosage**; tolerance or drug dependence may result from extended use

Pregnancy Risk Factor C; D (if used for prolonged periods)

Adverse Reactions

Percentage unknown: Increased liver enzymes, may increase LFTs; may decrease glucose, urinary 17-OHCS

>10%:

Cardiovascular: Hypotension

Central nervous system: Dizziness, lightheadedness, sedation, paradoxical excitement and insomnia, fatigue, drowsiness

Gastrointestinal: Nausea, vomiting, constipation

Neuromuscular & skeletal: Weakness

1% to 10%:

Central nervous system: Nervousness, headache, restlessness, malaise, confusion

Gastrointestinal: Anorexia, stomach cramps, xerostomia, biliary spasm

Genitourinary: Decreased urination, ureteral spasms

Respiratory: Dyspnea, shortness of breath

<1%: Histamine release, increased intracranial pressure, mental depression hallucinations, paradoxical CNS stimulation, paralytic ileus, psychologic and physical dependence with prolonged use, rash, urticaria

Drug Interactions CYP3A3/4 enzyme inhibitor

Decreased effect with charcoal, cigarette smoking

Increased toxicity: CNS depressants may potentiate pharmacologic effects; propoxyphene may inhibit the metabolism and increase the serum concentrations of carbamazepine, phenobarbital, MAO inhibitors, tricyclic antidepressants, and warfarin

Alcohol Interactions Avoid use (may increase central nervous system depression)

Onset Onset of effect: Oral: Within 0.5-1 hour

Duration 4-6 hours

Half-Life Parent drug: 8-24 hours (mean: ~15 hours); Norpropoxyphene: 34 hours

Education and Monitoring Issues

Patient Education: Take as directed; do not take a larger dose or more often than prescribed. Do not use alcohol, other prescription or OTC sedatives, tranquilizers, antihistamines, or pain medications without consulting prescriber. May cause dizziness, drowsiness, or impaired judgment; avoid driving or engaging in tasks requiring alertness until response to drug is known. If you experience vomiting or loss of appetite, frequent mouth care, small frequent meals, chewing gum, or sucking lozenges may help. Increased fluid intake, exercise, fiber in diet may help with constipation (if unresolved consult prescriber). Report unresolved nausea or vomiting, difficulty breathing or shortness of breath, or unusual weakness.

Dietary Considerations:

Food: May decrease rate of absorption, but may slightly increase bioavailability

Glucose may cause hyperglycemia; monitor blood glucose concentrations

Monitoring Parameters: Pain relief, respiratory and mental status, blood pressure

Reference Range:

Therapeutic: Ranges published vary between laboratories and may not correlate with clinical effect

Therapeutic concentration: 0.1-0.4 μg/mL (SI: 0.3-1.2 μmol/L)

Toxic: >0.5 μg/mL (SI: >1.5 μmol/L)

Related Information

Lipid-Lowering Agents Comparison *on page 1243*

Narcotic Agonists Comparison *on page 1244*

Propoxyphene and Acetaminophen *on page 786*

Propoxyphene and Aspirin *on page 786*

Propoxyphene and Acetaminophen

(proe POKS i feen & a seet a MIN oh fen)

Pharmacologic Class Analgesic, Combination (Narcotic)

U.S. Brand Names Darvocet-N®; Darvocet-N® 100; Genagesic®; Propacet®; Wygesic®

Use Management of mild to moderate pain

Dosage Forms TAB: (Darvocet-N®): Propoxyphene napsylate 50 mg and acetaminophen 325 mg; (Darvocet-N® 100): Propoxyphene napsylate 100 mg and acetaminophen 650 mg; (Genagesic®, Wygesic®): Propoxyphene hydrochloride 65 mg and acetaminophen 650 mg

Alcohol Interactions Avoid use (may increase central nervous system depression)

Propoxyphene and Aspirin (proe POKS i feen & AS pir in)

Pharmacologic Class Analgesic, Combination (Narcotic)

U.S. Brand Names Bexophene®; Darvon® Compound-65 Pulvules®

Dosage Forms CAP: Propoxyphene hydrochloride 65 mg and aspirin 389 mg with caffeine 32.4 mg. **TAB** (Darvon-N® with A.S.A.): Propoxyphene napsylate 100 mg and aspirin 325 mg

Pregnancy Risk Factor D

Alcohol Interactions Avoid use (may increase central nervous system depression and enhance gastric mucosal irritation)

Propranolol (proe PRAN oh lole)

Pharmacologic Class Antiarrhythmic Agent, Class II; Beta Blocker, Nonselective

U.S. Brand Names Betachron E-R®; Inderal®; Inderal® LA

Generic Available Yes

Mechanism of Action Nonselective beta-adrenergic blocker (class II antiarrhythmic); competitively blocks response to beta$_1$- and beta$_2$-adrenergic stimulation which results in decreases in heart rate, myocardial contractility, blood pressure, and myocardial oxygen demand

Use Management of hypertension, angina pectoris, pheochromocytoma, essential tremor, tetralogy of Fallot cyanotic spells, and arrhythmias (such as atrial fibrillation and flutter, A-V nodal re-entrant tachycardias, and catecholamine-induced arrhythmias); prevention of myocardial infarction, migraine headache; symptomatic treatment of hypertrophic subaortic stenosis

Unlabeled use: Tremor due to Parkinson's disease, alcohol withdrawal, aggressive behavior, antipsychotic-induced akathisia, esophageal varices bleeding, anxiety, schizophrenia, acute panic, and gastric bleeding in portal hypertension

USUAL DOSAGE

Tachyarrhythmias:

Oral:

Children: Initial: 0.5-1 mg/kg/day in divided doses every 6-8 hours; titrate dosage upward every 3-7 days; usual dose: 2-4 mg/kg/day; higher doses may be needed; do not exceed 16 mg/kg/day or 60 mg/day

Adults: 10-30 mg/dose every 6-8 hours

Elderly: Initial: 10 mg twice daily; increase dosage every 3-7 days; usual dosage range: 10-320 mg given in 2 divided doses

I.V.:

Children: 0.01-0.1 mg/kg slow IVP over 10 minutes; maximum dose: 1 mg

Adults: 1 mg/dose slow IVP; repeat every 5 minutes up to a total of 5 mg

Hypertension: Oral:

Children: Initial: 0.5-1 mg/kg/day in divided doses every 6-12 hours; increase gradually every 3-7 days; maximum: 2 mg/kg/24 hours

Adults: Initial: 40 mg twice daily; increase dosage every 3-7 days; usual dose: ≤320 mg divided in 2-3 doses/day; maximum daily dose: 640 mg

Migraine headache prophylaxis: Oral:

Children: 0.6-1.5 mg/kg/day **or**

≤35 kg: 10-20 mg 3 times/day

>35 kg: 20-40 mg 3 times/day

Adults: Initial: 80 mg/day divided every 6-8 hours; increase by 20-40 mg/dose every 3-4 weeks to a maximum of 160-240 mg/day given in divided doses every 6-8 hours; if satisfactory response not achieved within 6 weeks of starting therapy, drug should be withdrawn gradually over several weeks

Tetralogy spells: Children:

Oral: 1-2 mg/kg/day every 6 hours as needed, may increase by 1 mg/kg/day to a maximum of 5 mg/kg/day, or if refractory may increase slowly to a maximum of 10-15 mg/kg/day

I.V.: 0.15-0.25 mg/kg/dose slow IVP; may repeat in 15 minutes

Thyrotoxicosis:

Adolescents and Adults: Oral: 10-40 mg/dose every 6 hours

Adults: I.V.: 1-3 mg/dose slow IVP as a single dose

Adults: Oral:

Angina: 80-320 mg/day in doses divided 2-4 times/day

Pheochromocytoma: 30-60 mg/day in divided doses

Myocardial infarction prophylaxis: 180-240 mg/day in 3-4 divided doses
Hypertrophic subaortic stenosis: 20-40 mg 3-4 times/day
Essential tremor: 40 mg twice daily initially; maintenance doses: usually 120-320 mg/day

Dosing adjustment in renal impairment:

Cl_{cr} 31-40 mL/minute: Administer every 24-36 hours or administer 50% of normal dose
Cl_{cr} 10-30 mL/minute: Administer every 24-48 hours or administer 50% of normal dose
Cl_{cr} <10 mL/minute: Administer every 40-60 hours or administer 25% of normal dose

Hemodialysis: Not dialyzable (0% to 5%); supplemental dose is not necessary
Peritoneal dialysis: Supplemental dose is not necessary

Dosing adjustment/comments in hepatic disease: Marked slowing of heart rate may occur in cirrhosis with conventional doses; low initial dose and regular heart rate monitoring

Dosage Forms CAP, sustained action: 60 mg, 80 mg, 120 mg, 160 mg. **INJ:** 1 mg/mL (1 mL). **SOLN, oral** (strawberry-mint flavor): 4 mg/mL (5 mL, 500 mL); 8 mg/mL (5 mL, 500 mL). **SOLN, oral, concentrate:** 80 mg/mL (30 mL). **TAB:** 10 mg, 20 mg, 40 mg, 60 mg, 80 mg

Contraindications Uncompensated congestive heart failure, cardiogenic shock, bradycardia or heart block, pulmonary edema, severe hyperactive airway disease or chronic obstructive lung disease, Raynaud's disease, hypersensitivity to beta-blockers

Warnings/Precautions Safety and efficacy in children have not been established; administer very cautiously to patients with CHF, asthma, diabetes mellitus, hyperthyroidism. Abrupt withdrawal of the drug should be avoided, drug should be discontinued over 1-2 weeks; do not use in pregnant or nursing women; may potentiate hypoglycemia in a diabetic patient and mask signs and symptoms.

Pregnancy Risk Factor C (per manufacturer); D (2nd and 3rd trimesters, based on expert analysis)

Pregnancy Implications

Clinical effects on the fetus: Crosses the placenta. IUGR, hypoglycemia, bradycardia, respiratory depression, hyperbilirubinemia, polycythemia, polydactyly reported. IUGR probably related to maternal hypertension. Preterm labor has been reported. Available evidence suggests safe use during pregnancy and breast-feeding. Monitor breast-fed infant for symptoms of beta-blockade.

Breast-feeding/lactation: Crosses into breast milk. American Academy of Pediatrics considers **compatible** with breast-feeding.

Adverse Reactions

Cardiovascular: Bradycardia, congestive heart failure, reduced peripheral circulation, thrombocytopenia, purpura, chest pain, hypotension, impaired myocardial contractility, worsening of A-V conduction disturbance, cardiogenic shock

Central nervous system: Mental depression, lightheadedness, amnesia, emotional lability, confusion, hallucinations, dizziness, insomnia, fatigue, vivid dreams, lethargy, cold extremities, vertigo, syncope, cognitive dysfunction, psychosis, hallucinations, hypersomnolence

Dermatologic: Rash, alopecia, exfoliative dermatitis, psoriasiform eruptions, eczematous eruptions, hyperkeratosis, nail changes, pruritus, urticaria, ulcerative lichenoid, contact dermatitis

Endocrine & metabolic: Hypoglycemia, hyperglycemia, lipid abnormal, hyperkalemia

Gastrointestinal: Diarrhea, nausea, vomiting, stomach discomfort, constipation, anorexia

Genitourinary: Impotence, proteinuria (rare), oliguria (rare), interstitial nephritis (rare)

Hematologic: Agranulocytosis, thrombocytopenia

Neuromuscular & skeletal: Weakness, carpal tunnel syndrome (rare), paresthesias, myotonus, polyarthritis arthropathy

Respiratory: Wheezing, pharyngitis, bronchospasm, pulmonary edema

Ocular: Hyperemia of the conjunctiva, decreased tear production, decreased visual acuity, mydriasis

Drug Interactions CYP1A2, 2C18, 2C19, and 2D6 enzyme substrate

Albuterol (and other $beta_2$ agonists): Effects may be blunted by nonspecific beta-blockers

Alpha-blockers (prazosin, terazosin): Concurrent use of beta-blockers may increase risk of orthostasis

Antipyrine's clearance is reduced by 30% to 40%

Cimetidine increases the plasma concentration of propranolol and its pharmacodynamic effects may be increased

Clonidine: Hypertensive crisis after or during withdrawal of either agent

Drugs which slow A-V conduction (digoxin): Effects may be additive with beta-blockers

Epinephrine (including local anesthetics with epinephrine): Propranolol may cause hypertension

Flecainide: Pharmacological activity of both agents may be increased when used concurrently

Fluoxetine may inhibit the metabolism of propranolol, resulting in cardiac toxicity

Glucagon: Propranolol may blunt hyperglycemic action

Haloperidol: Hypotensive effects may be potentiated

Hydralazine: The bioavailability propranolol (rapid release) and hydralazine may be enhanced with concurrent dosing

(Continued)

Propranolol *(Continued)*

Insulin: Propranolol inhibits recovery and may cause hypertension and bradycardia following insulin-induced hypoglycemia. Also masks the tachycardia that usually accompanies insulin-induced hypoglycemia.

NSAIDs (ibuprofen, indomethacin, naproxen, piroxicam) may reduce the antihypertensive effects of beta-blockers

Salicylates may reduce the antihypertensive effects of beta-blockers

Sulfonylureas: Beta-blockers may alter response to hypoglycemic agents

Verapamil or diltiazem may have synergistic or additive pharmacological effects when taken concurrently with beta-blockers; avoid concurrent I.V. use of both

Alcohol Interactions Limit use (may increase risk of hypotension or dizziness)

Onset Onset of beta blockade: Oral: Within 1-2 hours

Duration ~6 hours

Half-Life 4-6 hours

Education and Monitoring Issues

Patient Education: Take exactly as directed; do not increase, decrease, or discontinue without consulting prescriber. Take at the same time each day. Tablets may be crushed and taken with liquids. Do not alter dietary intake of protein or carbohydrates without consulting prescriber. You may experience orthostatic hypotension, dizziness, drowsiness, or blurred vision (use caution when driving, climbing stairs, or changing position - rising from sitting or lying to standing - or engaging in tasks requiring alertness until response to drug is known); nausea, vomiting, or stomach discomfort (small frequent meals, frequent mouth care, chewing gum, or sucking lozenges may help); decreased sexual ability (reversible). If diabetic, monitor serum glucose closely. Report unusual swelling of extremities, difficulty breathing, unresolved cough, or unusual weight gain, cold extremities, persistent diarrhea, confusion, hallucinations, headache, nervousness, lack of improvement, or worsening of condition.

Monitoring Parameters: Blood pressure, EKG, heart rate, CNS and cardiac effects

Reference Range: Therapeutic: 50-100 ng/mL (SI: 190-390 nmol/L) at end of dose interval

Related Information

Beta-Blockers Comparison *on page 1233*
Propranolol and Hydrochlorothiazide *on page 788*

Propranolol and Hydrochlorothiazide

(proe PRAN oh lole & hye droe klor oh THYE a zide)

Pharmacologic Class Antihypertensive Agent, Combination

U.S. Brand Names Inderide®

Dosage Forms CAP, long-acting (Inderide® LA): 80/50 Propranolol hydrochloride 80 mg and hydrochlorothiazide 50 mg; 120/50 Propranolol hydrochloride 120 mg and hydrochlorothiazide 50 mg; 160/50 Propranolol hydrochloride 160 mg and hydrochlorothiazide 50 mg. **TAB** (Inderide®): 40/25 Propranolol hydrochloride 40 mg and hydrochlorothiazide 25 mg; 80/25 Propranolol hydrochloride 80 mg and hydrochlorothiazide 25 mg

Pregnancy Risk Factor C

Alcohol Interactions Limit use (may increase risk of hypotension or dizziness)

♦ **Propulsid®** *see* Cisapride *on page 201*

Propylthiouracil (proe pil thye oh YOOR a sil)

Pharmacologic Class Antithyroid Agent

Generic Available Yes

Mechanism of Action Inhibits the synthesis of thyroid hormones by blocking the oxidation of iodine in the thyroid gland; blocks synthesis of thyroxine and triiodothyronine

Use Palliative treatment of hyperthyroidism as an adjunct to ameliorate hyperthyroidism in preparation for surgical treatment or radioactive iodine therapy and in the management of thyrotoxic crisis. The use of antithyroid thioamides is as effective in elderly as they are in younger adults; however, the expense, potential adverse effects, and inconvenience (compliance, monitoring) make them undesirable. The use of radioiodine, due to ease of administration and less concern for long-term side effects and reproduction problems, makes it a more appropriate therapy.

USUAL DOSAGE Oral: Administer in 3 equally divided doses at approximately 8-hour intervals. Adjust dosage to maintain T_3, T_4, and TSH levels in normal range; elevated T_3 may be sole indicator of inadequate treatment. Elevated TSH indicates excessive antithyroid treatment.

Children: Initial: 5-7 mg/kg/day **or** 150-200 mg/m²/day in divided doses every 8 hours

or

6-10 years: 50-150 mg/day

>10 years: 150-300 mg/day

Maintenance: Determined by patient response **or** 1/3 to 2/3 of the initial dose in divided doses every 8-12 hours. This usually begins after 2 months on an effective initial dose.

Adults: Initial: 300 mg/day in divided doses every 8 hours. In patients with severe hyperthyroidism, very large goiters, or both, the initial dosage is usually 450 mg/day; an occasional patient will require 600-900 mg/day; maintenance: 100-150 mg/day in divided doses every 8-12 hours

Elderly: Use lower dose recommendations; Initial: 150-300 mg/day

Withdrawal of therapy: Therapy should be withdrawn gradually with evaluation of the patient every 4-6 weeks for the first 3 months then every 3 months for the first year after discontinuation of therapy to detect any reoccurrence of a hyperthyroid state.

Dosing adjustment in renal impairment: Adjustment is not necessary

Dosage Forms TAB: 50 mg

Contraindications Hypersensitivity to propylthiouracil or any component

Warnings/Precautions Use with caution in patients >40 years of age because PTU may cause hypoprothrombinemia and bleeding, use with extreme caution in patients receiving other drugs known to cause agranulocytosis; may cause agranulocytosis, thyroid hyperplasia, thyroid carcinoma (usage >1 year); breast-feeding (enters breast milk)

Pregnancy Risk Factor D

Adverse Reactions

>10%:

- Central nervous system: Fever
- Dermatologic: Skin rash
- Hematologic: Leukopenia

1% to 10%:

- Central nervous system: Dizziness
- Gastrointestinal: Nausea, vomiting, loss of taste perception, stomach pain
- Hematologic: Agranulocytosis
- Miscellaneous: SLE-like syndrome

<1%: Alopecia, aplastic anemia, arthralgia, bleeding, cholestatic jaundice, constipation, cutaneous vasculitis, drowsiness, drug fever, edema, exfoliative dermatitis, goiter, headache, hepatitis, nephritis, neuritis, paresthesia, pruritus, swollen salivary glands, thrombocytopenia, urticaria, vertigo, weight gain

Drug Interactions Increased effect: Increases anticoagulant activity

Onset For significant therapeutic effects 24-36 hours are required. Peak effect: Remissions of hyperthyroidism do not usually occur before 4 months of continued therapy.

Half-Life 1.5-5 hours; End-stage renal disease: 8.5 hours

Education and Monitoring Issues

Patient Education: Take as directed, at the same time each day around-the-clock; do not miss doses or make up missed doses. This drug will need to be taken for an extended period of time to achieve appropriate results. You may experience nausea or vomiting (small frequent meals may help), dizziness or drowsiness (use caution when driving or engaging in tasks that require alertness until response to drug is known). Report rash, fever, unusual bleeding or bruising, unresolved headache, yellowing of eyes or skin, or changes in color of urine or feces, unresolved malaise.

Monitoring Parameters: CBC with differential, prothrombin time, liver function tests, thyroid function tests (TSH, T_3, T_4); periodic blood counts are recommended chronic therapy

Reference Range: See table.

Laboratory Ranges

	Normal Values
Total T_4	5-12 µg/dL
Serum T_3	90-185 ng/dL
Free thyroxine index (FT_4I)	6-10.5
TSH	0.5-4.0 µIU/mL

- **Propyl-Thyracil®** *see* Propylthiouracil *on page 788*
- **Prorazin®** *see* Prochlorperazine *on page 773*
- **Prorex®** *see* Promethazine *on page 779*
- **Proscar®** *see* Finasteride *on page 364*
- **Prosedyl** *see* Quinidine *on page 802*
- **ProSom™** *see* Estazolam *on page 326*
- **Prostaphlin®** *see* Oxacillin *on page 683*
- **ProStep® Patch** *see* Nicotine *on page 651*
- **Prostigmin®** *see* Neostigmine *on page 645*
- **Prostin E₂® Vaginal Suppository** *see* Dinoprostone *on page 281*
- **Prostin VR** *see* Alprostadil *on page 38*
- **Prostin VR Pediatric® Injection** *see* Alprostadil *on page 38*

Protamine Sulfate (PROE ta meen SUL fate)

Pharmacologic Class Antidote

Generic Available Yes

Mechanism of Action Combines with strongly acidic heparin to form a stable complex (salt) neutralizing the anticoagulant activity of both drugs

Use Treatment of heparin overdosage; neutralize heparin during surgery or dialysis procedures

USUAL DOSAGE Protamine dosage is determined by the dosage of heparin; 1 mg of protamine neutralizes 90 USP units of heparin (lung) and 115 USP units of heparin (intestinal); maximum dose: 50 mg

In the situation of heparin overdosage, since blood heparin concentrations decrease rapidly **after** administration, adjust the protamine dosage depending upon the duration of time since heparin administration as follows:

Time Elapsed	Dose of Protamine (mg) to Neutralize 100 units of Heparin
Immediate	1-1.5
30-60 min	0.5-0.75
>2 h	0.25-0.375

If heparin administered by deep S.C. injection, use 1-1.5 mg protamine per 100 units heparin; this may be done by a portion of the dose (eg, 25-50 mg) given slowly I.V. followed by the remaining portion as a continuous infusion over 8-16 hours (the expected absorption time of the S.C. heparin dose)

Dosage Forms INJ: 10 mg/mL (5 mL, 10 mL, 25 mL)

Contraindications Hypersensitivity to protamine or any component

Warnings/Precautions May not be totally effective in some patients following cardiac surgery despite adequate doses; may cause hypersensitivity reaction in patients with a history of allergy to fish (have epinephrine 1:1000 available) and in patients sensitized to protamine (via protamine zinc insulin); too rapid administration can cause severe hypotensive and anaphylactoid-like reactions. Heparin rebound associated with anticoagulation and bleeding has been reported to occur occasionally; symptoms typically occur 8-9 hours after protamine administration, but may occur as long as 18 hours later.

Pregnancy Risk Factor C

Adverse Reactions

>10%:

Cardiovascular: Sudden fall in blood pressure, bradycardia

Respiratory: Dyspnea

1% to 10%: Hematologic: Hemorrhage

<1%: Flushing, hypersensitivity reactions, hypotension, lassitude, nausea, pulmonary hypertension, vomiting

Onset I.V. injection: Heparin neutralization occurs within 5 minutes

Education and Monitoring Issues

Patient Education: Report any difficulty breathing, rash or flushing, feeling of warmth, tingling or numbness, dizziness, or disorientation.

Monitoring Parameters: Coagulation test, APTT or ACT, cardiac monitor and blood pressure monitor required during administration

- **Prothazine-DC®** *see* Promethazine and Codeine *on page 780*
- **Protilase®** *see* Pancrelipase *on page 698*
- **Protonix®** *see* Pantoprazole *on page 701*
- **Protostat® Oral** *see* Metronidazole *on page 597*
- **Pro-Trin®** *see* Co-Trimoxazole *on page 230*

Protriptyline (proe TRIP ti leen)

Pharmacologic Class Antidepressant, Tricyclic (Secondary Amine)

U.S. Brand Names Vivactil®

Generic Available No

Mechanism of Action Increases the synaptic concentration of serotonin and/or norepinephrine in the central nervous system by inhibition of their reuptake by the presynaptic neuronal membrane

Use Treatment of various forms of depression, often in conjunction with psychotherapy

USUAL DOSAGE Oral:

Adolescents: 15-20 mg/day

Adults: 15-60 mg in 3-4 divided doses

Elderly: 15-20 mg/day

Dosage Forms TAB: 5 mg, 10 mg

Contraindications Narrow-angle glaucoma, hypersensitivity to protriptyline or any component

Warnings/Precautions Use with caution in patients with cardiac conduction disturbances, history of hyperthyroid, seizure disorders, or decreased renal function; safe use of tricyclic antidepressants in children <12 years of age has not been established; protriptyline should not be abruptly discontinued in patients receiving high doses for prolonged periods

Pregnancy Risk Factor C

Adverse Reactions

Cardiovascular: Arrhythmias, hypotension, myocardial infarction, stroke, heart block, hypertension, tachycardia, palpitations

Central nervous system: Dizziness, drowsiness, headache, confusion, delirium, hallucinations, restlessness, insomnia, nightmares, fatigue, delusions, anxiety, agitation, hypomania, exacerbation of psychosis, panic, seizures, incoordination, ataxia, EPS

Dermatologic: Alopecia, photosensitivity, rash, petechiae, urticaria, itching

Endocrine & metabolic: Breast enlargement, galactorrhea, SIADH, gynecomastia, increased or decreased libido

Gastrointestinal: Xerostomia, constipation, unpleasant taste, weight gain, increased appetite, nausea, diarrhea, heartburn, vomiting, anorexia, weight loss, trouble with gums, decreased lower esophageal sphincter tone may cause GE reflux

Genitourinary: Difficult urination, impotence, testicular edema

Hematologic: Agranulocytosis, leukopenia, eosinophilia, thrombocytopenia, purpura

Hepatic: Cholestatic jaundice, increased liver enzymes

Neuromuscular & skeletal: Fine muscle tremors, weakness, tremor, numbness, tingling

Ocular: Blurred vision, eye pain, increased intraocular pressure

Otic: Tinnitus

Miscellaneous: Diaphoresis (excessive), allergic reactions

Drug Interactions

Carbamazepine, phenobarbital, and rifampin may increase the metabolism of protriptyline resulting in decreased effect of protriptyline

Protriptyline inhibits the antihypertensive response to bethanidine, clonidine, debrisoquin, guanadrel, guanethidine, guanabenz, guanfacine; monitor BP; consider alternate antihypertensive agent

Abrupt discontinuation of clonidine may cause hypertensive crisis, protriptyline may enhance the response

Use with altretamine may cause orthostatic hypertension

Protriptyline may be additive with or may potentiate the action of other CNS depressants (sedatives, hypnotics, or ethanol); with MAO inhibitors, hyperpyrexia, hypertension, tachycardia, confusion, seizures, and **deaths have been reported** (serotonin syndrome), this combination should be avoided

Protriptyline may increase the prothrombin time in patients stabilized on warfarin

Cimetidine and methylphenidate may decrease the metabolism of protriptyline

Additive anticholinergic effects seen with other anticholinergic agents

The SSRIs, to varying degrees, inhibit the metabolism of TCAs and clinical toxicity may result

Use of lithium with a TCA may increase the risk for neurotoxicity

Phenothiazines may increase concentration of some TCAs and TCAs may increase concentration of phenothiazines; monitor for altered clinical response

TCAs may enhance the hypoglycemic effects of tolazamide, chlorpropamide, or insulin; monitor for changes in blood glucose levels

Cholestyramine and colestipol may bind TCAs and reduce their absorption; monitor for altered response

TCAs may enhance the effect of amphetamines; monitor for adverse CV effects

Verapamil and diltiazem appear to decrease the metabolism of imipramine and potentially other TCAs; monitor for increased TCA concentrations. The pressor response to I.V. epinephrine, norepinephrine, and phenylephrine may be enhanced in patients receiving TCAs, this combination is best avoided.

Indinavir, ritonavir may inhibit the metabolism of clomipramine and potentially other TCAs; monitor for altered effects; a decrease in TCA dosage may be required

Quinidine may inhibit the metabolism of TCAs; monitor for altered effect

Combined use of anticholinergics with TCAs may produce additive anticholinergic effects; combined use of beta-agonists with TCAs may predispose patients to cardiac arrhythmias

Alcohol Interactions Avoid use (may increase central nervous system depression)

Onset Maximum antidepressant effect: 2 weeks of continuous therapy is commonly required

Half-Life 54-92 hours, averaging 74 hours

Education and Monitoring Issues

Patient Education: Take exactly as directed (do not increase dose or frequency); may take 2-3 weeks to achieve desired results; may cause physical and/or psychological dependence. Avoid excessive alcohol, caffeine, and other prescription or OTC medications not approved by prescriber. Maintain adequate hydration (2-3 L/day of fluids unless instructed to restrict fluid intake). You may experience drowsiness, lightheadedness, impaired coordination, dizziness, or blurred vision (use caution when driving or engaging in tasks requiring alertness until response to drug is known); nausea, vomiting, altered taste, dry mouth (small frequent meals, frequent mouth care, chewing gum, or sucking lozenges may help); constipation (increased exercise, fluids, or dietary fruit and fiber may help); diarrhea (buttermilk, yogurt, or boiled milk may help);

(Continued)

Protriptyline *(Continued)*

increased appetite (monitor dietary intake to avoid excess weight gain); postural hypotension (use caution when climbing stairs or changing position from lying or sitting to standing); urinary retention (void before taking medication); or sexual dysfunction (reversible). Report persistent CNS effects (eg, insomnia, nervousness, restlessness, hallucinations, daytime sedation, impaired cognitive function); muscle cramping or tremors; chest pain, palpitations, rapid heartbeat, swelling of extremities, or severe dizziness; blurred vision or eye pain; yellowing of eyes or skin; pale stools/dark urine; or worsening of condition.

Dietary Considerations: Grapefruit juice may potentially inhibit the metabolism of TCAs

Reference Range: Therapeutic: 70-250 ng/mL (SI: 266-950 nmol/L); Toxic: >500 ng/mL (SI: >1900 nmol/L)

Related Information

Antidepressant Agents Comparison *on page 1231*

- **Protropin® Injection** *see* Human Growth Hormone *on page 438*
- **Proventil®** *see* Albuterol *on page 27*
- **Proventil® HFA** *see* Albuterol *on page 27*
- **Provera®** *see* Medroxyprogesterone Acetate *on page 558*
- **Provigil®** *see* Modafinil *on page 612*
- **Proviodine** *see* Povidone-Iodine *on page 756*
- **Provisc®** *see* Sodium Hyaluronate *on page 859*
- **Provocholine®** *see* Methacholine *on page 575*
- **Proxigel® Oral [OTC]** *see* Carbamide Peroxide *on page 139*
- **Prozac®** *see* Fluoxetine *on page 378*
- **Pseudo-Car® DM** *see* Carbinoxamine, Pseudoephedrine, and Dextromethorphan *on page 140*

Pseudoephedrine (soo doe e FED rin)

Pharmacologic Class Alpha/Beta Agonist

U.S. Brand Names Actifed® Allergy Tablet (Day) [OTC]; Afrin® Tablet [OTC]; Cenafed® [OTC]; Children's Silfedrine® [OTC]; Decofed® Syrup [OTC]; Drixoral® Non-Drowsy [OTC]; Efidac/24® [OTC]; Neofed® [OTC]; PediaCare® Oral; Sudafed® [OTC]; Sudafed® 12 Hour [OTC]; Sufedrin® [OTC]; Triaminic® AM Decongestant Formula [OTC]

Generic Available Yes

Mechanism of Action Directly stimulates alpha-adrenergic receptors of respiratory mucosa causing vasoconstriction; directly stimulates beta-adrenergic receptors causing bronchial relaxation, increased heart rate and contractility

Use Temporary symptomatic relief of nasal congestion due to common cold, upper respiratory allergies, and sinusitis; also promotes nasal or sinus drainage

USUAL DOSAGE Oral:

Children:

- <2 years: 4 mg/kg/day in divided doses every 6 hours
- 2-5 years: 15 mg every 6 hours; maximum: 60 mg/24 hours
- 6-12 years: 30 mg every 6 hours; maximum: 120 mg/24 hours

Adults: 30-60 mg every 4-6 hours, sustained release: 120 mg every 12 hours; maximum: 240 mg/24 hours

Dosing adjustment in renal impairment: Reduce dose

Dosage Forms

Pseudoephedrine hydrochloride: **CAP:** 60 mg; Timed release: 120 mg. **DROPS, oral:** 7.5 mg/0.8 mL (15 mL). **LIQ:** 15 mg/5 mL (120 mL); 30 mg/5 mL (120 mL, 240 mL, 473 mL). **SYR:** 15 mg/5 mL (118 mL). **TAB:** 30 mg, 60 mg; Timed release: 120 mg

Pseudoephedrine sulfate: **TAB:** Extended release: 120 mg, 240 mg

Contraindications Hypersensitivity to pseudoephedrine or any component; MAO inhibitor therapy

Warnings/Precautions Use with caution in patients >60 years of age; administer with caution to patients with hypertension, hyperthyroidism, diabetes mellitus, cardiovascular disease, ischemic heart disease, increased intraocular pressure, or prostatic hypertrophy. Elderly patients are more likely to experience adverse reactions to sympathomimetics. Overdosage may cause hallucinations, seizures, CNS depression, and death.

Pregnancy Risk Factor C

Adverse Reactions

>10%:

- Cardiovascular: Tachycardia, palpitations, arrhythmias
- Central nervous system: Nervousness, transient stimulation, insomnia, excitability, dizziness, drowsiness
- Neuromuscular & skeletal: Tremor

1% to 10%:

- Central nervous system: Headache
- Neuromuscular & skeletal: Weakness
- Miscellaneous: Diaphoresis

<1%: Convulsions, dyspnea, dysuria, hallucinations, nausea, shortness of breath, vomiting

Drug Interactions

Decreased effect of methyldopa, reserpine

Increased toxicity: MAO inhibitors may increase blood pressure effects of pseudoephedrine; propranolol, sympathomimetic agents may increase toxicity

Onset Decongestant effect: Oral: 15-30 minutes

Duration 4-6 hours (up to 12 hours with extended release formulation administration)

Half-Life 9-16 hours

Education and Monitoring Issues

Patient Education: Take only as prescribed; do not exceed prescribed dose or frequency. Do not chew or crush timed release capsules. Maintain adequate hydration (2-3 L/day of fluids unless instructed to restrict fluid intake). You may experience nervousness, insomnia, dizziness, or drowsiness (use caution when driving or engaging in tasks requiring alertness until response to drug is known). Report persistent CNS changes (dizziness, sedation, tremor, agitation, or convulsions); difficulty breathing; chest pain, palpitations, or rapid heartbeat; muscle tremor; or lack of improvement or worsening of condition.

Related Information

Acrivastine and Pseudoephedrine *on page 21*
Azatadine and Pseudoephedrine *on page 84*
Carbinoxamine and Pseudoephedrine *on page 140*
Carbinoxamine, Pseudoephedrine, and Dextromethorphan *on page 140*
Chlorpheniramine, Pseudoephedrine, and Codeine *on page 187*
Fexofenadine and Pseudoephedrine *on page 362*
Guaifenesin, Pseudoephedrine, and Codeine *on page 425*
Hydrocodone and Pseudoephedrine *on page 446*
Hydrocodone, Pseudoephedrine, and Guaifenesin *on page 446*
Loratadine and Pseudoephedrine *on page 541*
Triprolidine, Pseudoephedrine, and Codeine *on page 958*

♦ **Psorcon™ E** *see* Diflorasone *on page 270*

♦ **Psorion® Cream** *see* Betamethasone *on page 103*

Psyllium (SIL i yum)

Pharmacologic Class Laxative, Bulk-Producing

U.S. Brand Names Effer-Syllium® [OTC]; Fiberall® Powder [OTC]; Fiberall® Wafer [OTC]; Hydrocil® [OTC]; Konsyl-D® [OTC]; Konsyl® [OTC]; Metamucil® [OTC]; Metamucil® Instant Mix [OTC]; Modane® Bulk [OTC]; Perdiem® Plain [OTC]; Reguloid® [OTC]; Serutan® [OTC]; Syllact® [OTC]; V-Lax® [OTC]

Use Treatment of chronic atonic or spastic constipation and in constipation associated with rectal disorders; management of irritable bowel syndrome

USUAL DOSAGE Oral (administer at least 3 hours before or after drugs):

Children 6-11 years: (Approximately ½ adult dosage) ½ to 1 rounded teaspoonful in 4 oz glass of liquid 1-3 times/day

Adults: 1-2 rounded teaspoonfuls or 1-2 packets or 1-2 wafers in 8 oz glass of liquid 1-3 times/day

Contraindications Fecal impaction, GI obstruction, hypersensitivity to psyllium or any component

Pregnancy Risk Factor B

♦ **Pulmicort®** *see* Budesonide *on page 115*

♦ **Pulmicort® Turbuhaler®** *see* Budesonide *on page 115*

♦ **Purinol®** *see* Allopurinol *on page 34*

♦ **PVF® K** *see* Penicillin V Potassium *on page 713*

♦ **P-V-Tussin®** *see* Hydrocodone, Phenylephrine, Pyrilamine, Phenindamine, Chlorpheniramine, and Ammonium Chloride *on page 446*

♦ **P_xE_x® Ophthalmic** *see* Pilocarpine and Epinephrine *on page 736*

Pyrantel Pamoate (pi RAN tel PAM oh ate)

Pharmacologic Class Anthelmintic

U.S. Brand Names Antiminth® [OTC]; Pin-Rid® [OTC]; Pin-X® [OTC]; Reese's® Pinworm Medicine [OTC]

Generic Available No

Mechanism of Action Causes the release of acetylcholine and inhibits cholinesterase; acts as a depolarizing neuromuscular blocker, paralyzing the helminths

Use Treatment of pinworms (*Enterobius vermicularis*), whipworms (*Trichuris trichiura*), roundworms (*Ascaris lumbricoides*), and hookworms (*Ancylostoma duodenale*)

USUAL DOSAGE Children and Adults (purgation is not required prior to use): Oral:

Roundworm, pinworm, or trichostrongyliasis: 11 mg/kg administered as a single dose; maximum dose: 1 g. (**Note:** For pinworm infection, dosage should be repeated in 2 weeks and all family members should be treated).

Hookworm: 11 mg/kg administered once daily for 3 days

(Continued)

Pyrantel Pamoate *(Continued)*

Dosage Forms CAP: 180 mg. **LIQ:** 50 mg/mL (30 mL); 144 mg/mL (30 mL). **SUSP, oral** (caramel-currant flavor): 50 mg/mL (60 mL)

Contraindications Known hypersensitivity to pyrantel pamoate

Warnings/Precautions Use with caution in patients with liver impairment, anemia, malnutrition, or pregnancy. Since pinworm infections are easily spread to others, treat all family members in close contact with the patient.

Pregnancy Risk Factor C

Adverse Reactions

1% to 10%: Gastrointestinal: Anorexia, nausea, vomiting, abdominal cramps, diarrhea

<1%: Dizziness, drowsiness, elevated liver enzymes, headache, insomnia, rash, tenesmus, weakness

Drug Interactions Decreased effect with piperazine

Education and Monitoring Issues

Patient Education: May mix drug with milk or fruit juice; strict hygiene is essential to prevent reinfection

Monitoring Parameters: Stool for presence of eggs, worms, and occult blood, serum AST and ALT

Pyrazinamide (peer a ZIN a mide)

Pharmacologic Class Antitubercular Agent

Generic Available No

Mechanism of Action Converted to pyrazinoic acid in susceptible strains of *Mycobacterium* which lowers the pH of the environment; exact mechanism of action has not been elucidated

Use Adjunctive treatment of tuberculosis in combination with other antituberculosis agents

USUAL DOSAGE Oral (calculate dose on ideal body weight rather than total body weight):

Note: A four-drug regimen (isoniazid, rifampin, pyrazinamide, and either streptomycin or ethambutol) is preferred for the initial, empiric treatment of TB. When the drug susceptibility results are available, the regimen should be altered as appropriate.

Children and Adults:

- Daily therapy: 15-30 mg/kg/day (maximum: 2 g/day)
- Directly observed therapy (DOT): Twice weekly: 50-70 mg/kg (maximum: 4 g)
- DOT: 3 times/week: 50-70 mg/kg (maximum: 3 g)

Elderly: Start with a lower daily dose (15 mg/kg) and increase as tolerated

Dosing adjustment in renal impairment: Cl_{cr} <50 mL/minute: Avoid use or reduce dose to 12-20 mg/kg/day

Dosing adjustment in hepatic impairment: Reduce dose

Dosage Forms TAB: 500 mg

Contraindications Severe hepatic damage; hypersensitivity to pyrazinamide or any component; acute gout

Warnings/Precautions Use with caution in patients with renal failure, chronic gout, diabetes mellitus, or porphyria

Pregnancy Risk Factor C

Adverse Reactions

1% to 10%:

- Central nervous system: Malaise
- Gastrointestinal: Nausea, vomiting, anorexia
- Neuromuscular & skeletal: Arthralgia, myalgia

<1%: Acne, dysuria, fever, gout, hepatotoxicity, interstitial nephritis, itching, photosensitivity, porphyria, rash, thrombocytopenia

Half-Life 9-10 hours, increased with reduced renal or hepatic function; End-stage renal disease: 9 hours

Education and Monitoring Issues

Patient Education: Take with food for full length of therapy. Do not miss doses and do not discontinue without consulting prescriber. You will need regular medical follow-up while taking this medication. You may experience nausea or loss of appetite; small frequent meals, frequent mouth care, sucking lozenges, or chewing gum may help. Report unusual fever, unresolved nausea or vomiting, change in color of urine, pale stools, easy bruising or bleeding, blood in urine or difficulty urinating, yellowing of skin or eyes, or extreme joint pain.

Monitoring Parameters: Periodic liver function tests, serum uric acid, sputum culture, chest x-ray 2-3 months into treatment and at completion

Related Information

Antimicrobial Drugs of Choice *on page 1182*
Rifampin, Isoniazid, and Pyrazinamide *on page 822*
Tuberculosis Treatment Guidelines *on page 1213*

Pyrethrins (pye RE thrins)

Pharmacologic Class Scabicides/Pediculicides

U.S. Brand Names A-200™ Shampoo [OTC]; Barc™ Liquid [OTC]; End Lice® Liquid [OTC]; Lice-Enz® Shampoo [OTC]; Pronto® Shampoo [OTC]; Pyrinex® Pediculicide Shampoo [OTC]; Pyrinyl II® Liquid [OTC]; Pyrinyl Plus® Shampoo [OTC]; R & C® Shampoo [OTC]; RID® Shampoo [OTC]; Tisit® Blue Gel [OTC]; Tisit® Liquid [OTC]; Tisit® Shampoo [OTC]; Triple X® Liquid [OTC]

Use Treatment of *Pediculus humanus* infestations (head lice, body lice, pubic lice and their eggs)

USUAL DOSAGE Application of pyrethrins: Topical:

Apply enough solution to completely wet infested area, including hair
Allow to remain on area for 10 minutes
Wash and rinse with large amounts of warm water
Use fine-toothed comb to remove lice and eggs from hair
Shampoo hair to restore body and luster
Treatment may be repeated if necessary once in a 24-hour period
Repeat treatment in 7-10 days to kill newly hatched lice

Contraindications Known hypersensitivity to pyrethrins, ragweed, or chrysanthemums

Pregnancy Risk Factor C

- **Pyribenzamine** *see* Tripelennamine *on page 957*
- **Pyridiate®** *see* Phenazopyridine *on page 721*
- **Pyridium®** *see* Phenazopyridine *on page 721*

Pyridostigmine (peer id oh STIG meen)

Pharmacologic Class Acetylcholinesterase Inhibitor (Peripheral)

U.S. Brand Names Mestinon®; Mestinon® Time-Span®; Regonol® Injection

Generic Available No

Mechanism of Action Inhibits destruction of acetylcholine by acetylcholinesterase which facilitates transmission of impulses across myoneural junction

Use Symptomatic treatment of myasthenia gravis; also used as an antidote for nondepolarizing neuromuscular blockers; not a cure; patient may develop resistance to the drug

USUAL DOSAGE Normally, sustained release dosage form is used at bedtime for patients who complain of morning weakness

Myasthenia gravis:
- Oral:
  - Children: 7 mg/kg/day in 5-6 divided doses
  - Adults: Initial: 60 mg 3 times/day with maintenance dose ranging from 60 mg to 1.5 g/day; sustained release formulation should be dosed at least every 6 hours (usually 12-24 hours)
- I.M., I.V.:
  - Children: 0.05-0.15 mg/kg/dose (maximum single dose: 10 mg)
  - Adults: 2 mg every 2-3 hours or 1/30th of oral dose

Reversal of nondepolarizing neuromuscular blocker: I.M., I.V.:
- Children: 0.1-0.25 mg/kg/dose preceded by atropine
- Adults: 10-20 mg preceded by atropine

Dosing adjustment in renal impairment: Lower doses may be required

Dosage Forms INJ: 5 mg/mL (2 mL, 5 mL). **SYR** (raspberry flavor): 60 mg/5 mL (480 mL). **TAB:** 60 mg; Sustained release: 180 mg

Contraindications Hypersensitivity to pyridostigmine, bromides, or any component; GI or GU obstruction

Warnings/Precautions Use with caution in patients with epilepsy, asthma, bradycardia, hyperthyroidism, cardiac arrhythmias, or peptic ulcer; adequate facilities should be available for cardiopulmonary resuscitation when testing and adjusting dose for myasthenia gravis; have atropine and epinephrine ready to treat hypersensitivity reactions; overdosage may result in cholinergic crisis, this must be distinguished from myasthenic crisis; anticholinesterase insensitivity can develop for brief or prolonged periods

Pregnancy Risk Factor C

Adverse Reactions

>10%:
- Gastrointestinal: Diarrhea, nausea, stomach cramps, mouth watering
- Miscellaneous: Diaphoresis (increased)

1% to 10%:
- Genitourinary: Urge to urinate
- Ocular: Small pupils, lacrimation
- Respiratory: Increased bronchial secretions

<1%: A-V block, bradycardia, diplopia, drowsiness, dysphoria, headache, hyper-reactive cholinergic responses, hypersensitivity, laryngospasm, miosis, muscle spasms, respiratory paralysis, seizures, thrombophlebitis, weakness

Drug Interactions

Increased effect of depolarizing neuromuscular blockers (succinylcholine)
Increased toxicity with edrophonium

(Continued)

Pyridostigmine *(Continued)*

Onset Oral: 15-30 minutes; I.M.: 15-30 minutes; I.V.: 2-5 minutes

Duration Oral: Up to 6-8 hours (due to slow absorption); I.V.: 2-3 hours

Education and Monitoring Issues

Patient Education: This drug will not cure myasthenia gravis, but may help reduce symptoms. Use as directed; do not increase dose or discontinue without consulting prescriber. Take extended release tablets at bedtime; do not chew or crush extended release tablets. Maintain adequate hydration (2-3 L/day of fluids unless instructed to restrict fluid intake). May cause dizziness, drowsiness, or hypotension (rise slowly from sitting or lying position and use caution when driving or climbing stairs); vomiting or loss of appetite (frequent small meals, frequent mouth care, chewing gum, or sucking lozenges may help); or diarrhea (boiled milk, yogurt, or buttermilk may help). Report persistent abdominal discomfort; significantly increased salivation, sweating, tearing, or urination; flushed skin; chest pain or palpitations; acute headache; unresolved diarrhea; excessive fatigue, insomnia, dizziness, or depression; increased muscle, joint, or body pain; vision changes or blurred vision; or shortness of breath or wheezing.

Pyridoxine (peer i DOKS een)

Pharmacologic Class Antidote; Vitamin, Water Soluble

U.S. Brand Names Nestrex®

Generic Available Yes

Mechanism of Action Precursor to pyridoxal, which functions in the metabolism of proteins, carbohydrates, and fats; pyridoxal also aids in the release of liver and muscle-stored glycogen and in the synthesis of GABA (within the central nervous system) and heme

Use Prevents and treats vitamin B_6 deficiency, pyridoxine-dependent seizures in infants, adjunct to treatment of acute toxicity from isoniazid, cycloserine, or hydralazine overdose

USUAL DOSAGE

Recommended daily allowance (RDA):
- Children:
  - 1-3 years: 0.9 mg
  - 4-6 years: 1.3 mg
  - 7-10 years: 1.6 mg
- Adults:
  - Male: 1.7-2.0 mg
  - Female: 1.4-1.6 mg

Pyridoxine-dependent Infants:
- Oral: 2-100 mg/day
- I.M., I.V., S.C.: 10-100 mg

Dietary deficiency: Oral:
- Children: 5-25 mg/24 hours for 3 weeks, then 1.5-2.5 mg/day in multiple vitamin product
- Adults: 10-20 mg/day for 3 weeks

Drug-induced neuritis (eg, isoniazid, hydralazine, penicillamine, cycloserine): Oral:
- Children:
  - Treatment: 10-50 mg/24 hours
  - Prophylaxis: 1-2 mg/kg/24 hours
- Adults:
  - Treatment: 100-200 mg/24 hours
  - Prophylaxis: 25-100 mg/24 hours

Treatment of seizures and/or coma from acute isoniazid toxicity, a dose of pyridoxine hydrochloride equal to the amount of INH ingested can be given I.M./I.V. in divided doses together with other anticonvulsants; if the amount INH ingested is not known, administer 5 g I.V. pyridoxine

Treatment of acute hydralazine toxicity, a pyridoxine dose of 25 mg/kg in divided doses I.M./I.V. has been used

Dosage Forms INJ: 100 mg/mL (10 mL, 30 mL). **TAB:** 25 mg, 50 mg, 100 mg; Extended release: 100 mg

Contraindications Hypersensitivity to pyridoxine or any component

Warnings/Precautions Dependence and withdrawal may occur with doses >200 mg/day

Pregnancy Risk Factor A; C (if dose exceeds RDA recommendation)

Pregnancy Implications

Clinical effects on the fetus: Crosses the placenta; available evidence suggests safe use during pregnancy and breast-feeding

Breast-feeding/lactation: Crosses into breast milk; possible inhibition of lactation at doses >600 mg/day. American Academy of Pediatrics considers **compatible** with breast-feeding.

Adverse Reactions <1%: Allergic reactions have been reported decreased serum folic acid secretions, headache, increased AST, nausea, paresthesia, seizures have occurred following I.V. administration of very large doses, sensory neuropathy

Drug Interactions Decreased serum levels of levodopa, phenobarbital, and phenytoin

Half-Life 15-20 days

Education and Monitoring Issues

Patient Education: Take exactly as directed. Do not take more than recommended. Do not chew or crush extended release tablets. Do not exceed recommended intake of dietary B6 (eg, red meat, bananas, potatoes, yeast, lima beans, and whole grain cereals). You may experience burning or pain at injection site; notify prescriber if this persists.

Reference Range: Over 50 ng/mL (SI: 243 nmol/L) (varies considerably with method). A broad range is ~25-80 ng/mL (SI: 122-389 nmol/L). HPLC method for pyridoxal phosphate has normal range of 3.5-18 ng/mL (SI: 17-88 nmol/L).

Related Information

Epilepsy Guidelines *on page 1091*

Pyrimethamine (peer i METH a meen)

Pharmacologic Class Antimalarial Agent

U.S. Brand Names Daraprim®

Generic Available No

Mechanism of Action Inhibits parasitic dihydrofolate reductase, resulting in inhibition of vital tetrahydrofolic acid synthesis

Use Prophylaxis of malaria due to susceptible strains of plasmodia; used in conjunction with quinine and sulfadiazine for the treatment of uncomplicated attacks of chloroquine-resistant *P. falciparum* malaria; used in conjunction with fast-acting schizonticide to initiate transmission control and suppression cure; synergistic combination with sulfonamide in treatment of toxoplasmosis

USUAL DOSAGE

Malaria chemoprophylaxis (for areas where chloroquine-resistant *P. falciparum* exists):
- Begin prophylaxis 2 weeks before entering endemic area:
- Children: 0.5 mg/kg once weekly; not to exceed 25 mg/dose
  - **or**
- Children:
  - <4 years: 6.25 mg once weekly
  - 4-10 years: 12.5 mg once weekly
- Children >10 years and Adults: 25 mg once weekly
- Dosage should be continued for all age groups for at least 6-10 weeks after leaving endemic areas

Chloroquine-resistant *P. falciparum* malaria (when used in conjunction with quinine and sulfadiazine):
- Children:
  - <10 kg: 6.25 mg/day once daily for 3 days
  - 10-20 kg: 12.5 mg/day once daily for 3 days
  - 20-40 kg: 25 mg/day once daily for 3 days
- Adults: 25 mg twice daily for 3 days

Toxoplasmosis:
- Infants for congenital toxoplasmosis: Oral: 1 mg/kg once daily for 6 months with sulfadiazine then every other month with sulfa, alternating with spiramycin.
- Children: Loading dose: 2 mg/kg/day divided into 2 equal daily doses for 1-3 days (maximum: 100 mg/day) followed by 1 mg/kg/day divided into 2 doses for 4 weeks; maximum: 25 mg/day
  - With sulfadiazine or trisulfapyrimidines: 2 mg/kg/day divided every 12 hours for 3 days followed by 1 mg/kg/day once daily or divided twice daily for 4 weeks given with trisulfapyrimidines or sulfadiazine
- Adults: 50-75 mg/day together with 1-4 g of a sulfonamide for 1-3 weeks depending on patient's tolerance and response, then reduce dose by 50% and continue for 4-5 weeks **or** 25-50 mg/day for 3-4 weeks

In HIV, life-long suppression is necessary to prevent relapse; leucovorin (5-10 mg/day) is given concurrently

Dosage Forms TAB: 25 mg

Contraindications Megaloblastic anemia secondary to folate deficiency; known hypersensitivity to pyrimethamine, chloroguanide; resistant malaria

Warnings/Precautions When used for more than 3-4 days, it may be advisable to administer leucovorin to prevent hematologic complications; monitor CBC and platelet counts every 2 weeks; use with caution in patients with impaired renal or hepatic function or with possible G-6-PD

Pregnancy Risk Factor C

Adverse Reactions

1% to 10%:
- Gastrointestinal: Anorexia, abdominal cramps, vomiting
- Hematologic: Megaloblastic anemia, leukopenia, thrombocytopenia, agranulocytosis

<1%: Abnormal skin pigmentation, anaphylaxis, atrophic glossitis, depression, dermatitis, diarrhea, erythema multiforme, fever, insomnia, lightheadedness, malaise, pulmonary eosinophilia, rash, seizures, Stevens-Johnson syndrome, xerostomia

Drug Interactions

Decreased effect: Pyrimethamine effectiveness decreased by acid

(Continued)

Pyrimethamine *(Continued)*

Increased effect: Sulfonamides (synergy), methotrexate, TMP/SMX may increase the risk of bone marrow suppression; mild hepatotoxicity with lorazepam

Onset Within 1 hour

Half-Life 80-95 hours

Education and Monitoring Issues

Patient Education: Take on schedule as directed and take full course of therapy. If used for prophylaxis, begin 2 weeks before traveling to endemic areas, continue during travel period, and for 6-10 weeks following return. Regular blood tests will be necessary during therapy. You may experience GI distress (frequent small meals may help). You may experience dizziness, changes in mentation, insomnia, headache, or visual disturbances (use caution when driving or operating dangerous machinery). Report unresolved nausea or vomiting, anorexia, skin rash, fever, sore throat, unusual bleeding or bruising, yellowing of skin or eyes, and change in color of urine or stool.

Monitoring Parameters: CBC, including platelet counts

- **Pyrinex® Pediculicide Shampoo [OTC]** *see* Pyrethrins *on page 795*
- **Pyrinyl II® Liquid [OTC]** *see* Pyrethrins *on page 795*
- **Pyrinyl Plus® Shampoo [OTC]** *see* Pyrethrins *on page 795*
- **Pyronium®** *see* Phenazopyridine *on page 721*
- **PZI Iletin** *see* Insulin Preparations *on page 472*

Quazepam (KWAY ze pam)

Pharmacologic Class Benzodiazepine

U.S. Brand Names Doral®

Use Treatment of insomnia; more likely than triazolam to cause daytime sedation and fatigue; is classified as a long-acting benzodiazepine hypnotic (like flurazepam - Dalmane®), this long duration of action may prevent withdrawal symptoms when therapy is discontinued

USUAL DOSAGE Adults: Oral: Initial: 15 mg at bedtime, in some patients the dose may be reduced to 7.5 mg after a few nights

Dosing adjustment in hepatic impairment: Dose reduction may be necessary

Dosage Forms TAB: 7.5 mg, 15 mg

Contraindications Narrow-angle glaucoma, pregnancy, known hypersensitivity to quazepam

Pregnancy Risk Factor X

Drug Interactions

Decreased therapeutic effect: Carbamazepine, rifampin, rifabutin may enhance the metabolism of quazepam and decrease its therapeutic effect; consider using an alternative sedative/hypnotic agent

Increased toxicity: Cimetidine, ciprofloxacin, clarithromycin, clozapine, CNS depressants, diltiazem, disulfiram, digoxin, erythromycin, ethanol, fluconazole, fluoxetine, fluvoxamine, isoniazid, itraconazole, ketoconazole, labetalol, levodopa, loxapine, metoprolol, metronidazole, miconazole, nefazodone, omeprazole, phenytoin, rifabutin, rifampin, troleandomycin, valproic acid, verapamil may increase the serum level and/or toxicity of quazepam; monitor for altered benzodiazepine response

Alcohol Interactions Avoid use (may increase central nervous system depression)

Half-Life 25-41 hours; Metabolite: 40-114 hours

Education and Monitoring Issues

Dietary Considerations: Grapefruit juice may increase the serum level and/or toxicity

Manufacturer Wallace Laboratories

Related Information

Pharmaceutical Manufacturers Directory *on page 1020*

- **Queltuss®** *see* Guaifenesin and Dextromethorphan *on page 424*
- **Questran®** *see* Cholestyramine Resin *on page 192*
- **Questran® Light** *see* Cholestyramine Resin *on page 192*

Quetiapine (kwe TYE a peen)

Pharmacologic Class Antipsychotic Agent, Dibenzothiazepine

U.S. Brand Names Seroquel®

Mechanism of Action Mechanism of action of quetiapine, as with other antipsychotic drugs, is unknown. However, it has been proposed that this drug's antipsychotic activity is mediated through a combination of dopamine type 2 (D_2) and serotonin type 2 ($5\text{-}HT_2$) antagonism. However, it is an antagonist at multiple neurotransmitter receptors in the brain: serotonin $5\text{-}HT_{1A}$ and $5\text{-}HT_2$, dopamine D_1 and D_2, histamine H_1, and adrenergic $alpha_1$- and $alpha_2$-receptors; but appears to have no appreciable affinity at cholinergic muscarinic and benzodiazepine receptors.

Antagonism at receptors other than dopamine and $5\text{-}HT_2$ with similar receptor affinities may explain some of the other effects of quetiapine. The drug's antagonism of histamine H_1 receptors may explain the somnolence observed with it. The drug's antagonism of adrenergic $alpha_1$-receptors may explain the orthostatic hypotension observed with it.

Use Treatment of acute exacerbations of schizophrenia or other psychotic disorders. Like other atypical antipsychotics, quetiapine is probably best tried in cases for which typical antipsychotic drugs have proven ineffective.

USUAL DOSAGE Adults: Oral: 25-100 mg 2-3 times/day; usual starting dose: 25 mg twice daily and then increased in increments of 25-50 mg 2-3 times/day on the second or third day; by day 4, the dose should be in the range of 300-400 mg/day in 2-3 divided doses. Make further adjustments as needed at intervals of at least 2 days in adjustments of 25-50 mg twice daily. The usual maintenance range is 150-750 mg/day; maximum dose: 800 mg/day.

Dosing comments in elderly patients: 40% lower mean oral clearance of quetiapine in adults >65 years of age; higher plasma levels expected and, therefore, dosage adjustment may be needed

Dosing comments in hepatic insufficiency: 30% lower mean oral clearance of quetiapine than normal subjects; higher plasma levels expected in hepatically impaired subjects; dosage adjustment may be needed

Dosage Forms TAB: 25 mg, 100 mg, 200 mg

Contraindications Known hypersensitivity to this drug or any of its ingredients

Warnings/Precautions May induce orthostatic hypotension associated with dizziness, tachycardia, and, in some cases, syncope, especially during the initial dose titration period. Should be used with particular caution in patients with known cardiovascular disease (history of MI or ischemic heart disease, heart failure, or conduction abnormalities), cerebrovascular disease, or conditions that predispose to hypotension. Development of cataracts has been observed in animal studies, therefore, lens examinations should be made upon initiation of therapy and every 6 months thereafter.

Neuroleptic malignant syndrome (NMS) is a potentially fatal symptom complex that has been reported in association with administration of antipsychotic drugs. Clinical manifestations of NMS are hyperpyrexia, muscle rigidity, altered mental status, and evidence of autonomic instability (irregular pulse or blood pressure, tachycardia, diaphoresis, and cardiac dysrhythmia). Management of NMS should include immediate discontinuation of antipsychotic drugs and other drugs not essential to concurrent therapy, intensive symptomatic treatment and medication monitoring, and treatment of any concomitant medical problems for which specific treatment are available.

Tardive dyskinesia; caution in patients with a history of seizures, decreases in total free thyroxine, pre-existing hyperprolactinemia, elevations of liver enzymes, cholesterol levels and/or triglyceride increases.

Pregnancy Risk Factor C

Adverse Reactions

>10%:
- Central nervous system: Headache, somnolence
- Gastrointestinal: Weight gain

1% to 10%:
- Cardiovascular: Postural hypotension, tachycardia, palpitations
- Central nervous system: Dizziness, hypotension
- Dermatologic: Rash
- Gastrointestinal: Abdominal pain, constipation, xerostomia, dyspepsia, anorexia
- Hematologic: Leukopenia
- Neuromuscular & skeletal: Dysarthria, back pain, weakness
- Respiratory: Rhinitis, pharyngitis, cough, dyspnea
- Miscellaneous: Diaphoresis

<1%: Abnormal dreams, anemia, bradycardia, diabetes, elevated alkaline phosphatase, elevated GGT, epistaxis, hyperlipidemia, hypothyroidism, increased appetite, increased salivation, involuntary movements, leukocytosis, Q-T prolongation, rash, tardive dyskinesia, vertigo

Drug Interactions CYP3A4 enzyme substrate; CYP2D6 substrate (minor); CYP2C9 substrate (minor)

Caution with other centrally acting drugs; avoid alcohol

May enhance effects of antihypertensive agents; may antagonize levodopa, dopamine agonists

Increased clearance when given with phenytoin (5-fold) or thioridazine (65%), caution with other liver enzyme inducers (carbamazepine, barbiturates, rifampin, glucocorticoids)

Although data is not yet available, caution is advised with inhibitors of CYP3A4 (eg, ketoconazole, erythromycin)

Cimetidine in combination with quetiapine decreased quetiapine's clearance by 20%

Lorazepam's clearance is reduced 20% in the presence of quetiapine

Alcohol Interactions Avoid use (may cause excessive impairment in cognition/motor function)

Half-Life 6 hours

Education and Monitoring Issues

Patient Education: Use exactly as directed (do not increase dose or frequency); may cause physical and/or psychological dependence. It may take 2-3 weeks to achieve desired results; do not discontinue without consulting prescriber. Avoid excess alcohol or caffeine and other prescription or OTC medications not approved by prescriber. Maintain adequate hydration (2-3 L/day of fluids unless instructed to restrict fluid

(Continued)

Quetiapine *(Continued)*

intake). You may experience excess drowsiness, restlessness, dizziness, or blurred vision (use caution driving or when engaging in tasks requiring alertness until response to drug is known); mouth sores or GI upset (small frequent meals, frequent mouth care, chewing gum, or sucking lozenges may help); constipation (increased exercise, fluids, or dietary fruit and fiber may help); or postural hypotension (use caution climbing stairs or when changing position from lying or sitting to standing). Report persistent CNS effects (eg, somnolence, agitation, insomnia); severe dizziness; vision changes; difficulty breathing; or worsening of condition.

Dietary Considerations: In healthy volunteers, administration of quetiapine with food resulted in an increase in the AUC (by ~15%) compared to the fasting state; can be taken without regard to food

Monitoring Parameters: Patients should have eyes checked every 6 months for cataracts while on this medication

Manufacturer AstraZeneca

Related Information

Pharmaceutical Manufacturers Directory *on page 1020*

- **Quibron®** *see* Theophylline and Guaifenesin *on page 906*
- **Quibron®-T** *see* Theophylline Salts *on page 906*
- **Quibron®-T/SR** *see* Theophylline Salts *on page 906*
- **Quiess®** *see* Hydroxyzine *on page 455*
- **Quinaglute** *see* Quinidine *on page 802*
- **Quinaglute® Dura-Tabs®** *see* Quinidine *on page 802*
- **Quinalan®** *see* Quinidine *on page 802*

Quinapril (KWIN a pril)

Pharmacologic Class Angiotensin-Converting Enzyme (ACE) Inhibitors

U.S. Brand Names Accupril®

Generic Available No

Mechanism of Action Competitive inhibitor of angiotensin-converting enzyme (ACE); prevents conversion of angiotensin I to angiotensin II, a potent vasoconstrictor; results in lower levels of angiotensin II which causes an increase in plasma renin activity and a reduction in aldosterone secretion; a CNS mechanism may also be involved in hypotensive effect as angiotensin II increases adrenergic outflow from CNS; vasoactive kallikreins may be decreased in conversion to active hormones by ACE inhibitors, thus reducing blood pressure

Use Management of hypertension and treatment of congestive heart failure; increase circulation in Raynaud's phenomenon; idiopathic edema; believed to improve survival in heart failure

Unlabeled use: Hypertensive crisis, diabetic nephropathy, rheumatoid arthritis, diagnosis of anatomic renal artery stenosis, hypertension secondary to scleroderma renal crisis, diagnosis of aldosteronism, Bartter's syndrome, postmyocardial infarction for prevention of ventricular failure

USUAL DOSAGE

Adults: Oral: Initial: 10 mg once daily, adjust according to blood pressure response at peak and trough blood levels; in general, the normal dosage range is 20-80 mg/day for hypertension and 20-40 mg/day for edema in single or divided doses

Elderly: Initial: 2.5-5 mg/day; increase dosage at increments of 2.5-5 mg at 1- to 2-week intervals

Dosing adjustment in renal impairment:

Cl_{cr} >60 mL/minute: Administer 10 mg/day

Cl_{cr} 30-60 mL/minute: 5 mg/day

Cl_{cr} 10-30 mL/minute: 2.5 mg/day

Dosing comments in hepatic impairment: In patients with alcoholic cirrhosis, hydrolysis of quinapril to quinaprilat is impaired; however, the subsequent elimination of quinaprilat is unaltered

Dosage Forms TAB: 5 mg, 10 mg, 20 mg, 40 mg

Contraindications Hypersensitivity to quinapril or history of angioedema induced by other ACE inhibitors

Warnings/Precautions Use with caution in patients with renal insufficiency, autoimmune disease, renal artery stenosis; excessive hypotension may be more likely in volume-depleted patients, the elderly, and following the first dose (first dose phenomenon); quinapril should be discontinued if laryngeal stridor or angioedema of the face, tongue, or glottis is observed

Pregnancy Risk Factor C (1st trimester); D (2nd and 3rd trimesters)

Adverse Reactions Note: Frequency ranges include data from hypertension and heart failure trials. Higher rates of adverse reactions have generally been noted in patients with congestive heart failure. However, the frequency of adverse effects associated with placebo is also increased in this population.

1% to 10%:

Cardiovascular: Hypotension (2.9%), chest pain (2.4%), first-dose hypotension (up to 2.5%)

Central nervous system: Dizziness (3.9 to 7.7%), headache (1.7% to 5.6%), fatigue (2.6%)

Dermatologic: Rash (1.2%)

Endocrine and metabolic: Hyperkalemia (2%)

Gastrointestinal: Vomiting/nausea (1.4% to 2.4%), diarrhea (1.7%)

Neuromuscular and Skeletal: Myalgias (1.5% to 5%), back pain (1.2%)

Renal: Increased BUN/serum creatinine (2% - transient elevations may occur with a higher frequency), worsening of renal function (in patients with bilateral renal artery stenosis or hypovolemia)

Respiratory: Upper respiratory symptoms, cough (2% to 4.3%; up to 13% in some studies), dyspnea (1.9%)

<1% (limited to important or life-threatening symptoms): Angioedema, back pain, malaise, viral infection, palpitation, vasodilation, tachycardia, heart failure, hyperkalemia, myocardial infarction, cerebrovascular accident, hypertensive crisis, angina, orthostatic hypotension, arrhythmia, shock, hemolytic anemia, xerostomia, constipation, gastrointestinal hemorrhage, pancreatitis, abnormal liver function tests, somnolence, vertigo, syncope, nervousness, depression, insomnia, paresthesia, alopecia, increased sweating, pemphigus, pruritus, exfoliative dermatitis, photosensitivity, dermatopolymyositis, impotence, acute renal failure, eosinophilic pneumonitis, amblyopia, pharyngitis, agranulocytosis, hepatitis, thrombocytopenia.

A syndrome which may include fever, myalgia, arthralgia, interstitial nephritis, vasculitis, rash, eosinophilia and positive ANA, and elevated ESR has been reported with ACE inhibitors. In addition, pancreatitis and agranulocytosis (particularly in patients with collagen-vascular disease or renal impairment) have been associated with many ACE inhibitors.

Drug Interactions

Alpha$_1$ blockers: Hypotensive effect increased.

Aspirin and NSAIDs may decrease ACE inhibitor efficacy and/or increase risk of adverse renal effects.

Diuretics: Hypovolemia due to diuretics may precipitate acute hypotensive events or acute renal failure.

Insulin: Risk of hypoglycemia may be increased.

Lithium: Risk of lithium toxicity may be increased; monitor lithium levels, especially the first 4 weeks of therapy.

Mercaptopurine: Risk of neutropenia may be increased.

Potassium-sparing diuretics (amiloride, spironolactone, triamterene): Increased risk of hyperkalemia.

Potassium supplements may increase the risk of hyperkalemia.

Quinolones: Absorption may be decreased by quinapril; separate administration by at least 2-4 hours.

Tetracyclines: Absorption may be reduced by quinapril; separate administration by at least 2-4 hours.

Trimethoprim (high dose) may increase the risk of hyperkalemia.

Alcohol Interactions Avoid use (may increase risk of hypotension or dizziness)

Onset 1 hour

Duration 24 hours

Half-Life Quinapril: 0.8 hours; Quinaprilat: 2 hours

Education and Monitoring Issues

Patient Education: Take exactly as directed; do not discontinue without consulting prescriber. Take first dose at bedtime. Take all doses on an empty stomach (30 minutes before or 2 hours after meals). This drug does not eliminate need for diet or exercise regimen as recommended by prescriber. May cause dizziness, fainting, lightheadedness (use caution when driving or engaging in tasks requiring alertness until response to drug is known); postural hypotension (use caution when rising from lying or sitting position or climbing stairs); nausea, vomiting, altered taste, abdominal pain, dry mouth, or transient loss of appetite (small frequent meals, frequent mouth care, sucking lozenges, or chewing gum may help) - report if these persist. Report chest pain or palpitations; mouth sores; fever or chills; swelling of extremities; skin rash; numbness, tingling, or pain in muscles; difficulty in breathing or unusual cough; or other persistent adverse reactions.

Manufacturer Parke-Davis

Related Information

Angiotensin-Related Agents Comparison *on page 1226*

Heart Failure Guidelines *on page 1099*

Pharmaceutical Manufacturers Directory *on page 1020*

Quinapril and Hydrochlorothiazide

(KWIN a pril & hye droe klor oh THYE a zide)

Pharmacologic Class Angiotensin-Converting Enzyme (ACE) Inhibitors; Diuretic, Thiazide

U.S. Brand Names Accuretic®

(Continued)

Quinapril and Hydrochlorothiazide *(Continued)*

Dosage Forms TAB: Quinapril hydrochloride 10 mg and hydrochlorothiazide 12.5 mg; Quinapril hydrochloride 20 mg and hydrochlorothiazide 12.5 mg; Quinapril hydrochloride 20 mg and hydrochlorothiazide 25 mg

Alcohol Interactions Avoid use (may increase risk of hypotension or dizziness)

Manufacturer Parke-Davis

Related Information

Pharmaceutical Manufacturers Directory *on page 1020*

- **Quinate** *see* Quinidine *on page 802*
- **Quinidex®** *see* Quinidine *on page 802*
- **Quinidex® Extentabs®** *see* Quinidine *on page 802*

Quinidine (KWIN i deen)

Pharmacologic Class Antiarrhythmic Agent, Class I-A

U.S. Brand Names Cardioquin®; Quinaglute® Dura-Tabs®; Quinalan®; Quinidex® Extentabs®; Quinora®

Generic Available Yes

Mechanism of Action Class 1A antiarrhythmic agent; depresses phase O of the action potential; decreases myocardial excitability and conduction velocity, and myocardial contractility by decreasing sodium influx during depolarization and potassium efflux in repolarization; also reduces calcium transport across cell membrane

Use Prophylaxis after cardioversion of atrial fibrillation and/or flutter to maintain normal sinus rhythm; also used to prevent reoccurrence of paroxysmal supraventricular tachycardia, paroxysmal A-V junctional rhythm, paroxysmal ventricular tachycardia, paroxysmal atrial fibrillation, and atrial or ventricular premature contractions; also has activity against *Plasmodium falciparum* malaria

USUAL DOSAGE Dosage expressed in terms of the salt: 267 mg of quinidine gluconate = 200 mg of quinidine sulfate

Children: Test dose for idiosyncratic reaction (sulfate, oral or gluconate, I.M.): 2 mg/kg or 60 mg/m^2

Oral (quinidine sulfate): 15-60 mg/kg/day in 4-5 divided doses or 6 mg/kg every 4-6 hours; usual 30 mg/kg/day or 900 mg/m^2/day given in 5 daily doses

I.V. **not** recommended (quinidine gluconate): 2-10 mg/kg/dose given at a rate ≤10 mg/minute every 3-6 hours as needed

Adults: Test dose: Oral, I.M.: 200 mg administered several hours before full dosage (to determine possibility of idiosyncratic reaction)

Oral (for malaria):

Sulfate: 100-600 mg/dose every 4-6 hours; begin at 200 mg/dose and titrate to desired effect (maximum daily dose: 3-4 g)

Gluconate: 324-972 mg every 8-12 hours

I.M.: 400 mg/dose every 2-6 hours; initial dose: 600 mg (gluconate)

I.V.: 200-400 mg/dose diluted and given at a rate ≤10 mg/minute; may require as much as 500-750 mg

Dosing adjustment in renal impairment: Cl_{cr} <10 mL/minute: Administer 75% of normal dose

Hemodialysis: Slightly hemodialyzable (5% to 20%); 200 mg supplemental dose posthemodialysis is recommended

Peritoneal dialysis: Not dialyzable (0% to 5%)

Dosing adjustment/comments in hepatic impairment: Larger loading dose may be indicated, reduce maintenance doses by 50% and monitor serum levels closely

Dosage Forms

Quinidine gluconate: **INJ:** 80 mg/mL (10 mL). **TAB, sustained release:** 324 mg

Quinidine polygalacturonate: **TAB:** 275 mg

Quinidine sulfate: **TAB:** 200 mg, 300 mg; Sustained action: 300 mg

Contraindications Patients with complete A-V block with an A-V junctional or idioventricular pacemaker; patients with intraventricular conduction defects (marked widening of QRS complex); patients with cardiac-glycoside induced A-V conduction disorders; hypersensitivity to the drug or cinchona derivatives; concurrent use of sparfloxacin or ritonavir

Warnings/Precautions Use with caution in patients with myocardial depression, sick-sinus syndrome, incomplete A-V block, hepatic and/or renal insufficiency, myasthenia gravis; hemolysis may occur in patients with G-6-PD (glucose-6-phosphate dehydrogenase) deficiency; quinidine-induced hepatotoxicity, including granulomatous hepatitis can occur, increased serum AST and alkaline phosphatase concentrations, and jaundice may occur; use with caution in nursing women and elderly

Pregnancy Risk Factor C

Adverse Reactions

Incidence not determined: Hypotension, syncope

>10%:

Cardiovascular: QT_c prolongation (modest prolongation is common, however excessive prolongation is rare and indicates toxicity)

Central nervous system: Lightheadedness (15%)

Gastrointestinal: Diarrhea (35%), upper GI distress, bitter taste, diarrhea, anorexia, nausea, vomiting, stomach cramping (22%)

1% to 10%:

Cardiovascular: Angina (6%), palpitation (7%), new or worsened arrhythmias (proarrhythmic effect)

Central nervous system: Syncope(1% to 8%), headache (7%), fatigue (7%), weakness (5%), sleep disturbance (3%), tremor (2%), nervousness (2%), incoordination (1%)

Dermatologic: Rash (5%)

Ocular: Blurred vision

Otic: Tinnitus

Respiratory: Wheezing

<1% (limited to important or life-threatening symptoms): Tachycardia, QT_c prolongation (excessive), torsade de pointes, heart block, ventricular fibrillation, ventricular tachycardia, paradoxical increase in ventricular rate during atrial fibrillation/flutter, exacerbated bradycardia (in sick sinus syndrome), vascular collapse, confusion, delirium, vertigo, impaired hearing, respiratory depression, pneumonitis, bronchospasm, fever, urticaria, flushing, exfoliative rash, psoriaform rash, pruritus, lymphadenopathy, hemolytic anemia, vasculitis, thrombocytopenic purpura, thrombocytopenia, pancytopenia, uveitis, angioedema, agranulocytosis, sicca syndrome, arthralgia, myalgia, increased CPK, drug-induced lupus-like syndrome, cerebral hypoperfusion (possibly resulting in ataxia, apprehension and seizures), acute psychotic reactions, depression, hallucinations, mydriasis, disturbed color perception, night blindness, scotoma, optic neuritis, visual field loss, photosensitivity, abnormal pigmentation, granulomatous hepatitis, hepatotoxic reaction (rare), eczematous dermatitis, livedo reticularis

Case reports: Melanin pigmentation of the hard palate, esophagitis, nephropathy, cholestasis, pneumonitis, lichen planus

Note: Cinchonism, a syndrome which may include tinnitus, high-frequency hearing loss, deafness, vertigo, blurred vision, diplopia, photophobia, headache, confusion, and delirium has been associated with quinidine use. Usually associated with chronic toxicity, this syndrome has also been described after brief exposure to a moderate dose in sensitive patients. Vomiting and diarrhea may also occur as isolated reactions to therapeutic quinidine levels.

Drug Interactions CYP3A3/4 substrate/inhibitor, CYP2D6 inhibitor

Inhibitors of CYP3A3/4 (clarithromycin, erythromycin, itraconazole, ketoconazole, troleandomycin) may increase quinidine blood levels

Amiloride may cause prolonged ventricular conduction leading to arrhythmias

Amiodarone may increase quinidine blood levels; monitor quinidine levels

Amprenavir may increase the toxicity effects for quinidine

Cimetidine: Increase quinidine blood levels; closely monitor levels or use an alternative H_2 antagonist

Cisapride and quinidine may increase risk of malignant arrhythmias; concurrent use is contraindicated

Codeine: Analgesic efficacy may be reduced

Digoxin blood levels may be increased. Monitor digoxin blood levels

Enzyme inducers (aminoglutethimide, carbamazepine, phenobarbital, phenytoin, primidone, rifabutin, rifampin) may decrease quinidine blood levels

Metoprolol: Increased metoprolol blood levels

Mexiletine blood levels may be increased

Nifedipine blood levels may be increased by quinidine; nifedipine may decrease quinidine blood levels

Drugs which prolong the Q-T interval include amiodarone, amitriptyline, bepridil, disopyramide, erythromycin, haloperidol, imipramine, pimozide, procainamide, sotalol, and thioridazine. Effects may be additive; use with caution.

Propafenone blood levels may be increased

Propranolol blood levels may be increased

Ritonavir and nelfinavir may increase quinidine levels and toxicity; concurrent use is contraindicated

Sparfloxacin, gatifloxacin, and moxifloxacin may result in additional prolongation of the Q-T interval; concurrent use is contraindicated

Timolol blood levels may be increased

Urinary alkalinizers (antacids, sodium bicarbonate, acetazolamide) increase quinidine blood levels

Verapamil and diltiazem increase quinidine blood levels

Warfarin effects may be increased by quinidine; monitor INR closely during addition or withdrawal of quinidine

Half-Life 6-8 hours; increased half-life with elderly, cirrhosis, and congestive heart failure

Education and Monitoring Issues

Patient Education: Take exactly as directed, around-the-clock; do not take additional doses or discontinue without consulting prescriber. Do not crush, chew, or break sustained release capsules. You will need regular cardiac checkups and blood tests while taking this medication. You may experience dizziness, drowsiness, or visual changes (use caution when driving or engaging in tasks requiring alertness until response to drug is known); abnormal taste, nausea or vomiting, or loss of appetite (small frequent meals, frequent mouth care, chewing gum, or sucking lozenges may

(Continued)

Quinidine *(Continued)*

help); headaches (prescriber may recommend mild analgesic); or diarrhea (exercise, yogurt, or boiled milk may help - if persistent consult prescriber). Report chest pain, palpitation, or erratic heartbeat; difficulty breathing or wheezing; CNS changes (confusion, delirium, fever, consistent dizziness); skin rash; sense of fullness or ringing in ears; or changes in vision.

Monitoring Parameters: Cardiac monitor required during I.V. administration; CBC, liver and renal function tests, should be routinely performed during long-term administration

Reference Range: Therapeutic: 2-5 μg/mL (SI: 6.2-15.4 μmol/L). Patient dependent therapeutic response occurs at levels of 3-6 μg/mL (SI: 9.2-18.5 μmol/L). Optimal therapeutic level is method dependent; >6 μg/mL (SI: >18 μmol/L).

Quinine (KWYE nine)

Pharmacologic Class Antimalarial Agent

U.S. Brand Names Formula Q®

Generic Available Yes

Mechanism of Action Depresses oxygen uptake and carbohydrate metabolism; intercalates into DNA, disrupting the parasite's replication and transcription; affects calcium distribution within muscle fibers and decreases the excitability of the motor end-plate region; cardiovascular effects similar to quinidine

Use In conjunction with other antimalarial agents, suppression or treatment of chloroquine-resistant *P. falciparum* malaria; treatment of *Babesia microti* infection in conjunction with clindamycin; prevention and treatment of nocturnal recumbency leg muscle cramps

USUAL DOSAGE Oral:

Children:

- Treatment of chloroquine-resistant malaria: 25-30 mg/kg/day in divided doses every 8 hours for 5-7 days in conjunction with another agent
- Babesiosis: 25 mg/kg/day divided every 8 hours for 7 days

Adults:

- Treatment of chloroquine-resistant malaria: 260-650 mg every 8 hours for 6-12 days in conjunction with another agent
- Suppression of malaria: 325 mg twice daily and continued for 6 weeks after exposure
- Babesiosis: 650 mg every 6-8 hours for 7 days
- Leg cramps: 200-300 mg at bedtime

Dosing interval/adjustment in renal impairment:

- Cl_{cr} 10-50 mL/minute: Administer every 8-12 hours or 75% of normal dose
- Cl_{cr} <10 mL/minute: Administer every 24 hours or 30% to 50% of normal dose

Dialysis: Not removed

Peritoneal dialysis: Dose as for Cl_{cr} <10 mL/min

Continuous arteriovenous or venovenous hemodiafiltration (CAVH) effects: Dose for Cl_{cr} 10-50 mL/minute

Dosage Forms CAP: 200 mg, 260 mg, 325 mg. **TAB:** 260 mg

Contraindications Tinnitus, optic neuritis, G-6-PD deficiency, hypersensitivity to quinine or any component, history of black water fever, and thrombocytopenia with quinine or quinidine

Warnings/Precautions Use with caution in patients with cardiac arrhythmias (quinine has quinidine-like activity) and in patients with myasthenia gravis

Pregnancy Risk Factor X

Adverse Reactions

Percentage unknown: Cinchonism (risk of cinchonism is directly related to dose and duration of therapy): Severe headache, nausea, vomiting, diarrhea, blurred vision, tinnitus

<1%: Anginal symptoms, diplopia, epigastric pain, fever, flushing of the skin, hemolysis in G-6-PD deficiency, hepatitis, hypersensitivity reactions, hypoglycemia, impaired hearing, nightblindness, optic atrophy, pruritus, rash, thrombocytopenia

Drug Interactions CYP3A3/4 enzyme substrate; CYP3A3/4 enzyme inhibitor

Decreased effect: Phenobarbital, phenytoin, aluminum salt antacids, and rifampin may decrease quinine serum concentrations

Increased toxicity:

- To avoid risk of seizures and cardiac arrest, delay mefloquine dosing at least 12 hours after last dose of quinine
- Beta-blockers + quinine may increase bradycardia
- Quinine may enhance coumarin anticoagulants and potentiate nondepolarizing and depolarizing muscle relaxants
- Quinine may inhibit metabolism of astemizole resulting in toxic levels and potentially life-threatening cardiotoxicity
- Quinine may increase plasma concentration of digoxin by as much as twofold; closely monitor digoxin concentrations and decrease digoxin dose with initiation of quinine by ½
- Verapamil, amiodarone, urinary alkalinizing agents, and cimetidine may increase quinine serum concentrations

Half-Life 8-14 hours

Education and Monitoring Issues

Patient Education: Take on schedule as directed, with full 8 oz of water. Do not chew or crush sustained release tablets. You will need to return for follow-up blood tests. You may experience GI distress (taking medication with food, and frequent small meals may help). You may experience dizziness, changes in mentation, insomnia, headache, or visual disturbances (use caution when driving or engaging in tasks requiring alertness until response to drug is known). May discolor urine (black/brown/dark). Report persistent sore throat, fever, chills, flu-like signs, ringing in ears, vision disturbances, or unusual bruising or bleeding. Seek emergency help for palpitations or chest pain.

Reference Range: Toxic: >10 µg/mL

- **Quinobarb** *see* Quinidine *on page 802*
- **Quinora®** *see* Quinidine *on page 802*
- **Quinsana Plus® [OTC]** *see* Tolnaftate *on page 931*
- **Quintasa** *see* Mesalamine *on page 568*
- **QYS®** *see* Hydroxyzine *on page 455*

Rabeprazole (ra BE pray zole)

Pharmacologic Class Gastric Acid Secretion Inhibitor

U.S. Brand Names Aciphex™

Mechanism of Action Potent proton pump inhibitor; suppresses gastric acid secretion by inhibiting the parietal cell H+/K+ ATP pump

Use Short-term (4-8 weeks) treatment and maintenance of erosive or ulcerative gastroesophageal reflux disease (GERD); short-term (up to 4 weeks) treatment of duodenal ulcers; long-term treatment of pathological hypersecretory conditions, including Zollinger-Ellison syndrome. Also, possibly used for *H. pylori* eradication, symptomatic GERD, maintenance of healing of GERD, and maintenance of duodenal ulcer

USUAL DOSAGE Adults >18 years and Elderly:

GERD: 20 mg once daily for 4-8 weeks; maintenance: 20 mg once daily

Duodenal ulcer: 20 mg/day after breakfast for 4 weeks

Hypersecretory conditions: 60 mg once daily; dose may need to be adjusted as necessary. Doses as high as 100 mg and 60 mg twice daily have been used.

Dosage Forms TAB, delayed release (enteric coated): 20 mg

Contraindications Contraindicated in patients with known hypersensitivity to rabeprazole, substituted benzimidazoles, or to any component of the formulation

Warnings/Precautions Severe hepatic impairment; relief of symptoms with rabeprazole does not preclude the presence of a gastric malignancy

Pregnancy Risk Factor B

Pregnancy Implications Not recommended

Adverse Reactions

1% to 10%: Central nervous system: Headache

<1%:

Body as a whole: Weakness, fever, allergic reaction, chills, malaise, chest pain substernal, neck rigidity, photosensitivity reaction

Rare: Abdomen enlarged, face edema, hangover effect

Cardiovascular system: Hypertension, myocardial infarction, electrocardiogram abnormal, migraine, syncope, angina pectoris, bundle branch block, palpitation, sinus bradycardia, tachycardia

Rare: Bradycardia, pulmonary embolus, supraventricular tachycardia

Central nervous system: Insomnia, anxiety, dizziness, depression, nervousness, somnolence, hypertonia, neuralgia, vertigo, convulsions, abnormal dreams, libido decreased, neuropathy, paresthesia, tremor

Rare: Agitation, amnesia, confusion, extrapyramidal syndrome, hyperkinesia

Digestive system: Diarrhea, nausea, abdominal pain, vomiting, dyspepsia, flatulence, constipation, dry mouth, eructation, gastroenteritis, rectal hemorrhage, melena, anorexia, cholelithiasis, mouth ulceration, stomatitis, dysphagia, gingivitis, cholecystitis, increased appetite, abnormal stools, colitis, esophagitis, glossitis, pancreatitis, proctitis

Rare: Bloody diarrhea, cholangitis, duodenitis, gastrointestinal hemorrhage, hepatic encephalopathy, hepatitis, hepatoma, liver fatty deposit, salivary gland enlargement, thirst

Endocrine system: Hyperthyroidism, hypothyroidism

Hemic & lymphatic system: Anemia, ecchymosis, lymphadenopathy, hypochromic anemia

Metabolic & nutritional disorders: Peripheral edema, edema, weight gain, gout, dehydration, weight loss

Neuromuscular & skeletal: Myalgia, arthritis, leg cramps, bone pain, arthrosis, bursitis

Rare: Twitching

Respiratory system: Dyspnea, asthma, epistaxis, laryngitis, hiccups, hyperventilation

Rare: Apnea, hypoventilation

Skin & appendages: Rash, pruritus, sweating, urticaria, alopecia

Rare: Dry skin, herpes zoster, psoriasis, skin discoloration

(Continued)

Rabeprazole *(Continued)*

Special senses: Cataract, amblyopia, glaucoma, dry eyes, abnormal vision, tinnitus, otitis media

Rare: Corneal opacity, blurry vision, diplopia, deafness, eye pain, retinal degeneration, strabismus

Urogenital system: Cystitis, urinary frequency, dysmenorrhea, dysuria, kidney calculus, metrorrhagia, polyuria

Rare: Breast enlargement, hematuria, impotence, leukorrhea, menorrhagia, orchitis, urinary incontinence

Drug Interactions Cytochrome P-450 inhibitor (extremely high concentrations); may alter the absorption of pH-dependent drugs (eg, ketoconazole, itraconazole, digoxin)

Alcohol Interactions Avoid use (may enhance gastric mucosal irritation)

Onset 1 hour

Duration >24 hours

Half-Life 2 hours

Education and Monitoring Issues

Patient Education: Take as directed. Swallow whole, do not crush or chew. Follow recommended diet and activity instructions. You may experience headache (use of mild analgesic may help) or other side effects. Report these to prescriber if they persist.

Manufacturer Janssen Pharmaceutical, Inc

Related Information

Pharmaceutical Manufacturers Directory *on page 1020*

Rabies Immune Globulin (Human)

(RAY beez i MYUN GLOB yoo lin HYU man)

Pharmacologic Class Immune Globulin

U.S. Brand Names Hyperab®; Imogam®

Generic Available No

Mechanism of Action Rabies immune globulin is a solution of globulins dried from the plasma or serum of selected adult human donors who have been immunized with rabies vaccine and have developed high titers of rabies antibody. It generally contains 10% to 18% of protein of which not less than 80% is monomeric immunoglobulin G.

Use Part of postexposure prophylaxis of persons with rabies exposure who lack a history or pre-exposure or postexposure prophylaxis with rabies vaccine or a recently documented neutralizing antibody response to previous rabies vaccination; although it is preferable to administer RIG with the first dose of vaccine, it can be given up to 8 days after vaccination

USUAL DOSAGE Children and Adults: I.M.: 20 units/kg in a single dose (RIG should always be administered as part of rabies vaccine (HDCV)) regimen (as soon as possible after the first dose of vaccine, up to 8 days); infiltrate ½ of the dose locally around the wound; administer the remainder I.M.

Note: Persons known to have an adequate titer or who have been completely immunized with rabies vaccine should not receive RIG, only booster doses of HDCV

Dosage Forms INJ: 150 units/mL (2 mL, 10 mL)

Contraindications Inadvertent I.V. administration; allergy to thimerosal or any component

Warnings/Precautions Use with caution in individuals with thrombocytopenia, bleeding disorders, or prior allergic reactions to immune globulins

Pregnancy Risk Factor C

Adverse Reactions

1% to 10%:

Central nervous system: Fever (mild)

Local: Soreness at injection site

<1%: Anaphylactic shock, angioedema, soreness of muscles, stiffness, urticaria

Drug Interactions Decreased effect: Live virus vaccines (eg, MMR, rabies) may have delayed or diminished antibody response with immune globulin administration; should not be administered within 3 months unless antibody titers dictate as appropriate

Related Information

Animal and Human Bites Guidelines *on page 1177*

♦ **Radiostol®** *see* Ergocalciferol *on page 321*

Raloxifene (ral OX i feen)

Pharmacologic Class Selective Estrogen Receptor Modulator (SERM)

U.S. Brand Names Evista®

Mechanism of Action A selective estrogen receptor modulator, meaning that it affects some of the same receptors that estrogen does, but not all, and in some instances, it antagonizes or blocks estrogen; it acts like estrogen to prevent bone loss and improve lipid profiles, but it has the potential to block some estrogen effects such as those that lead to breast cancer and uterine cancer

Use Prevention and treatment of osteoporosis in postmenopausal women

USUAL DOSAGE Adults: Female: Oral: 60 mg/day which may be administered any time of the day without regard to meals

Dosage Forms TAB: 60 mg

Contraindications Pregnancy; prior hypersensitivity to raloxifene; active thromboembolic disorder; not intended for use in premenopausal women

Warnings/Precautions History of venous thromboembolism/pulmonary embolism; patients with cardiovascular disease; history of cervical/uterine carcinoma; renal/hepatic insufficiency (however, pharmacokinetic data are lacking); concurrent use of estrogens

Pregnancy Risk Factor X

Pregnancy Implications Raloxifene should not be used by pregnant women or by women planning to become pregnant in the immediate future

Adverse Reactions ≥2%:

Cardiovascular: Chest pain
Central nervous system: Migraine, depression, insomnia, fever
Dermatologic: Rash
Endocrine & metabolic: Hot flashes
Gastrointestinal: Nausea, dyspepsia, vomiting, flatulence, gastroenteritis, weight gain
Genitourinary: Vaginitis, urinary tract infection, cystitis, leukorrhea
Neuromuscular & skeletal: Leg cramps, arthralgia, myalgia, arthritis
Respiratory: Sinusitis, pharyngitis, cough, pneumonia, laryngitis
Miscellaneous: Infection, flu syndrome, diaphoresis

Drug Interactions Decreased effects: Ampicillin and cholestyramine decreases raloxifene absorption

Onset 8 weeks

Half-Life 28-32.5 hours

Education and Monitoring Issues

Patient Education: May be taken at any time of day without regard to meals. This medication is given to reduce incidence of osteoporosis; it will not reduce hot flashes or flushing. You may experience flu-like symptoms at beginning of therapy (these may resolve with use). Mild analgesics may reduce joint pain. Rest and cool environment may reduce hot flashes. Report fever; acute migraine; insomnia or emotional depression; unusual weight gain; unresolved gastric distress; urinary infection or vaginal burning or itching; chest pain; or swelling, warmth, or pain in calves.

Monitoring Parameters: Radiologic evaluation of bone mineral density (BMD) is the best measure of the treatment of osteoporosis; to monitor for the potential toxicities of raloxifene, complete blood counts should be evaluated periodically.

Manufacturer Eli Lilly and Co

Related Information

Pharmaceutical Manufacturers Directory *on page 1020*

Ramipril (ra MI pril)

Pharmacologic Class Angiotensin-Converting Enzyme (ACE) Inhibitors

U.S. Brand Names Altace™

Generic Available No

Mechanism of Action Ramipril is an angiotensin-converting enzyme (ACE) inhibitor which prevents the formation of angiotensin II from angiotensin I and exhibits pharmacologic effects that are similar to captopril. Ramipril must undergo enzymatic saponification by esterases in the liver to its biologically active metabolite, ramiprilat. The pharmacodynamic effects of ramipril result from the high-affinity, competitive, reversible binding of ramiprilat to angiotensin-converting enzyme thus preventing the formation of the potent vasoconstrictor angiotensin II. This isomerized enzyme-inhibitor complex has a slow rate of dissociation, which results in high potency and a long duration of action; a CNS mechanism may also be involved in the hypotensive effect as angiotensin II increases adrenergic outflow from CNS; vasoactive kallikreins may be decreased in conversion to active hormones by ACE inhibitors, thus reducing blood pressure

Use Treatment of hypertension, alone or in combination with thiazide diuretics; treatment of congestive heart failure within the first few days after myocardial infarction (**Note:** This indication is based on a study involving 2006 patients; a decrease by 26% in all-cause mortality was observed when ramipril was administered 3-10 days after a myocardial infarction)

USUAL DOSAGE Adults: Oral:

Hypertension: 2.5-5 mg once daily, maximum: 20 mg/day

Heart failure postmyocardial infarction: Initial: 2.5 mg twice daily titrated upward, if possible, to 5 mg twice daily

Note: The dose of any concomitant diuretic should be reduced; if the diuretic cannot be discontinued, initiate therapy with 1.25 mg; after the initial dose, the patient should be monitored carefully until blood pressure has stabilized

Dosing adjustment in renal impairment:

Cl_{cr} <40 mL/minute: Administer 25% of normal dose
Renal failure and hypertension: 1.25 mg once daily, titrated upward as possible
Renal failure and heart failure: 1.25 mg once daily, increasing to 1.25 mg twice daily up to 2.5 mg twice daily as tolerated

Dosage Forms CAP: 1.25 mg, 2.5 mg, 5 mg, 10 mg

Contraindications Hypersensitivity to ramipril or ramiprilat, or history of angioedema with any other angiotensin-converting enzyme inhibitors

(Continued)

Ramipril *(Continued)*

Warnings/Precautions Use with caution and modify dosage in patients with renal impairment (especially renal artery stenosis), severe congestive heart failure; severe hypotension may occur in the elderly and patients who are sodium and/or volume depleted, initiate lower doses and monitor closely when starting therapy in these patients; should be discontinued if laryngeal stridor or angioedema of the face, tongue, or glottis is observed

Pregnancy Risk Factor C (1st trimester); D (2nd and 3rd trimesters)

Adverse Reactions Note: Frequency ranges include data from hypertension and heart failure trials. Higher rates of adverse reactions have generally been noted in patients with congestive heart failure. However, the frequency of adverse effects associated with placebo is also increased in this population.

>10%: Respiratory: Cough (increased) (7.6% to 12%)

1% to 10%: Central nervous system: Headache (1.2% to 5.4%), dizziness (2.2% to 4.1%), fatigue (2%), vertigo (1.5%)

Cardiovascular: Hypotension (10.7%), angina (2.9%), postural hypotension (2.2%), syncope (2.1%)

Endocrine and metabolic: Hyperkalemia (1% to 10%)

Gastrointestinal: Nausea/vomiting (1.1% to 2.2%)

Neuromuscular & skeletal: Chest pain (noncardiac) (1.1%)

Renal: Renal dysfunction (1.2%), elevation in serum creatinine (1.2% to 1.5%), increased BUN (0.5% to 3%); transient elevations of creatinine and/or BUN may occur more frequently

Respiratory: Cough (estimated 1% to 10%)

<1% (limited to important or life-threatening symptoms): Anaphylactoid reaction, symptomatic hypotension, syncope, angina, arrhythmia, palpitation, myocardial infarction, cerebrovascular events, pancytopenia, hemolytic anemia, thrombocytopenia, angioedema, pancreatitis, abdominal pain, anorexia, constipation, diarrhea, xerostomia, dyspepsia, dysphagia, gastroenteritis, hepatitis, increased salivation, taste disturbance, hypersensitivity reactions (urticaria, rash, fever), erythema multiforme, pemphigus, photosensitivity, purpura, anxiety, amnesia, convulsions, depression, hearing loss, insomnia, nervousness, neuralgia, neuropathy, paresthesia, somnolence, tinnitus, tremor, vertigo, vision disturbances, arthralgia, arthritis, dyspnea, edema, epistaxis, impotence, increased sweating, malaise, myalgia, weight gain, decreased hemoglobin, decreased hematocrit, elevated transaminase levels, hyponatremia, eosinophilia, proteinuria.

Case reports: Agitation

Worsening of renal function may occur in patients with bilateral renal artery stenosis or in hypovolemia. In addition, a syndrome which may include fever, myalgia, arthralgia, interstitial nephritis, vasculitis, rash, eosinophilia and positive ANA, and elevated ESR has been reported with ACE inhibitors. Pancreatitis and agranulocytosis (particularly in patients with collagen vascular disease or renal impairment) have been associated with ACE inhibitors.

Drug Interactions

Alpha$_1$ blockers: Hypotensive effect increased

Aspirin and NSAIDs may decrease ACE inhibitor efficacy and/or increase risk of adverse renal effects

Diuretics: Hypovolemia due to diuretics may precipitate acute hypotensive events or acute renal failure

Insulin: Risk of hypoglycemia may be increased

Lithium: Risk of lithium toxicity may be increased; monitor lithium levels, especially the first 4 weeks of therapy

Mercaptopurine: Risk of neutropenia may be increased

Potassium-sparing diuretics (amiloride, spironolactone, triamterene): Increased risk of hyperkalemia

Potassium supplements may increase the risk of hyperkalemia

Trimethoprim (high dose) may increase the risk of hyperkalemia

Alcohol Interactions Avoid use (may increase risk of hypotension or dizziness)

Onset 1-2 hours

Duration 24 hours

Half-Life Ramiprilat: >50 hours

Education and Monitoring Issues

Patient Education: Take exactly as directed; do not discontinue without consulting prescriber. Take first dose at bedtime. This drug does not eliminate need for diet or exercise regimen as recommended by prescriber. Do not take potassium supplements or salt substitutes containing potassium without consulting prescriber. May cause dizziness, fainting, lightheadedness (use caution when driving or engaging in tasks requiring alertness until response to drug is known); postural hypotension (use caution when rising from lying or sitting position or climbing stairs); nausea or vomiting (small frequent meals, frequent mouth care, sucking lozenges, or chewing gum may help) - report if these persist. Report chest pain or palpitations; difficulty in breathing or unusual cough; or other persistent adverse reactions.

Manufacturer Monarch Pharmaceuticals

Related Information

Angiotensin-Related Agents Comparison *on page 1226*
Heart Failure Guidelines *on page 1099*
Pharmaceutical Manufacturers Directory *on page 1020*

Ranitidine Bismuth Citrate (ra NI ti deen BIZ muth SIT rate)

Pharmacologic Class Histamine H_2 Antagonist

U.S. Brand Names Tritec®

Mechanism of Action As a complex of ranitidine and bismuth citrate, gastric acid secretion is inhibited by histamine-blocking activity at the parietal cell and the structural integrity of *H. pylori* organisms is disrupted; additionally bismuth reduces the adherence of *H. pylori* to epithelial cells of the stomach and may exert a cytoprotectant effect, inhibiting pepsin, as well. Adequate eradication of *Helicobacter pylori* is achieved with the combination of clarithromycin.

Use In combination with clarithromycin for the treatment of active duodenal ulcer associated with *H. pylori* infection; not to be used as monotherapy

USUAL DOSAGE Adults: Oral: 400 mg twice daily for 4 weeks with clarithromycin 500 mg 2 times/day for first 2 week

Dosing adjustment in renal impairment: Not recommended with Cl_{cr} <25 mL/minute

Dosing adjustment in hepatic impairment: No dosage change necessary

Note: Most patients not eradicated of *H. pylori* following an adequate course of therapy that includes clarithromycin will have clarithromycin-resistant isolates and should be treated with an alternative multiple drug regimen

Dosage Forms TAB: 400 mg (ranitidine 162 mg, trivalent bismuth 128 mg, and citrate 110 mg)

Contraindications Hypersensitivity to ranitidine or bismuth compounds or components; acute porphyria

Warnings/Precautions Avoid use in patients with Cl_{cr} <25 mL/minute; do not use for maintenance therapy or for >16 weeks/year

Pregnancy Risk Factor C

Adverse Reactions

>1%:

Central nervous system: Headache (14%), dizziness (1% to 2%)

Gastrointestinal: Diarrhea (5%), nausea/vomiting (3%), constipation (2%), abdominal pain, gastric upset (<10%), darkening of the tongue and/or stool (60% to 70%), taste disturbance (11%)

Miscellaneous: Flu-like symptoms (2%)

<1%: Anemia, elevated LFTs, pruritus, rash, thrombocytopenia

Drug Interactions See individual monographs

Increased effect: Optimal antimicrobial effects of ranitidine bismuth citrate occur when the drug is taken with food

Alcohol Interactions Avoid use (may enhance gastric mucosal irritation)

Half-Life Bismuth: 11-28 days; Ranitidine: 3 hours; Complex: 5-8 days

Education and Monitoring Issues

Patient Education: Take as directed, with food. Do not supplement therapy with OTC medications. This drug may cause darkening of tongue or stool and may change your taste sensation. Report unresolved headache (prescriber may recommend something for relief), dizziness, diarrhea, constipation (prescriber may recommend something for relief), weakness, or loss of appetite.

Dietary Considerations: May be taken without regard to food

Monitoring Parameters: (13) C-urea breath tests to detect *H. pylori*, endoscopic evidence of ulcer healing, CBCs, LFTs, renal function tests

Manufacturer GlaxoWellcome

Related Information

Helicobacter pylori Treatment *on page 1107*
Pharmaceutical Manufacturers Directory *on page 1020*

Ranitidine Hydrochloride (ra NI ti deen hye droe KLOR ide)

Pharmacologic Class Histamine H_2 Antagonist

U.S. Brand Names Zantac®; Zantac® 75 [OTC]

Generic Available No

Mechanism of Action Competitive inhibition of histamine at H_2-receptors of the gastric parietal cells, which inhibits gastric acid secretion, gastric volume and hydrogen ion concentration reduced

Use Short-term treatment of active duodenal ulcers and benign gastric ulcers in children 1 month to 16 years of age and adults; long-term prophylaxis of duodenal ulcer and gastric hypersecretory states, gastroesophageal reflux, recurrent postoperative ulcer, upper GI bleeding, prevention of acid-aspiration pneumonitis during surgery, and prevention of stress-induced ulcers; causes fewer interactions than cimetidine

USUAL DOSAGE Giving oral dose at 6 PM may be better than 10 PM bedtime, the highest acid production usually starts at approximately 7 PM, thus giving at 6 PM controls acid secretion better

(Continued)

Ranitidine Hydrochloride *(Continued)*

Children 1 month to 16 years:
Treatment of gastric/duodenal ulcer: 2-4 mg/kg/day
Maintenance: 1-2 mg/kg/day (maximum: 150 mg/day)
Erosive esophagitis: 5-10 mg/kg/day (usually in 2 divided doses)
Children 1-16 years:
Oral: 1.25-2.5 mg/kg/dose every 12 hours; maximum: 300 mg/day
I.M., I.V.: 0.75-1.5 mg/kg/dose every 6-8 hours, maximum daily dose: 400 mg
Continuous infusion: 0.1-0.25 mg/kg/hour (preferred for stress ulcer prophylaxis in patients with concurrent maintenance I.V.s or TPNs)
Adults:
Short-term treatment of ulceration: 150 mg/dose twice daily or 300 mg at bedtime
Prophylaxis of recurrent duodenal ulcer: Oral: 150 mg at bedtime
Gastric hypersecretory conditions:
Oral: 150 mg twice daily, up to 600 mg/day
I.M., I.V.: 50 mg/dose every 6-8 hours (dose not to exceed 400 mg/day)
I.V.: 50 mg/dose IVPB every 6-8 hours (dose not to exceed 400 mg/day)
or
Continuous I.V. infusion: Initial: 50 mg IVPB, followed by 6.25 mg/hour titrated to gastric pH >4.0 for prophylaxis or >7.0 for treatment; **continuous I.V. infusion is preferred in patients with active bleeding**
Gastric hypersecretory conditions: Doses up to 2.5 mg/kg/hour (220 mg/hour) have been used
Dosing adjustment in renal impairment:
Cl_{cr} 10-50 mL/minute: Administer at 75% of normal dose or administer every 18-24 hours
Cl_{cr} <10 mL/minute: Administer at 50% of normal dose or administer every 18-24 hours
Hemodialysis: Slightly dialyzable (5% to 20%)
Dosing adjustment/comments in hepatic disease: Unchanged

Dosage Forms CAP (GELdose™): 150 mg, 300 mg. **GRANULES, effervescent** (EFFERdose™): 150 mg. **INF** in NaCl 0.45% (preservative free): 1 mg/mL (50 mL). **INJ:** 25 mg/mL (2 mL, 10 mL, 40 mL). **SYR** (peppermint flavor): 15 mg/mL (473 mL). **TAB:** 75 mg [OTC]; 150 mg, 300 mg; Effervescent (EFFERdose™): 150 mg

Contraindications Hypersensitivity to ranitidine or any component

Warnings/Precautions Use with caution in patients with liver and renal impairment; dosage modification required in patients with renal impairment; long-term therapy may cause vitamin B_{12} deficiency

Pregnancy Risk Factor B

Adverse Reactions
1% to 10%:
Central nervous system: Dizziness, sedation, malaise, headache, drowsiness
Dermatologic: Rash
Gastrointestinal: Constipation, nausea, vomiting, diarrhea
<1%: Agranulocytosis, arthralgia, bradycardia, bronchospasm, confusion, fever, gynecomastia, hepatitis, neutropenia, tachycardia, thrombocytopenia

Drug Interactions CYP2D6 and 3A3/4 enzyme inhibitor
Decreased effect: Variable effects on warfarin; antacids may decrease absorption of ranitidine; ketoconazole and itraconazole absorptions are decreased; may produce altered serum levels of procainamide and ferrous sulfate; decreased effect of nondepolarizing muscle relaxants, cefpodoxime, cyanocobalamin (decreased absorption), diazepam, oxaprozin
Decreased toxicity of atropine
Increased toxicity of cyclosporine (increased serum creatinine), gentamicin (neuromuscular blockade), glipizide, glyburide, midazolam (increased concentrations), metoprolol, pentoxifylline, phenytoin, quinidine

Alcohol Interactions Avoid use (may enhance gastric mucosal irritation)

Onset 1-2 hours

Duration 8-12 hours

Half-Life Adults: 2-2.5 hours; End-stage renal disease: 6-9 hours

Education and Monitoring Issues

Patient Education: Take exactly as directed (at meals and bedtime); do not increase dose - may take several days before you notice relief. If antacids are approved by prescriber, allow 1 hour between antacid and ranitidine. Avoid OTC medications, especially cold or cough medication and aspirin or anything containing aspirin. Follow diet as prescriber recommends. You may experience constipation or diarrhea (request assistance from prescriber); nausea or vomiting (frequent small meals, frequent mouth care, sucking lozenges, or chewing gum may help); impotence or loss of libido (reversible when drug is discontinued); drowsiness, dizziness, or fatigue (use caution when driving or engaging in tasks requiring alertness until response to drug is known). Report skin rash, fever, sore throat, tarry stools, changes in CNS, muscle or joint pain, yellowing of skin or eyes, and change in color of urine or stool.

Monitoring Parameters: AST, ALT, serum creatinine; when used to prevent stress-related GI bleeding, measure the intragastric pH and try to maintain pH >4; signs and symptoms of peptic ulcer disease, occult blood with GI bleeding, monitor renal function to correct dose; monitor for side effects

- **Rapamune®** *see* Sirolimus *on page 853*
- **R & C® Shampoo [OTC]** *see* Pyrethrins *on page 795*
- **Reactine** *see* Cetirizine *on page 172*
- **Rea-Lo® [OTC]** *see* Urea *on page 962*
- **Rebetol®** *see* Ribavirin *on page 818*
- **Rebetron™** *see* Interferon Alfa-2b and Ribavirin Combination Pack *on page 477*
- **Rectocort** *see* Hydrocortisone *on page 447*
- **Red Away** *see* Naphazoline *on page 636*
- **Redisol®** *see* Cyanocobalamin *on page 233*
- **Redoxon®** *see* Ascorbic Acid *on page 72*
- **Redoxon** *see* Sodium Ascorbate *on page 856*
- **Redutemp® [OTC]** *see* Acetaminophen *on page 17*
- **Reese's® Pinworm Medicine [OTC]** *see* Pyrantel Pamoate *on page 793*
- **Regitine®** *see* Phentolamine *on page 726*
- **Reglan®** *see* Metoclopramide *on page 592*
- **Regonol®** *see* Pyridostigmine *on page 795*
- **Regonol® Injection** *see* Pyridostigmine *on page 795*
- **Regranex®** *see* Becaplermin *on page 93*
- **Regular (Concentrated) Iletin® II U-500** *see* Insulin Preparations *on page 472*
- **Regular Iletin® I** *see* Insulin Preparations *on page 472*
- **Regular Insulin** *see* Insulin Preparations *on page 472*
- **Regular Purified Pork Insulin** *see* Insulin Preparations *on page 472*
- **Regular Strength Bayer® Enteric 500 Aspirin [OTC]** *see* Aspirin *on page 72*
- **Regulax SS® [OTC]** *see* Docusate *on page 290*
- **Regulex®** *see* Docusate *on page 290*
- **Reguloid® [OTC]** *see* Psyllium *on page 793*
- **Rela®** *see* Carisoprodol *on page 141*
- **Relafen®** *see* Nabumetone *on page 627*
- **Relaxadon®** *see* Hyoscyamine, Atropine, Scopolamine, and Phenobarbital *on page 456*
- **Relenza®** *see* Zanamivir *on page 990*
- **Relief® Ophthalmic Solution** *see* Phenylephrine *on page 727*
- **Relisorm** *see* Gonadorelin *on page 419*
- **Remeron®** *see* Mirtazapine *on page 609*
- **Remicade™** *see* Infliximab *on page 470*

Remifentanil (rem i FEN ta nil)

Pharmacologic Class Analgesic, Narcotic

U.S. Brand Names Ultiva™

Mechanism of Action Binds with stereospecific mu-opioid receptors at many sites within the CNS, increases pain threshold, alters pain reception, inhibits ascending pain pathways

Use Analgesic for use during general anesthesia for continued analgesia

USUAL DOSAGE Adults: I.V. continuous infusion:

During induction: 0.5-1 mcg/kg/minute

During maintenance:

With nitrous oxide (66%): 0.4 mcg/kg/minute (range: 0.1-2 mcg/kg/min)

With isoflurane: 0.25 mcg/kg/minute (range: 0.05-2 mcg/kg/min)

With propofol: 0.25 mcg/kg/minute (range: 0.05-2 mcg/kg/min)

Continuation as an analgesic in immediate postoperative period: 0.1 mcg/kg/minute (range: 0.025-0.2 mcg/kg/min)

Dosage Forms **POWDER for inj, lyophilized:** 1 mg/3 mL vial, 2 mg/5 mL vial, 5 mg/10 mL vial

Contraindications Not for intrathecal or epidural administration, due to the presence of glycine in the formulation, it is also contraindicated in patients with a known hypersensitivity to remifentanil, fentanyl or fentanyl analogs; interruption of an infusion will result in offset of effects within 5-10 minutes; the discontinuation of remifentanil infusion should be preceded by the establishment of adequate postoperative analgesia orders, especially for patients in whom postoperative pain is anticipated

Warnings/Precautions Remifentanil is not recommended as the sole agent in general anesthesia, because the loss of consciousness cannot be assured and due to the high incidence of apnea, hypotension, tachycardia and muscle rigidity; it should be administered by individuals specifically trained in the use of anesthetic agents and should not be used in diagnostic or therapeutic procedures outside the monitored anesthesia setting; resuscitative and intubation equipment should be readily available

Pregnancy Risk Factor C

(Continued)

Remifentanil *(Continued)*

Adverse Reactions

>10%: Gastrointestinal: Nausea, vomiting

1% to 10%:

Cardiovascular: Hypotension, bradycardia, tachycardia, hypertension

Central nervous system: Dizziness, headache, agitation, fever

Dermatologic: Pruritus

Ocular: Visual disturbances

Respiratory: Respiratory depression, apnea, hypoxia

Miscellaneous: Shivering, postoperative pain

Onset 1-3 minutes

Half-Life 10 minutes

Education and Monitoring Issues

Monitoring Parameters: Respiratory and cardiovascular status, blood pressure, heart rate

Manufacturer GlaxoWellcome

Related Information

Lipid-Lowering Agents Comparison *on page 1243*

Narcotic Agonists Comparison *on page 1244*

Pharmaceutical Manufacturers Directory *on page 1020*

- **Renagel®** *see* Sevelamer *on page 848*
- **Renal Function Tests** *see page 1049*
- **Renedil®** *see* Felodipine *on page 352*
- **Renova™** *see* Tretinoin, Topical *on page 944*
- **Rentamine®** *see* Chlorpheniramine, Ephedrine, Phenylephrine, and Carbetapentane *on page 186*

Repaglinide (re PAG li nide)

Pharmacologic Class Antidiabetic Agent (Miscellaneous)

U.S. Brand Names Prandin™

Mechanism of Action Nonsulfonylurea hypoglycemic agent of the meglitinide class (the nonsulfonylurea moiety of glyburide) used in the management of type 2 diabetes mellitus; stimulates insulin release from the pancreatic beta cells

Use Management of noninsulin-dependent diabetes mellitus (type II)

An adjunct to diet and exercise to lower the blood glucose in patients with type 2 diabetes mellitus whose hyperglycemia cannot be controlled satisfactorily by diet and exercise alone

In combination with metformin to lower blood glucose in patients whose hyperglycemia cannot be controlled by exercise, diet and either agent alone

USUAL DOSAGE Adults: Oral: Should be taken within 15 minutes of the meal, but time may vary from immediately preceding the meal to as long as 30 minutes before the meal

Initial: For patients not previously treated or whose Hb A_{1c} is <8%, the starting dose is 0.5 mg. For patients previously treated with blood glucose-lowering agents whose Hb A_{1c} is ≥8%, the initial dose is 1 or 2 mg before each meal.

Dose adjustment: Determine dosing adjustments by blood glucose response, usually fasting blood glucose. Double the preprandial dose up to 4 mg until satisfactory blood glucose response is achieved. At least 1 week should elapse to assess response after each dose adjustment.

Dose range: 0.5-4 mg taken with meals. Repaglinide may be dosed preprandial 2, 3 or 4 times/day in response to changes in the patient's meal pattern. Maximum recommended daily dose: 16 mg.

Patients receiving other oral hypoglycemic agents: When repaglinide is used to replace therapy with other oral hypoglycemic agents, it may be started the day after the final dose is given. Observe patients carefully for hypoglycemia because of potential overlapping of drug effects. When transferred from longer half-life sulfonylureas (eg, chlorpropamide), close monitoring may be indicated for up to ≥1 week.

Combination therapy: If repaglinide monotherapy does not result in adequate glycemic control, metformin may be added. Or, if metformin therapy does not provide adequate control, repaglinide may be added. The starting dose and dose adjustments for combination therapy are the same as repaglinide monotherapy. Carefully adjust the dose of each drug to determine the minimal dose required to achieve the desired pharmacologic effect. Failure to do so could result in an increase in the incidence of hypoglycemic episodes. Use appropriate monitoring of FPG and Hb A_{1c} measurements to ensure that the patient is not subjected to excessive drug exposure or increased probability of secondary drug failure. If glucose is not achieved after a suitable trial of combination therapy, consider discontinuing these drugs and using insulin.

Dosing adjustment/comments in renal impairment: Initial dosage adjustment does not appear to be necessary, but make subsequent increases carefully in patients with renal function impairment or renal failure requiring hemodialysis

Dosing adjustment in hepatic impairment: Use conservative initial and maintenance doses and avoid use in severe disease

Dosage Forms TAB: : 0.5 mg, 1 mg, 2 mg

Contraindications Diabetic ketoacidosis, with or without coma (treat with insulin); type 1 diabetes; hypersensitivity to the drug or its inactive ingredients

Warnings/Precautions Use with caution in patients with hepatic impairment. The administration of oral hypoglycemic drugs is associated with increased cardiovascular mortality as compared with treatment with diet alone or diet plus insulin. All oral hypoglycemic agents are capable of producing hypoglycemia. Proper patient selection, dosage, and instructions to the patients are important to avoid hypoglycemic episodes. It may be necessary to discontinue repaglinide and administer insulin if the patient is exposed to stress (fever, trauma, infection, surgery).

Pregnancy Risk Factor C

Pregnancy Implications Clinical effects on the fetus: Safety in pregnant women has not been established. Use during pregnancy only if clearly needed. Insulin is the drug of choice for the control of diabetes mellitus during pregnancy. It is not known whether repaglinide is excreted in breast milk. Because the potential for hypoglycemia in nursing infants may exist, decide whether to discontinue repaglinide or discontinue breast-feeding. If repaglinide is discontinued and if diet alone is inadequate for controlling blood glucose, consider insulin therapy.

Adverse Reactions

>10%:

Central nervous system: Headache

Endocrine & metabolic: Hyperglycemia, hypoglycemia, related symptoms

1% to 10%:

Cardiovascular: Chest pain

Gastrointestinal: Nausea, epigastric fullness, heartburn, constipation, diarrhea, anorexia, tooth disorder

Genitourinary: Urinary tract infection

Neuromuscular: Arthralgia, back pain, paresthesia

Miscellaneous: Allergy

Drug Interactions CYP3A4 enzyme substrate

Decreased effect: Drugs that induce CYP3A4 may increase metabolism of repaglinide (rifampin, barbiturates, carbamazepine). Certain drugs (thiazides, diuretics, corticosteroids, phenothiazines, thyroid products, estrogens, oral contraceptives, phenytoin, nicotinic acid, sympathomimetics, calcium channel blockers, isoniazid) tend to produce hyperglycemia and may lead to loss of glycemic control.

Increased effect: Agents that inhibit CYP3A4 (ketoconazole, miconazole) and antibacterial agents (erythromycin) may increase repaglinide concentrations

Increased toxicity: Since this agent is highly protein bound, the toxic potential is increased when given concomitantly with other highly protein bound drugs (ie, phenylbutazone, oral anticoagulants, hydantoins, salicylates, NSAIDs, sulfonamides) - increase hypoglycemic effect

Alcohol Interactions Avoid use (may cause hypoglycemia)

Onset Insulin levels increase within 15-60 minutes

Duration Up to 24 hours

Education and Monitoring Issues

Patient Education: Take this medication exactly as directed - 3-4 times a day, 15-30 minutes prior to a meal. If you skip a meal (or add an extra meal) skip (or add) a dose for that meal. Do not change dosage or discontinue without first consulting prescriber. It is important to follow dietary and lifestyle recommendations of prescriber. You will be instructed in signs of hypo-/hyperglycemia by prescriber or diabetic educator; be alert for adverse hypoglycemia (tachycardia, profuse perspiration, tingling of lips and tongue, seizures, or change in sensorium) and follow prescriber's instructions for intervention. You may experience mild side effects during first weeks of therapy (eg, headache, diarrhea, constipation, bloating); if these do not diminish, notify prescriber. Increasing dietary fiber or fluids and increasing exercise may reduce constipation (for persistent diarrhea consult prescriber). Mild analgesics may reduce headaches. Frequent mouth care, small frequent meals, chewing gum, sucking lozenges may help reduce nausea, vomiting, or heartburn. Report chest pain, palpitations, or irregular heartbeat; respiratory difficulty or symptoms of upper respiratory infection; urinary tract infection (burning or itching on urination); muscle pain or back pain; or persistent GI problems.

Dietary Considerations:

Food: When given with food, the AUC of repaglinide is decreased; administer repaglinide before meals

Glucose: Decreases blood glucose concentration. Hypoglycemia may occur. Educate patients how to detect and treat hypoglycemia. Monitor for signs and symptoms of hypoglycemia. Administer glucose if necessary. Evaluate patient's diet and exercise regimen. May need to decrease or discontinue dose of sulfonylurea.

Monitoring Parameters: Periodically monitor fasting blood glucose and glycosylated hemoglobin (Hb A_{1c}) levels with a goal of decreasing these levels towards the normal range. During dose adjustment, fasting glucose can be used to determine response.

Reference Range: Target range: Adults:

Fasting blood glucose: <120 mg/dL

Glycosylated hemoglobin: <7%

(Continued)

Repaglinide *(Continued)*

Manufacturer Novo Nordisk Pharm, Inc

Related Information

Hypoglycemic Drugs and Thiazolidinedione Information *on page 1240*

Pharmaceutical Manufacturers Directory *on page 1020*

- **Repan®** *see* Butalbital Compound *on page 123*
- **Reposans-10® Oral** *see* Chlordiazepoxide *on page 180*
- **Repronex™** *see* Menotropins *on page 562*
- **Requip™** *see* Ropinirole *on page 832*
- **Resa®** *see* Reserpine *on page 814*
- **Rescaps-D® S.R. Capsule** *see* Caramiphen and Phenylpropanolamine *on page 137*
- **Rescriptor®** *see* Delavirdine *on page 250*
- **Resectisol® Irrigation Solution** *see* Mannitol *on page 554*

Reserpine (re SER peen)

Pharmacologic Class Rauwolfia Alkaloid

U.S. Brand Names Resa®; Serpalan®; Serpasil®; Serpatabs®

Use Management of mild to moderate hypertension

Unlabeled use: Management of tardive dyskinesia

USUAL DOSAGE Oral (full antihypertensive effects may take as long as 3 weeks):

Children: 0.01-0.02 mg/kg/24 hours divided every 12 hours; maximum dose: 0.25 mg/day (not recommended in children)

Adults:

Hypertension: 0.1-0.25 mg/day in 1-2 doses; initial: 0.5 mg/day for 1-2 weeks; maintenance: reduce to 0.1-0.25 mg/day

Psychiatric: Initial: 0.5 mg/day; usual range: 0.1-1 mg

Elderly: Initial: 0.05 mg once daily, increasing by 0.05 mg every week as necessary

Dosing adjustment in renal impairment: Cl_{cr} <10 mL/minute: Avoid use

Dialysis: Not removed by hemo or peritoneal dialysis; supplemental dose is not necessary

Contraindications Any ulcerative condition, mental depression, hypersensitivity to reserpine or any component

Pregnancy Risk Factor C

Related Information

Chlorothiazide and Reserpine *on page 185*

Hydralazine, Hydrochlorothiazide, and Reserpine *on page 442*

Hydrochlorothiazide and Reserpine *on page 443*

- **Respa®-DM** *see* Guaifenesin and Dextromethorphan *on page 424*
- **Respa-GF®** *see* Guaifenesin *on page 423*
- **Respbid®** *see* Theophylline Salts *on page 906*
- **RespiGam™** *see* Respiratory Syncytial Virus Immune Globulin (Intravenous) *on page 814*

Respiratory Syncytial Virus Immune Globulin (Intravenous)

(RES peer rah tor ee sin SISH al VYE rus i MYUN GLOB yoo lin in tra VEE nus)

Pharmacologic Class Immune Globulin

U.S. Brand Names RespiGam™

Mechanism of Action RSV-IGIV is a sterile liquid immunoglobulin G containing neutralizing antibody to respiratory syncytial virus. It is effective in reducing the incidence and duration of RSV hospitalization and the severity of RSV illness in high risk infants.

Use Prevention of serious lower respiratory infection caused by respiratory syncytial virus (RSV) in children <24 months of age with bronchopulmonary dysplasia (BPD) or a history of premature birth (≤35 weeks gestation)

USUAL DOSAGE I.V.: 750 mg/kg/month according to the following infusion schedule:

1.5 mL/kg/hour for 15 minutes, then at 3 mL/kg/hour for the next 15 minutes if the clinical condition does not contraindicate a higher rate, and finally, administer at 6 mL/kg/hour until completion of dose

Dosage Forms INJ: 2500 mg RSV immunoglobulin/50 mL vial

Contraindications Selective IgA deficiency; history of severe prior reaction to any immunoglobulin preparation

Warnings/Precautions Use caution to avoid fluid overload in patients, particularly infants with bronchopulmonary dysplasia (BPD), when administering RSV-IGIV; hypersensitivity including anaphylaxis or angioneurotic edema may occur; keep epinephrine 1:1000 readily available during infusion; rare occurrences of aseptic meningitis syndrome have been associated with IGIV treatment, particularly with high doses; observe carefully for signs and symptoms of such and treat promptly

Pregnancy Risk Factor C

Adverse Reactions

1% to 10%:

Dermatologic: Rash (1%)

Cardiovascular: Tachycardia (1%), hypertension (1%), hypotension

Central nervous system: Fever (6%)

Endocrine & metabolic: Fluid overload (1%)
Gastrointestinal: Vomiting (2%), diarrhea (1%), gastroenteritis (1%)
Local: Injection site inflammation (1%)
Respiratory: Respiratory distress (2%), wheezing (2%), rales, hypoxia (1%), tachypnea (1%)

<1%: Abdominal cramps, anxiety, arthralgia, chest tightness, cough, cyanosis, dizziness, dyspnea, eczema, edema, flushing, heart murmur, myalgia, pallor, palpitations, pruritus, rhinorrhea

Drug Interactions

Decreased toxicity: Antibodies present in IVIG preparations may interfere with the immune response to live virus vaccines (eg, MMR); reimmunization is recommended if such vaccines are administered within 10 months following RSV-IVIG treatment; additionally, it is advised that booster doses of oral polio, DPT, and HIB be considered 3-4 months after the last dose of RSV-IVIG in order to ensure immunity

Education and Monitoring Issues

Monitoring Parameters: Monitor for symptoms of allergic reaction; check vital signs, cardiopulmonary status after each rate increase and thereafter at 30-minute intervals until 30 minutes following completion of the infusion

♦ **Restoril®** *see* Temazepam *on page 894*
♦ **Retavase™** *see* Reteplase *on page 815*

Reteplase (RE ta plase)

Pharmacologic Class Thrombolytic Agent

U.S. Brand Names Retavase™

Mechanism of Action Reteplase is a nonglycosylated form of tPA produced by recombinant DNA technology using *E. coli*; it initiates local fibrinolysis by binding to fibrin in a thrombus (clot) and converts entrapped plasminogen to plasmin

Use Improvement of ventricular function following acute myocardial infarction, for the reduction of the incidence of CHF and the reduction of mortality associated with acute myocardial infarction

Unlabeled uses (being evaluated): Peripheral arterial obstruction and central venous catheter clearance

USUAL DOSAGE

Children: Not recommended

Adults: 10 units I.V. over 2 minutes, followed by a second dose 30 minutes later of 10 units I.V. over 2 minutes

Withhold second dose if serious bleeding or anaphylaxis occurs

Dosage Forms INJ: Powder in vials; each vial contains reteplase 10.8 units; supplied with 2 mL diluent (preservative free)

Contraindications Active internal bleeding, history of cerebrovascular accident, recent intracranial or intraspinal surgery or trauma, intracranial neoplasm, arteriovenous malformations or aneurysm, known bleeding diathesis, severe uncontrolled hypertension, history of severe allergic reactions to reteplase, alteplase, anistreplase or streptokinase

Pregnancy Risk Factor C

Adverse Reactions Bleeding is the most frequent adverse effect associated with reteplase. Heparin and aspirin have been administered concurrently with reteplase in clinical trials. The incidence of adverse events is a reflection of these combined therapies, and are comparable with comparison thrombolytics.

>10%: Local: Injection site bleeding (4.6% to 48.6%)

1% to 10%:
Hematologic: Anemia (0.9% to 2.6%)
Gastrointestinal: Bleeding (1.8% to 9.0%)
Genitourinary: Bleeding (0.9% to 9.5%)

<1% (limited to important or life-threatening symptoms): Intracranial hemorrhage (0.8%), allergic/anaphylactoid reactions, cholesterol embolization

Other adverse effects noted are frequently associated with myocardial infarction (and therefore may or may not be attributable to Retavase™) and include arrhythmias, hypotension, cardiogenic shock, pulmonary edema, cardiac arrest, reinfarction, pericarditis, tamponade, thrombosis, and embolism

Drug Interactions

Aminocaproic acid (antifibrinolytic agent) may decrease effectiveness

Drugs which affect platelet function (eg, NSAIDs, dipyridamole, ticlopidine, clopidogrel, IIb/IIIa antagonists) may potentiate the risk of hemorrhage; use with caution

Heparin and aspirin: Use with aspirin and heparin may increase bleeding. However, aspirin and heparin were used concomitantly with reteplase in the majority of patients in clinical studies.

Warfarin or oral anticoagulants: Risk of bleeding may be increased during concurrent therapy

Onset 30-90 minutes

Half-Life In serum, 13-16 minutes

(Continued)

Reteplase *(Continued)*

Education and Monitoring Issues

Patient Education: This medication can only be administered I.V. You will have a tendency to bleed easily following this medication; use caution to prevent injury (use electric razor, use soft toothbrush, use caution with sharps). If bleeding occurs, apply pressure to bleeding spot until bleeding stops completely. Report unusual bruising or bleeding (eg, blood in urine, stool, or vomitus; bleeding gums; vaginal bleeding; nosebleeds); dizziness or changes in vision; back pain; skin rash; swelling of face, mouth, or throat; or difficulty breathing.

Monitoring Parameters: Monitor for signs of bleeding (hematuria, GI bleeding, gingival bleeding)

Manufacturer Centocor, Inc

Related Information

Pharmaceutical Manufacturers Directory *on page 1020*

- **Retin-A™ Micro Topical** *see* Tretinoin, Topical *on page 944*
- **Retin-A™ Topical** *see* Tretinoin, Topical *on page 944*
- **Retisol-A®** *see* Tretinoin, Topical *on page 944*
- **Retrovir®** *see* Zidovudine *on page 991*
- **Reversol® Injection** *see* Edrophonium *on page 306*
- **Revex®** *see* Nalmefene *on page 632*
- **Rev-Eyes** *see* Dapiprazole *on page 248*
- **ReVia®** *see* Naltrexone *on page 634*
- **Revimine** *see* Dopamine *on page 294*
- **Revitalose-C-1000®** *see* Ascorbic Acid *on page 72*
- **Rezine®** *see* Hydroxyzine *on page 455*
- **Rezulin®** *see* Troglitazone *WITHDRAWN FROM MARKET 3/21/2000 on page 958*
- **R-Gen®** *see* Iodinated Glycerol *on page 480*
- **Rheumatrex®** *see* Methotrexate *on page 582*
- **Rhinalar®** *see* Flunisolide *on page 373*
- **Rhinall® Nasal Solution [OTC]** *see* Phenylephrine *on page 727*
- **Rhinaris®-F** *see* Flunisolide *on page 373*
- **Rhinatate® Tablet** *see* Chlorpheniramine, Pyrilamine, and Phenylephrine *on page 187*
- **Rhindecon®** *see* Phenylpropanolamine *on page 729*
- **Rhinocort®** *see* Budesonide *on page 115*
- **Rhinocort® Aqua™** *see* Budesonide *on page 115*
- **Rhino-Mex-N** *see* Naphazoline *on page 636*
- **Rhinosyn-DMX® [OTC]** *see* Guaifenesin and Dextromethorphan *on page 424*
- **Rhodialax** *see* Lactulose *on page 506*
- **Rhodialose** *see* Lactulose *on page 506*

$Rh_o(D)$ Immune Globulin (Intramuscular)

(ar aych oh (dee) i MYUN GLOB yoo lin in tra MUS kue lar)

Pharmacologic Class Immune Globulin

U.S. Brand Names Gamulin® Rh; HypRho®-D; HypRho®-D Mini-Dose; MICRhoGAM™; Mini-Gamulin® Rh; RhoGAM™

Generic Available No

Mechanism of Action Suppresses the immune response and antibody formation of Rh-negative individuals to Rh-positive red blood cells

Use Prevention of isoimmunization in Rh-negative individuals exposed to Rh-positive blood during delivery of an Rh-positive infant, as a result of an abortion, following amniocentesis or abdominal trauma, or following a transfusion accident; prevention of hemolytic disease of the newborn if there is a subsequent pregnancy with an Rh-positive fetus

USUAL DOSAGE Adults (administered I.M. to mothers **not** to infant) I.M.:

Obstetrical usage: 1 vial (300 mcg) prevents maternal sensitization if fetal packed red blood cell volume that has entered the circulation is <15 mL; if it is more, give additional vials. The number of vials = RBC volume of the calculated fetomaternal hemorrhage divided by 15 mL

Postpartum prophylaxis: 300 mcg within 72 hours of delivery

Antepartum prophylaxis: 300 mcg at approximately 26-28 weeks gestation; followed by 300 mcg within 72 hours of delivery if infant is Rh-positive

Following miscarriage, abortion, or termination of ectopic pregnancy at up to 13 weeks of gestation: 50 mcg ideally within 3 hours, but may be given up to 72 hours after; if pregnancy has been terminated at 13 or more weeks of gestation, administer 300 mcg

Dosage Forms INJ: Each package contains one single dose 300 mcg of Rh_o (D) immune globulin; Microdose: Each package contains one single dose of microdose, 50 mcg of Rh_o (D) immune globulin

Contraindications $Rh_o(D)$-positive patient; known hypersensitivity to immune globulins or to thimerosal; transfusion of $Rh_o(D)$-positive blood in previous 3 months; prior sensitization to $Rh_o(D)$

Warnings/Precautions Use with caution in patients with thrombocytopenia or bleeding disorders, patients with IgA deficiency; do not inject I.V.; do not administer to neonates. $Rh_0(D)$-positive ITP patients should be monitored for signs and/or symptoms of intravascular hemolysis, clinically compromising anemia, and renal insufficiency.

Pregnancy Risk Factor C

Adverse Reactions <1%: Elevated bilirubin, lethargy, myalgia, pain at the injection site, splenomegaly, temperature elevation

Education and Monitoring Issues

Patient Education: Acetaminophen may be taken to ease minor discomfort after vaccination

$Rh_0(D)$ Immune Globulin (Intravenous-Human)

(ar aych oh (dee) i MYUN GLOB yoo lin in tra VEE nus-HYU man)

Pharmacologic Class Immune Globulin

U.S. Brand Names WinRho SD®

Mechanism of Action The $Rh_0(D)$ antigen is responsible for most cases of Rh sensitization, which occurs when Rh-positive fetal RBCs enter the maternal circulation of an Rh-negative woman. Injection of anti-D globulin results in opsonization of the fetal RBCs, which are then phagocytized in the spleen, preventing immunization of the mother. Injection of anti-D into an Rh-positive patient with ITP coats the patient's own D-positive RBCs with antibody and, as they are cleared by the spleen, they saturate the capacity of the spleen to clear antibody-coated cells, sparing antibody-coated platelets. Other proposed mechanisms involve the generation of cytokines following the interaction between antibody-coated RBCs and macrophages.

Use

Prevention of Rh isoimmunization in nonsensitized $Rh_0(D)$ antigen-negative women within 72 hours after spontaneous or induced abortion, amniocentesis, chorionic villus sampling, ruptured tubal pregnancy, abdominal trauma, transplacental hemorrhage, or in the normal course of pregnancy unless the blood type of the fetus or father is known to be $Rh_0(D)$ antigen-negative.

Suppression of Rh isoimmunization in $Rh_0(D)$ antigen-negative female children and female adults in their childbearing years transfused with $Rh_0(D)$ antigen-positive RBCs or blood components containing $Rh_0(D)$ antigen-positive RBCs

Treatment of idiopathic thrombocytopenic purpura (ITP) in nonsplenectomized $Rh_0(D)$ antigen-positive patients

USUAL DOSAGE

Prevention of Rh isoimmunization: I.V.: 1500 units (300 mcg) at 28 weeks gestation or immediately after amniocentesis if before 34 weeks gestation or after chorionic villus sampling; repeat this dose every 12 weeks during the pregnancy. Administer 600 units (120 mcg) at delivery (within 72 hours) and after invasive intrauterine procedures such as abortion, amniocentesis, or any other manipulation if at >34 weeks gestation. **Note:** If the Rh status of the baby is not known at 72 hours, administer $Rh_0(D)$ immune globulin to the mother at 72 hours after delivery. If >72 hours have elapsed, do not withhold $Rh_0(D)$ immune globulin, but administer as soon as possible, up to 28 days after delivery.

I.M.: Reconstitute vial with 1.25 mL and administer as above

Transfusion: Administer within 72 hours after exposure for treatment of incompatible blood transfusions or massive fetal hemorrhage as follows:

I.V.: 3000 units (600 mcg) every 8 hours until the total dose is administered (45 units [9 mcg] of Rh-positive blood/mL blood; 90 units [18 mcg] Rh-positive red cells/mL cells)

I.M.: 6000 units [1200 mcg] every 12 hours until the total dose is administered (60 units [12 mcg] of Rh-positive blood/mL blood; 120 units [24 mcg] Rh-positive red cells/mL cells)

Treatment of ITP: I.V.: Initial: 25-50 mcg/kg depending on the patient's Hgb concentration; maintenance: 25-60 mcg/kg depending on the clinical response

Dosage Forms **INJ:** 600 units [120 mcg], 1500 units [300 mcg] with 2.5 mL diluent

Contraindications Hypersensitivity to immune globulin or any component, IgA deficiency

Warnings/Precautions Anaphylactic hypersensitivity reactions can occur; studies indicate that there is no discernible risk of transmitting HIV or hepatitis B; do not administer by S.C. route; use only the I.V. route when treating ITP. $Rh_0(D)$-positive ITP patients should be monitored for signs and/or symptoms of intravascular hemolysis, clinically compromising anemia, and renal insufficiency

Pregnancy Risk Factor C

Adverse Reactions 1% to 10%:

Central nervous system: Headache (2%), fever (1%), chills (<2%)

Hematologic: Hemolysis (Hgb decrease of >2 g/dL in 5% to 10% of ITP patients)

Local: Slight edema and pain at the injection site

Drug Interactions Increased toxicity: Live virus, vaccines (measles, mumps, rubella); do not administer within 3 months after administration of these vaccines

Education and Monitoring Issues

Monitoring Parameters: Signs and/or symptoms of intravascular hemolysis, clinically compromising anemia, and renal insufficiency

♦ **Rhodis®** *see* Ketoprofen *on page 500*

- ♦ **Rhodis-EC®** *see* Ketoprofen *on page 500*
- ♦ **RhoGAM™** *see* Rh_0(D) Immune Globulin (Intramuscular) *on page 816*
- ♦ **Rhoprolene** *see* Betamethasone *on page 103*
- ♦ **Rhoprosone** *see* Betamethasone *on page 103*
- ♦ **Rhotral** *see* Acebutolol *on page 16*
- ♦ **Rhotrimine®** *see* Trimipramine *on page 955*
- ♦ **Rhulicaine® [OTC]** *see* Benzocaine *on page 98*
- ♦ **Rhythmin®** *see* Procainamide *on page 769*

Ribavirin (rye ba VYE rin)

Pharmacologic Class Antiviral Agent

U.S. Brand Names Rebetol®; Virazole® Aerosol

Generic Available No

Mechanism of Action Inhibits replication of RNA and DNA viruses; inhibits influenza virus RNA polymerase activity and inhibits the initiation and elongation of RNA fragments resulting in inhibition of viral protein synthesis

Use Inhalation: Treatment of patients with respiratory syncytial virus (RSV) infections; may also be used in other viral infections including influenza A and B and adenovirus; specially indicated for treatment of severe lower respiratory tract RSV infections in patients with an underlying compromising condition (prematurity, bronchopulmonary dysplasia and other chronic lung conditions, congenital heart disease, immunodeficiency, immunosuppression), and recent transplant recipients

Oral capsules: The combination therapy of oral ribavirin with interferon alfa-2b, recombinant (Intron® A) injection is indicated for the treatment of chronic hepatitis C in patients with compensated liver disease who have relapsed after alpha interferon therapy.

USUAL DOSAGE Infants, Children, and Adults:

Aerosol inhalation: Use with Viratek® small particle aerosol generator (SPAG-2) at a concentration of 20 mg/mL (6 g reconstituted with 300 mL of sterile water without preservatives)

Aerosol only: 12-18 hours/day for 3 days, up to 7 days in length

Dosage Forms CAP: 200 mg (available only in Rebetron® combination package). **POWDER for aero:** 6 g (100 mL)

Contraindications Females of childbearing age; hypersensitivity to ribavirin; patients with autoimmune hepatitis

Warnings/Precautions Use with caution in patients requiring assisted ventilation because precipitation of the drug in the respiratory equipment may interfere with safe and effective patient ventilation; monitor carefully in patients with COPD and asthma for deterioration of respiratory function. Ribavirin is potentially mutagenic, tumor-promoting, and gonadotoxic. Anemia has been observed in patients receiving the interferon/ribavirin combination. Severe psychiatric events have also occurred including depression and suicidal behavior during combination therapy; avoid use in patients with a psychiatric history.

Pregnancy Risk Factor X

Adverse Reactions

Inhalation:

1% to 10%:

Central nervous system: Fatigue, headache, insomnia

Gastrointestinal: Nausea, anorexia

Hematologic: Anemia

<1%: Apnea, cardiac arrest, conjunctivitis, digitalis toxicity, hypotension, mild bronchospasm, rash, skin irritation, worsening of respiratory function

Note: Incidence of adverse effects in healthcare workers approximate 51% headache; 32% conjunctivitis; 10% to 20% rhinitis, nausea, rash, dizziness, pharyngitis, and lacrimation

Oral: (All adverse reactions are documented while receiving combination therapy with interferon alpha-2b)

>10%:

Cardiovascular: Chest pain

Central nervous system: Dizziness, headache, fatigue, fever, insomnia, irritability, depression, emotional lability, impaired concentration

Dermatologic: Alopecia, rash, pruritus

Gastrointestinal: Nausea, anorexia, dyspepsia, vomiting

Hematologic: Decreased hemoglobin and WBC

Neuromuscular & skeletal: Myalgia, arthralgia, musculoskeletal pain, weakness, rigors

Respiratory: Dyspnea, sinusitis

Miscellaneous: Flu-like syndrome

1% to 10%:

Central nervous system: Nervousness

Endocrine & metabolic: Thyroid function test abnormalities

Gastrointestinal: Taste perversion

Drug Interactions Decreased effect of zidovudine

Half-Life 24 hours, much longer in the erythrocyte (16-40 days), which can be used as a marker for intracellular metabolism

Education and Monitoring Issues

Patient Education: Take as directed, for full course of therapy; do not discontinue even if feeling better. Use aerosol device as instructed. Maintain adequate fluid intake and report any swelling of ankles or feet, difficulty breathing, persistent lethargy, acute headache, insomnia, severe nausea or anorexia, confusion, fever, chills, sore throat, easy bruising or bleeding, mouth sores, or worsening of respiratory condition.

Monitoring Parameters: Respiratory function, CBC, reticulocyte count, I & O

Riboflavin (RYE boe flay vin)

Pharmacologic Class Vitamin, Water Soluble

U.S. Brand Names Riobin®

Generic Available Yes

Mechanism of Action Component of flavoprotein enzymes that work together, which are necessary for normal tissue respiration; also needed for activation of pyridoxine and conversion of tryptophan to niacin

Use Prevent riboflavin deficiency and treat ariboflavinosis

USUAL DOSAGE Oral:

Riboflavin deficiency:
- Children: 2.5-10 mg/day in divided doses
- Adults: 5-30 mg/day in divided doses

Recommended daily allowance:
- Children: 0.4-1.8 mg
- Adults: 1.2-1.7 mg

Dosage Forms TAB: 25 mg, 50 mg, 100 mg

Warnings/Precautions Riboflavin deficiency often occurs in the presence of other B vitamin deficiencies

Pregnancy Risk Factor A; C (if dose exceeds RDA recommendation)

Drug Interactions Decreased absorption with probenecid

Half-Life Biologic: 66-84 minutes

Education and Monitoring Issues

Patient Education: Take with food. Large doses may cause bright yellow or orange urine.

- ♦ **Rid-A-Pain® [OTC]** *see* Benzocaine *on page 98*
- ♦ **Ridaura®** *see* Auranofin *on page 82*
- ♦ **Ridene** *see* Nicardipine *on page 649*
- ♦ **Ridenol® [OTC]** *see* Acetaminophen *on page 17*
- ♦ **RID® Shampoo [OTC]** *see* Pyrethrins *on page 795*

Rifabutin (rif a BYOO tin)

Pharmacologic Class Antibiotic, Miscellaneous; Antitubercular Agent

U.S. Brand Names Mycobutin®

Mechanism of Action Inhibits DNA-dependent RNA polymerase at the beta subunit which prevents chain initiation

Use Prevention of disseminated *Mycobacterium avium* complex (MAC) in patients with advanced HIV infection; also utilized in multiple drug regimens for treatment of MAC

USUAL DOSAGE Oral:

Children: Efficacy and safety of rifabutin have not been established in children; a limited number of HIV-positive children with MAC have been given rifabutin for MAC prophylaxis; doses of 5 mg/kg/day have been useful

Adults: 300 mg once daily; for patients who experience gastrointestinal upset, rifabutin can be administered 150 mg twice daily with food

Dosage Forms CAP: 150 mg

Contraindications Hypersensitivity to rifabutin or any other rifamycins; rifabutin is contraindicated in patients with a WBC $<1000/mm^3$ or a platelet count $<50,000/mm^3$; concurrent use with ritonavir

Warnings/Precautions Rifabutin as a single agent must not be administered to patients with active tuberculosis since its use may lead to the development of tuberculosis that is resistant to both rifabutin and rifampin; rifabutin should be discontinued in patients with AST >500 units/L or if total bilirubin is >3 mg/dL. Use with caution in patients with liver impairment; modification of dosage should be considered in patients with renal impairment.

Pregnancy Risk Factor B

Adverse Reactions

>10%:
- Dermatologic: Rash (11%)
- Genitourinary: Discolored urine (30%)
- Hematologic: Neutropenia (25%), leukopenia (17%)

1% to 10%:
- Central nervous system: Headache (3%)

(Continued)

Rifabutin *(Continued)*

Gastrointestinal: Vomiting/nausea (3%), abdominal pain (4%), diarrhea (3%), anorexia (2%), flatulence (2%), eructation (3%)

Hematologic: Anemia, thrombocytopenia (5%)

Hepatic: Increased AST/ALT (7% to 9%)

Neuromuscular & skeletal: Myalgia

<1%: Chest pain, dyspepsia, fever, insomnia, taste perversion, uveitis

Drug Interactions CYP3A3/4 enzyme inducer

Decreased plasma concentration (due to induction of liver enzymes) of verapamil, methadone, digoxin, cyclosporine, corticosteroids, oral anticoagulants, theophylline, barbiturates, chloramphenicol, ketoconazole, oral contraceptives, quinidine, halothane, protease inhibitors, non-nucleoside reverse transcriptase inhibitors, and perhaps clarithromycin

Increased concentration by indinavir; reduce to 1/2 standard dose when used with indinavir

Increased risk of rifabutin-induced hematologic and ocular toxicity (uveitis) with concurrent administration of drug that inhibits CYP-450 enzymes such as protease inhibitors, erythromycin, clarithromycin, ketoconazole, and itraconazole. Ritonavir increases rifabutin metabolite concentrations (reduce rifabutin dose to 150 mg every other day).

Half-Life 45 hours (range: 16-69 hours)

Education and Monitoring Issues

Patient Education: May take with food if GI upset occurs. Will discolor urine, stool, saliva, tears, sweat, and other body fluid a red-brown color. Stains on clothing or contact lenses are permanent. Report skin rash, vomiting, fever, chills, flu-like symptoms, dark urine or pale stools, unusual bleeding or bruising, or unusual confusion, depression, or fatigue.

Monitoring Parameters: Periodic liver function tests, CBC with differential, platelet count

Manufacturer Pharmacia & Upjohn

Related Information

Antimicrobial Drugs of Choice *on page 1182*

Pharmaceutical Manufacturers Directory *on page 1020*

Tuberculosis Test Recommendations and Prophylaxis *on page 1163*

Tuberculosis Treatment Guidelines *on page 1213*

♦ **Rifadin®** *see* Rifampin *on page 820*

♦ **Rifadin® Injection** *see* Rifampin *on page 820*

♦ **Rifadin® Oral** *see* Rifampin *on page 820*

♦ **Rifamate®** *see* Rifampin and Isoniazid *on page 822*

Rifampin (RIF am pin)

Pharmacologic Class Antibiotic, Miscellaneous; Antitubercular Agent

U.S. Brand Names Rifadin® Injection; Rifadin® Oral; Rimactane® Oral

Generic Available Yes

Mechanism of Action Inhibits bacterial RNA synthesis by binding to the beta subunit of DNA-dependent RNA polymerase, blocking RNA transcription

Use Management of active tuberculosis in combination with other agents; eliminate meningococci from asymptomatic carriers; prophylaxis of *Haemophilus influenzae* type b infection; used in combination with other anti-infectives in the treatment of staphylococcal infections

USUAL DOSAGE Oral (I.V. infusion dose is the same as for the oral route):

Tuberculosis therapy:

Note: A four-drug regimen (isoniazid, rifampin, pyrazinamide, and either streptomycin or ethambutol) is preferred for the initial, empiric treatment of TB. When the drug susceptibility results are available, the regimen should be altered as appropriate.

Infants and Children <12 years:

Daily therapy: 10-20 mg/kg/day usually as a single dose (maximum: 600 mg/day)

Directly observed therapy (DOT): Twice weekly: 10-20 mg/kg (maximum: 600 mg); 3 times/week: 10-20 mg/kg (maximum: 600 mg)

Adults:

Daily therapy: 10 mg/kg/day (maximum: 600 mg/day)

Directly observed therapy (DOT): Twice weekly: 10 mg/kg (maximum: 600 mg); 3 times/week: 10 mg/kg (maximum: 600 mg)

H. influenzae **prophylaxis:**

Infants and Children: 20 mg/kg/day every 24 hours for 4 days, not to exceed 600 mg/dose

Adults: 600 mg every 24 hours for 4 days

Meningococcal prophylaxis:

<1 month: 10 mg/kg/day in divided doses every 12 hours for 2 days

Infants and Children: 20 mg/kg/day in divided doses every 12 hours for 2 days

Adults: 600 mg every 12 hours for 2 days

Nasal carriers of *Staphylococcus aureus*:

Children: 15 mg/kg/day divided every 12 hours for 5-10 days in combination with other antibiotics

Adults: 600 mg/day for 5-10 days in combination with other antibiotics

Synergy for *Staphylococcus aureus* infections: Adults: 300-600 mg twice daily with other antibiotics

Dosing adjustment in hepatic impairment: Dose reductions may be necessary to reduce hepatotoxicity

Dosage Forms CAP: 150 mg, 300 mg; **POWDER for inj:** 600 mg (contains a sulfite)

Contraindications Hypersensitivity to any rifamycins or any component; concurrent use of amprenavir

Warnings/Precautions Use with caution and modify dosage in patients with liver impairment; observe for hyperbilirubinemia; discontinue therapy if this in conjunction with clinical symptoms or any signs of significant hepatocellular damage develop; since rifampin has enzyme-inducing properties, porphyria exacerbation is possible; use with caution in patients with porphyria; do not use for meningococcal disease, only for short-term treatment of asymptomatic carrier states

Monitor for compliance and effects including hypersensitivity, decreased thrombocytopenia in patients on intermittent therapy; urine, feces, saliva, sweat, tears, and CSF may be discolored to red/orange; do not administer I.V. form via I.M. or S.C. routes; restart infusion at another site if extravasation occurs; remove soft contact lenses during therapy since permanent staining may occur; regimens of 600 mg once or twice weekly have been associated with a high incidence of adverse reactions including a flu-like syndrome

Pregnancy Risk Factor C

Pregnancy Implications Clinical effects on the fetus: Teratogenicity has occurred in rodents given may times the adult human dose

Adverse Reactions

Percentage unknown: Flushing, edema headache, drowsiness, dizziness, confusion, numbness, behavioral changes, pruritus, urticaria, pemphigoid reaction, eosinophilia, leukopenia, hemolysis, hemolytic anemia, thrombocytopenia (especially with high-dose therapy), hepatitis (rare), ataxia, myalgia, weakness, osteomalacia, visual changes, exudative conjunctivitis

1% to 10%:

Dermatologic: Rash (1% to 5%)

Gastrointestinal: (1% to 2%): Epigastric distress, anorexia, nausea, vomiting, diarrhea, cramps, pseudomembranous colitis, pancreatitis

Hepatic: Increased LFTs (up to 14%)

Drug Interactions CYP3A3/4 enzyme substrate; CYP1A2, 2C9, 2C18, 2C19, 3A3/4, and 3A5-7 enzyme inducer

Decreased effect: Rifampin induces liver enzymes which may decrease the plasma concentration of calcium channel blockers (verapamil, diltiazem, nifedipine), methadone, digitalis, cyclosporine, corticosteroids, oral anticoagulants, haloperidol, theophylline, barbiturates, chloramphenicol, imidazole antifungals, oral or systemic hormonal contraceptives, acetaminophen, benzodiazepines, hydantoins, sulfa drugs, enalapril, beta-blockers, chloramphenicol, clofibrate, dapsone, antiarrhythmics (disopyramide, mexiletine, quinidine, tocainide), diazepam, doxycycline, fluoroquinolones, levothyroxine, nortriptyline, progestins, tacrolimus, zidovudine, protease inhibitors (amprenavir contraindicated), and non-nucleoside reverse transcriptase inhibitors. Coadministration of rifampin with antacids may reduce absorption.

Increased effect/toxicity. Coadministration with INH or halothane may result in additive hepatotoxicity. Increased effect: Co-trimoxazole and probenecid may increase rifampin levels. Ritonavir increase serum concentrations of rifampin metabolites

Alcohol Interactions Avoid use (may increase risk of hepatotoxicity)

Half-Life 3-4 hours, prolonged with hepatic impairment; End-stage renal disease: 1.8-11 hours

Education and Monitoring Issues

Patient Education: Take per recommended schedule. Complete full course of therapy; do not skip doses. Take on an empty stomach (1 hour before or 2 hours after meals). Maintain adequate hydration (2-3 L/day of fluids unless instructed to restrict fluid intake). Will discolor urine, stool, saliva, tears, sweat, and other body fluids red-brown. Stains on clothing or contact lenses are permanent. Report persistent vomiting; fever, chill, or flu-like symptoms; unusual bruising or bleeding; or other persistent adverse effects.

Dietary Considerations: Food: Rifampin is best taken on an empty stomach since food decreases the extent of absorption

Monitoring Parameters: Periodic (baseline and every 2-4 weeks during therapy) monitoring of liver function (AST, ALT, bilirubin BSD), CBC; hepatic status and mental status, sputum culture, chest x-ray 2-3 months into treatment

Related Information

Antibiotic Treatment of Adults With Infective Endocarditis *on page 1179*
Antimicrobial Drugs of Choice *on page 1182*
Prophylaxis for Patients Exposed to Common Communicable Diseases *on page 1161*
Rifampin and Isoniazid *on page 822*
(Continued)

Rifampin *(Continued)*

Rifampin, Isoniazid, and Pyrazinamide *on page 822*
Tuberculosis Test Recommendations and Prophylaxis *on page 1163*
Tuberculosis Treatment Guidelines *on page 1213*

Rifampin and Isoniazid (RIF am pin & eye soe NYE a zid)

Pharmacologic Class Antibiotic, Miscellaneous

U.S. Brand Names Rifamate®

Dosage Forms CAP: Rifampin 300 mg and isoniazid 150 mg

Pregnancy Risk Factor C

Rifampin, Isoniazid, and Pyrazinamide

(RIF am pin, eye soe NYE a zid, & peer a ZIN a mide)

Pharmacologic Class Antibiotic, Miscellaneous

U.S. Brand Names Rifater®

Dosage Forms TAB: Rifampin 120 mg, isoniazid 50 mg, and pyrazinamide 300 mg

Pregnancy Risk Factor C

Rifapentine (RIF a pen teen)

Pharmacologic Class Antitubercular Agent

U.S. Brand Names Priftin®

Mechanism of Action Inhibits DNA-dependent RNA polymerase in susceptible strains of *Mycobacterium tuberculosis* (but not in mammalian cells). Rifapentine is bactericidal against both intracellular and extracellular MTB organisms. MTB resistant to other rifamycins including rifampin are likely to be resistant to rifapentine. Cross-resistance does not appear between rifapentine and other nonrifamycin antimycobacterial agents.

Use Treatment of pulmonary tuberculosis (indication is based on the 6-month follow-up treatment outcome observed in controlled clinical trial). Rifapentine must always be used in conjunction with at least one other antituberculosis drug to which the isolate is susceptible; it may also be necessary to add a third agent (either streptomycin or ethambutol) until susceptibility is known.

USUAL DOSAGE

Children: No dosing information available

Adults: **Rifapentine should not be used alone**; initial phase should include a 3- to 4-drug regimen

Intensive phase of short-term therapy: 600 mg (four 150 mg tablets) given weekly (every 72 hours); following the intensive phase, treatment should continue with rifapentine 600 mg once weekly for 4 months in combination with INH or appropriate agent for susceptible organisms

Dosing adjustment in renal or hepatic impairment: Unknown

Dosage Forms TAB, film-coated: 150 mg

Contraindications Patients with a history of hypersensitivity to rifapentine, rifampin, rifabutin, and any rifamycin analog

Warnings/Precautions Compliance with dosing regimen is absolutely necessary for successful drug therapy. patients with abnormal liver tests and/or liver disease should only be given rifapentine when absolutely necessary and under strict medical supervision. Monitoring of liver function tests should be carried out prior to therapy and then every 2-4 weeks during therapy if signs of liver disease occur or worsen, rifapentine should be discontinued. Pseudomembranous colitis has been reported to occur with various antibiotics including other rifamycins. If this is suspected, rifapentine should be stopped and the patient treated with specific and supportive treatment. Experience in treating TB in HIV-infected patients is limited.

Rifapentine may produce a red-orange discoloration of body tissues/fluids including skin, teeth, tongue, urine, feces, saliva, sputum, tears, sweat, and cerebral spinal fluid. Contact lenses may become permanently stained. All patients treated with rifapentine should have baseline measurements of liver function tests and enzymes, bilirubin, and a complete blood count. patients should be seen monthly and specifically questioned regarding symptoms associated with adverse reactions. Routine laboratory monitoring in people with normal baseline measurements is generally not necessary.

Pregnancy Risk Factor C

Pregnancy Implications Has been shown to be teratogenic in rats and rabbits. Rat offspring showed cleft palates, right aortic arch, and delayed ossification and increased number of ribs. Rabbits displayed ovarian agenesis, pes varus, arhinia, microphthalmia, and irregularities of the ossified facial tissues. Rat studies also show decreased fetal weight, increased number of stillborns, and decreased gestational survival. No adequate well-controlled studies in pregnant women are available. Rifapentine should be used during pregnancy only if the potential benefits justifies the potential risk to the fetus.

Adverse Reactions

>10%: Endocrine & metabolic: Hyperuricemia (most likely due to pyrazinamide from initiation phase combination therapy)

1% to 10%:

Cardiovascular: Hypertension

Central nervous system: Headache, dizziness
Dermatologic: Rash, pruritus, acne
Gastrointestinal: Anorexia, nausea, vomiting, dyspepsia, diarrhea
Hematologic: Neutropenia, lymphopenia, anemia, leukopenia, thrombocytosis
Hepatic: Increased ALT/AST
Neuromuscular & skeletal: Arthralgia, pain
Renal: Pyuria, proteinuria, hematuria, urinary casts
Respiratory: Hemoptysis

<1%: Aggressive reaction, arthrosis, bilirubinemia, constipation, esophagitis, fatigue, gastritis, gout, hematoma, hepatitis, hyperkalemia, hypovolemia, increased alkaline phosphatase, increased LDH, leukocytosis, neutrophilia, pancreatitis, peripheral edema, purpura, skin discoloration, thrombocytopenia, urticaria

Drug Interactions CYP3A4 and 2C8/9 inducer. Rifapentine may increase the metabolism of coadministered drugs that are metabolized by these enzymes. Enzymes are induced within 4 days after the first dose and returned to baseline 14 days after discontinuation of rifapentine. The magnitude of enzyme induction is dose and frequency dependent. Rifampin has been shown to accelerate the metabolism and may reduce activity of the following drugs (therefore, rifapentine may also do the same): Phenytoin, disopyramide, mexiletine, quinidine, tocainide, chloramphenicol, clarithromycin, dapsone, doxycycline, fluoroquinolones, warfarin, fluconazole, itraconazole, ketoconazole, barbiturates, benzodiazepines, beta-blockers, diltiazem, nifedipine, verapamil, corticosteroids, cardiac glycoside preparations, clofibrate, oral or other systemic hormonal contraceptives, haloperidol, HIV protease inhibitors, sulfonylureas, cyclosporine, tacrolimus, levothyroxine, methadone, progestins, quinine, delavirdine, zidovudine, sildenafil, theophylline, amitriptyline, and nortriptyline.

Rifapentine should be used with extreme caution, if at all, in patients who are also taking protease inhibitors

Patients using oral or other systemic hormonal contraceptives should be advised to change to nonhormonal methods of birth control when receiving concomitant rifapentine.

Rifapentine metabolism is mediated by esterase activity, therefore, there is minimal potential for rifapentine metabolism to be affected by other drug therapy.

Half-Life Rifapentine: 14-17 hours; 25-desacetyl rifapentine: 13 hours

Education and Monitoring Issues

Patient Education: Best to take on an empty stomach (1 hour before or 2 hours after meals); however, may be taken with food if GI upset occurs. Follow recommended dosing schedule exactly; do not increase dose or skip doses. You will need to be monitored on a regular basis while taking this medication. This medication will stain urine, stool, saliva, tears, sweat, and other body fluids a red-brown color. Stains on clothing or contact lenses are permanent. Report vomiting; fever, chills or flu-like symptoms; muscle weakness or unusual fatigue; dark urine, pale stools, or unusual bleeding or bruising; yellowing skin or eyes; skin rash; swelling of extremities; chest pain or palpitations; or persistent gastrointestinal upset.

Dietary Considerations: Food increases AUC and maximum serum concentration by 43% and 44% respectively as compared to fasting conditions

Monitoring Parameters: Patients with pre-existing hepatic problems should have liver function tests monitored every 2-4 weeks during therapy

♦ **Rifater®** *see* Rifampin, Isoniazid, and Pyrazinamide *on page 822*

♦ **Rilutek®** *see* Riluzole *on page 823*

Riluzole (RIL yoo zole)

Pharmacologic Class Glutamate Inhibitor

U.S. Brand Names Rilutek®

Use Amyotrophic lateral sclerosis (ALS): Treatment of patients with ALS; riluzole can extend survival or time to tracheostomy

USUAL DOSAGE Adults: Oral: 50 mg every 12 hours; no increased benefit can be expected from higher daily doses, but adverse events are increased

Dosage adjustment in smoking: Cigarette smoking is known to induce CYP 1A2; patients who smoke cigarettes would be expected to eliminate riluzole faster. There is no information, however, on the effect of, or need for, dosage adjustment in these patients.

Dosage adjustment in special populations: Females and Japanese patients may possess a lower metabolic capacity to eliminate riluzole compared with male and Caucasian subjects, respectively

Dosage adjustment in renal impairment: Use with caution in patients with concomitant renal insufficiency

Dosage adjustment in hepatic impairment: Use with caution in patients with current evidence or history of abnormal liver function indicated by significant abnormalities in serum transaminase, bilirubin or GGT levels. Baseline elevations of several LFTs (especially elevated bilirubin) should preclude use of riluzole.

Contraindications Severe hypersensitivity reactions to riluzole or any of the tablet components

(Continued)

Riluzole *(Continued)*

Pregnancy Risk Factor C

- **Rimactane®** *see* Rifampin *on page 820*
- **Rimactane® Oral** *see* Rifampin *on page 820*

Rimantadine (ri MAN ta deen)

Pharmacologic Class Antiviral Agent

U.S. Brand Names Flumadine®

Mechanism of Action Exerts its inhibitory effect on three antigenic subtypes of influenza A virus (H1N1, H2N2, H3N2) early in the viral replicative cycle, possibly inhibiting the uncoating process; it has no activity against influenza B virus and is two- to eightfold more active than amantadine

Use Prophylaxis (adults and children >1 year) and treatment (adults) of influenza A viral infection

USUAL DOSAGE Oral:

Prophylaxis:

Children <10 years: 5 mg/kg once daily; maximum: 150 mg

Children >10 years and Adults: 100 mg twice daily; decrease to 100 mg/day in elderly or in patients with severe hepatic or renal impairment (Cl_{cr} ≤10 mL/minute)

Treatment: Adults: 100 mg twice daily; decrease to 100 mg/day in elderly or in patients with severe hepatic or renal impairment (Cl_{cr} ≤10 mL/minute)

Dosage Forms SYR: 50 mg/5 mL (60 mL, 240 mL, 480 mL). **TAB:** 100 mg

Contraindications Hypersensitivity to drugs of the adamantine class, including rimantadine and amantadine

Warnings/Precautions Use with caution in patients with renal and hepatic dysfunction; avoid use, if possible, in patients with recurrent and eczematoid dermatitis, uncontrolled psychosis, or severe psychoneurosis. An increase in seizure incidence may occur in patients with seizure disorders; discontinue drug if seizures occur; consider the development of resistance during rimantadine treatment of the index case as likely if failure of rimantadine prophylaxis among family contact occurs and if index case is a child; viruses exhibit cross-resistance between amantadine and rimantadine.

Pregnancy Risk Factor C

Pregnancy Implications

Clinical effects on the fetus: Embryotoxic in high dose rat studies

Breast-feeding/lactation: Avoid use in nursing mothers due to potential adverse effect in infants; rimantadine is concentrated in milk

Adverse Reactions 1% to 10%:

Cardiovascular: Orthostatic hypotension, edema

Central nervous system: Dizziness (1.9%), confusion, headache (1.4%), insomnia (2.1%), difficulty in concentrating, anxiety (1.3%), restlessness, irritability, hallucinations; incidence of CNS side effects may be less than that associated with amantadine

Gastrointestinal: Nausea (2.8%), vomiting (1.7%), xerostomia (1.5%), abdominal pain (1.4%), anorexia (1.6%)

Genitourinary: Urinary retention

Drug Interactions

Acetaminophen: Reduction in AUC and peak concentration of rimantadine

Aspirin: Peak plasma and AUC concentrations of rimantadine are reduced

Cimetidine: Rimantadine clearance is decreased (~16%)

Half-Life 25.4 hours (increased in the elderly)

Education and Monitoring Issues

Patient Education: Take as directed, for full course of therapy. Use caution when changing position (rising from sitting or lying) until response is known. Report CNS changes (eg, confusion, insomnia, anxiety, restlessness, irritability, hallucinations), difficulty urinating, or severe nausea or vomiting.

Monitoring Parameters: Monitor for CNS or GI effects in elderly or patients with renal or hepatic impairment

Manufacturer Forest Pharmaceutical, Inc

Related Information

Pharmaceutical Manufacturers Directory *on page 1020*

Rimexolone (ri MEKS oh lone)

Pharmacologic Class Adrenal Corticosteroid

U.S. Brand Names Vexol® Ophthalmic Suspension

Use Treatment of inflammation after ocular surgery and the treatment of anterior uveitis

USUAL DOSAGE Adults: Ophthalmic: Instill 1 drop in conjunctival sac 2-4 times/day up to every 4 hours; may use every 1-2 hours during first 1-2 days

Contraindications Fungal, viral, or untreated pus-forming bacterial ocular infections; hypersensitivity to any component

Pregnancy Risk Factor C

- **Riobin®** *see* Riboflavin *on page 819*
- **Riphenidate** *see* Methylphenidate *on page 588*

Risedronate (ris ED roe nate)

Pharmacologic Class Bisphosphonate Derivative

U.S. Brand Names Actonel™

Mechanism of Action A bisphosphonate which inhibits bone resorption via actions on osteoclasts or on osteoclast precursors; decreases the rate of bone resorption direction, leading to an indirect decrease in bone formation

Use Paget's disease of the bone

Unlabeled use: Osteoporosis in postmenopausal women

USUAL DOSAGE Oral:

Adults (patients with Paget's disease should receive supplemental calcium and vitamin D if dietary intake is inadequate):

Paget's disease of bone: 30 mg once daily for 2 months

Elderly: No dosage adjustment is necessary

Dosage adjustment in renal impairment: Cl_{cr} <30 mL/minute: **Not** recommended

Dosage Forms TAB: 30 mg

Contraindications Hypersensitivity to risedronate, bisphosphonates, or any component; hypocalcemia; abnormalities of the esophagus which delay esophageal emptying such as stricture or achalasia; inability to stand or sit upright for at least 30 minutes

Warnings/Precautions Use caution in patients with renal impairment; concomitant hormone replacement therapy with risedronate for osteoporosis in postmenopausal women is not recommended; hypocalcemia must be corrected before therapy initiation with risedronate; ensure adequate calcium and vitamin D intake to provide for enhanced needs in patients with Paget's disease in whom the pretreatment rate of bone turnover may be greatly elevated.

Pregnancy Risk Factor C

Adverse Reactions

>10%:

- Dermatological: Rash
- Gastrointestinal: Abdominal pain, diarrhea
- Neuromuscular & skeletal: Arthralgia

1% to 10%:

- Cardiovascular: Chest pain
- Central nervous system: Headache, dizziness
- Gastrointestinal: Belching, colitis, constipation, nausea
- Neuromuscular & skeletal: Bone pain, leg cramps, myasthenia
- Respiratory: Bronchitis, rales/rhinitis

Drug Interactions Decreased effect: Calcium supplements and antacids interfere with the absorption of risedronate

Onset May require weeks

Half-Life Terminal: 220 hours

Education and Monitoring Issues

Patient Education: In order to be effective, this drug must be taken exactly as prescribed. Take 30 minutes before first food of the day with 6-8 ounces of water and avoid lying down for 30 minutes after ingestion. You may experience headache (request analgesic); skin rash; or abdominal pain, diarrhea, or constipation (report if persistent). Report unresolved muscle or bone pain or leg cramps; acute abdominal pain; chest pain, palpitations, or swollen extremities; disturbed vision or excessively dry eyes; ringing in the ears; or persistent flu-like symptoms.

Dietary Considerations: Mean oral bioavailability is decreased when given with food. Take ≥30 minutes before the first food or drink of the day other than water.

Monitoring Parameters: Alkaline phosphatase should be periodically measured; serum calcium, phosphorus, and possibly potassium due to its drug class; use of absorptiometry may assist in noting benefit in osteoporosis; monitor pain and fracture rate

Reference Range: Calcium (total): Adults: 9.0-11.0 mg/dL (2.05-2.54 mmol/L), may slightly decrease with aging; phosphorus: 2.5-4.5 mg/dL (0.81-1.45 mmol/L)

♦ **Risperdal®** *see* Risperidone *on page 825*

Risperidone (ris PER i done)

Pharmacologic Class Antipsychotic Agent, Benzisoxazole

U.S. Brand Names Risperdal®

Mechanism of Action Risperidone is a benzisoxazole derivative, mixed serotonin-dopamine antagonist; binds to 5-HT_2-receptors in the CNS and in the periphery with a very high affinity; binds to dopamine-D_2 receptors with less affinity. The binding affinity to the dopamine-D_2 receptor is 20 times lower than the 5-HT_2 affinity. The addition of serotonin antagonism to dopamine antagonism (classic neuroleptic mechanism) is thought to improve negative symptoms of psychoses and reduce the incidence of extrapyramidal side effects.

Use Management of psychotic disorders (eg, schizophrenia); nonpsychotic symptoms associated with dementia in elderly

USUAL DOSAGE Recommended starting dose: 1 mg twice daily; slowly increase to the optimum range of 4-6 mg/day; daily dosages >6 mg does not appear to confer any

(Continued)

Risperidone *(Continued)*

additional benefit, and the incidence of extrapyramidal reactions is higher than with lower doses

Dosing adjustment in renal, hepatic impairment: Starting dose of 0.25-0.5 mg twice daily is advisable

Dosing adjustment in elderly patients; A starting dose of 0.5 mg twice daily is recommended, and titration should progress slowly. Additional monitoring or renal function and orthostatic blood pressure may be warranted. If once-a-day dosing in the elderly or debilitated patient is considered, a twice daily regimen should be used to titrate to the target dose, and this dose should be maintained for 2-3 days prior to attempts to switch to a once-daily regimen.

Dosage Forms SOLN, oral: 1 mg/mL (100 mL). **TAB:** 0.25 mg, 0.5 mg, 1 mg, 2 mg, 3 mg, 4 mg

Contraindications Known hypersensitivity to any component of the product

Pregnancy Risk Factor C

Adverse Reactions

1% to 10%:

Cardiovascular: Hypotension (especially orthostatic), tachycardia, arrhythmias, abnormal T waves with prolonged ventricular repolarization; EKG changes, syncope

Central nervous system: Sedation (occurs at daily doses ≥20 mg/day), headache, dizziness, restlessness, anxiety, extrapyramidal reactions, dystonic reactions, pseudoparkinson signs and symptoms, tardive dyskinesia, neuroleptic malignant syndrome, altered central temperature regulation

Dermatologic: Photosensitivity (rare)

Endocrine & metabolic: Amenorrhea, galactorrhea, gynecomastia sexual dysfunction (up to 60%)

Gastrointestinal: Constipation, adynamic ileus, GI upset, xerostomia (problem for denture user), nausea and anorexia, weight gain

Genitourinary: Urinary retention, overflow incontinence, priapism

Hematologic: Agranulocytosis, leukopenia (usually in patients with large doses for prolonged periods)

Hepatic: Cholestatic jaundice

Ocular: Blurred vision, retinal pigmentation, decreased visual acuity (may be irreversible)

<1%: Seizures

Drug Interactions CYP2D6 enzyme substrate and weak inhibitor; CYP3A4 substrate

Risperidone may enhance the hypotensive effects of antihypertensive agents

Risperidone may antagonize effects of levodopa; carbamazepine decreases risperidone serum concentrations; clozapine decreases clearance of risperidone

Alcohol Interactions Avoid use (may increase central nervous system depression)

Half-Life 24 hours (risperidone and its active metabolite)

Education and Monitoring Issues

Patient Education: Use exactly as directed (do not increase dose or frequency); may cause physical and/or psychological dependence. It may take 2-3 weeks to achieve desired results; do not discontinue without consulting prescriber. Dilute solution with water, milk, orange or grapefruit juice; do not dilute with beverages containing caffeine, tannin, or pactinate (eg, coffee, colas, tea, or apple juice). Avoid excess alcohol or caffeine and other prescription or OTC medications not approved by prescriber. Maintain adequate hydration (2-3 L/day of fluids unless instructed to restrict fluid intake). You may experience excess sedation, drowsiness, restlessness, dizziness, or blurred vision (use caution driving or when engaging in tasks requiring alertness until response to drug is known); dry mouth, nausea, or GI upset (small frequent meals, frequent mouth care, chewing gum, or sucking lozenges may help); postural hypotension (use caution climbing stairs or when changing position from lying or sitting to standing); or urinary retention (void before taking medication). Report persistent CNS effects (eg, trembling fingers, altered gait or balance, excessive sedation, seizures, unusual muscle or skeletal movements, anxiety, abnormal thoughts, confusion, personality changes); chest pain, palpitations, rapid heartbeat, severe dizziness; swelling or pain in breasts (male and female), altered menstrual pattern, sexual dysfunction; pain or difficulty on urination; vision changes; skin rash or yellowing of skin; difficulty breathing; or worsening of condition.

Manufacturer Janssen Pharmaceutical, Inc

Related Information

Pharmaceutical Manufacturers Directory *on page 1020*

♦ **Ritalin®** *see* Methylphenidate *on page 588*

♦ **Ritalin-SR®** *see* Methylphenidate *on page 588*

Ritodrine (RI toe dreen)

Pharmacologic Class $Beta_2$ Agonist

U.S. Brand Names Pre-Par®; Yutopar®

Generic Available No

Mechanism of Action Tocolysis due to its uterine beta$_2$-adrenergic receptor stimulating effects; this agent's beta$_2$ effects can also cause bronchial relaxation and vascular smooth muscle stimulation

Use Inhibits uterine contraction in preterm labor

USUAL DOSAGE Adults: I.V.: 50-100 mcg/minute; increase by 50 mcg/minute every 10 minutes; continue for 12 hours after contractions have stopped

Hemodialysis: Removed by hemodialysis

Dosage Forms INF: 0.3 mL (500 mL). **INJ:** 10 mg/mL (5 mL), 15 mg/mL (10 mL)

Contraindications Do not use before 20th week of pregnancy, cardiac arrhythmias, pheochromocytoma

Warnings/Precautions Monitor hydration status and blood glucose concentrations; fatal maternal pulmonary edema has been reported, sometimes after delivery; fluid overload must be avoided, hydration levels should be monitored closely; if pulmonary edema occurs, the drug should be discontinued; use with caution in patients with moderate pre-eclampsia, diabetes, or migraine; some products may contain sulfites; maternal deaths have been reported in patients treated with ritodrine and concurrent corticosteroids (pulmonary edema)

Pregnancy Risk Factor B

Adverse Reactions

>10%:

Cardiovascular: Increases in maternal and fetal heart rates and maternal hypertension, palpitations

Endocrine & metabolic: Temporary hyperglycemia

Gastrointestinal: Nausea, vomiting

Neuromuscular & skeletal: Tremor

1% to 10%:

Cardiovascular: Chest pain

Central nervous system: Nervousness, anxiety, restlessness

<1%: Anaphylactic shock, impaired LFTs, ketoacidosis

Drug Interactions

Decreased effect with beta-blockers

Increased effect/toxicity with meperidine, sympathomimetics, diazoxide, magnesium, betamethasone (pulmonary edema), potassium-depleting diuretics, general anesthetics

Half-Life 15 hours

Education and Monitoring Issues

Patient Education:

I.V.: Remain in left lateral position during infusion; do not get out of bed. Report rapid heartbeat, dizziness, difficulty breathing, nervousness or restlessness, skin itching or rash.

Oral: Take as directed and follow instruction of prescriber for physical activity. Report palpitations or chest pain, acute nausea or vomiting, difficulty breathing, skin irritation or rash, abdominal cramping, vaginal discharge, or other signs of labor.

Monitoring Parameters: Hematocrit, serum potassium, glucose, colloidal osmotic pressure, heart rate, and uterine contractions

Ritonavir (rye TON a veer)

Pharmacologic Class Antiretroviral Agent, Protease Inhibitor

U.S. Brand Names Norvir®

Use Treatment of HIV infection; should always be used as part of a multidrug regimen (at least 3 antiretroviral agents)

USUAL DOSAGE Oral:

Children: 250 mg/m^2 twice daily; titrate dose upward to 400 mg/m^2 twice daily (maximum: 600 mg twice daily)

Adults: 600 mg twice daily; dose escalation tends to avoid nausea that many patients experience upon initiation of full dosing. Escalate the dose as follows: 300 mg twice daily for 1 day, 400 mg twice daily for 2 days, 500 mg twice daily for 1 day, then 600 mg twice daily. Ritonavir may be better tolerated when used in combination with other antiretrovirals by initiating the drug alone and subsequently adding the second agent within 2 weeks.

If used in combination with saquinavir, dose is 400 mg twice daily

Ritonavir is being studied with a number of other antiretroviral agents to utilize its enzyme-inhibiting properties to increase serum concentrations of the coadministered agent. Ritonavir dosing ranges from 100-400 mg twice daily in these regimens.

Dosing adjustment in renal impairment: None necessary

Dosing adjustment in hepatic impairment: Not determined; caution advised with severe impairment

Contraindications Patients with known hypersensitivity to ritonavir or any ingredients; coadministration with ergotamine as dihydroergotamine has been associated with acute ergot toxicity

Contraindicated drugs:

Antiarrhythmics: Amiodarone, bepridil, flecainide, propafenone, quinidine

Antihistamines: Astemizole, terfenadine

Antimigraine: Dihydroergotamine, ergotamine

(Continued)

Ritonavir *(Continued)*

GI motility drugs: Cisapride
Neuroleptics: Pimozide
Sedatives/hypnotics: Midazolam, triazolam

Warnings/Precautions Use caution in patients with hepatic insufficiency; safety and efficacy have not been established in children <16 years of age; use caution with benzodiazepines, antiarrhythmics (flecainide, encainide, bepridil, amiodarone, quinidine) and certain analgesics (meperidine, piroxicam, propoxyphene); see Drug Interactions

Pregnancy Risk Factor B

Adverse Reactions Protease inhibitors cause dyslipidemia which includes elevated cholesterol and triglycerides and a redistribution of body fat centrally to cause "protease paunch", buffalo hump, facial atrophy, and breast enlargement. These agents also cause hyperglycemia, and new onset diabetes mellitus has been reported.

>10%:

Gastrointestinal: Diarrhea, nausea, vomiting, taste perversion
Endocrine & metabolic: Increased triglycerides, hypercholesterolemia
Hematologic: Anemia, decreased WBCs
Hepatic: Increased GGT
Neuromuscular & skeletal: Weakness

1% to 10%:

Cardiovascular: Vasodilation
Central nervous system: Fever, headache, malaise, dizziness, insomnia, somnolence, thinking abnormally
Dermatologic: Rash
Endocrine & metabolic: Hyperlipidemia, increased uric acid, increased glucose
Gastrointestinal: Abdominal pain, anorexia, constipation, dyspepsia, flatulence, local throat irritation
Hematologic: Neutropenia, eosinophilia, neutrophilia, prolonged PT, leukocytosis
Hepatic: Increased LFTs
Neuromuscular & skeletal: Increased CPK, myalgia, paresthesia
Respiratory: Pharyngitis
Miscellaneous: Diaphoresis, increased potassium, increased calcium

Drug Interactions CYP1A2, 2A6, 2C9, 2C19, 2E1, and 3A3/4 enzyme substrate, CYP2D6 enzyme substrate (minor); CYP1A2 enzyme inducer; CYP2A6, 2C9, 1A2, 2C19, 2D6, 2E1, and 3A3/4 inhibitor

Increased effect/toxicity:

Amprenavir AUC is increased by ritonavir
Antiarrhythmics (amiodarone, bepridil, flecainide, propafenone, quinidine) toxicity may be greatly increased - concurrent use of ritonavir is contraindicated
Astemizole and terfenadine - cardiac toxicity (arrhythmia) is increased - concurrent use is contraindicated
Benzodiazepines (clorazepate, diazepam, estazolam, flurazepam midazolam, triazolam) toxicity may be increased - concurrent use of midazolam and triazolam is specifically contraindicated
Cisapride toxicity (arrhythmia) may be increased by ritonavir - concurrent use is contraindicated
Clarithromycin serum concentrations are increased by ritonavir
Desipramine (and possibly other TCA's) serum levels may be increased by ritonavir, (requiring dosage adjustment)
Ergot alkaloids (dihydroergotamine, ergotamine) toxicity is increased by ritonavir - concurrent use is contraindicated
HMG CoA reductase inhibitors (atorvastatin, cerivastatin, lovastatin, simvastatin) serum concentrations may be increased by ritonavir, increasing the risk of myopathy/rhabdomyolysis
Indinavir serum concentrations are increased by ritonavir
Ketoconazole serum concentrations are increased by ritonavir
Meperidine: serum concentrations of metabolite (normeperidine) are increased by ritonavir, which may increase the risk of CNS toxicity
Pimozide toxicity is significantly increased by ritonavir - concurrent use is contraindicated
Rifampin and rifabutin metabolite serum concentrations may be increased by ritonavir; reduce rifabutin dose to 150 mg every other day
Sildenafil serum concentrations may be increased by ritonavir - do not exceed maximum 25mg in a 48 hour period

Ritonavir may also increase the serum concentrations of the following drugs–dose decrease may be needed: bupropion, carbamazepine, clonazepam, clorazepate, cyclosporin, dexamethasone, diltiazem, disopyramide, dronabinol, ethosuximide, fluoxetine (and other SSRI's), lidocaine, methamphetamine, metoprolol, mexiletine, nifedipine, nefazodone, perphenazine, prednisone, propoxyphene, quinine, risperidone, tacrolimus, tramadol, thioridazine, timolol, verapamil, zolpidem

Decreased effect:

Ethinyl estradiol serum concentrations may be decreased (may also decrease effectiveness of combo products)

Methadone serum concentrations are decreased by ritonavir
Theophylline serum concentrations may be decreased by ritonavir

In addition, ritonavir may decrease the serum concentrations of the following drugs--dose increase may be needed: atovaquone, divalproex, lamotrigine, phenytoin, warfarin

Manufacturer Abbott Laboratories (Pharmaceutical Product Division)

Related Information

Antiretroviral Therapy for HIV Infection *on page 1190*
Pharmaceutical Manufacturers Directory *on page 1020*

♦ **Rivotril®** *see* Clonazepam *on page 214*

Rizatriptan (rye za TRIP tan)

Pharmacologic Class Serotonin 5-HT_{1D} Receptor Agonist

U.S. Brand Names Maxalt®; Maxalt-MLT™

Mechanism of Action Selective agonist for serotonin (5-HT_{1D} receptor) in cranial arteries to cause vasoconstriction and reduce sterile inflammation associated with antidromic neuronal transmission correlating with relief of migraine

Use Acute treatment of migraine with or without aura

USUAL DOSAGE Oral: 5-10 mg, repeat after 2 hours if significant relief is not attained; maximum: 30 mg in a 24-hour period (use 5 mg dose in patients receiving propranolol with a maximum of 15 mg in 24 hours)

Dosage Forms TAB, as benzoate: (Maxalt®): 5 mg, 10 mg; (Maxalt-MLT™) (orally disintegrating): 5 mg, 10 mg

Contraindications Prior hypersensitivity to rizatriptan; documented ischemic heart disease or Prinzmetal's angina; uncontrolled hypertension; basilar or hemiplegic migraine; during or within 2 weeks of MAO inhibitors; during or within 24 hours of treatment with another 5HT-1 agonist, or an ergot-containing or ergot-type medication (eg, methysergide, dihydroergotamine)

Warnings/Precautions Use only in patients with a clear diagnosis of migraine; use with caution in elderly or patients with hepatic or renal impairment, history of hypersensitivity to sumatriptan or adverse effects from sumatriptan, and in patients at risk of coronary artery disease. Do not use with ergotamines. May increase blood pressure transiently; may cause coronary vasospasm (less than sumatriptan); avoid in patients with signs/symptoms suggestive of reduced arterial flow (ischemic bowel, Raynaud's) which could be exacerbated by vasospasm. Phenylketonurics (tablets contain phenylalanine).

Patients who experience sensations of chest pain/pressure/tightness or symptoms suggestive of angina following dosing should be evaluated for coronary artery disease or Prinzmetal's angina before receiving additional doses.

Caution in dialysis patients or hepatically impaired. Reconsider diagnosis of migraine if no response to initial dose. Long-term effects on vision have not been evaluated.

Pregnancy Risk Factor C

Adverse Reactions

1% to 10%:

Cardiovascular: Systolic/diastolic blood pressure increases (5-10 mm Hg), chest pain (5%)
Central nervous system: Dizziness, drowsiness, fatigue (13% to 30% - dose related)
Dermatologic: Skin flushing
Endocrine & metabolic: Mild increase in growth hormone, hot flashes
Gastrointestinal: Nausea, vomiting, abdominal pain, dry mouth (<5%)
Respiratory: Dyspnea

<1%: Arthralgia, blurred vision, bradycardia, chills, decreased mental activity, diaphoresis, dry eyes, eye pain, facial edema, hangover, heat sensitivity, muscle weakness, myalgia, nasopharyngeal irritation, neck pain/stiffness, neurological/psychiatric abnormalities, palpitation, polyuria, pruritus, syncope, tachycardia, tinnitus

Drug Interactions

Use within 24 hours of another selective 5-HT_1 agonist or ergot-containing drug should be avoided due to possible additive vasoconstriction

Propranolol: Plasma concentration of rizatriptan increased 70%

SSRIs: In one study, no effects on rizatriptan concentrations were observed where paroxetine (an SSRI) was given concurrently with rizatriptan; rarely, concurrent use of an SSRI with rizatriptan has resulted in weakness and incoordination; monitor closely

MAO inhibitors and nonselective MAO inhibitors increase concentration of rizatriptan

Onset Within 30 minutes

Duration 14-16 hours

Half-Life 2-3 hours

Education and Monitoring Issues

Patient Education: Administration of orally disintegrating tablets: Do not open blister pack before using. Open with dry hands. Do not crush, chew, or swallow tablet; allow to dissolve on tongue. Take as prescribed; do not increase dosing schedule. May repeat one time after 2 hours, if first dose is ineffective. Do not ever take more than two doses without consulting prescriber. You may experience dizziness or drowsiness (use caution when driving, climbing stairs, or engaging in tasks requiring alertness until

(Continued)

Rizatriptan *(Continued)*

response to drug is known); skin flushing or hot flashes (cool clothes or a cool environment may help); mild abdominal discomfort or nausea or vomiting. Report severe dizziness, acute headache, chest pain or palpitation, stiff or painful neck or facial swelling, muscle weakness or pain, changes in mental acuity, blurred vision, eye pain, or excessive perspiration or urination.

Dietary Considerations: Food delays the absorption

Monitoring Parameters: Headache severity, signs/symptoms suggestive of angina; consider monitoring blood pressure, heart rate, and/or EKG with first dose in patients with likelihood of unrecognized coronary disease, such as patients with significant hypertension, hypercholesterolemia, obese patients, diabetics, smokers with other risk factors or strong family history of coronary artery disease

Manufacturer Merck & Co

Related Information

Pharmaceutical Manufacturers Directory *on page 1020*

- ♦ **RMS® Rectal** *see* Morphine Sulfate *on page 618*
- ♦ **Robafen® AC** *see* Guaifenesin and Codeine *on page 424*
- ♦ **Robafen DM® [OTC]** *see* Guaifenesin and Dextromethorphan *on page 424*
- ♦ **Robaxin®** *see* Methocarbamol *on page 581*
- ♦ **Robaxisal®** *see* Methocarbamol and Aspirin *on page 582*
- ♦ **Robicillin® VK** *see* Penicillin V Potassium *on page 713*
- ♦ **Robidrine®** *see* Pseudoephedrine *on page 792*
- ♦ **Robinul®** *see* Glycopyrrolate *on page 417*
- ♦ **Robinul® Forte** *see* Glycopyrrolate *on page 417*
- ♦ **Robitussin® [OTC]** *see* Guaifenesin *on page 423*
- ♦ **Robitussin® A-C** *see* Guaifenesin and Codeine *on page 424*
- ♦ **Robitussin®-DAC** *see* Guaifenesin, Pseudoephedrine, and Codeine *on page 425*
- ♦ **Robitussin®-DM [OTC]** *see* Guaifenesin and Dextromethorphan *on page 424*
- ♦ **Robomol®** *see* Methocarbamol *on page 581*
- ♦ **Rocaltrol®** *see* Calcitriol *on page 129*
- ♦ **Rocephin®** *see* Ceftriaxone *on page 164*
- ♦ **RO-Dexsone** *see* Dexamethasone *on page 256*
- ♦ **Rofact®** *see* Rifampin *on page 820*

Rofecoxib (roe fe COX ib)

Pharmacologic Class Nonsteroidal Anti-Inflammatory Agent (NSAID)

U.S. Brand Names Vioxx®

Mechanism of Action Inhibits prostaglandin synthesis by decreasing the activity of the enzyme, cyclo-oxygenase-2 (COX-2), which results in decreased formation of prostaglandin precursors. Rofecoxib does not inhibit cyclo-oxygenase-1 (COX-1) at therapeutic concentrations.

Use Relief of the signs and symptoms of osteoarthritis; management of acute pain in adults; treatment of primary dysmenorrhea

USUAL DOSAGE Adult: Oral:

Osteoarthritis: 12.5 mg once daily; may be increased to a maximum of 25 mg once daily

Acute pain and management of dysmenorrhea: 50 mg once daily as needed (use for longer than 5 days is not recommended)

Dosing comment in renal impairment: Use in advanced renal disease is not recommended

Dosing adjustment in hepatic impairment: No specific dosage adjustment is recommended (AUC may be increased by 69%)

Elderly: No specific adjustment is recommended. However, the AUC in elderly patients may be increased by 34% as compared to younger subjects. Use the lowest recommended dose.

Dosage Forms SUSP, oral: 12.5 mg/5 mL, 25 mg/5 mL. **TAB:** 12.5 mg, 25 mg

Contraindications Hypersensitivity to rofecoxib or any component, aspirin, or other nonsteroidal anti-inflammatory drugs (NSAIDs)

Warnings/Precautions Gastrointestinal irritation, ulceration, bleeding, and perforation may occur with NSAIDs (it is unclear whether rofecoxib is associated with rates of these events which are similar to nonselective NSAIDs). Use with caution in patients with a history of GI disease (bleeding or ulcers), decreased renal function, hepatic disease, congestive heart failure, hypertension, or asthma. Anaphylactoid reactions may occur, even with no prior exposure to rofecoxib.

Pregnancy Risk Factor C; D (after 34 weeks gestation or close to delivery)

Pregnancy Implications In late pregnancy may cause premature closure of the ductus arteriosus. In animal studies, rofecoxib has been found to be excreted in milk. It is not known whether rofecoxib is excreted in human milk. Because many drugs are excreted in milk, and the potential for serious adverse reactions exists, a decision should be made whether to discontinue nursing or discontinue the drug, taking into account the importance of the drug to the mother.

Adverse Reactions

2% to 10%:

Cardiovascular: Peripheral edema (3.7%), hypertension (3.5%)

Central nervous system: Headache (4.7%), dizziness (3%), weakness (2.2%)

Gastrointestinal: Diarrhea (6.5%), nausea (5.2%), heartburn (4.2%), epigastric discomfort (3.8%), dyspepsia (3.5%), abdominal pain (3.4%)

Genitourinary: Urinary tract infection (2.8%)

Neuromuscular & skeletal: Back pain (2.5%)

Respiratory: Upper respiratory infection (8.5%), bronchitis (2.0%), sinusitis (2.7%)

Miscellaneous: Flu-like syndrome (2.9%)

0.1% to 2%:

Cardiovascular: Chest pain, upper extremity edema, atrial fibrillation, bradycardia, arrhythmia, palpitation, tachycardia, venous insufficiency, fluid retention

Central nervous system: Anxiety, depression, decreased mental acuity, hypesthesia, insomnia, neuropathy, migraine, paresthesia, somnolence, vertigo, fever, pain

Dermatologic: Alopecia, atopic dermatitis, basal cell carcinoma, contact dermatitis, pruritus, rash, erythema, urticaria, dry skin

Endocrine & metabolic: Weight gain, hypercholesteremia

Gastrointestinal: Reflux, abdominal distension, abdominal tenderness, constipation, dry mouth, esophagitis, flatulence, gastritis, gastroenteritis, hematochezia, hemorrhoids, oral ulceration, dental caries, aphthous stomatitis

Genitourinary: Breast mass, cystitis, dysuria, menopausal disorder, nocturia, urinary retention, vaginitis, pelvic pain

Hematologic: Hematoma

Neuromuscular & skeletal: Muscle spasm, sciatica, arthralgia, bursitis, cartilage trauma, joint swelling, muscle cramps, muscle weakness, myalgia, tendonitis, traumatic arthropathy, fracture (wrist)

Ocular: Blurred vision, conjunctivitis

Otic: Otic pain, otitis media, tinnitus

Respiratory: Asthma, cough, dyspnea, pneumonia, respiratory infection, pulmonary congestion, rhinitis, epistaxis, laryngitis, dry throat, pharyngitis, tonsillitis, diaphragmatic hernia

Miscellaneous: Allergy, fungal infection, insect bite reaction, syncope, viral syndrome, herpes simplex, herpes zoster, increased sweating

<0.1% (limited to severe): Breast cancer, cerebrovascular accident, cholecystitis, colitis, colonic neoplasm, congestive heart failure, deep venous thrombosis, duodenal ulcer, gastrointestinal bleeding, intestinal obstruction, lymphoma, myocardial infarction, pancreatitis, prostatic cancer, transient ischemic attack, unstable angina, urolithiasis

Drug Interactions CYP3A4 enzyme inducer (mild)

Increased effect: Cimetidine increases AUC of rofecoxib by 23%. Rofecoxib may increase plasma concentrations of methotrexate and lithium. Rofecoxib may be used with low-dose aspirin, however rates of gastrointestinal bleeding may be increased with coadministration. Rofecoxib may increase the INR in patients receiving warfarin and may increase the risk of bleeding complications.

Decreased effects: Efficacy of thiazide diuretics, loop diuretics (furosemide) or ACE-inhibitors may be diminished by rofecoxib. Rifampin reduces the serum concentration of rofecoxib by approximately 50%. Antacids may reduce rofecoxib absorption.

Alcohol Interactions Avoid use (may enhance gastric mucosal irritation)

Onset 45 minutes

Duration Up to >24 hours

Half-Life 17 hours

Education and Monitoring Issues

Patient Education: Do not take more than recommended dose. May be taken with food to reduce GI upset. Do not take with antacids. Avoid alcohol, aspirin, or OTC medication unless approved by prescriber. You may experience dizziness, confusion, or blurred vision (avoid driving or engaging in tasks requiring alertness until response to drug is known); anorexia, nausea, vomiting, taste disturbance, gastric distress (small frequent meals, frequent mouth care, sucking lozenges, or chewing gum may help). Stop taking medication and report immediately stomach pain or cramping, unusual bleeding or bruising, or blood in vomitus, stool, or urine. Report persistent insomnia; skin rash; unusual fatigue or easy bruising or bleeding; muscle pain, tremors, or weakness; sudden weight gain; changes in hearing (ringing in ears); changes in vision; changes in urination pattern; or respiratory difficulty.

Dietary Considerations: Time to peak concentrations are delayed when taken with a high-fat meal; however, peak concentration and AUC are unchanged. Rofecoxib may be taken without regard to meals.

Manufacturer Merck & Co

Related Information

Nonsteroidal Anti-Inflammatory Agents Comparison *on page 1248*
Pharmaceutical Manufacturers Directory *on page 1020*

- **Roferon-A®** *see* Interferon Alfa-2a *on page 474*
- **Rogaine®** *see* Minoxidil *on page 607*
- **Rogaine® Extra Strength for Men [OTC]** *see* Minoxidil *on page 607*

- **Rogaine® for Men [OTC]** *see* Minoxidil *on page 607*
- **Rogaine® for Women [OTC]** *see* Minoxidil *on page 607*
- **RO-Gentycin** *see* Gentamicin *on page 408*
- **Rogitine®** *see* Phentolamine *on page 726*
- **Rolaids® Calcium Rich [OTC]** *see* Calcium Carbonate *on page 130*
- **Rolatuss® Plain Liquid** *see* Chlorpheniramine and Phenylephrine *on page 186*
- **Romazicon™ Injection** *see* Flumazenil *on page 371*
- **RO-Naphz** *see* Naphazoline *on page 636*
- **Rondamine-DM® Drops** *see* Carbinoxamine, Pseudoephedrine, and Dextromethorphan *on page 140*
- **Rondec®-DM** *see* Carbinoxamine, Pseudoephedrine, and Dextromethorphan *on page 140*
- **Rondec® Drops** *see* Carbinoxamine and Pseudoephedrine *on page 140*
- **Rondec® Filmtab®** *see* Carbinoxamine and Pseudoephedrine *on page 140*
- **Rondec® Syrup** *see* Carbinoxamine and Pseudoephedrine *on page 140*
- **Rondec-TR®** *see* Carbinoxamine and Pseudoephedrine *on page 140*
- **RO-Parcaine** *see* Proparacaine *on page 782*

Ropinirole (roe PIN i role)

Pharmacologic Class Anti-Parkinson's Agent

U.S. Brand Names Requip™

Mechanism of Action Ropinirole has a high relative *in vitro* specificity and full intrinsic activity at the D_2 and D_3 dopamine receptor subtypes, binding with higher affinity to D_3 than to D_2 or D_4 receptor subtypes. Although precise mechanism of action of ropinirole is unknown, it is believed to be due to stimulation of postsynaptic dopamine D_2-type receptors within the caudate-putamen in the brain.

Use Treatment of idiopathic Parkinson's disease; in patients with early Parkinson's disease who were not receiving concomitant levodopa therapy as well as in patients with advanced disease on concomitant levodopa

USUAL DOSAGE Adults: Oral: Dosage should be increased to achieve a maximum therapeutic effect, balanced against the principle side effects of nausea, dizziness, somnolence, and dyskinesia

Recommended starting dose: 0.25 mg 3 times/day; based on individual patient response, the dosage should be titrated with weekly increments as described below:

Week 1: 0.25 mg 3 times/day; total daily dose: 0.75 mg
Week 2: 0.5 mg 3 times/day; total daily dose: 1.5 mg
Week 3: 0.75 mg 3 times/day; total daily dose: 2.25 mg
Week 4: 1 mg 3 times/day; total daily dose: 3 mg

After week 4, if necessary, daily dosage may be increased by 1.5 mg/day on a weekly basis up to a dose of 9 mg/day, and then by up to 3 mg/day weekly to a total of 24 mg/day

Dosage Forms TAB: 0.25 mg, 0.5 mg, 1 mg, 2 mg, 5 mg

Contraindications Hypersensitivity to ropinirole

Warnings/Precautions Syncope, sometimes associated with bradycardia, was observed in association with ropinirole in both early Parkinson's disease (without L-dopa) patients and advanced Parkinson's disease (with L-dopa) patients. Dopamine agonists appear to impair the systemic regulation of blood pressure resulting in postural hypotension, especially during dose escalation. Parkinson's disease patients appear to have an impaired capacity to respond to a postural challenge. Parkinson's patients being treated with dopaminergic agonists ordinarily require careful monitoring for signs and symptoms of postural hypotension, especially during dose escalation, and should be informed of this risk. In patients with Parkinson's disease who were not treated with L-dopa, 5.2% of those treated with ropinirole reported hallucinations as compared to 1.4% on a placebo.

Pregnancy Risk Factor C

Adverse Reactions

Early Parkinson's disease:

Cardiovascular: Syncope, dependent/leg edema, orthostatic symptoms, flushing, chest pain, hypotension, hypertension, tachycardia, palpitations

Central nervous system: Dizziness (40%), somnolence (40%), headache, fatigue, pain, confusion, hallucinations, amnesia, malaise, hypoesthesia, vertigo, yawning

Gastrointestinal: Nausea (60%), dyspepsia, abdominal pain, xerostomia, anorexia, flatulence, vomiting

Genitourinary: Impotence

Neuromuscular & skeletal: Weakness

Ocular: Abnormal vision

Respiratory: Pharyngitis, dyspnea, rhinitis, sinusitis

Miscellaneous: Viral infection, diaphoresis (increased)

Advanced Parkinson's disease (with levodopa):

Cardiovascular: Hypotension (2%), syncope (3%)

Central nervous system: Dizziness (26%), aggravated parkinsonism, somnolence, headache (17%), insomnia, hallucinations, confusion (9%), pain (5%), paresis (3%), amnesia (5%), anxiety (6%), abnormal dreaming (3%)

Gastrointestinal: Nausea (30%), abdominal pain (9%), vomiting (7%), constipation (6%), diarrhea (5%), dysphagia (2%), flatulence (2%), increased salivation (2%), xerostomia, weight loss (2%)
Genitourinary: Urinary tract infections
Neuromuscular & skeletal: Dyskinesias (34%), falls (10%), hypokinesia (5%), paresthesia (5%), tremor (6%), arthralgia (7%), arthritis (3%)
Respiratory: Upper respiratory tract infection
Miscellaneous: Injury, increased diaphoresis (7%), viral infection, increased drug level (7%)

Endocrine & metabolic: Hypoglycemia, increased LDH, hyperphosphatemia, hyperuricemia, diabetes mellitus, hypokalemia, hypercholesterolemia, hyperkalemia, acidosis, hyponatremia, dehydration, hypochloremia
Gastrointestinal: Weight increase
Hepatic: Increased alkaline phosphatase
Neuromuscular & skeletal: Increased CPK
Renal: Elevated BUN, glycosuria
Miscellaneous: Thirst, increased lactate dehydrogenase (LDH)

Drug Interactions CYP1A2 enzyme substrate

Ciprofloxacin and enoxacin may inhibit the metabolism of ropinirole; consider using ofloxacin or lomefloxacin
CYP1A2 inducers or inhibitors may alter ropinirole's clearance
Estrogens reduced the oral clearance of ropinirole by 36%; dosage adjustments may be needed
Dopamine antagonists (antipsychotics, metoclopramide) may diminish the effects of ropinirole

Education and Monitoring Issues

Patient Education: Ropinirole can be taken with or without food. Hallucinations can occur and elderly are at a higher risk than younger patients with Parkinson's disease. Postural hypotension may develop with or without symptoms such as dizziness, nausea, syncope, and sometimes sweating. Hypotension and/or orthostatic symptoms may occur more frequently during initial therapy or with an increase in dose at any time. Use caution when rising rapidly after sitting or lying down, especially after having done so for prolonged periods and especially at the initiation of treatment with ropinirole. Because of additive sedative effects, caution should be used when taking CNS depressants (eg, benzodiazepines, antipsychotics, antidepressants) in combination with ropinirole.

Manufacturer SmithKline Beecham Pharmaceuticals

Related Information

Parkinson's Disease Dosing *on page 1249*
Pharmaceutical Manufacturers Directory *on page 1020*

Ropivacaine (roe PIV a kane)

Pharmacologic Class Local Anesthetic

U.S. Brand Names Naropin™

Mechanism of Action Blocks both the initiation and conduction of nerve impulses by decreasing the neuronal membrane's permeability to sodium ions, which results in inhibition of depolarization with resultant blockade of conduction

Use Local anesthetic (injectable) for use in surgery, postoperative pain management, and obstetrical procedures when local or regional anesthesia is needed. It can be administered via local infiltration, epidural block and epidural infusion, or intermittent bolus.

USUAL DOSAGE Dose varies with procedure, onset and depth of anesthesia desired, vascularity of tissues, duration of anesthesia, and condition of patient

Adults:
Lumbar epidural for surgery: 15-30 mL of 0.5% to 1%
Lumbar epidural block for cesarean section: 20-30 mL of 0.5%
Thoracic epidural block for postoperative pain relief: 5-15 mL of 0.5%
Major nerve block: 35-50 mL dose of 0.5% (175-250 mg)
Field block: 1-40 mL dose of 0.5% (5-200 mg)
Lumbar epidural for labor pain: Initial: 10-20 mL 0.2%; continuous infusion dose: 6-14 mL/hour of 0.2% with incremental injections of 10-15 mL/hour of 0.2% solution

Dosage Forms INF: 2 mg/mL (100 mL, 200 mL). **INJ** (single dose): 2 mg/mL (20 mL), 5 mg/mL (30 mL), 7.5 mg/mL (10 mL, 20 mL), 10 mg/mL (10 mL, 20 mL)

Contraindications Hypersensitivity to amide-type local anesthetics (eg, bupivacaine, mepivacaine, lidocaine); septicemia, severe hypotension and for spinal anesthesia, in the presence of complete heart block

Warnings/Precautions Use with caution in patients with liver disease, cardiovascular disease, neurological or psychiatric disorders; it is not recommended for use in emergency situations where rapid administration is necessary

Pregnancy Risk Factor B

Adverse Reactions

>10% (dose and route related):
Cardiovascular: Hypotension, bradycardia
Gastrointestinal: Nausea, vomiting

(Continued)

Ropivacaine *(Continued)*

Neuromuscular & skeletal: Back pain
Miscellaneous: Shivering

1% to 10% (dose related):
Cardiovascular: Hypertension, tachycardia
Central nervous system: Headache, dizziness, anxiety, lightheadedness
Neuromuscular & skeletal: Hypoesthesia, paresthesia, circumoral paresthesia
Otic: Tinnitus
Respiratory: Apnea

Drug Interactions CYP2D6 enzyme substrate

Increased effect: Other local anesthetics or agents structurally related to the amide-type anesthetics

Increased toxicity (possible but not yet reported): Drugs that decrease CYP1A enzyme function

Onset 3-15 minutes

Duration 3-15 hours

Half-Life 5-7 hours

Manufacturer AstraZeneca

Related Information

Pharmaceutical Manufacturers Directory *on page 1020*

Rosiglitazone (roe si GLI ta zone)

Pharmacologic Class Antidiabetic Agent (Thiazolidinedione)

U.S. Brand Names Avandia®

Mechanism of Action Thiazolidinedione antidiabetic agent that lowers blood glucose by improving target cell response to insulin, without increasing pancreatic insulin secretion. It has a mechanism of action that is dependent on the presence of insulin for activity.

Use

Type II diabetes, monotherapy: Improve glycemic control as an adjunct to diet and exercise

Type II diabetes, combination therapy: In combination with metformin when diet, exercise and metformin alone or diet, exercise and rosiglitazone alone do not result in adequate glycemic control.

USUAL DOSAGE

Adults: Oral: Initial: 4 mg daily as a single daily dose or in divided doses twice daily. If response is inadequate after 12 weeks of treatment, the dosage may be increased to 8 mg daily as a single daily dose or in divided doses twice daily. In clinical trials, the 4 mg twice-daily regimen resulted in the greatest reduction in fasting plasma glucose and HbA_{1c}.

Changing patients from troglitazone to rosiglitazone: For patients with normal hepatic enzymes who are switched from troglitazone to rosiglitazone, a 1-week washout is recommended before initiating therapy with rosiglitazone.

Elderly: No dosage adjustment is recommended

Dosage adjustment in renal impairment: No dosage adjustment is required

Dosage comment in hepatic impairment: Clearance is significantly lower in hepatic impairment. Therapy should not be initiated if the patient exhibits active liver disease of increased transaminases (>2.5 times the upper limit of normal) at baseline.

Dosage Forms TAB: 2 mg, 4 mg, 8 mg

Contraindications Hypersensitivity to rosiglitazone or any component of the formulation; active liver disease (transaminases >2.5 times the upper limit of normal at baseline)

Warnings/Precautions Should not be used in diabetic ketoacidosis. Mechanism requires the presence of insulin, therefore use in type 1 diabetes is not recommended. Use with caution in premenopausal, anovulatory women; may result in resumption of ovulation, increasing the risk of pregnancy. May result in hormonal imbalance; development of menstrual irregularities should prompt reconsideration of therapy. Use with caution in patients with anemia or depressed leukocyte counts (may reduce hemoglobin, hematocrit, and/or WBC). Use with caution in patients with heart failure or edema; may increase in plasma volume and/or increase cardiac hypertrophy. In general, use should be avoided in patients with NYHA class 3 or 4 heart failure. Use with caution in patients with elevated transaminases (AST or ALT); see Contraindications and Monitoring. Idiosyncratic hepatotoxicity has been reported with another thiazolidinedione agent (troglitazone). Monitoring should include periodic determinations of liver function.

Pregnancy Risk Factor C

Pregnancy Implications Treatment during mid-late gestation was associated with fetal death and growth retardation in animal models. In animal studies, rosiglitazone has been found to be excreted in milk. It is not known whether rosiglitazone is excreted in human milk. Should not be administered to a nursing woman.

Adverse Reactions Two cases of hepatocellular injury have been reported in men in their 60s within 2-3 weeks after initiation of rosiglitazone therapy. LFTs in these patients revealed severe hepatocellular injury which responded with rapid improvement of liver function and resolution of symptoms upon discontinuation of rosiglitazone. Both patients were also receiving other hepatotoxic medications (*Ann Intern Med*, 2000, 132:121-4; 132:164-6).

>10%: Endocrine and Metabolic: Weight gain, increase in total cholesterol, increased LDL cholesterol, increased HDL cholesterol

1% to 10%:

Cardiovascular: Edema (4.8%)
Central nervous system: Headache (5.9%), fatigue (3.6%)
Endocrine & metabolic: Hyperglycemia (3.9%), hypoglycemia (0.5% to 1.6%)
Gastrointestinal: Diarrhea (2.3%)
Hematologic: Anemia (1.9%)
Neuromuscular & skeletal: Back pain (4%)
Respiratory: Upper respiratory tract infection (9.9%), sinusitis (3.2%)
Miscellaneous: Injury (7.6%)

<1%: Elevated transaminases, increased bilirubin

Drug Interactions CYP2C8 and 2C9 (minor) isoenzyme substrate; minor metabolism by CYP2C9

When rosiglitazone was coadministered with glyburide, metformin, digoxin, warfarin, ethanol, or ranitidine, no significant pharmacokinetic alterations were observed

Alcohol Interactions Avoid use (may cause hypoglycemia)

Onset Delayed, may require several weeks to reach maximum effect

Duration >24 hours

Half-Life 3-4 hours

Education and Monitoring Issues

Patient Education: May be taken without regard to meals. Follow directions of prescriber. If dose is missed at the usual meal, take it with next meal; do not double dose if daily dose is missed completely. Monitor urine or serum glucose as recommended by prescriber. More frequent monitoring is required during periods of stress, trauma, surgery, pregnancy, or increased activity or exercise. Avoid alcohol. You may gain weight (small nutritious meals, increased exercise may help - consult prescriber). Report chest pain, rapid heartbeat or palpitations, acute hyper- or hypoglycemic reactions, or persistent headache or back pain.

Dietary Considerations: Management of type 2 diabetes should include diet control. Peak concentrations are lower by 28% and delayed when administered with food, but these effects are not believed to be clinically significant. Rosiglitazone may be taken without regard to meals.

Monitoring Parameters: Hemoglobin A_{1c} liver enzymes (prior to initiation of therapy, every 2 months for the first year of therapy, then periodically thereafter). Patients with an elevation in ALT >3 times the upper limit of normal should be re-checked as soon as possible. If the ALT levels remain >3 times the upper limit of normal, therapy with rosiglitazone should be discontinued.

Manufacturer SmithKline Beecham Pharmaceuticals

Related Information

Hypoglycemic Drugs and Thiazolidinedione Information *on page 1240*
Pharmaceutical Manufacturers Directory *on page 1020*

- **RO-Tropamide** *see* Tropicamide *on page 958*
- **Roubac®** *see* Co-Trimoxazole *on page 230*
- **Rouhex-G** *see* Chlorhexidine Gluconate *on page 181*
- **Rowasa® Rectal** *see* Mesalamine *on page 568*
- **Roxanol™ Oral** *see* Morphine Sulfate *on page 618*
- **Roxanol Rescudose®** *see* Morphine Sulfate *on page 618*
- **Roxanol SR™ Oral** *see* Morphine Sulfate *on page 618*
- **Roxicet® 5/500** *see* Oxycodone and Acetaminophen *on page 692*
- **Roxicodone™** *see* Oxycodone *on page 691*
- **Roxilox™** *see* Oxycodone and Acetaminophen *on page 692*
- **Roxiprin®** *see* Oxycodone and Aspirin *on page 692*
- **Roychlor** *see* Potassium Chloride *on page 751*
- **R-Tannamine® Tablet** *see* Chlorpheniramine, Pyrilamine, and Phenylephrine *on page 187*
- **R-Tannate® Tablet** *see* Chlorpheniramine, Pyrilamine, and Phenylephrine *on page 187*
- **Rubramin®** *see* Cyanocobalamin *on page 233*
- **Rubramin-PC®** *see* Cyanocobalamin *on page 233*
- **Rum-K®** *see* Potassium Chloride *on page 751*
- **Ru-Tuss®** *see* Chlorpheniramine, Phenylephrine, Phenylpropanolamine, and Belladonna Alkaloids *on page 187*
- **Ru-Tuss® Liquid** *see* Chlorpheniramine and Phenylephrine *on page 186*
- **Ru-Vert-M®** *see* Meclizine *on page 556*
- **Ryna-C® Liquid** *see* Chlorpheniramine, Pseudoephedrine, and Codeine *on page 187*
- **Rynacrom®** *see* Cromolyn Sodium *on page 231*
- **Ryna-CX®** *see* Guaifenesin, Pseudoephedrine, and Codeine *on page 425*
- **Rynatan®** *see* Azatadine and Pseudoephedrine *on page 84*

- **Rynatan® Pediatric Suspension** *see* Chlorpheniramine, Pyrilamine, and Phenylephrine *on page 187*
- **Rynatan® Tablet** *see* Chlorpheniramine, Pyrilamine, and Phenylephrine *on page 187*
- **Rynatuss® Pediatric Suspension** *see* Chlorpheniramine, Ephedrine, Phenylephrine, and Carbetapentane *on page 186*
- **Rythmodan** *see* Disopyramide *on page 287*
- **Rythmol®** *see* Propafenone *on page 781*
- **S** *see* Flurazepam *on page 383*
- **Sabulin®** *see* Albuterol *on page 27*
- **Safe Tussin® 30 [OTC]** *see* Guaifenesin and Dextromethorphan *on page 424*
- **Saizen® Injection** *see* Human Growth Hormone *on page 438*
- **Salagen® Oral** *see* Pilocarpine *on page 736*
- **Saleto-200® [OTC]** *see* Ibuprofen *on page 458*
- **Saleto-400®** *see* Ibuprofen *on page 458*
- **Salflex®** *see* Salsalate *on page 837*
- **Salgesic®** *see* Salsalate *on page 837*

Salicylic Acid and Lactic Acid (sal i SIL ik AS id & LAK tik AS id)

Pharmacologic Class Keratolytic Agent

U.S. Brand Names Duofilm® Solution

Dosage Forms SOLN, top: Salicylic acid 16.7% and lactic acid 16.7% in flexible collodion (15 mL)

Pregnancy Risk Factor C

Salicylic Acid and Propylene Glycol

(sal i SIL ik AS id & PROE pi leen GLYE cole)

Pharmacologic Class Keratolytic Agent

U.S. Brand Names Keralyt® Gel

Dosage Forms GEL, top: Salicylic acid 6% and propylene glycol 60% in ethyl alcohol 19.4% with hydroxypropyl methylcellulose and water (30 g)

Pregnancy Risk Factor C

- **SalineX® [OTC]** *see* Sodium Chloride *on page 858*

Salmeterol (sal ME te role)

Pharmacologic Class $Beta_2$ Agonist

U.S. Brand Names Serevent®; Serevent® Diskus®

Mechanism of Action Relaxes bronchial smooth muscle by selective action on $beta_2$-receptors with little effect on heart rate; because salmeterol acts locally in the lung, therapeutic effect is not predicted by plasma levels

Use Maintenance treatment of asthma and in prevention of bronchospasm in patients >12 years of age with reversible obstructive airway disease, including patients with symptoms of nocturnal asthma, who require regular treatment with inhaled, short-acting $beta_2$ agonists; prevention of exercise-induced bronchospasm; treatment of COPD-induced bronchospasm

USUAL DOSAGE

Inhalation: 42 mcg (2 puffs) twice daily (12 hours apart) for maintenance and prevention of symptoms of asthma

Prevention of exercise-induced asthma: 42 mcg (2 puffs) 30-60 minutes prior to exercise; additional doses should not be used for 12 hours

COPD: Adults: For maintenance treatment of bronchospasm associated with COPD (including chronic bronchitis and emphysema): 2 inhalations (42 mcg) twice daily (morning and evening - 12 hours apart); do not use a spacer with the inhalation powder

Dosage Forms AERO, oral: 21 mcg/spray [60 inhalations] (6.5 g), [120 inhalations] (13 g). **INH:** 25 mcg/metered inhalation. **POWDER for inhalation, oral** (Serevent® Diskus®): 50 mcg [46 mcg/inhalation] (60 doses)

Contraindications Hypersensitivity to salmeterol, adrenergic amines or any ingredients; need for acute bronchodilation; within 2 weeks of MAO inhibitor use

Warnings/Precautions Salmeterol is not meant to relieve acute asthmatic symptoms. Acute episodes should be treated with short-acting $beta_2$ agonist. Do not increase the frequency of salmeterol. Cardiovascular effects are not common with salmeterol when used in recommended doses. All beta agonists may cause elevation in blood pressure, heart rate, and result in excitement (CNS). Use with caution in patients with prostatic hypertrophy, diabetes, cardiovascular disorders, convulsive disorders, thyrotoxicosis, or others who are sensitive to the effects of sympathomimetic amines. Paroxysmal bronchospasm (which can be fatal) has been reported with this and other inhaled agents. If this occurs, discontinue treatment. The elderly may be at greater risk of cardiovascular side effects; safety and efficacy have not been established in children <12 years of age.

Pregnancy Risk Factor C

Adverse Reactions

>10%:

Central nervous system: Headache

Respiratory: Pharyngitis

1% to 10%:

Cardiovascular: Tachycardia, palpitations, elevation or depression of blood pressure, cardiac arrhythmias

Central nervous system: Nervousness, CNS stimulation, hyperactivity, insomnia, malaise, dizziness

Gastrointestinal: GI upset, diarrhea, nausea

Neuromuscular & skeletal: Tremors (may be more common in the elderly), myalgias, back pain, arthralgia

Respiratory: Upper respiratory infection, cough, bronchitis

<1%: Immediate hypersensitivity reactions (rash, urticaria, bronchospasm)

Drug Interactions CYP3A3/4 enzyme substrate

Decreased effect: Beta-adrenergic blockers (eg, propranolol)

Increased toxicity (cardiovascular): MAO inhibitors, tricyclic antidepressants

Onset 5-20 minutes (average 10 minutes); Peak effect: 2-4 hours

Duration 12 hours

Half-Life 3-4 hours

Education and Monitoring Issues

Patient Education: Use exactly as directed. Do not use more often than recommended (excessive use may result in tolerance, overdose may result in serious adverse effects) and do not discontinue without consulting prescriber. Do not use for acute attacks. Maintain adequate hydration (2-3 L/day of fluids unless instructed to restrict fluid intake). You may experience nervousness, dizziness, or fatigue (use caution when driving or engaging in tasks requiring alertness until response to drug is known); or dry mouth, stomach upset (frequent small meals, frequent mouth care, chewing gum, or sucking hard candy may help). Report unresolved GI upset; dizziness or fatigue; vision changes; chest pain, rapid heartbeat, or palpitations; insomnia; nervousness or hyperactivity; muscle cramping, tremors, or pain; unusual cough; or skin rash.

Monitoring Parameters: Pulmonary function tests, blood pressure, pulse, CNS stimulation

Manufacturer GlaxoWellcome

Related Information

Bronchodilators Comparison *on page 1235*

Pharmaceutical Manufacturers Directory *on page 1020*

♦ **Salmonine® Injection** *see* Calcitonin *on page 128*

♦ **Salofalk** *see* Mesalamine *on page 568*

Salsalate (SAL sa late)

Pharmacologic Class Salicylate

U.S. Brand Names Argesic®-SA; Artha-G®; Disalcid®; Marthritic®; Mono-Gesic®; Salflex®; Salgesic®; Salsitab®

Generic Available Yes

Mechanism of Action Inhibits prostaglandin synthesis, acts on the hypothalamus heat-regulating center to reduce fever, blocks prostaglandin synthetase action which prevents formation of the platelet-aggregating substance thromboxane A_2

Use Treatment of minor pain or fever; arthritis

USUAL DOSAGE Adults: Oral: 3 g/day in 2-3 divided doses

Dosing comments in renal impairment: In patients with end-stage renal disease undergoing hemodialysis: 750 mg twice daily with an additional 500 mg after dialysis

Dosage Forms CAP: 500 mg. **TAB:** 500 mg, 750 mg

Contraindications GI ulcer or bleeding, known hypersensitivity to salsalate

Warnings/Precautions Use with caution in patients with platelet and bleeding disorders, renal dysfunction, erosive gastritis, or peptic ulcer disease, previous nonreaction does not guarantee future safe taking of medication; do not use aspirin in children <16 years of age for chickenpox or flu symptoms due to the association with Reye's syndrome

Pregnancy Risk Factor C

Adverse Reactions

>10%: Gastrointestinal: Nausea, heartburn, stomach pains, dyspepsia

1% to 10%:

Central nervous system: Fatigue

Dermatologic: Rash

Gastrointestinal: Gastrointestinal ulceration

Hematologic: Hemolytic anemia

Neuromuscular & skeletal: Weakness

Respiratory: Dyspnea

Miscellaneous: Anaphylactic shock

<1%: Bronchospasm, does not appear to inhibit platelet aggregation, hepatotoxicity, impaired renal function, insomnia, iron deficiency anemia, jitters, leukopenia, nervousness, occult bleeding, thrombocytopenia

Drug Interactions

Decreased effect with urinary alkalinizers, antacids, corticosteroids; decreased effect of uricosurics, spironolactone

(Continued)

Salsalate *(Continued)*

Increased effect/toxicity of oral anticoagulants, hypoglycemics, methotrexate

Alcohol Interactions Avoid use (may enhance gastric mucosal irritation)

Onset Therapeutic effects occur within 3-4 days of continuous dosing

Half-Life 7-8 hours

Education and Monitoring Issues

Patient Education: Take this medication exactly as directed; do not increase dose without consulting prescriber. Do not crush tablets or break capsules. Take with food or milk to reduce GI distress. Maintain adequate fluid intake (2-3 L/day of fluids unless instructed to restrict fluid intake). Do not use alcohol, aspirin, or aspirin-containing medication, or any other anti-inflammatory medications without consulting prescriber. You may experience drowsiness (use caution when driving or engaging in tasks requiring alertness until response to drug is known); nausea or heartburn (frequent small meals, frequent mouth care, sucking lozenges, or chewing gum may help). GI bleeding, ulceration, or perforation can occur with or without pain; discontinue medication and contact prescriber if persistent abdominal pain, cramping, or blood in stool occurs. Report breathlessness or difficulty breathing; unusual bruising/bleeding; blood in urine, stool, mouth, or vomitus; unusual fatigue; skin rash or itching; change in urinary pattern; or change in hearing or ringing in ears.

♦ **Salsitab®** *see* Salsalate *on page 837*

SAMe

Pharmacologic Class Nutraceutical

Mechanism of Action S-adenosyl methionine is involved in several primary biochemical pathways. It functions as a methyl donor in synthetic pathways which form nucleic acids (DNA and RNA), proteins, phospholipids, and neurotransmitters. SAMe's role in phospholipid synthesis may influence membrane fluidity. It has also been noted to protect neuronal anoxia and promote myelination of nerve fibers. It is involved in trans-sulfuration reactions, regulating formation of sulfur-containing amino acids such as cysteine, glutathione, and taurine. Of note, glutathione is an important antioxidant, involved in the detoxification of a number of physiologic and environmental toxins. SAMe is also a cofactor in the synthesis of polyamines, which include spermidine, puescine, and spermine. Polyamines are essential for cellular growth and differentiation by virtue of their effects on gene expression, protein phosphorylation, neuron regeneration, and the DNA repair.

Use

Cardiovascular disease (Loehrer, 1996)
Depression (Kagan, 1990; Fava, 1995; Bressa, 1994; Rosenbaum, 1990)
Fibromyalgia (Jacobsen, 1991)
Insomnia (Sitaram, 1995)
Liver disease (Miglio, 1975)
Osteoarthritis (di Padova, 1987)
Rheumatoid arthritis (Polli, 1975)

USUAL DOSAGE Oral: Dosage range: 400-1600 mg/day

Dosage Forms S-adenosyl methionine

Adverse Reactions

Drug/Nutrient Interactions: May potentiate activity and/or toxicities of MAO inhibitors, tricyclic antidepressants, or SSRIs (not documented)

Nutrient/Nutrient Interactions: May potentiate the antidepressant effects of 5-HTP, tryptophan, and St John's wort

♦ **Sandimmune® Injection** *see* Cyclosporine *on page 237*
♦ **Sandimmune® Oral** *see* Cyclosporine *on page 237*
♦ **Sandoglobulin®** *see* Immune Globulin, Intravenous *on page 465*
♦ **Sandostatin®** *see* Octreotide Acetate *on page 670*
♦ **Sandostatin LAR® Depot** *see* Octreotide Acetate *on page 670*
♦ **Sang® CyA** *see* Cyclosporine *on page 237*
♦ **Sansert®** *see* Methysergide *on page 592*
♦ **Santyl®** *see* Collagenase *on page 227*
♦ **Sapoderm** *see* Hexachlorophene *on page 436*

Saquinavir (sa KWIN a veer)

Pharmacologic Class Antiretroviral Agent, Protease Inhibitor

U.S. Brand Names Fortovase®; Invirase®

Use Treatment of HIV infection in selected patients; used in combination with at least two other antiretroviral agents

USUAL DOSAGE Adults: Oral:

Fortovase®: Six 200 mg capsules (1200 mg) 3 times/day within 2 hours after a meal in combination with a nucleoside analog

Invirase®: Three 200 mg capsules (600 mg) 3 times/day within 2 hours after a full meal in combination with a nucleoside analog

Dose of either Fortovase® or Invirase® in combination with ritonavir: 400 mg twice daily

Contraindications Hypersensitivity to saquinavir or any components; exposure to direct sunlight without sunscreen or protective clothing; coadministration with terfenadine, cisapride, astemizole, triazolam, midazolam, or ergot derivatives

Warnings/Precautions The indication for saquinavir for the treatment of HIV infection is based on changes in surrogate markers. At present, there are no results from controlled clinical trials evaluating its effect on patient survival or the clinical progression of HIV infection (ie, occurrence of opportunistic infections or malignancies); use caution in patients with hepatic insufficiency; safety and efficacy have not been established in children <16 years of age. May exacerbate pre-existing hepatic dysfunction; use with caution in patients with hepatitis B or C and in cirrhosis

Pregnancy Risk Factor B

Adverse Reactions Protease inhibitors cause dyslipidemia which includes elevated cholesterol and triglycerides and a redistribution of body fat centrally to cause "protease paunch", buffalo hump, facial atrophy, and breast enlargement. These agents also cause hyperglycemia.

1% to 10%:

- Dermatologic: Rash
- Endocrine & metabolic: Hyperglycemia
- Gastrointestinal: Diarrhea, abdominal discomfort, nausea, abdominal pain, buccal mucosa ulceration
- Neuromuscular & skeletal: Paresthesia, weakness, increased CPK

<1%: Acute myeloblastic leukemia, altered AST/ALT/bilirubin/Hgb, ascites, ataxia, bullous skin eruption, confusion, elevated LFTs, exacerbation of chronic liver disease, headache, hemolytic anemia, hyper- and hypokalemia, hypoglycemia, jaundice, low serum amylase, pain, polyarthritis, portal hypertension, seizures, Stevens-Johnson syndrome, thrombocytopenia, thrombophlebitis, upper quadrant abdominal pain

Drug Interactions CYP3A3/4 enzyme substrate; CYP3A3/4 enzyme inhibitor

Decreased effect: Rifampin may decrease saquinavir's plasma levels and AUC by 40% to 80%; other enzyme inducers may induce saquinavir's metabolism (eg, phenobarbital, phenytoin, dexamethasone, carbamazepine); may decrease delavirdine concentrations

Increased effect: Ketoconazole significantly increases plasma levels and AUC of saquinavir; as a known, although not potent inhibitor of the cytochrome P-450 system, saquinavir may decrease the metabolism of terfenadine and astemizole, as well as cisapride, ergot derivatives, midazolam, and triazolam (and result in rare but serious effects including cardiac arrhythmias or prolonged sedation); other drugs which may have increased adverse effects if coadministered with saquinavir include calcium channel blockers, clindamycin, dapsone, and quinidine. Both clarithromycin and saquinavir levels/effects may be increased with coadministration. Delavirdine may increase concentration; ritonavir may increase AUC >17-fold; concurrent administration of nelfinavir results in increase in nelfinavir (18%) and saquinavir (mean: 392%).

Saquinavir increased serum concentrations of simvastatin and atorvastatin. Use cautiously with HMG-CoA reductase inhibitors. Avoid use with simvastatin.

Manufacturer Roche Laboratories

Related Information

Antiretroviral Therapy for HIV Infection *on page 1190*
Management of Healthcare Worker Exposures to HIV *on page 1151*
Pharmaceutical Manufacturers Directory *on page 1020*

Sargramostim (sar GRAM oh stim)

Pharmacologic Class Colony Stimulating Factor

U.S. Brand Names Leukine™

Generic Available No

Mechanism of Action Sargramostim induces partially committed progenitor cells in the granulocyte-macrophage pathway to divide and differentiate, resulting in proliferation, differentiation, and increased functional activity of neutrophils, eosinophils, monocytes, and macrophages

Use

Stimulation of myeloid regeneration following:

- Allogenic bone marrow transplantation
- Autologous bone marrow transplantation
- Peripheral blood progenitor cell (PBPC) transplantation

Stimulation of PBPC production in patients undergoing PBPC collection

Stimulation of granulocyte production in patients receiving myelosuppressive therapy associated with a significant risk of neutropenia

Shorten neutrophil recovery time following induction therapy for acute myelogenous leukemia (AML)

Engraftment delay or failure, following bone marrow transplantation

USUAL DOSAGE

Children and Adults: I.V. infusion over ≥2 hours or S.C.

Existing clinical data suggest that starting GM-CSF between 24 and 72 hours subsequent to chemotherapy may provide optimal neutrophil recover; continue therapy until the occurrence of an absolute neutrophil count of 10,000/μL after the neutrophil nadir

(Continued)

Sargramostim *(Continued)*

The available data suggest that rounding the dose to the nearest vial size may enhance patient convenience and reduce costs without clinical detriment

Myeloid reconstitution after peripheral stem cell, allogeneic or autologous bone marrow transplant: I.V.: 250 mcg/m²/day for 21 days to begin 2-4 hours after the marrow infusion on day 0 of autologous bone marrow transplant or ≥24 hours after chemotherapy or 12 hours after last dose of radiotherapy

If a severe adverse reaction occurs, reduce or temporarily discontinue the dose until the reaction abates

If blast cells appear or progression of the underlying disease occurs, disrupt treatment

Interrupt or reduce the dose by half if ANC is >20,000 cells/mm³

Patients should not receive sargramostim until the postmarrow infusion ANC is <500 cells/mm³

Neutrophil recovery following chemotherapy in AML: I.V.: 250 mg/m²/day over a 4-hour period starting ~day 11 or 4 days following the completion of induction chemotherapy, if day 10 bone marrow is hypoblastic with <5% blasts

If a second cycle of chemotherapy is necessary, administer ~4 days after the completion of chemotherapy if the bone marrow is hypoblastic with <5% blasts

Continue sargramostim until ANC is >1500 cells/mm³ for consecutive days or a maximum of 42 days

Discontinue sargramostim immediately if leukemic regrowth occurs

If a severe adverse reaction occurs, reduce the dose by 50% or temporarily discontinue the dose until the reaction abates

Mobilization of peripheral blood progenitor cells: I.V.: 250 mcg/m²/day over 24 hours or S.C. once daily

Continue the same dose through the period of PBPC collection

The optimal schedule for PBPC collection has not been established (usually begun by day 5 and performed daily until protocol specified targets are achieved)

If WBC >50,000 cells/mm³, reduce the dose by 50%

If adequate numbers of progenitor cells are not collected, consider other mobilization therapy

Postperipheral blood progenitor cell transplantation: I.V.: 250 mcg/m²/day over 24 hours or S.C. once daily beginning immediately following infusion of progenitor cells and continuing until ANC is >1500 for 3 consecutive days is attained

BMT failure or engraftment delay: I.V.: 250 mcg/m²/day for 14 days as a 2-hour infusion

The dose can be repeated after 7 days off therapy if engraftment has not occurred

If engraftment still has not occurred, a third course of 500 mcg/m²/day for 14 days may be tried after another 7 days off therapy; if there is still no improvement, it is unlikely that further dose escalation will be beneficial

If a severe adverse reaction occurs, reduce or temporarily discontinue the dose until the reaction abates

If blast cells appear or disease progression occurs, discontinue treatment

Dosage Forms INJ: 250 mcg, 500 mcg

Contraindications GM-CSF is contraindicated in the following instances:

Patients with excessive myeloid blasts (>10%) in the bone marrow or peripheral blood

Patients with known hypersensitivity to GM-CSF, yeast-derived products, or any known component of the product

Warnings/Precautions Simultaneous administration with cytotoxic chemotherapy or radiotherapy or administration 24 hours preceding or following chemotherapy is recommended. Use with caution in patients with pre-existing cardiac problems, hypoxia, fluid retention, pulmonary infiltrates or congestive heart failure, renal or hepatic impairment.

Rapid increase in peripheral blood counts: If ANC >20,000/mm³ or platelets >500,000/mm³, decrease dose by 50% or discontinue drug (counts will fall to normal within 3-7 days after discontinuing drug)

Growth factor potential: Use with caution with myeloid malignancies. Precaution should be exercised in the usage of GM-CSF in any malignancy with myeloid characteristics. GM-CSF can potentially act as a growth factor for any tumor type, particularly myeloid malignancies. Tumors of nonhematopoietic origin may have surface receptors for GM-CSF.

There is a "first-dose effect" (refer to Adverse Reactions for details) which is rarely seen with the first dose and does not usually occur with subsequent doses.

Pregnancy Risk Factor C

Pregnancy Implications Clinical effects to the fetus: Animal reproduction studies have not been conducted. It is not known whether sargramostim can cause fetal harm when administered to a pregnant woman or can affect reproductive capability. Sargramostim should be given to a pregnant woman only if clearly needed.

Adverse Reactions

>10%:

"First-dose" effects: Fever, hypotension, tachycardia, rigors, flushing, nausea, vomiting, dyspnea

Central nervous system: Neutropenic fever

Dermatologic: Alopecia

Endocrine & metabolic: Polydipsia
Gastrointestinal: Nausea, vomiting, diarrhea, stomatitis, GI hemorrhage, mucositis
Neuromuscular & skeletal: Bone pain, myalgia

1% to 10%:
Cardiovascular: Chest pain, peripheral edema, capillary leak syndrome
Central nervous system: Headache
Dermatologic: Rash
Endocrine & metabolic: Fluid retention
Gastrointestinal: Anorexia, sore throat, stomatitis, constipation
Hematologic: Leukocytosis
Local: Pain at injection site
Neuromuscular & skeletal: Weakness
Respiratory: Dyspnea, cough

<1%: Anaphylactic reaction, flushing, hypotension, malaise, pericardial effusion, pericarditis, thrombophlebitis, transient supraventricular arrhythmias

Drug Interactions
Increased toxicity: Lithium, corticosteroids may potentiate myeloproliferative effects

Onset Increase in WBC in 7-14 days

Duration WBC will return to baseline within 1 week after discontinuing drug.

Half-Life 2 hours

Education and Monitoring Issues

Patient Education: You may experience bone pain (request analgesic), nausea and vomiting (small frequent meals may help), hair loss (reversible). Report fever, chills, unhealed sores, severe bone pain, difficulty breathing, fluid retention, increased weight, swelling or pain at infusion site. Avoid crowds or exposure to infected persons; you will be susceptible to infection.

Monitoring Parameters: To avoid potential complications of excessive leukocytosis (WBC >50,000 cells/mm^3, ANC >20,000 cells/mm^3) a CBC with differential is recommended twice weekly during therapy. Sargramostim therapy should be interrupted or the dose reduced by half if the ANC is >20,000 cells/mm^3. Monitoring of renal and hepatic function in patients displaying renal or hepatic dysfunction prior to initiation of treatment is recommended and at least biweekly during sargramostim administration.

Reference Range: Excessive leukocytosis: ANC >20,000/mm^3 or WBC >50,000 cells/mm^3

Manufacturer Immunex Corp

Related Information
Filgrastim *on page 363*
Pharmaceutical Manufacturers Directory *on page 1020*

♦ **Sarna HC** *see* Hydrocortisone *on page 447*

Sassafras Oil

Pharmacologic Class Herbal

Mechanism of Action Contains safrole (up to 80%) which inhibits liver microsomal enzymes; its metabolite may cause hepatic tumors

Use Banned by FDA in food since 1960; has been used as a mild counterirritant on the skin (ie, for lice or insect bites); should not be ingested

USUAL DOSAGE Sassafras tea can contain as much as 200 mg (3 mg/kg) of safrole
Lethal dose: ~5 mL
Toxic dose: 0.66 mg/kg is considered to be toxic to humans based on rodent studies

Adverse Reactions (Primarily related to sassafras oil and safrole)
Cardiovascular: Tachycardia, flushing, hypotension, sinus tachycardia
Central nervous system: Anxiety, hallucinations, vertigo, aphasia
Dermatologic: Contact dermatitis
Gastrointestinal: Vomiting
Hepatic: Fatty changes of the liver, hepatic necrosis
Ocular: Mydriasis
Miscellaneous: Diaphoresis

Little documentation of adverse effects due to ingestion of herbal tea

Education and Monitoring Issues

Patient Education: Considered unsafe by the FDA

Saw Palmetto

Pharmacologic Class Herbal

Mechanism of Action Liposterolic extract of the berries may inhibit the enzymes 5α-reductase, along with cyclo-oxygenase and 5-lipoxygenase, thus exhibiting antiandrogen and anti-inflammatory effects; does not reduce prostatic enlargement but may help increase urinary flow (not FDA approved)

Use Benign prostatic hyperplasia

USUAL DOSAGE Adults: Dried fruit: 0.5-1 g 3 times/day

Contraindications Pregnancy and breast-feeding

Pregnancy Implications Do not use

(Continued)

Saw Palmetto *(Continued)*

Adverse Reactions

Central nervous system: Headache
Endocrine & metabolic: Gynecomastia
Gastrointestinal: Stomach problems (in rare cases) per Commission E

- ♦ **Scabene®** *see* Lindane *on page 531*
- ♦ **Scalpicin®** *see* Hydrocortisone *on page 447*
- ♦ **Scheinpharm Testone-Cyp** *see* Testosterone *on page 898*
- ♦ **Scheinpharm Triamcine-A** *see* Triamcinolone *on page 944*
- ♦ **Scholl Athlete's Foot Preparations** *see* Tolnaftate *on page 931*
- ♦ **Sclavo-PPD Solution®** *see* Tuberculin Purified Protein Derivative *on page 960*
- ♦ **Sclavo-PPD Solution®** *see* Tuberculin Tests *on page 960*
- ♦ **Sclavo Test-PPD®** *see* Tuberculin Purified Protein Derivative *on page 960*
- ♦ **Sclavo Test-PPD®** *see* Tuberculin Tests *on page 960*
- ♦ **Scopace™ Tablet** *see* Scopolamine *on page 842*

Scopolamine (skoe POL a meen)

Pharmacologic Class Anticholinergic Agent

U.S. Brand Names Isopto® Hyoscine Ophthalmic; Scopace™ Tablet; Transderm Scop® Patch

Generic Available Yes

Mechanism of Action Blocks the action of acetylcholine at parasympathetic sites in smooth muscle, secretory glands and the CNS; increases cardiac output, dries secretions, antagonizes histamine and serotonin

Use Preoperative medication to produce amnesia and decrease salivary and respiratory secretions; to produce cycloplegia and mydriasis; treatment of iridocyclitis; prevention of motion sickness; prevention of nausea/vomiting associated with anesthesia or opiate analgesia (patch); symptomatic treatment of postencephalitic parkinsonism and paralysis agitans (oral); inhibits excessive motility and hypertonus of the gastrointestinal tract in such conditions as the irritable colon syndrome, mild dysentery, diverticulitis, pylorospasm, and cardiospasm; it may also prevent motion sickness (oral)

USUAL DOSAGE

Preoperatively:

Children: I.M., S.C.: 6 mcg/kg/dose (maximum: 0.3 mg/dose) or 0.2 mg/m^2 may be repeated every 6-8 hours **or** alternatively:
4-7 months: 0.1 mg
7 months to 3 years: 0.15 mg
3-8 years: 0.2 mg
8-12 years: 0.3 mg

Adults:
I.M., I.V., S.C.: 0.3-0.65 mg; may be repeated every 4-6 hours
Transdermal patch: Apply 2.5 cm^2 patch to hairless area behind ear the night before surgery (the patch should be applied no sooner than 1 hour before surgery for best results)

Motion sickness: Transdermal: Children >12 years and Adults: Apply 1 disc behind the ear at least 4 hours prior to exposure and every 3 days as needed; effective if applied as soon as 2-3 hours before anticipated need, best if 12 hours before

Ophthalmic:

Refraction:
Children: Instill 1 drop of 0.25% to eye(s) twice daily for 2 days before procedure
Adults: Instill 1-2 drops of 0.25% to eye(s) 1 hour before procedure

Iridocyclitis:
Children: Instill 1 drop of 0.25% to eye(s) up to 3 times/day
Adults: Instill 1-2 drops of 0.25% to eye(s) up to 4 times/day

Oral: 0.4 to 0.8 mg as a range; the dosage may be cautiously increased in parkinsonism and spastic states.

Dosage Forms DISC, transdermal: 1.5 mg/disc (4's). **INJ:** 0.3 mg/mL (1 mL), 0.4 mg/mL (0.5 mL, 1 mL), 0.86 mg/mL (0.5 mL), 1 mg/mL (1 mL). **SOLN, ophth:** 0.25% (5 mL, 15 mL). **TAB:** 0.4 mg

Contraindications Hypersensitivity to scopolamine or any component; narrow-angle glaucoma; acute hemorrhage, gastrointestinal or genitourinary obstruction, thyrotoxicosis, tachycardia secondary to cardiac insufficiency, paralytic ileus

Warnings/Precautions Use with caution with hepatic or renal impairment since adverse CNS effects occur more often in these patients; use with caution in infants and children since they may be more susceptible to adverse effects of scopolamine; use with caution in patients with GI obstruction; anticholinergic agents are not well tolerated in the elderly and their use should be avoided when possible

Pregnancy Risk Factor C

Adverse Reactions

Ophthalmic:
>10%: Ocular: Blurred vision, photophobia

1% to 10%:

Ocular: Local irritation, increased intraocular pressure

Respiratory: Congestion

<1%: Vascular congestion, edema, drowsiness, eczematoid dermatitis, follicular conjunctivitis, exudate

Systemic:

>10%:

Dermatologic: Dry skin

Gastrointestinal: Constipation, xerostomia, dry throat

Local: Irritation at injection site

Respiratory: Dry nose

Miscellaneous: Diaphoresis (decreased)

1% to 10%:

Dermatologic: Increased sensitivity to light

Endocrine & metabolic: Decreased flow of breast milk

Gastrointestinal: Dysphagia

<1%: Ataxia, bloated feeling, blurred vision, confusion, drowsiness, dysuria, fatigue, headache, increased intraocular pain, loss of memory, nausea, orthostatic hypotension, palpitations, rash, tachycardia, ventricular fibrillation, vomiting, weakness

Note: Systemic adverse effects have been reported following ophthalmic administration

Drug Interactions

Decreased effect of acetaminophen, levodopa, ketoconazole, digoxin, riboflavin, potassium chloride in wax matrix preparations

Increased toxicity: Additive adverse effects with other anticholinergic agents; GI absorption of the following drugs may be affected: acetaminophen, levodopa, ketoconazole, digoxin, riboflavin, potassium chloride wax-matrix preparations

Onset Onset of effect: Oral, I.M.: 0.5-1 hour; I.V.: 10 minutes

Duration Oral, I.M.: 4-6 hours; I.V.: 2 hours; Transdermal: 3 days

Education and Monitoring Issues

Patient Education: Take as directed. You may experience drowsiness, confusion, impaired judgment, or vision changes (use caution when driving or engaging in tasks requiring alertness until response to drug is known); dry mouth, nausea, or vomiting (small frequent meals, frequent mouth care, chewing gum, or sucking lozenges may help); orthostatic hypotension (use caution when climbing stairs and when rising from lying or sitting position); constipation (increased exercise, fluid, or dietary fiber may reduce constipation; if not effective consult prescriber); increased sensitivity to heat and decreased perspiration (avoid extremes of heat, reduce exercise in hot weather); decreased milk if breast-feeding. Report hot, dry, flushed skin; blurred vision or vision changes; difficulty swallowing; chest pain, palpitations, or rapid heartbeat; painful or difficult urination; increased confusion, depression, or loss of memory; rapid or difficult respirations; muscle weakness or tremors; or eye pain.

Ophthalmic: Instill as often as recommended. Wash hands before using. Sit or lie down, open eye, look at ceiling, and instill prescribed amount of solution. Do not blink for 30 seconds, close eye and roll eye in all directions, and apply gentle pressure to inner corner of eye for 1-2 minutes. Do not let tip of applicator touch eye or contaminate tip of applicator. Temporary stinging or blurred vision may occur.

Related Information

Hyoscyamine, Atropine, Scopolamine, Kaolin, Pectin, and Opium *on page 457*

Phenylephrine and Scopolamine *on page 729*

- **Scot-Tussin® [OTC]** *see* Guaifenesin *on page 423*
- **Scot-Tussin® Senior Clear [OTC]** *see* Guaifenesin and Dextromethorphan *on page 424*
- **SeaMist® [OTC]** *see* Sodium Chloride *on page 858*
- **Sebizon® Topical Lotion** *see* Sulfacetamide Sodium *on page 876*
- **Secran®** *see* Vitamins, Multiple *on page 981*
- **Sectral®** *see* Acebutolol *on page 16*
- **Sedapap-10®** *see* Butalbital Compound *on page 123*
- **Selax®** *see* Docusate *on page 290*
- **Selecor®** *see* Celiprolol *on page 168*
- **Selectol®** *see* Celiprolol *on page 168*

Selegiline (seh LEDGE ah leen)

Pharmacologic Class Antidepressant, Monoamine Oxidase Inhibitor; Anti-Parkinson's Agent (Monoamine Oxidase Inhibitor)

U.S. Brand Names Eldepryl®

Generic Available No

Mechanism of Action Potent monoamine oxidase (MAO) type-B inhibitor; MAO-B plays a major role in the metabolism of dopamine; selegiline may also increase dopaminergic activity by interfering with dopamine reuptake at the synapse

Use Adjunct in the management of parkinsonian patients in which levodopa/carbidopa therapy is deteriorating

Unlabeled use: Early Parkinson's disease

Investigational: Alzheimer's disease

(Continued)

Selegiline *(Continued)*

Selegiline is also being studied in Alzheimer's disease. Small studies have shown some improvement in behavioral and cognitive performance in patients, however, further study is needed.

USUAL DOSAGE Oral:

Adults: 5 mg twice daily with breakfast and lunch or 10 mg in the morning

Elderly: Initial: 5 mg in the morning, may increase to a total of 10 mg/day

Dosage Forms CAP (Eldepryl®): 5 mg. **TAB:** 5 mg

Contraindications Known hypersensitivity to selegiline, concomitant use of meperidine

Warnings/Precautions Increased risk of nonselective MAO inhibition occurs with doses >10 mg/day; is a monoamine oxidase inhibitor type "B", there should **not** be a problem with tyramine-containing products as long as the typical doses are employed

Pregnancy Risk Factor C

Adverse Reactions

Cardiovascular: Orthostatic hypotension, hypertension, arrhythmias, palpitations, angina, tachycardia, peripheral edema, bradycardia, syncope

Central nervous system: Hallucinations, dizziness, confusion, anxiety, depression, drowsiness, behavior/mood changes, dreams/nightmares, fatigue, delusions

Dermatologic: Rash, photosensitivity

Gastrointestinal: Xerostomia, nausea, vomiting, constipation, weight loss, anorexia, diarrhea, heartburn

Genitourinary: Nocturia, prostatic hypertrophy, urinary retention, sexual dysfunction

Neuromuscular & skeletal: Tremor, chorea, loss of balance, restlessness, bradykinesia

Ocular: Blepharospasm, blurred vision

Miscellaneous: Diaphoresis (increased)

Drug Interactions CYP2D6 enzyme substrate

Concurrent use of selegiline (high dose) in combination with dextroamphetamine, methylphenidate, dextromethorphan, fenfluramine, meperidine, sibutramine, and venlafaxine may result in serotonin syndrome; these combinations are best avoided

Concurrent use of selegiline with an SSRI may result in mania or hypertension; it is generally best to avoid these combinations

Selegiline (>10 mg/day) in combination with tyramine (cheese, ethanol) may increase the pressor response; avoid high tyramine-containing foods in patients receiving >10 mg/day of selegiline

Alcohol Interactions Avoid use if taking >10 mg of selegiline/day (may increase risk of severe hypertension)

Onset Onset of therapeutic effects: Within 1 hour

Duration 24-72 hours

Half-Life 9 minutes

Education and Monitoring Issues

Patient Education: Take exactly as directed (may be prescribed in conjunction with levodopa/carbidopa) when used for parkinsonism; do not change dosage or discontinue without consulting prescriber. Therapeutic effects may take several weeks or months to achieve and you may need frequent monitoring during first weeks of therapy. Take with meals if GI upset occurs, before meals if dry mouth occurs, after eating if drooling or nausea occurs. Take at the same time each day. Avoid tyramine-containing foods. Maintain adequate hydration (2-3 L/day of fluids unless instructed to restrict fluid intake); void before taking medication. Do not use alcohol and prescription or OTC sedatives or CNS depressants without consulting prescriber. You may experience drowsiness, dizziness, confusion, or vision changes (use caution when driving, climbing stairs, or engaging in tasks requiring alertness until response to drug is known); orthostatic hypotension (use caution when changing position - rising to standing from sitting or lying); constipation (increased exercise, fluids, or dietary fruit and fiber may help); runny nose or flu-like symptoms (consult prescriber for appropriate relief); nausea, vomiting, loss of appetite, or stomach discomfort (small frequent meals, frequent mouth care, chewing gum, or sucking lozenges may help). Report unresolved constipation or vomiting; chest pain, palpitations, irregular heartbeat; CNS changes (hallucination, loss of memory, seizures, acute headache, nervousness, etc); painful or difficult urination; increased muscle spasticity, rigidity, or involuntary movements; skin rash; or significant worsening of condition.

Monitoring Parameters: Blood pressure, symptoms of parkinsonism

Related Information

Parkinson's Disease Dosing *on page 1249*

Selenium (se LEE nee um)

Pharmacologic Class Trace Element, Parenteral

U.S. Brand Names Sele-Pak®; Selepen®

Generic Available Yes

Mechanism of Action Part of glutathione peroxidase which protects cell components from oxidative damage due to peroxidases produced in cellular metabolism

Use Trace metal supplement

USUAL DOSAGE I.V. in TPN solutions:

Children: 3 mcg/kg/day

Adults:

Metabolically stable: 20-40 mcg/day

Deficiency from prolonged TPN support: 100 mcg/day for 24 and 21 days

Dosage Forms INJ: 40 mcg/mL (10 mL, 30 mL)

Contraindications Known hypersensitivity to selenium or any component

Pregnancy Risk Factor C

Adverse Reactions 1% to 10%:

Central nervous system: Lethargy

Dermatologic: Alopecia or hair discoloration

Gastrointestinal: Vomiting following long-term use on damaged skin; abdominal pain, garlic breath

Local: Irritation

Neuromuscular & skeletal: Tremor

Miscellaneous: Diaphoresis

Alcohol Interactions Avoid use (may increase central nervous system depression)

Selenium Sulfide (se LEE nee um SUL fide)

Pharmacologic Class Antiseborrheic Agent, Topical

U.S. Brand Names Exsel®; Head & Shoulders® Intensive Treatment [OTC]; Selsun®; Selsun Blue® [OTC]; Selsun Gold® for Women [OTC]

Use Treatment of itching and flaking of the scalp associated with dandruff, to control scalp seborrheic dermatitis; treatment of tinea versicolor

USUAL DOSAGE Topical:

Dandruff, seborrhea: Massage 5-10 mL into wet scalp, leave on scalp 2-3 minutes, rinse thoroughly, and repeat application; shampoo twice weekly for 2 weeks initially, then use once every 1-4 weeks as indicated depending upon control

Tinea versicolor: Apply the 2.5% lotion to affected area and lather with small amounts of water; leave on skin for 10 minutes, then rinse thoroughly; apply every day for 7 days

Contraindications Known hypersensitivity to selenium or any component

Pregnancy Risk Factor C

♦ **Sele-Pak®** *see* Selenium *on page 844*

♦ **Selepen®** *see* Selenium *on page 844*

♦ **Selsun®** *see* Selenium Sulfide *on page 845*

♦ **Selsun Blue® [OTC]** *see* Selenium Sulfide *on page 845*

♦ **Selsun Gold® for Women [OTC]** *see* Selenium Sulfide *on page 845*

♦ **Semilente® Insulin** *see* Insulin Preparations *on page 472*

♦ **Semprex®-D** *see* Acrivastine and Pseudoephedrine *on page 21*

Senna

Pharmacologic Class Herbal

Use Catharsis

USUAL DOSAGE

Sennosides:

Children >6 years: 20 mg at bedtime

Adults: 20-40 mg with water at bedtime

Senna granules: 2.5-5 mL (163-326 mg) at bedtime; maximum dose: 10 mL (652 mg)/day

Senna tablets:

Children >60 pounds: 1 tablet (187 mg) at bedtime; maximum daily dose: 2 tablets

Adults: 1-2 tablets (187-374 mg) at bedtime; maximum daily dose: 4 tablets (Note: Extra strength senna tablets contain 374 mg each)

Senna syrup:

Children

1 month to 1 year: 1.25-2.5 mL (55-109 mg) at bedtime up to 5 mL/day

1-5 years: 2.5-5 mL (109-218 mg) at bedtime, up to 10 mL/day

5-15 years: 5-10 mL (218-436 mg) at bedtime, up to 20 mL/day

Adults: 10-15 mL (436-654 mg); maximum daily dose: 30 mL (1308 mg)

Senna suppositories:

Children >60 pounds: $1/2$ suppository (326 mg)

Adults: 1 suppository (652 mg) at bedtime; can repeat in 2 hours

Tea: $1/2$ to 2 teaspoons of leaves (0.5-4 g of the herb)

Contraindications Per Commission E: Intestinal obstruction, acute intestinal inflammation (eg, Crohn's disease), colitis ulcerosa, appendicitis, abdominal pain of unknown origin, children <12 years, and pregnancy

♦ **Sensorcaine®** *see* Bupivacaine *on page 118*

♦ **Sensorcaine®-MPF** *see* Bupivacaine *on page 118*

♦ **Sential** *see* Urea and Hydrocortisone *on page 963*

♦ **Septa® Topical Ointment [OTC]** *see* Bacitracin, Neomycin, and Polymyxin B *on page 90*

♦ **Septisol®** *see* Hexachlorophene *on page 436*

♦ **Septra®** *see* Co-Trimoxazole *on page 230*
♦ **Septra® DS** *see* Co-Trimoxazole *on page 230*
♦ **Ser-Ap-Es®** *see* Hydralazine, Hydrochlorothiazide, and Reserpine *on page 442*
♦ **Serentil®** *see* Mesoridazine *on page 569*
♦ **Serevent®** *see* Salmeterol *on page 836*
♦ **Serevent® Diskus®** *see* Salmeterol *on page 836*

Sermorelin Acetate (ser moe REL in AS e tate)

Pharmacologic Class Diagnostic Agent

U.S. Brand Names Geref® Injection

Generic Available No

Use For the evaluation of short children whose height is at least 2 standard deviations below the mean height for their chronological age and sex, presenting with low basal serum levels of IGF-1 and IGF-1-BP3. A single intravenous injection of sermorelin is indicated for evaluating the ability of the somatotroph of the pituitary gland to secrete growth hormone (GH). A normal plasma GH response demonstrates that the somatotroph is intact.

Orphan drug: Sermorelin has been designated an orphan product for use in the treatment of growth hormone deficiencies, AIDS-associated catabolism or weight loss, and as an adjunct to gonadotropin on ovulation induction.

USUAL DOSAGE I.V.: As a single dose in the morning following an overnight fast:

Children and Adults:

<50 kg: Draw venous blood samples for GH determinations 15 minutes before and immediately prior to administration, then administer 1 mcg/kg followed by a 3 mL normal saline flush, draw blood samples again for GH determinations

>50 kg: Determine the number of ampuls needed based on a dose of 1 mcg/kg, draw venous blood samples for GH determinations 15 minutes before and immediately prior to administration, then administer 1 mcg/kg followed by a 3 mL normal saline flush, draw blood samples again for GH determinations

Dosage Forms POWDER for inj, lyophilized: 50 mcg

Contraindications Known hypersensitivity to sermorelin acetate, mannitol, or albumin

Warnings/Precautions Not used for the diagnosis of acromegaly; subnormal GH response may cause obesity, hyperglycemia, and elevated plasma fatty acids

Pregnancy Risk Factor C

Pregnancy Implications Clinical effects on the fetus: Sermorelin has been shown to produce minor variations in fetuses of rats and rabbits when given in S.C. doses of 50, 150, and 500 mcg/kg. In the rat teratology study, external malformations (thin tail) were observed in the higher dose groups, and there was an increase in minor skeletal variants at the high dose. Some visceral malformations (hydroureter) were observed in all treatment groups, with the incidence greatest in the high-dose group. In rabbits, minor skeletal anomalies were significantly greater in the treated animals than in the controls. There are no adequate and well-controlled studies in pregnant women.

Adverse Reactions 1% to 10%:

Cardiovascular: Tightness in the chest
Central nervous system: Headache
Dermatologic: Transient flushing of the face
Gastrointestinal: Nausea, vomiting
Local: Pain, redness, and/or swelling at the injection site

Drug Interactions The test should not be conducted in the presence of drugs that directly affect the pituitary secretion of somatotropin. These include preparations that contain or release somatostatin, insulin, glucocorticoids, or cyclo-oxygenase inhibitors such as ASA or indomethacin. Somatotropin levels may be transiently elevated by clonidine, levodopa, and insulin-induced hypoglycemia. Response to sermorelin may be blunted in patients who are receiving muscarinic antagonists (atropine) or who are hypothyroid or being treated with antithyroid medications such as propylthiouracil. Obesity, hyperglycemia, and elevated plasma fatty acids generally are associated with subnormal GH responses to sermorelin. Exogenous growth hormone therapy should be discontinued at least 1 week before administering the test.

Education and Monitoring Issues

Reference Range: Peak growth hormone levels of >7-10 mcg/L are rarely achieved upon provocation in patients with classic growth hormone deficiency; a marked growth hormone response in these patients (>10-12 mcg/L) is strongly suggestive of hypothalamic dysfunction, as opposed to pituitary dysfunction

♦ **Seromycin** *see* Cycloserine *on page 237*
♦ **Seromycin® Pulvules®** *see* Cycloserine *on page 237*
♦ **Serophene®** *see* Clomiphene *on page 212*
♦ **Seroquel®** *see* Quetiapine *on page 798*
♦ **Serostim® Injection** *see* Human Growth Hormone *on page 438*
♦ **Serpalan®** *see* Reserpine *on page 814*
♦ **Serpasil®** *see* Reserpine *on page 814*
♦ **Serpasil-Esidrix** *see* Hydrochlorothiazide and Reserpine *on page 443*

♦ **Serpatabs®** *see* Reserpine *on page 814*
♦ **Sertan®** *see* Primidone *on page 766*

Sertraline (SER tra leen)

Pharmacologic Class Antidepressant, Selective Serotonin Reuptake Inhibitor

U.S. Brand Names Zoloft®

Generic Available No

Mechanism of Action Antidepressant with selective inhibitory effects on presynaptic serotonin (5-HT) reuptake

Use Treatment of major depression and post-traumatic stress disorder; also being studied for use in obesity and obsessive-compulsive disorder

USUAL DOSAGE Oral:

Adults: Start with 50 mg/day in the morning and increase by 50 mg/day increments every 2-3 days if tolerated to 100 mg/day; additional increases may be necessary; maximum dose: 200 mg/day. If somnolence is noted, administer at bedtime.

Elderly: Start treatment with 25 mg/day in the morning and increase by 25 mg/day increments every 2-3 days if tolerated to 75-100 mg/day; additional increases may be necessary; maximum dose: 200 mg/day

Hemodialysis: Not removed by hemodialysis

Dosage comments in hepatic impairment: Sertraline is extensively metabolized by the liver; caution should be used in patients with hepatic impairment

Dosage Forms CONC, oral: 20 mg/mL. **TAB:** 25 mg, 50 mg, 100 mg

Contraindications Hypersensitivity to sertraline or any component

Warnings/Precautions Do not use in combination with monoamine oxidase inhibitor or within 14 days of discontinuing treatment or initiating treatment with a monoamine oxidase inhibitor due to the risk of serotonin syndrome; use with caution in patients with pre-existing seizure disorders, patients in whom weight loss is undesirable, patients with recent myocardial infarction, unstable heart disease, hepatic or renal impairment, patients taking other psychotropic medications, agitated or hyperactive patients as drug may produce or activate mania or hypomania; because the risk of suicide is inherent in depression, patient should be closely monitored until depressive symptoms remit and prescriptions should be written for minimum quantities to reduce the risk of overdose

Pregnancy Risk Factor C

Adverse Reactions

>10%:

- Central nervous system: Insomnia, somnolence, dizziness, headache, fatigue
- Gastrointestinal: Xerostomia, diarrhea, nausea
- Genitourinary: Ejaculatory disturbances

1% to 10%:

- Cardiovascular: Palpitations
- Central nervous system: Agitation, anxiety, nervousness
- Dermatologic: Rash
- Endocrine & metabolic: Decreased libido
- Gastrointestinal: Constipation, anorexia, dyspepsia, flatulence, vomiting
- Genitourinary: Micturition disorders
- Neuromuscular & skeletal: Tremors, paresthesia
- Ocular: Visual difficulty, abnormal vision
- Otic: Tinnitus
- Miscellaneous: Diaphoresis (increased)

Drug Interactions CYP3A3/4 enzyme substrate, CYP2D6 enzyme substrate (minor); CYP1A2 and 2D6 enzyme inhibitor (weak); CYP2C9, 2C19, and 3A3/4 enzyme inhibitor. **All serotonin reuptake inhibitors are capable of inhibiting CYP2D6 isoenzyme system.** The drugs metabolized by this system include desipramine, dextromethorphan, encainide, haloperidol, imipramine, metoprolol, perphenazine, propafenone, and thioridazine

Increased toxicity:

- MAO inhibitors and possibly with sumatriptan, lithium or tricyclic antidepressants → **serotonin syndrome**, serotonergic hyperstimulation with the following clinical features: mental status changes, restlessness, myoclonus, hyper-reflexia, diaphoresis, diarrhea, shivering, and tremor
- May decrease metabolism/plasma clearance of some drugs (diazepam, tolbutamide) to result in increased duration and pharmacological effects
- May displace highly plasma protein bound drugs from binding sites (eg, warfarin) to result in increased effect

Drug-Herb interaction: A number of case reports of serotonin syndrome have occurred as a result of concurrent use of sertraline and St John's wort (hypericum); to avoid the increased risk of hypertension, hyperthermia, myoclonus, and mental status changes associated with serotonin syndrome, patients should be warned against using hypericum concurrently

Alcohol Interactions Avoid use. Although alcohol may not cause central nervous system depression here, depressed patients should avoid/limit intake.

Onset Steady-state: 7 days; therapeutic effect: >2 weeks

(Continued)

Sertraline *(Continued)*

Half-Life Parent: 24 hours; Metabolites: 66 hours

Education and Monitoring Issues

Patient Education: Take exactly as directed (do not increase dose or frequency); may take 2-3 weeks to achieve desired results; may cause physical and/or psychological dependence. Take in the morning to reduce the incidence of insomnia. Avoid alcohol, caffeine, and other prescription or OTC medications not approved by prescriber. Maintain adequate hydration (2-3 L/day of fluids unless instructed to restrict fluid intake). You may experience drowsiness, dizziness, or lightheadedness (use caution when driving or engaging in tasks requiring alertness until response to drug is known); nausea, vomiting, anorexia, or dry mouth (small frequent meals, frequent mouth care, chewing gum, or sucking lozenges may help); postural hypotension (use caution when climbing stairs or changing position from sitting or lying to standing); urinary pattern changes (void before taking medication); or male sexual dysfunction (reversible). Report persistent insomnia or daytime sedation, agitation, nervousness, fatigue; muscle cramping, tremors, weakness, or change in gait; chest pain, palpitations, or swelling of extremities; vision changes or eye pain; changes in hearing or ringing in ears; difficulty breathing or breathlessness; skin rash or irritation; or worsening of condition.

Manufacturer Merck & Co

Related Information

Antidepressant Agents Comparison *on page 1231*
Pharmaceutical Manufacturers Directory *on page 1020*

- **Serutan® [OTC]** *see* Psyllium *on page 793*
- **Serzone®** *see* Nefazodone *on page 640*

Sevelamer (se VEL a mer)

Pharmacologic Class Phosphate Binder

U.S. Brand Names Renagel®

Mechanism of Action Sevelamer (a polymeric compound) binds phosphate within the intestinal lumen, limiting absorption and decreasing serum phosphate concentrations without altering calcium, aluminum, or bicarbonate concentrations

Use Reduction of serum phosphorous in patients with end-stage renal disease

USUAL DOSAGE Adults: Oral: 2-4 capsules 3 times/day with meals; the initial dose may be based on serum phosphorous:

(Phosphorous: Initial Dose)
>6.0 mg/dL and <7.5 mg/dL: 2 capsules 3 times/day
>7.5 mg/dL and <9.0 mg/dL: 3 capsules 3 times/day
≥9.0 mg/dL: 4 capsules 3 times/day

Dosage should be adjusted based on serum phosphorous concentration, with a goal of lowering to <6.0 mg/dL; maximum daily dose studied was 30 capsules/day.

Dosage Forms CAP: 403 mg

Contraindications Hypersensitivity to sevelamer or any component of the formulation, hypophosphatemia, or bowel obstruction

Warnings/Precautions Use with caution in patients with gastrointestinal disorders including dysphagia, swallowing disorders, severe gastrointestinal motility disorders, or major gastrointestinal surgery. May cause reductions in vitamin D, E, K, and folic acid absorption. Long-term studies of carcinogenic potential have not been completed. Capsules should not be taken apart or chewed.

Pregnancy Risk Factor C

Pregnancy Implications It is not known whether sevelamer is excreted in human milk. Because sevelamer may cause a reduction in the absorption of some vitamins, it should be used with caution in pregnant and/or nursing women.

Adverse Reactions

>10%:
Cardiovascular: Hypotension (11%), thrombosis (10%)
Central nervous system: Headache (10%)
Endocrine and metabolic: Decreased absorption of vitamins D, E, K and folic acid
Gastrointestinal: Diarrhea (16%), dyspepsia (5% to 11%), vomiting (12%)
Neuromuscular and skeletal: Pain (13%)
Miscellaneous: Infection (15%)

1% to 10%:
Cardiovascular: Hypertension (9%)
Gastrointestinal: Nausea (7%), flatulence (4%), diarrhea (4%), constipation (2%)
Respiratory: Cough (4%)

Drug Interactions No formal drug interaction studies have been undertaken. Sevelamer may bind to some drugs in the gastrointestinal tract and decrease their absorption. When changes in absorption of oral medications may have significant clinical consequences (such as antiarrhythmic and antiseizure medications), these medications should be taken at least 1 hour before or 3 hours after a dose of sevelamer.

Education and Monitoring Issues

Patient Education: Take as directed, with meals. Do not break or chew capsule. You may experience headache or dizziness (use caution when driving or engaging in tasks requiring alertness until response to drug is known); upset stomach, nausea, or vomiting (frequent small meals, frequent mouth care, or sucking hard candy may help); diarrhea (yogurt or buttermilk may help); hypotension (use caution when rising from sitting or lying position or when climbing stairs or bending over); or mild neuromuscular pain or stiffness (mild analgesic may help). Report persistent adverse reactions.

Monitoring Parameters: Serum phosphorus

Manufacturer Genzyme Corp

Related Information

Pharmaceutical Manufacturers Directory *on page 1020*

Sibutramine (si BYOO tra meen)

Pharmacologic Class Anorexiant

U.S. Brand Names Meridia®

Mechanism of Action Blocks the neuronal reuptake of norepinephrine and, to a lesser extent, serotonin and dopamine

Use Management of obesity, including weight loss and maintenance of weight loss, and should be used in conjunction with a reduced calorie diet; see "Guidelines for Treatment of Obesity" in Appendix

USUAL DOSAGE Adults ≥16 years: Initial: 10 mg once daily; after 4 weeks may titrate up to 15 mg once daily as needed and tolerated; doses >15 mg/day are not recommended

Dosage Forms CAP: 5 mg, 10 mg, 15 mg

Contraindications During or within 2 weeks of MAO inhibitors (eg, phenelzine, selegiline) or concomitant centrally-acting appetite suppressants. Use is not recommended in patients with anorexia nervosa; uncontrolled or poorly controlled hypertension, congestive heart failure, coronary heart disease, conduction disorders (arrhythmias) or stroke.

Warnings/Precautions Use with caution in severe renal impairment or severe hepatic dysfunction, seizure disorder, hypertension, narrow-angle glaucoma, nursing mothers, elderly patients

Pregnancy Risk Factor C

Adverse Reactions

>10%:

Central nervous system: Headache, insomnia

Gastrointestinal: Anorexia, xerostomia, constipation

Respiratory: Rhinitis

1% to 10%:

Cardiovascular: Tachycardia, vasodilation, hypertension, palpitations, chest pain, edema

Central nervous system: Migraine, dizziness, nervousness, anxiety, depression, somnolence, CNS stimulation, emotional liability

Dermatologic: Rash

Endocrine & metabolic: Dysmenorrhea

Gastrointestinal: Increased appetite, nausea, dyspepsia, gastritis, vomiting, taste perversion, abdominal pain

Neuromuscular & skeletal: Weakness, arthralgia, back pain

Respiratory: Pharyngitis, sinusitis, cough, laryngitis

Miscellaneous: Diaphoresis, flu-like syndrome, allergic reactions, thirst

Drug Interactions CYP3A3/4 enzyme substrate

Caution with other CNS active agents, avoid concurrent use with other serotonergic agents such as venlafaxine, selective serotonin reuptake inhibitors (eg, fluoxetine, fluvoxamine, paroxetine, sertraline), sumatriptan, dihydroergotamine, lithium, tryptophan, some opioid/analgesics (eg, dextromethorphan, tramadol). Other drugs that can raise the blood pressure can worsen the possibility of sibutramine-associated cardiovascular complications (eg, decongestants, centrally acting weight loss products, amphetamines, and amphetamine-like compounds). Possible interaction with ketoconazole, erythromycin, and other agents metabolized by the CYP3A4 enzyme system.

Alcohol Interactions Avoid concurrent excess alcohol ingestion

Education and Monitoring Issues

Patient Education: Take exactly as directed (do not increase dose or frequency without consulting prescriber). May be taken with meals (do not take at bedtime). Avoid alcohol, caffeine, or OTC medications that act as stimulants. You may experience restlessness, dizziness, sleepiness (use caution when driving or engaging in tasks requiring alertness until response to drug is known); insomnia (taking medication early in morning may help, warm milk, and quiet environment at bedtime may help); increased appetite, nausea or vomiting (small frequent meals, frequent mouth care may help); constipation (increased exercise, dietary fiber, fruit, or fluid may help); diarrhea (buttermilk, boiled milk, or yogurt may help); or altered menstrual periods (reversible when drug is discontinued). Report chest pain, palpitations, or irregular heartbeat; excessive nervousness, excitation, or sleepiness; back pain, muscle weakness, or tremors; CNS changes (acute headache, aggressiveness, restlessness, excitation, sleep disturbances); menstrual pattern changes; rash; blurred vision; runny nose, sinusitis, cough, or difficulty breathing.

Dietary Considerations: Sibutramine, as an appetite suppressant, is the most effective when combined with a low calorie diet and behavior modification counseling

(Continued)

Sibutramine *(Continued)*

Monitoring Parameters: Do initial blood pressure and heart rate evaluation and then monitor regularly during therapy. If patient has sustained increases in either blood pressure or pulse rate, consider discontinuing or reducing the dose of the drug.

Manufacturer Knoll Pharmaceutical Company

Related Information

Pharmaceutical Manufacturers Directory *on page 1020*

♦ **Siladryl® Oral [OTC]** *see* Diphenhydramine *on page 282*

Sildenafil (sil DEN a fil)

Pharmacologic Class Phosphodiesterase Enzyme Inhibitor

U.S. Brand Names Viagra®

Mechanism of Action Does not directly cause penile erections, but affects the response to sexual stimulation. The physiologic mechanism of erection of the penis involves release of nitric oxide (NO) in the corpus cavernosum during sexual stimulation. NO then activates the enzyme guanylate cyclase, which results in increased levels of cyclic guanosine monophosphate (cGMP), producing smooth muscle relaxation and inflow of blood to the corpus cavernosum. Sildenafil enhances the effect of NO by inhibiting phosphodiesterase type 5 (PDE5), which is responsible for degradation of cGMP in the corpus cavernosum; when sexual stimulation causes local release of NO, inhibition of PDE5 by sildenafil causes increased levels of cGMP in the corpus cavernosum, resulting in smooth muscle relaxation and inflow of blood to the corpus cavernosum; at recommended doses, it has no effect in the absence of sexual stimulation.

Use Treatment of erectile dysfunction

USUAL DOSAGE Adults: Oral: For most patients, the recommended dose is 50 mg taken as needed, approximately 1 hour before sexual activity. However, sildenafil may be taken anywhere from 30 minutes to 4 hours before sexual activity. Based on effectiveness and tolerance, the dose may be increased to a maximum recommended dose of 100 mg or decreased to 25 mg. The maximum recommended dosing frequency is once daily.

Dosage adjustment for patients >65 years of age, hepatic impairment (cirrhosis), severe renal impairment (Cl_{cr} <30 mL/minute), or concomitant use of potent CYP3A4 inhibitors (erythromycin, ketoconazole, itraconazole, saquinavir): Higher plasma levels have been associated which may result in increase in efficacy and adverse effects and, therefore, a starting dose of 25 mg should be considered

Dosage adjustment for patients receiving ritonavir: Based on the pharmacokinetic data, it is recommended not to exceed a maximum single dose of 25 mg of sildenafil in a 48-hour period

Dosage Forms TAB: 25 mg, 50 mg, 100 mg

Contraindications In patients with a known hypersensitivity to any component of the tablet; has been shown to potentiate the hypotensive effects of nitrates, and its administration to patients who are concurrently using organic nitrates in any form is contraindicated

Warnings/Precautions There is a degree of cardiac risk associated with sexual activity; therefore, prescribers may wish to consider the cardiovascular status of their patients prior to initiating any treatment for erectile dysfunction. Agents for the treatment of erectile dysfunction should be used with caution in patients with anatomical deformation of the penis (angulation, cavernosal fibrosis, or Peyronie's disease), or in patients who have conditions which may predispose them to priapism (sickle cell anemia, multiple myeloma, leukemia).

The safety and efficacy of sildenafil with other treatments for erectile dysfunction have not been studied and are, therefore, not recommended as combination therapy.

A minority of patients with retinitis pigmentosa have generic disorders of retinal phosphodiesterases. There is no safety information on the administration of sildenafil to these patients and sildenafil should be administered with caution.

Pregnancy Risk Factor B

Adverse Reactions

>10%:
- Central nervous system: Headache
- Cardiovascular: Flushing

1% to 10%:
- Central nervous system: Dizziness
- Dermatologic: Rash
- Gastrointestinal: Dyspepsia, diarrhea
- Genitourinary: Urinary tract infection
- Ocular: Abnormal vision
- Respiratory: Nasal congestion

Drug Interactions CYP3A3/4 enzyme substrate (major); CYP2C9 enzyme substrate (minor)

Increased effect/toxicity: Cimetidine, erythromycin, ketoconazole, itraconazole, protease inhibitors

Amprenavir and ritonavir have been found to substantially increase sildenafil serum concentrations and may decrease blood pressure; syncope and prolonged erection were reported; to reduce the chance of adverse events in patients taking ritonavir, a reduction in sildenafil dosage is recommended (not to exceed 25 mg in a 48-hour period).

Decreased effect: Rifampin

Onset ~60 minutes

Duration 2-4 hours

Half-Life 4 hours

Education and Monitoring Issues

Patient Education: Inform prescriber of all other medications you are taking; serious side effects can result when sildenafil is used with nitrates and some other medications. Do not combine sildenafil with other approaches to treating erectile dysfunction without consulting prescriber. Note that sildenafil provides no protection against sexually transmitted diseases, including HIV. You may experience headache, flushing, or abnormal vision (blurred or increased sensitivity to light); use caution when driving at night or in poorly lit environments. Report immediately acute allergic reactions, chest pain or palpitations, persistent dizziness, sign of urinary tract infection, rash, respiratory difficulties, genital swelling, or other adverse reactions.

Manufacturer Pfizer U.S. Pharmaceutical Group

Related Information

Pharmaceutical Manufacturers Directory *on page 1020*

- **Silphen® Cough [OTC]** *see* Diphenhydramine *on page 282*
- **Siltussin® [OTC]** *see* Guaifenesin *on page 423*
- **Siltussin DM® [OTC]** *see* Guaifenesin and Dextromethorphan *on page 424*
- **Silvadene®** *see* Silver Sulfadiazine *on page 852*

Silver Nitrate (SIL ver NYE trate)

Pharmacologic Class Antibiotic, Ophthalmic; Antibiotic, Topical; Cauterizing Agent, Topical; Topical Skin Product, Antibacterial

U.S. Brand Names Dey-Drop® Ophthalmic Solution

Generic Available Yes

Mechanism of Action Free silver ions precipitate bacterial proteins by combining with chloride in tissue forming silver chloride; coagulates cellular protein to form an eschar; silver ions or salts or colloidal silver preparations can inhibit the growth of both gram-positive and gram-negative bacteria. This germicidal action is attributed to the precipitation of bacterial proteins by liberated silver ions. Silver nitrate coagulates cellular protein to form an eschar, and this mode of action is the postulated mechanism for control of benign hematuria, rhinitis, and recurrent pneumothorax.

Use Prevention of gonococcal ophthalmia neonatorum; cauterization of wounds and sluggish ulcers, removal of granulation tissue and warts; aseptic prophylaxis of burns

USUAL DOSAGE

Neonates: Ophthalmic: Instill 2 drops immediately after birth (no later than 1 hour after delivery) into conjunctival sac of each eye as a single dose, allow to sit for ≥30 seconds; do not irrigate eyes following instillation of eye drops

Children and Adults:

Ointment: Apply in an apertured pad on affected area or lesion for approximately 5 days

Sticks: Apply to mucous membranes and other moist skin surfaces only on area to be treated 2-3 times/week for 2-3 weeks

Topical solution: Apply a cotton applicator dipped in solution on the affected area 2-3 times/week for 2-3 weeks

Dosage Forms APPLICATOR sticks, top: 75% with potassium nitrate 25% (6"). **OINT, top:** 10% (30 g). **SOLN:** Ophth: 1% (wax ampuls); Top: 10% (30 mL), 25% (30 mL), 50% (30 mL)

Contraindications Not for use on broken skin or cuts; hypersensitivity to silver nitrate or any component

Warnings/Precautions Do not use applicator sticks on the eyes; repeated applications of the ophthalmic solution into the eye can cause cauterization of the cornea and blindness

Pregnancy Risk Factor C

Adverse Reactions

>10%:

Dermatologic: Burning and skin irritation

Ocular: Chemical conjunctivitis

1% to 10%:

Dermatologic: Staining of the skin

Hematologic: Methemoglobinemia

Ocular: Cauterization of the cornea, blindness

Drug Interactions Decreased effect: Sulfacetamide preparations are **incompatible**

Education and Monitoring Issues

Patient Education: Use as directed; do not use more often than instructed. Store container in dry, dark place.

Ointment: Wear disposable gloves. Apply on pad to affected area for 4-5 days.

Sticks: Wear disposable gloves. Apply to mucous membranes and other moist skin surfaces to be treated 2-3 times each week for 2-3 weeks.

(Continued)

Silver Nitrate *(Continued)*

Solution: Wear disposable gloves. Apply to affected area with cotton applicator dipped in solution 2-3 times each week for 2-3 weeks.

Handle with care; silver nitrate stains skin, clothing, and utensils. Discontinue and contact prescriber if treated areas worsen or if redness, or irritation develops in surrounding area.

Monitoring Parameters: With prolonged use, monitor methemoglobin levels

Silver Sulfadiazine (SIL ver sul fa DYE a zeen)

Pharmacologic Class Antibiotic, Topical

U.S. Brand Names Silvadene®; SSD® AF; SSD® Cream; Thermazene®

Generic Available No

Mechanism of Action Acts upon the bacterial cell wall and cell membrane. Bactericidal for many gram-negative and gram-positive bacteria and is effective against yeast. Active against *Pseudomonas aeruginosa, Pseudomonas maltophilia, Enterobacter* species, *Klebsiella* species, *Serratia* species, *Escherichia coli, Proteus mirabilis, Morganella morganii, Providencia rettgeri, Proteus vulgaris, Providencia* species, *Citrobacter* species, *Acinetobacter calcoaceticus, Staphylococcus aureus, Staphylococcus epidermidis, Enterococcus* species, *Candida albicans, Corynebacterium diphtheriae,* and *Clostridium perfringens*

Use Prevention and treatment of infection in second and third degree burns

USUAL DOSAGE Children and Adults: Topical: Apply once or twice daily with a sterile-gloved hand; apply to a thickness of $^{1}/_{16}$"; burned area should be covered with cream at all times

Dosage Forms CRM, top: 1% [10 mg/g] (20 g, 50 g, 100 g, 400 g, 1000 g)

Contraindications Hypersensitivity to silver sulfadiazine or any component; premature infants or neonates <2 months of age because sulfonamides compete with bilirubin for protein binding sites which may displace bilirubin and cause kernicterus, pregnant women approaching or at term

Warnings/Precautions Use with caution in patients with G-6-PD deficiency, renal impairment, or history of allergy to other sulfonamides; sulfadiazine may accumulate in patients with impaired hepatic or renal function; fungal superinfection may occur; use of analgesic might be needed before application; systemic absorption is significant and adverse reactions may occur

Pregnancy Risk Factor B

Adverse Reactions

1% to 10%:

Dermatologic: Itching, rash, erythema multiforme, discoloration of skin

Hematologic: Hemolytic anemia, leukopenia, agranulocytosis, aplastic anemia

Hepatic: Hepatitis

Renal: Interstitial nephritis

Miscellaneous: Allergic reactions may be related to sulfa component

<1%: Photosensitivity

Drug Interactions Decreased effect: Topical proteolytic enzymes are inactivated

Education and Monitoring Issues

Patient Education: Usually applied by professional in burn care setting. Patient instruction should be appropriate to extent of burn, patient understanding, etc.

Monitoring Parameters: Serum electrolytes, urinalysis, renal function tests, CBC in patients with extensive burns on long-term treatment

♦ **Simron® [OTC]** *see* Ferrous Gluconate *on page 359*

♦ **Simulect®** *see* Basiliximab *on page 92*

Simvastatin (SIM va stat in)

Pharmacologic Class Antilipemic Agent (HMG-CoA Reductase Inhibitor)

U.S. Brand Names Zocor®

Generic Available No

Mechanism of Action Simvastatin is a methylated derivative of lovastatin that acts by competitively inhibiting 3-hydroxy-3-methylglutaryl-coenzyme A (HMG-CoA) reductase, the enzyme that catalyzes the rate-limiting step in cholesterol biosynthesis

Use "Secondary prevention" in patients with coronary heart disease and hypercholesterolemia to reduce the risk of total mortality by reducing coronary death; reduce the risk of nonfatal myocardial infarction; reduce the risk of undergoing myocardial revascularization procedures; and reduce the risk of stroke or transient ischemic attack

Adjunct to dietary therapy to decrease elevated serum total and LDL cholesterol, apolipoprotein B (apo-B), and triglyceride levels, and to increase HDL cholesterol in patients with primary hypercholesterolemia (heterozygous, familial and nonfamilial) and mixed dyslipidemia (Fredrickson types IIa and IIb); treatment of homozygous familial hypercholesterolemia; treatment of isolated hypertriglyceridemia (Fredrickson type IV) and type III hyperlipoproteinemia; to reduce the risk of myocardial infarction, stroke, or TIA

USUAL DOSAGE Oral:

Adults:

Initial: 20 mg once daily in the evening; patients who require only a moderate reduction of LDL cholesterol may be started at 10 mg

Maintenance: Recommended dosing range: 5-80 mg/day as a single dose in the evening; doses should be individualized according to the baseline LDL-C levels, the recommended goal of therapy, and the patient's response

Adjustments: Should be made at intervals of 4 weeks or more

Patients with homozygous familial hypercholesteremia: Adults: 40 mg in the evening or 80 mg/day in 3 divided doses of 20 mg, 20 mg, and an evening dose of 40 mg

Elderly: Maximum reductions in LDL-cholesterol may be achieved with daily dose of ≤20 mg

Patients who are concomitantly receiving cyclosporine: Initial: 5 mg, should not exceed 10 mg/day

Patients receiving concomitant fibrates or niacin: Dose should **not** exceed 10 mg/day

Dosing adjustment/comments in renal impairment: Because simvastatin does not undergo significant renal excretion, modification of dose should not be necessary in patients with mild to moderate renal insufficiency

Severe renal impairment: Cl_{cr} <10 mL/minute: Initial: 5 mg/day with close monitoring

Dosage Forms TAB: 5 mg, 10 mg, 20 mg, 40 mg, 80 mg

Contraindications Previous hypersensitivity to simvastatin or lovastatin or other HMG-CoA reductase inhibitors; active liver disease or unexplained elevations of serum transaminases; pregnancy and lactation

Pregnancy Risk Factor X

Adverse Reactions

1% to 10%:

Central nervous system: Headache (3.5%)

Gastrointestinal: Flatulence (1.9%), abdominal cramps (3.2%), diarrhea (1.9%), constipation (2.3%), nausea/vomiting (1.3%), dyspepsia/heartburn (1.1%)

Neuromuscular & skeletal: Myalgia, weakness (1.6%), increased CPK

Respiratory: Upper respiratory infection (2.1%)

<1%: Abnormal taste, blurred vision, lenticular opacities

Drug Interactions CYP3A3/4 enzyme substrate

Inhibitors of CYP3A3/4 (amprenavir, clarithromycin, cyclosporine, danazol, diltiazem, fluvoxamine, erythromycin, fluconazole, indinavir, itraconazole, ketoconazole, miconazole, nefazodone, nelfinavir, ritonavir, saquinavir, troleandomycin, and verapamil) increase simvastatin blood levels; may increase the risk of simvastatin-induced myopathy and rhabdomyolysis

Increased effect of warfarin and digoxin possible with simvastatin or other HMG-CoA reductase inhibitors

Concurrent use of clofibrate, fenofibrate, gemfibrozil, cyclosporine, and niacin with HMG-CoA reductase inhibitors may result in rhabdomyolysis

Decreased antihyperlipidemic activity possible with rifampin, nicotinic acid (fluvastatin) and isradipine (lovastatin)

Onset >3 days; maximal effects after 2 weeks

Education and Monitoring Issues

Patient Education: Take this medication as directed, with meals, 1 hour prior to or after any other medications. You may experience nausea, flatulence, dyspepsia (small frequent meals may help), headache, muscle or joint pain (will probably lessen with continued use), and light sensitivity (use sunblock and wear protective clothing). Report severe and unresolved gastric upset, any vision changes, changes in color of urine or stool, yellowing of skin or eyes, and any unusual bruising.

Monitoring Parameters: Creatine phosphokinase levels due to possibility of myopathy; serum cholesterol (total and fractionated)

Manufacturer Merck & Co

Related Information

Pharmaceutical Manufacturers Directory *on page 1020*

- **Sinarest® Nasal Solution [OTC]** *see* Phenylephrine *on page 727*
- **Sinemet®** *see* Levodopa and Carbidopa *on page 521*
- **Sinemet® CR** *see* Levodopa and Carbidopa *on page 521*
- **Sinequan® Oral** *see* Doxepin *on page 298*
- **Singulair®** *see* Montelukast *on page 616*
- **Sinubid®** *see* Phenyltoloxamine, Phenylpropanolamine, and Acetaminophen *on page 730*
- **Sinumist®-SR Capsulets®** *see* Guaifenesin *on page 423*
- **Sinupan®** *see* Guaifenesin and Phenylephrine *on page 425*
- **Sinutab® SA** *see* Phenyltoloxamine, Phenylpropanolamine, and Acetaminophen *on page 730*

Sirolimus (sir OH li mus)

Pharmacologic Class Immunosuppressant Agent

U.S. Brand Names Rapamune®

(Continued)

Sirolimus *(Continued)*

Mechanism of Action Sirolimus inhibits T-lymphocyte activation and proliferation in response to antigenic and cytokine stimulation. Its mechanism differs from other immunosuppressants. It inhibits acute rejection of allografts and prolongs graft survival.

Use Prophylaxis of organ rejection in patients receiving renal transplants, in combination with cyclosporin and corticosteroids

Unlabeled use: Prophylaxis of organ rejection in solid organ transplant patients in combination with tacrolimus and corticosteroids

USUAL DOSAGE Oral:

Adults ≥40 kg: Loading dose: For *de novo* transplant recipients, a loading dose of 3 times the daily maintenance dose should be administered on day 1 of dosing. Maintenance dose: 2 mg/day. Doses should be taken 4 hours after cyclosporine, and should be taken consistently either with or without food.

Children ≥13 years or Adults <40 kg: Loading dose: 3 mg/m^2 (day 1); followed by a maintenance of 1 mg/m^2/day.

Dosage adjustment in renal impairment: No dosage adjustment is necessary in renal impairment

Dosage adjustment in hepatic impairment: Reduce maintenance dose by approximately 33% in hepatic impairment. Loading dose is unchanged.

Dosage Forms SOLN, oral: 1 mg/mL (1 mL, 2 mL, 5mL, 60 mL, 150 mL)

Contraindications Hypersensitivity to sirolimus or any component of the formulation

Warnings/Precautions Immunosuppressive agents, including sirolimus, increase the risk of infection and may be associated with the development of lymphoma. Only prescribers experienced in the management of organ transplant patients should prescribe sirolimus. May increase serum lipids (cholesterol and triglycerides). Use with caution in patients with hyperlipidemia. May decrease GFR and increase serum creatinine. Use caution in patients with renal impairment, or when used concurrently with medications which may alter renal function. Has been associated with an increased risk of lymphocele. Avoid concurrent use of ketoconazole.

Pregnancy Risk Factor C

Pregnancy Implications Embryotoxicity and fetotoxicity may occur, as evidenced by increased mortality, reduced fetal weights and delayed ossification. Effective contraception must be initiated before therapy with sirolimus and continued for 12 weeks after discontinuation. Excretion in breast milk unknown. Breast-feeding is not recommended.

Adverse Reactions Incidence of many adverse effects are dose related

>20%:

Cardiovascular: Hypertension (39% to 49%), peripheral edema (54% to 64%), edema (16% to 24%), chest pain (16% to 24%)

Central nervous system: Fever (23% to 34%), headache (23% to 34%), pain (24% to 33%), insomnia (13% to 22%)

Dermatologic: Acne (20% to 31%), rash (10% to 20%)

Endocrine & metabolic: Hypercholesterolemia (38% to 46%), hyperkalemia (12% to 17%), hypokalemia (11% to 21%), hypophosphatemia (15% to 23%), hyperlipidemia (38% to 57%)

Gastrointestinal: Abdominal pain (28% to 36%), nausea (25% to 36%), vomiting (19% to 25%), diarrhea (25% to 42%), constipation (28% to 38%), dyspepsia (17% to 25%), weight gain (8% to 21%)

Genitourinary: Urinary tract infection (20% to 33%)

Hematologic: Anemia (23% to 37%), leukopenia (9% to 15%), thrombocytopenia (13% to 40%)

Neuromuscular & skeletal: Arthralgia (25% to 31%), weakness (22% to 40%), back pain (16% to 26%), tremor (21% to 31%)

Renal: Increased serum creatinine (35% to 40%)

Respiratory: Dyspnea (22% to 30%), upper respiratory infection (20% to 26%), pharyngitis (16% to 21%)

3% to 20%:

Cardiovascular: Atrial fibrillation, congestive heart failure, hypervolemia, hypotension, palpitation, peripheral vascular disorder, postural hypotension, syncope, tachycardia, thrombosis, vasodilation

Central nervous system: Chills, malaise, anxiety, confusion, depression, dizziness, emotional lability, hypesthesia, hypotonia, insomnia, neuropathy, somnolence

Dermatologic: Dermatitis (fungal), hirsutism, pruritus, skin hypertrophy, dermal ulcer, ecchymosis, cellulitis

Endocrine & metabolic: Cushing's syndrome, diabetes mellitus, glycosuria, acidosis, dehydration, hypercalcemia, hyperglycemia, hyperphosphatemia, hypocalcemia, hypoglycemia, hypomagnesemia, hyponatremia

Gastrointestinal: Enlarged abdomen, anorexia, dysphagia, eructation, esophagitis, flatulence, gastritis, gastroenteritis, gingivitis, gingival hyperplasia, ileus, mouth ulceration, oral moniliasis, stomatitis, weight loss

Genitourinary: Pelvic pain, scrotal edema, testis disorder, impotence

Hematologic: Leukocytosis, polycythemia, TTP, hemolytic-uremic syndrome, hemorrhage

Hepatic: Abnormal liver function tests, increased alkaline phosphatase, increased LDH, increased transaminases, ascites

Local: Thrombophlebitis

Neuromuscular & skeletal: Increased CPK, arthrosis, bone necrosis, leg cramps, myalgia, osteoporosis, tetany, hypertonia, paresthesia

Ocular: Abnormal vision, cataract, conjunctivitis

Otic: Ear pain, deafness, otitis media, tinnitus

Renal: Increased BUN, increased serum creatinine, albuminuria, bladder pain, dysuria, hematuria, hydronephrosis, kidney pain, tubular necrosis, nocturia, oliguria, pyuria, nephropathy (toxic), urinary frequency, urinary incontinence, urinary retention

Respiratory: Asthma, atelectasis, bronchitis, cough, epistaxis, hypoxia, lung edema, pleural effusion, pneumonia, rhinitis, sinusitis

Miscellaneous: Abscess, facial edema, flu-like syndrome, hernia, infection, lymphadenopathy, lymphocele, peritonitis, sepsis, diaphoresis

Drug Interactions CYP3A4 substrate and P-glycoprotein substrate

Increased effect/toxicity:

Cyclosporine increases C_{max} and AUC of sirolimus during concurrent therapy, and cyclosporine clearance may be reduced during concurrent therapy. Sirolimus should be taken 4 hours after cyclosporine oral solution and/or capsules.

Diltiazem and ketoconazole increase serum concentrations or sirolimus; clearance of sirolimus is increased by rifampin

Other inhibitors of CYP3A4 (eg, calcium channel blockers, antifungal agents, macrolide antibiotics, gastrointestinal prokinetic agents, HIV-protease inhibitors) are likely to increase sirolimus concentrations

Decreased effect: Inducers of CYP3A4 (eg, rifampin, phenobarbital, carbamazepine, rifabutin, phenytoin) are likely to decrease serum concentrations of sirolimus

Half-Life Mean: 62 hours

Education and Monitoring Issues

Patient Education: Take as directed; do not alter dose or discontinue without consulting prescriber. Do not ever mix sirolimus solution with anything other than water. Consult prescriber about timing of any other prescribed or OTC medications. Maintain adequate hydration (2-3 L/day of fluid, unless instructed to restrict fluids) during entire course of therapy. You will be susceptible to infection (avoid crowds and people with infectious or contagious diseases). If you are diabetic, monitor glucose levels closely (may alter glucose levels). You may experience nausea, vomiting, loss of appetite (small frequent meals, good mouth care, chewing gum, or sucking hard candy may help); constipation (increase exercise or dietary fiber and fluids); diarrhea (yogurt or buttermilk); muscle or back pain (mild analgesic). Inform prescriber of any adverse effects including, but not limited to, unresolved GI problems; difficulty breathing, cough, infection; skin rash or irritation; headache, insomnia, anxiety, confusion, emotional lability; changes in voiding pattern, burning, itching, or pain on urination; persistent bone, joint, or muscle cramping, pain or weakness; chest pain, palpitations, swelling of extremities; changes in vision or hearing, or any other adverse reactions.

Dietary Considerations: Do not administer with grapefruit juice - may decrease clearance of sirolimus. Ingestion with high-fat meals decreases peak concentrations but increases AUC by 35%. Sirolimus should be taken consistently either with or without food to minimize variability.

Monitoring Parameters: Monitor sirolimus levels in pediatric patients, patients with hepatic impairment, or on concurrent inhibitors or inducers of CYP3A4, and/or if cyclosporine dosing is markedly reduced or discontinued. Also monitor serum cholesterol and triglycerides, blood pressure, and serum creatinine. Routine therapeutic drug level monitoring is not required in most patients.

Reference Range: Mean serum trough concentrations: 9 ng/mL for the 2 mg/day treatment groups and 17 ng/mL in the 5 mg/day group

Manufacturer Wyeth-Ayerst Laboratories

Related Information

Pharmaceutical Manufacturers Directory *on page 1020*

♦ **Sirop Dentition** *see* Benzocaine *on page 98*

♦ **Skelaxin®** *see* Metaxalone *on page 573*

♦ **Skelid®** *see* Tiludronate *on page 921*

Skin Test Antigens, Multiple (skin test AN tee gens, MUL ti pul)

Pharmacologic Class Diagnostic Agent

U.S. Brand Names Multitest CMI®

Use Detection of nonresponsiveness to antigens by means of delayed hypersensitivity skin testing

USUAL DOSAGE Select only test sites that permit sufficient surface area and subcutaneous tissue to allow adequate penetration of all eight points, avoid hairy areas. Press loaded unit into the skin with sufficient pressure to puncture the skin and allow adequate penetration of all points, maintain firm contact for at least 5 seconds, during application the device should not be "rocked" back and forth and side to side without removing any of the test heads from the skin sites.

(Continued)

Skin Test Antigens, Multiple *(Continued)*

If adequate pressure is applied it will be possible to observe:

1. The puncture marks of the nine tines on each of the eight test heads
2. An imprint of the circular platform surrounding each test head
3. Residual antigen and glycerin at each of the eight sites

If any of the above three criteria are not fully followed, the test results may not be reliable.

Reading should be done in good light, read the test sites at both 24 and 48 hours, the largest reaction recorded from the two readings at each test site should be used. If two readings are not possible, a single 48 hour is recommended. A positive reaction from any of the seven delayed hypersensitivity skin test antigens is **induration ≥2 mm** providing there is no induration at the negative control site. The size of the induration reactions with this test may be smaller than those obtained with other intradermal procedures.

Contraindications Infected or inflamed skin, known hypersensitivity to skin test antigens; do not apply at sites involving acneiform, infected or inflamed skin; although severe systemic reactions are rare to diphtheria and tetanus antigens, persons known to have a history of systemic reactions should be tested with this test only after the test heads containing these antigens have been removed

Pregnancy Risk Factor C

- **Sleep-eze 3® Oral [OTC]** *see* Diphenhydramine *on page 282*
- **Sleepinal® [OTC]** *see* Diphenhydramine *on page 282*
- **Sleepwell 2-nite® [OTC]** *see* Diphenhydramine *on page 282*
- **Slim-Mint® [OTC]** *see* Benzocaine *on page 98*
- **Slo-bid™** *see* Theophylline Salts *on page 906*
- **Slo-Niacin® [OTC]** *see* Niacin *on page 647*
- **Slo-Phyllin®** *see* Theophylline Salts *on page 906*
- **Slo-Phyllin® GG** *see* Theophylline and Guaifenesin *on page 906*
- **Slow FE® [OTC]** *see* Ferrous Sulfate *on page 360*
- **Slow-K®** *see* Potassium Chloride *on page 751*
- **Slow-Mag® (Chloride)** *see* Magnesium Salts (Other) *on page 551*

Sodium Acetate (SOW dee um AS e tate)

Pharmacologic Class Alkalinizing Agent; Electrolyte Supplement, Oral

Use Sodium source in large volume I.V. fluids to prevent or correct hyponatremia in patients with restricted intake; used to counter acidosis through conversion to bicarbonate

USUAL DOSAGE Sodium acetate is metabolized to bicarbonate on an equimolar basis outside the liver; administer in large volume I.V. fluids as a sodium source. Refer to Sodium Bicarbonate monograph.

Maintenance electrolyte requirements of sodium in parenteral nutrition solutions:
- Daily requirements: 3-4 mEq/kg/24 hours or 25-40 mEq/1000 kcal/24 hours
- Maximum: 100-150 mEq/24 hours

Contraindications Alkalosis, hypocalcemia, low sodium diets, edema, cirrhosis

Pregnancy Risk Factor C

Sodium Ascorbate (SOW dee um a SKOR bate)

Pharmacologic Class Vitamin, Water Soluble

U.S. Brand Names Cenolate®

Use Prevention and treatment of scurvy and to acidify urine

USUAL DOSAGE Oral, I.V., S.C.:

Infants:
- Daily protective requirement: 30 mg
- Treatment: 100-300 mg/day (75-100 mg in premature infants)

Children:
- Scurvy: 100-300 mg/day in divided doses for at least 2 weeks
- Urinary acidification: 500 mg every 6-8 hours
- Dietary supplement: 35-45 mg/day

Adults:
- Scurvy: 100-250 mg 1-2 times/day for at least 2 weeks
- Urinary acidification: 4-12 g/day in divided doses
- Dietary supplement: 50-60 mg/day (RDA: 60 mg)
- Prevention and treatment of cold: 1-3 g/day

Dosage Forms CRYSTALS: 1020 mg per 1/4 teaspoonful [ascorbic acid 900 mg]. **INJ:** 250 mg/mL [ascorbic acid 222 mg/mL] (30 mL), 562.5 mg/mL [ascorbic acid 500 mg/mL] (1 mL, 2 mL). **TAB:** 585 mg [ascorbic acid 500 mg]

Contraindications Large doses during pregnancy

Pregnancy Risk Factor C

Sodium Bicarbonate (SOW dee um bye KAR bun ate)

Pharmacologic Class Alkalinizing Agent; Antacid; Electrolyte Supplement, Oral; Electrolyte Supplement, Parenteral

U.S. Brand Names Neut® Injection

Generic Available Yes

Mechanism of Action Dissociates to provide bicarbonate ion which neutralizes hydrogen ion concentration and raises blood and urinary pH

Use Management of metabolic acidosis; gastric hyperacidity; as an alkalinization agent for the urine; treatment of hyperkalemia

USUAL DOSAGE

Cardiac arrest: **Routine use of $NaHCO_3$ is not recommended and should be given only after adequate alveolar ventilation has been established and effective cardiac compressions are provided**

Infants and Children: I.V.: 0.5-1 mEq/kg/dose repeated every 10 minutes or as indicated by arterial blood gases; rate of infusion should not exceed 10 mEq/minute; neonates and children <2 years of age should receive 4.2% (0.5 mEq/mL) solution

Adults: I.V.: Initial: 1 mEq/kg/dose one time; maintenance: 0.5 mEq/kg/dose every 10 minutes or as indicated by arterial blood gases

Metabolic acidosis: Dosage should be based on the following formula if blood gases and pH measurements are available:

Infants and Children:

HCO_3^-(mEq) = 0.3 x weight (kg) x base deficit (mEq/L) **or**

HCO_3^-(mEq) = 0.5 x weight (kg) x [24 - serum HCO_3^- (mEq/L)]

Adults:

HCO_3^-(mEq) = 0.2 x weight (kg) x base deficit (mEq/L) **or**

HCO_3^-(mEq) = 0.5 x weight (kg) x [24 - serum HCO_3^- (mEq/L)]

If acid-base status is not available: Dose for older Children and Adults: 2-5 mEq/kg I.V. infusion over 4-8 hours; subsequent doses should be based on patient's acid-base status

Chronic renal failure: Oral: Initiate when plasma HCO_3^- <15 mEq/L

Children: 1-3 mEq/kg/day

Adults: Start with 20-36 mEq/day in divided doses, titrate to bicarbonate level of 18-20 mEq/L

Renal tubular acidosis: Oral:

Distal:

Children: 2-3 mEq/kg/day

Adults: 0.5-2 mEq/kg/day in 4-5 divided doses

Proximal: Children: Initial: 5-10 mEq/kg/day; maintenance: Increase as required to maintain serum bicarbonate in the normal range

Urine alkalinization: Oral:

Children: 1-10 mEq (84-840 mg)/kg/day in divided doses every 4-6 hours; dose should be titrated to desired urinary pH

Adults: Initial: 48 mEq (4 g), then 12-24 mEq (1-2 g) every 4 hours; dose should be titrated to desired urinary pH; doses up to 16 g/day (200 mEq) in patients <60 years and 8 g (100 mEq) in patients >60 years

Antacid: Adults: Oral: 325 mg to 2 g 1-4 times/day

Dosage Forms INJ: 4% [40 mg/mL = 2.4 mEq/5 mL] (5 mL); 4.2% [42 mg/mL = 5 mEq/10 mL] (10 mL); 7.5% [75 mg/mL = 8.92 mEq/10 mL] (10 mL, 50 mL); 8.4% [84 mg/mL = 10 mEq/10 mL] (10 mL, 50 mL). **POWDER:** 120 g, 480 g. **TAB:** 300 mg [3.6 mEq]; 325 mg [3.8 mEq]; 520 mg [6.3 mEq]; 600 mg [7.3 mEq]; 650 mg [7.6 mEq]

Contraindications Alkalosis, hypernatremia, severe pulmonary edema, hypocalcemia, unknown abdominal pain

Warnings/Precautions Rapid administration in neonates and children <2 years of age has led to hypernatremia, decreased CSF pressure and intracranial hemorrhage. **Use of I.V. $NaHCO_3$ should be reserved for documented metabolic acidosis and for hyperkalemia-induced cardiac arrest.** Routine use in cardiac arrest is not recommended. Avoid extravasation, tissue necrosis can occur due to the hypertonicity of $NaHCO_3$. May cause sodium retention especially if renal function is impaired; not to be used in treatment of peptic ulcer; use with caution in patients with CHF, edema, cirrhosis, or renal failure. Not the antacid of choice for the elderly because of sodium content and potential for systemic alkalosis.

Pregnancy Risk Factor C

Adverse Reactions Percentage unknown: Aggravation of congestive heart failure, belching, cerebral hemorrhage, edema, flatulence (with oral), gastric distension, hypernatremia, hyperosmolality, hypocalcemia, hypokalemia, increased affinity of hemoglobin for oxygen-reduced pH in myocardial tissue necrosis when extravasated; intracranial acidosis, metabolic alkalosis, milk alkali syndrome (especially with renal dysfunction), pulmonary edema, tetany

Drug Interactions

Decreased effect/levels of lithium, chlorpropamide, methotrexate, tetracyclines, and salicylates due to urinary alkalinization

Increased toxicity/levels of amphetamines, anorexiants, mecamylamine, ephedrine, pseudoephedrine, flecainide, quinidine, quinine due to urinary alkalinization

Onset Oral: Rapid; I.V.: 15 minutes

Duration Oral: 8-10 minutes; I.V.: 1-2 hours

(Continued)

Sodium Bicarbonate *(Continued)*

Education and Monitoring Issues

Patient Education: Do not use for chronic gastric acidity. Take as directed. Chew tablets thoroughly and follow with a full glass of water, preferably on an empty stomach (2 hours before or after food). Take at least 2 hours before or after any other medications. Report CNS effects (eg, irritability, confusion); muscle rigidity or tremors; swelling of feet or ankles; difficulty breathing; chest pain or palpitations; respiratory changes; or tarry stools.

Sodium Chloride (SOW dee um KLOR ide)

Pharmacologic Class Electrolyte Supplement, Oral; Lubricant, Ocular

U.S. Brand Names Adsorbonac® Ophthalmic [OTC]; Afrin® Saline Mist [OTC]; AK-NaCl® [OTC]; Ayr® Saline [OTC]; Breathe Free® [OTC]; Dristan® Saline Spray [OTC]; HuMist® Nasal Mist [OTC]; Muro 128® Ophthalmic [OTC]; Muroptic-5® [OTC]; NāSal™ [OTC]; Nasal Moist® [OTC]; Ocean Nasal Mist [OTC]; Pretz® [OTC]; SalineX® [OTC]; SeaMist® [OTC]

Use Parenteral restoration of sodium ion in patients with restricted oral intake (especially hyponatremia states or low salt syndrome). In general, parenteral saline uses:

Normal saline: Restores water/sodium losses
Hypotonic sodium chloride: Hydrating solution
Hypertonic sodium chloride: For severe hyponatremia and hypochloremia
Bacteriostatic sodium chloride: Dilution or dissolving drugs for I.M./I.V./S.C. injections
Concentrated sodium chloride: Additive for parenteral fluid therapy
Pharmaceutical aid/diluent for infusion of compatible drug additives

USUAL DOSAGE

Newborn electrolyte requirement:
- Premature: 2-8 mEq/kg/24 hours
- Term:
  - 0-48 hours: 0-2 mEq/kg/24 hours
  - >48 hours: 1-4 mEq/kg/24 hours
- Children: I.V.: Hypertonic solutions (>0.9%) should only be used for the initial treatment of acute serious symptomatic hyponatremia; maintenance: 3-4 mEq/kg/day; maximum: 100-150 mEq/day; dosage varies widely depending on clinical condition
- Replacement: Determined by laboratory determinations mEq
  - Sodium deficiency (mEq/kg) = [% dehydration (L/kg)/100 x 70 (mEq/L)] + [0.6 (L/kg) x (140 - serum sodium) (mEq/L)]
- Nasal: Use as often as needed

Adults:
- GU irrigant: 1-3 L/day by intermittent irrigation
- Heat cramps: Oral: 0.5-1 g with full glass of water, up to 4.8 g/day
- Replacement I.V.: Determined by laboratory determinations mEq
- Sodium deficiency (mEq/kg) = [% dehydration (L/kg)/100 x 70 (mEq/L)] + [0.6 (L/kg) x (140 - serum sodium) (mEq/L)]
- To correct acute, serious hyponatremia: mEq sodium = [desired sodium (mEq/L) - actual sodium (mEq/L)] x [0.6 x wt (kg)]; for acute correction use 125 mEq/L as the desired serum sodium; acutely correct serum sodium in 5 mEq/L/dose increments; more gradual correction in increments of 10 mEq/L/day is indicated in the asymptomatic patient
- Chloride maintenance electrolyte requirement in parenteral nutrition: 2-4 mEq/kg/24 hours or 25-40 mEq/1000 kcals/24 hours; maximum: 100-150 mEq/24 hours
- Sodium maintenance electrolyte requirement in parenteral nutrition: 3-4 mEq/kg/24 hours or 25-40 mEq/1000 kcals/24 hours; maximum: 100-150 mEq/24 hours. See table.

Approximate Deficits of Water and Electrolytes in Moderately Severe Dehydration

Condition	Water (mL/kg)	Sodium (mEq/kg)
Fasting and thirsting	100-120	5-7
Diarrhea		
isonatremic	100-120	8-10
hypernatremic	100-120	2-4
hyponatremic	100-120	10-12
Pyloric stenosis	100-120	8-10
Diabetic acidosis	100-120	9-10

*A **negative** deficit indicates total body **excess** prior to treatment.

Adapted from Behrman RE, Kleigman RM, Nelson WE, et al, eds, *Nelson Textbook of Pediatrics*, 14th ed, WB Saunders Co, 1992.

Ophthalmic:
- Ointment: Apply once daily or more often

Solution: Instill 1-2 drops into affected eye(s) every 3-4 hours

Abortifacient: 20% (250 mL) administered by transabdominal intra-amniotic instillation

Contraindications Hypertonic uterus, hypernatremia, fluid retention

Pregnancy Risk Factor C

Sodium Citrate and Citric Acid (SOW dee um SIT rate & SI trik AS id)

Pharmacologic Class Alkalinizing Agent

U.S. Brand Names Bicitra®; Oracit®

Use Treatment of metabolic acidosis; alkalinizing agent in conditions where long-term maintenance of an alkaline urine is desirable

USUAL DOSAGE Oral:

Infants and Children: 2-3 mEq/kg/day in divided doses 3-4 times/day **or** 5-15 mL with water after meals and at bedtime

Adults: 15-30 mL with water after meals and at bedtime

Contraindications Severe renal insufficiency, sodium-restricted diet

Pregnancy Risk Factor C

Sodium Citrate and Potassium Citrate Mixture

(SOW dee um SIT rate & poe TASS ee um SIT rate MIKS chur)

Pharmacologic Class Alkalinizing Agent

U.S. Brand Names Polycitra®

Dosage Forms SYR: Sodium citrate 500 mg, potassium citrate 550 mg, with citric acid 334 mg per 5 mL [sodium 1 mEq, potassium 1 mEq, bicarbonate 2 mEq]

Pregnancy Risk Factor Not established

Sodium Hyaluronate (SOW dee um hye al yoor ON ate)

Pharmacologic Class Ophthalmic Agent, Viscoelastic

U.S. Brand Names AMO Vitrax®; Amvisc®; Amvisc® Plus; Healon®; Healon® GV; Hyalgan®; Provisc®

Use Surgical aid in cataract extraction, intraocular implantation, corneal transplant, glaucoma filtration, and retinal attachment surgery; relief of mild to moderate pain due to osteoarthritis of the knee

USUAL DOSAGE Depends upon procedure (slowly introduce a sufficient quantity into eye)

Osteoarthritis (knee): Injection (not for I.V. use): Intra-articular injection once weekly into affected joint for a total of 5 weeks

Contraindications Hypersensitivity to hyaluronate

Pregnancy Risk Factor C

Sodium Hypochlorite Solution

(SOW dee um hye poe KLOR ite soe LOO shun)

Pharmacologic Class Disinfectant, Antibacterial (Topical)

Generic Available No

Use Treatment of athlete's foot (0.5%); wound irrigation (0.5%); disinfect utensils and equipment (5%)

USUAL DOSAGE Topical irrigation

Dosage Forms SOLN: 5% (4000 mL); Modified Dakin's solution: Full strength: 0.5% (1000 mL); Half strength: 0.25% (1000 mL); Quarter strength: 0.125% (1000 mL)

Contraindications Hypersensitivity

Warnings/Precautions For external use only; avoid eye or mucous membrane contact; do not use on open wounds

Pregnancy Risk Factor C

Adverse Reactions 1% to 10%:

Dermatologic: Irritating to skin

Hematologic: Dissolves blood clots, delays clotting

Education and Monitoring Issues

Patient Education: Use exactly as directed; do not overuse. Avoid contact with eyes. Report worsening of condition or lack of healing.

♦ **Sodium P.A.S.** *see* Aminosalicylate Sodium *on page 48*

Sodium Phenylacetate and Sodium Benzoate

(SOW dee um fen il AS e tate & SOW dee um BENZ oh ate)

Pharmacologic Class Ammonium Detoxicant

U.S. Brand Names Ucephan®

Dosage Forms SOLN: Sodium phenylacetate 100 mg and sodium benzoate 100 mg per mL (100 mL)

Pregnancy Risk Factor C

Sodium Phenylbutyrate (SOW dee um fen il BYOO ti rate)

Pharmacologic Class Urea Cycle Disorder (UCD) Treatment Agent

U.S. Brand Names Buphenyl®

(Continued)

Sodium Phenylbutyrate *(Continued)*

Mechanism of Action Sodium phenylbutyrate is a prodrug that, when given orally, is rapidly converted to phenylacetate, which is in turn conjugated with glutamine to form the active compound phenylacetyglutamine; phenylacetyglutamine serves as a substitute for urea and is excreted in the urine whereby it carries with it 2 moles of nitrogen per mole of phenylacetyglutamine and can thereby assist in the clearance of nitrogenous waste in patients with urea cycle disorders

Use Adjunctive therapy in the chronic management of patients with urea cycle disorder involving deficiencies of carbamoylphosphate synthetase, ornithine transcarbamylase, or argininosuccinic acid synthetase

USUAL DOSAGE

Powder: Patients weighing <20 kg: 450-600 mg/kg/day or 9.9-13 g/m^2/day, administered in equally divided amounts with each meal or feeding, four to six times daily; safety and efficacy of doses >20 g/day has not been established

Tablet: Children >20 kg and Adults: 450-600 mg/kg/day or 9.9-13 g/m^2/day, administered in equally divided amounts with each meal; safety and efficacy of doses >20 g/day have not been established

Dosage Forms POWDER: 3.2 g [sodium phenylbutyrate 3 g] per teaspoon (500 mL, 950 mL), 9.1 g [sodium phenylbutyrate 8.6 g] per tablespoon (500 mL, 950 mL). **TAB:** 500 mg

Contraindications Previous hypersensitivity to phenylbutyrate, severe hypertension, heart failure or renal dysfunction; phenylbutyrate is not indicated in the treatment of acute hyperammonemia

Warnings/Precautions Since no studies have been conducted in pregnant women, sodium phenylbutyrate should be used cautiously during pregnancy; each 1 gram of drug contains 125 mg of sodium and, therefore, should be used cautiously, if at all, in patients who must maintain a low sodium intake

Pregnancy Risk Factor C

Adverse Reactions

>10%: Endocrine & metabolic: Amenorrhea, menstrual dysfunction

1% to 10%:

Gastrointestinal: Anorexia, abnormal taste

Miscellaneous: Offensive body odor

Education and Monitoring Issues

Patient Education: It is important that patients understand and follow the dietary restrictions required when treating this disorder, the medication must be taken in strict accordance with the prescribed regimen and the patient should avoid altering the dosage without the prescriber's knowledge; the powder formulation has a very salty taste

Sodium Polystyrene Sulfonate

(SOW dee um pol ee STYE reen SUL fon ate)

Pharmacologic Class Antidote

U.S. Brand Names Kayexalate®; SPS®

Generic Available Yes

Mechanism of Action Removes potassium by exchanging sodium ions for potassium ions in the intestine before the resin is passed from the body; exchange capacity is 1 mEq/g *in vivo*, and *in vitro* capacity is 3.1 mEq/g, therefore, a wide range of exchange capacity exists such that close monitoring of serum electrolytes is necessary

Use Treatment of hyperkalemia

USUAL DOSAGE

Children:

Oral: 1 g/kg/dose every 6 hours

Rectal: 1 g/kg/dose every 2-6 hours (In small children and infants, employ lower doses by using the practical exchange ratio of 1 mEq K^+/g of resin as the basis for calculation)

Adults:

Oral: 15 g (60 mL) 1-4 times/day

Rectal: 30-50 g every 6 hours

Dosage Forms Oral or rectal: **POWDER for susp:** 454 g. **SUSP:** 1.25 g/5 mL with sorbitol 33% and alcohol 0.3% (60 mL, 120 mL, 200 mL, 500 mL)

Contraindications Hypernatremia, hypersensitivity to any component

Warnings/Precautions Use with caution in patients with severe congestive heart failure, hypertension, edema, or renal failure; avoid using the commercially available liquid product in neonates due to the preservative content; large oral doses may cause fecal impaction (especially in elderly); enema will reduce the serum potassium faster than oral administration, but the oral route will result in a greater reduction over several hours.

Pregnancy Risk Factor C

Adverse Reactions 1% to 10%:

Endocrine & metabolic: Hypokalemia, hypocalcemia, hypomagnesemia, sodium retention

Gastrointestinal: Fecal impaction, constipation, loss of appetite, nausea, vomiting

Drug Interactions Systemic alkalosis and seizure has occurred after cation-exchange resins were administered with nonabsorbable cation-donating antacids and laxatives (eg, magnesium hydroxide, aluminum carbonate)

Onset Within 2-24 hours

Education and Monitoring Issues

Patient Education: Emergency instructions depend on patient's condition. You will be monitored for effects of this medication and frequent blood tests may be necessary. Oral: Take as directed. Mix well with a full glass of liquid (not orange juice). You may experience nausea or vomiting (small frequent meals, frequent mouth care, chewing gum, or sucking lozenges may help); or constipation or fecal impaction (increased dietary fluids and exercise may help). Report persistent constipation or gastrointestinal distress; chest pain or rapid heartbeat; or mental confusion or muscle weakness.

Monitoring Parameters: Serum electrolytes (potassium, sodium, calcium, magnesium), EKG

Reference Range: Serum potassium: Adults: 3.5-5.2 mEq/L

- **Sodium Sulamyd** *see* Sulfacetamide Sodium *on page 876*
- **Sodium Sulamyd® Ophthalmic** *see* Sulfacetamide Sodium *on page 876*

Sodium Tetradecyl (SOW dee um tetra DEK il)

Pharmacologic Class Sclerosing Agent

U.S. Brand Names Sotradecol®

Use Treatment of small, uncomplicated varicose veins of the lower extremities; endoscopic sclerotherapy in the management of bleeding esophageal varices

USUAL DOSAGE I.V.: Test dose: 0.5 mL given several hours prior to administration of larger dose; 0.5-2 mL in each vein, maximum: 10 mL per treatment session; 3% solution reserved for large varices

Contraindications Arterial disease, thrombophlebitis, hypersensitivity to sodium tetradecyl or any component, valvular or deep vein incompetence, phlebitis, migraines, cellulitis, acute infections; bedridden patients; patients with uncontrolled systemic disease such as diabetes, toxic hyperthyroidism, tuberculosis, asthma, neoplasm, sepsis, blood dyscrasias, and acute respiratory or skin diseases

Pregnancy Risk Factor C

Sodium Thiosulfate (SOW dee um thye oh SUL fate)

Pharmacologic Class Antidote; Antifungal Agent

U.S. Brand Names Tinver® Lotion

Generic Available Yes

Mechanism of Action

Cyanide toxicity: Increases the rate of detoxification of cyanide by the enzyme rhodanese by providing an extra sulfur

Cisplatin toxicity: Complexes with cisplatin to form a compound that is nontoxic to either normal or cancerous cells

Use

Parenteral: Used alone or with sodium nitrite or amyl nitrite in cyanide poisoning or arsenic poisoning; reduce the risk of nephrotoxicity associated with cisplatin therapy

Topical: Treatment of tinea versicolor

USUAL DOSAGE

Cyanide and nitroprusside antidote: I.V.:

Children <25 kg: 50 mg/kg after receiving 4.5-10 mg/kg sodium nitrite; a half dose of each may be repeated if necessary

Children >25 kg and Adults: 12.5 g after 300 mg of sodium nitrite; a half dose of each may be repeated if necessary

Cyanide poisoning: I.V.: Dose should be based on determination as with nitrite, at rate of 2.5-5 mL/minute to maximum of 50 mL. See table.

Variation of Sodium Nitrite and Sodium Thiosulfate Dose With Hemoglobin Concentration*

Hemoglobin (g/dL)	Initial Dose Sodium Nitrite (mg/kg)	Initial Dose Sodium Nitrite 3% (mL/kg)	Initial Dose Sodium Thiosulfate 25% (mL/kg)
7	5.8	0.19	0.95
8	6.6	0.22	1.10
9	7.5	0.25	1.25
10	8.3	0.27	1.35
11	9.1	0.30	1.50
12	10.0	0.33	1.65
13	10.8	0.36	1.80
14	11.6	0.39	1.95

*Adapted from Berlin DM Jr, "The Treatment of Cyanide Poisoning in Children," *Pediatrics*, 1970, 46:793.

Cisplatin rescue should be given before or during cisplatin administration: I.V. infusion (in sterile water): 12 g/m^2 over 6 hours or 9 g/m^2 I.V. push followed by 1.2 g/m^2 continuous infusion for 6 hours

(Continued)

Sodium Thiosulfate *(Continued)*

Arsenic poisoning: I.V.: 1 mL first day, 2 mL second day, 3 mL third day, 4 mL fourth day, 5 mL on alternate days thereafter

Children and Adults: Topical: 20% to 25% solution: Apply a thin layer to affected areas twice daily

Dosage Forms INJ: 100 mg/mL (10 mL), 250 mg/mL (50 mL). **LOT:** 25% with salicylic acid 1% and isopropyl alcohol 10% (120 mL, 180 mL)

Contraindications Hypersensitivity to any component

Warnings/Precautions Safety in pregnancy has not been established; discontinue topical use if irritation or sensitivity occurs; rapid I.V. infusion has caused transient hypotension and EKG changes in dogs; can increase risk of thiocyanate intoxication

Pregnancy Risk Factor C

Adverse Reactions 1% to 10%:

Cardiovascular: Hypotension

Central nervous system: Coma, CNS depression secondary to thiocyanate intoxication, psychosis, confusion

Dermatologic: Contact dermatitis, local irritation

Neuromuscular & skeletal: Weakness

Otic: Tinnitus

Onset Rapid

Education and Monitoring Issues

Patient Education: Avoid topical application near the eyes, mouth, or other mucous membranes; notify prescriber if condition worsens or burning or irritation occurs; shake well before using

Monitoring Parameters: Monitor for signs of thiocyanate toxicity

- **Sodol®** *see* Carisoprodol *on page 141*
- **SoFlax®** *see* Docusate *on page 290*
- **Solagé™ Topical Solution** *see* Mequinol and Tretinoin *on page 566*
- **Solaquin® [OTC]** *see* Hydroquinone *on page 450*
- **Solaquin Forte®** *see* Hydroquinone *on page 450*
- **Solarcaine® [OTC]** *see* Benzocaine *on page 98*
- **Solarcaine® Aloe Extra Burn Relief [OTC]** *see* Lidocaine *on page 527*
- **Solatene®** *see* Beta-Carotene *on page 103*
- **Solazine** *see* Trifluoperazine *on page 950*
- **Solfoton®** *see* Phenobarbital *on page 723*
- **Solganal®** *see* Aurothioglucose *on page 83*
- **Solium®** *see* Chlordiazepoxide *on page 180*
- **Solu-Cortef®** *see* Hydrocortisone *on page 447*
- **Solu-Medrol® Injection** *see* Methylprednisolone *on page 589*
- **Solurex L.A.®** *see* Dexamethasone *on page 256*
- **Soluver Plus** *see* Salicylic Acid and Lactic Acid *on page 836*
- **Soma®** *see* Carisoprodol *on page 141*
- **Soma® Compound** *see* Carisoprodol and Aspirin *on page 142*
- **Soma® Compound w/Codeine** *see* Carisoprodol, Aspirin, and Codeine *on page 142*
- **Sominex® Oral [OTC]** *see* Diphenhydramine *on page 282*
- **Somnol®** *see* Flurazepam *on page 383*
- **Sonata®** *see* Zaleplon *on page 989*
- **Sopamycetin** *see* Chloramphenicol *on page 178*
- **Soprodol®** *see* Carisoprodol *on page 141*

Sorbitol (SOR bi tole)

Pharmacologic Class Genitourinary Irrigant; Laxative, Miscellaneous

Use Genitourinary irrigant in transurethral prostatic resection or other transurethral resection or other transurethral surgical procedures; diuretic; humectant; sweetening agent; hyperosmotic laxative; facilitate the passage of sodium polystyrene sulfonate through the intestinal tract

USUAL DOSAGE Hyperosmotic laxative (as single dose, at infrequent intervals):

Children 2-11 years:

Oral: 2 mL/kg (as 70% solution)

Rectal enema: 30-60 mL as 25% to 30% solution

Children >12 years and Adults:

Oral: 30-150 mL (as 70% solution)

Rectal enema: 120 mL as 25% to 30% solution

Adjunct to sodium polystyrene sulfonate: 15 mL as 70% solution orally until diarrhea occurs (10-20 mL/2 hours) or 20-100 mL as an oral vehicle for the sodium polystyrene sulfonate resin

When administered with charcoal:

Oral:

Children: 4.3 mL/kg of 35% sorbitol with 1 g/kg of activated charcoal

Adults: 4.3 mL/kg of 70% sorbitol with 1 g/kg of activated charcoal every 4 hours until first stool containing charcoal is passed

Topical: 3% to 3.3% as transurethral surgical procedure irrigation

Contraindications Anuria

- **Sorbitrate®** *see* Isosorbide Dinitrate *on page 490*
- **Soridol®** *see* Carisoprodol *on page 141*
- **Sotacor®** *see* Sotalol *on page 863*

Sotalol (SOE ta lole)

Pharmacologic Class Antiarrhythmic Agent, Class II; Antiarrhythmic Agent, Class III; Beta Blocker, $Beta_1$ Selective

U.S. Brand Names Betapace®; Betapace AF®

Mechanism of Action

Beta-blocker which contains both beta-adrenoreceptor-blocking (Vaughan Williams Class II) and cardiac action potential duration prolongation (Vaughan Williams Class III) properties

Class II effects: Increased sinus cycle length, slowed heart rate, decreased A-V nodal conduction, and increased A-V nodal refractoriness

Class III effects: Prolongation of the atrial and ventricular monophasic action potentials, and effective refractory prolongation of atrial muscle, ventricular muscle, and atrioventricular accessory pathways in both the antegrade and retrograde directions

Sotalol is a racemic mixture of *d*- and *l*-sotalol; both isomers have similar Class III antiarrhythmic effects while the *l*-isomer is responsible for virtually all of the beta-blocking activity

Sotalol has both $beta_1$- and $beta_2$-receptor blocking activity

The beta-blocking effect of sotalol is a noncardioselective [half maximal at about 80 mg/day and maximal at doses of 320-640 mg/day]. Significant beta-blockade occurs at oral doses as low as 25 mg/day.

The Class III effects are seen only at oral doses ≥160 mg/day

Use Treatment of documented ventricular arrhythmias (ie, sustained ventricular tachycardia), that in the judgment of the prescriber are life-threatening; maintenance of normal sinus rhythm in patients with symptomatic atrial fibrillation and atrial flutter who are currently in sinus rhythm

Unlabeled use: Supraventricular arrhythmias

USUAL DOSAGE Sotalol should be initiated and doses increased in a hospital with facilities for cardiac rhythm monitoring and assessment. Proarrhythmic events can occur after initiation of therapy and with each upward dosage adjustment.

Children: Oral: The safety and efficacy of sotalol in children have not been established

Supraventricular arrhythmias: 2-4 mg/kg/24 hours was given in 2 equal doses every 12 hours to 18 infants (≤2 months of age). All infants, except one with chaotic atrial tachycardia, were successfully controlled with sotalol. Ten infants discontinued therapy between the ages of 7-18 months when it was no longer necessary. Median duration of treatment was 12.8 months.

Adults: Oral:

Ventricular arrhythmias (Betapace®):

Initial: 80 mg twice daily

Dose may be increased (gradually allowing 2-3 days between dosing increments in order to attain steady-state plasma concentrations and to allow monitoring of QT intervals) to 240-320 mg/day.

Most patients respond to a total daily dose of 160-320 mg/day in 2-3 divided doses.

Some patients, with life-threatening refractory ventricular arrhythmias, may require doses as high as 480-640 mg/day; however, these doses should only be prescribed when the potential benefit outweighs the increased of adverse events.

Atrial fibrillation or atrial flutter (Betapace AF®): Initial: 80 mg twice daily

If the initial dose does not reduce the frequency of relapses of atrial fibrillation/flutter and is tolerated without excessive QT prolongation (not >520 msec) after 3 days, the dose may be increased to 120 mg twice daily This may be further increased to 160 mg twice daily if response is inadequate and QT prolongation is not excessive.

Elderly: Age does not significantly alter the pharmacokinetics of sotalol, but impaired renal function in elderly patients can increase the terminal half-life, resulting in increased drug accumulation

Dosage adjustment in renal impairment: Impaired renal function can increase the terminal half-life, resulting in increased drug accumulation. Sotalol (Betapace AF®) is contraindicated per the manufacturer for treatment of atrial fibrillation/flutter in patients with a Cl_{cr} <40 mL/minute.

Ventricular arrhythmias (Betapace®):

Cl_{cr} >60 mL/minute: Administer every 12 hours

Cl_{cr} 10-30 mL/minute: Administer every 24 hours

Cl_{cr} 10-30 mL/minute: Administer every 36-48 hours

Cl_{cr} <10 mL/minute: Individualize dose

Atrial fibrillation/flutter (Betapace AF®):

Cl_{cr} >60 mL/minute: Administer every 12 hours

Cl_{cr} 40-60 mL/minute: Administer every 24 hours

(Continued)

Sotalol *(Continued)*

Cl_{cr} <40 mL/minute: Use is contraindicated

Dialysis: Hemodialysis would be expected to reduce sotalol plasma concentrations because sotalol is not bound to plasma proteins and does not undergo extensive metabolism; administer dose postdialysis or administer supplemental 80 mg dose; peritoneal dialysis does not remove sotalol; supplemental dose is not necessary

Dosage Forms TAB: (Betapace®): 80 mg, 120 mg, 160 mg, 320 mg; (Betapace AF®): 80 mg, 120 mg, 160 mg

Contraindications Bronchial asthma, sinus bradycardia, second and third degree A-V block (unless a functioning pacemaker is present), congenital or acquired long Q-T syndromes, cardiogenic shock, uncontrolled congestive heart failure, and previous evidence of hypersensitivity to sotalol; concurrent use with sparfloxacin. Betapace AF® is contraindicated in patients with significantly reduced renal filtration (Cl_{cr} <40 mL/minute).

Warnings/Precautions Use with caution in patients with congestive heart failure, peripheral vascular disease, hypokalemia, hypomagnesemia, renal dysfunction, sick-sinus syndrome; abrupt withdrawal may result in return of life-threatening arrhythmias; sotalol can provoke new or worsening ventricular arrhythmias

Pregnancy Risk Factor B

Pregnancy Implications Clinical effects on the fetus: Although there are no adequate and well controlled studies in pregnant women, sotalol has been shown to cross the placenta, and is found in amniotic fluid. There has been a report of subnormal birth weight with sotalol, therefore, sotalol should be used during pregnancy only if the potential benefit outweighs the potential risk.

Adverse Reactions

>10%:

- Cardiovascular: Bradycardia (16%), chest pain (16%), palpitations (14%)
- Central nervous system: Fatigue (20%), dizziness (20%), lightheadedness (12%)
- Neuromuscular & skeletal: Weakness (13%)
- Respiratory: Dyspnea (21%)

1% to 10%:

- Cardiovascular: Congestive heart failure (5%), reduced peripheral circulation, peripheral vascular disorders (3%) (3%), edema (8%), abnormal EKG (7%), hypotension (6%), proarrhythmia (5%), syncope (5%)
- Central nervous system: Mental confusion (6%), anxiety (4%), headache (8%), sleep problems (8%), depression (4%)
- Dermatologic: Itching/rash (5%)
- Endocrine & metabolic: Decreased sexual ability (3%)
- Gastrointestinal: Diarrhea (7%), nausea/vomiting (10%), stomach discomfort (3% to 6%), flatulence (2%)
- Hematologic: Bleeding (2%)
- Neuromuscular & skeletal: Paresthesia (4%), extremity pain (7%), back pain (3%)
- Ocular: Visual problems (5%)
- Respiratory: Upper respiratory problems (5% to 8%), asthma (2%)
- Genitourinary: Impotence (2%)

<1% (limited to important or life-threatening symptoms): Raynaud's phenomenon, red crusted skin, skin necrosis after extravasation, phlebitis, diaphoresis, cold extremities, increased serum transaminases, emotional lability, clouded sensorium, incoordination, vertigo, paralysis, thrombocytopenia, eosinophilia, leukopenia, photosensitivity reaction, fever, pulmonary edema, hyperlipidemia, myalgia, pruritus, alopecia, xerostomia

Case reports: Leukocytoclastic vasculitis, retroperitoneal fibrosis, bronchiolitis obliterans with organized pneumonia

Drug Interactions

Antacids (aluminum/magnesium) decrease sotalol blood levels - separate by 2 hours

Cisapride and sotalol increases malignant arrhythmias; concurrent use is contraindicated

Clonidine: Sotalol may cause rebound hypertension after discontinuation of clonidine

Drugs which prolong the Q-T interval include amiodarone, amitriptyline, bepridil, disopyramide, erythromycin, haloperidol, imipramine, quinidine, pimozide, procainamide, and thioridazine. Effect/toxicity may be increased; use with caution.

Sparfloxacin, gatifloxacin, and moxifloxacin may result in additional prolongation of the Q-T interval; concurrent use is contraindicated

Alcohol Interactions Limit use (may increase risk of hypotension or dizziness)

Onset Rapid, 1-2 hours; Peak effect: 2.5-4 hours

Duration 8-16 hours

Half-Life 12 hours

Education and Monitoring Issues

Patient Education: Take exactly as directed; do not take additional doses or discontinue without consulting prescriber. You will need regular cardiac checkups and blood tests while taking this medication. You may experience dizziness, drowsiness, or visual changes (use caution when driving or engaging in tasks requiring alertness until response to drug is known); orthostatic hypotension (use caution when climbing stairs or when changing position - rising from lying or sitting position); abnormal taste, nausea or vomiting, or loss of appetite (small frequent meals, frequent mouth care, chewing gum, or sucking lozenges may help); decreased sexual ability (reversible); or constipation (increased exercise, dietary fiber, fruit, or fluid may help). Report chest pain, palpitation, or erratic heartbeat; difficulty breathing or unusual cough; mental depression or persistent insomnia (hallucinations); or changes in vision.

Monitoring Parameters: Serum magnesium, potassium, EKG

Manufacturer Berlex Laboratories, Inc

Related Information

Beta-Blockers Comparison *on page 1233*
Pharmaceutical Manufacturers Directory *on page 1020*

♦ **Sotradecol®** *see* Sodium Tetradecyl *on page 861*
♦ **Soyacal®** *see* Fat Emulsion *on page 351*
♦ **Span-FF® [OTC]** *see* Ferrous Fumarate *on page 359*

Sparfloxacin (spar FLOKS a sin)

Pharmacologic Class Antibiotic, Quinolone

U.S. Brand Names Zagam®

Mechanism of Action Inhibits DNA-gyrase in susceptible organisms; inhibits relaxation of supercoiled DNA and promotes breakage of double-stranded DNA

Use Treatment of adults with community-acquired pneumonia caused by *C. pneumoniae, H. influenzae, H. parainfluenza, M. catarrhalis, M. pneumoniae* or *S. pneumoniae*; treatment of acute bacterial exacerbations of chronic bronchitis caused by *C. pneumoniae, E. cloacae, H. influenzae, H. parainfluenza, K. pneumoniae, M. catarrhalis, S. aureus* or *S. pneumoniae*

USUAL DOSAGE Adults: Oral:

Loading dose: 2 tablets (400 mg) on day 1

Maintenance: 1 tablet (200 mg) daily for 10 days total therapy (total 11 tablets)

Dosing adjustment in renal impairment: Cl_{cr} <50 mL/minute: Administer 400 mg on day 1, then 200 mg every 48 hours for a total of 9 days of therapy (total 6 tablets)

Dosage Forms TAB: 200 mg

Contraindications Hypersensitivity to sparfloxacin, any component, or other quinolones; a concurrent administration with drugs which increase the Q-T interval including: amiodarone, bepridil, bretylium, disopyramide, furosemide, procainamide, quinidine, sotalol, albuterol, astemizole, chloroquine, cisapride, halofantrine, phenothiazines, prednisone, terfenadine, and tricyclic antidepressants; contraindicated in patients with known Q-T prolongation

Warnings/Precautions Not recommended in children <18 years of age, other quinolones have caused transient arthropathy in children; CNS stimulation may occur (tremor, restlessness, confusion, and very rarely hallucinations or seizures); use with caution in patients with known or suspected CNS disorder or renal dysfunction; prolonged use may result in superinfection; if an allergic reaction (itching, urticaria, dyspnea, pharyngeal or facial edema, loss of consciousness, tingling, cardiovascular collapse) occurs, discontinue the drug immediately; use caution to avoid possible photosensitivity reactions during and for several days following fluoroquinolone therapy; pseudomembranous colitis may occur and should be considered in patients who present with diarrhea

Pregnancy Risk Factor C

Pregnancy Implications

Clinical effects on the fetus: Avoid use in pregnant women unless the benefit justifies the potential risk to the fetus

Breast-feeding/lactation: Quinolones are known to distribute well into breast milk; consequently use during lactation should be avoided if possible

Adverse Reactions

>1%:

Central nervous system: Insomnia, agitation, sleep disorders, anxiety, delirium
Gastrointestinal: Diarrhea, abdominal pain, vomiting
Hematologic: Leukopenia, eosinophilia, anemia
Hepatic: Increased LFTs

<1%: Arthralgia, myalgia, photosensitivity, rash

Drug Interactions

Decreased effect: Decreased absorption with antacids containing aluminum, magnesium, and/or calcium, products containing zinc and iron salts, and didanosine when administered concurrently; phenytoin serum levels may be reduced by quinolones; antineoplastic agents may also decrease serum levels of fluoroquinolones

Increased toxicity/serum levels: Quinolones cause increased levels of caffeine, warfarin, cyclosporine, and theophylline (although one study indicates that sparfloxacin may not affect theophylline metabolism), cimetidine and probenecid increase quinolone levels; an increased incidence of seizures may occur with foscarnet. Avoid use with drugs which increase Q-T interval as significant risk of cardiotoxicity may occur. Use with cisapride may increase the risk of malignant arrhythmias, concurrent use is contraindicated.

Half-Life 16 hours

(Continued)

Sparfloxacin *(Continued)*

Education and Monitoring Issues

Patient Education: Take per recommended schedule around-the-clock. Maintain adequate hydration (2-3 L/day of fluids unless instructed to restrict fluid intake). Take complete prescription and do not skip doses; if dose is missed take as soon as possible, do not double doses. Do not take with antacids. You may experience dizziness, lightheadedness, anxiety, insomnia, or confusion; use caution when driving or engaging in tasks that require alertness until response to drug is known. Small frequent meals, frequent mouth care, sucking lozenges, or chewing gum may reduce nausea, vomiting, or taste disturbances. You may experience photosensitivity; use sunscreen, wear protective clothing and eyewear, and avoid direct sunlight. Report palpitations or chest pain; persistent diarrhea or GI disturbances or abdominal pain; muscle tremor or pain; pain, inflammation, or rupture of tendon; yellowing of eyes or skin, easy bruising or bleeding; unusual fatigue; fever, chills, signs of infection; or worsening of condition.

Monitoring Parameters: Evaluation of organ system functions (renal, hepatic, ophthalmologic, and hematopoietic) is recommended periodically during therapy; the possibility of crystalluria should be assessed; WBC and signs and symptoms of infection

Manufacturer Bertek Pharmaceuticals, Inc

Related Information

Antimicrobial Drugs of Choice *on page 1182*
Community Acquired Pneumonia in Adults *on page 1200*
Pharmaceutical Manufacturers Directory *on page 1020*

- **Sparine®** *see* Promazine *on page 777*
- **Spaslin®** *see* Hyoscyamine, Atropine, Scopolamine, and Phenobarbital *on page 456*
- **Spasmolin®** *see* Hyoscyamine, Atropine, Scopolamine, and Phenobarbital *on page 456*
- **Spasmophen®** *see* Hyoscyamine, Atropine, Scopolamine, and Phenobarbital *on page 456*
- **Spasquid®** *see* Hyoscyamine, Atropine, Scopolamine, and Phenobarbital *on page 456*
- **Spec-T® [OTC]** *see* Benzocaine *on page 98*
- **Spectam®** *see* Spectinomycin *on page 866*
- **Spectazole™ Topical** *see* Econazole *on page 305*

Spectinomycin (spek ti noe MYE sin)

Pharmacologic Class Antibiotic, Miscellaneous

U.S. Brand Names Spectam®; Trobicin®

Generic Available No

Mechanism of Action A bacteriostatic antibiotic that selectively binds to the 30s subunits of ribosomes, and thereby inhibiting bacterial protein synthesis

Use Treatment of uncomplicated gonorrhea

USUAL DOSAGE I.M.:

Children:

<45 kg: 40 mg/kg/dose 1 time (ceftriaxone preferred)
≥45 kg: See adult dose

Children >8 years who are allergic to PCNS/cephalosporins may be treated with oral tetracycline

Adults:

Uncomplicated urethral endocervical or rectal gonorrhea: 2 g deep I.M. or 4 g where antibiotic resistance is prevalent 1 time; 4 g (10 mL) dose should be given as two 5 mL injections, followed by doxycycline 100 mg twice daily for 7 days

Disseminated gonococcal infection: 2 g every 12 hours

Dosing adjustment in renal impairment: None necessary

Hemodialysis: 50% removed by hemodialysis

Dosage Forms POWDER for inj: 2 g, 4 g

Contraindications Hypersensitivity to spectinomycin or any component

Pregnancy Risk Factor B

Adverse Reactions <1%: Chills, dizziness, headache, nausea, pain at injection site, pruritus, rash, urticaria, vomiting

Duration Up to 8 hours

Half-Life 1.7 hours

Education and Monitoring Issues

Patient Education: This medication can only be administered I.M. You will need to return for follow-up blood tests. Report chills, nausea, vomiting, abdominal pain, unresolved headache, or dizziness.

Related Information

Antimicrobial Drugs of Choice *on page 1182*
Treatment of Sexually Transmitted Diseases *on page 1210*

- **Spectrobid®** *see* Bacampicillin *on page 89*
- **Spectro Gram** *see* Chlorhexidine Gluconate *on page 181*
- **Spersadex** *see* Dexamethasone *on page 256*

Spironolactone (speer on oh LAK tone)

Pharmacologic Class Diuretic, Potassium Sparing

U.S. Brand Names Aldactone®

Generic Available Yes

Mechanism of Action Competes with aldosterone for receptor sites in the distal renal tubules, increasing sodium chloride and water excretion while conserving potassium and hydrogen ions; may block the effect of aldosterone on arteriolar smooth muscle as well

Use Management of edema associated with excessive aldosterone excretion; hypertension; primary hyperaldosteronism; hypokalemia; treatment of hirsutism; cirrhosis of liver accompanied by edema or ascites. The benefits of spironolactone were additive to the benefits of angiotensin-converting enzyme inhibition in patients with severe CHF (further reducing mortality by 30% over 2 years) in RALES - a large controlled clinical trial.

USUAL DOSAGE Administration with food increases absorption. To reduce delay in onset of effect, a loading dose of 2 or 3 times the daily dose may be administered on the first day of therapy. Oral:

Neonates: Diuretic: 1-3 mg/kg/day divided every 12-24 hours

Children:

- Diuretic, hypertension: 1.5-3.5 mg/kg/day **or** 60 mg/m^2/day in divided doses every 6-24 hours
- Diagnosis of primary aldosteronism: 125-375 mg/m^2/day in divided doses
- Vaso-occlusive disease: 7.5 mg/kg/day in divided doses twice daily (not FDA approved)

Adults:

- Edema, hypertension, hypokalemia: 25-200 mg/day in 1-2 divided doses
- Diagnosis of primary aldosteronism: 100-400 mg/day in 1-2 divided doses
- Hirsutism in women: 50-200 mg/day in 1-2 divided doses
- CHF, patients with severe heart failure already using an ACE inhibitor and a loop diuretic ±digoxin: 25 mg/day, increased or reduced depending on individual response and evidence of hyperkalemia

Elderly: Initial: 25-50 mg/day in 1-2 divided doses, increasing by 25-50 mg every 5 days as needed

Dosing interval in renal impairment:

- Cl_{cr} 10-50 mL/minute: Administer every 12-24 hours
- Cl_{cr} <10 mL/minute: Avoid use

Dosage Forms TAB: 25 mg, 50 mg, 100 mg

Contraindications Hypersensitivity to spironolactone or any components, hyperkalemia, renal failure, anuria, patients receiving other potassium-sparing diuretics or potassium supplements

Warnings/Precautions Use with caution in patients with dehydration, hepatic disease, hyponatremia, renal sufficiency; it is recommended the drug may be discontinued several days prior to adrenal vein catheterization; shown to be tumorigenic in toxicity studies using rats at 25-250 times the usual human dose

Pregnancy Risk Factor D

Pregnancy Implications

Clinical effects on the fetus: No data available on crossing the placenta. 1 report of oral cleft. Generally, use of diuretics during pregnancy is avoided due to risk of decreased placental perfusion.

Breast-feeding/lactation: Crosses into breast milk. American Academy of Pediatrics considers **compatible** with breast-feeding.

Adverse Reactions Percentage unknown: Arrhythmia, ataxia, breast tenderness in females, chills, confusion, cough or hoarseness, decreased sexual ability, deepening of voice in females, diaphoresis, diarrhea, dizziness, drowsiness, dryness of mouth, dyspnea, dysuria, enlargement of breast in males, fever, headache, hyperkalemia, inability to achieve or maintain an erection, increased hair growth in females, increased thirst, lack of energy, lower back or side pain, menstrual changes, nausea, nervousness, numbness or paresthesia in hands/feet/lips, painful urination, shortness of breath, skin rash, stomach cramps, unusual fatigue, vomiting, weakness

Drug Interactions

Angiotensin-converting enzyme inhibitors and angiotensin-receptor antagonists can cause hyperkalemia, especially in patients with renal impairment, potassium-rich diets, or on other drugs causing hyperkalemia; avoid concurrent use or monitor closely

Cholestyramine can cause hyperchloremic acidosis in cirrhotic patients; avoid concurrent use

Digoxin's positive inotropic effect may be reduced; serum levels of digoxin may increase

Mitotane loses its effect; avoid concurrent use

Potassium supplements may increase potassium retention and cause hyperkalemia; avoid concurrent use

Salicylates may interfere with the natriuretic action of spironolactone

Half-Life 78-84 minutes

Education and Monitoring Issues

Patient Education: Take as directed, with meals or milk. This diuretic does not cause potassium loss; avoid excessive potassium intake (eg, salt substitutes, low-salt foods, bananas, nuts). Weigh yourself weekly at the same time, in the same clothes, and

(Continued)

Spironolactone *(Continued)*

report weight loss more than 5 lb/week. You may experience dizziness, drowsiness, headache; use caution when driving or engaging in tasks requiring alertness until response to drug is known. Small frequent meals, frequent mouth care, sucking lozenges, or chewing gum may reduce dry mouth, nausea, or vomiting. You may experience decreased sexual ability (reversible with discontinuing of medication). Report mental confusion; clumsiness; persistent fatigue, chills, numbness, or muscle weakness in hands, feet, or face; acute persistent diarrhea; breast tenderness or increased body hair in females; breast enlargement or inability to achieve erection in males; chest pain, rapid heartbeat or palpitations; or difficulty breathing.

Monitoring Parameters: Blood pressure, serum electrolytes (potassium, sodium), renal function, I & O ratios and daily weight throughout therapy

Related Information

Heart Failure Guidelines *on page 1099*
Hydrochlorothiazide and Spironolactone *on page 443*

- **Sporanox®** *see* Itraconazole *on page 495*
- **SPS®** *see* Sodium Polystyrene Sulfonate *on page 860*
- **S-P-T** *see* Thyroid *on page 915*
- **SRC® Expectorant** *see* Hydrocodone, Pseudoephedrine, and Guaifenesin *on page 446*
- **SSD® AF** *see* Silver Sulfadiazine *on page 852*
- **SSD® Cream** *see* Silver Sulfadiazine *on page 852*
- **SSKI®** *see* Potassium Iodide *on page 754*
- **Stadol®** *see* Butorphanol *on page 125*
- **Stadol® NS** *see* Butorphanol *on page 125*
- **Stagesic®** *see* Hydrocodone and Acetaminophen *on page 444*
- **Stahist®** *see* Chlorpheniramine, Phenylephrine, Phenylpropanolamine, and Belladonna Alkaloids *on page 187*

Stanozolol (stan OH zoe lole)

Pharmacologic Class Anabolic Steroid

U.S. Brand Names Winstrol®

Generic Available No

Mechanism of Action Synthetic testosterone derivative with similar androgenic and anabolic actions

Use Prophylactic use against hereditary angioedema

USUAL DOSAGE

Children: Acute attacks:
- <6 years: 1 mg/day
- 6-12 years: 2 mg/day

Adults: Oral: Initial: 2 mg 3 times/day, may then reduce to a maintenance dose of 2 mg/day or 2 mg every other day after 1-3 months

Dosing adjustment in hepatic impairment: Stanozolol is **not** recommended for patients with severe liver dysfunction

Dosage Forms TAB: 2 mg

Contraindications Nephrosis, carcinoma of breast or prostate, pregnancy, hypersensitivity to any component

Warnings/Precautions May stunt bone growth in children; anabolic steroids may cause peliosis hepatis, liver cell tumors, and blood lipid changes with increased risk of arteriosclerosis; monitor diabetic patients carefully; use with caution in elderly patients, they may be at greater risk for prostatic hypertrophy; use with caution in patients with cardiac, renal, or hepatic disease or epilepsy

Pregnancy Risk Factor X

Adverse Reactions

Male:

Postpubertal:
- >10%:
  - Dermatologic: Acne
  - Endocrine & metabolic: Gynecomastia
  - Genitourinary: Bladder irritability, priapism
- 1% to 10%:
  - Central nervous system: Insomnia, chills
  - Endocrine & metabolic: Decreased libido, hepatic dysfunction
  - Gastrointestinal: Nausea, diarrhea
  - Genitourinary: Prostatic hypertrophy (elderly)
  - Hematologic: Iron deficiency anemia, suppression of clotting factors
- <1%: Hepatic necrosis, hepatocellular carcinoma

Prepubertal:
- >10%:
  - Dermatologic: Acne
  - Endocrine & metabolic: Virilism

1% to 10%:
Central nervous system: Chills, insomnia, factors
Dermatologic: Hyperpigmentation
Gastrointestinal: Diarrhea, nausea
Hematologic: Iron deficiency anemia, suppression of clotting
<1%: Hepatic necrosis, hepatocellular carcinoma

Female:
>10%: Endocrine & metabolic: Virilism
1% to 10%:
Central nervous system: Chills, insomnia
Endocrine & metabolic: Hypercalcemia
Gastrointestinal: Nausea, diarrhea
Hematologic: Iron deficiency anemia, suppression of clotting factors
Hepatic: Hepatic dysfunction
<1%: Hepatic necrosis, hepatocellular carcinoma

Drug Interactions Increased toxicity: ACTH, adrenal steroids may increase risk of edema and acne; stanozolol enhances the hypoprothrombinemic effects of oral anticoagulants; enhances the hypoglycemic effects of insulin and sulfonylureas (oral hypoglycemics)

Education and Monitoring Issues

Patient Education: Take as directed; do not exceed recommended dosage. Diabetics should monitor serum glucose closely and notify prescriber of changes; this medication can alter glucose response. You may experience decrease of libido or impotence (usually reversible); nausea, vomiting, or GI distress (frequent small meals, frequent mouth care, chewing gum, or sucking lozenges may help); or diarrhea (buttermilk, boiled milk, yogurt may help). Report persistent GI distress or diarrhea; change in color of urine or stool; unusual bruising, bleeding, or yellowing of eyes or skin; fluid retention (swelling of ankles, feet, or hands, difficulty breathing, or sudden weight gain); unresolved CNS changes (insomnia or chills); menstrual irregularity; excessive growth of body hair; or other adverse reactions.

Manufacturer Sanofi Winthrop Pharmaceuticals

Related Information

Pharmaceutical Manufacturers Directory *on page 1020*

- **Staphcillin®** *see* Methicillin *on page 580*
- **Statex®** *see* Morphine Sulfate *on page 618*

Stavudine (STAV yoo deen)

Pharmacologic Class Antiretroviral Agent, Reverse Transcriptase Inhibitor (Nucleoside)

U.S. Brand Names Zerit®

Use Treatment of adults with HIV infection in combination with other antiretroviral agents

USUAL DOSAGE Oral:
Children: 2 mg/kg/day
Adults:
≥60 kg: 40 mg every 12 hours
<60 kg: 30 mg every 12 hours
Dose may be cut in half if symptoms of peripheral neuropathy occur

Dosing adjustment in renal impairment:
Cl_{cr} >50 mL/minute:
≥60 kg: 40 mg every 12 hours
<60 kg: 30 mg every 12 hours
Cl_{cr} 26-50 mL/minute:
≥60 kg: 20 mg every 12 hours
<60 kg: 15 mg every 12 hours
Hemodialysis:
≥60 kg: 20 mg every 24 hours
<60 kg: 15 mg every 24 hours

Contraindications Hypersensitivity to stavudine

Warnings/Precautions Use with caution in patients who demonstrate previous hypersensitivity to zidovudine, didanosine, zalcitabine, pre-existing bone marrow suppression, renal insufficiency, or peripheral neuropathy. Peripheral neuropathy may be the dose-limiting side effect. Zidovudine should not be used in combination with stavudine. Potentially fatal lactic acidosis and hepatomegaly have been reported, use with caution in patients at risk of hepatic disease

Pregnancy Risk Factor C

Adverse Reactions All adverse reactions reported below were similar to comparative agent, zidovudine, except for peripheral neuropathy, which was greater for stavudine.

>10%:
Central nervous system: Headache, chills/fever, malaise, insomnia, anxiety, depression, pain
Dermatologic: Rash
Gastrointestinal: Nausea, vomiting, diarrhea, pancreatitis, abdominal pain
Neuromuscular & skeletal: Peripheral neuropathy (15% to 21%)

(Continued)

Stavudine *(Continued)*

1% to 10%:
Hematologic: Neutropenia, thrombocytopenia
Hepatic: Increased hepatic transaminases, increased bilirubin
Neuromuscular & skeletal: Myalgia, back pain, weakness
<1%: Anemia, hepatic failure, hepatomegaly, lactic acidosis, pancreatitis

Manufacturer Bristol-Myers Squibb Company (Pharmaceutical Division)

Related Information
Antiretroviral Therapy for HIV Infection *on page 1190*
Pharmaceutical Manufacturers Directory *on page 1020*

- **S-T Cort®** *see* Hydrocortisone *on page 447*
- **Stelazine®** *see* Trifluoperazine *on page 950*
- **Sterapred®** *see* Prednisone *on page 763*
- **Stieva-A®** *see* Tretinoin, Topical *on page 944*
- **Stieva-A® Forte** *see* Tretinoin, Topical *on page 944*
- **Stilphostrol®** *see* Diethylstilbestrol *on page 269*
- **Stimate™ Nasal** *see* Desmopressin Acetate *on page 254*

Stinging Nettle

Pharmacologic Class Herb

Mechanism of Action

Root: Stinging nettle root is reported to inhibit binding to cytosolic androgen receptors within prostatic tissues. It also inhibits the effects of estrogen and should be avoided in pregnancy due to potential uterine stimulation. Stinging nettle root is claimed to influence the binding of 5 alpha-dihydrotestosterone with its receptors.

Stinging nettle leaf is used to increase the renal excretion of uric acid and mobilizes tissue stores. Freeze-dried stinging nettle leaf has been reported to have antihistaminic properties and may be useful for symptoms of allergic rhinitis.

Use
Leaf: Allergic rhinitis (Mittman, 1990)
Leaf: Increases uric acid excretion (Bradley, 1992)
Root: Benign prostatic hyperplasia (BPH) (Krzeski, 1993; Wagner, 1989)

USUAL DOSAGE Oral:
Leaf: 300-1200 mg 2-4 times/day as needed of freeze-dried leaf
Root: 250 mg 1-3 times/day, standardized to contain 1% to 2% plant silica per dose

Contraindications Use of stinging nettle is contraindicated in pregnancy (uterine stimulation in animal studies, Brinker, 1997). Use with caution in individuals with renal insufficiency or disease (due to silica content in leaf). Prostate exam and laboratory testing should be performed to rule out cancer prior to use for symptoms of BPH. Based on pharmacological activity, use with caution in individuals with gout or a history of uric acid renal stones.

Warnings/Precautions Use all herbal supplements with extreme caution in children <2 years of age and in pregnancy or lactation. Some herbs are contraindicated in pregnancy or lactation; make sure to observe warnings. Use with caution in individuals on medication and with pre-existing medical conditions. Always review for potential herb-drug interactions (HDIs) and other warnings. Large and prolonged doses may increase the potential for adverse effects. Herbs may cause transient adverse effects such as nausea, vomiting, and GI distress due to a variety of chemical constituents. Caution should be used in individuals having known allergies to plants.

Drug Interactions None known. At high intakes, may alter response to warfarin (due to vitamin K content).

St Johns Wort

Pharmacologic Class Herbal

Mechanism of Action Active ingredients are xanthones flavonoids (hypericin) which can act as monoamine oxidase inhibitors, although *in vitro* activity is minimal; majority of activity appears to be related to GABA modulation; may be related to dopamine, serotonin norepinephrine modulation also

Use Mild to moderate depression; also used traditionally for treatment of stress, anxiety, insomnia; used topically for vitiligo; also a popular drug for AIDS patients due to possible antiretroviral activity; used topically for wound healing
Per Commission E: Psychovegetative disorders, depressive moods, anxiety and/or nervous unrest; oily preparations for dyspeptic complaints; oily preparations externally for treatment of post-therapy of acute and contused injuries, myalgia, first degree burns

USUAL DOSAGE Based on hypericin extract content
Oral: 300 mg 3 times daily (not to be used longer than 8 weeks)
Herb: 2-4 g 3 times daily
Liquid extract: 2-4 mL 3 times/day
Tincture: 2-4 mL 3 times/day
Topical: Crushed leaves and flowers are applied to affected area after cleansing with soap and water

Per Commission E: 2-4 g drug (dried herb) or 0.2-1 mg of total hypericin in other forms of drug application

Contraindications Endogenous depression, pregnancy, children <2 years of age (not confirmed in animal models, *in vitro* only).

Warnings/Precautions May be photosensitizing

Pregnancy Implications Do not use

Adverse Reactions

Cardiovascular: Sinus tachycardia

Dermatologic: Photosensitization is possible, especially in fair-skinned persons (per Commission E)

Gastrointestinal: Stomach pains, abdominal pain

Drug Interactions Avoid amphetamines or other stimulants; use with caution in patients taking MAO inhibitors, levodopa, and 5-hydroxytryptophan; avoid tyramine-containing foods due to presence of hypercin although human data of this potential drug interaction is lacking; avoid concurrent use with SSRI or other antidepressants

♦ **St Joseph® Adult Chewable Aspirin [OTC]** *see* Aspirin *on page 72*

♦ **St. Joseph® Measured Dose Nasal Solution [OTC]** *see* Phenylephrine *on page 727*

♦ **Stop® [OTC]** *see* Fluoride *on page 376*

♦ **Streptase®** *see* Streptokinase *on page 871*

Streptokinase (strep toe KYE nase)

Pharmacologic Class Thrombolytic Agent

U.S. Brand Names Kabikinase®; Streptase®

Generic Available No

Mechanism of Action Activates the conversion of plasminogen to plasmin by forming a complex, exposing plasminogen-activating site, and cleaving a peptide bond that converts plasminogen to plasmin; plasmin degrades fibrin, fibrinogen and other procoagulant proteins into soluble fragments; effective both outside and within the formed thrombus/embolus

Use Thrombolytic agent used in treatment of recent severe or massive deep vein thrombosis, pulmonary emboli, myocardial infarction, and occluded arteriovenous cannulas

USUAL DOSAGE I.V.:

Children: Safety and efficacy not established; limited studies have used 3500-4000 units/kg over 30 minutes followed by 1000-1500 units/kg/hour

Clotted catheter: 25,000 units, clamp for 2 hours then aspirate contents and flush with normal saline

Adults: Antibodies to streptokinase remain for at least 3-6 months after initial dose: Administration requires the use of an infusion pump

An intradermal skin test of 100 units has been suggested to predict allergic response to streptokinase. If a positive reaction is not seen after 15-20 minutes, a therapeutic dose may be administered.

Guidelines for acute myocardial infarction (AMI): 1.5 million units over 60 minutes

Administration:

Dilute two 750,000 unit vials of streptokinase with 5 mL dextrose 5% in water (D_5W) each, gently swirl to dissolve

Add this dose of the 1.5 million units to 150 mL D_5W

This should be infused over 60 minutes; an in-line filter ≥0.45 micron should be used

Monitor for the first few hours for signs of anaphylaxis or allergic reaction. **Infusion should be slowed if lowering of 25 mm Hg in blood pressure or terminated if asthmatic symptoms appear.**

Begin heparin 5000-10,000 unit bolus followed by 1000 units/hour approximately 3-4 hours after completion of streptokinase infusion or when PTT is <100 seconds

Guidelines for acute pulmonary embolism (APE): 3 million unit dose over 24 hours

Administration:

Dilute four 750,000 unit vials of streptokinase with 5 mL dextrose 5% in water (D_5W) each, gently swirl to dissolve

Add this dose of 3 million units to 250 mL D_5W, an in-line filter ≥0.45 micron should be used

Administer 250,000 units (23 mL) over 30 minutes followed by 100,000 units/hour (9 mL/hour) for 24 hours

Monitor for the first few hours for signs of anaphylaxis or allergic reaction. **Infusion should be slowed if blood pressure is lowered by 25 mm Hg or if asthmatic symptoms appear.**

Begin heparin 1000 units/hour about 3-4 hours after completion of streptokinase infusion or when PTT is <100 seconds

Monitor PT, PTT, and fibrinogen levels during therapy

Thromboses: 250,000 units to start, then 100,000 units/hour for 24-72 hours depending on location

Cannula occlusion: 250,000 units into cannula, clamp for 2 hours, then aspirate contents and flush with normal saline

Dosage Forms POWDER for inj: 250,000 units (5 mL, 6.5 mL), 600,000 units (5 mL), 750,000 units (6 mL, 6.5 mL), 1,500,000 units (6.5 mL, 10 mL, 50 mL)

(Continued)

Streptokinase *(Continued)*

Contraindications Hypersensitivity to streptokinase or any component; recent streptococcal infection within the last 6 months; any internal bleeding; brain carcinoma; pregnancy; cerebrovascular accident or transient ischemic attack, gastrointestinal bleeding, trauma or surgery, prolonged external cardiac massage, intracranial or intraspinal surgery or trauma within 1 month; arteriovenous malformation or aneurysm; bleeding diathesis; severe hepatic or renal disease; subacute bacterial endocarditis; pericarditis; hemostatic defects; suspected aortic dissection, severe uncontrolled hypertension (BP systolic ≥180 mm Hg, BP diastolic ≥110 mm Hg)

Warnings/Precautions Avoid I.M. injections; use with caution in patients >75 years of age, patients with a history of cardiac arrhythmias, septic thrombophlebitis or occluded A-V cannula at seriously infected site, patients with a high likelihood of left heart thrombus, (eg, mitral stenosis with atrial fibrillation), major surgery within last 10 days, GI bleeding, diabetic hemorrhagic retinopathy, subacute bacterial endocarditis, cerebrovascular disease, recent trauma including cardiopulmonary resuscitation, or severe hypertension (systolic BP >180 mm Hg and/or diastolic BP >110 mm Hg); antibodies to streptokinase remain for 3-6 months after initial dose, use another thrombolytic enzyme (ie, alteplase) if thrombolytic therapy is indicated in patients with prior streptokinase therapy

Streptokinase is not indicated for restoration of patency of intravenous catheters. Serious adverse events relating to the use of streptokinase in the restoration of patency of occluded intravenous catheters have involved the use of high doses of streptokinase in small volumes (250,000 international units in 2 mL). Uses of lower doses of streptokinase in infusions over several hours, generally into partially occluded catheters, or local instillation into the catheter lumen and subsequent aspiration, have been described in the medical literature. Healthcare providers should consider the risk for potentially life-threatening reactions (eg, hypotension, hypersensitivity reactions, apnea, bleeding) associated with the use of streptokinase in the management of occluded intravenous catheters.

Pregnancy Risk Factor C

Adverse Reactions As with all drugs which may affect hemostasis, bleeding is the major adverse effect associated with streptokinase. Hemorrhage may occur at virtually any site. Risk is dependent on multiple variables, including the dosage administered, concurrent use of multiple agents which alter hemostasis, and patient predisposition (including hypertension). Rapid lysis of coronary artery thrombi by thrombolytic agents may be associated with reperfusion-related atrial and/or ventricular arrhythmias.

>10%:
- Cardiovascular: Hypotension
- Local: Injection site bleeding

1% to 10%:
- Central nervous system: Fever (1% to 4%)
- Dermatologic: Bruising, rash, pruritus
- Gastrointestinal: Gastrointestinal hemorrhage, nausea, vomiting
- Genitourinary: Genitourinary hemorrhage
- Hematologic: Anemia
- Miscellaneous: Diaphoresis
- Neuromuscular and skeletal: Muscle pain
- Ocular: Eye hemorrhage, periorbital edema
- Respiratory: Bronchospasm, epistaxis

<1%: Intracranial hemorrhage, retroperitoneal hemorrhage, pericardial hemorrhage, gingival hemorrhage, epistaxis, allergic reactions, anaphylaxis, anaphylactic shock, angioneurotic edema, anaphylactoid reactions, laryngeal edema, urticaria, back pain (during infusion), elevated transaminases, respiratory depression, morbilliform, erysipelas-like rash, hemarthrosis

Case reports: Guillain-Barré syndrome, Parsonage-Turner syndrome, splenic rupture, acute tubular necrosis, cholesterol embolization, ARDS

Additional cardiovascular events associated with use in myocardial infarction: A-V block, cardiogenic shock, heart failure, cardiac arrest, recurrent ischemia/infarction, myocardial rupture, electromechanical dissociation, pericardial effusion, pericarditis, mitral regurgitation, cardiac tamponade, thromboembolism, pulmonary edema, asystole, ventricular tachycardia

Drug Interactions

Aminocaproic acid (antifibrinolytic agent) may decrease effectiveness

Drugs which affect platelet function (eg, NSAIDs, dipyridamole, ticlopidine, clopidogrel, IIb/IIIa antagonists) may potentiate the risk of hemorrhage; use with caution

Heparin and aspirin: Use with aspirin and heparin may increase bleeding over aspirin and heparin alone. However, aspirin and heparin were used concurrently in the majority of patients in some major clinical studies of streptokinase.

Warfarin or oral anticoagulants: Risk of bleeding may be increased during concurrent therapy

Onset Activation of plasminogen occurs almost immediately

Duration Fibrinolytic effects last only a few hours, while anticoagulant effects can persist for 12-24 hours.

Half-Life 83 minutes

Education and Monitoring Issues

Patient Education: Following infusion, absolute bedrest is important; call for assistance changing position. You will have increased tendency to bleed; avoid razors, scissors or sharps, and use soft toothbrush or cotton swabs. Report back pain, abdominal pain, muscle cramping, acute onset headache, or chest pain.

Monitoring Parameters: Blood pressure, PT, APTT, platelet count, hematocrit, fibrinogen concentration, signs of bleeding

Reference Range:

Partial thromboplastin time (PTT) activated: 20.4-33.2 seconds
Prothrombin time (PT): 10.9-13.7 seconds (same as control)
Fibrinogen: 200-400 mg/dL

Streptomycin (strep toe MYE sin)

Pharmacologic Class Antibiotic, Aminoglycoside; Antitubercular Agent

Generic Available Yes

Mechanism of Action Inhibits bacterial protein synthesis by binding directly to the 30S ribosomal subunits causing faulty peptide sequence to form in the protein chain

Use Part of combination therapy of active tuberculosis; used in combination with other agents for treatment of streptococcal or enterococcal endocarditis, mycobacterial infections, plague, tularemia, and brucellosis

USUAL DOSAGE

Children:
- Daily therapy: 20-30 mg/kg/day (maximum: 1 g/day)
- Directly observed therapy (DOT): Twice weekly: 25-30 mg/kg (maximum: 1.5 g)
- DOT: 3 times/week: 25-30 mg/kg (maximum: 1 g)

Adults:
- Daily therapy: 15 mg/kg/day (maximum: 1 g)
- Directly observed therapy (DOT): Twice weekly: 25-30 mg/kg (maximum: 1.5 g)
- DOT: 3 times/week: 25-30 mg/kg (maximum: 1 g)
- Enterococcal endocarditis: 1 g every 12 hours for 2 weeks, 500 mg every 12 hours for 4 weeks in combination with penicillin
- Streptococcal endocarditis: 1 g every 12 hours for 1 week, 500 mg every 12 hours for 1 week
- Tularemia: 1-2 g/day in divided doses for 7-10 days or until patient is afebrile for 5-7 days
- Plague: 2-4 g/day in divided doses until the patient is afebrile for at least 3 days

Elderly: 10 mg/kg/day, not to exceed 750 mg/day; dosing interval should be adjusted for renal function; some authors suggest not to give more than 5 days/week or give as 20-25 mg/kg/dose twice weekly

Dosing interval in renal impairment:
- Cl_{cr} 10-50 mL/minute: Administer every 24-72 hours
- Cl_{cr} <10 mL/minute: Administer every 72-96 hours

Removed by hemo and peritoneal dialysis: Administer dose postdialysis

Dosage Forms INJ: 400 mg/mL (2.5 mL)

Contraindications Hypersensitivity to streptomycin or any component

Warnings/Precautions Use with caution in patients with pre-existing vertigo, tinnitus, hearing loss, neuromuscular disorders, or renal impairment; modify dosage in patients with renal impairment; aminoglycosides are associated with significant nephrotoxicity or ototoxicity; the ototoxicity is directly proportional to the amount of drug given and the duration of treatment; tinnitus or vertigo are indications of vestibular injury and impending bilateral irreversible damage; renal damage is usually reversible

Pregnancy Risk Factor D

Adverse Reactions

1% to 10%:
- Central nervous system: Neurotoxicity
- Renal: Nephrotoxicity
- Otic: Ototoxicity (auditory), ototoxicity (vestibular)

<1%: Anemia, arthralgia, difficulty in breathing, drowsiness, drug fever, eosinophilia, headache, hypotension, nausea, paresthesia, skin rash, tremor, vomiting, weakness

Drug Interactions

Increased/prolonged effect: Depolarizing and nondepolarizing neuromuscular blocking agents

Increased toxicity: Concurrent use of amphotericin may increase nephrotoxicity

Half-Life 2-4.7 hours, prolonged with renal impairment

Education and Monitoring Issues

Patient Education: This medication can only be given by intramuscular injection. Therapy for TB or HIV will generally last several months. Do not discontinue even if you are feeling better. Maintain adequate hydration (2-3 L/day of fluids unless instructed to restrict fluid intake). You may experience headache or dizziness (use caution when driving or engaging in tasks requiring alertness until response to drug is known); nausea, vomiting, or loss of appetite (frequent small meals, frequent mouth care, sucking lozenges, or chewing gum may help). Report immediately any rash, joint or back pain, or difficulty breathing; swelling of extremities or weight gain greater than 5 lb/

(Continued)

Streptomycin *(Continued)*

week; fever, chills, mouth sores, vaginal itching or drainage, or foul-smelling stool; change in hearing, ringing or sense of fullness in ears; numbness, loss of sensation, clumsiness, change in strength, or altered gait.

Monitoring Parameters: Hearing (audiogram), BUN, creatinine; serum concentration of the drug should be monitored in all patients; eighth cranial nerve damage is usually preceded by high-pitched tinnitus, roaring noises, sense of fullness in ears, or impaired hearing and may persist for weeks after drug is discontinued

Reference Range: Therapeutic: Peak: 20-30 µg/mL; Trough: <5 µg/mL; Toxic: Peak: >50 µg/mL; Trough: >10 µg/mL

Related Information

Antimicrobial Drugs of Choice *on page 1182*

Tuberculosis Treatment Guidelines *on page 1213*

- **Stresstabs® 600 Advanced Formula Tablets [OTC]** *see* Vitamins, Multiple *on page 981*
- **Stromectol®** *see* Ivermectin *on page 496*

Strontium-89 (STRON shee um-atey nine)

Pharmacologic Class Radiopharmaceutical

U.S. Brand Names Metastron®

Use Relief of bone pain in patients with skeletal metastases

USUAL DOSAGE Adults: I.V.: 148 megabecquerel (4 millicurie) administered by slow I.V. injection over 1-2 minutes or 1.5-2.2 megabecquerel (40-60 microcurie)/kg; repeated doses are generally not recommended at intervals <90 days; measure the patient dose by a suitable radioactivity calibration system immediately prior to administration

Dosage Forms INJ: 10.9-22.6 mg/mL [148 megabecquerel, 4 millicurie] (10 mL)

Contraindications Patients with a history of hypersensitivity to any strontium-containing compounds, or any other component; pregnancy, lactation

Warnings/Precautions Use caution in patients with bone marrow compromise; incontinent patients may require urinary catheterization. Body fluids may remain radioactive up to one week after injection. Not indicated for use in patients with cancer not involving bone and should be used with caution in patients whose platelet counts fall <60,000 or whose white blood cell counts fall <2400. A small number of patients have experienced a transient increase in bone pain at 36-72 hours postdose; this reaction is generally mild and self-limiting. It should be handled cautiously, in a similar manner to other radioactive drugs. Appropriate safety measures to minimize radiation to personnel should be instituted.

Pregnancy Risk Factor D

Adverse Reactions Most severe reactions of marrow toxicity can be managed by conventional means

Percentage unknown: Fever and chills (rare), flushing (most common after rapid injection), increase in bone pain may occur (10% to 20% of patients), leukopenia, thrombocytopenia

Education and Monitoring Issues

Patient Education: Eat and drink normally, there is no need to avoid alcohol or caffeine unless already advised to do so; may be advised to take analgesics until Metastron® begins to become effective; the effect lasts for several months, if pain returns before that, notify medical personnel

Monitoring Parameters: Routine blood tests

- **Stuartnatal® 1 + 1** *see* Vitamins, Multiple *on page 981*
- **Stuart Prenatal® [OTC]** *see* Vitamins, Multiple *on page 981*
- **Sublimaze® Injection** *see* Fentanyl *on page 355*

Sucralfate (soo KRAL fate)

Pharmacologic Class Gastrointestinal Agent, Miscellaneous

U.S. Brand Names Carafate®

Generic Available No

Mechanism of Action Forms a complex by binding with positively charged proteins in exudates, forming a viscous paste-like, adhesive substance. This selectively forms a protective coating that protects the lining against peptic acid, pepsin, and bile salts.

Use Short-term management of duodenal ulcers

Unlabeled use: Gastric ulcers; maintenance of duodenal ulcers; suspension may be used topically for treatment of stomatitis due to cancer chemotherapy and other causes of esophageal and gastric erosions; GERD, esophagitis; treatment of NSAID mucosal damage; prevention of stress ulcers; postsclerotherapy for esophageal variceal bleeding

USUAL DOSAGE Oral:

Children: Dose not established, doses of 40-80 mg/kg/day divided every 6 hours have been used

Stomatitis: 2.5-5 mL (1 g/10 mL suspension), swish and spit or swish and swallow 4 times/day

Adults:
Stress ulcer prophylaxis: 1 g 4 times/day
Stress ulcer treatment: 1 g every 4 hours
Duodenal ulcer:
Treatment: 1 g 4 times/day on an empty stomach and at bedtime for 4-8 weeks, or alternatively 2 g twice daily; treatment is recommended for 4-8 weeks in adults, the elderly may require 12 weeks
Maintenance: Prophylaxis: 1 g twice daily
Stomatitis: 1 g/10 mL suspension, swish and spit or swish and swallow 4 times/day

Dosage comment in renal impairment: Aluminum salt is minimally absorbed (<5%), however, may accumulate in renal failure

Dosage Forms SUSP, oral: 1 g/10 mL (420 mL). **TAB:** 1 g

Contraindications Hypersensitivity to sucralfate or any component

Warnings/Precautions Successful therapy with sucralfate should not be expected to alter the posthealing frequency of recurrence or the severity of duodenal ulceration; use with caution in patients with chronic renal failure who have an impaired excretion of absorbed aluminum. Because of the potential for sucralfate to alter the absorption of some drugs, separate administration (take other medication 2 hours before sucralfate) should be considered when alterations in bioavailability are believed to be critical

Pregnancy Risk Factor B

Pregnancy Implications

Clinical effects on the fetus: No data available; available evidence suggests safe use during pregnancy and breast-feeding

Breast-feeding/lactation: No data available. American Academy of Pediatrics has NO RECOMMENDATION.

Adverse Reactions

1% to 10%: Gastrointestinal: Constipation

<1%: Back pain diarrhea, dizziness, gastric discomfort, indigestion, insomnia, nausea, pruritus, rash, sleepiness, vertigo, vomiting, xerostomia

Drug Interactions Decreased effect: Digoxin, phenytoin (hydantoins), warfarin, ketoconazole, quinidine, ciprofloxacin, norfloxacin (quinolones), tetracycline, theophylline; because of the potential for sucralfate to alter the absorption of some drugs, separate administration (take other medications 2 hours before sucralfate) should be considered when alterations in bioavailability are believed to be critical

Note: When given with aluminum-containing antacids, may increase serum/body aluminum concentrations (see Warnings/Precautions)

Alcohol Interactions Avoid or limit use (may enhance gastric mucosal irritation)

Onset Paste formation and ulcer adhesion occur within 1-2 hours.

Duration Up to 6 hours

Education and Monitoring Issues

Patient Education: Take recommended dose before meals or on an empty stomach. Take any other medications at least 2 hours before taking sucralfate. Do not take antacids within 30 minutes of taking sucralfate. May cause constipation; increased exercise, increased dietary fiber, fruit or fluids, or mild stool softener may be helpful. If constipation or gastric distress persists, consult prescriber.

- **Sucrets® [OTC]** *see* Dyclonine *on page 304*
- **Sucrets® for Kids** *see* Dyclonine *on page 304*
- **Sudafed® [OTC]** *see* Pseudoephedrine *on page 792*
- **Sudafed® 12 Hour [OTC]** *see* Pseudoephedrine *on page 792*
- **Sufedrin® [OTC]** *see* Pseudoephedrine *on page 792*
- **Sular®** *see* Nisoldipine *on page 657*

Sulconazole (sul KON a zole)

Pharmacologic Class Antifungal Agent

U.S. Brand Names Exelderm®

Use Treatment of superficial fungal infections of the skin, including tinea cruris (jock itch), tinea corporis (ringworm), tinea versicolor, and possibly tinea pedis (athlete's foot - cream only)

USUAL DOSAGE Adults: Topical: Apply a small amount to the affected area and gently massage once or twice daily for 3 weeks (tinea cruris, tinea corporis, tinea versicolor) to 4 weeks (tinea pedis).

Contraindications Known hypersensitivity to sulconazole

Pregnancy Risk Factor C

- **Sulcrate** *see* Sucralfate *on page 874*
- **Sulf-10® Ophthalmic** *see* Sulfacetamide Sodium *on page 876*

Sulfabenzamide, Sulfacetamide, and Sulfathiazole

(sul fa BENZ a mide, sul fa SEE ta mide, & sul fa THYE a zole)

Pharmacologic Class Antibiotic, Vaginal

U.S. Brand Names Femguard®; Gyne-Sulf®; Sulfa-Gyn®; Sulfa-Trip®; Sultrin™; Trysul®; Vagilia®; V.V.S.®

(Continued)

Sulfabenzamide, Sulfacetamide, and Sulfathiazole *(Continued)*

Use Treatment of *Haemophilus vaginalis* vaginitis

USUAL DOSAGE Adults:

Cream: Insert one applicatorful in vagina twice daily for 4-6 days; dosage may then be decreased to ½ to ¼ of an applicatorful twice daily

Tablet: Insert one intravaginally twice daily for 10 days

Contraindications Hypersensitivity to sulfabenzamide, sulfacetamide, sulfathiazole or any component, renal dysfunction

Pregnancy Risk Factor C (avoid near term)

Sulfacetamide Sodium (sul fa SEE ta mide SOW dee um)

Pharmacologic Class Antibiotic, Ophthalmic; Antibiotic, Sulfonamide Derivative

U.S. Brand Names AK-Sulf® Ophthalmic; Bleph®-10 Ophthalmic; Cetamide® Ophthalmic; Isopto® Cetamide® Ophthalmic; Klaron® Lotion; Ocusulf-10® Ophthalmic; Sebizon® Topical Lotion; Sodium Sulamyd® Ophthalmic; Sulf-10® Ophthalmic

Use Treatment and prophylaxis of conjunctivitis due to susceptible organisms; corneal ulcers; adjunctive treatment with systemic sulfonamides for therapy of trachoma; topical application in scaling dermatosis (seborrheic); bacterial infections of the skin

USUAL DOSAGE

Children >2 months and Adults: Ophthalmic:

Ointment: Apply to lower conjunctival sac 1-4 times/day and at bedtime

Solution: Instill 1-3 drops several times daily up to every 2-3 hours in lower conjunctival sac during waking hours and less frequently at night

Children >12 years and Adults: Topical:

Seborrheic dermatitis: Apply at bedtime and allow to remain overnight; in severe cases, may apply twice daily

Secondary cutaneous bacterial infections: Apply 2-4 times/day until infection clears

Contraindications Hypersensitivity to sulfacetamide or any component, sulfonamides; infants <2 months of age

Pregnancy Risk Factor C

Related Information

Sulfacetamide Sodium and Fluorometholone *on page 876*
Sulfacetamide Sodium and Phenylephrine *on page 876*
Sulfacetamide Sodium and Prednisolone *on page 876*
Sulfur and Sulfacetamide Sodium *on page 883*

Sulfacetamide Sodium and Fluorometholone

(sul fa SEE ta mide SOW dee um & flure oh METH oh lone)

Pharmacologic Class Antibiotic/Corticosteroid, Ophthalmic

U.S. Brand Names FML-S® Ophthalmic Suspension

Dosage Forms SUSP, ophth: Sulfacetamide sodium 10% and fluorometholone 0.1% (5 mL, 10 mL)

Pregnancy Risk Factor C

Sulfacetamide Sodium and Phenylephrine

(sul fa SEE ta mide SOW dee um & fen il EF rin)

Pharmacologic Class Antibiotic, Ophthalmic

U.S. Brand Names Vasosulf® Ophthalmic

Dosage Forms SOLN, ophth: Sulfacetamide sodium 15% and phenylephrine hydrochloride 0.125% (5 mL, 15 mL)

Pregnancy Risk Factor C

Sulfacetamide Sodium and Prednisolone

(sul fa SEE ta mide SOW dee um & pred NIS oh lone)

Pharmacologic Class Antibiotic/Corticosteroid, Ophthalmic

U.S. Brand Names AK-Cide® Ophthalmic; Blephamide® Ophthalmic; Cetapred® Ophthalmic; Isopto® Cetapred® Ophthalmic; Metimyd® Ophthalmic; Vasocidin® Ophthalmic

Use Treatment of superficial ocular infections

Dosage Forms OINT, ophth: (AK-Cide®, Metimyd®, Vasocidin®): Sulfacetamide sodium 10% and prednisolone acetate 0.5% (3.5 g); (Blephamide®): Sulfacetamide sodium 10% and prednisolone acetate 0.2% (3.5 g); (Cetapred®): Sulfacetamide sodium 10% and prednisolone acetate 0.25% (3.5 g). **SUSP, ophth:** Sulfacetamide sodium 10% and prednisolone sodium phosphate 0.25% (5 mL); (AK-Cide®, Metimyd®): Sulfacetamide sodium 10% and prednisolone acetate 0.5% (5 mL); (Blephamide®): Sulfacetamide sodium 10% and prednisolone acetate 0.2% (2.5 mL, 5 mL, 10 mL); (Isopto® Cetapred®): Sulfacetamide sodium 10% and prednisolone acetate 0.25% (5 mL, 15 mL); (Vasocidin®): Sulfacetamide sodium 10% and prednisolone sodium phosphate: 0.25% (5 mL, 10 mL)

♦ **Sulfacet-R** *see* Sulfur and Sulfacetamide Sodium *on page 883*

♦ **Sulfacet-R® Topical** *see* Sulfur and Sulfacetamide Sodium *on page 883*

Sulfadiazine (sul fa DYE a zeen)

Pharmacologic Class Antibiotic, Sulfonamide Derivative

U.S. Brand Names Microsulfon®

Generic Available Yes

Mechanism of Action Interferes with bacterial growth by inhibiting bacterial folic acid synthesis through competitive antagonism of PABA

Use Treatment of urinary tract infections and nocardiosis, rheumatic fever prophylaxis; adjunctive treatment in toxoplasmosis; uncomplicated attack of malaria

USUAL DOSAGE Oral:

Congenital toxoplasmosis:

Newborns and Children <2 months: 100 mg/kg/day divided every 6 hours in conjunction with pyrimethamine 1 mg/kg/day once daily and supplemental folinic acid 5 mg every 3 days for 6 months

Children >2 months: 25-50 mg/kg/dose 4 times/day

Toxoplasmosis:

Children >2 months: Loading dose: 75 mg/kg; maintenance dose: 120-150 mg/kg/day, maximum dose: 6 g/day; divided every 4-6 hours in conjunction with pyrimethamine 2 mg/kg/day divided every 12 hours for 3 days followed by 1 mg/kg/day once daily (maximum: 25 mg/day) with supplemental folinic acid

Adults: 2-4 g/day divided every 4-8 hours in conjunction with pyrimethamine 25 mg/day and with supplemental folinic acid

Prevention of recurrent attacks of rheumatic fever:

>30 kg: 1 g/day

<30 kg: 0.5 g/day

Dosage Forms TAB: 500 mg

Contraindications Porphyria, hypersensitivity to any sulfa drug or any component, pregnancy at term, children <2 months of age unless indicated for the treatment of congenital toxoplasmosis, sunscreens containing PABA, nursing mothers

Warnings/Precautions Use with caution in patients with impaired hepatic function or impaired renal function, G-6-PD deficiency; dosage modification required in patients with renal impairment; fluid intake should be maintained ≥1500 mL/day, or administer sodium bicarbonate to keep urine alkaline; more likely to cause crystalluria because it is less soluble than other sulfonamides

Pregnancy Risk Factor B; D (at term)

Adverse Reactions

>10%:

Central nervous system: Fever, dizziness, headache

Dermatologic: Itching, rash, photosensitivity

Gastrointestinal: Anorexia, nausea, vomiting, diarrhea

1% to 10%:

Dermatologic: Lyell's syndrome, Stevens-Johnson syndrome

Hematologic: Granulocytopenia, leukopenia, thrombocytopenia, aplastic anemia, hemolytic anemia

Hepatic: Hepatitis

<1%: Acute nephropathy, crystalluria, hematuria, interstitial nephritis, jaundice, serum sickness-like reactions, thyroid function disturbance

Drug Interactions Decreased effect with PABA or PABA metabolites of drugs (eg, procaine, proparacaine, tetracaine, sunscreens); increased effect of oral anticoagulants and oral hypoglycemic agents

Half-Life 10 hours

Education and Monitoring Issues

Patient Education: Take as directed, at regular intervals around-the-clock. Take 1 hour before or 2 hours after meals with full glass of water. Complete full course of therapy even if you are feeling better. Avoid aspirin or aspirin-containing products and avoid large quantities of vitamin C. It is very important to maintain adequate hydration (2-3 L/day of fluids unless instructed to restrict fluid intake) to prevent kidney damage. You may experience dizziness or headache (use caution when driving or engaging in tasks requiring alertness until response to drug is known); photosensitivity (use sunblock, wear protective clothing and eyewear, avoid direct sunlight); nausea, vomiting, or loss of appetite (small frequent meals, frequent mouth care, sucking lozenges, or chewing gum may help). Report skin rash, persistent diarrhea, persistent or severe sore throat, fever, vaginal itching or discharge, unusual bruising or bleeding, fatigue, persistent headache or abdominal pain, or difficulty breathing.

Sulfadiazine, Sulfamethazine, and Sulfamerazine

(sul fa DYE a zeen, sul fa METH a zeen, & sul fa MER a zeen)

Pharmacologic Class Sulfonamide

Generic Available No

Mechanism of Action Interferes with microbial folic acid synthesis and growth via inhibition of para-aminobenzoic acid metabolism

Use Treatment of toxoplasmosis and other susceptible organisms, however, other agents are preferred

USUAL DOSAGE Adults: Oral: 2-4 g to start, then 2-4 g/day in 3-6 divided doses

(Continued)

Sulfadiazine, Sulfamethazine, and Sulfamerazine *(Continued)*

Dosage Forms TAB: Sulfadiazine 167 mg, sulfamethazine 167 mg, and sulfamerazine 167 mg

Contraindications Porphyria, known hypersensitivity to any sulfa drug or any component

Pregnancy Risk Factor B; D (at term)

Education and Monitoring Issues

Patient Education: Drink plenty of fluids

Sulfadoxine and Pyrimethamine (sul fa DOKS een & peer i METH a meen)

Pharmacologic Class Antimalarial Agent

U.S. Brand Names Fansidar®

Generic Available No

Mechanism of Action Sulfadoxine interferes with bacterial folic acid synthesis and growth via competitive inhibition of para-aminiobenzoic acid; pyrimethamine inhibits microbial dihydrofolate reductase, resulting in inhibition of tetrahydrofolic acid synthesis

Use Treatment of *Plasmodium falciparum* malaria in patients in whom chloroquine resistance is suspected; malaria prophylaxis for travelers to areas where chloroquine-resistant malaria is endemic

USUAL DOSAGE Children and Adults: Oral:

Treatment of acute attack of malaria: A single dose of the following number of Fansidar® tablets is used in sequence with quinine or alone:

- 2-11 months: 1/4 tablet
- 1-3 years: 1/2 tablet
- 4-8 years: 1 tablet
- 9-14 years: 2 tablets
- >14 years: 2-3 tablets

Malaria prophylaxis:

The first dose of Fansidar® should be taken 1-2 days before departure to an endemic area (CDC recommends that therapy be initiated 1-2 weeks before such travel), administration should be continued during the stay and for 4-6 weeks after return. Dose = pyrimethamine 0.5 mg/kg/dose and sulfadoxine 10 mg/kg/dose up to a maximum of 25 mg pyrimethamine and 500 mg sulfadoxine/dose weekly.

- 2-11 months: 1/8 tablet weekly **or** 1/4 tablet once every 2 weeks
- 1-3 years: 1/4 tablet once weekly **or** 1/2 tablet once every 2 weeks
- 4-8 years: 1/2 tablet once weekly **or** 1 tablet once every 2 weeks
- 9-14 years: 3/4 tablet once weekly **or** 1 1/2 tablets once every 2 weeks
- >14 years: 1 tablet once weekly **or** 2 tablets once every 2 weeks

Dosage Forms TAB: Sulfadoxine 500 mg and pyrimethamine 25 mg

Contraindications Known hypersensitivity to any sulfa drug, pyrimethamine, or any component; porphyria, megaloblastic anemia, severe renal insufficiency; children <2 months of age due to competition with bilirubin for protein binding sites

Warnings/Precautions Use with caution in patients with renal or hepatic impairment, patients with possible folate deficiency, and patients with seizure disorders, increased adverse reactions are seen in patients also receiving chloroquine; fatalities associated with sulfonamides, although rare, have occurred due to severe reactions including Stevens-Johnson syndrome, toxic epidermal necrolysis, hepatic necrosis, agranulocytosis, aplastic anemia and other blood dyscrasias; discontinue use at first sign of rash or any sign of adverse reaction; hemolysis occurs in patients with G-6-PD deficiency; leucovorin should be administered to reverse signs and symptoms of folic acid deficiency

Pregnancy Risk Factor C

Adverse Reactions

>10%:

- Central nervous system: Ataxia, seizures, headache
- Dermatologic: Photosensitivity
- Gastrointestinal: Atrophic glossitis, vomiting, gastritis
- Hematologic: Megaloblastic anemia, leukopenia, thrombocytopenia, pancytopenia
- Neuromuscular & skeletal: Tremors
- Miscellaneous: Hypersensitivity

1% to 10%:

- Dermatologic: Stevens-Johnson syndrome
- Hepatic: Hepatitis

<1%: Anorexia, crystalluria, erythema multiforme, glossitis, hepatic necrosis, rash, respiratory failure, thyroid function dysfunction, toxic epidermal necrolysis

Drug Interactions

Decreased effect with PABA or PABA metabolites of local anesthetics

Increased toxicity with methotrexate, other sulfonamides, co-trimoxazole

Education and Monitoring Issues

Patient Education: Begin prophylaxis at least 2 days before departure; drink plenty of fluids; avoid prolonged exposure to the sun; notify prescriber if rash, sore throat, pallor, or glossitis occurs

Monitoring Parameters: CBC, including platelet counts, and urinalysis should be performed periodically

- **Sulfa-Gyn®** *see* Sulfabenzamide, Sulfacetamide, and Sulfathiazole *on page 875*
- **Sulfalax® [OTC]** *see* Docusate *on page 290*

Sulfamethoxazole (sul fa meth OKS a zole)

Pharmacologic Class Antibiotic, Sulfonamide Derivative

U.S. Brand Names Gantanol®; Urobak®

Generic Available Yes: Tablet

Mechanism of Action Interferes with bacterial growth by inhibiting bacterial folic acid synthesis through competitive antagonism of PABA

Use Treatment of urinary tract infections, nocardiosis, toxoplasmosis, acute otitis media, and acute exacerbations of chronic bronchitis due to susceptible organisms

USUAL DOSAGE Oral:

Children >2 months: 50-60 mg/kg as single dose followed by 50-60 mg/kg/day divided every 12 hours; maximum: 3 g/24 hours or 75 mg/kg/day

Adults: Initial: 2 g, then 1 g 2-3 times/day; maximum: 3 g/24 hours

Dosing adjustment/interval in renal impairment:

Cl_{cr} 10-50 mL/minute: Administer every 12-24 hours

Cl_{cr} <10 mL/minute: Administer every 24 hours

Hemodialysis: Moderately dialyzable (20% to 50%)

Dosage Forms SUSP, oral (cherry flavor): 500 mg/5 mL (480 mL). **TAB:** 500 mg

Contraindications Porphyria, hypersensitivity to any sulfa drug or any component, pregnancy during 3rd trimester, children <2 months of age unless indicated for the treatment of congenital toxoplasmosis, sunscreens containing PABA

Warnings/Precautions Maintain adequate fluid intake to prevent crystalluria; use with caution in patients with renal or hepatic impairment, and patients with G-6-PD deficiency; should not be used for group A beta-hemolytic streptococcal infections

Pregnancy Risk Factor B; D (at term)

Adverse Reactions

>10%:

Central nervous system: Fever, dizziness, headache

Dermatologic: Itching, rash, photosensitivity

Gastrointestinal: Anorexia, nausea, vomiting, diarrhea

1% to 10%:

Dermatologic: Lyell's syndrome, Stevens-Johnson syndrome

Hematologic: Granulocytopenia, leukopenia, thrombocytopenia, aplastic anemia, hemolytic anemia

Hepatic: Hepatitis

<1%: Acute nephropathy, crystalluria, hematuria, interstitial nephritis, jaundice, serum sickness-like reactions, thyroid function disturbance, vasculitis

Drug Interactions

Decreased effect with PABA or PABA metabolites of drugs (ie, procaine, proparacaine, tetracaine); cyclosporine levels may be decreased

Increased effect/toxicity of oral anticoagulants, oral hypoglycemic agents, hydantoins, uricosuric agents, methotrexate when administered with sulfonamides

Increased toxicity of sulfonamides with diuretics, indomethacin, methenamine, probenecid, and salicylates

Half-Life 9-12 hours, prolonged with renal impairment

Education and Monitoring Issues

Patient Education: Take as directed, at regular intervals around-the-clock. Take 1 hour before or 2 hours after meals with a full glass of water. Take full course of therapy even if you feeling better. Avoid aspirin or aspirin-containing products and avoid large quantities of vitamin C. It is very important to maintain adequate hydration (2-3 L/day of fluids unless instructed to restrict fluid intake) to prevent kidney damage. You may experience dizziness or headache (use caution when driving or engaging in tasks requiring alertness until response to drug is known); photosensitivity (use sunscreen, wear protective clothing and eyewear, avoid direct sunlight); nausea, vomiting, or loss of appetite (small frequent meals, frequent mouth care, sucking lozenges, or chewing gum may help). Report skin rash, persistent diarrhea, persistent or severe sore throat, fever, vaginal itching or discharge, unusual bruising or bleeding, fatigue, persistent headache or abdominal pain, blackened stool, or difficulty breathing.

Monitoring Parameters: Monitor urine output

Related Information

Sulfamethoxazole and Phenazopyridine *on page 879*

Sulfamethoxazole and Phenazopyridine

(sul fa meth OKS a zole & fen az oh PEER i deen)

Pharmacologic Class Antibiotic, Sulfonamide Derivative

Dosage Forms TAB: Sulfamethoxazole 500 mg and phenazopyridine 100 mg

Pregnancy Risk Factor B (D at term)

- **Sulfamylon® Topical** *see* Mafenide *on page 550*

Sulfanilamide (sul fa NIL a mide)

Pharmacologic Class Antifungal Agent, Vaginal

U.S. Brand Names AVC™ Cream; AVC™ Suppository; Vagitrol®

Generic Available No

Mechanism of Action Interferes with microbial folic acid synthesis and growth via inhibition of para-aminiobenzoic acid metabolism; exerts a bacteriostatic action

Use Treatment of vulvovaginitis caused by *Candida albicans*

USUAL DOSAGE Adults: Female: Insert one applicatorful intravaginally once or twice daily continued through 1 complete menstrual cycle or insert one suppository intravaginally once or twice daily for 30 days

Dosage Forms CRM, vag (AVC™, Vagitrol®): 15% [150 mg/g] (120 g with applicator). **SUPP, vag** (AVC™): 1.05 g (16s)

Contraindications Hypersensitivity to sulfanilamide or any component

Warnings/Precautions Since sulfonamides may be absorbed from vaginal mucosa, the same precaution for oral sulfonamides apply (eg, blood dyscrasias); if a rash develops, terminate therapy immediately. Use vaginal applicators very cautiously after the 7th month of pregnancy.

Pregnancy Risk Factor C; D (if near term)

Adverse Reactions Percentage unknown: Rarely, systemic reactions occur; allergic reactions, burning, increased discomfort, Stevens-Johnson syndrome (infrequent)

Education and Monitoring Issues

Patient Education: Complete full course of therapy as directed. Insert vaginally as directed by prescriber or see package insert. You may be sensitive to direct sunlight (wear protective clothing, use sunblock, and avoid excessive exposure to direct sunlight). Sexual partner may experience irritation of penis; best to refrain from intercourse during period of treatment. Report persistent vaginal burning, itching, or irritation; rash; yellowing of eyes or skin, dark urine, or pale stool; unresolved nausea or vomiting; or painful urination.

Sulfasalazine (sul fa SAL a zeen)

Pharmacologic Class 5-Aminosalicylic Acid Derivative

U.S. Brand Names Azulfidine®; Azulfidine® EN-tabs®

Generic Available Yes

Mechanism of Action Acts locally in the colon to decrease the inflammatory response and systemically interferes with secretion by inhibiting prostaglandin synthesis

Use Management of ulcerative colitis; enteric coated tablets are used for for rheumatoid arthritis in patients who inadequately respond to analgesics and NSAIDs

USUAL DOSAGE Oral:

Children >2 years: Initial: 40-60 mg/kg/day in 3-6 divided doses; maintenance dose: 20-30 mg/kg/day in 4 divided doses

Adults: Initial: 1 g 3-4 times/day, 2 g/day maintenance in divided doses; may initiate therapy with 0.5-1 g/day enteric-coated tablets

Dosing interval in renal impairment:

Cl_{cr} 10-30 mL/minute: Administer twice daily

Cl_{cr} <10 mL/minute: Administer once daily

Dosing adjustment in hepatic impairment: Avoid use

Dosage Forms TAB: 500 mg; Enteric coated: 500 mg

Contraindications Hypersensitivity to sulfasalazine, sulfa drugs, or any component; porphyria, GI or GU obstruction; hypersensitivity to salicylates; children <2 years of age

Warnings/Precautions Use with caution in patients with renal impairment; impaired hepatic function or urinary obstruction, blood dyscrasias severe allergies or asthma, or G-6-PD deficiency; may cause folate deficiency (consider providing 1 mg/day folate supplement)

Pregnancy Risk Factor B; D (at term)

Adverse Reactions

>10%:

Central nervous system: Dizziness, headache (33%)

Dermatologic: Photosensitivity

Gastrointestinal: Anorexia, nausea, vomiting, diarrhea (33%)

Genitourinary: Reversible oligospermia (33%)

<3%:

Dermatologic: Urticaria/pruritus (<3%)

Hematologic: Hemolytic anemia (<3%), Heinz body anemia (<3%)

<0.1%: Acute nephropathy, aplastic anemia, crystalluria, granulocytopenia, hematuria, interstitial nephritis, jaundice, leukopenia, Lyell's syndrome, serum sickness-like reactions, Stevens-Johnson syndrome, thrombocytopenia, thyroid function disturbance

Drug Interactions

Decreased effect of iron, digoxin, folic acid, and like other sulfa drugs PABA or PABA metabolites of drugs (ie, procaine, proparacaine, tetracaine)

Increased effect of oral anticoagulants, methotrexate, and oral hypoglycemic agents as with other sulfa drugs

Half-Life 5.7-10 hours

Education and Monitoring Issues

Patient Education: Do not crush, chew, or dissolve coated tablets. Shake suspension well before use. Do not take on an empty stomach or with antacids. Maintain adequate hydration (2-3 L/day of fluids unless instructed to restrict fluid intake) to prevent kidney damage. Increased dietary iron may be recommended. You may experience nervousness or dizziness (use caution when driving or engaging in hazardous activities until response to drug is known). You may experience photosensitivity (use sunscreen, wear protective clothing and eyewear, avoid direct sunlight). Orange-yellow color of urine, sweat, tears is normal and will stain contact lenses and clothing. Report rash, persistent nausea or anorexia, or lack of improvement in symptoms (after 1-2 months).

♦ **Sulfatrim®** *see* Co-Trimoxazole *on page 230*

♦ **Sulfa-Trip®** *see* Sulfabenzamide, Sulfacetamide, and Sulfathiazole *on page 875*

♦ **Sulfex** *see* Sulfacetamide Sodium *on page 876*

Sulfinpyrazone (sul fin PEER a zone)

Pharmacologic Class Uricosuric Agent

U.S. Brand Names Anturane®

Generic Available Yes

Mechanism of Action Acts by increasing the urinary excretion of uric acid, thereby decreasing blood urate levels; this effect is therapeutically useful in treating patients with acute intermittent gout, chronic tophaceous gout, and acts to promote resorption of tophi; also has antithrombic and platelet inhibitory effects

Use Treatment of chronic gouty arthritis and intermittent gouty arthritis

Unlabeled use: To decrease the incidence of sudden death postmyocardial infarction

USUAL DOSAGE Adults: Oral: 100-200 mg twice daily; maximum daily dose: 800 mg

Dosing adjustment in renal impairment: Cl_{cr} <50 mL/minute: Avoid use

Dosage Forms CAP: 200 mg. **TAB:** 100 mg

Contraindications Active peptic ulcers, hypersensitivity to sulfinpyrazone, phenylbutazone, or other pyrazoles, GI inflammation, blood dyscrasias

Warnings/Precautions Safety and efficacy not established in children <18 years of age, use with caution in patients with impaired renal function and urolithiasis

Pregnancy Risk Factor C (per manufacturer); D (if near term, per expert analysis)

Adverse Reactions

1% to 10%: Gastrointestinal: Nausea, vomiting, stomach pain

<1%: Anemia, dermatitis, dizziness, flushing, headache, hepatic necrosis, increased bleeding time (decreased platelet aggregation), leukopenia, nephrotic syndrome, polyuria, rash, uric acid stones

Drug Interactions CYP2C and 3A3/4 enzyme inducer; CYP2C9 enzyme inhibitor

Decreased effect/levels of theophylline, verapamil; decreased uricosuric activity with salicylates, niacins

Increased effect of oral anticoagulants

Risk of acetaminophen hepatotoxicity is increased, but therapeutic effects may be reduced

Half-Life 2.7-6 hours

Education and Monitoring Issues

Patient Education: Take as directed, with meals or antacids and a full glass of water. Avoid aspirin, aspirin-containing medications, or acetaminophen products and avoid large quantities of vitamin C. It is very important to maintain adequate hydration (2-3 L/day of fluids unless instructed to restrict fluid intake) to prevent kidney damage. You may experience nausea or vomiting (small frequent meals, frequent mouth care, chewing gum, or sucking lozenges may help). Report skin rash, persistent stomach pain, painful urination or bloody urine, unusual bruising or bleeding, fatigue, or yellowing of eyes or skin.

Monitoring Parameters: Serum and urinary uric acid, CBC

Sulfisoxazole (sul fi SOKS a zole)

Pharmacologic Class Antibiotic, Sulfonamide Derivative

Generic Available Yes

Mechanism of Action Interferes with bacterial growth by inhibiting bacterial folic acid synthesis through competitive antagonism of PABA

Use Treatment of urinary tract infections, otitis media, *Chlamydia*; nocardiosis; treatment of acute pelvic inflammatory disease in prepubertal children; often used in combination with trimethoprim

USUAL DOSAGE Not for use in patients <2 months of age:

Children >2 months: Oral: Initial: 75 mg/kg, followed by 120-150 mg/kg/day in divided doses every 4-6 hours; not to exceed 6 g/day

Pelvic inflammatory disease: 100 mg/kg/day in divided doses every 6 hours; used in combination with ceftriaxone

Chlamydia trachomatis: 100 mg/kg/day in divided doses every 6 hours

Adults: Oral: Initial: 2-4 g, then 4-8 g/day in divided doses every 4-6 hours

Pelvic inflammatory disease: 500 mg every 6 hours for 21 days; used in combination with ceftriaxone

(Continued)

Sulfisoxazole *(Continued)*

Chlamydia trachomatis: 500 mg every 6 hours for 10 days

Dosing interval in renal impairment:

Cl_{cr} 10-50 mL/minute: Administer every 8-12 hours

Cl_{cr} <10 mL/minute: Administer every 12-24 hours

Hemodialysis: >50% removed by hemodialysis

Children and Adults: Ophthalmic:

Solution: Instill 1-2 drops to affected eye every 2-3 hours

Ointment: Apply small amount to affected eye 1-3 times/day and at bedtime

Dosage Forms SOLN, ophthalmic, as diolamine: 4% [40 mg/mL] (15 mL). **SUSP, oral, pediatric,** as acetyl (raspberry flavor): 500 mg/5 mL (480 mL). **TAB:** 500 mg

Contraindications Hypersensitivity to any sulfa drug or any component, porphyria, pregnancy during 3rd trimester, infants <2 months of age (sulfas compete with bilirubin for protein binding sites), patients with urinary obstruction, sunscreens containing PABA

Warnings/Precautions Use with caution in patients with G-6-PD deficiency (hemolysis may occur), hepatic or renal impairment; dosage modification required in patients with renal impairment; risk of crystalluria should be considered in patients with impaired renal function

Pregnancy Risk Factor B; D (at term)

Adverse Reactions

>10%:

Central nervous system: Fever, dizziness, headache

Dermatologic: Itching, rash, photosensitivity

Gastrointestinal: Anorexia, nausea, vomiting, diarrhea

1% to 10%:

Dermatologic: Lyell's syndrome, Stevens-Johnson syndrome

Hematologic: Granulocytopenia, leukopenia, thrombocytopenia, aplastic anemia, hemolytic anemia

Hepatic: Hepatitis

<1%: Acute nephropathy, crystalluria, hematuria, interstitial nephritis, jaundice, serum sickness-like reactions, thyroid function disturbance, vasculitis

Drug Interactions

Decreased effect with PABA or PABA metabolites of drugs (ie, procaine, proparacaine, tetracaine); cyclosporine levels may be decreased

Increased effect/toxicity of oral anticoagulants, oral hypoglycemic agents, hydantoins, uricosuric agents, methotrexate when administered with sulfonamides

Increased toxicity of sulfonamides with diuretics, indomethacin, methenamine, probenecid, and salicylates

Half-Life 4-7 hours, prolonged with renal impairment

Education and Monitoring Issues

Patient Education: Take as directed, at regular intervals around-the-clock. Take 1 hour before or 2 hours after meals with a full glass of water. Take full course of therapy even if you are feeling better. Avoid aspirin or aspirin-containing products and avoid large quantities of vitamin C. It is very important to maintain adequate hydration (2-3 L/day of fluids unless instructed to restrict fluid intake) to prevent kidney damage. You may experience dizziness or headache (use caution when driving or engaging in tasks requiring alertness until response to drug is known); photosensitivity (use sunscreen, wear protective clothing and eyewear, avoid direct sunlight); nausea, vomiting, or loss of appetite (small frequent meals, frequent mouth care, sucking lozenges, or chewing gum may help). Diabetics: Drug may cause false tests with Clinitest® urine glucose monitoring; use of glucose oxidase methods (Clinistix®) or serum glucose monitoring is preferable. Report persistent nausea, vomiting, diarrhea, or abdominal pain; skin rash; persistent or severe sore throat, mouth sores, fever, or vaginal itching or discharge; unusual bruising or bleeding; blackened stool; fatigue; or difficulty breathing.

Ophthalmic: Instill as often as recommended. Wash hands before using. Sit or lie down, open eye, look at ceiling, and instill prescribed amount of solution. Ointment: Pull lower lid down gently and instill thin ribbon of ointment inside lid. Close eye and roll eye in all directions, and apply gentle pressure to inner corner of eye for 1-2 minutes. Do not let tip of applicator touch eye or contaminate tip of applicator. Temporary stinging or blurred vision may occur. Report persistent pain, redness, burning, double vision, severe headache, or respiratory congestion.

Monitoring Parameters: CBC, urinalysis, renal function tests, temperature

Related Information

Antimicrobial Drugs of Choice *on page 1182*

Sulfisoxazole and Phenazopyridine *on page 882*

Treatment of Sexually Transmitted Diseases *on page 1210*

Sulfisoxazole and Phenazopyridine

(sul fi SOKS a zole & fen az oh PEER i deen)

Pharmacologic Class Antibiotic, Sulfonamide Derivative; Local Anesthetic

U.S. Brand Names Azo-Sulfisoxazole

Use Treatment of urinary tract infections and nocardiosis

Dosage Forms TAB: Sulfisoxazole 500 mg and phenazopyridine 50 mg
Pregnancy Risk Factor B; D (at term)

♦ **Sulfizole®** *see* Sulfisoxazole *on page 881*

Sulfur and Sulfacetamide Sodium

(SUL fur & sul fa SEE ta mide SOW dee um)

Pharmacologic Class Antiseborrheic Agent, Topical

U.S. Brand Names Novacet® Topical; Sulfacet-R® Topical

Dosage Forms LOT, top: Sulfur colloid 5% and sulfacetamide sodium 10% (30 mL)

Sulindac (sul IN dak)

Pharmacologic Class Nonsteroidal Anti-Inflammatory Agent (NSAID)

U.S. Brand Names Clinoril®

Generic Available Yes

Mechanism of Action Inhibits prostaglandin synthesis by decreasing the activity of the enzyme, cyclo-oxygenase, which results in decreased formation of prostaglandin precursors

Use Management of inflammatory disease, rheumatoid disorders; acute gouty arthritis; structurally similar to indomethacin but acts like aspirin; safest NSAID for use in mild renal impairment

USUAL DOSAGE Maximum therapeutic response may not be realized for up to 3 weeks

Oral:

Children: Dose not established

Adults: 150-200 mg twice daily or 300-400 mg once daily; not to exceed 400 mg/day

Dosing adjustment in hepatic impairment: Dose reduction is necessary

Dosage Forms TAB: 150 mg, 200 mg

Contraindications Hypersensitivity to sulindac, any component, aspirin or other nonsteroidal anti-inflammatory drugs (NSAIDs)

Warnings/Precautions Use with caution in patients with peptic ulcer disease, GI bleeding, bleeding abnormalities, impaired renal or hepatic function, congestive heart failure, hypertension, and patients receiving anticoagulants

Pregnancy Risk Factor B; D (at term)

Adverse Reactions

>10%:

Central nervous system: Dizziness

Dermatologic: Rash

Gastrointestinal: Abdominal cramps, heartburn, indigestion, nausea

1% to 10%:

Central nervous system: Headache, nervousness

Dermatologic: Itching

Endocrine & metabolic: Fluid retention

Gastrointestinal: Vomiting

Otic: Tinnitus

<1%: Acute renal failure, agranulocytosis, allergic rhinitis, anemia, angioedema, arrhythmias, aseptic meningitis, blurred vision, bone marrow suppression, confusion, congestive heart failure, conjunctivitis, cystitis, decreased hearing, drowsiness, dry eyes, epistaxis, erythema multiforme, gastritis, GI ulceration, hallucinations, hemolytic anemia, hepatitis, hot flashes, hypertension, insomnia, leukopenia, mental depression, peripheral neuropathy, polydipsia, polyuria, shortness of breath, Stevens-Johnson syndrome, tachycardia, thrombocytopenia, toxic amblyopia, toxic epidermal necrolysis, urticaria

Drug Interactions

Decreased effect of diuretics, beta-blockers, hydralazine, captopril

Increased toxicity with probenecid, NSAIDs; increased toxicity of digoxin, methotrexate, lithium, aminoglycosides antibiotics (reported in neonates), cyclosporine (increased nephrotoxicity), potassium-sparing diuretics (hyperkalemia), anticoagulants

Alcohol Interactions Avoid use (may enhance gastric mucosal irritation)

Onset Analgesic: ~1 hour

Duration 12-24 hours

Half-Life Parent drug: 7 hours; Active metabolite: 18 hours

Education and Monitoring Issues

Patient Education: Take this medication exactly as directed; do not increase dose without consulting prescriber. Take with food or milk to reduce GI distress. Maintain adequate fluid intake (2-3 L/day of fluids unless instructed to restrict fluid intake). Do not use alcohol, aspirin, or aspirin-containing medication, and all other anti-inflammatory medications without consulting prescriber. With long-term use of NSAIDs, you are advised to schedule regular ophthalmic exams. You may experience dizziness, nervousness, or headache (use caution when driving or engaging in tasks requiring alertness until response to drug is known); nausea, vomiting, or heartburn (frequent small meals, frequent mouth care, sucking lozenges, or chewing gum may help); constipation (increased exercise, fluids, or dietary fruit and fiber may help). GI bleeding, ulceration, or perforation can occur with or without pain; discontinue medication and

(Continued)

Sulindac *(Continued)*

contact prescriber if persistent abdominal pain or cramping, or blood in stool occurs. Report breathlessness or difficulty breathing; unusual bruising/bleeding; blood in urine, stool, mouth, or vomitus; unusual fatigue; skin rash or itching; change in urinary pattern; or change in hearing or ringing in ears.

Dietary Considerations: Food: May decrease the rate but not the extent of oral absorption. Drug may cause GI upset, bleeding, ulceration, perforation; take with food or milk to minimize GI upset.

Monitoring Parameters: Liver enzymes, BUN, serum creatinine, CBC, blood pressure

Related Information

Nonsteroidal Anti-Inflammatory Agents Comparison *on page 1248*

♦ **Sultrin™** *see* Sulfabenzamide, Sulfacetamide, and Sulfathiazole *on page 875*

Sumatriptan Succinate (SOO ma trip tan SUKS i nate)

Pharmacologic Class Serotonin 5-HT_{1D} Receptor Agonist

U.S. Brand Names Imitrex®

Mechanism of Action Selective agonist for serotonin (5-HT_{1D} receptor) in cranial arteries to cause vasoconstriction and reduces sterile inflammation associated with antidromic neuronal transmission correlating with relief of migraine

Use Acute treatment of migraine with or without aura

Sumatriptan injection: Acute treatment of cluster headache episodes

USUAL DOSAGE Adults:

Oral: 25 mg (taken with fluids); maximum recommended dose is 100 mg. If a satisfactory response has not been obtained at 2 hours, a second dose of up to 100 mg may be given. Efficacy of this second dose has not been examined. If a headache returns, additional doses may be taken at intervals of at least 2 hours up to a daily maximum of 300 mg. There is no evidence that an initial dose of 100 mg provides substantially greater relief than 25 mg.

Intranasal: A single dose of 5, 10 or 20 mg administered in one nostril. A 10 mg dose may be achieved by administering a single 5 mg dose in each nostril. If headache returns, the dose maybe be repeated once after 2 hours not to exceed a total daily dose of 40 mg. The safety of treating an average of >4 headaches in a 30-day period has not been established.

S.C.: 6 mg; a second injection may be administered at least 1 hour after the initial dose, but not more than 2 injections in a 24-hour period. If side effects are dose-limiting, lower doses may be used.

Dosage Forms INJ: 12 mg/mL (0.5 mL, 2 mL). **SPRAY, intranasal:** 5 mg (100 µL); 20 mg (100 µL). **TAB:** 25 mg, 50 mg

Contraindications Intravenous administration; use in patients with ischemic heart disease or Prinzmetal angina, patients with signs or symptoms of ischemic heart disease, uncontrolled HTN; use with ergotamine derivatives (within 24 hours of); use with in 24 hours of another 5-HT_1 agonist; concurrent administration or within 2 weeks of discontinuing an MAOI; hypersensitivity to any component; management of hemiplegic or basilar migraine

Warnings/Precautions

Sumatriptan is indicated only in patient populations with a clear diagnosis of migraine or cluster headache

Cardiac events (coronary artery vasospasm, transient ischemia, myocardial infarction, ventricular tachycardia/fibrillation, cardiac arrest and death) have been reported with 5-HT_1 agonist administration. Significant elevation in blood pressure, including hypertensive crisis, has also been reported on rare occasions in patients with and without a history of hypertension. Vasospasm-related reactions have been reported other than coronary artery vasospasm. Peripheral vascular ischemia and colonic ischemia with abdominal pain and bloody diarrhea have occurred.

Pregnancy Risk Factor C

Adverse Reactions

>10%:

- Central nervous system: Dizziness
- Endocrine & metabolic: Hot flashes
- Local: Injection site reaction
- Neuromuscular & skeletal: Paresthesia

1% to 10%:

- Cardiovascular: Tightness in chest
- Central nervous system: Drowsiness, headache
- Dermatologic: Burning sensation
- Gastrointestinal: Abdominal discomfort, mouth discomfort
- Neuromuscular & skeletal: Myalgia, numbness, weakness, neck pain, jaw discomfort
- Miscellaneous: Diaphoresis

<1%: Dehydration, dysmenorrhea, dyspnea, dysuria, hiccups, polydipsia, rashes, renal calculus, thirst

Drug Interactions Increased toxicity: Ergot-containing drugs, MAOIs, SSRIs can lead to symptoms of hyper-reflexia, weakness, and incoordination; if concomitant treatment with sumatriptan and an SSRI is clinically warranted, appropriate observation of the patient is advised

Alcohol Interactions Avoid use (may cause or worsen headaches)

Onset Within 30 minutes

Half-Life After S.C. administration: Distribution: 15 minutes; Terminal: 115 minutes

Education and Monitoring Issues

Patient Education: Take at first sign of migraine attack. This drug is to be used to reduce your migraine, not to prevent or reduce number of attacks. Oral: If headache returns or is not fully resolved after first dose, the dose may be repeated after 2 hours. **Do not exceed 300 mg in 24 hours.** S.C.: If headache returns or is not fully resolved after first dose, the dose may be repeated after 1 hour. **Do not exceed two injections in 24 hours. Do not take within 24 hours of any other migraine medication without first consulting prescriber.** You may experience some dizziness (use caution); hot flashes (cool room may help); nausea or vomiting (frequent small meals, frequent mouth care, sucking lozenges, or chewing gum may help); pain at injection site (lasts about 1 hour, will resolve); or excess sweating (will resolve). Report chest tightness or pain; excessive drowsiness; acute abdominal pain; skin rash or burning sensation; muscle weakness, soreness, or numbness; or respiratory difficulty.

Manufacturer GlaxoWellcome

Related Information

Pharmaceutical Manufacturers Directory *on page 1020*

- **Summer's Eve® Medicated Douche [OTC]** *see* Povidone-Iodine *on page 756*
- **Sumycin® Oral** *see* Tetracycline *on page 903*
- **Supeudol®** *see* Oxycodone *on page 691*
- **Suplasyn** *see* Sodium Hyaluronate *on page 859*
- **Supprelin™ Injection** *see* Histrelin *on page 437*
- **Suprax®** *see* Cefixime *on page 152*
- **Supres** *see* Chlorothiazide and Methyldopa *on page 185*

Suprofen (soo PROE fen)

Pharmacologic Class Nonsteroidal Anti-inflammatory Drug (NSAID)

U.S. Brand Names Profenal®

Generic Available No

Mechanism of Action Inhibits prostaglandin synthesis, acts on the hypothalamus heat-regulating center to reduce fever, blocks prostaglandin synthetase action which prevents formation of the platelet-aggregating substance thromboxane A_2; decreases pain receptor sensitivity.

Use Inhibition of intraoperative miosis

USUAL DOSAGE Adults: On day of surgery, instill 2 drops in conjunctival sac at 3, 2, and 1 hour prior to surgery; or 2 drops in sac every 4 hours, while awake, the day preceding surgery

Dosage Forms SOLN, ophth: 1% (2.5 mL)

Contraindications Previous hypersensitivity or intolerance to suprofen; epithelial herpes simplex keratitis; history of hypersensitivity reactions to aspirin or other nonsteroidal anti-inflammatory agents

Warnings/Precautions Use with caution in patients sensitive to acetylsalicylic acid and other NSAIDs; some systemic absorption occurs; use with caution in patients with bleeding tendencies; perform ophthalmic evaluation for those who develop eye complaints during therapy (blurred vision, diminished vision, changes in color vision, retinal changes)

Pregnancy Risk Factor C

Adverse Reactions

1% to 10%: Topical: Transient burning or stinging, redness, iritis

<1%: Chemosis, discomfort, pain, photophobia, punctate epithelial staining

Drug Interactions Decreased effect: When used concurrently with suprofen, acetylcholine chloride and carbachol may be ineffective

Half-Life 2-4 hours

Education and Monitoring Issues

Patient Education: Avoid aspirin and aspirin-containing products while taking this medication; get instructions on administration of eye drops

- **Surfak® [OTC]** *see* Docusate *on page 290*
- **Surmontil®** *see* Trimipramine *on page 955*
- **Survanta®** *see* Beractant *on page 102*
- **Susano®** *see* Hyoscyamine, Atropine, Scopolamine, and Phenobarbital *on page 456*
- **Suspected Organisms by Site of Infection for Empiric Therapy** *see page 1209*
- **Sustaire®** *see* Theophylline Salts *on page 906*
- **Sustiva™** *see* Efavirenz *on page 307*
- **Syllact® [OTC]** *see* Psyllium *on page 793*
- **Symadine®** *see* Amantadine *on page 42*
- **Symmetrel®** *see* Amantadine *on page 42*

- **Synacol® CF [OTC]** *see* Guaifenesin and Dextromethorphan *on page 424*
- **Synacort®** *see* Hydrocortisone *on page 447*
- **Synacthen Depot** *see* Cosyntropin *on page 229*
- **Synagis®** *see* Palivizumab *on page 696*
- **Synalar®** *see* Fluocinolone *on page 374*
- **Synalar-HP®** *see* Fluocinolone *on page 374*
- **Synalgos®-DC** *see* Dihydrocodeine Compound *on page 276*
- **Synamol** *see* Fluocinolone *on page 374*
- **Synarel®** *see* Nafarelin *on page 629*
- **Syn-Diltiazem** *see* Diltiazem *on page 278*
- **Synemol®** *see* Fluocinolone *on page 374*
- **Syn-Flunisolide** *see* Flunisolide *on page 373*
- **Syn-Minocycline** *see* Minocycline *on page 607*
- **Syn-Nadolol** *see* Nadolol *on page 628*
- **Synphasic** *see* Ethinyl Estradiol and Norethindrone *on page 342*
- **Syn-Pi** *see* Pindolol *on page 738*
- **Synthroid®** *see* Levothyroxine *on page 526*
- **Syprine®** *see* Trientine *on page 949*
- **Syracol-CF® [OTC]** *see* Guaifenesin and Dextromethorphan *on page 424*
- **Syrup DM-E** *see* Guaifenesin and Dextromethorphan *on page 424*
- **Sytobex®** *see* Cyanocobalamin *on page 233*
- **222® Tablets** *see* Aspirin and Codeine *on page 75*
- **282® Tablets** *see* Aspirin and Codeine *on page 75*
- **292® Tablets** *see* Aspirin and Codeine *on page 75*
- **624® Tablets** *see* Propoxyphene *on page 784*
- **Tac™-3** *see* Triamcinolone *on page 944*
- **Tac™-40** *see* Triamcinolone *on page 944*
- **TACE®** *see* Chlorotrianisene *on page 185*

Tacrine (TAK reen)

Pharmacologic Class Acetylcholinesterase Inhibitor (Central)

U.S. Brand Names Cognex®

Use Treatment of mild to moderate dementia of the Alzheimer's type

USUAL DOSAGE Adults: Initial: 10 mg 4 times/day; may increase by 40 mg/day adjusted every 6 weeks; maximum: 160 mg/day; best administered separate from meal times; see table.

Dose Adjustment Based Upon Transaminase Elevations

ALT	Regimen
≤3 x ULN*	Continue titration
>3 to ≤5 x ULN	Decrease dose by 40 mg/day, resume when ALT returns to normal
>5 x ULN	Stop treatment, may rechallenge upon return of ALT to normal

*ULN = upper limit of normal.

Patients with clinical jaundice confirmed by elevated total bilirubin (>3 mg/dL) should not be rechallenged with tacrine

Dosage Forms CAP: 10 mg, 20 mg, 30 mg, 40 mg

Contraindications Patients previously treated with the drug who developed jaundice and in those who are hypersensitive to tacrine or acridine derivatives

Warnings/Precautions The use of tacrine has been associated with elevations in serum transaminases; serum transaminases (specifically ALT) must be monitored throughout therapy; use extreme caution in patients with current evidence of a history of abnormal liver function tests; use caution in patients with bladder outlet obstruction, asthma, and sick-sinus syndrome (tacrine may cause bradycardia). Also, patients with cardiovascular disease, asthma, or peptic ulcer should use cautiously.

Pregnancy Risk Factor C

Adverse Reactions

>10%

Central nervous system: Headache, dizziness
Gastrointestinal: Nausea, vomiting, diarrhea
Miscellaneous: Elevated transaminases

1% to 10%

Cardiovascular: Flushing
Central nervous system: Confusion, ataxia, insomnia, somnolence, depression, anxiety, fatigue
Dermatologic: Rash
Gastrointestinal: Dyspepsia, anorexia, abdominal pain, flatulence, constipation, weight loss

Neuromuscular & skeletal: Myalgia, tremor
Respiratory: Rhinitis

Drug Interactions CYP1A2 enzyme substrate; CYP1A2 inhibitor

Tacrine in combination with other cholinergic agents (eg, ambenonium, edrophonium, neostigmine, pyridostigmine, bethanechol), will likely produce additive cholinergic effects

Tacrine in combination with beta blockers may produce additive bradycardia

Smoking may reduce tacrine plasma levels via enzyme induction (CYP1A2)

Fluvoxamine, enoxacin, and cimetidine increase tacrine concentrations via enzyme inhibition (CYP1A2)

Tacrine may worsen Parkinson's disease and inhibit the effects of levodopa

Tacrine may prolong the effect of succinylcholine

Tacrine may inhibit the metabolism of theophylline resulting in elevated plasma levels; dose adjustment will likely be needed

Tacrine may antagonize the therapeutic effect of anticholinergic agents (benztropine, trihexphenidyl)

Onset May require weeks of treatment

Half-Life 2-4 hours

Education and Monitoring Issues

Patient Education: This medication will not cure the disease, but may help reduce symptoms. Use as directed; do not increase dose or discontinue without consulting prescriber. Maintain adequate hydration (2-3 L/day of fluids unless instructed to restrict fluid intake). May cause dizziness, sedation, or hypotension (rise slowly from sitting or lying position and use caution when driving or climbing stairs); vomiting or loss of appetite (frequent small meals, frequent mouth care, or chewing gum, or sucking lozenges may help); or diarrhea (boiled milk, yogurt, or buttermilk may help). Report persistent abdominal discomfort; significantly increased salivation, sweating, tearing, or urination; flushed skin; chest pain or palpitations; acute headache; unresolved diarrhea; excessive fatigue, insomnia, dizziness, or depression; increased muscle, joint, or body pain; vision changes or blurred vision; shortness of breath or wheezing; or signs of jaundice (yellowing of eyes or skin, dark colored urine or light colored stool, abdominal pain, or easy fatigue).

Monitoring Parameters: ALT (SGPT) levels and other liver enzymes weekly for at least the first 18 weeks, then monitor once every 3 months

Reference Range: In clinical trials, serum concentrations >20 ng/mL were associated with a much higher risk of development of symptomatic adverse effects

Manufacturer Parke-Davis

Related Information

Pharmaceutical Manufacturers Directory *on page 1020*

Tacrolimus (ta KROE li mus)

Pharmacologic Class Immunosuppressant Agent

U.S. Brand Names Prograf®

Mechanism of Action Binds to 40 FK binding protein resulting in inhibition of calcium-dependent signal transduction pathway in T cells, thereby blocking the secretion of IL-2 and other cytokines

Use Potent immunosuppressive drug used in liver, kidney, heart, lung, small bowel transplant recipients; immunosuppressive drug for peripheral stem cell/bone marrow transplantation

USUAL DOSAGE

Children: Patients without pre-existing renal or hepatic dysfunction have required and tolerated higher doses than adults to achieve similar blood concentrations. It is recommended that therapy be initiated at high end of the recommended adult I.V. and oral dosing ranges.

Oral: 0.3 mg/kg/day divided every 12 hours; children generally require higher maintenance dosages on a mg/kg basis than adults

I.V. continuous infusion: 0.05-0.15 mg/kg/day

Adults:

Oral (usually 3-4 times the I.V. dose): 0.15-0.30 mg/kg/day in two divided doses administered every 12 hours and given 8-12 hours after discontinuation of the I.V. infusion. Lower tacrolimus doses may be sufficient as maintenance therapy.

Solid organ transplantation: Oral: 0.15-0.30 mg/kg/day in two divided doses administered every 12 hours; lower tacrolimus doses may be sufficient as maintenance therapy

Peripheral stem cell/bone marrow transplantation: Oral (usually ~2-3 times the intravenous dose): 0.06-0.09 mg/kg/day (maximum: 0.12 mg/kg/day) in two divided doses administered every 12 hours and given 8-12 hours after discontinuation of the intravenous infusion; adjust doses based on trough serum concentrations

I.V.:

Solid organ transplantation: Initial (given at least 6 hours after transplantation): 0.05-0.10 mg/kg/day; corticosteroid therapy is advised to enhance immunosuppression. Patients should be switched to oral therapy as soon as possible (within 2-3 days).

(Continued)

Tacrolimus *(Continued)*

Peripheral stem cell/bone marrow transplantation: Initial: 0.03 mg/kg/day as a continuous intravenous infusion

Dosing adjustment in renal impairment: Evidence suggests that lower doses should be used; patients should receive doses at the lowest value of the recommended I.V. and oral dosing ranges; further reductions in dose below these ranges may be required

Tacrolimus therapy should usually be delayed up to 48 hours or longer in patients with postoperative oliguria

Hemodialysis: Not removed by hemodialysis; supplemental dose is not necessary

Peritoneal dialysis: Significant drug removal is unlikely based on physiochemical characteristics

Dosing adjustment in hepatic impairment: Use of tacrolimus in liver transplant recipients experiencing post-transplant hepatic impairment may be associated with increased risk of developing renal insufficiency related to high whole blood levels of tacrolimus. The presence of moderate-to-severe hepatic dysfunction (serum bilirubin >2 mg/dL) appears to affect the metabolism of FK506. The half-life of the drug was prolonged and the clearance reduced after I.V. administration. The bioavailability of FK506 was also increased after oral administration. The higher plasma concentrations as determined by ELISA, in patients with severe hepatic dysfunction are probably due to the accumulation of FK506 metabolites of lower activity. These patients should be monitored closely and dosage adjustments should be considered. Some evidence indicates that lower doses could be used in these patients. See table.

Dosing Tacrolimus

Condition	Tacrolimus
Switch from I.V. to oral therapy	Threefold increase in dose
T-tube clamping	No change in dose
Pediatric patients	About 2 times higher dose compared to adults
Liver dysfunction	Decrease I.V. dose; decrease oral dose
Renal dysfunction	Does not affect kinetics; decrease dose to decrease levels if renal dysfunction is related to the drug
Dialysis	Not removed
Inhibitors of hepatic metabolism	Decrease dose
Inducers of hepatic metabolism	Monitor drug level; increase dose

Dosage Forms CAP: 1 mg, 5 mg. **INJ,** with alcohol and surfactant: 5 mg/mL (1 mL)

Contraindications Hypersensitivity to tacrolimus or any component; hypersensitivity to HCO-60 polyoxyl 60 hydrogenated castor oil (used in the parenteral dosage formulation) is a contraindication to parenteral tacrolimus therapy

Warnings/Precautions Increased susceptibility to infection and the possible development of lymphoma may occur after administration of tacrolimus; it should not be administered simultaneously with cyclosporine; since the pharmacokinetics show great inter- and intrapatient variability over time, monitoring of serum concentrations (trough for oral therapy) is essential to prevent organ rejection and reduce drug-related toxicity; tonic clonic seizures may have been triggered by tacrolimus. Injection contains small volume of ethanol.

Pregnancy Risk Factor C

Pregnancy Implications

Tacrolimus crosses the placenta and reaches concentrations four times greater than maternal plasma concentrations

Tacrolimus concentrations in breast milk are equivalent to plasma concentrations; breast-feeding is not advised while therapy is ongoing

Adverse Reactions

>10%:

- Cardiovascular: Hypertension, peripheral edema
- Central nervous system: Headache, insomnia, pain, fever
- Dermatologic: Pruritus
- Endocrine & metabolic: Hypo-/hyperkalemia, hyperglycemia, hypomagnesemia
- Gastrointestinal: Diarrhea, nausea, anorexia, vomiting, abdominal pain
- Hematologic: Anemia, leukocytosis
- Hepatic: LFT abnormalities, ascites
- Neuromuscular & skeletal: Tremors, paresthesias, back pain, weakness
- Renal: Nephrotoxicity, increased BUN/creatinine
- Respiratory: Pleural effusion, atelectasis, dyspnea
- Miscellaneous: Infection

1% to 10%:

- Central nervous system: Seizures
- Dermatologic: Rash
- Endocrine & metabolic: Hyperphosphatemia, hyperuricemia, pancreatitis
- Gastrointestinal: Constipation

Genitourinary: Urinary tract infection
Hematologic: Thrombocytopenia
Neuromuscular & skeletal: Myoclonus
Renal: Oliguria

<1%: Anaphylaxis, arthralgia, expressive aphasia, hemolytic uremic syndrome, hypertrophic cardiomyopathy, myalgia, photophobia, secondary malignancy

Drug Interactions CYP3A3/4 enzyme substrate

Decreased effect: Separate administration of antacids and Carafate® from tacrolimus by at least 2 hours

Increased effect: Cyclosporine is associated with synergistic immunosuppression and increased nephrotoxicity

Increased toxicity: Nephrotoxic antibiotics, NSAIDs and amphotericin B potentially increase nephrotoxicity

See table.

Drug Interactions With Tacrolimus

Drugs Which May INCREASE Tacrolimus Blood Levels		
Calcium Channel Blockers	**Antibiotic/Antifungal Agents**	**Other Drugs**
Diltiazem Nicardipine Verapamil	Clotrimazole Erythromycin Fluconazole Itraconazole Ketoconazole	Bromocriptine Cimetidine Clarithromycin Cyclosporine Danazol Methylprednisolone Metoclopramide Grapefruit juice
Drugs Which May DECREASE Tacrolimus Blood Levels		
Anticonvulsants	**Antibiotics**	
Carbamazepine Phenobarbital Phenytoin	Rifabutin Rifampin	

Half-Life 12 hours (range: 4-40 hours)

Education and Monitoring Issues

Patient Education: Take as directed, preferably 30 minutes before or 30 minutes after meals. Do not take within 2 hours before or after antacids. Do not alter dose and do not discontinue without consulting prescriber. Maintain adequate hydration (2-3 L/day of fluids unless instructed to restrict fluid intake) during entire course of therapy. You will be susceptible to infection (avoid crowds and people with infections or contagious diseases). If you are diabetic, monitor glucose levels closely (may alter glucose levels). You may experience nausea, vomiting, loss of appetite (frequent small meals, frequent mouth care may help); diarrhea (boiled milk, yogurt, or buttermilk may help); constipation (increased exercise or dietary fruit, fluid, or fiber may help, if not consult prescriber); muscle or back pain (mild analgesics may be recommended). Report chest pain; acute headache or dizziness; symptoms of respiratory infection, cough, or difficulty breathing; unresolved gastrointestinal effects; fatigue, chills, fever, unhealed sores, white plaques in mouth, irritation in genital area; unusual bruising or bleeding; pain or irritation on urination or change in urinary patterns; rash or skin irritation; or other unusual effects related to this medication.

Monitoring Parameters: Renal function, hepatic function, serum electrolytes, glucose and blood pressure, hypersensitivity indicators, neurological responses, and other clinical parameters; monitoring of serum concentrations (trough for oral therapy), see Warnings/Precautions; measure 3 times/week for first few weeks, then gradually decrease frequency as patient stabilizes

Reference Range:

Whole blood: Trough level: 7-20 ng/mL (ELISA). Plasma levels are generally 0.02-0.2 times whole blood levels; increased precision with whole blood levels.

Plasma: Trough levels: 0.5-2 ng/mL (ELISA, plasma, extracted at 37°C) for all transplant procedures (liver, heart, lung, kidney, small bowel) whole blood measurements produce concentration 5-40 times higher than those in serum due to high binding to RBCs (therapeutic range: 5-10 ng/mL, although levels >20 mg/mL may be desirable for short periods to prevent rejection)

Manufacturer Fujisawa Healthcare, Inc

Related Information

Pharmaceutical Manufacturers Directory *on page 1020*

- **Tagamet®** *see* Cimetidine *on page 198*
- **Tagamet® HB [OTC]** *see* Cimetidine *on page 198*
- **Talwin®** *see* Pentazocine *on page 715*
- **Talwin® NX** *see* Pentazocine *on page 715*
- **Tambocor™** *see* Flecainide *on page 366*

♦ **Tamiflu™** *see* Oseltamivir *on page 682*
♦ **Tamofen®** *see* Tamoxifen *on page 890*
♦ **Tamone®** *see* Tamoxifen *on page 890*

Tamoxifen (ta MOKS i fen)

Pharmacologic Class Antineoplastic Agent, Miscellaneous

U.S. Brand Names Nolvadex®

Generic Available No

Mechanism of Action Tamoxifen competes with estrogen for estrogen receptors on tumor cells, inhibiting estrogen's ability to stimulate tumor growth, and decreasing DNA synthesis. Inhibition of messenger RNA by the tamoxifen-estrogen receptor complex within tumor cells is also postulated. Cells tend to accumulate in the G_0 and G_1 phase of the cycle. Tamoxifen appears to be more a cytostatic, rather than cytocidal, agent.

Use Palliative or adjunctive treatment of advanced breast cancer; reduce the incidence of breast cancer in women at high risk (taking into account age, number of first-degree relatives with breast cancer, previous breast biopsies, age at first live birth, age at first menstrual period, and a history of lobular carcinoma *in situ*)

Unlabeled use: Treatment of mastalgia, gynecomastia, male breast cancer, and pancreatic carcinoma. Studies have shown tamoxifen to be effective in the treatment of primary breast cancer in elderly women. Comparative studies with other antineoplastic agents in elderly women with breast cancer had more favorable survival rates with tamoxifen. Initiation of hormone therapy rather than chemotherapy is justified for elderly patients with metastatic breast cancer who are responsive.

USUAL DOSAGE Oral (refer to individual protocols):

Adults: Oral: 10-20 mg twice daily in the morning and evening
20 mg/day
40 mg 4 times/day for 1 day, then 10 mg twice daily
10 mg 3 times/day

Dosage Forms TAB: 10 mg, 20 mg

Contraindications Hypersensitivity to tamoxifen

Warnings/Precautions Use with caution in patients with leukopenia, thrombocytopenia, or hyperlipidemias; ovulation may be induced; "hot flashes" may be countered by Bellergal-S® tablets; decreased visual acuity, retinopathy and corneal changes have been reported with use for more than 1 year at doses above recommended; hypercalcemia in patients with bone metastasis; hepatocellular carcinomas have been reported in animal studies; endometrial hyperplasia and polyps have occurred

Pregnancy Risk Factor D

Adverse Reactions

>10%:

Cardiovascular: Flushing

Dermatologic: Skin rash

Gastrointestinal: Little to mild nausea (10%), vomiting, weight gain

Hematologic: Myelosuppressive: Transient thrombocytopenia occurs in ~24% of patients receiving 10-20 mg/day; platelet counts return to normal within several weeks in spite of continued administration; leukopenia has also been reported and does resolve during continued therapy; anemia has also been reported

WBC: Rare

Platelets: None

Hepatic: Hepatotoxicity

Neuromuscular & skeletal: Increased bone and tumor pain and local disease flare shortly after starting therapy; this will subside rapidly, but patients should be aware of this since many may discontinue the drug due to the side effects

1% to 10%:

Cardiovascular: Thromboembolism: Tamoxifen has been associated with the occurrence of venous thrombosis and pulmonary embolism; arterial thrombosis has also been described in a few case reports

Central nervous system: Lightheadedness, depression, dizziness, headache, lassitude, mental confusion

Dermatologic: Rash

Endocrine & metabolic: Hypercalcemia may occur in patients with bone metastases; galactorrhea and vitamin deficiency, menstrual irregularities

Genitourinary: Vaginal bleeding or discharge, endometriosis, priapism, possible endometrial cancer

Neuromuscular & skeletal: Weakness

Ocular: Ophthalmologic effects (visual acuity changes, cataracts, or retinopathy), corneal opacities

Drug Interactions CYP1A2, 2A6, 2B6, 2C, 2D6, 2E1, and 3A3/4 enzyme substrate

Increased toxicity: Allopurinol results in exacerbation of allopurinol-induced hepatotoxicity; cyclosporine may result in increase in cyclosporine serum levels; warfarin results in significant enhancement of the anticoagulant effects of warfarin

Half-Life 7 days

Education and Monitoring Issues

Patient Education: Take as directed, morning and night and maintain adequate hydration (2-3 L/day of fluids unless instructed to restrict fluid intake). You may experience menstrual irregularities, vaginal bleeding, hot flashes, loss of libido (these will subside when treatment is completed). Bone pain may indicate a good therapeutic responses (consult prescriber for mild analgesics). For nausea, vomiting small, frequent meals, chewing gum, or sucking lozenges may help. You may experience photosensitivity (use sunscreen, wear protective clothing and eyewear, avoid direct sunlight). Report unusual bleeding or bruising, severe weakness, sedation, mental changes, swelling or pain in calves, difficulty breathing, or any changes in vision.

Monitoring Parameters: Monitor WBC and platelet counts, tumor

Manufacturer AstraZeneca

Related Information

Pharmaceutical Manufacturers Directory *on page 1020*

Tamsulosin (tam SOO loe sin)

Pharmacologic Class Alpha$_1$ Blockers

U.S. Brand Names Flomax®

Mechanism of Action An antagonist of alpha$_{1A}$ adrenoceptors in the prostate. Three subtypes identified: alpha$_{1A}$, alpha$_{1B}$, alpha$_{1D}$ have distribution that differs between human organs and tissue. Approximately 70% of the alpha$_1$-receptors in human prostate are of alpha$_{1A}$ subtype. The symptoms associated with benign prostatic hyperplasia (BPH) are related to bladder outlet obstruction, which is comprised of two underlying components: static and dynamic. Static is related to an increase in prostate size, partially caused by a proliferation of smooth muscle cells in the prostatic stroma. Severity of BPH symptoms and the degree of urethral obstruction do not correlate well with the size of the prostate. Dynamic is a function of an increase in smooth muscle tone in the prostate and bladder neck leading to constriction of the bladder outlet. Smooth muscle tone is mediated by the sympathetic nervous stimulation of alpha$_1$ adrenoceptors, which are abundant in the prostate, prostatic capsule, prostatic urethra, and bladder neck. Blockade of these adrenoceptors can cause smooth muscles in the bladder neck and prostate to relax, resulting in an improvement in urine flow rate and a reduction in symptoms of BPH.

Use Treatment of signs and symptoms of benign prostatic hyperplasia (BPH)

USUAL DOSAGE Oral: Adults: 0.4 mg once daily approximately 30 minutes after the same meal each day

Dosage Forms CAP: 0.4 mg

Warnings/Precautions Not intended for use as an antihypertensive drug; may cause orthostasis (ie, postural hypotension, dizziness, vertigo); patients should avoid situations where injury could result if syncope occurs; rule out the presence of carcinoma of prostate before beginning tamsulosin therapy

Pregnancy Risk Factor B

Adverse Reactions

Central nervous system: Headache, dizziness (0.4 mg: 14.9%; 0.8 mg: 17.1%), somnolence (0.4 mg: 3.0%; 0.8 mg: 4.3%), insomnia

Endocrine & metabolic: Decreased libido

Gastrointestinal: Diarrhea, nausea, tooth disorder

Genitourinary: Ejaculation disturbances

Neuromuscular & skeletal: Back pain, chest pain, asthenia

Ocular: Amblyopia

Respiratory: Rhinitis, pharyngitis, increased cough, sinusitis

Miscellaneous: Infections, allergic-type reactions such as skin rash, pruritus, angioedema, and urticaria have been reported upon drug rechallenge

Drug Interactions Use caution with concomitant administration of warfarin and tamsulosin; no dosage adjustments necessary if administered with atenolol, enalapril, or Procardia XL®; cimetidine resulted in a significant decrease (26%) in the clearance of tamsulosin which resulted in a moderate increase in tamsulosin AUC (44%); therefore, use with caution when used in combination with cimetidine (especially doses >0.4 mg); do not use in combination with other alpha-adrenergic blocking agents

Half-Life Healthy volunteers: 9-13 hours; target population: 14-15 hours

Education and Monitoring Issues

Patient Education: Take as directed 30 minutes, after same meal each day. Do not skip dose or discontinue without consulting prescriber. You may experience drowsiness, dizziness, or impaired judgment (use caution when driving or engaging in tasks that require alertness until response to drug is known); postural hypotension (use caution when rising from sitting or lying position or when climbing stairs); nausea (frequent mouth care or sucking lozenges may help); urinary incontinence (void before taking medication); ejaculatory disturbance (reversible, may resolve with continued use); diarrhea (boiled milk or yogurt may help); palpitations or rapid heartbeat; difficulty breathing, unusual cough, or sore throat; or other persistent side effects.

Dietary Considerations: The time to maximum concentration (T_{max}) is reached by 4-5 hours under fasting conditions and by 6-7 hours when administered with food. Taking it under fasted conditions results in a 30% increase in bioavailability and 40% to 70% increase in peak concentrations (C_{max}) compared to fed conditions.

(Continued)

Tamsulosin *(Continued)*

Manufacturer Boehringer Ingelheim, Inc

Related Information

Pharmaceutical Manufacturers Directory *on page 1020*

- **Tanac® [OTC]** *see* Benzocaine *on page 98*
- **Tanoral® Tablet** *see* Chlorpheniramine, Pyrilamine, and Phenylephrine *on page 187*
- **Tantaphen®** *see* Acetaminophen *on page 17*
- **Tapazole®** *see* Methimazole *on page 580*
- **Tarka®** *see* Trandolapril and Verapamil *on page 938*
- **Taro-Atenol®** *see* Atenolol *on page 76*
- **Taro-Cloxacillin®** *see* Cloxacillin *on page 220*
- **Taro-Sone** *see* Betamethasone *on page 103*
- **Tasmar®** *see* Tolcapone *on page 928*
- **Tavist®** *see* Clemastine *on page 207*
- **Tavist®-1 [OTC]** *see* Clemastine *on page 207*
- **Tavist-D®** *see* Clemastine and Phenylpropanolamine *on page 207*

Tazarotene (taz AR oh teen)

Pharmacologic Class Keratolytic Agent

U.S. Brand Names Tazorac®

Use Topical treatment of facial acne vulgaris; topical treatment of stable plaque psoriasis of up to 20% body surface area involvement

USUAL DOSAGE Children >12 years and Adults: Topical:

Acne: Cleanse the face gently. After the skin is dry, apply a thin film of tazarotene (2 mg/cm^2) once daily, in the evening, to the skin where the acne lesions appear. Use enough to cover the entire affected area. Tazarotene was investigated ≤12 weeks during clinical trials for acne.

Psoriasis: Apply tazarotene once daily, in the evening, to psoriatic lesions using enough (2 mg/cm^2) to cover only the lesion with a thin film to no more than 20% of body surface area. If a bath or shower is taken prior to application, dry the skin before applying the gel. Because unaffected skin may be more susceptible to irritation, avoid application of tazarotene to these areas. Tazarotene was investigated for up to 12 months during clinical trials for psoriasis.

Contraindications Hypersensitivity to tazarotene and other retinoids or vitamin A derivatives (isotretinoin, tretinoin, etretinate); pregnancy

Pregnancy Risk Factor X

- **Tazicef®** *see* Ceftazidime *on page 161*
- **Tazidime®** *see* Ceftazidime *on page 161*
- **Tazocin** *see* Piperacillin and Tazobactam Sodium *on page 741*
- **Tazorac®** *see* Tazarotene *on page 892*
- **Tebamide®** *see* Trimethobenzamide *on page 953*
- **Tebrazid** *see* Pyrazinamide *on page 794*
- **Teczem®** *see* Enalapril and Diltiazem *on page 311*
- **Tedral®** *see* Theophylline, Ephedrine, and Phenobarbital *on page 906*
- **Teejel** *see* Choline Salicylate *on page 194*
- **Teething Syrup** *see* Benzocaine *on page 98*
- **Tegison** *see* Etretinate *on page 348*
- **Tegopen®** *see* Cloxacillin *on page 220*
- **Tegretol®** *see* Carbamazepine *on page 137*
- **Tegretol®-XR** *see* Carbamazepine *on page 137*
- **Tegrin®-HC [OTC]** *see* Hydrocortisone *on page 447*
- **Teladar®** *see* Betamethasone *on page 103*

Telmisartan (tel mi SAR tan)

Pharmacologic Class Angiotensin II Antagonists

U.S. Brand Names Micardis®

Mechanism of Action Angiotensin II acts as a vasoconstrictor. In addition to causing direct vasoconstriction, angiotensin II also stimulates the release of aldosterone. Once aldosterone is released, sodium as well as water are reabsorbed. The end result is an elevation in blood pressure. Telmisartan is a nonpeptide AT1 angiotensin II receptor antagonist. This binding prevents angiotensin II from binding to the receptor thereby blocking the vasoconstriction and the aldosterone secreting effects of angiotensin II.

Use Alone or in combination with other antihypertensive agents in treating essential hypertension

USUAL DOSAGE Adults: Oral: Initial: 40 mg once daily; may be administered with or without food; usual maintenance dose range: 20-80 mg/day

Patients with volume depletion: Should be initiated on a lower dosage with close supervision or the condition should be corrected prior to initiating therapy or the use of an alternative ATII antagonist during initiation of therapy is warranted

Dosing in the elderly: No initial dose adjustment is required

Dosing in hepatic/biliary impairment: Supervise patients closely

Dosing in renal impairment: No initial dosing adjustment is necessary; patients on dialysis may develop orthostatic hypotension

Dosage Forms TAB: 40 mg, 80 mg

Contraindications Hypersensitivity to telmisartan or any component (telmisartan, sodium hydroxide, meglumine, povidone, sorbitol, magnesium stearate); sensitivity to other A-II receptor antagonists; pregnancy

Warnings/Precautions Avoid use or use smaller dose in volume-depleted patients. Drugs which alter renin-angiotensin system have been associated with deterioration in renal function, including oliguria, acute renal failure, and progressive azotemia. Use with caution in patients with renal artery stenosis (unilateral or bilateral) to avoid decrease in renal function; use caution in patients with pre-existing renal insufficiency (may decrease renal perfusion); the major route of elimination for telmisartan is via biliary elimination and as a result, patients with biliary obstruction can be expected to have reduced clearance and, therefore, telmisartan should be used with caution.

Pregnancy Risk Factor C (1st trimester); D (2nd and 3rd trimesters)

Pregnancy Implications Avoid use in the nursing mother, if possible, since telmisartan may be excreted in breast milk. The drug should be discontinued as soon as possible when pregnancy is detected. Drugs which act directly on renin-angiotensin can cause fetal and neonatal morbidity and death.

Adverse Reactions May be associated with worsening of renal function in patients dependent on renin-angiotensin-aldosterone system.

1% to 10%:

- Cardiovascular: Hypertension (1%), chest pain (1%), peripheral edema (1%)
- Central nervous system: Headache (1%), dizziness (1%), pain (1%), fatigue (1%)
- Gastrointestinal: Diarrhea (3%), dyspepsia (1%), nausea (1%), abdominal pain (1%)
- Genitourinary: Urinary tract infection (1%)
- Neuromuscular & skeletal: Back pain (3%), myalgia (1%)
- Respiratory: Upper respiratory infection (7%), sinusitis (3%), pharyngitis (1%), cough (1.6%)
- Miscellaneous: Flu-like syndrome (1%)

<1% (limited to important or life-threatening symptoms): Angioedema, allergic reaction, elevated liver enzymes, decrease in hemoglobin, increased serum creatinine and BUN, impotence, sweating, flushing, fever, malaise, palpitations, angina, tachycardia, abnormal EKG, insomnia, anxiety, nervousness, migraine, vertigo, depression, somnolence, paresthesia, involuntary muscle contractions, constipation, flatulence, dry mouth, hemorrhoids, gastroenteritis, enteritis, reflux, toothache, gout, hypercholesterolemia, diabetes mellitus, arthritis, arthralgia, leg cramps, fungal infection, abscess, otitis media, asthma, dyspnea, bronchitis, rhinitis, epistaxis, dermatitis, eczema, pruritus, rash, frequent urination, cystitis, abnormal vision, conjunctivitis, tinnitus, earache, cerebrovascular disorder

Drug Interactions

Digoxin levels may be increased

Lithium: Risk of toxicity may be increased by telmisartan; monitor lithium levels

Potassium-sparing diuretics (amiloride, potassium, spironolactone, triamterene): Increased risk of hyperkalemia

Potassium supplements may increase the risk of hyperkalemia

Trimethoprim (high dose) may increase the risk of hyperkalemia

Warfarin serum concentrations may be decreased (not associated with alteration in INR); monitor INR closely

Onset 1-2 hours

Duration Up to 24 hours

Half-Life Terminal: ~24 hours

Education and Monitoring Issues

Patient Education: Take exactly as directed. Do not miss doses, alter dosage, or discontinue without consulting prescriber. Do not alter salt or potassium intake without consulting prescriber. Monitor blood pressure on a regular basis as recommended by prescriber; at the same time each day. You may experience postural hypotension (change position slowly when rising from sitting or lying, when climbing stairs, or bending over); or transient nervousness, headache, or dizziness (use caution when driving or engaging in tasks requiring alertness until response to drug is known). Report unusual weight gain or swelling of ankles and hands; swelling of face, lips, throat, or tongue; persistent fatigue; dry cough or difficulty breathing; palpitations or chest pain; CNS changes; gastrointestinal disturbances; muscle or bone pain, cramping, or tremors; change in urinary pattern; or changes in hearing or vision.

Dietary Considerations: May be administered without regard to food

Monitoring Parameters: Supine blood pressure, electrolytes, serum creatinine, BUN, urinalysis, symptomatic hypotension, and tachycardia

Manufacturer Boehringer Ingelheim, Inc

(Continued)

Telmisartan *(Continued)*

Related Information

Angiotensin-Related Agents Comparison *on page 1226*

Pharmaceutical Manufacturers Directory *on page 1020*

Temazepam (te MAZ e pam)

Pharmacologic Class Benzodiazepine

U.S. Brand Names Restoril®

Generic Available Yes

Mechanism of Action Benzodiazepine anxiolytic sedative that produces CNS depression at the subcortical level, except at high doses, whereby it works at the cortical level; causes minimal change in REM sleep patterns

Use Treatment of anxiety and as an adjunct in the treatment of depression; also may be used in the management of panic attacks; transient insomnia and sleep latency

USUAL DOSAGE Adults: Oral: 15-30 mg at bedtime; 15 mg in elderly or debilitated patients

Dosage Forms CAP: 7.5 mg, 15 mg, 30 mg

Contraindications Hypersensitivity to temazepam or any component, severe uncontrolled pain, pre-existing CNS depression, or narrow-angle glaucoma; not to be used in pregnancy or lactation

Warnings/Precautions Safety and efficacy in children <18 years of age have not been established; do not use in pregnant women; may cause drug dependency; avoid abrupt discontinuance in patients with prolonged therapy or seizure disorders; use with caution in patients receiving other CNS depressants, in patients with hepatic dysfunction, and the elderly

Pregnancy Risk Factor X

Adverse Reactions

1% to 10%:

Central nervous system: Confusion, dizziness, drowsiness, fatigue, anxiety, headache, lethargy, hangover, euphoria, vertigo

Dermatologic: Rash

Endocrine & metabolic: Decreased libido

Gastrointestinal: Diarrhea

Neuromuscular & skeletal: Dysarthria, weakness

Otic: Blurred vision

Miscellaneous: Diaphoresis

<1%: Amnesia, anorexia, ataxia, back pain, blood dyscrasias, drug dependence, increased dreaming, menstrual irregularities, palpitations, paradoxical reactions, reflex slowing, tremor, vomiting

Drug Interactions CYP3A3/4 enzyme substrate

Alcohol and other CNS depressants may increase the CNS effects of temazepam

Oral contraceptives may increase the clearance of temazepam

Temazepam may decrease the antiparkinsonian efficacy of levodopa

Theophylline and other CNS stimulants may antagonize the sedative effects of temazepam

Alcohol Interactions Avoid use (may increase central nervous system depression)

Half-Life 9.5-12.4 hours

Education and Monitoring Issues

Patient Education: Use exactly as directed (do not increase dose or frequency or discontinue without consulting prescriber); may cause physical and/or psychological dependence. May take with food to decrease GI upset. While using this medication, do not use alcohol or other prescription or OTC medications (especially, pain medications, sedatives, antihistamines, or hypnotics) without consulting prescriber. Maintain adequate hydration (2-3 L/day of fluids unless instructed to restrict fluid intake). You may experience drowsiness, dizziness, lightheadedness, or blurred vision (use caution when driving or engaging in tasks requiring alertness until response to drug is known); or dry mouth or gastrointestinal discomfort (small frequent meals, frequent mouth care, chewing gum, or sucking lozenges may help). Report CNS changes (confusion, depression, increased sedation, excitation, headache, abnormal thinking, insomnia, or nightmares, memory impairment, impaired coordination); muscle pain or weakness; difficulty breathing; persistent dizziness, chest pain, or palpitations; alterations in normal gait; vision changes; or ineffectiveness of medication.

Monitoring Parameters: Respiratory and cardiovascular status

Reference Range: Therapeutic: 26 ng/mL after 24 hours

- **Temovate® Topical** *see* Clobetasol *on page 210*
- **Tempra® [OTC]** *see* Acetaminophen *on page 17*
- **Tenex®** *see* Guanfacine *on page 426*
- **Ten-K®** *see* Potassium Chloride *on page 751*
- **Tenoretic®** *see* Atenolol and Chlorthalidone *on page 78*
- **Tenormin®** *see* Atenolol *on page 76*
- **Tensilon® Injection** *see* Edrophonium *on page 306*

- **Tenuate®** *see* Diethylpropion *on page 268*
- **Tenuate® Dospan®** *see* Diethylpropion *on page 268*
- **Tequin™** *see* Gatifloxacin *on page 405*
- **Terak® Ophthalmic Ointment** *see* Oxytetracycline and Polymyxin B *on page 695*
- **Terazol® Vaginal** *see* Terconazole *on page 898*

Terazosin (ter AY zoe sin)

Pharmacologic Class Alpha$_1$ Blockers

U.S. Brand Names Hytrin®

Generic Available No

Mechanism of Action Alpha$_1$-specific blocking agent with minimal alpha$_2$ effects; this allows peripheral postsynaptic blockade, with the resultant decrease in arterial tone, while preserving the negative feedback loop which is mediated by the peripheral presynaptic alpha$_2$-receptors; terazosin relaxes the smooth muscle of the bladder neck, thus reducing bladder outlet obstruction

Use Management of mild to moderate hypertension; used alone or in combination with other agents such as diuretics or beta-blockers; benign prostate hypertrophy

USUAL DOSAGE Adults: Oral:

Hypertension: Initial: 1 mg at bedtime; slowly increase dose to achieve desired blood pressure, up to 20 mg/day; usual dose: 1-5 mg/day

Dosage reduction may be needed when adding a diuretic or other antihypertensive agent; if drug is discontinued for greater than several days, consider beginning with initial dose and retitrate as needed; dosage may be given on a twice daily regimen if response is diminished at 24 hours and hypotensive is observed at 2-4 hours following a dose

Benign prostatic hypertrophy: Initial: 1 mg at bedtime, increasing as needed; most patients require 10 mg day; if no response after 4-6 weeks of 10 mg/day, may increase to 20 mg/day

Dosage Forms CAP: 1 mg, 2 mg, 5 mg, 10 mg. **TAB:** 1 mg, 2 mg, 5 mg, 10 mg

Contraindications Hypersensitivity to terazosin, other alpha-adrenergic antagonists, or any component

Warnings/Precautions Marked orthostatic hypotension, syncope, and loss of consciousness may occur with first dose ("first dose phenomenon"). This reaction is more likely to occur in patients receiving beta-blockers, diuretics, low sodium diets, or first doses >1 mg/dose in adults; avoid rapid increase in dose; use with caution in patients with renal impairment.

Pregnancy Risk Factor C

Adverse Reactions

>10%:

Central nervous system: Dizziness (9% to 19%), headache (5% to 16%)

Neuromuscular & skeletal: Weakness (7.4% to 11.3%)

1% to 10%:

Cardiovascular: Peripheral edema (5.5%), palpitations (0.9% to 4.3%), postural hypotension (0.6% to 3.9%), tachycardia (1.9%)

Central nervous system: Fatigue, nervousness (2.3%)

Gastrointestinal: Xerostomia, nausea (4.4%), vomiting (1%), diarrhea/constipation (1%), abdominal pain (1%), flatulence (1%)

Neuromuscular & skeletal: Paresthesia (2.9%)

Respiratory: Dyspnea (1.7% to 3.1%), nasal congestion (1.9% to 5.9%)

<1%: Angina (~1%), arthritis, blurred vision, bronchospasm, conjunctivitis, decreased libido, depression, epistaxis, flu-like symptoms, insomnia, myalgia, pharyngitis, polyuria, priapism, rash, sexual dysfunction, syncope, tinnitus

Drug Interactions

Decreased antihypertensive response with NSAIDs and alpha$_1$-blockers; decreased clonidine effects

Increased hypotensive effect with diuretics and antihypertensive medications (especially beta-blockers)

Alcohol Interactions Use with caution (may increase risk of hypotension or dizziness)

Onset 1-2 hours

Half-Life 9.2-12 hours

Education and Monitoring Issues

Patient Education: Take as directed, at bedtime. Do not skip dose or discontinue without consulting prescriber. Follow recommended diet and exercise program. Do not use alcohol or OTC medications which may affect blood pressure (eg, cough or cold remedies, diet pills, stay-awake medications) without consulting prescriber. You may experience drowsiness, dizziness, or impaired judgment (use caution when driving or engaging in tasks that require alertness until response to drug is known); postural hypotension (use caution when rising from sitting or lying position or when climbing stairs); dry mouth or nausea (frequent mouth care or sucking lozenges may help); urinary incontinence (void before taking medication); or sexual dysfunction (reversible, may resolve with continued use). Report altered CNS status (eg, fatigue, lethargy, confusion, nervousness); sudden weight gain (weigh yourself in the same clothes at the same time of day once a week); unusual or persistent swelling of ankles, feet, or

(Continued)

Terazosin *(Continued)*

extremities; palpitations or rapid heartbeat; difficulty breathing; muscle weakness; or other persistent side effects.

Monitoring Parameters: Standing and sitting/supine blood pressure, especially following the initial dose at 2-4 hours following the dose and thereafter at the trough point to ensure adequate control throughout the dosing interval; urinary symptoms

Manufacturer Abbott Laboratories (Pharmaceutical Product Division)

Related Information

Pharmaceutical Manufacturers Directory *on page 1020*

Terbinafine (TER bin a feen)

Pharmacologic Class Antifungal Agent, Topical

U.S. Brand Names Daskil®; Lamisil® [OTC]; Lamisil® Dermgel®

Mechanism of Action Synthetic alkylamine derivative which inhibits squalene epoxidase, a key enzyme in sterol biosynthesis in fungi. This results in a deficiency in ergosterol within the fungal cell wall and results in fungal cell death.

Use Active against most strains of *Trichophyton mentagrophytes*, *Trichophyton rubrum*; may be effective for infections of *Microsporum gypseum* and *M. nanum*, *Trichophyton verrucosum*, *Epidermophyton floccosum*, *Candida albicans*, and *Scopulariopsis brevicaulis*

Oral: Onychomycosis of the toenail or fingernail due to susceptible dermatophytes

Topical: Antifungal for the treatment of tinea pedis (athlete's foot), tinea cruris (jock itch), tinea corporis (ringworm), and tinea versicolor

USUAL DOSAGE Adults:

Oral:

Superficial mycoses: Fingernail: 250 mg/day for up to 6 weeks; toenail: 250 mg/day for 12 weeks; doses may be given in two divided doses

Systemic mycosis: 250-500 mg/day for up to 16 months

Topical:

Athlete's foot: Apply to affected area twice daily for at least 1 week, not to exceed 4 weeks

Ringworm and jock itch: Apply to affected area once or twice daily for at least 1 week, not to exceed 4 weeks

Topical gel: Apply to affected area once daily for 7 days

Dosing adjustment in renal impairment: Although specific guidelines are not available, dose reduction in significant renal insufficiency (GFR <50 mL/minute) is recommended

Dosage Forms CRM: 1% (15 g, 30 g). **GEL, top:** 1% (5 g, 15 g, 30 g). **TAB:** 250 mg

Contraindications Hypersensitivity to terbinafine, naftifine or any component; pre-existing liver or renal disease (≤50 mL/minute GFR)

Warnings/Precautions While rare, the following complications have been reported and may require discontinuation of therapy: Changes in the ocular lens and retina, pancytopenia, neutropenia, Stevens-Johnson syndrome, toxic epidermal necrolysis. Discontinue if symptoms or signs of hepatobiliary dysfunction or cholestatic hepatitis develop. If irritation/sensitivity develop with topical use, discontinue therapy. Use caution in writing/filling prescriptions; confusion between Lamictal® (lamotrigine) and Lamisil® (terbinafine) has occurred.

Pregnancy Risk Factor B

Pregnancy Implications

Clinical effects on the fetus: Avoid use in pregnancy since treatment of onychomycosis is postponable

Breast-feeding/lactation: Although minimal concentrations of terbinafine cross into breast milk after topical use, oral or topical treatment during lactation should be avoided

Adverse Reactions

Oral: 1% to 10%:

Central nervous system: Headache, dizziness, vertigo

Dermatologic: Rash, pruritus, and alopecia with oral therapy

Gastrointestinal: Nausea, diarrhea, dyspepsia, abdominal pain, appetite decrease, taste disturbance

Hematologic: Neutropenia, lymphocytopenia

Hepatic: Cholestasis, jaundice, hepatitis, liver enzyme elevations

Ocular: Visual disturbance

Miscellaneous: Allergic reaction

Topical: 1% to 10%:

Dermatologic: Pruritus, contact dermatitis, irritation, burning, dryness

Local: Irritation, stinging

Drug Interactions

Decreased effect: Cyclosporine clearance is increased (~15%) with concomitant terbinafine; rifampin increases terbinafine clearance (100%)

Increased effect: Terbinafine clearance is decreased by cimetidine (33%) and terfenadine (16%); caffeine clearance is decreased by terfenadine (19%)

Half-Life 22-26 hours

Education and Monitoring Issues

Patient Education: Topical: Avoid contact with eyes, nose, or mouth during treatment with cream; nursing mothers should not use on breast tissue; advise prescriber if eyes or skin becomes yellow or if irritation, itching, or burning develops. Do not use occlusive dressings concurrent with therapy. Full clinical effect may require several months due to the time required for a new nail to grow.

Monitoring Parameters: CBC and LFTs at baseline and repeated if use is for >6 weeks

Manufacturer Novartis

Related Information

Pharmaceutical Manufacturers Directory *on page 1020*

Terbutaline (ter BYOO ta leen)

Pharmacologic Class $Beta_2$ Agonist

U.S. Brand Names Brethaire® Inhalation Aerosol; Brethine® Injection; Brethine® Oral; Bricanyl® Injection; Bricanyl® Oral

Generic Available No

Mechanism of Action Relaxes bronchial smooth muscle by action on $beta_2$-receptors with less effect on heart rate

Use Bronchodilator in reversible airway obstruction and bronchial asthma

USUAL DOSAGE

Children <12 years:

Oral: Initial: 0.05 mg/kg/dose 3 times/day, increased gradually as required; maximum: 0.15 mg/kg/dose 3-4 times/day or a total of 5 mg/24 hours

S.C.: 0.005-0.01 mg/kg/dose to a maximum of 0.3 mg/dose every 15-20 minutes for 3 doses

Nebulization: 0.01-0.03 mg/kg/dose every 4-6 hours

Inhalation: 1-2 inhalations every 4-6 hours

Children >12 years and Adults:

Oral:

12-15 years: 2.5 mg every 6 hours 3 times/day; not to exceed 7.5 mg in 24 hours

>15 years: 5 mg/dose every 6 hours 3 times/day; if side effects occur, reduce dose to 2.5 mg every 6 hours; not to exceed 15 mg in 24 hours

S.C.: 0.25 mg/dose repeated in 15-30 minutes for one time only; a total dose of 0.5 mg should not be exceeded within a 4-hour period

Nebulization: 0.01-0.03 mg/kg/dose every 4-6 hours

Inhalation: 2 inhalations every 4-6 hours; wait 1 minute between inhalations

Dosing adjustment/comments in renal impairment:

Cl_{cr} 10-50 mL/minute: Administer at 50% of normal dose

Cl_{cr} <10 mL/minute: Avoid use

Dosage Forms AERO, oral: 0.2 mg/actuation (10.5 g). **INJ:** 1 mg/mL (1 mL). **TAB:** 2.5 mg, 5 mg

Contraindications Hypersensitivity to terbutaline or any component, cardiac arrhythmias associated with tachycardia, tachycardia caused by digitalis intoxication

Warnings/Precautions Excessive or prolonged use may lead to tolerance; paradoxical bronchoconstriction may occur with excessive use; if it occurs, discontinue terbutaline immediately

Pregnancy Risk Factor B

Adverse Reactions

>10%:

Central nervous system: Nervousness, restlessness

Neuromuscular & skeletal: Trembling

1% to 10%:

Cardiovascular: Tachycardia, hypertension

Central nervous system: Dizziness, drowsiness, headache, insomnia

Gastrointestinal: Xerostomia, nausea, vomiting, bad taste in mouth

Neuromuscular & skeletal: Muscle cramps, weakness

Miscellaneous: Diaphoresis

<1%: Arrhythmias, chest pain, paradoxical bronchospasm

Drug Interactions

Decreased effect with beta-blockers

Increased toxicity with MAO inhibitors, TCAs

Onset Oral: 30-45 minutes; S.C.: Within 6-15 minutes

Half-Life 11-16 hours

Education and Monitoring Issues

Patient Education: Use exactly as directed. Do not use more often than recommended (excessive use may result in tolerance, overdose may result in serious adverse effects) and do not discontinue without consulting prescriber. Maintain adequate hydration (2-3 L/day of fluids unless instructed to restrict fluid intake). You may experience nervousness, dizziness, or fatigue (use caution when driving or engaging in tasks requiring alertness until response to drug is known); or dry mouth, stomach upset (frequent small meals, frequent mouth care, chewing gum, or sucking hard candy may help). Report unresolved GI upset; dizziness or fatigue; vision changes; chest pain, rapid heartbeat,

(Continued)

Terbutaline *(Continued)*

or palpitations; insomnia, nervousness, or hyperactivity; muscle cramping, tremors, or pain; unusual cough; or rash (hypersensitivity).

Preterm labor: Notify prescriber immediately if labor resumes or adverse side effects are noted.

Monitoring Parameters: Serum potassium, heart rate, blood pressure, respiratory rate

Related Information

Bronchodilators Comparison *on page 1235*

Terconazole (ter KONE a zole)

Pharmacologic Class Antifungal Agent, Vaginal

U.S. Brand Names Terazol® Vaginal

Use Local treatment of vulvovaginal candidiasis

USUAL DOSAGE Adults: Female: Insert 1 applicatorful intravaginally at bedtime for 7 consecutive days

Contraindications Known hypersensitivity to terconazole or components of the vaginal cream or suppository

Pregnancy Risk Factor C

Related Information

Treatment of Sexually Transmitted Diseases *on page 1210*

- ♦ **Terfluzine** *see* Trifluoperazine *on page 950*

Terpin Hydrate and Codeine (TER pin HYE drate & KOE deen)

Pharmacologic Class Antitussive/Expectorant

Dosage Forms ELIX: Terpin hydrate 85 mg and codeine 10 mg per 5 mL with alcohol 42.5%

Pregnancy Risk Factor C

- ♦ **Terra-Cortril® Ophthalmic Suspension** *see* Oxytetracycline and Hydrocortisone *on page 695*
- ♦ **Terramycin® I.M. Injection** *see* Oxytetracycline *on page 695*
- ♦ **Terramycin® Ophthalmic Ointment** *see* Oxytetracycline and Polymyxin B *on page 695*
- ♦ **Terramycin® Oral** *see* Oxytetracycline *on page 695*
- ♦ **Terramycin® w/Polymyxin B Ophthalmic Ointment** *see* Oxytetracycline and Polymyxin B *on page 695*
- ♦ **Teslac®** *see* Testolactone *on page 898*
- ♦ **Tessalon®** *see* Benzonatate *on page 99*
- ♦ **Tessalon® Perles** *see* Benzonatate *on page 99*
- ♦ **Testex®** *see* Testosterone *on page 898*
- ♦ **Testoderm® Transdermal System** *see* Testosterone *on page 898*

Testolactone (tes toe LAK tone)

Pharmacologic Class Androgen

U.S. Brand Names Teslac®

Use Palliative treatment of advanced disseminated breast carcinoma

USUAL DOSAGE Adults: Female: Oral: 250 mg 4 times/day for at least 3 months; desired response may take as long as 3 months

Contraindications In men for the treatment of breast cancer; known hypersensitivity to testolactone

Pregnancy Risk Factor C

- ♦ **Testopel® Pellet** *see* Testosterone *on page 898*

Testosterone (tes TOS ter one)

Pharmacologic Class Androgen

U.S. Brand Names Androderm® Transdermal System; AndroGel®; Andro-L.A.® Injection; Andropository® Injection; Delatest® Injection; Delatestryl® Injection; depAndro® Injection; Depotest® Injection; Depo®-Testosterone Injection; Duratest® Injection; Durathate® Injection; Everone® Injection; Histerone® Injection; Testex®; Testoderm® Transdermal System; Testopel® Pellet

Generic Available Yes

Mechanism of Action Principal endogenous androgen responsible for promoting the growth and development of the male sex organs and maintaining secondary sex characteristics in androgen-deficient males

Use Androgen replacement therapy in the treatment of delayed male puberty; postpartum breast pain and engorgement; inoperable breast cancer; male hypogonadism

USUAL DOSAGE

Children: I.M.:

Male hypogonadism:

Initiation of pubertal growth: 40-50 mg/m^2/dose (cypionate or enanthate ester) monthly until the growth rate falls to prepubertal levels

Terminal growth phase: 100 mg/m^2/dose (cypionate or enanthate ester) monthly until growth ceases

Maintenance virilizing dose: 100 mg/m^2/dose (cypionate or enanthate ester) twice monthly

Delayed puberty: 40-50 mg/m^2/dose monthly (cypionate or enanthate ester) for 6 months

Adults: Inoperable breast cancer: I.M.: 200-400 mg every 2-4 weeks

Male: Short-acting formulations: Testosterone Aqueous/Testosterone Propionate (in oil): I.M.:

Androgen replacement therapy: 10-50 mg 2-3 times/week

Male hypogonadism: 40-50 mg/m^2/dose monthly until the growth rate falls to prepubertal levels (~5 cm/year); during terminal growth phase: 100 mg/m^2/dose monthly until growth ceases; maintenance virilizing dose: 100 mg/m^2/dose twice monthly or 50-400 mg/dose every 2-4 weeks

Male: Long-acting formulations: Testosterone enanthate (in oil)/testosterone cypionate (in oil): I.M.:

Male hypogonadism: 50-400 mg every 2-4 weeks

Male with delayed puberty: 50-200 mg every 2-4 weeks for a limited duration

Male ≥18 years: Transdermal: Primary hypogonadism **or** hypogonadotropic hypogonadism:

Testoderm®: Apply 6 mg patch daily to scrotum (if scrotum is inadequate, use a 4 mg daily system)

Testoderm-TSS®: Apply 5 mg patch daily to clean, dry area of skin on the arm, back or upper buttocks. **Do not apply Testoderm-TSS® to the scrotum**

Androderm®: Apply 2 systems nightly to clean, dry area on the back, abdomen, upper arms or thighs for 24 hours for a total of 5 mg/day

AndroGel®: Males >18 years of age: 5 g (to deliver 50 mg of testosterone) applied once daily (preferably in the morning) to clean, dry, intact skin of the shoulder and upper arms and/or abdomen. Upon opening the packet(s), the entire contents should be squeezed into the palm of the hand and immediately applied to the application site(s). Application sites should be allowed to dry for a few minutes prior to dressing. Hands should be washed with soap and water after application. **Do not apply AndroGel® to the genitals**

Dosing adjustment/comments in hepatic disease: Reduce dose

Dosage Forms INJ: Aqueous susp: 25 mg/mL (10 mL, 30 mL), 50 mg/mL (10 mL, 30 mL), 100 mg/mL (10 mL, 30 mL); In oil, as cypionate: 100 mg/mL (1 mL, 10 mL), 200 mg/mL (1 mL, 10 mL); In oil, as enanthate: 100 mg/mL (1 mL< 5 mL, 10 mL), 200 mg/mL (1 mL, 5 mL, 10 mL); In oil, as propionate: 50 mg/mL (10 mL, 30 mL), 100 mg/mL (10 mL, 30 mL). **PELLET:** 75 mg (1 pellet per vial). **TRANSDERMAL system:** 2.5 mg/day; 4 mg/day, 5 mg/day, 6 mg/day. **TRANSDERMAL GEL:** AndroGel®: 1%: 50 mg (5 g gel); 75 mg (7.5 g gel)

Contraindications Severe renal or cardiac disease, benign prostatic hypertrophy with obstruction, undiagnosed genital bleeding, males with carcinoma of the breast or prostate; hypersensitivity to testosterone or any component; pregnancy

Warnings/Precautions Perform radiographic examination of the hand and wrist every 6 months to determine the rate of bone maturation; may accelerate bone maturation without producing compensating gain in linear growth; has both androgenic and anabolic activity, the anabolic action may enhance hypoglycemia. Transfer of testosterone to another person can occur when vigorous skin-to-skin contact is made with the application site; see Nursing Implications for recommended precautions.

Pregnancy Risk Factor X

Pregnancy Implications AndroGel® is not indicated for women and must not be used in women

Adverse Reactions

>10%:

Dermatologic: Acne

Endocrine & metabolic: Menstrual problems (amenorrhea), virilism, breast soreness

Genitourinary: Epididymitis, priapism, bladder irritability

1% to 10%:

Cardiovascular: Flushing, edema

Central nervous system: Excitation, aggressive behavior, sleeplessness, anxiety, mental depression, headache

Dermatologic: Hirsutism (increase in pubic hair growth)

Gastrointestinal: Nausea, vomiting, GI irritation

Genitourinary: Prostatic hypertrophy, prostatic carcinoma, impotence, testicular atrophy

Hepatic: Hepatic dysfunction

<1%: Cholestatic hepatitis, gynecomastia, hepatic necrosis, hypercalcemia, hypersensitivity reactions, hypoglycemia, leukopenia, polycythemia, suppression of clotting factors

Drug Interactions CYP3A3/4 and 3A5-7 enzyme substrate

Increased toxicity: Effects of oral anticoagulants may be enhanced

Duration Based upon the route of administration and which testosterone ester is used; cypionate and enanthate esters have the longest duration, up to 2-4 weeks after I.M. administration.

Half-Life 10-100 minutes

(Continued)

Testosterone *(Continued)*

Education and Monitoring Issues

Patient Education: Diabetics should monitor serum glucose closely and notify prescriber of changes; this medication may alter glycemic response. You may experience acne, growth of body hair, loss of libido, impotence, or menstrual irregularity (usually reversible); nausea or vomiting (small frequent meals, frequent mouth care, sucking lozenges, or chewing gum may help). Report changes in menstrual pattern; enlarged or painful breasts; deepening of voice or unusual growth of body hair; persistent penile erection; fluid retention (swelling of ankles, feet, or hands, difficulty breathing or sudden weight gain); unresolved changes in CNS (nervousness, chills, insomnia, depression, aggressiveness); altered urinary patterns; change in color of urine or stool; yellowing of eyes or skin; unusual bruising or bleeding; or other persistent adverse reactions.

Topical: Apply to clean, dry scrotal skin. Dry shave scrotal hair for optimal skin contact. Do not use chemical depilatories.

Monitoring Parameters: Periodic liver function tests, radiologic examination of wrist and hand every 6 months (when using in prepubertal children); serum testosterone levels should be measured approximately 14 days after initiation of therapy to ensure proper dosing. If the serum testosterone concentration is below the normal range, or if the desired clinical response is not achieved, the daily AndroGel® 1% dose may be increased from 5 g to 7.5 g and from 7.5 g to 10 g as instructed by the prescriber.

Reference Range: Testosterone, urine: Male: 100-1500 ng/24 hours; Female: 100-500 ng/24 hours

Related Information

Estradiol and Testosterone *on page 329*

♦ **Testred®** *see* Methyltestosterone *on page 591*

Tetanus Antitoxin (TET a nus an tee TOKS in)

Pharmacologic Class Antitoxin

Generic Available No

Mechanism of Action Provides passive immunization; solution of concentrated globulins containing antitoxic antibodies obtained from horse serum after immunization against tetanus toxin

Use Tetanus prophylaxis or treatment of active tetanus only when tetanus immune globulin (TIG) is not available; tetanus immune globulin (Hyper-Tet®) is the preferred tetanus immunoglobulin for the treatment of active tetanus; may be given concomitantly with tetanus toxoid adsorbed when immediate treatment is required, but active immunization is desirable

USUAL DOSAGE

Prophylaxis: I.M., S.C.:

Children <30 kg: 1500 units

Children and Adults ≥30 kg: 3000-5000 units

Treatment: Children and Adults: Inject 10,000-40,000 units into wound; administer 40,000-100,000 units

Dosage Forms INJ (equine): Not less than 400 units/mL (12.5 mL, 50 mL)

Contraindications Patients sensitive to equine-derived preparations

Warnings/Precautions Tetanus antitoxin is not the same as tetanus immune globulin; sensitivity testing should be conducted in all individuals regardless of clinical history; have epinephrine 1:1000 available

Pregnancy Risk Factor D

Adverse Reactions ≥10%: Skin eruptions, erythema, urticaria, local pain, numbness, arthralgia, serum sickness may develop up to several weeks after injection, anaphylaxis

Tetanus Immune Globulin (Human)

(TET a nus i MYUN GLOB yoo lin HYU man)

Pharmacologic Class Immune Globulin

U.S. Brand Names Hyper-Tet®

Generic Available No

Mechanism of Action Passive immunity toward tetanus

Use Passive immunization against tetanus; tetanus immune globulin is preferred over tetanus antitoxin for treatment of active tetanus; part of the management of an unclean, wound in a person whose history of previous receipt of tetanus toxoid is unknown or who has received less than three doses of tetanus toxoid; elderly may require TIG more often than younger patients with tetanus infection due to declining antibody titers with age

USUAL DOSAGE I.M.:

Prophylaxis of tetanus:

Children: 4 units/kg; some recommend administering 250 units to small children

Adults: 250 units

Treatment of tetanus:

Children: 500-3000 units; some should infiltrate locally around the wound

Adults: 3000-6000 units

Dosage Forms INJ: 250 units/mL

Contraindications Hypersensitivity to tetanus immune globulin, thimerosal, or any immune globulin product or component; patients with IgA deficiency; I.V. administration

Warnings/Precautions Have epinephrine 1:1000 available for anaphylactic reactions; do not administer I.V.

Pregnancy Risk Factor C

Adverse Reactions

>10%: Local: Pain, tenderness, erythema at injection site

1% to 10%:

Central nervous system: Fever (mild)

Dermatologic: Urticaria, angioedema

Neuromuscular & skeletal: Muscle stiffness

Miscellaneous: Anaphylaxis reaction

<1%: Sensitization to repeated injections

Drug Interactions Never administer tetanus toxoid and TIG in same syringe (toxoid will be neutralized); toxoid may be given at a separate site; concomitant administration with Td may decrease its immune response, especially in individuals with low prevaccination antibody titers

Related Information

Animal and Human Bites Guidelines *on page 1177*

Tetanus Toxoid, Adsorbed (TET a nus TOKS oyd, ad SORBED)

Pharmacologic Class Toxoid

Generic Available No

Mechanism of Action Tetanus toxoid preparations contain the toxin produced by virulent tetanus bacilli (detoxified growth products of *Clostridium tetani*). The toxin has been modified by treatment with formaldehyde so that it has lost toxicity but still retains ability to act as antigen and produce active immunity; the aluminum salt, a mineral adjuvant, delays the rate of absorption and prolongs and enhances its properties; duration ~10 years.

Use Selective induction of active immunity against tetanus in selected patients. **Note:** Tetanus and diphtheria toxoids for adult use (Td) is the preferred immunizing agent for most adults and for children after their seventh birthday. Young children should receive trivalent DTwP or DTaP (diphtheria/tetanus/pertussis - whole cell or acellular), as part of their childhood immunization program, unless pertussis is contraindicated, then TD is warranted.

USUAL DOSAGE Adults: I.M.:

Primary immunization: 0.5 mL; repeat 0.5 mL at 4-8 weeks after first dose and at 6-12 months after second dose

Routine booster doses are recommended only every 5-10 years

Dosage Forms INJ, adsorbed: Tetanus 5 Lf units per 0.5 mL dose (0.5 mL, 5 mL); Tetanus 10 Lf units per 0.5 mL dose (0.5 mL, 5 mL)

Contraindications Hypersensitivity to tetanus toxoid or any component (may use the fluid tetanus toxoid to immunize the rare patient who is hypersensitive to aluminum adjuvant); avoid use with chloramphenicol or if neurological signs or symptoms occurred after prior administration; poliomyelitis outbreaks require deferral of immunizations; acute respiratory infections or other active infections may dictate deferral of administration of routine primary immunizing but not emergency doses

Warnings/Precautions Not equivalent to tetanus toxoid fluid; the tetanus toxoid adsorbed is the preferred toxoid for immunization and Td, TD or DTaP/DTwP are the preferred adsorbed forms; avoid injection into a blood vessel; have epinephrine (1:1000) available; not for use in treatment of tetanus infection nor for immediate prophylaxis of unimmunized individuals; immunosuppressive therapy or other immunodeficiencies may diminish antibody response, however it is recommended for routine immunization of symptomatic and asymptomatic HIV-infected patients; deferral of immunization until immunosuppression is discontinued or administration of an additional dose >1 month after treatment is recommended; allergic reactions may occur; epinephrine 1:1000 must be available; use in pediatrics should be deferred until >1 year of age when a history of a CNS disorder is present; elderly may not mount adequate antibody titers following immunization

Pregnancy Risk Factor C

Adverse Reactions

>10%: Local: Induration/redness at injection site

1% to 10%:

Central nervous system: Chills, fever

Local: Sterile abscess at injection site

Miscellaneous: Allergic reaction

<1%: Arthus-type hypersensitivity reactions, blistering at injection site, fever >103°F, malaise, neurological disturbances

Drug Interactions Decreased response: If primary immunization is started in individuals receiving an immunosuppressive agent or corticosteroids, serologic testing may be needed to ensure adequate antibody response; concurrent use of TIG and tetanus toxoid may delay the development of active immunity by several days

(Continued)

Tetanus Toxoid, Adsorbed *(Continued)*

Education and Monitoring Issues

Patient Education: A nodule may be palpable at the injection site for a few weeks. DT, Td and T vaccines cause few problems; they may cause mild fever or soreness, swelling, and redness where the shot was given. These problems usually last 1-2 days, but this does not happen nearly as often as with DTP vaccine. Sometimes, adults who get these vaccines can have a lot of soreness and swelling where the shot was given.

Related Information

Animal and Human Bites Guidelines *on page 1177*

Tetanus Toxoid, Fluid (TET a nus TOKS oyd, FLOO id)

Pharmacologic Class Toxoid

Generic Available No

Mechanism of Action Tetanus toxoid preparations contain the toxin produced by virulent tetanus bacilli (detoxified growth products of *Clostridium tetani*). The toxin has been modified by treatment with formaldehyde so that is has lost toxicity but still retains ability to act as antigen and produce active immunity.

Use Detection of delayed hypersensitivity and assessment of cell-mediated immunity; active immunization against tetanus in the rare adult or child who is allergic to the aluminum adjuvant (a product containing adsorbed tetanus toxoid is preferred)

USUAL DOSAGE

Anergy testing: Intradermal: 0.1 mL

Primary immunization (**Note:** Td, TD, DTaP/DTwP are recommended): Adults: Inject 3 doses of 0.5 mL I.M. or S.C. at 4- to 8-week intervals; administer fourth dose 6-12 months after third dose

Booster doses: I.M., S.C.: 0.5 mL every 10 years

Dosage Forms INJ, fluid: Tetanus 4 Lf units per 0.5 mL dose (7.5 mL); Tetanus 5 Lf units per 0.5 mL dose (0.5 mL, 7.5 mL)

Contraindications Hypersensitivity to tetanus toxoid or any product components

Warnings/Precautions Epinephrine 1:1000 should be readily available; skin test responsiveness may be delayed or reduced in elderly patients

Pregnancy Risk Factor C

Adverse Reactions Percentage unknown: Very hypersensitive persons may develop a local reaction at the injection site; anaphylactic reactions, death, shock, urticaria are possible

Drug Interactions Increased effect: Cimetidine may augment delayed hypersensitivity responses to skin test antigens

Related Information

Animal and Human Bites Guidelines *on page 1177*

Tetracaine (TET ra kane)

Pharmacologic Class Local Anesthetic

U.S. Brand Names Pontocaine®

Generic Available Yes

Mechanism of Action Ester local anesthetic blocks both the initiation and conduction of nerve impulses by decreasing the neuronal membrane's permeability to sodium ions, which results in inhibition of depolarization with resultant blockade of conduction

Use Spinal anesthesia; local anesthesia in the eye for various diagnostic and examination purposes; topically applied to nose and throat for various diagnostic procedures; **approximately 10 times more potent than procaine**

USUAL DOSAGE Maximum adult dose: 50 mg

Children: Safety and efficacy have not been established

Adults:

- Ophthalmic (not for prolonged use):
  - Ointment: Apply ½" to 1" to lower conjunctival fornix
  - Solution: Instill 1-2 drops
- Spinal anesthesia:
  - High, medium, low, and saddle blocks: 0.2% to 0.3% solution
  - Prolonged (2-3 hours): 1% solution
  - Subarachnoid injection: 5-20 mg
  - Saddle block: 2-5 mg; a 1% solution should be diluted with equal volume of CSF before administration
- Topical mucous membranes (2% solution): Apply as needed; dose should not exceed 20 mg
- Topical for skin: Ointment/cream: Apply to affected areas as needed

Dosage Forms CRM: 1% (28 g). **INJ:** 1% [10 mg/mL] (2 mL); With dextrose 6%: 0.2% [2 mg/mL] (2 mL), 0.3% [3 mg/mL] (5 mL). **OINT:** Ophth: 0.5% [5 mg/mL] (3.75 g); Top: 0.5% [5 mg/mL] (28 g). **POWDER for inj:** 20 mg. **SOLN:** Ophth: 0.5% [5 mg/mL] (1 mL, 2 mL, 15 mL, 59 mL); Top: 2% [20 mg/mL] (30 mL, 118 mL)

Contraindications Hypersensitivity to tetracaine or any component; ophthalmic secondary bacterial infection, patients with liver disease, CNS disease, meningitis (if used for epidural or spinal anesthesia), myasthenia gravis

Warnings/Precautions No pediatric dosage recommendations; ophthalmic preparations may delay wound healing; use with caution in patients with cardiac disease and hyperthyroidism

Pregnancy Risk Factor C

Adverse Reactions

1% to 10%: Dermatologic: Contact dermatitis, burning, stinging, angioedema

<1%: Methemoglobinemia in infants, tenderness, urticaria, urethritis

Drug Interactions Decreased effect: Aminosalicylic acid, sulfonamides effects may be antagonized

Onset Onset of anesthetic effect:

Ophthalmic instillation: Within 60 seconds

Topical or spinal injection: Within 3-8 minutes after applied to mucous membranes or when saddle block administered for spinal anesthesia

Duration Topical: 1.5-3 hours

Education and Monitoring Issues

Patient Education: Topical or ophthalmic anesthesia effects may last for some time following use; you will need to observe appropriate safety precautions to prevent injury.

Ophthalmic: Do not rub or touch your eye, scratch your nose, or attempt to apply eye makeup until all sensation returns. May cause temporary rash or stinging when used. Report any ringing in ears, feeling of weakness or faintness, chest pain or palpitation, or increased restlessness.

Topical: Do not eat or drink anything until full sensation returns to lips, mouth, and throat. Use caution with heat or cold; you will not have accurate hot or cold sensation until full effects of anesthesia have worn off.

Related Information

Benzocaine, Butyl Aminobenzoate, Tetracaine, and Benzalkonium Chloride *on page 99*

Tetracaine and Dextrose *on page 903*

Tetracaine and Dextrose (TET ra kane & DEKS trose)

Pharmacologic Class Local Anesthetic

U.S. Brand Names Pontocaine® With Dextrose Injection

Dosage Forms INJ: Tetracaine hydrochloride 0.2% and dextrose 6% (2 mL); tetracaine hydrochloride 0.3% and dextrose 6% (5 mL)

Pregnancy Risk Factor C

♦ **Tetracap® Oral** *see* Tetracycline *on page 903*

Tetracycline (tet ra SYE kleen)

Pharmacologic Class Antibiotic, Ophthalmic; Antibiotic, Tetracycline Derivative; Antibiotic, Topical

U.S. Brand Names Achromycin® Ophthalmic; Achromycin® Topical; Nor-tet® Oral; Panmycin® Oral; Sumycin® Oral; Tetracap® Oral; Topicycline® Topical

Generic Available Yes

Mechanism of Action Inhibits bacterial protein synthesis by binding with the 30S and possibly the 50S ribosomal subunit(s) of susceptible bacteria; may also cause alterations in the cytoplasmic membrane

Use Treatment of susceptible bacterial infections of both gram-positive and gram-negative organisms; also infections due to *Mycoplasma*, *Chlamydia*, and *Rickettsia*; indicated for acne, exacerbations of chronic bronchitis, and treatment of gonorrhea and syphilis in patients that are allergic to penicillin; used concomitantly with metronidazole, bismuth subsalicylate and an H_2-antagonist for the treatment of duodenal ulcer disease induced by *H. pylori*

USUAL DOSAGE

Children >8 years: Oral: 25-50 mg/kg/day in divided doses every 6 hours

Children >8 years and Adults:

Ophthalmic:

Ointment: Instill every 2-12 hours

Suspension: Instill 1-2 drops 2-4 times/day or more often as needed

Topical: Apply to affected areas 1-4 times/day

Adults: Oral: 250-500 mg/dose every 6 hours

Helicobacter pylori: Clinically effective treatment regimens include triple therapy with amoxicillin or tetracycline, metronidazole, and bismuth subsalicylate; amoxicillin, metronidazole, and H_2-receptor antagonist; or double therapy with amoxicillin and omeprazole. Adult dose: 850 mg 3 times/day to 500 mg 4 times/day

Dosing interval in renal impairment:

Cl_{cr} 50-80 mL/minute: Administer every 8-12 hours

Cl_{cr} 10-50 mL/minute: Administer every 12-24 hours

Cl_{cr} <10 mL/minute: Administer every 24 hours

Dialysis: Slightly dialyzable (5% to 20%) via hemo- and peritoneal dialysis nor via continuous arteriovenous or venovenous hemofiltration (CAVH/CAVHD); no supplemental dosage necessary

Dosing adjustment in hepatic impairment: Avoid use or maximum dose is 1 g/day

(Continued)

Tetracycline *(Continued)*

Dosage Forms CAP: 100 mg, 250 mg, 500 mg. **OINT:** Ophth: 1% [10 mg/mL] (3.5 g); Top: 3% [30 mg/mL] (14.2 g, 30 g). **SOLN, top:** 2.2 mg/mL (70 mL). **SUSP:** Ophth: 1% [10 mg/mL] (0.5 mL, 1 mL, 4 mL); Oral: 125 mg/5 mL (60 mL, 480 mL). **TAB:** 250 mg, 500 mg

Contraindications Hypersensitivity to tetracycline or any component; do not administer to children ≤8 years of age

Warnings/Precautions Use of tetracyclines during tooth development may cause permanent discoloration of the teeth and enamel, hypoplasia and retardation of skeletal development and bone growth with risk being the greatest for children <4 years and those receiving high doses; use with caution in patients with renal or hepatic impairment (eg, elderly) and in pregnancy; dosage modification required in patients with renal impairment since it may increase BUN as an antianabolic agent; pseudotumor cerebri has been reported with tetracycline use (usually resolves with discontinuation); outdated drug can cause nephropathy; superinfection possible; use protective measure to avoid photosensitivity

Pregnancy Risk Factor D; B (topical)

Pregnancy Implications Breast-feeding/lactation: Excreted in breast milk; avoid use if possible in lactating mothers

Adverse Reactions

>10%: Gastrointestinal: Discoloration of teeth and enamel hypoplasia (young children)

1% to 10%:

Dermatologic: Photosensitivity

Gastrointestinal: Nausea, diarrhea

<1%: Abdominal cramps, acute renal failure, anaphylaxis, anorexia, antibiotic-associated pseudomembranous colitis, azotemia, bulging fontanels in infants, candidal superinfection, dermatologic effects, diabetes insipidus syndrome, esophagitis, exfoliative dermatitis, hepatotoxicity, hypersensitivity reactions, increased intracranial pressure, paresthesia, pericarditis, pigmentation of nails, pruritus, pseudotumor cerebri, renal damage, staphylococcal enterocolitis, superinfections, thrombophlebitis, vomiting

Drug Interactions

Decreased effect: Calcium, magnesium or aluminum-containing antacids, oral contraceptives, iron, zinc, sodium bicarbonate, penicillins, cimetidine may decrease tetracycline absorption

Although no clinical evidence exists, may bind with bismuth or calcium carbonate, an excipient in bismuth subsalicylate, during treatment for *H. pylori*

Increased toxicity: Methoxyflurane anesthesia when concurrent with tetracycline may cause fatal nephrotoxicity; warfarin with tetracyclines may result in increased anticoagulation; tetracyclines may rarely increase digoxin serum levels

Drug-Herb interactions: Berberine is a chemical extracted from **goldenseal** (*Hydrastis canadensis*), **barberry** (*Berberis vulgaris*), and **Oregon grape** (*Berberis aquifolium*), which has been shown to have antibacterial activity. One double-blind study found that giving berberine concurrently with tetracycline reduced the efficacy of tetracycline in the treatment of cholera. Berberine may decrease absorption of tetracycline. Another double-blind trial did not find that berberine interfered with tetracycline in cholera patients. Until more studies are completed, berberine-containing herbs should not be taken concomitantly with tetracyclines.

Half-Life Normal renal function: 8-11 hours; End-stage renal disease: 57-108 hours

Education and Monitoring Issues

Patient Education: Take this medication exactly as directed. Take all of the prescription even if you see an improvement in your condition. Do not use more or more often than recommended.

Oral: Preferable to take on an empty stomach (1 hour before or 2 hours after meals). Take at regularly scheduled times, around-the-clock. Avoid antacids, iron, or dairy products within 2 hours of taking tetracycline. You may experience photosensitivity (use sunscreen, wear protective clothing and eyewear, avoid direct sunlight); dizziness or lightheadedness (use caution when driving or engaging in tasks requiring alertness until response to drug is known); nausea/vomiting (frequent small meals, frequent mouth care, chewing gum, or sucking lozenges may help). Effect of oral contraceptives may be reduced; use barrier contraception. Report rash or intense itching, yellowing of skin or eyes, fever or chills, blackened stool, vaginal itching or discharge, foul-smelling stools, excessive thirst or urination, acute headache, unresolved diarrhea, difficulty breathing, condition does not improve, or worsening of condition.

Ophthalmic: Sit down, tilt head back, instill solution or drops inside lower eyelid, and roll eyeball in all directions. Close eye and apply gentle pressure to inner corner of eye for 30 seconds. Do not touch tip of applicator to eye or any contaminated surface. May experience temporary stinging or blurred vision. Inform prescriber if condition worsens or does not improve in 3-4 days.

Topical: Wash area and pat dry (unless contraindicated). Avoid getting in mouth or eyes. You may experience temporary stinging or burning which will resolve quickly. Treated skin may turn yellow; this will wash off. May stain clothing (permanent). Report rash. Inform prescriber if condition worsens or does not improve in a few days.

Dietary Considerations: Food: Dairy products decrease effect of tetracycline

Monitoring Parameters: Renal, hepatic, and hematologic function test, temperature, WBC, cultures and sensitivity, appetite, mental status

Related Information

Antimicrobial Drugs of Choice *on page 1182*

Bismuth Subsalicylate, Metronidazole, and Tetracycline *on page 109*

Helicobacter pylori Treatment *on page 1107*

- **Teveten®** *see* Eprosartan *on page 320*
- **Texacort** *see* Hydrocortisone *on page 447*
- **T-Gen®** *see* Trimethobenzamide *on page 953*
- **T-Gesic®** *see* Hydrocodone and Acetaminophen *on page 444*
- **Thalaris** *see* Sodium Chloride *on page 858*

Thalidomide (tha LI doe mide)

Pharmacologic Class Immunosuppressant Agent

U.S. Brand Names Thalomid®

Mechanism of Action A derivative of glutethimide; mode of action for immunosuppression is unclear; inhibition of neutrophil chemotaxis and decreased monocyte phagocytosis may occur; may cause 50% to 80% reduction of tumor necrosis factor - alpha

Use Treatment of erythema nodosum leprosum

Orphan status: Crohn's disease

Investigational: Treatment or prevention of graft-versus-host reactions after bone marrow transplantation; in aphthous ulceration in HIV-positive patients; Langerhans cell histocytosis, Behçet's syndrome; hypnotic agent; also may be effective in rheumatoid arthritis, discoid lupus, and erythema multiforme; useful in type 2 lepra reactions, but not type 1; can assist in healing mouth ulcers in AIDS patients

USUAL DOSAGE

Leprosy: Up to 400 mg/day; usual maintenance dose: 50-100 mg/day

Behçet's syndrome: 100-400 mg/day

Graft-vs-host reactions:

Children: 3 mg/kg 4 times/day

Adults: 100-1600 mg/day; usual initial dose: 200 mg 4 times/day for use up to 700 days

AIDS-related aphthous stomatitis: 200 mg twice daily for 5 days, then 200 mg/day for up to 8 weeks

Discoid lupus erythematosus: 100-400 mg/day; maintenance dose: 25-50 mg

Contraindications Pregnancy or women in childbearing years, neuropathy (peripheral), thalidomide hypersensitivity

Warnings/Precautions Liver, hepatic, neurological disorders, constipation, congestive heart failure, hypertension

Pregnancy Risk Factor X

Pregnancy Implications Embryotoxic with limb defects noted from the 27th to 40th gestational day of exposure; all cases of phocomelia occur from the 27th to 42nd gestational day; fetal cardiac, gastrointestinal, and genitourinary tract abnormalities have also been described

Adverse Reactions Percentage unknown: Alopecia, amenorrhea, clonus, constipation, dizziness, edema, fever, headache, irritability, lethargy, leukopenia, myoclonus, nausea, pruritus, sensory neuropathy (peripheral) (after prolonged therapy due to neuronal degeneration), sexual dysfunction, sinus tachycardia, tachycardia, vomiting, xerostomia

Half-Life 8.7 hours

Education and Monitoring Issues

Patient Education: You will be given oral and written instructions about the necessity of using two methods of contraception and and the necessity of keeping return visits for pregnancy testing. You may experience sleepiness, dizziness, lack of concentration (use caution when driving, climbing stairs, or engaging in tasks requiring alertness until response to drug is known); nausea or vomiting or loss of appetite (small frequent meals, frequent mouth care, chewing gum, or sucking lozenges may help); constipation or diarrhea; oral thrush (frequent mouth care is necessary); sexual dysfunction (reversible). Report any of the above if persistent or severe. Report chest pain or palpitations or swelling of extremities; back, neck, or muscle pain or stiffness; skin rash or eruptions; increased nervousness, anxiety, or insomnia; or any other symptom of adverse reactions.

Reference Range: Therapeutic plasma thalidomide levels in graft-vs-host reactions are 5-8 μg/mL, although it has been suggested that lower plasma levels (0.5-1.5 μg/mL) may be therapeutic; peak serum thalidomide level after a 200 mg dose: 1.2 μg/mL

Manufacturer Celgene Corp

Related Information

Pharmaceutical Manufacturers Directory *on page 1020*

- **Thalitone®** *see* Chlorthalidone *on page 191*
- **Thalomid®** *see* Thalidomide *on page 905*
- **Theo-24®** *see* Theophylline Salts *on page 906*
- **Theobid®** *see* Theophylline Salts *on page 906*

- **Theochron®** *see* Theophylline Salts *on page 906*
- **Theoclear® L.A.** *see* Theophylline Salts *on page 906*
- **Theo-Dur®** *see* Theophylline Salts *on page 906*
- **Theo-Dur® Sprinkle** *see* Theophylline Salts *on page 906*
- **Theolair™** *see* Theophylline Salts *on page 906*
- **Theon®** *see* Theophylline Salts *on page 906*

Theophylline and Guaifenesin (thee OF i lin & gwye FEN e sin)

Pharmacologic Class Theophylline Derivative

U.S. Brand Names Bronchial®; Glycerol-T®; Quibron®; Slo-Phyllin® GG

Dosage Forms CAP: Theophylline 150 mg and guaifenesin 90 mg, theophylline 300 mg and guaifenesin 180 mg. **ELIX:** Theophylline 150 mg and guaifenesin 90 mg per 15 mL (480 mL)

Pregnancy Risk Factor C

Theophylline, Ephedrine, and Hydroxyzine

(thee OF i lin, e FED rin, & hye DROKS i zeen)

Pharmacologic Class Theophylline Derivative

U.S. Brand Names Hydrophed®; Marax®

Dosage Forms SYR (dye free): Theophylline 32.5 mg, ephedrine 6.25 mg, and hydroxyzine 2.5 mg per 5 mL. **TAB:** Theophylline 130 mg, ephedrine 25 mg, and hydroxyzine 10 mg

Pregnancy Risk Factor C

Theophylline, Ephedrine, and Phenobarbital

(thee OF i lin, e FED rin, & fee noe BAR bi tal)

Pharmacologic Class Theophylline Derivative

U.S. Brand Names Tedral®

Dosage Forms SUSP: Theophylline 65 mg, ephedrine sulfate 12 mg, and phenobarbital 4 mg per 5 mL. **TAB:** Theophylline 118 mg, ephedrine sulfate 25 mg, and phenobarbital 11 mg; theophylline 130 mg, ephedrine sulfate 24 mg, and phenobarbital 8 mg

Pregnancy Risk Factor D

Theophylline Salts (thee OFF i lin salts)

Pharmacologic Class Bronchodilator; Theophylline Derivative

U.S. Brand Names Aerolate®; Aerolate III®; Aerolate JR®; Aerolate SR®; Aminophyllin™; Aquaphyllin®; Asmalix®; Bronkodyl®; Choledyl®; Constant-T®; Duraphyl™; Elixophyllin®; Elixophyllin® SR; LaBID®; Phyllocontin®; Quibron®-T; Quibron®-T/SR; Respbid®; Slo-bid™; Slo-Phyllin®; Sustaire®; Theo-24®; Theobid®; Theochron®; Theoclear® L.A.; Theo-Dur®; Theo-Dur® Sprinkle; Theolair™; Theon®; Theospan®-SR; Theovent®; Truphylline®

Generic Available Yes

Mechanism of Action Causes bronchodilatation, diuresis, CNS and cardiac stimulation, and gastric acid secretion by blocking phosphodiesterase which increases tissue concentrations of cyclic adenine monophosphate (cAMP) which in turn promotes catecholamine stimulation of lipolysis, glycogenolysis, and gluconeogenesis and induces release of epinephrine from adrenal medulla cells

Use Bronchodilator in reversible airway obstruction due to asthma, chronic bronchitis, and emphysema; for neonatal apnea/bradycardia

USUAL DOSAGE Use ideal body weight for obese patients

Approximate I.V. Theophylline Dosage for Treatment of Acute Bronchospasm

Group	Dosage for Next 12 h*	Dosage After 12 h*
Infants 6 wk - 6 mo	0.5 mg/kg/h	
Children 6 mo - 1 y	0.6-0.7 mg/kg/h	
Children 1-9 y	0.95 mg/kg/h (1.2 mg/kg/h)	0.79 mg/kg/h (1 mg/kg/h)
Children 9-16 y and young adult smokers	0.79 mg/kg/h (1 mg/kg/h)	0.63 mg/kg/h (0.8 mg/kg/h)
Healthy, nonsmoking adults	0.55 mg/kg/h (0.7 mg/kg/h)	0.39 mg/kg/h (0.5 mg/kg/h)
Older patients and patients with cor pulmonale	0.47 mg/kg/h (0.6 mg/kg/h)	0.24 mg/kg/h (0.3 mg/kg/h)
Patients with congestive heart failure or liver failure	0.39 mg/kg/h (0.5 mg/kg/h)	0.08-0.16 mg/kg/h (0.1-0.2 mg/kg/h)

*Equivalent hydrous aminophylline dosage indicated in parentheses.

Neonates:

Apnea of prematurity: Oral, I.V.: Loading dose: 4 mg/kg (theophylline); 5 mg/kg (aminophylline)

There appears to be a delay in theophylline elimination in infants <1 year of age, especially neonates; both the initial dose and maintenance dosage should be conservative

I.V.: Initial: Maintenance infusion rates:

Neonates:

≤24 days: 0.08 mg/kg/hour theophylline

>24 days: 0.12 mg/kg/hour theophylline

Infants 6-52 weeks: 0.008 (age in weeks) + 0.21 mg/kg/hour theophylline

Children >1 year and Adults:

Treatment of acute bronchospasm: I.V.: Loading dose (in patients not currently receiving aminophylline or theophylline): 6 mg/kg (based on aminophylline) given I.V. over 20-30 minutes; administration rate should not exceed 25 mg/minute (aminophylline). See table on previous page

Approximate I.V. maintenance dosages are based upon continuous infusions; bolus dosing (often used in children <6 months of age) may be determined by multiplying the hourly infusion rate by 24 hours and dividing by the desired number of doses/day; see table.

Maintenance Dose for Acute Symptoms

Population Group	Oral Theophylline (mg/kg/day)	I.V. Aminophylline
Premature infant or newborn - 6 wk (for apnea/bradycardia)	4	5 mg/kg/day
6 wk - 6 mo	10	12 mg/kg/day or continuous I.V. infusion*
Infants 6 mo - 1 y	12-18	15 mg/kg/day or continuous I.V. infusion*
Children 1-9 y	20-24	1 mg/kg/h
Children 9-12 y, and adolescent daily smokers of cigarettes or marijuana, and otherwise healthy adult smokers <50 y	16	0.9 mg/kg/h
Adolescents 12-16 y (nonsmokers)	13	0.7 mg/kg/h
Otherwise healthy nonsmoking adults (including elderly patients)	10 (not to exceed 900 mg/day)	0.5 mg/kg/h
Cardiac decompensation, cor pulmonale and/or liver dysfunction	5 (not to exceed 400 mg/day)	0.25 mg/kg/h

*For continuous I.V. infusion divide total daily dose by 24 = mg/kg/h.

Dosage should be adjusted according to serum level measurements during the first 12- to 24-hour period; see table.

Dosage Adjustment After Serum Theophylline Measurement

Serum Theophylline		Guidelines
Within normal limits	10-20 mcg/mL	Maintain dosage if tolerated. Recheck serum theophylline concentration at 6- to 12-month intervals.*
Too high	20-25 mcg/mL	Decrease doses by about 10%. Recheck serum theophylline concentration after 3 days and then at 6- to 12-month intervals.*
	25-30 mcg/mL	Skip next dose and decrease subsequent doses by about 25%. Recheck serum theophylline.
	>30 mcg/mL	Skip next 2 doses and decrease subsequent doses by 50%. Recheck serum theophylline.
Too low	7.5-10 mcg/mL	Increase dose by about 25%.† Recheck serum theophylline concentration after 3 days and then at 6- to 12-month intervals.*
	5-7.5 mcg/mL	Increase dose by about 25% to the nearest dose increment† and recheck serum theophylline for guidance in further dosage adjustment (another increase will probably be needed, but this provides a safety check).

*Finer adjustments in dosage may be needed for some patients.

†Dividing the daily dose into 3 doses administered at 8-hour intervals may be indicated if symptoms occur repeatedly at the end of a dosing interval.

From Weinberger M and Hendeles L, "Practical Guide to UsingTheophylline," *J Resp Dis*, 1981,2:12-27.

(Continued)

Theophylline Salts *(Continued)*

Oral theophylline: Initial dosage recommendation: Loading dose (to achieve a serum level of about 10 mcg/mL; loading doses should be given using a rapidly absorbed oral product **not** a sustained release product):

If no theophylline has been administered in the previous 24 hours: 4-6 mg/kg theophylline

If theophylline has been administered in the previous 24 hours: administer ½ loading dose or 2-3 mg/kg theophylline can be given in emergencies when serum levels are not available

On the average, for every 1 mg/kg theophylline given, blood levels will rise 2 mcg/mL

Ideally, defer the loading dose if a serum theophylline concentration can be obtained rapidly. However, if this is not possible, exercise clinical judgment. If the patient is not experiencing theophylline toxicity, this is unlikely to result in dangerous adverse effects.

See table.

Oral Theophylline Dosage for Bronchial Asthma*

Age	Initial 3 Days	Second 3 Days	Steady-State Maintenance
<1 y	0.2 x (age in weeks) + 5		0.3 x (age in weeks) + 8
1-9 y	16 up to a maximum of 400 mg/24 h	20	22
9-12 y	16 up to a maximum of 400 mg/24 h	16 up to a maximum of 600 mg/24 h	20 up to a maximum of 800 mg/24 h
12-16 y	16 up to a maximum of 400 mg/24 h	16 up to a maximum of 600 mg/24 h	18 up to a maximum of 900 mg/24 h
Adults	400 mg/24 h	600 mg/24 h	900 mg/24 h

*Dose in mg/kg/24 hours of theophylline.

Increasing dose: The dosage may be increased in approximately 25% increments at 2- to 3-day intervals so long as the drug is tolerated or until the maximum dose is reached

Maintenance dose: In newborns and infants, a fast-release oral product can be used. The total daily dose can be divided every 12 hours in newborns and every 6-8 hours in infants. In children and healthy adults, a slow-release product can be used. The total daily dose can be divided every 8-12 hours.

These recommendations, based on mean clearance rates for age or risk factors, were calculated to achieve a serum level of 10 mcg/mL (5 mcg/mL for newborns with apnea/bradycardia)

Dosage should be adjusted according to serum level

Oral oxtriphylline:

Children 1-9 years: 6.2 mg/kg/dose every 6 hours

Children 9-16 years and Adult smokers: 4.7 mg/kg/dose every 6 hours

Adult nonsmokers: 4.7 mg/kg/dose every 8 hours

Dose should be further adjusted based on serum levels

Dosing adjustment/comments in hepatic disease: Higher incidence of toxic effects including seizures in cirrhosis; plasma levels should be monitored closely during long-term administration in cirrhosis and during acute hepatitis, with dose adjustment as necessary

Hemodialysis: Administer dose posthemodialysis or administer supplemental 50% dose

Peritoneal dialysis: Supplemental dose is not necessary

Continuous arteriovenous or venovenous hemodiafiltration (CAVH/CAVHD) effects: Supplemental dose is not necessary

Dosage Forms

Aminophylline (79% theophylline): **INJ:** 25 mg/mL (10 mL, 20 mL); 250 mg (equivalent to 187 mg theophylline) per 10 mL, 500 mg (equivalent to 394 mg theophylline) per 20 mL. **LIQ, oral:** 105 mg (equivalent to 90 mg theophylline) per 5 mL (240 mL, 500 mL). **SUPP, rectal:** 250 mg (equivalent to 198 mg theophylline), 500 mg (equivalent to 395 mg theophylline). **TAB:** 100 mg (equivalent to 79 mg theophylline), 200 mg (equivalent to 158 mg theophylline); Cont release: 225 mg (equivalent to 178 mg theophylline)

Oxtriphylline (64% theophylline): **ELIX:** 100 mg (equivalent to 64 mg theophylline)/5 mL (5 mL, 10 mL, 473 mL). **SYR:** 50 mg (equivalent to 32 mg theophylline)/5 mL (473 mL). **TAB:** 100 mg (equivalent to 64 mg theophylline); 200 mg (equivalent to 127 mg theophylline); Sustained release: 400 mg (equivalent to 254 mg theophylline); 600 mg (equivalent to 382 mg theophylline)

Theophylline: **CAP:** Immediate release: 100 mg, 200 mg; Sustained release (8-12 hours): 50 mg, 60 mg, 65 mg, 75 mg, 100 mg, 125 mg, 130 mg, 200 mg, 250 mg, 260 mg, 300 mg; Timed release (12 hours): 50 mg, 75 mg, 125 mg, 130 mg, 200 mg, 250 mg, 260 mg; Timed release (24 hours): 100 mg, 200 mg, 300 mg. **INJ:** Theophylline in 5% dextrose: 200 mg/container (50 mL, 100 mL), 400 mg/container (100 mL, 250 mL, 500 mL, 1000 mL), 800 mg/container (250 mL, 500 mL, 1000 mL). **ELIX, oral:** 80 mg/15 mL (15 mL, 30 mL, 500 mL, 4000 mL). **SOLN, oral:** 80 mg/15 mL (15 mL, 18.75 mL, 30 mL, 120 mL, 500 mL, 4000 mL), 150 mg/15 mL (480 mL). **SYR, oral:** 80 mg/15 mL (5 mL, 15 mL, 30 mL, 120 mL, 500 mL, 4000 mL), 150 mg/15 mL (480 mL). **TAB:** Immediate release: 100 mg, 125 mg, 200 mg, 250 mg, 300 mg; Timed release (8-12 hours): 100 mg, 200 mg, 250 mg, 300 mg, 500 mg; Timed release (8-24 hours): 100 mg, 200 mg, 300 mg, 450 mg; Timed release (12-24 hours): 100 mg, 200 mg, 300 mg; Timed release (24 hours): 400 mg

Contraindications Uncontrolled arrhythmias, hyperthyroidism, peptic ulcers, uncontrolled seizure disorders, hypersensitivity to xanthines or any component

Warnings/Precautions Use with caution in patients with peptic ulcer, hyperthyroidism, hypertension, tachyarrhythmias, and patients with compromised cardiac function; do not inject I.V. solution faster than 25 mg/minute; elderly, acutely ill, and patients with severe respiratory problems, pulmonary edema, or liver dysfunction are at greater risk of toxicity because of reduced drug clearance

Although there is a great intersubject variability for half-lives of methylxanthines (2-10 hours), elderly as a group have slower hepatic clearance. Therefore, use lower initial doses and monitor closely for response and adverse reactions. Additionally, elderly are at greater risk for toxicity due to concomitant disease (eg, CHF, arrhythmias), and drug use (eg, cimetidine, ciprofloxacin, etc).

Pregnancy Risk Factor C

Pregnancy Implications

Clinical effects on the fetus: Crosses the placenta. Transient tachycardia, irritability, vomiting in newborn especially if maternal serum concentrations >20 mcg/mL. Apneic spells attributed to withdrawal in newborn exposed throughout gestation period. Available evidence suggests safe use during pregnancy.

Breast-feeding/lactation: Crosses into breast milk

Clinical effects on the infant: Irritability reported in infants. American Academy of Pediatrics considers **compatible** with breast-feeding.

Adverse Reactions See table.

Theophylline Serum Levels (mcg/mL)*	Adverse Reactions
15-25	GI upset, diarrhea, N/V, abdominal pain, nervousness, headache, insomnia, agitation, dizziness, muscle cramp, tremor
25-35	Tachycardia, occasional PVC
>35	Ventricular tachycardia, frequent PVC, seizure

*Adverse effects do not necessarily occur according to serum levels. Arrhythmia and seizure can occur without seeing the other adverse effects.

Uncommon at serum theophylline concentrations ≤20 mcg/mL

1% to 10%:
- Cardiovascular: Tachycardia
- Central nervous system: Nervousness, restlessness
- Gastrointestinal: Nausea, vomiting

<1%: Allergic reactions, gastric irritation, insomnia, irritability, rash, seizures, tremor

Drug Interactions CYP1A2 and 3A3/4 enzyme substrate, CYP2E enzyme substrate (minor)

Decreased effect/increased toxicity: Changes in diet may affect the elimination of theophylline; charcoal-broiled foods may increase elimination, reducing half-life by 50%; see table for factors affecting serum levels.

Drug-Herb interactions: St John's wort (hypericum) can induce CYP1A2 enzymes and as a result may explain why theophylline serum levels have decreased when given concurrently. Theophylline dosages may need to be increased in patients concurrently receiving theophylline and St John's wort to retain theophylline's clinical efficacy.

Onset Oral: 1-2 hours; I.V.: <30 minutes

Half-Life Variable; dependent on age, liver function, cardiac function, lung disease, and smoking history; range: 4-30 hours

Education and Monitoring Issues

Patient Education: Oral preparations should be taken with a full glass of water; capsule forms may be opened and sprinkled on soft foods; do not chew beads; notify prescriber if nausea, vomiting, severe GI pain, restlessness, or irregular heartbeat occurs; do not drink or eat large quantities of caffeine-containing beverages or food (colas, coffee, chocolate); remain in bed for 15-20 minutes after inserting suppository; do not chew or crush enteric coated or sustained release products; take at regular intervals; notify prescriber if insomnia, nervousness, irritability, palpitations, seizures occur; do not change brands or doses without consulting prescriber

Monitoring Parameters: Heart rate, CNS effects (insomnia, irritability); respiratory rate (COPD patients often have resting controlled respiratory rates in low 20s), serum theophylline level, arterial or capillary blood gases (if applicable)

(Continued)

Theophylline Salts *(Continued)*

Factors Reported to Affect Theophylline Serum Levels

Decreased Theophylline Level	Increased Theophylline Level
Aminoglutethimide	Allopurinol (>600 mg/d)
Barbiturates	Beta-blockers
Carbamazepine	Calcium channel blockers
Charcoal	Carbamazepine
High protein/low carbohydrate diet	CHF
Hydantoins	Cimetidine
Hypericum (St John's wort)	Ciprofloxacin
Isoniazid	Cor pulmonale
I.V. isoproterenol	Corticosteroids
Ketoconazole	Disulfiram
Loop diuretics	Ephedrine
Phenobarbital	Erythromycin
Phenytoin	Fever/viral illness
Rifampin	Hepatic cirrhosis
Smoking (cigarettes, marijuana)	Influenza virus vaccine
Sulfinpyrazone	Interferon
Sympathomimetics	Isoniazid
	Loop diuretics
	Macrolides
	Mexiletine
	Oral contraceptives
	Propranolol
	Quinolones
	Thiabendazole
	Thyroid hormones
	Troleandomycin

Reference Range:

Sample size: 0.5-1 mL serum (red top tube)
Saliva levels are approximately equal to 60% of plasma levels

Therapeutic levels: 10-20 μg/mL
Neonatal apnea 6-13 μg/mL
Pregnancy: 3-12 μg/mL
Toxic concentration: >20 μg/mL

Timing of serum samples: If toxicity is suspected, draw a level any time during a continuous I.V. infusion, or 2 hours after an oral dose; if lack of therapeutic is effected, draw a trough immediately before the next oral dose; see table.

Guidelines for Drawing Theophylline Serum Levels

Dosage Form	Time to Draw Level
I.V. bolus	30 min after end of 30 min infusion
I.V. continuous infusion	12-24 h after initiation of infusion
P.O. liquid, fast-release tab	Peak: 1 h postdose after at least 1 day of therapy Trough: Just before a dose after at least one day of therapy
P.O. slow-release product	Peak: 4 h postdose after at least 1 day of therapy Trough: Just before a dose after at least one day of therapy

Related Information

Theophylline and Guaifenesin *on page 906*
Theophylline, Ephedrine, and Hydroxyzine *on page 906*
Theophylline, Ephedrine, and Phenobarbital *on page 906*

- **Theospan®-SR** *see* Theophylline Salts *on page 906*
- **Theovent®** *see* Theophylline Salts *on page 906*
- **Therabid® [OTC]** *see* Vitamins, Multiple *on page 981*
- **Thera-Flur®** *see* Fluoride *on page 376*
- **Thera-Flur-N®** *see* Fluoride *on page 376*
- **Theragran® [OTC]** *see* Vitamins, Multiple *on page 981*
- **Theragran® Hematinic®** *see* Vitamins, Multiple *on page 981*
- **Theragran® Liquid [OTC]** *see* Vitamins, Multiple *on page 981*
- **Theragran-M® [OTC]** *see* Vitamins, Multiple *on page 981*
- **Thermazene®** *see* Silver Sulfadiazine *on page 852*

Thiabendazole (thye a BEN da zole)

Pharmacologic Class Anthelmintic
U.S. Brand Names Mintezol®

Generic Available No

Mechanism of Action Inhibits helminth-specific mitochondrial fumarate reductase

Use Treatment of strongyloidiasis, cutaneous larva migrans, visceral larva migrans, dracunculiasis, trichinosis, and mixed helminthic infections

USUAL DOSAGE Purgation is not required prior to use; drinking of fruit juice aids in expulsion of worms by removing the mucous to which the intestinal tapeworms attach themselves.

Children and Adults: Oral: 50 mg/kg/day divided every 12 hours (if >68 kg: 1.5 g/dose); maximum dose: 3 g/day
- Strongyloidiasis, ascariasis, uncinariasis, trichuriasis: For 2 consecutive days
- Cutaneous larva migrans: For 2-5 consecutive days
- Visceral larva migrans: For 5-7 consecutive days
- Trichinosis: For 2-4 consecutive days
- Dracunculosis: 50-75 mg/kg/day divided every 12 hours for 3 days

Dosing comments in renal/hepatic impairment: Use with caution

Dosage Forms SUSP, oral: 500 mg/5 mL (120 mL). **TAB, chewable** (orange flavor): 500 mg

Contraindications Known hypersensitivity to thiabendazole

Warnings/Precautions Use with caution in patients with renal or hepatic impairment, malnutrition or anemia, or dehydration

Pregnancy Risk Factor C

Adverse Reactions

>10%:
- Central nervous system: Seizures, hallucinations, delirium, dizziness, drowsiness, headache
- Gastrointestinal: Anorexia, diarrhea, nausea, vomiting, drying of mucous membranes
- Neuromuscular & skeletal: Numbness
- Otic: Tinnitus

1% to 10%: Dermatologic: Rash, Stevens-Johnson syndrome

<1%: Blurred or yellow vision, chills, hepatotoxicity, hypersensitivity reactions, leukopenia, lymphadenopathy, malodor of urine, nephrotoxicity

Drug Interactions Increased levels of theophylline and other xanthines

Half-Life 1.2 hours

Education and Monitoring Issues

Patient Education: Take exactly as directed for full course of medication. Tablets may be chewed, swallowed whole, or crushed and mixed with food. Increase dietary intake of fruit juices. All family members and close friends should also be treated. To reduce possibility of reinfection, wash hands and scrub nails carefully with soap and hot water before handling food, before eating, and before and after toileting. Keep hands out of mouth. Disinfect toilet daily and launder bed lines, undergarments, and nightclothes daily with hot water and soap. Do not go barefoot and do not sit directly on grass or ground. May cause dizziness, fainting, lightheadedness (use caution when driving or engaging in tasks requiring alertness until response to drug is known); abdominal pain, nausea, dry mouth, or vomiting (frequent small meals, frequent mouth care, sucking lozenges, or chewing gum may help). Report skin rash or itching, unresolved diarrhea or vomiting, CNS changes (hallucinations, delirium, acute headache), change in color of urine or stool, or easy bruising or unusual bleeding.

♦ **Thiamilate®** *see* Thiamine *on page 911*

Thiamine (THYE a min)

Pharmacologic Class Vitamin, Water Soluble

U.S. Brand Names Thiamilate®

Generic Available Yes

Mechanism of Action An essential coenzyme in carbohydrate metabolism by combining with adenosine triphosphate to form thiamine pyrophosphate

Use Treatment of thiamine deficiency including beriberi, Wernicke's encephalopathy syndrome, and peripheral neuritis associated with pellagra, alcoholic patients with altered sensorium; various genetic metabolic disorders

USUAL DOSAGE

Recommended daily allowance:
- <6 months: 0.3 mg
- 6 months to 1 year: 0.4 mg
- 1-3 years: 0.7 mg
- 4-6 years: 0.9 mg
- 7-10 years: 1 mg
- 11-14 years: 1.1-1.3 mg
- >14 years: 1-1.5 mg

Thiamine deficiency (beriberi):
- Children: 10-25 mg/dose I.M. or I.V. daily (if critically ill), or 10-50 mg/dose orally every day for 2 weeks, then 5-10 mg/dose orally daily for 1 month
- Adults: 5-30 mg/dose I.M. or I.V. 3 times/day (if critically ill); then orally 5-30 mg/day in single or divided doses 3 times/day for 1 month

(Continued)

Thiamine *(Continued)*

Wernicke's encephalopathy: Adults: Initial: 100 mg I.V., then 50-100 mg/day I.M. or I.V. until consuming a regular, balanced diet

Dietary supplement (depends on caloric or carbohydrate content of the diet):

Infants: 0.3-0.5 mg/day

Children: 0.5-1 mg/day

Adults: 1-2 mg/day

Note: The above doses can be found in multivitamin preparations

Metabolic disorders: Oral: Adults: 10-20 mg/day (dosages up to 4 g/day in divided doses have been used)

Dosage Forms INJ: 100 mg/mL (1 mL, 2 mL, 10 mL, 30 mL); 200 mg/mL (30 mL). **TAB:** 50 mg, 100 mg, 250 mg, 500 mg; Enteric coated: 20 mg

Contraindications Hypersensitivity to thiamine or any component

Warnings/Precautions Use with caution with parenteral route (especially I.V.) of administration

Pregnancy Risk Factor A; C (if dose exceeds RDA recommendation)

Adverse Reactions <1%: Angioedema, cardiovascular collapse and death, paresthesia, rash, warmth

Education and Monitoring Issues

Patient Education: Take exactly as directed; do not discontinue without consulting prescriber (deficiency state can occur in as little as 3 weeks). Follow dietary instructions (dietary sources include legumes, pork, beef, whole grains, yeast, fresh vegetables).

Reference Range: Therapeutic: 1.6-4 mg/dL

Thiethylperazine (thye eth il PER a zeen)

Pharmacologic Class Phenothiazine Derivative

U.S. Brand Names Norzine®; Torecan®

Generic Available No

Mechanism of Action Blocks postsynaptic mesolimbic dopaminergic receptors in the brain; exhibits a strong alpha-adrenergic blocking effect and depresses the release of hypothalamic and hypophyseal hormones; acts directly on chemoreceptor trigger zone and vomiting center

Use Relief of nausea and vomiting

Unlabeled use: Treatment of vertigo

USUAL DOSAGE Children >12 years and Adults:

Oral, I.M., rectal: 10 mg 1-3 times/day as needed

I.V. and S.C. routes of administration are not recommended

Hemodialysis: Not dialyzable (0% to 5%)

Dosing comments in hepatic impairment: Use with caution

Dosage Forms INJ: 5 mg/mL (2 mL). **SUPP, rectal:** 10 mg. **TAB:** 10 mg

Contraindications Comatose states, hypersensitivity to thiethylperazine or any component; pregnancy, cross-sensitivity to other phenothiazines may exist

Warnings/Precautions Reduce or discontinue if extrapyramidal effects occur; safety and efficacy in children <12 years of age have not been established; postural hypotension may occur after I.M. injection; the injectable form contains sulfite which may cause allergic reactions in some patients; use caution in patients with narrow-angle glaucoma

Pregnancy Risk Factor X

Adverse Reactions

>10%:

Central nervous system: Drowsiness, dizziness

Gastrointestinal: Xerostomia

Respiratory: Dry nose

1% to 10%:

Cardiovascular: Tachycardia, orthostatic hypotension

Central nervous system: Confusion, convulsions, extrapyramidal effects, tardive dyskinesia, fever, headache

Hematologic: Agranulocytosis

Hepatic: Cholestatic jaundice

Otic: Tinnitus

Drug Interactions Increased effect/toxicity with CNS depressants (eg, anesthetics, opiates, tranquilizers, alcohol), lithium, atropine, epinephrine, MAO inhibitors, TCAs

Onset Onset of antiemetic effect: Within 30 minutes

Duration ~4 hours

Education and Monitoring Issues

Patient Education: May cause drowsiness, impair judgment and coordination; may cause photosensitivity; avoid excessive sunlight; notify prescriber of involuntary movements or feelings of restlessness

Thioridazine (thye oh RID a zeen)

Pharmacologic Class Antipsychotic Agent, Phenothazine, Piperidine

U.S. Brand Names Mellaril®; Mellaril-S®

Generic Available Yes

Mechanism of Action Blocks postsynaptic mesolimbic dopaminergic receptors in the brain; exhibits a strong alpha-adrenergic blocking effect and depresses the release of hypothalamic and hypophyseal hormones

Use Management of manifestations of psychotic disorders; depressive neurosis; alcohol withdrawal; dementia in elderly; behavioral problems in children

USUAL DOSAGE Oral:

Children >2 years: Range: 0.5-3 mg/kg/day in 2-3 divided doses; usual: 1 mg/kg/day; maximum: 3 mg/kg/day

Behavior problems: Initial: 10 mg 2-3 times/day, increase gradually

Severe psychoses: Initial: 25 mg 2-3 times/day, increase gradually

Adults:

Psychoses: Initial: 50-100 mg 3 times/day with gradual increments as needed and tolerated; maximum: 800 mg/day in 2-4 divided doses; if >65 years, initial dose: 10 mg 3 times/day

Depressive disorders, dementia: Initial: 25 mg 3 times/day; maintenance dose: 20-200 mg/day

Hemodialysis: Not dialyzable (0% to 5%)

Dosage Forms CONC, oral: 30 mg/mL (120 mL); 100 mg/mL (3.4 mL, 120 mL). **SUSP, oral:** 25 mg/5 mL (480 mL); 100 mg/5 mL (480 mL). **TAB:** 10 mg, 15 mg, 25 mg, 50 mg, 100 mg, 150 mg, 200 mg

Contraindications Severe CNS depression, hypersensitivity to thioridazine or any component; cross-sensitivity to other phenothiazines may exist

Warnings/Precautions Oral formulations may cause stomach upset; may cause thermoregulatory changes; use caution in patients with narrow-angle glaucoma, severe liver or cardiac disease; doses of 1 g/day frequently cause pigmentary retinopathy

Pregnancy Risk Factor C

Adverse Reactions

Cardiovascular: Hypotension, orthostatic hypotension, peripheral edema, EKG changes

Central nervous system: EPS (pseudoparkinsonism, akathisia, dystonias, tardive dyskinesia), dizziness, drowsiness, neuroleptic malignant syndrome (NMS), impairment of temperature regulation, lowering of seizures threshold

Dermatologic: Increased sensitivity to sun, rash, discoloration of skin (blue-gray)

Endocrine & metabolic: Changes in menstrual cycle, changes in libido, breast pain, galactorrhea, amenorrhea

Gastrointestinal: Constipation, weight gain, nausea, vomiting, stomach pain, xerostomia, nausea, vomiting, diarrhea

Genitourinary: Difficulty in urination, ejaculatory disturbances, urinary retention, priapism

Hematologic: Agranulocytosis, leukopenia

Hepatic: Cholestatic jaundice, hepatotoxicity

Neuromuscular & skeletal: Tremor

Ocular: Pigmentary retinopathy, blurred vision, cornea and lens changes

Respiratory: Nasal congestion

Drug Interactions CYP1A2 and 2D6 enzyme substrate; CYP2D6 enzyme inhibitor

Phenothiazines inhibit the ability of bromocriptine to lower serum prolactin concentrations

Benztropine (and other anticholinergics) may inhibit the therapeutic response to thioridazine and excess anticholinergic effects may occur

Chloroquine may increase thioridazine concentrations

Cigarette smoking may enhance the hepatic metabolism of thioridazine. Larger doses may be required compared to a nonsmoker.

Concurrent use of thioridazine with an antihypertensive may produce additive hypotensive effects

Antihypertensive effects of guanethidine and guanadrel may be inhibited by thioridazine

Concurrent use with TCA may produce increased toxicity or altered therapeutic response

Thioridazine may inhibit the antiparkinsonian effect of levodopa; avoid this combination

Thioridazine plus lithium may rarely produce neurotoxicity

Barbiturates may reduce thioridazine concentrations

Propranolol may increase thioridazine concentrations

Sulfadoxine-pyrimethamine may increase thioridazine concentrations

Thioridazine and possibly other low potency antipsychotics may reverse the pressor effects of epinephrine

Thioridazine and CNS depressants (ethanol, narcotics) may produce additive CNS depressant effects

Thioridazine and trazodone may produce additive hypotensive effects

Phenylpropanolamine in combination with thioridazine may result in cardiac arrhythmias; monitor

Naltrexone in combination with thioridazine has been reported to cause lethargy and somnolence

Alcohol Interactions Avoid use (may increase central nervous system depression)

Duration 4-5 days

Half-Life 21-25 hours

Education and Monitoring Issues

Patient Education: Use exactly as directed (do not increase dose or frequency); may cause physical and/or psychological dependence. Do not discontinue without

(Continued)

Thioridazine *(Continued)*

consulting prescriber. Tablets/capsules may be taken with food. Mix oral solution with 2-4 ounces of liquid (eg, juice, milk, water, pudding). Do not take within 2 hours of any antacid. Store away from light. Avoid excess alcohol or caffeine and other prescription or OTC medications not approved by prescriber. Maintain adequate hydration (2-3 L/day of fluids unless instructed to restrict fluid intake). Avoid skin contact with liquid medication; may cause contact dermatitis (wash immediately with warm, soapy water). May turn urine red-brown (normal). You may experience excess drowsiness, lightheadedness, dizziness, or blurred vision (use caution driving or when engaging in tasks requiring alertness until response to drug is known); nausea, vomiting, or dry mouth (small frequent meals, frequent mouth care, chewing gum, or sucking lozenges may help); constipation (increased exercise, fluids, or dietary fruit and fiber may help); postural hypotension (use caution climbing stairs or when changing position from lying or sitting to standing); urinary retention (void before taking medication); ejaculatory dysfunction (reversible); decreased perspiration (avoid strenuous exercise in hot environments); photosensitivity (use sunscreen, wear protective clothing and eyewear, avoid direct sunlight). Report persistent CNS effects (eg, trembling fingers, altered gait or balance, excessive sedation, seizures, unusual movements, anxiety, abnormal thoughts, confusion, personality changes); chest pain, palpitations, rapid heartbeat, severe dizziness; unresolved urinary retention or changes in urinary pattern; altered menstrual pattern, change in libido, swelling or pain in breasts (male or female); vision changes; skin rash, irritation, or changes in color of skin (gray-blue); or worsening of condition.

Monitoring Parameters: For patients on prolonged therapy: CBC, ophthalmologic exam, blood pressure, liver function tests

Reference Range: Therapeutic: 1.0-1.5 μg/mL (SI: 2.7-4.1 μmol/L); Toxic: >10 μg/mL (SI: >27 μmol/L)

Thiothixene (thye oh THIKS een)

Pharmacologic Class Antipsychotic Agent, Thioxanthene Derivative

U.S. Brand Names Navane®

Generic Available Yes

Mechanism of Action Elicits antipsychotic activity by postsynaptic blockade of CNS dopamine receptors resulting in inhibition of dopamine-mediated effects; also has alpha-adrenergic blocking activity

Use Management of psychotic disorders

USUAL DOSAGE

Children <12 years: Oral: 0.25 mg/kg/24 hours in divided doses (dose not well established)

Children >12 years and Adults: Mild to moderate psychosis:

Oral: 2 mg 3 times/day, up to 20-30 mg/day; more severe psychosis: Initial: 5 mg 2 times/day, may increase gradually, if necessary; maximum: 60 mg/day

I.M.: 4 mg 2-4 times/day, increase dose gradually; usual: 16-20 mg/day; maximum: 30 mg/day; change to oral dose as soon as able

Hemodialysis: Not dialyzable (0% to 5%)

Dosage Forms CAP: 1 mg, 2 mg, 5 mg, 10 mg, 20 mg. **POWDER, for inj:** 5 mg/mL (2 mL)

Contraindications Hypersensitivity to thiothixene or any component; cross-sensitivity with other phenothiazines may exist, lactation

Warnings/Precautions Watch for hypotension when administering I.M. or I.V.; safety in children <6 months of age has not been established; use with caution in patients with narrow-angle glaucoma, bone marrow suppression, severe liver or cardiac disease, seizures

Pregnancy Risk Factor C

Adverse Reactions

Cardiovascular: Hypotension, tachycardia, syncope, nonspecific EKG changes

Central nervous system: Extrapyramidal signs (pseudoparkinsonism, akathisia, dystonias, lightheadedness, tardive dyskinesia), dizziness, drowsiness, restlessness, agitation, insomnia

Dermatologic: Discoloration of skin (blue-gray), rash, pruritus, urticaria, photosensitivity

Endocrine & metabolic: Changes in menstrual cycle, changes in libido, breast pain, galactorrhea, lactation, amenorrhea, gynecomastia, hyperglycemia, hypoglycemia

Gastrointestinal: Weight gain, nausea, vomiting, stomach pain, constipation, xerostomia, increased salivation

Genitourinary: Difficulty in urination, ejaculatory disturbances, impotence

Hematologic: Leukopenia, leukocytes

Neuromuscular & skeletal: Tremors

Ocular: Pigmentary retinopathy, blurred vision

Respiratory: Nasal congestion

Miscellaneous: Diaphoresis

Drug Interactions CYP1A2 enzyme substrate

Antipsychotics inhibit the ability of bromocriptine to lower serum prolactin concentrations

Benztropine (and other anticholinergics) may inhibit the therapeutic response to thiothixene and excess anticholinergic effects may occur

Chloroquine may increase thiothixene concentrations
Cigarette smoking may enhance the hepatic metabolism of thiothixene. Larger doses may be required compared to a nonsmoker.
Concurrent use of thiothixene with an antihypertensive may produce additive hypotensive effects
Antihypertensive effects of guanethidine and guanadrel may be inhibited by thiothixene
Concurrent use with TCA may produce increased toxicity or altered therapeutic response
Thiothixene may inhibit the antiparkinsonian effect of levodopa; avoid this combination
Thiothixene plus lithium may rarely produce neurotoxicity
Barbiturates may reduce thiothixene concentrations
Propranolol may increase thiothixene concentrations
Sulfadoxine-pyrimethamine may increase thiothixene concentrations
Thiothixene and low potency antipsychotics may reverse the pressor effects of epinephrine
Thiothixene and CNS depressants (ethanol, narcotics) may produce additive CNS depressant effects
Thiothixene and trazodone may produce additive hypotensive effects

Alcohol Interactions Avoid use (may increase central nervous system depression)

Half-Life >24 hours with chronic use

Education and Monitoring Issues

Patient Education: Use exactly as directed (do not increase dose or frequency); may cause physical and/or psychological dependence. Do not discontinue without consulting prescriber. Tablets/capsules may be taken with food. Mix oral solution with 2-4 ounces of liquid (eg, juice, milk, water, pudding). Do not take within 2 hours of any antacid. Avoid excess alcohol or caffeine and other prescription or OTC medications not approved by prescriber. Maintain adequate hydration (2-3 L/day of fluids unless instructed to restrict fluid intake). May turn urine red-brown (normal). You may experience excess drowsiness, lightheadedness, dizziness, or blurred vision (use caution driving or when engaging in tasks requiring alertness until response to drug is known); nausea or vomiting (small frequent meals, frequent mouth care, chewing gum, or sucking lozenges may help); constipation (increased exercise, fluids, or dietary fruit and fiber may help); postural hypotension (use caution climbing stairs or when changing position from lying or sitting to standing); urinary retention (void before taking medication); ejaculatory dysfunction (reversible); decreased perspiration (avoid strenuous exercise in hot environments); photosensitivity (use sunscreen, wear protective clothing and eyewear, avoid direct sunlight). Report persistent CNS effects (eg, trembling fingers, altered gait or balance, excessive sedation, seizures, unusual movements, anxiety, abnormal thoughts, confusion, personality changes); chest pain, palpitations, rapid heartbeat, severe dizziness; unresolved urinary retention or changes in urinary pattern; altered menstrual pattern, change in libido, swelling or pain in breasts (male or female); vision changes; skin rash, irritation, or changes in color of skin (gray-blue); or worsening of condition.

Monitoring Parameters: Liver function tests; for patients on prolonged therapy: CBC, ophthalmologic exam

♦ **Thorazine®** *see* Chlorpromazine *on page 187*
♦ **Thromboject** *see* Sodium Tetradecyl *on page 861*
♦ **Thymoglobulin®** *see* Antithymocyte Globulin (Rabbit) *on page 67*
♦ **Thyrar®** *see* Thyroid *on page 915*
♦ **Thyro-Block®** *see* Potassium Iodide *on page 754*
♦ **Thyrogen®** *see* Thyrotropin Alpha *on page 916*

Thyroid (THYE royd)

Pharmacologic Class Thyroid Product

U.S. Brand Names Armour® Thyroid; S-P-T; Thyrar®; Thyroid Strong®

Use Replacement or supplemental therapy in hypothyroidism; pituitary TSH suppressants (thyroid nodules, thyroiditis, multinodular goiter, thyroid cancer), thyrotoxicosis, diagnostic suppression tests

Dosage Forms CAP, pork source in soybean oil (S-P-T): 60 mg, 120 mg, 180 mg, 300 mg. **TAB:** (Armour® Thyroid): 15 mg, 30 mg, 60 mg, 90 mg, 120 mg, 180 mg, 240 mg, 300 mg; (Thyrar®) (bovine source): 30 mg, 60 mg, 120 mg; (Thyroid Strong®) (60 mg is equivalent to 90 mg thyroid USP): Regular: 30 mg, 60 mg, 120 mg; Sugar coated: 30 mg, 60 mg, 120 mg, 180 mg; Thyroid USP: 15 mg, 30 mg, 60 mg, 120 mg, 180 mg, 300 mg

Pregnancy Risk Factor A

Half-Life Liothyronine: 1-2 days; Thyroxine: 6-7 days

Education and Monitoring Issues

Patient Education: Thyroid replacement therapy is generally for life. Take as directed, in the morning before breakfast. Do not change brands and do not discontinue without consulting prescriber. Consult prescriber if drastically increasing or decreasing intake of goitrogenic food (eg, asparagus, cabbage, peas, turnip greens, broccoli, spinach, brussels sprouts, lettuce, soybeans). Report chest pain, rapid heart rate, palpitations, heat intolerance, excessive sweating, increased nervousness, agitation, or lethargy.

♦ **Thyroid Strong®** *see* Thyroid *on page 915*

Thyrotropin (thye roe TROE pin)

Pharmacologic Class Diagnostic Agent, Thyroid Function

U.S. Brand Names Thytropar®

Generic Available No

Mechanism of Action Stimulates formation and secretion of thyroid hormone, increases uptake of iodine by thyroid gland

Use Diagnostic aid to differentiate thyroid failure; diagnosis of decreased thyroid reserve, to differentiate between primary and secondary hypothyroidism and between primary hypothyroidism and euthyroidism in patients receiving thyroid replacement

USUAL DOSAGE Adults: I.M., S.C.: 10 units/day for 1-3 days; follow by a radioiodine study 24 hours past last injection, no response in thyroid failure, substantial response in pituitary failure

Dosage Forms **INJ:** 10 units

Contraindications Coronary thrombosis, untreated Addison's disease, hypersensitivity to thyrotropin or any component

Warnings/Precautions Use with caution in patients with angina pectoris or cardiac failure, patients with hypopituitarism, adrenal cortical suppression as may be seen with corticosteroid therapy; may cause thyroid hyperplasia

Pregnancy Risk Factor C

Adverse Reactions <1%: Anaphylaxis with repeated administration, fever, headache, increased bowel motility, menstrual irregularities, nausea, tachycardia, vomiting

Half-Life 35 minutes, dependent upon thyroid state

Education and Monitoring Issues

Patient Education: You will receive this medication for 3 days prior to the radiologic studies. You may experience some nausea or vomiting. Report dizziness, faintness, palpitations, or any respiratory difficulties.

Thyrotropin Alpha (thye roe TROE pin AL fa)

Pharmacologic Class Diagnostic Agent

U.S. Brand Names Thyrogen®

Mechanism of Action An exogenous source of human TSH that offers an additional diagnostic tool in the follow-up of patients with a history of well-differentiated thyroid cancer. Binding of thyrotropin alpha to TSH receptors on normal thyroid epithelial cells or on well-differentiated thyroid cancer tissue stimulates iodine uptake and organification and synthesis and secretion of thyroglobulin, triiodothyronine, and thyroxine.

Use As an adjunctive diagnostic tool for serum thyroglobulin (Tg) testing with or without radioiodine imaging in the follow-up of patients with well-differentiated thyroid cancer

Potential clinical uses:

1. Patients with an undetectable Tg on thyroid hormone suppressive therapy to exclude the diagnosis of residual or recurrent thyroid cancer
2. Patients requiring serum Tg testing and radioiodine imaging who are unwilling to undergo thyroid hormone withdrawal testing and whose treating prescriber believes that use of a less sensitive test is justified
3. Patients who are either unable to mount an adequate endogenous TSH response to thyroid hormone withdrawal or in whom withdrawal is medically contraindicated

USUAL DOSAGE Children >16 years and Adults: I.M.: 0.9 mg every 24 hours for 2 doses or every 72 hours for 3 doses. For radioiodine imaging, radioiodine administration should be given 24 hours following the final Thyrogen® injection. Scanning should be performed 48 hours after radioiodine administration (72 hours after the final injection of Thyrogen®).

Dosage Forms **KITS** containing two 1.1 mg vials (>4 international units) of thyrogen® and two 10 mL vials of sterile water for injection

Contraindications Hypersensitivity to any component

Warnings/Precautions Caution should be exercised when administered to patients who have been previously treated with bovine TSH and, in particular, to those patients who have experienced hypersensitivity reactions to bovine TSH

Considerations in the use of Thyrogen®:

1. There remains a meaningful risk of a diagnosis of thyroid cancer or of an underestimating the extent of disease when Thyrogen®-stimulated Tg testing is performed and in combination with radioiodine imaging
2. Thyrogen® Tg levels are generally lower than, and do not correlate with, Tg levels after thyroid hormone withdrawal
3. Newly detectable Tg level or a Tg level rising over time after Thyrogen® or a high index of suspicion of metastatic disease, even in the setting of a negative or low-stage Thyrogen® radioiodine scan, should prompt further evaluation such as thyroid hormone withdrawal to definitively establish the location and extent of thyroid cancer.
4. Decision to perform a Thyrogen® radioiodine scan in conjunction with a Thyrogen® serum Tg test and whether or when to withdraw a patient from thyroid hormones are complex. Pertinent factors in this decision include the sensitivity of the Tg assay used, the Thyrogen® Tg level obtained, and the index of suspicion of recurrent or persistent local or metastatic disease.
5. Thyrogen® is not recommended to stimulate radioiodine uptake for the purposes of ablative radiotherapy of thyroid cancer

6. The signs and symptoms of hypothyroidism which accompany thyroid hormone withdrawal are avoided with Thyrogen® use

Pregnancy Risk Factor C

Adverse Reactions 1% to 10%:

Central nervous system: Headache, chills, fever, flu-like syndrome, dizziness
Gastrointestinal: Nausea, vomiting
Neuromuscular & skeletal: Weakness, paresthesia

Half-Life Mean: 25 hours

♦ **Thytropar®** *see* Thyrotropin *on page 916*
♦ **Tiacid** *see* Salicylic Acid and Lactic Acid *on page 836*

Tiagabine (tye AG a bene)

Pharmacologic Class Anticonvulsant, Miscellaneous

U.S. Brand Names Gabitril®

Mechanism of Action The exact mechanism by which tiagabine exerts antiseizure activity is not definitively known; however, *in vitro* experiments demonstrate that it enhances the activity of gamma aminobutyric acid (GABA), the major neuroinhibitory transmitter in the nervous system. It is thought that binding to the GABA uptake carrier inhibits the uptake of GABA into presynaptic neurons, allowing an increased amount of GABA to be available to postsynaptic neurons. Based on *in vitro* studies, tiagabine does not inhibit the uptake of dopamine, norepinephrine, serotonin, glutamate, or choline.

Use Adjunctive therapy in adults and children ≥12 years of age in the treatment of partial seizures

USUAL DOSAGE Take with food; Oral:

Children 12-18 years: 4 mg once daily for 1 week; may increase to 8 mg daily in 2 divided doses for 1 week; then may increase by 4-8 mg weekly to response or up to 32 mg daily in 2-4 divided doses

Adults: 4 mg once daily for 1 week; may increase by 4-8 mg weekly to response or up to 56 mg daily in 2-4 divided doses

Dosage Forms TAB: 4 mg, 12 mg, 16 mg, 20 mg

Contraindications Patients who have demonstrated hypersensitivity to the drug or any of its ingredients

Warnings/Precautions Anticonvulsants should not be discontinued abruptly because of the possibility of increasing seizure frequency; tiagabine should be withdrawn gradually to minimize the potential of increased seizure frequency, unless safety concerns require a more rapid withdrawal

Pregnancy Risk Factor C

Adverse Reactions All adverse effects are dose-related

>1%:

Central nervous system: Dizziness, headache, somnolence, CNS depression, memory disturbance, ataxia, confusion
Neuromuscular & skeletal: Tremors, weakness, myalgia

Drug Interactions CYP2D6 and 3A3/4 enzyme substrate

Primidone, phenobarbital, phenytoin, and carbamazepine increase tiagabine clearance by 60%

Valproate increased free tiagabine concentrations by 40%

Half-Life Volunteers: 7-9 hours; in patients receiving enzyme-inducing drugs: 4-7 hours

Education and Monitoring Issues

Patient Education: Take exactly as directed (do not increase dose or frequency or discontinue without consulting prescriber). While using this medication, do not use alcohol and other prescription or OTC medications (especially pain medications, sedatives, antihistamines, or hypnotics) without consulting prescriber. Maintain adequate hydration (2-3 L/day of fluids unless instructed to restrict fluid intake). You may experience drowsiness, dizziness, disturbed concentration, or blurred vision (use caution when driving or engaging in tasks requiring alertness until response to drug is known); nausea, vomiting, or loss of appetite (small frequent meals, frequent mouth care, chewing gum, or sucking lozenges may help). Wear identification of epileptic status and medications. Report behavioral or CNS changes; skin rash; muscle cramping, weakness, tremors, changes in gait; vision difficulties; persistent GI distress (cramping, pain, vomiting); chest pain, irregular heartbeat, or palpitations; cough or difficulty breathing; worsening of seizure activity, or loss of seizure control.

Monitoring Parameters: A reduction in seizure frequency is indicative of therapeutic response to tiagabine in patients with partial seizures. Complete blood counts, renal function tests, liver function tests, and routine blood chemistry should be monitored periodically during therapy.

Reference Range: Maximal plasma level after a 24 mg/dose: 552 ng/mL

Manufacturer Abbott Laboratories (Pharmaceutical Product Division)

Related Information

Anticonvulsants by Seizure Type Comparison *on page 1230*
Pharmaceutical Manufacturers Directory *on page 1020*

♦ **Tiamate®** *see* Diltiazem *on page 278*
♦ **Tiamol** *see* Fluocinonide *on page 375*

♦ **Tiazac™** *see* Diltiazem *on page 278*
♦ **Ticar®** *see* Ticarcillin *on page 918*

Ticarcillin (tye kar SIL in)

Pharmacologic Class Antibiotic, Penicillin

U.S. Brand Names Ticar®

Generic Available No

Mechanism of Action Inhibits bacterial cell wall synthesis by binding to one or more of the penicillin binding proteins (PBPs); which in turn inhibits the final transpeptidation step of peptidoglycan synthesis in bacterial cell walls, thus inhibiting cell wall biosynthesis. Bacteria eventually lyse due to ongoing activity of cell wall autolytic enzymes (autolysins and murein hydrolases) while cell wall assembly is arrested.

Use Treatment of susceptible infections such as septicemia, acute and chronic respiratory tract infections, skin and soft tissue infections, and urinary tract infections due to susceptible strains of *Pseudomonas*, and other gram-negative bacteria

USUAL DOSAGE Ticarcillin is generally given I.V., I.M. injection is only for the treatment of uncomplicated urinary tract infections and dose should not exceed 2 g/injection when administered I.M.

Neonates: I.M., I.V.:
- Postnatal age <7 days:
  - <2000 g: 75 mg/kg/dose every 12 hours
  - >2000 g: 75 mg/kg/dose every 8 hours
- Postnatal age >7 days:
  - <1200 g: 75 mg/kg/dose every 12 hours
  - 1200-2000 g: 75 mg/kg/dose every 8 hours
  - >2000 g: 75 mg/kg/dose every 6 hours

Infants and Children:
- Systemic infections: I.V.: 200-300 mg/kg/day in divided doses every 4-6 hours
- Urinary tract infections: I.M., I.V.: 50-100 mg/kg/day in divided doses every 6-8 hours
- Maximum dose: 24 g/day

Adults: I.M., I.V.: 1-4 g every 4-6 hours, usual dose: 3 g I.V. every 4-6 hours

Dosing adjustment in renal impairment: Adults:
- Cl_{cr} 30-60 mL/minute: 2 g every 4 hours or 3 g every 8 hours
- Cl_{cr} 10-30 mL/minute: 2 g every 8 hours or 3 g every 12 hours
- Cl_{cr} <10 mL/minute: 2 g every 12 hours

Moderately dialyzable (20% to 50%)

Continuous arteriovenous or venovenous hemodiafiltration (CAVH) effects: Dose as for Cl_{cr} 10-50 mL/minute

Dosage Forms POWDER for inj: 1 g, 3 g, 6 g, 20 g, 30 g

Contraindications Hypersensitivity to ticarcillin or any component or penicillins

Warnings/Precautions Due to sodium load and adverse effects (anemia, neuropsychological changes), use with caution and modify dosage in patients with renal impairment; serious and occasionally severe or fatal hypersensitivity (anaphylactoid) reactions have been reported in patients on penicillin therapy (especially with a history of beta-lactam hypersensitivity and/or a history of sensitivity to multiple allergens); use with caution in patients with seizures

Pregnancy Risk Factor B

Adverse Reactions Percentage unknown: Acute interstitial nephritis, anaphylaxis, bleeding, confusion, convulsions, drowsiness, electrolyte imbalance, eosinophilia, fever, hemolytic anemia, hypersensitivity reactions, Jarisch-Herxheimer reaction, myoclonus, positive Coombs' reaction, rash, thrombophlebitis

Drug Interactions

Decreased effect:
- Tetracyclines may decrease penicillin effectiveness
- Aminoglycosides → physical inactivation of aminoglycosides in the presence of high concentrations of ticarcillin
- Decreased effectiveness of oral contraceptives

Increased effect:
- Probenecid may increase penicillin levels
- Neuromuscular blockers may increase duration of blockade
- Potential toxicity in patients with with mild to moderate renal dysfunction
- Aminoglycosides → synergistic efficacy
- Increased bleeding risk with large I.V. doses and anticoagulants

Half-Life 1-1.3 hours, prolonged with renal impairment and/or hepatic impairment

Education and Monitoring Issues

Patient Education: This medication will be administered I.V. or I.M. Maintain adequate hydration (2-3 L/day of fluids unless instructed to restrict fluid intake). Small frequent meals, frequent mouth care, sucking lozenges, or chewing gum may reduce nausea or dry mouth. Maintain good oral and vaginal hygiene to reduce incidence of opportunistic infection. If diabetic, drug may cause false tests with Clinitest® urine glucose monitoring; use of glucose oxidase methods (Clinistix®) or serum glucose monitoring is preferable. This drug may interfere with oral contraceptives; an alternate form of birth control should be used. Report persistent diarrhea or abdominal pain (do not use antidiarrhea medication without consulting prescriber), fever, chills, unhealed sores, bloody urine or stool, muscle pain, mouth sores, difficulty breathing, or skin rash.

Monitoring Parameters: Serum electrolytes, bleeding time, and periodic tests of renal, hepatic, and hematologic function; monitor for signs of anaphylaxis during first dose

Manufacturer SmithKline Beecham Pharmaceuticals

Related Information

Antimicrobial Drugs of Choice *on page 1182*
Community Acquired Pneumonia in Adults *on page 1200*
Pharmaceutical Manufacturers Directory *on page 1020*

Ticarcillin and Clavulanate Potassium

(tye kar SIL in & klav yoo LAN ate poe TASS ee um)

Pharmacologic Class Antibiotic, Penicillin

U.S. Brand Names Timentin®

Generic Available No

Mechanism of Action Inhibits bacterial cell wall synthesis by binding to one or more of the penicillin binding proteins (PBPs); which in turn inhibits the final transpeptidation step of peptidoglycan synthesis in bacterial cell walls, thus inhibiting cell wall biosynthesis. Bacteria eventually lyse due to ongoing activity of cell wall autolytic enzymes (autolysins and murein hydrolases) while cell wall assembly is arrested.

Use Treatment of infections of lower respiratory tract, urinary tract, skin and skin structures, bone and joint, and septicemia caused by susceptible organisms. Clavulanate expands activity of ticarcillin to include beta-lactamase producing strains of *S. aureus*, *H. influenzae*, *Bacteroides* species, and some other gram-negative bacilli

USUAL DOSAGE I.V.:

Children and Adults <60 kg: 200-300 mg of ticarcillin component/kg/day in divided doses every 4-6 hours

Children >60 kg and Adults: 3.1 g (ticarcillin 3 g plus clavulanic acid 0.1 g) every 4-6 hours; maximum: 24 g/day

Urinary tract infections: 3.1 g every 6-8 hours

Dosing adjustment in renal impairment:

Cl_{cr} 30-60 mL/minute: Administer 2 g every 4 hours or 3.1 g every 8 hours

Cl_{cr} 10-30 mL/minute: Administer 2 g every 8 hours or 3.1 g every 12 hours

Cl_{cr} <10 mL/minute: Administer 2 g every 12 hours

Moderately dialyzable (20% to 50%)

Continuous arteriovenous or venovenous hemodiafiltration (CAVH) effects: Dose as for Cl_{cr} 10-50 mL/minute

Dosage Forms INF, premixed (frozen): Ticarcillin disodium 3 g and clavulanate potassium 0.1 g (100 mL). **POWDER for inj:** Ticarcillin disodium 3 g and clavulanate potassium 0.1 g (3.1 g, 31 g)

Contraindications Known hypersensitivity to ticarcillin, clavulanate, or any penicillin

Warnings/Precautions Not approved for use in children <12 years of age; use with caution and modify dosage in patients with renal impairment; use with caution in patients with a history of allergy to cephalosporins and in patients with CHF due to high sodium load

Pregnancy Risk Factor B

Adverse Reactions Percentage unknown: Acute interstitial nephritis, anaphylaxis, bleeding, confusion, convulsions, drowsiness, electrolyte imbalance, fever, hemolytic anemia, hypersensitivity reactions, Jarisch-Herxheimer reaction, myoclonus, positive Coombs' reaction, rash, thrombophlebitis

Drug Interactions

Decreased effect:

Tetracyclines may decrease penicillin effectiveness

Aminoglycosides → physical inactivation of aminoglycosides in the presence of high concentrations of ticarcillin

Decreased effectiveness of oral contraceptives

Increased effect:

Probenecid may increase penicillin levels

Neuromuscular blockers may increase duration of blockade

Potential toxicity in patients with with mild to moderate renal dysfunction

Aminoglycosides → synergistic efficacy

Increased bleeding risk with large I.V. doses and anticoagulants

Half-Life

Clavulanate: 66-90 minutes

Ticarcillin: 66-72 minutes in patients with normal renal function; clavulanic acid does not affect the clearance of ticarcillin

Renal failure: Ticarcillin: ~13 hours

Education and Monitoring Issues

Patient Education: This medication will be administered I.V. or I.M. Maintain adequate hydration (2-3 L/day of fluids unless instructed to restrict fluid intake). Small frequent meals, frequent mouth care, sucking lozenges, or chewing gum may reduce nausea or dry mouth. Maintain good oral and vaginal hygiene to reduce incidence of opportunistic

(Continued)

Ticarcillin and Clavulanate Potassium *(Continued)*

infection. If diabetic, drug may cause false tests with Clinitest® urine glucose monitoring; use of glucose oxidase methods (Clinistix®) or serum glucose monitoring is preferable. This drug may interfere with oral contraceptives; an alternate form of birth control should be used. Report persistent diarrhea or abdominal pain (do not use antidiarrhea medication without consulting prescriber), fever, chills, unhealed sores, bloody urine or stool, muscle pain, mouth sores, difficulty breathing, or skin rash.

Monitoring Parameters: Observe signs and symptoms of anaphylaxis during first dose

Manufacturer SmithKline Beecham Pharmaceuticals

Related Information

Antimicrobial Drugs of Choice *on page 1182*
Community Acquired Pneumonia in Adults *on page 1200*
Pharmaceutical Manufacturers Directory *on page 1020*

♦ **Ticlid®** *see* Ticlopidine *on page 920*

Ticlopidine (tye KLOE pi deen)

Pharmacologic Class Antiplatelet Agent

U.S. Brand Names Ticlid®

Generic Available No

Mechanism of Action Ticlopidine is an inhibitor of platelet function with a mechanism which is different from other antiplatelet drugs. The drug significantly increases bleeding time. This effect may not be solely related to ticlopidine's effect on platelets. The prolongation of the bleeding time caused by ticlopidine is further increased by the addition of aspirin in *ex vivo* experiments. Although many metabolites of ticlopidine have been found, none have been shown to account for *in vivo* activity.

Use Platelet aggregation inhibitor that reduces the risk of thrombotic stroke in patients who have had a stroke or stroke precursors

Unlabeled use: Protection of aortocoronary bypass grafts, diabetic microangiopathy, ischemic heart disease, prevention of postoperative DVT, reduction of graft loss following renal transplant; reduction of postoperative reocclusion in patients receiving PTCA with stents

USUAL DOSAGE Adults: Oral: 1 tablet twice daily with food

Dosage Forms TAB: 250 mg

Contraindications Hypersensitivity to ticlopidine; active bleeding disorders; neutropenia or thrombocytopenia; severe liver impairment

Warnings/Precautions Patients predisposed to bleeding such as those with gastric or duodenal ulcers; patients with underlying hematologic disorders; patients receiving oral anticoagulant therapy or nonsteroidal anti-inflammatory agents (including aspirin); liver disease; patients undergoing lumbar puncture or surgical procedure. Ticlopidine should be discontinued if the absolute neutrophil count falls to $<1200/mm^3$ or if the platelet count falls to $<80,000/mm^3$. If possible, ticlopidine should be discontinued 10-14 days prior to surgery. Use caution when phenytoin or propranolol is used concurrently.

Pregnancy Risk Factor B

Adverse Reactions As with all drugs which may affect hemostasis, bleeding is associated with ticlopidine. Hemorrhage may occur at virtually any site. Risk is dependent on multiple variables, including the use of multiple agents which alter hemostasis and patient susceptibility.

>10%: Gastrointestinal: Diarrhea (12.5%)

1% to 10%: Central nervous system: Dizziness (1.1%)

Dermatologic: Rash (5.1%), purpura (2.2%), pruritus (1.3%)

Gastrointestinal: Nausea (7%), dyspepsia (7%), gastrointestinal pain (3.7%), vomiting (1.9%), flatulence (1.5%), anorexia (1%)

Hematologic: Neutropenia (2.4%)

Hepatic: Abnormal liver function test (1%)

<1% (limited to important or life-threatening symptoms): Thrombotic thrombocytopenic purpura (TTP), thrombocytopenia (immune), agranulocytosis, eosinophilia, pancytopenia, thrombocytosis, bone marrow suppression, gastrointestinal bleeding, ecchymosis, epistaxis, hematuria, menorrhagia, conjunctival bleeding, intracranial bleeding (rare), urticaria, exfoliative dermatitis, Stevens-Johnson syndrome, erythema multiforme, maculopapular rash, erythema nodosum, headache, weakness, pain, tinnitus, hemolytic anemia, aplastic anemia, hepatitis, jaundice, hepatic necrosis, peptic ulcer, renal failure, nephrotic syndrome, hyponatremia, vasculitis, sepsis, pneumonitis (allergic), angioedema, positive ANA, systemic lupus erythematosus, peripheral neuropathy, serum sickness, arthropathy, myositis

Case reports: Chronic diarrhea, increase in serum creatinine, bronchiolitis obliterans-organized pneumonia

Drug Interactions CYP2C19 inhibitor; CYP1A2 inhibitor

Antacids reduce absorption of ticlopidine (~18%)

Anticoagulants or other antiplatelet agents may increase the risk of bleeding; use with caution

Carbamazepine blood levels may be increased by ticlopidine

Cimetidine increases ticlopidine levels

Cyclosporine blood levels may be reduced by ticlopidine
Digoxin blood levels may be decreased by ticlopidine
Phenytoin blood levels may be increased by ticlopidine
Theophylline blood levels may be increased by ticlopidine

Onset Within 6 hours; Peak: Achieved after 3-5 days of oral therapy; serum levels do not correlate with clinical antiplatelet activity.

Half-Life 24 hours

Education and Monitoring Issues

Patient Education: Take exact dosage prescribed, with food. Do not use aspirin, aspirin-containing medications, or OTC medications without consulting prescriber. You may experience easy bleeding or bruising (use soft toothbrush or cotton swabs and frequent mouth care, use electric razor, avoid sharp knives or scissors). Report unusual bleeding or bruising or persistent fever or sore throat; blood in urine, stool, or vomitus; delayed healing of any wounds; skin rash; yellowing of skin or eyes; changes in color of urine of stool; pain or burning on urination; respiratory difficulty; or skin rash.

Monitoring Parameters: Signs of bleeding; CBC with differential every 2 weeks starting the second week through the third month of treatment; more frequent monitoring is recommended for patients whose absolute neutrophil counts have been consistently declining or are 30% less than baseline values. Liver function tests (alkaline phosphatase and transaminases) should be performed in the first 4 months of therapy if liver dysfunction is suspected.

Manufacturer Roche Laboratories

Related Information

Pharmaceutical Manufacturers Directory *on page 1020*

- **Ticon®** *see* Trimethobenzamide *on page 953*
- **Tigan®** *see* Trimethobenzamide *on page 953*
- **Tikosyn™** *see* Dofetilide *on page 291*
- **Tilade® Inhalation Aerosol** *see* Nedocromil Sodium *on page 639*

Tiludronate (tye LOO droe nate)

Pharmacologic Class Bisphosphonate Derivative

U.S. Brand Names Skelid®

Mechanism of Action Inhibition of normal and abnormal bone resorption. Inhibits osteoclasts through at least two mechanisms: disruption of the cytoskeletal ring structure, possibly by inhibition of protein-tyrosine-phosphatase, thus leading to the detachment of osteoclasts from the bone surface area and the inhibition of the osteoclast proton pump.

Use Treatment of Paget's disease of the bone (1) who have a level of serum alkaline phosphatase (SAP) at least twice the upper limit of normal, (2) or who are symptomatic, (3) or who are at risk for future complications of their disease

USUAL DOSAGE Tiludronate should be taken with 6-8 oz of plain water and not taken within 2 hours of food

Adults: Oral: 400 mg (2 tablets of tiludronic acid) daily for a period of 3 months; allow an interval of 3 months to assess response

Dosing adjustment in renal impairment: Cl_{cr} <30 mL/minute: **Not recommended**

Dosing adjustment in hepatic impairment: Adjustment is not necessary

Dosage Forms TAB: 240 mg [tiludronic acid 200 mg]; dosage is expressed in terms of tiludronic acid

Contraindications Hypersensitivity to biphosphonates or any component of the product

Warnings/Precautions Not recommended in patients with severe renal impairment (Cl_{cr} <30 mL/minute). Use with caution in patients with active upper GI problems (eg, dysphagia, symptomatic esophageal diseases, gastritis, duodenitis, ulcers).

Pregnancy Risk Factor C

Adverse Reactions 1% to 10%:

Cardiovascular: Flushing
Central nervous system: Vertigo, involuntary muscle contractions, anxiety, nervousness
Dermatologic: Pruritus, increased sweating, Stevens-Johnson type syndrome (rare)
Gastrointestinal: Xerostomia, gastritis
Genitourinary: Urinary tract infection
Neuromuscular & skeletal: Weakness, pathological fracture
Respiratory: Bronchitis
Miscellaneous: Increased diaphoresis

Drug Interactions

Decreased effect:

Calcium supplements, antacids interfere with the bioavailability (decreased 60%) when administered 1 hour before tiludronate

Aspirin decreases the bioavailability of tiludronate by up to 50% when taken 2 hours after tiludronate

Increased effect/toxicity: Indomethacin increases the bioavailability of tiludronate two- to fourfold

Onset Delayed, may require several weeks

Half-Life Healthy volunteers: 50 hours; Pagetic patients: 150 hours

(Continued)

Tiludronate *(Continued)*

Education and Monitoring Issues

Patient Education: In order to be effective this drug must be taken exactly as prescribed: Take 2 hours before or 2 hours after meals, aspirin, indomethacin, or calcium, magnesium, or aluminum containing medications such as antacids. Take with 6-8 oz. of water. Do not remove medication from foil strip until ready to be used. You may experience mild skin rash; abdominal pain, diarrhea, or constipation (report if persistent). Report unresolved muscle or bone pain or leg cramps; acute abdominal pain; chest pain, palpitations, or swollen extremities; disturbed vision or excessively dry eyes; ringing in the ears; persistent rash or skin disorder; unusual weakness or increased perspiration.

Dietary Considerations: In single-dose studies, the bioavailability of tiludronate was reduced by 90% when an oral dose was administered with, or 2 hours after, a standard breakfast compared to the same dose administered after an overnight fast and 4 hours before a standard breakfast; therefore, do not take within 2 hours of food

Manufacturer Sanofi Winthrop Pharmaceuticals

Related Information

Pharmaceutical Manufacturers Directory *on page 1020*

♦ **Timentin** *see* Ticarcillin and Clavulanate Potassium *on page 919*

Timolol (TYE moe lole)

Pharmacologic Class Beta Blocker, Nonselective; Ophthalmic Agent, Antiglaucoma

U.S. Brand Names Betimol® Ophthalmic; Blocadren® Oral; Timoptic® OcuDose®; Timoptic® Ophthalmic; Timoptic-XE® Ophthalmic

Generic Available No

Mechanism of Action Blocks both beta$_1$- and beta$_2$-adrenergic receptors, reduces intraocular pressure by reducing aqueous humor production or possibly outflow; reduces blood pressure by blocking adrenergic receptors and decreasing sympathetic outflow, produces a negative chronotropic and inotropic activity through an unknown mechanism

Use Ophthalmic dosage form used to treat elevated intraocular pressure such as glaucoma or ocular hypertension; orally for treatment of hypertension and angina and reduce mortality following myocardial infarction and prophylaxis of migraine

USUAL DOSAGE

Children and Adults: Ophthalmic: Initial: 0.25% solution, instill 1 drop twice daily; increase to 0.5% solution if response not adequate; decrease to 1 drop/day if controlled; do not exceed 1 drop twice daily of 0.5% solution

Adults: Oral:

Hypertension: Initial: 10 mg twice daily, increase gradually every 7 days, usual dosage: 20-40 mg/day in 2 divided doses; maximum: 60 mg/day

Prevention of myocardial infarction: 10 mg twice daily initiated within 1-4 weeks after infarction

Migraine headache: Initial: 10 mg twice daily, increase to maximum of 30 mg/day

Dosage Forms

Timolol hemihydrate: **SOLN, ophth** (Betimol®): 0.25% (2.5 mL, 5 mL, 10 mL, 15 mL), 0.5% (2.5 mL, 5 mL, 10 mL, 15 mL)

Timolol maleate: **GEL, ophth** (Timoptic-XE®): 0.25% (2.5 mL, 5 mL); 0.5% (2.5 mL, 5 mL). **SOLN, ophth** (Timoptic®): 0.25% (2.5 mL, 5 mL, 10 mL, 15 mL); 0.5% (2.5 mL, 5 mL, 10 mL, 15 mL); Preservative free, single use (Timoptic® OcuDose®): 0.25%, 0.5%; **TAB (Blocadren®):** 5 mg, 10 mg, 20 mg

Contraindications Uncompensated congestive heart failure, cardiogenic shock, bradycardia or heart block, severe chronic obstructive pulmonary disease, asthma, hypersensitivity to beta-blockers

Warnings/Precautions Some products contain sulfites which can cause allergic reactions; tachyphylaxis may develop; use with a miotic in angle-closure glaucoma; use with caution in patients with decreased renal or hepatic function (dosage adjustment required); severe CNS, cardiovascular and respiratory adverse effects have been seen following ophthalmic use; patients with a history of asthma, congestive heart failure, or bradycardia appear to be at a higher risk

Pregnancy Risk Factor C (per manufacturer); D (2nd and 3rd trimester, based on expert analysis)

Adverse Reactions

Ophthalmic:

1% to 10%:

Dermatologic: Alopecia

Ocular: Burning, stinging of eyes

<1%: Rash, blepharitis, conjunctivitis, keratitis, vision disturbances

Oral:

>10%: Endocrine & metabolic: Decreased sexual ability

1% to 10%:

Cardiovascular: Bradycardia, arrhythmia, reduced peripheral circulation

Central nervous system: Dizziness, fatigue

Dermatologic: Itching

Neuromuscular & skeletal: Weakness
Ocular: Burning eyes, stinging of eyes
Respiratory: Dyspnea

<1%: Anxiety, chest pain, congestive heart failure, diarrhea, dry sore eyes, hallucinations, mental depression, nausea, nightmares, numbness in toes and fingers, skin rash, stomach discomfort, vomiting

Drug Interactions CYP2D6 enzyme substrate

Decreased effect of beta-blockers with aluminum salts, barbiturates, calcium salts, cholestyramine, colestipol, NSAIDs, penicillins (ampicillin), rifampin, salicylates and sulfinpyrazone due to decreased bioavailability and plasma levels

Beta-blockers may decrease the effect of sulfonylureas

Increased effect/toxicity of beta-blockers with calcium blockers (diltiazem, felodipine, nicardipine), contraceptives, flecainide, propafenone (metoprolol, propranolol), quinidine (in extensive metabolizers), ciprofloxacin

Beta-blockers may increase the effect/toxicity of flecainide, phenothiazines, acetaminophen, clonidine (hypertensive crisis after or during withdrawal of either agent), epinephrine (initial hypertensive episode followed by bradycardia), nifedipine and verapamil lidocaine, ergots (peripheral ischemia), prazosin (postural hypotension)

Beta-blockers may affect the action or levels of ethanol, disopyramide, nondepolarizing muscle relaxants and theophylline although the effects are difficult to predict

Alcohol Interactions Limit use (may increase risk of hypotension or dizziness)

Onset Onset of hypotensive effect: Oral: Within 15-45 minutes; Peak effect: Within 0.5-2.5 hours

Duration ~4 hours; intraocular effects persist for 24 hours after ophthalmic instillation

Half-Life 2-2.7 hours; prolonged with reduced renal function

Education and Monitoring Issues

Patient Education:

Oral: Take exact dose prescribed; do not increase, decrease, or discontinue dosage without consulting prescriber. Take at the same time each day. Does not replace recommended diet or exercise program. If diabetic, monitor serum glucose closely. May cause postural hypotension (use caution when rising from sitting or lying position or climbing stairs); dizziness, drowsiness, or blurred vision (use caution when driving or engaging in tasks requiring alertness until response to drug is known); decreased sexual ability (reversible); or nausea or vomiting (small frequent meals or frequent mouth care may help). Report swelling of extremities, respiratory difficulty, or new cough; weight gain (>3 lb/week); unresolved diarrhea or vomiting; or cold blue extremities.

Ophthalmic: For ophthalmic use only. Apply prescribed amount as often as directed. Wash hands before using and do not touch tip of applicator to eye or contaminate tip of applicator. Tilt head back and look upward. Gently pull down lower lid and put drop(s) inside lower eyelid at inner corner. Close eye and roll eyeball in all directions. Do not blink for ½ minute. Apply gentle pressure to inner corner of eye for 30 seconds. Wipe away excess from skin around eye. Do not use any other eye preparation for at least 10 minutes. Do not share medication with anyone else. Temporary stinging or blurred vision may occur. Immediately report any adverse cardiac or CNS effects (usually signifies overdose). Report persistent eye pain, redness, burning, watering, dryness, double vision, puffiness around eye, vision disturbances, other adverse eye response, worsening of condition or lack of improvement. Inform prescriber if you are or intend to be pregnant. Consult prescriber if breast-feeding.

Monitoring Parameters: Blood pressure, apical and radial pulses, fluid I & O, daily weight, respirations, mental status, and circulation in extremities before and during therapy

Related Information

Beta-Blockers Comparison *on page 1233*

- **Timoptic® OcuDose®** *see* Timolol *on page 922*
- **Timoptic® Ophthalmic** *see* Timolol *on page 922*
- **Timoptic-XE® Ophthalmic** *see* Timolol *on page 922*
- **Tinactin® [OTC]** *see* Tolnaftate *on page 931*
- **Tinactin® for Jock Itch [OTC]** *see* Tolnaftate *on page 931*
- **Tine Test PPD** *see* Tuberculin Purified Protein Derivative *on page 960*
- **Tine Test PPD** *see* Tuberculin Tests *on page 960*
- **Ting® [OTC]** *see* Tolnaftate *on page 931*
- **Tinver® Lotion** *see* Sodium Thiosulfate *on page 861*

Tioconazole (tye oh KONE a zole)

Pharmacologic Class Antifungal Agent, Vaginal

U.S. Brand Names Vagistat® Vaginal

Use Local treatment of vulvovaginal candidiasis

USUAL DOSAGE Adults: Vaginal: Insert 1 applicatorful in vagina, just prior to bedtime, as a single dose; therapy may extend to 7 days

Contraindications Known hypersensitivity to tioconazole

Pregnancy Risk Factor C

(Continued)

Tioconazole *(Continued)*

Related Information

Treatment of Sexually Transmitted Diseases *on page 1210*

- **Tisit® Blue Gel [OTC]** *see* Pyrethrins *on page 795*
- **Tisit® Liquid [OTC]** *see* Pyrethrins *on page 795*
- **Tisit® Shampoo [OTC]** *see* Pyrethrins *on page 795*
- **Titralac** *see* Calcium Carbonate *on page 130*
- **Ti-U-Lac HC** *see* Urea and Hydrocortisone *on page 963*
- **TOBI™ Inhalation Solution** *see* Tobramycin *on page 924*
- **Tobradex** *see* Tobramycin and Dexamethasone *on page 925*
- **TobraDex® Ophthalmic** *see* Tobramycin and Dexamethasone *on page 925*

Tobramycin (toe bra MYE sin)

Pharmacologic Class Antibiotic, Aminoglycoside; Antibiotic, Ophthalmic

U.S. Brand Names AKTob® Ophthalmic; Nebcin® Injection; TOBI™ Inhalation Solution; Tobrex® Ophthalmic

Generic Available Yes

Mechanism of Action Interferes with bacterial protein synthesis by binding to 30S and 50S ribosomal subunits resulting in a defective bacterial cell membrane

Use Treatment of documented or suspected infections caused by susceptible gram-negative bacilli including *Pseudomonas aeruginosa*; topically used to treat superficial ophthalmic infections caused by susceptible bacteria. Tobramycin solution for inhalation is indicated for the management of cystic fibrosis patients (>6 years of age) with *Pseudomonas aeruginosa*.

USUAL DOSAGE Individualization is critical because of the low therapeutic index

Use of ideal body weight (IBW) for determining the mg/kg/dose appears to be more accurate than dosing on the basis of total body weight (TBW)

In morbid obesity, dosage requirement may best be estimated using a dosing weight of IBW + 0.4 (TBW - IBW)

Initial and periodic peak and trough plasma drug levels should be determined, particularly in critically ill patients with serious infections or in disease states known to significantly alter aminoglycoside pharmacokinetics (eg, cystic fibrosis, burns, or major surgery). Two to three serum level measurements should be obtained after the initial dose to measure the half-life in order to determine the frequency of subsequent doses.

Infants and Children <5 years: I.M., I.V.: 2.5 mg/kg/dose every 8 hours
Children >5 years: 1.5-2.5 mg/kg/dose every 8 hours
Note: Some patients may require larger or more frequent doses if serum levels document the need (ie, cystic fibrosis or febrile granulocytopenic patients).
Adults: I.M., I.V.:
- Severe life-threatening infections: 2-2.5 mg/kg/dose
- Urinary tract infection: 1.5 mg/kg/dose
- Synergy (for gram-positive infections): 1 mg/kg/dose

Children and Adults: Ophthalmic: Instill 1-2 drops of solution every 4 hours; apply ointment 2-3 times/day; for severe infections apply ointment every 3-4 hours, or solution 2 drops every 30-60 minutes initially, then reduce to less frequent intervals
Inhalation:
- Standard aerosolized tobramycin:
  - Children: 40-80 mg 2-3 times/day
  - Adults: 60-80 mg 3 times/day
- High-dose regimen: Children ≥6 years and Adults with cystic fibrosis and *Pseudomonas aeruginosa*: 300 mg every 12 hours (do not administer doses <6 hours apart); administer in repeated cycles of 28 days on drug followed by 28 days off drug

Some clinicians suggest a daily dose of 4-7 mg/kg for all patients with normal renal function. This dose is at least as efficacious with similar, if not less, toxicity than conventional dosing

Dosing interval in renal impairment:
- Cl_{cr} ≥60 mL/minute: Administer every 8 hours
- Cl_{cr} 40-60 mL/minute: Administer every 12 hours
- Cl_{cr} 20-40 mL/minute: Administer every 24 hours
- Cl_{cr} 10-20 mL/minute: Administer every 48 hours
- Cl_{cr} <10 mL/minute: Administer every 72 hours

Hemodialysis: Dialyzable; 30% removal of aminoglycosides occurs during 4 hours of HD - administer dose after dialysis and follow levels
Continuous arteriovenous or venovenous hemofiltration (CAVH/CAVHD): Dose as for Cl_{cr} of 10-40 mL/minute and follow levels
- Administration in CAPD fluid:
  - Gram-negative infection: 4-8 mg/L (4-8 mcg/mL) of CAPD fluid
  - Gram-positive infection (ie, synergy): 3-4 mg/L (3-4 mcg/mL) of CAPD fluid
- Administration IVPB/I.M.: Dose as for Cl_{cr} <10 mL/minute and follow levels

Dosing adjustment/comments in hepatic disease: Monitor plasma concentrations

Dosage Forms INJ (Nebcin®): 10 mg/mL (2 mL), 40 mg/mL (1.5 mL, 2 mL). **OINT, ophth** (Tobrex®): 0.3% (3.5 g). **POWDER for inj** (Nebcin®): 40 mg/mL (1.2 g vials). **SOLN, inhal:** (TOBI™): 60 mg/mL (5 mL) **SOLN, ophth:** 0.3% (5 mL); (AKTob®, Tobrex®): 0.3% (5 mL)

Contraindications Hypersensitivity to tobramycin or other aminoglycosides or components

Warnings/Precautions Use with caution in patients with renal impairment; pre-existing auditory or vestibular impairment; and in patients with neuromuscular disorders; dosage modification required in patients with impaired renal function; (I.M. & I.V.) Aminoglycosides are associated with significant nephrotoxicity or ototoxicity; the ototoxicity is directly proportional to the amount of drug given and the duration of treatment; tinnitus or vertigo are indications of vestibular injury; ototoxicity is often irreversible; renal damage is usually reversible

Pregnancy Risk Factor C

Adverse Reactions

1% to 10%:

Renal: Nephrotoxicity

Neuromuscular & skeletal: Neurotoxicity (neuromuscular blockade)

Otic: Ototoxicity (auditory), ototoxicity (vestibular)

<1%: Anemia, arthralgia, drowsiness, drug fever, dyspnea, edema of the eyelid, eosinophilia, headache, hypotension, itching eyes, keratitis, lacrimation, nausea, paresthesia, rash, tremor, vomiting, weakness

Drug Interactions

Increased effect: Extended spectrum penicillins (synergistic)

Increased toxicity:

Neuromuscular blockers increase neuromuscular blockade

Amphotericin B, cephalosporins, loop diuretics, and vancomycin may increase risk of nephrotoxicity

Half-Life 2-3 hours, directly dependent upon glomerular filtration rate; Adults with impaired renal function: 5-70 hours

Education and Monitoring Issues

Patient Education:

Systemic: Maintain adequate hydration (2-3 L/day of fluids unless instructed to restrict fluid intake). Report decreased urine output, swelling of extremities, difficulty breathing, vaginal itching or discharge, rash, diarrhea, oral thrush, unhealed wounds, dizziness, change in hearing acuity or ringing in ears, or worsening of condition.

Ophthalmic: Use as frequently as recommended; do not overuse. Sit down, tilt head back, instill solution or drops inside lower eyelid, and roll eyeball in all directions. Close eye and apply gentle pressure to inner corner of eye for 30 seconds. Do not touch tip of applicator to eye or any contaminated surface. May experience temporary stinging or blurred vision. Do not use any other eye preparation for 10 minutes. Inform prescriber if condition worsens or does not improve in 3-4 days.

Dietary Considerations: Calcium, magnesium, potassium: Renal wasting may cause hypocalcemia, hypomagnesemia, and/or hypokalemia

Monitoring Parameters: Urinalysis, urine output, BUN, serum creatinine, peak and trough plasma tobramycin levels; be alert to ototoxicity; hearing should be tested before and during treatment

Reference Range:

Timing of serum samples: Draw peak 30 minutes after 30-minute infusion has been completed or 1 hour following I.M. injection or beginning of infusion; draw trough immediately before next dose

Therapeutic levels:

Peak:

Serious infections: 6-8 μg/mL (SI: 12-17 mg/L)

Life-threatening infections: 8-10 μg/mL (SI: 17-21 mg/L)

Urinary tract infections: 4-6 μg/mL (SI: 7-12 mg/L)

Synergy against gram-positive organisms: 3-5 μg/mL

Trough:

Serious infections: 0.5-1 μg/mL

Life-threatening infections: 1-2 μg/mL

Monitor serum creatinine and urine output; obtain drug levels after the third dose unless otherwise directed

Related Information

Antimicrobial Drugs of Choice *on page 1182*

Tobramycin and Dexamethasone *on page 925*

Tobramycin and Dexamethasone

(toe bra MYE sin & deks a METH a sone)

Pharmacologic Class Antibiotic/Corticosteroid, Ophthalmic

U.S. Brand Names TobraDex® Ophthalmic

Use Treatment of blepharitis, conjunctivitis, or keratitis caused by susceptible organisms

(Continued)

Tobramycin and Dexamethasone *(Continued)*

Dosage Forms OINT, ophth: Tobramycin 0.3% and dexamethasone 0.1% (3.5 g). **SUSP, ophth:** Tobramycin 0.3% and dexamethasone 0.1% (2.5 mL, 5 mL)

♦ **Tobrex® Ophthalmic** *see* Tobramycin *on page 924*

Tocainide (toe KAY nide)

Pharmacologic Class Antiarrhythmic Agent, Class I-B

U.S. Brand Names Tonocard®

Generic Available No

Mechanism of Action Class 1B antiarrhythmic agent; suppresses automaticity of conduction tissue, by increasing electrical stimulation threshold of ventricle, HIS-Purkinje system, and spontaneous depolarization of the ventricles during diastole by a direct action on the tissues; blocks both the initiation and conduction of nerve impulses by decreasing the neuronal membrane's permeability to sodium ions, which results in inhibition of depolarization with resultant blockade of conduction

Use Suppress and prevent symptomatic life-threatening ventricular arrhythmias

Unlabeled use: Trigeminal neuralgia

USUAL DOSAGE Adults: Oral: 1200-1800 mg/day in 3 divided doses, up to 2400 mg/day

Dosing adjustment in renal impairment: Cl_{cr} <30 mL/minute: Administer 50% of normal dose or 600 mg once daily

Hemodialysis: Moderately dialyzable (20% to 50%)

Dosing adjustment in hepatic impairment: Maximum daily dose: 1200 mg

Dosage Forms TAB: 400 mg, 600 mg

Contraindications Second or third degree A-V block without a pacemaker, hypersensitivity to tocainide, amide-type anesthetics, or any component

Warnings/Precautions May exacerbate some arrhythmias (ie, atrial fibrillation/flutter); use with caution in CHF patients; administer with caution in patients with pre-existing bone marrow failure, cytopenia, severe renal or hepatic disease

Pregnancy Risk Factor C

Adverse Reactions

>10%:

Central nervous system: Dizziness (8% to 15%)

Gastrointestinal: Nausea (14% to 15%)

1% to 10%:

Cardiovascular: Tachycardia (3%), bradycardia/angina/palpitations (0.5% to 1.8%), hypotension (3%)

Central nervous system: Nervousness (0.5% to 1.5%), confusion (2% to 3%), headache (4.6%), anxiety, incoordination, giddiness, vertigo

Dermatologic: Rash (0.5% to 8.4%)

Gastrointestinal: Vomiting (4.5%), diarrhea (4% to 5%), anorexia (1% to 2%), loss of taste

Neuromuscular & skeletal: Paresthesia (3.5% to 9%), tremor (dose-related: 2.9% to 8.4%), ataxia (dose-related: 2.9% to 8.4%), hot and cold sensations

Ocular: Blurred vision (~1.5%), nystagmus (1%)

<1% (limited to important or life-threatening symptoms): Hypersensitivity reactions, increased ANA, sinoatrial block, syncope, vasovagal episodes, diaphoresis, edema, fever, chills, cinchonism, asthenia, malaise, A-V block, hypertension, increased QRS duration, prolonged Q-T interval, right bundle branch block, cardiomegaly, angina, pulmonary embolism, sinus arrest, vasculitis, orthostatic hypotension, pericarditis, hepatitis, jaundice, abnormal liver function tests, pancreatitis, abdominal pain, constipation, dysphagia, dyspepsia, stomatitis, xerostomia, muscle cramps, neck pain, depression, psychosis, psychic disturbances, agitation, decreased mental acuity, dysarthria, impaired memory, slurred speech, sleep disturbance, insomnia, local anesthesia, myasthenia gravis, convulsions, coma, pneumonia, interstitial pneumonitis, fibrosing alveolitis, pulmonary fibrosis, dyspnea, hiccup, yawning, pulmonary edema, respiratory arrest, urticaria, alopecia, pallor, pruritus, erythema multiforme, exfoliative dermatitis, Stevens-Johnson syndrome, diplopia, earache, taste perversion, urinary retention, polyuria, hallucinations, delirium

Case reports: Pericarditis, immune complex glomerulonephritis, granulomatous hepatitis

Note: Rare, potentially severe hematologic reactions, have occurred (generally within the first 12 weeks of therapy). These may include agranulocytosis, bone marrow depression, aplastic anemia, hypoplastic anemia, hemolytic anemia, anemia, leukopenia, neutropenia, thrombocytopenia, and eosinophilia.

Drug Interactions

Decreased plasma levels: Phenobarbital, phenytoin, rifampin, and other hepatic enzyme inducers, cimetidine and drugs which make the urine acidic

Increased toxicity/levels of caffeine and theophylline

Increased effects with metoprolol

Half-Life 11-14 hours, prolonged with renal and hepatic impairment with half-life increased to 23-27 hours

Education and Monitoring Issues

Patient Education: Take exactly as directed, with food. If dose is missed, take as soon as possible, do not double next dose. Do not discontinue without consulting prescriber. You will need regular cardiac checkups while taking this medication. You may experience dizziness, nervousness, or visual changes (use caution when driving or engaging in tasks requiring alertness until response to drug is known); nausea or vomiting, or loss of appetite (frequent small meals, frequent mouth care, chewing gum, or sucking lozenges may help); mild muscle discomfort (analgesics may be recommended). Report chest pain, palpitations, or erratic heartbeat; difficulty breathing or unusual cough; mental confusion or depression; muscle tremor, weakness, or pain; or changes in vision.

Reference Range: Therapeutic: 5-12 µg/mL (SI: 22-52 µmol/L)

Manufacturer AstraZeneca

Related Information

Pharmaceutical Manufacturers Directory *on page 1020*

♦ **Toesen®** *see* Oxytocin *on page 695*
♦ **Tofranil®** *see* Imipramine *on page 462*
♦ **Tofranil-PM®** *see* Imipramine *on page 462*

Tolazamide (tole AZ a mide)

Pharmacologic Class Antidiabetic Agent, Oral

U.S. Brand Names Tolinase®

Use Adjunct to diet for the management of mild to moderately severe, stable, noninsulin-dependent (type II) diabetes mellitus

USUAL DOSAGE Oral (doses >1000 mg/day normally do not improve diabetic control):

Adults:

Initial: 100-250 mg/day with breakfast or the first main meal of the day
- Fasting blood sugar <200 mg/dL: 100 mg/day
- Fasting blood sugar >200 mg/dL: 250 mg/day
- Malnourished, underweight, elderly, or patient who is not eating properly: 100 mg/day

Adjust dose in increments of 100-250 mg/day at weekly intervals to response. If >500 mg/day is required, give in divided doses twice daily; maximum daily dose: 1 g (doses >1 g/day are not likely to improve control)

Conversion from insulin → tolazamide
- 10 units day = 100 mg/day
- 20-40 units/day = 250 mg/day
- >40 units/day = 250 mg/day and 50% of insulin dose

Doses >500 mg/day should be given in 2 divided doses

Dosing adjustment in renal impairment: Conservative initial and maintenance doses are recommended because tolazamide is metabolized to active metabolites, which are eliminated in the urine

Dosing comments in hepatic impairment: Conservative initial and maintenance doses and careful monitoring of blood glucose are recommended

Elderly: Patients are prone to develop renal insufficiency, which may put them at risk of hypoglycemia; dose selection should include assessment of renal function

Contraindications Type I diabetes therapy (IDDM), hypersensitivity to sulfonylureas, diabetes complicated by ketoacidosis

Pregnancy Risk Factor D

Related Information

Hypoglycemic Drugs and Thiazolidinedione Information *on page 1240*

Tolazoline (tole AZ oh leen)

Pharmacologic Class $Alpha_1$ Blockers

U.S. Brand Names Priscoline®

Generic Available No

Mechanism of Action Competitively blocks alpha-adrenergic receptors to produce brief antagonism of circulating epinephrine and norepinephrine; reduces hypertension caused by catecholamines and causes vascular smooth muscle relaxation (direct action); results in peripheral vasodilation and decreased peripheral resistance

Use Treatment of persistent pulmonary vasoconstriction and hypertension of the newborn (persistent fetal circulation), peripheral vasospastic disorders

USUAL DOSAGE

Neonates: Initial: I.V.: 1-2 mg/kg over 10-15 minutes via scalp vein or upper extremity; maintenance: 1-2 mg/kg/hour; use lower maintenance doses in patients with decreased renal function. Also used in neonates for acute vasospasm "cath toes" at 0.25 mg/kg/hour (no load); maximum dose: 6-8 mg/kg/hour.

Dosing interval in renal impairment in newborns: Urine output <0.9 mL/kg/hour: Decrease dose to 0.08 mg/kg/hour for every 1 mg/kg of loading dose

Adults: Peripheral vasospastic disorder: I.M., I.V., S.C.: 10-50 mg 4 times/day

Dosage Forms INJ: 25 mg/mL (4 mL)

Contraindications Hypersensitivity to tolazoline; known or suspected coronary artery disease

(Continued)

Tolazoline *(Continued)*

Warnings/Precautions Stimulates gastric secretion and may activate stress ulcers; therefore, use with caution in patients with gastritis, peptic ulcer; use with caution in patients with mitral stenosis

Pregnancy Risk Factor C

Adverse Reactions 1% to 10%:

Cardiovascular: Hypotension, peripheral vasodilation, tachycardia, hypertension, arrhythmias
Endocrine & metabolic: Hypochloremic alkalosis
Gastrointestinal: GI bleeding, abdominal pain, nausea, diarrhea
Hematologic: Thrombocytopenia, increased agranulocytosis, pancytopenia
Local: Burning at injection site
Neuromuscular & skeletal: Increased pilomotor activity
Ocular: Mydriasis
Renal: Acute renal failure, oliguria
Respiratory: Pulmonary hemorrhage
Miscellaneous: Increased secretions

Drug Interactions

Decreased effect (vasopressor) of epinephrine followed by a rebound increase in blood pressure
Increased toxicity: Disulfiram reaction may possibly be seen with concomitant ethanol use

Alcohol Interactions Avoid use

Education and Monitoring Issues

Patient Education: Side effects decrease with continued therapy; avoid alcohol

Monitoring Parameters: Vital signs, blood gases, cardiac monitor

Tolbutamide (tole BYOO ta mide)

Pharmacologic Class Antidiabetic Agent (Sulfonylurea)

U.S. Brand Names Orinase® Diagnostic Injection; Orinase® Oral

Use Adjunct to diet for the management of mild to moderately severe, stable, noninsulin-dependent (type II) diabetes mellitus

USUAL DOSAGE Divided doses may increase gastrointestinal side effects

Adults:

Oral: Initial: 1-2 g/day as a single dose in the morning or in divided doses throughout the day. Total doses may be taken in the morning; however, divided doses may allow increased gastrointestinal tolerance. Maintenance dose: 0.25-3 g/day; however, a maintenance dose >2 g/day is seldom required.

I.V. bolus: 1 g over 2-3 minutes

Elderly: Oral: Initial: 250 mg 1-3 times/day; usual: 500-2000 mg; maximum: 3 g/day

Dosing adjustment in renal impairment: Adjustment is not necessary

Hemodialysis: Not dialyzable (0% to 5%)

Dosing adjustment in hepatic impairment: Reduction of dose may be necessary in patients with impaired liver function

Contraindications Diabetes complicated by ketoacidosis, therapy of IDDM, hypersensitivity to sulfonylureas

Pregnancy Risk Factor D

Related Information

Hypoglycemic Drugs and Thiazolidinedione Information *on page 1240*

Tolcapone (TOLE ka pone)

Pharmacologic Class Anti-Parkinson's Agent (COMT Inhibitor)

U.S. Brand Names Tasmar®

Mechanism of Action A reversible inhibitor of catechol-O-methyltransferase (COMT). COMT is the major route of metabolism for levodopa. When tolcapone is taken with levodopa the pharmacokinetics are altered, resulting in more sustained levodopa serum levels compared to levodopa taken alone. The resulting levels of levodopa provide for increased concentrations available for absorption across the blood-brain barrier, thereby providing for increased CNS levels of dopamine, the active metabolite of levodopa.

Use An adjunct to levodopa/carbidopa for the treatment of signs and symptoms of Parkinson's disease

USUAL DOSAGE Oral: 100 mg 3 times/day always given as an adjunct to levodopa/carbidopa. The first dose of the day should be given with the first dose of the day of levodopa/carbidopa, and then administer the next 2 doses 6 and 12 hours later. Because increased liver enzymes occur more frequently with 200 mg 3 times/day, only increase to 200 mg if clinically justified.

Note: Many patients will require a decrease in levodopa dosage to avoid increased dopaminergic side effects

Dosing adjustment in renal impairment: Generally, no adjustment necessary; however, in patients with severe renal failure, treat with caution and do not exceed 100 mg 3 times/day

Dosing adjustment in hepatic impairment: Do not use if the patient has evidence of active liver disease or the AST or ALT are greater than the upper limit of normal

Dosage Forms TAB: 100 mg, 200 mg

Contraindications Hypersensitivity to tolcapone or other ingredients, including tolcapone, lactose monohydrate, cellulose, povidone, sodium starch glycolate, talc, and/or magnesium stearate; patients with liver disease or who had increased LFTs on tolcapone; patients with a history of nontraumatic rhabdomyolysis or hyperpyrexia and confusion possibly related to medication

Warnings/Precautions Note: Due to reports of fatal liver injury associated with use of this drug, the manufacturer is advising that tolcapone be reserved for use only in patients who do not have severe movement abnormalities and who do not respond to or who are not appropriate candidates for other available treatments. Before initiating therapy with tolcapone, the risks should be discussed with the patient, and the patient can provide written informed consent (form available from Roche).

It is not recommended that patients receive tolcapone concomitantly with nonselective MAO inhibitors (see Drug Interactions). Selegiline is a selective MAO-B inhibitor and can be taken with tolcapone.

Patients receiving tolcapone are predisposed to orthostatic hypotension, diarrhea (usually within the first 6-12 weeks of therapy), transient hallucinations (most commonly within the first 2 weeks of therapy), and new onset or worsened dyskinesia. Use with caution in patients with severe renal failure. Tolcapone is secreted into maternal milk in rats and may be excreted into human milk; until more is known, tolcapone should be considered **incompatible** with breast-feeding.

Pregnancy Risk Factor C

Adverse Reactions Patients receiving tolcapone are predisposed to orthostatic hypotension. Inform the patient and explain methods to manage the symptoms. Patients may experience diarrhea, most commonly 6-12 weeks after tolcapone is started. Diarrhea is sometimes associated with anorexia. Patients may experience hallucinations shortly after starting therapy, most commonly within the first 2 weeks. Hallucinations may diminish or resolve with a decrease in the levodopa dose. Hallucinations commonly accompany confusion and sometimes insomnia or excessive dreaming. Tolcapone may exacerbate or induce dyskinesia; lowering the levodopa dose may help. Use tolcapone with caution in patients with severe renal or hepatic failure.

>10%:

- Cardiovascular: Orthostasis
- Central nervous system: Sleep disorder, excessive dreaming, headache, dizziness, somnolence, confusion
- Gastrointestinal: Nausea, anorexia, diarrhea
- Neuromuscular & skeletal: Dyskinesia, dystonia, muscle cramps

1% to 10%:

- Cardiovascular: Hypotension, chest pain, syncope
- Central nervous system: Hallucination, fatigue
- Gastrointestinal: Vomiting, constipation, dry mouth, dyspepsia, abdominal pain, flatulence
- Genitourinary: Urine discoloration
- Neuromuscular & skeletal: Hyperkinesia, stiffness, arthritis
- Respiratory: Dyspnea

<1%: Allergic reaction, amnesia, anemia, angina pectoris, arteriosclerosis, bradycardia, bronchitis, cellulitis, cerebrovascular accident, cholecystitis, colitis, coronary artery disorder, delirium, duodenal ulcer, encephalopathy, epistaxis, extrapyramidal syndrome, fatal liver injury, gastrointestinal hemorrhage, heart arrest, hematuria, hemiplegia, hypercholesteremia, hypertension, hyperventilation, leukemia, manic reaction, meningitis, myocardial infarct, myocardial ischemia, myoclonus, neuralgia, psychosis, thrombocytopenia, thrombosis, uterine hemorrhage, vasodilation

Drug Interactions Theoretically, nonselective MAO inhibitors (phenelzine and tranylcypromine) taken with tolcapone may inhibit the major metabolic pathways of catecholamines, which may result in excessive adverse effects possibly due to levodopa accumulation. Concomitant therapy is not recommended.

Half-Life 2-3 hours

Education and Monitoring Issues

Patient Education: Take exactly as directed (may be prescribed in conjunction with levodopa/carbidopa); do not change dosage or discontinue without consulting prescriber. Therapeutic effects may take several weeks or months to achieve and you may need frequent monitoring during first weeks of therapy. Best to take 2 hours before or after a meal; however, may be taken with meals if GI upset occurs. Take at the same time each day. Maintain adequate hydration (2-3 L/day of fluids unless instructed to restrict fluid intake). Do not use alcohol and prescription or OTC sedatives or CNS depressants without consulting prescriber. Urine or perspiration may appear darker. You may experience drowsiness, dizziness, confusion, or vision changes (use caution when driving, climbing stairs, or engaging in tasks requiring alertness until response to drug is known); orthostatic hypotension (use caution when changing position - rising to standing from sitting or lying); increased susceptibility to heat stroke, decreased perspiration (use caution in hot weather - maintain adequate fluids and reduce exercise activity); constipation (increased exercise, fluids, or dietary fruit and fiber may help); dry

(Continued)

Tolcapone *(Continued)*

skin or nasal passages (consult prescriber for appropriate relief); nausea, vomiting, loss of appetite, or stomach discomfort (small frequent meals, frequent mouth care, chewing gum, or sucking lozenges may help). Report unresolved constipation or vomiting; chest pain or irregular heartbeat; difficulty breathing; acute headache or dizziness; CNS changes (hallucination, loss of memory, nervousness, etc); painful or difficult urination; abdominal pain or blood in stool; increased muscle spasticity, rigidity, or involuntary movements; skin rash; or significant worsening of condition.

Dietary Considerations: Tolcapone taken with food within 1 hour before or 2 hours after the dose decreases bioavailability by 10% to 20%

Monitoring Parameters: Blood pressure, symptoms of Parkinson's disease, liver enzymes at baseline and then every 2 weeks for the first year of therapy, every 4 weeks for the next 6 months, then every 8 weeks thereafter. If the dose is increased to 200 mg 3 times/day, reinitiate LFT monitoring at the previous frequency. Discontinue therapy if the ALT or AST exceeds the upper limit of normal or if the clinical signs and symptoms suggest the onset of liver failure.

Manufacturer Roche Laboratories, Inc

Related Information

Parkinson's Disease Dosing *on page 1249*
Pharmaceutical Manufacturers Directory *on page 1020*

♦ **Tolectin® 200** *see* Tolmetin *on page 930*
♦ **Tolectin® 400** *see* Tolmetin *on page 930*
♦ **Tolectin® DS** *see* Tolmetin *on page 930*
♦ **Tolinase®** *see* Tolazamide *on page 927*

Tolmetin (TOLE met in)

Pharmacologic Class Nonsteroidal Anti-Inflammatory Agent (NSAID)

U.S. Brand Names Tolectin® 200; Tolectin® 400; Tolectin® DS

Generic Available No

Mechanism of Action Inhibits prostaglandin synthesis by decreasing the activity of the enzyme, cyclo-oxygenase, which results in decreased formation of prostaglandin precursors

Use Treatment of rheumatoid arthritis and osteoarthritis, juvenile rheumatoid arthritis

USUAL DOSAGE Oral:

Children ≥2 years:

Anti-inflammatory: Initial: 20 mg/kg/day in 3 divided doses, then 15-30 mg/kg/day in 3 divided doses

Analgesic: 5-7 mg/kg/dose every 6-8 hours

Adults: 400 mg 3 times/day; usual dose: 600 mg to 1.8 g/day; maximum: 2 g/day

Dosage Forms CAP (Tolectin® DS): 400 mg. **TAB** (Tolectin®): 200 mg, 600 mg

Contraindications Known hypersensitivity to tolmetin or any component, aspirin, or other nonsteroidal anti-inflammatory drugs (NSAIDs)

Warnings/Precautions Use with caution in patients with upper GI disease, impaired renal function, congestive heart failure, hypertension, and patients receiving anticoagulants; if GI upset occurs with tolmetin, take with antacids other than sodium bicarbonate

Pregnancy Risk Factor C; D (at term)

Adverse Reactions

>10%:

Central nervous system: Dizziness
Dermatologic: Rash
Gastrointestinal: Abdominal cramps, heartburn, indigestion, nausea

1% to 10%:

Central nervous system: Headache, nervousness
Dermatologic: Itching
Endocrine & metabolic: Fluid retention
Gastrointestinal: Vomiting
Otic: Tinnitus

<1%: Acute renal failure, agranulocytosis, allergic rhinitis, anemia, angioedema, arrhythmias, aseptic meningitis, blurred vision, bone marrow suppression, confusion, congestive heart failure, conjunctivitis, cystitis, decreased hearing, drowsiness, dry eyes, epistaxis, erythema multiforme, gastritis, GI ulceration, hallucinations, hemolytic anemia, hepatitis, hot flashes, hypertension, insomnia, leukopenia, mental depression, peripheral neuropathy, polydipsia, polyuria, shortness of breath, Stevens-Johnson syndrome, tachycardia, thrombocytopenia, toxic amblyopia, toxic epidermal necrolysis, urticaria

Drug Interactions

Decreased effect with aspirin; decreased effect of thiazides, furosemide

Increased toxicity of digoxin, methotrexate, cyclosporine, lithium, insulin, sulfonylureas, potassium-sparing diuretics, aspirin

Alcohol Interactions Avoid use (may enhance gastric mucosal irritation)

Onset Analgesic: 1-2 hours; Anti-inflammatory: Days - weeks

Half-Life Biphasic: rapid: 2 hours; slow: 5 hours

Education and Monitoring Issues

Patient Education: Take this medication exactly as directed; do not increase dose without consulting prescriber. Do not crush tablets or break capsules. Take with food or milk to reduce GI distress. Maintain adequate fluid intake (2-3 L/day of fluids unless instructed to restrict fluid intake). You should have regular ophthalmic evaluations when using NSAIDs for long periods of time. Do not use alcohol, aspirin, or aspirin-containing medication, and all other anti-inflammatory medications without consulting prescriber. You may experience dizziness, nervousness, or headache (use caution when driving or engaging in tasks requiring alertness until response to drug is known); nausea, vomiting, or heartburn (frequent small meals, frequent mouth care, sucking lozenges, or chewing gum may help); constipation (increased exercise, fluids, or dietary fruit and fiber may help). GI bleeding, ulceration, or perforation can occur with or without pain; discontinue medication and contact prescriber if persistent abdominal pain or cramping, or blood in stool occurs. Report chest pain or palpitations; breathlessness or difficulty breathing; unusual bruising/bleeding; blood in urine, stool, mouth, or vomitus; unusual fatigue; skin rash or itching; unusual weight gain or swelling of extremities; change in urinary pattern; or change in vision or hearing or ringing in ears.

Monitoring Parameters: Occult blood loss, CBC, liver enzymes, BUN, serum creatinine, periodic liver function test

Related Information

Nonsteroidal Anti-Inflammatory Agents Comparison *on page 1248*

Tolnaftate (tole NAF tate)

Pharmacologic Class Antifungal Agent

U.S. Brand Names Absorbine® Antifungal [OTC]; Absorbine® Jock Itch [OTC]; Absorbine Jr.® Antifungal [OTC]; Aftate® for Athlete's Foot [OTC]; Aftate® for Jock Itch [OTC]; Blis-To-Sol® [OTC]; Breezee® Mist Antifungal [OTC]; Dr Scholl's Athlete's Foot [OTC]; Dr Scholl's Maximum Strength Tritin [OTC]; Genaspor® [OTC]; NP-27® [OTC]; Quinsana Plus® [OTC]; Tinactin® [OTC]; Tinactin® for Jock Itch [OTC]; Ting® [OTC]; Zeasorb-AF® Powder [OTC]

Use Treatment of tinea pedis, tinea cruris, tinea corporis, tinea manuum, tinea versicolor infections

USUAL DOSAGE Children and Adults: Topical: Wash and dry affected area; apply 1-3 drops of solution or a small amount of cream or powder and rub into the affected areas 2-3 times/day for 2-4 weeks

Contraindications Known hypersensitivity to tolnaftate; nail and scalp infections

Pregnancy Risk Factor C

Tolterodine (tole TER oh dine)

Pharmacologic Class Anticholinergic Agent

U.S. Brand Names Detrol™

Mechanism of Action Tolterodine is a competitive antagonist of muscarinic receptors. In animal models, tolterodine demonstrates selectivity for urinary bladder receptors over salivary receptors. Urinary bladder contraction is mediated by muscarinic receptors. Tolterodine increases residual urine volume and decreases detrusor muscle pressure.

Use Treatment of patients with an overactive bladder with symptoms of urinary frequency, urgency, or urge incontinence

USUAL DOSAGE Adults: Oral: Initial: 2 mg twice daily; the dose may be lowered to 1 mg twice daily based on individual response and tolerability

Dosing adjustment in patients concurrently taking CYP3A4 inhibitors: 1 mg twice daily

Dosing adjustment in renal impairment: Use with caution

Dosing adjustment in hepatic impairment: Administer 1 mg twice daily

Dosage Forms TAB: 1 mg, 2 mg

Contraindications Urinary retention or gastric retention; uncontrolled narrow-angle glaucoma; demonstrated hypersensitivity to tolterodine or ingredients

Warnings/Precautions Caution in patients with bladder flow obstruction, pyloric stenosis or other GI obstruction, narrow-angle glaucoma (controlled), reduced hepatic/renal function

Pregnancy Risk Factor C

Adverse Reactions

>10%: Central nervous system: Headache

1% to 10%:

- Cardiovascular: Chest pain, hypertension (1.5%)
- Central nervous system: Vertigo (8.6%), nervousness (1.1%), somnolence (3.0%)
- Dermatologic: Pruritus (1.3%), rash (1.9%), dry skin (1.7%)
- Gastrointestinal: Abdominal pain (7.6%), constipation (6.5%), diarrhea (4.0%), dyspepsia (5.9%), flatulence (1.3%), nausea (4.2%), vomiting (1.7%), weight gain (1.5%)
- Genitourinary: Dysuria (2.5%), polyuria (1.1%), urinary retention (1.7%), urinary tract infection (5.5%)
- Neuromuscular & skeletal: Back pain, falling (1.3%), paresthesia (1.1%)
- Ocular: Vision abnormalities (4.7%), dry eyes (3.8%)

(Continued)

Tolterodine *(Continued)*

Respiratory: Bronchitis (2.1%), cough (2.1%), pharyngitis (1.5%), rhinitis (1.1%), sinusitis (1.1%), upper respiratory infection (5.9%)

Miscellaneous: Flu-like symptoms (4.4%), infection (2.1%)

Drug Interactions CYP3A3/4 substrate; CYP2D6 substrate

Increased toxicity: Macrolide antibiotics/azole antifungal agents may inhibit the metabolism of tolterodine. Doses of tolterodine >1 mg twice daily should not be exceeded.

Fluoxetine, which inhibits CYP2D6, increases concentration 4.8 times. Other drugs which inhibit this isoenzyme may also interact. Studies with inhibitors of cytochrome isoenzyme 3A4 have not been performed.

Onset 1-2 hours

Duration ~12 hours

Education and Monitoring Issues

Patient Education: Take as directed, preferably with food. You may experience headache (a mild analgesic may help); dizziness, nervousness, or sleepiness (use caution when driving, climbing stairs, or engaging in tasks requiring alertness until response to drug is known); abdominal discomfort, diarrhea, constipation, nausea or vomiting (small frequent meals, increased exercise, adequate fluid intake may help). Report back pain, muscle spasms, alteration in gait, or numbness of extremities; unresolved or persistent constipation, diarrhea, or vomiting; or symptoms of upper respiratory infection or flu. Report immediately any chest pain or palpitations; difficulty urinating or pain on urination.

Dietary Considerations: Food increases bioavailability (~53% increase)

Manufacturer Pharmacia & Upjohn

Related Information

Pharmaceutical Manufacturers Directory *on page 1020*

- **Tolu-Sed® DM [OTC]** *see* Guaifenesin and Dextromethorphan *on page 424*
- **Tonocard®** *see* Tocainide *on page 926*
- **Topamax®** *see* Topiramate *on page 932*
- **Topicaine** *see* Benzocaine *on page 98*
- **Topicort** *see* Desoximetasone *on page 256*
- **Topicort®-LP** *see* Desoximetasone *on page 256*
- **Topicycline® Topical** *see* Tetracycline *on page 903*
- **Topilene** *see* Betamethasone *on page 103*

Topiramate (toe PYE ra mate)

Pharmacologic Class Anticonvulsant, Miscellaneous

U.S. Brand Names Topamax®

Mechanism of Action Mechanism is not fully understood, it is thought to decrease seizure frequency by blocking sodium channels in neurons, enhancing GABA activity and by blocking glutamate activity

Use Adjunctive therapy for partial onset seizures in adults and pediatric patients (ages 2-16 years)

Unlabeled use: Bipolar disorder

Orphan drug: Topiramate has also been granted orphan drug status for the treatment of Lennox-Gastaut syndrome

USUAL DOSAGE

Adults: Initial: 50 mg/day; titrate by 50 mg/day at 1-week intervals to target dose of 200 mg twice daily; usual maximum dose: 1600 mg/day

Children 2-16 years: Partial seizures (adjunctive therapy): Initial dose titration should begin at 25 mg (or less, based on a range of 1-3 mg/kg/day) nightly for the first week. Dosage may be increased in increments of 1-3 mg/kg/day (administered in two divided doses) at 1- or 2-week intervals to a total daily dose of 5-9 mg/kg/day.

Dosing adjustment in renal impairment: Cl_{cr} <70 mL/minute: Administer 50% dose and titrate more slowly

Dosing adjustment in hepatic impairment: Clearance may be minimally reduced

Dosage Forms CAP, sprinkle: 15 mg, 25 mg. **TAB:** 25 mg, 100 mg, 200 mg

Contraindications Patients with a known hypersensitivity to any components of this drug

Warnings/Precautions Avoid abrupt withdrawal of topiramate therapy, it should be withdrawn slowly to minimize the potential of increased seizure frequency; the risk of kidney stones is about 2-4 times that of the untreated population, the risk of this event may be reduced by increasing fluid intake; use cautiously in patients with hepatic or renal impairment, during pregnancy or in nursing mothers.

Pregnancy Risk Factor C

Pregnancy Implications Breast-feeding/lactation: In studies of rats topiramate has been shown to be secreted in milk; however, it has not been studied in humans

Adverse Reactions

>10%:

Central nervous system: Fatigue, dizziness, ataxia, somnolence, psychomotor slowing, nervousness, memory difficulties, speech problems

Gastrointestinal: Nausea
Neuromuscular & skeletal: Paresthesia, tremor
Ocular: Nystagmus
Respiratory: Upper respiratory infections

1% to 10%:
Cardiovascular: Chest pain, edema
Central nervous system: Language problems, abnormal coordination, confusion, depression, difficulty concentrating, hypoesthesia
Endocrine & metabolic: Hot flashes
Gastrointestinal: Dyspepsia, abdominal pain, anorexia, constipation, xerostomia, gingivitis, weight loss
Neuromuscular & skeletal: Myalgia, weakness, back pain, leg pain, rigors
Otic: Decreased hearing
Renal: Nephrolithiasis
Respiratory: Pharyngitis, sinusitis, epistaxis
Miscellaneous: Flu-like symptoms

Drug Interactions CYP2C19 enzyme substrate; CYP2C19 enzyme inhibitor

Decreased effect: Phenytoin can decrease topiramate levels by as much as 48%, carbamazepine reduces it by 40% and valproic acid reduces topiramate by 14%; digoxin levels and norethindrone blood levels are decreased when coadministered with topiramate

Increased toxicity: Concomitant administration with other CNS depressants will increase its sedative effects; coadministration with other carbonic anhydrase inhibitors may increase the chance of nephrolithiasis

Alcohol Interactions Avoid use (may increase central nervous system depression)

Half-Life Mean: 21 hours

Education and Monitoring Issues

Patient Education: Take exactly as directed; do not increase dose or frequency or discontinue without consulting prescriber. While using this medication, do not use alcohol and other prescription or OTC medications (especially pain medications, sedatives, antihistamines, or hypnotics) without consulting prescriber. Maintain adequate hydration (2-3 L/day of fluids unless instructed to restrict fluid intake). You may experience drowsiness, dizziness, disturbed concentration, memory changes, or blurred vision (use caution when driving or engaging in tasks requiring alertness until response to drug is known); mouth sores, nausea, vomiting, or loss of appetite (small frequent meals, frequent mouth care, chewing gum, or sucking lozenges may help). Wear identification of epileptic status and medications. Report behavioral or CNS changes; skin rash; muscle cramping, weakness, tremors, changes in gait; chest pain, irregular heartbeat, or palpitations; hearing loss; cough or difficulty breathing; worsening of seizure activity, or loss of seizure control.

Manufacturer Ortho-McNeil Pharmaceutical

Related Information

Anticonvulsants by Seizure Type Comparison *on page 1230*
Pharmaceutical Manufacturers Directory *on page 1020*

- **Topisone** *see* Betamethasone *on page 103*
- **Toprol XL®** *see* Metoprolol *on page 595*
- **Topsyn** *see* Fluocinonide *on page 375*
- **Toradol** *see* Ketorolac Tromethamine *on page 501*
- **Toradol® Injection** *see* Ketorolac Tromethamine *on page 501*
- **Toradol® Oral** *see* Ketorolac Tromethamine *on page 501*
- **Torecan** *see* Thiethylperazine *on page 912*

Toremifene (TORE em i feen)

Pharmacologic Class Antineoplastic Agent, Miscellaneous

U.S. Brand Names Fareston®

Mechanism of Action Nonsteroidal, triphenylethylene derivative. Competitively binds to estrogen receptors on tumors and other tissue targets, producing a nuclear complex that decreases DNA synthesis and inhibits estrogen effects. Nonsteroidal agent with potent antiestrogenic properties which compete with estrogen for binding sites in breast and other tissues; cells accumulate in the G_0 and G_1 phases; therefore, tamoxifen is cytostatic rather than cytocidal.

Use Treatment of metastatic breast cancer in postmenopausal women with estrogen-receptor (ER) positive or ER unknown tumors

USUAL DOSAGE Refer to individual protocols

Adults: Oral: 60 mg once daily, generally continued until disease progression is observed
60-240 mg/day
200-300 mg/day
60 mg for 3 days, then 20 mg/day

Dosage adjustment in renal impairment: No dosage adjustment necessary

Dosage adjustment in hepatic impairment: Toremifene is extensively metabolized in the liver and dosage adjustments may be indicated in patients with liver disease; however, no specific guidelines have been developed

(Continued)

Toremifene *(Continued)*

Dosage Forms TAB: 60 mg

Contraindications Hypersensitivity to toremifene

Warnings/Precautions Hypercalcemia and tumor flare have been reported in some breast cancer patients with bone metastases during the first weeks of treatment. Tumor flare is a syndrome of diffuse musculoskeletal pain and erythema with increased size of tumor lesions that later regress. It is often accompanied by hypercalcemia. Tumor flare does not imply treatment failure or represent tumor progression. Institute appropriate measures if hypercalcemia occurs, and if severe, discontinue treatment. Drugs that decrease renal calcium excretion (eg, thiazide diuretics) may increase the risk of hypercalcemia in patients receiving toremifene.

Patients with a history of thromboembolic disease should generally not be treated with toremifene

Pregnancy Risk Factor D

Adverse Reactions

>10%:

Endocrine & metabolic: Vaginal discharge, hot flashes

Gastrointestinal: Nausea

Miscellaneous: Diaphoresis

1% to 10%:

Cardiovascular: Thromboembolism: Tamoxifen has been associated with the occurrence of venous thrombosis and pulmonary embolism; arterial thrombosis has also been described in a few case reports; cardiac failure, myocardial infarction, edema

Central nervous system: Dizziness

Endocrine & metabolic: Hypercalcemia may occur in patients with bone metastases; galactorrhea and vitamin deficiency, menstrual irregularities

Gastrointestinal: Vomiting

Genitourinary: Vaginal bleeding or discharge, endometriosis, priapism, possible endometrial cancer

Ocular: Ophthalmologic effects (visual acuity changes, cataracts, or retinopathy), corneal opacities, dry eyes

Drug Interactions CYP3A3/4 enzyme substrate

Decreased effect: CYP3A4 enzyme inducers: Phenobarbital, phenytoin and carbamazepine increase the rate of toremifene metabolism and lower the steady state concentration in serum

Increased toxicity:

CYP3A4-6 enzyme inhibitors (ketoconazole, erythromycin) inhibit the metabolism of toremifene

Warfarin results in significant enhancement of the anticoagulant effects of warfarin; has been speculated that a decrease in antitumor effect of tamoxifen may also occur due to alterations in the percentage of active tamoxifen metabolites

Half-Life ~5 days

Education and Monitoring Issues

Patient Education: Take as directed, without regard to food. You may experience an initial "flare" of this disease (increased bone pain and hot flashes) which will subside with continued use. You may experience nausea, vomiting, or loss of appetite (frequent mouth care, frequent small meals, chewing gum, or sucking lozenges may help); dizziness (use caution when driving, climbing stairs, or engaging in tasks requiring alertness until response to drug is known); or loss of hair (will grow back). Report vomiting that occurs immediately after taking medication; chest pain, palpitations or swollen extremities; vaginal bleeding, hot flashes, or excessive perspiration; chest pain, unusual coughing, or difficulty breathing; or any changes in vision or dry eyes.

Monitoring Parameters: Obtain periodic complete blood counts, calcium levels, and liver function tests. Closely monitor patients with bone metastases for hypercalcemia during the first few weeks of treatment. Leukopenia and thrombocytopenia have been reported rarely; monitor leukocyte and platelet counts during treatment.

♦ **Tornalate®** *see* Bitolterol *on page 110*

Torsemide (TOR se mide)

Pharmacologic Class Diuretic, Loop

U.S. Brand Names Demadex®

Mechanism of Action Inhibits reabsorption of sodium and chloride in the ascending loop of Henle and distal renal tubule, interfering with the chloride-binding cotransport system, thus causing increased excretion of water, sodium, chloride, magnesium, and calcium; does not alter GFR, renal plasma flow, or acid-base balance

Use Management of edema associated with congestive heart failure and hepatic or renal disease; used alone or in combination with antihypertensives in treatment of hypertension; I.V. form is indicated when rapid onset is desired

USUAL DOSAGE Adults: Oral, I.V.:

Congestive heart failure: 10-20 mg once daily; may increase gradually for chronic treatment by doubling dose until the diuretic response is apparent (for acute treatment, I.V. dose may be repeated every 2 hours with double the dose as needed)

Chronic renal failure: 20 mg once daily; increase as described above

Hepatic cirrhosis: 5-10 mg once daily with an aldosterone antagonist or a potassium-sparing diuretic; increase as described above

Hypertension: 5 mg once daily; increase to 10 mg after 4-6 weeks if an adequate hypotensive response is not apparent; if still not effective, an additional antihypertensive agent may be added

Dosage Forms **INJ:** 10 mg/mL (2 mL, 5 mL). **TAB:** 5 mg, 10 mg, 20 mg, 100 mg

Contraindications Anuria; hypersensitivity to torsemide or any component, or other sulfonylureas; safety in children <18 years has not been established

Warnings/Precautions Excessive diuresis may result in dehydration, acute hypotensive or thromboembolic episodes and cardiovascular collapse; rapid injection, renal impairment, or excessively large doses may result in ototoxicity; SLE may be exacerbated; sudden alterations in electrolyte balance may precipitate hepatic encephalopathy and coma in patients with hepatic cirrhosis and ascites; monitor carefully for signs of fluid or electrolyte imbalances, especially hypokalemia in patients at risk for such (eg, digitalis therapy, history of ventricular arrhythmias, elderly, etc), hyperuricemia, hypomagnesemia, or hypocalcemia; use caution with exposure to ultraviolet light.

Pregnancy Risk Factor B

Pregnancy Implications Clinical effect on the fetus: A decrease in fetal weight, an increase in fetal resorption, and delayed fetal ossification has occurred in animal studies

Adverse Reactions

>10%: Cardiovascular: Orthostatic hypotension

1% to 10%:

- Central nervous system: Headache, dizziness, vertigo, pain
- Dermatologic: Photosensitivity, urticaria
- Endocrine & metabolic: Electrolyte imbalance, dehydration, hyperuricemia
- Gastrointestinal: Diarrhea, loss of appetite, stomach cramps
- Ocular: Blurred vision

<1%: Agranulocytosis, anemia, gout, hepatic dysfunction, interstitial nephritis, leukopenia, nausea, nephrocalcinosis, ototoxicity, pancreatitis, prerenal azotemia, rash, redness at injection site, thrombocytopenia

Drug Interactions CYP2C9 enzyme substrate

ACE inhibitors: Hypotensive effects and/or renal effects are potentiated by hypovolemia

Aminoglycosides: Ototoxicity may be increased

Anticoagulant activity is enhanced

Antidiabetic agents: Glucose tolerance may be decreased

Antihypertensive agents: Effects may be enhanced

Beta-blockers: Plasma concentrations of beta-blockers may be increased with torsemide

Chloral hydrate: Transient diaphoresis, hot flashes, hypertension may occur

Cisplatin: Ototoxicity may be increased

Digitalis: Arrhythmias may occur with diuretic-induced electrolyte disturbances

Enzyme inducers (phenytoin, phenobarbital, carbamazepine) theoretically may reduce efficacy of torsemide

Lithium: Plasma concentrations of lithium may be increased; monitor lithium levels

NSAIDs: Torsemide efficacy may be decreased

Probenecid: Torsemide action may be reduced

Salicylates: Diuretic action may be impaired in patients with cirrhosis and ascites

Thiazides: Synergistic effects may result

Onset Onset of diuresis: 30-60 minutes; Peak effect: 1-4 hours

Duration ~6 hours

Half-Life 2-4; 7-8 hours in cirrhosis (dose modification appears unnecessary)

Education and Monitoring Issues

Patient Education: Take recommended dosage with food or milk at the same time each day (preferably not in the evening to avoid sleep interruption). Do not miss doses, alter dosage, or discontinue without consulting prescriber. Include orange juice or bananas (or other potassium-rich foods) in daily diet; do not take potassium supplements without consulting prescriber. Do not use alcohol or OTC medications without consulting prescriber. You may experience postural hypotension; change position slowly when rising from sitting or lying. May cause transient drowsiness, blurred vision, or dizziness; avoid driving or engaging in tasks that require alertness until response to drug is known. You may have reduced tolerance to heat (avoid strenuous activity in hot weather or excessively hot showers). Increased exercise and increased dietary fiber, fruit, and fluids may reduce constipation. Report unusual weight gain or loss (>5 lb/week), swelling of ankles and hands, persistent fatigue, unresolved constipation or diarrhea, weakness, fatigue, dizziness, vomiting, cramps, change in hearing, or chest pain or palpitations.

Monitoring Parameters: Renal function, electrolytes, and fluid status (weight and I & O), blood pressure

Manufacturer Roche Laboratories

Related Information

Pharmaceutical Manufacturers Directory *on page 1020*

♦ **Totacillin®** *see* Ampicillin *on page 59*

♦ **Totacillin®-N** *see* Ampicillin *on page 59*

♦ **Touro Ex®** *see* Guaifenesin *on page 423*

Tramadol (TRA ma dole)

Pharmacologic Class Analgesic, Non-narcotic

U.S. Brand Names Ultram®

Mechanism of Action Binds to μ-opiate receptors in the CNS causing inhibition of ascending pain pathways, altering the perception of and response to pain; also inhibits the reuptake of norepinephrine and serotonin, which also modifies the ascending pain pathway

Use Relief of moderate to moderately severe pain

USUAL DOSAGE Adults: Oral: 50-100 mg every 4-6 hours, not to exceed 400 mg/day

Initiation of low dose followed by titration in increments of 50 mg/day every 3 days to effective dose (not >400 mg/day) may minimize dizziness and vertigo

Dosage Forms TAB: 50 mg, 100 mg

Contraindications Previous hypersensitivity to tramadol or any components; do not give to opioid-dependent patients; concurrent use of monoamine oxidase inhibitors; acute alcohol intoxication; concurrent use of centrally acting analgesics, opioids, or psychotropic drugs

Warnings/Precautions Elderly patients and patients with chronic respiratory disorders may be at greater risk of adverse events; liver disease; patients with myxedema, hypothyroidism, or hypoadrenalism should use tramadol with caution and at reduced dosages; not recommended during pregnancy or in nursing mothers; increased incidence of seizures may occur in patients receiving concurrent tricyclic antidepressants; tolerance or drug dependence may result from extended use

Pregnancy Risk Factor C

Adverse Reactions

>1%:

Central nervous system: Dizziness, headache, somnolence, stimulation, restlessness

Gastrointestinal: Nausea, diarrhea, constipation, vomiting, dyspepsia

Neuromuscular & skeletal: Weakness

Miscellaneous: Diaphoresis

<1%: Palpitations, respiratory depression, seizures, suicidal tendency

Drug Interactions CYP2D6 enzyme substrate

Decreased effects: Carbamazepine (decreases half-life by 33% to 50%)

Increased toxicity: Monoamine oxidase inhibitors and tricyclic antidepressants (seizures); quinidine (inhibits CYP2D6, thereby increases tramadol serum concentrations); cimetidine (tramadol half-life increased 20% to 25%)

Alcohol Interactions Avoid use (may increase central nervous system depression)

Onset 1 hour

Half-Life 6.3-7.4 hours

Education and Monitoring Issues

Patient Education: If self-administered, use exactly as directed (do not increase dose or frequency); may cause physical and/or psychological dependence. Take with food or milk. While using this medication, do not use alcohol and other prescription or OTC medications (especially pain medications, sedatives, antihistamines, or cough preparations) without consulting prescriber. Maintain adequate hydration (2-3 L/day of fluids unless instructed to restrict fluid intake). You may experience drowsiness, dizziness, or blurred vision (use caution when driving or engaging in tasks requiring alertness until response to drug is known); nausea, vomiting, or loss of appetite (small frequent meals, frequent mouth care, chewing gum, or sucking lozenges may help); constipation (increased exercise, fluids, or dietary fruit and fiber may help). Report severe unresolved constipation; difficulty breathing or shortness of breath; excessive sedation or increased insomnia and restlessness; changes in urinary pattern or menstrual pattern; muscle weakness or tremors; or chest pain or palpitations.

Monitoring Parameters: Monitor patient for pain, respiratory rate, and look for signs of tolerance and, therefore, abuse potential; monitor blood pressure and pulse rate, especially in patients on higher doses

Reference Range: 100-300 ng/mL; however, serum level monitoring is not required

Manufacturer Ortho-McNeil Pharmaceutical

Related Information

Pharmaceutical Manufacturers Directory *on page 1020*

♦ **Trandate®** *see* Labetalol *on page 503*

Trandolapril (tran DOE la pril)

Pharmacologic Class Angiotensin-Converting Enzyme (ACE) Inhibitors

U.S. Brand Names Mavik®

Generic Available No

Mechanism of Action Trandolapril is an angiotensin-converting enzyme (ACE) inhibitor which prevents the formation of angiotensin II from angiotensin I. Trandolapril must undergo enzymatic hydrolysis, mainly in liver, to its biologically active metabolite, trandolaprilat. A CNS mechanism may also be involved in the hypotensive effect as angiotensin

II increases adrenergic outflow from the CNS. Vasoactive kallikrein's may be decreased in conversion to active hormones by ACE inhibitors, thus, reducing blood pressure.

Use Treatment of hypertension (alone or in combination with other antihypertensive medications such as hydrochlorothiazide). For stable patients who have evidence of left-ventricular systolic dysfunction (identified by wall motion abnormalities) or who are symptomatic from CHF within the first few days after sustaining acute myocardial infarction. Administration to Caucasians decreases the risk of death (principally cardiovascular death) and decreases the risk of heart failure-related admissions.

USUAL DOSAGE Adults: Oral:

Hypertension: Initial dose in patients not receiving a diuretic: 1 mg/day (2 mg/day in black patients). Adjust dosage according to the blood pressure response. Make dosage adjustments at intervals of ≥1 week. Most patients have required dosages of 2-4 mg/day. There is a little experience with doses >8 mg/day. Patients inadequately treated with once daily dosing at 4 mg may be treated with twice daily dosing. If blood pressure is not adequately controlled with trandolapril monotherapy, a diuretic may be added.

Heart failure postmyocardial infarction or left-ventricular dysfunction postmyocardial infarction: Initial: 1 mg/day; titrate patients (as tolerated) towards the target dose of 4 mg/day. If a 4 mg dose is not tolerated, patients can continue therapy with the greatest tolerated dose.

Dosing adjustment in renal impairment: Cl_{cr} ≤30 mL/minute: Recommended starting dose: 0.5 mg/day

Dosing adjustment in hepatic impairment: Cirrhosis: Recommended starting dose: 0.5 mg/day

Dosage Forms TAB: 1 mg, 2 mg, 4 mg

Contraindications Hypersensitivity to trandolapril, other ACE inhibitors, in patients with a history of angioedema related to previous treatment with an ACE inhibitor, or any component

Warnings/Precautions Neutropenia, agranulocytosis, angioedema, decreased renal function (hypertension, renal artery stenosis, CHF), hepatic dysfunction (elimination, activation), proteinuria, first-dose hypotension (hypovolemia, CHF, dehydrated patients at risk, eg, diuretic use, elderly), elderly (due to renal function changes); use with caution and modify dosage in patients with renal impairment; use with caution in patients with collagen vascular disease, CHF, hypovolemia, valvular stenosis, hyperkalemia (>5.7 mEq/L), anesthesia

Patients taking diuretics are at risk for developing hypotension on initial dosing; to prevent this, discontinue diuretics 2-3 days prior to initiating trandolapril; may restart diuretics if blood pressure is not controlled by trandolapril alone

Pregnancy Risk Factor C (1st trimester); D (2nd and 3rd trimesters)

Adverse Reactions Note: Frequency ranges include data from hypertension and heart failure trials. Higher rates of adverse reactions have generally been noted in patients with congestive heart failure. However, the frequency of adverse effects associated with placebo is also increased in this population.

>1%:

Cardiovascular: Hypotension (<1% to 11%), bradycardia (<1% to 4.7%), intermittent claudication (3.8%), stroke (3.3%)

Central nervous system: Dizziness (1.3% to 23%), syncope (5.9%), asthenia (3.3%)

Endocrine & metabolic: Elevated uric acid (15%), hyperkalemia (5.3%), hypocalcemia (4.7%)

Gastrointestinal: Dyspepsia (6.4%), gastritis (4.2%)

Neuromuscular & skeletal: Myalgia (4.7%)

Renal: Elevated BUN (9%), elevated serum creatinine (1.1% to 4.7%) Respiratory: Cough (1.9% to 35%)

<1% (limited to important or life-threatening symptoms): Chest pain, A-V block (first-degree), edema, flushing, palpitations, drowsiness, insomnia, paresthesia, vertigo, pruritus, rash, pemphigus, epistaxis, pharyngitis, upper respiratory tract infection, anxiety, impotence, decreased libido, abdominal distension, abdominal pain, constipation dyspepsia, diarrhea, vomiting, pancreatitis, leukopenia, neutropenia, thrombocytopenia, increased serum creatinine, increased ALT, muscle pain, gout, dyspnea, angioedema, laryngeal edema, symptomatic hypotension, transaminase elevation, increased bilirubin. Worsening of renal function may occur in patients with bilateral renal artery stenosis or in hypovolemic patients. In addition, a syndrome which may include fever, myalgia, arthralgia, interstitial nephritis, vasculitis, rash, eosinophilia and positive ANA, and elevated ESR has been reported with ACE inhibitors.

Drug Interactions

$Alpha_1$ blockers: Hypotensive effect increased

Aspirin and NSAIDs may decrease ACE inhibitor efficacy

Diuretics: Hypovolemia due to diuretics may precipitate acute hypotensive events or acute renal failure

Insulin: Risk of hypoglycemia may be increased

Lithium: Risk of lithium toxicity may be increased; monitor lithium levels, especially the first 4 weeks of therapy

Mercaptopurine: Risk of neutropenia may be increased

(Continued)

Trandolapril *(Continued)*

Potassium-sparing diuretics (amiloride, potassium, spironolactone, triamterene): Increased risk of hyperkalemia
Potassium supplements may increase the risk of hyperkalemia
Trimethoprim (high dose) may increase the risk of hyperkalemia

Alcohol Interactions Avoid use (may increase risk of hypotension or dizziness)

Onset 1-2 hours

Duration Trandolaprilat (active metabolite) is very lipophilic in comparison to other ACE inhibitors which may contribute to its prolonged duration of action (72 hours after a single dose)

Half-Life Parent: 6 hours; Active metabolite trandolaprilat: 10 hours

Education and Monitoring Issues

Patient Education: Take exactly as directed; do not discontinue without consulting prescriber. Take first dose at bedtime. This drug does not eliminate need for diet or exercise regimen as recommended by prescriber. May cause dizziness, fainting, lightheadedness (use caution when driving or engaging in tasks requiring alertness until response to drug is known); diarrhea (buttermilk, boiled milk, yogurt may help). Report chest pain or palpitations; swelling of extremities, mouth or tongue; skin rash; difficulty in breathing or unusual cough; or other persistent adverse reactions.

Monitoring Parameters: Serum potassium, renal function, serum creatinine, BUN, CBC

Manufacturer Knoll Pharmaceutical Company

Related Information

Angiotensin-Related Agents Comparison *on page 1226*
Pharmaceutical Manufacturers Directory *on page 1020*
Trandolapril and Verapamil *on page 938*

Trandolapril and Verapamil (tran DOE la pril & ver AP a mil)

Pharmacologic Class Antihypertensive Agent, Combination

U.S. Brand Names Tarka®

Dosage Forms TAB: Trandolapril 1 mg and verapamil hydrochloride 240 mg; Trandolapril 2 mg and verapamil hydrochloride 180 mg; Trandolapril 2 mg and verapamil hydrochloride 240 mg; Trandolapril 4 mg and verapamil hydrochloride 240 mg

Pregnancy Risk Factor C (1st trimester); D (2nd and 3rd trimesters)

Alcohol Interactions Avoid use (may increase risk of hypotension or dizziness)

Manufacturer Knoll Pharmaceutical Company

Related Information

Pharmaceutical Manufacturers Directory *on page 1020*

- **Transdermal-NTG® Patch** *see* Nitroglycerin *on page 659*
- **Transderm-Nitro®** *see* Nitroglycerin *on page 659*
- **Transderm-Nitro® Patch** *see* Nitroglycerin *on page 659*
- **Transderm Scop® Patch** *see* Scopolamine *on page 842*
- **Transderm-V** *see* Scopolamine *on page 842*
- **Tranxene®** *see* Clorazepate *on page 218*

Tranylcypromine (tran il SIP roe meen)

Pharmacologic Class Antidepressant, Monoamine Oxidase Inhibitor

U.S. Brand Names Parnate®

Generic Available No

Mechanism of Action Inhibits the enzymes monoamine oxidase A and B which are responsible for the intraneuronal metabolism of norepinephrine and serotonin and increasing their availability to postsynaptic neurons; decreased firing rate of the locus ceruleus, reducing norepinephrine concentration in the brain; agonist effects of serotonin

Use Symptomatic treatment of depressed patients refractory to or intolerant to tricyclic antidepressants or electroconvulsive therapy; has a more rapid onset of therapeutic effect than other MAO inhibitors, but causes more severe hypertensive reactions

USUAL DOSAGE Adults: Oral: 10 mg twice daily, increase by 10 mg increments at 1- to 3-week intervals; maximum: 60 mg/day

Dosing comments in hepatic impairment: Use with care and monitor plasma levels and patient response closely

Dosage Forms TAB: 10 mg

Contraindications Uncontrolled hypertension, known hypersensitivity to tranylcypromine, pheochromocytoma, cardiovascular disease, severe renal or hepatic impairment, pheochromocytoma

Warnings/Precautions Safety in children <16 years of age has not been established; use with caution in patients who are hyperactive, hyperexcitable, or who have glaucoma, suicidal tendencies, diabetes, elderly

Pregnancy Risk Factor C

Adverse Reactions

Cardiovascular: Orthostatic hypotension, edema

Central nervous system: Dizziness, headache, drowsiness, sleep disturbances, fatigue, hyper-reflexia, twitching, ataxia, mania
Dermatologic: Rash, pruritus
Endocrine & metabolic: Decreased sexual ability (anorgasmia, ejaculatory disturbances, impotence), hypernatremia, hypermetabolic syndrome
Gastrointestinal: Xerostomia, constipation, weight gain
Genitourinary: Urinary retention
Hematologic: Leukopenia
Hepatic: Hepatitis
Neuromuscular & skeletal: Weakness, tremor, myoclonus
Ocular: Blurred vision, glaucoma
Miscellaneous: diaphoresis

Drug Interactions CYP2A6 and 2C19 enzyme inhibitor

In general, the combined use of tranylcypromine with TCAs, venlafaxine, trazodone, and SSRIs should be divided due to the potential for severe adverse reactions (serotonin syndrome, death)
MAOIs may inhibit the metabolism of barbiturates and prolong their effect
MAOIs in combination with dexfenfluramine, sibutramine, meperidine, fenfluramine, and dextromethorphan may cause serotonin syndrome; these combinations are best avoided
MAOIs in combination with amphetamines, other stimulants (methylphenidate), metaraminol, and decongestants (pseudoephedrine) may result in severe hypertensive reaction; these combinations are best avoided
Foods (eg, cheese) and beverages (eg, ethanol) containing tyramine, should be avoided in patients receiving an MAOI; hypertensive crisis may result
MAOIs inhibit the antihypertensive response to guanadrel or guanethidine; use an alternative antihypertensive agent
MAOIs in combination with levodopa and reserpine may result in hypertensive reactions; monitor
MAOIs in combination with lithium have resulted in malignant hyperpyrexia; this combination is best avoided
MAOIs may increase the pressor response of norepinephrine; monitor
MAOIs may prolong the muscle relaxation produced by succinylcholine via decreased plasma pseudocholinesterase
Tramadol may increase the risk of seizures and serotonin in patients receiving an MAOI
MAOIs may produce hypoglycemia in patients with diabetes; monitor
MAOIs may produce delirium in patients receiving disulfiram; monitor

Alcohol Interactions Avoid use (alcoholic beverages containing tyramine may induce a severe hypertensive response)

Onset 2-3 weeks of continued dosing are required to obtain full therapeutic effect

Duration May continue to have a therapeutic effect and interactions 2 weeks after discontinuing therapy

Half-Life 90-190 minutes

Education and Monitoring Issues

Patient Education: Take exactly as directed (do not increase dose or frequency); may take 2-3 weeks to achieve desired results; may cause physical and/or psychological dependence. Take in the morning to reduce the incidence of insomnia. Avoid excessive alcohol, caffeine, and other prescription or OTC medications not approved by prescriber. Avoid tyramine-containing foods (eg pickles, aged cheese, wine); see prescriber for complete list of foods to be avoided. Maintain adequate hydration (2-3 L/day of fluids unless instructed to restrict fluid intake). You may experience drowsiness, dizziness, or blurred vision (use caution when driving or engaging in tasks requiring alertness until response to drug is known); anorexia or dry mouth (small frequent meals, frequent mouth care, chewing gum, or sucking lozenges may help); constipation (increased exercise, fluids, or dietary fruit and fiber may help); diarrhea (buttermilk, yogurt, or boiled milk may help); orthostatic hypotension (use caution when climbing stairs or changing position from lying or sitting to standing); or altered sexual ability (reversible). Report persistent excessive sedation; muscle cramping, tremors, weakness, or change in gait; chest pain, palpitations, rapid heartbeat, or swelling of extremities; vision changes; or worsening of condition.

Dietary Considerations: Food: Avoid tyramine-containing foods

Monitoring Parameters: Blood pressure, blood glucose

Manufacturer SmithKline Beecham Pharmaceuticals

Related Information

Antidepressant Agents Comparison *on page 1231*
Pharmaceutical Manufacturers Directory *on page 1020*

Trastuzumab (tras TU zoo mab)

Pharmacologic Class Antineoplastic Agent, Miscellaneous

U.S. Brand Names Herceptin®

Mechanism of Action Trastuzumab is a monoclonal antibody which binds to the extracellular domain of the human epidermal growth factor receptor 2 protein (HER2); it mediates antibody-dependent cellular cytotoxicity against cells which overproduce HER2

(Continued)

Trastuzumab *(Continued)*

Use

Single agent for the treatment of patients with metastatic breast cancer whose tumors overexpress the HER2/neu protein and who have received one or more chemotherapy regimens for their metastatic disease

Combination therapy with paclitaxel for the treatment of patients with metastatic breast cancer whose tumors overexpress the HER2/neu protein and who have not received chemotherapy for their metastatic disease

Note: HER2/neu protein overexpression or amplification has been noted in ovarian, gastric, colorectal, endometrial, lung, bladder, prostate, and salivary gland tumors. It is not yet known whether trastuzumab may be effective in these other carcinomas which overexpress HER2/neu protein.

USUAL DOSAGE I.V. infusion:

Adults:

Initial loading dose: 4 mg/kg intravenous infusion over 90 minutes

Maintenance dose: 2 mg/kg intravenous infusion over 90 minutes (can be administered over 30 minutes if prior infusions are well tolerated) weekly until disease progression

Dosing adjustment in renal impairment: Data suggest that the disposition of trastuzumab is not altered based on age or serum creatinine (up to 2 mg/dL); however, no formal interaction studies have been performed

Dosing adjustment in hepatic impairment: No data is currently available

Dosage Forms POWDER for inj: 440 mg

Contraindications None known

Warnings/Precautions Congestive heart failure associated with trastuzumab may be severe and has been associated with disabling cardiac failure, death, mural thrombus, and stroke. Left ventricular function should be evaluated in all patients prior to and during treatment with trastuzumab. Discontinuation should be strongly considered in patients who develop a clinically significant decrease in ejection fraction during therapy. Combination therapy which includes anthracyclines and cyclophosphamide increases the incidence and severity of cardiac dysfunction. Extreme caution should be used when treating patients with pre-existing cardiac disease or dysfunction, and in patients with previous exposure to anthracyclines. Advanced age may also predispose to cardiac toxicity. Hypersensitivity to hamster ovary cell proteins or any component of this product.

Pregnancy Risk Factor B

Pregnancy Implications It is not known whether trastuzumab is secreted in human milk; because many immunoglobulins are secreted in milk, and the potential for serious adverse reactions exists, patients should discontinue nursing during treatment and for 6 months after the last dose

Adverse Reactions

>10%:

Central nervous system: Pain (47%), fever (36%), chills (32%), headache (26%)

Dermatologic: Rash (18%)

Neuromuscular & skeletal: Weakness (42%), back pain (22%)

Gastrointestinal: Nausea (33%), diarrhea (25%), vomiting (23%), abdominal pain (22%), anorexia (14%)

Respiratory: Cough (26%), dyspnea (22%), rhinitis (14%), pharyngitis (12%)

Miscellaneous: Infection (20%)

1% to 10%:

Cardiovascular: Peripheral edema (10%), congestive heart failure (7%), tachycardia (5%)

Central nervous system: Insomnia (14%), dizziness (13%), paresthesia (9%), depression (6%), peripheral neuritis (2%), neuropathy (1%)

Dermatologic: Herpes simplex (2%), acne (2%)

Gastrointestinal: Nausea and vomiting (8%)

Genitourinary: Urinary tract infection (5%)

Hematologic: Anemia (4%), leukopenia (3%)

Neuromuscular & skeletal: Bone pain (7%), arthralgia (6%)

Respiratory: Sinusitis (9%)

Miscellaneous: Flu syndrome (10%), accidental injury (6%), allergic reaction (3%)

<1%: Acute leukemia, amblyopia, anaphylactoid reaction, arrhythmia, ascites, cardiac arrest, cellulitis, coagulopathy, colitis, deafness, esophageal ulcer, gastroenteritis, hematemesis, hemorrhage, hepatic failure, hepatitis, hydrocephalus, hypotension, hypothyroidism, ileus, intestinal obstruction, lymphangitis, pancreatitis, pancytopenia, pericardial effusion, radiation injury, shock, stomatitis, syncope, vascular thrombosis

Drug Interactions Increased effect: Paclitaxel may result in a decrease in clearance of trastuzumab, increasing serum concentrations

Half-Life Mean: 5.8 days (range: 1-32 days)

Education and Monitoring Issues

Patient Education: This medication can only be administered by infusion. Report immediately any adverse reactions during infusion (eg, chills, fever, headache, backache, or nausea/vomiting) so appropriate medication can be administered. You will be susceptible to infection (avoid crowds or exposure to persons with infections or contagious diseases). You may experience dizziness or weakness (use caution when driving or engaging in tasks requiring alertness until response to drug is known); nausea or vomiting (small frequent meals, frequent mouth care, chewing gum, or sucking lozenges may help); diarrhea (boiled milk, yogurt, or buttermilk may help); or headache, back or joint pain (mild analgesics may offer relief). Report persistent gastrointestinal effects; sore throat, runny nose, or difficulty breathing; chest pain, irregular heartbeat, palpitations, swelling of extremities, or unusual weight gain; muscle or joint weakness, numbness, or pain; skin rash or irritation; itching or pain on urination; unhealed sores, white plaques in mouth or genital area, unusual bruising or bleeding; or other unusual effects related to this medication.

Monitoring Parameters: Signs and symptoms of cardiac dysfunction

Manufacturer Genentech, Inc

Related Information

Pharmaceutical Manufacturers Directory *on page 1020*

♦ **Trasylol®** *see* Aprotinin *on page 70*

Trazodone (TRAZ oh done)

Pharmacologic Class Antidepressant, Serotonin Reuptake Inhibitor/Antagonist

U.S. Brand Names Desyrel®

Generic Available Yes

Mechanism of Action Inhibits reuptake of serotonin and norepinephrine by the presynaptic neuronal membrane and desensitization of adenyl cyclase, down regulation of beta-adrenergic receptors, and down regulation of serotonin receptors

Use Treatment of depression

USUAL DOSAGE Oral: Therapeutic effects may take up to 4 weeks to occur; therapy is normally maintained for several months after optimum response is reached to prevent recurrence of depression

Children 6-18 years: Initial: 1.5-2 mg/kg/day in divided doses; increase gradually every 3-4 days as needed; maximum: 6 mg/kg/day in 3 divided doses

Adolescents: Initial: 25-50 mg/day; increase to 100-150 mg/day in divided doses

Adults: Initial: 150 mg/day in 3 divided doses (may increase by 50 mg/day every 3-7 days); maximum: 600 mg/day

Elderly: 25-50 mg at bedtime with 25-50 mg/day dose increase every 3 days for inpatients and weekly for outpatients, if tolerated; usual dose: 75-150 mg/day

Dosage Forms TAB: 50 mg, 100 mg, 150 mg, 300 mg

Contraindications Hypersensitivity to trazodone or any component

Warnings/Precautions Safety and efficacy in children <18 years of age have not been established; monitor closely and use with extreme caution in patients with cardiac disease or arrhythmias. Very sedating, but little anticholinergic effects; therapeutic effects may take up to 4 weeks to occur; therapy is normally maintained for several months after optimum response is reached to prevent recurrence of depression.

Pregnancy Risk Factor C

Adverse Reactions

>10%:

Central nervous system: Dizziness, headache, sedation

Gastrointestinal: Nausea, xerostomia

1% to 10%:

Cardiovascular: Syncope, hypertension, hypotension, edema

Central nervous system: Confusion, decreased concentration, fatigue, incoordination

Gastrointestinal: Diarrhea, constipation, weight gain or loss

Neuromuscular & skeletal: Tremor, myalgia

Ocular: Blurred vision

Respiratory: Nasal congestion

<1%: Agitation, bradycardia, extrapyramidal reactions, hepatitis, priapism, rash, seizures, tachycardia, urinary retention

Drug Interactions CYP2D6 and 3A3/4 enzyme substrate

Trazodone in combination with other serotonergic agents (buspirone, MAOIs) may produce additive serotonergic effects

Trazodone in combination with other psychotropics (low potency antipsychotics) may result in additional hypotension

Trazodone in combination with ethanol may result in additive sedation and impairment of motor skills

Fluoxetine may inhibit the metabolism of trazodone resulting in elevated plasma levels

Alcohol Interactions Avoid use (may increase central nervous system depression)

Onset Therapeutic effects take 1-3 weeks to appear

Half-Life 4-7.5 hours, 2 compartment kinetics

Education and Monitoring Issues

Patient Education: Take exactly as directed (do not increase dose or frequency); may take 2-4 weeks to achieve desired results; may cause physical and/or psychological dependence. Take after meals. Avoid excessive alcohol, caffeine, and other prescription or OTC medications not approved by prescriber. Maintain adequate hydration (2-3 L/day of fluids unless instructed to restrict fluid intake). You may experience drowsiness, lightheadedness, dizziness (use caution when driving or engaging in tasks

(Continued)

Trazodone *(Continued)*

requiring alertness until response to drug is known); postural hypotension (use caution when climbing stairs or changing position from lying or sitting to standing); nausea, dry mouth (small frequent meals, frequent mouth care, chewing gum, or sucking lozenges may help); constipation (increased exercise, fluids, or dietary fruit and fiber may help); or diarrhea (buttermilk, yogurt, or boiled milk may help). Report persistent dizziness or headache; muscle cramping, tremors, or altered gait; blurred vision or eye pain; chest pain or irregular heartbeat; or worsening of condition.

Reference Range:

Plasma levels do not always correlate with clinical effectiveness

Therapeutic: 0.5-2.5 µg/mL

Potentially toxic: >2.5 µg/mL

Toxic: >4 µg/mL

Related Information

Antidepressant Agents Comparison *on page 1231*

- **Treatment of Cardiovascular Disease in the Diabetic** *see page 1136*
- **Treatment of Sexually Transmitted Diseases** *see page 1210*
- **Trecator®-SC** *see* Ethionamide *on page 345*
- **Tremytoine®** *see* Phenytoin *on page 730*
- **Trendar® [OTC]** *see* Ibuprofen *on page 458*
- **Trental®** *see* Pentoxifylline *on page 715*

Tretinoin, Oral (TRET i noyn, oral)

Pharmacologic Class Antineoplastic Agent, Miscellaneous

U.S. Brand Names Vesanoid®

Mechanism of Action Retinoid that induces maturation of acute promyelocytic leukemia (APL) cells in cultures; induces cytodifferentiation and decreased proliferation of APL cells

Use Acute promyelocytic leukemia (APL): Induction of remission in patients with APL, French American British (FAB) classification M3 (including the M3 variant), characterized by the presence of the t(15;17) translocation or the presence of the PML/RARα gene who are refractory to or who have relapsed from anthracycline chemotherapy, or for whom anthracycline-based chemotherapy is contraindicated. Tretinoin is for the induction of remission only. All patients should receive an accepted form of remission consolidation or maintenance therapy for APL after completion of induction therapy with tretinoin.

USUAL DOSAGE Oral:

Children: There are limited clinical data on the pediatric use of tretinoin. Of 15 pediatric patients (age range: 1-16 years) treated with tretinoin, the incidence of complete remission was 67%. Safety and efficacy in pediatric patients <1 year of age have not been established. Some pediatric patients experience severe headache and pseudotumor cerebri, requiring analgesic treatment and lumbar puncture for relief. Increased caution is recommended. Consider dose reduction in children experiencing serious or intolerable toxicity; however, the efficacy and safety of tretinoin at doses <45 mg/m^2/day have not been evaluated.

Adults: 45 mg/m^2/day administered as two evenly divided doses until complete remission is documented. Discontinue therapy 30 days after achievement of complete remission or after 90 days of treatment, whichever occurs first. If after initiation of treatment the presence of the t(15;17) translocation is not confirmed by cytogenetics or by polymerase chain reaction studies and the patient has not responded to tretinoin, consider alternative therapy.

Note: Tretinoin is for the induction of remission only. Optimal consolidation or maintenance regimens have not been determined. All patients should therefore receive a standard consolidation or maintenance chemotherapy regimen for APL after induction therapy with tretinoin unless otherwise contraindicated.

Dosage Forms CAP: 10 mg

Contraindications Sensitivity to parabens, vitamin A, or other retinoids

Warnings/Precautions Patients with acute promyelocytic leukemia (APL) are at high risk and can have severe adverse reactions to tretinoin. Administer under the supervision of a prescriber who is experienced in the management of patients with acute leukemia and in a facility with laboratory and supportive services sufficient to monitor drug tolerance and to protect and maintain a patient compromised by drug toxicity, including respiratory compromise.

About 25% of patients with APL, who have been treated with tretinoin, have experienced a syndrome called the retinoic acid-APL (RA-APL) syndrome which is characterized by fever, dyspnea, weight gain, radiographic pulmonary infiltrates and pleural or pericardial effusions. This syndrome has occasionally been accompanied by impaired myocardial contractility and episodic hypotension. It has been observed with or without concomitant leukocytosis. Endotracheal intubation and mechanical ventilation have been required in some cases due to progressive hypoxemia, and several patients have expired with multiorgan failure. The syndrome usually occurs during the first month of treatment, with some cases reported following the first dose.

Management of the syndrome has not been defined, but high-dose steroids given at the first suspicion of RA-APL syndrome appear to reduce morbidity and mortality. At the first signs suggestive of the syndrome, immediately initiate high-dose steroids (dexamethasone 10 mg I.V.) every 12 hours for 3 days or until resolution of symptoms, regardless of the leukocyte count. The majority of patients do not require termination of tretinoin therapy during treatment of the RA-APL syndrome.

During treatment, ~40% of patients will develop rapidly evolving leukocytosis. Rapidly evolving leukocytosis is associated with a higher risk of life-threatening complications.

If signs and symptoms of the RA-APL syndrome are present together with leukocytosis, initiate treatment with high-dose steroids immediately. Consider adding full-dose chemotherapy (including an anthracycline, if not contraindicated) to the tretinoin therapy on day 1 or 2 for patients presenting with a WBC count of $>5 \times 10^9$/L or immediately, for patients presenting with a WBC count of $<5 \times 10^9$/L, if the WBC count reaches $\geq 6 \times 10^9$/L by day 5, or $\geq 10 \times 10^9$/L by day 10 or $\geq 15 \times 10^9$/L by day 28.

Not to be used in women of childbearing potential unless the woman is capable of complying with effective contraceptive measures; therapy is normally begun on the second or third day of next normal menstrual period; two reliable methods of effective contraception must be used during therapy and for 1 month after discontinuation of therapy, unless abstinence is the chosen method. Within one week prior to the institution of tretinoin therapy, the patient should have blood or urine collected for a serum or urine pregnancy test with a sensitivity of at least 50 mIU/L. When possible, delay tretinoin therapy until a negative result from this test is obtained. When a delay is not possible, place the patient on two reliable forms of contraception. Repeat pregnancy testing and contraception counseling monthly throughout the period of treatment.

Initiation of therapy with tretinoin may be based on the morphological diagnosis of APL. Confirm the diagnosis of APL by detection of the t(15;17) genetic marker by cytogenetic studies. If these are negative, PML/RARα fusion should be sought using molecular diagnostic techniques. The response rate of other AML subtypes to tretinoin has not been demonstrated.

Retinoids have been associated with pseudotumor cerebri (benign intracranial hypertension), especially in children. Early signs and symptoms include papilledema, headache, nausea, vomiting and visual disturbances.

Up to 60% of patients experienced hypercholesterolemia or hypertriglyceridemia, which were reversible upon completion of treatment.

Elevated liver function test results occur in 50% to 60% of patients during treatment. Carefully monitor liver function test results during treatment and give consideration to a temporary withdrawal of tretinoin if test results reach >5 times the upper limit of normal.

Pregnancy Risk Factor D

Adverse Reactions Virtually all patients experience some drug-related toxicity, especially headache, fever, weakness and fatigue. These adverse effects are seldom permanent or irreversible nor do they usually require therapy interruption

>10%:
- Cardiovascular: Arrhythmias, flushing, hypotension, hypertension, peripheral edema, chest discomfort, edema
- Central nervous system: Dizziness, anxiety, insomnia, depression, confusion, malaise, pain
- Dermatologic: Burning, redness, cheilitis, inflammation of lips, dry skin, pruritus, photosensitivity
- Endocrine & metabolic: Increased serum concentration of triglycerides
- Gastrointestinal: GI hemorrhage, abdominal pain, other GI disorders, diarrhea, constipation, dyspepsia, abdominal distention, weight gain or loss, xerostomia
- Hematologic: Hemorrhage, disseminated intravascular coagulation
- Local: Phlebitis, injection site reactions
- Neuromuscular & skeletal: Bone pain, arthralgia, myalgia, paresthesia
- Ocular: Itching of eye
- Renal: Renal insufficiency
- Respiratory: Upper respiratory tract disorders, dyspnea, respiratory insufficiency, pleural effusion, pneumonia, rales, expiratory wheezing, dry nose
- Miscellaneous: Infections, shivering

1% to 10%:
- Cardiovascular: Cardiac failure, cardiac arrest, myocardial infarction, enlarged heart, heart murmur, ischemia, stroke, myocarditis, pericarditis, pulmonary hypertension, secondary cardiomyopathy, cerebral hemorrhage, pallor
- Central nervous system: Intracranial hypertension, agitation, hallucination, agnosia, aphasia, cerebellar edema, cerebellar disorders, convulsions, coma, CNS depression, encephalopathy, hypotaxia, no light reflex, neurologic reaction, spinal cord disorder, unconsciousness, dementia, forgetfulness, somnolence, slow speech, hypothermia
- Dermatologic: Skin peeling on hands or soles of feet, rash, cellulitis
- Endocrine & metabolic: Fluid imbalance, acidosis
- Gastrointestinal: Hepatosplenomegaly, ulcer

(Continued)

Tretinoin, Oral *(Continued)*

Genitourinary: Dysuria, polyuria, enlarged prostate
Hepatic: Ascites, hepatitis
Neuromuscular & skeletal: Tremor, leg weakness, hyporeflexia, dysarthria, facial paralysis, hemiplegia, flank pain, asterixis, abnormal gait
Ocular: Dry eyes, photophobia
Renal: Acute renal failure, renal tubular necrosis
Respiratory: Lower respiratory tract disorders, pulmonary infiltration, bronchial asthma, pulmonary/larynx edema, unspecified pulmonary disease
Miscellaneous: Face edema, lymph disorders

<1%: Alopecia, anorexia, bleeding of gums, cataracts, conjunctivitis, corneal opacities, decrease in hemoglobin and hematocrit, hyperuricemia, increase in erythrocyte sedimentation rate, inflammatory bowel syndrome, mood changes, nausea, optic neuritis, pseudomotor cerebri, vomiting

Drug Interactions CYP3A3/4 enzyme substrate

Metabolized by the hepatic cytochrome P-450 system; therefore, all drugs that induce or inhibit this system would be expected to interact with tretinoin CYP2C9 substrate

Increased toxicity: Ketoconazole increases the mean plasma AUC of tretinoin

Half-Life Parent drug: 0.5-2 hours

Education and Monitoring Issues

Patient Education: Take with food. Do not crush, chew, or dissolve capsules. You will need frequent blood tests while taking this medication. Maintain adequate hydration (2-3 L/day of fluids unless instructed to restrict fluid intake), avoid alcohol and foods containing vitamin A, and foods with high fat content. You may experience lethargy, dizziness, visual changes, confusion, anxiety (avoid driving or engaging in tasks requiring alertness until response to drug is known). For nausea and vomiting, loss of appetite, or dry mouth small, frequent meals, chewing gum, or sucking lozenges may help. You may experience photosensitivity (use sunscreen, wear protective clothing and eyewear, avoid direct sunlight). You may experience dry, itchy, skin, and dry or irritated eyes (avoid contact lenses). Report persistent vomiting or diarrhea, difficulty breathing, unusual bleeding or bruising, acute GI pain, bone pain, or vision changes immediately.

Dietary Considerations: Absorption of retinoids has been shown to be enhanced when taken with food

Monitoring Parameters: Monitor the patient's hematologic profile, coagulation profile, liver function test results and triglyceride and cholesterol levels frequently

Tretinoin, Topical (TRET i noyn, TOP i kal)

Pharmacologic Class Retinoic Acid Derivative

U.S. Brand Names Avita®; Renova™; Retin-A™ Micro Topical; Retin-A™ Topical

Use Treatment of acne vulgaris, photodamaged skin, and some skin cancers

USUAL DOSAGE Children >12 years and Adults: Topical: Begin therapy with a weaker formulation of tretinoin (0.025% cream or 0.01% gel) and increase the concentration as tolerated; apply once daily before retiring or on alternate days; if stinging or irritation develop, decrease frequency of application

Contraindications Hypersensitivity to tretinoin or any component; sunburn

Pregnancy Risk Factor C

- **Triacet™** *see* Triamcinolone *on page 944*
- **Triacin-C®** *see* Triprolidine, Pseudoephedrine, and Codeine *on page 958*
- **Triad®** *see* Butalbital Compound *on page 123*
- **Triadapin®** *see* Doxepin *on page 298*
- **Triaderm** *see* Triamcinolone *on page 944*
- **Triam-A®** *see* Triamcinolone *on page 944*

Triamcinolone (trye am SIN oh lone)

Pharmacologic Class Corticosteroid, Oral Inhaler; Corticosteroid, Nasal; Corticosteroid, Parenteral

U.S. Brand Names Amcort®; Aristocort®; Aristocort® A; Aristocort® Forte; Aristocort® Intralesional; Aristospan® Intra-Articular; Aristospan® Intralesional; Atolone®; Azmacort™; Delta-Tritex®; Flutex®; Kenacort®; Kenaject-40®; Kenalog®; Kenalog-10®; Kenalog-40®; Kenalog® H; Kenalog® in Orabase®; Kenonel®; Nasacort®; Nasacort® AQ; Tac™-3; Tac™-40; Triacet™; Triam-A®; Triam Forte®; Triderm®; Tri-Kort®; Trilog®; Trilone®; Tri-nasal®; Tristoject®

Generic Available Yes

Mechanism of Action Decreases inflammation by suppression of migration of polymorphonuclear leukocytes and reversal of increased capillary permeability; suppresses the immune system by reducing activity and volume of the lymphatic system; suppresses adrenal function at high doses

Use

Inhalation: Control of bronchial asthma and related bronchospastic conditions.
Nasal spray: Treatment of the nasal symptoms of seasonal and perennial allergic rhinitis

Systemic: Adrenocortical insufficiency, rheumatic disorders, allergic states, respiratory diseases, systemic lupus erythematosus, and other diseases requiring anti-inflammatory or immunosuppressive effects

Topical: Inflammatory dermatoses responsive to steroids

USUAL DOSAGE In general, single I.M. dose of 4-7 times oral dose will control patient from 4-7 days up to 3-4 weeks

Children 6-12 years:

Oral inhalation: 1-2 inhalations 3-4 times/day, not to exceed 12 inhalations/day

I.M. (acetonide or hexacetonide): 0.03-0.2 mg/kg at 1- to 7-day intervals

Intra-articular, intrabursal, or tendon-sheath injection: 2.5-15 mg, repeated as needed

Children >12 years and Adults:

Intranasal: 2 sprays in each nostril once daily; may increase after 4-7 days up to 4 sprays once daily or 1 spray 4 times/day in each nostril

Topical: Apply a thin film 2-3 times/day. Therapy should be discontinued when control is achieved; if no improvement is seen, reassessment of diagnosis may be necessary.

Oral: 4-48 mg/day

I.M. (acetonide or hexacetonide): 60 mg (of 40 mg/mL), additional 20-100 mg doses (usual: 40-80 mg) may be given when signs and symptoms recur, best at 6-week intervals to minimize HPA suppression

Intra-articular (hexacetonide): 2-20 mg every 3-4 weeks

Intralesional (diacetate or acetonide - use 10 mg/mL): 1 mg/injection site, may be repeated one or more times/week depending upon patient's response; maximum: 30 mg at any one time; may use multiple injections if they are more than 1 cm apart

Intra-articular, intrasynovial, and soft-tissue (diacetate or acetonide - use 10 mg/mL or 40 mg/mL) 2.5-40 mg depending upon location, size of joints, and degree of inflammation; repeat when signs and symptoms recur

Sublesionally (as acetonide): Up to 1 mg per injection site and may be repeated one or more times weekly; multiple sites may be injected if they are 1 cm or more apart, not to exceed 30 mg

See table.

Triamcinolone Dosing

	Acetonide	Diacetate	Hexacetonide
Intrasynovial	2.5-40 mg	5-40 mg	
Intralesional	2.5-40 mg	5-48 mg	Up to 0.5 mg/sq inch affected area
Sublesional	1-30 mg		
Systemic I.M.	2.5-60 mg/d	~40 mg/wk	20-100 mg
Intra-articular		5-40 mg	2-20 mg average
large joints	5-15 mg		10-20 mg
small joints	2.5-5 mg		2-6 mg
Tendon sheaths	10-40 mg		
Intradermal	1 mg/site		

Oral inhalation: 2 inhalations 3-4 times/day, not to exceed 16 inhalations/day

Dosage Forms AERO: Oral inh: 100 mcg/metered spray (2 oz); Nasal: 55 mcg per actuation (15 mL). **OINT, oral:** 0.1% (5 g). **SYR:** 2 mg/5 mL (120 mL), 4 mg/5 mL (120 mL). **TAB:** 1 mg, 2 mg, 4 mg, 8 mg

Triamcinolone acetonide: **AERO, top:** 0.2 mg/2 second spray (23 g, 63 g). **CRM:** 0.025% (15 g, 60 g, 80 g, 240 g, 454 g), 0.1% (15 g, 30 g, 60 g, 80 g, 90 g, 120 g, 240 g), 0.5% (15 g, 20 g, 30 g, 240 g). **INJ:** 10 mg/mL (5 mL); 40 mg/mL (1 mL, 5 mL, 10 mL). **LOT:** 0.025% (60 mL), 0.1% (15 mL, 60 mL). **OINT, top:** 0.025% (15 g, 30 g, 60 g, 80 g, 120 g, 454 g), 0.1% (15 g, 30 g, 60 g, 80 g, 120 g, 240 g, 454 g), 0.5% (15 g, 20 g, 30 g, 240 g). **SPRAY, nasal:** 55 mcg per actuation in aqueous base (16.5 g)

Triamcinolone diacetate: **INJ:** 25 mg/mL (5 mL), 40 mg/mL (1 mL, 5 mL, 10 mL)

Triamcinolone hexacetonide: **INJ:** 5 mg/mL (5 mL), 20 mg/mL (1 mL, 5 mL)

Contraindications Known hypersensitivity to triamcinolone; systemic fungal infections; serious infections (except septic shock or tuberculous meningitis); primary treatment of status asthmaticus

Warnings/Precautions Fatalities have occurred due to adrenal insufficiency in asthmatic patients during and after transfer from systemic corticosteroids to aerosol steroids; several months may be required for recovery from this syndrome; during this period, aerosol steroids do **not** provide the increased systemic steroid requirement needed to treat patients having trauma, surgery or infections; avoid using higher than recommended dose

Use with caution in patients with hypothyroidism, cirrhosis, nonspecific ulcerative colitis and patients at increased risk for peptic ulcer disease; do not use occlusive dressings on weeping or exudative lesions and general caution with occlusive dressings should be observed; discontinue if skin irritation or contact dermatitis should occur; do not use in patients with decreased skin circulation; avoid the use of high potency steroids on the face

(Continued)

Triamcinolone *(Continued)*

Because of the risk of adverse effects, systemic corticosteroids should be used cautiously in the elderly, in the smallest possible dose, and for the shortest possible time. Azmacort™ (metered dose inhaler) comes with its own spacer device attached and may be easier to use in older patients. Controlled clinical studies have shown that inhaled and intranasal corticosteroids may cause a reduction in growth velocity in pediatric patients. Growth velocity provides a means of comparing the rate of growth among children of the same age.

In studies involving inhaled corticosteroids, the average reduction in growth velocity was approximately 1 cm (about 1/3 of an inch) per year. It appears that the reduction is related to dose and how long the child takes the drug.

FDA's Pulmonary and Allergy Drugs and Metabolic and Endocrine Drugs advisory committees discussed this issue at a July 1998 meeting. They recommended that the agency develop class-wide labeling to inform healthcare providers so they would understand this potential side effect and monitor growth routinely in pediatric patients who are treated with inhaled corticosteroids, intranasal corticosteroids or both.

Long-term effects of this reduction in growth velocity on final adult height are unknown. Likewise, it also has not yet been determined whether patients' growth will "catch up" if treatment in discontinued. Drug manufacturers will continue to monitor these drugs to learn more about long-term effects. Children are prescribed inhaled corticosteroids to treat asthma. Intranasal corticosteroids are generally used to prevent and treat allergy-related nasal symptoms.

Patients are advised not to stop using their inhaled or intranasal corticosteroids without first speaking to their healthcare providers about the benefits of these drugs compared to their risks.

Pregnancy Risk Factor C

Pregnancy Implications

Clinical effects on the fetus: No data on crossing the placenta or effect on fetus

Breast-feeding/lactation: No data on crossing into breast milk or clinical effects on the infant

Adverse Reactions

>10%:

Central nervous system: Insomnia, nervousness

Gastrointestinal: Increased appetite, indigestion

1% to 10%:

Ocular: Cataracts

Endocrine & metabolic: Diabetes mellitus, hirsutism

Neuromuscular & skeletal: Arthralgia

Respiratory: Epistaxis

<1%: Abdominal distention, acne, amenorrhea, bone growth suppression, bruising, burning, cough, Cushing's syndrome, delirium, dry throat, euphoria, fatigue, hallucinations, headache, hoarseness, hyperglycemia, hyperpigmentation, hypersensitivity reactions, hypertrichosis, hypopigmentation, itching, mood swings, muscle wasting, oral candidiasis, osteoporosis, pancreatitis, peptic ulcer, seizures, skin atrophy, sodium and water retention, ulcerative esophagitis, wheezing, xerostomia

Drug Interactions

Decreased effect: Barbiturates, phenytoin, rifampin ↑ metabolism of triamcinolone; vaccine and toxoid effects may be reduced

Increased toxicity: Salicylates may increase risk of GI ulceration

Alcohol Interactions Avoid use (may enhance gastric mucosal irritation)

Duration Oral: 8-12 hours

Half-Life Biologic: 18-36 hours

Education and Monitoring Issues

Patient Education: Take exactly as directed; do not increase dose or discontinue abruptly without consulting prescriber. Take oral medication with or after meals. Limit intake of caffeine or stimulants. Prescriber may recommend increased dietary vitamins, minerals, or iron. Diabetics should monitor glucose levels closely (antidiabetic medication may need to be adjusted). Inform prescriber if you are experiencing greater than normal levels of stress (medication may need adjustment). Some forms of this medication may cause GI upset (oral medication may be taken with meals to reduce GI upset; small frequent meals and frequent mouth care may reduce GI upset). You may be more susceptible to infection (avoid crowds and persons with contagious or infective conditions). Report promptly excessive nervousness or sleep disturbances; any signs of infection (sore throat, unhealed injuries); excessive growth of body hair or loss of skin color; changes in vision; excessive or sudden weight gain (>3 lb/week); swelling of face or extremities; difficulty breathing; muscle weakness; change in color of stools (black or tarry) or persistent abdominal pain; or worsening of condition or failure to improve.

Topical: For external use only. Not for eyes or mucous membranes or open wounds. Apply in very thin layer to occlusive dressing. Apply dressing to area being treated. Avoid prolonged or excessive use around sensitive tissues, genital, or rectal areas.

Inform prescriber if condition worsens (swelling, redness, irritation, pain, open sores) or fails to improve.

Aerosol: Not for use during acute asthmatic attack. Follow directions that accompany product. Rinse mouth and throat after use to prevent candidiasis. Do not use intranasal product if you have a nasal infection, nasal injury, or recent nasal surgery. If using two products, consult prescriber in which order to use the two products. Inform prescriber if condition worsens or does not improve.

Related Information

Asthma Guidelines *on page 1077*
Corticosteroids Comparison *on page 1237*
Nystatin and Triamcinolone *on page 670*

- **Triam Forte®** *see* Triamcinolone *on page 944*
- **Triaminic** *see* Pheniramine, Phenylpropanolamine, and Pyrilamine *on page 723*
- **Triaminic® AM Decongestant Formula [OTC]** *see* Pseudoephedrine *on page 792*
- **Triaminic® Oral Infant Drops** *see* Pheniramine, Phenylpropanolamine, and Pyrilamine *on page 723*

Triamterene (trye AM ter een)

Pharmacologic Class Diuretic, Potassium Sparing

U.S. Brand Names Dyrenium®

Generic Available No

Mechanism of Action Interferes with potassium/sodium exchange (active transport) in the distal tubule, cortical collecting tubule and collecting duct by inhibiting sodium, potassium-ATPase; decreases calcium excretion; increases magnesium loss

Use Alone or in combination with other diuretics to treat edema and hypertension; decreases potassium excretion caused by kaliuretic diuretics

USUAL DOSAGE Adults: Oral: 100-300 mg/day in 1-2 divided doses; maximum dose: 300 mg/day

Dosing comments in renal impairment: Cl_{cr} <10 mL/minute: Avoid use

Dosing adjustment in hepatic impairment: Dose reduction is recommended in patients with cirrhosis

Dosage Forms CAP: 50 mg, 100 mg

Contraindications Hyperkalemia, renal impairment, diabetes, hypersensitivity to triamterene or any component; do not administer to patients receiving spironolactone, amiloride, or potassium supplementation unless the patient has documented evidence of hypokalemia unresponsive to either agent alone

Warnings/Precautions Use with caution in patients with severe hepatic encephalopathy, patients with diabetes, renal dysfunction, a history of renal stones, or those receiving potassium supplements, potassium-containing medications, blood or ACE inhibitors

Pregnancy Risk Factor B (per manufacturer); D (based on expert analysis)

Pregnancy Implications

Clinical effects on the fetus: No data available. Generally, use of diuretics during pregnancy is avoided due to risk of decreased placental perfusion.

Breast-feeding/lactation: No data available

Adverse Reactions

1% to 10%:

Cardiovascular: Hypotension, edema, congestive heart failure, bradycardia
Central nervous system: Dizziness, headache, fatigue
Dermatologic: Rash
Gastrointestinal: Constipation, nausea
Respiratory: Dyspnea

<1%: Dehydration, flushing, gynecomastia, hyperkalemia, hyperchloremic hyponatremia, inability to achieve or maintain an erection, metabolic acidosis, postmenopausal bleeding

Drug Interactions

Angiotensin-converting enzyme inhibitors can cause hyperkalemia, especially in patients with renal impairment, potassium-rich diets, or on other drugs causing hyperkalemia; avoid concurrent use or monitor closely.

Potassium supplements may further increase potassium retention and cause hyperkalemia; avoid concurrent use.

Onset Diuresis occurs within 2-4 hours

Duration 7-9 hours

Education and Monitoring Issues

Patient Education: Take in the morning; take the last dose of multiple doses no later than 6 PM unless instructed otherwise; take after meals; notify prescriber if weakness, headache or nausea occurs; avoid excessive ingestion of food high in potassium or use of salt substitute; may increase blood glucose; may impart a blue fluorescence color to urine

Monitoring Parameters: Blood pressure, serum electrolytes (especially potassium), renal function, weight, I & O

Related Information

Heart Failure Guidelines *on page 1099*

(Continued)

Triamterene *(Continued)*

Hydrochlorothiazide and Triamterene *on page 443*

- **Triapin®** *see* Butalbital Compound *on page 123*
- **Triavil®** *see* Amitriptyline and Perphenazine *on page 52*

Triazolam (trye AY zoe lam)

Pharmacologic Class Benzodiazepine

U.S. Brand Names Halcion®

Generic Available No

Mechanism of Action Depresses all levels of the CNS, including the limbic and reticular formation, probably through the increased action of gamma-aminobutyric acid (GABA), which is a major inhibitory neurotransmitter in the brain

Use Short-term treatment of insomnia

USUAL DOSAGE Onset of action is rapid, patient should be in bed when taking medication

Oral:

Children <18 years: Dosage not established

Adults: 0.125-0.25 mg at bedtime

Dosing adjustment/comments in hepatic impairment: Reduce dose or avoid use in cirrhosis

Dosage Forms TAB: 0.125 mg, 0.25 mg

Contraindications Hypersensitivity to triazolam, or any component, cross-sensitivity with other benzodiazepines may occur; severe uncontrolled pain; pre-existing CNS depression; concurrent use of amprenavir, nelfinavir, or ritonavir; narrow-angle glaucoma; not to be used in pregnancy or lactation

Warnings/Precautions May cause drug dependency; avoid abrupt discontinuance in patients with prolonged therapy or seizure disorders; not considered a drug of choice in the elderly

Pregnancy Risk Factor X

Adverse Reactions

>10%:

Cardiovascular: Tachycardia, chest pain

Central nervous system: Drowsiness, fatigue, ataxia, lightheadedness, memory impairment, insomnia, anxiety, depression, headache

Dermatologic: Rash

Endocrine & metabolic: Decreased libido

Gastrointestinal: Xerostomia, decreased salivation, constipation, nausea, vomiting, diarrhea, increased or decreased appetite

Neuromuscular & skeletal: Dysarthria

Ocular: Blurred vision

Miscellaneous: Diaphoresis

1% to 10%:

Cardiovascular: Syncope, hypotension

Central nervous system: Confusion, nervousness, dizziness, akathisia

Dermatologic: Dermatitis

Gastrointestinal: Weight gain or loss, increased salivation, muscle cramps

Neuromuscular & skeletal: Rigidity, tremor

Otic: Tinnitus

Respiratory: Nasal congestion, hyperventilation

<1%: Blood dyscrasias, drug dependence, menstrual irregularities, reflex slowing

Drug Interactions CYP3A3/4 and 3A5-7 enzyme substrate

Carbamazepine, rifampin, and rifabutin may enhance the metabolism of triazolam and decrease its therapeutic effect; consider using an alternative sedative/hypnotic agent

Protease inhibitors (amprenavir, nelfinavir, ritonavir) increase the toxicity of triazolam - avoid concurrent use

Cimetidine, ciprofloxacin, clarithromycin, clozapine, CNS depressants, diltiazem, disulfiram, digoxin, erythromycin, ethanol, fluconazole, fluoxetine, fluvoxamine, isoniazid, itraconazole, ketoconazole, labetalol, levodopa, loxapine, metoprolol, metronidazole, miconazole, nefazodone, omeprazole, phenytoin, rifabutin, rifampin, troleandomycin, valproic acid, verapamil may increase the serum level and/or toxicity of triazolam; monitor for altered benzodiazepine response

Alcohol Interactions Avoid use (may increase central nervous system depression)

Onset Onset of hypnotic effect: Within 15-30 minutes

Duration 6-7 hours

Half-Life 1.7-5 hours

Education and Monitoring Issues

Patient Education: Take exactly as directed (do not increase dose or frequency); may take 2-3 weeks to achieve desired results; may cause physical and/or psychological dependence. Do not use excessive alcohol or other prescription or OTC medications (especially pain medications, sedatives, antihistamines, or hypnotics) without consulting prescriber. Maintain adequate hydration (2-3 L/day of fluids unless instructed to restrict fluid intake). You may experience drowsiness, lightheadedness, impaired coordination, dizziness, or blurred vision (use caution when driving or engaging in tasks requiring alertness until response to drug is known); nausea, vomiting, or dry mouth (small frequent meals, frequent mouth care, chewing gum, or sucking lozenges may help); constipation (increased exercise, fluids, or dietary fruit and fiber may help); altered sexual drive or ability (reversible); or photosensitivity (use sunscreen, wear protective clothing and eyewear, avoid direct sunlight). Report persistent CNS effects (eg, memory impairment, confusion, depression, increased sedation, excitation, headache, agitation, insomnia or nightmares, dizziness, fatigue, impaired coordination, changes in personality, or changes in cognition); changes in urinary pattern; muscle cramping, weakness, tremors, or rigidity; ringing in ears or visual disturbances; chest pain, palpitations, or rapid heartbeat; excessive perspiration; excessive GI symptoms (cramping, constipation, vomiting, anorexia); or worsening of condition.

Dietary Considerations: Grapefruit juice may increase the serum level and/or toxicity

Monitoring Parameters: Respiratory and cardiovascular status

♦ **Triban®** *see* Trimethobenzamide *on page 953*

Trichlormethiazide (trye klor meth EYE a zide)

Pharmacologic Class Diuretic, Thiazide

U.S. Brand Names Metahydrin®; Naqua®

Use Management of mild to moderate hypertension; treatment of edema in congestive heart failure and nephrotic syndrome

USUAL DOSAGE Adults: Oral: 1-4 mg/day; initially doses may be given twice daily

Dosing adjustment in renal impairment: Reduced dosage is necessary

Contraindications Hypersensitivity to trichlormethiazide, other thiazides and sulfonamides, or any component

Pregnancy Risk Factor D

♦ **TriCor™** *see* Fenofibrate *on page 353*

♦ **Tricosal®** *see* Choline Magnesium Trisalicylate *on page 193*

♦ **Tri-Cyclen** *see* Ethinyl Estradiol and Norgestimate *on page 344*

♦ **Triderm®** *see* Triamcinolone *on page 944*

♦ **Tridesilon® Topical** *see* Desonide *on page 255*

♦ **Tridil® Injection** *see* Nitroglycerin *on page 659*

Trientine (TRYE en teen)

Pharmacologic Class Chelating Agent

U.S. Brand Names Syprine®

Generic Available No

Mechanism of Action Trientine hydrochloride is an oral chelating agent structurally dissimilar from penicillamine and other available chelating agents; an effective oral chelator of copper used to induce adequate cupriuresis

Use Treatment of Wilson's disease in patients intolerant to penicillamine

USUAL DOSAGE Oral (administer on an empty stomach):

Children <12 years: 500-750 mg/day in divided doses 2-4 times/day; maximum: 1.5 g/day

Adults: 750-1250 mg/day in divided doses 2-4 times/day; maximum dose: 2 g/day

Dosage Forms CAP: 250 mg

Contraindications Rheumatoid arthritis, biliary cirrhosis, cystinuria, known hypersensitivity to trientine

Warnings/Precautions May cause iron deficiency anemia; monitor closely; use with caution in patients with reactive airway disease

Pregnancy Risk Factor C

Adverse Reactions Percentage unknown: Anemia, epigastric pain, heartburn, iron deficiency, malaise, muscle cramps, systemic lupus erythematosus (SLE), tenderness, thickening and fissuring of skin

Drug Interactions Decreased effect with iron and possibly other mineral supplements

Education and Monitoring Issues

Patient Education: Take 1 hour before or 2 hours after meals and at least 1 hour apart from any drug, food, or milk; do not chew capsule, swallow whole followed by a full glass of water; notify prescriber of any fever or skin changes; any skin exposed to the contents of a capsule should be promptly washed with water

Manufacturer Merck & Co

Related Information

Pharmaceutical Manufacturers Directory *on page 1020*

Triethanolamine Polypeptide Oleate-Condensate

(trye eth a NOLE a meen pol i PEP tide OH lee ate-KON den sate)

Pharmacologic Class Otic Agent, Cerumenolytic

U.S. Brand Names Cerumenex® Otic

Use Removal of ear wax (cerumen)

USUAL DOSAGE Children and Adults: Otic: Fill ear canal, insert cotton plug; allow to remain 15-30 minutes; flush ear with lukewarm water as a single treatment; if a second application is needed for unusually hard impactions, repeat the procedure

(Continued)

Triethanolamine Polypeptide Oleate-Condensate *(Continued)*

Contraindications Perforated tympanic membrane or otitis media, hypersensitivity to product or any component

Pregnancy Risk Factor C

◆ **Trifed-C®** *see* Triprolidine, Pseudoephedrine, and Codeine *on page 958*

Trifluoperazine (trye floo oh PER a zeen)

Pharmacologic Class Antipsychotic Agent, Phenothazine, Piperazine

U.S. Brand Names Stelazine®

Generic Available Yes

Mechanism of Action Blocks postsynaptic mesolimbic dopaminergic receptors in the brain; exhibits a strong alpha-adrenergic blocking effect and depresses the release of hypothalamic and hypophyseal hormones

Use Treatment of psychoses and management of nonpsychotic anxiety

USUAL DOSAGE

Children 6-12 years: Psychoses:

Oral: Hospitalized or well supervised patients: Initial: 1 mg 1-2 times/day, gradually increase until symptoms are controlled or adverse effects become troublesome; maximum: 15 mg/day

I.M.: 1 mg twice daily

Adults:

Psychoses:

Outpatients: Oral: 1-2 mg twice daily

Hospitalized or well supervised patients: Initial: 2-5 mg twice daily with optimum response in the 15-20 mg/day range; do not exceed 40 mg/day

I.M.: 1-2 mg every 4-6 hours as needed up to 10 mg/24 hours maximum

Nonpsychotic anxiety: Oral: 1-2 mg twice daily; maximum: 6 mg/day; therapy for anxiety should not exceed 12 weeks; do not exceed 6 mg/day for longer than 12 weeks when treating anxiety; agitation, jitteriness, or insomnia may be confused with original neurotic or psychotic symptoms

Hemodialysis: Not dialyzable (0% to 5%)

Dosage Forms CONC, oral: 10 mg/mL (60 mL). **INJ:** 2 mg/mL (10 mL). **TAB:** 1 mg, 2 mg, 5 mg, 10 mg

Contraindications Hypersensitivity to trifluoperazine or any component, cross-sensitivity with other phenothiazines may exist, coma, circulatory collapse, history of blood dyscrasias

Warnings/Precautions Safety in children <6 months of age has not been established; use with caution in patients with cardiovascular disease, seizures, hepatic dysfunction, narrow-angle glaucoma, or bone marrow suppression; watch for hypotension when administering I.M. or I.V.; use with caution in patients with myasthenia gravis or Parkinson's disease

Pregnancy Risk Factor C

Adverse Reactions

Cardiovascular: Hypotension, orthostatic hypotension, cardiac arrest

Central nervous system: Extrapyramidal signs (pseudoparkinsonism, akathisia, dystonias, tardive dyskinesia), dizziness, headache, neuroleptic malignant syndrome (NMS), impairment of temperature regulation, lowering of seizures threshold

Dermatologic: Increased sensitivity to sun, rash, discoloration of skin (blue-gray)

Endocrine & metabolic: Changes in menstrual cycle, changes in libido, breast pain, hyperglycemia, hypoglycemia, gynecomastia, lactation, galactorrhea

Gastrointestinal: Constipation, weight gain, nausea, vomiting, stomach pain, xerostomia

Genitourinary: Difficulty in urination, ejaculatory disturbances, urinary retention, priapism

Hematologic: Agranulocytosis, leukopenia, pancytopenia, thrombocytopenic purpura, eosinophilia, hemolytic anemia, aplastic anemia

Hepatic: Cholestatic jaundice, hepatotoxicity

Neuromuscular & skeletal: Tremor

Ocular: Pigmentary retinopathy, cornea and lens changes

Respiratory: Nasal congestion

Drug Interactions CYP1A2 enzyme substrate

Phenothiazines inhibit the ability of bromocriptine to lower serum prolactin concentrations

Benztropine (and other anticholinergics) may inhibit the therapeutic response to trifluoperazine and excess anticholinergic effects may occur

Chloroquine may increase trifluoperazine concentrations

Cigarette smoking may enhance the hepatic metabolism of trifluoperazine. Larger doses may be required compared to a nonsmoker.

Concurrent use of trifluoperazine with an antihypertensive may produce additive hypotensive effects

Antihypertensive effects of guanethidine and guanadrel may be inhibited by trifluoperazine

Concurrent use with TCA may produce increased toxicity or altered therapeutic response

Trifluoperazine may inhibit the antiparkinsonian effect of levodopa; avoid this combination

Trifluoperazine plus lithium may rarely produce neurotoxicity

Barbiturates may reduce trifluoperazine concentrations
Propranolol may increase trifluoperazine concentrations
Sulfadoxine-pyrimethamine may increase trifluoperazine concentrations
Trifluoperazine and low potency antipsychotics may reverse the pressor effects of epinephrine
Trifluoperazine and CNS depressants (ethanol, narcotics) may produce additive CNS depressant effects
Trifluoperazine and trazodone may produce additive hypotensive effects

Alcohol Interactions Avoid use (may increase central nervous system depression)

Half-Life >24 hours with chronic use

Education and Monitoring Issues

Patient Education: Use exactly as directed (do not increase dose or frequency); may cause physical and/or psychological dependence. Do not discontinue without consulting prescriber. Tablets/capsules may be taken with food. Mix oral solution with 2-4 ounces of liquid (eg, juice, milk, water, pudding). Do not take within 2 hours of any antacid. Avoid excess alcohol or caffeine and other prescription or OTC medications not approved by prescriber. Maintain adequate hydration (2-3 L/day of fluids unless instructed to restrict fluid intake). Avoid skin contact with liquid medication; may cause contact dermatitis (wash immediately with warm, soapy water). You may experience excess drowsiness, lightheadedness, dizziness, or blurred vision (use caution driving or when engaging in tasks requiring alertness until response to drug is known); nausea or vomiting (small frequent meals, frequent mouth care, chewing gum, or sucking lozenges may help); constipation (increased exercise, fluids, or dietary fruit and fiber may help); postural hypotension (use caution climbing stairs or when changing position from lying or sitting to standing); urinary retention (void before taking medication); ejaculatory dysfunction (reversible); decreased perspiration (avoid strenuous exercise in hot environments); photosensitivity (use sunscreen, wear protective clothing and eyewear, avoid direct sunlight). Report persistent CNS effects (eg, trembling fingers, altered gait or balance, excessive sedation, seizures, unusual movements, anxiety, abnormal thoughts, confusion, personality changes); chest pain, palpitations, rapid heartbeat, severe dizziness; unresolved urinary retention or changes in urinary pattern; altered menstrual pattern, changes in libido, swelling or pain in breasts (male or female); vision changes; skin rash, irritation, or changes in color of skin (gray-blue); or worsening of condition.

Reference Range: Therapeutic response and blood levels have not been established

Trifluridine (trye FLURE i deen)

Pharmacologic Class Antiviral Agent, Ophthalmic

U.S. Brand Names Viroptic® Ophthalmic

Generic Available No

Mechanism of Action Interferes with viral replication by incorporating into viral DNA in place of thymidine, inhibiting thymidylate synthetase resulting in the formation of defective proteins

Use Treatment of primary keratoconjunctivitis and recurrent epithelial keratitis caused by herpes simplex virus types I and II

USUAL DOSAGE Adults: Instill 1 drop into affected eye every 2 hours while awake, to a maximum of 9 drops/day, until re-epithelialization of corneal ulcer occurs; then use 1 drop every 4 hours for another 7 days; do **not** exceed 21 days of treatment; if improvement has not taken place in 7-14 days, consider another form of therapy

Dosage Forms SOLN, ophth: 1% (7.5 mL)

Contraindications Known hypersensitivity to trifluridine or any component

Warnings/Precautions Mild local irritation of conjunctival and cornea may occur when instilled but usually transient effects

Pregnancy Risk Factor C

Adverse Reactions

1% to 10%: Local: Burning, stinging
<1%: Epithelial keratopathy, hyperemia, hypersensitivity reactions, increased intraocular pressure, keratitis, palpebral edema, stromal edema

Education and Monitoring Issues

Patient Education: For ophthalmic use only. Store in refrigerator; do not use discolored solution. Apply prescribed amount as often as directed. Wash hands before using and do not let tip of applicator touch eye or contaminate tip of applicator. Tilt head back and look upward. Gently pull down lower lid and put drop(s) in inner corner of eye. Close eye and roll eyeball in all directions. Do not blink for 1/2 minute. Apply gentle pressure to inner corner of eye for 30 seconds. Wipe away excess from skin around eye. Do not use any other eye preparation for at least 10 minutes. Do not touch tip of applicator to eye or contaminate tip of applicator. Do not share medication with anyone else. May cause sensitivity to bright light (dark glasses may help); temporary stinging or blurred vision may occur. Inform prescriber if you experience eye pain, redness, burning, watering, dryness, double vision, puffiness around eye, vision disturbances, or other adverse eye response; worsening of condition or lack of improvement within 7-14 days.

♦ **Trihexy®** *see* Trihexyphenidyl *on page 952*

Trihexyphenidyl (trye heks ee FEN i dil)

Pharmacologic Class Anticholinergic Agent; Anti-Parkinson's Agent (Anticholinergic)

U.S. Brand Names Artane®; Trihexy®

Generic Available Yes: Tablet

Mechanism of Action Thought to act by blocking excess acetylcholine at cerebral synapses; many of its effects are due to its pharmacologic similarities with atropine

Use Adjunctive treatment of Parkinson's disease; also used in treatment of drug-induced extrapyramidal effects and acute dystonic reactions

USUAL DOSAGE Adults: Oral: Initial: 1-2 mg/day, increase by 2 mg increments at intervals of 3-5 days; usual dose: 5-15 mg/day in 3-4 divided doses

Dosage Forms CAP, sustained release: 5 mg. **ELIX:** 2 mg/5 mL (480 mL). **TAB:** 2 mg, 5 mg

Contraindications Hypersensitivity to trihexyphenidyl or any component, patients with narrow-angle glaucoma; pyloric or duodenal obstruction, stenosing peptic ulcers; bladder neck obstructions; achalasia; myasthenia gravis

Warnings/Precautions Use with caution in hot weather or during exercise. Elderly patients require strict dosage regulation. Use with caution in patients with tachycardia, cardiac arrhythmias, hypertension, hypotension, prostatic hypertrophy or any tendency toward urinary retention, liver or kidney disorders, and obstructive disease of the GI or GU tract. May exacerbate mental symptoms when used to treat extrapyramidal reactions. When given in large doses or to susceptible patients, may cause weakness.

Pregnancy Risk Factor C

Adverse Reactions

>10%:
- Dermatologic: Dry skin
- Gastrointestinal: Constipation, xerostomia, dry throat
- Respiratory: Dry nose
- Miscellaneous: Diaphoresis (decreased)

1% to 10%:
- Dermatologic: Increased sensitivity to light
- Endocrine & metabolic: Decreased flow of breast milk
- Gastrointestinal: Dysphagia

<1%: Ataxia, bloated feeling, blurred vision, confusion, drowsiness, dysuria, fatigue, headache, increased intraocular pain, loss of memory, nausea, orthostatic hypotension, palpitations, rash, tachycardia, ventricular fibrillation, vomiting, weakness

Drug Interactions

Decreased effect: May increase gastric degradation of levodopa and decrease the amount of levodopa absorbed by delaying gastric emptying; the opposite may be true for digoxin

Therapeutic effects of cholinergic agents (tacrine, donepezil) and neuroleptics may be antagonized

Increased toxicity: Central and/or peripheral anticholinergic syndrome can occur when administered with amantadine, rimantadine, narcotic analgesics, phenothiazines and other antipsychotics (especially with high anticholinergic activity), tricyclic antidepressants, quinidine and some other antiarrhythmics, and antihistamines

Alcohol Interactions Avoid use (may increase central nervous system depression)

Onset Peak effect: Within 1 hour

Half-Life 3.3-4.1 hours

Education and Monitoring Issues

Patient Education: Take exactly as directed; with meals if GI upset occurs, before meals if dry mouth occurs, after eating if drooling or if nausea occurs. Take at the same time each day. Maintain adequate hydration (2-3 L/day of fluids unless instructed to restrict fluid intake); void before taking medication. Do not use alcohol and all prescription or OTC sedatives or CNS depressants without consulting prescriber. You may experience drowsiness, confusion, or vision changes (use caution when driving, climbing stairs, or engaging in tasks requiring alertness until response to drug is known); increased susceptibility to heat stroke, decreased perspiration (use caution in hot weather - maintain adequate fluids and reduce exercise activity); constipation (increased exercise, fluids, or dietary fruit and fiber may help); dry skin or nasal passages (consult prescriber for appropriate relief). Report unresolved constipation, chest pain or palpitations, difficulty breathing, CNS changes (hallucination, loss of memory, nervousness, etc), painful or difficult urination, increased muscle spasticity or rigidity, skin rash, or significant worsening of condition.

Monitoring Parameters: IOP monitoring and gonioscopic evaluations should be performed periodically

- ♦ **TriHIBIT®** *see Haemophilus* b Conjugate Vaccine *on page 427*
- ♦ **Tri-K®** *see* Potassium Acetate, Potassium Bicarbonate, and Potassium Citrate *on page 751*
- ♦ **Tri-Kort®** *see* Triamcinolone *on page 944*
- ♦ **Trilafon®** *see* Perphenazine *on page 719*
- ♦ **Trileptal®** *see* Oxcarbazepine *on page 687*
- ♦ **Tri-Levlen®** *see* Ethinyl Estradiol and Levonorgestrel *on page 341*

- **Trilisate®** *see* Choline Magnesium Trisalicylate *on page 193*
- **Trilog®** *see* Triamcinolone *on page 944*
- **Trilone®** *see* Triamcinolone *on page 944*
- **Trimazide®** *see* Trimethobenzamide *on page 953*

Trimethobenzamide (trye meth oh BEN za mide)

Pharmacologic Class Anticholinergic Agent; Antiemetic

U.S. Brand Names Arrestin®; Pediatric Triban®; Tebamide®; T-Gen®; Ticon®; Tigan®; Triban®; Trimazide®

Generic Available No

Mechanism of Action Acts centrally to inhibit the medullary chemoreceptor trigger zone

Use Control of nausea and vomiting (especially for long-term antiemetic therapy); less effective than phenothiazines but may be associated with fewer side effects

USUAL DOSAGE Rectal use is contraindicated in neonates and premature infants

Children:

Rectal: <14 kg: 100 mg 3-4 times/day

Oral, rectal: 14-40 kg: 100-200 mg 3-4 times/day

Adults:

Oral: 250 mg 3-4 times/day

I.M., rectal: 200 mg 3-4 times/day

Dosage Forms CAP: 100 mg, 250 mg. **INJ:** 100 mg/mL (2 mL, 20 mL). **SUPP, rectal:** 100 mg, 200 mg

Contraindications Hypersensitivity to trimethobenzamide, benzocaine, or any component; injection contraindicated in children and suppositories are contraindicated in premature infants or neonates

Warnings/Precautions May mask emesis due to Reye's syndrome or mimic CNS effects of Reye's syndrome in patients with emesis of other etiologies; use in patients with acute vomiting should be avoided

Pregnancy Risk Factor C

Adverse Reactions

>10%: Central nervous system: Drowsiness

1% to 10%:

Cardiovascular: Hypotension

Central nervous system: Dizziness, headache

Gastrointestinal: Diarrhea

Neuromuscular & skeletal: Muscle cramps

<1%: Blood dyscrasias, convulsions, hepatic impairment, hypersensitivity skin reactions, mental depression, opisthotonus

Drug Interactions Antagonism of oral anticoagulants may occur

Onset Onset of antiemetic effect: Oral: Within 10-40 minutes; I.M.: Within 15-35 minutes

Duration 3-4 hours

Education and Monitoring Issues

Patient Education: Take as directed before meals; do not increase dose and do not discontinue without consulting prescriber. You may experience drowsiness or blurred vision (use caution when driving or engaging in tasks that require alertness until response to drug is known) or diarrhea (buttermilk or yogurt may help). Report chest pain or palpitations, persistent dizziness or blurred vision, or CNS changes (disorientation, depression, confusion).

Trimethoprim (trye METH oh prim)

Pharmacologic Class Antibiotic, Miscellaneous

U.S. Brand Names Proloprim®; Trimpex®

Generic Available Yes

Mechanism of Action Inhibits folic acid reduction to tetrahydrofolate, and thereby inhibits microbial growth

Use Treatment of urinary tract infections due to susceptible strains of *E. coli*, *P. mirabilis*, *K. pneumoniae*, *Enterobacter* sp and coagulase-negative *Staphylococcus* including *S. saprophyticus*; acute otitis media in children; acute exacerbations of chronic bronchitis in adults; in combination with other agents for treatment of toxoplasmosis, *Pneumocystis carinii*; treatment of superficial ocular infections involving the conjunctiva and cornea

USUAL DOSAGE Oral:

Children: 4 mg/kg/day in divided doses every 12 hours

Adults: 100 mg every 12 hours or 200 mg every 24 hours; in the treatment of *Pneumocystis carinii* pneumonia; dose may be as high as 15-20 mg/kg/day in 3-4 divided doses

Dosing interval in renal impairment: Cl_{cr} 15-30 mL/minute: Administer 50 mg every 12 hours

Hemodialysis: Moderately dialyzable (20% to 50%)

Dosage Forms SOLN, oral: 50 mg (base)/5 mL **TAB:** 100 mg, 200 mg

Contraindications Hypersensitivity to trimethoprim or any component, megaloblastic anemia due to folate deficiency

Warnings/Precautions Use with caution in patients with impaired renal or hepatic function or with possible folate deficiency

(Continued)

Trimethoprim *(Continued)*

Pregnancy Risk Factor C

Adverse Reactions

1% to 10%:

Dermatologic: Rash (3% to 7%), pruritus

Hematologic: Megaloblastic anemia (with chronic high doses)

<1%: Cholestatic jaundice, elevated BUN/serum creatinine, epigastric distress, exfoliative dermatitis, fever, hyperkalemia, increased LFTs, leukopenia, nausea, neutropenia, thrombocytopenia, vomiting

Drug Interactions Increased effect/toxicity/levels of phenytoin; increased myelosuppression with methotrexate; may increase levels of digoxin

Half-Life 8-14 hours, prolonged with renal impairment

Education and Monitoring Issues

Patient Education: Take per recommended schedule. Complete full course of therapy; do not skip doses. Do not chew or crush tablets; swallow whole with milk or food. Maintain adequate hydration (2-3 L/day of fluids unless instructed to restrict fluid intake). You may experience nausea, vomiting, or GI upset (small frequent meals, frequent mouth care, sucking lozenges, or chewing gum may help). Report skin rash, redness, or irritation; feelings of acute fatigue or weakness; unusual bleeding or bruising; or other persistent adverse effects.

Reference Range: Therapeutic: Peak: 5-15 mg/L; Trough: 2-8 mg/L

Related Information

Trimethoprim and Polymyxin B *on page 954*

Trimethoprim and Polymyxin B (trye METH oh prim & pol i MIKS in bee)

Pharmacologic Class Antibiotic, Ophthalmic

U.S. Brand Names Polytrim® Ophthalmic

Dosage Forms SOLN, ophth: Trimethoprim sulfate 1 mg and polymyxin B sulfate 10,000 units per mL (10 mL)

Pregnancy Risk Factor C

Trimetrexate Glucuronate (tri me TREKS ate gloo KYOOR oh nate)

Pharmacologic Class Antineoplastic Agent, Miscellaneous

U.S. Brand Names Neutrexin® Injection

Mechanism of Action Exerts an antimicrobial effect through potent inhibition of the enzyme dihydrofolate reductase (DHFR)

Use Alternative therapy for the treatment of moderate-to-severe *Pneumocystis carinii* pneumonia (PCP) in immunocompromised patients, including patients with acquired immunodeficiency syndrome (AIDS), who are intolerant of, or are refractory to, co-trimoxazole therapy or for whom co-trimoxazole and pentamidine are contraindicated. **Concurrent folinic acid (leucovorin) must always be administered.**

USUAL DOSAGE Adults: I.V.: 45 mg/m^2 once daily over 60 minutes for 21 days; it is necessary to reduce the dose in patients with liver dysfunction, although no specific recommendations exist; concurrent folinic acid 20 mg/m^2 every 6 hours orally or I.V. for 24 days

Dosage Forms POWDER for inj: 25 mg

Contraindications Previous hypersensitivity to trimetrexate or methotrexate, severe existing myelosuppression

Warnings/Precautions Must be administered with concurrent leucovorin to avoid potentially serious or life-threatening toxicities; leucovorin therapy must extend for 72 hours past the last dose of trimetrexate; use with caution in patients with mild myelosuppression, severe hepatic or renal dysfunction, hypoproteinemia, hypoalbuminemia, or previous extensive myelosuppressive therapies

Pregnancy Risk Factor D

Adverse Reactions 1% to 10%:

Central nervous system: Seizures, fever

Dermatologic: Rash

Gastrointestinal: Stomatitis, nausea, vomiting

Hematologic: Neutropenia, thrombocytopenia, anemia

Hepatic: Elevated LFTs

Neuromuscular & skeletal: Peripheral neuropathy

Renal: Increased serum creatinine

Miscellaneous: Flu-like illness, hypersensitivity reactions

Drug Interactions

Decreased effect of pneumococcal vaccine

Increased toxicity (infection rates) of yellow fever vaccine

Half-Life 15-17 hours

Education and Monitoring Issues

Patient Education: This medication can only be administered I.V. Frequent blood tests will be required to assess effectiveness of therapy. Avoid aspirin, and aspirin-containing medication unless approved by prescriber. Report persistent fever, chills, joint pain, numbness or tingling of extremities, vomiting or nausea (antiemetic medications may be needed), acute abdominal pain, mouth sores, increased bruising or bleeding, blood in urine or stool, changes in sensorium (eg, confusion, hallucinations, seizures), increased difficulty breathing, or acute persistent malaise or weakness.

Monitoring Parameters: Check and record patient's temperature daily; absolute neutrophil counts (ANC), platelet count, renal function tests (serum creatinine, BUN), hepatic function tests (ALT, AST, alkaline phosphatase)

Trimipramine (trye MI pra meen)

Pharmacologic Class Antidepressant, Tricyclic (Tertiary Amine)

U.S. Brand Names Surmontil®

Generic Available Yes

Mechanism of Action Increases the synaptic concentration of serotonin and/or norepinephrine in the central nervous system by inhibition of their reuptake by the presynaptic neuronal membrane

Use Treatment of various forms of depression, often in conjunction with psychotherapy

USUAL DOSAGE Adults: Oral: 50-150 mg/day as a single bedtime dose up to a maximum of 200 mg/day outpatient and 300 mg/day inpatient

Dosage Forms CAP: 25 mg, 50 mg, 100 mg

Contraindications Narrow-angle glaucoma; avoid use during pregnancy and lactation

Warnings/Precautions Use with caution in patients with cardiovascular disease, conduction disturbances, seizure disorders, urinary retention, hyperthyroidism or those receiving thyroid replacement; avoid use during lactation; use with caution in pregnancy; do not discontinue abruptly in patients receiving chronic high-dose therapy

Pregnancy Risk Factor C

Adverse Reactions

Cardiovascular: Arrhythmias, hypotension, hypertension, tachycardia, palpitations, heart block, stroke, myocardial infarction

Central nervous system: Headache, exacerbation of psychosis, confusion, delirium, hallucinations, nervousness, restlessness, delusions, agitation, insomnia, nightmares, anxiety, seizures

Dermatologic: Photosensitivity, rash, petechiae, itching

Endocrine & metabolic: Sexual dysfunction, breast enlargement, galactorrhea, SIADH

Gastrointestinal: Xerostomia, constipation, increased appetite, nausea, unpleasant taste, weight gain, diarrhea, heartburn, vomiting, anorexia, trouble with gums, decreased lower esophageal sphincter tone may cause GE reflux

Genitourinary: Difficult urination, urinary retention, testicular edema

Hematologic: Agranulocytosis, eosinophilia, purpura, thrombocytopenia

Hepatic: Cholestatic jaundice, increased liver enzymes

Neuromuscular & skeletal: Tremors, numbness, tingling, paresthesia, incoordination, ataxia, peripheral neuropathy, extrapyramidal symptoms

Ocular: Blurred vision, eye pain, disturbances in accommodation, mydriasis, increased intraocular pressure

Otic: Tinnitus

Miscellaneous: Allergic reactions

Drug Interactions CYP2D6 enzyme substrate

Carbamazepine, phenobarbital, and rifampin may increase the metabolism of trimipramine resulting in decreased effect of trimipramine

Trimipramine inhibits the antihypertensive response to bethanidine, clonidine, debrisoquin, guanadrel, guanethidine, guanabenz, guanfacine; monitor BP; consider alternate antihypertensive agent

Abrupt discontinuation of clonidine may cause hypertensive crisis, trimipramine may enhance the response

Use with altretamine may cause orthostatic hypertension

Trimipramine may be additive with or may potentiate the action of other CNS depressants (sedatives, hypnotics, or ethanol); with MAO inhibitors, hyperpyrexia, hypertension, tachycardia, confusion, seizures, and **deaths have been reported** (serotonin syndrome), this combination should be avoided

Trimipramine may increase the prothrombin time in patients stabilized on warfarin

Cimetidine and methylphenidate may decrease the metabolism of trimipramine

Additive anticholinergic effects seen with other anticholinergic agents

The SSRIs, to varying degrees, inhibit the metabolism of TCAs and clinical toxicity may result

Use of lithium with a TCA may increase the risk for neurotoxicity

Phenothiazines may increase concentration of some TCAs and TCAs may increase concentration of phenothiazines; monitor for altered clinical response

TCAs may enhance the hypoglycemic effects of tolazamide, chlorpropamide, or insulin; monitor for changes in blood glucose levels

Cholestyramine and colestipol may bind TCAs and reduce their absorption; monitor for altered response

TCAs may enhance the effect of amphetamines; monitor for adverse CV effects

Verapamil and diltiazem appear to decrease the metabolism of imipramine and potentially other TCAs; monitor for increased TCA concentrations. The pressor response to I.V.

(Continued)

Trimipramine *(Continued)*

epinephrine, norepinephrine, and phenylephrine may be enhanced in patients receiving TCAs, this combination is best avoided.

Indinavir, ritonavir may inhibit the metabolism of clomipramine and potentially other TCAs; monitor for altered effects; a decrease in TCA dosage may be required

Quinidine may inhibit the metabolism of TCAs; monitor for altered effect

Combined use of anticholinergics with TCAs may produce additive anticholinergic effects; combined use of beta-agonists with TCAs may predispose patients to cardiac arrhythmias

Alcohol Interactions Avoid use (may increase central nervous system depression)

Onset Oral: Therapeutic effects require >2 weeks

Half-Life 20-26 hours

Education and Monitoring Issues

Patient Education: Take exactly as directed (do not increase dose or frequency); may take 2-3 weeks to achieve desired results; may cause physical and/or psychological dependence. Take at bedtime. Avoid excessive alcohol, caffeine, and other prescription or OTC medications not approved by prescriber. Maintain adequate hydration (2-3 L/day of fluids unless instructed to restrict fluid intake). You may experience drowsiness, lightheadedness, dizziness, or blurred vision (use caution when driving or engaging in tasks requiring alertness until response to drug is known); nausea, altered taste, dry mouth (small frequent meals, frequent mouth care, chewing gum, or sucking lozenges may help); constipation (increased exercise, fluids, or dietary fruit and fiber may help); diarrhea (buttermilk, yogurt, or boiled milk may help); increased appetite (monitor dietary intake to avoid excess weight gain); postural hypotension (use caution when climbing stairs or changing position from lying or sitting to standing); urinary retention (void before taking medication); or sexual dysfunction (reversible). Report persistent CNS effects (eg, insomnia, restlessness, fatigue, anxiety, impaired cognitive function, seizures); muscle cramping or tremors; chest pain, palpitations, rapid heartbeat, swelling of extremities, or severe dizziness; unresolved urinary retention; vision changes or eye pain; yellowing of eyes or skin; pale stools/dark urine; or worsening of condition.

Dietary Considerations: Grapefruit juice may potentially inhibit the metabolism of TCAs

Monitoring Parameters: Blood pressure and pulse rate prior to and during initial therapy; evaluate mental status; monitor weight

Related Information

Antidepressant Agents Comparison *on page 1231*

- **Trimox®** *see* Amoxicillin *on page 56*
- **Trimpex®** *see* Trimethoprim *on page 953*
- **Trinalin®** *see* Azatadine and Pseudoephedrine *on page 84*
- **Tri-nasal®** *see* Triamcinolone *on page 944*
- **Tri-Norinyl®** *see* Ethinyl Estradiol and Norethindrone *on page 342*
- **Triotann® Tablet** *see* Chlorpheniramine, Pyrilamine, and Phenylephrine *on page 187*

Trioxsalen (trye OKS a len)

Pharmacologic Class Psoralen

U.S. Brand Names Trisoralen®

Generic Available No

Mechanism of Action Psoralens are thought to form covalent bonds with pyrimidine bases in DNA which inhibit the synthesis of DNA. This reaction involves excitation of the trioxsalen molecule by radiation in the long-wave ultraviolet light (UVA) resulting in transference of energy to the trioxsalen molecule producing an excited state. Binding of trioxsalen to DNA occurs only in the presence of ultraviolet light. The increase in skin pigmentation produced by trioxsalen and UVA radiation involves multiple changes in melanocytes and interaction between melanocytes and keratinocytes. In general, melanogenesis is stimulated but the size and distribution of melanocytes is unchanged.

Use In conjunction with controlled exposure to ultraviolet light or sunlight for repigmentation of idiopathic vitiligo; increasing tolerance to sunlight with albinism; enhance pigmentation

USUAL DOSAGE Children >12 years and Adults: Oral: 10 mg/day as a single dose, 2-4 hours before controlled exposure to UVA (for 15-35 minutes) or sunlight; do not continue for longer than 14 days

Dosage Forms TAB: 5 mg

Contraindications Hypersensitivity to psoralens, melanoma, a history of melanoma, or other diseases associated with photosensitivity; porphyria, acute lupus erythematosus; patients <12 years of age

Warnings/Precautions Serious burns from UVA or sunlight can occur if dosage or exposure schedules are exceeded; patients must wear protective eye wear to prevent cataracts; use with caution in patients with severe hepatic or cardiovascular disease

Pregnancy Risk Factor C

Adverse Reactions

>10%:

Dermatologic: Itching

Gastrointestinal: Nausea

1% to 10%:

Central nervous system: Dizziness, headache, mental depression, insomnia, nervousness

Dermatologic: Severe burns from excessive sunlight or ultraviolet exposure

Gastrointestinal: Gastric discomfort

Onset Peak photosensitivity: 2 hours

Duration Skin sensitivity to light remains for 8-12 hours

Half-Life ~2 hours

Education and Monitoring Issues

Patient Education: This medication is used in conjunction with specific ultraviolet treatment. Follow prescriber's directions exactly for oral medication which can be taken with food or milk to reduce nausea. Avoid use of any other skin treatments unless approved by prescriber. You must wear protective eyewear during treatments. Control exposure to direct sunlight as per prescriber's instructions. If sunlight cannot be avoided, use sunblock (consult prescriber for specific SPF level), wear protective clothing, and wrap-around protective eyewear. Consult prescriber immediately if burning, blistering, or skin irritation occur.

Tripelennamine (tri pel EN a meen)

Pharmacologic Class Antihistamine

Generic Available Yes

Mechanism of Action Competes with histamine for H_1-receptor sites on effector cells in the gastrointestinal tract, blood vessels, and respiratory tract

Use Perennial and seasonal allergic rhinitis and other allergic symptoms including urticaria

USUAL DOSAGE Oral:

Infants and Children: 5 mg/kg/day in 4-6 divided doses, up to 300 mg/day maximum

Adults: 25-50 mg every 4-6 hours, extended release tablets 100 mg morning and evening up to 100 mg every 8 hours

Dosage Forms TAB, as hydrochloride: 50 mg

Contraindications Hypersensitivity to tripelennamine or any component

Warnings/Precautions Use with caution in patients with narrow-angle glaucoma, bladder neck obstruction, symptomatic prostate hypertrophy, asthmatic attacks, and stenosing peptic ulcer

Pregnancy Risk Factor B

Adverse Reactions

>10%:

Central nervous system: Slight to moderate drowsiness

Respiratory: Thickening of bronchial secretions

1% to 10%:

Central nervous system: Headache, fatigue, nervousness, dizziness

Gastrointestinal: Appetite increase, weight gain, nausea, diarrhea, abdominal pain, xerostomia

Neuromuscular & skeletal: Arthralgia

Respiratory: Pharyngitis

<1%: Angioedema, blurred vision, bronchospasm, depression, edema, epistaxis, hepatitis, hypotension, insomnia, myalgia, palpitations, paradoxical excitement, paresthesia, photosensitivity, rash, sedation, tremor, urinary retention

Drug Interactions Increased effect/toxicity with alcohol, CNS depressants, MAO inhibitors

Alcohol Interactions Avoid use (may increase central nervous system depression)

Onset Onset of antihistaminic effect: Within 15-30 minutes

Duration 4-6 hours (up to 8 hours with PBZ-SR®)

Education and Monitoring Issues

Patient Education: Take as directed; do not exceed recommended dose. Avoid use of other depressants, alcohol, or sleep-inducing medications unless approved by prescriber. You may experience drowsiness or dizziness (use caution when driving or engaging in tasks requiring alertness until response to drug is known); or dry mouth, nausea, or abdominal discomfort (frequent small meals, frequent mouth care, chewing gum, or sucking hard candy may help). Report persistent dizziness, sedation, or agitation; chest pain, rapid heartbeat, or palpitations; difficulty breathing; changes in urinary pattern; yellowing of skin or eyes; dark urine or pale stool; or lack of improvement or worsening of condition.

- **Triphasil®** *see* Ethinyl Estradiol and Levonorgestrel *on page 341*
- **Tri-Phen-Chlor®** *see* Chlorpheniramine, Phenyltoloxamine, Phenylpropanolamine, and Phenylephrine *on page 187*
- **Triple Antibiotic® Topical** *see* Bacitracin, Neomycin, and Polymyxin B *on page 90*
- **Triple X® Liquid [OTC]** *see* Pyrethrins *on page 795*

Triprolidine, Pseudoephedrine, and Codeine

(trye PROE li deen, soo doe e FED rin, & KOE deen)

Pharmacologic Class Antihistamine/Decongestant/Antitussive

U.S. Brand Names Actagen-C®; Allerfrin® w/Codeine; Aprodine® w/C; Triacin-C®; Trifed-C®

Dosage Forms SYR: Triprolidine hydrochloride 1.25 mg, pseudoephedrine hydrochloride 30 mg, and codeine phosphate 10 mg per 5 mL with alcohol 4.3%

Pregnancy Risk Factor C

- ♦ **Triptil®** *see* Protriptyline *on page 790*
- ♦ **Triquilar** *see* Ethinyl Estradiol and Levonorgestrel *on page 341*
- ♦ **Trisoralen®** *see* Trioxsalen *on page 956*
- ♦ **Tri-Statin® II Topical** *see* Nystatin and Triamcinolone *on page 670*
- ♦ **Tristoject®** *see* Triamcinolone *on page 944*
- ♦ **Trisulfa®** *see* Co-Trimoxazole *on page 230*
- ♦ **Trisulfa-S®** *see* Co-Trimoxazole *on page 230*
- ♦ **Tri-Tannate Plus®** *see* Chlorpheniramine, Ephedrine, Phenylephrine, and Carbetapentane *on page 186*
- ♦ **Tri-Tannate® Tablet** *see* Chlorpheniramine, Pyrilamine, and Phenylephrine *on page 187*
- ♦ **Tritec®** *see* Ranitidine Bismuth Citrate *on page 809*
- ♦ **Tritin** *see* Tolnaftate *on page 931*
- ♦ **Tri-Vi-Flor®** *see* Vitamins, Multiple *on page 981*
- ♦ **Trobicin®** *see* Spectinomycin *on page 866*
- ♦ **Trocaine® [OTC]** *see* Benzocaine *on page 98*

Troglitazone *WITHDRAWN FROM MARKET 3/21/2000*

(TROE gli to zone)

Pharmacologic Class Antidiabetic Agent (Thiazolidinedione)

U.S. Brand Names Rezulin®

Dosage Forms TAB: 200 mg, 400 mg

Onset Generally requires >3 weeks

Half-Life 16-34 hours

- ♦ **Tromboject** *see* Sodium Tetradecyl *on page 861*
- ♦ **Trombovar** *see* Sodium Tetradecyl *on page 861*
- ♦ **Tropicacyl®** *see* Tropicamide *on page 958*

Tropicamide (troe PIK a mide)

Pharmacologic Class Anticholinergic Agent

U.S. Brand Names Mydriacyl®; Opticyl®; Tropicacyl®

Use Short-acting mydriatic used in diagnostic procedures; as well as preoperatively and postoperatively; treatment of some cases of acute iritis, iridocyclitis, and keratitis

USUAL DOSAGE Children and Adults (individuals with heavily pigmented eyes may require larger doses):

Cycloplegia: Instill 1-2 drops (1%); may repeat in 5 minutes

Exam must be performed within 30 minutes after the repeat dose; if the patient is not examined within 20-30 minutes, instill an additional drop

Mydriasis: Instill 1-2 drops (0.5%) 15-20 minutes before exam; may repeat every 30 minutes as needed

Contraindications Glaucoma, hypersensitivity to tropicamide or any component

Pregnancy Risk Factor C

Related Information

Hydroxyamphetamine and Tropicamide *on page 451*

- ♦ **Trosyd** *see* Tioconazole *on page 923*

Trovafloxacin (TROE va flox a sin)

Pharmacologic Class Antibiotic, Quinolone

U.S. Brand Names Trovan™

Mechanism of Action Inhibits DNA-gyrase in susceptible organisms; inhibits relaxation of supercoiled DNA and promotes breakage of double-stranded DNA

Use Should be used only in life- or limb-threatening infections. Trovafloxacin is now restricted for distribution to only hospitals and long-term care facilities.

Treatment of nosocomial pneumonia, community-acquired pneumonia, complicated intra-abdominal infections, gynecologic/pelvic infections, complicated skin and skin structure infections

USUAL DOSAGE Adults:

Nosocomial pneumonia: I.V.: 300 mg single dose followed by 200 mg/day orally for a total duration of 10-14 days

Community-acquired pneumonia: Oral, I.V.: 200 mg/day for 7-14 days

Complicated intra-abdominal infections, including postsurgical infections/gynecologic and pelvic infections: I.V.: 300 mg as a single dose followed by 200 mg/day orally for a total duration of 7-14 days

Skin and skin structure infections, complicated, including diabetic foot infections: Oral, I.V.: 200 mg/day for 10-14 days

Dosage adjustment in renal impairment: No adjustment is necessary

Dosage adjustment for hemodialysis: None required; trovafloxacin not sufficiently removed by hemodialysis

Dosage adjustment in hepatic impairment:

Mild to moderate cirrhosis:

Initial dose for normal hepatic function: 300 mg I.V.; 200 mg I.V. or oral; 100 mg oral

Reduced dose: 200 mg I.V.; 100 mg I.V. or oral; 100 mg oral

Severe cirrhosis: No data available

Dosage Forms **INJ** (alatrofloxacin): 5 mg/mL (40 mL, 60 mL). **TAB** (trovafloxacin): 100 mg, 200 mg

Contraindications History of hypersensitivity to trovafloxacin, alatrofloxacin, quinolone antimicrobial agents or any other components of these products

Warnings/Precautions For use only in serious life- or limb-threatening infections. Initiation of therapy must occur in an inpatient healthcare facility. May alter GI flora resulting in pseudomembranous colitis due to *Clostridium difficile*; use with caution in patients with seizure disorders or severe cerebral atherosclerosis; discontinue if skin rash or pain, inflammation, or rupture of a tendon; photosensitivity; CNS stimulation may occur which may lead to tremor, restlessness, confusion, hallucinations, paranoia, depression, nightmares, insomnia, or lightheadedness. Hepatic reactions have resulted in death. Risk of hepatotoxicity is increased if therapy exceeds 14 days.

Pregnancy Risk Factor C

Adverse Reactions **Note:** Fatalities have occurred in patients developing hepatic necrosis

<10%:

Central nervous system: Dizziness, lightheadedness, headache

Dermatologic: Rash, pruritus

Gastrointestinal: Nausea, vomiting, diarrhea, abdominal pain

Genitourinary: Vaginitis

Hepatic: Increased LFTs

Local: Injection site reaction, pain, or inflammation

<1%: Anaphylaxis, hepatic necrosis, pancreatitis, Stevens-Johnson syndrome

Drug Interactions Decreased effect of oral trovafloxacin:

Antacids containing magnesium or aluminum, sucralfate, citric acid buffered with sodium citrate, and metal cations: Administer oral trovafloxacin doses at least 2 hours before or 2 hours after

Morphine: Administer I.V. morphine at least 2 hours after oral trovafloxacin in the fasting state and at least 4 hours after oral trovafloxacin when taken with food

Half-Life 9.1-12.7 hours

Education and Monitoring Issues

Patient Education: Take per recommended schedule; complete full course of therapy and do not skip doses. Take on an empty stomach (1 hour before or 2 hours after meals, dairy products, antacids, or other medication). Dizziness may be reduced if taken at bedtime with food. Maintain adequate hydration (2-3 L/day of fluids unless instructed to restrict fluid intake). You may experience dizziness or lightheadedness (use caution when driving or engaging in tasks that require alertness until response to drug is known); nausea or GI upset (small frequent meals, frequent mouth care, sucking lozenges, or chewing gum may help). Report CNS disturbances (hallucinations, gait disturbances); chest pain or palpitations; persistent GI disturbances; signs of opportunistic infection (sore throat, chills, fever, burning, itching on urination, vaginal discharge, white plaques in mouth); tendon pain, swelling, or redness; difficulty breathing, or worsening of condition.

Dietary Considerations: Dairy products such as milk and yogurt reduce the absorption of oral trovafloxacin - avoid concurrent use. The bioavailability may also be decreased by enteral feedings.

Monitoring Parameters: Periodic assessment of liver function tests should be considered

Manufacturer Pfizer U.S. Pharmaceutical Group

Related Information

Pharmaceutical Manufacturers Directory *on page 1020*

- **Trovan™** *see* Trovafloxacin *on page 958*
- **Truphylline®** *see* Theophylline Salts *on page 906*
- **Trusopt®** *see* Dorzolamide *on page 295*

Trypsin, Balsam Peru, and Castor Oil

(TRIP sin, BAL sam pe RUE, & KAS tor oyl)

Pharmacologic Class Protectant, Topical

U.S. Brand Names Granulex

(Continued)

Trypsin, Balsam Peru, and Castor Oil *(Continued)*

Dosage Forms AERO, top: Trypsin 0.1 mg, balsam Peru 72.5 mg, and castor oil 650 mg per 0.82 mL (60 g, 120 g)

- ♦ **Trysul®** *see* Sulfabenzamide, Sulfacetamide, and Sulfathiazole *on page 875*
- ♦ **Tubasal®** *see* Aminosalicylate Sodium *on page 48*

Tuberculin Purified Protein Derivative

(too BER kyoo lin PUR eh fyed PRO teen de RI va tive)

Pharmacologic Class Diagnostic Agent

U.S. Brand Names Aplisol®; Aplitest®; Sclavo-PPD Solution®; Sclavo Test-PPD®; Tine Test PPD; Tubersol®

Generic Available No

Mechanism of Action Tuberculosis results in individuals becoming sensitized to certain antigenic components of the *M. tuberculosis* organism. Culture extracts called tuberculins are contained in tuberculin skin test preparations. Upon intracutaneous injection of these culture extracts, a classic delayed (cellular) hypersensitivity reaction occurs. This reaction is characteristic of a delayed course (peak occurs >24 hours after injection, induration of the skin secondary to cell infiltration, and occasional vesiculation and necrosis). Delayed hypersensitivity reactions to tuberculin may indicate infection with a variety of nontuberculosis mycobacteria, or vaccination with the live attenuated mycobacterial strain of *M. bovis* vaccine, BCG, in addition to previous natural infection with *M. tuberculosis.*

Use Skin test in diagnosis of tuberculosis, cell-mediated immunodeficiencies

USUAL DOSAGE Children and Adults: Intradermal: 0.1 mL about 4" below elbow; use 1/4" to 1/2" or 26- or 27-gauge needle; significant reactions are ≥5 mm in diameter

Interpretation of induration of tuberculin skin test injections: Positive: ≥10 mm; inconclusive: 5-9 mm; negative: <5 mm

Interpretation of induration of Tine test injections: Positive: >2 mm and vesiculation present; inconclusive: <2 mm (give patient Mantoux test of 5 TU/0.1 mL - base decisions on results of Mantoux test); negative: <2 mm or erythema of any size (no need for retesting unless person is a contact of a patient with tuberculosis or there is clinical evidence suggestive of the disease)

Dosage Forms INJ: First test strength: 1 TU/0.1 mL (1 mL); Intermediate test strength: 5 TU/0.1 mL (1 mL, 5 mL, 10 mL); Second test strength: 250 TU/0.1 mL (1 mL). **TINE:** 5 TU each test

Contraindications 250 TU strength should not be used for initial testing

Warnings/Precautions Do not administer I.V. or S.C.; epinephrine (1:1000) should be available to treat possible allergic reactions

Pregnancy Risk Factor C

Adverse Reactions 1% to 10%:

Dermatologic: Ulceration, necrosis, vesiculation

Local: Pain at injection site

Drug Interactions Decreased effect: Reaction may be suppressed in patients receiving systemic corticosteroids, aminocaproic acid, or within 4-6 weeks following immunization with live or inactivated viral vaccines

Education and Monitoring Issues

Patient Education: Return to prescriber for reaction interpretation at 48-72 hours

Related Information

Prophylaxis for Patients Exposed to Common Communicable Diseases *on page 1161*

Tuberculin Tests (too BER kyoo lin tests)

Pharmacologic Class Vaccine

U.S. Brand Names Aplisol®; Aplitest®; Sclavo-PPD Solution®; Sclavo Test-PPD®; Tine Test PPD; Tubersol®

Generic Available No

Mechanism of Action Tuberculosis results in individuals becoming sensitized to certain antigenic components of the *M. tuberculosis* organism. Culture extracts called tuberculins are contained in tuberculin skin test preparations. Upon intracutaneous injection of these culture extracts, a classic delayed (cellular) hypersensitivity reaction occurs. This reaction is characteristic of a delayed course (peak occurs >24 hours after injection, induration of the skin secondary to cell infiltration, and occasional vesiculation and necrosis). Delayed hypersensitivity reactions to tuberculin may indicate infection with a variety of nontuberculosis mycobacteria, or vaccination with the live attenuated mycobacterial strain of *M. bovis* vaccine, BCG, in addition to previous natural infection with *M. tuberculosis.*

Use Skin test in diagnosis of tuberculosis, cell-mediated immunodeficiencies

USUAL DOSAGE Children and Adults: Intradermal: 0.1 mL about 4" below elbow; use 1/4" to 1/2" or 26- or 27-gauge needle; significant reactions are ≥5 mm in diameter

Interpretation of induration of tuberculin skin test injections: Positive: ≥10 mm; inconclusive: 5-9 mm; negative: <5 mm

Interpretation of induration of Tine test injections: Positive: >2 mm and vesiculation present; inconclusive: <2 mm (give patient Mantoux test of 5 TU/0.1 mL - base decisions on results of Mantoux test); negative: <2 mm or erythema of any size (no need for retesting unless person is a contact of a patient with tuberculosis or there is clinical evidence suggestive of the disease)

Dosage Forms INJ: First test strength: 1 TU/0.1 mL (1 mL); Intermediate test strength: 5 TU/0.1 mL (1 mL, 5 mL, 10 mL); Second test strength: 250 TU/0.1 mL (1 mL). **TINE:** 5 TU each test

Contraindications 250 TU strength should not be used for initial testing

Warnings/Precautions Do not administer I.V. or S.C.; epinephrine (1:1000) should be available to treat possible allergic reactions

Pregnancy Risk Factor C

Adverse Reactions 1% to 10%:

Dermatologic: Ulceration, vesiculation

Local: Pain at injection site

Miscellaneous: Necrosis

Drug Interactions Decreased effect: Reaction may be suppressed in patients receiving systemic corticosteroids, aminocaproic acid, or within 4-6 weeks following immunization with live or inactivated viral vaccines

Education and Monitoring Issues

Patient Education: Return to prescriber for reaction interpretation at 48-72 hours

- **Tuberculosis Test Recommendations and Prophylaxis** *see page 1163*
- **Tuberculosis Treatment Guidelines** *see page 1213*
- **Tubersol®** *see* Tuberculin Purified Protein Derivative *on page 960*
- **Tubersol®** *see* Tuberculin Tests *on page 960*
- **Tums® [OTC]** *see* Calcium Carbonate *on page 130*
- **Tums® E-X Extra Strength Tablet [OTC]** *see* Calcium Carbonate *on page 130*
- **Tums® Extra Strength Liquid [OTC]** *see* Calcium Carbonate *on page 130*
- **Tusibron® [OTC]** *see* Guaifenesin *on page 423*
- **Tusibron-DM® [OTC]** *see* Guaifenesin and Dextromethorphan *on page 424*
- **Tussafed® Drops** *see* Carbinoxamine, Pseudoephedrine, and Dextromethorphan *on page 140*
- **Tussafin® Expectorant** *see* Hydrocodone, Pseudoephedrine, and Guaifenesin *on page 446*
- **Tuss-Allergine® Modified T.D. Capsule** *see* Caramiphen and Phenylpropanolamine *on page 137*
- **Tussar® SF Syrup** *see* Guaifenesin, Pseudoephedrine, and Codeine *on page 425*
- **Tuss-DM® [OTC]** *see* Guaifenesin and Dextromethorphan *on page 424*
- **Tussigon®** *see* Hydrocodone and Homatropine *on page 445*
- **Tussionex®** *see* Hydrocodone and Chlorpheniramine *on page 445*
- **Tussi-Organidin® DM NR** *see* Guaifenesin and Dextromethorphan *on page 424*
- **Tussi-Organidin® NR** *see* Guaifenesin and Codeine *on page 424*
- **Tussogest® Extended Release Capsule** *see* Caramiphen and Phenylpropanolamine *on page 137*
- **Tusstat® Syrup** *see* Diphenhydramine *on page 282*
- **Twilite® Oral [OTC]** *see* Diphenhydramine *on page 282*
- **Twin-K®** *see* Potassium Citrate and Potassium Gluconate *on page 753*
- **Two-Dyne®** *see* Butalbital Compound *on page 123*
- **Tylenol® [OTC]** *see* Acetaminophen *on page 17*
- **Tylenol® Extended Relief [OTC]** *see* Acetaminophen *on page 17*
- **Tylenol® With Codeine** *see* Acetaminophen and Codeine *on page 18*
- **Tylox®** *see* Oxycodone and Acetaminophen *on page 692*
- **Tyrodone® Liquid** *see* Hydrocodone and Pseudoephedrine *on page 446*
- **UAD® Otic** *see* Neomycin, Polymyxin B, and Hydrocortisone *on page 644*
- **Ucephan®** *see* Sodium Phenylacetate and Sodium Benzoate *on page 859*
- **U-Cort™** *see* Hydrocortisone *on page 447*
- **Ultiva™** *see* Remifentanil *on page 811*
- **Ultracef®** *see* Cefadroxil *on page 148*
- **Ultradol** *see* Etodolac *on page 347*
- **Ultralente® Insulin** *see* Insulin Preparations *on page 472*
- **Ultram®** *see* Tramadol *on page 936*
- **Ultra Mide® Topical** *see* Urea *on page 962*
- **Ultramop** *see* Methoxsalen *on page 585*
- **Ultraquin®** *see* Hydroquinone *on page 450*
- **Ultrase® MT12** *see* Pancrelipase *on page 698*
- **Ultrase® MT20** *see* Pancrelipase *on page 698*
- **Ultravate** *see* Halobetasol *on page 429*
- **Ultravate™ Topical** *see* Halobetasol *on page 429*
- **Unasyn®** *see* Ampicillin and Sulbactam *on page 60*
- **Unguentine® [OTC]** *see* Benzocaine *on page 98*

- **Uni-Ace® [OTC]** *see* Acetaminophen *on page 17*
- **Uni-Bent® Cough Syrup** *see* Diphenhydramine *on page 282*
- **Unicap® [OTC]** *see* Vitamins, Multiple *on page 981*
- **Unicort** *see* Hydrocortisone *on page 447*
- **Uni-Decon®** *see* Chlorpheniramine, Phenyltoloxamine, Phenylpropanolamine, and Phenylephrine *on page 187*
- **Unipen®** *see* Nafcillin *on page 630*
- **Unipen® Injection** *see* Nafcillin *on page 630*
- **Unipen® Oral** *see* Nafcillin *on page 630*
- **Uni-Pro® [OTC]** *see* Ibuprofen *on page 458*
- **Uniretic™** *see* Moexipril and Hydrochlorothiazide *on page 614*
- **Unitrol® [OTC]** *see* Phenylpropanolamine *on page 729*
- **Uni-Tussin® [OTC]** *see* Guaifenesin *on page 423*
- **Uni-tussin® DM [OTC]** *see* Guaifenesin and Dextromethorphan *on page 424*
- **Univasc®** *see* Moexipril *on page 613*
- **Urabeth®** *see* Bethanechol *on page 106*

Uracil Mustard (YOOR a sil MUS tard)

Pharmacologic Class Antineoplastic Agent, Alkylating Agent

Generic Available No

Mechanism of Action Polyfunctional alkylating agent, but exact mechanism of action has not been determined; it is a cell cycle-phase nonspecific antineoplastic agent

Use Palliative treatment in symptomatic chronic lymphocytic leukemia; non-Hodgkin's lymphomas, chronic myelocytic leukemia, mycosis fungoides, thrombocytosis, polycythemia vera, ovarian carcinoma

USUAL DOSAGE Oral (do not administer until 2-3 weeks after maximum effect of any previous x-ray or cytotoxic drug therapy of the bone marrow is obtained):

Children: 0.3 mg/kg in a single weekly dose for 4 weeks

Adults: 0.15 mg/kg in a single weekly dose for 4 weeks

Thrombocytosis: 1-2 mg/day for 14 days

Dosage Forms CAP: 1 mg

Contraindications Severe leukopenia, thrombocytopenia, aplastic anemia; in patients whose bone marrow is infiltrated with malignant cells; hypersensitivity to any component; pregnancy

Warnings/Precautions The U.S. Food and Drug Administration (FDA) currently recommends that procedures for proper handling and disposal of antineoplastic agents be considered. Impaired kidney or liver function. The drug should be discontinued if intractable vomiting or diarrhea, precipitous falls in leukocyte or platelet count, or myocardial ischemia occurs. Use with caution in patients who have had high-dose pelvic radiation or previous use of alkylating agents. Patient should be hospitalized during initial course of therapy; may impair fertility in men and women; use with caution in patients with pre-existing marrow suppression.

Pregnancy Risk Factor X

Adverse Reactions

>10%:

Gastrointestinal: Nausea, vomiting, diarrhea

Hematologic: Myelosuppressive; leukopenia and thrombocytopenia nadir: 2-4 weeks, anemia

1% to 10%:

Central nervous system: Mental depression, nervousness

Dermatologic: Hyperpigmentation, alopecia

Endocrine & metabolic: Hyperuricemia

<1%: Hepatotoxicity, pruritus, stomatitis

Education and Monitoring Issues

Patient Education: This drug may take weeks or months for effectiveness to become apparent. Do not discontinue without consulting prescriber. Maintain adequate hydration (2-3 L/day of fluids unless instructed to restrict fluid intake). For nausea or vomiting, loss of appetite, or dry mouth, small frequent meals, chewing gum, or sucking lozenges may help. You may experience hair loss (reversible); diarrhea (if persistent, consult prescriber); nervousness, irritability, shakiness, amenorrhea, altered sperm production (usually reversible). Report persistent nausea or vomiting, fever, sore throat, chills, unusual bleeding or bruising, consistent feelings of tiredness or weakness, or yellowing of skin or eyes.

- **Urasal®** *see* Methenamine *on page 579*

Urea (yoor EE a)

Pharmacologic Class Diuretic, Osmotic; Keratolytic Agent; Topical Skin Product

U.S. Brand Names Amino-Cerv™ Vaginal Cream; Aquacare® Topical [OTC]; Carmol® Topical [OTC]; Gormel® Creme [OTC]; Lanaphilic® Topical [OTC]; Nutraplus® Topical

[OTC]; Rea-Lo® [OTC]; Ultra Mide® Topical; Ureacin®-20 Topical [OTC]; Ureacin®-40; Ureaphil® Injection

Use Reduces intracranial pressure and intraocular pressure; topically promotes hydration and removal of excess keratin in hyperkeratotic conditions and dry skin; mild cervicitis

USUAL DOSAGE

Children: I.V. slow infusion:
- <2 years: 0.1-0.5 g/kg
- >2 years: 0.5-1.5 g/kg

Adults:
- I.V. infusion: 1-1.5 g/kg by slow infusion (1-2½ hours); maximum: 120 g/24 hours
- Topical: Apply 1-3 times/day
- Vaginal: Insert 1 applicatorful in vagina at bedtime for 2-4 weeks

Contraindications Severely impaired renal function, hepatic failure; active intracranial bleeding, sickle cell anemia, topical use in viral skin disease

Pregnancy Risk Factor C

Related Information

Urea and Hydrocortisone *on page 963*

Urea and Hydrocortisone (yoor EE a & hye droe KOR ti sone)

Pharmacologic Class Corticosteroid, Topical

U.S. Brand Names Carmol-HC® Topical

Dosage Forms CRM, top: Urea 10% and hydrocortisone acetate 1% in a water-washable vanishing cream base (30 g)

Pregnancy Risk Factor C

- ♦ **Ureacin®-20 Topical [OTC]** *see* Urea *on page 962*
- ♦ **Ureacin®-40** *see* Urea *on page 962*
- ♦ **Ureaphil® Injection** *see* Urea *on page 962*
- ♦ **Urecholine®** *see* Bethanechol *on page 106*
- ♦ **Uremol®** *see* Urea *on page 962*
- ♦ **Uremol-HC** *see* Urea and Hydrocortisone *on page 963*
- ♦ **Urex®** *see* Methenamine *on page 579*
- ♦ **Uridon®** *see* Chlorthalidone *on page 191*
- ♦ **Urisec®** *see* Urea *on page 962*
- ♦ **Urispas®** *see* Flavoxate *on page 365*
- ♦ **Uri-Tet® Oral** *see* Oxytetracycline *on page 695*
- ♦ **Uritol®** *see* Furosemide *on page 399*
- ♦ **Urobak®** *see* Sulfamethoxazole *on page 879*
- ♦ **Urodine®** *see* Phenazopyridine *on page 721*
- ♦ **Uro Gantanol** *see* Sulfamethoxazole and Phenazopyridine *on page 879*
- ♦ **Urogesic®** *see* Phenazopyridine *on page 721*

Urokinase (yoor oh KIN ase)

Pharmacologic Class Thrombolytic Agent

U.S. Brand Names Abbokinase® Injection

Generic Available No

Mechanism of Action Promotes thrombolysis by directly activating plasminogen to plasmin, which degrades fibrin, fibrinogen, and other procoagulant plasma proteins

Use Thrombolytic agent used in treatment of recent severe or massive deep vein thrombosis, pulmonary emboli, myocardial infarction, and occluded arteriovenous cannulas; not useful on thrombi over 1 week old

USUAL DOSAGE

Children and Adults: Deep vein thrombosis: I.V.: Loading: 4400 units/kg over 10 minutes, then 4400 units/kg/hour for 12 hours

Adults:

Myocardial infarction: Intracoronary: 750,000 units over 2 hours (6000 units/minute over up to 2 hours)

Occluded I.V. catheters:

5000 units (use only Abbokinase® Open Cath) in each lumen over 1-2 minutes, leave in lumen for 1-4 hours, then aspirate; may repeat with 10,000 units in each lumen if 5000 units fails to clear the catheter; **do not infuse into the patient**; volume to instill into catheter is equal to the volume of the catheter

I.V. infusion: 200 units/kg/hour in each lumen for 12-48 hours at a rate of at least 20 mL/hour

Dialysis patients: 5000 units is administered in each lumen over 1-2 minutes; leave urokinase in lumen for 1-2 days, then aspirate

Clot lysis (large vessel thrombi): Loading: I.V.: 4400 units/kg over 10 minutes, increase to 6000 units/kg/hour; maintenance: 4400-6000 units/kg/hour adjusted to achieve clot lysis or patency of affected vessel; doses up to 50,000 units/kg/hour have been used. **Note:** Therapy should be initiated as soon as possible after diagnosis of thrombi and continued until clot is dissolved (usually 24-72 hours).

Acute pulmonary embolism: Three treatment alternatives: 3 million unit dosage

(Continued)

Urokinase *(Continued)*

Alternative 1: 12-hour infusion: 4400 units/kg (2000 units/lb) bolus over 10 minutes followed by 4400 units/kg/hour (2000 units/lb); begin heparin 1000 units/hour approximately 3-4 hours after completion of urokinase infusion or when PTT is <100 seconds

Alternative 2: 2-hour infusion: 1 million unit bolus over 10 minutes followed by 2 million units over 110 minutes; begin heparin 1000 units/hour approximately 3-4 hours after completion of urokinase infusion or when PTT is <100 seconds

Alternative 3: Bolus dose only: 15,000 units/kg over 10 minutes; begin heparin 1000 units/hour approximately 3-4 hours after completion of urokinase infusion or when PTT is <100 seconds

Dosage Forms POWDER, for inj: 250,000 units (5 mL); Catheter clear: 5000 units (1 mL)

Contraindications Active internal bleeding, history of a cerebrovascular accident, recent intracranial or intraspinal surgery (within prior two months), recent trauma including cardiopulmonary resuscitation, intracranial neoplasm, A-V malformation or aneurysm, known bleeding diathesis, or severe uncontrolled arterial hypertension; hypersensitivity to urokinase or any component

Warnings/Precautions Use with caution in patients with recent (within 10 days) major surgery, obstetrical delivery, organ biopsy, previous puncture of noncompressible vessels, recent serious GI bleeding, high likelihood of left heart thrombus (eg, mitral stenosis with A-fib), subacute bacterial endocarditis, hemostatic defects including those secondary to severe hepatic or renal disease, pregnancy, cerebrovascular disease, diabetic hemorrhagic retinopathy, or any other condition in which bleeding might constitute a significant hazard or be particularly difficult to manage because of its location

The FDA is recommending (1/25/99) that Abbokinase® be reserved for only those situations where a prescriber has considered the alternatives and has determined that the use of urokinase is critical to the care of a specific patient in a specific situation; Abbokinase® is produced from primary cultures of kidney cells harvested postmortem from human neonates. Products manufactured from human source materials have the potential to transmit infectious agents. While some procedures to help control such risks in products of human source are in place, recent manufacturing inspections revealed deficiencies in some of the procedures used by Abbott and its supplier of the human neonatal kidney cells that could increase the risk of transmitting infectious agents. In considering this risk, the prescriber should be aware of the following information regarding currently available lots of urokinase; the kidney cells used in the manufacture of this product were harvested postmortem from human neonates from a population at high risk for a variety of infectious diseases, including tropical diseases. The screening of potential donors did not include the questioning of the mothers to determine infectious disease status or specific risk factors for infectious diseases; neither the mothers nor the neonate donors were tested for hepatitis C virus (HCV) infection; Abbott has recently instituted a test for HCV in the kidney cells used in the manufacture of Abbokinase® and negative test results have been obtained for currently available lots; however, Abbott has not validated this test; prior to use in the manufacture of Abbokinase®, the human kidney cells were harvested, stored and handled in a manner which may have permitted contamination with infectious agents; the FDA is not aware of any cases of infectious diseases that can be attributed to the use of Abbokinase®; however, the likelihood that cases of infectious diseases caused by Abbokinase®, if any, would have been recognized as such and reported to FDA is probably very low; therefore, the actual risk to patients of developing an infectious disease as a result of using Abbokinase® is unknown; for each setting in which the use of Abbokinase® is being contemplated, we encourage you to consider the appropriateness of other treatment options; FDA approved indications for Abbokinase® are: pulmonary embolism, coronary artery thrombosis, and I.V. catheter clearance; it should also be noted that the FDA has not approved the use of Abbokinase® for clearance of peripheral venous and arterial obstructions or for clearance of arterio-venous cannulas; other thrombolytic products on the U.S. market with well-described experience in multiple indications include Streptase® (Streptokinase), Kabikinase® (Streptokinase), Activase® (Alteplase), Eminase® (Anistreplase), and Retavase™ (Reteplase). We encourage all prescribers to consider the appropriateness of other treatment options

Pregnancy Risk Factor B

Adverse Reactions

>10%:

Cardiovascular: Hypotension, arrhythmias

Hematologic: Bleeding, especially at sites of percutaneous trauma

Ocular: Periorbital swelling

Respiratory: Dyspnea

<1%: Anaphylaxis, anemia, bronchospasm, chills, diaphoresis, epistaxis, eye hemorrhage, headache, nausea, rash, vomiting

Drug Interactions Increased toxicity (increased bleeding) with anticoagulants, antiplatelet drugs, aspirin, indomethacin, dextran

Onset I.V.: Fibrinolysis occurs rapidly

Duration 4 or more hours

Half-Life 10-20 minutes

Education and Monitoring Issues

Patient Education: You will require frequent blood tests. Report any signs of unusual bleeding. Use electric razor and soft toothbrush.

Monitoring Parameters: CBC, reticulocyte count, platelet count, DIC panel (fibrinogen, plasminogen, FDP, D-dimer, PT, PTT), thrombosis panel (AT-III, protein C), urinalysis, ACT

Manufacturer Abbott Laboratories (Pharmaceutical Product Division)

Related Information

Pharmaceutical Manufacturers Directory *on page 1020*

- **Uro-KP-Neutral®** *see* Potassium Phosphate and Sodium Phosphate *on page 755*
- **Urolene Blue®** *see* Methylene Blue *on page 587*
- **Urozide®** *see* Hydrochlorothiazide *on page 442*

Ursodiol (ER soe dye ole)

Pharmacologic Class Gallstone Dissolution Agent

U.S. Brand Names Actigall™

Generic Available No

Mechanism of Action Decreases the cholesterol content of bile and bile stones by reducing the secretion of cholesterol from the liver and the fractional reabsorption of cholesterol by the intestines

Use Gallbladder stone dissolution

USUAL DOSAGE Adults: Oral: 8-10 mg/kg/day in 2-3 divided doses; use beyond 24 months is not established; obtain ultrasound images at 6-month intervals for the first year of therapy; 30% of patients have stone recurrence after dissolution

Dosage Forms CAP: 300 mg

Contraindications Not to be used with cholesterol, radiopaque, bile pigment stones, or stones >20 mm in diameter; allergy to bile acids

Warnings/Precautions Gallbladder stone dissolution may take several months of therapy; complete dissolution may not occur and recurrence of stones within 5 years has been observed in 50% of patients; use with caution in patients with a nonvisualizing gallbladder and those with chronic liver disease; not recommended for children

Pregnancy Risk Factor B

Adverse Reactions

1% to 10%: Gastrointestinal: Diarrhea

<1%: Abdominal pain, biliary pain, constipation, dyspepsia, fatigue, headache, metallic taste, nausea, pruritus, rash, vomiting

Drug Interactions Decreased effect with aluminum-containing antacids, cholestyramine, colestipol, clofibrate, oral contraceptives (estrogens)

Half-Life 100 hours

Education and Monitoring Issues

Patient Education: Frequent blood work will be necessary to follow drug effects. Drug will need to be taken for 1-3 months after stone is dissolved. Stones may recur. Report any persistent nausea, vomiting, abdominal pain, or yellowing of skin or eyes.

Monitoring Parameters: ALT, AST, sonogram

- **Ursofalk** *see* Ursodiol *on page 965*
- **USPHS/IDSA Guidelines for the Prevention of Opportunistic Infections in Persons Infected With HIV** *see page 1165*
- **Vagifem®** *see* Estradiol *on page 327*
- **Vagilia®** *see* Sulfabenzamide, Sulfacetamide, and Sulfathiazole *on page 875*
- **Vaginex** *see* Tripelennamine *on page 957*
- **Vagistat® Vaginal** *see* Tioconazole *on page 923*
- **Vagitrol®** *see* Sulfanilamide *on page 880*

Valacyclovir (val ay SYE kloe veer)

Pharmacologic Class Antiviral Agent, Ophthalmic

U.S. Brand Names Valtrex®

Mechanism of Action Valacyclovir is rapidly and nearly completely converted to acyclovir by intestinal and hepatic metabolism. Acyclovir is converted to acyclovir monophosphate by virus-specific thymidine kinase then further converted to acyclovir triphosphate by other cellular enzymes. Acyclovir triphosphate inhibits DNA synthesis and viral replication by competing with deoxyguanosine triphosphate for viral DNA polymerase and being incorporated into viral DNA.

Use Treatment of herpes zoster (shingles) in immunocompetent patients; episodic treatment or prophylaxis of recurrent genital herpes in immunocompetent patients; for first episode genital herpes

USUAL DOSAGE Oral: Adults:

Shingles: 1 g 3 times/day for 7 days

Genital herpes:

Episodic treatment: 500 mg twice daily for 5 days

Prophylaxis: 500-1000 mg once daily

(Continued)

Valacyclovir *(Continued)*

Dosing interval in renal impairment:

Cl_{cr} 30-49 mL/minute: 1 g every 12 hours
Cl_{cr} 10-29 mL/minute: 1 g every 24 hours
Cl_{cr} <10 mL/minute: 500 mg every 24 hours

Hemodialysis: 33% removed during 4-hour session

Dosage Forms CAPLET: 500 mg, 1000 mg

Contraindications Hypersensitivity to the drug or any component

Warnings/Precautions Thrombotic thrombocytopenic purpura/hemolytic uremic syndrome has occurred in immunocompromised patients; use caution and adjust the dose in elderly patients or those with renal insufficiency; safety and efficacy in children have not been established

Pregnancy Risk Factor B

Pregnancy Implications

Clinical effects on the fetus: Teratogenicity registry, thus far, has shown no increased rate of birth defects than that of the general population; however, the registry is small and use during pregnancy is only warranted if the potential benefit to the mother justifies the risk of the fetus

Breast-feeding/lactation: Avoid use in breast-feeding, if possible, since the drug distributes in high concentrations in breast milk

Adverse Reactions

>10%:

Central nervous system: Headache (13% to 17%)
Gastrointestinal: Nausea (8% to 16%)

1% to 10%:

Central nervous system: Dizziness (2% to 4%)
Dermatologic: Pruritus
Gastrointestinal: Diarrhea (4% to 5%), constipation (1% to 5%), abdominal pain (2% to 3%), anorexia (≤3%), vomiting (≤7%)
Neuromuscular & skeletal: Weakness (2% to 4%)
Ocular: Photophobia

Drug Interactions Decreased toxicity: Cimetidine and/or probenecid has decreased the rate but not the extent of valacyclovir conversion to acyclovir

Half-Life

Normal renal function: 2.5-3.3 hours (acyclovir); ~30 minutes (valacyclovir)

End-stage renal disease: 14 hours removed partially by hemodialysis, half-life during dialysis: 4 hours; liver disease may decrease rate but not extent of conversion to acyclovir (half-life not affected)

Education and Monitoring Issues

Patient Education: Begin use as soon as possible following development of signs of herpes zoster. Take with plenty of fluids. May take without regard to meals.

Monitoring Parameters: Urinalysis, BUN, serum creatinine, liver enzymes, and CBC

Manufacturer GlaxoWellcome

Related Information

Pharmaceutical Manufacturers Directory *on page 1020*

♦ **Valergen® Injection** *see* Estradiol *on page 327*

Valerian

Pharmacologic Class Herbal

Mechanism of Action Most pharmacologic activity located in fresh root or dried rhizome; the plant contains essential oils (valerenic acid and valenol, valepotriates, and alkaloids <0.2% concentration) which may affect neurotransmitter levels (serotonin, GABA, and norepinephrine); also has antispasmodic properties

Use Herbal medicine use as a sleep-promoting agent and minor tranquilizer (similar to benzodiazepines); used in anxiety, panic attacks, intestinal cramps, headaches

Per Commission E: Restlessness, sleep disorders based on nervous conditions

USUAL DOSAGE Adults:

Sedative: 1-3 g (1-3 mL of tincture)
Sleep aid: 1-3 mL of tincture at bedtime
Dried root: 0.3-1 g

Adverse Reactions

Cardiovascular: Cardiac disturbances (unspecified)
Central nervous system: Lightheadedness, restlessness, fatigue
Gastrointestinal: Nausea
Neuromuscular & skeletal: Tremor
Ocular: Blurred vision

Drug Interactions Not synergistic with alcohol; potentiation of other CNS depressants is possible

♦ **Valertest No.1® Injection** *see* Estradiol and Testosterone *on page 329*
♦ **Valisone®** *see* Betamethasone *on page 103*
♦ **Valium® Injection** *see* Diazepam *on page 261*

♦ **Valium® Oral** *see* Diazepam *on page 261*
♦ **Valpin® 50** *see* Anisotropine *on page 65*

Valproic Acid and Derivatives (val PROE ik AS id & dah RIV ah tives)

Pharmacologic Class Anticonvulsant, Miscellaneous

U.S. Brand Names Depacon™; Depakene®; Depakote®

Generic Available Yes

Mechanism of Action Causes increased availability of gamma-aminobutyric acid (GABA), an inhibitory neurotransmitter, to brain neurons or may enhance the action of GABA or mimic its action at postsynaptic receptor sites

Use Management of simple and complex absence seizures; mixed seizure types; myoclonic and generalized tonic-clonic (grand mal) seizures; may be effective in partial seizures, infantile spasms, bipolar disorder; prevention of migraine headaches

USUAL DOSAGE Children and Adults:

Oral: Initial: 10-15 mg/kg/day in 1-3 divided doses; increase by 5-10 mg/kg/day at weekly intervals until therapeutic levels are achieved; maintenance: 30-60 mg/kg/day in 2-3 divided doses

Children receiving more than 1 anticonvulsant (ie, polytherapy) may require doses up to 100 mg/kg/day in 3-4 divided doses

I.V.: Administer as a 60 minute infusion (≤20 mg/min) with the same frequency as oral products; switch patient to oral products as soon as possible

Rectal: Dilute syrup 1:1 with water for use as a retention enema; loading dose: 17-20 mg/kg one time; maintenance: 10-15 mg/kg/dose every 8 hours

Not dialyzable (0% to 5%)

Dosing adjustment/comments in hepatic impairment: Reduce dose

Dosage Forms

Divalproex sodium: **CAP, sprinkle** (Depakote® Sprinkle®): 125 mg. **TAB, delayed release** (Depakote®): 125 mg, 250 mg, 500 mg

Valproic acid: **CAP** (Depakene®): 250 mg

Valproate sodium: **INJ** (Depacon™): 100 mg/mL (5 mL). **SYR** (Depakene®): 250 mg/5 mL (5 mL, 50 mL, 480 mL)

Contraindications Hypersensitivity to valproic acid or derivatives or any component; hepatic dysfunction

Warnings/Precautions Hepatic failure resulting in fatalities has occurred in patients; children <2 years of age are at considerable risk; monitor patients closely for appearance of malaise, weakness, facial edema, anorexia, jaundice, and vomiting; may cause severe thrombocytopenia, bleeding; hepatotoxicity has been reported after 3 days to 6 months of therapy; tremors may indicate overdosage; use with caution in patients receiving other anticonvulsants

Pregnancy Risk Factor D

Pregnancy Implications

Clinical effects on the fetus: Crosses the placenta. Neural tube, cardiac, facial (characteristic pattern of dysmorphic facial features), skeletal, multiple other defects reported. Epilepsy itself, number of medications, genetic factors, or a combination of these probably influence the teratogenicity of anticonvulsant therapy. Risk of neural tube defects with use during first 30 days of pregnancy warrants discontinuation prior to pregnancy and through this period of possible.

Breast-feeding/lactation: Crosses into breast milk. American Academy of Pediatrics considers **compatible** with breast-feeding.

Adverse Reactions

>10%:

- Central nervous system: Somnolence, dizziness, headache
- Gastrointestinal: Nausea, vomiting, diarrhea
- Neuromuscular & skeletal: Weakness
- Ocular: Diplopia, blurred vision

1% to 10%:

- Cardiovascular: Peripheral edema
- Central nervous system: Ataxia, emotional lability, abnormal thinking, amnesia, insomnia, nervousness
- Dermatologic: Rash, alopecia
- Endocrine & metabolic: Change in menstrual cycle
- Gastrointestinal: Abdominal pain, anorexia, dyspepsia, increased appetite, constipation, weight gain or loss
- Hematologic: Thrombocytopenia
- Neuromuscular & skeletal: Tremor
- Ocular: Nystagmus
- Otic: Tinnitus
- Respiratory: Flu syndrome, rhinitis

<1%: Erythema multiforme, hyperammonemia, liver failure, pancreatitis, prolongation of bleeding time, transient increased liver enzymes

Drug Interactions CYP2C19 enzyme substrate; CYP2C9 and 2D6 enzyme inhibitor, CYP3A3/4 enzyme inhibitor (weak)

Absence seizures have been reported in patients receiving VPA and clonazepam

(Continued)

Valproic Acid and Derivatives *(Continued)*

Valproic acid may displace clozapine from protein binding site resulting in decreased clozapine serum concentrations

Carbamazepine, lamotrigine, and phenytoin may induce the metabolism of valproic acid; monitor

Valproic acid may increase, decrease, or have no effect on carbamazepine and phenytoin levels

Valproic acid may increase serum concentrations of carbamazepine - epoxide (active metabolite); monitor

Cholestyramine may bind VPA in GI tract; monitor

Clarithromycin, erythromycin, troleandomycin, felbamate, and isoniazid may inhibit the metabolism of VPA; monitor

VPA inhibits the metabolism of lamotrigine; monitor

VPA appears to inhibit the metabolism of nimodipine and phenobarbital; monitor

Alcohol Interactions Avoid or limit use (may increase central nervous system depression)

Half-Life 8-17 hours

Education and Monitoring Issues

Patient Education: When used to treat generalized seizures, patient instructions are determined by patient's condition and ability to understand.

Oral: Take as directed; do not alter dose or timing of medication. Do not increase dose or take more than recommended. Do not crush or chew capsule or enteric-coated pill. While using this medication, do not use alcohol and other prescription or OTC medications (especially pain medications, sedatives, antihistamines, or hypnotics) without consulting prescriber. Maintain adequate hydration (2-3 L/day of fluids unless instructed to restrict fluid intake). Diabetics should monitor serum glucose closely (valproic acid will alter results of urine ketones). Report alterations in menstrual cycle; abdominal cramps, unresolved diarrhea, vomiting, or constipation; skin rash; unusual bruising or bleeding; blood in urine, stool or vomitus; malaise; weakness; facial swelling; yellowing of skin or eyes; excessive sedation; or restlessness.

Dietary Considerations:

Food:

Valproic acid may cause GI upset; take with large amount of water or food to decrease GI upset. May need to split doses to avoid GI upset.

Food may delay but does not affect the extent of absorption

Coated particles of divalproex sodium may be mixed with semisolid food (eg, applesauce or pudding) in patients having difficulty swallowing; particles should be swallowed and not chewed

Valproate sodium oral solution will generate valproic acid in carbonated beverages and may cause mouth and throat irritation; do not mix valproate sodium oral solution with carbonated beverages

Milk: No effect on absorption; may take with milk

Sodium: SIADH and water intoxication; monitor fluid status. May need to restrict fluid.

Monitoring Parameters: Liver enzymes, CBC with platelets

Reference Range: Therapeutic: 50-100 μg/mL (SI: 350-690 μmol/L); Toxic: >200 μg/mL (SI: >1390 μmol/L). Seizure control may improve at levels >100 μg/mL (SI: 690 μmol/L), but toxicity may occur at levels of 100-150 μg/mL (SI: 690-1040 μmol/L).

Related Information

Anticonvulsants by Seizure Type Comparison *on page 1230*
Epilepsy Guidelines *on page 1091*

Valsartan (val SAR tan)

Pharmacologic Class Angiotensin II Antagonists

U.S. Brand Names Diovan™

Mechanism of Action As a prodrug, valsartan produces direct antagonism of the angiotensin II (AT2) receptors, unlike the angiotensin-converting enzyme inhibitors. It displaces angiotensin II from the AT1 receptor and produces its blood pressure lowering effects by antagonizing AT1-induced vasoconstriction, aldosterone release, catecholamine release, arginine vasopressin release, water intake, and hypertrophic responses. This action results in more efficient blockade of the cardiovascular effects of angiotensin II and fewer side effects than the ACE inhibitors.

Use Alone or in combination with other antihypertensive agents in treating essential hypertension; may have an advantage over losartan due to minimal metabolism requirements and consequent use in mild to moderate hepatic impairment

USUAL DOSAGE Adults: 80 mg/day; may be increased to 160 mg if needed (maximal effects observed in 4-6 weeks)

Dosing adjustment in renal impairment: No dosage adjustment necessary if Cl_{cr} >10 mL/minute

Dosing adjustment in hepatic impairment (mild - moderate): ≤80 mg/day

Dialysis: Not significantly removed

Dosage Forms CAP: 80 mg, 160 mg

Contraindications Hypersensitivity to valsartan or any components, pregnancy, severe hepatic insufficiency, biliary cirrhosis or biliary obstruction, primary hyperaldosteronism, bilateral renal artery stenosis

Warnings/Precautions Use extreme caution with concurrent administration of potassium-sparing diuretics or potassium supplements, in patients with mild to moderate hepatic dysfunction (adjust dose), in those who may be sodium/water depleted (eg, on high-dose diuretics), and in the elderly; avoid use in patients with congestive heart failure, unilateral renal artery stenosis, aortic/mitral valve stenosis, coronary artery disease, or hypertrophic cardiomyopathy, if possible

Pregnancy Risk Factor C (1st trimester); D (2nd and 3rd trimesters)

Pregnancy Implications Breast-feeding/lactation: Although no human data exist, valsartan is known to be excreted in animal breast milk and should be avoided in lactating mothers if possible

Adverse Reactions Similar incidence to placebo; independent of race, age, and gender.

>1%:

Central nervous system: Dizziness (2% to 9%), drowsiness (2.1%), ataxia (1.4%), fatigue (2%)

Cardiovascular: Hypotension (6.9%)

Endocrine & metabolic: Increased serum potassium (4.4%)

Gastrointestinal: Abdominal pain (2%), dysgeusia (1.4%)

Hematologic: Neutropenia (1.9%)

Hepatic: Increased LFTs

Respiratory: Cough (2.9% versus 1.5% in placebo)

Miscellaneous: Viral infection (3%)

>1% but frequency ≤ placebo: Headache, alopecia, upper respiratory infection, cough, diarrhea, rhinitis, sinusitis, nausea, pharyngitis, edema, arthralgia

<1% (limited to important or life-threatening symptoms): Anemia, increased creatinine (0.8%), orthostatic effects, allergic reactions, asthenia, palpitations, pruritus, rash, constipation, xerostomia, dyspepsia, flatulence, back pain, muscle cramps, myalgia, anxiety, insomnia, paresthesia, somnolence, dyspnea, vertigo, impotence, chest pain, syncope, anorexia, vomiting, angioedema, decreased hematocrit, decreased hemoglobin, increased serum transaminases, increased total bilirubin, tachycardia, depression, neuralgia, polyuria, conjunctivitis, epistaxis, joint pain. May be associated with worsening of renal function in patients dependent on renin-angiotensin-aldosterone system.

Case report: Antisynthetase syndrome without myositis

Drug Interactions

Lithium: Risk of toxicity may be increased by valsartan; monitor lithium levels

Potassium-sparing diuretics (amiloride, potassium, spironolactone, triamterene): Increased risk of hyperkalemia

Potassium supplements may increase the risk of hyperkalemia

Trimethoprim (high dose) may increase the risk of hyperkalemia

Half-Life 9 hours

Education and Monitoring Issues

Patient Education: Take exactly as directed; do not discontinue without consulting prescriber. Take first dose at bedtime. This drug does not eliminate need for diet or exercise regimen as recommended by prescriber. May cause dizziness, fainting, lightheadedness (use caution when driving or engaging in tasks requiring alertness until response to drug is known); mild hypotension use caution when changing position (rising from sitting or lying position) until response to therapy is established; decreased libido (will resolve). Report chest pain or palpitations; unrelenting headache; swelling of extremities, face, or tongue; muscle weakness or pain; difficulty in breathing or unusual cough; flu-like symptoms; or other persistent adverse reactions.

Monitoring Parameters: Baseline and periodic electrolyte panels, renal and liver function tests, urinalysis; symptoms of hypotension or hypersensitivity

Manufacturer Novartis

Related Information

Angiotensin-Related Agents Comparison *on page 1226*

Pharmaceutical Manufacturers Directory *on page 1020*

Valsartan and Hydrochlorothiazide *on page 969*

Valsartan and Hydrochlorothiazide

(val SAR tan & hye droe klor oh THYE a zide)

Pharmacologic Class Antihypertensive Agent, Combination

U.S. Brand Names Diovan™ HCT

Dosage Forms TAB: Valsartan 80 mg and hydrochlorothiazide 12.5 mg; valsartan 160 mg and hydrochlorothiazide 12.5 mg

Manufacturer Novartis

Related Information

Pharmaceutical Manufacturers Directory *on page 1020*

♦ **Valtrex®** *see* Valacyclovir *on page 965*

♦ **Vamate®** *see* Hydroxyzine *on page 455*

♦ **Vancenase® AQ Inhaler** *see* Beclomethasone *on page 94*
♦ **Vancenase® Nasal Inhaler** *see* Beclomethasone *on page 94*
♦ **Vanceril® Oral Inhaler** *see* Beclomethasone *on page 94*
♦ **Vancocin®** *see* Vancomycin *on page 970*
♦ **Vancocin® CP** *see* Vancomycin *on page 970*
♦ **Vancoled®** *see* Vancomycin *on page 970*

Vancomycin (van koe MYE sin)

Pharmacologic Class Antibiotic, Miscellaneous

U.S. Brand Names Lyphocin®; Vancocin®; Vancoled®

Generic Available Yes

Mechanism of Action Inhibits bacterial cell wall synthesis by blocking glycopeptide polymerization through binding tightly to D-alanyl-D-alanine portion of cell wall precursor

Use Treatment of patients with infections caused by staphylococcal species and streptococcal species; used orally for staphylococcal enterocolitis or for antibiotic-associated pseudomembranous colitis produced by *C. difficile*

USUAL DOSAGE Initial dosage recommendation: I.V.:

Neonates:
- Postnatal age ≤7 days:
  - <1200 g: 15 mg/kg/dose every 24 hours
  - 1200-2000 g: 10 mg/kg/dose every 12 hours
  - >2000 g: 15 mg/kg/dose every 12 hours
- Postnatal age >7 days:
  - <1200 g: 15 mg/kg/dose every 24 hours
  - ≥1200 g: 10 mg/kg/dose divided every 8 hours

Infants >1 month and Children:
- 40 mg/kg/day in divided doses every 6 hours
- Prophylaxis for bacterial endocarditis:
  - Dental, oral, or upper respiratory tract surgery: 20 mg/kg 1 hour prior to the procedure
  - GI/GU procedure: 20 mg/kg plus gentamicin 2 mg/kg 1 hour prior to surgery

Infants >1 month and Children with staphylococcal central nervous system infection: 60 mg/kg/day in divided doses every 6 hours

Adults:
- With normal renal function: 1 g **or** 10-15 mg/kg/dose every 12 hours
- Prophylaxis for bacterial endocarditis:
  - Dental, oral, or upper respiratory tract surgery: 1 g 1 hour before surgery
  - GI/GU procedure: 1 g plus 1.5 mg/kg gentamicin 1 hour prior to surgery

Dosing interval in renal impairment (vancomycin levels should be monitored in patients with any renal impairment):
- Cl_{cr} >60 mL/minute: Start with 1 g or 10-15 mg/kg/dose every 12 hours
- Cl_{cr} 40-60 mL/minute: Start with 1 g or 10-15 mg/kg/dose every 24 hours
- Cl_{cr} <40 mL/minute: Will need longer intervals; determine by serum concentration monitoring

Hemodialysis: Not dialyzable (0% to 5%); generally not removed; exception minimal-moderate removal by some of the newer high-flux filters; dose may need to be administered more frequently; monitor serum concentrations
- Continuous ambulatory peritoneal dialysis (CAPD): Not significantly removed; administration via CAPD fluid: 15-30 mg/L (15-30 mcg/mL) of CAPD fluid
- Continuous arteriovenous hemofiltration: Dose as for Cl_{cr} 10-40 mL/minute

Antibiotic lock technique (for catheter infections): 2 mg/mL in SWI/NS or D_5W; instill 3-5 mL into catheter port as a flush solution instead of heparin lock (**Note:** Do not mix with any other solutions)

Intrathecal: Vancomycin is available as a powder for injection and may be diluted to 1-5 mg/mL concentration in preservative-free 0.9% sodium chloride for administration into the CSF
- Neonates: 5-10 mg/day
- Children: 5-20 mg/day
- Adults: Up to 20 mg/day

Oral: Pseudomembranous colitis produced by *C. difficile*:
- Neonates: 10 mg/kg/day in divided doses
- Children: 40 mg/kg/day in divided doses, added to fluids
- Adults: 125 mg 4 times/day for 10 days

Dosage Forms CAP: 125 mg, 250 mg. **POWDER:** For oral soln: 1 g, 10 g; For inj: 500 mg, 1 g, 2 g, 5 g, 10 g

Contraindications Hypersensitivity to vancomycin or any component; avoid in patients with previous severe hearing loss

Warnings/Precautions Use with caution in patients with renal impairment or those receiving other nephrotoxic or ototoxic drugs; dosage modification required in patients with impaired renal function (especially elderly)

Pregnancy Risk Factor C

Adverse Reactions

Oral:
- >10%: Gastrointestinal: Bitter taste, nausea, vomiting

1% to 10%:
Central nervous system: Chills, drug fever
Hematologic: Eosinophilia
<1%: Interstitial nephritis, ototoxicity, renal failure, thrombocytopenia, vasculitis
Parenteral:
>10%:
Cardiovascular: Hypotension accompanied by flushing
Dermatologic: Erythematous rash on face and upper body (red neck or red man syndrome - infusion rate related)
1% to 10%:
Central nervous system: Chills, drug fever
Dermatologic: Rash
Hematologic: Eosinophilia, reversible neutropenia
<1%: Ototoxicity (especially with large doses), renal failure (especially with renal dysfunction or pre-existing hearing loss) Stevens-Johnson syndrome, thrombocytopenia, vasculitis

Drug Interactions Increased toxicity: Anesthetic agents; other ototoxic or nephrotoxic agents

Half-Life Half-life (biphasic): Terminal: Adults: 5-11 hours, prolonged significantly with reduced renal function; End-stage renal disease: 200-250 hours

Education and Monitoring Issues

Patient Education:

Oral: Take per recommended schedule. Complete full course of therapy; do not skip doses. Maintain adequate hydration (2-3 L/day of fluids unless instructed to restrict fluid intake). You may experience nausea, vomiting, or GI upset (small frequent meals, frequent mouth care, sucking lozenges, or chewing gum may help).

Oral/I.V.: Report chills or pain at infusion site, skin rash or redness, decrease in urine output, chest pain or palpitations, persistent GI disturbances, signs of opportunistic infection (sore throat, chills, fever, burning, itching on urination, vaginal discharge, white plaques in mouth), difficulty breathing, changes in hearing or fullness in ears, or worsening of condition.

Monitoring Parameters: Periodic renal function tests, urinalysis, serum vancomycin concentrations, WBC, audiogram

Reference Range:

Timing of serum samples: Draw peak 1 hour after 1-hour infusion has completed; draw trough just before next dose
Therapeutic levels: Peak: 25-40 μg/mL; Trough: 5-12 μg/mL
Toxic: >80 μg/mL (SI: >54 μmol/L)

Related Information

Antibiotic Treatment of Adults With Infective Endocarditis *on page 1179*
Antimicrobial Drugs of Choice *on page 1182*
Prevention of Bacterial Endocarditis *on page 1154*

♦ **Vanoxide-HC®** *see* Benzoyl Peroxide and Hydrocortisone *on page 100*
♦ **Vansil™** *see* Oxamniquine *on page 684*
♦ **Vantin®** *see* Cefpodoxime *on page 159*
♦ **Vapocet®** *see* Hydrocodone and Acetaminophen *on page 444*
♦ **Vapo-Iso®** *see* Isoproterenol *on page 488*

Varicella-Zoster Immune Globulin (Human)

(var i SEL a-ZOS ter i MYUN GLOB yoo lin HYU man)

Pharmacologic Class Immune Globulin

Generic Available No

Mechanism of Action The exact mechanism has not been clarified but the antibodies in varicella-zoster immune globulin most likely neutralize the varicella-zoster virus and prevent its pathological actions

Use Passive immunization of susceptible immunodeficient patients after exposure to varicella; most effective if begun within 96 hours of exposure; there is no evidence VZIG modifies established varicella-zoster infections.

Restrict administration to those patients meeting the following criteria:

Neoplastic disease (eg, leukemia or lymphoma)
Congenital or acquired immunodeficiency
Immunosuppressive therapy with steroids, antimetabolites or other immunosuppressive treatment regimens
Newborn of mother who had onset of chickenpox within 5 days before delivery or within 48 hours after delivery
Premature (≥28 weeks gestation) whose mother has no history of chickenpox
Premature (<28 weeks gestation or ≤1000 g VZIG) regardless of maternal history

One of the following types of exposure to chickenpox or zoster patient(s) may warrant administration:

Continuous household contact
Playmate contact (>1 hour play indoors)

(Continued)

Varicella-Zoster Immune Globulin (Human) *(Continued)*

Hospital contact (in same 2-4 bedroom or adjacent beds in a large ward or prolonged face-to-face contact with an infectious staff member or patient)

Susceptible to varicella-zoster

Age <15 years; administer to immunocompromised adolescents and adults and to other older patients on an individual basis

An acceptable alternative to VZIG prophylaxis is to treat varicella, if it occurs, with high-dose I.V. acyclovir

Age is the most important risk factor for reactivation of varicella zoster; persons <50 years of age have incidence of 2.5 cases per 1000, whereas those 60-79 have 6.5 cases per 1000 and those >80 years have 10 cases per 1000

USUAL DOSAGE High risk susceptible patients who are exposed again more than 3 weeks after a prior dose of VZIG should receive another full dose; there is no evidence VZIG modifies established varicella-zoster infections.

I.M.: Administer by deep injection in the gluteal muscle or in another large muscle mass. Inject 125 units/10 kg (22 lb); maximum dose: 625 units (5 vials); minimum dose: 125 units; do not administer fractional doses. Do not inject I.V. See table.

VZIG Dose Based on Weight

Weight of Patient		Dose	
kg	lb	Units	No. of Vials
0-10	0-22	125	1
10.1-20	22.1-44	250	2
20.1-30	44.1-66	375	3
30.1-40	66.1-88	500	4
>40	>88	625	5

Dosage Forms INJ: 125 units of antibody in single dose vials

Contraindications Not for prophylactic use in immunodeficient patients with history of varicella, unless patient's immunosuppression is associated with bone marrow transplantation; **not** recommended for nonimmunodeficient patients, including pregnant women, because the severity of chickenpox is much less than in immunosuppressed patients; allergic response to gamma globulin or anti-immunoglobulin; sensitivity to thimerosal; persons with IgA deficiency; do not administer to patients with thrombocytopenia or coagulopathies

Warnings/Precautions VZIG is not indicated for prophylaxis or therapy of normal adults who are exposed to or who develop varicella; it is not indicated for treatment of herpes zoster. Do not inject I.V.

Pregnancy Risk Factor C

Adverse Reactions

1% to 10%: Local: Discomfort at the site of injection (pain, redness, edema)

<1%: Anaphylactic shock, angioedema, GI symptoms, headache, malaise, rash, respiratory symptoms

Drug Interactions Decreased effect: Live virus vaccines (do not administer within 3 months of immune globulin administration)

Related Information

Prophylaxis for Patients Exposed to Common Communicable Diseases *on page 1161*

- **Vascor®** *see* Bepridil *on page 101*
- **Vaseretic®** *see* Enalapril and Hydrochlorothiazide *on page 311*
- **Vaseretic® 10-25** *see* Enalapril and Hydrochlorothiazide *on page 311*
- **Vasocidin®** *see* Sulfacetamide Sodium and Prednisolone *on page 876*
- **Vasocidin® Ophthalmic** *see* Sulfacetamide Sodium and Prednisolone *on page 876*
- **VasoClear® [OTC]** *see* Naphazoline *on page 636*
- **Vasocon** *see* Naphazoline *on page 636*
- **Vasocon Regular®** *see* Naphazoline *on page 636*

Vasopressin (vay soe PRES in)

Pharmacologic Class Antidiuretic Hormone Analog; Hormone, Posterior Pituitary

U.S. Brand Names Pitressin® Injection

Generic Available No

Mechanism of Action Increases cyclic adenosine monophosphate (cAMP) which increases water permeability at the renal tubule resulting in decreased urine volume and increased osmolality; causes peristalsis by directly stimulating the smooth muscle in the GI tract

Use Treatment of diabetes insipidus; prevention and treatment of postoperative abdominal distention; differential diagnosis of diabetes insipidus

Unlabeled use: Adjunct in the treatment of GI hemorrhage and esophageal varices

USUAL DOSAGE

Diabetes insipidus (highly variable dosage; titrated based on serum and urine sodium and osmolality in addition to fluid balance and urine output):

I.M., S.C.:

Children: 2.5-10 units 2-4 times/day as needed

Adults: 5-10 units 2-4 times/day as needed (dosage range 5-60 units/day)

Continuous I.V. infusion: Children and Adults: 0.5 milliunit/kg/hour (0.0005 unit/kg/hour); double dosage as needed every 30 minutes to a maximum of 0.01 unit/kg/hour

Intranasal: Administer on cotton pledget or nasal spray

Abdominal distention (aqueous): Adults: I.M.: 5 mg stat, 10 mg every 3-4 hours

GI hemorrhage: I.V. infusion: Dilute aqueous in NS or D_5W to 0.1-1 unit/mL

Children: Initial: 0.002-0.005 units/kg/minute; titrate dose as needed; maximum: 0.01 unit/kg/minute; continue at same dosage (if bleeding stops) for 12 hours, then taper off over 24-48 hours

Adults: Initial: 0.2-0.4 unit/minute, then titrate dose as needed, if bleeding stops; continue at same dose for 12 hours, taper off over 24-48 hours

Dosing adjustment in hepatic impairment: Some patients respond to much lower doses with cirrhosis

Dosage Forms INJ, aqueous: 20 pressor units/mL (0.5 mL, 1 mL)

Contraindications Hypersensitivity to vasopressin or any component

Warnings/Precautions Use with caution in patients with seizure disorders, migraine, asthma, vascular disease, renal disease, cardiac disease; chronic nephritis with nitrogen retention. Goiter with cardiac complications, arteriosclerosis; I.V. infiltration may lead to severe vasoconstriction and localized tissue necrosis; also, gangrene of extremities, tongue, and ischemic colitis. Elderly patients should be cautioned not to increase their fluid intake beyond that sufficient to satisfy their thirst in order to avoid water intoxication and hyponatremia; under experimental conditions, the elderly have shown to have a decreased responsiveness to vasopressin with respect to its effects on water homeostasis

Pregnancy Risk Factor B

Adverse Reactions

1% to 10%:

Cardiovascular: Increased blood pressure, bradycardia, arrhythmias, venous thrombosis, vasoconstriction with higher doses, angina

Central nervous system: Pounding in the head, fever, vertigo

Dermatologic: Urticaria, circumoral pallor

Gastrointestinal: Flatulence, abdominal cramps, nausea, vomiting

Neuromuscular & skeletal: Tremor

Miscellaneous: Diaphoresis

<1%: Allergic reaction, myocardial infarction, water intoxication

Drug Interactions

Decreased effect: Lithium, epinephrine, demeclocycline, heparin, and alcohol block antidiuretic activity to varying degrees

Increased effect: Chlorpropamide, phenformin, urea and fludrocortisone potentiate antidiuretic response

Onset Nasal: 1 hour

Duration Nasal: 3-8 hours; Parenteral: I.M., S.C.: 2-8 hours

Half-Life Nasal: 15 minutes; Parenteral: 10-20 minutes

Education and Monitoring Issues

Patient Education: Side effects such as abdominal cramps and nausea may be reduced by drinking a glass of water with each dose. Avoid alcohol use. Report chest pain, dizziness, pounding in head, itching, abdominal pain, persistent nausea or vomiting, unexplained sweating, and tremors. Report burning or stinging at I.V. site.

Monitoring Parameters: Serum and urine sodium, urine output, fluid input and output, urine specific gravity, urine and serum osmolality

Reference Range: Plasma: 0-2 pg/mL (SI: 0-2 ng/L) if osmolality <285 mOsm/L; 2-12 pg/mL (SI: 2-12 ng/L) if osmolality >290 mOsm/L

- **Vasosulf® Ophthalmic** *see* Sulfacetamide Sodium and Phenylephrine *on page 876*
- **Vasotec®** *see* Enalapril *on page 309*
- **Vasotec® I.V.** *see* Enalapril *on page 309*
- **V-Cillin K®** *see* Penicillin V Potassium *on page 713*
- **Veetids®** *see* Penicillin V Potassium *on page 713*
- **Velosef®** *see* Cephradine *on page 170*
- **Velosulin® BR Human (Buffered)** *see* Insulin Preparations *on page 472*
- **Velosulin® Human** *see* Insulin Preparations *on page 472*
- **Velosulin® (Regular)** *see* Insulin Preparations *on page 472*
- **Velvelan®** *see* Urea *on page 962*

Venlafaxine (VEN la faks een)

Pharmacologic Class Antidepressant, Serotonin/Norepinephrine Reuptake Inhibitor

U.S. Brand Names Effexor®; Effexor® XR

(Continued)

Venlafaxine *(Continued)*

Mechanism of Action Venlafaxine and its active metabolite o-desmethylvenlafaxine (ODV) are potent inhibitors of neuronal serotonin and norepinephrine reuptake and weak inhibitors of dopamine reuptake; causes beta-receptor down regulation and reduces adenylcyclase coupled beta-adrenergic systems in the brain

Use Treatment of depression in adults

Unapproved use: Obsessive-compulsive disorder

USUAL DOSAGE Adults: Oral:

Immediate-release tablets: 75 mg/day, administered in 2 or 3 divided doses, taken with food; dose may be increased in 75 mg/day increments at intervals of at least 4 days, up to 225-375 mg/day

Extended-release capsules: 75 mg once daily taken with food; for some new patients, it may be desirable to start at 37.5 mg/day for 4-7 days before increasing to 75 mg once daily; dose may be increased by up to 75 mg/day increments every 4 days as tolerated, up to a maximum of 225 mg/day

Dosing adjustment in renal impairment: Cl_{cr} 10-70 mL/minute: Decrease dose by 25%; decrease total daily dose by 50% if dialysis patients; dialysis patients should receive dosing after completion of dialysis

Dosing adjustment in moderate hepatic impairment: Reduce total daily dosage by 50%

Dosage Forms CAP, extended release: 37.5 mg, 75 mg, 150 mg. **TAB:** 25 mg, 37.5 mg, 50 mg, 75 mg, 100 mg

Contraindications Do not use concomitantly with MAO inhibitors, contraindicated in patients with hypersensitivity to venlafaxine or other components

Warnings/Precautions Venlafaxine is associated with sustained increases in blood pressure (10-15 mm Hg SDBP); venlafaxine may actuate mania or hypomania and seizures. Concurrent therapy with a monoamine oxidase inhibitor may result in serious or fatal reactions; at least 14 days should elapse between treatment with an MAO inhibitor and venlafaxine. Patients with cardiovascular disorders or a recent myocardial infarction probably should only receive venlafaxine if the benefits of therapy outweigh the risks.

Pregnancy Risk Factor C

Adverse Reactions

≥10%:

- Central nervous system: Headache, somnolence, dizziness, insomnia, nervousness
- Gastrointestinal: Nausea, xerostomia, constipation, anorexia
- Genitourinary: Abnormal ejaculation
- Neuromuscular & skeletal: Weakness
- Miscellaneous: Diaphoresis

1% to 10%:

- Cardiovascular: Hypertension, sinus tachycardia, postural hypotension, vasodilation
- Central nervous system: Anxiety, abnormal dreams, agitation, confusion, abnormal thinking, yawning
- Dermatologic: Rash, pruritus
- Endocrine & metabolic: Decreased libido
- Gastrointestinal: Weight loss, vomiting, diarrhea, dyspepsia, flatulence, taste perversion
- Genitourinary: Impotence, urinary retention
- Neuromuscular & skeletal: Tremor, hypertonia, paresthesia
- Ocular: Blurred vision, mydriasis
- Otic: Tinnitus

Drug Interactions CYP2D6, 2E1, and 3A3/4 enzyme substrate; CYP2D6 enzyme inhibitor (weak)

Increased toxicity: Cimetidine MAO inhibitors (hyperpyrexic crisis); TCAs, fluoxetine, sertraline, phenothiazine, class 1C antiarrhythmics, warfarin; venlafaxine is a weak inhibitor of CYP2D6, which is responsible for metabolizing antipsychotics, antiarrhythmics, TCAs, and beta-blockers. Therefore, interactions with these agents are possible, however, less likely than with more potent enzyme inhibitors such as the SSRIs.

Alcohol Interactions Avoid use (may increase central nervous system depression)

Onset Therapeutic effects: >2 weeks

Half-Life Active metabolite: 11-13 hours; Venlafaxine: 3-7 hours

Education and Monitoring Issues

Patient Education: Take exactly as directed (do not increase dose or frequency); may take 2-3 weeks to achieve desired results; may cause physical and/or psychological dependence. Take with food. Avoid excessive alcohol, caffeine, and other prescription or OTC medications not approved by prescriber. Maintain adequate hydration (2-3 L/day of fluids unless instructed to restrict fluid intake). You may experience excess drowsiness, lightheadedness, dizziness, or blurred vision (use caution when driving or engaging in tasks requiring alertness until response to drug is known); nausea, vomiting, anorexia, altered taste, dry mouth (small frequent meals, frequent mouth care, chewing gum, or sucking lozenges may help); constipation (increased exercise, fluids, or dietary fruit and fiber may help); diarrhea (buttermilk, yogurt, or boiled milk may help); postural hypotension (use caution when climbing stairs or changing position from lying or sitting to standing); urinary retention (void before taking medication); or sexual dysfunction (reversible). Report persistent CNS effects (eg, insomnia, restlessness, fatigue, anxiety, abnormal thoughts, confusion, personality changes, impaired cognitive function); muscle cramping or tremors; chest pain, palpitations, rapid heartbeat, swelling of extremities, or severe dizziness; unresolved urinary retention; vision changes or eye pain; hearing changes or ringing in ears; skin rash or irritation; or worsening of condition.

Dietary Considerations: Food: May be taken without regard to food

Monitoring Parameters: Blood pressure should be regularly monitored, especially in patients with a high baseline blood pressure

Reference Range: Peak serum level of 163 ng/mL (325 ng/mL of ODV metabolite) obtained after a 150 mg oral dose

Manufacturer Wyeth-Ayerst Laboratories

Related Information

Antidepressant Agents Comparison *on page 1231*

Pharmaceutical Manufacturers Directory *on page 1020*

- **Venoglobulin®-I** *see* Immune Globulin, Intravenous *on page 465*
- **Venoglobulin®-S** *see* Immune Globulin, Intravenous *on page 465*
- **Ventolin®** *see* Albuterol *on page 27*
- **Ventolin® Rotocaps®** *see* Albuterol *on page 27*

Verapamil (ver AP a mil)

Pharmacologic Class Antiarrhythmic Agent, Class IV; Calcium Channel Blocker

U.S. Brand Names Calan®; Calan® SR; Covera-HS®; Isoptin®; Isoptin® SR; Verelan®

Generic Available Yes

Mechanism of Action Inhibits calcium ion from entering the "slow channels" or select voltage-sensitive areas of vascular smooth muscle and myocardium during depolarization; produces a relaxation of coronary vascular smooth muscle and coronary vasodilation; increases myocardial oxygen delivery in patients with vasospastic angina; slows automaticity and conduction of A-V node.

Use Orally used for treatment of angina pectoris (vasospastic, chronic stable, unstable) and hypertension; I.V. for supraventricular tachyarrhythmias (PSVT, atrial fibrillation, atrial flutter); only Covera-HS® is approved for both hypertension and angina as a sustained release product

USUAL DOSAGE

Children: SVT:

I.V.:

<1 year: 0.1-0.2 mg/kg over 2 minutes; repeat every 30 minutes as needed

1-15 years: 0.1-0.3 mg/kg over 2 minutes; maximum: 5 mg/dose, may repeat dose in 15 minutes if adequate response not achieved; maximum for second dose: 10 mg/dose

Oral (dose not well established):

1-5 years: 4-8 mg/kg/day in 3 divided doses **or** 40-80 mg every 8 hours

>5 years: 80 mg every 6-8 hours

Adults:

SVT: I.V.: 5-10 mg (approximately 0.075-0.15 mg/kg), second dose of 10 mg (~0.15 mg/kg) may be given 15-30 minutes after the initial dose if patient tolerates, but does not respond to initial dose

Angina: Oral: Initial dose: 80-120 mg 3 times/day (elderly or small stature: 40 mg 3 times/day); range: 240-480 mg/day in 3-4 divided doses

Hypertension: 80 mg 3 times/day or 240 mg/day (sustained release); range: 240-480 mg/day; 120 mg/day in the elderly or small patients (no evidence of additional benefit in doses >360 mg/day)

Note: One time per day dosing is recommended at bedtime with Covera-HS®

Dosing adjustment in renal impairment: Cl_{cr} <10 mL/minute: Administer at 50% to 75% of normal dose

Dialysis: Not dialyzable (0% to 5 %) via hemo or peritoneal dialysis; supplemental dose is not necessary

Dosing adjustment/comments in hepatic disease: Reduce dose in cirrhosis, reduce dose to 20% to 50% of normal and monitor EKG

Dosage Forms CAP, sustained release (Verelan®): 120 mg, 180 mg, 240 mg, 360 mg. **INJ:** 2.5 mg/mL (2 mL, 4 mL); (Isoptin®): 2.5 mg/mL (2 mL, 4 mL). **TAB:** 40 mg, 80 mg, 120 mg; (Calan®, Isoptin®): 40 mg, 80 mg, 120 mg; Sustained release: 180 mg, 240 mg; (Calan® SR, Isoptin® SR): 120 mg, 180 mg, 240 mg; (Covera-HS®): 180 mg, 240 mg

Contraindications Sinus bradycardia; advanced heart block; ventricular tachycardia; cardiogenic shock; hypersensitivity to verapamil or any component; atrial fibrillation or flutter associated with accessory conduction pathways

Warnings/Precautions Use with caution in sick-sinus syndrome, severe left ventricular dysfunction, hepatic or renal impairment, hypertrophic cardiomyopathy (especially obstructive), abrupt withdrawal may cause increased duration and frequency of chest pain; avoid I.V. use in neonates and young infants due to severe apnea, bradycardia, or hypotensive reactions; elderly may experience more constipation and hypotension. (Continued)

Verapamil *(Continued)*

Monitor EKG and blood pressure closely in patients receiving I.V. therapy particularly in patients with supraventricular tachycardia.

Pregnancy Risk Factor C

Pregnancy Implications

Clinical effects on the fetus: Use in pregnancy only when clearly needed and when the benefits outweigh the potential hazard to the fetus. Crosses the placenta. 1 report of suspected heart block when used to control fetal supraventricular tachycardia. May exhibit tocolytic effects.

Breast-feeding/lactation: Crosses into breast milk. American Academy of Pediatrics considers **compatible** with breast-feeding.

Adverse Reactions Oral (P.O.), intravenous (I.V.):

> 10%:

Gastrointestinal: Gingival hyperplasia (19%)

1% to 10%

Cardiovascular: Bradycardia (1.4% P.O., 1.2% I.V.), first-, second-, or third-degree A-V block (1.2% P.O., unknown I.V.), congestive heart failure (1.8% P.O.), hypotension (2.5% P.O., 3% I.V.), peripheral edema (1.9% P.O.), symptomatic hypotension (1.5% I.V.), severe tachycardia (1% I.V.)

Central nervous system: Dizziness (3.3% P.O., 1.2% I.V.), fatigue (1.7% P.O.), headache (2.2% P.O., 1.2% I.V.)

Dermatologic: Rash (1.2% P.O.)

Gastrointestinal: Constipation (12% up to 42% in clinical trials), nausea (2.7% P.O., 0.9% I.V.)

Respiratory: Dyspnea (1.4% P.O.)

<1% (P.O.) (limited to important or life-threatening symptoms): Angina, atrioventricular dissociation, chest pain, claudication, myocardial infarction, palpitations, purpura (vasculitis), syncope, diarrhea, dry mouth, gastrointestinal distress, gingival hyperplasia, ecchymosis, bruising, cerebrovascular accident, confusion, equilibrium disorders, insomnia, muscle cramps, paresthesia, psychotic symptoms, shakiness, somnolence, arthralgia, rash, exanthema, hair loss, hyperkeratosis, macules, sweating, urticaria, Stevens-Johnson syndrome, erythema multiforme, blurred vision, tinnitus, gynecomastia, galactorrhea/hyperprolactinemia, increased urination, spotty menstruation, impotence, flushing, abdominal discomfort

<1% (I.V.) (limited to important or life-threatening symptoms): Bronchi/laryngeal spasm, itching, urticaria, emotional depression, rotary nystagmus, sleepiness, vertigo, muscle fatigue, diaphoresis, respiratory failure, myoclonus

Case reports: Stevens-Johnson syndrome, erythema multiforme, exfoliative dermatitis, EPS, gynecomastia, eosinophilia, ventricular fibrillation, asystole, EMD, shock. myoclonus, Parkinsonian syndrome, GI obstruction, pulmonary edema, respiratory failure, hair color change

Drug Interactions CYP3A3/4 and 1A2 enzyme substrate; CYP3A3/4 inhibitor

Alfentanil's plasma concentration is increased. Fentanyl and sufentanil may be affected similarly

Amiodarone use may lead to bradycardia and decreased cardiac output; monitor closely if using together

Aspirin and concurrent verapamil use may increase bleeding times; monitor closely, especially if on other antiplatelet agents or anticoagulants

Azole antifungals may inhibit the calcium channel blocker's metabolism; avoid this combination. Try an antifungal like terbinafine (if appropriate) or monitor closely for altered effect of the calcium channel blocker.

Barbiturates reduce the plasma concentration of verapamil; may require much higher dose of verapamil

Beta-blockers may have increased pharmacodynamic interactions with verapamil

Buspirone's serum concentration may increase; may require dosage adjustment

Calcium may reduce the calcium channel blocker's effects, particularly hypotension

Carbamazepine's serum concentration is increased and toxicity may result; avoid this combination

Cimetidine reduced verapamil's metabolism; consider an alternative H_2 antagonist

Cyclosporine's serum concentrations are increased by verapamil; avoid this combination. Use another calcium channel blocker or monitor cyclosporine trough levels and renal function closely.

Digoxin's serum concentration is increased; reduce digoxin's dose when adding verapamil

Doxorubicin's clearance was reduced; monitor for altered doxorubicin's effect

Erythromycin may increase verapamil's effects; monitor altered verapamil effect

Ethanol's effects may be increased by verapamil; reduce ethanol consumption

Flecainide may have additive negative effects on conduction and inotropy

HMG-CoA reductase inhibitors (atorvastatin, cerivastatin, lovastatin, simvastatin): Serum concentration will likely be increased; consider pravastatin/fluvastatin or a dihydropyridine calcium channel blocker

Lithium neurotoxicity may result when verapamil is added; monitor lithium levels

Midazolam's plasma concentration is increased by verapamil; monitor for prolonged CNS depression

Nafcillin decreases plasma concentration of verapamil; avoid this combination

Nondepolarizing muscle relaxant's neuromuscular blockade is prolonged; monitor closely

Prazosin's serum concentration increases; monitor blood pressure

Quinidine's serum concentration is increased; adjust quinidine's dose as necessary

Rifampin increases the metabolism of calcium channel blockers; adjust the dose of the calcium channel blocker to maintain efficacy

Tacrolimus's serum concentrations are increased by verapamil; avoid the combination. Use another calcium channel blocker or monitor tacrolimus trough levels and renal function closely.

Theophylline's serum concentration may be increased by verapamil. Those at increased risk include children and cigarette smokers.

Alcohol Interactions Avoid or limit use (may increase alcohol levels)

Onset Oral (nonsustained tablets): Peak effect: 2 hours; I.V.: Peak effect: 1-5 minutes

Duration Oral (nonsustained tablets): 6-8 hours; I.V.: 10-20 minutes

Half-Life Single dose: 2-8 hours, increased up to 12 hours with multiple dosing; increased half-life with hepatic cirrhosis

Education and Monitoring Issues

Patient Education: Oral: Take as directed, around-the-clock. Do not alter dosage or discontinue therapy without consulting prescriber. Do not crush or chew extended release form. Avoid (or limit) alcohol and caffeine. You may experience dizziness or lightheadedness (use caution when driving or engaging in tasks requiring alertness until response to drug is known); nausea or vomiting (small frequent meals, frequent mouth care, chewing gum, or sucking lozenges may help); constipation (increased exercise, dietary fiber, fruit, or fluids may help); diarrhea (buttermilk, boiled milk, or yogurt may help). Report chest pain, palpitations, or irregular heartbeat; unusual cough, difficulty breathing, or swelling of extremities (feet/ankles); muscle tremors or weakness; confusion or acute lethargy; or skin irritation or rash.

Monitoring Parameters: Monitor blood pressure closely

Reference Range: Therapeutic: 50-200 ng/mL (SI: 100-410 nmol/L) for parent; under normal conditions norverapamil concentration is the same as parent drug. Toxic: >90 μg/mL

Related Information

Calcium Channel Blocking Agents Comparison *on page 1236*

Trandolapril and Verapamil *on page 938*

- ♦ **Verazinc® [OTC]** *see* Zinc Supplements *on page 993*
- ♦ **Vercyte®** *see* Pipobroman *on page 743*
- ♦ **Verelan®** *see* Verapamil *on page 975*
- ♦ **Vergon® [OTC]** *see* Meclizine *on page 556*
- ♦ **Veriga** *see* Piperazine *on page 742*
- ♦ **Verimex** *see* Piperazine *on page 742*
- ♦ **Vermizine®** *see* Piperazine *on page 742*
- ♦ **Vermox®** *see* Mebendazole *on page 555*
- ♦ **Verrex-C&M®** *see* Podophyllin and Salicylic Acid *on page 746*
- ♦ **Versed®** *see* Midazolam *on page 602*
- ♦ **Versel** *see* Selenium Sulfide *on page 845*
- ♦ **Versol** *see* Piperazine *on page 742*
- ♦ **Vesanoid®** *see* Tretinoin, Oral *on page 942*
- ♦ **Vexol** *see* Rimexolone *on page 824*
- ♦ **Vexol® Ophthalmic Suspension** *see* Rimexolone *on page 824*
- ♦ **Viadur®** *see* Leuprolide Acetate *on page 514*
- ♦ **Viagra®** *see* Sildenafil *on page 850*
- ♦ **Vibazine®** *see* Buclizine *on page 114*
- ♦ **Vibramycin®** *see* Doxycycline *on page 300*
- ♦ **Vibramycin® IV** *see* Doxycycline *on page 300*
- ♦ **Vibra-Tabs®** *see* Doxycycline *on page 300*
- ♦ **Vicks® 44E [OTC]** *see* Guaifenesin and Dextromethorphan *on page 424*
- ♦ **Vicks® Children's Chloraseptic® [OTC]** *see* Benzocaine *on page 98*
- ♦ **Vicks® Chloraseptic® Sore Throat [OTC]** *see* Benzocaine *on page 98*
- ♦ **Vicks® Pediatric Formula 44E [OTC]** *see* Guaifenesin and Dextromethorphan *on page 424*
- ♦ **Vicks® Sinex® Nasal Solution [OTC]** *see* Phenylephrine *on page 727*
- ♦ **Vicodin®** *see* Hydrocodone and Acetaminophen *on page 444*
- ♦ **Vicodin® ES** *see* Hydrocodone and Acetaminophen *on page 444*
- ♦ **Vicodin® HP** *see* Hydrocodone and Acetaminophen *on page 444*
- ♦ **Vicon Forte®** *see* Vitamins, Multiple *on page 981*
- ♦ **Vicon® Plus [OTC]** *see* Vitamins, Multiple *on page 981*
- ♦ **Vicoprofen®** *see* Hydrocodone and Ibuprofen *on page 445*

Vidarabine (vye DARE a been)

Pharmacologic Class Antiviral Agent, Ophthalmic

U.S. Brand Names Vira-A® Ophthalmic

Generic Available No

Mechanism of Action Inhibits viral DNA synthesis by blocking DNA polymerase

Use Treatment of acute keratoconjunctivitis and epithelial keratitis due to herpes simplex virus type 1 and 2; superficial keratitis caused by herpes simplex virus

USUAL DOSAGE Children and Adults: Ophthalmic: Keratoconjunctivitis: Instill ½" of ointment in lower conjunctival sac 5 times/day every 3 hours while awake until complete re-epithelialization has occurred, then twice daily for an additional 7 days

Dosage Forms OINT, ophth: 3% [30 mg/mL = 28 mg/mL base] (3.5 g)

Contraindications Hypersensitivity to vidarabine or any component; sterile trophic ulcers

Warnings/Precautions Not effective against RNA virus, adenoviral ocular infections, bacterial fungal or chlamydial infections of the cornea, or trophic ulcers; temporary visual haze may be produced; neoplasia has occurred with I.M. vidarabine-treated animals; although *in vitro* studies have been inconclusive, they have shown mutagenesis

Pregnancy Risk Factor C

Adverse Reactions Percentage unknown: Burning eyes, foreign body sensation, keratitis, lacrimation, photophobia, uveitis

Education and Monitoring Issues

Patient Education: For ophthalmic use only. Store in refrigerator. Apply prescribed amount as often as directed. Wash hands before using and do not let tip of applicator touch eye or contaminate tip of applicator. Tilt head back and look upward. Gently pull down lower lid and put drop(s) in inner corner of eye. Close eye and roll eyeball in all directions. Do not blink for ½ minute. Apply gentle pressure to inner corner of eye for 30 seconds. Wipe away excess from skin around eye. Do not use any other eye preparation for at least 10 minutes. Do not touch tip of applicator to eye or contaminate tip of applicator. Do not share medication with anyone else. May cause sensitivity to bright light (dark glasses may help); temporary stinging or blurred vision may occur. Inform prescriber if you experience eye pain, redness, burning, watering, dryness, double vision, puffiness around eye, vision disturbances, or other adverse eye response; worsening of condition or lack of improvement within 7-14 days.

- **Vi-Daylin® [OTC]** *see* Vitamins, Multiple *on page 981*
- **Vi-Daylin/F®** *see* Vitamins, Multiple *on page 981*
- **Videx®** *see* Didanosine *on page 267*
- **Vioform® [OTC]** *see* Clioquinol *on page 209*
- **Viokase®** *see* Pancrelipase *on page 698*
- **Vioxx®** *see* Rofecoxib *on page 830*
- **Vira-A® Ophthalmic** *see* Vidarabine *on page 978*
- **Viracept®** *see* Nelfinavir *on page 641*
- **Viramune®** *see* Nevirapine *on page 647*
- **Virazole® Aerosol** *see* Ribavirin *on page 818*
- **Virilon®** *see* Methyltestosterone *on page 591*
- **Viroptic® Ophthalmic** *see* Trifluridine *on page 951*
- **Viscoat®** *see* Chondroitin Sulfate-Sodium Hyaluronate *on page 195*
- **Visken®** *see* Pindolol *on page 738*
- **Vistacon-50®** *see* Hydroxyzine *on page 455*
- **Vistaject-25®** *see* Hydroxyzine *on page 455*
- **Vistaject-50®** *see* Hydroxyzine *on page 455*
- **Vistaquel®** *see* Hydroxyzine *on page 455*
- **Vistaril®** *see* Hydroxyzine *on page 455*
- **Vistazine®** *see* Hydroxyzine *on page 455*
- **Vistide®** *see* Cidofovir *on page 197*
- **Vita-C® [OTC]** *see* Ascorbic Acid *on page 72*
- **VitaCarn® Oral** *see* Levocarnitine *on page 519*
- **Vita-E** *see* Vitamin E *on page 980*

Vitamin A (VYE ta min aye)

Pharmacologic Class Vitamin, Fat Soluble

U.S. Brand Names Aquasol A®; Del-Vi-A®; Palmitate-A® 5000 [OTC]

Generic Available Yes

Mechanism of Action Needed for bone development, growth, visual adaptation to darkness, testicular and ovarian function, and as a cofactor in many biochemical processes

Use Treatment and prevention of vitamin A deficiency

USUAL DOSAGE

RDA:

<1 year: 375 mcg
1-3 years: 400 mcg
4-6 years: 500 mcg*

7-10 years: 700 mcg*
>10 years: 800-1000 mcg*
Male: 1000 mcg
Female: 800 mcg
* mcg retinol equivalent (0.3 mcg retinol = 1 unit vitamin A)

Vitamin A supplementation in measles (recommendation of the World Health Organization): Children: Oral: Administer as a single dose; repeat the next day and at 4 weeks for children with ophthalmologic evidence of vitamin A deficiency:
6 months to 1 year: 100,000 units
>1 year: 200,000 units

Note: Use of vitamin A in measles is recommended only for patients 6 months to 2 years of age hospitalized with measles and its complications **or** patients >6 months of age who have any of the following risk factors and who are not already receiving vitamin A: immunodeficiency, ophthalmologic evidence of vitamin A deficiency including night blindness, Bitot's spots or evidence of xerophthalmia, impaired intestinal absorption, moderate to severe malnutrition including that associated with eating disorders, or recent immigration from areas where high mortality rates from measles have been observed

Note: Monitor patients closely; dosages >25,000 units/kg have been associated with toxicity

Severe deficiency with xerophthalmia: Oral:
Children 1-8 years: 5000-10,000 units/kg/day for 5 days or until recovery occurs
Children >8 years and Adults: 500,000 units/day for 3 days, then 50,000 units/day for 14 days, then 10,000-20,000 units/day for 2 months

Deficiency (without corneal changes): Oral:
Infants <1 year: 100,000 units every 4-6 months
Children 1-8 years: 200,000 units every 4-6 months
Children >8 years and Adults: 100,000 units/day for 3 days then 50,000 units/day for 14 days

Malabsorption syndrome (prophylaxis): Children >8 years and Adults: Oral: 10,000-50,000 units/day of water miscible product

Dietary supplement: Oral:
Infants up to 6 months: 1500 units/day
Children:
6 months to 3 years: 1500-2000 units/day
4-6 years: 2500 units/day
7-10 years: 3300-3500 units/day
Children >10 years and Adults: 4000-5000 units/day

Dosage Forms CAP: 10,000 units [OTC], 25,000 units, 50,000 units. **DROPS, oral** (water miscible) [OTC]: 5000 units/0.1 mL (30 mL). **INJ:** 50,000 units/mL (2 mL). **TAB** [OTC]: 5000 units

Contraindications Hypervitaminosis A, hypersensitivity to vitamin A or any component; pregnancy if dose exceeds RDA recommendations

Warnings/Precautions Evaluate other sources of vitamin A while receiving this product; patients receiving >25,000 units/day should be closely monitored for toxicity

Pregnancy Risk Factor A; X (if dose exceeds RDA recommendation)

Pregnancy Implications Clinical effect on the fetus: Excessive use of vitamin A shortly before and during pregnancy could be harmful to babies

Adverse Reactions 1% to 10%:
Central nervous system: Irritability, vertigo, lethargy, malaise, fever, headache
Dermatologic: Drying or cracking of skin
Endocrine & metabolic: Hypercalcemia
Gastrointestinal: Weight loss
Ocular: Visual changes
Miscellaneous: Hypervitaminosis A

Drug Interactions
Decreased effect: Cholestyramine decreases absorption of vitamin A; neomycin and mineral oil may also interfere with vitamin A absorption
Increased toxicity: Retinoids may have additive adverse effects

Education and Monitoring Issues
Patient Education: Take exactly as directed; do not take more than the recommended dose. Take with meals. Do not use mineral oil or other vitamin A supplements without consulting prescriber. Report persistent nausea, vomiting, or loss of appetite; excessively dry skin or lips; headache or CNS irritability; loss of hair; or changes in vision.
Reference Range: 1 RE = 1 retinol equivalent; 1 RE = 1 µg retinol or 6 µg beta-carotene; Normal levels of Vitamin A in serum = 80-300 units/mL

Vitamin B Complex With Vitamin C and Folic Acid

(VYE ta min bee KOM pleks with VYE ta min see & FOE lik AS id)

Pharmacologic Class Vitamin, Water Soluble

U.S. Brand Names Berocca®; Nephrocaps®

(Continued)

Vitamin B Complex With Vitamin C and Folic Acid
(Continued)

Dosage Forms CAP

Vitamin E (VYE ta min ee)

Pharmacologic Class Vitamin, Fat Soluble

U.S. Brand Names Amino-Opti-E® [OTC]; Aquasol E® [OTC]; E-Complex-600® [OTC]; E-Vitamin® [OTC]; Vita-Plus® E Softgels® [OTC]; Vitec® [OTC]; Vite E® Creme [OTC]

Generic Available Yes

Mechanism of Action Prevents oxidation of vitamin A and C; protects polyunsaturated fatty acids in membranes from attack by free radicals and protects red blood cells against hemolysis

Use Prevention and treatment hemolytic anemia secondary to vitamin E deficiency; dietary supplement

Investigational: To reduce the risk of bronchopulmonary dysplasia or retrolental fibroplasia in infants exposed to high concentrations of oxygen

USUAL DOSAGE One unit of vitamin E = 1 mg *dl*-alpha-tocopherol acetate. Oral:

Vitamin E deficiency:

Children (with malabsorption syndrome): 1 unit/kg/day of water miscible vitamin E (to raise plasma tocopherol concentrations to the normal range within 2 months and to maintain normal plasma concentrations)

Adults: 60-75 units/day

Prevention of vitamin E deficiency: Adults: 30 units/day

Prevention of retinopathy of prematurity or BPD secondary to O_2 therapy: (American Academy of Pediatrics considers this use investigational and routine use is not recommended):

Retinopathy prophylaxis: 15-30 units/kg/day to maintain plasma levels between 1.5-2 µg/mL (may need as high as 100 units/kg/day)

Cystic fibrosis, beta-thalassemia, sickle cell anemia may require higher daily maintenance doses:

Cystic fibrosis: 100-400 units/day

Beta-thalassemia: 750 units/day

Sickle cell: 450 units/day

Recommended daily allowance:

Premature infants ≤3 months: 17 mg (25 units)

Infants:

≤6 months: 3 mg (4.5 units)

6-12 months: 4 mg (6 units)

Children:

1-3 years: 6 mg (9 units)

4-10 years: 7 mg (10.5 units)

Children >11 years and Adults:

Male: 15 mg (22 int. units)

Female: 15 mg (22 int. units)

Topical: Apply a thin layer over affected area

Dosage Forms CAP: 100 units, 200 units, 330 mg, 400 units, 500 units, 600 units, 1000 units; Water miscible: 73.5 mg, 147 mg, 165 mg, 330 mg, 400 units. **CRM:** 50 mg/g (15 g, 30 g, 60 g, 75 g, 120 g, 454 g). **DROPS, oral:** 50 mg/mL (12 mL, 30 mL). **LIQ, top:** 10 mL, 15 mL, 30 mL, 60 mL. **LOT:** 120 mL. **OIL:** 15 mL, 30 mL, 60 mL. **OINT, top:** 30 mg/g (45 g, 60 g). **TAB:** 200 units, 400 units

Contraindications Hypersensitivity to drug or any components; I.V. route

Warnings/Precautions May induce vitamin K deficiency; necrotizing enterocolitis has been associated with oral administration of large dosages (eg, >200 units/day) of a hyperosmolar vitamin E preparation in low birth weight infants

Pregnancy Risk Factor A; C (if dose exceeds RDA recommendation)

Adverse Reactions <1%: Blurred vision, contact dermatitis with topical preparation, diarrhea, fatigue, gonadal dysfunction, headache, intestinal cramps, nausea, weakness

Drug Interactions

Vitamin E may impair the hematologic response to iron in children with iron-deficiency anemia; monitor

Vitamin E may alter the effect of vitamin K actions on clotting factors resulting in an increase hypoprothrombinemic response to warfarin; monitor

Education and Monitoring Issues

Patient Education: Take exactly as directed; do not take more than the recommended dose. Do not use mineral oil or other vitamin E supplements without consulting prescriber. Report persistent nausea, vomiting, or cramping; or gonadal dysfunction.

Reference Range: Therapeutic: 0.8-1.5 mg/dL (SI: 19-35 µmol/L), some method variation

Vitamins, Multiple (VYE ta mins, MUL ti pul)

Pharmacologic Class Vitamin

Multivitamin Products Comparison

Product	Content Given Per	A IU	D IU	E IU	C mg	FA mg	B_1 mg	B_2 mg	B_3 mg	B_6 mg	B_{12} mcg	Other
Theragran®	5 mL liquid	10,000	400		200		10	10	100	4.1	5	B_5 21.4 mg
Vi-Daylin®	1 mL drops	1500	400	4.1	35		0.5	0.6	8	0.4	1.5	Alcohol <0.5%
Vi-Daylin® Iron	1 mL	1500	400	4.1	35		0.5	0.6	8	0.4		Fe 10 mg
Albee® with C	tablet				300		15	10.2		5		Niacinamide 50 mg, pantothenic acid 10 mg
Vitamin B complex	tablet					400 mcg	1.5	1.7		2	6	Niacinamide 20 mg
Hexavitamin	cap/tab	5000	400		75		2	3	20			
Iberet-Folic-500®	tablet				500	0.8	6	6	30	5	25	B_5 10 mg, Fe 105 mg
Stuartnatal® 1+1	tablet	4000	400	11	120	1	1.5	3	20	10	12	Cu, Zn 25 mg, Fe 65 mg, Ca 200 mg
Theragran-M®	tablet	5000	400	30	90	0.4	3	3.4	30	3	9	Cl, Cr, I, K, B_5 10 mg, Mg, Mn, Mo, P, Se, Zn 15 mg, Fe 27 mg, biotin 30 mcg, beta-carotene 1250 IU
Vi-Daylin®	tablet	2500	400	15	60	0.3	1.05	1.2	13.5	1.05	4.5	
M.V.I.®-12 injection	5 mL	3300	200	10	100	0.4	3	3.6	40	4	5	B_5 15 mg, biotin 60 mcg
M.V.I.®-12 unit vial	20 mL											
M.V.I.® pediatric powder	5 mL	2300	400	7	80	0.14	1.2	1.4	17	1	1	B_5 5 mg, biotin 20 mcg, vitamin K 200 mcg

(Continued)

Vitamins, Multiple *(Continued)*

U.S. Brand Names Adeflor®; Allbee® With C; Becotin® Pulvules®; Cefol® Filmtab®; Chromagen® OB [OTC]; Eldercaps® [OTC]; Filibon® [OTC]; Florvite®; Iberet-Folic-500®; LKV-Drops® [OTC]; Mega-B® [OTC]; Multi Vit® Drops [OTC]; M.V.I.®; M.V.I.®-12; M.V.I.® Concentrate; M.V.I.® Pediatric; Natabec® [OTC]; Natabec® FA [OTC]; Natabec® Rx; Natalins® [OTC]; Natalins® Rx; NeoVadrin® [OTC]; Niferex®-PN; Poly-Vi-Flor®; Poly-Vi-Sol® [OTC]; Pramet® FA; Pramilet® FA; Prenavite® [OTC]; Secran®; Stresstabs® 600 Advanced Formula Tablets [OTC]; Stuartnatal® 1 + 1; Stuart Prenatal® [OTC]; Therabid® [OTC]; Theragran® [OTC]; Theragran® Hematinic®; Theragran® Liquid [OTC]; Theragran-M® [OTC]; Tri-Vi-Flor®; Unicap® [OTC]; Vicon Forte®; Vicon® Plus [OTC]; Vi-Daylin® [OTC]; Vi-Daylin/F®

Use Dietary supplement

USUAL DOSAGE

Infants 1.5-3 kg: I.V.: 3.25 mL/24 hours (M.V.I.® Pediatric)
Children:
Oral:
≤2 years: Drops: 1 mL/day (premature infants may get 0.5-1 mL/day)
>2 years: Chew 1 tablet/day
≥4 years: 5 mL/day liquid
I.V.: >3 kg and <11 years: 5 mL/24 hours (M.V.I.® Pediatric)
Adults:
Oral: 1 tablet/day or 5 mL/day liquid
I.V.: >11 years: 5 mL of vials 1 and 2 (M.V.I.®-12)/one TPN bag/day
I.V. solutions: 10 mL/24 hours (M.V.I.®-12)

Dosage Forms See table.

Contraindications Hypersensitivity to product components

Warnings/Precautions RDA values are not requirements, but are recommended daily intakes of certain essential nutrients; periodic dental exams should be performed to check for dental fluorosis; use with caution in patients with severe renal or liver failure

Pregnancy Risk Factor A; C (if used in doses above RDA recommendation)

Adverse Reactions 1% to 10%: Hypervitaminosis; refer to individual vitamin entries for individual reactions

Education and Monitoring Issues

Patient Education: Take only amount prescribed

Reference Range: Recommended daily allowances are published by Food and Nutrition Board, National Research Council - National Academy of Sciences and are revised periodically. RDA quantities apply only to healthy persons and are not intended to cover therapeutic nutrition requirements in disease or other abnormal states (ie, metabolic disorders, weight reduction, chronic disease, drug therapy).

- **Vita-Plus® E Softgels® [OTC]** *see* Vitamin E *on page 980*
- **Vitec® [OTC]** *see* Vitamin E *on page 980*
- **Vite E® Creme [OTC]** *see* Vitamin E *on page 980*
- **Vito Reins®** *see* Phenazopyridine *on page 721*
- **Vitrasert®** *see* Ganciclovir *on page 402*
- **Vitravene™** *see* Fomivirsen *on page 393*
- **Vivactil®** *see* Protriptyline *on page 790*
- **Vivelle** *see* Estradiol *on page 327*
- **Vivol®** *see* Diazepam *on page 261*
- **V-Lax® [OTC]** *see* Psyllium *on page 793*
- **Volmax®** *see* Albuterol *on page 27*
- **Voltaren® Ophthalmic** *see* Diclofenac *on page 263*
- **Voltaren® Oral** *see* Diclofenac *on page 263*
- **Voltaren Rapide®** *see* Diclofenac *on page 263*
- **Voltaren®-XR Oral** *see* Diclofenac *on page 263*
- **VōSol®** *see* Acetic Acid *on page 19*
- **VōSol® HC Otic** *see* Acetic Acid, Propylene Glycol Diacetate, and Hydrocortisone *on page 20*
- **V.V.S.®** *see* Sulfabenzamide, Sulfacetamide, and Sulfathiazole *on page 875*
- **Vytone® Topical** *see* Iodoquinol and Hydrocortisone *on page 481*

Warfarin (WAR far in)

Pharmacologic Class Anticoagulant, Coumarin Derivative

U.S. Brand Names Coumadin®

Generic Available Yes: Tablet

Mechanism of Action Interferes with hepatic synthesis of vitamin K-dependent coagulation factors (II, VII, IX, X)

Use Prophylaxis and treatment of venous thrombosis, pulmonary embolism and thromboembolic disorders; atrial fibrillation with risk of embolism and as an adjunct in the prophylaxis of systemic embolism after myocardial infarction

Unlabeled use: Prevention of recurrent transient ischemic attacks and to reduce risk of recurrent myocardial infarction

USUAL DOSAGE Oral:

Infants and Children: 0.05-0.34 mg/kg/day; infants <12 months of age may require doses at or near the high end of this range; consistent anticoagulation may be difficult to maintain in children <5 years of age

Adults: 5-15 mg/day for 2-5 days, then adjust dose according to results of prothrombin time; usual maintenance dose ranges from 2-10 mg/day

I.V. (administer as a slow bolus injection): 2-5 mg/day

Dosing adjustment/comments in hepatic disease: Monitor effect at usual doses; the response to oral anticoagulants may be markedly enhanced in obstructive jaundice (due to reduced vitamin K absorption) and also in hepatitis and cirrhosis (due to decreased production of vitamin K-dependent clotting factors); prothrombin index should be closely monitored

Dosage Forms POWDER for inj, lyophilized: 2 mg, 5 mg. **TAB:** 1 mg, 2 mg, 2.5 mg, 3 mg, 4 mg, 5 mg, 6 mg, 7.5 mg, 10 mg

Contraindications Hypersensitivity to warfarin or any component; severe liver or kidney disease; open wounds; uncontrolled bleeding; GI ulcers; neurosurgical procedures; malignant hypertension, pregnancy

Warnings/Precautions

Do not switch brands once desired therapeutic response has been achieved

Use with caution in patients with active tuberculosis or diabetes

Concomitant use with vitamin K may decrease anticoagulant effect; monitor carefully

Concomitant use with NSAIDs or aspirin may cause severe GI irritation and also increase the risk of bleeding due to impaired platelet function

Salicylates may further increase warfarin's effect by displacing it from plasma protein binding sites

Patients with protein C or S deficiency are at increased risk of skin necrosis syndrome

Before committing an elderly patient to long-term anticoagulation therapy, their risk for bleeding complications secondary to falls, drug interactions, living situation, and cognitive status should be considered. The risk for bleeding complications decreases with the duration of therapy and may increase with advancing age.

If a patient is to undergo an invasive surgical procedure (dental to actual minor/major surgery), warfarin should be stopped 3 days before the scheduled surgery date and the INR/PT should be checked prior to the procedure

Pregnancy Risk Factor D

Pregnancy Implications

Clinical effects on the fetus: Oral anticoagulants cross the placenta and produce fetal abnormalities. Warfarin should not be used during pregnancy because of significant risks. Adjusted-dose heparin can be given safely throughout pregnancy in patients with venous thromboembolism.

Breast-feeding/lactation: Warfarin does not pass into breast milk and can be given to nursing mothers

Adverse Reactions

1% to 10%:

Dermatologic: Skin lesions, alopecia, skin necrosis

Gastrointestinal: Anorexia, nausea, vomiting, stomach cramps, diarrhea

Hematologic: Hemorrhage, leukopenia, unrecognized bleeding sites (eg, colon cancer) may be uncovered by anticoagulation

Respiratory: Hemoptysis

<1%: Agranulocytosis, anorexia, discolored toes (blue or purple), fever, hepatotoxicity, mouth ulcers, rash, renal damage

Drug Interactions CYP1A2 enzyme substrate (minor), CYP2C8, 2C9, 2C18, 2C19, and 3A3/4 enzyme substrate; CYP2C9 enzyme inhibitor

Decrease Anticoagulant Effects

Increased Warfarin Metabolism	Increased Procoagulant Factors	Decreased Drug Absorption	Other
Barbiturates Carbamazepine Dicloxacillin Glutethimide Griseofulvin Nafcillin Phenytoin Rifampin	Estrogens Oral contraceptives Vitamin K (including nutritional supplements)	Aluminum hydroxide Cholestyramine* Colestipol*	Ethchlorvynol Griseofulvin Spironolactone† Sucralfate

*Cholestyramine and colestipol may increase the anticoagulant effect by binding vitamin K in the gut; yet, the decreased drug absorption appears to be of more concern.

†Diuretic-induced hemoconcentration with subsequent concentration of clotting factors has been reported to decrease the effects of oral anticoagulants.

(Continued)

Warfarin *(Continued)*

Increased Bleeding Tendency

Inhibit Platelet Aggregation	Inhibit Procoagulant Factors	Ulcerogenic Drugs
Cephalosporins Dipyridamole Indomethacin Oxyphenbutazone Penicillin, parenteral Phenylbutazone Salicylates Sulfinpyrazone	Antimetabolites Quinidine Quinine Salicylates	Adrenal corticosteroids Indomethacin Oxyphenbutazone Phenylbutazone Potassium products Salicylates

Use of these agents with oral anticoagulants may increase the chances of hemorrhage.

Enhanced Anticoagulant Effects

Decrease Vitamin K	Displace Anticoagulant	Inhibit Metabolism	Other
Oral antibiotics: Can ↑/↓ INR Check INR 3 days after a patient begins antibiotics to see the INR value and adjust the warfarin dose accordingly	Chloral hydrate Clofibrate Diazoxide Ethacrynic acid Miconazole Nalidixic acid Phenylbutazone Salicylates Sulfonamides Sulfonylureas	Alcohol (acute ingestion)* Allopurinol Amiodarone Azole antifungals Chloramphenicol Chlorpropamide Cimetidine Ciprofloxacin Co-trimoxazole Disulfiram Flutamide Isoniazid Metronidazole Norfloxacin Ofloxacin Omperazole Phenylbutazone Phenytoin Propafenone Propoxyphene Protease inhibitors Quinidine Sulfinpyrazone Sulfonamides Tamoxifen Tolbutamide Zafirlukast Zileuton	Acetaminophen Anabolic steroids Clarithromycin Clofibrate Danazol Erythromycin Gemfibrozil Glucagon Influenza vaccine Propranolol Propylthiouracil Ranitidine SSRIs Sulindac Tetracycline Thyroid drugs Vitamin E (≥400 int. units)

* The hypoprothrombinemic effect of oral anticoagulants has been reported to be both increased and decreased during chronic and excessive alcohol ingestion. Data are insufficient to predict the direction of this interaction in alcoholic patients.

Drug-Herb interactions:

Ginseng (*Panax ginseng*) has been associated with vaginal bleeding in two case reports and with a decrease in warfarin activity in another case report

Dan shen (*Salvia miltiorrhiza*), a Chinese herb, was associated with increased warfarin activity in two cases

Devil's claw (*Harpagophytum procumbens*) was associated with purpura in a patient treated with warfarin

Garlic (*Allium sativum*) extracts have been associated with reports of bleeding and two cases of increased warfarin activity

Ginkgo biloba extracts have been associated with cases of spontaneous bleeding, although the ginkgo extracts were not definitively shown to be the cause of the problem, and one case report of a patient taking warfarin in whom bleeding occurred, has been reported after the addition of ginkgo

Although there are no specific studies demonstrating interactions with anticoagulants, the following herbs containing coumarin-like substances that may interact with warfarin and may cause bleeding include dong quai, fenugreek, horse chestnut, red clover, sweet clover, and sweet woodruff

Alcohol Interactions Avoid use. Acute alcohol ingestion (binge drinking) decreases the metabolism of warfarin and increases PT/INR. Chronic daily alcohol use increases the metabolism of warfarin and decreases PT/INR.

Onset INR may increase within 36-72 hours; full therapeutic effect is not established until 5-7 days

Half-Life 3-5 days, highly variable among individuals

Education and Monitoring Issues

Patient Education: Take exactly as directed; if dose is missed, take as soon as possible. Do not double doses. Do not take any medication your prescriber is not aware of and follow diet and activity as recommended by prescriber. You may have a tendency to bleed easily while taking this drug; brush teeth with soft brush, floss with waxed floss, use electric razor, and avoid scissors or sharp knives and potentially harmful activities. You may experience nausea or vomiting (small frequent meals, frequent mouth care, sucking lozenges, or chewing gum may help). May discolor urine or stool. Report skin rash or irritation, unusual fever, persistent nausea or GI upset, unusual bleeding or bruising (bleeding gums, nosebleed, blood in urine, dark stool, bloody emesis), pain in joints or back, swelling or pain at injection site.

Dietary Considerations:

Food:

Vitamin K: Foods high in vitamin K (eg, beef liver, pork liver, green tea and leafy green vegetables) inhibit anticoagulant effect. Do not change dietary habits once stabilized on warfarin therapy; a balanced diet with a consistent intake of vitamin K is essential; avoid large amounts of alfalfa, asparagus, broccoli, Brussels sprouts, cabbage, cauliflower, green teas, kale, lettuce, spinach, turnip greens, watercress. It is recommended that the diet contain a CONSISTENT vitamin K content of 70-140 mcg/day. Check with prescriber before changing diet.

Vitamin E: May increase warfarin effect; do not change dietary habits or vitamin supplements once stabilized on warfarin therapy

Monitoring Parameters: Prothrombin time, hematocrit, INR

Reference Range:

Therapeutic: 2-5 μg/mL (SI: 6.5-16.2 μmol/L)

Prothrombin time should be 1½ to 2 times the control or INR should be ↑ 2 to 3 times based upon indication

Normal prothrombin time: 10-13 seconds

INR Ranges Based Upon Indication

Diagnosis	Targeted INR Range	Targeted INR
Acute myocardial infarction with risk factors*	2.0-3.0	2.5
Atrial fibrillation	2.0-3.0	2.5
Bileaflet mechanical aortic valve		
Atrial fibrillation	2.5-3.5	3.0
or		
Atrial fibrillation with ASA 80-100 mg/day	2.0-3.0	2.5
Bileaflet mechanical aortic valve		
NL LA, NSR, NL EF	2.0-3.0	2.5
Bileaflet or tilting disk mechanical mitral valve	2.5-3.5	3.0
or		
Bileaflet or tilting disk mechanical mitral valve with ASA 80-100 mg/day	2.0-3.0	2.5
Bioprosthetic mitral or aortic valve		
Atrial fibrillation	2.0-3.0	2.5
NSR	2.0-3.0†	2.5†
Cardioembolic cerebral ischemic events	2.0-3.0	2.5
Mechanical heart valve (caged ball, caged disk) with ASA 80-100 mg/day	2.5-3.5	3.0
Mechanical prosthetic valve with systemic embolism (adequate anticoagulation)	2.5-3.5‡	3.0‡
Venous thromboembolism	2.0-3.0	2.5

*Anterior Q-wave infarction, severe left-ventricular dysfunction, mural thrombus on 2D echo, atrial fibrillation, history of systemic or pulmonary embolism, congestive heart failure

†Maintained for up to 3 months

‡Add ASA 100 mg/day

For a complete discussion, see *Chest*, 1998, 114(5 Suppl):439S-759S.

Warfarin levels are not used for monitoring degree of anticoagulation. They may be useful if a patient with unexplained coagulopathy is using the drug surreptitiously or if it is unclear whether clinical resistance is due to true drug resistance or lack of drug intake.

Normal prothrombin time (PT): 10.9-12.9 seconds. Healthy premature newborns have prolonged coagulation test screening results (eg, PT, APTT, TT) which return to normal adult values at approximately 6 months of age. Healthy prematures, however, do not develop spontaneous hemorrhage or thrombotic complications because of a balance between procoagulants and inhibitors

(Continued)

Warfarin *(Continued)*

The World Health Organization (WHO), in cooperation with other regulatory-advisory bodies, has developed system of standardizing the reporting of PT values through the determination of the International Normalized Ratio (INR). The INR involves the standardization of the PT by the generation of two pieces of information: the PT ratio and the International Sensitivity Index (ISI)

Therapeutic ranges are now available or being developed to assist practicing prescribers in their treatment of patients with a wide variety of thrombotic disorders

Related Information

Anticoagulation Guidelines *on page 1068*

- **Warfilone®** *see* Warfarin *on page 982*
- **Wellbutrin®** *see* Bupropion *on page 120*
- **Wellbutrin® SR** *see* Bupropion *on page 120*
- **Wellcovorin®** *see* Leucovorin *on page 513*
- **Westcort®** *see* Hydrocortisone *on page 447*
- **Wigraine®** *see* Ergotamine *on page 323*
- **40 Winks® [OTC]** *see* Diphenhydramine *on page 282*
- **WinRho SD®** *see* Rh_0(D) Immune Globulin (Intravenous-Human) *on page 817*
- **Winstrol®** *see* Stanozolol *on page 868*
- **Wycillin®** *see* Penicillin G Procaine *on page 712*
- **Wydase® Injection** *see* Hyaluronidase *on page 440*
- **Wygesic®** *see* Propoxyphene and Acetaminophen *on page 786*
- **Wymox®** *see* Amoxicillin *on page 56*
- **Wytensin®** *see* Guanabenz *on page 425*
- **Xalatan®** *see* Latanoprost *on page 510*
- **Xanax®** *see* Alprazolam *on page 37*
- **Xenical®** *see* Orlistat *on page 680*
- **Xopenex™** *see* Levalbuterol *on page 515*
- **Xylocaine®** *see* Lidocaine *on page 527*
- **Xylocaine®** *see* Lidocaine and Epinephrine *on page 529*
- **Xylocaine® With Epinephrine** *see* Lidocaine and Epinephrine *on page 529*
- **Xylocard®** *see* Lidocaine *on page 527*
- **Yeast-Gard® Medicated Douche** *see* Povidone-Iodine *on page 756*
- **Yodoxin®** *see* Iodoquinol *on page 480*

Yohimbe

Pharmacologic Class Herb

Mechanism of Action The alkaloid yohimbine has central nervous system stimulatory activity. Also, yohimbine has selective $alpha_2$ adrenergic blocking properties, which is the basis for its use in erectile dysfunction. Yohimbine also blocks peripheral 5-HT receptors. Aphrodisiac activity may be due to enlargement of the vasculature in the genitals, increase of nerve impulses to genital tissue, and an increased transmission of reflex excitability in the sacral region of the spinal cord.

Use May increase sexual vitality in men and women; used in male erectile dysfunction (Riley, 1994)

USUAL DOSAGE Oral: 500-750 mg twice daily

Contraindications Contraindicated in pregnancy. Do not use in individuals taking MAO inhibitors or antihypertensives; do not use in hypertensive individuals (De Smet 1994) or cardiovascular disease. Toxic doses may trigger psychosis, hypotension, and cardiac failure. Based on pharmacological activity, use with caution in individuals receiving $alpha_2$ blockers. Based on pharmacological activity, may cause CNS stimulation (anxiety, insomnia), hypertension, and tachycardia.

Warnings/Precautions Use all herbal supplements with extreme caution in children <2 years of age and in pregnancy or lactation. Some herbs are contraindicated in pregnancy or lactation; make sure to observe warnings. Use with caution in individuals on medication and with pre-existing medical conditions. Always review for potential herb-drug interactions (HDIs) and other warnings. Large and prolonged doses may increase the potential for adverse effects. Herbs may cause transient adverse effects such as nausea, vomiting, and GI distress due to a variety of chemical constituents. Caution should be used in individuals having known allergies to plants.

Drug Interactions MAO inhibitors, antihypertensives, naloxone, tricyclic antidepressants, $alpha_2$ blockers, sympathomimetics

- **Yutopar®** *see* Ritodrine *on page 826*
- **Zaditor™** *see* Ketotifen *on page 502*

Zafirlukast (za FIR loo kast)

Pharmacologic Class Leukotriene Receptor Antagonist

U.S. Brand Names Accolate®

Mechanism of Action Zafirlukast is a selectively and competitive leukotriene-receptor antagonist (LTRA) of leukotriene D4 and E4 (LTD4 and LTE4), components of slow-reacting substance of anaphylaxis (SRSA). Cysteinyl leukotriene production and receptor occupation have been correlated with the pathophysiology of asthma, including airway edema, smooth muscle constriction and altered cellular activity associated with the inflammatory process, which contribute to the signs and symptoms of asthma.

Use Prophylaxis and chronic treatment of asthma in adults and children ≥7 years of age

USUAL DOSAGE Oral:

Children <7 years: Safety and effectiveness has not been established

Children 7-11 years: 10 mg twice daily

Adults: 20 mg twice daily

Elderly: The mean dose (mg/kg) normalized AUC and C_{max} increase and plasma clearance decreases with increasing age. In patients >65 years of age, there is an 2-3 fold greater C_{max} and AUC compared to younger adults.

Dosing adjustment in renal impairment: There are no apparent differences in the pharmacokinetics between renally impaired patients and normal subjects.

Dosing adjustment in hepatic impairment: In patients with hepatic impairment (ie, biopsy-proven cirrhosis), there is a 50% to 60% greater C_{max} and AUC compared to normal subjects.

Dosage Forms TAB: 10 mg, 20 mg

Contraindications Hypersensitivity to zafirlukast or any of its inactive ingredients

Warnings/Precautions The clearance of zafirlukast is reduced in patients with stable alcoholic cirrhosis such that the C_{max} and AUC are approximately 50% to 60% greater than those of normal adults.

Zafirlukast is not indicated for use in the reversal of bronchospasm in acute asthma attacks, including status asthmaticus. Therapy with zafirlukast can be continued during acute exacerbations of asthma.

An increased proportion of zafirlukast patients >55 years old reported infections as compared to placebo-treated patients. these infections were mostly mild or moderate in intensity and predominantly affected the respiratory tract. Infections occurred equally in both sexes, were dose-proportional to total milligrams of zafirlukast exposure and were associated with coadministration of inhaled corticosteroids.

Although the frequency of hepatic transaminase elevations was comparable between zafirlukast and placebo-treated patients, a single case of symptomatic hepatitis and hyperbilirubinemia, without other attributable cause, occurred in patient who had received 40 mg/day of zafirlukast for 100 days. In this patient, the liver enzymes returned to normal within 3 months of stopping zafirlukast.

Pregnancy Risk Factor B

Pregnancy Implications

Clinical effects on the fetus: At 2,000 mg/kg/day in rats, maternal toxicity and deaths were seen with increased incidence of early fetal resorption. Spontaneous abortions occurred in cynomolgus monkeys at a maternally toxic dose of 2,000 mg/kg/day orally. There are no adequate and well controlled trials in pregnant women.

Breast-feeding/lactation: Zafirlukast is excreted in breast milk; do not administer to nursing women

Adverse Reactions

>10%: Central nervous system: Headache (12.9%)

1% to 10%:

- Central nervous system: Dizziness, pain, fever
- Gastrointestinal: Nausea, diarrhea, abdominal pain, vomiting, dyspepsia
- Neuromuscular & skeletal: Myalgia, weakness

Drug Interactions CYP2C9 enzyme substrate; CYP2C9 and 3A3/4 enzyme inhibitor

Decreased effect:

Erythromycin: Coadministration of a single dose of zafirlukast with erythromycin to steady state results in decreased mean plasma levels of zafirlukast by 40% due to a decrease in zafirlukast bioavailability.

Terfenadine: Coadministration of zafirlukast with terfenadine to steady state results in a decrease in the mean C_{max} (66%) and AUC (54%) of zafirlukast. No effect of zafirlukast on terfenadine plasma concentrations or EKG parameters was seen.

Theophylline: Coadministration of zafirlukast at steady state with a single dose of liquid theophylline preparations results in decreased mean plasma levels of zafirlukast by 30%, but no effects on plasma theophylline levels were observed.

Increased effect: Aspirin: Coadministration of zafirlukast with aspirin results in mean increased plasma levels of zafirlukast by 45%

Increased toxicity: Warfarin: Coadministration of zafirlukast with warfarin results in a clinically significant increase in prothrombin time (PT). Closely monitor prothrombin times of patients on oral warfarin anticoagulant therapy and zafirlukast, and adjust anticoagulant dose accordingly.

Onset Peak concentrations: 3 hours

Half-Life 10 hours

(Continued)

Zafirlukast *(Continued)*

Education and Monitoring Issues

Patient Education: Do not use during acute bronchospasm. Take regularly as prescribed, even during symptom-free periods. Do not take more than recommended or discontinue use without consulting prescriber. Do not stop taking other antiasthmatic medications unless instructed by prescriber. Avoid aspirin or aspirin-containing medications unless approved by prescriber. You may experience headache, drowsiness, dizziness, or blurred vision (use caution when driving or engaging in tasks requiring alertness until response to drug is known); gastric upset, nausea, or vomiting (small frequent meals, frequent mouth care, chewing gum, or sucking lozenges may help). Report persistent CNS or GI symptoms; muscle or back pain; weakness, fever, chills; yellowing of skin or eyes; dark urine, or pale stool; skin rash; or worsening of condition.

Manufacturer Zeneca Pharmaceuticals

Related Information

Pharmaceutical Manufacturers Directory *on page 1020*

♦ **Zagam®** *see* Sparfloxacin *on page 865*

Zalcitabine (zal SITE a been)

Pharmacologic Class Antiretroviral Agent, Reverse Transcriptase Inhibitor (Nucleoside)

U.S. Brand Names Hivid®

Use In combination with at least two other antiretrovirals in the treatment of patients with HIV infection; it is not recommended that zalcitabine be given in combination with didanosine, stavudine, or lamivudine due to overlapping toxicities, virologic interactions, or lack of clinical data

USUAL DOSAGE Oral:

Children <13 years: Safety and efficacy have not been established

Adults: Daily dose: 0.75 mg every 8 hours

Dosing adjustment in renal impairment: Adults:

Cl_{cr} 10-40 mL/minute: 0.75 mg every 12 hours

Cl_{cr} <10 mL/minute: 0.75 mg every 24 hours

Moderately dialyzable (20% to 50%)

Contraindications Hypersensitivity to zalcitabine or any component

Warnings/Precautions Careful monitoring of pancreatic enzymes and liver function tests in patients with a history of pancreatitis, increased amylase, those on parenteral nutrition or with a history of ethanol abuse; discontinue use immediately if pancreatitis is suspected; lactic acidosis and severe hepatomegaly and failure have rarely occurred with zalcitabine resulting in fatality; some cases may possibly be related to underlying hepatitis B; use with caution in patients on digitalis, congestive heart failure, renal failure, hyperphosphatemia; zalcitabine can cause severe peripheral neuropathy; avoid use, if possible, in patients with pre-existing neuropathy

Pregnancy Risk Factor C

Adverse Reactions

>10%:

- Central nervous system: Fever (5% to 17%), malaise (2% to 13%)
- Neuromuscular & skeletal: Peripheral neuropathy (28.3%)

1% to 10%:

- Central nervous system: Headache (2.1%), dizziness (1.1%), fatigue (3.8%), seizures (1.3%)
- Endocrine & metabolic: Hypoglycemia (1.8% to 6.3%), hyponatremia (3.5%), hyperglycemia (1% to 6%)
- Hematologic: Anemia (occurs as early as 2-4 weeks), granulocytopenia (usually after 6-8 weeks)
- Dermatologic: Rash (2% to 11%), pruritus (3% to 5%)
- Gastrointestinal: Nausea (3%), dysphagia (1% to 4%), anorexia (3.9%), abdominal pain (3% to 8%), vomiting (1% to 3%), diarrhea (0.4% to 9.5%), weight loss, oral ulcers (3% to 7%), increased amylase (3% to 8%)
- Hepatic: Abnormal hepatic function (8.9%), hyperbilirubinemia (2% to 5%)
- Neuromuscular & skeletal: Myalgia (1% to 6%), foot pain
- Respiratory: Pharyngitis (1.8%), cough (6.3%), nasal discharge (3.5%)

<1%: Atrial fibrillation, chest pain, constipation, edema, epistaxis, heart racing, hepatitis, hepatic failure, hepatomegaly, hypertension, hypocalcemia, jaundice, myositis, night sweats, pain, palpitations, pancreatitis, syncope, tachycardia, weakness

Drug Interactions

Decreased effect: Magnesium/aluminum-containing antacids and metoclopramide may reduce zalcitabine absorption

Increased toxicity:

- Amphotericin, foscarnet, cimetidine, probenecid, and aminoglycosides may potentiate the risk of developing peripheral neuropathy or other toxicities associated with zalcitabine by interfering with the renal elimination of zalcitabine
- Other drugs associated with peripheral neuropathy which should be avoided, if possible, include chloramphenicol, cisplatin, dapsone, disulfiram, ethionamide,

glutethimide, didanosine, gold, hydralazine, iodoquinol, isoniazid, metronidazole, nitrofurantoin, phenytoin, ribavirin, and vincristine

It is not recommended that zalcitabine be given in combination with didanosine, stavudine, or lamivudine due to overlapping toxicities, virologic interactions, or lack of clinical data

Manufacturer Roche Laboratories

Related Information

Antiretroviral Therapy for HIV Infection *on page 1190*

Pharmaceutical Manufacturers Directory *on page 1020*

Zaleplon (ZAL e plon)

Pharmacologic Class Hypnotic, Nonbenzodiazepine

U.S. Brand Names Sonata®

Mechanism of Action Zaleplon is unrelated to benzodiazepines, barbiturates, or other hypnotics. However, it interacts with the benzodiazepine GABA receptor complex. Nonclinical studies have shown that it binds selectively to the brain omega-1 receptor situated on the alpha subunit of the GABA-A receptor complex.

Use Short-term treatment of insomnia

USUAL DOSAGE

Adults: Oral: 10 mg at bedtime (range: 5-20 mg)

Elderly: 5 mg at bedtime

Dosage adjustment in renal impairment: No adjustment for mild to moderate renal impairment; use in severe renal impairment has not been adequately studied

Dosage adjustment in hepatic impairment: Mild to moderate impairment: 5 mg; not recommended for use in patients with severe hepatic impairment

Dosage Forms CAP: 5 mg, 10 mg

Contraindications Known hypersensitivity to zaleplon or any component

Warnings/Precautions Symptomatic treatment of insomnia should be initiated only after careful evaluation of potential causes of sleep disturbance. Failure of sleep disturbance to resolve after 7-10 days may indicate psychiatric and/or medical illness.

Use with caution in patients with depression, particularly if suicidal risk may be present. Use with caution in patients with a history of drug dependence. Abrupt discontinuance may lead to withdrawal symptoms. May impair physical and mental capabilities. Patients must be cautioned about performing tasks which require mental alertness (operating machinery or driving). Use with caution in patients receiving other CNS depressants or psychoactive medications. Effects with other sedative drugs or ethanol may be potentiated.

Use with caution in the elderly, those with compromised respiratory function, or renal and hepatic impairment. Because of the rapid onset of action, zaleplon should be administered immediately prior to bedtime or after the patient has gone to bed and is having difficulty falling asleep.

Pregnancy Risk Factor C

Pregnancy Implications Not recommended

Adverse Reactions

>10%: Central nervous system: Headache

1% to 10%:

Cardiovascular: Peripheral edema

Central nervous system: Amnesia, anxiety, depersonalization, dizziness, hallucinations, hypesthesia, somnolence, vertigo, malaise, depression, lightheadedness, impaired coordination

Dermatologic: Photosensitivity reaction, rash, pruritus

Gastrointestinal: Abdominal pain, anorexia, colitis, dyspepsia, nausea, constipation, xerostomia

Genitourinary: Dysmenorrhea (2% to 4%)

Neuromuscular & skeletal: Paresthesia, tremor, myalgia, weakness

Ocular: Abnormal vision, eye pain

Otic: Hyperacusis

Respiratory: Epistaxis

Miscellaneous: Parosmia

Drug Interactions CYP3A4 substrate (minor metabolic pathway)

Zaleplon potentiates the CNS effects of alcohol, imipramine, and thioridazine

CYP3A4 inducers (eg, phenytoin, carbamazepine, phenobarbital) could lead to ineffectiveness of zaleplon (rifampin decreased AUC 80%); consider an alternative hypnotic

Cimetidine inhibits both aldehyde oxidase and CYP3A4 leading to an 85% increase in C_{max} and AUC of zaleplon. Use 5 mg zaleplon as starting dose in patient receiving cimetidine.

Alcohol Interactions Avoid use (may increase central nervous system depression)

Onset Rapid

Duration 6-8 hours

Half-Life 1 hour

(Continued)

Zaleplon *(Continued)*

Education and Monitoring Issues

Patient Education: Take exactly as directed; immediately before bedtime, or when you cannot fall asleep. Do not alter dosage or frequency, may be habit forming. Avoid alcohol and other prescription or OTC medications (especially medications to relieve pain, induce sleep, reduce anxiety, treat or prevent cold, coughs, or allergies) unless approved by prescriber. You may experience drowsiness, dizziness, somnolence, vertigo, lightheadedness, blurred vision (avoid driving or engaging in activities that require alertness until response to drug is known); photosensitivity (avoid exposure to direct sunlight, wear protective clothing, and sunscreen); nausea or GI discomfort (small frequent meals, good mouth care, chewing gum, or sucking hard candy may help); constipation (increase exercise or dietary fiber and fluids); menstrual disturbances (reversible when drug is discontinued). Discontinue drug and report any severe CNS disturbances (hallucinations, acute nervousness or anxiety, persistent sleepiness or lethargy, impaired coordination, amnesia, or impaired thought processes); skin rash or irritation; eye pain or major vision changes; difficulty breathing; chest pain; ear pain; muscle weakness or pain.

Dietary Considerations: High fat meal prolonged absorption; delayed t_{max} by 2 hours, and reduced C_{max} by 35%

Monitoring Parameters: Cardiac, mental status, and respiratory

Manufacturer Wyeth-Ayerst Laboratories

Related Information

Pharmaceutical Manufacturers Directory *on page 1020*

Zanamivir (za NA mi veer)

Pharmacologic Class Neuraminidase Inhibitor

U.S. Brand Names Relenza®

Mechanism of Action Zanamivir inhibits influenza virus neuraminidase enzymes, potentially altering virus particle aggregation and release

Use Treatment of uncomplicated acute illness due to influenza virus in adults and adolescents 12 years of age or older. Treatment should only be initiated in patients who have been symptomatic for no more than 2 days.

Investigational use: Prophylaxis against influenza A/B infections

USUAL DOSAGE Adolescents ≥12 years and Adults: 2 inhalations (10 mg total) twice daily for 5 days. Two doses should be taken on the first day of dosing, regardless of interval, while doses should be spaced by approximately 12 hours on subsequent days.

Prophylaxis (investigational use): 2 inhalations (10 mg) once daily for duration of exposure period (6 weeks has been used in clinical trial)

Dosage Forms POWDER, for inhal: (Rotadisk®): 5 mg per blister

Contraindications Hypersensitivity to zanamivir or any component of the formulation

Warnings/Precautions Patients must be instructed in the use of the delivery system. No data are available to support the use of this drug in patients who begin treatment after 48 hours of symptoms, as a prophylactic treatment for influenza, or in patients with significant underlying medical conditions. Use with caution in patients with underlying respiratory disease - bronchospasm may be provoked. Not a substitute for other flu shot; consider primary or concomitant bacterial infections.

Pregnancy Risk Factor B

Pregnancy Implications Zanamivir has been shown to cross the placenta in animal models, however, no evidence of fetal malformations has been demonstrated. Zanamivir has been shown to be excreted in the milk of animals, but its excretion in human milk is unknown. Caution should be used when zanamivir is administered to a nursing mother.

Adverse Reactions Most adverse reactions occurred at a frequency which was equal to the control (lactose vehicle)

>1.5%:

Central nervous system: Headache (2%), dizziness (2%)

Gastrointestinal: Nausea (3%), diarrhea (3%), vomiting (1%)

Respiratory: Sinusitis (3%), bronchitis (2%), cough (2%)

Miscellaneous: Infection (ear, nose and throat) (2%)

<1.5%: Malaise, fatigue, fever, abdominal pain, myalgia, arthralgia, and urticaria

Drug Interactions No clinically significant pharmacokinetic interactions are predicted

Half-Life 2.5-5 hours

Education and Monitoring Issues

Patient Education: Use only as directed; 2 doses daily, 12 hours apart. Two doses should be taken on the first day of dosing, regardless of time interval. Follow exact directions for inhalation device as found on product insert. You may experience headache (use mild analgesic); nausea or vomiting (small frequent meals, good mouth care, chewing gum or sucking hard candy may help). If dizziness occurs, use caution when driving or engaging in tasks which require alertness. Discontinue medication and notify healthcare provider if you experience acute or persistent side effects such as difficulty breathing; chest pains; ear, nose, or throat infection; or acute abdominal pain.

Manufacturer GlaxoWellcome

Related Information

Pharmaceutical Manufacturers Directory *on page 1020*

- ♦ **Zantac®** *see* Ranitidine Hydrochloride *on page 809*
- ♦ **Zantac® 75 [OTC]** *see* Ranitidine Hydrochloride *on page 809*
- ♦ **Zantryl®** *see* Phentermine *on page 726*
- ♦ **Zarontin®** *see* Ethosuximide *on page 346*
- ♦ **Zaroxolyn®** *see* Metolazone *on page 594*
- ♦ **ZeaSorb AF** *see* Tolnaftate *on page 931*
- ♦ **Zeasorb-AF® Powder [OTC]** *see* Miconazole *on page 600*
- ♦ **Zeasorb-AF® Powder [OTC]** *see* Tolnaftate *on page 931*
- ♦ **Zebeta®** *see* Bisoprolol *on page 109*
- ♦ **Zefazone®** *see* Cefmetazole *on page 153*
- ♦ **Zemplar™** *see* Paricalcitol *on page 704*
- ♦ **Zenapax®** *see* Daclizumab *on page 242*
- ♦ **Zerit®** *see* Stavudine *on page 869*
- ♦ **Zestoretic®** *see* Lisinopril and Hydrochlorothiazide *on page 534*
- ♦ **Zestril®** *see* Lisinopril *on page 532*
- ♦ **Ziac™** *see* Bisoprolol and Hydrochlorothiazide *on page 110*
- ♦ **Ziagen™** *see* Abacavir *on page 14*

Zidovudine (zye DOE vyoo deen)

Pharmacologic Class Antiretroviral Agent, Reverse Transcriptase Inhibitor (Nucleoside)

U.S. Brand Names Retrovir®

Use Management of patients with HIV infections in combination with at least two other antiretroviral agents; for prevention of maternal/fetal HIV transmission as monotherapy

USUAL DOSAGE

Prevention of maternal-fetal HIV transmission:

Neonatal: Oral: 2 mg/kg/dose every 6 hours for 6 weeks beginning 8-12 hours after birth; infants unable to receive oral dosing may receive 1.5 mg/kg I.V. infused over 30 minutes every 6 hours

Maternal (>14 weeks gestation): Oral: 100 mg 5 times/day until the start of labor; during labor and delivery, administer zidovudine I.V. at 2 mg/kg over 1 hour followed by a continuous I.V. infusion of 1 mg/kg/hour until the umbilical cord is clamped

Children 3 months to 12 years for HIV infection:

Oral: 160 mg/m^2/dose every 8 hours; dosage range: 90 mg/m^2/dose to 180 mg/m^2/dose every 6-8 hours; some Working Group members use a dose of 180 mg/m^2 every 12 hours when using in drug combinations with other antiretroviral compounds, but data on this dosing in children is limited

I.V. continuous infusion: 20 mg/m^2/hour

I.V. intermittent infusion: 120 mg/m^2/dose every 6 hours

Adults:

Oral: 300 mg twice daily or 200 mg 3 times/day

I.V.: 1-2 mg/kg/dose (infused over 1 hour) administered every 4 hours around-the-clock (6 doses/day)

Prevention of HIV following needlesticks: 200 mg 3 times/day plus lamivudine 150 mg twice daily; a protease inhibitor (eg, indinavir) may be added for high risk exposures; begin therapy within 2 hours of exposure if possible

Patients should receive I.V. therapy only until oral therapy can be administered

Dosing interval in renal impairment: Cl_{cr} <10 mL/minute: May require minor dose adjustment

Hemodialysis: At least partially removed by hemo- and peritoneal dialysis; administer dose after hemodialysis or administer 100 mg supplemental dose; during CAPD, dose as for Cl_{cr} <10 mL/minute

Continuous arteriovenous or venovenous hemodiafiltration (CAVH) effects: Administer 100 mg every 8 hours

Dosing adjustment in hepatic impairment: Reduce dose by 50% or double dosing interval in patients with cirrhosis

Contraindications Life-threatening hypersensitivity to zidovudine or any component

Warnings/Precautions Often associated with hematologic toxicity including granulocytopenia and severe anemia requiring transfusions; zidovudine has been shown to be carcinogenic in rats and mice

Pregnancy Risk Factor C

Adverse Reactions

>10%:

Central nervous system: Severe headache (42%), fever (16%)

Dermatologic: Rash (17%)

Gastrointestinal: Nausea (46% to 61%), anorexia (11%), diarrhea (17%), pain (20%), vomiting (6% to 25%)

Hematologic: Anemia (23% in children), leukopenia, granulocytopenia (39% in children)

Neuromuscular & skeletal: Weakness (19%)

(Continued)

Zidovudine *(Continued)*

1% to 10%:

Central nervous system: Malaise (8%), dizziness (6%), insomnia (5%), somnolence (8%)

Dermatologic: Hyperpigmentation of nails (bluish-brown)

Gastrointestinal: Dyspepsia (5%)

Hematologic: Changes in platelet count

Neuromuscular & skeletal: Paresthesia (6%)

<1%: Bone marrow suppression, cholestatic jaundice, confusion, granulocytopenia, hepatotoxicity, mania, myopathy, neurotoxicity, pancytopenia, seizures, tenderness, thrombocytopenia

Drug Interactions

Decreased effect: Acetaminophen may decrease AUC of zidovudine as can the rifamycins

Increased toxicity: Coadministration with drugs that are nephrotoxic (amphotericin B), cytotoxic (flucytosine, Adriamycin®, vincristine, vinblastine, doxorubicin, interferon), inhibit glucuronidation or excretion (acetaminophen, cimetidine, indomethacin, lorazepam, probenecid, aspirin), or interfere with RBC/WBC number or function (acyclovir, ganciclovir, pentamidine, dapsone); although the AUC was unaffected, the rate of absorption and peak plasma concentrations were increased significantly when zidovudine was administered with clarithromycin (n=18); valproic acid increased AZT's AUC by 80% and decreased clearance by 38% (believed due to inhibition first pass metabolism); fluconazole may increase zidovudine's AUC and half-life, concomitant interferon alfa may increase hematologic toxicities and phenytoin, trimethoprim, and interferon beta-1b may increase zidovudine levels

Manufacturer GlaxoWellcome

Related Information

Antiretroviral Therapy for HIV Infection *on page 1190*

Management of Healthcare Worker Exposures to HIV *on page 1151*

Pharmaceutical Manufacturers Directory *on page 1020*

Zidovudine and Lamivudine *on page 992*

Zidovudine and Lamivudine (zye DOE vyoo deen & la MI vyoo deen)

Pharmacologic Class Antiretroviral Agent, Reverse Transcriptase Inhibitor (Non-Nucleoside); Antiretroviral Agent, Reverse Transcriptase Inhibitor (Nucleoside)

U.S. Brand Names Combivir™

Use Management of patients with HIV infections in combination with at least one other antiretroviral agent

Dosage Forms TAB: Zidovudine 300 mg and lamivudine 150 mg

Manufacturer GlaxoWellcome

Related Information

Pharmaceutical Manufacturers Directory *on page 1020*

♦ **Zilactin®-B Medicated [OTC]** *see* Benzocaine *on page 98*

♦ **Zilactin-L® [OTC]** *see* Lidocaine *on page 527*

Zileuton (zye LOO ton)

Pharmacologic Class 5-Lipoxygenase Inhibitor

U.S. Brand Names Zyflo™

Mechanism of Action Specific inhibitor of 5-lipoxygenase and thus inhibits leukotriene (LTB1, LTC1, LTD1 and LTE1) formation. Leukotrienes are substances that induce numerous biological effects including augmentation of neutrophil and eosinophil migration, neutrophil and monocyte aggregation, leukocyte adhesion, increased capillary permeability and smooth muscle contraction.

Use Prophylaxis and chronic treatment of asthma in adults and children ≥12 years of age

USUAL DOSAGE Oral:

Adults: 600 mg 4 times/day with meals and at bedtime

Elderly: Zileuton pharmacokinetics were similar in healthy elderly subjects (>65 years) compared with healthy younger adults (18-40 years)

Dosing adjustment in renal impairment: Dosing adjustment is not necessary in renal impairment or renal failure (even during dialysis)

Dosing adjustment in hepatic impairment: Contraindicated in patients with active liver disease

Dosage Forms TAB: 600 mg

Contraindications Active liver disease or transaminase elevations greater than or equal to three times the upper limit of normal (≥3 x ULN), hypersensitivity to zileuton or any of its active ingredients

Warnings/Precautions Elevations of one or more liver function tests may occur during therapy. These laboratory abnormalities may progress, remain unchanged or resolve with continued therapy. Use with caution in patients who consume substantial quantities of alcohol or have a past history of liver disease. Zileuton is not indicated for use in the reversal of bronchospasm in acute asthma attacks, including status asthmaticus. Zileuton can be continued during acute exacerbations of asthma.

Pregnancy Risk Factor C

Pregnancy Implications

Clinical effects on the fetus: Developmental studies indicated adverse effects (reduced body weight and increased skeletal variations) in rats at an oral dose of 300 mg/kg/day. There are no adequate and well controlled studies in pregnant women.

Breast-feeding/lactation: Zileuton and its metabolites are excreted in rat milk; it is not known if zileuton is excreted in breast milk

Adverse Reactions

>10%:

Central nervous system: Headache (24.6%)

Hepatic: Increased ALT (12%)

1% to 10%:

Cardiovascular: Chest pain

Central nervous system: Pain, dizziness, fever, insomnia, malaise, nervousness, somnolence

Gastrointestinal: Dyspepsia, nausea, abdominal pain, constipation, flatulence

Hematologic: Low white blood cell count

Neuromuscular & skeletal: Myalgia, arthralgia, weakness

Ocular: Conjunctivitis

Drug Interactions CYP1A2, 2C9, and 3A3/4 enzyme substrate; CYP1A2 and 3A3/4 inhibitor

Increased toxicity:

Propranolol: Doubling of propranolol AUC and consequent increased beta-blocker activity

Terfenadine: Decrease in clearance of terfenadine leading to increase in AUC

Theophylline: Doubling of serum theophylline concentrations - reduce theophylline dose and monitor serum theophylline concentrations closely.

Warfarin: Clinically significant increases in prothrombin time (PT) - monitor PT closely

Onset Peak concentrations: 1-2 hours

Half-Life 2.5 hours

Education and Monitoring Issues

Patient Education: This medication is not for an acute asthmatic attack; in acute attack, follow instructions of prescriber. Do not stop other asthma medication unless advised by prescriber. Take with meals and at bedtime on a continuous bases; do not discontinue even if feeling better (this medication may help reduce incidence of acute attacks). Avoid alcohol and other medications unless approved by your prescriber. You may experience mild headache (mild analgesic may help); fatigue or dizziness (use caution when driving); or nausea or heartburn (small frequent meals, frequent mouth care, sucking lozenges, or chewing gum may help). Report persistent headache, chest pain, rapid heartbeat, or palpitations; skin rash or itching; unusual bleeding (eg, tarry stools, easy bruising, or blood in stool, urine, or mouth); skin rash or irritation; muscle weakness or tremors; redness, irritation, or infections of the eye; or worsening of asthmatic condition.

Monitoring Parameters: Evaluate hepatic transaminases at initiation of and during therapy with zileuton. Monitor serum ALT before treatment begins, once-a-month for the first 3 months, every 2-3 months for the remainder of the first year, and periodically thereafter for patients receiving long-term zileuton therapy. If symptoms of liver dysfunction (right upper quadrant pain, nausea, fatigue, lethargy, pruritus, jaundice or "flu-like" symptoms) develop or transaminase elevations >5 times the ULN occur, discontinue therapy and follow transaminase levels until normal.

Manufacturer Abbott Laboratories (Pharmaceutical Product Division)

Related Information

Pharmaceutical Manufacturers Directory *on page 1020*

- **Zinacef® Injection** *see* Cefuroxime *on page 165*
- **Zinca-Pak®** *see* Zinc Supplements *on page 993*
- **Zincate®** *see* Zinc Supplements *on page 993*

Zinc Gelatin (zingk JEL ah tin)

Pharmacologic Class Protectant, Topical

U.S. Brand Names Gelucast®

Generic Available Yes

Use As a protectant and to support varicosities and similar lesions of the lower limbs

USUAL DOSAGE Apply externally as an occlusive boot

Dosage Forms BANDAGE: 3" x 10 yards, 4" x 10 yards

Contraindications Hypersensitivity to any component

Adverse Reactions 1% to 10%: Local: Irritation

Zinc Supplements (zink SUP la ments)

Pharmacologic Class Mineral, Oral; Mineral, Parenteral; Trace Element

U.S. Brand Names Eye-Sed® [OTC]; Orazinc® [OTC]; Verazinc® [OTC]; Zinca-Pak®; Zincate®

(Continued)

Zinc Supplements *(Continued)*

Use Cofactor for replacement therapy to different enzymes helps maintain normal growth rates, normal skin hydration and senses of taste and smell; zinc supplement (oral and parenteral); may improve wound healing in those who are deficient. May be useful to promote wound healing in patients with pressure sores.

USUAL DOSAGE Clinical response may not occur for up to 6-8 weeks

Zinc sulfate:

RDA: Oral:

Birth to 6 months: 3 mg elemental zinc/day

6-12 months: 5 mg elemental zinc/day

1-10 years: 10 mg elemental zinc/day (44 mg zinc sulfate)

≥11 years: 15 mg elemental zinc/day (65 mg zinc sulfate)

Zinc deficiency: Oral:

Infants and Children: 0.5-1 mg elemental zinc/kg/day divided 1-3 times/day; somewhat larger quantities may be needed if there is impaired intestinal absorption or an excessive loss of zinc

Adults: 110-220 mg zinc sulfate (25-50 mg elemental zinc)/dose 3 times/day

Parenteral: TPN: I.V. infusion (chloride or sulfate): Supplemental to I.V. solutions (clinical response may not occur for up to 6-8 weeks):

Premature Infants <1500 g, up to 3 kg: 300 mcg/kg/day

Full-term Infants and Children ≤5 years: 100 mcg/kg/day

or

Premature Infants: 400 mcg/kg/day

Term <3 months: 250 mcg/kg/day

Term >3 months: 100 mcg/kg/day

Children: 50 mcg/kg/day

Adults:

Stable with fluid loss from small bowel: 12.2 mg zinc/liter TPN or 17.1 mg zinc/kg (added to 1000 mL I.V. fluids) of stool or ileostomy output

Metabolically stable: 2.5-4 mg/day, add 2 mg/day for acute catabolic states

Contraindications Hypersensitivity to any component

Pregnancy Risk Factor A

- **Zithromax™** *see* Azithromycin *on page 86*
- **Zocor®** *see* Simvastatin *on page 852*
- **Zofran®** *see* Ondansetron *on page 676*
- **Zoladex** *see* Goserelin *on page 420*
- **Zoladex® Implant** *see* Goserelin *on page 420*
- **Zolicef®** *see* Cefazolin *on page 149*

Zolmitriptan (zohl mi TRIP tan)

Pharmacologic Class Serotonin 5-HT_{1D} Receptor Agonist

U.S. Brand Names Zomig®

Mechanism of Action Selective agonist for serotonin (5-HT_{1B} and 5-HT_{1D} receptors) in cranial arteries to cause vasoconstriction and reduce sterile inflammation associated with antidromic neuronal transmission correlating with relief of migraine

Use Acute treatment of migraine with or without auras

USUAL DOSAGE Adults:

Oral: Initial recommended dose: 2.5 mg or lower (achieved by manually breaking a 2.5 mg tablet in half). If the headache returns, the dose may be repeated after 2 hours, not to exceed 10 mg within a 24-hour period. Response is greater following the 2.5 or 5 mg dose compared with 1 mg, with little added benefit and increased side effects associated with the 5 mg dose.

Dosage adjustment in hepatic impairment: Administer with caution in patients with liver disease, generally using doses <2.5 mg. Patients with moderate-to-severe hepatic impairment may have decreased clearance of zolmitriptan, and significant elevation in blood pressure was observed in some patients.

Dosage Forms TAB: 2.5 mg, 5 mg

Contraindications

Use in patients with ischemic heart disease or Prinzmetal angina, patients with signs or symptoms of ischemic heart disease, uncontrolled hypertension; use in patients with symptomatic Wolff-Parkinson-White syndrome or arrhythmias associated with other cardiac accessory conduction pathway disorders

Use with ergotamine derivatives (within 24 hours of); use within 24 hours of another 5-HT_1 agonist; concurrent administration or within 2 weeks of discontinuing an MAOI; hypersensitivity to any component; management of hemiplegic or basilar migraine

Warnings/Precautions Zolmitriptan is indicated only in patient populations with a clear diagnosis of migraine. Cardiac events (coronary artery vasospasm, transient ischemia, myocardial infarction, ventricular tachycardia/fibrillation, cardiac arrest, and death) have been reported with 5-HT_1 agonist administration. Significant elevation in blood pressure, including hypertensive crisis, has also been reported on rare occasions in patients with and without a history of hypertension. Vasospasm-related reactions have been reported other than coronary artery vasospasm. Peripheral vascular ischemia and colonic ischemia with abdominal pain and bloody diarrhea have occurred. Use with caution in patients with hepatic impairment.

Pregnancy Risk Factor C

Adverse Reactions

>10%:

Central nervous system: Dizziness
Endocrine & metabolic: Hot flashes
Neuromuscular & skeletal: Paresthesia

1% to 10%:

Cardiovascular: Tightness in chest
Central nervous system: Drowsiness, headache
Dermatologic: Burning sensation
Gastrointestinal: Abdominal discomfort, mouth discomfort
Neuromuscular & skeletal: Myalgia, numbness, weakness, neck pain, jaw discomfort
Miscellaneous: Diaphoresis

<1%: Dehydration, dysmenorrhea, dyspnea, dysuria, hiccups, polydipsia, rashes, renal calculus, thirst

Drug Interactions Increased toxicity: Ergot-containing drugs, MAOIs, cimetidine, oral contraceptives, SSRIs

Alcohol Interactions Avoid use (may cause or worsen headaches)

Onset Within 30 minutes to 1 hour

Half-Life 3 hours

Education and Monitoring Issues

Patient Education: This drug is to be used to reduce your migraine, not to prevent or reduce number of attacks. If first dose brings relief, second dose may be taken anytime after 2 hours if migraine returns. If you have no relief with first dose, do not take a second dose without consulting prescriber. Do not exceed 10 mg in 24 hours. You may experience some dizziness or drowsiness; use caution when driving or engaging in tasks requiring alertness until response to drug is known. Frequent mouth care and sucking on lozenges may relieve dry mouth. Report immediately any chest pain, heart throbbing or tightness in throat; swelling of eyelids, face, or lips; skin rash or hives; easy bruising; blood in urine, stool, or vomitus; pain or itching with urination; or pain, warmth, or numbness in extremities.

Manufacturer Zeneca Pharmaceuticals

Related Information

Pharmaceutical Manufacturers Directory *on page 1020*

♦ **Zoloft®** *see* Sertraline *on page 847*

Zolpidem (zole PI dem)

Pharmacologic Class Hypnotic, Miscellaneous

U.S. Brand Names Ambien™

Mechanism of Action Structurally dissimilar to benzodiazepine, however, has much or all of its actions explained by its effects on benzodiazepine (BZD) receptors, especially the omega-1 receptor; retains hypnotic and much of the anxiolytic properties of the BZD, but has reduced effects on skeletal muscle and seizure threshold.

Use Short-term treatment of insomnia

USUAL DOSAGE Duration of therapy should be limited to 7-10 days

Adults: Oral: 10 mg immediately before bedtime; maximum dose: 10 mg
Elderly: 5 mg immediately before bedtime
Hemodialysis: Not dialyzable
Dosing adjustment in hepatic impairment: Decrease dose to 5 mg

Dosage Forms TAB: 5 mg, 10 mg

Contraindications Lactation

Warnings/Precautions Closely monitor elderly or debilitated patients for impaired cognitive or motor performance; not recommended for use in children <18 years of age. Use caution in compromised respiratory function (has decreased oxygen saturation) in sleep apnea patients.

Pregnancy Risk Factor B

Adverse Reactions

1% to 10%:

Central nervous system: Headache, drowsiness, dizziness
Gastrointestinal: Nausea, diarrhea
Neuromuscular & skeletal: Myalgia

<1%: Amnesia, confusion, falls, tremor, vomiting

Drug Interactions CYP3A3/4 enzyme substrate

Decreased effect: Rifampin
Increased effect/toxicity with alcohol, CNS depressants, sertraline

Alcohol Interactions Avoid use (may increase central nervous system depression)

Onset 30 minutes

Duration 6-8 hours

Half-Life 2-2.6 hours, in cirrhosis increased to 9.9 hours

(Continued)

Zolpidem *(Continued)*

Education and Monitoring Issues

Patient Education: Use exactly as directed (do not increase dose or frequency or discontinue without consulting prescriber); may cause physical and/or psychological dependence. While using this medication, do not use alcohol or other prescription or OTC medications (especially, pain medications, sedatives, antihistamines, or hypnotics) without consulting prescriber. Maintain adequate hydration (2-3 L/day of fluids unless instructed to restrict fluid intake). You may experience drowsiness, dizziness, or blurred vision (use caution when driving or engaging in tasks requiring alertness until response to drug is known); nausea (small frequent meals, frequent mouth care, chewing gum, or sucking lozenges may help); or diarrhea (buttermilk, boiled milk, yogurt may help). Report CNS changes (confusion, depression, increased sedation, excitation, headache, abnormal thinking, insomnia, or nightmares); muscle pain or weakness; difficulty breathing; chest pain or palpitations; or ineffectiveness of medication.

Monitoring Parameters: Respiratory, cardiac and mental status

Reference Range: 80-150 ng/mL

Manufacturer Searle

Related Information

Pharmaceutical Manufacturers Directory *on page 1020*

- **Zomig®** *see* Zolmitriptan *on page 994*
- **Zonalon® Topical Cream** *see* Doxepin *on page 298*
- **Zone-A Forte®** *see* Pramoxine and Hydrocortisone *on page 758*
- **Zonegam™** *see* Zonisamide *on page 996*

Zonisamide (zoe NIS ay mide)

Pharmacologic Class Anticonvulsant, Miscellaneous

U.S. Brand Names Zonegam™

Mechanism of Action The exact mechanism of action is not known. May stabilize neuronal membranes and suppress neuronal hypersynchronization through action at sodium and calcium channels; does not affect GABA activity.

Use Adjunct treatment of partial seizures in adults with epilepsy

USUAL DOSAGE Children >16 years and Adults: Oral: Adjunctive treatment of partial seizures: Initial dose: 100 mg/day; dose may be increased to 200 mg/day after two weeks. Further dosage increases to 300 mg and 400 mg/day can then be made with a minimum of 2 weeks between adjustments, in order to reach steady-state at each dosage level. Doses of up to 600 mg/day have been studied, however, there is no evidence of increased response with doses >400 mg/day.

Dosage adjustment in renal/hepatic impairment: Slower titration and frequent monitoring are indicated in patients with renal or hepatic disease. Do not use if $Cl_{[cr}$ <50 mL/min.

Elderly: Data from clinical trials insufficient for patients >65 years of age; begin dosing at the low end of the dosing range

Dosage Forms CAP: 100 mg

Contraindications Hypersensitivity to sulfonamides or zonisamide

Warnings/Precautions Rare, but potentially fatal sulfonamide reactions have occurred following the use of zonisamide. These reactions include Stevens-Johnson syndrome and toxic epidermal necrolysis, usually appearing within 2-16 weeks of drug initiation. Discontinue zonisamide if rash develops. Decreased sweating and hyperthermia requiring hospitalizaiton have been reported in children. The safety and efficacy in children <16 years of age have not been established. Discontinue zonisamide in patients who develop acute renal failure or a significant sustained increase in creatinine/BUN concentration. Kidney stones have been reported. Use cautiously in patients with renal or hepatic dysfunction. Do not use if estimated Cl_{cr} <50 mL/min. Significant CNS effects include psychiatric symptoms, psychomotor slowing, and fatigue or somnolence. Fatigue and somnolence occur within the first month of treatment, most commonly at doses of 300-500 mg/day. Abrupt withdrawal may precipitate seizures; discontinue or reduce doses gradually.

Pregnancy Risk Factor C

Pregnancy Implications Fetal abnormalities and death have been reported in animals; however, there are no studies in pregnant women. It is not known if zonisamide is excreted in human milk. Use during pregnancy/lactation only if the potential benefits outweigh potential risks.

Adverse Reactions Adjunctive therapy: Frequencies noted in patients receiving other anticonvulsants:

>10%:

Central nervous system: Somnolence (17%), dizziness (13%)

Gastrointestinal: Anorexia (13%)

1% to 10%:

Central nervous system: Headache (10%), agitation/irritability (9%), fatigue (8%), tiredness (7%), ataxia (6%), confusion (6%), decreased concentration (6%), memory impairment (6%), depression (6%), insomnia (6%), speech disorders (5%), mental slowing (4%), anxiety (3%), nervousness (2%), schizophrenic/schizophreniform behavior (2%), difficulty in verbal expression (2%), status epilepticus (1%)

Dermatologic: Rash (3%), bruising (2%)

Gastrointestinal: Nausea (9%), abdominal pain (6%), diarrhea (5%), dyspepsia (3%), weight loss (3%), constipation (2%), dry mouth (2%), taste perversion (2%)

Neuromuscular & skeletal: Paresthesia (4%)

Ocular: Diplopia (6%), nystagmus (4%)

Respiratory: Rhinitis (2%)

Miscellaneous: Flu-like syndrome (4%)

Additional adverse effects have been reported as Frequent (occur in at least 1:100 patients), Infrequent (occur in 1:100 to 1:1000 patients) or Rare (occur in less than 1:1000 patients):

Frequent: Tremor, convulsion, hyperesthesia, incoordination, pruritus, vomiting, weakness, abnormal gait, accidental injury, amblyopia, tinnitus, pharyngitis, increased cough

Infrequent: Flank pain, malaise, abnormal dreams, vertigo, movement disorder, hypotonia, euphoria, chest pain, facial edema, palpitation, tachycardia, vascular insufficiency, hypotension, hypertension, syncope, bradycardia, peripheral edema, edema, cerebrovascular accident, maculopapular rash, acne, alopecia, dry skin, eczema, urticaria, hirsutism, pustular rash, vesiculobullous rash, dehydration, decreased libido, amenorrhea, flatulence, gingivitis, gum hyperplasia, gastritis, gastroenteritis, stomatitis, glossitis, melena, ulcerative stomatitis, gastro-duodenal ulcer, dysphagia, weight gain, urinary frequency, dysuria, urinary incontinence, impotence, urinary retention, urinary urgency, polyuria, nocturia, rectal hemorrhage, gum hemorrhage, leukopenia, anemia, cholelithiasis, thrombophlebitis, neck rigidity, leg cramps, myalgia, myasthenia, arthralgia, arthritis, hypertonia, neuropathy, twitching, hyperkinesia, dysarthria, peripheral neuritis, parathesia, increased reflexes, allergic reaction, lymphadenopathy, immunodeficiency, thirst, sweating, parosmia, conjunctivitis, visual field defect, glaucoma, deafness, hematuria, dyspnea

Rare: Dystonia, encephalopathy, hyperesthesia, atrial fibrillation, heart failure, ventricular extrasystoles, petechia, hypoglycemia, hyponatremia, gynocomastia, mastitis, menorrhagia, cholangitis, hematemesis, colitis, duodenitis, esophagitis, fecal incontinence, mouth ulceration, enuresis, bladder pain, bladder calculus, thrombocytopenia, microcytic anemia, cholecystitis, cholestatic jaundice, increase SGOT, increase SGPT, circumoral paresthesia, dyskinesia, facial paralysis, hypokinesia, myoclonus, lupus erythematosus, increase lactic dehydrogenase, oculogyric crisis, photophobia, iritis, albuminuria, pulmonary embolus, apnea, hemoptysis

Case reports: Stevens Johnson Syndrome, toxic epidermal necrolysis, aplastic anemia, agranulocytosis, kidney stones, increase BUN, increase serum creatinine, increase serum alkaline phosphatase

Drug Interactions CYP3A4 enzyme substrate

Zonisamide did not affect steady-state levels of carbamazepine, phenytoin, or valproate

Zonisamide's half-life is decreased by carbamazepine, phenytoin, phenobarbital, and valproate. Other medications that induce or inhibit CYP3A4 would also be expected to alter serum levels of zonisamide.

Cimetidine: Single dose zonisamide levels were not altered by cimetidine

Alcohol Interactions Avoid use (may increase central nervous system depression)

Education and Monitoring Issues

Patient Education: May cause drowsiness, especially at higher doses. Do not drive a car or operate other complex machinery until effects on performance can be determined. Avoid alcohol and other CNS depressants. Contact healthcare provider immediately if seizures worsen or for any of the following: skin rash; sudden back pain, abdominal pain, blood in the urine; fever, sore throat, oral ulcers or easy bruising. Contact healthcare provider before becoming pregnant or breast-feeding. Swallow capsules whole, do not bite or break. It is important to drink 6-8 glasses of water each day while using this medication. Do not stop taking this or other seizure medications without talking to your healthcare professional first.

Dietary Considerations: Food delays time to maximum concentration, but does not affect bioavailability; may be taken with or without food

Monitoring Parameters: BUN and serum creatinine

Manufacturer Elan Pharmaceuticals

Related Information

Epilepsy Guidelines *on page 1091*

Pharmaceutical Manufacturers Directory *on page 1020*

- **ZORprin®** *see* Aspirin *on page 72*
- **Zosyn™** *see* Piperacillin and Tazobactam Sodium *on page 741*
- **Zovia®** *see* Ethinyl Estradiol and Ethynodiol Diacetate *on page 341*
- **Zovirax®** *see* Acyclovir *on page 22*
- **Zyban™** *see* Bupropion *on page 120*
- **Zydone®** *see* Hydrocodone and Acetaminophen *on page 444*
- **Zyflo™** *see* Zileuton *on page 992*
- **Zyloprim®** *see* Allopurinol *on page 34*

- ♦ **Zymase®** *see* Pancrelipase *on page 698*
- ♦ **Zyprexa™** *see* Olanzapine *on page 673*
- ♦ **Zyrtec®** *see* Cetirizine *on page 172*
- ♦ **Zyvox™** *see* Linezolid *on page 532*

APPENDIX

Miscellaneous

Abbreviations and Measurements

Disease State Management and Therapeutic Guidelines

General Medicine

Immunizations and Vaccinations

APPENDIX *(Continued)*

Infectious Disease – Prophylaxis

Infectious Disease – Treatment

Maternal and Fetal Guidelines

Comparative Drug Charts

Herbal/Nutritional Information

PATIENT EDUCATION FOR MANAGEMENT OF COMMON SIDE EFFECTS

MANAGEMENT OF DRUG-RELATED PROBLEMS

Patients may experience some type of side effect or adverse drug reaction as a result of their drug therapy. The type of effect, the severity, and the frequency of occurrence is dependent on the medication and dose being used, as well as the individual's response to therapy. The following information is presented as helpful tips to assist the patient through these drug-related problems. Pharmacological support may also be required for their management.

Alopecia

- Your hair loss is temporary. Hair usually will begin to grow within 3-6 months of completing drug therapy.
- Your hair may come back with a different texture, color, or thickness.
- Avoid excessive shampooing and hair combing, or harsh hair care products.
- Avoid excessive drying of hair.
- Avoid use of permanents, dyes, or hair sprays.
- Always cover head in cold weather or sunshine.

Anemia

- Observe all bleeding precautions (see Thrombocytopenia).
- Get adequate sleep and rest.
- Be alert for potential for dizziness, fainting, or extreme fatigue.
- Maintain adequate nutrition and hydration.
- Have laboratory tests done as recommended.
- If unusual bleeding occurs, notify prescriber.

Anorexia

- Small frequent meals containing favorite foods may tempt appetite.
- Eat simple foods such as toast, rice, bananas, mashed potatoes, scrambled eggs.
- Eat in a pleasant environment conducive to eating.
- When possible, eat with others.
- Avoid noxious odors when eating.
- Use nutritional supplements high in protein and calories.
- Freezing nutritional supplements sometimes makes them more palatable.
- A small glass of wine (if not contraindicated) may stimulate appetite.
- Mild exercise or short walks may stimulate appetite.
- Request antiemetic medication to reduce nausea or vomiting.

Diarrhea

- Include fiber, high protein foods, and fruits in dietary intake.
- Drink plenty of liquids.
- Buttermilk, yogurt, or boiled milk may be helpful.
- Antidiarrheal agents may be needed. Consult your prescriber.
- Include regular rest periods in your activities.
- Institute skin care regimen to prevent breakdown and promote comfort.

Fluid Retention/Edema

- Elevate legs when sitting.
- Wear support hose.
- Increase physical exercise.
- Maintain adequate hydration; avoiding fluids will not reduce edema.
- Weigh yourself regularly.
- If your prescriber has advised you to limit your salt intake, avoid foods such as ham, bacon, processed meats, and canned foods. Many foods are high in salt content. Read labels carefully.
- Report to prescriber if any of the following occur: sudden weight gain, decrease in urination, swelling of hands or feet, increase in waist size, wet cough, or difficulty breathing.

Headache

- Lie down.
- Use cool cloth on forehead.
- Avoid caffeine.
- Use mild analgesics. Consult prescriber.

Leukopenia/Neutropenia

- Monitor for signs of infections: persistent sore throat, fever, chills, fatigue, headache, flu-like symptoms, vaginal discharge, foul-smelling stools.
- Prevent infection. Maintain strict handwashing at all times. Avoid crowds when possible. Avoid exposure to infected persons.
- Avoid exposure to temperature changes.
- Maintain adequate nutrition and hydration.
- Maintain good personal hygiene.
- Avoid injury or skin breaks.
- Avoid vaccinations (unless recommended by healthcare provider).
- Avoid sunburn.

Nausea and Vomiting

- Eat food served cold or at room temperature. Ice chips are sometimes helpful.
- Drink clear liquids in severe cases of nausea. Avoid carbonated beverages.
- Sip liquids slowly.
- Avoid spicy food. Bland foods are easier to digest.
- Rinse mouth with lemon water. Practice good oral hygiene.
- Avoid sweet, fatty, salty foods and foods with strong odors.
- Eat small frequent meals rather than heavy meals.
- Use relaxation techniques and guided imagery.
- Use distractions such as meals, television, reading, games, etc.
- Sleep during intense periods of nausea.
- Chew gum or suck on hard candy or lozenges.
- Eat in an upright (sitting position), rather than semirecumbant.
- Avoid tight constrictive clothing at meal time.
- Use some mild exercise following light meals rather than lying down.
- Request antiemetic medication to reduce nausea or vomiting.

Postural Hypotension

- Use care and rise slowly from sitting or lying position to standing.
- Use care when climbing stairs.
- Initiate ambulation slowly. Get your bearings before you start walking.
- Do not bend over; always squat slowly if you must pick up something from floor.
- Use caution when showering or bathing (use secure handrails).

Stomatitis

- Perform good oral hygiene frequently, especially before and after meals.
- Avoid use of strong or alcoholic commercial mouthwashes.
- Keep lips well lubricated.
- Avoid tobacco or other products that are irritating to the oral mucosa.
- Avoid hot, spicy, excessively salty foods.
- Eat soft foods and drink adequate fluids.
- Request topical or systemic analgesics for painful ulcerations.
- Be alert for and report signs of oral fungal infections.

Thrombocytopenia

- Avoid aspirin and aspirin-containing products.
- Use electric or safety razor and blunt scissors.
- Use soft toothbrush or cotton swabs for oral care. Avoid use of dental floss.
- Avoid use of enemas, cathartics, and suppositories unless approved by prescriber.
- Avoid valsalva maneuvers such as straining at stool.
- Use stool softeners if necessary to prevent constipation. Consult prescriber.
- Avoid blowing nose forcefully.
- Never go barefoot, wear protective foot covering.

PATIENT EDUCATION FOR MANAGEMENT OF COMMON SIDE EFFECTS *(Continued)*

- Use care when trimming nails (if necessary).
- Maintain safe environment; arrange furniture to provide safe passageway.
- Maintain adequate lighting in darkened areas to avoid bumping into objects.
- Avoid handling sharp tools or instruments.
- Avoid contact sports or activities that might result in injury.
- Promptly report signs of bleeding; abdominal pain; blood in stool, urine, or vomitus; unusual fatigue; easy bruising; bleeding around gums; or nose-bleeds.
- If injection or bloodsticks are necessary, inform healthcare provider that you may have excess bleeding.

Vertigo

- Observe postural hypotension precautions.
- Use caution when driving or using any machinery.
- Avoid sudden position shifts; do not "rush".
- Utilize appropriate supports (eg, cane, walker) to prevent injury.

FDA PREGNANCY CATEGORIES

Throughout this book there is a field labeled Pregnancy Risk Factor (PRF) and the letter A, B, C, D or X immediately following which signifies a category. The FDA has established these five categories to indicate the potential of a systemically absorbed drug for causing birth defects. The key differentiation among the categories rests upon the reliability of documentation and the risk:benefit ratio. Pregnancy Category X is particularly notable in that if any data exists that may implicate a drug as a teratogen and the risk:benefit ratio is clearly negative, the drug is contraindicated during pregnancy.

These categories are summarized as follows:

- A Controlled studies in pregnant women fail to demonstrate a risk to the fetus in the first trimester with no evidence of risk in later trimesters. The possibility of fetal harm appears remote.
- B Either animal-reproductive studies have not demonstrated a fetal risk but there are no controlled studies in pregnant women, or animal-reproduction studies have shown an adverse effect (other than a decrease in fertility) that was not confirmed in controlled studies in women in the first trimester and there is no evidence of a risk in later trimesters.
- C Either studies in animals have revealed adverse effects on the fetus (teratogenic or embryocidal effects or other) and there are no controlled studies in women, or studies in women and animals are not available. Drugs should be given only if the potential benefits justify the potential risk to the fetus.
- D There is positive evidence of human fetal risk, but the benefits from use in pregnant women may be acceptable despite the risk (eg, if the drug is needed in a life-threatening situation or for a serious disease for which safer drugs cannot be used or are ineffective).
- X Studies in animals or human beings have demonstrated fetal abnormalities or there is evidence of fetal risk based on human experience, or both, and the risk of the use of the drug in pregnant women clearly outweighs any possible benefit. The drug is contraindicated in women who are or may become pregnant.

DRUGS IN PREGNANCY

Analgesics

- **Acceptable:** Acetaminophen, meperidine, methadone
- **Controversial:** Codeine, propoxyphene
- **Unacceptable:** Nonsteroidal anti-inflammatory agents, salicylates, phenazopyridine

Antimicrobials

- **Acceptable:** Penicillins, 1st and 2nd generation cephalosporins, erythromycin (base and EES), clotrimazole, miconazole, nystatin, isoniazid*, lindane, acyclovir, metronidazole
- **Controversial:** 3rd generation cephalosporins, aminoglycosides, nitrofurantoin†
- **Unacceptable:** Erythromycin estolate, chloramphenicol, sulfa, tetracyclines

ENT

- **Acceptable:** Diphenhydramine*, dextromethorphan
- **Controversial:** Pseudoephedrine
- **Unacceptable:** Brompheniramine, cyproheptadine, dimenhydrinate

GI

- **Acceptable:** Trimethobenzamide, antacids*, simethicone, other H_2-blockers, psyllium, bisacodyl, docusate
- **Controversial:** Metoclopramide, prochlorperazine

Neurologic

- **Controversial:** Phenytoin, phenobarbital
- **Unacceptable:** Carbamazepine, valproic acid, ergotamine

Pulmonary

- **Acceptable:** Theophylline, metaproterenol, terbutaline, inhaled steroids
- **Unacceptable:** Epinephrine, oral steroids

Psych

- **Acceptable:** Hydroxyzine*, lithium*, haloperidol
- **Controversial:** Benzodiazepines, tricyclics, phenothiazines

Other

- **Acceptable:** Heparin, insulin
- **Unacceptable:** Warfarin, sulfonylureas

*Do not use in first trimester
†Do not use in third trimester

PENDING DRUGS OR DRUGS IN CLINICAL TRIALS

Brand Name	Generic Name	Use
Advair® Diskus®	salmeterol/fluticasone	Asthma
Alredase®	tolrestat	Controlling late complications of diabetes
Arkin-Z®	vesnarinone	Congestive heart failure agent
Baypress®	nitrendipine	Calcium channel blocker for hypertension
Berotec®	fenoterol	Beta-2 agonist for asthma
Catatrol®	viloxazine	Bicyclic antidepressant
Cipralan®	cifenline succinate	Antiarrhythmic agent
Cytolex®	pexiganan	Diabetic foot ulcers
Decabid®	indecainide hydrochloride	Antiarrhythmic agent
Delaprem®	hexoprenaline sulfate	Tocolytic agent
Dirame®	propiram	Opioid analgesic
Enable®	tenidap sodium	Arthritis
Exelom®	rivastigmine	Alzheimer's disease
Fareston®	toremifene citrate	Antiestrogen for breast cancer
Freedox®	triliazad mesylate	Prevents progressive neuronal degeneration
Frisium®	clobazam	Benzodiazepine
Gastrozepine®	pirenzepine	Antiulcer drug
Inhibace®	cilazapril	ACE inhibitor
Isoprinosine®	inosiplex	Immunomodulating drug
Lacipil®	lacidipine	Hypertension
Lunelle®	medroxyprogesterone/estradiol	Contraceptive
Malarone®	atavaquone/proguanil	Malaria
Maxicam®	isoxicam	NSAID
Mentane®	velnacrine	Alzheimer's disease agent
Micturin®	terodiline hydrochloride	Agent for urinary incontinence
Mobic®	meloxicam	Arthritis
Mogadon®	nitrazepam	Benzodiazepine
Motilium®	domperidone	Antiemetic
Napa®	acecainide	Antiarrhythmic agent
Natrecor®	nesiritide	Congestive heart failure
NovoLog®	insulin agent	Diabetes
Orzel®	tegafur/uracil	Colorectal cancer
Pindac®	pinacidil	Antihypertensive
Prothiaden®	dothiepin hydrochloride	Tricyclic antidepressant
Protonix®	pantopraxole	Proton pump inhibitor
Qvar®	beclomethasone	Asthma
Rimadyl®	caprofen	NSAID
Roxiam®	remoxipride	Antipsychotic agent
Selecor®	celiprolol hydrochloride	Beta-adrenergic blocker
Spexil®	trospectomycin	Antibiotic, a spectinomycin analog
Targocoid®	teicoplanin	Antibiotic, similar to vancomycin
Unicard®	dilevalol	Beta-adrenergic blocker
Visudyne®	vertaporfin	Macular degeneration

NEW DRUGS INTRODUCED OR APPROVED BY THE FDA IN 1999

Brand Name	Generic Name	Use
Aciphex™	rabeprazole	Reflux ulcer and duodenal ulcer
Actos®	pioglitazone	Type II diabetes
Agenerase™	amprenavir	HIV
Aggrenox®	dipyridamole & aspirin	Reduce risk of nonfatal stroke
Alamast®	pemirolast	Allergic conjunctivitis
Alocril™	nedocromil (ophthalmic)	Allergic conjunctivitis
Antagon™	ganirelix	Prevent premature LH surges
Aromasin®	exemestane	Breast cancer
Avandia®	rosiglitazone	Type II diabetes
Avapro® HCT	irbesartan and hydrochlorothiazide	Hypertension
Avelox™	moxifloxacin	Antibiotic
Busulfex®	busalfan	Chronic myelogenous leukemia
Cafcit®	caffeine, citrated	Idiopathic apnea of prematurity
Cenestin®	synthetic conj. estrogens, A	Symptoms of menopause
Chirocaine®	levobupivacaine	Local or regional anesthesia
Comtan®	entacapone	Parkinson's disease
Comvax®	*Haemophilus* B conjugate and hepatitis B vaccine	Vaccination
Curosurf®	poractant alfa	Respiratory distress syndrome (RDS)
DepoCyt™	cytarabine (liposomal)	Lymphomatous meningitis
Ellence™	epirubicin	Antineoplastic
Ferrlecit®	sodium ferric gluconate complex	Iron deficiency in dialysis patient
Hectoral™	doxercalciferol	Hyperparathyroidism
INOmax™	nitric oxide	Hypoxic respiratory failure associated with pulmonary hypertension
Keppra™	levetiracetam	Epilepsy
Levulan® Kerastick™	aminolevulenic acid	Nonhyperkeratotic actinic keratoses
Nabi-HB®	hepatitis B immune globulin	Hepatitis B
NovoSeven®	recombinant factor VIIa	Hemophilia A or B
Ontak®	denileukin diftitox	Cutaneous T-cell lymphoma (CTCL)
Panretin™	alitretinoin	AIDS-related Kaposi's sarcoma
Pletal®	cilostazol	Intermittent claudication
Precedex™	dexmedetomidine	Sedation
Preveon®	adefovir	HIV
Rapamune™	sirolimus	Immunosuppressant
Raplan®	rapacuronium	Neuromuscular blocking agent
Relenza®	zanamivir	Influenza
Solagé™	mequinol and tretinoin	Treatment of solar lentigines
Sonata®	zaleplon	Hypnotic agent
Sucraid™	sacrosidase	Congenital sucrase-isomaltase deficiency
Synercid®	quinupristin/dalfopristin	Antibiotic (vancomycin-resistant bacteria)
Tamiflu™	oseltamivir	Type A & B influenza
Targretin®	bexarotene	Cutaneous T-cell lymphoma

NEW DRUGS INTRODUCED OR APPROVED BY THE FDA IN 1999 *(Continued)*

Brand Name	Generic Name	Use
Tequin™	gatifloxacin	Antibiotic
Teveten®	eprosartan	Hypertension
Temodar®	temozolomide	Alkylating agent
Thyrogen®	thyrotropin alpha	Diagnostic agent
Tikosyn®	dofetilide	Antiarrhythmic agent
Trileptal™	oxcarabine	Epilespy
Vioxx®	rofecoxib	Osteoarthritis, pain, dysmenorrhea
Vitravene™	fomivirsen	Cytomegalovirus
Xenical®	orlistat	Obesity
Xopenex®	levalbuterol	Bronchospasm
Zaditor®	ketotifen fumarate	Allergic conjunctivitis
Ziagen™	abacavir	HIV

DRUG PRODUCTS NO LONGER AVAILABLE IN THE U.S.

Brand Name	Generic Name
Achromycin® Parenteral	tetracycline
Achromycin® V Capsule	tetracycline
Achromycin® V Oral Suspension	tetracycline
ACTH-40®	corticotropin
Actidil®	triprolidine
Actifed® Syrup	triprolidine and pseudoephedrine
Actifed® With Codeine	triprolidine, pseudoephedrine, and codeine
Adapin®	doxepin
Adalat® 20 mg	nifedipine
Adipex-P®	phentermine (all products)
Adipost®	phendimetrazine tartrate
Adphen®	phendimetrazine tartrate
Adrin®	nylidrin hydrochloride
Aerolate® Oral Solution	theophylline
Aerosporin® Injection	polymyxin B
Agoral® Plain	mineral oil
Akarpine® Ophthalmic	pilocarpine
AKbeta® 0.25%	levobunolol
AK-Neo-Dex®	neomycin and dexamethasone
Akoline® C.B. Tablet	vitamin
AK-Pentolate® 2%	cyclopentolate
Ak-Zol®	acetazolamide
Ala-Tet®	tetracycline
Alupent® Syrup	metaproterenol
Amin-Aid®	amino acid
Amonidrin® Tablet	guaifenesin
Anacin-3® (all products)	acetaminophen
Anaids® Tablet	alginic acid and sodium bicarbonate
Anergan® 25 Injection	promethazine hydrochloride
Anoxine-AM® Capsule	phentermine hydrochloride
Antabuse® 500 mg	disulfiram
Antinea® Cream	benzoic acid and salicylic acid
Antivert® Chewable Tablet	meclizine hydrochloride
Antrocol® Capsule & Tablet	atropine and belladonna
Apomorphine	apomorphine (now available as an orphan drug only)
Arcotinic® Tablet	iron and liver combination
Arduan®	pipecuronium
Argyrol® S.S.	silver protein, mild
Arlidin®	nylidrin (all products)
Arthritis Foundation® Ibuprofen	ibuprofen
Arthritis Foundation® Nighttime	acetaminophen and diphenhydramine
Arthritis Foundation® Pain Reliever, Aspirin Free	acetaminophen
Arthritis Strength Bufferin®	aspirin (buffered)
Articulose-50® Injection	prednisolone
Asbron-G® Elixir	theophylline and guaifenesin
Asbron-G® Tablet	theophylline and guaifenesin
Asproject®	sodium thiosalicylate
Atabrine® Tablet	quinacrine hydrochloride

DRUG PRODUCTS NO LONGER AVAILABLE IN THE U.S.
(Continued)

Brand Name	Generic Name
Atropine Soluble Tablet	atropine soluble tablet
Aureomycin®	chlortetracycline
Axotal®	butalbital compound and aspirin
Azlin® Injection	azlocillin
Azo Gantanol®	sulfamethoxazole and phenazopyridine
Azo Gantrisin®	sulfisoxazole and phenazopyridine
Azulfidine® Suspension	sulfasalazine
B-A-C®	butalbital compound with aspirin
Bactocill®	oxacillin
Bancap®	butalbital compound with acetaminophen
Banesin®	acetaminophen
Bantron®	lobeline (all products)
Baypress®	nitrendipine
Becomject-100®	vitamin B complex
Beesix®	pyridoxine hydrochloride
Bellafoline®	levorotatory alkaloids of belladonna (all products)
Bemote®	dicyclomine
Bena-D®	diphenhydramine
Benadryl® 50 mg Capsule	diphenhydramine hydrochloride
Benadryl® Cold/Flu	acetaminophen, diphenhydramine, and pseudoephedrine
Benahist® Injection	diphenhydramine hydrochloride
Benoject®	diphenhydramine hydrochloride
Betapen-VK®	penicillin V potassium
Beta-Val® Ointment	betamethasone
Biamine® Injection	thiamine hydrochloride
Bilezyme® Tablet	pancrelipase
Biomox®	amoxicillin
Biphetamine®	amphetamine and dextroamphetamine
Blanex® Capsule	chloroxazone and acetaminophen
Bretylol®	bretylium
Bronkephrine®	ethylnorepinephrine hydrochloride
Buffered®, Tri-buffered	aspirin
Bufferin® Arthritis Strength	aspirin
Bufferin® Extra Strength	aspirin
Buf-Puf® Acne Cleansing Bar	salicylic acid
Butace®	butalbital compound
Caladryl® Spray	diphenhydramine and calamine
Calciparine® Injection	heparin calcium
Camalox® Suspension & Tablet	aluminum hydroxide, calcium carbonate, and magnesium hydroxide
Cantharone®	cantharidin
Cantharone Plus®	cantharidin
Caroid®	cascara sagrada and phenolphthalein
Catarase® 1:5000	chymotrypsin (all products)
Ceclor Suspension 187 mg/5 mL (50 mL)	cefaclor
Ceclor Suspension 375 mg/5 mL (50 mL)	cefaclor
Cedilanid-D® Injection	deslanoside
Cenocort® A-40	triamcinolone
Cenocort® Forte	triamcinolone

Brand Name	Generic Name
Centrax® Capsule & Tablet	prazepam
Cerespan®	papaverine hydrochloride
Cetane®	ascorbic acid
Chenix® Tablet	chenodiol
Chlorgest-HD® Elixir	chlorpheniramine, phenylephrine, and hydrocodone
Chlorofon-A® Tablet	chlorzoxazone
Chloromycetin® Cream	chloramphenicol
Chloromycetin® Kapseals®	chloramphenicol
Chloromycetin® Ophthalmic	chloramphenicol
Chloromycetin® Otic	chloramphenicol
Chloromycetin® Palmitate Oral Suspension	chloramphenicol
Chloroserpine®	reserpine and hydrochorothiazide
Chlortab®	chlorpheniramine maleate
Choledyl®	oxtriphylline
Chymex®	bentiromide (all products)
Cipralan®	cifenline
Cithalith-S® Syrup	lithium citrate
Citro-Nesia® Solution	magnesium citrate
Clistin® Tablet	carbinoxamine maleate
Clorpactin® XCB Powder	oxychlorosene sodium
Cobalasine® Injection	adenosine phosphate
Codimal-A® Injection	brompheniramine maleate
Codimal® Expectorant	guaifenesin and phenylpropanolamine
Coly-Mycin® S Oral	colistin sulfate
Constant-T® Tablet	theophylline
Control-L®	pyrethrins
Cortaid® Ointment	hydrocortisone
Cortrophin-Zinc®	corticotropin
Crinone® Vaginal Gel	progesterone
Crysticillin® 300 A.S.	penicillin G procaine
Crysticillin® 600 A.S.	penicillin G procaine
Crystodigin® 0.05 mg & 0.15 mg Tablet	digitoxin
Cyclospasmol®	cyclandelate (all products)
Cycrin® 10 mg Tablet	medroxyprogesterone acetate
D-Amp®	ampicillin
Danex® Shampoo	pyrithione zinc
Dapex-37.5®	phentermine hydrochloride
Darbid® Tablet	isopropamide iodide (all products)
Daricon®	oxyphencyclimine (all products)
Darvon® 32 mg Capsule	propoxyphene hydrochloride
Darvon-N® Oral Suspension	propoxyphene napsylate
Datril® Extra Strength	acetaminophen
Decadron® 0.25 mg and 6 mg Tablets	dexamethasone
Decaspray®	dexamethasone
Dehist®	brompheniramine maleate
Deltalin® Capsule	ergocalciferol
Depo-Provera® 100 mg/mL	medroxyprogesterone
Deprol®	meprobamate and benactyzine hydrochloride
Dermoxyl® Gel	benzoyl peroxide
Despec® Liquid	guaifenesin, phenylpropanolamine, and phenylephrine
Dexacen-4®	dexamethasone

DRUG PRODUCTS NO LONGER AVAILABLE IN THE U.S. *(Continued)*

Brand Name	Generic Name
Dexacen® LA-8	dexamethasone
Dexedrine® Elixir	dextroamphetamine sulfate
Dialose® Capsule	docusate sodium
Diaparene® Cradol®	methylbenzethonium
Dilantin-30® Pediatric Suspension	phenytoin
Dilantin® With Phenobarbital	phenytoin with phenobarbital
Dilaudid® 1 mg & 3 mg Tablet	hydromorphone hydrochloride
Dimetane®	brompheniramine maleate
Dispos-a-Med® Isoproterenol	isoproterenol
Diupress®	chlorothiazide and reserpine
Dizymes® Tablet	pancreatin
Dommanate® Injection	dimenhydrinate
Donphen® Tablet	hyoscyamine, atropine, scopolamine, and phenobarbital
Dopastat® Injection	dopamine hydrochloride
Doriden® Tablet	glutethimide
Doxinate® Capsule	docusate sodium
Dramamine® Injection	dimenhydrinate
Dramocen®	dimenhydrinate
Dramoject®	dimenhydramine
Drize®	chlorpheniramine and phenylpropanolamine
D-S-S Plus®	docusate and casanthranol
Duo-Medihaler®	isoproterenol and phenylephrine
Duracid®	aluminum hydroxide, magnesium carbonate, and calcium carbonate
Duract®	bromfenac (all products)
Dyflex-400® Tablet	dyphylline
Dymelor®	acetohexamide
Elase® Ointment	fibrinolysin and desoxyribonuclease (all products)
Elase®-Chloromycetin® Ointment	fibrinolysin and desoxyribonuclease
Eldepryl® Tablet	selegiline
Eldoquin® Lotion	hydroquinone
Elixophyllin SR®	theophylline
E-Lor® Tablet	propoxyphene and acetaminophen
Emete-Con® Injection	benzquinamide
Emetine Hydrochloride	emetine hydrochloride
Endep®	amitriptyline hydrochloride
Enduron® 2.5 mg Tablet	methyclothiazide
Enkaid®	encainide
Enovid®	mestranol and norethynodrel
E.N.T.®	brompheniramine and phenylpropanolamine
Entozyme®	pancreatin
E.P. Mycin® Capsule	oxytetracycline
Ergostat®	ergotamine
Ergotrate® Maleate	ergonovine maleate
Eridium®	phenazopyridine hydrochloride
Ery-Sol® Topical Solution	erythromycin, topical
Esidrix® 100 mg Tablet	hydrochlorothiazide
Estradurin® Injection	polyestradiol phosphate
Estroject-2® Injection	estradiol

Brand Name	Generic Name
Estroject-L.A.® Injection	estradiol
Estronol® Injection	estrone
Estrovis®	quinestrol
Ethaquin®	ethaverine hydrochloride
Ethatab®	ethaverine hydrochloride
Ethavex-100®	ethaverine hydrochloride
Euthroid® Tablet	liotrix
Fansidar®	sulfadoxine and pyrimethamine
Fastin®	phentermine (all products)
FemCare®	clotrimazole
Femstat®	butoconazole nitrate
Fergon Plus®	iron with vitamin B
Fer-In-Sol® Capsule	ferrous sulfate
Fermalox®	ferrous sulfate, magnesium hydroxide, and docusate
Ferndex	dextroamphetamine sulfate
Flonase® 9 g	fluticasone
Folex® Injection	methotrexate
Gamastan®	immune globulin, intramuscular
Gammagard® Injection	immune globulin, intravenous
Gammar®	immune globulin, intramuscular
Gantrisin® Ophthalmic	sulfisoxazole
Gantrisin® Tablet	sulfisoxazole
Gelusil® Liquid	aluminum hydroxide, magnesium hydroxide, and simethicone
Gen-D-phen®	diphenhydramine hydrochloride
GlaucTabs®	methazolamide
Grisactin®	griseofulvin
Gynogen® Injection	estradiol
Halazone Tablet	halazone
Halenol® Tablet	acetaminophen
Harmonyl®	deserpidine
HemFe®	iron with vitamins
Hep-B-Gammagee®	hepatitis B immune globulin
Herplex®	idoxuridine
Hetrazan®	diethylcarbamazine citrate
Hismanal®	astemizole
Histalet® Syrup	chlorpheniramine and pseudoephedrine
Histalet® X	guaifenesin and pseudoephedrine
Histaject®	brompheniramine maleate
Histamine Phosphate Injection	histamine phosphate
Hydeltra-T.B.A.®	prednisolone
Hydramine®	diphenhydramine hydrochloride
Hydrobexan® Injection	hydroxocobalamin
Hydropres® 25 mg Tablet	hydrochlorothiazide and reserpine
Hydroxacen®	hydroxyzine
Ilosone®	erythromycin estolate
Intal® Inhalation Capsule	cromolyn sodium
Intercept®	nonoxynol 9
Iodo-Niacin® Tablet	potassium iodide and niacinamide hydroiodide
Ionamin®	phentermine (all products)
Iophen®	iodinated glycerol
Iophen-C®	iodinated glycerol and codeine

DRUG PRODUCTS NO LONGER AVAILABLE IN THE U.S. *(Continued)*

Brand Name	Generic Name
Iophen-DM®	iodinated glycerol and dextromethorphan (all products)
Iophylline®	iodinated glycerol and theophylline
Iotuss®	iodinated glycerol and codeine
Iotuss-DM®	iodinated glycerol and dextromethorphan (all products)
Iso-Bid®	isosorbide dinitrate
Isopto® P-ES	pilocarpine and physostigmine
Isovex®	ethaverine hydrochloride
Isuprel® Glossets®	isoproterenol
Kaopectate® Children's Tablet	attapulgite
Kato® Powder	potassium chloride
Keflin®	cephalothin sodium
Kestrin® Injection	estrone
Klorvess® Liquid	potassium chloride
Koate®-HS Injection	antihemophilic factor (human)
Koate®-HT Injection	antihemophilic factor (human)
Kolyum® Powder	potassium chloride and potassium gluconate
Konyne-HT® Injection	factor IX complex (human)
Kwell®	lindane
Lamprene® 100 mg	clofazimine
Laniazid® Tablet	isoniazid
Lasan® Topical	anthralin
Lasan® HP-1 Topical	anthralin
Ledercillin VK®	penicillin V potassium
Libritabs® 5 mg	chlordiazepoxide
Listerex® Scrub	salicylic acid
Lorcet®	hydrocodone and acetaminophen
Lorelco®	probucol
Malatal®	hyoscyamine, atropine, scopolamine, and phenobarbital
Malotuss® Syrup	guaifenesin
Mandelamine® Tablet	methenamine
Mantadil® Cream	chlorcyclizine
Marezine® Injection	cyclizine hydrochloride
Marplan®	isocarboxazid
Max-Caro®	beta-carotene
Meclomen®	meclofenamate sodium
Medihaler-Epi®	epinephrine
Medihaler Ergotamine®	ergotamine
Medrapred®	prednisolone and atropine
Medrol® Acetate Topical	methylprednisolone
Melfiat® Tablet	phendimetrazine tartrate
Meprospan®	meprobamate
Mesantoin®	mephenytoin
Metaprel® Aerosol	metaproterenol sulfate
Metaprel® Inhalation Solution	metaproterenol sulfate
Metaprel® Tablet	metaproterenol sulfate
Metizol® Tablet	metronidazole
Metopirone® Tablet	metyrapone tartrate
Metra®	phendimetrazine tartrate

Brand Name	Generic Name
Miflex® Tablet	chlorzoxazone and acetaminophen
Milprem®	meprobamate and conjugated estrogens
Minocin® Tablet	minocycline
Miochol®	acetylcholine
Moisturel® Lotion	dimethicone
Monocete® Topical Liquid	monochloroacetic acid
Moxam® Injection	moxalactam
Mus-Lax®	chlorzoxazone
Mylaxen® Injection	hexafluorenium bromide
Myochrysine®	gold sodium thiomalate
Nafcil®	nafcillin
Nalfon® Tablet	fenoprofen calcium
Nandrobolic® Injection	nandrolone phenpropionate
Narcan® 1 mg/mL Injection	naloxone hydrochloride
Navane® Concentrate & Injection	thiothixene
N-B-P® Ointment	bacitracin, neomycin, and polymyxin B
Neo-Castaderm®	resorcinol, boric acid, acetone
Neo-Cortef® Topical	neomycin and hydrocortisone
NeoDecadron® Topical	neomycin and dexamethasone
Neo-Medrol® Acetate Topical	methylprednisolone and neomycin
Neoquess® Injection	dicyclomine hydrochloride
Neoquess® Tablet	hyoscyamine sulfate
Neo-Synalar® Topical	neomycin and fluocinolone
Neo-Synephrine® 12 Hour Nasal Solution	oxymetazoline hydrochloride
Neurontin® 600 mg & 800 mg	gabapentin
Neutra-Phos® Capsule	potassium phosphate and sodium phosphate
Niac®	niacin
Niacels®	niacin
Niclocide®	niclosamide
Nidryl®	diphenhydramine hydrochloride
Niferex Forte®	iron with vitamins
Niloric®	ergoloid mesylates
Nipride® Injection	nitroprusside sodium
Nisaval®	pyrilamine maleate
Nitro-Bid® Oral	nitroglycerin
Nitrocine® Oral	nitroglycerin
Nitrostat® 0.15 mg Tablet	nitroglycerin
Noctec®	chloral hydrate
Noludar®	methyprylon
Norlutate®	norethindrone
Norlutin®	norethindrone
Novafed®	pseudoephedrine
Novahistine DH® Liquid	chlorpheniramine, pseudoephedrine, and codeine
Novahistine DMX® Liquid	guaifenesin, pseudoephedrine, and dextromethorphan
Novahistine® Elixir	chlorpheniramine and phenylephrine
Novahistine® Expectorant	guaifenesin, pseudoephedrine, and codeine
Nursoy®	enteral nutritional therapy
Nydrazid® Injection	isoniazid
Obe-Nix® 30	phentermine (all products)
Obephen®	phentermine (all products)
Obermine®	phentermine (all products)

DRUG PRODUCTS NO LONGER AVAILABLE IN THE U.S. *(Continued)*

Brand Name	Generic Name
Obestin-30®	phentermine (all products)
Ophthaine®	proparacaine
Ophthocort®	chloramphenicol, polymyxin B, and hydrocortisone
Oradex-C®	dyclonine
Oratect®	benzocaine
Oreticyl®	deserpidine and hydrochlorothiazide
Organidin®	iodinated glycerol
Otic Tridesilon®	desonide and acetic acid
Oxsoralen® Oral	methoxsalen
Panwarfin®	warfarin sodium
Paplex®	salicylic acid
Paradione®	paramethadione
Para-Hist AT®	promethazine, phenylephrine, and codeine
Pargen Fortified®	chlorzoxazone
Par Glycerol®	iodinated glycerol
Parmine®	phentermine hydrochloride
Parsidol®	ethopropazine (all products)
Pavabid HP®	papaverine hydrochloride
Pavasule®	papaverine hydrochloride
Pavatym®	papaverine hydrochloride
Pavesed®	papaverine hydrochloride
PBZ® Elixir	tripelennamine
PBZ® Tablet	tripelennamine
PBZ-SR® Tablet	tripelennamine
Pentids®	penicillin G potassium, oral (all products)
Pfizerpen-AS®	penicillin G procaine
Phenaphen®	acetaminophen
Phenaphen®/Codeine #4	acetaminophen and codeine
Phenaseptic®	phenol
Phencen-50®	promethazine
Phenetron®	chlorpheniramine
Phentrol®	phentermine (all products)
Phenurone®	phenacemide
Phos-Ex® 62.5	calcium acetate
Phos-Ex® 125	calcium acetate
Phos-Ex® 167	calcium acetate
Phos-Ex® 250	calcium acetate
pHos-pHaid®	ammonium biphosphate, sodium biphosphate, and sodium acid pyrophosphate
Phosphaljel®	aluminum phosphate
Pindac®	pinacidil
Plasma-Plex®	plasma protein fraction
Polargen®	dexchlorpheniramine maleate
Poliovax® Injection	poliovirus vaccine, inactivated
Polycillin® Oral	ampicillin
Polycillin-N® Injection	ampicillin
Polycillin-PRB®	ampicillin and probenecid (all products)
Polyflex® Tablet	chlorzoxazone
Polygam® Injection	immune globulin, intravenous

Brand Name	Generic Name
Polymox®	amoxicillin
Pondimin®	fenfluramine
Posicor®	mibefradil (all products)
Predaject-50®	prednisolone
Predalone®	prednisolone
Predicort-50®	prednisolone
Preludin®	phenmetrazine hydrochloride
Premarin® Vaginal Cream	conjugated estrogens
Proampacin®	ampicillin and probenecid (all products)
Procan SR®	procainamide
Profilate-HP®	antihemophilic factor (human)
Projestaject® Injection	progesterone
Prokine® Injection	sargramostim
Prolamine®	phenylpropanolamine
Proloid®	thyroglobulin
Prometh®	promethazine
Proplex® SX-T Injection	factor IX complex (human)
Pro-Sof®	docusate sodium
Prostaphlin®	oxacillin
Protopam® Tablet	pralidoxime chloride
Provatene®	beta-carotene
Pyridium Plus®	phenazopyridine, hyoscyamine, and butabarbital
Questran® Tablet	cholestyramine resin
Quinamm®	quinine sulfate
Quiphile®	quinine sulfate
Q-vel®	quinine sulfate
Raxar®	grepafloxacin
Rectacort® suppository	hydrocortisone
Redux®	dexfenfluramine
Regutol®	docusate
Rep-Pred®	methylprednisolone
Rezulin®	troglitazone
R-Gen®	iodinated glycerol
Rhesonativ® Injection	Rh_o(D) immune globulin
Rhindecon®	phenylpropanolamine
Rhinolar®	chlorpheniramine, phenylpropanolamine, and methscopolamine
Rhuli® Cream	benzocaine, calamine, and camphor
Robicillin® Tablet	penicillin V potassium
Robitet®	tetracycline
Romycin® Solution	erythromycin, topical
Rondomycin® Capsule	methacycline hydrochloride (all products)
Rufen®	ibuprofen
Scabene®	lindane
Sclavo - PPD® Solution	tuberculin purified protein derivative
Sclavo Test-PPD®	tuberculin purified protein derivative
Sebulex®	sulfur and salicylic acid
Sebulon®	pyrithione zinc
Seconal™ Oral	secobarbital sodium
Seldane®	terfenadine
Seldane-D®	terfenadine and pseudoephedrine
Selecor®	celiprolol
Selestoject®	betamethasone

DRUG PRODUCTS NO LONGER AVAILABLE IN THE U.S. *(Continued)*

Brand Name	Generic Name
Senolax®	senna
Serax®	oxazepam
Serpasil®	reserpine
Siblin®	psyllium
Skelex®	chlorzoxazone
Slo-Salt®	salt substitute
Sodium P.A.S.®	aminosalicylate sodium
Sofarin®	warfarin sodium
Solatene®	beta-carotene
Spasmoject®	dicyclomine
Spectrobid® Oral Suspension	bacampicillin
Staphcillin®	methicillin (all products)
Statobex®	phendimetrazine tartrate
Sterapred®	prednisone
Streptomycin	streptomycin
Sucostrin®	succinylcholine chloride
Sudafed® Children	pseudoephedrine
Sudafed® Cough	guaifenesin, pseudoephedrine, and dextromethorphan
Sudafed® Plus Liquid	chlorpheniramine and pseudoephedrine
Superchar®	charcoal
Superchar® With Sorbitol	charcoal
Surital®	thiamylal sodium
Symmetrel® Capsule	amantadine hydrochloride
Synkayvite®	menadiol sodium
Syntocinon®	oxytocin
Tabron®	vitamins, multiple
Tacaryl®	methdilazine hydrochloride (all products)
Taractan®	chlorprothixene
T-Caine® Lozenge	benzocaine
Tegopen®	cloxacillin
Teline®	tetracycline
Temaril®	trimeprazine tartrate
Tepanil®	diethylpropion hydrochloride
Tepanil® TenTabs®	diethylpropion hydrochloride
Tes-Tape®	diagnostic aids (*in vitro*), urine
Tetralan®	tetracycline
Tetram®	tetracycline
Theelin® Aqueous Injection	estrone
Theobid® Jr Duracaps®	theophylline
Theo-Dur® Sprinkle®	theophylline
Theolair-SR® 250 mg Tablet	theophylline
Theo-Organidin®	iodinated glycerol and theophylline
Theramin® Expectorant	guaifenesin and phenylpropanolamine
Thiacide®	methenamine and potassium acid phosphate
Tiject-20®	trimethobenzamide
Tindal®	acetophenazine maleate
Torecan® Suppository	thiethylperazine
Totacillin-N®	ampicillin
Tral®	hexocyclium methylsulfate

Brand Name	Generic Name
Travase®	sutilains
Tridione® Suppository	trimethadione
Trimox® 500 mg	amoxicillin
Trofan®	L-tryptophan
Trofan DS®	L-tryptophan
Tryptacin®	L-tryptophan
Tucks® Cream	witch hazel
Tusal®	sodium thiosalicylate
Tussi-Organidin®	iodinated glycerol and codeine
Tussi-Organidin® DM	iodinated glycerol and dextromethorphan (all products)
Tusso-DM®	iodinated glycerol and dextromethorphan (all products)
Tuss-Ornade®	caramiphen and phenylpropanolamine
Ultralente® U	insulin zinc suspension, extended
Ultrase® MT24	pancrelipase
Unipen®	nafcillin
Unipres®	hydralazine, hydrochlorothiazide, and reserpine
Ureacin®-40 Topical	urea
Uri-Tet®	oxytetracycline
Urobiotic-25®	oxytetracycline and sulfamethizole
Uticort®	betamethasone (all products)
Valadol®	acetaminophen
Valergen® Injection	estradiol
Valmid® Capsule	ethinamate
Valpin® 50	anisotropine methylbromide
Valrelease®	diazepam
Vanex-LA®	guaifenesin and phenylpropanolamine
Vanseb-T® Shampoo	coal tar, sulfur, and salicylic acid
V-Cillin K®	penicillin V potassium
Velsar® Injection	vinblastine sulfate
Vercyte®	pipobroman
Verr-Canth®	cantharidin
Verrex®	podophyllin and salicylic acid
Verrusol®	salicylic acid, podophyllin, and cantharidin
V-Gan® Injection	promethazine hydrochloride
Vicks® Vatronol®	ephedrine
Vioform®-Hydrocortisone Topical	clioquinol and hydrocortisone
Visine®	tetrahydrozoline hydrochloride
Vistaject-25®	hydroxyzine
Vistaject-50®	hydroxyzine
Vontrol®	diphenidol
Wehamine® Injection	dimenhydrinate
Wehdryl®	diphenhydramine
Wesprin® Buffered	aspirin
Wyamycin S®	erythromycin
Zebrax®	clidinium and chlordiazepoxide
Zetran®	diazepam
Zolyse®	chymotrypsin alpha (all products)
Zyban® 100 mg	bupropion

PHARMACEUTICAL MANUFACTURERS DIRECTORY

Abbott Laboratories
(Abbott Diagnostic Division)
One Abbott Park Road
Abbott Park, IL 60064-3500
www.abbott.com

Abbott Laboratories
(Hospital Products Division)
200 Abbott Park Road
Abbott Park, IL 60064-3537

Abbott Laboratories
(Pharmaceutical Product Division)
100 Abbott Park Road
Abbott Park, IL 60064-3500
(800) 633-9110
www.abbott.com

Able Laboratories
6 Hollywood Court
South Plainfield, NJ 07080

Adams (see Medeva)

Adria (see Pharmacia)

Agouron Pharmaceuticals, Inc
10350 North Torrey Pines Road
La Jolla, CA 92037-1020
(800) 585-6050
www.agouron.com

Akorn, Inc
2500 Millbrook Drive
Buffalo Grove, IL 60089
www.akorn.com

Alcon Laboratories, Inc
6201 South Freeway
Ft Worth, TX 76134
(800) 862-5266
www.alconlabs.com

Allerderm Laboratories
PO Box 2070
Petaluma, CA 94953-2070

Allergan Herbert (see Allergan)

Allergan, Inc
2525 DuPont Drive
Irvine, CA 92612
(800) 347-4500
www.allergan.com

Alpha Therapeutic Corp
5555 Valley Boulevard
Los Angeles, CA 90032

Alpharma
(U.S. Pharmaceuticals Division)
7205 Windsor Boulevard
Baltimore, MD 21244

Alra Labs, Inc
3850 Clearview Court
Gurnee, IL 60031

Alto Pharmaceuticals, Inc
PO Box 1910
Land O'Lakes, FL 34639-1910
altopharm@aol.com

Alza Corp
950 Page Mill Road
PO Box 10950
Palo Alto, CA 94303-0802
(800) 634-8977
www.alza.com

Ambix Labs, Inc
210 Orchard Street
East Rutherford, NJ 07073

American Drug Industries, Inc
5810 South Perry Avenue
Chicago, IL 60621

American Pharmaceutical, Co
12 Dwight Place
Fairfield, NJ 07004-3434

American Regent Laboratories Inc
1 Luitpold Drive
Shirley, NY 11967

Ames (see Miles Biological Products)

Amgen, Inc
One Amgen Center Drive
Thousand Oaks, CA 91320-1789
(800) 772-6436
www.amgen.com

Amide Pharmaceuticals, Inc
101 East Main Street
Little Falls, NJ 07424

Anaquest (see Ohmeda)

ANDRX Pharmaceuticals, Inc
4001 South West 47th Avenue
Fort Lauderdale, FL 33314

Angelini Pharmaceuticals, Inc
70 Grand Avenue
River Edge, NJ 07661
dapp@nac.net

Apotex Corp
50 Lakeview Parkway
Suite 127
Vernon Hills, IL 60061

Apothecary Products, Inc
11531 Rupp Drive
Burnsville, MN 55337-1295
pillminder@aol.com

Apothecon Products
(A Bristol-Myers Squibb Company)
PO Box 4500
Princeton, NJ 08543-4500
www.apothecon.com

Applied Genetics Inc
205 Buffalo Avenue
Freeport, NY 11520
www.agiderm.com

Arcola Laboratories
500 Arcola Road
Collegeville, PA 19426-0107
www.rpr.rpna.com

AstraZeneca (see Zeneca)

Baker Norton Pharmaceuticals, Inc
4400 Biscayne Boulevard
Miami, FL 33137

Banner Pharmacaps, Inc
4125 Premier Drive
PO Box 2210
High Point, NC 27261-2210

Barr Laboratories, Inc
Box 2900
Pomona, NY 10970-0519
www.barrlabs.com

Bausch & Lomb Pharmaceuticals
8500 Hidden River Parkway
Tampa, FL 33637
(800) 323-0000
www.bausch.com

Bausch & Lomb Surgical
555 West Arrow Highway
Claremont, CA 91711
www.blsurgical.com

Baxter Healthcare Corporation
One Baxter Parkway DF4-1W
Deerfield, IL 60015
www.baxter.com

Baxter Healthcare Corporation
(I.V. Systems Division)
One Baxter Parkway
Deerfield, IL 60015
www.baxter.com

Baxter Pharmaceutical Products, Inc
95 Spring Street
New Providence, NJ 07974
(800) 262-3784

Bayer Corporation
N 3525 Regal Street
Box 3145
Spokane, WA 99220

Bayer Corporation
(Diagnostic Division)
430 South Beiger Street
PO Box 2004
Mishawaka, IN 46544-2004
www.bayerdiag.com

Bayer Corporation
(Biological and Pharmaceutical Division)
400 Morgan Lane
West Haven, CT 06516-4175
(800) 288-8371
www.bayer.com

Bayer, Inc
77 Belfield Road
Toronto, Ontario, Canada M9W 1G6
www.bayerdiag.com

Becton Dickinson and Company
One Becton Drive
Franklin Lakes, NJ 07417-1881
(888) 237-2762
www.bd.com

Becton Dickinson Microbiology Systems
(Division of Becton Dickinson and Company)
PO Box 999
7 Loveton Circle
Sparks, MD 21152
www.ms.bd.com

Bedford Laboratories
(Division of Ben Venue Laboratories)
300 Northfield Road
PO Box 46568
Bedford, OH 44146
www.boehringer-ingelheim.com

Beecham (see SmithKline Beecham)

Beiersdorf
PO Box 5529
Norwalk, CT 06856-5529

Beiersdorf Inc
187 Danbury Road
Wilton, CT 06897

Berlex Laboratories, Inc
300 Fairfield Road
Wayne, NJ 07470
(888) 237-5394
www.berlex.com

Berna Products, Corp
4216 Ponce de Leon Boulevard
Coral Gables, FL 33146
www.bernaproducts.com

Bertek Pharmaceuticals, Inc
PO Box 2006
Sugar Land, TX 77478
(800) 231-3052
www.dowhickam.com

Beta Dermaceuticals, Inc
PO Box 691106
San Antonio, TX 78216-1106

Beutlich Pharmaceuticals
1541 Shields Drive
Waukegan, IL 60085-8304
www.beutlich.com

PHARMACEUTICAL MANUFACTURERS DIRECTORY
(Continued)

Biocraft (see Teva USA)

Biogen
14 Cambridge Center
Cambridge, MA 02142
(800) 262-4363
www.biogen.com

Biopharmaceutics, Inc
990 Station Road
Bellport, NY 11713
www.feminique.com

Bio-Technology General Corp
70 Wood Avenue South
Iselin, NJ 08830

Blaine Company, Inc
1515 Production Drive
Burlington, KY 41005
www.blainepharma.com

Block Drug Co, Inc
257 Cornelison Avenue
Jersey City, NJ 07302
(800) 365-6500
www.blockdrug.com

Bock (see Sanofi Winthrop)

Boehringer Ingelheim, Inc
900 Ridgebury Road
Ridgefield, CT 06877-0368
(800) 542-6257
www.boehringer-ingelheim.com

Boots (see Knoll)

Braintree Laboratories, Inc
PO Box 850929
Braintree, MA 02185-0929

Brightstone Pharma
109 MacKenan Drive
Cary, NC 27511
www.brightstonepharma.com

Bristol-Myers Squibb (Oncology/Immunology Division)
PO Box 4500
Princeton, NJ 08543-4500
www.bms.com

Bristol-Myers Squibb (OTC Products)
225 High Ridge Road
Stanford, CT 06905
www.bms.com

Bristol-Myers Squibb Company (Pharmaceutical Division)
PO Box 4500
Princeton, NJ 08543-4500
(800) 321-1335
www.bms.com

BTG (see Bio-Technology General Corp)

Burroughs Wellcome
(see GlaxoWellcome)

C&M Pharmacal, Inc
1721 Maple Lane Avenue
Hazel Park, MI 48030-2696
www.glytone.com

Caraco Pharmaceutical Laboratories Ltd
1150 Elijah McCoy Drive
Detroit, MI 48202
www.caraco.com

Celgene Corporation
7 Powder Horn Drive
Warren, NJ 07059
(800) 890-4619

Centeon
1020 First Avenue
King of Prussia, PA 19406-1310
www.centeon.com/na

Center Labs
35 Channel Drive
Port Washington, NY 11050
www.centerpharm.com

Centers for Disease Control
1600 Clifton Road
Mail Stop D-09
Atlanta, GA 30333
(404) 639-3670
www.cdc.gov

Centocor, Inc
200 Great Valley Parkway
Malvern, PA 19355
(888) 874-3083
www.centocor.com

Century Pharmaceuticals, Inc
10377 Hague Road
Indianapolis, IN 46256

Chemrich Laboratories
5211 Telegraph Road
Los Angeles, CA 90022

Cheshire Drugs
6225 Shiloh Road, Suite D
Alpharetta, GA 30005
www.cpsrx.com

Chiron Therapeutics
4560 Horton Street
Emeryville, CA 94608
(800) 244-7668

Ciba-Geigy Pharmaceuticals (see Novartis)

Circa Pharmaceuticals, Inc
33 Ralph Avenue
PO Box 30
Copiague, NY 11726-0030
www.circapharm.com

Clay-Park Labs, Inc
Bathgate Industrial Park
1700 Bathgate Avenue
Bronx, NY 10457

Coast Labs, Inc
521 West 17th Street
Long Beach, CA 90813-1513

Copley Labs, Inc
25 John Road
Canton, MA 02021

COR Therapeutics
256 East Grand Avenue
South San Francisco, CA 94080
(888) 267-4633

Danbury Pharmacal, Inc
131 West Street
Danbury, CT 06810

Del-Ray Laboratories, Inc
22-20th Avenue North West
Birmingham, AL 35215

Denison Pharmaceuticals, Inc
60 Dunnell Lane
PO Box 1305
Pawtucket, RI 02862

Dermik Labs, Inc
500 Arcola Road
PO Box 1200
Collegeville, PA 19426-0107
www.rpr.rpna.com

Daiichi Pharmaceutical Corp
11 Philips Parkway
Montvale, NJ 07645
(877) 324-4244

Déy Laboratories
2751 Napa Valley Corporate Drive
Napa, CA 94558
www.deyinc.com

DuPont Merck Pharmaceutical
PO Box 80705
Wilmington, DE 19807
(800) 474-2762
www.dupontpharma.com

Dura Pharmaceuticals
7475 Lusk Boulevard
San Diego, CA 92121-4202
(800) 859-8585
www.durapharm.com

Duramed Pharmaceuticals
5040 Duramed Drive
Cincinnati, OH 45213
(800) 543-8338
www.duramed.com

DUSA Pharmaceuticals, Inc
Wilmington, MA 01887

Elan Pharmaceuticals
800 Gateway Boulevard
San Francisco, CA 94080
(888) 638-7605

Emrex/Economed Pharmaceuticals, Inc
4305 Sartin Road
PO Box 3303
Burlington, NC 27217

Endo Generic Products
223 Wilmington West Chester Pike
Chadds Ford, PA 19317
www.endo.com

Eon Labs Manufacturing, Inc
227-15 North Conduit Avenue
Laurelton, NY 11413

ESI Lederle
PO Box 41502
Philadelphia, PA 19101
www.AHP.com

Ethex Corp
10888 Metro Court
St Louis, MO 63043-2413
www.ethex.com

Falcon Opthalmics, Inc
6201 South Freeway
Fort Worth, TX 76134
Parent Company: Alcon Laboratories
www.alconlabs.com

Faulding/Purepac Pharmaceutical Co
200 Elmora Avenue
Elizabeth, NJ 07207
www.faulding.com.au

Ferndale Laboratories, Inc
780 West Eight Mile Road
Ferndale, MI 48220

Fisons (see Medeva)

Fisons (see Rhone-Poulenc Rorer)

C.B. Fleet Co, Inc
4615 Murray Place
P0 Box 11349
Lynchburg, VA 24506-1349

Forest/Inwood Laboratories, Inc
500 Commack Road
Commack, NY 11725-5000

Forest Pharmaceuticals, Inc
13600 Shoreline Drive
St Louis, MO 63045
(800) 678-1605
www.tiazac.com

Fougera
(Division of Altana Inc)
60 Baylis Road
Melville, NY 11747
www.fougera.com

Fujisawa Healthcare, Inc
Parkway Center North
Three Parkway North
Deerfield, IL 60015-2548
(800) 888-7704
www.fujisawa.com

PHARMACEUTICAL MANUFACTURERS DIRECTORY
(Continued)

Galderma Laboratories, Inc
PO Box 331329
Fort Worth, TX 76163
(800) 582-8225
www.galderma.com

Gebauer Company
9410 St Catherine Avenue
Cleveland, OH 44104
www.gebauerco.com

Geigy Pharmaceuticals (see Novartis)

GenDerm Corporation
600 Knightsbridge Parkway
Lincolnshire, IL 60069
www.genderm.com

Genentech, Inc
1 DNA Way
South San Francisco, CA 94080
(800) 225-1000
www.gene.com

Genetco, Inc
711 Union Parkway
Ronkonkoma, NY 11779

Genetics Institute
35 Cambridge Park Drive
Cambridge, MA 02140
(617) 503-7332

Geneva Pharmaceuticals, Inc
2655 West Midway Boulevard
PO Box 446
Broomfield, CO 80038-0446
www.genevarx.com

Gensia Automedics, Inc
9360 Town Center Drive
San Diego, CA 92121
www.gensia.com

GensiaSicor Pharmaceuticals, Inc
19 Hughes
Irvine, CA 92618-1902
www.gensiasicor.com

Genzyme Corp
One Kendall Square
Building 1400
Cambridge, MA 02139
(800) 326-7002
www.genzyme.com

Genzyme Genetics
5 Mountain Road
Framingham, MA 01701

Genzyme Tissue Repair
64 Sidney Street
Cambridge, MA 02139

Genzyme Transgenics
5 Mountain Road
Framingham, MA 01701

Gilead Sciences, Inc
333 Lakeside Drive
Foster City, CA 94404
(800) 445-3235
www.gilead.com

Glades Pharmaceuticals, Inc
500 Satellite Boulevard
Suwanee, GA 30024
www.glades.com

GlaxoWellcome
Five Moore Drive
Research Triangle Park, NC 27709
(888) 825-5249
www.glaxowellcome.com

Glenwood, LLC
83 North Summit Street
Tenafly, NJ 07670
www.glenwood-llc.com

Glenwood-Palisades
One New England Avenue
Piscataway, NJ 08855

Global Pharmaceutical Corp
Castor & Kensington Avenues
Philadelphia, PA 19124
www.globalphar.com

Gray Pharmaceutical Company
100 Connecticut Avenue
Norwalk, CT 06856

Great Southern Laboratories
10863 Rockley Road
Houston, TX 77099

Guardian Drug Co
72 Prince Street
Trenton, NJ 08638

G&W Laboratories, Inc
111 Coolidge Street
South Plainfield, NJ 07080-3895

Gynex (see BTG)

Halsey Drug Company, Inc
695 North Perryville Road
Rockford, IL 61107
www.halseydrug.com

The Harvard Drug Group
31778 Enterprise Drive
Lovonia, MI 48150

Healthpoint
2600 Airport Freeway
Forth Worth, TX 76111
www.healthpoint.com

Heartland Healthcare Services
4755 South Avenue
Toledo, OH 43615

H&H Laboratories
4701 25 Mile Road
Shelby Township, MI 48316

Hi-Tech Pharmacal Co, Inc
369 Bayview Avenue
Amityville, NY 11701
www.diabeticproducts.com

Hoechst-Marion Roussel
10236 Marion Park Drive
PO Box 9627
Kansas City, MO 64134-0627
(800) 362-7466
www.hmri.com

Hoechst-Roussel
(see Hoechst Marion Roussel)

ICI Pharma (see Zeneca)

ICN Pharmaceuticals, Inc
3300 Hyland Avenue
Costa Mesa, CA 92626
(800) 556-1937
www.icnpharm.com

Immunex Corp
51 University Street
Seattle, WA 98101
(800) 466-8639
www.immunex.com

ImmunoGen, Inc
148 Sidney Street
Cambridge, MA 02139

Immuno-U.S., Inc
1200 Parkdale Road
Rochester, MI 48307-1744

International Ethical Labs
Avenue America Miranda #1021
Reparto Metropolitano
Rio Piedras, Puerto Rico 00921

International Medication Systems, Ltd (IMS)
1886 Santa Anita Avenue
S El Monte, CA 91733

Interpharm, Inc
3 Fairchild Avenue
Plainview, NY 11803

Invamed, Inc
2400 Route 130 North
Dayton, NJ 08810

Ion Laboratories
7431 Pebble Drive
Fort Worth, TX 76118-6416

Janssen Pharmaceutical, Inc
P0 Box 200
Titusville, NJ 08560-0200
(800) 526-7736
www.us.janssen.com

Jerome Stevens Pharmaceuticals, Inc
60 Da Vinci Drive
Bohemia, NY 11716

Johnson & Johnson
Grandview Road
Skillman, NJ 08558-9418
(800) 635-6789
www.jnj.com

Jones Pharma
1945 Craig Road
PO Box 46903
St Louis, MO 63146
www.jmedpharma.com

Kabi (see Pharmacia)

Kenwood Laboratories
383 Route 46 West
Fairfield, NJ 07004-2402
www.bradpharm.com

Key Pharmaceutical
2000 Galloping Hill Road
Kenilworth, NJ 07033

King Pharmaceuticals, Inc
501 Fifth Street
Bristol, TN 37620
www.kingpharm.com

Knoll Pharmaceutical Company
3000 Continental Drive North
Mt Olive, NJ 07828-1234
(800) 526-0221
www.basf.com

Konsyl Pharmaceuticals, Inc
4200 South Hulen
Fort Worth, TX 76109
www.konsyl.com

Kremers Urban
PO Box 427
Mequon, WI 53092

Lannett Co, Inc
9000 State Road
Philadelphia, PA 19136-1615
www.lannett.com

Lederle Laboratories
401 North Middletown Road
Pearl River, NY 10965-1299
(800) 395-9938

Lemmon (see Teva USA)

Ligand Pharmaceuticals, Inc
10275 Science Center Drive
San Diego, CA 92121
(619) 550-7506
www.ligand.com

Eli Lilly and Company
Lilly Corporate Center
Indianapolis, IN 46285
(800) 545-5979
www.lilly.com

Liposome Company
One Research Way
Princeton, NJ 08540
(609) 452-7060
www.liposome.com

PHARMACEUTICAL MANUFACTURERS DIRECTORY
(Continued)

Liquipharm, Inc
PO Box D-3700
Pomona, NY 10970
www.liquipharm.com

L. Perrigo Company
515 Eastern Avenue
Allegan, MI 49010
www.perrigo.com

Lyphomed (see Fujisawa)

3M Pharmaceuticals
3M Center Building, 275-3W-01
St Paul, MN 55144-1000
(800) 328-0255
www.mmm.com

Mallinckrodt
675 McDonnell Boulevard
P0 Box 5840
St Louis, MO 63134
www.mkg.com
www.mallinckrodt.com

Marion Merrell Dow
(see Hoechst Marion Roussel)

Marlop Pharmaceuticals, Inc
5704 Mosholu Avenue
Bronx, NY 10471-0536

Marsam Pharmaceuticals Inc (Subsidiary of Schein Pharmaceutical, Inc)
P0 Box 1022
24 Olney Avenue, Bldg 31
Cherry Hill, NJ 08003
www.schein-rx.com

Martec Pharmaceutical, Inc
1800 North Topping Avenue
PO Box 33510
Kansas City, MO 64120-3510
Parent Company: Ratiopharm, GmbH
www.martec-kc.com

Mason Pharmaceuticals, Inc
4425 Jamboree Road
Suite 250
Newport Beach, CA 92660

McGaw, Inc
P0 Box 19791
Irvine, CA 92713-9791

McNeil Consumer Products Co
Camp Hill Road
Mail Stop 278
Ft Washington, PA 19034-2292
(215) 273-7000

McNeil Pharmaceutical
Route 202, PO Box 300
Raritan, NJ 08869-0602
www.ortho-mcneil.com

Mead Johnson (see Bristol-Myers Squibb)

Med-Derm Pharmaceuticals
PO Box 5193
Kingsport, TN 37663

Medeva Pharmaceuticals, Inc
PO Box 1710
755 Jefferson Road
Rochester, NY 14603-1710
www.medeva.com

Medimmune, Inc
35 West Watkins Mill Road
Gaithersburg, MD 20878
(800) 934-7426
www.medimmune.com

Medirex, Inc
20 Chapin Road
PO Box 731
Pine Brook, NJ 07058
Parent Company: Sidmak Laboratories

Merck & Co
P0 Box 4
West Point, PA 19486
(800) 672-6372
www.merck.com

Meridian Medical Technologies, Inc
10240 Old Columbia Road
Columbia, MD 21046
info@meridianmt.com
www.meridianmeds.com

Merrell Dow
(see Hoechst Marion Roussel)

Merz Pharmaceuticals, Inc
4215 Tudor Lane
Greensboro, NC 27410

MGI Pharma, Inc
9900 Bren Road East
Suite 300E, Opus Center
Minnetonka, MN 55343-9667

Mikart, Inc
1750 Chattahoochee Avenue
Atlanta, GA 30318
www.mikart.com

Miles (see Bayer)

Miles Allergy (see Bayer)

Monarch (see King Pharm)

Monarch Pharmaceuticals
355 Beecham Street
Bristol, TN 37620
(800) 776-3637
www.monarchpharm.com

Moore Medical
389 John Downey Drive
New Britain, CT 06050
www.mooremedical.com

Morton Grove Pharmaceuticals, Inc
6451 West Main Street
Morton Grove, IL 60053
www.mgp-online.com

Mova Pharmaceutical Corp
214 Carnegie Center
Suite 106
Princeton, NJ 08540

Muro Pharmaceuticals, Inc
890 East Street
Tewksbury, MA 01876

Mutual Pharmaceutical Co, Inc/ United Research Laboratories
1100 Orthodox Street
Philadelphia, PA 19124
www.mutual.com

Mylan Pharmaceuticals, Inc
781 Chestnut Ridge Road
P0 Box 4310
Morgantown, WV 26504-4310
www.mylan.com

Nabi
5800 Park of Commerce Boulevard NW
Boca Raton FL 33487
(800) 642-8874
www.nabi.com

Nephron Pharmaceuticals Corporation
4121 - 34th Street SW
Orlando, FL 32811-6458
www.hephronpharm.com
rwilburn@pharmacy.com

Nestle Clinical Nutrition
3 Parkway North, Suite 500
P0 Box 760
Deerfield, IL 60015

Neurex Corporation (see Elan)

Norwich Eaton (see Proctor & Gamble)

Novartis
59 Route 10
East Hanover, NJ 07936
(888) 344-8585
www.us.novartis.com

Novo Nordisk Pharmaceuticals, Inc
100 Overlook Center
Suite 200
Princeton, NJ 08540
(800) 727-6500
www.novo-nordisk.com

Novopharm USA, Inc
165 East Commerce Drive
Schaumburg, IL 60173-5326
(800) 426-0769
www.novopharmusa.com

Ohm Laboratories, Inc
PO Box 7397
North Brunswick, NJ 08902
Parent Company: Ranbaxy Pharmaceuticals
www.ranbaxy.com

Ohmeda
(see Baxter Pharmaceutical Products)

OMJ Pharmaceuticals, Inc
PO Box 367
San German, Puerto Rico 00683

Organon, Inc
375 Mt Pleasant Avenue
West Orange, NJ 07052
(800) 241-8812

Ortho Biotech, Inc
Route 202 South
P0 Box 670
Raritan, NJ 08869-0670
(800) 325-7504
www.procrit.com

Ortho-McNeil Pharmaceutical
Route 202
PO Box 600
Raritan, NJ 08869-0600
(800) 682-6532
www.ortho-mcneil.com

Otsuka America Pharmaceutical
2440 Research Boulevard
Suite 250
Rockville, MD 20850
(800) 562-3974
www.otsuka.com

Paddock Laboratories
P0 Box 27286
3940 Quebec Avenue North
Minneapolis, MN 55427
www.paddocklabs.com

PAR Pharmaceutical, Inc
One Ram Ridge Road
Spring Valley, NY 10977
Parent Company: Pharmaceutical Resources, Inc
www.parpharm.com

Parkedale Pharmaceuticals, Inc (Subsidiary of King Pharmaceuticals, Inc)
501 Fifth Street
Bristol, TN 37620
www.kingpharm.com

Parke-Davis (Division of Warner-Lambert Company)
201 Tabor Road
Morris Plains, NJ 07950
(800) 223-0432
www.parke-davis.com

PHARMACEUTICAL MANUFACTURERS DIRECTORY
(Continued)

Parmed Pharmaceuticals, Inc
4220 Hyde Park Boulevard
Niagra Falls, NY 14305-6714
Parent Company: Alpharma

Parnell Pharmaceuticals, Inc
1525 Francisco Boulevard
San Rafael, CA 94901
www.parnellpharm.com

Pasteur Merieux Connaught
Discovery Drive
Swiftwater, PA 18370-0187
www.us.pmc-vacc.com

PD-RX Pharmaceuticals
72 North Ann Arbor
Oklahoma City, OK 73127
www.pdrx.com

Pecos Pharmaceutical
25301 Cabot Road
Suites 212-213
Laguna Hills, CA 92653

Pedinol Pharmacal Inc
30 Banfi Plaza North
Farmingdale, NY 11735
www.pedinol.com

Person & Covey
616 Allen Avenue
Glendale, CA 91201

Pfizer U.S. Pharmaceutical Group
235 East 42nd Street
New York, NY 10017-5755
(800) 438-1985
www.pfizer.com

Pharma Tek, Inc
PO Box 1920
Huntington, NY 11743
www.pharma-tek.com

Pharmaceutical Formulations, Inc
460 Plainfield Avenue
Edison, NJ 08818

Pharmaceutical Laboratories
1170 West Corporate Drive
Suite 102
Arlington, TX 76006

Pharmaceutical Specialties, Inc
P0 Box 6298
2112 15th Street NW
Rochester, MN 55901
www.psico.com

Pharmacia & Upjohn Company (Ophthalmics Division)
701 East Milham Road
Kalamazoo, MI 49001
pnu.com

Pharmacia & Upjohn
7000 Portage Road
Kalamazoo, MI 49001
(800) 253-8600
www.pnu.com

Pharmacy Division of Bayer
400 Morgan Lane
Westhaven, Conneticut 06516-4175
www.bayer.com

Pharmakon Labs, Inc
6050 Jet Port Industrial Boulevard
Tampa, FL 33634

Pharmics, Inc
PO Box 27554
Salt Lake City, UT 84127
www.pharmics.com

Physician's Total Care
5415 South 125th East Avenue
Suite 205
Tulsa, OK 74146

Plantex USA, Inc
482 Hudson Terrace
Englewood Cliffs, NJ 07632

Pratt Pharmaceuticals Division
Pfizer Inc
U.S. Pharmaceuticals Group
235 East 42nd Street
New York, NY 10017-5755

Procter & Gamble Pharmaceuticals
P0 Box 231
Norwich, NY 13815-0231

Procter & Gamble Co
1 Procter & Gamble Plaza
Cincinnati, OH 45202
(800) 543-7270
www.pg.com

Purdue Frederick Co
100 Connecticut Avenue
Norwalk, CT 06850-3590
(203) 853-0123
www.pharma.com

PUREPAC Pharmaceutical Co
200 Elmora Avenue
Elizabeth, NJ 07207
Parent Company: F.H. Faulding and Company
www.Faulding.com

Qualitest Pharmaceuticals, Inc
1236 Jordan Road
Huntsville, AL 35811

Quality Research Pharmaceuticals, Inc
1117 Third Avenue South West
Carmel, IN 46032

Ranbaxy Pharmaceuticals, Inc
600 College Road East
Princeton, NJ 08540

Reckitt & Colman
1909 Huguenot Road
Suite 300
Richmond, VA 23235
(800) 444-7599
www.reckitt.com

Reed & Carnrick (see Schwarz Pharma)

Rhone-Poulenc Rorer Pharmaceuticals, Inc
500 Arcola Road
PO Box 1200
Collegeville, PA 19426
(800) 340-7502
www.rp-rorer.com

Richwood Pharmaceutical Company, Inc
7900 Tanners Gate Drive
Suite 200
Florence, KY 41042

R.I.D. Inc
609 North Mednik Avenue
Los Angeles, CA 90022

Roberts Pharmaceuticals
4 Industrial Way West
Eatontown, NJ 07724
(800) 828-2088
www.robertspharm.com

Robins (see Wyeth-Ayerst)

Roche Laboratories
340 Kingsland Street
Nutley, NJ 07110-1199
(800) 526-6367
www.rocheUSA.com

Roerig Division
Pfizer Inc
U.S. Pharmaceuticals Group
235 East 42nd Street
New York, NY 10017-5755

Rorer (see Rhone-Poulenc Rorer)

Rosemont Pharmaceutical Corp
301 South Cherokee Street
Denver, CO 80223
Parent Company: Akzo Nobel

Ross Laboratories
6480 Busch Boulevard
Columbus, OH 43229
(800) 624-7677

Roxane Laboratories, Inc
PO Box 16532
Columbus, OH 43216-6532
(800) 848-0120
www.roxane.com

Rugby Laboratories, Inc
2725 Northwoods Parkway
Norcross, GA 30071
Parent Company: Watson Laboratories

Sandoz Pharmaceuticals Corp
59 Route 10
East Hanover, NJ 07936
www.sandoz.com

Sanofi Winthrop Pharmaceuticals
90 Park Avenue
New York, NY 10016
(800) 223-1062

Savage Laboratories
(Division of Altana Inc)
60 Baylis Road
Melville, NY 11747
www.savagelabs.com

Scandipharm, Inc
22 Inverness Center Parkway
Suite 310
Birmingham, AL 35242
www.scandipharm.com

Schaffer Laboratories
1058 North Allen Avenue
Pasadina, CA 91104

Schein Pharmaceutical, Inc
100 Campus Drive
Florham Park, NJ 07932
www.schein-rx.com

Schering-Plough Corp
2000 Galloping Hill Road
Kenilworth, NJ 07033-0530
(800) 526-4099

Schwarz Pharma
6140 West Executive Dr
Mequon, WI 53092
(800) 558-5114
www.schwarzusa.com

Searle
5200 Old Orchard Road
Skokie, IL 60077
(847) 982-7000
www.searlehealthnet.com

Seneca Pharmaceutical, Inc
PO Box 25021
8621 Barefoot Industrial Road
Raleigh, NC 27613

Sequus Pharmaceuticals, Inc
980 Hamilton Court
Mento Park, CA 94025
www.sequus.com

Serono Laboratories, Inc
100 Longwater Circle
Norwell, MA 02061
www.seronousa.com

PHARMACEUTICAL MANUFACTURERS DIRECTORY
(Continued)

Sheffield Laboratories
170 Broad Street
New London, CT 06320
www.sheffield-labs.com

Shire Richwood, Inc
7900 Tanners Gate Drive
Suite 200
Florence, KY 41042
www.shiregroup.com

Sidmak Laboratories, Inc
17 West Street
PO Box 371
East Hanover, NJ 07936-0371
www.sidmaklab.com

Sigma-Tau Pharmaceuticals, Inc
800 South Frederick Avenue
Suite 300
Gaithersburg, MD 20877
(800) 447-0169
www.sigma-tau.it

SmithKline Beecham Pharmaceuticals
One Franklin Plaza
P0 Box 7929
Philadelphia, PA 19101
(800) 366-8900
www.sb.com

SmithKline Beecham Consumer Healthcare
P0 Box 1467
Pittsburgh, PA 15230
www.sb.com

Sola/Barnes (see Pilkington Barnes Hind)

SoloPak Pharmaceuticals Inc
6001 Broken Sound Parkway
Suite 600
Boca Raton, FL 33487

Solvay Pharmaceuticals
901 Sawyer Road
Marietta, GA 30062-2224
(800) 354-0026
www.solvay.com

Somerset Pharmaceuticals, Inc
P0 Box 30706
Tampa, FL 33630-3706

Southward Pharmaceuticals, Inc
33 Hammond Street
Suite 201
Irvine, CA 92718

Squibb (see Bristol-Myers Squibb)

Steris Laboratories, Inc
620 North 51st Avenue
Phoenix, AZ 85043-4705
Parent Company: Schein Pharmaceutical
www.schein-rx.com

Sterling (see Sanofi Winthrop)

Stratus Pharmaceuticals
14377 South West 142nd Street
Miami, FL 33186
www.stratuspharmaceuticals.com

Stuart (see Zeneca)

Superior Pharmaceutical Co
1385 Kemper Meadow Drive
Cincinnati, OH 45240-1635
www.superiorpharm.com

Survival (see Meridian Medical)

Syncor Pharmaceuticals, Inc
1313 Washington Avenue
Golden, CO 80401

Syntex (see Roche)

Takeda Pharmaceuticals America, Inc
475 Half Day Road
Suite 500
Lincolnshire, IL 60069
(877) 825-3327

Tap Pharmaceuticals
2355 Waukegan Road
Deerfield, IL 60015
(800) 348-2779
www.tapholdings.com

Taro Pharmaceuticals USA, Inc
5 Skyline Drive
Hawthorne, NY 10532
www.taropharma.com

Taylor Pharmaceuticals
1222 West Grand
Decatur, IL 62526

Teva Pharmaceuticals USA
151 Domorah Drive
Montgomeryville, PA 18936
www.tevapharmusa.com

Teva Pharmaceuticals USA
650 Cathill Road
Sellersville, PA 18960
www.tevapharmusa.com

Thames Pharmacal Co
2100 Fifth Avenue
Ronkonkoma, NY 11779

Triton (see Berlex)

UCB Pharmaceuticals, Inc
1950 Lake Park Drive
Atlanta, GA 30080
(800) 477-7877
www.ucb.be

UDL Laboratories, Inc
P0 Box 2629
Loves Park, IL 61132-2629

Unimed
2150 East Lake Cook Rd
Buffalo Grove, IL 60089
(800) 541-3492
www.unimed.com

Upjohn (see Pharmacia & Upjohn)

Upsher-Smith Laboratories, Inc
14905 23rd Avenue North
Minneapolis, MN 55447
www.upsher-smith.com

U.S. Bioscience
One Tower Bridge
100 Front Street Suite 400
West Conshohocken, PA 19428
(800) 447-3969
www.usbio.com

U.S. Pharmaceutical Corp
2401 Mellon Court
Suite C
Decatur, GA 30035

Value in Pharmaceuticals (VIP)
3000 Alt Boulevard
Grand Island, NY 14702
www.vippharm.com

Wallace Laboratories (Division of Carter-Wallace, Inc)
Half Acre Road
Cranbury, NJ 08512
(609) 655-6000
www.astelin.com

Warner Chilcott Laboratories
100 Enterprise Drive
Suite 280
Rockaway, NJ 07866
(800) 521-8813
www.wclabs.com

Warner Lambert Co
201 Tabor Road
Morris Plains, NJ 07950
(800) 223-0182
www.warner-lambert.com

Warrick Pharmaceuticals
1095 Morris Avenue
Union, NJ 07083-7137

Watson Laboratories, Inc
311 Bonnie Circle
Corona, CA 91720
www.watsonpharm.com

West-Ward
465 Industrial Way West
Eatontown, NJ 07724
Parent Company: Hikma Pharmaceuticals

Westwood-Squibb Pharmaceuticals
100 Forest Avenue
Buffalo, NY 14213
(800) 333-0950
www.westwood-squibb.com

Whitby (see UCB Pharma)

Winthrop (see Sanofi Winthrop)

Wyeth-Ayerst Laboratories
P0 Box 8299
Philadelphia, PA 19101
(800) 934-5556
www.ahp.com/wyeth

Zeneca Pharmaceuticals
1800 Concord Pike
Wilmington, DE 19897
(302) 886-8000
www.zeneca.com

Zenith Goldline Pharmaceuticals
4400 Biscayne Boulevard
Miami, FL 33137
(800) 327-4114
www.zenithgoldline.com

Zila Pharmaceuticals, Inc
5227 North 7th Street
Phoenix, AZ 85014-2817
www.zila.com

ABBREVIATIONS, ACRONYMS, AND SYMBOLS

Abbreviation	Meaning
$\overline{aa}$, aa	of each
AA	Alcoholics Anonymous
ac	before meals or food
ad	to, up to
a.d.	right ear
ADHD	attention-deficit/hyperactivity disorder
ADLs	activities of daily living
ad lib	at pleasure
AIMS	Abnormal Involuntary Movement Scale
a.l.	left ear
AM	morning
amp	ampul
amt	amount
aq	water
aq. dest.	distilled water
a.s.	left ear
ASAP	as soon as possible
a.u.	each ear
AUC	area under the curve
BDI	Beck Depression Inventory
bid	twice daily
bm	bowel movement
bp	blood pressure
BPRS	Brief Psychiatric Rating Scale
BSA	body surface area
c	a gallon
$\bar{c}$	with
cal	calorie
cap	capsule
CBT	cognitive behavioral therapy
cc	cubic centimeter
CGI	Clinical Global Impression
cm	centimeter
CIV	continuous I.V. infusion
comp	compound
cont	continue
CT	computed tomography
d	day
d/c	discontinue
dil	dilute
disp	dispense
div	divide
DSM-IV	Diagnostic and Statistical Manual
DTs	delirium tremens
dtd	give of such a dose
ECT	electroconvulsive therapy
EEG	electroencephalogram
elix, el	elixir
emp	as directed
EPS	extrapyramidal side effects
et	and
ex aq	in water
f, ft	make, let be made

Abbreviation	Meaning
FDA	Food and Drug Administration
g	gram
GA	Gamblers Anonymous
GAD	generalized anxiety disorder
GAF	Global Assessment of Functioning Scale
GABA	gamma-aminobutyric acid
GITS	gastrointestinal therapeutic system
gr	grain
gtt	a drop
h	hour
HAM-A	Hamilton Anxiety Scale
HAM-D	Hamilton Depression Scale
hs	at bedtime
I.M.	intramuscular
IU	international unit
I.V.	intravenous
kcal	kilocalorie
kg	kilogram
KIU	kallikrein inhibitor unit
L	liter
LAMM	L-α-acetyl methadol
liq	a liquor, solution
M	mix
MADRS	Montgomery Asbery Depression Rating Scale
MAOIs	monamine oxidase inhibitors
mcg	microgram
MDEA	3,4-methylene-dioxy amphetamine
m. dict	as directed
MDMA	3,4-methylene-dioxy methamphetamine
mEq	milliequivalent
mg	milligram
mixt	a mixture
mL	milliliter
mm	millimeter
MMSE	Mini-Mental State Examination
MPPP	l-methyl-4-proprionoxy-4-phenyl pyridine
MR	mental retardation
MRI	magnetic resonance imaging
NF	National Formulary
NMS	neuroleptic malignant syndrome
no.	number
noc	in the night
non rep	do not repeat, no refills
NPO	nothing by mouth
O, Oct	a pint
OCD	obsessive-compulsive disorder
o.d.	right eye
o.l.	left eye
o.s.	left eye
o.u.	each eye
PANSS	Positive and Negative Symptom Scale
pc, post cib	after meals
PCP	phencyclidine
per	through or by
PM	afternoon or evening
P.O.	by mouth
P.R.	rectally

ABBREVIATIONS, ACRONYMS, AND SYMBOLS *(Continued)*

Abbreviation	Meaning
prn	as needed
PTSD	post-traumatic stress disorder
pulv	a powder
q	every
qad	every other day
qd	every day
qh	every hour
qid	four times a day
qod	every other day
qs	a sufficient quantity
qs ad	a sufficient quantity to make
qty	quantity
qv	as much as you wish
REM	rapid eye movement
Rx	take, a recipe
rep	let it be repeated
$\overline{s}$	without
sa	according to art
sat	saturated
S.C.	subcutaneous
sig	label, or let it be printed
sol	solution
solv	dissolve
$\overline{ss}$	one-half
sos	if there is need
SSRIs	selective serotonin reuptake inhibitors
stat	at once, immediately
supp	suppository
syr	syrup
tab	tablet
tal	such
TCA	tricyclic antidepressant
TD	tardive dyskinesia
tid	three times a day
tr, tinct	tincture
trit	triturate
tsp	teaspoonful
ULN	upper limits of normal
ung	ointment
USAN	United States Adopted Names
USP	United States Pharmacopeia
u.d., ut dict	as directed
v.o.	verbal order
w.a.	while awake
x3	3 times
x4	4 times
YBOC	Yale Brown Obsessive-Compulsive Scale
YMRS	Young Mania Rating Scale

APOTHECARY/METRIC EQUIVALENTS

Approximate Liquid Measures

Basic equivalent: 1 fluid ounce = 30 mL

Examples:

1 gallon	3800 mL	1 gallon	128 fluid ounces
1 quart	960 mL	1 quart	32 fluid ounces
1 pint	480 mL	1 pint	16 fluid ounces
8 fluid oz	240 mL	15 minims	1 mL
4 fluid oz	120 mL	10 minims	0.6 mL

Approximate Household Equivalents

1 teaspoonful	5 mL	1 tablespoonful	15 mL

Weights

Basic equivalents:

1 oz	30 g	15 gr	1 g

Examples:

4 oz	120 g	1 gr	60 mg
2 oz	60 g	1/100 gr	600 mcg
10 gr	600 mg	1/150 gr	400 mcg
7½ gr	500 mg	1/200 gr	300 mcg
16 oz	1 lb		

Metric Conversions

Basic equivalents:

1 g	1000 mg	1 mg	1000 mcg

Examples:

5 g	5000 mg	5 mg	5000 mcg
0.5 g	500 mg	0.5 g	500 mcg
0.05 g	50 mg	0.05 mg	50 mcg

Exact Equivalents

1 g	=	15.43 gr	0.1 mg	=	1/600 gr
1 mL	=	16.23 minims	0.12 mg	=	1/500 gr
1 minim	=	0.06 mL	0.15 mg	=	1/400 gr
1 gr	=	64.8 mg	0.2 mg	=	1/300 gr
1 pint (pt)	=	473.2 mL	0.3 mg	=	1/200 gr
1 oz	=	28.35 g	0.4 mg	=	1/150 gr
1 lb	=	453.6 g	0.5 mg	=	1/120 gr
1 kg	=	2.2 lbs	0.6 mg	=	1/100 gr
1 qt	=	946.4 mL	0.8 mg	=	1/80 gr
			1 mg	=	1/65 gr

Solids*

¼ grain	=	15 mg
½ grain	=	30 mg
1 grain	=	60 mg
1½ grains	=	90 mg
5 grains	=	300 mg
10 grains	=	600 mg

*Use exact equivalents for compounding and calculations requiring a high degree of accuracy.

AVERAGE WEIGHTS AND SURFACE AREAS

Average Weight and Surface Area of Preterm Infants, Term Infants, and Children

Age	Average Weight (kg)*	Approximate Surface Area (m^2)
Weeks Gestation		
26	0.9-1	0.1
30	1.3-1.5	0.12
32	1.6-2	0.15
38	2.9-3	0.2
40 (term infant at birth)	3.1-4	0.25
Months		
3	5	0.29
6	7	0.38
9	8	0.42
Year		
1	10	0.49
2	12	0.55
3	15	0.64
4	17	0.74
5	18	0.76
6	20	0.82
7	23	0.90
8	25	0.95
9	28	1.06
10	33	1.18
11	35	1.23
12	40	1.34
Adult	70	1.73

*Weights from age 3 months and over are rounded off to the nearest kilogram.

BODY SURFACE AREA OF ADULTS AND CHILDREN

Calculating Body Surface Area in Children

In a child of average size, find weight and corresponding surface area on the boxed scale to the left; or, use the nomogram to the right. Lay a straightedge on the correct height and weight points for the child, then read the intersecting point on the surface area scale.

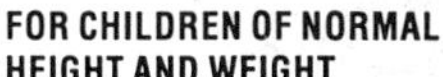

FOR CHILDREN OF NORMAL HEIGHT AND WEIGHT

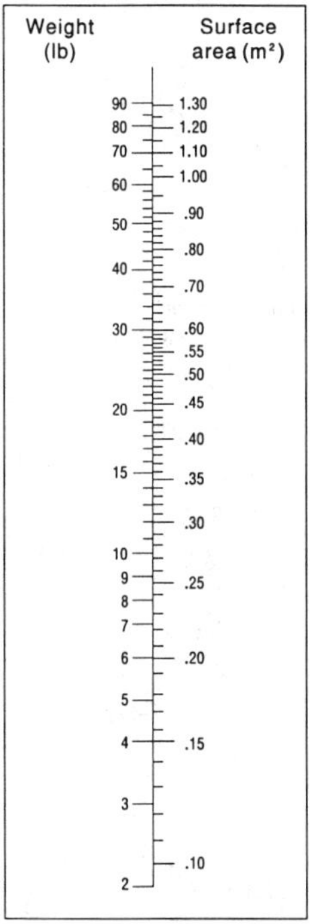

Weight (lb) — Surface area (m²)

90 — 1.30; 80 — 1.20; 70 — 1.10; 60; 1.00; 50; .90; .80; 40; .70; 30 — .60; .55; .50; 20; .45; .40; 15; .35; .30; 10; 9; .25; 8; 7; 6 — .20; 5; 4 — .15; 3; .10; 2

NOMOGRAM

Height (cm) (in) — Surface area (m²) — Weight (lb) (kg)

Height (cm): 240, 220, 200, 190, 180, 170, 160, 150, 140, 130, 120, 110, 100, 90, 80, 70, 60, 50, 40, 30

Height (in): 90, 85, 80, 75, 70, 65, 60, 55, 50, 45, 40, 35, 30, 28, 26, 24, 22, 20, 19, 18, 17, 16, 15, 14, 13, 12

Surface area (m²): 2.0, 1.9, 1.8, 1.7, 1.6, 1.5, 1.4, 1.3, 1.2, 1.1, 1.0, 0.9, 0.8, 0.7, 0.6, 0.5, 0.4, 0.3, 0.2, 0.1

Weight (lb): 180, 160, 140, 130, 120, 110, 100, 90, 80, 70, 60, 50, 45, 40, 35, 30, 25, 20, 18, 16, 14, 12, 10, 9, 8, 7, 6, 5, 4, 3

Weight (kg): 80, 70, 60, 50, 40, 30, 25, 20, 15, 10, 9.0, 8.0, 7.0, 6.0, 5.0, 4.0, 3.0, 2.5, 2.0, 1.5, 1.0

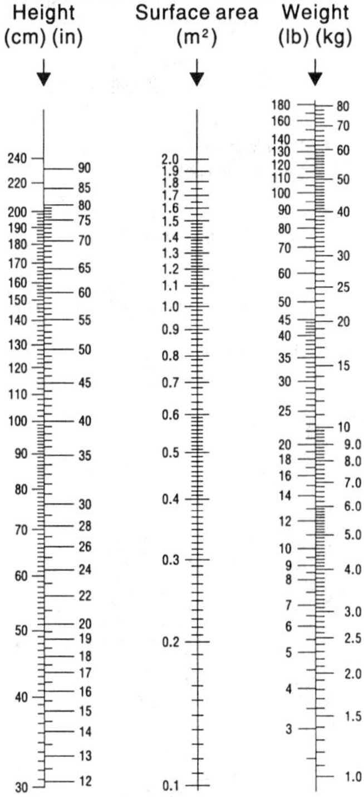

BODY SURFACE AREA FORMULA (Adult and Pediatric)

$$BSA\ (m^2) = \sqrt{\frac{Ht\ (in) \times Wt\ (lb)}{3131}}$$ or, in metric: $$BSA\ (m^2) = \sqrt{\frac{Ht\ (cm) \times Wt\ (kg)}{3600}}$$

References

Lam TK and Leung DT, "More on Simplified Calculation of Body Surface Area," *N Engl J Med*, 1988, 318(17):1130 (Letter).

Mosteller RD, "Simplified Calculation of Body Surface Area", *N Engl J Med*, 1987, 317(17):1098 (Letter).

IDEAL BODY WEIGHT CALCULATION

Adults (18 years and older)

IBW (male) = 50 + (2.3 x height in inches over 5 feet)
IBW (female) = 45.5 + (2.3 x height in inches over 5 feet)

*IBW is in kg.

Children

a. 1-18 years

$$IBW = \frac{(height^2 \times 1.65)}{1000}$$

*IBW is in kg.
Height is in cm.

b. 5 feet and taller

IBW (male) = 39 + (2.27 x height in inches over 5 feet)
IBW (female) = 42.2 + (2.27 x height in inches over 5 feet)

*IBW is in kg.

MILLIEQUIVALENT AND MILLIMOLE CALCULATIONS & CONVERSIONS

DEFINITIONS & CALCULATIONS

Definitions

mole	=	gram molecular weight of a substance (aka molar weight)
millimole (mM)	=	milligram molecular weight of a substance (a millimole is 1/1000 of a mole)
equivalent weight	=	gram weight of a substance which will combine with or replace one gram (one mole) of hydrogen; an equivalent weight can be determined by dividing the molar weight of a substance by its ionic valence
milliequivalent (mEq)	=	milligram weight of a substance which will combine with or replace one milligram (one millimole) of hydrogen (a milliequivalent is 1/1000 of an equivalent)

Calculations

$$\text{moles} = \frac{\text{weight of a substance (grams)}}{\text{molecular weight of that substance (grams)}}$$

$$\text{millimoles} = \frac{\text{weight of a substance (milligrams)}}{\text{molecular weight of that substance (milligrams)}}$$

equivalents = moles x valence of ion

milliequivalents = millimoles x valence of ion

$$\text{moles} = \frac{\text{equivalents}}{\text{valence of ion}}$$

$$\text{millimoles} = \frac{\text{milliequivalents}}{\text{valence of ion}}$$

millimoles = moles x 1000

milliequivalents = equivalents x 1000

Note: Use of equivalents and milliequivalents is valid only for those substances which have fixed ionic valences (eg, sodium, potassium, calcium, chlorine, magnesium bromine, etc). For substances with variable ionic valences (eg, phosphorous), a reliable equivalent value cannot be determined. In these instances, one should calculate millimoles (which are fixed and reliable) rather than milliequivalents.

MILLIEQUIVALENT CONVERSIONS

To convert mg/100 mL to mEq/L the following formula may be used:

$$\frac{\text{(mg/100 mL) x 10 x valence}}{\text{atomic weight}} = \text{mEq/L}$$

To convert mEq/L to mg/100 mL the following formula may be used:

$$\frac{\text{(mEq/L) x atomic weight}}{\text{10 x valence}} = \text{mg/100 mL}$$

To convert mEq/L to volume of percent of a gas the following formula may be used:

$$\frac{\text{(mEq/L) x 22.4}}{10} = \text{volume percent}$$

MILLIEQUIVALENT AND MILLIMOLE CALCULATIONS & CONVERSIONS *(Continued)*

Valences and Atomic Weights of Selected Ions

Substance	Electrolyte	Valence	Molecular Wt
Calcium	Ca^{++}	2	40
Chloride	Cl^{-}	1	35.5
Magnesium	Mg^{++}	2	24
Phosphate	HPO_4^{--} (80%)	1.8	96*
pH = 7.4	$H_2PO_4^{-}$ (20%)	1.8	96*
Potassium	K^{+}	1	39
Sodium	Na^{+}	1	23
Sulfate	SO_4^{--}	2	96*

*The molecular weight of phosphorus only is 31, and sulfur only is 32.

Approximate Milliequivalents — Weights of Selected Ions

Salt	mEq/g Salt	Mg Salt/mEq
Calcium carbonate ($CaCO_3$)	20	50
Calcium chloride ($CaCl_2 - 2H_2O$)	14	73
Calcium gluconate (Ca gluconate$_2$ – $1H_2O$)	4	224
Calcium lactate (Ca lactate$_2$ – $5H_2O$)	6	154
Magnesium sulfate ($MgSO_4$)	16	60
Magnesium sulfate ($MgSO_4 - 7H_2O$)	8	123
Potassium acetate (K acetate)	10	98
Potassium chloride (KCl)	13	75
Potassium citrate (K_3 citrate – $1H_2O$)	9	108
Potassium iodide (KI)	6	166
Sodium bicarbonate ($NaHCO_3$)	12	84
Sodium chloride (NaCl)	17	58
Sodium citrate (Na_3 citrate – $2H_2O$)	10	98
Sodium iodine (NaI)	7	150
Sodium lactate (Na lactate)	9	112

CORRECTED SODIUM

Corrected Na^+ = measured Na^+ + [1.5 x (glucose – 150 divided by 100)]

Note: Do not correct for glucose <150.

WATER DEFICIT

Water deficit = 0.6 x body weight [1 – (140 divided by Na^+)]

Note: Body weight is estimated weight in kg when fully hydrated; **Na^+** is serum or plasma sodium. Use corrected Na^+ if necessary. Consult medical references for recommendations for replacement of deficit.

TOTAL SERUM CALCIUM CORRECTED FOR ALBUMIN LEVEL

[(Normal albumin – patient's albumin) x 0.8] + patient's measured total calcium

ACID-BASE ASSESSMENT

Henderson-Hasselbalch Equation

$$pH = 6.1 + \log (HCO_3^- / (0.03)(pCO_2))$$

Alveolar Gas Equation

PIO_2	=	FiO_2 x (total atmospheric pressure – vapor pressure of H_2O at 37°C)
	=	FiO_2 x (760 mm Hg – 47 mm Hg)
PAO_2	=	$PIO_2 - PACO_2 / R$

Alveolar/arterial oxygen gradient = $PAO_2 - PaO_2$

Normal ranges:

Children	15-20 mm Hg
Adults	20-25 mm Hg

where:

PIO_2	=	Oxygen partial pressure of inspired gas (mm Hg) (150 mm Hg in room air at sea level)
FiO_2	=	Fractional pressure of oxygen in inspired gas (0.21 in room air)
PAO_2	=	Alveolar oxygen partial pressure
$PACO_2$	=	Alveolar carbon dioxide partial pressure
PaO_2	=	Arterial oxygen partial pressure
R	=	Respiratory exchange quotient (typically 0.8, increases with high carbohydrate diet, decreases with high fat diet)

Acid-Base Disorders

Acute metabolic acidosis (<12 h duration):

$$PaCO_2 \text{ expected} = 1.5\ (HCO_3^-) + 8 \pm 2$$

or

$$\text{expected change in pCO} = (1\text{-}1.5) \times \text{change in } HCO_3^-$$

Acute metabolic alkalosis (<12 h duration):

$$\text{expected change in } pCO_2 = (0.5\text{-}1) \times \text{change in } HCO_3^-$$

Acute respiratory acidosis (<6 h duration):

$$\text{expected change in } HCO_3^- = 0.1 \times pCO_2$$

Acute respiratory acidosis (>6 h duration):

$$\text{expected change in } HCO_3^- = 0.4 \times \text{change in } pCO_2$$

Acute respiratory alkalosis (<6 h duration):

$$\text{expected change in } HCO_3^- = 0.2 \times \text{change in } pCO_2$$

Acute respiratory alkalosis (>6 h duration):

$$\text{expected change in } HCO_3^- = 0.5 \times \text{change in } pCO_2$$

ACID-BASE EQUATION

H^+ (in mEq/L) = (24 x $PaCO_2$) divided by HCO_3^-

Aa GRADIENT

Aa gradient [(713)(FiO_2 – ($PaCO_2$ divided by 0.8))] – PaO_2

Aa gradient	=	alveolar-arterial oxygen gradient
FiO_2	=	inspired oxygen (expressed as a fraction)
$PaCO_2$	=	arterial partial pressure carbon dioxide (mm Hg)
PaO_2	=	arterial partial pressure oxygen (mm Hg)

MILLIEQUIVALENT AND MILLIMOLE CALCULATIONS & CONVERSIONS *(Continued)*

OSMOLALITY

Definition: The summed concentrations of all osmotically active solute particles.

Predicted serum osmolality =

2 Na^+ + glucose (mg/dL) / 18 + BUN (mg/dL) / 2.8

The normal range of serum osmolality is 285-295 mOsm/L.

Differential diagnosis of increased serum osmolal gap (>10 mOsm/L)

Medications and toxins

- Alcohols (ethanol, methanol, isopropanol, glycerol, ethylene glycol)
- Mannitol
- Paraldehyde

Calculated Osm

Osmolal gap = measured Osm – calculated Osm

0 to +10: Normal

>10: Abnormal

<0: Probable lab or calculation error

For drugs causing increased osmolar gap, see "Toxicology Information" section in this Appendix.

BICARBONATE DEFICIT

HCO_3^- deficit = (0.4 x wt in kg) x (HCO_3^- desired – HCO_3^- measured)

Note: In clinical practice, the calculated quantity may differ markedly from the actual amount of bicarbonate needed or that which may be safely administered.

ANION GAP

Definition: The difference in concentration between unmeasured cation and anion equivalents in serum.

Anion gap = Na^+ – (Cl^- + HCO_3^-)

(The normal anion gap is 10-14 mEq/L)

Differential Diagnosis of Increased Anion Gap Acidosis

Organic anions

- Lactate (sepsis, hypovolemia, seizures, large tumor burden)
- Pyruvate
- Uremia
- Ketoacidosis (β-hydroxybutyrate and acetoacetate)
- Amino acids and their metabolites
- Other organic acids

Inorganic anions

- Hyperphosphatemia
- Sulfates
- Nitrates

Differential Diagnosis of Decreased Anion Gap

Organic cations

- Hypergammaglobulinemia

Inorganic cations

- Hyperkalemia
- Hypercalcemia
- Hypermagnesemia

Medications and toxins

- Lithium

Hypoalbuminemia

RETICULOCYTE INDEX

(% retic divided by 2) x (patient's Hct divided by normal Hct) or (% retic divided by 2) x (patient's Hgb divided by normal Hgb)

Normal index: 1.0
Good marrow response: 2.0-6.0

PEDIATRIC DOSAGE ESTIMATIONS

Dosage Estimations Based on Weight:

Augsberger's rule:

$$\frac{(1.5 \times \text{weight in kg} + 10)}{\%\text{ of adult dose}} = \text{child's approximate dose}$$

Clark's rule:

$$\frac{\text{weight (in pounds)}}{150} \times \text{adult dose} = \text{child's approximate dose}$$

Dosage Estimations Based on Age:

Augsberger's rule:

$$\frac{(4 \times \text{age in years} + 20)}{\%\text{ of adult dose}} = \text{child's approximate dose}$$

Bastedo's rule:

$$\frac{\text{age in years} + 3}{30} \times \text{adult dose} = \text{child's approximate dose}$$

Cowling's rule:

$$\frac{\text{age at next birthday (in years)}}{24} \times \text{adult dose} = \text{child's approximate dose}$$

Dilling's rule:

$$\frac{\text{age (in years)}}{20} \times \text{adult dose} = \text{child's approximate dose}$$

Fried's rule for infants (younger than 1 year):

$$\frac{\text{age (in months)}}{150} \times \text{adult dose} = \text{infant's approximate dose}$$

Young's rule:

$$\frac{\text{age (in years)}}{\text{age} + 12} \times \text{adult dose} = \text{child's approximate dose}$$

POUNDS/KILOGRAMS CONVERSION

1 pound = 0.45359 kilograms
1 kilogram = 2.2 pounds

lb	= kg	lb	= kg	lb	= kg
1	0.45	70	31.75	140	63.50
5	2.27	75	34.02	145	65.77
10	4.54	80	36.29	150	68.04
15	6.80	85	38.56	155	70.31
20	9.07	90	40.82	160	72.58
25	11.34	95	43.09	165	74.84
30	13.61	100	45.36	170	77.11
35	15.88	105	47.63	175	79.38
40	18.14	110	49.90	180	81.65
45	20.41	115	52.16	185	83.92
50	22.68	120	54.43	190	86.18
55	24.95	125	56.70	195	88.45
60	27.22	130	58.91	200	90.72
65	29.48	135	61.24		

TEMPERATURE CONVERSION

Celsius to Fahrenheit = (°C x 9/5) + 32 = °F
Fahrenheit to Celsius = (°F – 32) x 5/9 = °C

°C	= °F	°C	= °F	°C	= °F
100.0	212.0	39.0	102.2	36.8	98.2
50.0	122.0	38.8	101.8	36.6	97.9
41.0	105.8	38.6	101.5	36.4	97.5
40.8	105.4	38.4	101.1	36.2	97.2
40.6	105.1	38.2	100.8	36.0	96.8
40.4	104.7	38.0	100.4	35.8	96.4
40.2	104.4	37.8	100.1	35.6	96.1
40.0	104.0	37.6	99.7	35.4	95.7
39.8	103.6	37.4	99.3	35.2	95.4
39.6	103.3	37.2	99.0	35.0	95.0
39.4	102.9	37.0	98.6	0	32.0
39.2	102.6				

LIVER DISEASE

Pugh's Modification of Child's Classification for Severity

Parameter	Points for Increasing Abnormality		
	1	2	3
Encephalopathy	None	1 or 2	3 or 4
Ascites	Absent	Slight	Moderate
Bilirubin (mg/dL)	<2.9	2.9-5.8	>5.8
Albumin (g/dL)	>3.5	2.8-3.5	<2.8
Prothrombin time (seconds over control)	1-4	4-6	>6

Scores:

Mild hepatic impairment = <6 points.
Moderate hepatic impairment = 6-10 points.
Severe hepatic impairment = >10 points.

Considerations for Drug Dose Adjustment

Extent of Change in Drug Dose	Conditions or Requirements to Be Satisfied
No or minor change	Mild liver disease
	Extensive elimination of drug by kidneys and no renal dysfunction
	Elimination by pathways of metabolism spared by liver disease
	Drug is enzyme-limited and given acutely
	Drug is flow/enzyme-sensitive and only given acutely by I.V. route
	No alteration in drug sensitivity
Decrease in dose up to 25%	Elimination by the liver does not exceed 40% of the dose; no renal dysfunction
	Drug is flow-limited and given by I.V. route, with no large change in protein binding
	Drug is flow/enzyme-limited and given acutely by oral route
	Drug has a large therapeutic ratio
>25% decrease in dose	Drug metabolism is affected by liver disease; drug administered chronically
	Drug has a narrow therapeutic range; protein binding altered significantly
	Drug is flow-limited and given orally
	Drug is eliminated by kidneys and renal function severely affected
	Altered sensitivity to drug due to liver disease

Reference

Arns PA, Wedlund PJ, and Branch RA, "Adjustment of Medications in Liver Failure," *The Pharmacologic Approach to the Critically Ill Patient*, 2nd ed, Chernow B, ed, Baltimore, MD: Williams & Wilkins, 1988, 85-111.

CREATININE CLEARANCE ESTIMATING METHODS IN PATIENTS WITH STABLE RENAL FUNCTION

These formulas provide an acceptable estimate of the patient's creatinine clearance **except** in the following instances.

- Patient's serum creatinine is changing rapidly (either up or down).
- Patients are markedly emaciated.

In above situations, certain assumptions have to be made.

- In patients with rapidly rising serum creatinines (ie, >0.5-0.7 mg/dL/day), it is best to assume that the patient's creatinine clearance is probably <10 mL/minute.
- In emaciated patients, although their actual creatinine clearance is less than their calculated creatinine clearance (because of decreased creatinine production), it is not possible to easily predict how much less.

Infants

Estimation of creatinine clearance using serum creatinine and body length (to be used when an adequate timed specimen cannot be obtained). **Note:** This formula may not provide an accurate estimation of creatinine clearance for infants younger than 6 months of age and for patients with severe starvation or muscle wasting.

$Cl_{cr} = K \times L/S_{cr}$

where:

Cl_{cr} = creatinine clearance in mL/minute/1.73 m^2
K = constant of proportionality that is age specific

Age	K
Low birth weight ≤1 y	0.33
Full-term ≤1 y	0.45
2-12 y	0.55
13-21 y female	0.55
13-21 y male	0.70

L = length in cm
S_{cr} = serum creatinine concentration in mg/dL

Reference

Schwartz GJ, Brion LP, and Spitzer A, "The Use of Plasma Creatinine Concentration for Estimating Glomerular Filtration Rate in Infants, Children and Adolescents," *Ped Clin N Amer*, 1987, 34:571-90.

Children (1-18 years)

Method 1: (Traub SL, Johnson CE, *Am J Hosp Pharm*, 1980, 37:195-201)

$$Cl_{cr} = \frac{0.48 \times (\text{height}) \times BSA}{S_{cr} \times 1.73}$$

where:

BSA = body surface area in m^2
Cl_{cr} = creatinine clearance in mL/min
S_{cr} = serum creatinine in mg/dL
Height = in cm

CREATININE CLEARANCE ESTIMATING METHODS IN PATIENTS WITH STABLE RENAL FUNCTION *(Continued)*

Method 2: Nomogram (Traub SL and Johnson CE, *Am J Hosp Pharm*, 1980, 37:195-201)

Children 1-18 Years

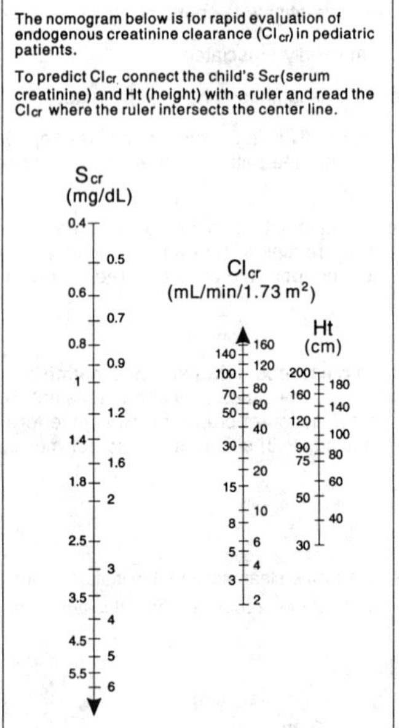

Adults (18 years and older)

Method: (Cockroft DW and Gault MH, *Nephron*, 1976, 16:31-41)

Estimated creatinine clearance (Cl_{cr}) (mL/min):

$$\text{Male} = \frac{(140 - \text{age})\ \text{IBW (kg)}}{72 \times S_{cr}}$$

$$\text{Female} = \text{estimated } Cl_{cr} \text{ male} \times 0.85$$

Note: The use of the patient's ideal body weight (IBW) is recommended for the above formula except when the patient's actual body weight is less than ideal. Use of the IBW is especially important in obese patients.

RENAL FUNCTION TESTS

Endogenous creatinine clearance vs age (timed collection)

Creatinine clearance (mL/min/1.73 m^2) = (Cr_uV/Cr_sT) (1.73/A)

where:

Cr_u	=	urine creatinine concentration (mg/dL)
V	=	total urine collected during sampling period (mL)
Cr_s	=	serum creatinine concentration (mg/dL)
T	=	duration of sampling period (min) (24 h = 1440 min)
A	=	body surface area (m^2)

Age-specific normal values

5-7 d	50.6 ± 5.8 mL/min/1.73 m^2
1-2 mo	64.6 ± 5.8 mL/min/1.73 m^2
5-8 mo	87.7 ± 11.9 mL/min/1.73 m^2
9-12 mo	86.9 ± 8.4 mL/min/1.73 m^2
≥18 mo	
male	124 ± 26 mL/min/1.73 m^2
female	109 ± 13.5 mL/min/1.73 m^2
Adults	
male	105 ± 14 mL/min/1.73 m^2
female	95 ± 18 mL/min/1.73 m^2

Note: In patients with renal failure (creatinine clearance <25 mL/min), creatinine clearance may be elevated over GFR because of tubular secretion of creatinine.

Calculation of Creatinine Clearance From a 24-Hour Urine Collection

Equation 1:

$$Cl_{cr} = \frac{U \times V}{P}$$

where:

Cl_{cr}	=	creatinine clearance
U	=	urine concentration of creatinine
V	=	total urine volume in the collection
P	=	plasma creatinine concentration

Equation 2:

$$Cl_{cr} = \frac{\text{(total urine volume [mL]) x (urine Cr concentration [mg/dL])}}{\text{(serum creatinine [mg/dL]) x (time of urine collection [minutes])}}$$

Occasionally, a patient will have a 12- or 24-hour urine collection done for direct calculation of creatinine clearance. Although a urine collection for 24 hours is best, it is difficult to do since many urine collections occur for a much shorter period. A 24-hour urine collection is the desired duration of urine collection because the urine excretion of creatinine is diurnal and thus the measured creatinine clearance will vary throughout the day as the creatinine in the urine varies. When the urine collection is less than 24 hours, the total excreted creatinine will be affected by the time of the day during which the collection is performed. A 24-hour urine collection is sufficient to be able to accurately average the diurnal creatinine excretion variations. If a patient has 24 hours of urine collected for creatinine clearance, equation 1 can be used for calculating the creatinine clearance. To use equation 1 to calculate the creatinine clearance, it will be necessary to know the duration of urine collection, the urine collection volume, the urine creatinine concentration, and the serum creatinine value that reflects the urine collection period. In most cases, a serum creatinine concentration is drawn anytime during the day, but it is best to have the value drawn halfway through the collection period.

RENAL FUNCTION TESTS *(Continued)*

Amylase/Creatinine Clearance Ratio*

$$\frac{\text{Amylase}_u \times \text{creatinine}_p}{\text{Amylase}_p \times \text{creatinine}_u} \times 100$$

u = urine; p = plasma

Serum BUN/Serum Creatinine Ratio

Serum BUN (mg/dL:serum creatinine (mg/dL))

Normal BUN:creatinine ratio is 10-15

BUN:creatinine ratio >20 suggests prerenal azotemia (also seen with high urea-generation states such as GI bleeding)

BUN:creatinine ratio <5 may be seen with disorders affecting urea biosynthesis such as urea cycle enzyme deficiencies and with hepatitis.

Fractional Sodium Excretion

Fractional sodium secretion (FENa) = $Na_uCr_s/Na_sCr_u \times 100\%$

where:

Na_u = urine sodium (mEq/L)
Na_s = serum sodium (mEq/L)
Cr_u = urine creatinine (mg/dL)
Cr_s = serum creatinine (mg/dL)

FENa <1% suggests prerenal failure

FENa >2% suggest intrinsic renal failure
(for newborns, normal FENa is approximately 2.5%)

Note: Disease states associated with a falsely elevated FENa include severe volume depletion (>10%), early acute tubular necrosis and volume depletion in chronic renal disease. Disorders associated with a lowered FENa include acute glomerulonephritis, hemoglobinuric or myoglobinuric renal failure, nonoliguric acute tubular necrosis and acute urinary tract obstruction. In addition, FENa may be <1% in patients with acute renal failure **and** a second condition predisposing to sodium retention (eg, burns, congestive heart failure, nephrotic syndrome).

Urine Calcium/Urine Creatinine Ratio (spot sample)

Urine calcium (mg/dL): urine creatinine (mg/dL)

Normal values <0.21 (mean values 0.08 males, 0.06 females)

Premature infants show wide variability of calcium:creatinine ratio, and tend to have lower thresholds for calcium loss than older children. Prematures without nephrolithiasis had mean Ca:Cr ratio of 0.75 ± 0.76. Infants with nephrolithiasis had mean Ca:Cr ratio of 1.32 ± 1.03 (Jacinto, et al, *Pediatrics,* vol 81, p 31.)

Urine Protein/Urine Creatinine Ratio (spot sample)

P_u/Cr_u	Total Protein Excretion ($mg/m^2/d$)
0.1	80
1	800
10	8000

where:

P_u = urine protein concentration (mg/dL)
Cr_u = urine creatinine concentration (mg/dL)

PEDIATRIC ALS ALGORITHMS

BRADYCARDIA

Fig. 1: Pediatric bradycardia decision tree. ABCs indicates airway, breathing, and circulation; ALS, advanced life support; E.T., endotracheal; I.O., intraosseous; and I.V., intravenous.

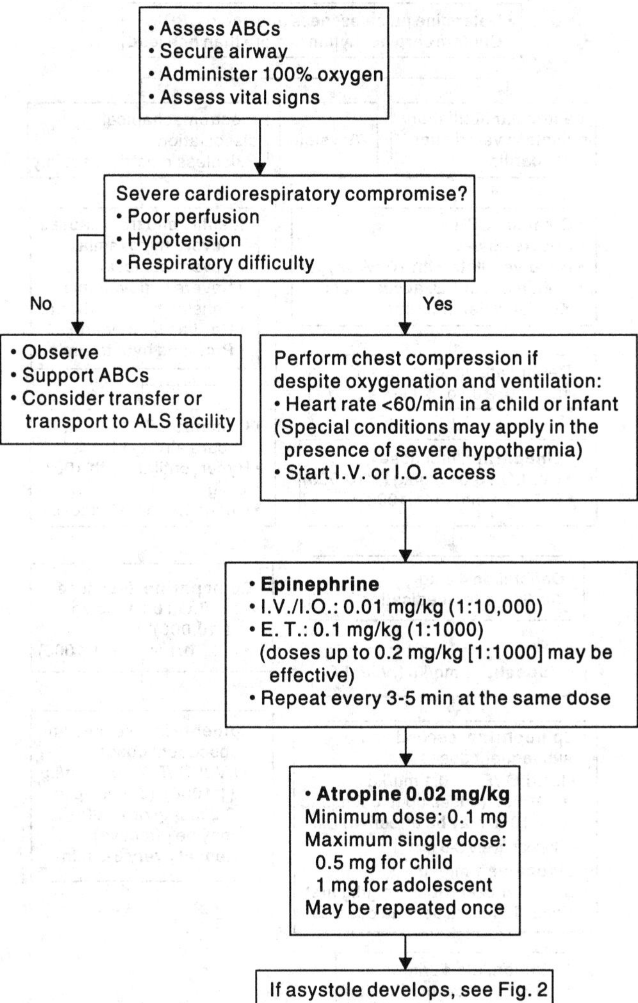

Used with permission: Emergency Cardiac Care Committee and Subcommittees, American Heart Association, "Guidelines for Cardiopulmonary Resuscitation and Emergency Care, IV: Pediatric Advanced Life Support," *JAMA*, 1992, 268:2262-75.

PEDIATRIC ALS ALGORITHMS *(Continued)*

ASYSTOLE AND PULSELESS ARREST

Fig. 2: Pediatric asystole and pulseless arrest decision tree. CPR indicates cardiopulmonary resuscitation; E.T, endotracheal; I.O., intraosseous; and I.V., intravenous.

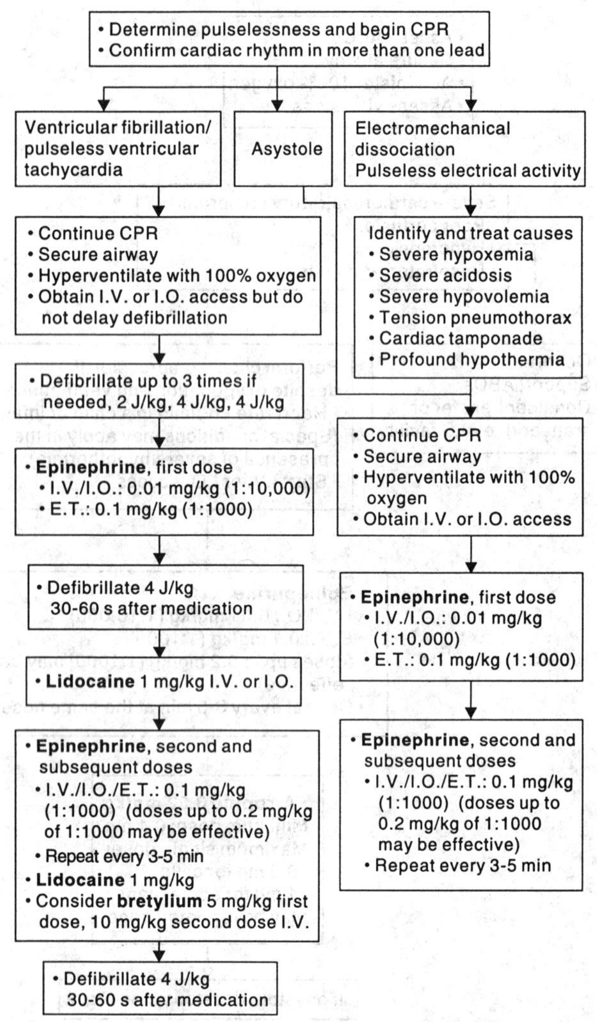

Used with permission: Emergency Cardiac Care Committee and Subcommittees, American Heart Association, "Guidelines for Cardiopulmonary Resuscitation and Emergency Care, IV: Pediatric Advanced Life Support," *JAMA*, 1992, 268:2262-75.

ADULT ACLS ALGORITHMS

EMERGENCY CARDIAC CARE

Fig. 1: Universal algorithm for adult emergency cardiac care (ECC)

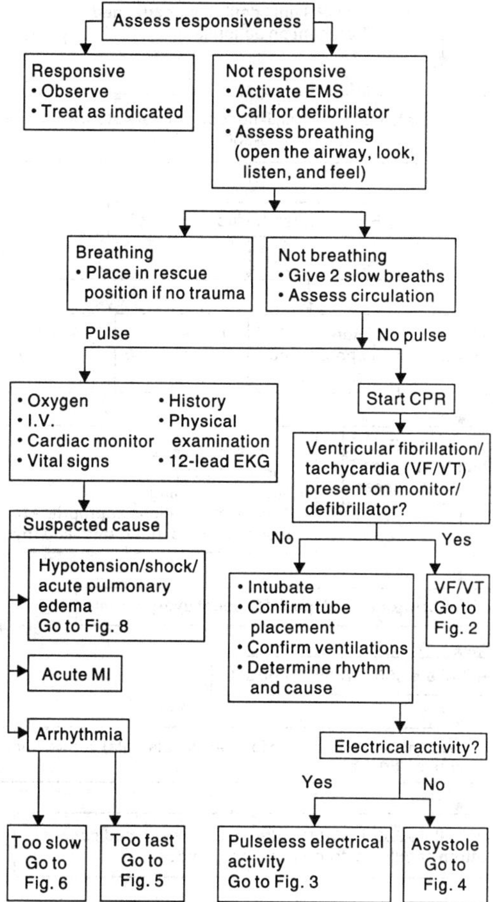

Used with permission: Emergency Cardiac Care Committee and Subcommittees, American Heart Association, "Guidelines for Cardiopulmonary Resuscitation and Emergency Care, III: Adult Advanced Cardiac Life Support," *JAMA*, 1992, 268:2199-2241.

ADULT ACLS ALGORITHMS *(Continued)*

V. FIB AND PULSELESS V. TACH

Fig. 2: Adult algorithm for ventricular fibrillation and pulseless ventricular tachycardia (VF/VT)

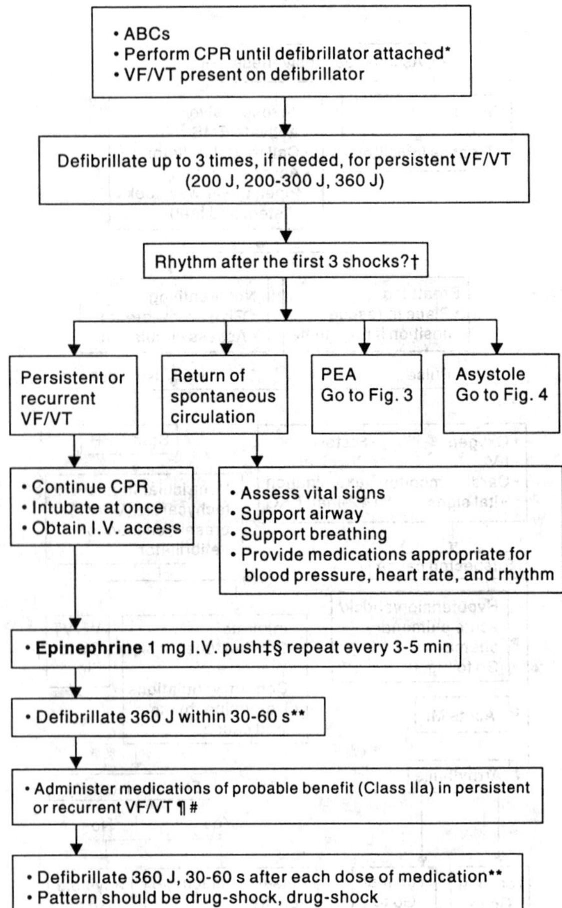

Class I: Definitely helpful
Class IIa: Acceptable, probably helpful
Class IIb: Acceptable, possibly helpful
Class III: Not indicated, may be harmful

* Precordial thump is a Class IIb action in witnessed arrest, no pulse, and no defibrillator immediately available.

† Hypothermic cardiac arrest is treated differently after this point.

‡ The recommended dose of **epinephrine** is 1 mg I.V. push every 3-5 min. If this approach fails, several Class IIb dosing regimens can be considered:

- Intermediate: **Epinephrine** 2-5 mg I.V. push, every 3-5 min
- Escalating: **Epinephrine** 1 mg-3 mg-5 mg I.V. push (3 min apart)
- High: **Epinephrine**: 0.1 mg/kg I.V. push, every 3-5 min

§ **Sodium bicarbonate (1 mEq/kg)** is Class I if patient has known pre-existing hyperkalemia

** Multiple sequenced shock (200 J, 200-300 J, 360 J) are acceptable here (Class I), especially when medications are delayed

¶ **Lidocaine** 1.5 mg/kg I.V. push. Repeat in 3-5 min to total loading dose of 3 mg/kg; then use

- **Bretylium** 5 mg/kg I.V. push. Repeat in 5 min at 10 mg/kg
- **Magnesium sulfate** 1-2 g I.V. in torsade de pointes or suspected hypo-magnesemic state or severe refractory VF
- **Procainamide** 30 mg/min in refractory VF (maximum total: 17 mg/kg)

\# **Sodium bicarbonate** (1 mEq/kg I.V.): Class IIa

- If known pre-existing bicarbonate-responsive acidosis
- If overdose with tricyclic antidepressants
- To alkalinize the urine in drug overdoses

Class IIb

- If intubated and continued long arrest interval
- Upon return of spontaneous circulation after long arrest interval

Class III

- Hypoxic lactic acidosis

Used with permission: Emergency Cardiac Care Committee and Subcommittees, American Heart Association, "Guidelines for Cardiopulmonary Resuscitation and Emergency Care, III: Adult Advanced Cardiac Life Support," *JAMA*, 1992, 268:2199-2241.

ADULT ACLS ALGORITHMS *(Continued)*

PULSELESS ELECTRICAL ACTIVITY

Fig. 3: Adult algorithm for pulseless electrical activity (PEA) (electromechanical dissociation [EMD]).

PEA includes:

- Electromechanical dissociation (EMD)
- Pseudo-EMD
- Idioventricular rhythms
- Ventricular escape rhythms
- Bradyasystolic rhythms
- Postdefibrillation idioventricular rhythms

- Continue CPR
- Intubate at once
- Obtain I.V. access
- Assess blood flow using Doppler ultrasound

↓

Consider possible causes (Parentheses = possible therapies and treatments)

- Hypovolemia (volume infusion)
- Hypoxia (ventilation)
- Cardiac tamponade (pericardiocentesis)
- Tension pneumothorax (needle decompression)
- Hypothermia
- Massive pulmonary embolism (surgery, **thrombolytics**)
- Drug overdoses such as tricyclics, digitalis, beta blockers, calcium channel blockers
- Hyperkalemia*
- Acidosis†
- Massive acute myocardial infarction

↓

Epinephrine 1 mg I.V. push*‡, repeat every 3-5 min

↓

- If absolute bradycardia (<60 beats/min) or relative bradycardia, give **atropine** 1 mg I.V.
- Repeat every 3-5 min up to a total of 0.04 mg/kg§

Class I: Definitely helpful
Class IIa: Acceptable, probably helpful
Class IIb: Acceptable, possibly helpful
Class III: Not indicated, may be harmful

* **Sodium bicarbonate** 1 mEq/kg is Class I if patient has known pre-existing hyperkalemia

† **Sodium bicarbonate** 1 mEq/kg:

Class IIa
- If known pre-existing bicarbonate-responsive acidosis
- If overdose with tricyclic antidepressants
- To alkalinize the urine in drug overdoses

Class IIb
- If intubated and long arrest interval
- Upon return of spontaneous circulation after long arrest interval

Class III
- Hypoxic lactic acidosis

‡ The recommended dose of **epinephrine** is 1 mg I.V. push every 3-5 min. If this approach fails, several Class IIb dosing regimens can be considered.
- Intermediate: **Epinephrine** 2-5 mg I.V. push every 3-5 min
- Escalating: **Epinephrine** 1 mg-3 mg-5 mg I.V. push (3 min apart)
- High: **Epinephrine** 0.1 mg/kg I.V. push every 3-5 min

§ Shorter **atropine** dosing intervals are possibly helpful in cardiac arrest (Class IIb)

ADULT ACLS ALGORITHMS *(Continued)*

ASYSTOLE

Fig. 4: Adult asystole treatment algorithm.

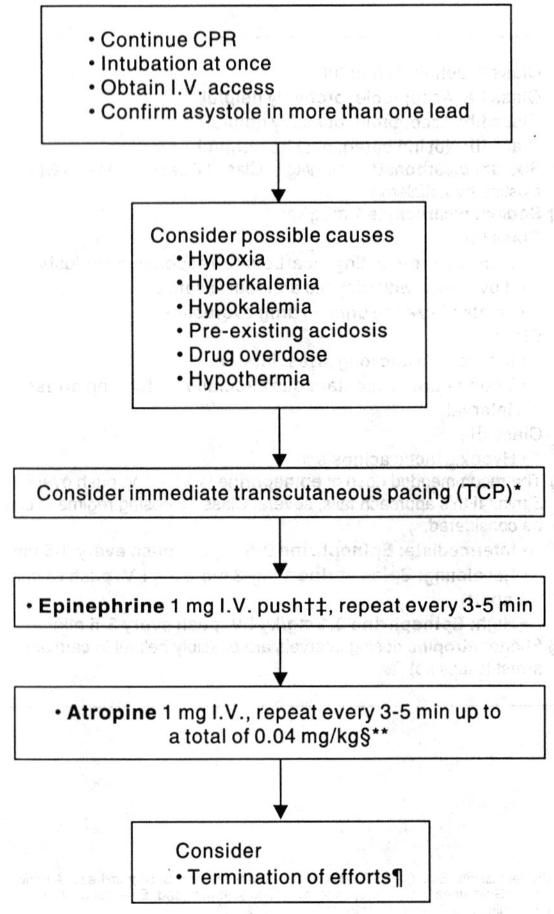

Class I: Definitely helpful
Class IIa: Acceptable, probably helpful
Class IIb: Acceptable, possibly helpful
Class III: Not indicated, may be harmful

* TCP is a Class IIb intervention. Lack of success may be due to delays in pacing. To be effective, TCP must be performed early, simultaneously with drugs. Evidence does not support routine use of TCP for asystole.

† The recommended dose of **epinephrine** is 1 mg I.V. push every 3-5 min. If this approach fails, several Class IIb dosing regimens can be considered:

- Intermediate: **Epinephrine** 2-5 mg I.V. push every 3-5 min
- Escalating: **Epinephrine** 1 mg-3 mg-5 mg I.V. push (3 min apart)
- High: **Epinephrine** 0.1 mg/kg I.V. push every 3-5 mim

‡ **Sodium bicarbonate** 1 mEq/kg is Class I if patient has known pre-existing hyperkalemia

§ Shorter **atropine** dosing intervals are Class IIb in asystolic arrest

****Sodium bicarbonate** 1 mEq/kg:

Class IIa
- If known pre-existing bicarbonate responsive acidosis
- If overdose with tricyclic antidepressants
- To alkalinize the urine in drug overdoses

Class IIb
- If intubated and continued long arrest interval
- Upon return of spontaneous circulation after long arrest interval

Class III
- Hypoxic lactic acidosis

¶ If patient remains in asystole or other agonal rhythms after successful intubation and initial medications and no reversible causes are identified, consider termination of resuscitative efforts by a physician. Consider interval since arrest.

ADULT ACLS ALGORITHMS *(Continued)*

TACHYCARDIA

Fig. 5: Adult tachycardia algorithm.

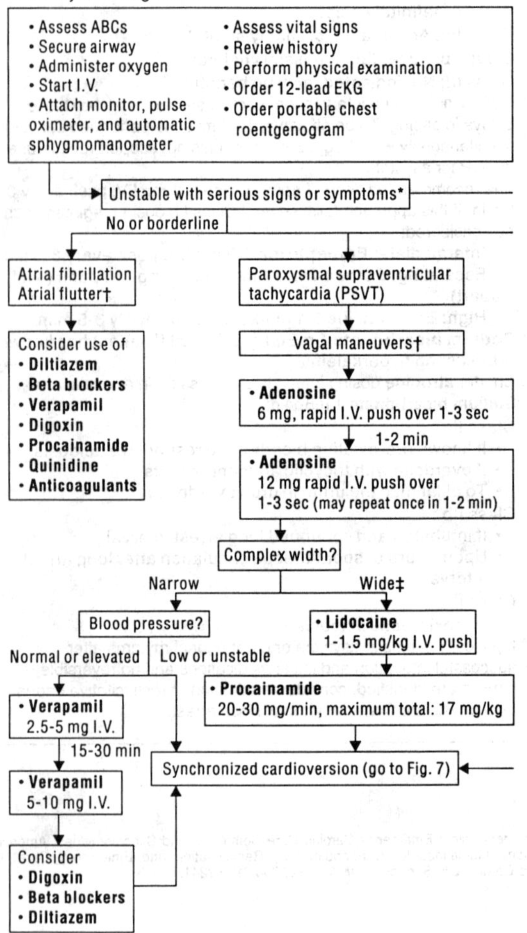

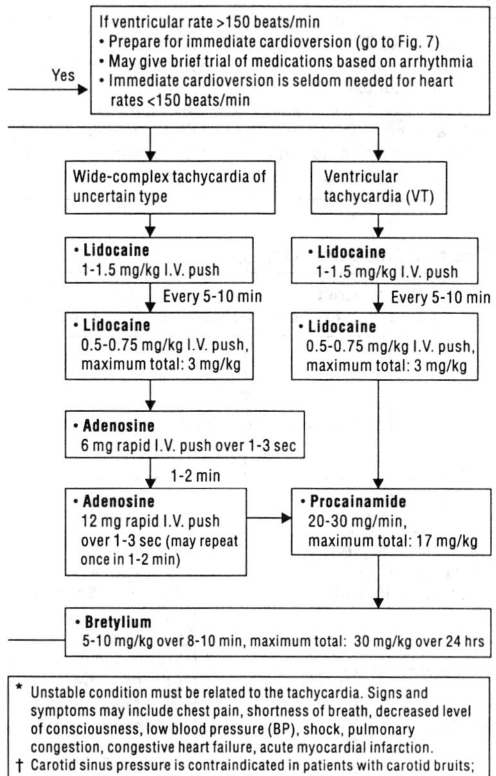

* Unstable condition must be related to the tachycardia. Signs and symptoms may include chest pain, shortness of breath, decreased level of consciousness, low blood pressure (BP), shock, pulmonary congestion, congestive heart failure, acute myocardial infarction.

† Carotid sinus pressure is contraindicated in patients with carotid bruits; avoid ice water immersion in patients with ischemic heart disease.

‡ If the wide-complex tachycardia is known with certainty to be PSVT and BP is normal/elevated, sequence can include **verapamil.**

Used with permission: Emergency Cardiac Care Committee and Subcommittees, American Heart Association, "Guidelines for Cardiopulmonary Resuscitation and Emergency Care, III: Adult Advanced Cardiac Life Support," *JAMA*, 1992, 268:2199-2241.

ADULT ACLS ALGORITHMS *(Continued)*

BRADYCARDIA

Fig. 6: Adult bradycardia algorithm (with the patient not in cardiac arrest).

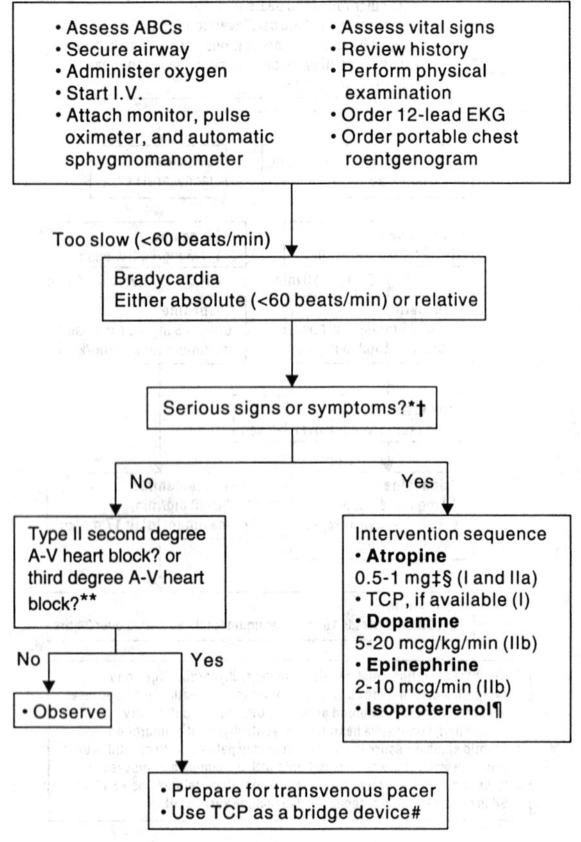

* Serious signs or symptoms must be related to the slow rate. Clinical manifestations include:
Symptoms (chest pain, shortness of breath, decreased level of consciousness), and
Signs (low BP, shock, pulmonary congestion, CHF, acute MI)

† Do not delay TCP while awaiting I.V. access or for **atropine** to take effect if patient is symptomatic.

‡ Denervated transplanted hearts will not respond to **atropine**. Go at once to pacing, **catecholamine** infusion, or both.

§ **Atropine** should be given in repeat doses in 3-5 min up to a total of 0.04 mg/kg. Consider shorter dosing intervals in severe clinical conditions. It has been suggested that atropine should be used with caution in atrioventricular (A-V) block at the His-Purkinje level (type II A-V block and new third degree block with wide QRS complexes) (Class IIb).

** Never treat third degree heart block plus ventricular escape beats with **lidocaine.**

¶ **Isoproterenol** should be used, if at all, with extreme caution. At low doses it is Class IIb (possibly helpful); at higher doses it is Class III (harmful).

Verify patient tolerance and mechanical capture. Use analgesia and sedation as needed.

Used with permission: Emergency Cardiac Care Committee and Subcommittees, American Heart Association, "Guidelines for Cardiopulmonary Resuscitation and Emergency Care, III: Adult Advanced Cardiac Life Support," *JAMA*, 1992, 268:2199-2241.

ADULT ACLS ALGORITHMS *(Continued)*

ELECTRICAL CONVERSION

Fig. 7: Adult electrical cardioversion algorithm (with the patient not in cardiac arrest).

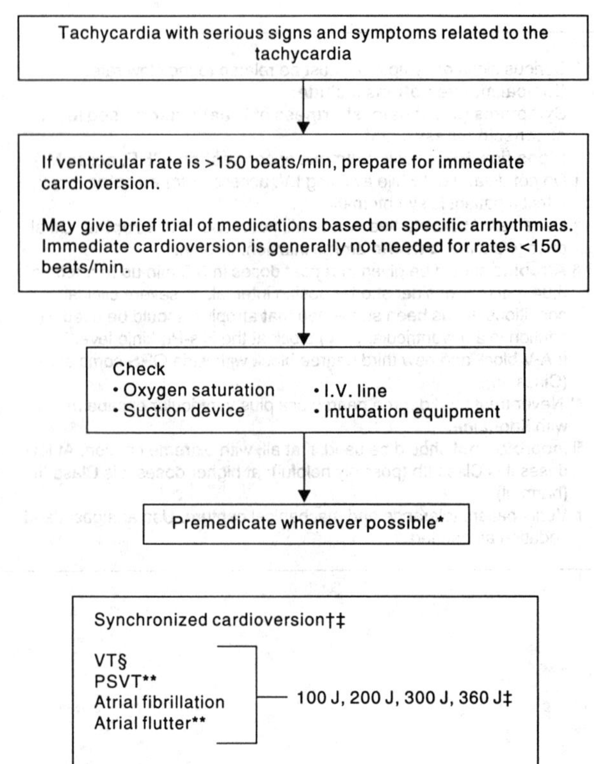

* Effective regimens have included a sedative (eg, **diazepam, midazolam, barbiturates, etomidate, ketamine, methohexital**) with or without an analgesic agent (eg, **fentanyl, morphine, meperidine**). Many experts recommend anesthesia if service is readily available.
† Note possible need to resynchronize after each cardioversion.
‡ If delays in synchronization occur and clinical conditions are critical, go to immediate unsynchronized shocks.
§ Treat polymorphic VT (irregular form and rate) like VF: 200 J, 200-300 J, 360 J.
**PSVT and atrial flutter often respond to lower energy levels (start with 50 J).

Used with permission: Emergency Cardiac Care Committee and Subcommittees, American Heart Association, "Guidelines for Cardiopulmonary Resuscitation and Emergency Care, III: Adult Advanced Cardiac Life Support," *JAMA*, 1992, 268:2199-2241.

ADULT ACLS ALGORITHMS *(Continued)*

HYPOTENSION, SHOCK

Fig. 8: Adult algorithm for hypotension, shock, and acute pulmonary edema.

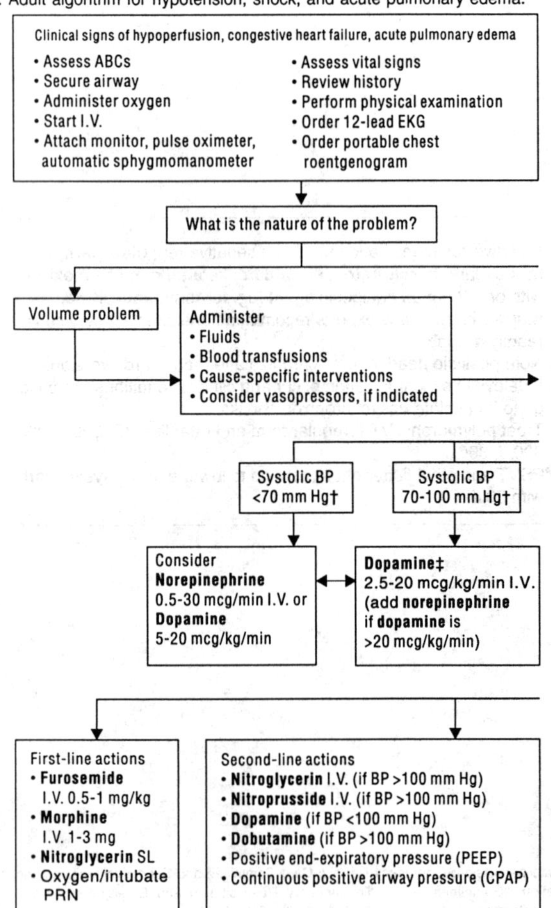

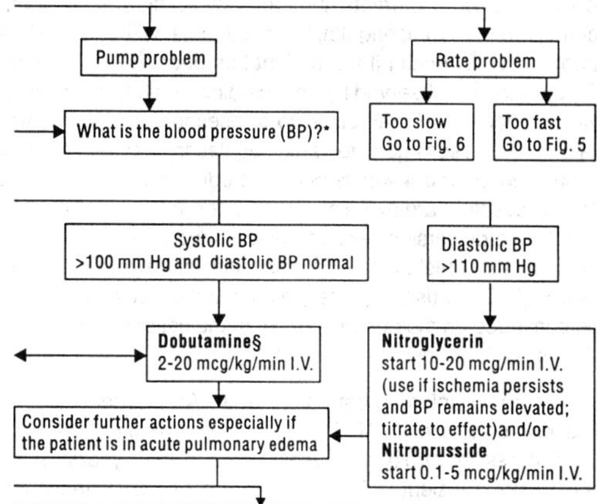

Third-line actions

- **Amrinone** 0.75 mg/kg then 5-15 mcg/kg/min (if other drugs fail)
- **Aminophylline** 5 mg/kg (if wheezing)
- **Thrombolytic** therapy (if not in shock)
- **Digoxin** (if atrial fibrillation, supraventricular tachycardias)
- Angioplasty (if drugs fail)
- Intra-aortic balloon pump (bridge to surgery)
- Surgical interventions (valves, coronary artery bypass grafts, heart transplant)

* Base management after this point on invasive hemodynamic monitoring if possible.
† Fluid bolus of 250-500 mL normal saline should be tried. If no response, consider sympathomimetics.
‡ Move to dopamine and stop **norepinephrine** when BP improves.
§ Add **dopamine** when BP improves. Avoid **dobutamine** when systolic BP <100 mm Hg.

Used with permission: Emergency Cardiac Care Committee and Subcommittees, American Heart Association, "Guidelines for Cardiopulmonary Resuscitation and Emergency Care, III: Adult Advanced Cardiac Life Support," *JAMA*, 1992, 268:2199-2241.

ANTICOAGULATION

This section focuses on treatment of atrial fibrillation and management of patients with prosthetic valves.

ATRIAL FIBRILLATION (AF)

The goal of anticoagulation in patients with AF is to prevent stroke and thromboembolic events and to promote thrombus dissolution, if present, prior to elective cardioversion. Anticoagulation in patients with atrial fibrillation is required prior to cardioversion if the patient has been in AF for more than 48 hours or if a thrombus is observed by echocardiography. Patients with a longer or unknown duration of AF may undergo transesophageal echocardiography (TEE) to aid in the assessment for anticoagulation therapy. Anticoagulation therapy is maintained for 3-4 weeks prior to cardioversion and continued for 4 weeks after successful cardioversion. It is important that anticoagulation be maintained after cardioversion because even though the atrium is electrically in sinus rhythm, the mechanical force is diminished and the likelihood of clotting is still high. Obviously, if there are other indications for anticoagulation, it should be continued. In the absence of contraindications, daily aspirin should be started after warfarin therapy is completed.

The need for chronic antithrombotic therapy in AF depends on patient risk factors. The risk of stroke in AF is approximately 6 times that of patients without AF. The risk for stroke increases with age (>60 years); if the patient has had a previous transient ischemic attack, stroke, or systemic embolus; if the patient has hypertension (treated or untreated); or with poor ventricular function, rheumatic mitral valve disease, or a prosthetic heart valve. These risk factors should be considered when deciding on the intensity of oral anticoagulation or when prescribing chronic antithrombotic therapy (see table). Patients with diabetes, coronary artery disease, or thyrotoxicosis are at a high risk for stroke. Patients with chronic or paroxysmal AF should be on chronic antithrombotic therapy. Warfarin (INR 2.0-3.0) and aspirin (325 mg daily) are considered first-line therapies for the prophylaxis of thromboembolic events in AF.

Recommendations for Atrial Fibrillation

Risk Factors*	Age	Recommended Therapy
None	<65 y	Aspirin
None	65-75 y	Aspirin or warfarin
≥1	<65 to 75 y	Warfarin
None or ≥1	>75 y	Warfarin

*Risk factors: Prior TIA or stroke, systemic embolus, hypertension (treated or untreated), poor left ventricular function, rheumatic mitral valve disease, or prosthetic heart valve.

Heparin Therapy

Heparin therapy may be initially started to anticoagulate patients with AF. Therapy may be switched to warfarin therapy on the first day if a therapeutic aPTT can be achieved. The aPTT should be evaluated at baseline and every 6 hours following the start of heparin therapy or if dosage adjustments are made. The optimal dose of heparin is achieved when aPTT is maintained between 1.5-2.5 times the patient's baseline aPPT.

Warfarin Therapy

The target INR range for warfarin therapy in AF is 2.0-3.0. Patients with mechanical heart valves may require a higher range (see below). Patients should **not** receive loading doses of warfarin (ie, 10 mg daily for 3 days then 5 mg daily) as the steady-state INR is not achieved more quickly. The intensity of anticoagulation therapy should be monitored closely until the patient has reached a stable PT/INR. Once the patient is stabilized on a fixed dose of warfarin, the PT/INR can be monitored on a monthly basis if the patient demonstrates a stable PT/INR on chronic therapy. If dosage adjustments are made, PT/INR should be evaluated in approximately 2 weeks. Supratherapeutic INR values are managed based on the presence and severity of bleeding (see table). Patients on warfarin should be warned to seek medical evaluation if they develop a very severe headache, abdominal pain, unusual bleeding, backache, or if they experience significant trauma, particularly head injuries.

Management of Supratherapeutic INR

INR	Patient Situation	Action
>3 and ≤5	No bleeding or need for rapid reversal (ie, no need for surgery)	Omit next few warfarin dose and/or restart at lower dose when INR approaches desired range. If only minimally above range, then no dosage reduction may be required.
>5 and <9.0	No bleeding or need for rapid reversal	Omit next 1-2 doses, monitor INR more frequently, and restart at lower dose when INR approaches target range **or** omit dose and give 1-2.5 mg vitamin K orally (use this if patient has risk factors for bleeding).
	No bleeding but reversal needed for surgery or dental extraction within 24 hours	Vitamin K 2-4 mg orally (expected reversal within 24 hours); give additional 1-2 mg if INR remains high at 24 hours.
>9.0 and <20.0	No bleeding	Stop warfarin, give vitamin K 3-5 mg orally; follow INR closely; repeat vitamin K if needed. Reassess need and dose of warfarin when INR approaches desirable range.
Rapid reversal required (ie, INR >20)	Serious bleeding or major warfarin overdose	Stop warfarin, give vitamin K 10 mg by slow I.V. infusion. May repeat vitamin K every 12 hours and give fresh plasma transfusion or prothrombin complex concentrate as needed. When appropriate, heparin can be given until the patient becomes responsive to warfarin.

ANTICOAGULATION *(Continued)*

Warfarin Interactions

Intensity of warfarin anticoagulation is affected by foods high in vitamin K, alcohol, diseases such as congestive heart failure, and by concomitant drug therapy. Drugs that inhibit or induce P-450 2C9 isoenzyme will have the greatest effect on INR (see following table). It is important to note that just as the therapeutic effect of warfarin requires several days to become apparent, treatment with vitamin K may also inhibit the effects of warfarin for several days. Foods high in vitamin K decrease PT/INR and include green leafy vegetables (eg, kale, broccoli, spinach, parsley, collard greens). Acute alcohol consumption can increase PT/INR while chronic ingestion can decrease PT/INR. Drug interactions with warfarin may occur by several mechanisms, including impairment of absorption, induction or inhibition of metabolism, competition for protein-binding sites, and platelet inhibition. Drugs that inhibit or induce P-450 2C9 (responsible for metabolism of S-warfarin) may have the greatest effect on INR. Select and important drug-drug interactions are depicted in the following table.

Selected Warfarin Drug Interactions

Drug	Effect on P-450	Isoenzyme		
		1A2	2C9	3A4
Amiodarone	Inhibit		X	X
Carbamazepine	Induce		X	X
Ciprofloxacin	Inhibit	X		
Cimetidine	Inhibit	X		
Dicloxacillin	Induce			
Erythromycin	Inhibit	X		X
Fluconazole	Inhibit		X	X
Metronidazole	Inhibit		X	
Nafcillin	Induce			
Omeprazole	Inhibit			X
Phenobarbital	Induce	X	X	X
Phenytoin	Induce	X	X	X
Rifampin	Induce	X	X	X
SSRI	Inhibit	X		
TMP/SMX (Bactrim®)	Inhibit		X	
Zileuton	Inhibit	X		
Zafirlukast	Inhibit		X	

PROSTHETIC HEART VALVES

Patients with mechanical prosthetic valves require life-long anticoagulation therapy. The optimal intensity of anticoagulation is not established. The risk of thromboembolism is greater in valve patients who have atrial fibrillation (AF); have an enlarged left atrium (>5.5 cm); have a history of systemic embolism, left ventricular systolic dysfunction, coronary artery disease, left atrial thrombus; have ball valve; or have more than one mechanical valve. The risk for thromboembolism is also higher for mechanical valves in the mitral position compared to aortic. These factors should be weighed in each patient before deciding the desired level of anticoagulation to prevent thromboembolism and to avoid bleeding complications. Ranges for anticoagulation intensity in patients with prosthetic valves are described in the following table.

Prosthetic Valves

Valve Location	Type	Recommended INR / Therapy
Mechanical	Mitral - bileaflet or tilting disk	2.5-3.5 or 2.0-3.0 plus aspirin 80-100 mg daily
	Mitral - cage disk or ball	2.5-3.5 plus aspirin (80-100 mg daily)
	Aortic - bileaflet (eg, St Jude, CarboMedics)	2.0-3.0 if normal left ventricular function, left atrial size, and sinus rhythm 2.5-3.5 or 2.0-3.0 plus aspirin (80-100 mg daily) if AF and high-risk patients
	Mitral or aortic valve and history of systemic embolism despite adequate warfarin therapy	2.5-3.5 plus aspirin 80-100 mg daily
Bioprosthetic	Mitral or aortic	2.0-3.0 for 3 months after insertion or indefinitely if patient has AF; left atrial thrombus or permanent pacemaker, duration uncertain; prior systemic embolism, duration of therapy should be increased to 3-12 months; chronic low-dose aspirin therapy (≤160 mg daily) after warfarin therapy

As a general rule, concomitant warfarin and aspirin therapy should be avoided, except in special situations. For patients with mechanical prosthetic valves who suffer a systemic thromboembolism despite adequate anticoagulation therapy, low-dose aspirin should be added and the INR should be maintained between 2.5 and 3.5. The combination of warfarin and low-dose aspirin in all mechanical valve patients is uncertain; patients at the highest risk for thromboembolism should be considered. For patients who cannot tolerate aspirin, dypyridamole 150 mg daily may be combined with warfarin therapy.

Resources

Guidelines

Proceedings of the American College of Chest Physicians – 5th Consensus Conference on Antithrombotic Therapy, *Chest*, 1998, 114(5 Suppl):439S-769S.

Drug Therapy

Albers GW, Yim JM, Belew KM, et al, "Status of Antithrombotic Therapy for Patients With Atrial Fibrillation in University Hospitals," *Arch Intern Med*, 1996, 156:2311-6.

Connolly SJ, Laupacis A, Gent M, et al, The CAFA Study Co-Investigators. Canadian Atrial Fibrillation Anticoagulation (CAFA) Study, *J Am Coll Cardiol*, 1991, 18:349-55.

Crowther MA, Ginsberg JB, Kearon C, et al, "A Randomized Trial Comparing 5 mg and 10 mg Warfarin Loading Doses," *Arch Intern Med*, 1999, 159:46-8.

EAFT Study Group, "European Atrial Fibrillation Trial: Secondary Prevention of Vascular Events in Patients With Nonrheumatic Atrial Fibrillation and a Recent Transient Ischaemic Attack or Minor Ischaemic Stroke," *Lancet*, 1993, 342:1255-62.

Eckman MH, Falk RH, and Pauker SG, "Cost-Effectiveness of Therapies for Patients With Nonvalvular Atrial Fibrillation," *Arch Intern Med*, 1998, 158:1669-77.

Ezekowitz MD, Bridgers SL, James KE, et al, "Warfarin in the Prevention of Stroke Associated With Nonrheumatic Atrial Fibrillation," *N Engl J Med*, 1992, 327:1406-12.

Gullov AL, Koefoed BG, and Petersen P, "Bleeding During Warfarin and Aspirin Therapy in Patients With Atrial Fibrillation: The AFASAK 2 Study," *Arch Intern Med*, 1999, 159(12):1322-8.

Gullov AL, Koefoed BG, Petersen P, et al, "Fixed Minidose Warfarin and Aspirin Alone and in Combination vs Adjusted-Dose Warfarin for Stroke Prevention in Atrial Fibrillation: Second Copenhagen Atrial Fibrillation, Aspirin, and Anticoagulation Study," *Arch Intern Med*, 1998, 158:1513-21.

Petersen P, Boysen G, Godtfredsen J, et al, "Placebo-Controlled, Randomised Trial of Warfarin and Aspirin for Prevention of Thromboembolic Complications in Chronic Atrial Fibrillation: The Copenhagen AFASAK Study," *Lancet*, 1989, 1:175-8.

ANTICOAGULATION *(Continued)*

Stroke Prevention in Atrial Fibrillation Investigators, "Stroke Prevention in Atrial Fibrillation Study: Final Results," *Circulation*, 1991, 84:527-39.

Stroke Prevention in Atrial Fibrillation Investigators, "Warfarin Versus Aspirin for Prevention of Thromboembolism in Atrial Fibrillation: Stroke Prevention in Atrial Fibrillation II Study," *Lancet*, 1994, 343:687-91.

The Boston Area Anticoagulation Trial for Atrial Fibrillation Investigators, "The Effect of Low-Dose Warfarin on the Risk of Stroke in Patients With Nonrheumatic Atrial Fibrillation," *N Engl J Med*, 1990, 323:1505-11.

ANTIEMETICS FOR CHEMOTHERAPY-INDUCED NAUSEA AND VOMITING

GENERAL PRINCIPLES FOR MANAGING NAUSEA AND VOMITING

1. Prophylaxis is **much** better than treatment of actual vomiting. For agents with a moderate-to-high (30% to 100%) incidence of nausea, patients should be pretreated with an antiemetic. Depending on the antiemetic agent(s) and route(s) of administration, pretreatment may range from 1 hour to 5 minutes prior to administration of the antineoplastic agent(s).

2. Doses and intervals of the antiemetic regimen need to be individualized for each patient. "PRN" regimens should **not** be used. A fixed schedule of drug administration is preferable.

3. If a patient has had no nausea for 24 hours while on their scheduled antiemetic regimen, it is usually possible to switch to a "PRN" regimen. The patient should be advised to resume the fixed schedule at the **first** sign of recurrent nausea, and continue it until they have had at least 24 hours without nausea.

4. Titrate antiemetic dose to patient tolerance.

5. In most cases, combination regimens are required for optimum control of nausea. Do not be afraid to use two or more agents, from different pharmacologic categories, to achieve optimal results.

6. To the extent possible, avoid duplication of agents from the same pharmacologic category.

7. Anticipatory nausea and vomiting can often be minimized if the patient receives effective prophylaxis against nausea from the first cycle of therapy.

8. If anticipatory nausea does develop, an anxiolytic agent is usually the drug of choice.

9. "If it's not broken - **don't** fix it!" Regardless of your own preferences, if the patient's current antiemetic regimen is working, don't change it.

10. For moderately emetogenic regimens, a steroid and dopamine blocker (eg, metoclopramide, prochlorperazine, thiethylperazine) may be the most cost-effective regimen.

11. For highly emetogenic regimens, a steroid and serotonin receptor blocker (eg, dolasetron, granisetron, ondansetron) combination is the preferred regimen.

12. A dopamine blocker (eg, metoclopramide, prochlorperazine, thiethylperazine) is a good first alternative if the serotonin blocker fails.

13. Although most nausea or vomiting develops within the first 24 hours after treatment, delayed reactions (1-7 days after chemotherapy) are not uncommon.

14. Other antiemetics (eg, cannabinoids, antihistamines, or anticholinergics) have limited use as initial therapy. They are best used in combination with more effective agents (steroids, dopamine, or serotonin blockers); or, as second- or third-line therapy.

15. Serotonin blockers are most effective in scheduled prophylactic regimens; rather than in "PRN" regimens to chase existing vomiting.

16. The serotonin blockers appear to have a "ceiling" dose, above which there is little or no added antiemetic effect.

ANTIEMETICS FOR CHEMOTHERAPY-INDUCED NAUSEA AND VOMITING *(Continued)*

Time Course of Nausea and Vomiting

Drug	Onset (h)	Duration (h)
Azacitidine	1-3	3-4
Carboplatin	2-6	1-48
Carmustine	2-6	4-6
Cisplatin	1-4	12-96
Cyclophosphamide	6-8	8-24
Cytarabine	1-3	3-8
Dacarbazine	1-2	2-4
Dactinomycin	2-5	4-24
Daunorubicin	1-3	4-24
Doxorubicin	1-3	4-24
Ifosfamide	2-3	12-72
Lomustine	2-6	4-6
Mechlorethamine	1-3	2-8
Mitomycin	1-2	48-72
Plicamycin	4-6	4-24
Procarbazine	24-27	Variable
Streptozocin	1-3	1-12

Emetogenic Potential of Single Chemotherapeutic Agents

Very High (>90%)

Cisplatin
Cytarabine (>2 g)
Dacarbazine
Didemnin-B
JM-216
Mechlorethamine
Melphalan (I.V.)
Streptozocin

High (60% to 90%)

Aldesleukin
Amifostine
Carmustine
Cyclophosphamide (>1 g)
Cytarabine (<2 g)
Dactinomycin
Elsamitrucin
Estramustine
Etoposide
Hydroxyurea
Idarubicin
Irinotecan
Lomustine
Mitotane
Mitomycin
Mitoxantrone
Semustine
Toremifene
Tretinoin

Moderate (30% to 60%)

Altretamine
Amonafide
Amsacrine
Asparaginase
Azacytidine
Carboplatin
Cladribine
Cyclophosphamide (<1 g)
Daunorubicin
Dexrazocane
Diazequone
Docetaxel
Doxorubicin
Epirubicin
Ifosfamide
Interferons
Interleukin-6
Mitoguazone
PALA
Pegaspergase
Pentostatin
Plicamycin
Procarbazine
Teniposide
Tomudex
Topotecan
Trimetrexate
Vinblastine
Vinorelbine

Low (10% to 30%)

Floxuridine
Fluorouracil
Flutamide
Gemcitabine
Levamisole
Melphalan (oral)
Methotrexate (high dose)
Steroids
Suramin
Tamoxifen
Thioguanine
Vindesine

Very Low (<10%)

Androgens
Aminoglutethimide
Anastrozole
Bicalutamide
Bleomycin
Busulfan
Chlorambucil
Estrogens
Fludarabine
Goserelin
Homoharringtonine
Leucovorin
Leuprolide
Megestrol
Mercaptopurine
Mesna
Methotrexate (low dose)
Paclitaxel
Thiotepa
Vincristine

Drugs With a High Incidence but Low Severity of Nausea/Vomiting

Amonafide
Carboplatin
Cyclophosphamide (<1 g)
Dexrazoxane
Docetaxel
Gemcitabine
Hydroxyurea
Interferons
Mitoguazone
Mitoxantrone
Tretinoin
Vinblastine

Drugs With a Low Incidence but High Severity of Nausea/Vomiting

Lomustine
Methotrexate (high dose)
Semustine

Potency of Antiemetic Drugs

Potency	Type of Antiemetic Drug
Active against highly emetogenic chemotherapy	Serotonin antagonist Substituted benzamide (high dose)
Active against mildly or moderately emetogenic chemotherapy	Butyrophenone Cannabinoid Corticosteroid Phenothiazine
Minimally active	Anticholinergic agent Antihistamine Benzodiazepine

REPRESENTATIVE ANTIEMETIC REGIMENS

Highly emetogenic chemotherapy

Dexamethasone 10-20 mg P.O. or I.V. + a serotonin antagonist daily 15-30 minutes before treatment on each day of chemotherapy

Recommended serotonin antagonist regimens:
- Dolasetron 100 mg P.O. once daily
- Granisetron 2 mg P.O. once daily
- Granisetron 1 mg P.O. every 12 hours
- Granisetron 10 mcg/kg I.V. once daily
- Granisetron 1 mg I.V. once daily
- Ondansetron 0.45 mg/kg I.V. once daily
- Ondansetron 24-32 mg I.V. once daily
- Ondansetron 0.15 mg/kg I.V. every 8 hours
- Ondansetron 8-10 mg I.V. every 8 hours

For continuous infusion therapy, carboplatin, and high-dose (>1 g/m^2) cyclophosphamide regimens, the following regimen may be preferred:

Dexamethasone 10 mg P.O. or I.V. + a serotonin antagonist every 12 hours

Recommended serotonin antagonist regimens:
- Granisetron 1 mg P.O.
- Granisetron 10 mcg/kg I.V.
- Ondansetron 10-16 mg I.V.
- Ondansetron 16-24 mg P.O.

Moderately emetogenic chemotherapy:

Dexamethasone 10 mg P.O. or I.V. + a serotonin antagonist daily 15-30 minutes before treatment on each day of chemotherapy

Recommended serotonin antagonist regimens:
- Granisetron 1 mg P.O. once daily
- Ondansetron 16 mg P.O. once daily
- Ondansetron 8-10 mg I.V. once daily

For continuous infusion therapy, the following regimen may be preferred:

ANTIEMETICS FOR CHEMOTHERAPY-INDUCED NAUSEA AND VOMITING *(Continued)*

Dexamethasone 4 mg P.O. or I.V. + ondansetron 8 mg P.O. or I.V. every 12 hours on each day of chemotherapy

Mildly emetogenic chemotherapy (all agents are given 15-30 minutes before treatment, and may be repeated every 4-6 hours if necessary. With the exceptions of dexamethasone (given over 5-15 minutes) and droperidol (given by I.V. push), intravenous doses should be given over 30 minutes.):

Dexamethasone 4 mg P.O./I.V./I.M.

Droperidol 1.25-5 mg I.M./I.V. push

Haloperidol 2 mg P.O./I.V./I.M.

Metoclopramide 30 mg P.O./I.V./I.M.

Prochlorperazine 10-20 mg P.O./I.V./I.M.

Thiethylperazine 10-20 mg P.O./I.V./I.M.

Delayed nausea and vomiting:

Dexamethasone + a dopamine or serotonin antagonist. Therapy should start within 12-24 hours of administration of the emetogenic chemotherapy.

Recommended regimens:

Dexamethasone

8 mg P.O. every 12 hours for 2 days, then 4 mg P.O. every 12 hours for 2 days **or**

20 mg P.O. 1 hour before chemotherapy; 10 mg P.O. 12 hours after chemotherapy, then 8 mg P.O. every 12 hours for 4 doses, then 4 mg P.O. every 12 hours for 4 doses

Recommended dopamine/serotonin antagonist regimens:

Droperidol 1.25-2.5 mg I.V./I.M. every 4 hours for 4 days

Metoclopramide 0.5 mg/kg P.O. every 6 hours for 4 days

Ondansetron 8 mg P.O. every 8 hours for 4 days

Prochlorperazine 10 mg P.O. every 6 hours for 4 days

Prochlorperazine 15 mg (sustained release) P.O. 1 hour before chemotherapy, then every 12 hours for 5 doses

Thiethylperazine 10 mg P.O. every 6 hours for 4 days

Recommended Doses of Serotonin ($5HT_3$) Antiemetics Prophylaxis of Acute Highly Emetogenic Chemotherapy-Induced Nausea/Vomiting

ASCO	ASHP	NCCN	MASCC
Dolasetron			
100 mg P.O.	100-200 mg P.O.	100 mg P.O.	100-200 mg P.O.
1.8 mg/kg* I.V.	1.8 mg/kg* I.V.	1.8 mg/kg* I.V.	1.8 mg/kg I.V.
Granisetron			
2 mg P.O.	2 mg P.O.	2 mg P.O.†	2 mg P.O.
10 mcg/kg‡ I.V	10 mcg/kg I.V.	10 mcg/kg§ I.V.	10 mcg/kg I.V.
Ondansetron			
12-24 mg P.O.	24 mg P.O.	8 mg P.O. bid	12-16 mg P.O.
8 mg I.V.¶	8 mg I.V.	8 mg I.V.#	8 mg I.V.

*Or 100 mg

†Or 100 mg

‡Or 1 mg

§Maximum: 1 mg

¶Or 0.15 mg/kg

#Maximum: 32 mg/24 hours

ASTHMA

Expert Panel Report II: Guidelines for the Diagnosis and Management of Asthma

Stepwise Approach for Managing Asthma in Adults and Children >5 Years of Age: Classify Severity

Goals of Asthma Treatment

- Prevent chronic and troublesome symptoms (eg, coughing or breathlessness in the night, in the early morning, or after exertion)
- Maintain (near) "normal" pulmonary function
- Maintain normal activity levels (ie, exercise and other physical activity)
- Prevent recurrent exacerbations of asthma and minimize the need for emergency department visits or hospitalizations
- Provide optimal pharmacotherapy with minimal or no adverse effects
- Meet patients' and families' expectations of and satisfaction with asthma care

Clinical Features Before Treatment*

Symptoms**	Night-time Symptoms	Lung Function
	STEP 4: Severe Persistent	
• Continual symptoms • Limited physical activity • Frequent exacerbations	Frequent	• FEV_1/PEF ≤60% predicted • PEF variability >30%
	STEP 3: Moderate Persistent	
• Daily symptoms • Daily use of inhaled short-acting $beta_2$-agonist • Exacerbations affect activity • Exacerbations ≥2 times/week may last days	>1 time/week	• FEV_1/PEF >60% - <80% predicted • PEF variability >30%
	STEP 2: Mild Persistent	
• Symptoms >2 times/week but <1 time/day • Exacerbations may affect activity	>2 times/month	• FEV_1/PEF ≥80% predicted • PEF variability 20% - 30%
	STEP 1: Mild Intermittent	
• Symptoms ≤2 times/week • Asymptomatic and normal PEF between exacerbations • Exacerbations brief (from a few hours to a few days); intensity may vary	≤2 times/month	• FEV_1/PEF ≥80% predicted • PEF variability ≤20%

*The presence of one of the features of severity is sufficient to place a patient in that category. An individual should be assigned to the most severe grade in which any feature occurs. The characteristics noted in this figure are general and may overlap because asthma is highly variable. Furthermore, an individual's classification may change over time.

**Patients at any level of severity can have mild, moderate, or severe exacerbations. Some patients with intermittent asthma experience severe and life-threatening exacerbations separated by long periods of normal lung function and no symptoms.

ASTHMA *(Continued)*

Stepwise Approach for Managing Infants and Young Children (≤5 Years of Age) With Acute or Chronic Asthma Symptoms

Long-Term Control	Quick Relief
STEP 4: Severe Persistent	
Daily anti-inflammatory medicine • High-dose inhaled corticosteroid with spacer/holding chamber and face mask • If needed, add systemic corticosteroids 2 mg/kg/day and reduce to lowest daily or alternate-day dose that stabilizes symptoms	• Bronchodilator as needed for symptoms (see step 1) up to 3 times/day
STEP 3: Moderate Persistent	
Daily anti-inflammatory medication. Either: • Medium-dose inhaled corticosteroid with spacer/holding chamber and face mask **or** Once control is established: • Medium-dose inhaled corticosteroid and nedocromil **or** • Medium-dose inhaled corticosteroid and long-acting bronchodilator (theophylline)	• Bronchodilator as needed for symptoms (see step 1) up to 3 times/day
STEP 2: Mild Persistent	
Daily anti-inflammatory medication. Either: • Cromolyn (nebulizer is preferred; or MDI) or nedocromil (MDI only) tid-qid • Infants and young children usually begin with a trial of cromolyn or nedocromil **or** • Low-dose inhaled corticosteroid with spacer/holding chamber and face mask	• Bronchodilator as needed for symptoms (see step 1)
STEP 1: Mild Intermittent	
No daily medication needed	• Bronchodilator as needed for symptoms <2 times/week. Intensity of treatment will depend upon severity of exacerbation (see "Managing Exacerbations"). Either: – Inhaled short-acting beta$_2$-agonist by nebulizer or face mask and spacer/holding chamber **or** – Oral beta$_2$-agonist for symptoms • With viral respiratory infection: – Bronchodilator q4-6h up to 24 hours (longer with physician consult) but, in general, repeat no more than once every 6 weeks – Consider systemic corticosteroid if current exacerbation is severe **or** Patient has history of previous severe exacerbations
↓ **Step Down** Review treatment every 1-6 months. If control is sustained for at least 3 months, a gradual stepwise reduction in treatment may be possible.	↑ **Step Up** If control is not achieved, consider step up. First: review patient medication technique, adherence, and environmental control (avoidance of allergens or other precipitant factors)

Notes:

- **The stepwise approach presents guidelines to assist clinical decision making. Asthma is highly variable; clinicians should tailor specific medication plans to the needs and circumstances of individual patients.**
- Gain control as quickly as possible; then decrease treatment to the least medication necessary to maintain control. Gaining control may be accomplished by either starting treatment at the step most appropriate to the initial severity of their condition or by starting at a higher level of therapy (eg, a course of systemic corticosteroids or higher dose of inhaled corticosteroids).
- A rescue course of systemic corticosteroid (prednisolone) may be needed at any time and step.
- In general, use of short-acting beta$_2$-agonist on a daily basis indicates the need for additional long-term control therapy.
- It is important to remember that there are very few studies on asthma therapy for infants.

- Consultation with an asthma specialist is recommended for patients with moderate or severe persistent asthma in this age group. Consider consultation for all patients with mild persistent asthma.

Stepwise Approach for Managing Asthma in Adults and Children >5 Years of Age: Treatment

(Preferred treatments are in **bold** print)

Long-Term Control	Quick Relief	Education
	STEP 4: Severe Persistent	
Daily medications: • **Anti-inflammatory: Inhaled corticosteroid (high dose) and** • Long-acting bronchodilator: Either **long-acting inhaled beta$_2$-agonist**, sustained-release theophylline, or long-acting beta$_2$-agonist tablets **and** • Corticosteroid tablets or syrup long term (2 mg/kg/day, generally do not exceed 60 mg per day).	• Short-acting bronchodilator: **Inhaled beta$_2$-agonists** as needed for symptoms. • Intensity of treatment will depend on severity of exacerbation; see "Managing Exacerbations" • Use of short-acting inhaled beta$_2$-agonists on a daily basis, or increasing use, indicates the need for additional long-term control therapy.	Steps 2 and 3 actions plus: • Refer to individual education/counseling
	STEP 3: Moderate Persistent	
Daily medication: • Either – **Anti-inflammatory: Inhaled corticosteroid (medium dose) or** – **Inhaled corticosteroid (low-medium dose)** and add a long-acting bronchodilator, especially for night-time symptoms: Either **long-acting inhaled beta$_2$-agonist**, sustained-release theophylline, or long-acting beta$_2$-agonist tablets. • If needed – Anti-inflammatory: **Inhaled corticosteroids (medium-high dose) and** – **Long-acting bronchodilator,** especially for nighttime symptoms; either **long-acting inhaled beta$_2$-agonist,** sustained release theophylline, or long-acting beta$_2$-agonist tablets.	• Short-acting bronchodilator: **Inhaled beta$_2$-agonists** as needed for symptoms. • Intensity of treatment will depend on severity of exacerbation; see "Managing Exacerbations." • Use of short-acting inhaled beta$_2$-agonists on a daily basis, or increasing use, indicates the need for additional long-term control therapy.	Step 1 actions plus: • Teach self-monitoring • Refer to group education if available • Review and update self-management plan
	STEP 2: Mild Persistent	
One daily medication: • **Anti-inflammatory:** Either **inhaled corticosteroid** (low doses) or **cromolyn or nedocromil** (children usually begin with a trial of cromolyn or nedocromil). • Sustained-release theophylline to serum concentration of 5-15 mcg/mL is an alternative, but not preferred, therapy. Zafirlukast or zileuton may also be considered for patients ≥12 years of age, although their position in therapy is not fully established.	• Short-acting bronchodilator: **Inhaled beta$_2$-agonists** as needed for symptoms. • Intensity of treatment will depend on severity of exacerbation; see "Managing Exacerbations." •Use of short-acting inhaled beta$_2$-agonists on a daily basis, or increasing use, indicates the need for additional long-term control therapy.	Step 1 actions plus: • Teach self-monitoring • Refer to group education if available • Review and update self-management plan

ASTHMA *(Continued)*

Long-Term Control	Quick Relief	Education
	STEP 1: Mild Intermittent	
No daily medication needed.	• Short-acting bronchodilator: **Inhaled beta$_2$-agonists** as needed for symptoms. • Intensity of treatment will depend on severity of exacerbation; see "Managing Exacerbations" • Use of short-acting inhaled beta$_2$-agonists more than 2 times/ week may indicate the need to initiate long-term control therapy	• Teach basic facts about asthma • Teach inhaler/spacer/ holding chamber technique • Discuss roles of medications •Develop self-management plan • Develop action plan for when and how to take rescue actions, especially for patients with a history of severe exacerbations • Discuss appropriate environmental control measures to avoid exposure to known allergens and irritants

↓ Step down
Review treatment every 1-6 months; a gradual stepwise reduction in treatment may be possible.

↑Step up
If control is not maintained, consider step up. First, review patient medication technique, adherence, and environmental control (avoidance of allergens or other factors that contribute to asthma severity.)

Notes:

- **The stepwise approach presents general guidelines to assist clinical decision making; it is not intended to be a specific prescription. Asthma is highly variable; clinicians should tailor specific medication plans to the needs and circumstances of individual patients.**
- Gain control as quickly as possible; then decrease treatment to the least medication necessary to maintain control. Gaining control may be accomplished by either starting treatment at the step most appropriate to the initial severity of the condition or starting at a higher level of therapy (eg, a course of systemic corticosteroids or higher dose of inhaled corticosteroids).
- A rescue course of systemic corticosteroids may be needed at any time and at any step.
- Some patients with intermittent asthma experience severe and life-threatening exacerbations separated by long periods of normal lung function and no symptoms. This may be especially common with exacerbations provoked by respiratory infections. A short course of systemic corticosteroids is recommended.
- At each step, patients should control their environment to avoid or control factors that make their asthma worse (eg, allergens, irritants); this requires specific diagnosis and education.

Management of Asthma Exacerbations: Home Treatment*

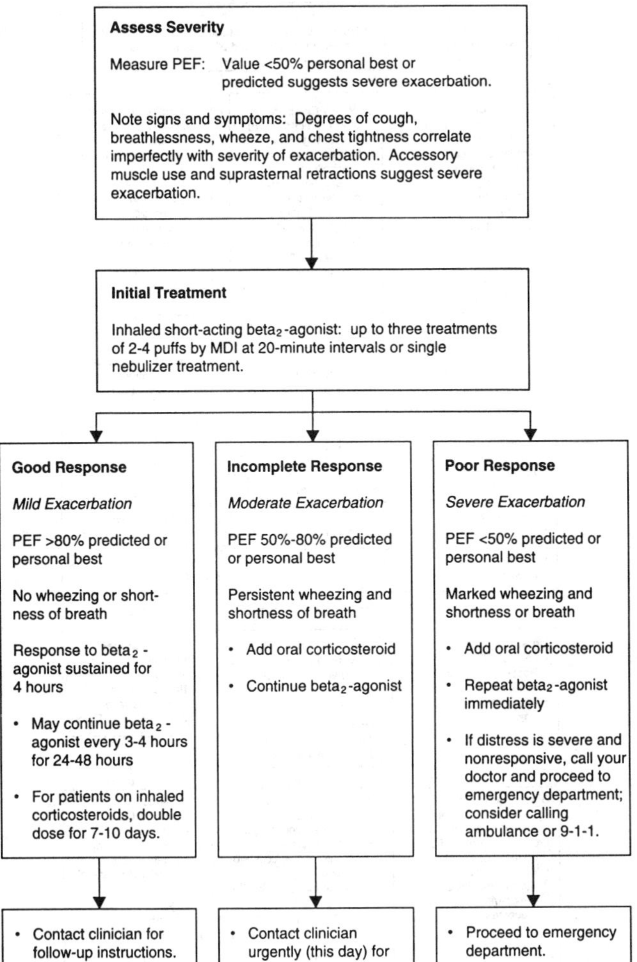

*Patients at high risk of asthma-related death should receive immediate clinical attention after initial treatment. Additional therapy may be required.

ASTHMA *(Continued)*

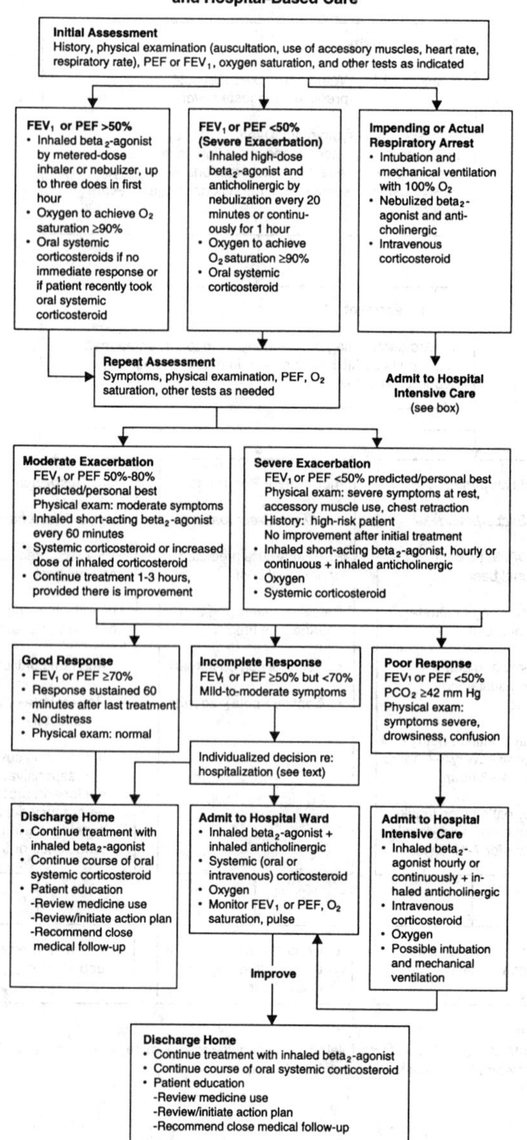

ESTIMATED COMPARATIVE DAILY DOSAGES FOR INHALED CORTICOSTEROIDS

Children

Drug	Low Dose	Medium Dose	High Dose
Beclomethasone dipropionate 42 mcg/puff 84 mcg/puff	84-336 mcg (2-8 puffs)	336-672 mcg (8-16 puffs)	>672 mcg (>16 puffs)
Budesonide Turbuhaler 200 mcg/dose	100-200 mcg	200-400 mcg (1-2 inhalations – 200 mcg)	>400 mcg (>2 inhalations – 200 mcg)
Flunisolide 250 mcg/puff	500-750 mcg (2-3 puffs)	1000-1250 mcg (4-5 puffs)	>1250 mcg (>5 puffs)
Fluticasone Metered dose inhaler: 44, 110, 220 mcg/puff	88-176 mcg (2-4 puffs – 44 mcg)	176-440 mcg (4-10 puffs – 44 mcg) or (2-4 puffs – 110 mcg)	>440 mcg (>4 puffs – 110 mcg)
Dry powder inhaler: 50, 100, 250 mcg/dose	(2-4 inhalations – 50 mcg)	(2-4 inhalations – 100 mcg)	(>4 inhalations – 100 mcg)
Triamcinolone acetonide 100 mcg/puff	400-800 mcg (4-8 puffs)	800-1200 mcg (8-12 puffs)	>1200 mcg (>12 puffs)

Adults

Drug	Low Dose	Medium Dose	High Dose
Beclomethasone dipropionate 42 mcg/puff	168-504 mcg (4-12 puffs – 42 mcg)	504-840 mcg (12-20 puffs – 42 mcg)	>840 mcg (>20 puffs – 42 mcg)
84 mcg/puff	(2-6 puffs – 84 mcg)	(6-10 puffs – 84 mcg)	(>10 puffs – 84 mcg)
Budesonide Turbuhaler 200 mcg/dose	200-400 mcg (1-2 inhalations)	400-600 mcg (2-3 inhalations)	>600 mcg (>3 inhalations)
Flunisolide 250 mcg/puff	500-1000 mcg (2-4 puffs)	1000-2000 mcg (4-8 puffs)	>2000 mcg (>8 puffs)
Fluticasone Metered dose inhaler: 44, 110, 220 mcg/puff	88-264 mcg (2-6 puffs – 44 mcg) or (2 puffs – 110 mcg)	264-660 mcg (2-6 puffs – 110 mcg)	>660 mcg (>6 puffs – 110 mcg) or (>3 puffs – 220 mcg)
Dry powder inhaler: 50, 100, 250 mcg/dose	(2-6 inhalations – 50 mcg)	(3-6 inhalations – 100 mcg)	(>6 inhalations – 100 mcg)
Triamcinolone acetonide 100 mcg/puff	400-1000 mcg (4-10 puffs)	1000-2000 mcg (10-20 puffs)	>2000 mcg (>20 puffs)

ASTHMA *(Continued)*

Notes:

- **The most important determinant of appropriate dosing is the clinician's judgment of the patient's response to therapy.** The clinician must monitor the patient's response on several clinical parameters and adjust the dose accordingly. The stepwise approach to therapy emphasizes that once control of asthma is achieved, the dose of mediation should be carefully titrated to the minimum dose required to maintain control, thus reducing the potential for adverse effect.
- The reference point for the range in the dosages for children is data on the safety on inhaled corticosteroids in children, which, in general, suggest that the dose ranges are equivalent to beclomethasone dipropionate 200-400 mcg/day (low dose), 400-800 mcg/day (medium dose), and >800 mcg/day (high dose).
- Some dosages may be outside package labeling.
- Metered-dose inhaler (MDI) dosages are expressed as the actuator dose (the amount of drug leaving the actuator and delivered to the patient), which is the labeling required in the United States. This is different from the dosage expressed as the valve dose (the amount of drug leaving the valve, all of which is not available to the patient), which is used in many European countries and in some of the scientific literature. Dry powder inhaler (DPI) doses (eg, Turbuhaler) are expressed as the amount of drug in the inhaler following activation.

ESTIMATED CLINICAL COMPARABILITY OF DOSES FOR INHALED CORTICOSTEROIDS

Data from *in vitro* and in clinical trials suggest that the different inhaled corticosteroid preparations are not equivalent on a per puff or microgram basis. However, it is not entirely clear what implications these differences have for dosing recommendations in clinical practice because there are few data directly comparing the preparations. Relative dosing for clinical comparability is affected by differences in topical potency, clinical effects at different doses, delivery device, and bioavailability. The Expert Panel developed recommended dose ranges for different preparations based on available data and the following assumptions and cautions about estimating relative doses needed to achieve comparable clinical effect.

- **Relative topical potency using human skin blanching**
  - Standard test for determining relative topical anti-inflammatory potency is the topical vasoconstriction (MacKenzie skin blanching) test.
  - The MacKenzie topical skin blanching test correlates with binding affinities and binding half-lives for human lung corticosteroid receptors (see following table) (Dahlberg, et al, 1984; Hogger and Rohdewald 1994).
  - The relationship between relative topical anti-inflammatory effect and clinical comparability in asthma management is not certain. However, recent clinical trials suggest that different *in vitro* measures of anti-inflammatory effect is not certain. However, recent clinical trials suggest that different in vitro measures of anti-inflammatory effect correlate with clinical efficacy (Barnes and Pedersen 1993; Johnson 1996; Kamada, et al, 1996; Ebden, et al, 1986; Leblanc, et al, 1994; Gustaffson, et al, 1993; Lundback, et al, 1993; Barnes, et al, 1993; Fabbri, et al, 1993; Langdon and Capsey, 1994; Ayres, et al, 1995; Rafferty, et al, 1985; Bjorkander, et al, 1982, Stiksa, et al, 1982; Willey, et al, 1982.)

Medication	Topical Potency (Skin Blanching)*	Corticosteroid Receptor Binding Half-Life	Receptor Binding Affinity
Beclomethasone dipropionate (BDP)	600	7.5 hours	13.5
Budesonide (BUD)	980	5.1 hours	9.4
Flunisolide (FLU)	330	3.5 hours	1.8
Fluticasone propionate (FP)	1200	10.5 hours	18.0
Triamcinolone acetonide (TAA)	330	3.9 hours	3.6

*Numbers are assigned in reference to dexamethasone, which has a value of "1" in the MacKenzie test.

- **Relative doses to achieve similar clinical effects**
  - Clinical effects are evaluated by a number of outcome parameters (eg, changes in spirometry, peak flow rates, symptom scores, quick-relief $beta_2$-agonist use, frequency of exacerbations, airway responsiveness).
  - The daily dose and duration of treatment may affect these outcome parameters differently (eg, symptoms and peak flow may improve at lower doses and over a shorter treatment time than bronchial reactivity) (van Essen-Zandvliet, et al, 1992; Haahtela, et al, 1991)
  - Delivery systems influence comparability. For example, the delivery device for budesonide (Turbuhaler) delivers approximately twice the amount of drug to the airway as the MDI, thus enhancing the clinical effect (Thorsson, et al, 1994); Agertoft and Pedersen, 1993).
  - Individual patients may respond differently to different preparations, as noted by clinical experience.
  - Clinical trials comparing effects in reducing symptoms and improving peak expiratory flow demonstrate:
  - BDP amd BUD achieved comparable effects at similar microgram doses by MDI (Bjorkander, et al, 1982; Ebden, et al, 1986; Rafferty, et al, 1985).
  - BDP achieved effects similar to twice the dose of TAA on a microgram basis.

Reference

National Asthma Education and Prevention Program, February 1997.

CONTRAST MEDIA REACTIONS, PREMEDICATION FOR PROPHYLAXIS

(American College of Radiology Guidelines for Use of Nonionic Contrast Media)

It is estimated that approximately 5% to 10% of patients will experience adverse reactions to administration of contrast dye (less for nonionic contrast). In approximately 1000-2000 administrations, a life-threatening reaction will occur.

A variety of premedication regimens have been proposed, both for pretreatment of "at risk" patients who require contrast media and before the routine administration of the intravenous high osmolar contrast media. Such regimens have been shown in clinical trials to decrease the frequency of all forms of contrast medium reactions. Pretreatment with a 2-dose regimen of methylprednisolone 32 mg, 12 and 2 hours prior to intravenous administration of HOCM (ionic), has been shown to decrease mild, moderate, and severe reactions in patients at increased risk and perhaps in patients without risk factors. Logistical and feasibility problems may preclude adequate premedication with this or any regimen for all patients It is unclear at this time that steroid pretreatment prior to administration of ionic contrast media reduces the incidence of reactions to the same extent or less than that achieved with the use of nonionic contrast media alone. Information about the efficacy of nonionic contrast media combined with a premedication strategy, including steroids, is preliminary or not yet currently available. For high-risk patients (ie, previous contrast reactors), the combination of a pretreatment regimen with nonionic contrast media has empirical merit and may warrant consideration. Oral administration of steroids appears preferable to intravascular routes, and the drug may be prednisone or methylprednisolone. Supplemental administration of H_1 and H_2 antihistamine therapies, orally or intravenously, may reduce the frequency of urticaria, angioedema, and respiratory symptoms. Additionally, ephedrine administration has been suggested to decrease the frequency of contrast reactions, but caution is advised in patients with cardiac disease, hypertension, or hyperthyroidism. No premedication strategy should be a substitute for the ABC approach to preadministration preparedness listed above. Contrast reactions do occur despite any and all premedication prophylaxis. The incidence can be decreased, however, in some categories of "at risk" patients receiving high osmolar contrast media plus a medication regimen. For patients with previous contrast medium reactions, there is a slight chance that recurrence may be more severe or the same as the prior reaction, however, it is more likely that there will be no recurrence.

A general premedication regimen is

Methylprednisolone	32 mg orally at 12 and 2 hours prior to procedure
Diphenhydramine	50 mg orally 1 hour prior to the procedure

An alternative premedication regimen is

Prednisone	50 mg orally 13, 7, and 1 hour before the procedure
Diphenhydramine	50 mg orally 1 hour before the procedure
Ephedrine	25 mg orally 1 hour before the procedure (except when contraindicated)

Indication for nonionic contrast are

Previous reaction to contrast — premedicate*
Known allergy to iodine or shellfish
Asthma, especially if on medication
Myocardial instability or CHF
Risk for aspiration or severe nausea and vomiting
Difficulty communicating or inability to give history
Patients taking beta-blockers
Small children at risk for electrolyte imbalance or extravasation
Renal failure with diabetes, sickle cell disease, or myeloma
At physician or patient request

*Life-threatening reactions (throat swelling, laryngeal edema, etc), consider omitting the intravenous contrast.

DEPRESSION

Criteria for Major Depressive Episode

A. Five (or more) of the following symptoms have been present during the same 2-week period and represent a change from previous functioning; at least one of the symptoms is either (1) depressed mood or (2) loss of interest or pleasure.

1. Depressed mood most of the day, nearly every day
2. Marked diminished interest or pleasure in all, or almost all, activities
3. Significant weight loss (not dieting) or weight gain, or decrease or increase in appetite nearly every day
4. Insomnia or hypersomnia nearly every day
5. Psychomotor agitation or retardation nearly every day
6. Fatigue or loss of energy nearly every day
7. Feelings of worthlessness or excessive or inappropriate guilt (may be delusional) nearly every day
8. Diminished ability to think or concentrate, or indecisiveness
9. Recurrent thoughts of death, recurrent suicidal ideation without a specific plan, or a suicide attempt or a specific suicide plan

B. The symptoms cause clinically significant distress or impairment in social, occupational or other important areas of functioning.

C. The symptoms are not due to the direct physiologic effects of a substance or a general medical condition (eg, hypothyroidism).

Medications That May Precipitate Depression

Anti-inflammatory & analgesic agents	Indomethacin, pentazocine, phenacetin, phenylbutazone
Antimicrobial agents	Cycloserine, ethambutol, sulfonamides, select gram-negative antibiotics
Cardiovascular/ antihypertensive agents	Clonidine, digitalis, diuretics, guanethidine, hydralazine, indapamide, methyldopa, prazocin, procainamide, propranolol, reserpine
CNS-agents	Alcohol, amantadine, amphetamine & derivatives, barbiturates, benzodiazepines, chloral hydrate, carbamazepine, cocaine, haloperidol, L-dopa, phenothiazines, succinimide derivatives, levetiracetam
Hormonal agents	ACTH, corticosteroids, estrogen, melatonin, oral contraceptives, progesterone
Miscellaneous	Antineoplastic agents, cimetidine, disulfiram, organic pesticides, physostigmine

Medical Disorders & Psychiatric Disorders Associated With Depression

Endocrine diseases	Acromegaly, Addison's disease, Cushing's disease, diabetes mellitus, hyperparathyroidism, hypoparathyroidism, hyperthyroidism, hypothyroidism, insulinoma, pheochromocytoma, pituitary dysfunction
Deficiency states	Pernicious anemia, severe anemia, Wernicke's encephalopathy
Infections	Encephalitis, fungal infections, meningitis, neurosyphilis, influenza, mononucleosis, tuberculosis, AIDS
Collagen disorders	Rheumatoid arthritis
Systemic lupus erythematosus	
Metabolic disorders	Electrolyte imbalance, hypokalemia, hyponatremia, hepatic encephalopathy, Pick's disease, uremia, Wilson's disease
Cardiovascular disease	Cerebral arteriosclerosis, chronic bronchitis, congestive heart failure, emphysema, myocardial infarction, paroxysmal dysrhythmias, pneumonia
Neurologic disorders	Alzheimer's disease, amyotrophic lateral sclerosis, brain tumors, chronic pain syndrome, Creutzfeldt-Jakob disease, Huntington's disease, multiple sclerosis, myasthenia gravis, Parkinson's disease, poststroke, trauma (postconcussion)
Malignant disease	Breast, gastrointestinal, lung, pancreas, prostate
Psychiatric disorders	Alcoholism, anxiety disorders, eating disorders, schizophrenia

DEPRESSION *(Continued)*

Somatic Treatments of Depression in the Patient With Medical Illness

Condition	First Choice	Second-Line Options	Alternatives
Thyroid Hypothyroid	Thyroid (T)	T_4 or T_3 + antidepressant (SSRIs , TCAs, new generation agents)	ECT, other antidepressants psychostimulants
Hyperthyroid	Antidepressant and antihyperthyroid medications	Select a different group of antidepressants	
Diabetes mellitus	SSRIs, other new generation antidepressants	TCAs (second amine or low-dose tertiary amine) MAOIs	ECT, buspirone, psychostimulants, thyroid supplements, mood stabilizers
Cardiovascular disorders	SSRIs, bupropion	ECT, psychostimulants B-blockers, buspirone	ECT, TCAs, MAOIs, mood stabilizers
Renal disease	Fluoxetine, sertraline	TCAs, other new generation antidepressants, psychostimulants	ECT, anticonvulsants, lithium (if dialysis or CLOSELY monitored)
Hepatic disease (reduced dose ALL)	Sertraline	Other new generation antidepressants, TCAs-secondary amines	TCAs-tertiary amines
HIV	Bupropion, SSRIs, psychostimulants	TCAs	ECT
Transplant	**Closely monitor.** See cardiovascular, renal, liver, pulmonary, new antidepressant agents, TCAs-secondary amines		
Neurologic	Newer generation antidepressants, TCAs-secondary amines	Selegiline, anticonvulsants	Bromocriptine
Malignancy	Newer generation antidepressants, TCAs-secondary amines psychostimulants	TCAs-tertiary amines of pain MAOIs	ECT
Respiratory	Activating antidepressants, buspirone		More sedating antidepressants, ECT
Gastrointestinal	TCAs-secondary amines, new generation antidepressants	TCAs-tertiary amines	ECT

DIABETES MELLITUS TREATMENT

INSULIN-DEPENDENT DIABETES MELLITUS

Treatment goals that emphasize glycemic control have been recommended by the American Diabetes Association (see table).

Glycemic Control for People With Diabetes

Biochemical Index	Nondiabetic	Goal	Action Suggested
Preprandial glucose	<115	80-120	<80 >140
Bedtime glucose (mg/dL)	<120	100-140	<100 >160
Hb A_{1C} (%)	<8	<7	>8

These values are for nonpregnant individuals. Action suggested depends on individual patient circumstances, Hb A_{1C} referenced to a nondiabetic range of 4% to 6% (mean 5%, SD 0.5%).

NONINSULIN-DEPENDENT DIABETES MELLITUS

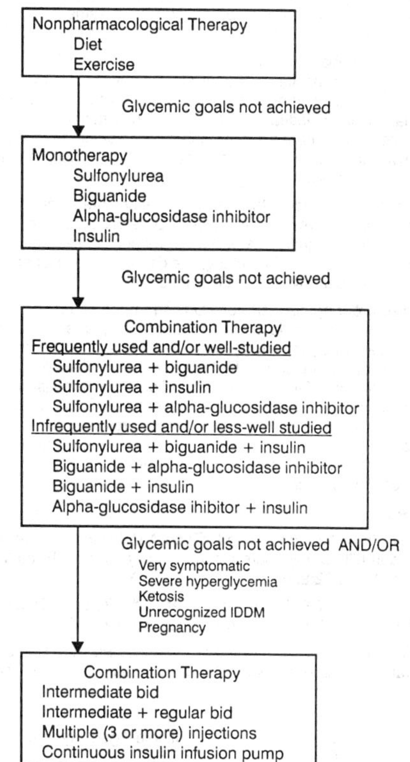

EMERGING RISK FACTORS FOR CORONARY ARTERY DISEASE

The traditional risk factors for cardiac disease are well established and thoroughly documented. These include hyperlipidemia, hypertension, smoking, and diabetes. Epidemiologic studies have also confirmed the important influence of family history, gender, and a sedentary lifestyle in the evolution of coronary artery disease.

With improvements in our ability to detect early cardiac ischemia, and more sophisticated approaches to cardiovascular epidemiology, there is emerging evidence of novel metabolic, behavioral, and inflammatory markers that may help identify those at increased risk for cardiovascular disease and more important, perhaps, allow for appropriate intervention.

There is currently great excitement over the possible contribution of increased plasma homocyst(e)ine to the development of vascular disease. Patients with high levels of homocyst(e)ine (often associated with abnormalities in methyltetrahydrofolate reductase activity) appear to develop vascular disease, beyond that which would be expected, based on the traditional risk factor profile. While the contribution of homocyst(e)ine to vascular disease has not been definitively established, the early evidence is promising. High homocyst(e)ine levels should be suspected in those patients with severe vascular disease in the absence of hyperlipidemia or other risk factors. Increased homocyst(e)ine levels are easily and safely reduced by oral intake of folic acid. However, it is unknown whether reducing plasma homocyst(e)ine by increasing folic acid intake also decreases the risk for vascular disease.

An additional metabolic variable that may be important in the development of cardiovascular disease is insulin. A recent study showed that over a 25-year follow-up of Finnish police, those with higher fasting insulin levels had a significantly increased risk for vascular disease, independent of other risk factors. The exact mechanisms by which insulin may enhance artherosclerotic or other degenerative processes is not known. Nevertheless, the association between hyperinsulinemia and other cardiovascular risk factors is widely recognized.

Behavioral characteristics that may be associated with adverse cardiovascular outcomes include depression and type A personality. Those patients with myocardial infarction who have significant depressive responses have more poor outcomes. Similarly, type A personality in the setting of existing cardiac ischemia may also be accompanied by poorer cardiovascular outcomes.

There is also great enthusiasm for studying the potential role of infectious and inflammatory processes in the development of coronary artery disease and other vascular disease. In particular, infections with *Chlamydia* have been linked to an increased prevalence of vascular disease. Using inflammatory markers (ie, C-reactive protein) as indirect evidence for infection, several studies have demonstrated that the incidence of cardiovascular events is increased in patients with high levels of C-reactive protein. Clearly, an infectious etiology contributing to cardiovascular events would suggest that the use of antimicrobial or anti-inflammatory therapy may enhance cardiovascular protection, and provides an intriguing avenue for future investigation of mechanisms mediating cardiovascular risk.

Resources

Gallacher J, Yarnell J, and Butland, "Type A Behavior and Prevalent Heart Disease in the Caerphilly Study: Increase in Risk or Symptom Reporting?" *J Epidem Comm Health*, 1988, 62:226.

Lagrand WK, Visser CA, Hermens WT, et al, "C-Reactive Protein as a Cardiovascular Risk Factor – More Than an Epiphenomenon?" *Circulation*, 1989, 100:96-102.

Nygard O, Nordrehaug JE, Refsum H, et al, "Plasma Homocyst(e)ine Levels and Mortality in Patients With Coronary Artery Disease," *N Engl J Med*, 1997, 337:230-6.

Vanhala MJ, Kumpusalo EA, Pitkajarvi TK, et al, "Hyperinsulinemia and Clustering of Cardiovascular Risk Factors in Middle-Aged Hypertensive Finnish Men and Women," *J Hyperten*, 1997, 15:475-81.

EPILEPSY

Antiepileptic Drugs for Children and Adolescents by Seizure Type and Epilepsy Syndrome

Seizure Type or Epilepsy Syndrome	First Line Therapy	Alternatives
Partial seizures (with or without secondary generalization)	Carbamazepine	Valproate, phenytoin, gabapentin, lamotrigine, vigabatrin, phenobarbital, primidone; consider clonazepam, clorazepate, acetazolamide, oxcarbazepine
Generalized tonic-clonic seizures	Valproate or carbamazepine	Phenytoin, phenobarbital, primidone; consider clonazepam
Childhood absence epilepsy		
Before 10 years of age	Ethosuximide or valproate	Methsuximide, acetazolamide, clonazepam, lamotrigine
After 10 years of age	Valproate	Ethosuximide, methsuximide, acetazolamide, clonazepam, lamotrigine; consider adding carbamazepine, phenytoin, or phenobarbital for generalized tonic-clonic seizures if valproate not tolerated
Juvenile myoclonic epilepsy	Valproate	Phenobarbital, primidone, clonazepam; consider carbamazepine, phenytoin, methsuximide, acetazolamide
Progressive myoclonic epilepsy	Valproate	Valproate plus clonazepam, phenobarbital
Lennox-Gastaut and related syndromes	Valproate	Clonazepam, phenobarbital, lamotrigine, ethosuximide, felbamate; consider methsuximide, ACTH or steroids, pyridoxine, ketogenic diet
Infantile spasms	ACTH or steroids	Valproate; consider clonazepam, vigabatrin (especially with tuberous sclerosis), pyridoxine
Benign epilepsy of childhood with centrotemporal spikes	Carbamazepine or valproate	Phenytoin; consider phenobarbital, primidone
Neonatal seizures	Phenobarbital	Phenytoin; consider clonazepam, primidone, valproate, pyridoxine

Adapted from Bourgeois BFD, "Antiepileptic Drugs in Pediatric Practice," *Epilepsia*, 1995, 36 (Suppl 2):S34-S45.

EPILEPSY *(Continued)*

FEBRILE SEIZURES

A febrile seizure is defined as a seizure occurring for no reason other than an elevated temperature. It does not have an infectious or metabolic origin within the CNS (ie, it is not caused by meningitis or encephalitis). Fever is usually >102°F rectally, but the more rapid the rise in temperature, the more likely a febrile seizure may occur. About 4% of children develop febrile seizures at one time of their life, usually occurring between 3 months and 5 years of age with the majority occurring at 6 months to 3 years of age. There are 3 types of febrile seizures:

1. **Simple** febrile seizures are nonfocal febrile seizures of less than 15 minutes duration. They do not occur in multiples.
2. **Complex** febrile seizures are febrile seizures that are either focal, have a focal component, are longer than 15 minutes in duration, or are multiple febrile seizures that occur within 30 minutes.
3. **Febrile status epilepticus** is a febrile seizure that is a generalized tonic-clonic seizure lasting longer than 30 minutes.

Note: Febrile seizures should not be confused with true epileptic seizures associated with fever or "seizure with fever." "Seizure with fever" includes seizures associated with acute neurologic illnesses (ie, meningitis, encephalitis).

Long-term prophylaxis with phenobarbital may reduce the risk of subsequent febrile seizures. The 1980 NIH Consensus paper stated that after the first febrile seizure, long-term prophylaxis should be considered under any of the following:

1. Presence of abnormal neurological development or abnormal neurological exam
2. Febrile seizure was complex in nature: duration >15 minutes focal febrile seizure followed by transient or persistent neurological abnormalities
3. Positive family history of afebrile seizures (epilepsy)

Also consider long-term prophylaxis in certain cases if:

1. the child has multiple febrile seizures
2. the child is <12 months of age

Anticonvulsant prophylaxis is usually continued for 2 years or 1 year after the last seizure, whichever is longer. With the identification of phenobarbital's adverse effects on learning and cognitive function, many physicians will not start long-term phenobarbital prophylaxis after the first febrile seizure unless the patient has more than one of the above risk factors. Most physicians would start long-term prophylaxis if the patient has a second febrile seizure.

Daily administration of phenobarbital and therapeutic phenobarbital serum concentrations ≥15 mcg/mL decrease recurrence rates of febrile seizures. Valproic acid is also effective in preventing recurrences of febrile seizures, but is usually reserved for patients who have significant adverse effects to phenobarbital. The administration of rectal diazepam (as a solution or suppository) at the time of the febrile illness has been shown to be as effective as daily phenobarbital in preventing recurrences of febrile seizures. However, these rectal dosage forms are not available in the United States. Some centers in the USA are using the injectable form of diazepam rectally. The solution for injection is filtered prior to use if drawn from an ampul. A recent study suggests that oral diazepam, 0.33 mg/kg/dose given every 8 hours only when the child has a fever, may reduce the risk of recurrent febrile seizures (see Rosman, et al). **Note**: A more recent study by Uhari (1995) showed that lower doses of diazepam, 0.2 mg/kg/dose, were not effective.) Carbamazepine and phenytoin are not effective in preventing febrile seizures.

References

Berg AT, Shinnar S, Hauser WA, et al, "Predictors of Recurrent Febrile Seizures: A Meta-Analytic Review," *J Pediatr*, 1990, 116 (3):329-37.

Camfield PR, Camfield CS, Gordon K, et al, "Prevention of Recurrent Febrile Seizures," *J Pediatr*, 1995, 126 (6):929-30.

NIH Consensus Statement, "Febrile Seizures: A Consensus of Their Significance, Evaluation and Treatment," *Pediatrics*, 1980, 66 (6):1009-12.

Rosman NP, Colton T, Labazzo J, et al, "A Controlled Trial of Diazepam Administration During Febrile Illnesses to Prevent Recurrence of Febrile Seizures," *N Engl J Med*, 1993, 329 (2):79-84.

Uhari M, Rantala H, Vainionpaa L, et al, "Effects of Acetaminophen and of Low Intermittent Doses of Diazepam on Prevention of Recurrences of Febrile Seizures," *J Pediatr*, 1995, 126(6):991-5.

CONVULSIVE STATUS EPILEPTICUS

Recommendations of the Epilepsy Foundation of America's Working Group on Status Epilepticus

(*JAMA*, 1993, 270:854-9)

Convulsive status epilepticus is an emergency that is associated with high morbidity and mortality. The outcome largely depends on etiology, but prompt and appropriate pharmacological therapy can reduce morbidity and mortality. Etiology varies in children and adults and reflects the distribution of disease in these age groups. Antiepileptic drug administration should be initiated whenever a seizure has lasted 10 minutes. Immediate concerns include supporting respiration, maintaining blood pressure, gaining intravenous access, and identifying and treating the underlying cause. Initial therapeutic and diagnostic measures are conducted simultaneously. The goal of therapy is rapid termination of clinical and electrical seizure activity; the longer a seizure continues, the greater the likelihood of an adverse outcome. Several drug protocols now in use will terminate status epilepticus. Common to all patients is the need for a clear plan, prompt administration of appropriate drugs in adequate doses, and attention to the possibility of apnea, hypoventilation, or other metabolic abnormalities.

EPILEPSY *(Continued)*

Figure 1. Algorithm for the Initial Management of Status Epilepticus

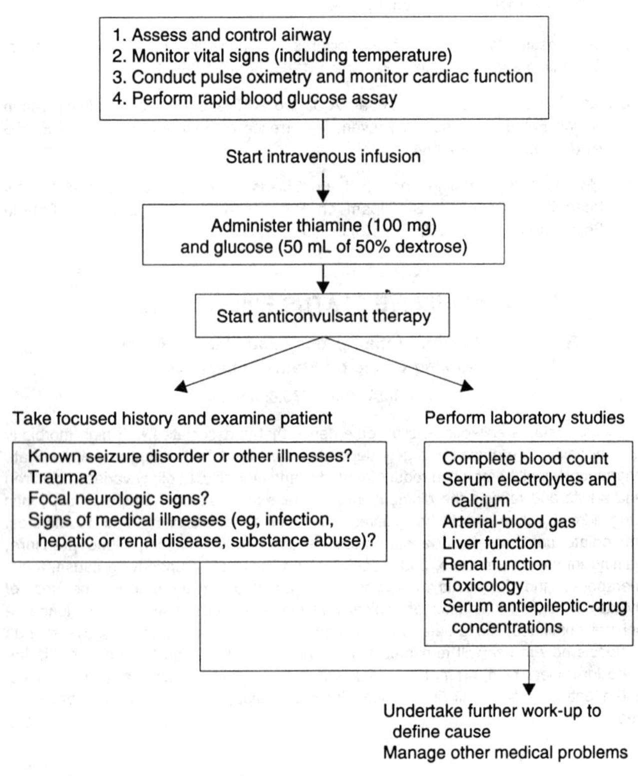

Adapted from Lowenstein A, "Current Concepts: Status Epilepticus," *N Engl J Med*, 1998, 338:970-6 with permission.

Figure 2. Antiepileptic Drug Therapy for Status Epilepticus

I.V. denotes intravenous and PE denoted phenytoin equivalents. The horizontal bars indicate the approximate duration of drug infusions

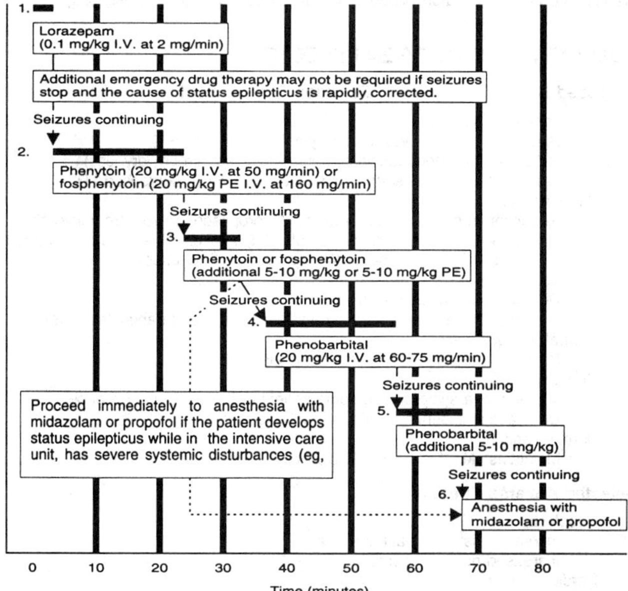

Adapted from Lowenstein A, "Current Concepts: Status Epilepticus," N Engl J Med, 1998, 338:970-6 with permission.

ESTROGEN REPLACEMENT THERAPY

HORMONAL REPLACEMENT WITH ESTROGEN

Estrogen replacement therapy has been demonstrated to have a number of beneficial effects in postmenopausal women. However, this therapy does carry a number of associated risks. The following table summarizes the benefits and risks of hormonal replacement therapy. Many controversies remain to be resolved. The scientific literature concerning these agents continues to develop, and the benefits and risks of therapy will, no doubt, continue to evolve. Current medical literature, individual monographs, and product literature, should also be consulted to guide prescribing.

SUMMARY OF ESTROGEN EFFECTS

Proposed Beneficial Effects of Estrogen Replacement

- Endocrine/metabolic
  - Blocks menopausal vasomotor symptoms (hot flashes)
  - Relief of other menopausal symptoms (vaginal atrophy/dryness)
  - Beneficial effects on serum lipids: increased HDL, decreased LDL
- Cardiovascular
  - Reduction in cardiovascular mortality* - proposed to result from lipid effects as well as vasodilatory, antiplatelet, and endothelial effects; current data (HERS trial) does not support beneficial effect
- Musculoskeletal
  - Decreases bone resorption
  - Increases bone mineral density (in both cortical and trabecular bone)
- Central nervous system
  - Improves memory in Alzheimer's disease†
- Genitourinary
  - May improve symptoms in some patients with stress incontinence
  - Decreases incidence of urinary tract infection
- Dermatologic
  - Maintains skin thickness and elasticity

Selected Adverse Effects

- Neoplastic
  - Increased risk of breast cancer‡
  - Increased risk of endometrial cancer§
- Cardiovascular
  - Hypertension
- Endocrine/metabolic
  - May increase serum glucose
  - May increase serum triglycerides§
- Hematologic
  - Increased risk of thromboembolism¶ - DVT, stroke, pulmonary embolism
- Gastrointestinal
  - Increased risk of gallbladder disease

*Controversial.
†Recent evidence suggests no benefits; sources: *JAMA* 2000, 283:1007-15; *Neurology*, 2000, 54:295-301.
‡Risk may be increased in with combination progestin.
§Attenuated by progestin.
¶Although baseline risk is low, risk is increased by 1-2 cases per 10,000 women per year.

ESTROGEN PRODUCTS

Estrogen is available in a variety of products. These products are differentiated based on their source (natural versus synthetic), number of estrogen compounds contained in the product, and the route of administration. The majority of beneficial effects have been demonstrated with conjugated estrogens from an equine source. Due to its chemical complexity (over 10 active estrogenic compounds have been identified), it is difficult to say whether all of the effects attributed to this product may be generalized to other estrogens. In addition, the route of administration may influence the systemic response. Finally, some of the physiologic changes correlated to menopause may result from cellular changes which are not reversed by exogenous hormonal replacement. The following table lists the available compounds, representative brand names, and notes concerning key clinical issues.

Estrogen Replacement Products

Agent and Source	Representative Brand Names	Form	Use	Notes
Multiple Component Products				
Conjugated estrogens (equine)	Premarin®	Tab Vaginal I.V.	Menopausal symptoms and prevention of osteoporosis	Contains at least 10 active estrogenic compounds
Conjugated estrogens with medroxyprogesterone	Prempro® Premphase®	TD	Menopausal symptoms and prevention of osteoporosis	Combination without cyclic effects
Conjugated estrogens (synthetic)	Cenestin®	Tab	Menopausal symptoms	Not biologically equivalent to Premarin®; consists of 9 active estrogenic compounds
Esterified estrogens	Estratab® Menest®	Tab	Menopausal symptoms and prevention of osteoporosis	
Estradiol with norethindrone	Activelle™ CombiPatch®	Tab TD	Menopausal symptoms	
Ethinyl estradiol with norethindrone	Femhrt®	Tab	Menopausal symptoms and prevention of osteoporosis	
Ethinyl estradiol with norgestimate	Ortho-Prefest™	Tab	Menopausal symptoms and prevention of osteoporosis	
Single Component Products				
Estradiol	Alora® Esclim® Estrace® Climera® Estraderm® FemPatch® Innofem® Vivelle®	TD TD Tab, vaginal TD TD TD Tab TD	Menopausal symptoms; Climera®: Prevention of osteoporosis	
Estropipate (piprazine estrone sulfate)	Ogen® Ortho-Est®	Tab	Menopausal symptoms and prevention of osteoporosis	
Dienestrol	DV® Cream	Vaginal	Relief of vaginal symptoms	
Selective Estrogen Receptor Modulator (SERM)				
Raloxifene	Evista®	Tab	Prevention and treatment of osteoporosis	

*Relative to menopausal management.

TD = transdermal.

ESTROGEN REPLACEMENT THERAPY *(Continued)*

SELECTIVE ESTROGEN RECEPTOR MODULATORS

Selective estrogen receptor modulators (SERMs) are nonsteroidal modulators of estrogen-receptor mediated reactions. The key difference between these agents and estrogen replacement therapies is the potential to exert tissue-specific effects. Due to their chemical differences, these agents retain some of estrogen's beneficial effects on bone metabolism and lipid levels, but differ in their actions on breast and endometrial tissues, potentially limiting adverse effects related to nonspecific hormone stimulation. Among the SERMs, tamoxifen and toremifene retain stimulatory effects in endometrial tissue, while raloxifene does not stimulate endometrial or breast tissue, limiting the potential for endometrial or breast cancer related to this agent. Presumably, because of this activity, tamoxifen is approved for breast cancer prevention in high-risk women as well as for adjuvant treatment of breast cancer. Toremifene is also indicated for the treatment of breast cancer. Raloxifene is the only SERM which has been approved by the FDA for osteoporosis prevention. Its role in breast cancer management or prevention continues to be defined. As with estrogen replacement, each of these therapies has been associated with an increased risk of thromboembolism, and is contraindicated in patients with a history of thromboembolic disease.

The following table briefly summarizes the comparative effects of agents used in hormonal replacement therapy.

Receptor Interactions/Effects

Agent	Endometrial	Breast	Bone	Lipids
Estrogens	Agonist	Agonist	Highest Increase*	↓ LDL ↑LDL
Tamoxifen	Agonist	Antagonist	Increased†	↓ LDL‡
Toremifene	Agonist	Antagonist	Increased	↓ LDL‡ Increased HDL
Raloxifene	Antagonist	Antagonist	Increased	↓ LDL‡

*In a comparative trial, conjugated estrogens increased hip mineral density by approximately two times that observed with raloxifene.

†May effect specific skeletal areas preferentially (lumbar versus radial).

‡Effects are less than with conjugated estrogens.

Note: Effects on HDL may vary based on product and/or route of administration.

It should be noted that the effects on bone observed with SERMs appears to be less than that observed with estrogen replacement. In one study, the effect of raloxifene on hip bone mineral density was approximately half of that observed with conjugated estrogens. In addition, the effects on lipid profiles are less than with estrogen replacement. Tamoxifen's effects on bone may be inconsistent, with one study noting some effect on lumbar density, while radial bone mineral density was not preserved. Some authors recommend the use of raloxifene in patients where carcinoma of the breast or endometrium are of concern. However, it has been noted that the limited ability to block some of the vasomotor symptoms of menopause may limit compliance.

OTHER HORMONAL THERAPY

Methyltestosterone has been used either as a sole agent or in combination with estrogen. Its primary effects are to block vasomotor symptoms and increase libido in postmenopausal women. When used in combination with estrogen, the beneficial effect on lipids is less than with estrogen alone. Increases in bone mineral density are observed with combination treatment.

HEART FAILURE

This chapter outlines a general approach to treatment of chronic systolic heart failure and highlights various aspects of drug therapy in this population. Patient assessment and management (see algorithm on following page) and select drug therapies for heart failure are listed (see following table), followed by general considerations for each class of drugs. Detailed consensus recommendations for the management of chronic heart failure are published (*Am J Cardiol* 1999, 83:1A-38A and *Circulation*, 1995, 92:2764-84).

Drug Therapy for Systolic Heart Failure

Drug Therapy*	Role	Benefit	Comment
ACEI	Standard therapy for patients with asymptomatic and symptomatic heart failure (NYHA class I-IV)	Improves morbidity and mortality	- Achieve target or maximum tolerated dose - Optimize diuretic therapy, if needed, prior to initiating ACEI therapy - Ramipril may improve cardiovascular morbidity and mortality in high-risk patients without heart failure
Beta-blockers	Standard therapy for patients with **stable** NYHA class II-III heart failure	Improves morbidity and mortality	- Beneficial effects specific to individual agents - Need close patient contact / follow-up
Diuretics	Standard therapy for the treatment of symptoms of heart failure	Improves symptoms; spironolactone improves mortality in severe (NYHA class IV) heart failure	- Achieve and maintain euvolemia - Combine with standard therapy - Consider spironolactone in severe heart failure
Digoxin	Patients with symptoms despite optimal standard therapy	Improves symptoms and frequency of hospitalizations for heart failure	- No beneficial impact on mortality - No therapeutic range for efficacy (toxicity >2 ng/mL) - Potential for drug interactions
Angiotensin-II receptor blockers	Patients intolerant to ACEI (angioedema or intractable cough)	Very limited data showing similar improvements in morbidity and mortality compared to ACEI	- Mechanistically similar to ACEI - Comparative and combination ACEI trials ongoing
Calcium channel blockers	None	None	- Amlodipine or felodipine may be used to treat hypertension or angina in patients with heart failure
Hydralazine/ISDN	Patients intolerant to ACEI	Improves mortality	- Requires frequent daily dosing - No outcome data for combined therapy with standard therapy

*See following information and also individual monographs.

HEART FAILURE *(Continued)*

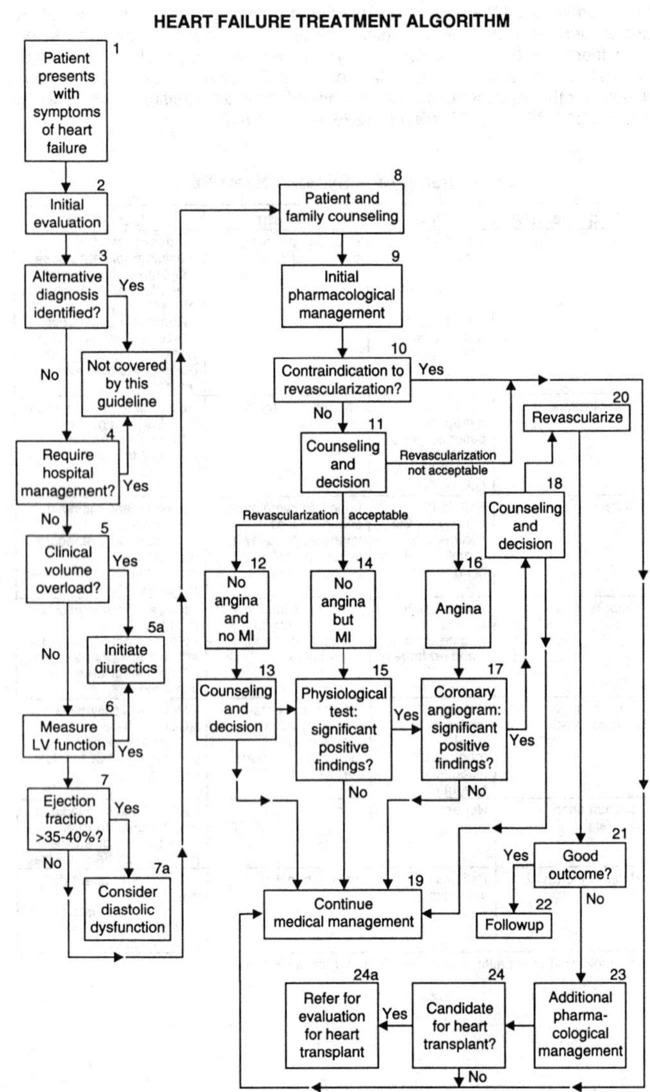

DRUG THERAPY

Angiotensin-Converting Enzyme Inhibitors (ACEI)

ACEI improve morbidity and mortality and are "standard therapy" for the treatment of systolic heart failure. All patients with symptomatic or asymptomatic systolic heart failure (NYHA class I-IV) should be on ACEI therapy unless contraindicated. Therapy should be initiated and titrated to the established target dose (see the following table) or to the maximum tolerated dose. Therapy should be continued long-term unless the patient cannot tolerate or develops a contraindication.

Contraindications for therapy include hypotension (systolic pressure <90 mm Hg; diastolic pressure <60 mm Hg), shock, angioedema, anuric renal failure, pregnancy, significant hyperkalemia, and bilateral renal artery stenosis. Patients on diuretic therapy or those with asymptomatic low blood pressure should be monitored more closely for signs of symptomatic hypotension with initiation of ACEI therapy. ACEIs should not be used to treat hemodynamically unstable heart failure. See specific ACEI monographs for drug and dosing information.

Dosing of ACEIs in Heart Failure*

ACEI	Initial Dose	Target Dose
Captopril	6.25-12.5 mg tid	50 mg tid
Enalapril	2.5 mg bid	10 mg bid
Fosinopril	10 mg daily	20-40 mg daily
Lisinopril	5 mg daily	20 mg daily
Quinapril	5 mg bid	20 mg bid
Ramipril	2.5 mg bid	5 mg bid
Trandolapril	1 mg daily	4 mg daily

*Doses are based on clinical trials and national guidelines.

Beta-Blockers

Carvedilol, sustained release metoprolol (CR/XL), and bisoprolol have demonstrated in clinical trials to decrease morbidity and mortality in patients with mild to moderate heart failure (NYHA class II-III) when combined with standard therapy (target doses of ACEI, diuretics, ± digoxin). Other beta-blockers (eg, bucindolol and celiprolol) have no benefit or may tend to increase mortality. Only carvedilol is FDA approved for the treatment of heart failure. (See individual drug monographs for carvedilol, metoprolol, and bisoprolol.)

All patients on standard therapy with **stable** NYHA class II-III systolic heart failure should be on beta-blocker therapy. Beta-blocker therapy may be considered for patients on standard therapy with mild systolic heart failure (NYHA class I). Patients with sympathetic nervous system activation (eg, heart rate >85 beats/minute) may derive greatest benefit. Beta-blocker therapy is not recommended for patients with unstable heart failure, NYHA class IV systolic heart failure, and in those that cannot tolerate therapy or where therapy is contraindicated.

Contraindications to beta-blockade include bradycardia, 2nd or 3rd degree AV block, hypotension (systolic pressure <90 mm Hg/diastolic pressure <60 mm Hg), decompensated heart failure, and noncompliance. Special consideration should be given in evaluating the risk versus benefit for beta blockade in patients with coexisting conditions, including poorly controlled diabetes, severe COPD, and severe reactive airway disease. These patients should be followed more frequently if beta-blocker therapy is prescribed.

In general, beta-blocker therapy should be initiated at low dose and titrated slowly, no faster than doubling the dose at weekly intervals to tolerated or target doses (see following table). Therapy should be initiated and titrated by practitioners or clinics with experience and capabilities for close patient contact and follow-up.

During the initiation and titration of beta-blocker therapy it is imperative that patients be frequently monitored for signs of worsening heart failure. Significant weight gain, increasing shortness of breath, edema, paroxysmal nocturnal dyspnea, and dyspnea on exertion may necessitate slowing or decreasing the dose of beta-blocker with dose adjustment of ACEI and diuretic therapies. Patients should be well educated on the potential signs of worsening heart failure, importance of diet and drug compliance, and the need to notify the practitioner or clinic immediately if symptoms of worsening heart failure occur.

HEART FAILURE *(Continued)*

Initial and Target Doses for Beta-Blocker Therapy in Heart Failure*

Beta-Blocker	Starting Dose	Target Dose	Comment
Bisoprolol	1.25 mg/day	10 mg/day	- β_1-selective: possible benefit in patients with reactive airway disease - Inconvenient dosage forms for initial dose titration
Carvedilol	3.125 mg/day	25-50 mg/day	- FDA approved for heart failure - Nonselective beta-blocker/α_1-blocker - Possible greater reduction in blood pressure (α-blocking effects) - Convenient dosages
Metoprolol XL/CR	12.5 mg/day	200 mg/day	- Compelling data for mortality benefit - β_1-selective: possible benefit in patients with reactive airway disease - Inconvenient dosage forms for initial dose titration - Less potential to decrease blood pressure (no α-blocking properties)

*Doses are those used in clinical trials.

Digoxin

Digoxin improves symptoms of heart failure and decreases hospitalizations for heart failure, but does not improve mortality. Digoxin should be used in patients who have symptoms despite optimal standard therapy (ACEIs, diuretics, beta-blocker). There is no compelling evidence for a target therapeutic serum level for digoxin in the treatment of heart failure.

Digoxin should be avoided in patients with sinus and AV block. Caution should be used with digoxin in patients with potential drug interactions, unstable renal function, hypokalemia, and hypomagnesemia.

Diuretics

Therapy should be initiated immediately in patients with heart failure who have signs of volume overload. Patients with mild volume overload can be managed adequately on thiazide diuretics. Patients with more severe volume overload, particularly in patients with a creatinine clearance <30 mL/minute should be started on a loop diuretic. Diuretic therapy should eliminate symptoms of heart failure (eg, edema) and may be monitored and dosed by changes in body weight. Resistance to therapy, as is seen in severe heart failure, may necessitate intravenous diuretic therapy or the use of more than one diuretic. See monographs for individual diuretics.

In the RALES study (*N Engl J Med*, 1999, 341:709-17), spironolactone at a daily dose of 25 mg decreased morbidity and mortality when combined with standard therapy in patients with severe heart failure. When combined with standard therapy (ACEI), serum potassium levels should be monitored. It is unknown if the beneficial effects of this therapy extend to patients with less severe heart failure. The RALES study gives further evidence that the renin-angiotensin-aldosterone system plays an important pathophysiologic role in heart failure. Blockade of this system may confer a cardiovascular benefit.

Diuretic Therapy for Heart Failure

Diuretic	Initial Dose (mg)	Target Dose (mg)	Recommended Maximal Dose (mg)	Comment
Thiazide Diuretics				
Chlorthalidone Hydrochlorothiazide	25 qd	As needed	50 qd	- Postural hypotension, hypokalemia, hyperglycemia, hyperuricemia, rash; rare severe reaction includes pancreatitis, bone marrow suppression, and anaphylaxis
Loop Diuretics				
Bumetanide Ethacrynic acid Furosemide	0.5-1 qd 50 qd 10-40 qd	As needed	10 qd 200 bid 240 bid	- Same as thiazide diuretics
Thiazide-Related Diuretic				
Metolazone	2.5*	As needed	10 qd	- Same as thiazide diuretics
Potassium-Sparing Diuretics				
Amiloride Spironolactone Triamterene	5 qd 25 qd 50 qd	As needed	40 qd 100 bid 100 bid	- Hyperkalemia (especially if administered with ACEI), rash, gynecomastia (spironolactone only) - Spironolactone (25 mg/day) decreases mortality in severe heart failure

*Given as a single test dose initially.

Adapted from U.S. Department of Health & Human Services, the Agency for Healthcare Policy and Research (ACHPR) Publication No. 94-0613, June, 1994.

HEART FAILURE *(Continued)*

Hydralazine/Isosorbide Dinitrate (ISDN)

The combination of hydralazine (initial dose 10 mg qid up to 75 mg qid) and isosorbide dinitrate (initial dose 5 mg tid up to 40 mg tid), has been shown to improve mortality in patients with heart failure not on ACEI therapy. ACEI therapy is superior compared to hydralazine/ISDN in improving mortality.

The combination of hydralazine/ISDN may be considered in patients intolerant to ACEI therapy. The combination is sometimes added to standard therapy if symptoms or fatigue persist. However, there is little data to suggest that the addition of hydralazine/ISDN to standard therapy further improves morbidity and mortality.

The chronic use of other direct vasodilators may increase morbidity and mortality in this population.

Angiotensin II Receptor Blockers (ARBs)

The renin-angiotensin-aldosterone system plays a key role in the progression of heart failure. For this reason, the role of ARBs in this patient population is being extensively evaluated. Mechanistically, angiotensin II is also produced through non-ACE systems and heart failure patients have "escape" of angiotensin II levels with chronic ACEI therapy. For these reasons, ARB therapy may confer a positive impact on morbidity and mortality by directly blocking the detrimental affects of angiotensin II. It is not established if ARB therapy provides similar mortality benefits as ACEIs or if there is an added benefit in combining an ABR to standard (ACEI) therapy.

In the Evaluation of Losartan in the Elderly (ELITE) trial, losartan and captopril therapy produced similar effects on renal function (primary study endpoint). The risk for cardiovascular events (secondary study endpoint) were significantly decreased in those treated with losartan. Preliminary findings of a follow-up study (ELITE-II) showed similar cardiovascular events and no differences in hospitalization rates between patients randomized to captopril or losartan. In another ARB trial (RESOLVD), candesartan and enalapril therapy alone and the combination of these two agents were evaluated. The findings of this trial showed no difference in clinical effects overall and a trend for improved left ventricular structure with ARB and ACEI combination therapy. Ongoing studies will give more data on the potential role of ARBs in the treatment of heart failure.

Current recommendations for ARB therapy is in those heart failure patients that are intolerant of ACEI therapy (see drug monographs).

Calcium Channel Blockers (CCBs)

CCBs do not improve mortality in patients with congestive heart failure. Amlodipine and felodipine therapy in heart failure trials do not increase or decrease mortality and may be used to treat angina and/or hypertension in this patient population. Other CCBs should be avoided in patients with heart failure, particularly in patients with edema, because of a tendency to increase cardiovascular morbidity and mortality.

Resources

Guidelines

Committee on Evaluation and Management of Heart Failure. Guidelines for the Evaluation and Management of Heart Failure. Report of the American College of Cardiology/American Heart Association Task Force on Practice Guidelines. *Circulation*, 1995, 92:2764-84.

Consensus recommendations for the management of chronic heart failure. On behalf of the membership of the advisory council to improve outcomes nationwide in heart failure, *Am J Cardiol*, 1999, 83(2A):1A-38A.

Standard Therapy

Australia/New Zealand Heart Failure Research Collaborative Group, "Randomised, Placebo-Controlled Trial of Carvedilol in Patients With Congestive Heart Failure Due it Ischaemic Heart Disease," *Lancet*, 1997, 349:375-80.

CIBIS II Investigators and Committee, " The Cardiac Insufficiency Bisoprolol Study II (CIBIS-II): A Randomised Trial," *Lancet*, 1999, 353:9-13.

CIBIS Investigators, "A Randomized Trial of Beta-Blockade in Heart Failure: The Cardiac Insufficiency Bisoprolol Study (CIBIS)," *Circulation*, 1994, 90:1765-1773.

Cohn JN, Archibald DG, Ziesche S, et al, "Effect of Vasodilator Therapy on Mortality in Chronic Congestive Heart Failure: Results of a Veterans Administration Cooperative Study," *N Engl J Med*, 1986, 314:1547-52.

Cohn JN, Johnson G, Ziesche S, et al, "A Comparison of Enalapril With Hydralazine-Isosorbide Dinitrate in the Treatment of Chronic Congestive Heart Failure," *N Engl J Med*, 1991, 325:303-10.

CONSENSUS Trial Study Group, "Effects of Enalapril on Mortality in Severe Congestive Heart Failure," *N Engl J Med*, 1987, 316:1429-35.

Eichhorn EJ and Bristow MR, "Practical Guidelines for Initiation of Beta Adrenergic Blockade in Patients With Chronic Heart Failure," *Am J Cardiol*, 1997, 79:794-8.

Hjalmarson A, Goldstein S, Fagerberg B, et al, "Effect of Metoprolol CR/XL in Chronic Heart Failure: Metoprolol CR XL Randomised Intervention Trial in Congestive Heart Failure (MERIT-HF)," *Lancet*, 1999, 353:2001-7.

Kukin ML, Kalman J, Charney RH, et al, "Prospective, Randomized Comparison of Effect of Long-Term Treatment With Metoprolol or Carvedilol on Symptoms, Exercise, Ejection Fraction, and Oxidative Stress in Heart Failure," *Circulation*, 1999, 99:2645-51.

MacDonald PS, Keogh AM, Aboyoun CL, et al, "Tolerability and Efficacy of Carvedilol in Patients With New York Heart Association Class IV Heart Failure," *J Am Coll Cardiol*, 1999, 33:924-31.

Packer M, Bristow MR, Cohn, et al, "The Effect of Carvedilol on Morbidity and Mortality in Patients With Chronic Heart Failure," *N Engl J Med*, 1996, 334:1349-55.

Packer M, Colucci WS, Sackner-Bernstein JD, et al, "Double-Blind, Placebo-Controlled Study of Effects of Carvedilol in Patients With Moderate to Severe Heart Failure: The PRECISE Trial," *Circulation*, 1996, 94:2793-9.

SOLVD Investigators, "Effect of Enalapril on Survival in Patients With Reduced Left-Ventricular Ejection Fractions and Congestive Heart Failure," *N Engl J Med*, 1991, 325:293-302.

The Digitalis Investigation Group, "The Effects of Digoxin on Mortality and Morbidity in Patients With Heart Failure," *N Engl J Med*, 1997, 336:525-33.

Vantrimpont P, Rouleau JL, Wun CC, et al, "Additive Beneficial Effects of Beta-Blockers to Angiotensin-Converting Enzyme Inhibitors in the Survival and Ventricular Enlargement (SAVE) Study. SAVE Investigators," *J Am Coll Cardiol*, 1997, 29:229-36.

Waagstein F, Bristow MR, Swedberg K, et al, "Beneficial Effects of Metoprolol in Idiopathic Dilated Cardiomyopathy. Metoprolol in Dilated Cardiomyopathy (MDC) Trial Study Group," *Lancet*, 1993, 342:1441-6.

Others

Cairns JA, Connolly SJ, Roberts R, et al , (for the CAMIAT Investigators), "Randomized Trial of Outcomes After Myocardial Infarction in Patients With Frequent or Repetitive Ventricular Premature Depolarizations: CAMIAT, "*Lancet*, 1997, 349:675-682.

Cohn JN, Levine TB, Olivari MT, et al, "Plasma Norepinephrine as a Guide to Prognosis in Patients With Chronic Congestive Heart Failure," *N Engl J Med*, 1984, 311:819-823.

Doval HY, Daniel N, Grancelli H, et al, "Randomized Trial of Low Dose Amiodarone in Severe Congestive Heart Failure," *Lancet*, 1994, 344:493-7.

Julian DG, Camm AJ, Frangin G, et al, (for the European Trial Investigators), "Randomized Trial of Effect of Amiodarone on Mortality in Patients With Left Ventricular Dysfunction After Recent Myocardial Infarction: EMAIT,"*Lancet*, 1997, 349:667-74.

Küpper AJ, Fintelman H, Huige MC, et al, "Cross-over Comparison of the Fixed Combination of Hydrochlorothiazide and Triamterene and the Free Combination of Furosemide and Triamterene in the Maintenance Treatment of Congestive Heart Failure," *Eur J Clin Pharmacol*, 1986, 30:341-3.

Massie BM, Fisher SG, Deedwania PC, et al, (for the CHF-STAT Investigators), "Effect of Amiodarone on Clinical Status and Left Ventricular Function in Patients With Congestive Heart Failure," *Circulation*, 1995, 93:2128-2134.

HEART FAILURE *(Continued)*

O'Connor CM, Gattis WA, Uretsky BF, et al, "Continuous Intravenous Dobutamine is Associated With an Increased Risk of Death in Patients With Advanced Heart Failure: Insights From the Flolan International Randomized Survival Trial (FIRST)," *Am Heart J*, 1999, 138:78-86.

Pitt B, Zannad F, Remme WJ et al (for the Randomized Aldactone Evaluation Study Investigators (RALES)), " The Effect of Spironolactone on Morbidity and Mortality in Patients With Severe Heart Failure," *N Engl J Med*, 1999, 341:709-17.

Sacher HL, Sacher ML, Landau SW, et al, "The Clinical and Hemodynamic Effects of Coenzyme Q10 in Congestive Cardiomyopathy," *Am J Ther*, 1997, 4:66-72.

Watson PS, Scalia GM, Galbraith A, et al, "Lack of Effect of Coenzyme Q on Left Ventricular Function in Patients With Congestive Heart Failure," *J Am Coll Cardiol*, 1999, 33:1549-1552.

HELICOBACTER PYLORI TREATMENT

Multiple Drug Regimens for the Treatment of *H. pylori* Infection

Drug	Dosages*	Duration of Therapy
Regimen 1†		
Bismuth subsalicylate (Pepto-Bismol®)	Two 262 mg tablets 4 times/day	2 weeks
plus		
Metronidazole (Flagyl®)	250 mg 3 or 4 times/day	2 weeks
plus		
Tetracycline (various) or amoxicillin (Amoxil®, others)	250-500 mg 4 times/day	2 weeks
plus		
Histamine H_2-receptor antagonist	Full dose‡ at bedtime	4-6 weeks
Regimen 2		
Metronidazole (Flagyl®)	500 mg 3 times/day	12-14 days
plus		
Amoxicillin (Amoxil®, others)	750 mg 3 times/day	12-14 days
plus		
Histamine H_2-receptor antagonist	Full dose† at bedtime	6-10 weeks
Regimen 3		
Bismuth subsalicylate (Pepto-Bismol®)	Two 262 mg tablets 4 times/day	2 weeks
plus		
Tetracycline (various)	500 mg 4 times/day	2 weeks
plus		
Clarithromycin (Biaxin™)	500 mg 3 times/day	2 weeks
plus		
Histamine H_2-receptor antagonist	Full dose† after evening meal	6 weeks
Regimen 4		
Omeprazole (Prilosec™)	20 mg twice daily	2 weeks
plus		
Amoxicillin (Amoxil®, others)	1 g twice daily or 500 mg 4 times/day	2 weeks
Regimen 5		
Omeprazole (Prilosec™)	20 mg twice daily	2 weeks
plus		
Clarithromycin (Biaxin™)	250 mg twice a day or 500 mg 2 or 3 times/day	2 weeks
or		
Lansoprazole (Prevacid®)	30 mg/day	
plus		
Amoxicillin (Amoxil®)	1 g twice daily	
plus		
Clarithromycin (Biaxin™)	500 mg twice daily	
Regimen 6		
Ranitidine bismuth citrate (Tritec™)	400 mg twice daily	4 weeks
plus		
Clarithromycin (Biaxin™)	500 mg 3 times/day	2 weeks

*All therapies are oral and begin concurrently.

†Marketed as Helidac®, a packet containing 262.4 mg bismuth subsalicylate, 250 mg metronidazole and 500 mg tetracycline; an H_2-antagonist must be purchased separately.

‡Full dose refers to the dosage used to treat acute ulcers, not to the maintenance dose.

HYPERGLYCEMIA- OR HYPOGLYCEMIA-CAUSING DRUGS

Hyperglycemia	Hypoglycemia	Hyperglycemia or Hypoglycemia
Caffeine	Anabolic steroids	Beta-blockers (also may mask symptoms of hypoglycemia)
Calcitonin	ACE inhibitors	Alcohol
Corticosteroids	Chloramphenicol	Lithium
Diltiazem	Clofibrate	Phenothiazines
Estrogens	Disopyramide	Rifampin
Isoniazid	MAO inhibitors	Octreotide
Morphine	Miconazole (oral form)	Fluoxetine
Nifedipine	Probenecid	
Nicotine	Pyridoxine	
Nicotinic acid	Salicylates	
Oral contraceptives	Sulfonamides	
Phenytoin	Tetracycline	
Sympathomimetic amines	Verapamil	
Theophylline	Warfarin	
Thiazide diuretics		
Thyroid products		

Adapted from American Association of Diabetes Educators, *A Core Curriculum for Diabetes Education*, 3rd ed, Vol 10, Chicago, IL: 1998, 338-41.

HYPERLIPIDEMIA

MORTALITY

There is a strong link between serum cholesterol and cardiovascular mortality. This association becomes stronger in patients with established coronary artery disease. Lipid-lowering trials show that reductions in LDL cholesterol are followed by reductions in mortality. In general, each 1% fall in LDL cholesterol confers a 2% reduction in cardiovascular events. The aim of therapy for hyperlipidemia is to decrease cardiovascular morbidity and mortality by lowering cholesterol to a target level using safe and cost-effective treatment modalities. The target LDL cholesterol is determined by the number of patient risk factors (see the following Risk Factors and Goal LDL Cholesterol tables). The goal is achieved through diet, lifestyle modification, and drug therapy (see Figures 1-3). The basis for these recommendations is provided by longitudinal interventional studies, demonstrating that lipid-lowering in patients with prior cardiovascular events (secondary prevention) and in patients with hyperlipidemia but no prior cardiac event (primary prevention) lowers the occurrence of future cardiovascular events, including stroke. In a recent randomized study of relatively low-risk patients with LDLs ≥115 mg/dL, who were referred for revascularization (angioplasty), those assigned to aggressive lipid-lowering therapy were at the same or lower risk for subsequent ischemic events than those who underwent angioplasty (*N Engl J Med*, 1999, 341:170-6).

Table 1. Risk Factors

Positive risk factors	Male ≥45 years
	Female ≥55 years or premature menopause without hormonal replacement therapy
	Family history of premature coronary heart disease, defined as myocardial infarction or sudden death before 55 years of age in father or other first degree relative, or before 65 years of age in mother or other first degree female relative
	Current cigarette smoking
	Hypertension (blood pressure ≥140/90 mm Hg) or taking antihypertensive medication
	Low HDL (<35 mg/dL [0.9 mmol/L])
	Diabetes mellitus
Negative risk factors	High HDL (≥60 mg/dL [1.6 mmol/L])*

*If HDL is ≥60 mg/dL, may subtract one positive risk factor.

Table 2. Goal LDL Cholesterol

Risk Factors	Target LDL Cholesterol
1 risk factor	<160 mg/dL
≥2 risk factors	<130 mg/dL
Established atherosclerotic disease (prior MI, angina, positive coronary angiogram, large vessel atherosclerotic disease, peripheral vascular disease)	<100 mg/dL
Diabetes (with or without established coronary artery disease)	<100 mg/dL

NONDRUG THERAPY

Dietary therapy and lifestyle modifications should be individualized for each patient. A Step I diet is recommended for all patients. Patients with established coronary artery disease may be initiated on a Step II diet (see the following table). Before drug therapy is initiated, dietary and lifestyle modifications should be tried for 6 months, if deemed appropriate. Nondrug and drug therapy should be initiated simultaneously in patients with very elevated cholesterol (>20% from their target LDL) and in those with established coronary artery disease. Increasing physical activity, especially in sedentary and overweight patients, and smoking cessation will aid in the treatment of hyperlipidemia and improve cardiovascular health.

HYPERLIPIDEMIA *(Continued)*

Table 3. NCEP Diet Recommendations

	Step I Diet	Step II Diet
Total fat	≤30% total calories	≤30% total calories
saturated fat	8% to 10% total calories	<7% total calories
polyunsaturated	≤10% total calories	≤10% total calories
monounsaturated	≤15% total calories	≤15% total calories
Carbohydrates	≥55% total calories	≥55% total calories
Protein	~15% total calories	~15% total calories
Cholesterol	<300 mg/day	<200 mg/day
Avg cholesterol reductions	3% to 14%	additional 3% to 7%

DRUG THERAPY

Drug therapy should be selected based on the patient's lipid profile, concomitant disease states, and the cost of therapy. The following table lists specific advantages and disadvantages for various classes of lipid-lowering medications. The cost and expected reduction in lipids with therapy are listed in the Lipid-Lowering Agents table on the following page. Refer to individual drug monographs for detailed information.

Table 4. Advantages and Disadvantages of Specific Lipid-Lowering Therapies

	Advantages	Disadvantages
Bile acid sequestrants	Good choice for ↑ LDL, especially when combined with a statin (↓ LDL ≤50%); low potential for systemic side effects; good choice for younger patients	Can increase triglycerides; higher incidence of adverse effects; moderately expensive; drug interactions; inconvenient dosing
Niacin	Good choice for almost any lipid abnormality; inexpensive; greatest increase in HDL	High incidence of adverse effects; may adversely affect NIDDM and gout; sustained release niacin may decrease the incidence of flushing and circumvent the need for multiple daily dosing; sustained release niacin may not increase HDL cholesterol or decrease triglycerides as well as immediate release niacin
HMG-CoA reductase inhibitors	Produces greatest ↓ in LDL; generally well-tolerated; convenient once-daily dosing; proven decrease in mortality	Expensive
Gemfibrozil	Good choice in patients with ↑ triglycerides where niacin is contraindicated or not well-tolerated; gemfibrozil is well tolerated	Variable effects on LDL

Table 5. Lipid-Lowering Agents

Drug	Dose/Day	Effect on LDL (%)	Effect on HDL (%)	Effect on TG (%)	Avg Wholesale Price/Mo ($)
HMG-CoA Reductase Inhibitors					
Atorvastatin	10 mg	-38	+6	-13	56
	20 mg	-46	+5	-20	87
	40 mg	-51	+5	-32	105
	80 mg (40 mg bid)	-54	+5	-37	210
Cerivastatin	0.2 mg	-25	+10	-11	43
	0.3 mg	-28	+10	-13	43
	0.4 mg	-34	+7	-16	43
Fluvastatin	20 mg	-17	+2	-5	38
	40 mg	-23	+3	-12	38
	40 mg bid	-32	+4	-12	76
Lovastatin	20 mg	-29	+7	-8	73
	40 mg	-31	+5	-2	131
	80 mg	-48	+8	-13	262
Pravastatin	10 mg	-20	+5	-3	63
	20 mg	-24	+3	-15	68
	40 mg	-34	+6	-10	112
Simvastatin	10 mg	-28	+7	-12	65
	20 mg	-35	+5	-17	114
	40 mg	-41	+10	-15	114
	80 mg	-47	+8	-24	228
Bile Acid Sequestrants					
Cholestyramine	8-24 g/day	-15 to -30	+3 to +5	+0 to +20	82-163
Colestipol	10-20 g/day	-15 to -30	+3 to +5	+0 to +20	102-204
Gemfibrozil	600 mg bid	-5 to -10*	+10 to +20	-40 to -60	11
Fenofibrate	67-201 mg/day	-20 to -25	+1 to -34	-30 to -50	62-186
Niacin	2-3 g/day	-21 to -27	+10 to +35	-10 to -50	4-8

*May increase LDL in some patients.

Table 6. Recommended Liver Function Monitoring for HMG-CoA Reductase Inhibitors

Agent	Initial and After Elevation in Dose	6 Weeks*	12 Weeks*	Semiannually
Atorvastatin	x	x	x	x
Cerivastatin	x	x	x	x
Fluvastatin	x	x	x	x
Lovastatin	x	x	x	x
Pravastatin	x		x	
Simvastatin	x			x

*After initiation of therapy or any elevation in dose.

COMBINATION DRUG THERAPY

If after at least 8 weeks of therapy at the maximum recommended or tolerated dose, the patient's LDL cholesterol is not at target, consider optimizing nondrug measures, prescribing a different lipid-lowering drug, or adding another lipid-lowering medication to the current therapy. Successful drug combinations include statin and niacin, statin and bile acid sequestrant, or niacin and bile acid sequestrant. At maximum recommended doses, LDL cholesterol may be decreased by 50% to 60% with combination therapy. This is the same reduction achieved by atorvastatin 40 mg twice daily. If a bile acid sequestrant is used with other lipid-lowering agents, space doses 1 hour before or 4 hours after the bile acid sequestrant administration. Statins combined with either fenofibrate or gemfibrozil increase the risk of rhabdomyolysis. In this situation, patient education (muscle pain/weakness) and careful follow-up are warranted.

HYPERLIPIDEMIA *(Continued)*

Summary of the Second Report of the National Cholesterol Education Program (NCEP) Expert Panel on Detection, Evaluation, and Treatment of High Blood Cholesterol in Adults (Adult Treatment Panel II)

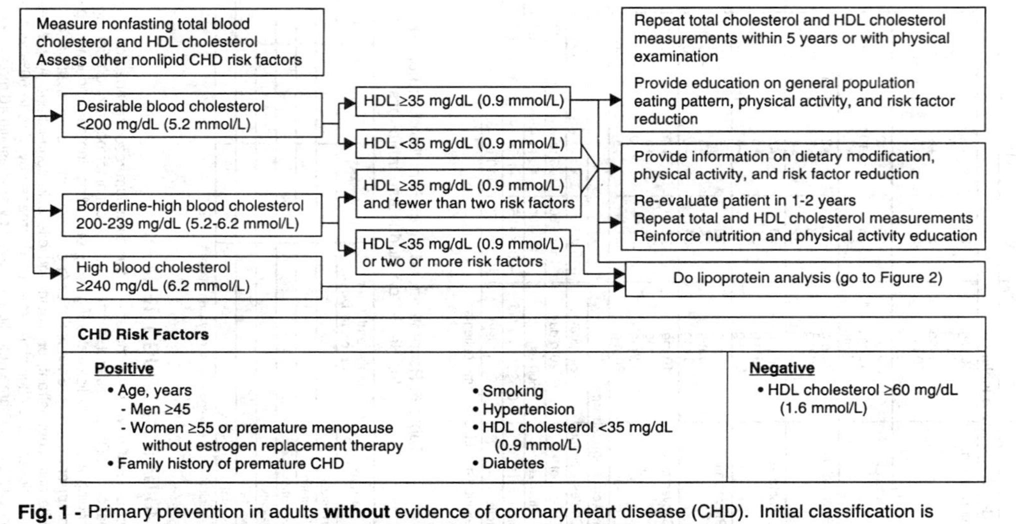

Fig. 1 - Primary prevention in adults **without** evidence of coronary heart disease (CHD). Initial classification is based on total cholesterol and high-density lipoprotein (HDL) cholesterol levels.

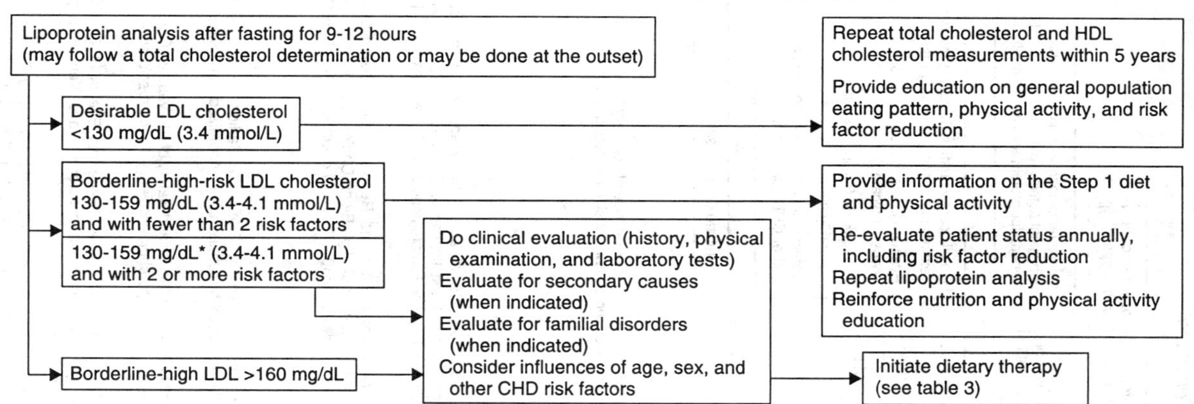

* On the basis of the average of two determinations. If the first two LDL cholesterol test results differ by more than 30 mg/dL (0.7 mmol/L), a third test result should be obtained within 1-8 weeks and the average value of the three tests used.

Fig. 2 - Primary prevention in adults **without** evidence of coronary heart disease (CHD). Subsequent classification is based on low-density lipoprotein (LDL) cholesterol level.

HYPERLIPIDEMIA *(Continued)*

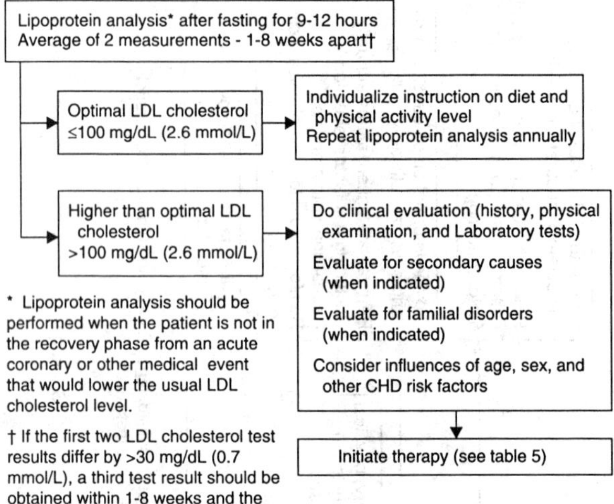

* Lipoprotein analysis should be performed when the patient is not in the recovery phase from an acute coronary or other medical event that would lower the usual LDL cholesterol level.

† If the first two LDL cholesterol test results differ by >30 mg/dL (0.7 mmol/L), a third test result should be obtained within 1-8 weeks and the average value of the 3 tests used.

Fig. 3 - Secondary prevention in adults **with** evidence of coronary heart disease (CHD). Classification is based on low-density lipoprotein (LDL) cholesterol level.

Resources

Guidelines

Gavin JR, Alberti KGMM, Davidson MB, et al, for the Members of the Expert Committee on the Diagnosis and Classification of Diabetes Mellitus, "American Diabetes Association: Clinical Practice Recommendations," *Diabetes Care*, 1999, 22(Suppl 1):S1-S114.

National Cholesterol Education Program, "Second Report of the Expert Panel on Detection, Evaluation, and Treatment of High Blood Cholesterol in Adults (Adult Treatment Panel II)," *JAMA*, 1993, 269:3015-23 or *Circulation*, 1994, 89(3):1329-445.

Others

Berthold HK, Sudhop T, and von Bergmann K, "Effect of a Garlic Oil Preparation on Serum Lipoproteins and Cholesterol Metabolism: A Randomized Controlled Trial," *JAMA*, 1998, 279:1900-2.

Bertolini S, Bon GB, Campbell LM, et al, "Efficacy and Safety of Atorvastatin Compared to Pravastatin in Patients With Hypercholesterolemia," *Atherosclerosis*, 1997, 130:191-7.

Blankenhorn DH, Nessim SA, Johnson RL, et al, "Beneficial Effects of Combined Colestipol-Niacin Therapy on Coronary Atherosclerosis and Venous Bypass Grafts," *JAMA*, 1987, 257:3233-40.

Brown G, Albers JJ, Fisher LD, et al, "Regression of Coronary Artery Disease as a Result of Intensive Lipid-Lowering Therapy in Men With High Levels of Apolipoprotein B," *N Engl J Med*, 1990, 323:1289-98.

Capuzzi DM, Guyton JR, Morgan JM, et al, "Efficacy and Safety of an Extended-Release Niacin (Niaspan®): A Long-Term Study," *Am J Cardiol*, 1998, 82:74U-81U.

Coronary Drug Project Research Program, "Clofibrate and Niacin in Coronary Heart Disease," *JAMA*, 1975, 231:360-81.

Dart A, Jerums G, Nicholson G, et al, "A Multicenter, Double-Blind, One-Year Study Comparing Safety and Efficacy of Atorvastatin Versus Simvastatin in Patients With Hypercholesterolemia," *Am J Cardiol*, 1997, 80:39-44.

Davidson M, McKenney J, Stein E, et al, "Comparison of One-Year Efficacy and Safety of Atorvastatin Versus Lovastatin in Primary Hypercholesterolemia," *Am J Cardiol*, 1997, 79:1475-81.

Frick MH, Heinonen OP, Huttunen JK, et al, "Helsinki Heart Study: Primary-Prevention Trial With Gemfibrozil in Middle-Aged Men With Dyslipidemia," *N Engl J Med*, 1987, 317:1237-45.

Garber AM, Browner WS, and Hulley SB, "Clinical Guideline, Part 2: Cholesterol Screening in Asymptomatic Adults, Revisited," *Ann Intern Med*, 1995, 124:518-31.

Johannesson M, Jonsson B, Kjekshus J, et al, "Cost-Effectiveness of Simvastatin Treatment to Lower Cholesterol Levels in Patients With Coronary Heart Disease. Scandinavian Simvastatin Survival Study Group," *N Engl N Med*, 1997, 336:332-6.

Jones P, Kafonek S, Laurora I, et al, "Comparative Dose Efficacy Study of Atorvastatin Versus Simvastatin, Pravastatin, Lovastatin, and Fluvastatin in Patients With Hypercholesterolemia," *Am J Cardiol*, 1998, 81:582-7.

Kasiske BL, Ma JZ, Kalil RS, et al, "Effects of Antihypertensive Therapy on Serum Lipids," *Ann Intern Med*, 1995, 133-41.

Lipid Research Clinics Program, "The Lipid Research Clinics Coronary Primary Prevention Trial Results: I. Reduction in Incidence of Coronary Heart Disease," *JAMA*, 1984, 251:351-64.

Multiple Risk Factor Intervention Trial Research Group, "Multiple Risk Factor Intervention Trial: Risk Factor Changes and Mortality Results," *JAMA*, 1982, 248:1465-77.

Pitt B, Waters D, Brown WV, et al, "Aggressive Lipid-Lowering Therapy Compared With Angioplasty in Stable Coronary Artery Disease. Atorvastatin Versus Revascularization Treatment Investigators," *N Engl J Med*, 1999, 341(2):70-6.

Ross SD, Allen IE, Connelly JE, et al, "Clinical Outcomes in Statin Treatment Trials: A Meta-Analysis," *Arch Intern Med*, 1999, 159:1793-802.

Sacks FM, Pfeffer MA, Moye LA, et al, "The Effect of Pravastatin on Coronary Events After Myocardial Infarction in Patients With Average Cholesterol Levels," *N Engl J Med*, 1996, 335:1001-9.

Scandinavian Simvastatin Survival Study, "Randomized Trial of Cholesterol Lowering in 4444 Patients With Coronary Heart Disease: The Scandinavian Simvastatin Survival Study (4S)," *Lancet*, 1994, 344:1383-9.

Schrott HG, Bittner V, Vittinghoff E, et al, "Adherence to National Cholesterol Education Program Treatment Goals in Postmenopausal Women With Heart Disease. The Heart and Estrogen/Progestin Replacement Study (HERS)," *JAMA*, 1997, 277:1281-6.

Shepherd J, Cobbe SM, Ford I, et al, "Prevention of Coronary Heart Disease With Pravastatin in Men With Hypercholesterolemia, The West of Scotland Coronary Prevention Study Group," *N Engl J Med*, 1995, 333:1301-7.

Stein EA, Davidson MH, Dobs AS, et al, "Efficacy and Safety of Simvastatin 80 mg/day in Hypercholesterolemic Patients. The Expanded Dose Simvastatin U.S. Study Group," *Am J Cardiol*, 1998, 82:311-6.

HYPERTENSION

The optimal blood pressure for adults is <120/80 mm Hg. Consistent systolic pressure ≥140 mm Hg or a diastolic pressure ≥90 mm Hg, in the absence of a secondary cause, define hypertension. Hypertension affects approximately 25% (50 million people) of the United States population. Of those patients on antihypertensive medication, only one in four patients have their blood pressure controlled (<140/90 mm Hg). Recent mortality rates for stroke and heart disease, in which hypertension is an antecedent, remain unchanged. The prevention, detection, evaluation, and treatment of high blood pressure is therefore paramount for each person and for all healthcare providers.

The Sixth Report of the Joint National Committee (JNC VI) is an excellent reference and guide for the treatment of hypertension (*Arch Intern Med*, 1997, 157:2413-46). Hypertension is classified in stages for adults (see Table 1).

Table 1. Adult Classification of Blood Pressure

Category	Systolic (mm Hg)		Diastolic (mm Hg)
Optimal	<120	and	<80
Normal	<130	and	<85
High normal	130-139	or	85-89
Hypertension			
Stage 1	140-159	or	90-99
Stage 2	160-179	or	100-109
Stage 3	≥180	or	≥110
Isolated systolic	≥140	and	<90

Adapted from the Sixth Report of the Joint National Committee on Prevention, Detection, Evaluation, and Treatment of High Blood Pressure, NIH Publication No. 98-4080, November 1997.

Table 2. Normal Blood Pressure in Children

Age (y)	Girls' SBP/DBP (mm Hg)		Boys' SBP/DBP (mm Hg)	
	50th Percentile for Height	75th Percentile for Height	50th Percentile for Height	75th Percentile for Height
1	104/58	105/59	102/57	104/58
6	111/73	112/73	114/74	115/75
12	123/80	124/81	123/81	125/82
17	129/84	130/85	136/87	138/88

SBP = systolic blood pressure.

DBP = diastolic blood pressure.

Adapted from the report by the NHBPEP Working Group on Hypertension Control in Children and Adolescents.

Initial follow up of adult patients is based on office blood pressure recordings (see Table 3).

Table 3. Blood Pressure Screening and Follow-up

Initial Screening BP (mm Hg)		Follow-up Recommended
Systolic	Diastolic	
<130	<85	Recheck in 2 years
130-139	85-89	Recheck in 1 year
140-159	90-99	Confirm within 2 months
160-179	100-109	Evaluate/treatment within 1 month
≥180	≥110	Evaluate/treatment immediately or within 1 week

Adapted from the Sixth Report of the Joint National Committee on Prevention, Detection, Evaluation, and Treatment of High Blood Pressure, NIH Publication No. 98-4080, November 1997.

Based on these initial assessments, treatment strategies for patients with hypertension are stratified based on their blood pressure and their risk group classification (see Table 4).

Table 4. Blood Pressure and Risk Stratification

Blood Pressure Stages	Risk Group A (no RF or TOD)	Risk Group B (≥1 RF, not including diabetes, no TOD)	Risk Group C (TOD and/or diabetes regardless of RF)
High normal (130-139/85-89 mm Hg)	Lifestyle modification	Lifestyle modification	Drug therapy* and lifestyle modification
Stage 1 (140-159/90-99 mm Hg)	Lifestyle modification (up to 12 mo)	Lifestyle modification (up to 6 mo)†	Drug therapy and lifestyle modification
Stages 2 and 3 (≥160/≥100 mm Hg)	Drug therapy and lifestyle modification	Drug therapy and lifestyle modification	Drug therapy and lifestyle modification

*For those with heart failure, renal insufficiency, or diabetes.

†For patients with multiple risk factors, consider starting both drug and lifestyle modification together.

RF = risk factor.

TOD = target-organ disease.

Adapted from the Sixth Report of the Joint National Committee on Prevention, Detection, Evaluation, and Treatment of High Blood Pressure, NIH Publication No. 98-4080, November 1997.

Patients in Risk **Group A** have no risk factors; **Group B**, at least one risk factor (other than diabetes), and no cardiovascular disease or target organ disease (see Table 5); **Group C**, have cardiovascular disease or diabetes or target organ disease (see Table 5). Risk factors include smoking, dyslipidemia, diabetes, age >60 years, male gender, postmenopausal women, and family history of cardiovascular disease (cardiovascular event in first degree female relatives <65 years and in first degree male relatives <55 years).

Table 5. Target-Organ Disease

Organ System	Manifestation
Cardiac	Clinical, EKG, or radiologic evidence of coronary artery disease; prior MI, angina, post-CABG; left ventricular hypertrophy (LVH); left ventricular dysfunction or cardiac failure
Cerebrovascular	Transient ischemic attack or stroke
Peripheral vascular	Absence of pulses in extremities (except dorsalis pedis), claudication, aneurysm
Renal	Serum creatinine ≥130 μmol/L (1.5 mg/dL); proteinuria (≥1+); microalbuminuria
Retinopathy	Hemorrhages or exudates, with or without papilledema

Adapted from the Sixth Report of the Joint National Committee on Prevention, Detection, Evaluation, and Treatment of High Blood Pressure, NIH Publication No. 98-4080, November 1997.

Treatment of hypertension should be individualized. Lower blood pressures should be achieved for patients with diabetes or renal disease. A treatment algorithm (see following page) may be used to select specific antihypertensives based on specific or compelling indications. Special consideration for starting combination therapy should be made in each patient. Starting drug therapy at a low dose and titrating upward if blood pressure is not controlled is recommended. The benefit of these strategies is to minimize the occurrence of adverse effects while achieving optimal blood pressure control. One caveat for starting at a low dose and then titrating upward is that patients and clinicians must commit to well-timed follow-up so that blood pressure is controlled in a timely manner. Lifestyle modification and risk reduction should be begun and continued throughout treatment.

Rationale for combination drug therapy is discussed on the following pages.

HYPERTENSION *(Continued)*

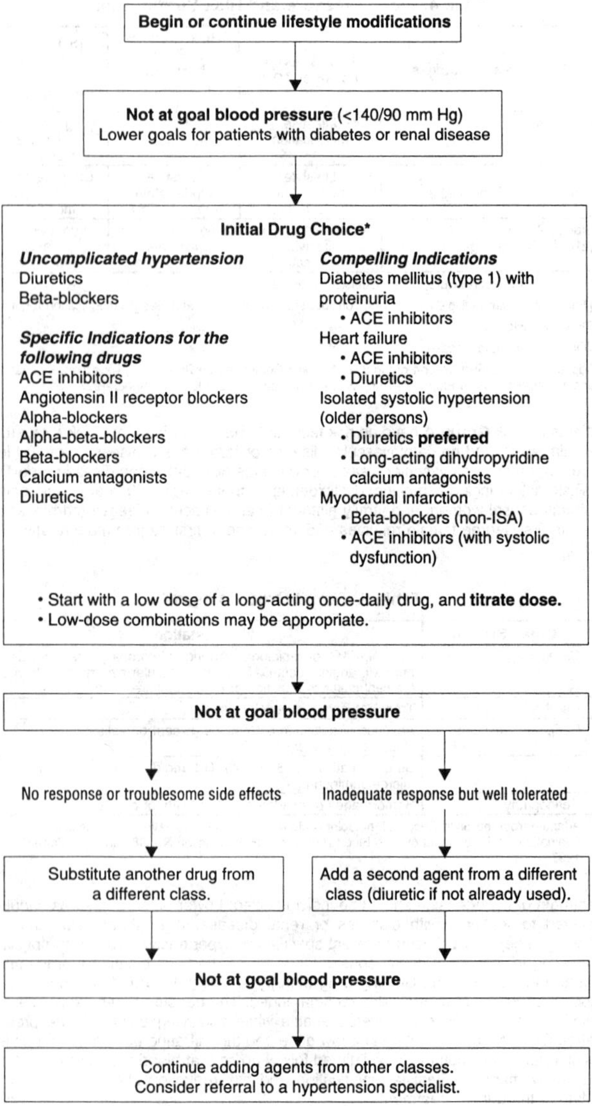

Begin or continue lifestyle modifications
Not at goal blood pressure (<140/90 mm Hg)
Lower goals for patients with diabetes or renal disease
Initial Drug Choice*
Uncomplicated hypertension
Diuretics
Beta-blockers
Specific Indications for the following drugs
ACE inhibitors
Angiotensin II receptor blockers
Alpha-blockers
Alpha-beta-blockers
Beta-blockers
Calcium antagonists
Diuretics
Compelling Indications
Diabetes mellitus (type 1) with proteinuria
• ACE inhibitors
Heart failure
• ACE inhibitors
• Diuretics
Isolated systolic hypertension (older persons)
• Diuretics preferred
• Long-acting dihydropyridine calcium antagonists
Myocardial infarction
• Beta-blockers (non-ISA)
• ACE inhibitors (with systolic dysfunction)
• Start with a low dose of a long-acting once-daily drug, and titrate dose.
• Low-dose combinations may be appropriate.
Not at goal blood pressure
No response or troublesome side effects
Inadequate response but well tolerated
Substitute another drug from a different class.
Add a second agent from a different class (diuretic if not already used).
Not at goal blood pressure
Continue adding agents from other classes.
Consider referral to a hypertension specialist.

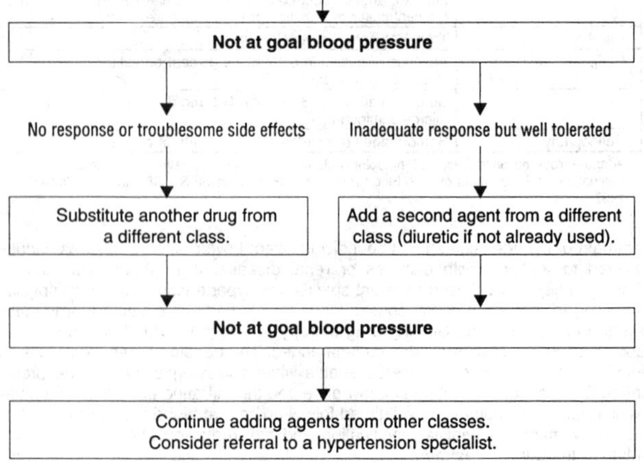

* Unless contraindicated. ACE indicates angiotensin-converting enzyme; ISA, intrinsic sympathomimetic activity. Based on randomized controlled trials.

COMBINATION THERAPY IN THE TREATMENT OF HYPERTENSION

Important concerns in treating hypertension are the efficacy and side effects of therapy. In the past, progressive increases in dosage of a single drug were used to improve blood pressure control. Historically (based on the Joint National Committee [JNC] recommendations), the maximum doses of recommended drugs have decreased from those proposed in earlier JNC reports.

More recently, the concept of combination therapy has begun to gain increasing favor. This is reflected most clearly in the report of the Sixth Joint National Committee on Detection, Evaluation, and Treatment of High Blood Pressure (JNC VI). Specifically, JNC VI endorses the use of low doses of two antihypertensive drugs in fixed-dose combinations as a possible route for initial treatment of hypertension. This recommendation extends earlier JNC V recognition that combining drugs with different modes of action may allow smaller doses of drugs to be used to achieve control, and minimize the potential for dose-dependent side effects.

Combination therapy thus constitutes the use of an additional antihypertensive medication before the first therapeutic agent is necessarily at maximum dose, or the use of two agents in low doses at the onset of antihypertensive treatment. The rationale, background, and experience with combination therapy are nicely reviewed in Kaplan NM and Sever PS, "Combination Therapy: A Key to Comprehensive Patient Care," *Am J Hyperten*, 1997, 10(7 part 2):127S and by Moser M and Black HR, "The Role of Combination Therapy in the Treatment of Hypertension," *Am J Hyperten*, 11:73S-8S).

Fundamental to the combination therapy approach are the following considerations.

- Drugs with different and complementary mechanisms of action may often produce synergistic reductions in blood pressure, classically evident in the use of diuretics and ACE inhibitors.
- Low doses of a single drug are less likely to induce side effects.
- More than 50% of all hypertensive patients will need more than one drug to achieve blood pressure control.

In effect, this therapeutic strategy allows exploitation of the steepest part of the antihypertensive dose response curve, achieving synergistic or additive therapeutic benefit while limiting potential for side effects. Disadvantages include first, the need to take two drugs, often resulting in taking two separate tablets. It is important to ensure that both therapeutic preparations have equivalent durations of action. Second, the cost of separate products may exceed that of increased doses of a single medication.

In mitigation, fixed-dose combinations of antihypertensive preparations are available with recent options, including Lexxel® (calcium channel blocker and ACE inhibitor), Hyzaar® (angiotensin receptor blocker and hydrochlorothiazide), Capozide® (ACE inhibitor and hydrochlorothiazide), and Ziac® (beta-blocker and hydrochlorothiazide). These combinations help address cost and convenience issues in combination therapy.

HYPERTENSION *(Continued)*

COMPELLING INDICATIONS FOR SPECIFIC THERAPIES

Indication	Drug Therapy
Compelling Indications Unless Contraindicated	
Diabetes mellitus (type I) with proteinuria	ACEI
Heart failure	ACEI, diuretics, BB (carvedilol, metoprolol XL/CR, bisoprolol, hydralazine + isosorbide dinitrate)
Isolated systolic hypertension (older patients)	Diuretics (preferred), CCB (long-acting)
Myocardial infarction	Beta-blockers (non-ISA), ACEI (with systolic dysfunction)
High-risk patients (CVD plus risk factors)	ACEI (ramipril)
May Have Favorable Effects on Comorbid Conditions	
Angina	Beta-blockers, CCB (long-acting)
Atrial tachycardia and fibrillation	Beta-blockers, CCB (non-DHP)
Cyclosporine-induced hypertension (caution with the dose of cyclosporine)	CCB
Diabetes mellitus (types I and II) with proteinuria	ACEI (preferred), CCB
Diabetes mellitus (type II)	Low-dose diuretics (≤25 mg HCTZ)
Dyslipidemia	Alpha-blockers
Essential tremor	Beta-blockers (noncardioselective)
Heart failure	Losartan, candesartan
Hyperthyroidism	Beta-blockers
Migraine	Beta-blockers (noncardioselective), CCB (long-acting) (non-DHP)
Myocardial infarction (non-Q-wave with normal systolic function and no edema)	Diltiazem, verapamil (long-acting)
Osteoporosis	Thiazides
Preoperative hypertension	Beta-blockers
Prostatism (BPH)	Alpha-blockers
Renal insufficiency (caution in renovascular hypertension and creatinine ≥265.2 mmol/L [3 mg/dL])	ACEI
May Have Unfavorable Effects on Comorbid Conditions*	
Bronchospastic disease	Beta-blockers†
Depression	Beta-blockers, central alpha-agonists, reserpine†
Diabetes mellitus (types I and II)	Beta-blockers, high-dose diuretics
Dyslipidemia	Beta-blockers (non-ISA), diuretics (high-dose)
Gout	Diuretics
Second or third degree heart block	Beta-blockers†, CCB (non-DHP)†
Heart failure	Beta-blockers (with high ISA), CCB (except amlodipine, felodipine)
Liver disease	Labetalol hydrochloride, methyldopa†
Peripheral vascular disease	Beta-blockers
Pregnancy	ACEI†, angiotensin II receptor blockers†
Renal insufficiency	Potassium-sparing agents
Renovascular disease	ACEI, angiotensin II receptor blockers

ACEI indicates angiotensin-converting enzyme inhibitors; BPH, benign prostatic hyperplasia; CCB, calcium antagonists; DHP, dihydropyridine; ISA, intrinsic sympathomimetic activity; MI, myocardial infarction; and non-CS, noncardioselective.

Conditions and drugs are listed in alphabetical order.

*These drugs may be used with special monitoring unless contraindicated.

†Contraindicated.

HYPERTENSION AND PREGNANCY

The report of the NHBPEP Working Group on High Blood Pressure in Pregnancy permits continuation of drug therapy in women with chronic hypertension (**except for ACE inhibitors**). In addition, angiotensin II receptor blockers should not be used during pregnancy. In women with chronic hypertension with diastolic levels ≥100 mm Hg (lower when end organ damage or underlying renal disease is present) and in women with acute hypertension when levels are ≥105 mm Hg, the following agents are suggested (see table).

Suggested Drug	Comments
Central alpha-agonists	Methyldopa (C) is the drug of choice recommended by the NHBPEP Working Group.
Beta-blockers	Atenolol (C) and metoprolol (C) appear to be safe and effective in late pregnancy. Labetalol (C) also appears to be effective (alpha- and beta-blockers).
Calcium antagonists	Potential synergism with magnesium sulfate may lead to precipitous hypotension. (C)
ACE inhibitors, angiotensin II receptor blockers	Fetal abnormalities, including death, can be caused, and these drugs **should not** be used in pregnancy. (D)
Diuretics	Diuretics (C) are recommended for chronic hypertension if prescribed before gestation or if patients appear to be salt-sensitive. They are not recommended in pre-eclampsia.
Direct vasodilators	Hydralazine (C) is the parenteral drug of choice based on its long history of safety and efficacy. (C)

Adapted from Sibai and Lindheimer. There are several other antihypertensive drugs for which there are very limited data. The U.S. Food and Drug Administration classifies pregnancy risk as follows: C = adverse effects in animals; no controlled trials in humans; use if risk appears justified; D = positive evidence of fetal risk. ACE = angiotensin-converting enzyme.

HYPERTENSION *(Continued)*

HYPERTENSIVE EMERGENCIES AND URGENCIES

General Treatment Principles in the Treatment of Hypertensive Emergencies

Principle	Considerations
Admit the patient to the hospital, preferably in the ICU. Monitor vital signs appropriately.	Establish I.V. access and place patient on a cardiac monitor. Place a femoral intra-arterial line and pulmonary arterial catheter, if indicated, to assess cardiopulmonary function and intravascular volume status.
Perform rapid but thorough history and physical examination.	Determine cause of, or precipitating factors to, hypertensive crisis if possible (remember to obtain a medication history including Rx, OTC, and illicit drugs). Obtain details regarding any prior history of hypertension (severity, duration, treatment), as well as other coexisting illnesses. Assess the extent of hypertensive end organ damage. Determine if a hypertensive urgency or emergency exists.
Determine goal blood pressure based on premorbid level, duration, severity and rapidity of increase of blood pressure, concomitant medical conditions, race, and age.	Acute decreases in blood pressure to normal or subnormal levels during the initial treatment period may reduce perfusion to the brain, heart, and kidneys, and must be avoided except in specific instances (ie, dissecting aortic aneurysm). Gradually establish a normal (or reasonable) blood pressure over the next 1-2 weeks.
Select an appropriate antihypertensive regimen depending on the individual patient and clinical setting.	Initiate a controlled decrease in blood pressure. Avoid concomitant administration of multiple agents that may cause precipitous falls in blood pressure. Select the agent with the best hemodynamic profile based on the primary treatment goal. Avoid diuretics and sodium restriction during the initial treatment period unless there is a clear clinical indication (ie, CHF, pulmonary edema). Avoid sedating antihypertensives in patients with hypertensive encephalopathy, CVA, or other CNS disorders in whom mental status must be monitored. Use caution with direct vasodilating agents that induce reflex tachycardia or increase cardiac output in patients with coronary heart disease, history of angina or myocardial infarction, or dissecting aortic aneurysm. Preferably choose an agent that does not adversely affect glomerular filtration rate or renal blood flow and also agents that have favorable effects on cerebral blood flow and its autoregulation, especially for patients with hypertensive encephalopathy or CVAs. Select the most efficacious agent with the fewest adverse effects based on the underlying cause of the hypertensive crisis and other individual patient factors.
Initiate a chronic antihypertensive regimen after the patient's blood pressure is stabilized	Begin oral antihypertensive therapy once goal blood pressure is achieved before gradually tapering parenteral medications. Select the best oral regimen based on cost, ease of administration, adverse effect profile, and concomitant medical conditions.

Oral Agents Used in the Treatment of Hypertensive Urgencies and Emergencies

Drug	Dose	Onset	Cautions
Captopril*	P.O.: 25 mg, repeat as required	15-30 min	Hypotension, renal failure in bilateral renal artery stenosis
Clonidine	P.O.: 0.1-0.2 mg, repeated every hour as needed to a total dose of 0.6 mg	30-60 min	Hypotension, drowsiness, dry mouth
Labetalol	P.O.: 200-400 mg, repeat every 2-3 h	30 min to 2 h	Bronchoconstriction, heart block, orthostatic hypotension

*There is no clearly defined clinical advantage in the use of sublingual over oral routes of administration with these agents.

Recommendations for the Use of Intravenous Antihypertensive Drugs in Selected Hypertensive Emergencies

Condition	Agent(s) of Choice	Agent(s) to Avoid or Use With Caution	General Treatment Principles
Hypertensive encephalopathy	Nitroprusside, labetalol, diazoxide	Methyldopa, reserpine	Avoid drugs with CNS-sedating effects
Acute intracranial or subarachnoid hemorrhage	Nicardipine*, nitroprusside, trimethaphan	Beta-blockers	Careful titration with a short-acting agent
Cerebral infarction	Nicardipine*, nitroprusside, labetalol, trimethaphan	Beta-blockers, minoxidil, diazoxide	Careful titration with a short-acting agent. Avoid agents that may decrease cerebral blood flow.
Head trauma	Esmolol, labetalol	Methyldopa, reserpine, nitroprusside, nitroglycerin, hydralazine	Avoid drugs with CNS sedating effects, or those that may increase intracranial pressure
Acute myocardial infarction, myocardial ischemia	Nitroglycerin, nicardipine* (calcium channel blockers), labetalol	Hydralazine, diazoxide, minoxidil	Avoid drugs which cause reflex tachycardia and increased myocardial oxygen consumption
Acute pulmonary edema	Nitroprusside, nitroglycerin, loop diuretics	Beta-blockers (labetalol), minoxidil, methyldopa	Avoid drugs which may cause sodium and water retention and edema exacerbation
Renal dysfunction	Hydralazine, calcium channel blockers	Nitroprusside, ACE inhibitors, beta-blockers (labetalol)	Avoid drugs with increased toxicity in renal failure and those that may cause decreased renal blood flow.
Eclampsia	Hydralazine, labetalol, nitroprusside†	Trimethaphan, diuretics, diazoxide (diazoxide may cause cessation of labor)	Avoid drugs that may cause adverse fetal effects, compromise placental circulation, or decrease cardiac output.
Pheochromo-cytoma	Phentolamine, nitroprusside, beta-blockers (eg, esmolol) only after alpha blockade (phentolamine)	Beta-blockers in the absence of alpha blockade, methyldopa, minoxidil	Use drugs of proven efficacy and specificity. Unopposed beta blockade may exacerbate hypertension.
Dissecting aortic aneurysm	Nitroprusside and beta blockade, trimethaphan	Hydralazine, diazoxide, minoxidil	Avoid drugs which may increase cardiac output.
Postoperative hypertension	Nitroprusside, nicardipine*, labetalol	Trimethaphan	Avoid drugs which may exacerbate postoperative ileus.

*The use of nicardipine in these situations is by the recommendation of the author based on a review of the literature.

†Reserve nitroprusside for eclamptic patients with life-threatening hypertension unresponsive to other agents due to the potential risk to the fetus (cyanide and thiocyanate metabolites may cross the placenta).

HYPERTENSION *(Continued)*

Selected Intravenous Agents for Hypertensive Emergencies

Drug	Dose*	Onset of Action	Duration of Action	Adverse Effects†	Special Indications
Vasodilators					
Sodium nitroprusside	0.25-10 mcg/kg/min as I.V. infusion‡ (max: 10 min only)	Immediate	1-2 min	Nausea, vomiting, muscle twitching, sweating, thiocyanate and cyanide intoxication	Most hypertensive emergencies; caution with high intracranial pressure or azotemia
Nicardipine hydrochloride	5-15 mg/h I.V.	5-10 min	1-4 h	Tachycardia, headache, flushing, local phlebitis	Most hypertensive emergencies except acute heart failure; caution with coronary ischemia
Fenoldopam mesylate	0.1-0.3 mcg/kg/min I.V. infusion	<5 min	30 min	Tachycardia, headache, nausea, flushing	Most hypertensive emergencies; caution with glaucoma
Nitroglycerin	5-100 mcg/min as I.V. infusion‡	2-5 min	3-5 min	Headache, vomiting, methemoglobinemia, tolerance with prolonged use	Coronary ischemia
Enalaprilat	1.25-5 mg every 6 hours I.V.	15-30 min	6 h	Precipitous fall in pressure in high-renin states; response variable	Acute left ventricular failure; avoid in acute myocardial infarction
Hydralazine hydrochloride	10-20 mg I.V. 10-50 mg I.M.	10-20 min 20-30 min	3-8 h	Tachycardia, flushing, headache, vomiting, aggravation of angina	Eclampsia
Diazoxide	50-100 mg I.V. bolus repeated, or 15-30 mg/min infusion	2-4 min	6-12 h	Nausea, flushing, tachycardia, chest pain	Now obsolete; when no intensive monitoring available
Adrenergic Inhibitors					
Labetalol hydrochloride	20-80 mg I.V. bolus every 10 min; 0.5-2 mg/min I.V. infusion	5-10 min	3-6 h	Vomiting, scalp tingling, burning in throat, dizziness, nausea, heart block, orthostatic hypotension	Most hypertensive emergencies except acute heart failure
Esmolol hydrochloride	250-500 mcg/kg/min for 1 min, then 50-100 mcg/kg/min for 4 min; may repeat	1-2 min	10-20 min	Hypotension, nausea	Aortic dissection, perioperative
Phentolamine	5-15 mg I.V.	1-2 min	3-10 min	Tachycardia, flushing, headache	Catecholamine excess

I.V. indicates intravenous; I.M., intramuscular

*These doses may vary from those in the *Physicians' Desk Reference* (51st edition).

†Hypotension may occur with all agents.

‡Require special delivery system.

Resources

Guidelines

1999 World Health Organization-International Society of Hypertension Guidelines for the Management of Hypertension. Guidelines Subcommittee, *J Hypertens*, 1999, 17:151-83.

National High Blood Pressure Education Program Working Group on Hypertension Control in Children and Adolescents. Update on the 1987 Task Force Report on High Blood Pressure in Children and Adolescents: A Working Group Report From the National High Blood Pressure Education Program, *Pediatrics*, 1996, 98:649-58.

National High Blood Pressure Education Program Working Group. 1995 Update of the Working Group Reports on Chronic Renal Failure and Renovascular Hypertension, *Arch Intern Med*, 1996, 156:1938-47.

"The Sixth Report of the National Committee on Detection, Evaluation, and Treatment of High Blood Pressure (JNC-VI)," *Arch Intern Med*, 1997, 157:2413-46.

Others

Appel LJ, Moore TJ, Obarzanek E, et al, "A Clinical Trial of the Effect of Dietary Patterns on Blood Pressure. The DASH Collaborative Research Group," *N Engl J Med*, 1997, 336:1117-24.

Epstein M and Bakris G, "Newer Approaches to Antihypertensive Therapy: Use of Fixed-Dose Combination Therapy," *Arch Intern Med*, 1996, 156:1969-78.

Estacio RO and Schrier RW, "Antihypertensive Therapy in Type II Diabetes: Implications of the Appropriate Blood Pressure Control in Diabetes (ABCD) Trial," *Am J Cardiol*, 1998, 82:9R-14R.

Flack JM, Neaton J, Grimm RJ, et al, "Blood Pressure and Mortality Among Men With Prior Myocardial Infarction. The Multiple Risk Factor Intervention Trial Research Group," *Circulation*, 1995, 92:2437-45.

Frishman WH, Bryzinski BS, Coulson LR, et al, "A Multifactorial Trial Design to Assess Combination Therapy in Hypertension: Treatment With Bisoprolol and Hydrochlorothiazide," *Arch Intern Med*, 1994, 154:1461-8.

Furberg CD, Psaty BM, and Meyer JV, "Nifedipine: Dose-Related Increase in Mortality in Patients With Coronary Heart Disease," *Circulation*, 1995, 92:1326-31.

Glynn RJ, Brock DB, Harris T, et al, "Use of Antihypertensive Drugs and Trends in Blood Pressure in the Elderly," *Arch Intern Med*, 1995, 155:1855-60.

Gradman AH, Cutler NR, Davis PJ, et al, "Combined Enalapril and Felodipine Extended Release (ER) for Systemic Hypertension. The Enalapril-Felodipine ER Factorial Study Group," *Am J Cardiol*, 1997, 79:431-5.

Grim RH Jr, Flack JM, Grandits GA, et al, "Long-Term Effects on Plasma Lipids of Diet and Drugs to Treat Hypertension. The Treatment of Mild Hypertension Study (TOMHS) Research Group," *JAMA*, 1996, 275:1549-56.

Grim RH Jr, Grandits GA, Cutler JA, et al, "Relationships of Quality-of-Life Measures to Long-Term Lifestyle and Drug Treatment in the Treatment of Mild Hypertension Study. The TOMHS Research Group," *Arch Intern Med*, 1997, 157:638-48.

Grossman E, Messerli FH, Grodzicki T, et al, "Should a Moratorium Be Placed on Sublingual Nifedipine Capsules Given for Hypertensive Emergencies and Pseudoemergencies?" *JAMA*, 1996, 276:1328-31.

Hansson L, Zanchetti A, Carruthers SG, et al, "Effects of Intensive Blood Pressure Lowering and Low-Dose Aspirin in Patients With Hypertension: Principal Results of the Hypertension Optimal Treatment (HOT) Randomized Trial. HOT Study Group," *Lancet*, 1998, 351:1755-62.

Kaplan NM and Gifford RW Jr, "Choice of Initial Therapy for Hypertension," *JAMA*, 1996, 275:1577-80.

Kasiske BL, Ma JZ, Kalil RSN, et al, "Effects of Antihypertensive Therapy in Serum Lipids," *Ann Intern Med*, 1995, 122:133-41.

Kostis JB, Davis BR, Cutler J, et al, "Prevention of Heart Failure by Antihypertensive Drug Treatment in Older Persons With Isolated Systolic Hypertension. SHEP Cooperative Research Group," *JAMA*, 1997, 278:212-6.

Lazarus JM, Bourgoignie JJ, Buckalew VM, et al, "Achievement and Safety of a Low Blood Pressure Goal in Chronic Renal Disease: The Modification of Diet in Renal Disease Study Group," *Hypertension*, 1997, 29:641-50.

Lindheimer MD, "Hypertension in Pregnancy," *Hypertension*, 1993, 22:127-37.

Materson BJ, Reda DJ, Cushman WC, et al, "Single-Drug Therapy for Hypertension in

HYPERTENSION *(Continued)*

Men: A Comparison of Six Antihypertensive Agents With Placebo. The Department of Veterans Affairs Cooperative Study Group on Antihypertensive Agents," *N Engl J Med*, 1993, 328:914-21.

Miller NH, Hill M, Kottke T, et al, "The Multi-Level Compliance Challenge: Recommendations for a Call to Action; A Statement for Healthcare Professionals," *Circulation*, 1997, 95:1085-90.

Neaton JD and Wentworth D, "Serum Cholesterol, Blood Pressure, Cigarette Smoking, and Death From Coronary Heart Disease: Overall Findings and Differences by Age for 316,099 White Men. The Multiple Risk Factor Intervention Trial Research Group," *Arch Intern Med*, 1992, 152:56-64.

Neaton JD, Grim RH, Prineas RJ, et al, "Treatment of Mild Hypertension Study (TOHMS). Final Results," *JAMA*, 1993, 270:721-31.

Oparil S, Levine JH, Zuschke CA, et al, "Effects of Candesartan Cilexetil in Patients With Severe Systemic Hypertension," *Am J Cardiol*, 1999, 84:289-93.

Perloff D, Grim C, Flack J, et al, "Human Blood Pressure Determination by Sphygmomanometry," *Circulation*, 1993, 88:2460-7.

Perry HM Jr, Bingham S, Horney A, et al, "Antihypertensive Efficacy of Treatment Regimens Used in Veterans Administration Hypertension Clinics. Department of Veterans Affairs Cooperative Study Group on Antihypertensive Agents," *Hypertension*, 1998, 31:771-9.

Preston RA, Materson BJ, Reda DJ, et al, "Age-Race Subgroup Compared With Renin Profile as Predictors of Blood Pressure Response to Antihypertensive Therapy," *JAMA*, 1998, 280:1168-72.

Psaty BM, Smith NL, Siscovick DS, et al, "Health Outcomes Associated With Antihypertensive Therapies Used as First-Line Agents. A Systemic Review and Meta-analysis," *JAMA*, 1997, 277:739-45.

Radevski IV, Valtchanova SP, Candy GP, et al, "Comparison of Acebutolol With and Without Hydrochlorothiazide Versus Carvedilol With and Without Hydrochlorothiazide in Black Patients With Mild to Moderate Systemic Hypertension," *Am J Cardiol*, 1999, 84(1):70-5.

Setaro JF and Black HR, "Refractory Hypertension," *N Engl J Med*, 1992, 327:543-7.

SHEP Cooperative Research Group, "Prevention of Stroke by Antihypertensive Drug Treatment in Older Persons With Isolated Systolic Hypertension: Final Results of the Systolic Hypertension in the Elderly Program (SHEP)," *JAMA*, 1991, 265:3255-64.

Sibai BM, "Treatment of Hypertension in Pregnant Women," *N Engl J Med*, 1996, 335:257-65.

Sowers JR, "Comorbidity of Hypertension and Diabetes: The Fosinopril Versus Amlodipine Cardiovascular Events Trial," *Am J Cardiol*, 1998, 82:15R-19R.

Sternberg H, Rosenthal T, Shamiss A, et al, "Altered Circadian Rhythm of Blood Pressure in Shift Workers," *J Hum Hypertens*, 1995, 9:349-53.

"The Hypertension Prevention Trial: Three-Year Effects of Dietary Changes on Blood Pressure. Hypertension Prevention Trial Research Group," *Arch Intern Med*, 1990, 150:153-62.

Trials of Hypertension Prevention Collaborative Research Group, "Effects of Weight Loss and Sodium Reduction Intervention on Blood Pressure and Hypertension Incidence in Overweight People With High-Normal Blood Pressure: The Trials of Hypertension Prevention, Phase II," *Arch Intern Med*, 1997, 157:657-67.

Tuomilehto J, Rastenyte D, Birkenhager WH, et al, "Effects of Calcium Channel Blockade in Older Patients With Diabetes and Systolic Hypertension," *N Engl J Med*, 1999, 340:677-84.

Veelken R and Schmieder RE, "Overview of Alpha-1 Adrenoceptor Antagonism and Recent Advances in Hypertensive Therapy," *Am J Hypertens*, 1996, 9:139S-49S.

White WB, Black HR, Weber MA, et al, "Comparison of Effects of Controlled Onset Extended Release Verapamil at Bedtime and Nifedipine Gastrointestinal Therapeutic System on Arising on Early Morning Blood Pressure, Heart Rate, and the Heart Rate-Blood Pressure Product," *Am J Cardiol*, 1998, 81:424-31.

OSTEOPOROSIS MANAGEMENT QUICK REFERENCE

PREVALENCE

Osteoporosis effects 25 million Americans of which 80% are women. 27% of American women >80 years of age have osteopenia and 70% of American women >80 years of age have osteoporosis.

CONSEQUENCES

1.3 million bone fractures annually (low impact/nontraumatic) and pain, pulmonary insufficiency, decreased quality of life, and economic costs; >250,000 hip fractures per year with a 20% mortality rate.

RISK FACTORS

Advanced age, female, chronic renal disease, hyperparathyroidism, Cushing's disease, hypogonadism/anorexia, hyperprolactinemia, cancer, large and prolonged dose heparin or glucocorticoids, anticonvulsants, hyperthyroidism (current or history, or excessive thyroid supplements), sedentary, excessive exercise, early menopause, oophorectomy without hormone replacement, excessive aluminum-containing antacid, smoking, methotrexate.

DIAGNOSIS/MONITORING

DXA bone density, history of fracture (low impact or nontraumatic), compressed vertebrae, decreased height, hump-back appearance. Osteomark™ urine assay measures bone breakdown fragments and may help assess therapy response earlier than DXA but diagnostic value is uncertain as Osteomark™ doesn't reveal extent of bone loss. Bone markers may be tested to evaluate effectiveness of antiresorptive urine therapy.

OSTEOPOROSIS PREVENTION

1. Adequate dietary calcium (eg, dairy products)
2. Vitamin D (eg, fortified dairy products, cod, fatty fish)
3. Weight-bearing exercise (eg, walking) as tolerated
4. Calcium supplement of 1000-1500 mg elemental calcium daily (divided in 500 mg increments); women >65 years on estrogen replacement therapy supplement 1000 mg elemental calcium; women >65 not receiving estrogens and men >55 years supplement 1500 mg elemental calcium. To minimize constipation add fiber and start with 500 mg/day for several months, then increase to 500 mg twice daily taken at different times than fiber. Chewable and liquid products are available. Calcium carbonate is given with food to enhance bioavailability. Calcium citrate may be given without regards to meals.
   - Contraindications: Hypercalcemia, ventricular fibrillation
   - Side effects: Constipation, anorexia
   - Drug interactions: Fiber, tetracycline, iron supplement, minerals
5. Vitamin D Supplement: 400-800 units daily (often satisfied by 1-2 multivitamins or fortified milk) in addition to calcium or a combined calcium and vitamin D supplement and/or >15 minutes direct sunlight/day. Some elderly, especially with significant renal or liver disease can't metabolize (activate) vitamin D and require calcitriol 0.25 mcg orally twice daily or adjusted per serum calcium level, the active form of vitamin D; can check 1,25 OH vitamin D level to confirm need for calcitriol.
   - Contraindications: Hypercalcemia (weakness, headache, drowsiness, nausea, diarrhea), hypercalciuria and renal stones
   - Side effects (uncommon): Hypercalcemia (see above)
   - Monitor 24-hour urine and serum calcium if using >1000 units/day

OSTEOPOROSIS MANAGEMENT QUICK REFERENCE
(Continued)

6. Estrogen: Especially useful if bone density <80% of average plus symptoms of estrogen deficiency or cardiac disease. Bone density increases over 1-2 years then plateaus. This is considered 1st line therapy unless contraindicated due to medicinal history (see below) or patient preference to avoid HRT (hormone replacement therapy).
   - Contraindications: Pregnancy, breast or estrogen-dependent cancer, undiagnosed abnormal genital bleeding, active thrombophlebitis, or history of thromboembolism during previous estrogen or oral contraceptive therapy or pregnancy. Pretreatment mammogram, gynecological exam are advised along with routine breast exam because of a possibly increased risk of breast cancer with long-term use.
   - Dose: Conjugated estrogen of 0.625 mg/day or its equivalent (continuous therapy preferred).
   - Side effects: Vaginal spotting/bleeding, nausea, vomiting, breast tenderness/enlargement, amenorrheic with extended use.
     Initiate therapy slowly (side effects are more common and severe in women without estrogen for many years). Administer with medroxyprogesterone acetate (MPA) 2.5-5 mg daily in women with uterus (unopposed estrogen can cause endometrial cancer). MPA can increase vaginal bleeding, increase weight, edema, mood changes.
   - Drug Interactions: May increase corticosteroid effect, monitor for need to decrease corticosteroid dose.

OSTEOPOROSIS TREATMENT

1. Calcium, vitamin D, exercise, and estrogen: As above
2. Alendronate (Fosamax®): Consider if patient is intolerant of, or refuses estrogen or it is contraindicated, especially if severe osteoporosis (ie, ≥2.5 standard deviations below average young adult bone density, T-score, or history of low impact or nontraumatic fracture). Increasing bone density of hip and spine observed for at least 3 years (ie, no plateau as seen with estrogen).
   - Contraindications: Hypocalcemia, not advised if existing gastrointestinal disorders (eg, esophageal disorders such as reflux, sensitive stomach).
   - Dose: 10 mg once daily (treatment dose for osteoporosis; not recommended if creatinine clearance <35 mL/minute) before breakfast on an empty stomach with 6-8 ounces tap water (not mineral water, coffee, or juice) and remain upright or raise head of bed for bedridden patients at least 30 degree angle for at least 30 minutes (otherwise may cause ulcerative esophagitis) before eating or drinking. Osteopenia: 5 mg per day for prevention.

   Therapy with calcium and vitamin D is advised, but must be given at a different time of day than alendronate.
   - Side effects (well tolerated): Difficulty swallowing, heartburn, abdominal discomfort, nausea (GI side effects increase with aspirin products), arthralgia/myalgia, constipation, diarrhea, headache, esophagitis.
   - Drug interactions: None known to date.
3. Etidronate: Not FDA approved for postmenopausal osteoporosis and can decrease the quality of bone formation, therefore, change to alendronate.
4. Calcitonin (nasal; Miacalcin®): Indicated if estrogen refused, intolerant, or contraindicated. Potential analgesic effect.
   - Contraindications: Hypersensitivity to salmon protein or gelatin diluent; 1 spray (200 units) into 1 nostril daily (alternate right and left nostril daily); 5 days on and 2 days off is also effective; alternate day administration not effective. If used only for pain, can decrease dose once pain is controlled.
   - Side effects (few): Nasal dryness and irritation (periodically inspect); adequate dietary or supplemental calcium + vitamin D is essential.

   Subcutaneous route (100 units daily): Many side effects (eg, nausea, flushing, anorexia) and the discomfort/inconvenience of injection.

5. Fall prevention: Minimize psychoactive and cardiovascular drugs (monitor BP for orthostasis), give diuretics early in the day, environmental safety check.

	% Elemental Calcium	Elemental Calcium
Calcium gluconate (various)	9	500 mg = 45 mg
Calcium glubionate (Neo-Calglucon®)	6.5	1.8 g = 115 g/5 mL
Calcium lactate (various)	13	325 mg = 42.25 mg
Calcium citrate (Citrical®)	21	950 mg = 200 mg
Effervescent tabs (Citrical Liquitab®)		2376 mg = 500 mg
Calcium acetate		
Phos-Ex 250®	25	1000 mg = 250 mg
Phos-Lo®		667 mg = 169 mg
Tricalcium phosphate (Posture®)	39	1565.2 mg = 600 mg
Calcium carbonate		
Tums®	40	1.2 g = 500 mg
Oscal-500® oral suspension		1.2 g/5 mL = 500 mg
Caltrate 600®		1.5 g = 600 mg

References

Ashworth L, "Focus on Alendronate. A Nonhormonal Option for the Treatment of Osteoporosis in Postmenopausal Women," *Formulary*, 1996, 31:23-30.

Johnson SR, "Should Older Women Use Estrogen Replacement," *J Am Geriatr Soc*, 1996, 44:89-90.

Liberman UA, Weiss SR, and Brool J, "Effect of Oral Alendronate on Bone-Mineral Density and the Incidence of Fracture in Postmenopausal Osteoporosis," *N Engl J Med*, 1995, 333:1437-43.

"New Drugs for Osteoporosis," *Med Lett Drugs Ther*, 1996, 38:1-3.

NIH Consensus Development Panel on Optimal Calcium Intake, *JAMA*, 1994, 272:1942-8.

PCA Osteoporosis Prevention and Treatment Video-Teleconference (March 1, April 2 and 3, 1996).

PARKINSON'S DISEASE MANAGEMENT

Management of Parkinson's Disease

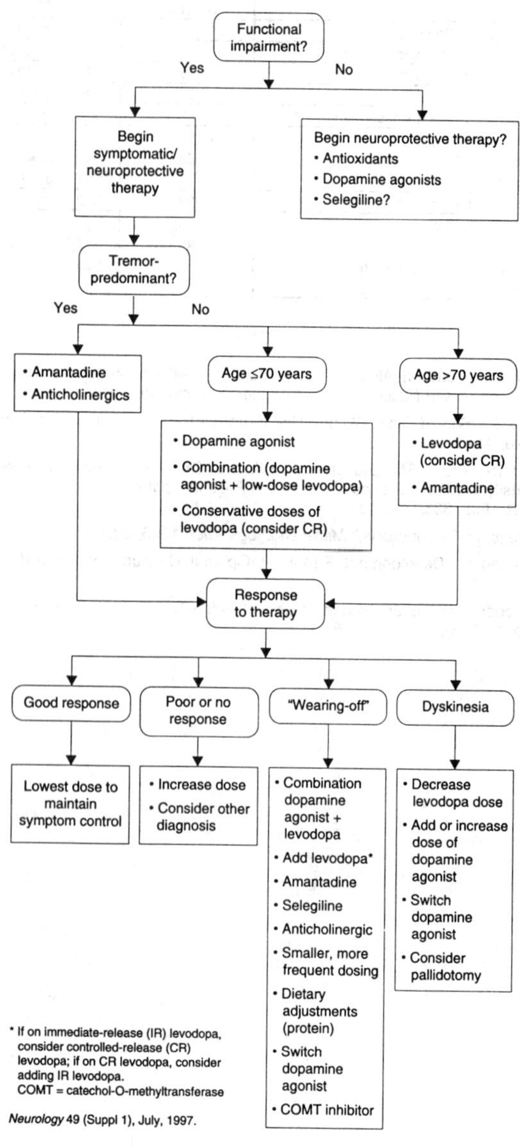

* If on immediate-release (IR) levodopa, consider controlled-release (CR) levodopa; if on CR levodopa, consider adding IR levodopa.
COMT = catechol-O-methyltransferase

Neurology 49 (Suppl 1), July, 1997.

PHARMACOTHERAPY OF URINARY INCONTINENCE

Incontinence Type	Drug Class	Drug Therapy	Adverse Effects and Precautions	Comments
Urge incontinence	Anticholinergic agents	Oxybutynin (2.5-5 mg bid-qid), propantheline (7.5-30 mg at least tid), dicyclomine (10-20 mg tid)	Dry mouth, visual disturbances, constipation, dry skin, confusion	Anticholinergics are the first-line drug therapy (oxybutynin is preferred); propantheline is a second-line therapy
		Tolterodine (1-2 mg bid)	Dry mouth, visual disturbances, constipation, dry skin, confusion	**Note:** Tolterodine was not included in practice guideline; no comment may be made concerning placement in therapy
	Tricyclic antidepressants (TCAs)	Imipramine, desipramine, nortriptyline (25-100 mg/day)	Anticholinergic effects (as above), orthostatic hypotension, and cardiac dysrhythmia	TCAs are generally reserved for patients with an additional indication (eg, depression, neuralgia) at an initial dose of 10-25 mg 1-3 times/day
Stress incontinence	Alpha-adrenergic agonists	Phenylpropanolamine (PPA) in sustained-release form (25-100 mg bid), pseudoephedrine (15-60 mg tid)	Anxiety, insomnia, agitation, respiratory difficulty, sweating, cardiac dysrhythmia, hypertension, tremor; should not be used in obstructive syndromes and/or hypertension	PPA (preferred) or pseudoephedrine are first-line therapy for women with no contraindication (notably hypertension)
Stress or combined urge/ stress incontinence	Estrogen replacement agents	Conjugated estrogens (0.3-0.625 mg/day orally or 1 g vaginal cream at bedtime)	Should not be used if suspected or confirmed breast or endometrial cancer, active or past thromboembolism with past oral contraceptive, estrogen, or pregnancy; headache, spotting, edema, breast tenderness, possible depression	Estrogen (oral or vaginal) is an adjunctive therapy for postmenopausal women as it augments alpha-agonists such as PPA or pseudoephedrine
			Give progesterone with estrogen if uterus is present; pretreatment/periodic mammogram, gynecologic, breast exam advised	Progestin (eg, medroxyprogesterone 2.5-10 mg/day) continuously or intermittently; combined oral or vaginal estrogen and PPA in postmenopausal women if single drug is inadequate; imipramine is an alternative therapy when first-line therapy is inadequate
	Imipramine (10-25 mg tid)		May worsen cardiac conduction abnormalities, postural hypotension, anticholinergic effects	
Overflow	Alpha-adrenergic antagonists	Terazosin (1 mg at bedtime with first dose in supine position and increase by 1 mg every 4 days to 5 mg/day)	Postural hypotension, dizziness, vertigo, heart palpitations, edema, headache, anticholinergic effects	Possible benefit in men with obstructive symptoms of benign prostatic hyperplasia; monitor postural vital signs with first dose/ each dose increase; may worsen female stress incontinence
		Doxazosin (1 mg at bedtime with first dose in supine position and increase by 1 mg every 7-14 days to 5 mg/day)	Same as terazosin (may be smaller incidence of hypotension)	Same as terazosin

"Urinary Incontinence," *Clinical Practice Guideline* , 1996, American Medical Directors Association, reprinted with permission. For more information call 1-800-876-2632.

SMOKING AND SMOKING CESSATION

Approximately 400,000 deaths each year may be attributed to cigarette smoking. Although the majority of an estimated 48 million smokers would like to stop smoking, they are unable to because of their psychological and physiological dependence. Cigarette smoking is associated with cardiovascular diseases including stroke, chronic obstructive lung disease, aortic aneurysm, and peripheral vascular diseases. Smoking is one of the most important and modifiable risk factors for cardiovascular disease, in particular for acute cardiac events such as myocardial infarction and sudden death. It is important to recognize that the adverse cardiovascular effects of tobacco use are magnified in the setting of other risk factors (ie, diabetes, hyperlipidemia, and hypertension). Cigar smoking is also associated with an increased risk for coronary heart disease. Cigarette and cigar smoking may also affect other organ systems and may contribute to other diseases, particularly cancer. The chemical constituents of cigarette smoke that elicit cardiovascular damage and carcinogenesis are unknown. The mechanism of the putative triggering effects of smoking is also unknown.

SMOKING AND THE SYMPATHETIC NERVOUS SYSTEM

Sympathetic activation with resultant release of the sympathetic neural transmitter, norepinephrine, within the myocardium has been shown to lower the ventricular fibrillation threshold in animals. The ventricular threshold was also lowered in animals forced to inhale cigarette smoke. Sympathetic vasoconstriction and tachycardia increase myocardial oxygen demand. In patients with coronary artery disease, smoking may induce coronary vasoconstriction through sympathetic activation. Sympathetic activation may have effects beyond those of increasing blood pressure and lowering the ventricular threshold. Tachycardia and decreased diastolic filling time may trigger cardiac ischemia in patients with coronary artery disease. Thus, there is a strong rationale for supposing that activation of the sympathetic nervous system, acting at one or several potential substrates, may precipitate acute cardiovascular events in patients with underlying coronary artery disease.

SMOKING AND ENDOTHELIAL FUNCTION

There is increasing evidence that endothelial function, specifically endothelium-mediated vasodilation, may be impaired in response to tobacco smoke exposure. This is apparent in smokers, and also in nonsmokers who are chronically exposed to passive cigarette smoke. The long-term implications of endothelial dysfunction are not clear, but may contribute to damage to blood vessels.

SMOKING CESSATION

The goals of therapy are to improve health and reduce mortality. All healthcare providers should encourage smoking cessation (see the following flowchart). Therapies for smoking cessation focus on educational efforts on the health consequences of smoking, behavioral counseling, support groups, and drug therapy. The most successful treatments for smoking cessation include those that combine both nondrug and drug therapies. Motivators for smoking cessation that should be reinforced in each smoker include the benefits of cessation, namely improvement in health, reduced risk of illness, financial savings, etc. The barriers smokers may face (eg, weight gain, failure to quit, peer pressure to continue to smoke, stress, fear of withdrawal symptoms) should also be discussed. As most insurance providers do not cover the cost of smoking cessation aids, the cost of therapy should be discussed with patients. In general, the costs associated with smoking cessation treatments are less than or equivalent to smoking 1-2 packs of cigarettes per day, and are far outweighed by the cost of treating smoking-related illnesses. Educational efforts and support in building on the motivators for cessation, while minimizing barriers, will help to optimize success rates. These measures should be carried out when candidates for smoking cessation are identified and at each follow-up visit. It is important for healthcare personnel and patients to recognize that the psychological addiction extends far beyond the physiological addiction, and may continue for years.

SMOKING CESSATION ALGORITHM

General Population
Clinician contact (Healthcare settings, worksites, others)
Screen for tobacco use
Never users
Primary prevention
Current users
Advise
Willingness to quit
Yes
Assess
Intervene
Follow-up procedures
Relapse
Abstinent
Return to general population
No
Promote Motivation to quit
Willing to quit
Remain unwilling
Ex-users
Relapse prevention

SMOKING AND SMOKING CESSATION *(Continued)*

Potential Withdrawal Symptoms

Symptom	Duration	Comments
Anxiety	2-4 wk	
Chest tightness	<2 wk	
Cigarette cravings	Intense for first several weeks then tapers but may last for years	Keep motivated, initiate drug therapy (nicotine, bupropion)
Constipation	4 wk	Increase fluid intake and fiber in diet
Cough	<2 wk	Drink water
Dizziness	1-2 d	Know it will be short-lived
Decreased concentration	2-4 wk	
Depression	2-4 wk	
Headache	Variable	Relax
Hunger	2-4 wk	Avoid high calorie foods
Sleeplessness/restlessness	<2 wk	Avoid stimulants (eg, caffeine) at bedtime

The goal of drug therapy is to reduce withdrawal symptoms and afford smokers the best chance to stop smoking. Drug therapy may also decrease associated weight gain. Nicotine replacement and bupropion are effective in smoking cessation. Drug therapy for smoking cessation should be discussed with each smoker and smoker preference used to help decide among the available products. Other drugs, including benzodiazepines, buspirone, clonidine, beta-blockers, and silver nitrate, have also been used in treatments for smoking cessation. However, the lack of efficacy and a paucity of clinical trials should limit their general use in the treatment of smoking cessation.

NICOTINE REPLACEMENT THERAPY

Nicotine replacement therapy is available as a transdermal patch, nasal spray, inhaler, and gum. Therapy is designed to "replace" a portion of the nicotine level produced by smoking to reduce cravings. Smoking produces nicotine levels as high as 40-50 ng/mL; nicotine replacement therapy maintains nicotine levels between 10 and 20 ng/mL. Patients with cardiovascular disease may be treated with nicotine replacement products. The risks of therapy are likely to be less than if the person continues to smoke. It is important that patients **do not** smoke during nicotine replacement therapy, particularly those patients with cardiocvascular disease.

Smoking Cessation Products

Products	Rx* Only	Dosage / Patch	Nicotine (mg)	Comments
NOREPINEPHRINE THERAPY				
Bupropion	X	300 mg/day		Use caution with seizures, alcoholism, history of head trauma, anorexia. Side effects include dry mouth, insomnia.
NICOTINE REPLACEMENT				
Transdermal Patches				
Habitrol™	X	21 mg/24 h 14 mg/24 h 7 mg/24 h	52.5 35 17.5	24-hour replacement
Nicoderm®	X	21 mg/24 h 14 mg/24 h 7 mg/24 h	114	24-hour replacement
Nicoderm® CQ		21 mg/24 h 14 mg/24 h 7 mg/24 h	75 36	24-hour replacement
Nicotrol®		15 mg/16 h 10 mg/16 h 5 mg/16 h	24.9 16.6 8.3	Nicotine free for 8 hours
Prostep®	X	22 mg/24 h 11 mg/24 h	30 15	24-hour replacement
Nasal Spray				
Nicotrol® NS	X	2 sprays	1	Mimics rapid increase in blood nicotine levels associated with smoking
Inhaler				
Nicotrol® Inhaler	X	1 inhalation	0.05	Buccal absorption
Chewing Gum				
Nicorette® Gum		2 mg/piece	1	Buccal absorption, special chewing instructions, therapy >11 months may be associated with hyperinsulinemia / insulin resistance
Nicorette® DS Gum		4 mg/piece	2	

*Rx = by prescription only.

BUPROPION

Bupropion is an antidepressant which may mimic some of the action of nicotine by central release of dopamine and norepinephrine. Therapy may be started 1 week before smoking cessation to reach steady state, and then continued for 7-12 weeks. A recent study reported that bupropion alone or in combination with a nicotine patch resulted in significantly higher longer-term rates of smoking cessation than either nicotine alone or placebo (*N Engl J Med*, 1999, 340:685-91).

Resources

Guidelines

"The Agency for Health Care Policy and Research Smoking Cessation Clinical Practice Guideline," *JAMA*, 1996, 275(16):1270-80.

"Practice Guideline for the Treatment of Patients With Nicotine Dependence. American Psychiatric Association," *Am J Psychiatry*, 1996, 153(10 Suppl):1-31.

Smoking Cessation Clinics/Specialists

Support Groups

Local chapters of the American Lung Association (1-800-586-4872), American Cancer Society (1-800-227-2345), or American Heart Association (1-800-242-8721).

Internet

www.quitnet.org

TREATMENT OF CARDIOVASCULAR DISEASE IN THE DIABETIC

TREATMENT OF HYPERTENSION

Diabetic patients are exposed to a wide range of adverse outcomes. These include cerebrovascular and cardiovascular events, retinopathy, nephropathy, neuropathy, and limb ischemia. The treatment of the diabetes itself is important in avoiding the development of hyperosmolar and ketoacidotic coma and also contributes, in the long-term, to improvements in outcome. Similarly, it is important that other risk factors such as tobacco use and hyperlipidemia be addressed very aggressively in diabetic patients.

There is increasing evidence that hypertension should also be aggressively treated in diabetics. The recent UKPDS study examined the effects of an ACE inhibitor or a beta-blocker in lowering blood pressure in diabetic patients. While there was no evidence that one class of drug was superior to the other in terms of outcome, what was very clear was that the reduction in blood pressure in diabetes, no matter how this was achieved, was a very powerful factor in attenuating the development of adverse events in diabetic patients. Thus, the blood pressure goals set for diabetic patients should be lower than those which we accept in the general management of the hypertensive patient. *The goal blood pressure in patients with diabetes is a systolic pressure <130 mm Hg and a diastolic pressure <85 mm Hg. Furthermore, in achieving blood pressure control, we should not feel restricted to a particular class of drugs.* Importantly, the UKPDS study also showed that, contrary to widespread belief, beta-blockers are not contraindicated in diabetic patients and, in fact, can be very beneficial.

The prevalence of hypertension is increased in diabetic patients, in part because of the widespread prevalence of each of these diseases, and in part because of the consequences of renal damage. In long-standing diabetics with established neuropathic and vascular disease, however, treatment of blood pressure may often be problematic. In these patients, orthostatic hypotension is often a problem so that blood pressures on lying flat are often high, but very low on standing, sometimes with symptomatic hypotension. Clearly, the problem with treating the high blood pressure in the supine position is that blood pressures on standing often fall to intolerably low levels. One approach to this is to minimize the duration and degree to which the patient lies flat, particularly during sleep. For example, it may be necessary to elevate the head of the bed to allow a slight orthostatic stress, even during sleep and recumbency, so that supine blood pressures are reduced.

TREATMENT OF CARDIAC ISCHEMIA

Diabetic patients are at high risk for ischemic heart disease. While stenoses are often evident in the large epicardial coronary arteries, diabetic patients are also susceptible to the development of microvascular disease. Thus, cardiac catheterization in diabetic patients with angina may sometimes show normal epicardial coronary arteries. This does not exclude the presence of decreased myocardial perfusion since because of microvascular disease, there is decreased myocardial flow reserve. In other words, while baseline myocardial blood flow in the diabetic patient may be similar to that evident in the normal subject, during stress, myocardial flow velocity in normal subjects may increase fourfold but only twofold in the diabetic patient. Similar microvascular problems in the absence of epicardial coronary artery disease may be evident in patients with hypertension and in smokers.

Another problem with ischemic heart disease in diabetic patients is the high incidence of silent ischemia. Thus, diabetic patients may often have significant cardiac ischemia in the absence of any chest pain. This ischemia, however, would be evident on more objective measures (ie, ST segment monitoring, echocardiographic evaluation, and radionuclide imaging).

The goal LDL cholesterol level in patients with diabetes is <100 mg/dL.

HIGH-RISK DIABETIC PATIENTS

In a recent study (HOPE), ramipril (10 mg/day) decreased cardiovascular morbidity and mortality (myocardial infarction, stroke, or death from cardiovascular causes) in high-risk patients without evidence of heart failure. This cardiovascular benefit was maintained in a subgroup analysis of diabetic patients with at least one other risk factor (hypertension, elevated total cholesterol, low HDL cholesterol, cigarette smoking, or documented microalbuminuria). In high-risk diabetic patients, there is therefore evidence that ramipril may contribute to improved cardiovascular outcomes.

Resources

Curb JD, Pressel SL, Cutler JA, et al, "Effect of Diuretic-Based Antihypertensive Treatment on Cardiovascular Disease in Older Diabetic Patients With Isolated Systolic Hypertension," *JAMA*, 1996, 276(23):1886-92.

Gavin JR, Alberti KGMM, Davidson MB, et al, for the Members of the Expert Committee on the Diagnosis and Classification of Diabetes Mellitus, "American Diabetes Association: Clinical Practice Recommendations," *Diabetes Care*, 1999, 22(Suppl 1):S1-S114.

"National High Blood Pressure Education Program Working Group Report on Hypertension in Diabetes," *Hypertension*, 1994, 23(2):145-58.

The Heart Outcomes Prevention Evaluation (HOPE) Study Investigators, "Effects of an Angiotensin-Converting-Enzyme Inhibitor, Ramipril, on Death From Cardiovascular Causes, Myocardial Infarction, and Stroke in High-Risk Patients," *N Engl J Med*, 2000, 342(3):145-53.

"Tight Blood Pressure Control and Risk of Macrovascular and Microvascular Complications in Type 2 Diabetes: UKPDS 38. UK Prospective Diabetes Study Group," *BMJ*, 1998, 317(7160):703-13.

Internet

Internet: www.diabetes.org

IMMUNIZATION RECOMMENDATIONS

Standards for Pediatric Immunization Practices

Standard 1.	Immunization services are readily available.
Standard 2.	There are no barriers or unnecessary prerequisites to the receipt of vaccines.
Standard 3.	Immunization services are available free or for a minimal fee.
Standard 4.	Providers utilize all clinical encounters to screen and, when indicated, immunize children.
Standard 5.	Providers educate parents and guardians about immunizations in general terms.
Standard 6.	Providers question parents or guardians about contraindications and, before immunizing a child, inform them in specific terms about the risks and benefits of the immunizations their child is to receive.
Standard 7.	Providers follow only true contraindications.
Standard 8.	Providers administer simultaneously all vaccine doses for which a child is eligible at the time of each visit.
Standard 9.	Providers use accurate and complete recording procedures.
Standard 10.	Providers co-schedule immunization appointments in conjunction with appointments for other child health services.
Standard 11.	Providers report adverse events following immunization promptly, accurately, and completely.
Standard 12.	Providers operate a tracking system.
Standard 13.	Providers adhere to appropriate procedures for vaccine management.
Standard 14.	Providers conduct semiannual audits to assess immunization coverage levels and to review immunization records in the patient populations they serve.
Standard 15.	Providers maintain up-to-date, easily retrievable medical protocols at all locations where vaccines are administered.
Standard 16.	Providers operate with patient-oriented and community-based approaches.
Standard 17.	Vaccines are administered by properly trained individuals.
Standard 18.	Providers receive ongoing education and training on current immunization recommendations.

Recommended by the National Vaccine Advisory Committee, April 1992.
Approved by the United States Public Health Service, May 1992.
Endorsed by the American Academy of Pediatrics, May 1992.

The Standards represent the consensus of the National Vaccine Advisory Committee (NVAC) and of a broad group of medical and public health experts about what constitutes the most desirable immunization practices. It is recognized by the NVAC that not all of the current immunization practices of public and private providers are in compliance with the Standards. Nevertheless, the Standards are expected to be useful as a means of helping providers to identify needed changes, to obtain resources if necessary, and to actually implement the desirable immunization practices in the future.

Recommended Childhood Immunization Schedule
United States, January - December 2000

Vaccines[1] are listed under the routinely recommended ages. Bars indicate range of recommended ages for immunization. Any dose not given at the recommended age should be given as a "catch up" immunization at any subsequent visit when indicated and feasible. (Ovals) indicate vaccines to be given if previously recommended doses were missed or given earlier than the recommended minimum age.

Age → / Vaccine ↓	Birth	1 mo	2 mo	4 mo	6 mo	12 mo	15 mo	18 mo	24 mo	4-6 y	11-12 y	14-16 y
Hepatitis B[2]	Hep B											
		Hep B			Hep B						(Hep B)	
Diphtheria, Tetanus, Pertussis[3]			DTaP	DTaP	DTaP		DTaP[3]			DTaP	Td	
H. influenzae type b[4]			Hib	Hib	Hib	Hib						
Polio[5]			IPV	IPV	IPV[5]					IPV[5]		
Measles, Mumps, Rubella[6]						MMR				MMR[6]	(MMR[6])	
Varicella[7]						Var					(Var[7])	
Hepatitis A[8]									Hep A[8] in selected areas			

1 This schedule indicates the recommended ages for routine administration of currently licensed childhood vaccines as of 11/1/99. Additional vaccines may be licensed and recommended during the year. Licensed combination vaccines may be used whenever any components of the combinations are indicated and its other components are not contraindicated. Providers should consult the manufacturers' package inserts for detailed recommendations.

2 Infants born to HBsAg-negative mothers should receive the 1st dose of hepatitis B (Hep B) vaccine by age 2 months. The 2nd dose should be at least one month after the 1st dose. The 3rd dose should be administered at least 4 months after the 1st dose and at least 2 months after the 2nd dose, but not before 6 months of age for infants.

Infants born to HBsAg-positive mothers should receive hepatitis B vaccine and 0.5 mL hepatitis B immune globulin (HBIG) within 12 hours of birth at separate sites. The 2nd dose is recommended at 1 month of age and the 3rd dose at 6 months of age.

Infants born to mothers whose HBsAg status is unknown should receive hepatitis B vaccine within 12 hours of birth. Maternal blood should be drawn at the time of delivery to determine the mother's HBsAg status; if the HBsAg test is positive, the infant should receive HBIG as soon as possible (no later than 1 week of age).

All children and adolescents (through 18 years of age) who have not been immunized against hepatitis B may begin the series during any visit. Special efforts should be made to immunize children who were born in or whose parents were born in areas of the world with moderate or high endemicity of hepatitis B virus infection.

3 The 4th dose of DTaP (diphtheria and tetanus toxoids and acellular pertussis vaccine) may be administered as early as 12 months of age, provided 6 months have elapsed since the 3rd dose and the child is unlikely to return to at age 15-18 months. Td (tetanus and diphtheria toxoids) is recommended at 11-12 years of age if at least 5 years have elapsed since the last dose of DTP, DTaP or DT. Subsequent routine Td boosters are recommended every 10 years.

4 Three *Haemophilus influenzae* type b (Hib) conjugate vaccines are licensed for infant use. If PRP-OMP (PedvaxHIB® and ComVax® [Merck]) is administered at 2 and 4 months of age, a dose at 6 months is not required. Because clinical studies in infants have demonstrated that using some combination products may induce a lower immune response to the Hib vaccine component, DTaP/Hib combination products should not be used for primary immunization in infants at 2, 4, or 6 months of age, unless FDA-approved for these ages.

5 To eliminate the risk of vaccine-associated paralytic polio (VAPP), an all-IPV schedule is now recommended for routine childhood polio vaccination in the United States. All children should receive four doses of IPV at 2 months, 4 months, 6-18 months, and 4-6 years. OPV (if available) may be used only for the following special circumstances: **1)** Mass vaccination campaigns to control outbreaks of paralytic polio. **2)** Unvaccinated children who will be traveling in <4 weeks to areas where polio is endemic or epidemic. **3)** Children of parents who do not accept the recommended number of vaccine injections. These children may receive OPV only for the third or fourth dose or both; in this situation, healthcare providers should administer OPV only after discussing the risk for VAPP with parents or caregivers. **4)** During the transition to an all-IPV schedule, recommendations for the use of remaining OPV supplies in physicians' offices and clinics have been issued by the American Academy of Pediatrics (see *Pediatrics*, December 1999).

6 The 2nd dose of measles, mumps, and rubella vaccine (MMR) is recommended routinely at 4-6 years of age but may be administered during any visit, provided at least 4 weeks have elapsed since receipt of the 1st dose and that both doses are administered beginning at or after 12 months of age. Those who have not previously received the second dose should complete the schedule by the 11 to 12-year-old visit.

7 Varicella (Var) vaccine is recommended at any visit on or after the first birthday for susceptible children, ie, those who lack a reliable history of chickenpox (as judged by a healthcare provider) and who have not been immunized. Susceptible persons 13 years of age or older should receive 2 doses, given at least 4 weeks apart.

8 Hepatitis A (Hep A) is shaded to indicate its recommended use in selected states and/or regions; consult your local public health authority. (Also see *MMWR,* Oct. 01, 1999/48(RR12); 1-37).

Adapted from the Advisory Committee on Immunization Practices (ACIP), the American Academy of Pediatrics (AAP), and the American Academy of Family Physicians (AAFP).

IMMUNIZATION RECOMMENDATIONS *(Continued)*

RECOMMENDATIONS OF THE ADVISORY COMMITTEE ON IMMUNIZATION PRACTICES (ACIP)

Recommendations for Measles Vaccination*

Category	Recommendations
Unvaccinated, no history of measles (12-15 mo)	A 2-dose schedule (with MMR) is recommended if born after 1956. The first dose is recommended at 12-15 mo; the second is recommended at 4-6 y
Children 12 mo in areas of recurrent measles transmission	Vaccinate; a second dose is indicated at 4-6 y (at school entry)
Children 6-11 mo in epidemic situations†	Vaccinate (with monovalent measles vaccine or, if not available, MMR); revaccination (with MMR) at 12-15 mo is necessary and a third dose is indicated at 4-6 y
Children 11-12 y who have received 1 dose of measles vaccine at ≥12 mo	Revaccinate (1 dose)
Students in college and other posthigh school institutions who have received 1 dose of measles vaccine at ≥12 mo	Revaccinate (1 dose)
History of vaccination before the first birthday	Consider susceptible and vaccinate (2 doses)
Unknown vaccine, 1963-1967	Consider susceptible and vaccinate (2 doses)
Further attenuated or unknown vaccine given with IG	Consider susceptible and vaccinate (2 doses)
Egg allergy	Vaccinate; no reactions likely
Neomycin allergy, nonanaphylactic	Vaccinate; no reactions likely
Tuberculosis	Vaccinate; vaccine does not exacerbate infection
Measles exposure	Vaccinate or give IG, depending on circumstances
HIV-infected	Vaccinate (2 doses) unless severely compromised
Immunoglobulin or blood product received	Vaccinate at the appropriate interval

*See text for details. MMR indicates measles-mumps-rubella vaccine; IG, immune globulin.

†See Outbreak Control.

Adapted from "Report of the Committee on Infectious Diseases," *1997 Red Book®*, 24th ed.

Recommended Immunization Schedule For HIV-Infected Children[1]

Age ➝ / Vaccine ↓	Birth	1 mo	2 mos	4 mos	6 mos	12 mos	15 mos	18 mos	24 mos	4-6 yrs	11-12 yrs	14-16 yrs
← Recommendations for these vaccines are the same as those for immunocompetent children ←												
Hepatitis B[2]	Hep B-1											
		Hep B-2			Hep B-3						Hep B[3]	
Diphtheria, Tetanus, Pertussis[4]			DTaP	DTaP	DTaP		DTaP			DTaP	Td	
Haemophilus influenzae type b[5]			Hib	Hib	Hib	Hib						
← Recommendations for these vaccines differ from those for immunocompetent children ←												
Polio[6]			IPV	IPV	IPV					IPV		
Measles, Mumps, Rubella[7]	Do not give to severely immunosuppressed (Category 3) children.					MMR	MMR					
Influenza[8]					Influenza (a dose is required every year)							
Streptococcus pneumoniae[9]									*pneumo-coccal*			
Varicella[10]	Give only to asymptomatic nonimmunosuppressed (Category 1) children. CONTRAINDICATED in all other HIV-infected children.					Varicella						
Rotavirus						**CONTRAINDICATED in <u>all</u> HIV-infected persons**						

Note: Modified from the immunization schedule for immunocompetent children. This schedule also applies to children born to HIV-infected mothers whose HIV infection status has not been determined. Once a child is known not to be HIV-infected, the schedule for immunocompetent children applies. This schedule indicates the recommended age for routine administration of currently licensed childhood vaccines. Some combination vaccines are available and may be used whenever administration of all componenets of the vaccine is indicated. Providers should consult the manufacturers' package inserts for detailed recommendations.

1 Vaccines are listed under the routinely recommended ages. Bars indicate range of acceptable ages for vaccination. Shaded bars indicate catch-up vaccination: at 11-12 years of age, hepatitis B vaccine should be administered to children not previously vaccinated.

2 ***Infants born to HBsAg-negative mothers*** should receive 2.5 mcg of Merch vaccine (Recombivax HB®) or 10 mcg of Smith Kline Beecham (SB) vaccine (Engerix-B®). The 2nd dose should be administered >1 mo after the 1st dose.

Infants born to HBsAg-positive mothers should receive 0.5 mL of hepatitis B immune globulin (HBIG) within 12 h of birth and either 5 mcg of Merck vaccine (Recombivax HB®) or 10 mcg of SB vaccine (Engerix-B®) at a separate site. The 2nd dose is recommended at 1-2 months of age and the 3rd dose at 6 months of age.

Infants born to mothers whose HBsAg status is unknown should receive either 5 mcg of Merck vaccine (Recombivax HB®) or 10 mcg of SB vaccine (Engerix-B®) within 12 h of birth. The 2nd dose of vaccine is recommended at 1 month of age and the 3rd dose at 6 of age. Blood should be drawn at the time of delivery to determine the mother's HBsAg status; if it is positive, the infant should receive HBIG as soon as possible (no later than 1 week of age). The dosage and timing of subsequent vaccine doses should be based upon the mother's HBsAg status.

3 Children and adolescents who have not been vaccinated against hepatitis B in infancy can begin the series during any childhood visit. Those who have not previously received 3 doses of hepatitis B vaccine should initiate or complete the series during the 11 to 12 year old visit. The 2nd dose should be administered at least 1 month after the 1st dose, and the 3rd dose should be administered at least 4 mos after the 1st dose and at 2 mos after 2nd dose.

4 DTaP (diphtheria and tetanus toxoids and acellular pertusssis vaccine) is the preferred vaccine for all doses in the vaccination series, including copletion of the series in children who have received >1 dose of whole-cell DtP vaccine. The 4th dose of DTaP may be administered as early as 12 months of age, provided 6 months have elapsed since the 3rd dose, and if the child is considered unlikely to return at 15-18 months of age. Td (tetanus and diphtheria toxoids, absorbed for adult use) is recommended at 11-12 years of age if at least 5 years have elapsed since the last dose of DTaP or DT. Subsequent routine Td boosters are recommended every 10 years.

5 Three H. influenzae type b (Hib) conjugate vaccines are licensed for infant use. If PRP-OMP (PedvaxHIB® [Merck]) is administered at 2 and 4 months of age, a dose at 6 months is not required. After the primary series has been completed, any Hib conjugate vaccine may be used as a booster.

6 Inactivated poliovirus vaccine (IPV) is the only polio vaccine recommended for HIV-infected persons and their household contacts. Although the third dose fo IPV is generally administered at 12-18 months, the 3rd dose of IPV has been approved to be administered as early as 6 months of age. Oral poliovirus vaccine (OPV) should NOT be administered to HIV-infected persons or their household contacts.

7 MMR should not be administered to severely immunocompromised children. HIV-infected children without severe immunosuppression should routinely receive their first dose of MMR as soon as possible upon reaching the first birthday. Consideration should be given to administering the 2nd dose of MMR vaccine as soon as one month (ie, minimum 28 days) after the first dose, rather than waiting until school entry.

8 Influenza virus vaccine should be administered to all HIV-infected children >6 months of age each year. Children aged 6 months to 8 years who are receiving influenza vaccine for the first time should receive two doses of split virus vaccine separated by at least one month. In subsequent years, a single dose of vaccine (split virus for persons ≥12 y of age, whole or split virus for persons >12 y of age) should be administered each year. The dose of vaccine for children aged 6-35 months is 0.25 mL: the dose for children aged ≥3 years is 0.5 mL.

9 The 23-valent pneumococcal vaccine should be administered to HIV-infected children at 24 months of age. Revaccination should generally be offered to HIV-infected children vaccinated 3-5 years (children aged ≤10 years) or >5 years (children aged >10 years) earlier.

10 Varicella zoster virus vaccine, 0.5 mL, is given as a subcutaneous dose between 12 mos and 12 y of age; a second dose should be given 3 mos later. The vaccine should be given only to asymptomatic, nonimmunosuppressed children.

Adapted from the American Academy of Pediatrics and American Academy of Family Practice Physicians, Advisory Committee on Immunization Practices and the Centers for Disease Control.

IMMUNIZATION RECOMMENDATIONS *(Continued)*

Licensed Vaccines and Toxoids Available in the United States, by Type and Recommended Routes of Administration

	Type	Route
Adenovirus*	Live virus	Oral
Anthrax†	Inactivated bacteria	Subcutaneous
Bacillus of Calmette and Guerin (BCG)	Live bacteria	Intradermal/percutaneous
Cholera	Inactivated bacteria	Subcutaneous, intramuscular, or intradermal‡
Diphtheria-tetanus-pertussis (DTP)	Toxoids and inactivated whole bacteria	Intramuscular
DTP-*Haemophilus influenzae* type b conjugate (DTP-Hib)	Toxoids, inactivated whole bacteria, and bacterial polysaccharide conjugated to protein	Intramuscular
Diphtheria-tetanus-acellular pertussis (DTaP)	Toxoids and inactivated bacterial components	Intramuscular
Hepatitis A	Inactivated virus	Intramuscular
Hepatitis B	Purified viral antigen	Intramuscular
Haemophilus influenzae type b conjugate (Hib)§	Bacterial polysaccharide conjugated to protein	Intramuscular
Influenza	Inactivated virus or viral components	Intramuscular
Japanese encephalitis	Inactivated virus	Subcutaneous
Lyme disease vaccine	Noninfectious lipoprotein	Intramuscular
Measles	Live virus	Subcutaneous
Measles-mumps-rubella (MMR)	Live virus	Subcutaneous
Meningococcal	Bacterial polysaccharides of serotypes A/C/Y/W-135	Subcutaneous
Mumps	Live virus	Subcutaneous
Pertussis†	Inactivated whole bacteria	Intramuscular
Plague	Inactivated bacteria	Intramuscular
Pneumococcal	Bacterial polysaccharides of 23 pneumococcal types	Intramuscular or subcutaneous
Poliovirus vaccine		
Inactivated (IPV)	Inactivated viruses of all 3 serotypes	Subcutaneous
Oral (OPV)	Live viruses of all 3 serotypes	Oral
Rabies	Inactivated virus	Intramuscular or intradermal¶
Rubella	Live virus	Subcutaneous
Tetanus	Inactivated toxin (toxoid)	Intramuscular#
Tetanus-diphtheria (Td or DT)•	Inactivated toxins (toxoids)	Intramuscular#
Typhoid		
Parenteral	Inactivated bacteria	Subcutaneous♦
Ty21a oral	Live bacteria	Oral
Varicella	Live virus	Subcutaneous
Yellow fever	Live virus	Subcutaneous

Modified from *MMWR Morb Mortal Wkly Rep*, 1994, 43(RR-1).

*Available only to the U.S. Armed Forces.

†Distributed by the Division of Biologic Products, Michigan Department of Public Health.

‡The intradermal dose is lower than the subcutaneous dose.

§The recommended schedule for infants depends on the vaccine manufacturer; consult the package insert and ACIP recommendations for specific products.

¶The intradermal dose of rabies vaccine, human diploid cell (HDCV), is lower than the intramuscular dose and is used only for pre-exposure vaccination. **Rabies vaccine, adsorbed (RVA) should not be used intradermally.**

#Preparations with adjuvants should be administered intramuscularly.

•Td-tetanus and diphtheria toxoids for use among persons ≥7 years of age. Td contains the same amount of tetanus toxoid as DTP or DT, but contains a smaller dose of diphtheria toxoid. DT = tetanus and diphtheria toxoids for use among children <7 years of age.

♦Booster doses may be administered intradermally unless vaccine that is acetone-killed and dried is used.

Immune Globulins and Antitoxins* Available in the United States, by Type of Antibodies and Indications for Use

Immunobiologic	Type	Indication(s)
Botulinum antitoxin	Specific equine antibodies	Treatment of botulism
Cytomegalovirus immune globulin, intravenous (CMV-IGIV)	Specific human antibodies	Prophylaxis for bone marrow and kidney transplant recipients
Diphtheria antitoxin	Specific equine antibodies	Treatment of respiratory diphtheria
Immune globulin (IG)	Pooled human antibodies	Hepatitis A pre- and postexposure prophylaxis; measles postexposure prophylaxis
Immune globulin, intravenous (IGIV)	Pooled human antibodies	Replacement therapy for antibody deficiency disorders; immune thrombocytopenic purpura (ITP); hypogammaglobulinemia in chronic lymphocytic leukemia; Kawasaki disease
Hepatitis B immune globulin (HBIG)	Specific human antibodies	Hepatitis B postexposure prophylaxis
Rabies immune globulin (HRIG)†	Specific human antibodies	Rabies postexposure management of persons not previously immunized with rabies vaccine
Tetanus immune globulin (TIG)	Specific human antibodies	Tetanus treatment; postexposure prophylaxis of persons not adequately immunized with tetanus toxoid
Vaccinia immune globulin (VIG)	Specific human antibodies	Treatment of eczema vaccinatum, vaccinia necrosum, and ocular vaccinia
Varicella-zoster immune globulin (VZIG)	Specific human antibodies	Postexposure prophylaxis of susceptible immunocompromised persons, certain susceptible pregnant women, and perinatally exposed newborn infants

Modified from *MMWR Morb Mortal Wkly Rep*, 1994, 43(RR-1).

*Immune globulin preparations and antitoxins are administered intramuscularly unless otherwise indicated.

†HRIG is administered around the wounds in addition to the intramuscular injection.

IMMUNIZATION RECOMMENDATIONS *(Continued)*

Suggested Intervals Between Administration of Immune Globulin Preparations for Various Indications and Vaccines Containing Live Measles Virus*

Indication	Dose (including mg IgG/kg)	Time Interval (mo) Before Measles Vaccination
Tetanus (TIG) prophylaxis	I.M.: 250 units (10 mg IgG/kg)	3
Hepatitis A (IG) prophylaxis		
Contact prophylaxis	I.M.: 0.02 mL/kg (3.3 mg IgG/kg)	3
International travel	I.M.: 0.06 mL/kg (10 mg IgG/kg)	3
Hepatitis B prophylaxis (HBIG)	I.M.: 0.06 mL/kg (10 mg IgG/kg)	3
Rabies immune globulin (HRIG)	I.M.: 20 IU/kg (22 mg IgG/kg)	4
Varicella prophylaxis (VZIG)	I.M.: 125 units/10 kg (20-40 mg IgG/kg) (max: 625 units)	5
Measles prophylaxis (IG)		
Standard (ie, nonimmunocompromised contact)	I.M.: 0.25 mL/kg (40 mg IgG/kg)	5
Immunocompromised contact	I.M.: 0.50 mL/kg (80 mg IgG/kg)	6
Blood transfusion		
RBCs, washed	I.V.: 10 mL/kg (negligible IgG/kg)	0
RBCs, adenine-saline added	I.V.: 10 mL/kg (10 mg IgG/kg)	3
Packed RBCs (Hct 65%)†	I.V.: 10 mL/kg (60 mg IgG/kg)	6
Whole blood cells (Hct 35%-50%)†	I.V.: 10 mL/kg (80-100 mg IgG/kg)	6
Plasma/platelet products	I.V.: 10 mL/kg (160 mg IgG/kg)	7
Replacement therapy for immune deficiencies	I.V.: 300-400 mg/kg (as IGIV)‡	8
Treatment of		
Immune thrombocytopenic purpura§	I.V.: 400 mg/kg (as IGIV)	8
Immune thrombocytopenic purpura§	I.V.: 1000 mg/kg (as IGIV)	10
Kawasaki disease	I.V.: 2 g/kg (as IGIV)	11

*This table is not intended for determining the correct indications and dosage for the use of immune globulin preparations. Unvaccinated persons may not be fully protected against measles during the entire suggested time interval, and additional doses of immune globulin and/or measles vaccine may be indicated after measles exposure. The concentration of measles antibody in a particular immune globulin preparation can vary by lot. The rate of antibody clearance after receipt of an immune globulin preparation also can vary. The recommended time intervals are extrapolated from an estimated half-life of 30 days of passively acquired antibody and an observed interference with the immune response to measles vaccine for 5 months after a dose of 80 mg IgG/kg.

†Assumes a serum IgG concentration of 16 mg/mL.

‡Measles vaccination is recommended for most HIV-infected children who do not have evidence of severe immunosuppression, but it is contraindicated for patients who have congenital disorders of the immune system.

§Formerly referred to as idiopathic thrombocytopenic purpura.

Modified from *MMWR Morb Mortal Wkly Rep*, 1996, 45(RR-12).

HAEMOPHILUS INFLUENZAE VACCINATION

Recommendations for *Haemophilus influenzae* Type b Conjugate Vaccination in Children Immunized Beginning at 2-6 Months of Age

Vaccine Product at Initiation*	Total No. of Doses to Be Administered	Currently Recommended Vaccine Regimens
HbOC or PRP-T	4	3 doses at 2-month intervals When feasible, same vaccine for doses 1-3 Fourth dose at 12-15 months of age Any conjugate vaccine for dose 4
PRP-OMP	3	2 doses at 2-month intervals When feasible, same vaccine for doses 1 and 2 Third dose at 12-15 months of age Any conjugate vaccine for dose 3†

Adapted from "Report of the Committee on Infectious Diseases," *1994 Red Book®*, 23rd ed, Montvale, NJ: Medical Economics Co, Inc.

*See text. The HbOC, PRP-T, or PRP-OMP should be given in a separate syringe and at a separate site from other immunizations unless specific combinations are approved by the FDA. HbOC is also available as a combination vaccine with DTP (HbOC-DTP). This combination can be used in infants scheduled to receive separate injections of DTP and HbOC. PRP-T may be reconstituted with DTP, made by Connaught Laboratories; other licensed formulations of DTP may not be used for this purpose.

†The safety and efficacy of PRP-OMP, PRP-D, PRP-T, and HbOC are likely to be equivalent in children 12 months and older.

Recommendations for *Haemophilus influenzae* Type b Conjugate Vaccination in Children in Whom Initial Vaccination Is Delayed Until 7 Months of Age or Older

Age at Initiation of Immunization (mo)	Vaccine Product at Initiation	Total No. of Doses to Be Administered	Currently Recommended Vaccine Regimens*
7-11	HbOC, PRP-T, or PRP-OMP	3	2 doses at 2-month intervals† When feasible, same vaccine for doses 1 and 2 Third dose at 12-18 months, given at least 2 months after dose 2 Any conjugate vaccine for dose 3‡
12-14	HbOC, PRP-T, PRP-OMP, or PRP-D	2	2-month interval between doses† Any conjugate vaccine for dose 2‡
15-59	HbOC, PRP-T, PRP-OMP, or PRP-D	1	Any conjugate vaccine
60 and older§	HbOC, PRP-T, PRP-OMP, or PRP-D	1 or 2¶	Any conjugate vaccine

Adapted from "Report of the Committee on Infectious Diseases," *1994 Red Book®*, 23rd ed, Montvale, NJ: Medical Economics Co, Inc.

*See text. HbOC, PRP-T, or PRP-OMP should be given in a separate syringe and at a separate site from other immunizations unless specific combinations are approved by the FDA. HbOC is also available as a combination vaccine with DTP (HbOC-DTP). This combination can be used in infants scheduled to receive separate injections of DTP and HbOC. PRP-T may be reconstituted with DTP, made by Connaught Laboratories; other licensed formulations of DTP may not be used for this purpose. In children 15 months or older eligible to receive DTaP (containing acellular pertussis vaccine), however, separate injections of conjugate vaccine and DTaP are acceptable because of the lower rate of febrile, minor local and systemic reactions associated with DTaP.

†For "catch up," a minimum of a 1-month interval between doses may be used.

‡The safety and efficacy of PRP-OMP, PRP-D, PRP-T, and HbOC are likely to be equivalent for use as a booster dose in children 12 months or older.

§Only for children with chronic illness known to be associated with an increased risk for *H. influenzae* type b disease (see text).

¶Two doses separated by 2 months are recommended by some experts for children with certain underlying diseases associated with increased risk of disease and impaired antibody responses to *H. influenzae* type conjugate vaccination (see text).

IMMUNIZATION RECOMMENDATIONS *(Continued)*

Recommendations for *Haemophilus influenzae* Type b Conjugate Vaccination in Children With a Lapse in Vaccination

Age at Presentation (mo)	Previous Vaccination History	Recommended Regimen
7-11	1 dose*	1 dose of conjugate at 7-11 months, with a booster dose given at least 2 months later, at 12-15 months†
	2 doses of HbOC or PRP-T	Same as above
12-14	2 doses before 12 months*	A single dose of any licensed conjugate‡
	1 dose before 12 months*	2 additional doses of any licensed conjugate, separated by 2 months‡
15-59	Any incomplete schedule	A single dose of any licensed conjugate‡

Adapted from "Report of the Committee on Infectious Diseases," *1994 Red Book®*, 23rd ed, Montvale, NJ: Medical Economics Co, Inc.

*PRP-OMP, PRP-T, or HbOC. HbOC is also available as a combination vaccine with DTP (HbOC-DTP), which may be used in infants scheduled to receive separate injections of DTP and HbOC. PRP-T may be reconstituted with DTP, made by Connaught Laboratories; other licensed formulations of DTP may not be used for this purpose. In children 15 months or older eligible to receive DTaP (containing acellular pertussis), however, separate injections of conjugate vaccine and DTaP may be given because of the lower rate of febrile, minor local and systemic reactions associated with DTaP.

†For the dose given at 7-11 months, when feasible, the same vaccine should be given as was used for the dose given at 2-6 months. For the dose given at 12-15 months, any licensed conjugate can be used.

‡The Academy considers that safety and efficacy of PRP-OMP, PRP-D, PRP-T, or HbOC are likely to be equivalent when used in children 12 months or older.

ADVERSE EVENTS AND VACCINATION

Reportable Events Following Vaccination*

These events are reportable by law to the Vaccine Adverse Event Reporting System (VAERS). In addition, individuals are encouraged to report any clinically significant or unexpected events (even if uncertain whether the vaccine caused the event) for any vaccine, whether or not it is listed in the table. Manufacturers also are required to report to the VAERS program all adverse events made known to them for any vaccine.

Vaccine/Toxoid		Event	Interval From Vaccination
Tetanus in any combination; DTaP, DTP, DTP-Hib, DT, Td, TT	A.	Anaphylaxis or anaphylactic shock	7 d
	B.	Briachial neuritis	28 d
	C.	Any sequela (including death) of above	No limit
	D.	Events described in manufacturer's package events insert as contraindications to additional doses of vaccine	See package insert
Pertussis in any combination; DTaP, DTP, DTP-Hib, P	A.	Anaphylaxis or anaphylactic shock	7 d
	B.	Encephalopathy (or encephalitis)	7 d
	C.	Any sequela (including death) of above events	No limit
	D.	Events described in manufacturer's package insert as contraindications to additional doses of vaccine	See package insert
Measles, mumps, and rubella in any combination; MMR, MR, M, R	A.	Anaphylaxis or anaphylactic shock	7 d
	B.	Encephalopathy (or encephalitis)	15 d
	C.	Any sequela (including death) of above events	No limit
	D.	Events described in manufacturer's package insert as contraindications to additional doses of vaccine	See package insert
Rubella in any combination; MMR, MR, R	A.	Chronic arthritis	42 d
	B.	Any sequela (including death) of above events	No limit
	C.	Events described in manufacturer's package insert as contraindications to additional doses of vaccine	See package insert
Measles in any combination; MMR, MR, M	A.	Thrombocytopenic purpura	30 d
	B.	Vaccine-strain measles viral infection in an immunodeficient recipient	6 mo
	C.	Any sequela (including death) of above events	No limit
	D.	Events described in manufacturer's package insert as contraindications to additional doses of vaccine	See package insert
Oral polio (OPV)	A.	Paralytic polio	
		• in a nonimmunodeficient recipient	30 d
		• in an immunodeficient recipient	6 mo
		• in a vaccine-associated community case	No limit
	B.	Vaccine-strain polio viral infection	
		• in a nonimmunodeficient recipient	30 d
		• in an immunodeficient recipient	6 mo
		• in a vaccine-associated community case	No limit
	C.	Any sequela (including death) of above events	No limit
	D.	Events described in manufacturer's package insert as contraindications to additional doses of vaccine	See package insert
Inactivated polio (IPV)	A.	Anaphylaxis or anaphylactic shock	7 d
	B.	Any sequela (including death) of above events	No limit
	C.	Events described in manufacturer's package insert as contraindications to additional doses of vaccine	See package insert
Hepatitis B	A.	Anaphylaxis or anaphylactic shock	7 d
	B.	Any sequela (including death) of above events	No limit
	C.	Events described in manufacturer's package insert as contraindications to additional doses of vaccine	See package insert
Haemophilus influenzae type b	A.	Early onset Hib disease	7 d
	B.	Any sequela (including death) of above events	No limit
	C.	Events described in manufacturer's package insert as contraindications to additional doses of vaccine	See package insert
Varicella	A.	No condition specified for compensation	Not applicable
	B.	Events described in manufacturer's package insert as contraindications to additional doses of vaccine	See package insert

*Effective March 24, 1997.

Adapted from "Report of the Committee on Infectious Diseases," *1997 Red Book®*, 24th ed.

IMMUNIZATION RECOMMENDATIONS *(Continued)*

PREVENTION OF HEPATITIS A THROUGH ACTIVE OR PASSIVE IMMUNIZATION

Recommendations of the Advisory Committee on Immunization Practices (ACIP)

December 27, 1996, Vol. 45, No. RR-15

PROPHYLAXIS AGAINST HEPATITIS A VIRUS INFECTION

Recommended Doses of Immune Globulin (IG) for Hepatitis A Pre-exposure and Postexposure Prophylaxis

Setting	Duration of Coverage	IG Dose*
Pre-exposure	Short-term (1-2 months)	0.02 mL/kg
	Long-term (3-5 months)	0.06 mL/kg†
Postexposure	—	0.02 mL/kg

*IG should be administered by intramuscular injection into either the deltoid or gluteal muscle. For children <24 months of age, IG can be administered in the anterolateral thigh muscle.

†Repeat every 5 months if continued exposure to HAV occurs.

Recommended Dosages of Havrix®*

Vaccinee's Age (y)	Dose (EL.U.)†	Volume (mL)	No. Doses	Schedule (mo)‡
2-18	720	0.5	2	0, 6-12
>18	1440	1.0	2	0, 6-12

*Hepatitis A vaccine, inactivated, SmithKline Beecham Biologicals.

†ELISA units.

‡0 months represents timing of the initial dose; subsequent numbers represent months after the initial dose.

Recommended Dosages of VAQTA®*

Vaccinee's Age (y)	Dose (units)	Volume (mL)	No. Doses	Schedule (mo)†
2-17	25	0.5	2	0, 6-18
>17	50	1.0	2	0, 6

*Hepatitis A vaccine, inactivated, Merck & Company, Inc.

†0 months represents timing of the initial dose; subsequent numbers represent months after the initial dose.

RECOMMENDATIONS FOR TRAVELERS

Recommended Immunizations for Travelers to Developing Countries*

Immunizations	Length of Travel[1]		
	Brief, <2 wk	Intermediate, 2 wk - 3 mo	Long-term Residential, >3 mo
Review and complete age-appropriate childhood schedule	+	+	+
• DTaP (or DTP) may be given at 4 wk intervals[2]			
• Poliovirus vaccine may be given at 4-8 wk intervals[2]			
• Measles: extra dose given if 6-11 mo old at 1st dose			
• Varicella			
• Hepatitis B[3]			
Yellow fever[4]	+	+	+
Typhoid fever[5]	±	+	+
Meningococcal meningitis[6]	±	±	±
Rabies[7]	+	+	+
Japanese encephalitis[4]	–	±	+

*See disease-specific chapters for details. For further sources of information, see text.

[1]+ indicates recommended; ± consider; and –, not recommended.

[2]If necessary to complete the recommended schedule before departure.

[3]If insufficient time to complete 6-month primary series, accelerated series can be given (see *Red Book®* for details).

[4]For endemic regions see *Health Information for International Travel*, page 2 of *Red Book®*.

[5]Indicated for travelers who will consume food at nontourist facilities.

[6]For endemic regions of central Africa and during local epidemics.

[7]Indicated for persons with high risk of wild animal exposure and for spelunkers.

Adapted from "Report of the Committee on Infectious Diseases," *1997 Red Book®*, 24th ed.

Recommendations for Pre-exposure Immunoprophylaxis of Hepatitis A Infection for Travelers*

Age (y)	Likely Exposure (mo)	Recommended Prophylaxis
<2	<3	IG 0.02 mL/kg†
	3-5	IG 0.06 mL/kg†
	Long term	IG 0.06 mL/kg at departure and every 5 mo thereafter†
≥2	<3‡	HAV vaccine§¶
		or
		IG 0.02 mL/kg†
	3-5‡	HAV vaccine§¶
		or
		IG 0.06 mL/kg†
		HAV vaccine§¶

*HAV, hepatitis A virus; IG, immune globulin.

†IG should be administered deep into a large muscle mass. Ordinarily no more than 5 mL should be administered in one site in an adult or large child; lesser amounts (maximum 3 mL) should be given to small children and infants.

‡Vaccine is preferable, but IG is an acceptable alternative.

§To ensure protection in travelers whose departure is imminent, IG also may be given (see text).

¶Dose and schedule of HAV vaccine as recommended according to age.

Adapted from "Report of the Committee on Infectious Diseases," *1997 Red Book®*, 24th ed.

IMMUNIZATION RECOMMENDATIONS *(Continued)*

Prevention of Malaria*

Drug†	Adult Dosage	Pediatric Dosage
	Chloroquine-Sensitive Areas	
Chloroquine phosphate	P.O.: 300 mg base (500 mg salt), once/week beginning 1 week before exposure, and continuing for 4 weeks after last exposure	5 mg/kg base (8.3 mg/kg salt) once/week (maximum 300 mg base)
	Chloroquine-Resistant Areas	
Mefloquine‡	P.O.: 250 mg salt (228 mg base), once/week, beginning 1 week before travel and continuing for 4 weeks after last exposure	15-19 kg: 1/4 tablet/wk 20-30 kg: 1/2 tablet/wk 31-45 kg: 3/4 tablet/wk >45 kg: 1 tablet/wk
Alternatives		
Doxycycline§	100 mg/d, starting 1-2 days before exposure and continuing for 4 weeks after last exposure	>8 y: P.O.: 2 mg/kg/d (maximum 100 mg/d)
or		
Chloroquine phosphate	Same as above	Same as above
with or without		
Proguanil#	200 mg daily during exposure and for 4 weeks after last exposure	<2 y: 50 mg/d 2-6 y: 100 mg/d 7-10 y: 150 mg/d >10 y: 200 mg/d
plus		
Pyrimethamine-sulfadoxine (Fansidar®) for presumptive treatment¶	Carry a single dose (3 tablets) for self-treatment of febrile illness when medical care is not immediately available	Used as for adults in the following doses: <1 y: 1/4 tablet 1-3 y: 1/2 tablet 4-8 y: 1 tablet 9-14 y: 2 tablets >14 y: 3 tablets

*Currently, no drug regimen guarantees protection against malaria. Travelers to countries with risk of malaria should be advised to avoid mosquito bites by using personal protective measures (see text).

†All drugs should be continued for 4 weeks after last exposure.

‡Mefloquine is not licensed by the Food and Drug Administration for children weighing <15 kg, but recent recommendations from the Centers for Disease Control and Prevention allow use of the drug to be considered in children without weight restrictions when travel to chloroquine-resistant *P. falciparum* areas cannot be avoided. Mefloquine is **contraindicated** for use by travelers with a known hypersensitivity to mefloquine and travelers with a history of epilepsy or severe psychiatric disorders. A review of available data suggests that a mefloquine may be administered to persons concurrently receiving β-blockers if they have no underlying arrhythmia. However, mefloquine is not recommended for persons with cardiac conduction abnormalities until additional data are available. Caution may be advised for persons involved in tasks requiring fine coordination and spatial discrimination, such as airline pilots. Quinidine or quinine may exacerbate the known side effects or mefloquine; patients not responding to mefloquine therapy or failing mefloquine prophylaxis should be closely monitored if they are treated with quinidine or quinine.

§Physicians who prescribe doxycycline as malaria chemoprophylaxis should advise patients to limit the exposure to direct sunlight to minimize the possibility of photosensitivity reaction. Use of doxycycline is contraindicated in pregnant women and usually in children <8 years. Physicians must weight the benefits of doxycycline therapy against the possibility of dental staining in children <8 years (see Antimicrobial and Related Therapy).

#Proguanil (chloroguanide hydrochloride) is not available in the United States but is widely available overseas. It is recommended primarily for use in Africa south of the Sahara. Failures in prophylaxis with chloroquine and chloroguanide have been reported commonly, however, as they are only 40% to 60% effective.

¶Use of Fansidar®, which contains 25 mg pyrimethamine and 500 mg sulfadoxine per tablet, is contraindicated in patients with a history of sulfonamide or pyrimethamine intolerance, in infants <2 months, and in pregnant women at term. Resistance to pyrimethamine-sulfadoxine has been reported from Southeast Asia and the Amazon Basin and therefore should not be used for treatment of malaria acquired in these area.

Adapted from "Report of the Committee on Infectious Diseases," *1997 Red Book®*, 24th ed.

MANAGEMENT OF HEALTHCARE WORKER EXPOSURES TO HIV

RECOMMENDATIONS FOR POSTEXPOSURE PROPHYLAXIS

Adapted from "Public Health Service Guidelines for the Management of Health-Care Worker Exposures to HIV and Recommendations for Postexposure Prophylaxis," *MMWR Morb Mortal Wkly Rep*, 1998, 47(RR-7)

Figure 1. Determining the need for HIV postexposure prophylaxis (PEP) after an occupational exposure*

Step 1: Determine the Exposure Code (EC)

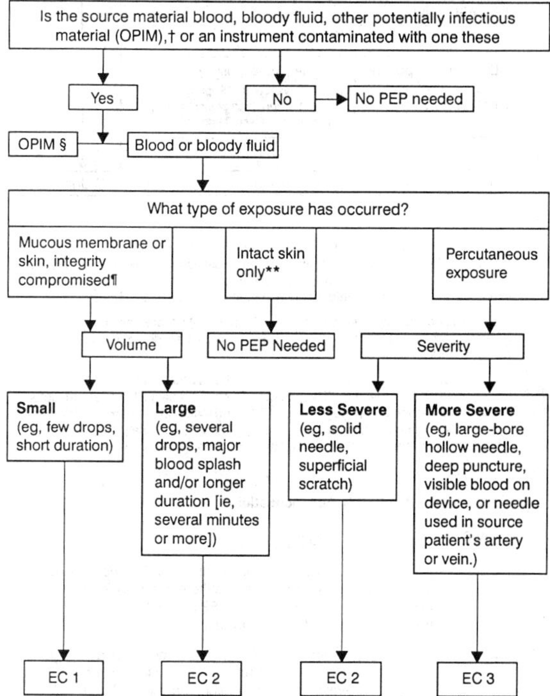

* This algorithm is intended to guide initial decisions about PEP and should be used in conjunction with other guidance provided in this report.

† Semen or vaginal secretions; cerebrospinal, synovial, pleural, peritoneal, pericardial, or amniotic fluids; or tissue

§ Exposure to OPIM must be evaluated on a case-by-case basis. In general, these body substances are considered a low risk for transmission in health-care settings. Any unprotected contact to concentrated HIV in a research laboratory or production facility is considered an occupational exposure that requires clinical evaluation to determine the need for PEP.

¶ Skin integrity is considered compromised if there is evidence of chapped skin, dermatitis, abrasion, or open wound.

** Contact with intact skin is not normally considered a risk for HIV transmission. However, if the exposure was to blood, and the circumstance suggests a higher volume exposure (eg, an extensive area of skin was exposed or there was prolonged contact with blood), the risk for HIV transmission should be considered.

†† The combination of these severity factors (eg, large-bore, hollow needle and deep puncture) contribute to an elevated risk for transmission if the source person is HIV-

MANAGEMENT OF HEALTHCARE WORKER EXPOSURES TO HIV *(Continued)*

Figure 1. Determining the need for HIV postexposure prophylaxis (PEP) after an occupational exposure* — Continued

Step 2: Determine the HIV Status Code (HIV SC)

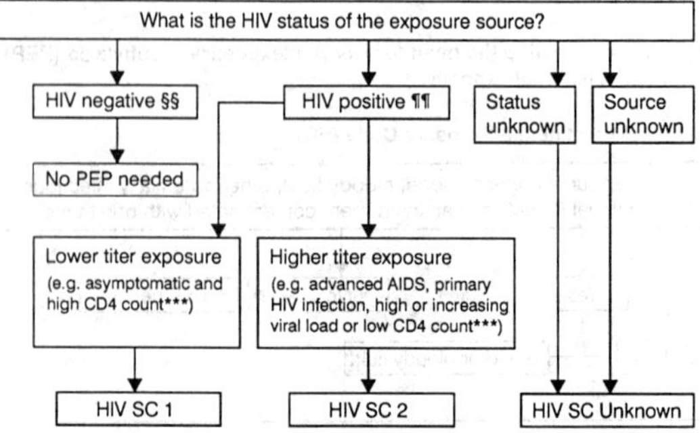

§§ A source is considered negative for HIV infection if there is laboratory documentation of a negative HIV antibody, HIV polymerase chain reaction (PCR), or HIV p24 antigen test result from a specimen collected at or near the time of exposure and there is no clinical evidence of recent retroviral-like illness.

¶¶ A source is considered infected with HIV (HIV positive) if there has been a positive laboratory result for HIV antibody, HIV PCR, or HIV p24 antigen or physician-diagnosed AIDS.

*** Examples are used as surrogates to estimates the HIV titer in an exposure source for purposes of considering PEP regimens and do not reflect all clinical situations that may be observed. Although a high HIV titer (HIV SC 2) in an exposure source has been associated with an increased risk for transmission, the possibility of transmission from a source with a low HIV titer also must be considered.

Step 3: Determine the PEP Recommendation

EC	HIV SC	PEP recommendation
1	1	PEP may not be warranted. Exposure type does not pose a known risk for HIV transmission. Whether the risk for drug toxicity outweighs the benefit of PEP should be decided by the exposed HCW and treating clinician.
1	2	Consider basic regimen. ††† Exposure type poses a negligible risk for HIV transmission. A high HIV titer in the source may justify consideration of PEP. Whether the risk for drug toxicity outweighs the benefit of PEP should be decided by the exposed HCW and treating clinician.
2	1	Recommended basic regimen. Most HIV exposures are in thes category; no increased risk for HIV transmission has been observed but use of PEP is appropriate.
2	1	Recommended expanded regimen. §§§ Exposure type represents an increased HIV transmission risk.
3	1 or 2	Recommended expanded regimen. Exposure type represents an increased HIV transmission risk.

††† Basic regimen is four weeks of zidovudine, 600 mg per day in two or three divided doses, and lamivudine, 150 mg twice daily.

§§§ Expanded regimen is the basic regimen plus either indinavir, 800 mg every 8 hours, or nelfinavir, 750 mg three times a day.

Basic and Expanded Postexposure Prophylaxis Regimens

Regimen Category	Application	Drug Regimen
Basic	Occupational HIV exposures for which there is a recognized transmission risk (see Figure 1)	4 weeks (28 days) of both zidovudine 600 mg every day in divided doses (ie, 300 mg 2 times/day, 200 mg 3 times/day, or 100 mg every 4 h) **and** lamivudine 150 mg 2 times/d.
Expanded	Occupational HIV exposures that pose an increased risk for transmission (eg, larger volume of blood and/or higher virus titer in blood; see Figure 1)	Basic regimen plus **either** indinavir 800 mg every 8 h **or** nelfinavir 750 mg 3 times/d*

*Indinavir should be taken on an empty stomach (ie, without food or with a light meal) and with increased fluid consumption (ie, drinking six 8 oz glasses of water throughout the day); nelfinavir should be taken with meals.

PREVENTION OF BACTERIAL ENDOCARDITIS

Recommendations by the American Heart Association (*JAMA*, 1997, 277:1794-801)

Consensus Process - The recommendations were formulated by the writing group after specific therapeutic regimens were discussed. The consensus statement was subsequently reviewed by outside experts not affiliated with the writing group and by the Science Advisory and Coordinating Committee of the American Heart Association. These guidelines are meant to aid practitioners but are not intended as the standard of care or as a substitute for clinical judgment.

Table 1. Cardiac Conditions*

Endocarditis Prophylaxis Recommended

High-risk Category

- Prosthetic cardiac valves, including bioprosthetic and homograft valves
- Previous bacterial endocarditis
- Complex cyanotic congenital heart disease (eg, single ventricle states, transposition of the great arteries, tetralogy of Fallot)
- Surgically constructed systemic pulmonary shunts or conduits

Moderate-risk Category

- Most other congenital cardiac malformations (other than above and below)
- Acquired valvar dysfunction (eg, rheumatic heart disease)
- Hypertrophic cardiomyopathy
- Mitral valve prolapse with valvar regurgitation and/or thickened leaflets

Endocarditis Prophylaxis Not Recommended

Negligible-risk Category (no greater risk than the general population)

- Isolated secundum atrial septal defect
- Surgical repair of atrial septal defect, ventricular septal defect, or patent ductus arteriosus (without residua beyond 6 months)
- Previous coronary artery bypass graft surgery
- Mitral valve prolapse without valvar regurgitation†
- Physiologic, functional, or innocent heart murmurs
- Previous Kawasaki disease without valvar dysfunction
- Previous rheumatic fever without valvar dysfunction
- Cardiac pacemakers (intravascular and epicardial) and implanted defibrillators

*This table lists selected conditions but is not meant to be all-inclusive.

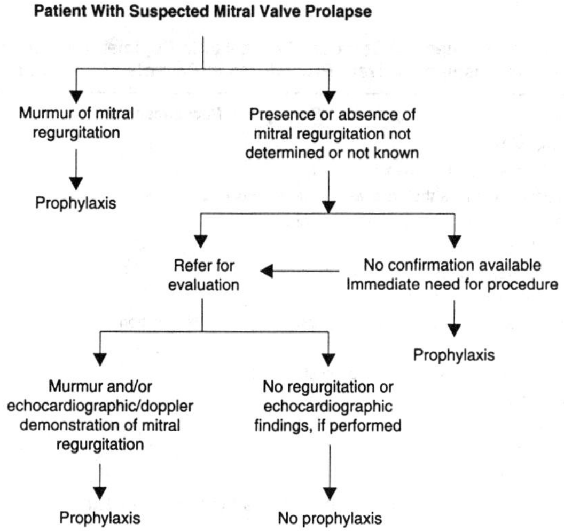

Patient With Suspected Mitral Valve Prolapse

- → Murmur of mitral regurgitation
  - → Prophylaxis
- → Presence or absence of mitral regurgitation not determined or not known
  - → Refer for evaluation
    - → Murmur and/or echocardiographic/doppler demonstration of mitral regurgitation
      - → Prophylaxis
    - → No regurgitation or echocardiographic findings, if performed
      - → No prophylaxis
  - → No confirmation available / Immediate need for procedure (→ Refer for evaluation)
    - → Prophylaxis

Table 2. Dental Procedures and Endocarditis Prophylaxis

Endocarditis Prophylaxis Recommended*
Dental extractions
Periodontal procedures including surgery, scaling and root planing, probing, and recall maintenance
Dental implant placement and reimplantation of avulsed teeth
Endodontic (root canal) instrumentation or surgery only beyond the apex
Subgingival placement of antibiotic fibers or strips
Initial placement of orthodontic bands but not brackets
Intraligamentary local anesthetic injections
Prophylactic cleaning of teeth or implants where bleeding is anticipated
Endocarditis Prophylaxis Not Recommended
Restorative dentistry† (operative and prosthodontic) with or without retraction cord‡
Local anesthetic injections (nonintraligamentary)
Intracanal endodontic treatment; post placement and buildup
Placement of rubber dams
Postoperative suture removal
Placement of removable prosthodontic or orthodontic appliances
Taking of oral impressions
Fluoride treatments
Taking of oral radiographs
Orthodontic appliance adjustment
Shedding of primary teeth

*Prophylaxis is recommended for patients with high- and moderate-risk cardiac conditions.

†This includes restoration of decayed teeth (filling cavities) and replacement of missing teeth.

‡Clinical judgment may indicate antibiotic use in selected circumstances that may create significant bleeding.

PREVENTION OF BACTERIAL ENDOCARDITIS *(Continued)*

Table 3. Recommended Standard Prophylactic Regimen for Dental, Oral, or Upper Respiratory Tract Procedures in Patients Who Are at Risk*

Endocarditis Prophylaxis Recommended

Respiratory Tract
- Tonsillectomy and/or adenoidectomy
- Surgical operations that involve respiratory mucosa
- Bronchoscopy with a rigid bronchoscope

Gastrointestinal Tract*
- Sclerotherapy for esophageal varices
- Esophageal stricture dilation
- Endoscopic retrograde cholangiography with biliary obstruction
- Biliary tract surgery
- Surgical operations that involve intestinal mucosa

Genitourinary Tract
- Prostatic surgery
- Cystoscopy
- Urethral dilation

Endocarditis Prophylaxis Not Recommended

Respiratory Tract
- Endotracheal intubation
- Bronchoscopy with a flexible bronchoscope, with or without biopsy†
- Tympanostomy tube insertion

Gastrointestinal Tract
- Transesophageal echocardiography†
- Endoscopy with or without gastrointestinal biopsy†

Genitourinary Tract
- Vaginal hysterectomy†
- Vaginal delivery†
- Cesarean section
- In uninfected tissues:
  - Urethral catheterization
  - Uterine dilatation and curettage
  - Therapeutic abortion
  - Sterilization procedures
  - Insertion or removal of intrauterine devices

Other
- Cardiac catheterization, including balloon angioplasty
- Implanted cardiac pacemakers, implanted defibrillators, and coronary stents
- Incision or biopsy or surgically scrubbed skin
- Circumcision

*Prophylaxis is recommended for high-risk patients, optional for medium-risk patients.

†Prophylaxis is optional for high-risk patients.

Table 4. Prophylactic Regimens for Dental, Oral, Respiratory Tract, or Esophageal Procedures

Situation	Agent	Regimen*	
		Adults	Children
Standard general prophylaxis	Amoxicillin	2 g P.O. 1 h before procedure	50 mg/kg P.O. 1 h before procedure
Unable to take oral medications	Ampicillin	2 g I.M./I.V. within 30 min before procedure	50 mg/kg I.M./I.V. within 30 min before procedure
Allergic to penicillin	Clindamycin or	600 mg P.O. 1 h before procedure	20 mg/kg P.O. 1 h before procedure
	Cephalexin† or cefadroxil† or	2 g P.O 1 h before procedure	50 mg/kg P.O. 1 h before procedure
	Azithromycin or clarithromycin	500 mg P.O. 1 h before procedure	15 mg/kg P.O. 1 h before procedure
Allergic to penicillin and unable to take oral medications	Clindamycin or	600 mg I.V. within 30 min before procedure	20 mg/kg I.V. within 30 min before procedure
	Cefazolin†	1 g I.M./I.V. within 30 min before procedure	25 mg/kg I.M./I.V. within 30 min before procedure

*Total children's dose should not exceed adult dose.

†Cephalosporins should not be used in individuals with immediate-type hypersensitivity reaction (urticaria, angioedema, or anaphylaxis) to penicillins

Table 5. Prophylactic Regimens for Genitourinary/Gastrointestinal (Excluding Esophageal) Procedures*

Situation	Agents*	Regimen†	
		Adults	Children
High-risk‡ patients	Ampicillin plus gentamicin	Ampicillin 2 g I.M. or I.V. plus gentamicin 1.5 mg/kg (not to exceed 120 mg) within 30 min of starting the procedure; 6 h later, ampicillin 1 g I.M./I.V. or amoxicillin 1 g orally	Ampicillin 50 mg/kg I.M./I.V. (not to exceed 2 g) plus gentamicin 1.5 mg/kg within 30 min of starting the procedure; 6 h later, ampicillin 25 mg/kg I.M./I.V. or amoxicillin 25 mg/kg orally
High-risk‡ patients allergic to ampicillin/ amoxicillin	Vancomycin plus gentamicin	Vancomycin 1 g I.V. over 1-2 h plus gentamicin 1.5 mg/kg I.M./I.V. (not to exceed 120 mg); complete injection/infusion within 30 min of starting the procedure	Vancomycin 20 mg/kg I.V. over 1-2 h plus gentamicin 1.5 mg/kg I.M./I.V.; complete injection/infusion within 30 min of starting the procedure
Moderate-risk§ patients	Amoxicillin or ampicillin	Amoxicillin 2 g orally 1 h before procedure, or ampicillin 2 g I.M./I.V within 30 min of starting the procedure	Amoxicillin 50 mg/kg orally 1 h before procedure, or ampicillin 50 mg/kg I.M./I.V. within 30 min of starting the procedure
Moderate-risk§ patients allergic to ampicillin/amoxicillin	Vancomycin	Vancomycin 1 g I.V. over 1-2 h; complete infusion within 30 min of starting the procedure	Vancomycin 20 mg/kg I.V. over 1-2 h; complete infusion within 30 min of starting the procedure

*Total children's dose should not exceed adult dose

†No second dose of vancomycin or gentamicin is recommended

‡High-risk: Patients are those who have prosthetic valves, a previous history of endocarditis (even in the absence of other heart disease, complex cyanotic congenital heart disease, or surgically constructed systemic pulmonary shunts or conduits).

§Moderate-risk: Individuals with certain other underlying cardiac defects. Congenital cardiac conditions include the following uncorrected conditions: Patent ductus arteriosus, ventricular septal defect, ostium primum atrial septal defect, coarctation of the aorta, and bicuspid aortic valve. Acquired valvar dysfunction and hypertrophic cardiomyopathy are also moderate risk conditions.

PREVENTION OF WOUND INFECTION & SEPSIS IN SURGICAL PATIENTS

Nature of Operation	Likely Pathogens	Recommended Drugs	Adult Dosage Before Surgery[1]
Cardiac			
Prosthetic valve, coronary artery bypass, other open-heart surgery, pacemaker or defibrillator implant	*S. epidermidis*, *S. aureus*, *Corynebacterium*, enteric gram-negative bacilli	Cefazolin	1-2 g I.V.[2]
		or cefuroxime	1-2 g I.V.[2]
		or vancomycin[3]	1 g I.V.
Gastrointestinal			
Esophageal, gastroduodenal	Enteric gram-negative bacilli, gram-positive cocci	*High risk[4] only:* cefazolin	1-2 g I.V.
Biliary tract	Enteric gram-negative bacilli, enterococci, clostridia	*High risk[5] only:* cefazolin	1-2 g I.V.
Colorectal	Enteric gram-negative bacilli, anaerobes, enterococci	*Oral:* neomycin + erythromycin base[6]	1-2 g I.V.
		Parenteral:	
		Cefoxitin	1-2 g I.V.
		or cefotetan	1-2 g I.V.
Appendectomy, nonperforated	Enteric gram-negative bacilli, anaerobes, enterococci	Cefoxitin	1-2 g I.V.
		or cefotetan	1-2 g I.V.
Genitourinary	Enteric gram-negative bacilli, enterococci	*High risk[7] only:* Ciprofloxacin	500 mg P.O. or 400 mg I.V.
Gynecologic and Obstetric			
Vaginal or abdominal hysterectomy	Enteric gram-negatives, anaerobes, group B streptococci, enterococci	Cefazolin	1-2 g I.V.
		or cefotetan	1-2 g I.V.
		or cefoxitin	1 g I.V.
Cesarean section	Same as for hysterectomy	*High risk[8] only:* Cefazolin	1 g I.V. after cord clamping
Abortion	Same as for hysterectomy	*First trimester, high-risk[9] only:* Aqueous penicillin G	2 mill units I.V.
		or doxycycline	300 mg P.O.[10]
		Second trimester: Cefazolin	1 g I.V.
Head and Neck			
Entering oral cavity or pharynx	*S. aureus*, streptococci, oral anaerobes	Cefazolin	1-2 g I.V.
		or clindamycin	600-900 mg I.V.
		± gentamicin	1.5 mg/kg I.V.
Neurosurgery			
Craniotomy	*S. aureus*, *S. epidermidis*	Cefazolin	1-2 g I.V.
		or vancomycin[3]	1 g I.V.
Ophthalmic	*S. aureus*, *S. epidermidis*, streptococci, enteric gram-negative bacilli, *Pseudomonas*	Gentamicin or tobramycin or neomycin-gramicidin-polymyxin B	Multiple drops topically over 2-24 h
		Cefazolin	100 mg subconjunctivally at end of procedure
Orthopedic			
Total joint replacement, internal fixation of fractures	*S. aureus*, *S. epidermidis*	Cefazolin	1-2 g I.V.
		or vancomycin[3]	1 g I.V.
Thoracic (Noncardiac)	*S. aureus*, *S. epidermidis*, streptococci, enteric gram-negative bacilli	Cefazolin	1-2 g I.V.
		or cefuroxime	1-2 g I.V.
		or vancomycin[3]	1 g I.V.

Nature of Operation	Likely Pathogens	Recommended Drugs	Adult Dosage Before Surgery[1]
Vascular			
Arterial surgery involving the abdominal aorta, a prosthesis, or a groin incision	*S. aureus*, *S. epidermidis*, enteric gram-negative bacilli	Cefazolin	1-2 g I.V.
		or vancomycin[3]	1 g I.V.
Lower extremity amputation for ischemia	*S. aureus*, *S. epidermidis*, enteric gram-negative bacilli, clostridia	Cefazolin	1-2 g I.V.
		or vancomycin[3]	1 g I.V.
CONTAMINATED SURGERY[11]			
Ruptured viscus	Enteric gram-negative bacilli, anaerobes, enterococci	Cefoxitin	1-2 g I.V. q6h
		or cefotetan	1-2 g I.V. q12h
		± gentamicin	1.5 mg/kg I.V. q8h
		or clindamycin	600 mg I.V. q6h
		+ gentamicin	1.5 mg/kg I.V. q8h
Traumatic wound	*S. aureus*, Group A strep, clostridia	Cefazolin[12]	1-2 g I.V. q8h

[1]Parenteral prophylactic antimicrobials can be given as a single intravenous dose just before the operation. For prolonged operations, additional intraoperative doses should be given every 4-8 hours for the duration of the procedure.

[2]Some consultants recommend an additional dose when patients are removed from bypass during open-heart surgery.

[3]For hospitals in which methicillin-resistant *S. aureus* and *S. epidermidis* are a frequent cause of postoperative wound infection, or for patients allergic to penicillins or cephalosporin. Rapid I.V. administration may cause hypotension, which could be especially dangerous during induction of anesthesia. Even if the drug is given over 60 minutes, hypotension may occur; treatment with diphenhydramine (Benadryl® and others) and further slowing of the infusion rate may be helpful (Maki DG et al, *J Thorac Cardiovasc Surg*, 1992, 104:1423). For procedures in which enteric gram-negative bacilli are likely pathogens, such as vascular surgery involving a groin incision, cefazolin should be included in the prophylaxis regimen for patients not allergic to cephalosporins.

[4]Morbid obesity, esophageal obstruction, decreased gastric acidity or gastrointestinal motility.

[5]Age >70 years, acute cholecystitis, nonfunctioning gall bladder, obstructive jaundice or common duct stones.

[6]After appropriate diet and catharsis, 1 g of each at 1 PM, 2 PM, and 11 PM the day before an 8 AM operation.

[7]Urine culture positive or unavailable, preoperative catheter.

[8]Active labor or premature rupture of membranes.

[9]Patients with previous pelvic inflammatory disease, previous gonorrhea or multiple sex partners.

[10]Divided into 100 mg one hour before the abortion and 200 mg one half hour after.

[11]For contaminated or "dirty" surgery, therapy should usually be continued for about 5 days.

[12]For bite wounds, in which likely pathogens may also include oral anaerobes, *Eikenella corrodens* (human) and *Pasteurella multocida* (dog and cat), some *Medical Letter* consultants recommend use of amoxicillin/clavulanic acid (Augmentin®) or ampicillin/sulbactam (Unasyn®)

Adapted with permission from *The Medical Letter*, 1997, 39(Issue 1012).

POSTEXPOSURE PROPHYLAXIS FOR HEPATITIS B*

Exposure	Hepatitis B Immune Globulin	Hepatitis B Vaccine
Perinatal	0.5 mL I.M. within 12 h of birth	0.5 mL† I.M. within 12 h of birth (no later than 7 d), and at 1 and 6 mo‡; test for HB_sAg and anti-HB_s at 12-15 mo
Sexual	0.06 mL/kg I.M. within 14 d of sexual contact; a second dose should be given if the index patient remains HB_sAg-positive after 3 mo and hepatitis B vaccine was not given initially	1 mL I.M. at 0, 1, and 6 mo for homosexual and bisexual men and regular sexual contacts of persons with acute and chronic hepatitis B
Percutaneous; exposed person unvaccinated		
Source known HB_sAg-positive	0.06 mL/kg I.M. within 24 h	1 mL I.M. within 7 d, and at 1 and 6 mo§
Source known, HB_sAg status not known	Test source for HB_sAg; if source is positive, give exposed person 0.06 mL/kg I.M. once within 7 d	1 mL I.M. within 7 d, and at 1 and 6 mo§
Source not tested or unknown	Nothing required	1 mL I.M. within 7 d, and at 1 and 6 mo
Percutaneous; exposed person vaccinated		
Source known HB_sAg-positive	Test exposed person for anti-HB_s¶. If titer is protective, nothing is required; if titer is not protective, give 0.06 mL/kg within 24 h	Review vaccination status#
Source known, HB_sAg status not known	Test source for HB_sAg and exposed person for anti-HB_s. If source is HB_sAg-negative, or if source is HB_sAg-positive but anti-HB_s titer is protective, nothing is required. If source is HB_sAg-positive and anti-HB_s titer is not protective or if exposed person is a known nonresponder, give 0.06 mL/kg I.M. within 24 h. A second dose of hepatitis B immune globulin can be given 1 mo later if a booster dose of hepatitis B vaccine is not given.	Review vaccination status#
Source not tested or unknown	Test exposed person for anti-HB_s. If anti-HB_s titer is protective, nothing is required. If anti-HB_s titer is not protective, 0.06 mL/kg may be given along with a booster dose of hepatitis B vaccine	Review vaccination status#

*HB_sAg = hepatitis B surface antigen; anti-HB_s = antibody to hepatitis B surface antigen; I.M. = intramuscularly; SRU = standard ratio units.

†Each 0.5 mL dose of plasma-derived hepatitis B vaccine contains 10 µg of HB_sAg; each 0.5 mL dose of recombinant hepatitis B vaccine contains 5 µg (Merck Sharp & Dohme) or 10 µg (SmithKline Beecham) of HB_sAg.

‡If hepatitis B immune globulin and hepatitis B vaccine are given simultaneously, they should be given at separate sites.

§If hepatitis B vaccine is not given, a second dose of hepatitis B immune globulin should be given 1 month later.

¶Anti-HB_s titers <10 SRU by radioimmunoassay or negative by enzyme immunoassay indicate lack of protection. Testing the exposed person for anti-HB_s is not necessary if a protective level of antibody has been shown within the previous 24 months.

#If the exposed person has not completed a three-dose series of hepatitis B vaccine, the series should be completed. Test the exposed person for anti-HB_s. If the antibody level is protective, nothing is required. If an adequate antibody response in the past is shown on retesting to have declined to an inadequate level, a booster dose (1 mL) of hepatitis B vaccine should be given. If the exposed person has inadequate antibody or is a known nonresponder to vaccination, a booster dose can be given along with one dose of hepatitis B immune globulin.

PROPHYLAXIS FOR PATIENTS EXPOSED TO COMMON COMMUNICABLE DISEASES

Disease	Exposure	Prophylaxis/Management
Invasive *Haemophilus influenzae* disease	Close contact with an infected child for more than 4 hours	Give rifampin 20 mg/kg orally once daily for 4 days (600 mg maximum daily dose) to entire family with at least one household contact less than 48 months old. Contraindication: Pregnant contacts.
Hepatitis A	Direct contact with an infected child, or sharing of food or utensils	Give 0.02 mL/kg immune globulin (IG) within 7 days of exposure.
Hepatitis B	Needlestick (used needle) Mucous membrane exposure with blood or body fluid Direct inoculation of blood or body fluid into open cut, lesion, or laceration	**Known source and employee status unknown: Test patient for HB_sAg and employee for anti-HB_s.** If patient is HB_sAg negative and the patient does not have non-A, non-B hepatitis, do nothing. If patient is HB_sAg negative and has non-A, non-B hepatitis, **offer** ISG (optional). If patient is HB_sAg positive, give HBIG and hepatitis B vaccine within 48 hours of exposure. Employee antibody status may not be available for up to a week, so the above should be given as soon as patient's antigen status is known. Occasionally, the patient's antigen status will be unavailable for more than 24 hours. In these cases, HBIG should be given if the patient is high risk (ie, Asian immigrants, institutionalized patients, homosexuals, intravenous drug abusers, hemodialysis patients, patients with a history of hepatitis). If the employee is anti-HB_s negative, give the second and third doses of hepatitis B vaccine. **Known source and employee documented anti-HB_s positive:** If source has non-A, non-B hepatitis, offer ISG (optional). If employee is believed to be anti-HB_s positive due to vaccination, has received 3 doses of vaccine, and has not had an anti-HB_s test done, draw serum for anti-HB_s
Measles	15 minutes or more in the same room with a child with measles from 2 days before the onset of symptoms to 4 days after the appearance of the rash	Children who have not been vaccinated and have not had natural infection should be isolated from the 7th through the 18th day after exposure and/or for 4 days after the rash appears. Those who have not been vaccinated should be vaccinated within 72 hours of exposure if no contraindication exists, or receive immune globulin (IG) 0.25 mL/kg I.M. for immunocompetent individuals and 0.5 mL/kg (maximum: 15 mL) for immunosuppressed individuals. Children who are younger than 15 months of age should be revaccinated at 15 months of age but at least 3 months after receipt of vaccine or IG. Older individuals who have received IG should be vaccinated 3 months later.
Meningococcal disease	Household contact or direct contact with secretions	Household, day care center, and nursery school children should receive rifampin prophylaxis for 2 days. Dosages are given every 12 hours for a total of 4 doses. Dosage is 10 mg/kg/dose for children ages 1 month to 12 years (maximum: 600 mg/dose), 5 mg/kg/dose for infants less than 1 month of age, and 600 mg/dose for adults. Contraindication: Pregnant contacts **Because prophylaxis is not always effective, exposed children should be monitored for symptoms.** **Employee exposure: Anyone who develops a febrile illness should receive prompt medical evaluation. If indicated, antimicrobial therapy should be administered.**

PROPHYLAXIS FOR PATIENTS EXPOSED TO COMMON COMMUNICABLE DISEASES *(Continued)*

Disease	Exposure	Prophylaxis/Management
Pertussis	Housed in the same room with an infected child or spent 15 minutes in the playroom with the infected child	**Prophylaxis:** Contacts less than 7 years old who have had at least 4 doses of pertussis vaccine should receive a booster dose of DTP, unless a dose has been given within the past 3 years, and should receive erythromycin 40-50 mg/kg/day orally for 14 days. Contacts less than 7 years old who are not immunized or who have received less than 4 doses of DTP should have DTP immunization initiated or continued according to the recommended schedule. Children who have received their third dose 6 months or more before exposure should be given their fourth dose at this time. Erythromycin should also be given for 14 days. Contacts 7 years of age and above should receive prophylactic erythromycin (maximum: 1 g/day) for 10-14 days. All exposed patients should be watched closely for respiratory symptoms for 14 days after exposure has stopped because immunity conferred by the vaccine is not absolute and the efficacy of erythromycin in prophylaxis has not been established.
Tuberculosis	Housed in the same room with a child with contagious tuberculosis (tuberculosis is contagious if the child has a cough plus AFB seen on smear plus cavitation on CXR)	Place PPD immediately and 10 weeks after exposure. Start on INH. Consult Infectious Diseases if seroconversion occurs.
Varicella-zoster	1 hour or more in the same room with a contagious child from 24 hours before vesicles appear to when all vesicles are crusted, which is usually 5 to 7 days after vesicles appear. In household exposure, communicability is 48 hours before vesicles appear.	**Immunocompetent** children who have not been vaccinated or had natural infection, should have titers drawn only if they will still be hospitalized for more than 10 days after exposure. If titers are negative, they should be isolated from 10 to 21 days after exposure and/or until all lesions are crusted and dry. If VZIG was given the child should be isolated from 10 to 28 days after exposure. **Immunocompromised** children who have not been vaccinated or had natural infection should first have titers drawn, and then receive VZIG (varicella-zoster immune globulin) **1 vial/10 kg I.M.** up to a maximum of 5 vials as soon as possible but at most 96 hours after exposure. Fractional doses are not recommended. If titers are positive, nothing further need be done. If titers are negative, the child should be isolated from 10 to 28 days after exposure and should be monitored very carefully for the appearance of vesicles so that treatment can be initiated. VZIG is available from the Blood Bank.

TUBERCULOSIS

Tuberculin Skin Test Recommendations*

Children for whom immediate skin testing is indicated:

- Contacts of persons with confirmed or suspected infectious tuberculosis (contact investigation); this includes children identified as contacts of family members or associates in jail or prison in the last 5 years
- Children with radiographic or clinical findings suggesting tuberculosis
- Children immigrating from endemic countries (eg, Asia, Middle East, Africa, Latin America)
- Children with travel histories to endemic countries and/or significant contact with indigenous persons from such countries

Children who should be tested annually for tuberculosis†:

- Children infected with HIV or living in household with HIV-infected persons
- Incarcerated adolescents

Children who should be tested every 2-3 years†:

- Children exposed to the following individuals: HIV-infected, homeless, residents of nursing homes, institutionalized adolescents or adults, users of illicit drugs, incarcerated adolescents or adults, and migrant farm workers. Foster children with exposure to adults in the preceding high-risk groups are included.

Children who should be considered for tuberculin skin testing at ages 4-6 and 11-16 years:

- Children whose parents immigrated (with unknown tuberculin skin test status) from regions of the world with high prevalence of tuberculosis; continued potential exposure by travel to the endemic areas and/or household contact with persons from the endemic areas (with unknown tuberculin skin test status) should be an indication for repeat tuberculin skin testing
- Children without specific risk factors who reside in high-prevalence areas; in general, a high-risk neighborhood or community does not mean an entire city is at high risk; rates in any area of the city may vary by neighborhood, or even from block to block; physicians should be aware of these patterns in determining the likelihood of exposure; public health officials or local tuberculosis experts should help clinicians identify areas that have appreciable tuberculosis rates

Children at increased risk of progression of infection to disease: Those with other medical risk factors, including diabetes mellitus, chronic renal failure, malnutrition, and congenital or acquired immunodeficiencies deserve special consideration. Without recent exposure, these persons are not at increased risk of acquiring tuberculosis infection. Underlying immune deficiencies associated with these conditions theoretically would enhance the possibility for progression to severe disease. Initial histories of potential exposure to tuberculosis should be included on all of these patients. If these histories or local epidemiologic factors suggest a possibility of exposure, immediate and periodic tuberculin skin testing should be considered. An initial Mantoux tuberculin skin test should be performed before initiation of immunosuppressive therapy in any child with an underlying condition that necessitates immunosuppressive therapy.

---

*BCG immunization is not a contraindication to tuberculin skin testing.

†Initial tuberculin skin testing is at the time of diagnosis or circumstance, beginning as early as at age 3 months.

TUBERCULOSIS *(Continued)*

Tuberculosis Prophylaxis

Specific Circumstances/ Organism	Comments	Regimen
Category I. Exposure (Household members and other close contacts of potentially infectious cases) (Exposee tuberculin test negative)*		
Neonate	Rx essential	INH (10 mg/kg/d) for 3 months, then repeat tuberculin test (TBnT). If mother's smear negative and infant's TBnT negative and chest x-ray (CXR) are normal, stop INH. In the United Kingdom, BCG is then given (*Lancet*, 1990, 2:1479), unless mother is HIV-positive. If infants repeat TBnT is positive and/or CXR abnormal (hilar adenopathy and/or infiltrate), administer INH + RIF (10-20 mg/kg/d) (or streptomycin) for a total of 6 months. If mother is being treated, separation from mother is not indicated.
Children <5 y	Rx indicated	As for neonate first 3 months. If repeat TBnT is negative, stop. If repeat TBnT is positive, continue INH for a total of 9 months. If INH is not given initially, repeat TBnT at 3 months; if positive, treat with INH for 9 months (see Category II below).
Older children and adults	No Rx	Repeat TBnT at 3 months, if positive, treat with INH for 6 months (see Category II below)
Category II. Infection Without Disease (Positive tuberculin test)*		
Regardless of age (see INH Preventive Therapy)	Rx indicated	INH (5 mg/kg/d, maximum: 300 mg/d for adults, 10 mg/kg/d not to exceed 300 mg/d for children). Results with 6 months of treatment are nearly as effective as 12 months (65% vs 75% reduction in disease). *Am Thoracic Society* (6 months), *Am Acad Pediatrics*, 1991 (9 months). If CXR is abnormal, treat for 12 months. In HIV-positive patient, treatment for a minimum of 12 months, some suggest longer. Monitor transaminases monthly (*MMWR Morb Mortal Wkly Rep* 1989, 38:247).
Age <35 y	Rx indicated	Reanalysis of earlier studies favors INH prophylaxis for 6 months (if INH-related hepatitis case fatality rate is <1% and TB case fatality is ≥6.7%, which appears to be the case, monitor transaminases monthly (*Arch Int Med*, 1990, 150:2517).
INH-resistant organisms likely	Rx indicated	Data on efficacy of alternative regimens is currently lacking. Regimens include ETB + RIF daily for 6 months. PZA + RIF daily for 2 months, then INH + RIF daily until sensitivities from index case (if available) known, then if INH-CR, discontinue INH and continue RIF for 9 months, otherwise INH + RIF for 9 months (this latter is *Am Acad Pediatrics*, 1991 recommendation).
INH + RIF resistant organisms likely	Rx indicated	Efficacy of alternative regimens is unknown; PZA (25-30 mg/kg/d P.O.) + ETB (15-25 mg/kg/d P.O.) (at 25 mg/kg ETB, monitoring for retrobulbar neuritis required), for 6 months unless HIV-positive, then 12 months; PZA + ciprofloxacin (750 mg P.O. bid) or ofloxacin (400 mg P.O. bid) x 6-12 months *(MMWR Morb Mortal Wkly Rep*, 1992, 41(RR11):68).

INH = isoniazid; RIF = rifampin; KM = kanamycin; ETB = ethambutol

SM = streptomycin; CXR = chest x-ray; Rx = treatment

See also guidelines for interpreting PPD in "Skin Testing for Delayed Hypersensitivity" in the Appendix.

*Tuberculin test (TBnT). The standard is the Mantoux test, 5 TU PPD in 0.1 mL diluent stabilized with Tween 80. Read at 48-72 hours measuring maximum diameter of induration. A reaction ≥5 mm is defined as positive in the following: positive HIV or risk factors, recent close case contacts, CXR consistent with healed TBc. ≥10 mm is positive in foreign-born in countries of high prevalence, injection drug users, low income populations, nursing home residents, patients with medical conditions which increase risk (see above, preventive treatment). ≥15 mm is positive in all others (*Am Rev Resp Dis*, 1990, 142:725). Two-stage TBnT: Use in individuals to be tested regularly (ie, healthcare workers). TBn reactivity may decrease over time but be boosted by skin testing. If unrecognized, individual may be incorrectly diagnosed as recent converter. If first TBnT is reactive but <10 mm, repeat 5 TU in 1 week, if then ≥10 mm = positive, not recent conversion (*Am Rev Resp Dis*, 1979, 119:587).

USPHS/IDSA GUIDELINES FOR THE PREVENTION OF OPPORTUNISTIC INFECTIONS IN PERSONS INFECTED WITH HIV

(From "1999 USPHS/IDSA Guidelines for the Prevention of Opportunistic Infections in Persons Infected With Human Immunodeficiency Virus. USPHS/IDSA Prevention of Opportunistic Infections Working Group," *MMWR Morb Mortal Wkly Rep*, 1999, 48(RR-10):1-59. Updated March 2000 from website www.hivatis.org.)

DRUG REGIMENS FOR ADULTS AND ADOLESCENTS

Prophylaxis for First Episode of Opportunistic Disease in HIV-Infected Adults and Adolescents

Pathogen	Indication	Preventive Regimens	
		First Choice	Alternatives
I. Strongly Recommended as Standard of Care			
*Pneumocystis carinii**	CD4⁺ count <200/µL *or* oropharyngeal candidiasis	TMP-SMZ, 1 DS P.O. once daily (AI); TMP-SMZ, 1 SS P.O. once daily (AI)	Dapsone, 50 mg P.O. twice daily *or* 100 mg P.O. once daily (BI); dapsone, 50 mg P.O. once daily *plus* pyrimethamine, 50 mg P.O. weekly *plus* leucovorin, 25 mg P.O. weekly (BI); dapsone, 200 mg P.O. *plus* pyrimethamine, 75 mg P.O. *plus* leucovorin, 25 mg P.O. weekly (BI); aerosolized pentamidine, 300 mg monthly via Respirgard II™ nebulizer (BI); atovaquone, 1500 mg P.O. once daily (BI); TMP-SMZ, 1 DS P.O. 3 times/week (BI)
Mycobacterium tuberculosis			
Isoniazid-sensitive†	TST reaction ≥5 mm *or* prior positive TST result without treatment *or* contact with case of active tuberculosis	Isoniazid, 300 mg P.O. *plus* pyridoxine, 50 mg P.O. once daily x 9 months (AII) *or* isoniazid, 900 mg P.O. *plus* pyridoxine, 100 mg P.O. twice a week x 9 months (BI); rifampin 600 mg *plus* pyrazinamide 20 mg/kg P.O. once daily x 2 months (AI)	Rifabutin, 300 mg P.O. once daily *plus* pyrazinamide 20 mg/kg P.O. once daily x 2 months (BIII); rifampin, 600 mg P.O. once daily x 4 months (BIII)
Isoniazid-resistant	Same; high probability of exposure to isoniazid-resistant tuberculosis	Rifampin, 600 mg *plus* pyrazinamide 20 mg/kg P.O. once daily x 2 months (AI)	Rifabutin, 300 mg *plus* pyrazinamide 20 mg/kg P.O. once daily x 2 months (BIII); rifampin, 600 mg P.O. once daily x 4 months (BIII); rifabutin, 300 mg P.O. once daily x 4 months (CIII)
Multidrug (isoniazid and rifampin)-resistant	Same; high probability of exposure to multidrug-resistant tuberculosis	Choice of drugs requires consultation with public health authorities	None

USPHS/IDSA GUIDELINES FOR THE PREVENTION OF OPPORTUNISTIC INFECTIONS IN PERSONS INFECTED WITH HIV *(Continued)*

Prophylaxis for First Episode of Opportunistic Disease in HIV-Infected Adults and Adolescents *(continued)*

Pathogen	Indication	Preventive Regimens	
		First Choice	Alternatives
Toxoplasma gondii§	IgG antibody to *Toxoplasma* and CD4+ count <100/µL	TMP-SMZ, 1 DS P.O. once daily (AII)	TMP-SMZ, 1 SS P.O. once daily (BIII); dapsone, 50 mg P.O. once daily *plus* pyrimethamine, 50 mg P.O. once weekly *plus* leucovorin, 25 mg P.O. once weekly (BI); atovaquone, 1500 mg P.O. once daily with or without pyrimethamine, 25 mg P.O. once daily *plus* leucovorin, 10 mg P.O. once daily (CIII)
Mycobacterium avium complex¶	CD4+ count <50/µL	Azithromycin, 1200 mg P.O. once weekly (AI) or clarithromycin, 500 mg P.O. twice daily (AI)	Rifabutin, 300 mg P.O. once daily (BI); azithromycin, 1200 mg P.O. once weekly *plus* rifabutin, 300 mg P.O. once daily (CI)
Varicella zoster virus (VZV)	Significant exposure to chickenpox or shingles for patients who have no history of either condition or, if available, negative antibody to VZV	Varicella zoster immune globulin (VZIG), 5 vials (1.25 mL each) I.M., administered ≤96 hours after exposure, ideally within 48 hours (AIII)	
II. Generally Recommended			
*Streptococcus pneumoniae***	All patients	Pneumococcal vaccine, 0.5 mL I.M. (CD4+ ≥200/µL [BII]; CD4+ <200/µL [CIII]) — may reimmunize if initial immunization was given when CD4+ <200/µL and if CD4+ increases to >200/µL on HAART (CIII)	None
Hepatitis B virus††	All susceptible (anti-HBc-negative) patients	Hepatitis B vaccine: 3 doses (BII)	None
Influenza virus††	All patients (annually, before influenza season)	Whole or split virus, 0.5 mL/year I.M. (BIII)	Rimantadine, 100 mg P.O. twice daily (CIII) *or* amantadine, 100 mg P.O. twice daily (CIII)
Hepatitis A virus ††	All susceptible (anti-HAV-negative) patients with chronic hepatitis C	Hepatitis A vaccine: 2 doses (BIII)	None
III. Not Routinely Indicated			
Bacteria	Neutropenia	Granulocyte-colony-stimulating factor (G-CSF), 5-10 mcg/kg S.C. once daily x 2-4 weeks *or* granulocyte-macrophage colony-stimulating factor (GM-CSF), 250 mcg/m² I.V. over 2 hours once daily x 2-4 weeks (CII)	None
Cryptococcus neoformans§§	CD4+ count <50/µL	Fluconazole, 100-200 mg P.O. once daily (CI)	Itraconazole capsule, 200 mg P.O. once daily (CIII)
Histoplasma capsulatum§§	CD4+ count <100/µL, endemic geographic area	Itraconazole, 200 mg P.O. once daily (CI)	None

Prophylaxis for First Episode of Opportunistic Disease in HIV-Infected Adults and Adolescents *(continued)*

Pathogen	Indication	Preventive Regimens	
		First Choice	Alternatives
Cytomegalovirus (CMV)¶¶	CD4⁺ count <50/μL and CMV antibody positivity	Oral ganciclovir, 1 g P.O. 3 times/day (CI)	None

Note: Information included in these guidelines may not represent Food and Drug Administration (FDA) approval or approved labeling for the particular products or indications in question. Specifically, the terms "safe" and "effective" may not be synonymous with the FDA-defined legal standards for product approval.

Abbreviations: Anti-HBc = antibody to hepatitis B core antigen; CMV = cytomegalovirus; DS = double-strength tablet; HAART = highly active antiretroviral therapy; HAV = hepatitis A virus; SS = single-strength tablet; TMP-SMZ = trimethoprim-sulfamethoxazole; and TST = tuberculin skin test. The Respirgard II™ nebulizer is manufactured by Marquest, Englewood, CO. Letters and Roman numerals in parentheses after regimens indicate the strength of the recommendation and the quality of evidence supporting it.

*Prophylaxis should also be considered for persons with a CD4⁺ percentage <14%, for persons with a history of an AIDS-defining illness, and possibly for those with CD4⁺ count >200 but <250 cells/μL. TMP-SMZ also reduces the frequency of toxoplasmosis and some bacterial infections. Patients receiving dapsone should be tested for glucose-6-phosphate dehydrogenase deficiency. A dosage of 50 mg once daily is probably less effective than that of 100 mg once daily. The efficacy of parenteral pentamidine (eg, 4 mg/kg/month) is uncertain. Fansidar® (sulfadoxine-pyrimethamine) is rarely used because of severe hypersensitivity reactions. Patients who are being administered therapy for toxoplasmosis with sulfadiazine-pyrimethamine are protected against *Pneumocystis carinii* pneumonia and do not need additional prophylaxis against PCP.

†Directly observed therapy recommended for isoniazid (INH), 900 mg twice weekly; INH regimens should include pyridoxine to prevent peripheral neuropathy. Rifampin should not be administered concurrently with protease inhibitors or non-nucleoside reverse transcriptase inhibitors. Rifabutin should not be given with hard-gel saquinavir or delavirdine; caution is also advised when the drug is coadministered with soft-gel saquinavir. Rifabutin may be administered at a reduced dose (150 mg once daily) with indinavir, nelfinavir, or amprenavir; at a reduced dose of 150 mg every other day (or 150 mg 3 times/week) with ritonavir; or at an increased dose (450 mg once daily) with efavirenz; information is lacking regarding coadministration of rifabutin with nevirapine. Exposure to multidrug-resistant tuberculosis may require prophylaxis with two drugs; consult public health authorities. Possible regimens include pyrazinamide plus either ethambutol or a fluoroquinolone.

§Protection against toxoplasmosis is provided by TMP-SMZ, dapsone plus pyrimethamine, and possibly by atovaquone. The latter may be used with or without pyrimethamine. Pyrimethamine alone probably provides little, if any, protection.

¶See footnote above (†) regarding use of rifabutin with protease inhibitors or non-nucleoside reverse transcriptase inhibitors.

**Vaccination should be offered to persons who have a CD4⁺ T-lymphocyte count <200 cells/μL, although the efficacy may be diminished. Revaccination 5 years after the first dose or sooner if the initial immunization was given when the CD4⁺ count was <200 cells/μL and if the CD4⁺ count has increased to >200 cells/μL on HAART is considered optional. Some authorities are concerned that immunizations may stimulate the replication of HIV. However, one study showed no adverse effect of pneumococcal vaccination on patient survival.

††These immunizations or chemoprophylactic regimens do not target pathogens traditionally classified as opportunistic but should be considered for use in HIV-infected patients as indicated. Data are inadequate concerning clinical benefit of these vaccines in this population, although it is logical to assume that those patients who develop antibody responses will derive some protection. Some authorities are concerned that immunizations may stimulate HIV replication, although for influenza vaccination, a large observational study of HIV-infected persons in clinical care showed no adverse effect of this vaccine, including multiple doses, on patient survival (J. Ward, CDC, personal communication). Hepatitis B vaccine has been recommended for all children and adolescents and for all adults with risk factors for hepatitis B virus (HBV). Rimantadine/amantadine are appropriate during outbreaks of influenza A. Because of the theoretical concern that increases in HIV plasma RNA following vaccination during pregnancy might increase the risk of perinatal transmission of HIV, providers may wish to defer vaccination until after antiretroviral therapy is initiated.

§§There may be a few unusual occupational or other circumstances under which to consider prophylaxis; consult a specialist.

¶¶Acyclovir is not protective against CMV. Valacyclovir is not recommended because of an unexplained trend toward increased mortality observed in persons with AIDS who were being administered this drug for prevention of CMV disease.

USPHS/IDSA GUIDELINES FOR THE PREVENTION OF OPPORTUNISTIC INFECTIONS IN PERSONS INFECTED WITH HIV *(Continued)*

Prophylaxis to Prevent Recurrence of Opportunistic Disease (After Chemotherapy for Acute Disease) in HIV-Infected Adults and Adolescents

Pathogen	Indication	Preventive Regimens	
		First Choice	Alternatives
I. Recommended for Life as Standard of Care			
Pneumocystis carinii	Prior *P. carinii* pneumonia	TMP-SMZ, 1 DS P.O. once daily (AI); TMP-SMZ, 1 SS P.O. once daily (AI)	Dapsone, 50 mg P.O. twice daily *or* 100 mg P.O. once daily (BI); dapsone, 50 mg P.O. once daily *plus* pyrimethamine, 50 mg P.O. weekly *plus* leucovorin, 25 mg P.O. weekly (BI); dapsone, 200 mg P.O. *plus* pyrimethamine, 75 mg P.O. *plus* leucovorin, 25 mg P.O. weekly (BI); aerosolized pentamidine, 300 mg monthly via Respirgard II™ nebulizer (BI); atovaquone, 1500 mg P.O. once daily (BI); TMP-SMZ, 1 DS P.O. 3 times/week (CI)
*Toxoplasma gondii**	Prior toxoplasmic encephalitis	Sulfadiazine, 500-1000 mg P.O. 4 times/day *plus* pyrimethamine 25-75 mg P.O. once daily *plus* leucovorin, 10-25 mg P.O. once daily (AI)	Clindamycin, 300-450 mg P.O. every 6-8 hours *plus* pyrimethamine, 25-75 mg P.O. once daily *plus* leucovorin, 10-25 mg P.O. once daily (BI); atovaquone, 750 mg P.O. every 6-12 hours with or without pyrimethamine, 25 mg P.O. once daily *plus* leucovorin 10 mg P.O. once daily (CIII)
Mycobacterium avium complex†	Documented disseminated disease	Clarithromycin, 500 mg P.O. twice daily (AI) *plus* ethambutol, 15 mg/kg P.O. once daily (AII); with or without rifabutin, 300 mg P.O. once daily (CI)	Azithromycin, 500 mg P.O. once daily (AII) *plus* ethambutol, 15 mg/kg P.O. once daily (AII); with or without rifabutin, 300 mg P.O. once daily (CI)
Cytomegalovirus	Prior end-organ disease	Ganciclovir, 5-6 mg/kg I.V. 5-7 days/week *or* 1000 mg P.O. 3 times/day (AI); *or* foscarnet, 90-120 mg/kg I.V. once daily (AI); *or* (for retinitis) ganciclovir sustained-release implant, every 6-9 months *plus* ganciclovir, 1-1.5 g P.O. 3 times/day (AI)	Cidofovir, 5 mg/kg I.V. every other week with probenecid 2 g P.O. 3 hours before the dose followed by 1 g P.O. given 2 hours after the dose, and 1 g P.O. 8 hours after the dose (total of 4 g) (AI); fomivirsen, 1 vial (330 mcg) injected into the vitreous, then repeated every 2-4 weeks (AI)
Cryptococcus neoformans	Documented disease	Fluconazole, 200 mg P.O. once daily (AI)	Amphotericin B, 0.6-1 mg/kg I.V. weekly to 3 times/week (AI); itraconazole, 200 mg P.O. once daily (BI)
Histoplasma capsulatum	Documented disease	Itraconazole capsule, 200 mg P.O. twice daily (AI)	Amphotericin B, 1 mg/kg I.V. weekly (AI)
Coccidioides immitis	Documented disease	Fluconazole, 400 mg P.O. once daily (AII)	Amphotericin B, 1 mg/kg I.V. weekly (AI); itraconazole, 200 mg P.O. twice daily (AII)
Salmonella species (non-*typhi*)§	Bacteremia	Ciprofloxacin, 500 mg P.O. twice daily for several months (BII)	Antibiotic chemoprophylaxis with another active agent (CIII)
II. Recommended Only if Subsequent Episodes Are Frequent or Severe			
Herpes simplex virus	Frequent/ severe recurrences	Acyclovir, 200 mg P.O. 3 times/ day *or* 400 mg P.O. twice daily (AI); famciclovir, 500 mg P.O. twice daily (AI)	Valacyclovir, 500 mg P.O. twice daily (CIII)
Candida (oropharyngeal or vaginal)	Frequent/ severe recurrences	Fluconazole, 100-200 mg P.O. once daily (CI)	Itraconazole solution, 200 mg P.O. once daily (CI); ketoconazole, 200 mg P.O. once daily (CIII)

Prophylaxis to Prevent Recurrence of Opportunistic Disease (After Chemotherapy for Acute Disease) in HIV-Infected Adults and Adolescents *(continued)*

Pathogen	Indication	Preventive Regimens	
		First Choice	**Alternatives**
Candida (esophageal)	Frequent/ severe recurrences	Fluconazole, 100-200 mg P.O. once daily (BI)	Itraconazole solution, 200 mg P.O. once daily (BI); ketoconazole, 200 mg P.O. once daily (CIII)

Note: Information included in these guidelines may not represent Food and Drug Administration (FDA) approval or approved labeling for the particular products or indications in question. Specifically, the terms "safe" and "effective" may not be synonymous with the FDA-defined legal standards for product approval.

DS = double-strength tablet; SS = single-strength tablet; and TMP-SMZ = trimethoprim-sulfamethoxazole. The Respirgard II™ nebulizer is manufactured by Marquest, Englewood, CO. Letters and Roman numerals in parentheses after regimens indicate the strength of the recommendation and the quality of the evidence supporting it.

* Pyrimethamine/sulfadiazine confers protection against PCP as well as toxoplasmosis; clindamycin-pyrimethamine does not.

† Many multiple-drug regimens are poorly tolerated. Drug interactions (eg, those seen with clarithromycin/rifabutin) can be problematic; rifabutin has been associated with uveitis, especially when administered at daily doses of >300 mg or concurrently with fluconazole or clarithromycin. Rifabutin should not be administered concurrently with hard-gel saquinavir, ritonavir, or delavirdine; caution is also advised when the drug is coadministered with soft-gel saquinavir. Rifabutin may be administered at reduced dose (150 mg once daily with indinavir, nelfinavir, or amprenavir; or 150 mg every other day with ritonavir) or at increased dose (450 mg once daily) with efavirenz. Information is lacking regarding coadministration of rifabutin with nevirapine.

§ Efficacy of eradication of *Salmonella* has been demonstrated only for ciprofloxacin.

Criteria for Discontinuing and Restarting Opportunistic Infection Prophylaxis for Adult Patients With HIV Infection*

Opportunistic Illness	Discontinuation Criteria for Prophylaxis		Criteria for Restarting Prophylaxis
	Primary	**Secondary**	
Pneumocystis carinii pneumonia	CD4⁺ >200 cells/µL for >3-6 months (CII)	No criteria recommended for stopping	Same as criteria for initiating (CIII)
Disseminated *Mycobacterium avium* complex	CD4⁺ >100 cells/µL for >3-6 months; sustained suppression of HIV plasma RNA (CIII)	No criteria recommended for stopping	Same as criteria for initiating (CIII)
Toxoplasmosis	No criteria recommended for stopping	No criteria recommended for stopping	NA
Cryptococcosis	NA	No criteria recommended for stopping	NA
Histoplasmosis	NA	No criteria recommended for stopping	NA
Coccidioidomycosis	NA	No criteria recommended for stopping	NA
Cytomegalovirus Retinitis	NA	• CD4⁺ >100-150 cells/µL for >3-6 months • Durable suppression of HIV plasma RNA • Nonsight-threatening lesion • Adequate vision in contralateral eye • Regular ophthalmic examination	Restart maintenance when CD4⁺ <50-100 cells/µL (CIII)

*The safety of discontinuing prophylaxis in children whose CD4+ counts have increased in response to HAART has not been studied.

USPHS/IDSA GUIDELINES FOR THE PREVENTION OF OPPORTUNISTIC INFECTIONS IN PERSONS INFECTED WITH HIV *(Continued)*

DRUG REGIMENS FOR INFANTS AND CHILDREN

Prophylaxis for First Episode of Opportunistic Disease in HIV-Infected Infants and Children

Pathogen	Indication	Preventive Regimens	
		First Choice	Alternatives
I. Strongly Recommended as Standard of Care			
*Pneumocystis carinii**	HIV-infected or HIV-indeterminate infants 1-12 months of age; HIV-infected children 1-5 years of age with CD4⁺ count <500/µL *or* CD4⁺ percentage <15%; HIV-infected children 6-12 years of age with CD4⁺ count <200/µL *or* CD4⁺ percentage <15%	TMP-SMZ, 150/750 mg/m²/day in 2 divided doses P.O. 3 times/week on consecutive days (AII); acceptable alternative dosage schedules: (AII) Single dose P.O. 3 times/week on consecutive days 2 divided doses P.O. once daily; 2 divided doses P.O. 3 times/week on alternate days	Dapsone (children ≥1 month of age), 2 mg/kg (max: 100 mg) P.O. once daily *or* 4 mg/kg (max: 200 mg) P.O. once weekly (CII); aerosolized pentamidine (children ≥5 years of age), 300 mg/month via Respirgard II™ nebulizer (CIII); atovaquone (children 1-3 months and >24 months of age, 30 mg/kg P.O. once daily; children 4-24 months of age, 45 mg/kg P.O. once daily) (CII)
Mycobacterium tuberculosis†			
Isoniazid-sensitive	TST reaction ≥5 mm *or* prior positive TST result without treatment *or* contact with case of active tuberculosis	Isoniazid, 10-15 mg/kg (max: 300 mg) P.O. once daily x 9 months (AII), *or* 20-30 mg/kg (max: 900 mg) P.O. twice weekly x 9 months (BIII)	Rifampin, 10-20 mg/kg (max: 600 mg) P.O. once daily x 4-6 months (BIII)
Isoniazid-resistant	Same as above; high probability of exposure to isoniazid-resistant tuberculosis	Rifampin, 10-20 mg/kg (max: 600 mg) P.O. once daily x 4-6 months (BIII)	Uncertain
Multidrug (isoniazid and rifampin)-resistant	Same as above; high probability of exposure to multidrug-resistant tuberculosis	Choice of drug requires consultation with public health authorities	None
Mycobacterium avium complex†	For children ≥6 years of age, CD4⁺ count <50/µL; 2-6 years of age, CD4⁺ count <75/µL; 1-2 years of age, CD4⁺ count <500/µL; <1 year of age, CD4⁺ count <750/µL	Clarithromycin, 7.5 mg/kg (max: 500 mg) P.O. twice daily (AII), *or* azithromycin, 20 mg/kg (max: 1200 mg) P.O. weekly (AII)	Azithromycin, 5 mg/kg (max: 250 mg) P.O. once daily (AII); children ≥6 years of age, rifabutin, 300 mg P.O. once daily (BI)
Varicella zoster virus§	Significant exposure to varicella or shingles with no history of chickenpox or shingles	Varicella zoster immune globulin (VZIG), 1 vial (1.25 mL)/10 kg (max: 5 vials) I.M., administered ≤96 hours after exposure, ideally within 48 hours (AII)	None
Vaccine-preventable pathogens¶	HIV exposure/infection	Routine immunizations	None
II. Generally Recommended			
*Toxoplasma gondii***	IgG antibody *Toxoplasma* and severe immunosuppression	TMP-SMZ, 150/750 mg/m²/d in 2 divided doses P.O. once daily (BIII)	Dapsone (children ≥1 month of age), 2 mg/kg *or* 15 mg/m² (max: 25 mg) P.O. once daily *plus* pyrimethamine, 1 mg/kg P.O. once daily *plus* leucovorin, 5 mg P.O. every 3 days (BIII); atovaquone (children 1-3 months and >24 months of age, 30 mg/kg P.O. once daily; children 14-24 months of age, 45 mg/kg P.O. once daily) (CIII)
Varicella zoster virus¶	HIV-infected children who are asymptomatic and not immunosuppressed	Varicella zoster vaccine (see vaccine-preventable pathogens) (BII)	None

Prophylaxis for First Episode of Opportunistic Disease in HIV-Infected Infants and Children *(continued)*

Pathogen	Indication	Preventive Regimens	
		First Choice	Alternatives
Influenza virus¶	All patients (annually, before influenza season)	Influenza vaccine (see vaccine-preventable pathogens) (BIII)	Rimantadine or amantadine (during outbreaks of influenza A); children 1-9 years of age, 5 mg/kg/day P.O. in 2 divided doses; ≥10 years of age, use adult doses (CIII)
III. Not Recommended for Most Children; Indicated for Use Only in Unusual Circumstances			
Invasive bacterial infections††	Hypogammaglobulinemia (ie, IgG <400 mg/dL)	IVIG (400 mg/kg every 2-4 weeks) (AI)	None
Cryptococcus neoformans	Severe immunosuppression	Fluconazole, 3-6 mg/kg P.O. once daily (CII)	Itraconazole, 2-5 mg/kg P.O. every 12-24 hours (CIII)
Histoplasma capsulatum	Severe immunosuppression, endemic geographic area	Itraconazole, 2-5 mg/kg P.O. every 12-24 hours (CIII)	None
Cytomegalovirus (CMV)§§	CMV antibody positivity and severe immunosuppression	Oral ganciclovir 30 mg/kg P.O. 3 times/day (CII)	None

Note: Information included in these guidelines may not represent Food and Drug Administration (FDA) approval or approved labeling for the particular products or indications in question. Specifically, the terms "safe" and "effective" may not be synonymous with the FDA-defined legal standards for product approval. CMV = cytomegalovirus; IVIG = intravenous immune globulin; TMP-SMZ = trimethoprim-sulfamethoxazole; and VZIG = varicella zoster immune globulin. The Respirgard II™ nebulizer is manufactured by Marquest, Englewood, CO. Letters and Roman numerals in parentheses after regimens indicate the strength of the recommendation and the quality of the evidence supporting it.

*Daily TMP-SMZ reduces the frequency of some bacterial infections. TMP-SMZ, dapsone-pyrimethamine, and possibly atovaquone (with or without pyrimethamine) appear to protect against toxoplasmosis, although data have not been prospectively collected. When compared with weekly dapsone, a recent study suggested that daily dapsone is associated with lower incidence of PCP but higher hematologic toxicity and mortality. The efficacy of parenteral pentamidine (eg, 4 mg/kg/every 2-4 weeks) is controversial. Patients receiving therapy for toxoplasmosis with sulfadiazine-pyrimethamine are protected against *Pneumocystis carinii* pneumonia (PCP) and do not need TMP-SMZ.

†Significant drug interactions may occur between rifamycins (rifampin and rifabutin) and protease inhibitors and non-nucleoside reverse transcriptase inhibitors. Consult a specialist.

§Children routinely being administered intravenous immune globulin (IVIG) should receive VZIG if the last dose of IVIG was administered >21 days before exposure.

¶HIV-infected and HIV-exposed children should be immunized according to the childhood immunization schedule, which has been adapted from the January-December 1999 schedule recommended for immunocompetent children by the Advisory Committee on Immunization Practices, the American Academy of Pediatrics, and the American Academy of Family Physicians. This schedule differs from that for immunocompetent children in that IPV replaces OPV, and vaccination against influenza (BIII) and *S. pneumoniae* (BII) should be offered. MMR should not be administered to severely immunocompromised children (DIII). Vaccination against varicella is indicated only for asymptomatic nonimmunosuppressed children (BII), and rotavirus vaccine is contraindicated in all HIV-infected children (EIII). Once an HIV-exposed child is determined not to be HIV infected, the schedule for immunocompetent children applies.

**Protection against toxoplasmosis is provided by the preferred antipneumocystis regimens and possibly by atovaquone. The latter may be used with or without pyrimethamine. Pyrimethamine alone probably provides little, if any, protection.

††Respiratory syncytial virus (RSV) IVIG (750 mg/kg), not monoclonal RSV antibody, may be substituted for IVIG during the RSV season to provide broad anti-infective protection, if this product is available.

§§Oral ganciclovir results in reduced CMV shedding in CMV-infected children. Acyclovir is not protective against CMV.

USPHS/IDSA GUIDELINES FOR THE PREVENTION OF OPPORTUNISTIC INFECTIONS IN PERSONS INFECTED WITH HIV *(Continued)*

Prophylaxis to Prevent Recurrence of Opportunistic Disease (After Chemotherapy for Acute Disease) in HIV-Infected Infants and Children

Pathogen	Indication	Preventive Regimens: First Choice	Preventive Regimens: Alternatives
I. Recommended for Life as Standard of Care			
Pneumocystis carinii	Prior *P. carinii* pneumonia	TMP-SMZ, 150/750 mg/m²/d in 2 divided doses P.O. 3 times/week on consecutive days (AII) Acceptable alternative schedules for same dosage (AII) Single dose P.O. 3 times/week on consecutive days; 2 divided doses P.O. daily; 2 divided doses P.O. 3 times/week on alternate days	Dapsone (children ≥1 month of age), 2 mg/kg (max: 100 mg) P.O. once daily *or* 4 mg/kg (max: 200 mg) P.O. weekly (CII); aerosolized pentamidine (children ≥5 years of age), 300 mg monthly via Respirgard II™ nebulizer (CIII); atovaquone (children 1-3 months and >24 months of age, 30 mg/kg P.O. once daily; children 4-24 months, 45 mg/kg P.O. once daily) (CII)
*Toxoplasma gondii**	Prior toxoplasmic encephalitis	Sulfadiazine, 85-120 mg/kg/d in 2-4 divided doses P.O. daily *plus* pyrimethamine, 1 mg/kg *or* 15 mg/m² (max: 25 mg) P.O. once daily *plus* leucovorin, 5 mg P.O. every 3 days (AI)	Clindamycin, 20-30 mg/kg/d in 4 divided doses P.O. once daily *plus* pyrimethamine, 1 mg/kg P.O. once daily *plus* leucovorin, 5 mg P.O. every 3 days (BI)
Mycobacterium avium complex†	Prior disease	Clarithromycin, 7.5 mg/kg (max: 500 mg) P.O. twice daily (AII) *plus* ethambutol, 15 mg/kg (max: 900 mg) P.O. once daily (AII); with or without rifabutin, 5 mg/kg (max: 300 mg) P.O. once daily (CII)	Azithromycin, 5 mg/kg (max: 250 mg) P.O. once daily (AII) *plus* ethambutol, 15 mg/kg (max: 900 mg) P.O. once daily (AII); with or without rifabutin, 5 mg/kg (max: 300 mg) P.O. once daily (CII)
Cryptococcus neoformans	Documented disease	Fluconazole, 3-6 mg/kg P.O. once daily (AII)	Amphotericin B, 0.5-1 mg/kg I.V. 1-3 times/week (AI); itraconazole, 2-5 mg/kg P.O. every 12-24 hours (BII);
Histoplasma capsulatum	Documented disease	Itraconazole, 2-5 mg/kg P.O. every 12-48 hours (AIII)	Amphotericin B, 1 mg/kg I.V. weekly (AIII)
Coccidioides immitis	Documented disease	Fluconazole, 6 mg/kg P.O. once daily (AIII)	Amphotericin B, 1 mg/kg I.V. weekly (AIII); itraconazole, 2-5 mg/kg P.O. every 12-48 hours (AIII)
Cytomegalovirus	Prior end-organ disease	Ganciclovir, 5 mg/kg I.V. once daily, *or* foscarnet, 90-120 mg/kg I.V. once daily (AI)	(For retinitis) — ganciclovir sustained-release implant, every 6-9 months *plus* ganciclovir, 30 mg/kg P.O. 3 times/d (BIII)
Salmonella species (non-*typhi*)§	Bacteremia	TMP-SMZ, 150/750 mg/m² in 2 divided doses P.O. once daily for several months (CIII)	Antibiotic chemoprophylaxis with another active agent (CIII)
II. Recommended Only if Subsequent Episodes Are Frequent or Severe			
Invasive bacterial infections¶	>2 infections in 1-year period	TMP-SMZ, 150/750 mg/m² in 2 divided doses P.O. once daily (BI); *or* IVIG, 400 mg/kg every 2-4 weeks (BI)	Antibiotic chemoprophylaxis with another active agent (BIII)
Herpes simplex virus	Frequent/severe recurrences	Acyclovir, 80 mg/kg/d in 3-4 divided doses P.O. daily (AII)	
Candida (oropharyngeal)	Frequent/severe recurrences	Fluconazole, 3-6 mg/kg P.O. once daily (CIII)	

Prophylaxis to Prevent Recurrence of Opportunistic Disease (After Chemotherapy for Acute Disease) in HIV-Infected Infants and Children *(continued)*

Pathogen	Indication	Preventive Regimens	
		First Choice	Alternatives
Candida (esophageal)	Frequent/ severe recurrences	Fluconazole, 3-6 mg/kg P.O. once daily (BIII)	Itraconazole solution, 5 mg/kg P.O. once daily (CIII); ketoconazole, 5-10 mg/kg P.O. every 12-24 hours (CIII)

Note: Information included in these guidelines may not represent Food and Drug Administration (FDA) approval or approved labeling for the particular products or indications in question. Specifically, the terms "safe" and "effective" may not be synonymous with the FDA-defined legal standards for product approval. IVIG = intravenous immune globulin and TMP-SMZ = trimethoprim-sulfamethoxazole. The Respirgard II™ nebulizer is manufactured by Marquest, Englewood, CO. Letters and Roman numerals in parentheses after regimens indicate the strength of the recommendations and the quality of the evidence supporting it.

* Only pyrimethamine plus sulfadiazine confers protection against PCP as well as toxoplasmosis. Although the clindamycin plus pyrimethamine regimen is the preferred alternative in adults, it has not been tested in children. However, these drugs are safe and are used for other infections.

†Significant drug interactions may occur between rifabutin and protease inhibitors and non-nucleoside reverse transcriptase inhibitors. Consult an expert.

§ Drug should be determined by susceptibilities of the organism isolated. Alternatives to TMP-SMZ include ampicillin, chloramphenicol, or ciprofloxacin. However, ciprofloxacin is not approved for use in persons aged <18 years; therefore, it should be used in children with caution and only if no alternatives exist.

¶ Antimicrobial prophylaxis should be chosen based on the microorganism and antibiotic sensitivities. TMP-SMZ, if used, should be administered daily. Providers should be cautious about using antibiotics solely for this purpose because of the potential for development of drug-resistant microorganisms. IVIG may not provide additional benefit to children receiving daily TMP-SMZ, but may be considered for children who have recurrent bacterial infections despite TMP-SMZ prophylaxis. Choice of antibiotic prophylaxis vs IVIG should also involve consideration of adherence, ease of intravenous access, and cost. If IVIG is used, RSV-IVIG (750 mg/kg), not monoclonal RSV antibody, may be substituted for IVIG during the RSV season to provide broad anti-infective protection, if this product is available.

INTERPRETATION OF GRAM'S STAIN RESULTS GUIDELINES

These guidelines are not definitive but presumptive for the identification of organisms on Gram's stain. Treatment will depend on the quality of the specimen and appropriate clinical evaluation.

Gram-Negative Bacilli (GNB)	**Example**
Enterobacteriaceae	*Escherichia coli* *Serratia* sp *Klebsiella* sp *Enterobacter* sp *Citrobacter* sp
Nonfermentative GNB	*Xanthomonas maltophilia*
Pseudomonas aeruginosa	
Bacteroides fragilis group	
If fusiform (long and pointed)	*Capnocytophaga* sp *Fusobacterium* sp
Gram-Negative Cocci (GNC)	
Diplococci, pairs	*Moraxella (Branhamella) catarrhalis* *Neisseria gonorrhoeae* *Neisseria meningitidis*
Coccobacilli	*Acinetobacter* sp *Haemophilus influenzae*
Gram-Positive Bacilli (GPB)	
Diphtheroids (small pleomorphic)	*Corynebacterium* sp *Propionibacterium*
Large, with spores	*Bacillus* sp *Clostridium* sp
Branching, beaded, rods	*Actinomyces* sp *Nocardia* sp
Other	*Lactobacillus* sp *Listeria* sp
Gram-Positive Cocci (GPC)	
Pairs, chains, clusters	*Enterococcus* sp *Staphylococcus* sp *Streptococcus* sp
Pairs, lancet-shaped	*Streptococcus pneumoniae*

KEY CHARACTERISTICS OF SELECTED BACTERIA

Gram-Negative Bacilli (GNB)	**Example**
Lactose-positive	*Citrobacter* sp* (Enterobacteriaceae) *Enterobacter* sp* (Enterobacteriaceae) *Escherichia coli* (Enterobacteriaceae) *Klebsiella pneumoniae* (Enterobacteriaceae)
Lactose-negative/oxidase-negative	*Acinetobacter* sp *Morganella morganii* *Proteus mirabilis*: indole-negative *Proteus vulgaris*: indole-positive *Providencia* sp *Salmonella* sp *Serratia* sp† (Enterobacteriaceae) *Shigella* sp *Xanthomonas maltophilia*
Lactose-negative/oxidase-positive	*Aeromonas hydrophila* (may be lactose positive) *Alcaligenes* sp *Flavobacterium* sp *Moraxella* sp‡ *Pseudomonas aeruginosa* Other *Pseudomonas* sp
Anaerobes	*Bacteroides* sp (*B. fragilis*) *Fusobacterium* sp
Other	*Haemophilus influenzae* (coccobacillus)
Gram-Positive Baccili (GPB)	
Anaerobes	*Lactobacillus* sp *Eubacterium* sp *Clostridium* sp (spores) *Bifidobacterium* sp *Actinomyces* sp (branching, filamentous) *Propionibacterium acnes*
Bacillus sp	*B. cereus, B. subtilis* (large with spores)
Branching, beaded; partial acid-fast positive	*Nocardia* sp
CSF, blood	*Listeria monocytogenes*
Rapidly growing mycobacteria	*M. fortuitum* *M. chelonei*
Vaginal flora, rarely blood	*Lactobacillus* sp
Often blood culture contaminants	Diphtheroids (may be *Corynebacterium* sp)
Resistant to many agents except vancomycin	*C. jeikeium*
Other	*Actinomyces* sp (branching, beaded)
Gram-Negative Cocci (GNC)	
Diplococci, pairs	*Capnocytophaga* sp *Fusobacterium* sp (fusiform) *Moraxella catarrhalis* *Neisseria meningitidis* *Neisseria gonorrhoeae*
Coccobacilli	*Acinetobacter* sp
Anaerobes	*Veillonella* sp
Gram-Positive Cocci (GPC)	
Catalase-negative	*Streptococcus* sp (chains) *Micrococcus* sp (usually insignificant)
Catalase-positive	*Staphylococcus* sp (pairs, chains, clusters)
Coagulase-negative	Coagulase-negative staphylococci (CNS)
Bloods	*S. epidermidis* or CNS
Urine	*S. saprophyticus* (CNS)
Coagulase-positive	*S. aureus*
Anaerobes	*Peptostreptococcus* sp

KEY CHARACTERISTICS OF SELECTED BACTERIA
(Continued)

Fungi	
Molds	
Sparsely septate hyphae	Zygomycetes (eg, *Rhizopus* sp and *Mucor*)
Septate hyphae brown pigment	Phaeohyphomycetes, for example, *Alternaria* sp *Bipolaris* sp *Curvularia* sp *Exserohilum* sp
Nonpigmented (hyaline)	Hyalophomycetes, for example *Aspergillus* sp (*A. fumigatus, A. flavus*) Dermatophytes *Fusarium* sp *Paecilomyces* sp *Penicillium* sp
Thermally dimorphic (yeast in tissue; mold *in vitro*)	*Blastomyces dermatitidis* *Coccidioides immitis* *Histoplasma capsulatum* (slow growing) *Paracoccidioides brasilliensis* *Sporothrix schenckii*
Yeast	*Candida* sp (germ tube positive = *C. albicans* *Cryptococcus* sp (no pseudohyphae) *C. neoformans* *Rhodotorula, Saccharomyces* sp *Torulopsis glabrata* *Trichosporon* sp
Virus	Influenza Hepatitis A, B, C, D Human immunodeficiency virus Rubella Herpes Cytomegalovirus Respiratory syncytial virus Epstein-Barr
Chlamydiae	*Chlamydia trachomatis* *Chlamydia pneumoniae* (TWAR) *Chlamydia psittaci*
Rickettsiae	
Ureaplasma	
Mycoplasma	*Mycoplasma pneumoniae* *Mycoplasma hominis*
Spirochetes	*Treponema pallidum* *Borrelia burgdorferi*
Mycobacteria	*Mycobacterium tuberculosis* *Mycobacterium intracellulare*

Most Common Blood Culture Contaminants

Alpha-hemolytic streptococci
Bacillus sp
Coagulase-negative staphylococci
Diphtheroids
Lactobacilli
Micrococcus sp
Propionibacterium sp

*May be lactose-negative.
†May produce red pigment and appear lactose-positive initially.
‡May be either bacillary or coccoid.

ANIMAL AND HUMAN BITES GUIDELINES

Wound Management

Irrigation: Critically important; irrigate all penetration wounds using 20 mL syringe, 19 gauge needle and >250 mL 1% povidone iodine solution. This method will reduce wound infection by a factor of 20. When there is high risk of rabies, use viricidal 1% benzalkonium chloride in addition to the 1% povidone iodine. Irrigate wound with normal saline after antiseptic irrigation.

Debridement: Remove all crushed or devitalized tissue remaining after irrigation; minimize removal on face and over thin skin areas or anywhere you would create a worse situation than the bite itself already has; do not extend puncture wounds surgically — rather, manage them with irrigation and antibiotics.

Suturing: Close most dog bites if <8 hours (<12 hours on face); do not routinely close puncture wounds, or deep or severe bites on the hands or feet, as these are at highest risk for infection. Cat and human bites should not be sutured unless cosmetically important. Wound edge freshening, where feasible, reduces infection; minimize sutures in the wound and use monofilament on the surface.

Immobilization: Critical in all hand wounds; important for infected extremities.

Hospitalization/I.V. Antibiotics: Admit for I.V. antibiotics all significant human bites to the hand, especially closed fist injuries, and bites involving penetration of the bone or joint (a high index of suspicion is needed). Consider I.V. antibiotics for significant established wound infections with cellulitis or lymphangitis, any infected bite on the hand, any infected cat bite, and any infection in an immunocompromised or asplenic patient. Outpatient treatment with I.V. antibiotics may be possible in selected cases by consulting with infectious disease.

Laboratory Assessment

Gram's Stain: Not useful prior to onset of clinically apparent infection; examination of purulent material may show a predominant organism in established infection, aiding antibiotic selection; not warranted unless results will change your treatment.

Culture: Not useful or cost effective prior to onset of clinically apparent infection.

X-Ray: Whenever you suspect bony involvement, especially in craniofacial dog bites in very small children or severe bite/crush in an extremity; cat bites with their long needle like teeth may cause osteomyelitis or a septic joint, especially in the hand or wrist.

Immunizations

Tetanus: All bite wounds are contaminated. If not immunized in last 5 years, or if not current in a child, give DPT, DT, Td, or TT as indicated. For absent or incomplete primary immunization, give 250 units tetanus immune globulin (TIG) in addition.

Rabies: In the U.S. 30,000 persons are treated each year in an attempt to prevent 1-5 cases. Domestic animals should be quarantined for 10 days to prove need for prophylaxis. High risk animal bites (85% of cases = bat, skunk, raccoon) usually receive treatment consisting of:

- human rabies immune globulin (HRIG): 20 units/kg I.M. (unless previously immunized with HDCV)
- human diploid cell vaccine (HDCV): 1 mL I.M. on days 0, 3, 7, 14, and 28 (unless previously immunized with HDCV - then give only first 2 doses)

Consult with Infectious Disease before ordering rabies prophylaxis.

ANIMAL AND HUMAN BITES GUIDELINES *(Continued)*

Bite Wounds and Prophylactic Antibiotics

Parenteral vs Oral: If warranted, consider an initial I.V. dose to rapidly establish effective serum levels, especially if high risk, delayed treatment, or if patient reliability is poor.

Dog Bite:

1. Rarely get infected (~5%)
2. Infecting organisms: Coagulase-negative staph, coagulase-positive staph, alpha strep, diphtheroids, beta strep, *Pseudomonas aeruginosa*, gamma strep, *Pasteurella multocida*
3. Prophylactic antibiotics are seldom indicated. Consider for high risk wounds such as distal extremity puncture wounds, severe crush injury, bites occurring in cosmetically sensitive areas (eg, face), or in immunocompromised or asplenic patients.

Cat Bite:

1. Often get infected (~25% to 50%)
2. Infecting organisms: *Pasteurella multocida* (first 24 hours), coagulase-positive staph, anaerobic cocci (after first 24 hours)
3. Prophylactic antibiotics are indicated in all cases.

Human Bite:

1. Intermediate infection rate (~15% to 20%)
2. Infecting organisms: Coagulase-positive staph, alpha, beta, gamma strep, *Haemophilus*, *Eikenella corrodens*, anaerobic streptococci, *Fusobacterium*, *Veillonella*, bacteroides.
3. Prophylactic antibiotics are indicated in almost all cases except superficial injuries.

Bite Wound Antibiotic Regimens

	Dog Bite	Cat Bite	Human Bite
Prophylactic Antibiotics			
Prophylaxis	No routine prophylaxis, consider if involves face or hand, or immunosuppressed or asplenic patients	Routine prophylaxis	Routine prophylaxis
Prophylactic antibiotic	Amoxicillin	Amoxicillin	Amoxicillin
Penicillin allergy	Doxycycline if >10 y or co-trimoxazole	Doxycycline if >10 y or co-trimoxazole	Doxycycline if >10 y or erythromycin and cephalexin*
Outpatient Oral Antibiotic Treatment (mild to moderate infection)			
Established infection	Amoxicillin and clavulanic acid	Amoxicillin and clavulanic acid	Amoxicillin and clavulanic acid
Penicillin allergy (mild infection only)	Doxycycline if >10 y	Doxycycline if >10 y	Cephalexin* or clindamycin
Outpatient Parenteral Antibiotic Treatment (moderate infections – single drug regimens)			
	Ceftriaxone	Ceftriaxone	Cefotetan
Inpatient Parenteral Antibiotic Treatment			
Established infection	Ampicillin + cefazolin	Ampicillin + cefazolin	Ampicillin + clindamycin
Penicillin allergy	Cefazolin*	Ceftriaxone*	Cefotetan* or imipenem
Duration of Prophylactic and Treatment Regimens			
Prophylaxis: 5 days			
Treatment: 10-14 days			

*Contraindicated if history of immediate hypersensitivity reaction (anaphylaxis) to penicillin.

ANTIBIOTIC TREATMENT OF ADULTS WITH INFECTIVE ENDOCARDITIS

Table 1. Suggested Regimens for Therapy of Native Valve Endocarditis Due to Penicillin-Susceptible Viridans Streptococci and *Streptococcus bovis* (Minimum Inhibitory Concentration ≤0.1 μg/mL)*

Antibiotic	Dosage and Route	Duration (wk)	Comments
Aqueous crystalline penicillin G sodium	12-18 million units/24 h I.V. either continuously or in 6 equally divided doses	4	Preferred in most patients older than 65 y and in those with impairment of the eighth nerve or renal function
or			
Ceftriaxone sodium	2 g once daily I.V. or I.M.†	4	
Aqueous crystalline penicillin G sodium	12-18 million units/24 h I.V. either continuously or in 6 equally divided doses	2	When obtained 1 hour after a 20- to 30-minute I.V. infusion or I.M. injection, serum concentration of gentamicin of approximately 3 μg/mL is desirable; trough concentration should be <1 μg/mL
With gentamicin sulfate‡	1 mg/kg I.M. or I.V. every 8 hours	2	
Vancomycin hydrochloride§	30 mg/kg/24 h I.V. in 2 equally divided doses, not to exceed 2 g/24 h unless serum levels are monitored	4	Vancomycin therapy is recommended for patients allergic to β-lactams; peak serum concentrations of vancomycin should be obtained 1 h after completion of the infusion and should be in the range of 30-45 μg/mL for twice-daily dosing

*Dosages recommended are for patients with normal renal function. For nutritionally variant streptococci, see Table 3. I.V. indicates intravenous; I.M., intramuscular.

†Patients should be informed that I.M. injection of ceftriaxone is painful.

‡Dosing of gentamicin on a mg/kg basis will produce higher serum concentrations in obese patients that in lean patients. Therefore, in obese patients, dosing should be based on ideal body weight. (Ideal body weight for men is 50 kg + 2.3 kg per inch over 5 feet, and ideal body weight for women is 45.5 kg + 2.3 kg per inch over 5 feet.) Relative contraindications to the use of gentamicin are age >65 years, renal impairment, or impairment of the eighth nerve. Other potentially nephrotoxic agents (eg, nonsteroidal anti-inflammatory drugs) should be used cautiously in patients receiving gentamicin.

§Vancomycin dosage should be reduced in patients with impaired renal function. Vancomycin given on a mg/kg basis will produce higher serum concentrations in obese patients than in lean patients. Therefore, in obese patients, dosing should be based on ideal body weight. Each dose of vancomycin should be infused over at least 1 h to reduce the risk of the histamine-release "red man" syndrome.

Table 2. Therapy for Native Valve Endocarditis Due to Strains of Viridans Streptococci and *Streptococcus bovis* Relatively Resistant to Penicillin G (Minimum Inhibitory Concentration >0.1 μg/mL and <0.5 μg/mL)*

Antibiotic	Dosage and Route	Duration (wk)	Comments
Aqueous crystalline penicillin G sodium	18 million units/24 h I.V. either continuously or in 6 equally divided doses	4	Cefazolin or other first-generation cephalosporins may be substituted for penicillin in patients whose penicillin hypersensitivity is not of the immediate type.
With gentamicin sulfate†	1 mg/kg I.M. or I.V. every 8 h	2	
Vancomycin hydrochloride§	30 mg/kg/24 h I.V. in 2 equally divided doses, not to exceed 2 g/24 h unless serum levels are monitored	4	Vancomycin therapy is recommended for patients allergic to β-lactams

*Dosages recommended are for patients with normal renal function. I.V. indicates intravenous; I.M., intramuscular.

†For specific dosing adjustment and issues concerning gentamicin (obese patients, relative contraindications), see Table 1 footnotes.

‡For specific dosing adjustment and issues concerning vancomycin (obese patients, length of infusion), see Table 1 footnotes.

ANTIBIOTIC TREATMENT OF ADULTS WITH INFECTIVE ENDOCARDITIS *(Continued)*

Table 3. Standard Therapy for Endocarditis Due to Enterococci*

Antibiotic	Dosage and Route	Duration (wk)	Comments
Aqueous crystalline penicillin G sodium	18-30 million units/24 h I.V. either continuously or in 6 equally divided doses	4-6	4-week therapy recommended for patients with symptoms <3 months in duration; 6-week therapy recommended for patients with symptoms >3 months in duration.
With gentamicin sulfate†	1 mg/kg I.M. or I.V. every 8 h	4-6	
Ampicillin sodium	12 g/24 h I.V. either continuously or in 6 equally divided doses	4-6	
With gentamicin sulfate†	1 mg/kg I.M. or I.V. every 8 hours	4-6	
Vancomycin hydrochloride†‡	30 mg/kg/24 h I.V. in 2 equally divided doses, not to exceed 2 g/ 24 h unless serum levels are monitored	4-6	Vancomycin therapy is recommended for patients allergic to β-lactams; cephalosporins are not acceptable alternatives for patients allergic to penicillin
With gentamicin sulfate†	1 mg/kg I.M. or I.V. every 8 h	4-6	

*All enterococci causing endocarditis must be tested for antimicrobial susceptibility in order to select optimal therapy. This table is for endocarditis due to gentamicin- or vancomycin-susceptible enterococci, viridans streptococci with a minimum inhibitory concentration of >0.5 μg/mL, nutritionally variant viridans streptococci, or prosthetic valve endocarditis caused by viridans streptococci or *Streptococcus bovis.* Antibiotic dosages are for patients with normal renal function. I.V. indicates intravenous; I.M., intramuscular.

†For specific dosing adjustment and issues concerning gentamicin (obese patients, relative contraindications), see Table 1 footnotes.

‡For specific dosing adjustment and issues concerning vancomycin (obese patients, length of infusion), see Table 1 footnotes.

Table 4. Therapy for Endocarditis Due to *Staphylococcus* in the Absence of Prosthetic Material*

Antibiotic	Dosage and Route	Duration	Comments
	Methicillin-Susceptible Staphylococci		
Regimens for non-β-lactam-allergic patients			
Nafcillin sodium or oxacillin sodium	2 g I.V. every 4 h	4-6 wk	Benefit of additional aminoglycosides has not been established
With optional addition of gentamicin sulfate†	1 mg/kg I.M. or I.V. every 8 h	3-5 d	
Regimens for β-lactam-allergic patients			
Cefazolin (or other first-generation cephalosporins in equivalent dosages)	2 g I.V. every 8 h	4-6 wk	Cephalosporins should be avoided in patients with immediate-type hypersensitivity to penicillin
With optional addition of gentamicin†	1 mg/kg I.M. or I.V. every 8 hours	3-5 d	
Vancomycin hydrochloride‡	30 mg/kg/24 h I.V. in 2 equally divided doses, not to exceed 2 g/ 24 h unless serum levels are monitored	4-6 wk	Recommended for patients allergic to penicillin
	Methicillin-Resistant Staphylococci		
Vancomycin hydrochloride‡	30 mg/kg/24 h I.V. in 2 equally divided doses; not to exceed 2 g/ 24 h unless serum levels are monitored	4-6 wk	

*For treatment of endocarditis due to penicillin-susceptible staphylococci (minimum inhibitory concentration ≤0.1 μg/mL), aqueous crystalline penicillin G sodium (Table 1, first regimen) can be used for 4-6 weeks instead of nafcillin or oxacillin. Shorter antibiotic courses have been effective in some drug addicts with right-sided endocarditis due to *Staphylococcus aureus.* I.V. indicates intravenous; I.M., intramuscular.

†For specific dosing adjustment and issues concerning gentamicin (obese patients, relative contraindications), see Table 1 footnotes.

‡For specific dosing adjustment and issues concerning vancomycin (obese patients, length of infusion), see Table 1 footnotes.

Table 5. Treatment of Staphylococcal Endocarditis in the Presence of a Prosthetic Valve or Other Prosthetic Material*

Antibiotic	Dosage and Route	Duration (wk)	Comments
	Regimen for Methicillin-Resistant Staphylococci		
Vancomycin hydrochloride†	30 mg/kg/24 h I.V. in 2 or 4 equally divided doses, not to exceed 2 g/24 h unless serum levels are monitored	≥6	
With rifampin‡	300 mg orally every 8 h	≥6	Rifampin increases the amount of warfarin sodium required for antithrombotic therapy.
And with gentamicin sulfate§¶	1 mg/kg I.M. or I.V. every 8 h	2	
	Regimen for Methicillin-Susceptible Staphylococci		
Nafcillin sodium or oxacillin sodium†	2 g I.V. every 4 h	≥6	First-generation cephalosporins or vancomycin should be used in patients allergic to β-lactam. Cephalosporins should be avoided in patients with immediate-type hypersensitivity to penicillin or with methicillin-resistant staphylococci.
With rifampin‡	300 mg orally every 8 h	≥6	
And with gentamicin sulfate§¶	1 mg/kg I.M. or I.V. every 8 h	2	

*Dosages recommended are for patients with normal renal function. I.V. indicates intravenous; I.M., intramuscular.

†For specific dosing adjustment and issues concerning gentamicin (obese patients, relative contraindications), see Table 1 footnotes.

‡Rifampin plays a unique role in the eradication of staphylococcal infection involving prosthetic material; combination therapy is essential to prevent emergence of rifampin resistance.

§For a specific dosing adjustment and issues concerning gentamicin (obese patients, relative contraindications), see Table 1 footnotes.

¶Use during initial 2 weeks.

Table 6. Therapy for Endocarditis Due to HACEK Microorganisms (*Haemophilus parainfluenzae, Haemophilus aphrophilus, Actinobacillus actinomycetemcomitans, Cardiobacterium hominus, Eikenella corrodens,* and *Kingella kingae*)*

Antibiotic	Dosage and Route	Duration (wk)	Comments
Ceftriaxone sodium†	2 g once daily I.V. or I.M.†	4	Cefotaxime sodium or other third-generation cephalosporins may be substituted
Ampicillin sodium‡	12 g/24 h I.V. either continuously or in 6 equally divided doses	4	
With gentamicin sulfate§	1 mg/kg I.M. or I.V. every 6 h	4	

*Antibiotic dosages are for patients with normal renal function. I.V. indicates intravenous; I.M. intramuscular.

†Patients should be informed that I.M. injection of ceftriaxone is painful.

‡Ampicillin should not be used if laboratory tests show β-lactamase production.

§For specific dosing adjustment and issues concerning gentamicin (obese patients, relative contraindications), see Table 1 footnotes.

Note: Tables 1-6 are from Wilson WR, Karchmer AW, Dajani AS, et al, "Antibiotic Treatment of Adults With Infective Endocarditis Due to Streptococci, Enterococci, Staphylococci, and HACEK Microorganisms," *JAMA*, 1995, 274(21):1706-13, with permission.

ANTIMICROBIAL DRUGS OF CHOICE

The following table lists the antibacterial drugs of choice for various infecting organisms. This table is reprinted with permission from *The Medical Letter*, 1999, 41(1064):99-104. Users should not assume that all antibiotics which are appropriate for a given organism are listed or that those not listed are inappropriate. The infection caused by the organism may encompass varying degrees of severity, and since the antibiotics listed may not be appropriate for the differing degrees of severity, or because of other patient-related factors, it cannot be assumed that the antibiotics listed for any specific organism are interchangeable. This table should not be used by itself without first referring to *The Medical Letter*, an infectious disease manual, or the infectious disease department. Therefore, only use this table as a tool for obtaining more information about the therapies available.

Infecting Organism	Drug of First Choice	Alternative Drugs
GRAM-POSITIVE COCCI		
**Enterococcus*[1]		
endocarditis or other severe infection	Penicillin G or ampicillin + gentamicin or streptomycin[2]	Vancomycin + gentamicin or streptomycin; quinupristin/dalfopristin; linezolid[3]
uncomplicated urinary tract infection	Ampicillin or amoxicillin	Nitrofurantoin; a fluoroquinolone[4]; fosfomycin
**Staphylococcus aureus* or *epidermidis*	A penicillinase-resistant penicillin[5]	A cephalosporin[6,7]; vancomycin; amoxicillin/clavulanic acid; ticarcillin/clavulanic acid; piperacillin/tazobactam; ampicillin/sulbactam; imipenem or meropenem; clindamycin; a fluoroquinolone[4]; penicillin G or V[8]
methicillin-resistant [9]	Vancomycin ± gentamicin ± rifampin	Trimethoprim-sulfamethoxazole; a fluoroquinolone[4]; minocycline[10]
Streptococcus pyogenes (group A) and groups C and G[11]	Penicillin G or V[8]	Clindamycin; erythromycin; a cephalosporin[6,7]; vancomycin; clarithromycin[12]; azithromycin
Streptococcus, group B	Penicillin G or ampicillin	A cephalosporin[6,7]; vancomycin; erythromycin
**Streptococcus*, viridans group[1]	Penicillin G ± gentamicin	A cephalosporin[6,7]; vancomycin
Streptococcus bovis	Penicillin G	A cephalosporin[6,7]; vancomycin
Streptococcus, anaerobic or *Peptostreptococcus*	Penicillin G	Clindamycin; a cephalosporin[6,7]; vancomycin
**Streptococcus pneumoniae*[13] (pneumococcus), penicillin-susceptible (MIC <0.1 mcg/mL)	Penicillin G or V[8]	A cephalosporin[6,7]; erythromycin; azithromycin; clarithromycin[12]; a fluoroquinolone[4]; meropenem; imipenem; trimethoprim-sulfamethoxazole; clindamycin; a tetracycline[10]
penicillin – intermediate resistance	Penicillin G I.V. (12 million units/day for adults) or ceftriaxone or cefotaxime	Levofloxacin; vancomycin; clindamycin
penicillin – high level resistance (MIC ≥2 mcg/mL)	**Meningitis:** Vancomycin + ceftriaxone or cefotaxime ± rifampin	Meropenem; imipenem; clindamycin
	Other Infections: Vancomycin + ceftriaxone or cefotaxime; or levofloxacin	Quinupristin/dalfopristin; linezolid[3]

Infecting Organism	Drug of First Choice	Alternative Drugs
GRAM-NEGATIVE COCCI		
Moraxella (Branhamella) catarrhalis	Trimethoprim-sulfamethoxazole	Amoxicillin/clavulanic acid; erythromycin; a tetracycline[10]; cefuroxime[6]; cefotaxime[6]; ceftizoxime[6]; ceftriaxone[6]; cefuroxime axetil[6]; cefixime[6]; cefpodoxime[6]; a fluoroquinolone[4]; clarithromycin[12]; azithromycin
**Neisseria gonorrhoeae* (gonococcus)[14]	Ceftriaxone[6] or cefixime[6] or ciprofloxacin[4] or ofloxacin[4]	Cefotaxime[6]; spectinomycin; penicillin G
Neisseria meningitidis[15] (meningococcus)	Penicillin G	Cefotaxime[6]; ceftizoxime[6]; ceftriaxone[6]; chloramphenicol[16]; a sulfonamide[17]; a fluoroquinolone[4]
GRAM-POSITIVE BACILLI		
Bacillus anthracis (anthrax)	Penicillin G	Erythromycin; a tetracycline[10]; ciprofloxacin[18]
Bacillus cereus, subtilis	Vancomycin	Imipenem or meropenem; clindamycin
Clostridium perfringens[19]	Penicillin G	Clindamycin; metronidazole; imipenem or meropenem; chloramphenicol[16]
Clostridium tetani[20]	Penicillin G	A tetracycline[10]
Clostridium difficile[21]	Metronidazole	Vancomycin (oral)
Corynebacterium diphtheriae[22]	Erythromycin	Penicillin G
Corynebacterium, JK group	Vancomycin	Penicillin G + gentamicin; erythromycin
**Erysipelothrix rhusiopethiae*	Penicillin G	Erythromycin, a cephalosporin[6,7]; a fluoroquinolone[4]
Listeria monocytogenes	Ampicillin ± gentamicin	Trimethoprim-sulfamethoxazole; trimethoprim
ENTERIC GRAM-NEGATIVE BACILLI		
**Bacteroides*	Metronidazole or clindamycin	Imipenem or meropenem; amoxicillin/clavulanic acid; ticarcillin/clavulanic acid; piperacillin/tazobactam; ampicillin/sulbactam; cefoxitin[6]; cefotetan[6]; chloramphenicol[16]; cefmetazole[6]; penicillin G
**Campylobacter fetus*	Imipenem or meropenem	Gentamicin
**Campylobacter jejuni*	Erythromycin or azithromycin; a fluoroquinolone[4]	A tetracycline[10]; gentamicin
**Citrobacter freundi*	Imipenem or meropenem[23]	A fluoroquinolone[4]; amikacin; tetracycline[10]; trimethoprim-sulfamethoxazole; cefotaxime[6,23]; ceftizoxime[6,23]; ceftriaxone[6,23]; cefepime[6,23]; or ceftazidime[6,23]
**Enterobacter*	Imipenem or meropenem[23]	Gentamicin, tobramycin, or amikacin; trimethoprim-sulfamethoxazole; ciprofloxacin[18]; ticarcillin[24]; mezlocillin[24] or piperacillin[24]; aztreonam[23]; cefotaxime[6,23]; ceftizoxime[6,23]; ceftriaxone[6,23]; cefepime[6,23]; or ceftazidime[6,23]

ANTIMICROBIAL DRUGS OF CHOICE *(Continued)*

Infecting Organism	Drug of First Choice	Alternative Drugs
**Escherichia coli*[25]	Cefotaxime, ceftizoxime, ceftriaxone, cefepime, or ceftazidime[6,23]	Ampicillin ± gentamicin, tobramycin or amikacin; carbenicillin[24]; ticarcillin[24]; mezlocillin[24] or piperacillin[24]; gentamicin, tobramycin or amikacin; amoxicillin/clavulanic acid[23]; ticarcillin/clavulanic acid[24]; piperacillin/tazobactam[24]; ampicillin/sulbactam[23]; trimethoprim/sulfamethoxazole; imipenem or meropenem[23]; aztreonam[23]; a fluoroquinolone[4]; another cephalosporin[6,7]
**Helicobacter pylori*[26]	Tetracycline hydrochloride[10] + metronidazole + bismuth subsalicylate	Tetracycline hydrochloride + clarithromycin[12] + bismuth subsalicylate; amoxicillin + metronidazole + bismuth subsalicylate; amoxicillin + clarithromycin[12]
**Klebsiella pneumoniae*[25]	Cefotaxime, ceftizoxime, ceftriaxone, cefepime, or ceftazidime[6,23]	Imipenem or meropenem[23]; gentamicin, tobramycin, or amikacin; amoxicillin/clavulanic acid[23]; ticarcillin/clavulanic acid[24]; piperacillin/tazobactam[24]; ampicillin/sulbactam[23]; trimethoprim-sulfamethoxazole; aztreonam[23]; a fluoroquinolone[4]; mezlocillin[24] or piperacillin[24]; another cephalosporin[6,7]
**Proteus mirabilis*[25]	Ampicillin[27]	A cephalosporin[6,7,23]; ticarcillin[24]; mezlocillin[24] or piperacillin[24]; gentamicin, tobramycin, or amikacin; trimethoprim-sulfamethoxazole; imipenem or meropenem[23]; aztreonam[23]; a fluoroquinolone[4]; chloramphenicol[16]
Proteus, indole-positive (including *Providencia rettgeri, Morganella morganii*, and *Proteus vulgaris*)	Cefotaxime, ceftizoxime, ceftriaxone, cefepime, or ceftazidime[6,23]	Imipenem or meropenem[23]; gentamicin, tobramycin, or amikacin; carbenicillin[24]; ticarcillin[24]; mezlocillin[24] or piperacillin[24]; amoxicillin/clavulanic acid[23]; ticarcillin/clavulanic acid[24]; piperacillin/tazobactam[24]; ampicillin/sulbactam[23]; aztreonam[23]; trimethoprim-sulfamethoxazole; a fluoroquinolone[4]
**Providencia stuartii*	Cefotaxime, ceftizoxime, ceftriaxone, cefepime, or ceftazidime[6,23]	Imipenem or meropenem[23]; ticarcillin/clavulanic acid[24]; piperacillin/tazobactam[24]; gentamicin, tobramycin, or amikacin; carbenicillin[24]; ticarcillin[24], mezlocillin[24], or piperacillin[24]; aztreonam[23]; trimethoprim-sulfamethoxazole; a fluoroquinolone[4]
**Salmonella typhi*[28]	A fluoroquinolone[4] or ceftriaxone[6]	Chloramphenicol[16]; trimethoprim-sulfamethoxazole; ampicillin; amoxicillin
*other *Salmonella*[29]	Cefotaxime[6] or ceftriaxone[6] or a fluoroquinolone[4]	Ampicillin or amoxicillin; trimethoprim-sulfamethoxazole; chloramphenicol[16]
**Serratia*	Imipenem or meropenem[23]	Gentamicin or amikacin; cefotaxime, ceftizoxime, ceftriaxone, cefepime or ceftazidime[6,23]; aztreonam[23]; trimethoprim-sulfamethoxazole; carbenicillin[30], ticarcillin[30], mezlocillin[30] or piperacillin[30]; a fluoroquinolone[4]
**Shigella*	A fluoroquinolone[4]	Azithromycin; trimethoprim-sulfamethoxazole; ampicillin; ceftriaxone[6]

Infecting Organism	Drug of First Choice	Alternative Drugs
**Yersinia enterocolitica*	Trimethoprim-sulfamethoxazole	A fluoroquinolone[4]; gentamicin, tobramycin, or amikacin; cefotaxime or ceftizoxime[6]
OTHER GRAM-NEGATIVE BACILLI		
**Acinetobacter*	Imipenem or meropenem[23]	Amikacin, tobramycin, or gentamicin; ciprofloxacin[18]; trimethoprim-sulfamethoxazole; ticarcillin[24], mezlocillin[24], or piperacillin[24]; ceftazidime[23]; minocycline[10]; doxycycline[10]
**Aeromonas*	Trimethoprim-sulfamethoxazole	Gentamicin or tobramycin; imipenem; a fluoroquinolone[4]
Bartonella		
Agent of bacillary angiomatosis *(Bartonella hensalae* or *quintana*)	Erythromycin	Doxycycline[10]; azithromycin
Cat scratch bacillus (*Bartonella henselae*)[31]	Ciprofloxacin[18]	Azithromycin; trimethoprim-sulfamethoxazole; gentamicin; rifampin
Bordetella pertussis (whooping cough)	Erythromycin	Trimethoprim-sulfamethoxazole
**Brucella*	A tetracycline[10] + rifampin	A tetracycline[10] + streptomycin or gentamicin; chloramphenicol[16] ± streptomycin; trimethoprim-sulfamethoxazole ± gentamicin; rifampin + a tetracycline[10]
**Burkholderia capacia*	Trimethoprim-sulfamethoxazole	Ceftazidime[6]; chloramphenicol[16]
Calymmatobacterium granulomatis (granuloma inguinale)	Trimethoprim-sulfamethoxazole	Doxycycline[10] or ciprofloxacin[18] ± gentamicin
Capnocytophaga canimorsus[32]	Penicillin G	Cefotaxime[6]; ceftizoxime[6]; ceftriaxone[6]; imipenem or meropenem; vancomycin; a fluoroquinolone[4]; clindamycin
**Eikenella corrodens*	Ampicillin	An erythromycin; a tetracyline[10]; amoxicillin/clavulanic acid; ampicillin/sulbactam; ceftriaxone[6]
**Francisella tularensis* (tularemia)	Streptomycin	Gentamicin; a tetracycline[10]; chloramphenicol[16]
**Fusobacterium*	Penicillin G	Metronidazole; clindamycin; cefoxitin[6]; chloramphenicol[16]
Gardnerella vaginalis (bacterial vaginosis)	Oral metronidazole[33]	Topical clindamycin or metronidazole; oral clindamycin
**Haemophilus ducreyi* (chancroid)	Azithromycin or ceftriaxone	Ciprofloxacin[18] or erythromycin
**Haemophilus influenzae*		
meningitis, epiglottitis, arthritis, and other serious infections	Cefotaxime or ceftriaxone[6]	Cefuroxime[6] (not for meningitis); chloramphenicol[16]; meropenem
upper respiratory infections and bronchitis	Trimethoprim-sulfamethoxazole	Cefuroxime[6]; amoxicillin/clavulanic acid; cefuroxime axetil[6]; cefpodoxime[6]; cefaclor[6]; cefotaxime[6]; ceftizoxime[6]; ceftriaxone[6]; cefixime[6]; a tetracycline[10]; clarithromycin[12]; azithromycin; a fluoroquinolone[4]; ampicillin or amoxicillin
Legionella species	Azithromycin or a fluoroquinolone[4] or erythromycin ± rifampin	Doxycycline[10] ± rifampin; trimethoprim-sulfamethoxazole
Leptotrichia buccalis	Penicillin G	A tetracycline[10]; clindamycin; erythromycin
Pasteurella multocida	Penicillin G	A tetracycline[10]; a cephalosporin[6,7]; amoxicillin/clavulanic acid; ampicillin/sulbactam

ANTIMICROBIAL DRUGS OF CHOICE *(Continued)*

Infecting Organism	Drug of First Choice	Alternative Drugs
**Pseudomonas aeruginosa*		
urinary tract infection	Ciprofloxacin[18]	Carbenicillin, ticarcillin, piperacillin, or mezlocillin; ceftazidime[6]; cefepime[5]; imipenem or meropenem; aztreonam; tobramycin; gentamicin; amikacin
other infections	Ticarcillin, mezlocillin, or piperacillin + tobramycin, gentamicin, or amikacin[34]	Ceftazidime[6], imipenem, meropenem, aztreonam, cefepime[6] + tobramycin, gentamicin, or amikacin; ciprofloxacin[18]
Pseudomonas mallei (glanders)	Streptomycin + a tetracycline[10]	Streptomycin + chloramphenicol[16]
**Pseudomonas pseudomallei* (melioidosis)	Ceftazidime[6]	Chloramphenicol[16] + doxycycline[10] + trimethoprim-sulfamethoxazole; amoxicillin/clavulanic acid; imipenem or meropenem
Spirillum minus (rat bite fever)	Penicillin G	A tetracycline[10]; streptomycin
**Stenotrophomonas maltophilia (Pseudomonas maltophilia)*	Trimethoprim-sulfamethoxazole	Minocycline[10]; ceftazidime[6]; a fluoroquinolone[4] ± ticarcillin-clavulanic acid
Streptobacillus moniliformis (rat bite fever, Haverhill fever)	Penicillin G	A tetracycline[10]; streptomycin
Vibrio cholerae (cholera)[35]	A tetracycline[10]	A fluoroquinolone[4]; trimethoprim-sulfamethoxazole
Vibrio vulnificus	A tetracycline[10]	Cefotaxime[6]
Yersinia pestis (plague)	Streptomycin ± a tetracycline[10]	Chloramphenicol[16]; gentamicin; trimethoprim-sulfamethoxazole
ACID-FAST BACILLI		
**Mycobacterium tuberculosis*	Isoniazid + rifampin + pyrazinamide ± ethambutol or streptomycin[16]	levofloxacin, ofloxacin or ciprofloxacin[18]; cycloserine[16]; capreomycin[16] or kanamycin[16] or amikacin[16]; ethionamide[16]; clofazimine[16]; aminosalicylic acid[16]
**Mycobacterium kansasii*	Isoniazid + rifampin ± ethambutol or streptomycin[16]	Clarithromycin[12]; ethionamide[16]; cycloserine[16]
**Mycobacterium avium* complex	Clarithromycin[12] or azithromycin + one or more of the following: ethambutol; rifabutin; ciprofloxacin[18]	Rifampin; amikacin[16]
prophylaxis	Clarithromycin[12] or azithromycin	Rifabutin
**Mycobacterium fortuitum/ chelonae* complex	Amikacin + clarithromycin[10]	Cefoxitin[6]; rifampin; a sulfonamide; doxycycline; ethambutol
Mycobacterium marinum (balnei)[36]	Minocycline[10]	Trimethoprim-sulfamethoxazole; rifampin; clarithromycin[12]; doxycycline[10]
Mycobacterium leprae (leprosy)	Dapsone + rifampin ± clofazimine	Minocycline[10]; ofloxacin[18]; sparfloxacin[18]; clarithromycin[12]
ACTINOMYCETES		
Actinomyces israelii (actinomycosis)	Penicillin G	A tetracycline[10]; erythromycin; clindamycin
Nocardia	Trimethoprim-sulfamethoxazole	Sulfisoxazole; amikacin[16]; a tetracycline[10]; imipenem or meropenem; cycloserine[16]
**Rhodococcus equi*	Vancomycin ± a fluoroquinolone[4], rifampin, imipenem or meropenem or amikacin	Erythromycin

Infecting Organism	Drug of First Choice	Alternative Drugs
Tropheryma whippelii (agent of Whipple's disease)	Trimethoprim-sulfamethoxazole	Penicillin G; a tetracycline[10]
CHLAMYDIA		
Chlamydia psittaci (psittacosis, ornithosis)	A tetracycline[10]	Chloramphenicol[16]
Chlamydia trachomatis		
(trachoma)	Azithromycin	A tetracycline[10] (topical plus oral); a sulfonamide (topical plus oral)
(inclusion conjunctivitis)	Erythromycin (oral or I.V.)	A sulfonamide
(pneumonia)	Erythromycin	A sulfonamide
(urethritis, cervicitis)	Azithromycin or doxycycline[10]	Erythromycin; ofloxacin[18]; amoxicillin
(lymphogranuloma venereum)	A tetracycline[10]	Erythromycin
Chlamydia pneumoniae (TWAR strain)	A tetracycline[10]	Erythromycin; clarithromycin[12]; azithromycin; a fluoroquinolone[4]
EHRLICHIA		
Ehrlichia chaffeensis	Doxycycline[10]	Chloramphenicol[16]
Ehrlichia ewingii	Doxycycline[10]	
Agent of human granulocytic ehrlichiosis	Doxycycline[10]	
MYCOPLASMA		
Mycoplasma pneumoniae	Erythromycin or a tetracycline[10] or clarithromycin[12] or azithromycin	A fluoroquinolone[4]
Ureaplasma urealyticum	Erythromycin	A tetracycline[10]; clarithromycin[12]; azithromycin; ofloxacin[18]
RICKETTSIA – Rocky Mountain spotted fever, endemic typhus (murine), epidemic typhus (louse-borne), scrub typhus, trench fever, Q fever	Doxycycline[10]	Chloramphenicol[16]; a fluoroquinolone[4]
SPIROCHETES		
Borrelia burgdorferi (Lyme disease)[37]	Doxycycline[10] or amoxicillin or cefuroxime axetil[6]	Ceftriaxone[6]; cefotaxime[6]; penicillin G; azithromycin; clarithromycin[12]
Borrelia recurrentis (relapsing fever)	A tetracycline[10]	Penicillin G
Leptospira	Penicillin G	A tetracycline[10]
Treponema pallidum (syphilis)	Penicillin G[8]	A tetracycline[10]; ceftriaxone[6]
Treponema pertenue (yaws)	Penicillin G	A tetracycline[10]

*Resistance may be a problem; susceptibility tests should be performed.

1. Disk sensitivity testing may not provide adequate information; beta-lactamase assays, "E" tests, and dilution tests for susceptibility should be used in serious infections.

2. Aminoglycoside resistance is increasingly common among enterococci. Treatment options include ampicillin 2 g I.V. q4h, continuous infusion of ampicillin, a combination of ampicillin plus a fluoroquinolone, or a combination of ampicillin, imipenem, and vancomycin (Tripodi MF et al, *Eur J Clin Microbiol Infect Dis*, 1998, 17:734; Antony SJ, *Scand J Infect Dis*, 1997, 29:628).

3. An investigational drug in the U.S.A. (*Zyvox* – Pharmacia & Upjohn).

4. Among the fluoroquinolones, levofloxacin, sparfloxacin, and grepafloxacin have the greatest *in vitro* activity against *S. pneumoniae*, including penicillin- and cephalosporin-resistant strains. Levofloxacin, sparfloxacin, and grepafloxacin also have good activity against many strains of *S. aureus*, but resistance has become frequent among methicillin-resistant strains. Ciprofloxacin has the greatest activity against *Pseudomonas aeruginosa*. Sparfloxacin has a substantial incidence of photosensitivity reactions. For urinary tract infections, norfloxacin, lomefloxacin, or enoxacin can be used. Ciprofloxacin, ofloxacin, and levofloxacin are available for intravenous use. None of these agents are recommended for children or pregnant women.

ANTIMICROBIAL DRUGS OF CHOICE *(Continued)*

Trovafloxacin has been associated with rare but fatal hepatitis and should be restricted to brief (<14 d) inpatient use with liver monitoring.

5. For oral use against staphylococci, cloxacillin or dicloxacillin is preferred; for severe infections, a parenteral formulation of nafcillin or oxacillin should be used. Ampicillin, amoxicillin, bacampicillin, carbenicillin, ticarcillin, mezlocillin, and piperacillin are not effective against penicillinase-producing staphylococci. The combination of clavulanic acid with amoxicillin or ticarcillin, sulbactam with ampicillin, and tazobactam with piperacillin may be active against these organisms.
6. The cephalosporins have been used as alternatives to penicillin in patients allergic to penicillins, but such patients may also have allergic reactions to cephalosporins.
7. For parenteral treatment of staphylococcal or nonenterococcal streptococcal infections, a first-generation cephalosporin such as cephalothin or cefazolin can be used. For oral therapy, cephalexin or cephradine can be used. The second-generation cephalosporins cefamandole, cefprozil, cefuroxime, cefuroxime axetil, cefonicid, cefotetan, cefmetazole, cefoxitin, and loracarbef are more active than the first-generation drugs against gram-negative bacteria. Cefuroxime is active against ampicillin-resistant strains of *H. influenzae*. Cefoxitin, cefotetan, and cefmetazole are the most active of the cephalosporins against *B. fragilis*, but cefotetan and cefmetazole have been associated with prothrombin deficiency. The third-generation cephalosporins cefotaxime, cefoperazone, ceftizoxime, ceftriaxone, and ceftazidime, and the fourth-generation cefepime have greater activity than the second-generation drugs against enteric gram-negative bacilli. Ceftazidime has poor activity against many gram-positive cocci and anaerobes, and ceftizoxime has poor activity against penicillin-resistant *S. pneumoniae*. Cefepime has *in vitro* activity against gram-positive cocci similar to cefotaxime and ceftriaxone and somewhat greater activity against enteric gram-negative bacilli. The activity of cefepime against *Pseudomonas aeruginosa* is similar to that of ceftazidime. Cefixime, cefpodoxime, cefdinir, and cefibuten are oral cephalosporins with more activity than second-generation cephalosporins against facultative gram-negative bacilli; they have no useful activity against anaerobes or *Pseudomonas aeruginosa*, and cefixime and ceftibuten have no useful activity against staphylococci. With the exception of cefoperazone (which, like cefamandole, can cause bleeding), ceftazidime and cefepime, the activity of all currently available cephalosporins against *Pseudomonas aeruginosa* is poor or inconsistent.
8. Penicillin V (or amoxicillin) is preferred for oral treatment of infections caused by nonpenicillinase-producing staphylococci and other gram-positive cocci. For initial therapy of severe infections, penicillin G, administered parenterally, is first choice. For somewhat longer action in less severe infections due to group A streptococci, pneumococci or *Treponema pallidum*, procaine penicillin G, an intramuscular formulation, is given once or twice daily, but is seldom used now. Benzathine penicillin G, a slowly absorbed preparation, is usually given in a single monthly injection for prophylaxis of rheumatic fever, once for treatment of group A streptococcal pharyngitis and once or more for treatment of syphilis.
9. Many strains of coagulase-positive staphylococci and coagulase-negative staphylococci are resistant to penicillinase-resistant penicillins; those strains are also resistant to cephalosporins, imipenem, and meropenem.
10. Tetracyclines are generally not recommended for pregnant women or children younger than 8 years old.
11. For serious soft-tissue infection due to group A streptococci, clindamycin may be more effective than penicillin. Group A streptococci may, however, be resistant to clindamycin; therefore, some *Medical Letter* consultants suggest using both clindamycin and penicillin, with or without I.V. immune globulin, to treat serious soft-tissue infections. Group A streptococci may also be resistant to erythromycin, azithromycin, and clarithromycin.
12. Not recommended for use in pregnancy.
13. Some strains of *S. pneumoniae* are resistant to erythromycin, clindamycin, trimethoprim-sulfamethoxazole, clarithromycin, azithromycin and chloramphenicol, and resistance to the newer fluoroquinolones is increasing (Chen DK et al, *N Engl J Med*, 1999, 341:233). Nearly all strains tested so far are susceptible to quinupristin/dalfopristin *in vitro*.
14. Patients with gonorrhea should be treated presumptively for coinfection with *C. trachomatis* with azithromycin or doxycycline.
15. Rare strains of *N. meningitidis* are resistant or relatively resistant to penicillin. Rifampin or a fluoroquinolone is recommended for prophylaxis after close contact with infected patients.
16. Because of the possibility of serious adverse effects, this drug should be used only for severe infections when less hazardous drugs are ineffective.
17. Sulfonamide-resistant strains are frequent in the U.S.A; sulfonamides should be used only when susceptibility is established by susceptibility tests.
18. Usually not recommended for use in children or pregnant women.
19. Debridement is primary. Large doses of penicillin G are required. Hyperbaric oxygen therapy may be a useful adjunct to surgical debridement in management of the spreading, necrotic type.
20. For prophylaxis, a tetanus toxoid booster and, for some patients, tetanus immune globulin (human) are required.
21. In order to decrease the emergence of vancomycin-resistant enterococci in hospitals, many clinicians now recommend use of metronidazole first in treatment of patients with

C. difficile colitis, with oral vancomycin used only for seriously ill patients or those who do not respond to metronidazole (Wilcox M, *J Antimicrob Chemother*, 1998 (41 Suppl) C:41).
22. Antitoxin is primary; antimicrobials are used only to halt further toxin production and to prevent the carrier state.
23. In severely ill patients, most *Medical Letter* consultants would add gentamicin, tobramycin, or amikacin.
24. In severely ill patients, most *Medical Letter* consultants would add gentamicin, tobramycin, or amikacin (but see footnote 34).
25. For an acute, uncomplicated urinary tract infection, before the infecting organism is known, the drug of first choice is trimethoprim-sulfamethoxazole.
26. Eradication of *H. pylori* with various antibacterial combinations, given concurrently with an H_2-receptor blocker or proton pump inhibitor, has led to rapid healing of active peptic ulcers and low recurrence rates (Taylor JL et al, *Arch Intern Med*, 1997, 157:87).
27. Large doses (6 g or more/day) are usually necessary for systemic infections. In severely ill patients, some *Medical Letter* consultants would add gentamicin, tobramycin, or amikacin.
28. A fluoroquinolone or amoxicillin is the drug of choice for *S. typhi* carriers.
29. Most cases of *Salmonella* gastroenteritis subside spontaneously without antimicrobial therapy.
30. In severely ill patients, most *Medical Letter* consultants would add gentamicin or amikacin (but see footnote 34).
31. Role of antibiotics is not clear (Chia JK et al, *Clin Infect Dis*, 1998, 26:193).
32. Pers C et al, *Clin Infect Dis*, 1996, 23:71.
33. Metronidazole is effective for bacterial vaginosis even though it is not usually active against *Gardnerella in vitro.*
34. Neither gentamicin, tobramycin, netilmicin, or amikacin should be mixed in the same bottle with carbenicillin, ticarcillin, mezlocillin, or piperacillin for intravenous administration. When used in high doses or in patients with renal impairment, these penicillins may inactivate the aminoglycosides.
35. Antibiotic therapy is an adjunct to and not a substitute for prompt fluid and electrolyte replacement.
36. Most infections are self-limited without drug treatment
37. For treatment of erythema migrans, facial nerve palsy, mild cardiac disease, and some cases of arthritis, oral therapy is satisfactory; for more serious neurologic or cardiac disease or arthritis, parenteral therapy with ceftriaxone, cefotaxime, or penicillin G is recommended (*Medical Letter*, 1997, 39:47).

ANTIRETROVIRAL THERAPY FOR HIV INFECTION

Report of the NIH Panel to Define Principles of Therapy of HIV Infection

GUIDELINES FOR THE USE OF ANTIRETROVIRAL AGENTS IN HIV-INFECTED ADULTS AND ADOLESCENTS

Adapted from *MMWR Morb Mortal Wkly Rep*, 1998, 47(RR-5) and *JAMA*, 1998, 280:78-86.
(Updated March 2000 from www.hivatis.org)

Indications for Plasma HIV RNA Testing*

Clinical Indication	Information	Use
Syndrome consistent with acute HIV infection	Establishes diagnosis when HIV antibody test is negative or indeterminate	Diagnosis†
Initial evaluation of newly diagnosed HIV infection	Baseline viral load "set point"	Decision to start or defer therapy
Every 3-4 months in patients not on therapy	Changes in viral load	Decision to start therapy
2-8 weeks after initiation of antiretroviral therapy	Initial assessment of drug efficacy	Decision to continue or change therapy
3-4 months after start of therapy	Maximal effect of therapy	Decision to continue or change therapy
Every 3-4 months in patients on therapy	Durability of antiretroviral effect	Decision to continue or change therapy
Clinical event or significant decline in CD4+ T cells	Association with changing or stable viral load	Decision to continue, initiate, or change therapy

*Acute illness (eg, bacterial pneumonia, tuberculosis, HSV, PCP) and immunizations can cause increases in plasma HIV RNA for 2-4 weeks; viral load testing should not be performed during this time. Plasma HIV RNA results should usually be verified with a repeat determination before starting or making changes in therapy.

†Diagnosis of HIV infection determined by HIV RNA testing should be confirmed by standard methods (eg, Western blot serology) performed 2-4 months after the initial indeterminate or negative test.

Risks and Benefits of Early Initiation of Antiretroviral Therapy in the Asymptomatic HIV-infected Patient

Potential Benefits

Control of viral replication and mutation; reduction of viral burden

Prevention of progressive immunodeficiency; potential maintenance or reconstitution of a normal immune system

Delayed progression to AIDS and prolongation of life

Decreased risk of selection of resistant virus

Decreased risk of drug toxicity

Possible decreased risk of viral transmission

Potential Risks

Reduction in quality of life from adverse drug effects and inconvenience of current maximally suppressive regimens

Earlier development of drug resistance

Transmission of drug-resistant virus

Limitation in future choices of antiretroviral agents due to development of resistance

Unknown long-term toxicity of antiretroviral drugs

Unknown duration of effectiveness of current antiretroviral therapies

Indications for the Initiation of Antiretroviral Therapy in the Chronically HIV-Infected Patient

Clinical Category	$CD4^+$ T-cell Count and HIV RNA	Recommendation
Symptomatic (AIDS, thrush, unexplained fever)	Any value	Treat
Asymptomatic	$CD4^+$ T cells <500/mm^3 **or** HIV RNA >10,000 (bDNA) or >20,000 (RT-PCR)	Treatment should be offered. Strength of recommendation is based on prognosis for disease-free survival and willingness of the patient to accept therapy*
Asymptomatic	$CD4^+$ T cells >500/mm^3 **and** HIV RNA <10,000 (bDNA) or <20,000 (RT-PCR)	Many experts would delay therapy and observe; however, some experts would treat

*Some experts would observe patients whose $CD4^+$ T cell counts are between 350-500/mm^3 and HIV RNA levels <10,000 (bDNA) or <20,000 (RT-PCR).

Recommended Antiretroviral Agents for Treatment of Established HIV Infection

Priority is given to regimens in which clinical trials data suggest sustained suppression of HIV plasma RNA and sustained increase in $CD4^+$T cell count, and favorable clinical outcome. Particular emphasis is given to regimens that have been compared directly with other regimens that perform sufficiently well with regard to these parameters to be included in the "strongly recommended" category. Additional consideration is given to the regimen's pill burden, dosing frequency, food requirements, convenience, toxicity, and drug interaction profile compared with other regimens.

One choice each from column A and column B. Drugs are listed in random, not priority, order:

	Column A	Column B
Strongly Recommended	Efavirenz Indinavir Nelfinavir Ritonavir + Saquinavir (SGC* or HGC*)	Stavudine + Lamivudine Stavudine + Didanosine Zidovudine + Lamivudine Zidovudine + Didanosine
Recommended as an Alternative	Abacavir Amprenavir Delavirdine Nelfinavir + Saquinavir - SGC Nevirapine Ritonavir Saquinavir - SGC	Didanosine + Lamivudine Zidovudine + Zalcitabine
No Recommendation; Insufficient Data†	Hydroxyurea in combination with other antiretroviral drugs Ritonavir + Indinavir Ritonavir + Nelfinavir	
Not Recommended; Should Not Be Offered (All monotherapies, whether from column A or B‡)	Saquinavir - HGC§	Stavudine + Zidovudine Zalcitabine + Lamivudine Zalcitabine + Stavudine Zalcitabine + Didanosine

*Saquinavir-SGC, soft-gel capsule (Fortovase®); Saquinavir-HGC, hard-gel capsule (Invirase®).

†This category includes drugs or combinations for which information is too limited to allow a recommendation for or against use.

‡Zidovudine monotherapy may be considered for prophylactic use in pregnant women with low viral load and high $CD4^+$ T cell counts to prevent perinatal transmission

§Use of saquinavir-HGC (Invirase®) is not recommended, except in combination with ritonavir

ANTIRETROVIRAL THERAPY FOR HIV INFECTION *(Continued)*

Recommendations for the Use of Drug Resistance Assays

Clinical Setting / Recommendation	Rationale
Recommended	
Virologic failure during HAART	Determine the role of resistance in drug failure and maximize the number of active drugs in the new regimen, if indicated.
Suboptimal suppression of viral load after initiation of antiretroviral therapy	Determine the role of resistance and maximize the number of active drugs in the new regimen, if indicated.
Consider	
Acute HIV infection	Determine if drug-resistant virus was transmitted and change regimen accordingly.
Not Generally Recommended	
Chronic HIV infection prior to initiation of therapy	Uncertain prevalence of resistant virus. Current assays may not detect minor drug-resistant species.
After discontinuation of drugs	Drug-resistant mutations may become minor species in the absence of selective drug pressure. Current assays may not detect minor drug-resistant species.
Plasma viral load <1000 HIV RNA copies/mL	Resistance assays cannot be reliably performed because of low coy number of HIV RNA.

Goals of HIV Therapy and Tools to Achieve Them

Goals of Therapy

Maximal and durable suppression of viral load

Restoration and/or preservation of immunologic function

Improvement of quality of life

Reduction of HIV-related morbidity and mortality

Tools to Achieve Goals of Therapy

Maximize adherence to the antiretroviral regimen

Rational sequencing of drugs

Preservation of future treatment options

Use of resistance testing in selected clinical settings

GUIDELINES FOR THE USE OF ANTIRETROVIRAL AGENTS IN PEDIATRIC HIV INFECTION

Adapted from *MMWR Morb Mort Wkly Rep*, 1998, 47(RR-4).
(Updated March 2000 from www.hivatis.org)

1994 Revised Human Immunodeficiency Virus Pediatric Classification System: Immune Categories Based on Age-specific CD4$^+$ T-lymphocyte and Percentage*

Immune Category	<12 (mo)		1-5 (y)		6-12 (y)	
	No./µL	%	No./µL	%	No./µL	%
Category 1 (no suppression)	≥1500	≥25	≥1000	≥25	≥500	≥25
Category 2 (moderate suppression)	750-1499	15-24	500-999	15-24	200-499	15-24
Category 3 (severe suppression)	<750	<15	<500	<15	<200	<15

*Modified from: CDC. 1994 Revised Classification System for Human Immunodeficiency Virus Infection in Children Less Than 13 Years of Age. *MMWR Morb Mort Wkly Rep*, 1994, 43(RR-12):1-10.

1994 Revised Human Immunodeficiency Virus Pediatric Classification System: Clinical Categories*

Category N: Not Symptomatic

Children who have no signs or symptoms considered to be the result of HIV infection or who have only **one** of the conditions listed in category A

Category A: Mildly Symptomatic

Children with **two** or more of the following conditions, but none of the conditions listed in categories B and C:

- Lymphadenopathy (≥0.5 cm at more than two sites; bilateral = one site)
- Hepatomegaly
- Splenomegaly
- Dermatitis
- Parotitis
- Recurrent or persistent upper respiratory infection, sinusitis, or otitis media

Category B: Moderately Symptomatic

Children who have symptomatic conditions other than those listed for category A or category C that are attributed to HIV infection. Examples of conditions in clinical category B include, but are not limited to, the following:

- Anemia (<8 g/dL), neutropenia (<1000/mm^3), or thrombocytopenia (<100,000/mm^3) persisting ≥30 days
- Bacterial meningitis, pneumonia, or sepsis (single episode)
- Candidiasis, oropharyngeal (ie, thrush) persisting for >2 months in children aged >6 months
- Cardiomyopathy
- Cytomegalovirus infection with onset before age 1 month
- Diarrhea, recurrent or chronic
- Hepatitis
- Herpes simplex virus (HSV) stomatitis, recurrent (ie, more than two episodes within 1 year)
- HSV bronchitis, pneumonitis, or esophagitis with onset before age 1 month
- Herpes zoster (ie, shingles) involving at least two distinct episodes or more than one dermatome
- Leiomyosarcoma
- Lymphoid interstitial pneumonia (LIP) or pulmonary lymphoid hyperplasia complex
- Nephropathy
- Nocardiosis
- Fever lasting >1 month
- Toxoplasmosis with onset before age 1 month
- Varicella, disseminated (ie, complicated chickenpox)

Category C: Severely Symptomatic

Children who have any condition listed in the 1987 surveillance case definition for acquired immunodeficiency syndrome, with the exception of LIP (which is a category B condition).

*Modified from: CDC. 1994 Revised Classification System for Human Immunodeficiency Virus Infection in Children Less Than 13 Years of Age. *MMWR Morb Mort Wkly Rep* 1994, 43(RR-12):1-10.

ANTIRETROVIRAL THERAPY FOR HIV INFECTION *(Continued)*

Association of Baseline CD4⁺ T-lymphocyte Percentage With Long-Term Risk for Death in Human Immunodeficiency Virus (HIV)-Infected Children*

Baseline (%)	No. Patients#	Deaths†	
		No.	%
<5	33	32	97
5-9	29	22	76
10-14	30	13	43
15-19	41	18	44
20-24	52	13	25
25-29	49	15	31
30-34	48	5	10
≥35	92	30	33

* Data from the National Institute of Child Health and Human Development Intravenous Immunoglobulin Clinical Trial.

† Mean follow-up: 5.1 years.

Includes 374 patients for whom baseline CD4⁺ T-lymphocyte percentage data were available.

Source: Mofenson L, Korelitz J, Meyer WA, et al, "The Relationship Between Serum Human Immunodeficiency Virus Type 1 (HIV-1) RNA Level, CD4 Lymphocyte Percent and Long-Term Mortality Risk in HIV-1 Infected Children," *J Infect Dis*, 1997, 175:1029-38.

Indications for Initiation of Antiretroviral Therapy in Children With Human Immunodeficiency Virus (HIV) Infection*

- Clinical symptoms associated with HIV infection (clinical categories A, B, or C)
- Evidence of immune suppression, indicated by CD4⁺ T-lymphocyte absolute number or percentage (ie, immune category 2 or 3)
- Age <12 months - regardless of clinical, immunologic, or virologic status
- For asymptomatic children ≥1 year of age with normal immune status, two options can be considered:
  - Preferred approach: Initiate therapy regardless of age or symptom status
  - Alternative approach: Defer treatment in situations in which the risk for clinical disease progression is low and other factors (eg, concern for the durability of response, safety, and adherence) favor postponing treatment. In such cases, the healthcare provider should regularly monitor virologic, immunologic, and clinical status. Factors to be considered in deciding to initiate therapy include the following:
    - High or increasing HIV RNA copy number
    - Rapidly declining CD4⁺ T-lymphocyte number or percentage to values approaching those indicative of moderate immune suppression (ie, immune category 2)
    - Development of clinical symptoms

*Indications for initiation of antiretroviral therapy in postpubertal HIV-infected adolescents should follow the adult guidelines (Office of Public Health and Science, Department of Health and Human Services. Availability of report of NIH panel to define principles of therapy of HIV infection and guidelines for the use of antiretroviral agents in HIV-infected adults. Federal Register, 1997, 62:33417-8).

Recommended Antiretroviral Regimens for Initial Therapy for Human Immunodeficiency Virus (HIV) Infection in Children

Strongly Recommended

Clinical trial evidence of clinical benefit and/or sustained suppression of HIV replication in adults and/or children.

- One highly active protease inhibitor plus two nucleoside analogue reverse transcriptase inhibitors (NRTIs)

  – Preferred protease inhibitor for infants and children who cannot swallow pills or capsules: nelfinavir or ritonavir; alternative for children who can swallow pills or capsules: indinavir

  – Recommended dual NRTI combinations: the most data on use in children are available for the combinations of zidovudine (ZDV) and dideoxyinosine (ddl) and for ZDV and lamivudine (3TC); more limited data is available for the combinations of stavudine (d4T) and ddl, d4T and 3TC, and ZDV and zalcitabine (ddC)*
- Alternative for children who can swallow capsules: Efavirenz (Sustiva®)** plus 2 NRTIs (see above) or efavirenz (Sustiva®) plus nelfinavir and 1 NRTI

Recommended as an Alternative

Clinical trial evidence of suppression of HIV replication, but durability may be less in adults and/or children than with strongly recommended regimens; or the durability of suppression is not yet defined; or evidence of efficacy may not outweigh potential adverse consequences (eg, toxicity, drug interactions, cost, etc).

- Nevirapine and two NRTIs
- Abacavir in combination with ZDV and 3TC

Offer Only in Special Circumstances

Clinical trial evidence of limited benefit for patients or data are inconclusive, but may be reasonably offered in special circumstances.

- Two NRTIs
- Amprenavir in combination with 2 NRTIs or abacavir

Not Recommended

Evidence against use because of overlapping toxicity and/or because use may be virologically undesirable

- Any monotherapy†
- d4T and ZDV
- ddC and ddl
- ddC and d4T
- ddC and 3TC

*ddC is not available in a liquid preparation commercially, although a liquid formulation is available through a compassionate use program of the manufacturer (Hoffman-LaRoche Inc, Nutley, New Jersey). ZDV and ddC is a less preferred choice for use in combination with a protease inhibitor.

**Efavirenz is currently available only in capsule form, but liquid preparation is currently being evaluated. There are currently no data on appropriate dosage of efavirenz in children <3 years of age.

†Except for ZDV, chemoprophylaxis administered to HIV-exposed infants during the first 6 weeks of life to prevent perinatal HIV transmission; if an infant is identified as HIV-infected while receiving ZDV prophylaxis, therapy should be changed to a combination antiretroviral drug regimen.

ANTIRETROVIRAL THERAPY FOR HIV INFECTION *(Continued)*

Considerations for Changing Antiretroviral Therapy for Human Immunodeficiency Virus (HIV)-Infected Children

Virologic Considerations*

- Less than a minimally acceptable virologic response after 8-12 weeks of therapy; for children receiving antiretroviral therapy with two nucleoside analogue reverse transcriptase inhibitors (NRTIs) and a protease inhibitor, such a response is defined as a <10-fold (1.0 $\log_{10}$) decrease from baseline HIV RNA levels; for children who are receiving less potent antiretroviral therapy (ie, dual NRTI combinations), an insufficient response is defined as a <5-fold (0.7 $\log_{10}$) decrease in HIV RNA levels from baseline
- HIV RNA not suppressed to undetectable levels after 4-6 months of antiretroviral therapy†
- Repeated detection of HIV RNA in children who initially responded to antiretroviral therapy with undetectable levels‡
- A reproducible increase in HIV RNA copy number among children who have had a substantial HIV RNA response, but still have low levels of detectable HIV RNA; such an increase would warrant change in therapy if, after initiation of the therapeutic regimen, a >3-fold (0.5 $\log_{10}$) increase in copy number for children ≥2 years of age and a >5-fold (0.7 $\log_{10}$) increase is observed for children <2 years of age

Immunologic Considerations*

- Change in immunologic classification§
- For children with $CD4^+$ T-lymphocyte percentages of <15% (ie, those in immune category 3), a persistent decline of five percentiles or more in $CD4^+$ cell percentage (eg, from 15% to 10%)
- A rapid and substantial decrease in absolute $CD4^+$ T-lymphocyte count (eg, a >30% decline in <6 months)

Clinical Considerations

- Progressive neurodevelopmental deterioration
- Growth failure defined as persistent decline in weight-growth velocity despite adequate nutritional support and without other explanation
- Disease progression defined as advancement from one pediatric clinical category to another (eg, from clinical category A to clinical category B)**

*At least two measurements (taken 1 week apart) should be performed before considering a change in therapy.

†The initial HIV RNA level of the child at the start of therapy and the level achieved with therapy should be considered when contemplating potential drug changes. For example, an immediate change in therapy may not be warranted if there is a sustained 1.5-2.0 $\log_{10}$ decrease in HIV RNA copy number, even if RNA remains detectable at low levels.

‡More frequent evaluation of HIV RNA levels should be considered if the HIV RNA increase is limited (eg, if when using an HIV RNA assay with a lower limit of detection of 1000 copies/mL, there is a ≤0.7 $\log_{10}$ increase from undetectable to approximately 5000 copies/mL in an infant <2 years of age).

§Minimal changes in $CD4^+$ T-lymphocyte percentile that may result in change in immunologic category (eg, from 26% to 24%, or 16% to 14%) may not be as concerning as a rapid substantial change in $CD4^+$ percentile within the same immunologic category (eg, a drop from 35% to 25%).

**In patients with stable immunologic and virologic parameters, progression from one clinical category to another may not represent an indication to change therapy. Thus, in patients whose disease progression is not associated with neurologic deterioration or growth failure, virologic and immunologic considerations are important in deciding whether to change therapy.

Guidelines for Changing an Antiretroviral Regimen for Suspected Drug Failure

- Criteria for changing therapy include a suboptimal reduction in plasma viremia after initiation of therapy, reappearance of viremia after suppression to undetectable, significant increases in plasma viremia from the nadir of suppression, and declining $CD4^+$ T cell numbers.
- When the decision to change therapy is based on viral load determination, it is preferable to confirm with a second viral load test.
- Distinguish between the need to change a regimen because of drug intolerance or inability to comply with the regimen versus failure to achieve the goal of sustained viral suppression; single agents can be changed in the event of drug intolerance.
- In general, do not change a single drug or add a single drug to a failing regimen; it is important to use at least two new drugs and preferably to use an entirely new regimen with at least three new drugs. If susceptibility testing indicates resistance to only one agent in a combination regimen, it may be possible to replace only that drug; however, this approach requires clinical validation.
- Many patients have limited options for new regimens of desired potency; in some of these cases, it is rational to continue the prior regimen if partial viral suppression was achieved.
- In some cases, regimens identified as suboptimal for initial therapy are rational due to limitations imposed by toxicity, intolerance, or nonadherence. This especially applies in late-stage disease. For patients with no rational alternative options who have virologic failure with return of viral load to baseline (pretreatment levels) and a declining $CD4^+$ T cell count, there should be consideration for discontinuation of antiretroviral therapy.
- Experience is limited with regimens using combinations of two protease inhibitors or combinations of protease inhibitors with NNRTIs; for patients with limited options due to drug intolerance or suspected resistance, these regimens provide possible alternative treatment options.

  There is limited information about the value of restarting a drug that the patient has previously received. Susceptibility testing may be useful in this situation if clinical evidence suggestive of the emergence of resistance is observed. However, testing for phenotypic or genotypic resistance in peripheral blood virus may fail to detect minor resistant variants. Thus, the presence of resistance is more useful information in altering treatment strategies than the absence of detectable resistance.
- Avoid changing from ritonavir to indinavir or vice versa for drug failure, because high-level cross-resistance is likely.
- Avoid changing among NNRTIs for drug failure, since high-level cross-resistance is likely.
- The decision to change therapy and the choice of a new regimen requires that the clinician have considerable expertise in the care of persons living with HIV. Physicians who are less experienced in the care of persons with HIV infection are strongly encouraged to obtain assistance through consultation with or referral to a clinician who has considerable expertise in the care of HIV-infected patients.

ANTIRETROVIRAL THERAPY FOR HIV INFECTION *(Continued)*

Acute Retroviral Syndrome: Associated Signs and Symptoms (Expected Frequency)

- Fever (96%)
- Lymphadenopathy (74%)
- Pharyngitis (70%)
- Rash (70%)
  - Erythematous maculopapular with lesions on face and trunk and sometimes extremities, including palms and soles
  - Mucocutaneous ulceration involving mouth, esophagus, or genitals
- Myalgia or arthralgia (54%)
- Diarrhea (32%)
- Headache (32%)
- Nausea and vomiting (27%)
- Hepatosplenomegaly (14%)
- Weight loss (13%)
- Thrush (12%)
- Neurologic symptoms (12%)
  - Meningoencephalitis or aseptic meningitis
  - Peripheral neuropathy or radiculopathy
  - Facial palsy
  - Guillain-Barré syndrome
  - Brachial neuritis
  - Cognitive impairment or psychosis

Zidovudine Perinatal Transmission Prophylaxis Regimen

Antepartum	Initiation at 14-34 weeks gestation and continued throughout pregnancy A. PACTG 076 regimen: ZDV 100 mg 5 times/day B. Acceptable alternative regimen: ZDV 200 mg 3 times/day or ZDV 300 mg twice daily
Intrapartum	During labor, ZDV 2 mg/kg I.V. over 1 hour, followed by a continuous infusion of 1 mg/kg I.V. until delivery
Postpartum	Oral administration of ZDV to the newborn (ZDV syrup, 2 mg/kg every 6 hours) for the first 6 weeks of life, beginning at 8-12 hours after birth

CLINICAL SYNDROMES ASSOCIATED WITH FOOD-BORNE DISEASES

Clinical Syndromes	Incubation Period (h)	Causes	Commonly Associated Vehicles
Nausea and vomiting	<1-6	*Staphylococcus aureus* (preformed toxins, A, B, C, D, E)	Ham, poultry, cream-filled pastries, potato and egg salad, mushrooms
		Bacillus cereus (emetic toxin)	Fried rice, pork
		Heavy metals (copper, tin, cadmium, zinc)	Acidic beverages
Histamine response and gastrointestinal (GI) tract	<1	Histamine (scombroid)	Fish (bluefish, bonito, mackerel, mahi-mahi, tuna)
Neurologic, including paresthesia and GI tract	0-6	Tetrodotoxin, ciguatera	Puffer fish
			Fish (amberjack, barracuda, grouper, snapper)
		Paralytic compounds	Shellfish (clams, mussels, oysters, scallops, other mollusks)
		Neurotoxic compounds	Shellfish
		Domoic acid	Mussels
		Monosodium glutamate	Chinese food
Neurologic and GI tract manifestations	0-2	Mushroom toxins (early onset)	Mushrooms
Moderate-to-severe abdominal cramps and watery diarrhea	8-16	*B. cereus* enterotoxin	Beef, pork, chicken, vanilla sauce
		Clostridium perfringens enterotoxin	Beef, poultry, gravy
	16-48	Caliciviruses	Shellfish, salads, ice
		Enterotoxigenic *Escherichia coli*	Fruits, vegetables
		Vibrio cholerae 01 and 0139	Shellfish
		V. cholerae non-01	Shellfish
Diarrhea, fever, abdominal cramps, blood and mucus in stools	16-72	*Salmonella*	Poultry, pork, eggs, dairy products, including ice cream, vegetables, fruit
		Shigella	Egg salad, vegetables
		Campylobacter jejuni	Poultry, raw milk
		Invasive *E. coli*	
		Yersinia enterocolitica	Pork chitterlings, tofu, raw milk
		Vibrio parahaemolyticus	Fish, shellfish
Bloody diarrhea, abdominal cramps	72-120	Enterohemorrhagic *E. coli*	Beef (hamburger), raw milk, roast beef, salami, salad dressings
Methemoglobin poisoning	6-12	Mushrooms (late onset)	Mushrooms
Hepatorenal failure	6-24	Mushrooms (late onset)	Mushrooms
Gastrointestinal then blurred vision, dry mouth, dysarthria, diplopia, descending paralysis	18-36	*Clostridium botulinum*	Canned vegetables, fruits and fish, salted fish, bottled garlic
Extraintestinal manifestations	Varied	Brainerd disease	Unpasteurized milk
		Brucella	Cheese, raw milk
		Group A *Streptococcus*	Egg and potato salad
		Listeria monocytogenes	Cheese, raw milk, hot dogs, cole slaw, cold cuts
		Trichinella spiralis	Pork
		Vibrio vulnificus	Shellfish

Adapted from "Report of the Committee on Infectious Diseases," *1997 Red Book®*, 24th ed.

COMMUNITY-ACQUIRED PNEUMONIA IN ADULTS

GUIDELINES FOR MANAGEMENT

Adapted from the Guidelines From the Infectious Diseases Society of America, *Clinical Infectious Diseases*, 1998, 26:811-38.

Algorithm

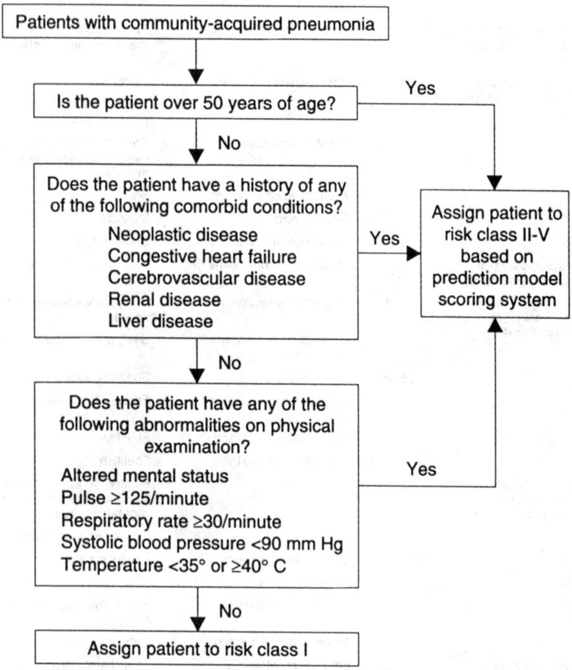

Patients with community-acquired pneumonia

↓

Is the patient over 50 years of age? — Yes → Assign patient to risk class II-V based on prediction model scoring system

↓ No

Does the patient have a history of any of the following comorbid conditions?
- Neoplastic disease
- Congestive heart failure
- Cerebrovascular disease
- Renal disease
- Liver disease

— Yes → Assign patient to risk class II-V based on prediction model scoring system

↓ No

Does the patient have any of the following abnormalities on physical examination?
- Altered mental status
- Pulse ≥125/minute
- Respiratory rate ≥30/minute
- Systolic blood pressure <90 mm Hg
- Temperature <35° or ≥40° C

— Yes → Assign patient to risk class II-V based on prediction model scoring system

↓ No

Assign patient to risk class I

Stratification of Risk Score

Risk	Risk class	Based on
Low	I	Algorithm
	II	≤ 70 total points
	III	71-90 total points
Moderate	IV	91-130 total points
High	V	> 130 total points

The table below is the prediction model for identification of patient risk for persons with community-acquired pneumonia. This model may be used to help guide the initial decision on site of care; however, its use may not be appropriate for all patients with this illness and, therefore, should be applied in conjunction with physician judgment.

Scoring System

Patient Characteristic	Points Assigned[1]
Demographic factors	
Age: Male	age (in years)
Female	age (in years) -10
Nursing home resident	+10
Comorbid illnesses	
Neoplastic disease	+30
Liver disease	+20
Congestive heart failure	+10
Cerebrovascular disease	+10
Renal disease	+10
Physical examination findings	
Altered mental status	+20
Respiratory rate ≥30/minute	+20
Systolic blood pressure <90 mm Hg	+20
Temperature <35°C or ≥40°C	+15
Pulse ≥125/minute	+10
Laboratory findings	
pH <7.35	+30
BUN >10.7 mmol/L	+20
Sodium <130 mEq/L	+20
Glucose >13.9 mmol/L	+10
Hematocrit <30%	+10
PO_2 <60 mm Hg[2]	+10
Pleural effusion	+10

[1] A risk score (reset point score) for a given patient is obtained by summing the patient age in years (age -10 for females) and the points for each applicable patient characteristic.

[2] Oxygen saturation <90% also was considered normal.

Risk-Class Mortality Rates for Patients With Pneumonia

		Validation Cohort		
Risk Class	No. of Points	No. of Patients	Mortality (%)	Recommendations for Site of Care
I	No predictors	3,034	0.1	Outpatient
II	≤70	5,778	0.6	Outpatient
III	71-90	6,790	2.8	Inpatient (briefly)
IV	91-130	13,104	8.2	Inpatient
V	>130	9,333	29.2	Inpatient

COMMUNITY-ACQUIRED PNEUMONIA IN ADULTS *(Continued)*

Epidemiological and Underlying Conditions Related to Specific Pathogens in Selected Patients With Community-Acquired Pneumonia

Conditions	Commonly Encountered Pathogens
Alcoholism	*Streptococcus pneumoniae*, anaerobes, gram-negative bacilli
COPD/smoker	*S. pneumoniae, Haemophilus influenzae, Moraxella catarrhalis, Legionella* species
Nursing home residency	*S. pneumoniae*, gram-negative bacilli, *H. influenzae, Staphylococcus aureus*, anaerobes, *Chlamydia pneumoniae*
Poor dental hygiene	Anaerobes
Epidemic Legionnaires' disease	*Legionella* species
Exposure to bats or soil enriched with bird droppings	*Histoplasma capsulatum*
Exposure to birds	*Chlamydia psittaci*
Exposure to rabbits	*Francisella tularensis*
HIV infection (early stage)	*S. pneumoniae, H. influenzae, Mycobacterium tuberculosis*
Travel to the southwestern United States	*Coccidioides immiris*
Exposure to farm animals or parturient cats	*Caxiella burnetii**
Influenza active in community	Influenza, *S. pneumoniae, S. aureus, Streptococcus pyogenes, H. influenzae*
Suspected large-volume aspiration	Anaerobes, chemical pneumonitis
Structural disease of the lung (bronchiectasis or cystic fibrosis)	*Pseudomonas aeruginosa, Burkholderia (Pseudomonas) cepacia*, or *S. aureus*
Injection drug use	*S. aureus*, anaerobes, *M. tuberculosis*
Airway obstruction	Anaerobes

*Agent of Q fever

COPD = chronic obstructive pulmonary disease

Flow Chart Approach to Treating Outpatients and Inpatients with Community-Acquired Pneumonia

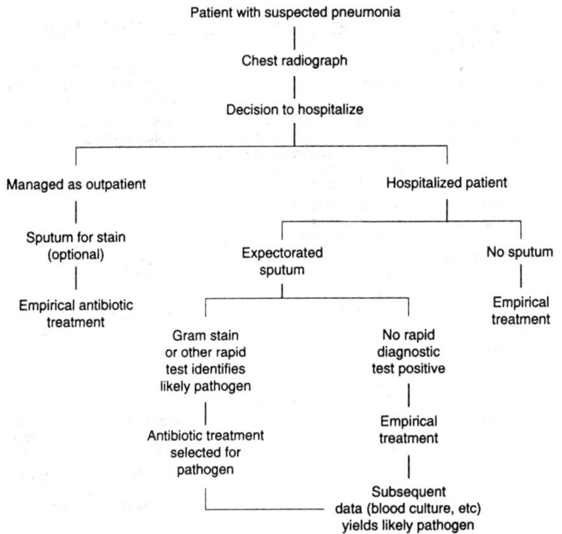

Community-Acquired Pneumonia

Possible reasons for failure of empirical treatment in patients with community-acquired pneumonia.

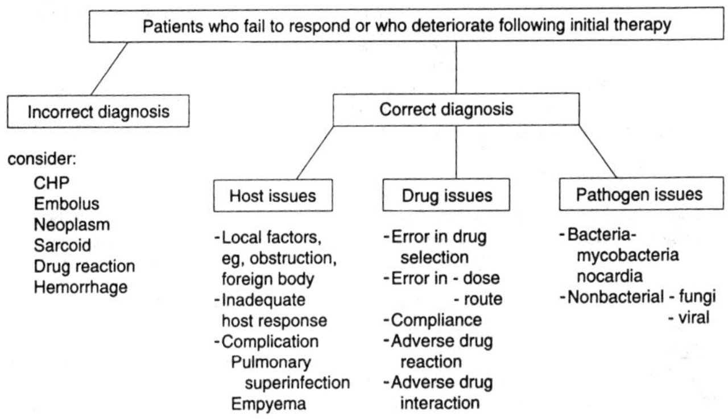

COMMUNITY-ACQUIRED PNEUMONIA IN ADULTS *(Continued)*

Treatment of Pneumonia According to Pathogen

Pathogen	Preferred Antimicrobial	Alternative Antimicrobial
Streptococcus pneumoniae		
Penicillin susceptible (MIC, <0.1 mcg/mL)	Penicillin G or penicillin V, amoxicillin	Cephalosporins,* macrolides,† clindamycin, fluoroquinolones,‡ doxycycline
Intermediately penicillin resistant (MIC, 0.1-1 mcg/mL)	Parenteral penicillin G, ceftriaxone or cefotaxime, amoxicillin, fluoroquinolones,‡ other agents based on *in vitro* susceptibility test results	Clindamycin, doxycycline, oral cephalosporins*
Highly penicillin-resistant¤ (MIC, ≥2 mcg/mL)	Agents based on *in vitro* susceptibility results, fluoroquinolones,‡ vancomycin	
Empirical selection	Fluoroquinolones,‡ selection based on susceptibility test results in community§	Clindamycin, doxycycline, vancomycin
	Penicillin¶	Cephalosporins,* macrolides,† amoxicillin, clindamycin
Haemophilus influenzae	Second- or third-generation cephalosporins, doxycycline, beta-lactam - beta-lactamase inhibitor, fluoroquinolones‡	Azithromycin, TMP-SMZ
Moraxella catarrhalis	Second- or third-generation cephalosporins, TMP-SMZ, amoxicillin/clavulanate	Macrolides,† fluoroquinolones,‡ beta-lactam - beta-lactamase inhibitor
Anaerobes	Clindamycin, penicillin plus metronidazole, beta-lactam - beta-lactamase inhibitor	Penicillin G or penicillin V, ampicillin/amoxicillin with or without metronidazole
Staphylococcus aureus¤		
Methicillin-suspectible	Nafcillin/oxacillin with or without rifampin or gentamicin¤	Cefazolin or cefuroxime, vancomycin, clindamycin, TMP-SMZ, fluoroquinolones‡
Methicillin-resistant	Vancomycin with or without rifampin or gentamicin	Requires *in vitro* testing; TMP-SMZ
Enterobacteriaceae (coliforms: *Escherichia coli, Klebsiella, Proteus, Enterobacter*)¤	Third-generation cephalosporin with or without an aminoglycoside, carbapenems**	Aztreonam, beta-lactam - beta-lactamase inhibitor, fluoroquinolones‡
Pseudomonas aeruginosa¤	Aminoglycoside plus antipseudomonal beta-lactam: ticarcillin, piperacillin, mezlocillin, cefazidime, cefepime, aztreonam, or carbapenems**	Aminoglycoside plus ciprofloxacin, ciprofloxacin plus antipseudomonal beta-lactam
Legionella species	Macrolides† with or without rifampin, fluoroquinolones‡	Doxycycline with or without rifampin
Mycoplasma pneumoniae	Doxycycline, macrolides,† fluoroquinolones‡	
Chlamydia pneumoniae	Doxycycline, macrolides,† fluoroquinolones‡	
Chlamydia psittaci	Doxycycline	Erythromycin, chloramphenicol
Nocardia species	Sulfonamide with or without minocycline or amikacin, TMP-SMZ	Imipenem with or without amikacin, doxycycline, or minocycline
Coxiella burnetii#	Tetracycline	Chloramphenicol
Influenza A	Amantadine or rimantadine	
Hantavirus	None††	

Note: TMP-SMZ = trimethoprim-sulfamethoxazole.

*Intravenous: Cefazolin, cefuroxime, cefotaxime, ceftriaxone; oral: cefpodoxime, cefprozil, cefuroxime.

†Erythromycin, clarithromycin, or azithromycin.

‡Levofloxacin, sparfloxacin, gatifloxacin, moxifloxacin, trovafloxacin, or another fluoroquinolone with enhanced activity against *S. pneumoniae*; ciprofloxacin is appropriate for *Legionella* species, fluoroquinolone-susceptible *S. aureus*, and most gram-negative bacilli.

¤*In vitro* susceptibility tests are required for optimal treatment; for *Enterobacter* species, the preferred antibiotics are fluoroquinolones and carbapenems.

§High rates of high-level penicillin resistance, susceptibility of community strains unknown, and/or patient is seriously ill.
¶Low rates of penicillin resistance in community and patient is at low risk for infection with resistant *S. pneumoniae*.
**Imipenem and meropenem.
#Agent of Q fever.
††Provide supportive care.

Empirical Antibiotic Selection for Patients With Community-Acquired Pneumonia

Outpatients

Generally preferred: Macrolides,* fluoroquinolones,† or doxycycline

Modifying factors

Suspected penicillin-resistant *Streptococcus pneumoniae*: Fluoroquinolones†

Young adult (>17-40 y): Doxycycline

Hospitalized patients

General medical ward

Generally preferred: Beta-lactam‡ with or without a macrolide* or a fluoroquinolone† (alone)

Alternatives: Cefuroxime with or without a macrolide* or azithromycin (alone)

Hospitalized in the intensive care unit for serious pneumonia

Generally preferred: Erythromycin, azithromycin, or a fluoroquinolone† plus cefotaxime, ceftriaxone, or a beta-lactam - beta-lactamase inhibitor¤

Modifying factors

Structural disease of the lung: Antipseudomonal penicillin, a carbapenem, or cefepime plus a macrolide* or a fluoroquinolone† plus an aminoglycoside

Penicillin allergy: A fluoroquinolone† with or without clindamycin

Suspected aspiration: A fluoroquinolone plus either clindamycin or metronidazole or a beta-lactam - beta-lactamase inhibitor¤

*Azithromycin, clarithromycin, or erythromycin

†Levofloxacin, sparfloxacin, gatifloxacin, moxifloxacin, trovafloxacin, or another fluoroquinolone with enhanced activity against *S. pneumoniae*

‡Cefotaxime, ceftriaxone, or a beta-lactam - beta-lactamase inhibitor

¤Ampicillin/sulbactam, or ticarcillin/clavulanate, or piperacillin/tazobactam (for structural disease of the lung, ticarcillin/clavulanate or piperacillin)

MALARIA TREATMENT

Drug	Adult Dosage	Pediatric Dosage
All *Plasmodium* species except chloroquine-resistant *Plasmodium falciparum*		
Oral Drug of Choice		
Chloroquine phosphate	600 mg base (1 g), then 300 mg base (500 mg) 6 h later, and 300 mg base (500 mg) at 24 and 48 h	10 mg base/kg (max: 600 mg base), then 5 mg base/kg 6 h later (max: 300 mg base), and 5 mg base/kg/d at 24 and 48 h (max: 300 mg base)
Parenteral Drug of Choice		
Quinidine gluconate*	10 mg/kg loading dose, I.V. (max: 600 mg) during 1-2 h, then 0.02 mg/kg/min continuous infusion until oral therapy can be started	Same as adult
or		
Quinine dihydrochloride*†	600 mg in 300 mL of normal saline I.V. during 2-4 h; repeat every 8 h (max: 1800 mg/d) until oral therapy can be started	30 mg/kg/d; give 1/3 of daily dose over 2-4 h; repeat every 8 h until oral therapy can be started (max: 1800 mg/d)
***P. falciparum* acquired in areas of known chloroquine resistance**		
Oral Regimen of Choice‡		
Quinine sulfate§	650 mg 3 times/d for 3-7 d	30 mg/kg/d in 3 doses for 3-7 d
plus		
Tetracycline‖	250 mg 4 times/d for 7 d	5 mg/kg 4 times/d for 7 d (max: 250 mg 4 times/d)
Alternative Regimen		
Oral: Quinine sulfate	650 mg 3 times/d for 3-7 d	30 mg/kg/d in 3 doses for 3-7 d
Parenteral: Quinidine gluconate*	Same as above	Same as above
or		
Quinine dihydrochloride*†	Same as above	Same as above
plus		
Pyrimethamine-sulfadoxine (Fansidar®)¶	Single dose of 3 tablets on last day of quinine therapy	<1 y of age, single dose of 1/4 tablet; 1-3 y of age, single dose of 1/2 tablet; 4-8 y of age, single dose of 1 tablet; 9-14 y of age, single dose of 2 tablets; >14 y of age, single dose of 3 tablets
or		
Mefloquine hydrochloride#**	Single dose of 15-25 mg/kg (max: 1250 mg)	15-25 mg/kg in a single dose (max: 1250 mg)
Prevention of relapses: *Plasmodium vivax* and *Plasmodium ovale* only		
Primaquine phosphate#	15 mg base (26.3 mg)/d for 14 d or 45 mg base (79 mg)/wk for 8 wk	0.3 mg base/kg/d for 14 d (max: 26.3 mg/d)

*Electrocardiogram monitoring is recommended to detect arrhythmias, widening QRS complex, or prolonged QT interval. Patients should also be monitored for hypotension. I.V. indicates intravenous.

†Not available in the United States.

‡The combination of quinine sulfate and tetracycline is the most efficacious regimen for all chloroquine-resistant *P. falciparum* infections.

§For treatment of *P. falciparum* infections acquired in Southeast Asia and possibility in other areas such as South America, quinine sulfate should be continued for 7 days.

‖Physicians must weigh the benefits of tetracycline therapy against the possibility of dental staining children younger than 8 years.

¶Use of Fansidar®, which contains 25 mg pyrimethamine and 500 mg sulfadoxine per tablet, is contraindicated in patients with a history of sulfonamide or pyrimethamine intolerance, in infants younger than 2 months and in pregnant women at term. Pregnant women should be administered chloroquine, or if chloroquine-resistant malaria is suspected, quinine or mefloquine. Resistance to pyrimethamine-sulfadoxine has been reported from Southeast Asia and the Amazon Basin, and therefore, this drug should not be used for treatment of malaria acquired in these areas.

#Mefloquine is not licensed by the Food and Drug Administration for children who weigh less than 15 kg, but recent Center for Disease Control and Prevention recommendations allow use of the drug to be considered in children without weight restrictions when travel to chloroquine-resistant *P. falciparum* areas cannot be avoided. Mefloquine is contraindicated for use by travelers with a known hypersensitivity to mefloquine, or for travelers with a history of epilepsy or severe psychiatric disorders. A review of available data suggests that mefloquine may be administered to persons concurrently receiving beta-blockers if they have no underlying arrhythmia. However, mefloquine is not recommended for persons with cardiac conduction abnormalities until additional data are available. Caution may be advised for persons involved in tasks requiring fine coordination and spatial discrimination, such as airline pilots. Quinidine or quinine may exacerbate the known side effects of mefloquine; patients not responding to mefloquine therapy or failing mefloquine prophylaxis should be monitored closely if they are treated with quinidine or quinine.

**For most patients, 15 mg/kg in a single dose is effective therapy, except for those who acquired infection in the areas of the Amazon basin, or the Thailand-Cambodian and Thailand-Myanmar borders (see ‡ footnote).

††Primaquine phosphate can cause hemolytic anemia in patients with glucose-6-phosphate dehydrogenase (G-6-PD) deficiency. A G-6-PD screen should be done before initiating treatment. Pregnant women should not be administered primaquine.

Adapted from "Report of the Committee on Infectious Diseases," *1997 Red Book®*, 24th ed.

RECOMMENDATIONS FOR PREVENTING THE SPREAD OF VANCOMYCIN RESISTANCE

Recommendations of the Hospital Infection Control Practices Advisory Committee (HICPAC)

(*MMWR Morb Mortal Wkly Rep*, 1995, 44(RR-12))

Prudent Vancomycin Use

Vancomycin use has been reported consistently as a risk factor for infection and colonization with VRE and may increase the possibility of the emergence of vancomycin-resistant *S. aureus* (VRSA) and/or vancomycin-resistant *S. epidermidis* (VRSE). Therefore, all hospitals and other healthcare delivery services, even those at which VRE have never been detected, should a) develop a comprehensive, antimicrobial-utilization plan to provide education for their medical staff (including medical students who rotate their training in different departments of the healthcare facility), b) oversee surgical prophylaxis, and c) develop guidelines for the proper use of vancomycin (as applicable to the institution).

Guideline development should be part of the hospital's quality-improvement program and should involve participation from the hospital's pharmacy and therapeutics committee; hospital epidemiologist; and infection-control, infectious-disease, medical, and surgical staffs. The guidelines should include the following considerations:

1. Situations in which the use of vancomycin is appropriate or acceptable
   - For treatment of serious infections caused by beta-lactam-resistant gram-positive microorganisms; vancomycin may be less rapidly bactericidal than are beta-lactam agents for beta-lactam-susceptible staphylococci
   - For treatment of infections caused by gram-positive microorganisms in patients who have serious allergies to beta-lactam antimicrobials
   - When antibiotic-associated colitis fails to respond to metronidazole therapy or is severe and potentially life-threatening
   - Prophylaxis, as recommended by the American Heart Association, for endocarditis following certain procedures in patients at high risk for endocarditis
   - Prophylaxis for major surgical procedures involving implantation of prosthetic materials or devices (eg, cardiac and vascular procedures and total hip replacement) at institutions that have a high rate of infections caused by MRSA or methicillin-resistant *S. epidermidis*. A single dose of vancomycin administered immediately before surgery is sufficient unless the procedure lasts >6 hours, in which case the dose should be repeated. Prophylaxis should be discontinued after a maximum of two doses.
2. Situations in which the use of vancomycin should be discouraged
   - Routine surgical prophylaxis other than in a patient who has a life-threatening allergy to beta-lactam antibiotics
   - Empiric antimicrobial therapy for a febrile neutropenic patient, unless initial evidence indicates that the patient has an infection caused by gram-positive microorganisms (eg, at an inflamed exit site of Hickman catheter) and the prevalence of infections caused by MRSA in the hospital is substantial
   - Treatment in response to a single blood culture positive for coagulase-negative *Staphylococcus*, if other blood cultures taken during the same time frame are

RECOMMENDATIONS FOR PREVENTING THE SPREAD OF VANCOMYCIN RESISTANCE *(Continued)*

negative (ie, if contamination of the blood culture is likely). Because contamination of blood cultures with skin flora (eg, *S. epidermidis*) could result in inappropriate administration of vancomycin, phlebotomists and other personnel who obtain blood cultures should be trained to minimize microbial contamination of specimens.

- Continued empiric use for presumed infections in patients whose cultures are negative for beta-lactam-resistant gram-positive microorganisms
- Systemic or local (eg, antibiotic lock) prophylaxis for infection or colonization of indwelling central or peripheral intravascular catheters
- Selective decontamination of the digestive tract
- Eradication of MRSA colonization
- Primary treatment of antibiotic-associated colitis
- Routine prophylaxis for very low-birthweight infants (ie, infants who weigh <1500 g [3 lbs 4 oz])
- Routine prophylaxis for patients on continuous ambulatory peritoneal dialysis or hemodialysis
- Treatment (chosen for dosing convenience) of infections caused by beta-lactam-sensitive gram-positive microorganisms in patients who have renal failure
- Use of vancomycin solution for topical application or irrigation

3. Enhancing compliance with recommendations
   - Although several techniques may be useful, further study is required to determine the most effective methods for influencing the prescribing practices of physicians
   - Key parameters of vancomycin use can be monitored through the hospital's quality assurance/improvement process or as part of the drug-utilization review of the Pharmacy and Therapeutics Committee and the medical staff

SUSPECTED ORGANISMS BY SITE OF INFECTION FOR EMPIRIC THERAPY

Site	Organisms
Urinary Tract	
Community acquired	*E. coli*, other gram-negative rods, *S. aureus*, *S. epidermidis*, *S. faecalis*
Nosocomial	Resistant gram-negative rods, enterococci
Respiratory Tract	
Pneumonia	
Community acquired	
normal adult	*S. pneumoniae*, virus, *Mycoplasma* (atypical)
normal child	*S. pneumoniae*, *H. influenzae*
aspiration	Aerobic and anaerobic mouth flora
alcoholic	*S. pneumoniae*, *Klebsiella*, anaerobes (below the belt)
COPD	*S. pneumoniae*, *H. influenzae*
Nosocomial	
aspiration	Mouth anaerobes, gram-negative aerobic rods, *S. aureus*
neutropenic	Fungi, gram-negative aerobic rods, *S. aureus*
HIV-infected	Fungi, *P. carinii*, *Legionella*, *Nocardia*, *S. pneumoniae*
Epiglottis	*H. influenzae*
Acute sinusitis	*S. pneumoniae*, *H. influenzae*, *M. catarrhalis* *(B. catarrhalis)*
Chronic sinusitis	Anaerobes, *S. aureus*
Bronchitis, otitis	*S. pneumoniae*, *H. influenzae*, *M. catarrhalis* *(B. catarrhalis)*
Pharyngitis	Group A streptococci
Skin and Soft Tissue	
Cellulitis	Group A streptococci, *S. aureus*
I.V. site	*S. aureus*, *S. epidermidis*
Surgical wound	*S. aureus*, gram-negative rods
Diabetic ulcer	*S. aureus*, gram-negative aerobic rods, anaerobes
Furuncle	*S. aureus*
Intra-abdominal	Anaerobes (*B. fragilis*), *E. coli*, enterococci
Cardiac	
Endocarditis	
subacute	*S. viridans*
acute	
I.V. drug user	*S. aureus*, gram-negative aerobic rods, *S. faecalis*, fungi
prosthetic valve	*S. epidermidis*
Gastric	
Gastroenteritis	*Salmonella*, *Shigella*, *H. pylori*, *C. difficile*, ameba, *G. lamblia*, viral, *E. coli*
Bone/Joint	
Osteomyelitis/septic arthritis	*S. aureus*, gram-negative aerobic rods
Central Nervous System	
Meningitis	
<2 mo	*E. coli*, group B streptococci, *Listeria*
2 mo to 12 y	*H. influenzae*, *S. pneumoniae*, *N. meningitidis*
adult and nosocomial	*S. pneumoniae*, *N. meningitidis*, gram-negative aerobic rods
postneurosurgery	*S. aureus*, gram-negative rods

TREATMENT OF SEXUALLY TRANSMITTED DISEASES

Type or Stage	Drug of Choice	Dosage	Alternatives
CHLAMYDIAL INFECTION AND RELATED CLINICAL SYNDROMES[1]			
Urethritis, cervicitis, conjunctivitis, or proctitis (except lymphogranuloma venereum)			
	Azithromycin OR	1 g oral once	Ofloxacin[3] 300 mg oral bid x 7 d
	Doxycycline[2,3]	100 mg oral bid x 7 d	Erythromycin[4] 500 mg oral qid x 7 d
Infection in pregnancy			
	Amoxicillin	500 mg oral tid x 10 d	Azithromycin[5] 1 g oral once Erythromycin[4] 500 mg oral qid x 7 d
Neonatal			
Ophthalmia	Erythromycin	12.5 mg/kg oral qid x 14 d	Azithromycin 20 mg/kg oral qd x 3 d
Pneumonia	Erythromycin	12.5 mg/kg oral or I.V. qid x 14 d	
Lymphogranuloma venereum			
	Doxycycline[2,3]	100 mg oral bid x 21 d	Erythromycin[4] 500 mg oral qid x 21 d
GONORRHEA[6]			
Urethral, cervical, rectal, or pharyngeal			
	Cefixime OR	400 mg oral once	Spectinomycin 2 g I.M. once[7]
	Ciprofloxacin[3] OR	500 mg oral once	
	Ofloxacin[3] OR	400 mg oral once	
	Ceftriaxone	125 mg I.M. once	
EPIDIDYMITIS	Ofloxacin	300 mg bid x 10 d	Ceftriaxone 250 mg I.M. once followed by doxycycline[2] 100 mg oral bid x 10 d
PELVIC INFLAMMATORY DISEASE			
- Inpatients	Cefotetan or	2 g I.V. q12h	Ofloxacin 400 mg I.V. q12h
	cefoxitin **plus** doxycycline[3]	2 g I.V. q6h 100 mg I.V. or oral q12h, until improved	**plus** metronidazole 500 mg I.V. q8h Ampicillin/sulbactam 3 g I.V. q6h **plus** doxycycline[3] 100 mg orally or I.V. q12h
	followed by doxycycline[3] OR	100 mg oral bid to complete 14 days	Ciprofloxacin 200 mg I.V. q12h **plus** doxycycline[3] 100 mg I.V. q12h
	Clindamycin **plus** gentamicin	900 mg I.V. q8h 2 mg/kg I.V. once, then 1.5 mg/kg I.V. q8h, until improved	**plus** metronidazole 500 mg I.V. q8h
	followed by doxycycline[3]	100 mg oral bid to complete 14 days	All continued until improved, then followed by doxycycline[3] 100 mg oral bid to complete 14 d[8]
- Outpatients	Ofloxacin[3] **plus** metronidazole	400 mg oral bid x 14 d 500 mg oral bid x 14 d	
	OR Ceftriaxone	250 mg I.M. once	

Type or Stage	Drug of Choice	Dosage	Alternatives
	OR Cefoxitin **plus** probenecid **either cephalosporin followed by** doxycycline[3,9]	2 g I.M. once 1 g oral once 100 mg oral bid x 14 d	
VAGINAL INFECTION			
Trichomoniasis			
	Metronidazole	2 g oral once	Metronidazole 375 mg or 500 mg oral bid x 7 d
Bacterial vaginosis			
	Metronidazole OR Metronidazole gel 0.75% OR Clindamycin 2% cream	500 mg oral bid x 7 d 5 g intravaginally once or twice daily x 5 d 5 g intravaginally qhs x 3-7 d	Metronidazole 250 mg oral tid x 7 d Clindamycin 300 mg oral bid x 7 d Metronidazole 2 g oral once[10]
Vulvovaginal candidiasis			
	Intravaginal butoconazole, clotrimazole, miconazole, terconazole, or tioconazole[11]		Nystatin 100,000 unit vaginal tablet once daily x 14 d
	OR Fluconazole	150 mg oral once	
SYPHILIS			
Early (primary, secondary, or latent <1 y)			
	Penicillin G benzathine	2.4 million units I.M. once[12]	Doxycycline[3] 100 mg oral bid x 14 d
Late (>1 year's duration, cardiovascular, gumma, late-latent)			
	Penicillin G benzathine	2.4 million units I.M. weekly x 3 wk	Doxycycline[3] 100 mg oral bid x 4 wk
Neurosyphilis[13]			
	Penicillin G	3-4 million units I.V. q4h x 10-14 d	Penicillin G procaine 2.4 million units I.M. daily, **plus** probenecid 500 mg qid oral, both x 10-14 d
Congenital			
	Penicillin G OR	50,000 units/kg I.V. q8-12h for 10-14 d	
	Penicillin G procaine	50,000 units/kg I.M. daily for 10-14 d	
CHANCROID[14]			
	Azithromycin OR	1 g oral once	Ciprofloxacin[3] 500 mg oral bid x 3 d
	Ceftriaxone	250 mg I.M. once	Erythromycin[4] 500 mg oral qid x 7 d
GENITAL HERPES			
First episode			
	Acyclovir OR Famciclovir OR Valacyclovir	400 mg oral tid x 7-10 d[15] 250 mg oral tid x 7-10 d 1 g oral bid x 7-10 d	Acyclovir 200 mg oral 5 times/d x 7-10 d[15]
Recurrent[16]			
	Acyclovir	400 mg oral tid x 5 d	
	OR Famciclovir	125 mg oral bid x 5 d	
	OR Valacyclovir	500 mg oral bid x 5 d	

TREATMENT OF SEXUALLY TRANSMITTED DISEASES *(Continued)*

Type or Stage	Drug of Choice	Dosage	Alternatives
Severe (hospitalized patients)			
	Acyclovir	5-10 mg/kg I.V. q8h x 5-7 d	
Suppression of recurrence[17]			
	Valacyclovir	500 mg - 1 g once daily[18]	Acyclovir 200 mg oral 2-5 times/day
	OR Acyclovir	400 mg oral bid	Famciclovir 250 mg oral bid

[1]Related clinical syndromes include nonchlamydial nongonococcal urethritis and cervicitis.
[2]Or tetracycline 500 mg oral qid or minocycline 100 mg oral bid.
[3]Contraindicated in pregnancy.
[4]Erythromycin estolate is contraindicated in pregnancy.
[5]Safety in pregnancy not established.
[6]All patients should also receive a course of treatment effective for *Chlamydia*.
[7]Recommended only for use during pregnancy in patients allergic to beta-lactams. Not effective for pharyngeal infection.
[8]Or clindamycin 450 mg oral qid to complete 14 days.
[9]Some experts would add metronidazole 500 mg bid
[10]Higher relapse rate with single dose, but useful for patients who may not comply with multiple-dose therapy.
[11]For preparations and dosage of topical products, see *Medical Letter*, 36:81,1994; single-dose therapy is not recommended.
[12]Some experts recommend repeating this regimen after 7 days, especially in patients with HIV infection.
[13]Patients allergic to penicillin should be desensitized.
[14]All regimens, especially single-dose ceftriaxone, are less effective in HIV-infected patients.
[15]For first-episode proctitis, use acyclovir 800 mg oral tid or 400 mg oral 5 times/day.
[16]Antiviral therapy is variably effective for treatment of recurrences; only effective if started early.
[17]Preventive treatment should be discontinued for 1-2 months once a year to reassess the frequency of recurrence.
[18]Use 500 mg qd in patients with <10 recurrences per year and 500 mg bid or 1 g daily in patients with ≥10 recurrences per year.

TUBERCULOSIS TREATMENT GUIDELINES

Recommended Treatment Regimens for Drug-Susceptible Tuberculosis in Infants, Children, and Adolescents*

Infection or Disease Category	Regimen	Remarks
Asymptomatic infection (positive skin test, no disease):		If daily therapy is not possible, therapy twice a week may be used for 6-9 months. HIV-infected children should be treated for 12 months.
• Isoniazid-susceptible	6-9 months of isoniazid once a day	
• Isoniazid-resistant	6-9 months of rifampin once a day	
• Isoniazid-rifampin-resistant*	Consult a tuberculosis specialist	
Pulmonary	**6-Month Regimens** 2 months of isoniazid, rifampin, and pyrazinamide once a day, followed by 4 months of isoniazid and rifampin daily	If possible drug resistance is a concern (see text), another drug (ethambutol or streptomycin) is added to the initial drug therapy until drug susceptibilities are determined.
	or	
	2 months of isoniazid, rifampin, and pyrazinamide daily, followed by 4 months of isoniazid and rifampin twice a week	Drugs can be given 2 or 3 times per week under direct observation in the initial phase if nonadherence is likely.
	9-Month Alternative Regimens (for hilar adenopathy only) 9 months of isoniazid and rifampin once a day **or** 1 month of isoniazid and rifampin once a day, followed by 8 months of isoniazid and rifampin twice a week	Regimens consisting of 6 months of isoniazid and rifampin once a day, and 1 month of isoniazid and rifampin once a day, followed by 5 months of isoniazid and rifampin twice a week, have been successful in areas where drug resistance is rare.
Extrapulmonary meningitis, disseminated (miliary), bone/joint disease	2 months of isoniazid, rifampin, pyrazinamide, and streptomycin once a day, followed by 10 months of isoniazid and rifampin once a day (12 months total)	Streptomycin is given with initial therapy until drug susceptibility is known.
	or	
	2 months of isoniazid, rifampin, pyrazinamide, and streptomycin once a day, followed by 10 months of isoniazid and rifampin twice a week (12 months total)	For patients who may have acquired tuberculosis in geographic areas where resistance to streptomycin is common, capreomycin (15-30 mg/kg/d) or kanamycin (15-30 mg/kg/d) may be used instead of streptomycin.
Other (eg, cervical lymphadenopathy)	Same as for pulmonary disease	See Pulmonary.

*Duration of therapy is longer in HIV-infected persons and additional drugs may be indicated.

Adapted from "Report of the Committee on Infectious Diseases," *1997 Red Book®*, 24th ed.

TUBERCULOSIS TREATMENT GUIDELINES *(Continued)*

Commonly Used Drugs for the Treatment of Tuberculosis in Infants, Children, and Adolescents

Drugs	Dosage Forms	Daily Dose (mg/kg/d)	Twice a Week Dose (mg/kg per dose)	Maximum Dose	Adverse Reactions
Ethambutol	Tablets 100 mg 400 mg	15-25	50	2.5 g	Optic neuritis (usually reversible), decreased visual acuity, decreased red-green color discrimination, gastrointestinal disturbances, hypersensitivity
Isoniazid*	Scored tablets 100 mg 300 mg Syrup 10 mg/mL	10-15†	20-30	Daily, 300 mg Twice a week, 900 mg	Mild hepatic enzyme elevation, hepatitis,† peripheral neuritis, hypersensitivity
Pyrazinamide*	Scored tablets 500 mg	20-40	50	2 g	Hepatotoxicity, hyperuricemia
Rifampin*	Capsules 150 mg 300 mg Syrup formulated in syrup from capsules	10-20	10-20	600 mg	Orange discoloration of secretions/urine, staining contact lenses, vomiting, hepatitis, flu-like reaction, and thrombocytopenia; may render birth-control pills ineffective
Streptomycin (I.M. administration)	Vials 1 g 4 g	20-40	20-40	1 g	Auditory and vestibular toxicity, nephrotoxicity, rash

*Rifamate® is a capsule containing 150 mg of isoniazid and 300 mg of rifampin. Two capsules provide the usual adult (>50 kg body weight) daily doses of each drug. Rifater® is a capsule containing 50 mg of isoniazid, 120 mg of rifampin, and 300 mg of pyrazinamide.

†When isoniazid in a dosage exceeding 10 mg/kg/day is used in combination with rifampin, the incidence of hepatotoxicity may be increased.

Adapted from "Report of the Committee on Infectious Diseases," *1997 Red Book®*, 24th ed.

Rifampin is a bactericidal agent. It is metabolized by the liver and affects the pharmacokinetics of many other drugs, affecting their serum concentrations. Mycobacterium tuberculosis, initially resistant to rifampin, remains relatively uncommon in most areas of the United States. Rifampin is excreted in bile and urine and can cause orange urine, sweat and tears. It can also cause discoloration of soft contact lenses and render oral contraceptives ineffective. Hepatotoxicity occurs rarely. Blood dyscrasia accompanied by influenza-like symptoms can occur if doses are taken sporadically.

Less Commonly Used Drugs for Treatment of Drug-Resistant Tuberculosis in Infants, Children, and Adolescents*

Drugs	Dosage Forms	Daily Dose (mg/kg/d)	Maximum Dose	Adverse Reactions
Capreomycin	Vials 1 g	15-30 (I.M. administration)	1 g	Ototoxicity, nephrotoxicity
Ciprofloxacin†	Tablets 250 mg 500 mg 750 mg	Adults 500-1500 mg total per day (twice a day)	1.5 g	Theoretical effect on growing cartilage, gastrointestinal tract disturbances, rash, headache
Cycloserine	Capsules 250 mg	10-20	1 g	Psychosis, personality changes, convulsions, rash
Ethionamide	Tablets 250 mg	15-20 given in 2 or 3 divided doses	1 g	Gastrointestinal tract disturbances, hepatotoxicity, hypersensitive reactions
Kanamycin	Vials 75 mg/2 mL 500 mg/2 mL 1 g/3 mL	15-30 (I.M. 1 g administration)	1 g	Auditory toxicity, nephrotoxicity, vestibular toxicity
Ofloxacin†	Tablets 200 mg 300 mg 400 mg	Adults 400-800 mg total per day (twice a day)	0.8 g	Theoretical effect on growing cartilage, gastrointestinal tract disturbances, rash, headache
Para-amino salicylic acid (PAS)	Tablets 500 mg	200-300 (3 or 4 times a day)	10 g	Gastrointestinal tract disturbances, hypersensitivity, hepatotoxicity

*These drugs should be used in consultation with a specialist in tuberculosis.

†Fluoroquinolones are not currently approved for use in persons younger than 18 years; their use in younger patients necessitates assessment of the potential risks and benefits (see Antimicrobials and Related Therapy).

Adapted from "Report of the Committee on Infectious Diseases," *1997 Red Book®*, 24th ed.

TUBERCULOSIS TREATMENT GUIDELINES *(Continued)*

TB Drugs in Special Situations

Drug	Pregnancy	CNS TB Disease	Renal Insufficiency
Isoniazid	Safe	Good penetration	Normal clearance
Rifampin	Safe	Fair penetration Penetrates inflamed meninges (10% to 20%)	Normal clearance
Pyrazinamide	Avoid	Good penetration	Clearance reduced Decrease dose or prolong interval
Ethambutol	Safe	Penetrates inflamed meninges only (4% to 64%)	Clearance reduced Decrease dose or prolong interval
Streptomycin	Avoid	Penetrates inflamed meninges only	Clearance reduced Decrease dose or prolong interval
Capreomycin	Avoid	Penetrates inflamed meninges only	Clearance reduced Decrease dose or prolong interval
Kanamycin	Avoid	Penetrates inflamed meninges only	Clearance reduced Decrease dose or prolong interval
Ethionamide	Do not use	Good penetration	Normal clearance
Para-aminosalicylic acid	Safe	Penetrates inflamed meninges only (10% to 50%)	Incomplete data on clearance
Cycloserine	Avoid	Good penetration	Clearance reduced Decrease dose or prolong interval
Ciprofloxacin	Do not use	Fair penetration (5% to 10%) Penetrates inflamed meninges (50% to 90%)	Clearance reduced Decrease dose or prolong interval
Ofloxacin	Do not use	Fair penetration (5% to 10%) Penetrates inflamed meninges (50% to 90%)	Clearance reduced Decrease dose or prolong interval
Amikacin	Avoid	Penetrates inflamed meninges only	Clearance reduced Decrease dose or prolong interval
Clofazimine	Avoid	Penetration unknown	Clearance probably normal

Safe = The drug has not been demonstrated to have teratogenic effects.

Avoid = Data on the drug's safety are limited, or the drug is associated with mild malformations (as in the aminoglycosides).

Do not use = Studies show an association between the drug and premature labor, congenital malformations, or teratogenicity.

Recommendations for Coadministering Different Antiretroviral Drugs With the Antimycobacterial Drugs Rifabutin and Rifampin

Antiretroviral	Use in Combination with Rifabutin	Use in Combination with Rifampin	Comments
Saquinavir#			
Hard-gel capsules (HGC)	Possibly†, if antiretroviral regimen also includes ritonavir	Possibly, if antiretroviral regimen also includes ritonavir	Coadministration of saquinavir SGC with usual-dose rifabutin (300 mg/day or 2-3 times/week) is a possibility. However, the pharmacokinetic data and clinical experience for this combination are limited.
Soft-gel capsules (SGC)	Probably§	Possibly, if antiretroviral regimen also includes ritonavir	The combination of saquinavir SGC or saquinavir HGC and ritonavir, coadministered with 1) usual-dose rifampin (600 mg/day or 2-3 times/ week), or 2) reduced-dose rifabutin (150 mg 2-3 times/week) is a possibility. However, the pharmacokinetic data and clinical experience for these combinations are limited. Coadministration of saquinavir or saquinavir SGC with rifampin is not recommended because rifampin markedly decreases concentrations of saquinavir.
Ritonavir	Probably	Probably	If the combination of ritonavir and rifabutin is used, then a substantially reduced-dose rifabutin regimen (150 mg 2-3 times/week) is recommended. Coadministration of ritonavir with usual-dose rifampin (600 mg/day or 2-3 times/week) is a possibility, though pharmacokinetic data and clinical experience are limited.
Indinavir	Yes	No	There is limited, but favorable, clinical experience with coadministration of indinavir¶ with a reduced daily dose of rifabutin (150 mg) or with the usual dose of rifabutin (300 mg 2-3 times/ week). Coadministration of indinavir with rifampin is not recommended because rifampin markedly decreases concentrations of indinavir.
Nelfinavir	Yes	No	There is limited, but favorable, clinical experience with coadministration of nelfinavir## with a reduced daily dose of rifabutin (150 mg) or with the usual dose of rifabutin (300 mg 2-3 times/ week). Coadministration of nelfinavir with rifampin is not recommended because rifampin markedly decreases concentrations of nelfinavir.
Amprenavir	Yes	No	Coadministration of amprenavir with a reduced daily dose of rifabutin (150 mg) or with the usual dose of rifabutin (300 mg 2-3 times/week) is a possibility, but there is no published clinical experience. Coadministration of amprenavir with rifampin is not recommended because rifampin markedly decreases concentrations of amprenavir.

TUBERCULOSIS TREATMENT GUIDELINES *(Continued)*

Recommendations for Coadministering Different Antiretroviral Drugs With the Antimycobacterial Drugs Rifabutin and Rifampin *(continued)*

Antiretroviral	Use in Combination with Rifabutin	Use in Combination with Rifampin	Comments
Nevirapine	Yes	Possibly	Coadministration of nevirapine with usual-dose rifabutin (300 mg/day or 2-3 times/week) is a possibility based on pharmacokinetic study data. However, there is no published clinical experience for this combination. Data are insufficient to assess whether dose adjustments are necessary when rifampin is coadministered with nevirapine. Therefore, rifampin and nevirapine should be used only in combination if clearly indicated and with careful monitoring.
Delavirdine	No	No	Contraindicated because of the marked decrease in concentrations of delavirdine when administered with either rifabutin or rifampin.
Efavirenz	Probably	Probably	Coadministration of efavirenz with increased-dose rifabutin (450 mg/day or 600 mg/day, or 600 mg 2-3 times/ week) is a possibility, though there is no published clinical experience. Coadministration of efavirenz†† with usual-dose rifampiin (600 mg/day or 2-3 times/week) is a possibility, though there is no published clinical experience.

Usual recommended doses are 400 mg twice daily for each of these protease inhibitors and 400 mg of ritonavir.

† Despite limited data and clinical experience, the use of this combination is potentially successful.

§ Based on available data and clinical experience, the successful use of this combination is likely.

¶ Usual recommended dose is 800 mg every 8 hours; some experts recommend increasing the indinavir dose to 1000 mg every 8 hours if indinavir is used in combination with rifabutin.

Usual recommended dose is 750 mg 3 times/day or 1250 mg twice daily; some experts recommend increasing the nelfinavir dose to 1000 mg if the 3-times/day dosing is used and nelfinavir is used in combination with rifabutin.

†† Usual recommended dose is 600 mg/day; some experts recommend increasing the efavirenz dose to 800 mg/day if efavirenz is used in combination with rifampin.

Updated March 2000 from www.hivatis.org -"Updated Guidelines for the Use of Rifabutin or Rifampin for the Treatment and Prevention of Tuberculosis Among HIV-Infected Patients Taking Protease Inhibitors or Nonnucleoside Reverse Transcriptase Inhibitors," *MMWR,* March 10, 2000, 49(09):185-9.

MATERNAL/FETAL MEDICATIONS

Adapted from Briggs GG, "Medication Use During the Perinatal Period," *J Am Pharm Assoc*, 1998, 38:717-27.

Antibiotics in Pregnancy

Antibiotics Which Are Generally Regarded as Safe	
Antibiotic	**Comments**
Aminoglycosides (limited use)	
Penicillins	
Cephalosporins	
Clindamycin	
Erythromycin	
Antibiotics to Be Avoided	
Tetracyclines	Staining of deciduous teeth (4th month through term)
Aminoglycosides (prolonged use)	Eighth cranial nerve damage (hearing loss, vestibulotoxicity)
Fluoroquinolones	Potentially mutagenic, cartilage damage, arthropathy, and teratogenicity
Erythromycin estolate	Hepatotoxic in mother
Ribavirin	Possibly fetotoxic

Treatment and Prevention of Infection

Prophylaxis	
Preterm premature rupture of membranes	Ampicillin, amoxicillin, cefazolin, amoxicillin/clavulanate, ampicillin/sulbactam, erythromycin
Prevention of bacterial endocarditis	Ampicillin 2 g and gentamicin 1.5 mg/kg (max 120 mg) within 30 min of delivery, followed by 1 g ampicillin (I.V.) or amoxicillin (oral) 6 hours later
Cesarean section	Cefazolin (I.V. or uterine irrigation) or clindamycin/gentamicin
Treatment	
Bacterial vaginosis	Clindamycin (oral or gel) in first trimester (gel has been associated with higher rate of preterm deliveries) Metronidazole (oral) for 7 days or gel for 5 days (after first trimester)
Chorioamnionitis	Ampicillin plus gentamicin (clindamycin, erythromycin, or vancomycin if PCN allergic)
Genital herpes	First episode: Oral acyclovir Near term treatment may reduce Cesarian sections I.V. therapy for disseminated infection
Group B streptococci	Penicillin G 5 million units once, then 2.5 million units q4h Ampicillin 2 g once, then 1 g q4h Clindamycin or erythromycin if PCN allergic
HIV	Zidovudine (limits maternal-fetal transmission) Oral dosing during pregnancy/I.V. prior to delivery Other antiretroviral agents - effects unknown
Postpartum endometritis	Ampicillin (vancomycin if PCN allergic) plus clindamycin (or metronidazole) plus gentamicin until afebrile
Pyelonephritis	Ampicillin-gentamicin Cefazolin Co-trimoxazole

MATERNAL/FETAL MEDICATIONS *(Continued)*

Treatment and Prevention of Infection *(continued)*

	Prophylaxis
Urinary tract infection	Amoxicillin/ampicillin (resistance has increased) Co-trimoxazole Nitrofurantoin Cephalexin
Vaginal candidiasis	Buconizole for 7 days Clotrimazole for 7 days Miconazole for 7 days Terconazole for 7 days

Preterm Labor: Tocolytic Agents

Drug Class	Route	Fetal/Neonatal Toxicities	Maternal Toxicities
Beta-adrenergic agonists Ritodrine, terbutaline	Oral, I.V., S.C.	Fetal tachycardia, intraventricular septal hypertrophy, neonatal hyperinsulinemia/ hypoglycemia	Pulmonary, edema, myocardial infarction, hypokalemia, hypotension, hyperglycemia, tachycardia
Magnesium	I.V.	Neurologic depression in newborn (loss of reflexes, hypotonia, respiratory depression(; fetal hypocalcemia and hypercalcuria; abnormal fetal bone mineralization and enamel hypoplasia	Hypotension, respiratory depression, ileus/ constipation, hypocalcemia, pulmonary edema, hypotension, headache/dizziness
NSAIDs Indomethacin	Oral, P.R.	Ductus arteriosis: premature closure, ricuspid regurgitation, primary pulmonary hypertension of the newborn, PDA; intraventricular hemorrhage, necrotizing enterocolitis, renal failure	GI bleeding, oligohydramnios, pulmonary edema, acute renal failure
Calcium channel blockers Nifedipine	Oral	Hypoxia secondary to maternal hypotension	Hypotension, flushing, tachycardia, headache
Nitrates Nitroglycerin	I.V./ S.L.	Hypoxia secondary to maternal hypotension	Hypotension, headache, dizziness

Pregnancy-Induced Hypertension*

Drug Class	Maternal/Fetal Effects
Antihypertensives Contraindicated in PIH	
Diuretics	Reduction of maternal plasma volume exacerbates disease; use in chronic hypertension acceptable (if no superimposed pregnancy-induced hypertension)
ACE-inhibitors	Teratogenic in second and third trimester; fetal/newborn anuria and hypotension, fetal oligohydramnios; neonatal death (congenital abnormalities of skull and renal failure)
Hypertension Treatment†	
Central-acting Methyldopa	Relatively safe in second/third trimester
Beta-blockers Acebutolol, atenolol, metoprolol, pindolol, propranolol	Increased risk of IUGR
Alpha-/beta-blocking Labetolol	See beta-blockers
Vasodilators Hydralazine	Relatively safe in second/third trimester
Nitrates Nitroglycerin	Relatively safe in second/third trimester
Calcium channel blockers Nifedipine	Relatively safe in second/third trimester

*Includes management of pre-eclampsia/eclampsia and HELLP syndrome. **Note:** Prevention may include low-dose aspirin (81 mg/day) or calcium supplementation (2 g/day).

†All agents must be carefully titrated to avoid fetal hypoxia.

Other Maternal-Fetal Drug Therapy

Drug	Dose/Route
Fetal Lung Maturation	
Betamethasone	Two 12 mg doses I.M. at a 24-hour interval
Dexamethasone	Four 6 mg doses I.M. at 12-hour intervals
Doses repeated weekly up to 34 weeks gestation	
Cervical Ripening	
Oxytocin	I.V. dosing - often ineffective
Hygroscopic cervical dilators	
Dinoprostone (prostaglandin E2)	Gel (0.5 mg) or vaginal insert (10 mg, releasing 0.3 mg/h)
Misoprostol (prostaglandin E1)	Oral tablets inserted intravaginally 25-50 mcg q3-4h for up to 24 hours; oral dosing is investigational
Analgesia During Labor	
Meperidine	25-50 mg I.V. q1-2h or 50-100 mg I.M. q2-4h
Fentanyl	50-100 mcg q1h
Butorphanol	No advantage over other agents
Nalbuphine	No advantage over other agents
Tramadol	No advantage over other agents
Postpartum Hemorrhage	
Oxytocin	I.V. usually; also I.M. or intramyometrially (IMM)
Methylergonovine	I.M. or I.M.M.; contraindicated in hypertension
Carboprost (PG F2 alpha)	Pyrexia is common; contraindicated in cardiac, pulmonary, renal, or hepatic disease
Misoprostil	Rectal administration has been investigated

MATERNAL/FETAL TOXICOLOGY

Drugs and Chemicals Proven to Be Teratogenic in Humans

Drug/ Chemical	Fetal Adverse Effects	Relative Risk for Teratogenicity	Clinical Intervention
Alcohol	**Fetal alcohol syndrome:** Mental retardation, microcephaly, poor coordination, hypotonia, hyperactivity, short upturned nose, micrognathia or retrognathia (infancy) or prognathia (adolescence), short palpebral fissures, hypoplastic philtrum, thinned upper lips, microphthalmia, antenatal/postnatal growth retardation, occasional pathologies of eyes, mouth, heart, kidneys, gonads, skin, muscle, and skeleton	In alcoholic women consuming >2 g/kg/d ethanol over first trimester: 2- to 3-fold higher risk for congenital malformations (about 10%)	To calculate accurate dose of alcohol: **Prospective:** To discontinue exposure; if woman is alcoholic, refer to addiction center **During pregnancy:** To alleviate fears in mild or occasional drinkers who may terminate pregnancy based on unrealistic perception of risk, level 2 ultrasound to rule out visible malformation
Alkylating agents (busulfan, chlorambucil, cyclophosphamide, mechlorethamine)	Growth retardation, cleft palate, microphthalmia hypoplastic ovaries, cloudy corneas, agenesis of kidney, malformations of digits, cardiac defects, multiple other anomalies	Based on case reports, between 10% and 50% of cases were malformed for different drugs. It is possible that adverse outcome was overrepresented.	Level 2 ultrasound to rule out visible malformations. Supplement folic acid to women receiving antifolates (eg, methotrexate).
Antimetabolite agents (aminopterin azauridine, cytarabine, 5-FU, 6-MP, methotrexate)	Hydrocephalus, meningoencephalocele, anencephaly, malformed skull, cerebral hypoplasia, growth retardation, eye and ear malformations, malformed nose and cleft palate, malformed extremities and fingers **Aminopterin syndrome:** Cranial dysostosis, hydrocephalus, hypertelorism, anomalies of external ear, micrognathia, posterior cleft palate	Based on case reports 7%-75% of cases were malformed. It is possible that adverse outcome was overrepresented.	Level 2 ultrasound to rule out visible malformations.
Carbamazepine	Increased risk for neural tube defects (NTDs)	NTDs estimated at 1% with carbamazepine	Periconceptional folate; maternal and/ or amniotic α-fetoprotein; ultrasound to rule out NTD.
Carbon monoxide	Cerebral atrophy, mental retardation, microcephaly, convulsions, spastic disorders, intrauterine or postnatal death	Based on case reports, when mother is severely poisoned, high risk for neurological sequelae; no increased risk in mild accidental exposures	Measure maternal carboxyhemoglobin levels. Treat with 100% oxygen for 5 hours after maternal carboxyhemoglobin returns to normal because fetal equilibration takes longer. If hyperbaric chamber available, should be used, as elimination half-life of CO is more rapid. Fetal monitoring by an obstetrician; sonographic follow-up.

Drugs and Chemicals Proven to Be Teratogenic in Humans *(continued)*

Drug/ Chemical	Fetal Adverse Effects	Relative Risk for Teratogenicity	Clinical Intervention
Diethylstilbestrol (DES)	**Female offspring:** Clear cell vaginal or cervical adenocarcinoma in young female adults exposed in utero (before 18th week); irregular menses (oligomenorrhea), reduced pregnancy rates, increased rate of preterm deliveries, increased perinatal mortality and spontaneous abortion **Male offspring:** Cysts of epididymis, cryptorchidism, hypogonadism, diminished spermatogenesis	Exposure before 18 weeks of gestation: ≤1.4/1000 of exposed female with carcinoma. Congenital morphological changes in vaginal epithelium in 39% of exposures.	**Diagnosis:** Direct observation of mucosa and Shiller's test. **Treatment:** Mechanical excision or destruction in relatively confined area. Surgery and radiotherapy for diffused tumor.
Lead	Lower scores in developmental tests	Higher risk when maternal lead is >10 μg/dL	**Maternal lead levels >10 μg/dL:** Investigate for possible source of contamination. **Levels >25 μg/dL:** Consider chelation
Lithium carbonate	Possibly higher risk for Ebstein's anomaly; no detectable higher risk for other malformations		Women who need lithium should continue therapy, with sonographic follow-up. Patients may need higher doses because of increased clearance rate.
Methyl mercury, mercuric sulfide	Microcephaly, eye malformations, cerebral palsy, mental retardation, malocclusion of teeth	Women of affected babies consumed 9-27 ppm mercury; greater risk when ingested at 6-8 gestational months. Relative risk was not elucidated, but 13/220 babies born in Minamata, Japan, at time of contamination had severe disease.	Good correlation between mercury concentrations in maternal hair follicles and neurological outcome of the fetus. Hair mercury content >50 ppm was used successfully as a cut point for termination. In acute poisoning, the fetus is 4-10 times more sensitive than the adult to methylmercury toxicity.

MATERNAL/FETAL TOXICOLOGY *(Continued)*

Drugs and Chemicals Proven to Be Teratogenic in Humans *(continued)*

Drug/ Chemical	Fetal Adverse Effects	Relative Risk for Teratogenicity	Clinical Intervention
PCBs	**Stillbirth** **Signs at birth:** White eye discharge, 30% (32/108); teeth present, 8.7% (11/127); irritated/swollen gums, 11% (11/99); hyperpigmentation ("cola" staining), 42.5% (54/127); deformed/small nails, 24.6% (30/122); acne, 12.8% (16/125) **Subsequent history:** Bronchitis or pneumonia, 27.2% (30/124); chipped or broken teeth, 35.5% (38/107); hair loss, 12.2% (14/115); acne scars, 9.6% (11/115); generalized itching, 27.8% (32/1150) **Developmental:** Do not meet milestones; lower scores than unexposed controls; evidence of CNS damage	4%-20% (6/159-8/39)	These figures, which are from cases poisoned by high consumption of PCB-contaminated rice oil, cannot be extrapolated to cases in which maternal poisoning has not been verified. Women working near PCBs (eg, hydroelectric facilities) should use effective protection.
Penicillamine	Skin hyperelastosis	Few case reports; risk unknown	
Phenytoin	**Fetal hydantoin syndrome:** Low nasal bridge, inner epicanthal folds, ptosis, strabismus, hypertelorism, low set or abnormal ears, wide mouth, large fontanels, anomalies and hypoplasia of distal phalanges and nails, skeletal abnormalities, microcephaly and mental retardation, growth deficiency, neuroblastoma, cardiac defects, cleft palate/lip	5%-10% of typical syndrome; about 30% of partial picture. Relative risk of 7 for offspring IQ ≤84.	Neurologist should consider changing to other medications. Keep phenytoin concentrations at lower effective levels. Level 2 ultrasound to rule out visible malformations, vitamin K to neonate. Epilepsy itself increases teratogenic risk.
Systemic retinoids (isotretinoin, etretinate)	Spontaneous abortions; deformities of cranium, ears, face, heart, limbs, liver; hydrocephalus, microcephalus, heart defects. Cognitive defects even without dysmorphology	For isotretinoin: 38% risk. 80% of malformation are CNS.	Treated women should have an effective method of contraception. Pregnancy termination. If diagnosed too late, sonographic follow-up to rule out confirmed malformations.
Tetracycline	Yellow, gray-brown, or brown staining of deciduous teeth, destruction of enamel	From 4 months of gestation and on, occurs in 50% of fetuses exposed to tetracycline; 12.5% to oxytetracycline	If exposure before 14-16 weeks of gestation, no known risk
Thalidomide	Limb phocomelia, amelia, hypoplasia, congenital heart defects, renal malformations, cryptorchidism, abducens paralysis, deafness, microtia, anotia	About 20% risk when exposure to drug occurs in days 34-50 of gestation.	Thalidomide is an effective drug for some forms of leprosy. Treated women should have an effective mode of contraception.

Drugs and Chemicals Proven to Be Teratogenic in Humans *(continued)*

Drug/ Chemical	Fetal Adverse Effects	Relative Risk for Teratogenicity	Clinical Intervention
Trimethadione	**Fetal trimethadione syndrome:** Intrauterine growth retardation, cardiac anomalies, microcephaly, cleft palate and lip, abnormal ears, dysmorphic face, mental retardation, tracheoesophageal fistula, postnatal death	Based on case reports: 83% risk; 32% infantile or neonatal death	No need for this antiepileptic to date
Valproic acid	Lumbosacral spina bifida with meningomyelocele; CNS defects, microcephaly, cardiac defects	1.2% risk of neural tube defects	Level 2 ultrasound and maternal α-fetoproteins or amniocentesis to rule out neural tube defects. Epilepsy itself increases teratogenic risk.
Warfarin	**Fetal warfarin syndrome:** Nasal hypoplasia, chondrodysplasia punctata, branchydactyly, skull defects, abnormal ears, malformed eyes, CNS malformations, microcephaly, hydrocephalus, skeletal deformities, mental retardation, optic atrophy, spasticity, Dandy Walker malformations	16% of exposed fetuses have malformation; another 3% hemorrhages; 8% stillbirths	**Prospective:** Switch to heparin for the first trimester. Deliver by a cesarean section. Women should be followed up in a high-risk perinatal unit.

Reprinted with permission from "Drugs and Chemicals Proven to Be Teratogenic in Humans," *Maternal-Fetal Toxicology: A Clinician's Guide*, 2nd ed, Koren G, ed, New York, NY: Marcel Dekker, Inc, 1994, 37-43.

ANGIOTENSIN-RELATED AGENTS

Comparisons of Indications and Adult Dosages

Drug	Hypertension	CHF	Renal Dysfunction	Dialyzable	Strengths (mg)
Benazepril	20-80 mg qd qd-bid Maximum: 80 mg qd	Not FDA approved	Cl_{cr} <30 mL/min: 5 mg/day initially Maximum: 40 mg qd	Yes	Tablets 5, 10, 20, 40
Candesartan†	8-32 mg qd qd-bid Maximum: 32 mg qd	Not FDA approved	No adjustment necessary	No	Tablets 4, 8, 16, 32
Captopril	25-150 mg qd bid-tid Maximum: 450 mg qd	6.25-100 mg tid Maximum: 450 mg qd	Cl_{cr} 10-50 mL/min: 75% of usual dose Cl_{cr} <10 mL/min: 50% of usual dose	Yes	Tablets 12.5, 25, 50, 100
Enalapril	5-40 mg qd qd-bid Maximum: 40 mg qd	2.5-20 mg bid Maximum: 20 mg bid	Cl_{cr} 30-80 mL/min: 5 mg/day initially Cl_{cr} <30 mL/min: 2.5 mg/day initially	Yes	Tablets 2.5, 5, 10, 20
(Enalaprilat*)	(0.625 mg, 1.25 mg, 2.5 mg q6h Maximum: 5 mg q6h)	(Not FDA approved)	Cl_{cr} <30 mL/min: 0.625 mg)	(Yes)	(2.5 mg/2 mL vial)
Eprosartan†	400-800 mg qd qd-bid	Not FDA approved	No dosage adjustment necessary	Unknown	Tablets 400, 600
Fosinopril	10-40 mg qd Maximum: 80 mg qd	10-40 mg qd	No dosage reduction necessary	Not well dialyzed	Tablets 10, 20
Irbesartan†	150 mg qd Maximum: 300 mg qd	Not FDA approved	No dosage reduction necessary	No	Tablets 75, 150, 300
Lisinopril	10-40 mg qd Maximum: 80 mg qd	5-20 mg qd	Cl_{cr} 10-30 mL/min: 5 mg/day initially Cl_{cr} <10 mL/min: 2.5 mg/day initially	Yes	Tablets 5, 10, 20, 40
Losartan†	25-100 mg qd or bid	Not FDA approved	No adjustment needed	No	Tablets 25, 50
Moexipril	7.5-30 mg qd qd-bid Maximum: 30 mg qd	Not FDA approved	Cl_{cr} <30 mL/min: 3.75 mg/day initially Maximum: 15 mg/day	Unknown	Tablets 7.5, 15
Perindopril	4-16 mg qd	4 mg qd (Not FDA approved)	Cl_{cr} 30-60 mL/min: 2 mg qd Cl_{cr} 15-29 mL/min: 2 mg qod Cl_{cr} <15 mL/min: 2 mg on dialysis days	Yes	Tablets 2, 4, 8
Quinapril	10-80 mg qd qd-bid	5-20 mg bid	Cl_{cr} 30-60 mL/min: 5 mg/day initially Cl_{cr} <10 mL/min: 2.5 mg qd initially	Not well dialyzed	Tablets 5, 10, 20, 40
Ramipril	2.5-20 mg qd qd-bid	2.5-20 mg qd	Cl_{cr} <40 mL/min: 1.25 mg/day Maximum: 5 mg qd	Unknown	Capsules 1.25, 2.5, 5

Comparisons of Indications and Adult Dosages *(continued)*

Drug	Hypertension	CHF	Renal Dysfunction	Dialyzable	Strengths (mg)
Telmisartan†	20-80 mg qd	Not FDA approved	No dosage reduction necessary	No	Tablets 40, 80
Trandolapril	2-4 mg qd maximum: 8 mg/d qd-bid	Not FDA approved	Cl_{cr} <30 mL/min: 0.5 mg/day initially	No	Tablets 1 mg, 2 mg, 4 mg
Valsartan†	80-160 mg qd	Not FDA approved	Decrease dose only if Cl_{cr} <10 mL/minute	No	Capsules 80, 160

*Enalaprilat is the only available ACEI in a parenteral formulation.

†Angiotensin II antagonist

Dosage is based on 70 kg adult with normal hepatic and renal function.

ANGIOTENSIN-RELATED AGENTS *(Continued)*

Comparative Pharmacokinetics

Drug	Prodrug	Lipid Solubility	Absorption (%)	Serum $t_{1/2}$ (h)	Serum Protein Binding (%)	Elimination	Onset of Hypotensive Action (h)	Peak Hypotensive Effects (h)	Duration of Hypotensive Effects (h)
Benazepril	Yes	No data	37	10-12	>95	Primarily renal, some biliary	0.5-1	0.5-1	24
Benazeprilat									
Captopril	No	Not very lipophilic	75	<2	25-30	Metabolism to disulfide, then renally	0.25-0.5	0.5-1.5	6-12
Enalapril	Yes	Lipophilic	60 (53-73)	1.3	50-60	Renal	1	4-6	24
Enalaprilat				11			0.25	3-4	~6
Fosinopril	Yes	Very lipophilic	36	12	>95	Renal 50% Hepatic 50%	1	~3	24
Fosinoprilat									
Lisinopril	No	Very hydrophilic	25 (6-60)	12	0	Renal	1	~7	24
Moexipril	Yes	No data		2-9	≥50	Urine 13% Feces 53%	1		24
Perindopril	Yes		65-95	1.5-3	10-20	Hepatic/Renal		1	
Perindoprilat				25-30	60			3-4	
Quinapril	Yes	No data	60	0.8	97	Renal 61% Hepatic 37%	1	1	24
Quinaprilat				2					
Ramipril	Yes	Somewhat lipophilic	50-100	1-2	73	Renal	1-2	1	24
Ramiprilat				13-17	56				
Trandolapril	Yes	Very lipophilic	10-70	0.6-1.1	80	Hepatic/Renal	0.5	2-4	≥24
Trandolaprilat			40-60	16-24	94				

Comparative Pharmacokinetics of Angiotensin II Receptor Antagonists

	Candesartan	Eprosartan	Irbesartan	Losartan	Telmisartan	Valsartan
Prodrug	Yes*	No	No	Yes†	No	No
Time to peak (h)	3-4	1-2	1.5-2	1 / 2-4†	0.5-1	2-4
Bioavailability (%)	15	13%	60-80	33	42-58	25
Food - Area-under-the-curve	No effect	No effect	No effect	9% to 10%	9.6% to 20%	9% to 40%
Elimination half-life (h)	9	5-9	11-15	2 / 6-9†	24	6
Elimination altered in renal dysfunction	Yes‡	No	No	No	No	No
Precautions in severe renal dysfunction	Yes	Yes	Yes	Yes	Yes	Yes
Elimination altered in hepatic dysfunction	No	No	No	Yes	Yes	Yes
Precautions in hepatic dysfunction	No	Yes	No	No	Yes	No
Protein binding (%)	>99	98	90	~99	>99.5	95

*Candesartan cilexetil: Active metabolite candesartan

†Losartan: Active metabolite EXP3174

‡Dosage adjustments are not necessary

ANTICONVULSANTS BY SEIZURE TYPE

Seizure Type	Age	Commonly Used	Alternatives
Primarily generalized tonic-clonic seizures	1-12 mo	Carbamazepine Phenytoin Phenobarbital	Valproate
	1-6 y	Carbamazepine Phenytoin Phenobarbital	Valproate
	6-11 y	Carbamazepine	Valproate Phenytoin Phenobarbital Lamotrigine†
Primarily generalized tonic-clonic seizures with absence or with myoclonic seizures	1 mo - 18 y	Valproate	Phenytoin‡ Phenobarbital‡ Carbamazepine‡
Absence seizures	Any age	Ethosuximide	Valproate Clonazepam Diamox Lamotrigine†
Myoclonic seizures	Any age	Valproate Clonazepam	Phenytoin† Phenobarbital†
Tonic and atonic seizures	Any age	Valproate	Phenytoin† Clonazepam Phenobarbital†
Partial seizures	1-12 mo	Phenobarbital	Carbamazepine Phenytoin
	1-6 y	Carbamazepine	Phenytoin Phenobarbital Valproate† Lamotrigine† Oxcarbazepine (4-6 y) Gabapentin
	6-18 y	Carbamazepine	Lamotrigine Phenytoin Phenobarbital Oxcarbazepine (6-16 y) Tiagabine Topiramate Valproate†
Infantile spasms		Corticotropin (ACTH)	Prednisone† Valproate† Clonazepam† Diazepam†

†Not FDA approved for this indication.

‡Phenytoin, phenobarbital, carbamazepine will not treat absence seizures. Addition of another anticonvulsant (ie, ethosuximide) would be needed.

ANTIDEPRESSANT AGENTS

Comparison of Usual Dosage, Mechanism of Action, and Adverse Effects of Antidepressants

Drug	Usual Dosage (mg/d)	Reuptake Inhibition		Adverse Effects					
		N	S	ACH	Drowsiness	Orthostatic Hypotension	Cardiac Arrhythmias	GI Distress	Weight Gain
First-Generation Antidepressants *Tricyclic Antidepressants*									
Amitriptyline (Elavil®, Endep®)	100-300	Moderate	High	4+	4+	4+	3+	1	4+
Clomipramine† (Anafranil®)	100-250	Moderate	High	4+	4+	2+	3+	1+	4+
Desipramine (Norpramin®, Pertofrane®)	100-300	High	Low	1+	2+	2+	2+	0	1+
Doxepin (Adapin®, Sinequan®)	100-300	Low	Moderate	3+	4+	2+	2+	0	4+
Imipramine (Janimine®, Tofranil®)	100-300	Moderate	Moderate	3+	3+	4+	3+	1+	4+
Nortriptyline (Aventyl®, Pamelor®)	50-200	Moderate	Low	2+	2+	1+	2+	0	1+
Protriptyline (Vivactil®)	15-60	Moderate	Low	2+	1+	2+	3+	0	0
Trimipramine (Surmontil®)	100-300	Low	Low	4+	4+	3+	3+	0	4+
Monoamine Oxidase Inhibitors									
Phenelzine (Nardil®)	15-90	—	—	2+	2+	2+	1+	1+	3+
Tranylcypromine (Parnate®)	10-40	—	—	2+	1+	2+	1+	1+	2+
Second-Generation Antidepressants *Older Second-Generation Antidepressants*									
Amoxapine (Asendin®)	100-400	Moderate	Low	2+	2+	2+	2+	0	2+
Maprotiline (Ludiomil®)	100-225	Moderate	Low	2+	3+	2+	2+	0	2+
Trazodone (Desyrel®)	150-500	Very low	Moderate	0	4+	3+	1+	1+	2+
Newer Second-Generation Antidepressants									
Bupropion (Wellbutrin®)	300-450‡	Very low§	Very low§	0	0	0	1+	1+	0

ANTIDEPRESSANT AGENTS *(Continued)*

Comparison of Usual Dosage, Mechanism of Action, and Adverse Effects of Antidepressants *(continued)*

Drug	Usual Dosage (mg/d)	Reuptake Inhibition		Adverse Effects					
		N	S	ACH	Drowsiness	Orthostatic Hypotension	Cardiac Arrhythmias	GI Distress	Weight Gain
Third-Generation Antidepressants *Selective Serotonin Reuptake Inhibitors*									
Citalopram (Celexa®)	20-60	Very low	Very high	0	0	0	0	3+¶	0
Fluoxetine (Prozac®)	10-40	Very low	High	0	0	0	0	3+¶	0
Fluvoxamine (Luvox®)	100-300	Very low	Very high	0	0	0	0	3+¶	0
Paroxetine (Paxil®)	20-50	Very low	Very high	1+	1+	0	0	3+¶	1+
Sertraline (Zoloft®)	50-150	Very low	Very high	0	0	0	0	3+¶	0
Serotonin/Norepinephrine Reuptake Inhibitors									
Venlafaxine# (Effexor®)	75-375	Very high	Very high	1+	1+	0	1+	3+¶	0
Atypical Antidepressants with 5HT2 Receptor Antagonist Properties									
Mirtazapine (Remeron®)**	15-45	Very low	Very low	1+	2+	0	0	0	3
Nefazodone (Serzone®)**	300-600	Very low	High	1+	1+	0	0	1+	0

Key: N = norepinephrine; S = serotonin; ACH = anticholinergic effects (dry mouth, blurred vision, urinary retention, constipation); 0 - 4+ = absent or rare - relatively common.

†Not approved by FDA for depression

‡Not to exceed 150 mg/dose to minimize seizure risk

§Norepinephrine and serotonin reuptake inhibition is minimal, but inhibits dopamine reuptake

¶Nausea is usually mild and transient

Comparative studies evaluating the adverse effects of venlafaxine in relation to other antidepressants have not been performed

** These agents work primarily through antagonizing the postsynaptic 5HT2 receptor.

BETA-BLOCKERS

Agent*	Adrenergic Receptor Blocking Activity	Lipid Solubility	Protein Bound (%)	Half-life (h)	Bioavailability (%)	Primary (Secondary) Route of Elimination	Starting Oral Daily Dose	Indications	Usual Dosage
Acebutolol (Sectral®)	$beta_1$	Low	15-25	3-4	40 7-fold†	Hepatic (renal)	400 mg	Hypertension Arrhythmias	P.O.: 400-1200 mg/d
Atenolol (Tenormin®)	$beta_1$	Low	<5-10	6-9‡	50-60 4-fold†	Renal (hepatic)	50 mg	Hypertension Angina pectoris Acute MI	P.O. 50-200 mg/d I.V.: 5 mg x 2 doses
Betaxolol (Kerlone®)	$beta_1$	Low	50	14-22	89	Hepatic (renal)	10 mg	Hypertension	P.O.: 10-20 mg
Bisoprolol (Zebeta™)	$beta_1$	Low	30	9-12	80	Renal	5 mg	Hypertension	P.O.: 10-20 mg
Carteolol (Cartrol®)	$beta_1$ $beta_2$	Low	23-30	6	85	Renal	2.5 mg	Hypertension	P.O.: 2.5-10 mg
Carvedilol (Coreg®)	$beta_1$ $beta_2$ $alpha_1$	High	95-98	6-10	25-35	Hepatic (bile)	6.25 mg bid	Hypertension CHF: Class II, III	Hypertension: 12.5-50 mg/d CHF: 3.125-25 mg bid (weight >85 kg: 50 mg bid)
Esmolol (Brevibloc®)	$beta_1$	Low	55	0.15	NA 5-fold†	Red blood cell	NA	Supraventricular tachycardia Sinus tachycardia	I.V. infusion: 50-200 mcg/kg/min
Labetalol (Trandate®, Normodyne®)	$alpha_1$ $beta_1$ $beta_2$	Moderate	50	5.5-8	18-30 10-fold†	Renal (hepatic)	200 mg	Hypertension	P.O.: 400-800 mg/d I.V.: 20-80 mg at 10-min intervals up to a maximum of 300 mg **or** continuous infusion of 2 mg/min
Metoprolol (Lopressor®)	$beta_1$	Moderate	10-12	3-7	50 10-fold†	Hepatic (renal)	50 mg	Hypertension Angina pectoris Acute MI	P.O.: 100-450 mg/d I.V.: Post-MI 15 mg Angina: 15 mg then 2-5 mg/h Arrhythmias: 0.2 mg/kg
Metoprolol (long-acting)					77				
Nadolol (Corgard®)	$beta_1$ $beta_2$	Low	25-30	20-24	30 5-8-fold†	Renal	80 mg	Hypertension Angina pectoris	P.O.: 40-320 mg/d
Penbutolol (Levatol®)	$beta_1$ $beta_2$	High	80-98	5	100	Hepatic (renal)	20 mg	Hypertension	P.O.: 20-40 mg

BETA-BLOCKERS *(Continued)*

Agent*	Adrenergic Receptor Blocking Activity	Lipid Solubility	Protein Bound (%)	Half-life (h)	Bioavailability (%)	Primary (Secondary) Route of Elimination	Starting Oral Daily Dose	Indications	Usual Dosage
Pindolol (Visken®)	$beta_1$ $beta_2$	Moderate	40	3-4§	90 4-fold†	Hepatic (renal)	20 mg	Hypertension	P.O.: 20-60 mg/d
Propranolol (Inderal®, various)	$beta_1$ $beta_2$	High	90	3-5	30 20-fold†	Hepatic	80 mg	Hypertension Angina pectoris Arrhythmias	P.O.: 40-320 mg/d I.V.: 1-5 mg
Propranolol long-acting (Inderal-LA®)				8-11				Hypertrophic subaortic stenosis Prophylaxis (post-MI)	P.O.: 180-240 mg/d
Sotalol (Betapace®)	$beta_1$ $beta_2$	Low	0	12	90-100	Renal	160 mg	Ventricular arrhythmias Atrial fibrillation	P.O.: 160-320 mg
Timolol (Blocadren®)	$beta_1$ $beta_2$	Low to moderate	<10	4	75 7-fold†	Hepatic (renal)	20 mg	Hypertension Prophylaxis (post-MI)	P.O.: 20-40 mg/d P.O.: 20 mg/d

†Interpatient variations in plasma levels.

‡Half-life increased to 16-27 hours in creatinine clearances of 15-35 mL/min and >27 hours in Cl_{cr} <15 mL/min.

§Half-life variable: 7-15 hours.

BRONCHODILATORS

Comparison of Inhaled Sympathomimetic Bronchodilators

Generic (Brand)	Adrenergic Receptor	Onset (min)	Duration Activity (h)
Albuterol (Proventil®)	$Beta_1 < Beta_2$	<5	3-8
Bitolterol (Tornalate®)	$Beta_1 < Beta_2$	3-4	5 > 8
Epinephrine (Bronkaid®)	Alpha and $Beta_1$ and $Beta_2$	1-5	1-3
Isoetharine (Bronkometer®)	$Beta_1 < Beta_2$	<5	1-3
Isoproterenol (Isuprel®)	$Beta_1$ and $Beta_2$	2-5	0.5-2
Levalbuterol	$Beta_1 < Beta_2$	10-17	5-6
Metaproterenol (Alupent®)	$Beta_1 < Beta_2$	5-30	2-6
Pirbuterol (Maxair®)	$Beta_1 < Beta_2$	<5	5
Salmeterol (Serevent®)	$Beta_1 < Beta_2$	5-14	12
Terbutaline (Brethaire®)	$Beta_1 < Beta_2$	5-30	3-6

CALCIUM CHANNEL BLOCKING AGENTS

	Amlodipine	Bepridil	Diltiazem	Felodipine	Isradipine	Nicardipine	Nifedipine	Nisoldipine	Verapamil
Bioavailability (%)	60-65	59	40	15	15-24	35	60-75	5	20-35
Protein binding (%)	95-98	>99	77-85	99	95	95	95	>99	83-92
Half-life	35-50 h	24 h	3.5-6 h (5-7 h in sustained released preparations)	10-16 h	8 h	2-4 h	2-5 h	7-12 h	Oral: One dose: 2.8-7.4 h Rep dose: 4.5-12 h I.V. (biphasic) Short phase: 4 min Long phase: 2-5 h
Onset of action	—	60 min	Oral: 60 min	2-5 h	120 min	20 min	Oral: 10-20 min	—	Oral: 30 min I.V.: 1-5 min
Peak	6-12 h	2-3 h	Oral: 2-3 h	2-4 h	1.5 h	0.5-2 h	Oral: 0.5-6 h	6-12 h	Oral: 1-2.2 h Oral, ext release: 5-7 h I.V.: 2 h
Duration of action	24 h	—	Ext release: 12 h Tablet: 6-8 h	24 h	—	8 h	12-24 h	—	Oral, ext release: 24 h Tablet: 8-10 h I.V.: 2 h
Elimination	Renal; fecal	Renal	Biliary/renal: 96%-98% (2%-4% unchanged)	Renal: 70% Biliary: 30%	Renal	Renal: 60% Biliary/fecal 35%	Renal: 80% Biliary/fecal 20%	Renal	Renal: 70% Biliary/fecal: 9%-16%
Solubility in water	—	—	Yes	—	—	Slightly	No	—	Yes
Maximum tolerated dosage (adult)	250 mg	—	12 g	—	—	600 mg (standard) 2160 mg (sustained)	900 mg	—	16 g (standard) 9.6 g (sustained)
Therapeutic dose	5-10 mg/day	200-400 mg/day	30-60 mg tid or qid for standard 180-400 mg daily for sustained release	2-10 mg/day	5-20 mg/day	20-40 mg tid for standard 30-60 mg bid for sustained release	10-40 mg tid or qid for standard 90-180 mg once daily for sustained release	20-60 mg/day	80-160 mg qid for standard 120-240 mg once daily for sustained release
Actions									
contractility	0	↓	↓	0/↑	0	↓	↑	0	↓↓
heart rate	0	↓	↓	↑	+/–	↑	↑	+/–	↓
cardiac output	0	0	↑	↑	↑	↑↑	↑	0	↓↑
peripheral vascular resistance	↓↓	↓	↓	↓↓	↓↓↓	↓↓↓	↓↓↓	↓↓↓	↓↓

ND = no data in humans. ++ = most frequent; + = less frequent; – = rare; 0 = no effect.

CORTICOSTEROIDS

Corticosteroids, Systemic Equivalencies

Glucocorticoid	Pregnancy Category	Approximate Equivalent Dose (mg)	Routes of Administration	Relative Anti-inflammatory Potency	Relative Mineralocorticoid Potency	Protein Binding (%)	Half-life	
							Plasma (min)	Biologic (h)
Short-Acting								
Cortisone	D	25	P.O., I.M.	0.8	2	90	30	8-12
Hydrocortisone	C	20	I.M., I.V.	1	2	90	80-118	8-12
Intermediate-Acting								
Methylprednisolone*	—	4	P.O., I.M., I.V.	5	0	—	78-188	18-36
Prednisolone	B	5	P.O., I.M., I.V., intra-articular, intradermal, soft tissue injection	4	1	90-95	115-212	18-36
Prednisone	B	5	P.O.	4	1	70	60	18-36
Triamcinolone*	C	4	P.O., I.M., intra-articular, intradermal, intrasynovial, soft tissue injection	5	0	—	200+	18-36
Long-Acting								
Betamethasone	C	0.6-0.75	P.O., I.M., intra-articular, intradermal, intrasynovial, soft tissue injection	25	0	64	300+	36-54
Dexamethasone	C	0.75	P.O., I.M., I.V., intra-articular, intradermal, soft tissue injection	25-30	0	—	110-210	36-54
Mineralocorticoids								
Fludrocortisone	C	—	P.O.	10	125	42	210+	18-36

*May contain propylene glycol as an excipient in injectable forms.

CORTICOSTEROIDS *(Continued)*

GUIDELINES FOR SELECTION AND USE OF TOPICAL CORTICOSTEROIDS

The quantity prescribed and the frequency of refills should be monitored to reduce the risk of adrenal suppression. In general, short courses of high-potency agents are preferable to prolonged use of low potency. After control is achieved, control should be maintained with a low potency preparation.

1. Low-to-medium potency agents are usually effective for treating thin, acute, inflammatory skin lesions; whereas, high or super-potent agents are often required for treating chronic, hyperkeratotic, or lichenified lesions.
2. Since the stratum corneum is thin on the face and intertriginous areas, low-potency agents are preferred but a higher potency agent may be used for 2 weeks.
3. Because the palms and sole shave a thick stratum corneum, high or super-potent agents are frequently required.
4. Low potency agents are preferred for infants and the elderly. Infants have a high body surface area to weight ratio; elderly patients have thing, fragile skin.
5. The vehicle in which the topical corticosteroid is formulated influences the absorption and potency of the drug. Ointment bases are preferred for thick, lichenified lesions; they enhance penetration of the drug. Creams are preferred for acute and subacute dermatoses; they may be used on moist skin areas or intertriginous areas. Solutions, gels, and sprays are preferred for the scalp or for areas where a nonoil-based vehicle is needed.
6. In general, super-potent agents should not be used for longer than 3 weeks unless the lesion is limited to a small body area. Medium-to-high potency agents usually cause only rare adverse effects when treatment is limited to 3 months or less, and use on the face and intertriginous areas are avoided. If long-term treatment is needed, intermittent vs continued treatment is recommended.
7. Most preparations are applied once or twice daily. More frequent application may be necessary for the palms or soles because the preparation is easily removed by normal activity and penetration is poor due to a thick stratum corneum. Every-other-day or weekend-only application may be effective for treating some chronic conditions.

Corticosteroids, Topical

Steroid		Vehicle
Very High Potency		
0.05%	Augmented betamethasone dipropionate	Ointment
0.05%	Clobetasol propionate	Cream, ointment
0.05%	Diflorasone diacetate	Ointment
0.05%	Halobetasol propionate	Cream, ointment
High Potency		
0.1%	Amcinonide	Cream, ointment, lotion
0.05%	Betamethasone dipropionate, augmented	Cream
0.05%	Betamethasone dipropionate	Cream, ointment
0.1%	Betamethasone valerate	Ointment
0.05%	Desoximetasone	Gel
0.25%	Desoximetasone	Cream, ointment
0.05%	Diflorasone diacetate	Cream, ointment
0.2%	Fluocinolone acetonide	Cream
0.05%	Fluocinonide	Cream, ointment, gel
0.1%	Halcinonide	Cream, ointment
0.5%	Triamcinolone acetonide	Cream, ointment

Corticosteroids, Topical *(continued)*

Steroid		Vehicle
Intermediate Potency		
0.025%	Betamethasone benzoate	Cream, gel, lotion
0.05%	Betamethasone dipropionate	Lotion
0.1%	Betamethasone valerate	Cream
0.1%	Clocortolone pivalate	Cream
0.05%	Desoximetasone	Cream
0.025%	Fluocinolone acetonide	Cream, ointment
0.05%	Flurandrenolide	Cream, ointment, lotion, tape
0.005%	Fluticasone propionate	Ointment
0.05%	Fluticasone propionate	Cream
0.1%	Hydrocortisone butyrate†	Ointment, solution
0.2%	Hydrocortisone valerate†	Cream, ointment
0.1%	Mometasone furoate†	Cream, ointment, lotion
0.025%	Triamcinolone acetonide	Cream, ointment, lotion
0.1%	Triamcinolone acetonide	Cream, ointment, lotion
Low Potency		
0.05%	Alclometasone dipropionate†	Cream, ointment
0.05%	Desonide	Cream
0.01%	Dexamethasone	Aerosol
0.04%	Dexamethasone	Aerosol
0.1%	Dexamethasone sodium phosphate	Cream
0.01%	Fluocinolone acetonide	Cream, solution
0.25%	Hydrocortisone†	Lotion
0.5%	Hydrocortisone†	Cream, ointment, lotion, aerosol
0.5%	Hydrocortisone acetate†	Cream, ointment
1%	Hydrocortisone acetate†	Cream, ointment
1%	Hydrocortisone	Cream, ointment, lotion, solution
2.5%	Hydrocortisone	Cream, ointment, lotion

†Not fluorinated.

HYPOGLYCEMIC DRUGS AND THIAZOLIDINEDIONE INFORMATION

Contraindications to Therapy and Potential Adverse Effects of Oral Antidiabetic Agents

	Sulfonylureas/ Meglitinide	Metformin	Acarbose/ Miglitol	Pioglitazone/ Rosiglitazone
Contraindications				
Insulin dependency	A	A	A*	
Pregnancy/lactation	A	A	A	
Hypersensitivity to the agent	A	A	A	A
Hepatic impairment	R	A	R	A
Renal impairment	R	A	R	
Congestive heart failure		A		R
Chronic lung disease		A		
Peripheral vascular disease		A		
Steroid-induced diabetes	R	R		
Inflammatory bowel disease		A	A	
Major recurrent illness	R	A		
Surgery	R	A		
Alcoholism	R	A		A
Adverse Effects				
Hypoglycemia	Yes	No	No	No
Body weight gain	Yes	No	No	Yes
Hypersensitivity	Yes	No	No	No
Drug interactions	Yes	No	No	Yes/No
Lactic acidosis	No	Yes	No	No
Gastrointestinal disturbances	No	Yes	Yes	No

*Can be used in conjunction with insulin.

A = absolute.

R = relative.

Comparative Pharmacokinetics

Drug	Duration of Action (h)	Dose and Frequency (mg)	Metabolism
Sulfonylureas – First Generation Agents			
Acetohexamide	12-24	250-1500 bid	Hepatic (60%) with active metabolite
Chlorpropamide	24-72	100-500 qd	Renal excretion (30%) and hepatic metabolism with active metabolites
Tolazamide	10-24	100-1000 qd or bid	Hepatic with active metabolites
Tolbutamide	6-24	500-3000 qd-tid	Hepatic
Sulfonylureas – Second Generation Agents			
Glimepiride	24	1-4 mg qd	Hepatic
Glipizide	12-24	2.5-40 qd or bid	Hepatic
Glipizide GITS	24	5-10 qd	Hepatic
Glyburide	16-24	1.25-20 qd or bid	Hepatic with active metabolites
Meglitinides			
Repaglinide	<4 hours (single dose)	0.4-4 mg administered with meals 2, 3, or 4 times/day	Hepatic to inactive metabolites

Comparative Thiazolidinedione Pharmacokinetics

Parameter	Pioglitazone (Actos®)	Rosiglitazone (Avandia®)
Absorption	Food slightly delays but does not alter the extent of absorption	Absolute bioavailability is 99% Food ↓ C_{max} and delays T_{max}, but not change in AUC
C_{max}	156-342 ng/mL	–
T_{max}	2 hours	1 hour
Distribution	0.63 ± 0.41 L/kg	17.6 L
Plasma protein binding	>99% to serum albumin	99.8% to serum albumin
Metabolism	Extensive liver metabolism by hydroxylation and oxidation. Some metabolites are pharmacologically active CYP2C8 and CYP3A4 metabolism	Extensive metabolism via N-demethylation and hydroxylation with no unchanged drug excreted in the urine CYP2C8 and some CYP2C9 metabolism
Excretion	Urine (15% to 30%) and bile	Urine (64%) and feces (23%)
Half-life	3-6 hours (pioglitazone) 16-24 hours (pioglitazone and metabolites)	3.15-3.59 hours
Effect of hemodialysis	Not removed	Not removed

(Package inserts: Actos®, 1999; Avandia®, 1999; Rezulin®, 1999; Plosker, 1999.)

HYPOGLYCEMIC DRUGS AND THIAZOLIDINEDIONE INFORMATION *(Continued)*

Approved Indications for Thiazolidinedione Derivatives

Indication	Pioglitazone (Actos®)	Rosiglitazone (Avandia®)
Monotherapy	X	X
Combination Therapy – Dual Therapy		
Combination with sulfonylureas	X	–
Combination therapy with Glucophage® (metformin)	X	X
Combination therapy with insulin	X	–
Combination Therapy – Triple Therapy		
Combination therapy with sulfonylureas and Glucophage® (metformin)	–	–

(Package inserts: Actos®, 1999; Avandia®, 1999; Rezulin®, 1999.)

Comparative Lipid Effects

Parameter	Pioglitazone (Actos®)	Rosiglitazone (Avandia®)
LDL	No significant change	↑ up to 12.1%
HDL	↑ up to 13%	↑ up to 18.5%
Total cholesterol	No significant change	↑
Total cholesterol/HDL ratio	–	–
LDL/HDL ratio	–	No change
Triglycerides	↓ up to 28%	Variable effects

(Package inserts: Actos®, 1999; Avandia®, 1999; Rezulin®, 1999; Plosker, 1999)

LIPID-LOWERING AGENTS

Effects on Lipoproteins

Drug	Total Cholesterol (%)	LDLC (%)	HDLC (%)	TG (%)
Bile-acid resins	↓20-25	↓20-35	→	↑5-20
Fibric acid derivatives	↓10	↓10 (↑)	↑10-25	↓40-55
HMG-CoA RI (statins)	↓15-35	↓20-40	↑2-15	↓7-25
Nicotinic acid	↓25	↓20	↑20	↓40
Probucol	↓10-15	↓<10	↓30	→

Comparative Dosages of Agents Used to Treat Hyperlipidemia

Antilipemic Agent*	Usual Daily Dose	Average Dosing Interval
Fibric Acid Derivatives		
Clofibrate	2000 mg	qid
Gemfibrozil	1200 mg	bid
Miscellaneous Agents		
Niacin	6 g	tid
Bile Acid Sequestrants		
Colestipol	max: 30 g	bid
Cholestyramine	max: 24 g	tid-qid

Dosage is based on 70 kg adult with normal hepatic and renal function.

Recommended Liver Function Monitoring for HMG-CoA Reductase Inhibitors

Agent	Initial and After Elevation in Dose	6 Weeks*	12 Weeks*	Semiannually
Atorvastatin	x	x	x	x
Cerivastatin	x	x	x	x
Fluvastatin	x	x	x	x
Lovastatin	x	x	x	x
Pravastatin	x		x	
Simvastatin	x			x

*After initiation of therapy or any elevation in dose.

Comparative Dosages of HMG-CoA Reductase Inhibitors

Agent	Daily Dosage
Atorvastatin (Lipitor®)	10 mg
Cerivastatin (Baycol®)	0.3 mg
Fluvastatin (Lescol®)	20 mg (dose recommended by manufacturer, but appears to be less effective than the recommended doses of atorvastatin, lovastatin, pravastatin, and simvastatin)
Lovastatin (Mevacor®)	20 mg
Pravastatin (Pravachol®)	20 mg
Simvastatin (Zocor®)	10 mg

NARCOTIC AGONISTS

Comparative Pharmacokinetics

Drug	Onset (min)	Peak (h)	Duration (h)	Half-Life (h)	Average Dosing Interval (h)		Equianalgesic Doses* (mg)	
							I.M.	Oral
Alfentanil	Immediate	ND	ND	1-2	—	—	ND	NA
Buprenorphine	15	1	4-8	2-3			0.4	—
Butorphanol	I.M.: 30-60; I.V.: 4-5	0.5-1	3-5	2.5-3.5	3	(3-6)	2	—
Codeine	P.O.: 30-60; I.M.: 10-30	0.5-1	4-6	3-4	3	(3-6)	120	200
Fentanyl	I.M.: 7-15 I.V.: Immediate	ND	1-2	1.5-6	1	(0.5-2)	0.1	NA
Hydrocodone	ND	ND	4-8	3.3-4.4	6	(4-8)	ND	ND
Hydromorphone	P.O.: 15-30	0.5-1	4-6	2-4	4	(3-6)	1.5	7.5
Levorphanol	P.O.: 10-60	0.5-1	4-8	12-16	6	(6-24)	2	4
Meperidine	P.O./I.M./S.C.: 10-15 I.V.: ≤5	0.5-1	2-4	3-4	3	(2-4)	75	300
Methadone	P.O.: 30-60; I.V.: 10-20	0.5-1	4-6 (acute); >8 (chronic)	15-30	8	(6-12)	10	20
Morphine	P.O.: 15-60 I.V.: ≤5	P.O./I.M./S.C.: 0.5-1; I.V.: 0.3	3-6	2-4	4	(3-6)	10	60# (acute); 30 (chronic)
Nalbuphine	I.M.: 30; I.V.: 1-3	1	3-6	5		—	10	—
Oxycodone	P.O.: 10-15	0.5-1	4-6	3-4	4	(3-6)	NA	30
Oxymorphone	5-15	0.5-1	3-6				1	10†
Pentazocine	15-20	0.25-1	3-4	2-3	3	(3-6)		

Comparative Pharmacokinetics *(continued)*

Drug	Onset (min)	Peak (h)	Duration (h)	Half-Life (h)	Average Dosing Interval (h)		Equianalgesic Doses* (mg)	
							I.M.	Oral
Propoxyphene	P.O.: 30-60	2-2.5	4-6	3.5-15	6	(4-8)	ND	130‡-200§
Remifentanil	1-3	<0.3	0.1-0.2	0.15-0.3	—	—	ND	ND
Sufentanil	1.3-3	ND	ND	2.5-3	—	—	0.02	NA

ND = no data available. NA = not applicable.

*Based on acute, short-term use. Chronic administration may alter pharmacokinetics and decrease the oral parenteral dose ratio. The morphine oral-parenteral ratio decreases to ~1.5-2.5:1 upon chronic dosing.

#Extensive survey data suggest that the relative potency of I.M.:P.O. morphine of 1:6 changes to 1:2-3 with chronic dosing.

†Rectal

‡HCl salt

§Napsylate salt

NARCOTIC AGONISTS *(Continued)*

Comparative Pharmacology

Drug	Analgesic	Antitussive	Constipation	Respiratory Depression	Sedation	Emesis
Phenanthrenes						
Codeine	+	+++	+	+	+	+
Hydrocodone	+	+++		+		
Hydromorphone	++	+++	+	++	+	+
Levorphanol	++	++	++	++	++	+
Morphine	++	+++	++	++	++	++
Oxycodone	++	+++	++	++	++	++
Oxymorphone	++	+	++	+++		+++
Phenylpiperidines						
Alfentanil	++					
Fentanyl	++			+		+
Meperidine	++	+	+	++	+	
Sufentanil	+++					
Diphenylheptanes						
Methadone	++	++	++	++	+	+
Propoxyphene	+			+	+	+
Agonist/Antagonist						
Buprenorphine	++	N/A	+++	+++	++	++
Butorphanol	++	N/A	+++	+++	++	+
Dezocine	++		+	++	+	++
Nalbuphine	++	N/A	+++	+++	++	++
Pentazocine	++	N/A	+	++	++ or stimulation	++

NICOTINE PRODUCTS

Dosage Form	Brand Name	Dosing	Recommended Treatment Duration	Strengths Available
Chewing gum	Nicorette® (OTC)	Chew 1 piece q1-2h for 6 wks, then decrease to 1 piece q2-4h for 3 wks, then 1 piece q4-8h for 3 wks, then discontinue	~12 wks	2 mg, 4 mg
Transdermal	Habitrol® (OTC)	One 21 mg/d patch qd for 4-8 wks, then one 14 mg/d patch qd for 2-4 wks, then one 7 mg/d patch qd for 2-4 wks, then discontinue Low-dose Regimen[1]: One 14 mg/d patch qd for 6 wks, then one 7 mg/d patch qd for 2-4 wks, then discontinue	~12 wks	Patch: 21 mg/d 14 mg/d 7 mg/d
	Nicoderm CQ® (OTC)	One 21 mg/d patch qd for 6 wks, then one 14 mg/d patch qd for 2 wks, then one 7 mg/d patch qd for 2 wks, then discontinue Low-dose Regimen[1]: One 14 mg/d patch qd for 6 wks, then one 7 mg/d patch qd for 2 wks, then discontinue	~10 wks	Patch: 21 mg/d 14 mg/d 7 mg/d
	Nicotrol®	One 15 mg patch qd, worn for 16 h/d and removed for 8 h/d for a total of 6 wks, then discontinue	~6 wks	15 mg/16 h patch
Nasal spray	Nicotrol® NS	One dose is 2 sprays (1 spray in each nostril) Initial dose: 1-2 sprays q1h, should not exceed 10 sprays (5 doses)/h or 80 sprays (40 doses)/d	~12 wks	10 mL spray 0.5/mg spray (200 actuations)
Inhaler	Nicotrol®	Inhaler releases 4 mg nicotine (the equivalent of 2 cigarettes smoked) for 20 min of active inhaler puffing Usual dose: 6-16 cartridges/d for up to 12 wks, then reduce dose gradually over ensuing 12 wks, then discontinue	~18-24 wks	10 mg/ cartridge: releases 4 mg/ cartridge

[1]Transdermal low-dose regimens are intended for patients <100 lbs, smoke <10 cigarettes/d, and/or have a history of cardiovascular disease.

NONSTEROIDAL ANTI-INFLAMMATORY AGENTS

Comparative Dosages and Pharmacokinetics

Drug	Maximum Recommended Daily Dose (mg)	Time to Peak Levels (h)*	Half-life (h)
Propionic Acids			
Fenoprofen (Nalfon®)	3200	1-2	2-3
Flurbiprofen (Ansaid®)	300	1.5	5.7
Ibuprofen	3200	1-2	1.8-2.5
Ketoprofen (Orudis®)	300	0.5-2	2-4
Naproxen (Naprosyn®)	1500	2-4	12-15
Naproxen sodium (Anaprox®)	1375	1-2	12-13
Oxaprozin	1800	3-5	42-50
Acetic Acids			
Diclofenac sodium delayed release (Voltaren®)	225	2-3	1-2
Diclofenac potassium immediate release (Cataflam®)	200	1	1-2
Etodolac (Lodine®)	1200	1-2	7.3
Indomethacin (Indocin®)	200	1-2	4.5
Indomethacin SR	150	2-4	4.5-6
Ketorolac (Toradol®)	I.M.: 120† P.O.: 40	0.5-1	3.8-8.6
Sulindac (Clinoril®)	400	2-4	7.8 (16.4)‡
Tolmetin (Tolectin®)	2000	0.5-1	1-1.5
Fenamates (Anthranilic Acids)			
Meclofenamate (Meclomen®)	400	0.5-1	2 (3.3)§
Mefenamic acid (Ponstel®)	1000	2-4	2-4
Nonacidic Agent			
Nabumetone (Relafen®)	2000	3-6	24
Oxicam			
Piroxicam (Feldene®)	20	3-5	30-86
Cox-2 Inhibitors			
Celecoxib (Celebrex®)	400	3	11
Rofecoxib (Vioxx®)	50	2-3	17

Dosage is based on 70 kg adult with normal hepatic and renal function.

*Food decreases the rate of absorption and may delay the time to peak levels.

†150 mg on the first day.

‡Half-life of active sulfide metabolite.

§Half-life with multiple doses.

PARKINSON'S DISEASE DOSING

Dosing of Drugs Used for the Treatment of Parkinson's Disease

Generic Drug (Brand Name)	Receptor Affinity	Initial Dose	Titration Schedule	Usual Daily Dosage Range	Recommended Dosing Schedule
Amantadine (Symmetrel®)	NMDA receptor antagonist and inhibits neuronal reuptake of dopamine	100 mg every other day	100 mg/dose every week, up to 300 mg 3 times/d	100-200 mg	Twice daily
Benztropine (Cogentin®)	Cholinergic receptors, also has antihistamine effects	0.5-2 mg/d in 1-4 divided doses	0.5 mg/dose every 5-6 d	2-6 mg	1-2 times/d
Bromocriptine (Parlodel®)	Moderate affinity for D_2 and D_3 dopamine receptors	1.25 mg twice daily	2.5 mg/d every 2-4 wks	2.5-100 mg	3 times/d
Cabergoline (Dostinex)*	Selective to D_2 dopamine receptors	0.5 mg once daily	0.25-0.5 mg/d every 4 wks	0.5-5 mg	Once daily
Entacapone (Comtan®)	COMT enzyme inhibitor	200 mg 3 times/day	Titrate down the doses of levodopa/carbidopa as required	600-1600 mg	3 times/d; up to 8 times/d
Levodopa/carbidopa (Sinemet® CR)	Converts to dopamine; binds to all CNS dopamine receptors	10/100-25/100 mg 2-4 times/d	One-half to 1 tablet (10/100 or 25/100) every 1-2 d	50/200 to 200/2000 mg (3-8 tablets)	3 times/d or twice daily (for controlled release)
Pergolide (Permax®)	Low affinity for D_1 and maximal affinity for D_2 and D_3 dopamine receptors	0.05 mg/night	0.1-0.15 mg/d every 3 d for 12 d, then 0.25 mg/d every 3 d	0.05-5 mg	3 times/d
Pramipexole (Mirapex®)	High affinity for D_2 and D_3 dopamine receptors	0.125 mg 3 times/d	0.125 mg/dose every 5-7 d	1.5-4.5 mg	3 times/d
Ropinirole (Requip®)	High affinity for D_2 and D_3 dopamine receptors	0.25 mg 3 times/d	0.25 mg/dose weekly for 4 wks, then 1.5 mg/d every week up to 9 mg/d; 3 mg/d up to a max of 24 mg/d	0.75-24 mg	3 times/d

PARKINSON'S DISEASE DOSING *(Continued)*

Dosing of Drugs Used for the Treatment of Parkinson's Disease *(continued)*

Generic Drug (Brand Name)	Receptor Affinity	Initial Dose	Titration Schedule	Usual Daily Dosage Range	Recommended Dosing Schedule
Selegiline (Eldepryl®)	No receptor effects, inhibits monoamine oxidase	5-10 mg twice daily	Titrate down the doses of levodopa/carbidopa as required	5-10 mg	Twice daily
Tolcapone (Tasmar®)	COMT enzyme inhibitor	100 mg 3 times/d	Titrate down the doses of levodopa/carbidopa as required	300-600 mg	3 times/d

*Cabergoline is not FDA approved for the treatment of Parkinson's disease.

HERBAL AND NUTRITIONAL PRODUCTS

TOP HERBAL PRODUCTS

This section contains general information on commonly encountered herbal or nutritional products. A more complete listing products follows.

Alpha-lipoic Acid

Synonyms: Alpha-lipoate; Lipoic Acid; Thioctic acid
Use: Glaucoma, neuropathies
Mechanism of Action/Effect: Alpha-lipoic acid is a sulfur-containing cofactor which is normally synthesized in humans. Alpha-lipoic acid functions as a potent antioxidant.
Warnings: Use with caution in individuals who may be predisposed to hypoglycemia (including individuals receiving antidiabetic agents)
Drug Interactions: Oral hypoglycemics or insulin
Adverse Reactions: Dermatologic reactions (rashes) have been reported with alpha-lipoic acid
Dosing: Oral: Range: 20-600 mg/day; common dosage: 25-50 mg twice daily

Androstenedione

Use: Increase strength and muscle mass
Mechanism of Action/Effect: Androstenedione is a weak androgenic steroid hormone. Androstenedione is believed to facilitate faster recovery from exercise and to promote muscle development in response to training.
Warnings: Use with caution in individuals with congestive heart failure; not to be used in individuals with hypertension. Caution should be used in prostate conditions and hormone-sensitive tumors. The FDA requires specific labeling on this supplement, noting that these supplements "contain steroid hormones that may cause breast enlargement, testicular shrinkage, and infertility in males, and increased facial and body hair, voice deepening and clitoral enlargement in females."
Drug Interactions: Estrogens and androgenic drugs
Dosing: Oral: 50-100 mg/day, usually about 1 hour before exercising

Arginine

Synonyms: L-Arginine
Use: Helps to lower elevated cholesterol, improve circulation, increase lean body mass, inflammatory bowel disease, immunity enhancement, male infertility, surgery and wound healing, sexual vitality and enhancement
Mechanism of Action/Effect: Arginine plays a key role in the urea cycle, which is the biochemical pathway that metabolized protein and other nitrogen-containing compounds. It has also has been found that arginine is the precursor to nitric oxide.
Contraindications: Caution in individuals with herpes simplex since arginine can stimulate the growth of this virus.
Drug Interactions: Nitroglycerin and sildenafil
Dosing: Oral: Dosage range: 3-6 g/day

Bifidobacterium bifidum / Lactobacillus acidophilus

Use:

B. bifidum: Crohn's disease, diarrhea, maintenance of anaerobic microflora in the colon, ulcerative colitis

L. acidophilus: Constipation, infant diarrhea, lactose intolerance, recolonization of the GI tract with beneficial bacteria during and after antibiotic use

Mechanism of Action/Effect: Natural components of colonic flora, used to facilitate recolonization with benign symbiotic organisms; promote vitamin K synthesis and absorption
Drug Interactions: Antibiotics eliminate *B. bifidum* and *L. acidophilus*
Adverse Reactions: No known toxicity or serious side effect
Dosing: Oral: 5-10 billion colony forming units (CFU) per day (dairy free); refrigerate to maintain optimum potency

Bilberry

Synonym: *Vaccinium myrtillus*
Use:

Ophthalmologic disorders: Macular degeneration, diabetic retinopathy, cataracts
Vascular disorders: Varicose veins, phlebitis

HERBAL AND NUTRITIONAL PRODUCTS *(Continued)*

Mechanism of Action/Effect: Bilberry reportedly inhibits a variety of inflammatory mediators, including histamine, proteases, leukotrienes, and prostaglandins. May decrease capillary permeability and inhibit platelet aggregation.
Contraindications: Contraindicated in individuals with active bleeding (eg, peptic ulcer, intracranial bleeding).
Warnings: Use with caution in individuals with a history of bleeding, hemostatic disorders, or drug-related hemostatic problems. Use with caution in individuals taking anticoagulant medications, including warfarin, aspirin, aspirin-containing products, NSAIDs, or antiplatelet agents (eg, ticlopidine, clopidogrel, dipyridamole). Discontinue use prior to dental or surgical procedures (generally at least 14 days before).
Drug Interactions: Oral hypoglycemics or insulin (effects may be altered)
Dosing: Oral: 80 mg 2-3 times/day

Black Cohosh

Synonym: *Cimicifuga racemosa*
Use: Vasomotor symptoms of menopause; premenstrual syndrome (PMS), mild depression, arthritis
Mechanism of Action/Effect: Contains multiple phytoestrogens and salicylic acid (small amounts)
Contraindications: Contraindicated in pregnancy (may stimulate uterine contractions) and lactation; contraindicated in individuals with a history of estrogen-dependent tumors or endometrial cancer
Warnings: Use with caution in individuals allergic to salicylates; it is not known whether the amount of salicylic acid is likely to affect platelet aggregation or have other effects associated with salicylates. Use with caution in individuals on hormone replacement therapy or oral contraceptives or a history of thromboembolic disease or stroke.
Drug Interactions: Oral contraceptives, hormonal replacement therapy
Adverse Reactions: May cause nausea, vomiting, headache and hypotension at higher dosages
Dosing: Oral: 20-40 mg twice daily

Chamomile

Synonyms: *Matricaria chamomilla*; *Matricaria recutita*
Use: Has been used for indigestion and its hypnotic properties; topical anti-inflammatory agent; used for hemorrhoids, irritable bowel, eczema, mastitis and leg ulcers; used to flavor cigarette tobacco
Mechanism of Action/Effect: Pharmacologic activities include antispasmodic, anti-inflammatory, antiulcer, and antibacterial effects; a sedative effect has also been documented
Contraindications: Hypersensitivity to *Asteraceae/Compositae* family or ragweed pollens
Warnings: Use with caution in asthmatics; cross sensitivity may occur in individuals allergic to ragweed pollens, asters, or chrysanthemums.
Drug Interactions: May increase effect of coumarin-type anticoagulants at high doses; may potentiate sedatives (benzodiazepines, barbiturates)
Adverse Reactions: Contact dermatitis, emesis (from dried flowering heads), anaphylaxis; can cause hypersensitivity reactions especially in atopic individuals
Dosing:

Tea: ±150 mL H_2O poured over heaping tablespoon (±3 g) of chamomile, covered and steeped 5-10 minutes; tea is used 3-4 times/day for GI upset

Liquid extract: 1-4 mL 3 times/day

Pregnancy Implications: Excessive use should be avoided due to potential teratogenicity.

Chasteberry

Synonyms: Chastetree; *Vitex agnus-castus*
Use: Acne vulgaris, corpus luteum insufficiency, hyperprolactinemia, insufficient lactation, menopause, menstrual disorders (amenorrhea, endometriosis, premenstrual syndrome)
Mechanism of Action/Effect: Noted to possess significant effect on pituitary function and has been demonstrated to have progesterone-like effects. In addition, it may stimulate luteinizing hormone (LH) and inhibit follicle-stimulating hormone (FSH).
Contraindications: Contraindicated in pregnancy and lactation, based on case reports of uterine stimulation and emmenagogue effects
Warnings: Use with caution in individuals receiving hormonal therapy.

Drug Interactions: Hormonal replacement therapy, oral contraceptives, dopamine antagonists such as metoclopramide and antipsychotics
Dosing: Oral: 400 mg/day (in the morning, preferably on an empty stomach)

Chondroitin Sulfate

Use: Osteoarthritis
Mechanism of Action/Effect: Chondroitin sulfate also inhibits synovial enzymes (elastase, hyaluronidase) which may contribute to cartilage destruction and loss of joint function. Although studes are not conclusive, chondroitin has been reported to act synergistically with glucosamine to support the maintenance of strong, healthy cartilage and maintain joint function.
Warnings: Chondroitin has no known toxicity or serious side effects.
Dosing: Oral: Dosage range: 300-1500 mg/day

Chromium

Use: Improves glycemic control; increases lean body mass; reduces obesity; improves lipid profile by decreasing total cholesterol and triglycerides, increasing HDL
Mechanism of Action/Effect: Chromium picolinate is the only active form of chromium. It appears that chromium, in its trivalent form, increases insulin sensitivity and improves glucose transport into cells. The mechanism by which this happens could include one or more of the following: Increase the number of insulin receptors, enhance insulin binding to target tissues, promote activation of insulin-receptor tyrosine dinase activity, enhance beta-cell sensitivity in the pancreas.
Drug Interactions: Any medications that may also affect blood sugars (eg, beta-blockers, thiazides, oral hypoglycemics, and insulin); discuss chromium use prior to initiating
Adverse Reactions: Nausea, loose stools, flatulence, changes in appetite; isolated reports of anemia, cognitive impairment, renal failure
Dosing: 50-600 mcg/day

Coenzyme Q_{10}

Synonym: Ubiquinone
Use: Angina, chronic fatigue syndrome, CHF, hypertension, muscular dystrophy, obesity, periodontal disease
Mechanism of Action/Effect: Coenzyme Q_{10} is involved in ATP generation, the primary source of energy in human physiology. Functions as a lipid-soluble antioxidant, providing protection against free radical damage. Dosages in excess of 300 mg per day have been reported to be of benefit in some conditions, including breast cancer, diabetes, and cardiovascular diseases.
Drug Interactions: Drugs which can cause depletion of CoQ_{10}: Hydralazine, thiazide diuretics, HMG-CoA reductase inhibitors, sulfonylureas, beta blockers, tricyclic antidepressants, chlorpromazine, clonidine, methyldopa, diazoxide, biguanides, haloperidol; CoQ_{10} may decrease response to warfarin
Dosing: Oral: Dosage range: 30-200 mg/day

Cranberry

Synonyms: *Vaccinium macrocarpon*
Use: Prevention of nephrolithiasis, urinary tract infection
Mechanism of Action/Effect: Although early research indicated that cranberry worked through urinary acidification, current research indicates that a cranberry-derived glycoprotein inhibits *E. coli.* adherence to the epithelial cells of the urinary tract.
Contraindications: None known
Drug Interactions: None known
Dosing: Oral: 300-400 mg twice daily or 8-16 ounces of cranberry juice daily; the use of 100% cranberry juice (not cranberry juice cocktail) is recommended.

Dehydroepiandosterone

Synonyms: DHEA
Use: Antiaging, depression, diabetes, fatigue, lupus
Mechanism of Action/Effect: DHEA is secreted by the adrenal glands, and is the precursor for the synthesis of over 50 additional hormones, including estrogen and testosterone. DHEA has also been shown to stimulate the production of insulin growth factor-1 (IGF-1). It has been reported to cause a change in the response to insulin, decreasing the insulin requirement in individuals with diabetes. Supplementation may also increase circulating testosterone levels.
Contraindications: Use is contraindicated in individuals with a history of prostate or breast cancer.

HERBAL AND NUTRITIONAL PRODUCTS *(Continued)*

Warnings: Use with caution in individuals with diabetes or in those who may be predisposed to hypoglycemia. Blood glucose should be closely monitored in individuals with diabetes, and the dosage of antidiabetic agents should be closely monitored among health care providers. Use with caution in individuals with hepatic dysfunction.
Drug Interactions: May interact with androgens, estrogens, corticosteroids, insulin, oral hypoglycemic agents
Adverse Reactions: No known toxicity or serious side effects, however, long-term human studies have not been conducted
Dosing: Oral: Dosage range: 5-50 mg/day; doses of 100 mg/day are sometimes used in elderly individuals

Dong Quai

Synonyms: *Angelica sinensis*; Chinese angelica
Use: Anemia, hypertension, improvement in energy (particularly in females), menopause, dysmenorrhea, PMS, amenorrhea
Mechanism of Action/Effect: Dong quai is rich in phytoestrogens, which may demonstrate similar pharmacological effects, but are less potent than pure estrogenic compounds. Dong quai has also been reported to cause vasodilation and may have hematopoietic properties.
Contraindications: Based on potential interference with platelet aggregation (observed with related species) may alter hemostasis. Contraindicated in individuals with active bleeding (eg, peptic ulcer, intracranial bleeding).
Warnings: Use with caution in individuals with a history of bleeding, hemostatic disorders, or drug-related hemostatic problems. May potentiate effects of warfarin. Use caution in individuals taking anticoagulant medications, including warfarin, aspirin, aspirin-containing products, NSAIDs, or antiplatelet agents (eg, ticlopidine, clopidogrel, dipyridamole). Discontinue use prior to dental or surgical procedures (generally at least 14 days before). Caution in pregnancy and lactation. May cause photosensitization; avoid prolonged exposure to sunlight or other sources of ultraviolet radiation (ie, tanning booths). Use with caution in individuals at risk of hypotension, or in those who would tolerate hypotension poorly (cerebrovascular or cardiovascular disease). Use with caution in individuals taking antihypertensive medications. Use with caution in individuals on hormone replacement therapy or oral contraceptives or with a history of estrogen-dependent tumors, endometrial cancer, thromboembolic disease, or stroke.
Drug Interactions: Antihypertensives, anticoagulants, antiplatelet drugs, hormonal replacement therapy, oral contraceptives, photosensitizing medications.
Dosing: Oral: 200 mg twice daily

Echinacea

Synonyms: American Coneflower; Black Susans; Comb Flower; *Echinacea angustifolia*; Indian Head; Purple Coneflower; Scury Root; Snakeroot
Use: Treatment of cold and flu; treatment of minor upper respiratory tract infections, urinary tract infections
Mechanism of Action/Effect: Caffeic acid glycosides and isolutylamides associated with the plant can cause immune stimulation (leukocyte phagocytosis and T-cell activation). Also has an antihyaluronidase and anti-inflammatory activity.
Contraindications: Autoimmune diseases, such as collagen vascular disease (lupus, RA), multiple sclerosis; allergy to sunflowers, daisies, ragweed; tuberculosis, HIV, AIDS, pregnancy (parenteral administration only contraindicated per Commission E, oral use of *Echinacea* is not contraindicated during pregnancy per Commission E)
Warnings: May alter immunosuppression; persons allergic to sunflowers may display cross-allergy potential; use as a preventative treatment should be discouraged. Long-term use may cause immunosuppression.
Drug Interactions: May alter response to immunosuppressive therapy
Adverse Reactions: Tingling sensation of tongue, allergic reactions (rare), none known for oral and external use per Commission E; may become immunosuppressive with continuous use over 6-8 weeks
Dosing: Continuous use should not exceed 8 weeks.

Per Commission E: Expressed juice (of fresh herb): 6-9 mL/day
Capsule/tablet or tea form: 500 mg to 2 g 3 times/day
Liquid extract: 0.25-1 mL 3 times/day
Tincture: 1-2 mL 3 times/day
May be applied topically.

Evening Primrose

Synonyms: Evening Primrose Oil; *Oenothera biennis*
Use: Diabetic neuropathy, endometriosis, hyperglycemia, irritable bowel syndrome, multiple sclerosis, omega-6-fatty acid supplementation, PMS, menopause, rheumatoid arthritis
Mechanism of Action/Effect: Evening primrose oil contains high amounts of gamma-linolenic acid, or GLA, which is an essential fatty acid (omega-6 fatty acid). Omega-6 fatty acids reportedly reduce generation of arachidonic acid metabolites in short-term use, improving symptoms of various inflammatory and immune conditions. The fatty acids found in evening primrose oil also have been reported to stimulate hormone synthesis.
Contraindications: Evening primrose oil may lower seizure threshold (based on animal studies); use is contraindicated in individuals with seizure disorders, schizophrenia, or in individuals receiving anticonvulsant or antipsychotic medications. May inhibit platelet aggregation; contraindicated in individuals with active bleeding (eg, peptic ulcer, intracranial bleeding).
Warnings: Use with caution in individuals with a history of bleeding, hemostatic disorders, or drug-related hemostatic problems. Use with caution in individuals taking warfarin, aspirin, aspirin-containing products, NSAIDs, or antiplatelet agents (eg, ticlopidine, clopidogrel, dipyridamole). Discontinue use prior to dental or surgical procedures (generally at least 14 days before).
Drug Interactions: Anticonvulsant medications (seizure threshold decreased); anticoagulants, aspirin, aspirin-containing products, NSAIDs, or antiplatelet agents
Dosing: Oral: 500 mg to 8 g/day

Feverfew

Synonyms: Altamisa; Bachelor's Buttons; Featherfew; Featherfoil; Nosebleed; *Tanacetum parthenium*; Wild Quinine
Lactation: Contraindicated
Use: Prophylaxis and treatment of migraine headaches; treatment of menstrual complaints and fever
Mechanism of Action/Effect: Active ingredient is parthenolide (~0.2% concentration), which is a serotonin antagonist; also, the plant may be an inhibitor of prostaglandin synthesis and platelet aggregation; may have spasmolytic activity
Contraindications: Pregnancy; children <2 years of age; allergies to feverfew and other members of Asteraceae, daisy, ragweed, chamomile
Warnings: Use with caution in patients taking medications with serotonergic properties.
Drug Interactions: Use with caution in patients taking aspirin or anticoagulants.
Adverse Reactions: Mouth ulcerations, contact dermatitis, abdominal pain, nausea, vomiting, loss of taste; postfeverfew syndrome on discontinuation (nervousness, insomnia, still joints, headache)
Dosing: 125 mg once or twice daily

Garlic

Synonyms: *Allium savitum*; Comphor of the Poor; Nectar of the Gods; Poor Mans Treacle; Rustic Treacle; Stinking Rose
Use: Lower LDL cholesterol and triglycerides and raise HDL cholesterol; hypertension; may lower blood glucose and decrease thrombosis; potential anti-inflammatory and antitumor effects
Mechanism of Action/Effect: Allinin garlic is converted to allicin (after the bulb is ground), which is odoriferous and may have some antioxidant activity; ajoene (a byproduct of allicin) has potent platelet inhibition effects; garlic can also decrease LDL cholesterol levels and increase fibrinolytic activity
Contraindications: Pregnancy
Warnings: Onset of cholesterol-lowering and hypotensive effects may require months. Use with caution in patients receiving treatment for hyperglycemia or hypertension.
Drug Interactions: Iodine uptake may be reduced with garlic ingestion; can exacerbate bleeding in patients taking aspirin or anticoagulant agents; may increase the risk of hypoglycemia; may increase response to antihypertensives
Adverse Reactions: Skin blistering, eczema, systemic contact dermatitis, immunologic contact urticaria, GI upset and changes in intestinal flora (rare) per Commission E, lacrimation, asthma (upon inhalation of garlic dust), allergic reactions (rare), change in odor of skin and breath (per Commission E)
Half-Life Elimination: N-acetyl-S-allyl-L-cysteine: 6 hours
Excretion: Pulmonary and renal
Dosing: Adults: 4-12 mg allicin/day

HERBAL AND NUTRITIONAL PRODUCTS *(Continued)*

Average daily dose for cardiovascular benefit: 0.25-1 g/kg or 1-4 cloves daily in an 80 kg individual in divided doses

Toxic dose: >5 cloves or >25 mL of extract can cause GI symptoms

Additional Information: 1% as active as penicillin as an antibiotic; number one over-the-counter medication in Germany; enteric-coated products may demonstrate best results.

Ginger

Synonyms: *Zingiber officinale*

Pregnancy Risk Factor: No administration for morning sickness during pregnancy per Commission E; however, some contradictory recommendations exist. High doses may be abortifacient.

Use: Digestive aid; treatment of nausea (antiemetic) and motion sickness; treatment of headaches, colds, and flu; ginger oil is used as a flavoring agent in beverages and mouthwashes; may be useful in some forms of arthritis

Mechanism of Action/Effect: Unknown; may increase GI motility; appears to decrease prostaglandin synthesis; may have cardiotonic activity; may inhibit platelet aggregation (very high doses)

Contraindications: Gallstones (per Commission E)

Warnings: Use with caution in diabetics, patients on cardiac glycosides, and those receiving anticoagulants.

Drug Interactions: May alter response to cardiotonic, hypoglycemic, anticoagulant, and antiplatelet agents.

Dosing:

Prevention of motion sickness or digestive aid: 1-4 g/day (250 mg of ginger root powder 3-4 times/day)

Per Commission E: 2-4 g/day or equivalent preparations

Ginkgo Biloba

Synonyms: Kew Tree; Maidenhair Tree

Use: Dilates blood vessels; plant/leaf extract has been used in Europe for intermittent claudication, arterial insufficiency, and cerebral vascular disease (dementia); tinnitus, visual disorders, traumatic brain injury, vertigo of vascular origin

Per Commission E: Demential syndromes including memory deficits, etc (tinnitus, headache); depressive emotional conditions, primary degenerative dementia, vascular dementia, or both

Investigational: Asthma, impotence (male)

Mechanism of Action/Effect: Inhibits platelet aggregation; ginkgo biloba leaf extract contain terpenoids and flavonoids which can allegedly inactivate oxygen-free radicals causing vasodilatation and antagonize effects of platelet activating factor (PAF); fruit pulp contains ginkolic acids which are allergens (seeds are not sensitizing)

Contraindications: Pregnancy; patients with clotting disorders; hypersensitivity to ginkgo biloba preparations (per Commission E)

Warnings: Use with caution following recent surgery or trauma. Effects may require 1-2 months.

Drug Interactions: Due to effects on PAF, use with caution in patients receiving anticoagulants or platelet inhibitors

Adverse Reactions: Palpitations, bilateral subdural hematomas, headache (very seldom per Commission E), dizziness, seizures (in children), restlessness, urticaria, cheilitis, nausea, diarrhea, vomiting, stomatitis, proctitis, stomach or intestinal upsets (very seldom per Commission E), hyphema, allergic skin reactions (very seldom per Commission E)

Onset of Effect: 1 hour

Peak Absorption: 2-3 hours

Duration of Action: 7 hours

Bioavailability: 70% to 100%

Half-life: Ginkgolide A: 4 hours; ginkgolide B: 10.6 hours; bilobalide: 3.2 hours

Dosing: Beneficial effects for cerebral ischemia in the elderly occur after 1 month of use.

Usual dosage: ~40 mg 3 times/day with meals; 60-80 mg twice daily to 3 times/day depending on indication; maximum dose: 360 mg/day

Cerebral ischemia: 120 mg/day in 2-3 divided doses (24% flavonoid-glycoside extract, 6% terpene glycosides)

Ginseng, Panax

Synonyms: Asian Ginseng; *Panax ginseng*
Use:
Mechanism of Action/Effect: Ginsenosides are believed to act via hormone receptors in the hypothalamus, pituitary glands, and other tissues. Ginsenosides stimulate secretion of adrenocorticotropic hormone (ACTH), leading to production of increased release of adrenal hormones, including cortisol. Specific triterpenoid saponins (diols) are claimed to be mediate improvements in endurance and learning. These compounds are also believed to contribute to sedative and antihypertensive properties. A second group (triols) reportedly increase blood pressure and function as central nervous system stimulants. *Panax ginseng* is reported to have immunostimulating effects. *Panax ginseng* has been claimed to facilitate adaptation to stress caused by chemotherapy and radiation.
Contraindications: Use is contraindicated in renal failure and acute infection. May alter hemostasis; contraindicated in individuals with active bleeding.
Warnings: Avoid in pregnancy and lactation. Use with caution in individuals receiving MAO inhibitors. Use caution with stimulant medications, including decongestants, caffeine, and caffeine-containing beverages. May cause diarrhea, hypertension, nervousness, dermatologic eruptions, and insomnia after prolonged use or high dosages (Ginseng Abuse Syndrome). May also cause mastalgia or vaginal breakthrough bleeding. May cause palpitations and tachycardia in sensitive individuals or in high doses. Use with caution in individuals with hypertension or hypotension. Use with caution in individuals with a history of bleeding, hemostatic disorders, or drug-related hemostatic problems. Discontinue use prior to dental or surgical procedures (generally at least 14 days before).
Drug Interactions: Antihypertensives, MAO inhibitors, central nervous stimulants (caffeine), sympathomimetics, and hormonal therapies; anticoagulant medications, including warfarin, aspirin, aspirin-containing products, NSAIDs, or antiplatelet agents (eg, ticlopidine, clopidogrel, dipyridamole).
Dosing: Oral: 100-600 mg/day in divided doses

Ginseng, Siberian

Synonyms: *Eleutherococcus senticosus;* Siberian Ginseng
Use: Adaptogen, beneficial in athletic performance, adaptation to stress (decreased fatigue), support of immune function
Mechanism of Action/Effect: Believed to facilitate adaptation to stress and to act as immune stimulant. Reported benefits include increased physical endurance, mental alertness, increased amount and quality of work performed, decreased sick days, and enhanced athletic performance.
Contraindications: Hemostasis may be affected; contraindicated in individuals with active bleeding (eg, peptic ulcer, intracranial bleeding).
Warnings: Use with caution in individuals with hypertension or in individuals receiving antihypertensive medications. Caution in individuals at risk of hypotension, elderly individuals, or those who would not tolerate transient hyper- or hypotensive episodes (ie, cerebrovascular or cardiovascular disease). May potentiate effects of antihypertensives. Use with caution in diabetes, and in individuals with a history of bleeding, hemostatic disorders, or drug-related hemostatic problems. Discontinue use prior to dental or surgical procedures (generally at least 14 days before). Extensive or prolonged use may heighten estrogenic activity (based on pharmacological activity).
Drug Interactions: Barbiturates, antihypertensives, insulin, oral hypoglycemics, digoxin, stimulants (including OTC stimulants); anticoagulant medications, including warfarin, aspirin, aspirin-containing products, NSAIDs, or antiplatelet agents (eg, ticlopidine, clopidogrel, dipyridamole).
Dosing: Oral: 100-200 mg twice daily

Glucosamine

Use: Osteoarthritis, rheumatoid arthritis, tendonitis, gout, bursitis
Mechanism of Action/Effect: Glucosamine is an amino sugar which is a key component in the synthesis of proteoglycans, a group of proteins found in cartilage. These proteoglycans are negatively charged, and attract water so they can produce synovial fluid in the joints. The theory is that supplying the body with these precursors will replenish important synovial fluid, and lead to production of new cartilage. Glucosamine also appears to inhibit cartilage-destroying enzymes (eg, collagenase and phospholipase A2), thus stopping the degenerative processes of osteoarthritis. A third mechanism may be glucosamine's ability to prevent production of damaging superoxide radicals, which may lead to cartilage destruction.
Adverse Reactions: Few effects (eg, flatulence, nausea)

HERBAL AND NUTRITIONAL PRODUCTS *(Continued)*

Warnings: Use caution in patients with diabetes; may cause insulin resistance
Drug Interactions: May increase effect of oral anticoagulants; may alter response to insulin or oral hypoglycemics
Dosing: 500 mg of the sulfate form 3 times/day

Golden Seal

Synonyms: Eye Balm; Eye Root; *Hydrastis canadensis*; Indian Eye; Jaundice Root; Orange Root; Tumeric Root; Yellow Indian Paint; Yellow Root
Lactation: Contraindicated
Use: Gastrointestinal and peripheral vascular activity; used in sterile eyewashes; used as a mouthwash, laxative, to treat hemorrhoids, and to stop postpartum hemorrhage. Efficacy not established in clinical studies; has been used to treat mucosal inflammation/gastritis.
Mechanism of Action/Effect: Contains the alkaloids hydrastine (4%) and berberine (6%), which at higher doses can cause vasoconstriction, hypertension, and mucosal irritation; berberine can produce hypotension
Contraindications: Pregnancy
Warnings: Should not be used in patients with hypertension, glaucoma, diabetes, history of stroke, or heart disease.
Drug Interactions: May interfere with vitamin B absorption
Adverse Reactions: With high doses: Stimulation/agitation, nausea, vomiting, diarrhea, mouth and throat irritation, extremity numbness, respiratory failure
Dosing:
Root: 0.5-1 g 3 times/day
Solid form: Usual dose: 5-10 grains

Green Tea

Synonyms: *Camellia sinensis*
Use: Anticarcinogenic activity, antioxidant, support in cancer prevention and cardiovascular disease, may lower cholesterol, platelet-aggregation inhibitor
Mechanism of Action/Effect: Green tea reportedly has antioxidant properties and protects against oxidative damage to cells and tissues. Demonstrated to increase HDL cholesterol, decrease LDL cholesterol, and decrease triglycerides. Green tea has also been reported to block the peroxidation of LDL, inhibit formation of thromboxane formation, and block platelet aggregation. Human studies have noted a correlation between consumption of green tea and improvement in prognosis in some forms of breast cancer.
Contraindications: Contraindicated in individuals with active bleeding (eg, peptic ulcer, intracerebral bleeding).
Warnings: Non-decaffeinated products should be used with caution in individuals with peptic ulcer disease or cardiovascular disease. Use with caution in individuals with a history of bleeding, hemostatic disorders, or drug-related hemostatic problems. aspirin, aspirin-containing products, NSAIDs, or antiplatelet agents (eg, ticlopidine, clopidogrel, dipyridamole). Discontinue use prior to dental or surgical procedures (generally at least 14 days before). Green tea has also been reported to antagonize the effects of warfarin. Use with caution when taking other stimulants such as caffeine and decongestants, unless a caffeine-free product is used. It is important to note that the addition of milk to any tea may significantly lower the antioxidant potential of this agent
Drug Interactions: Aspirin, aspirin-containing products, NSAIDs, or antiplatelet agents (eg, ticlopidine, clopidogrel, dipyridamole); avoid caffeine-containing products
Adverse Reactions: If product is not decaffeinated, caffeine may cause gastric irritation, decreased appetite, insomnia, tachycardia, palpitations, and nervousness in sensitive individuals.
Dosing: Oral: 250-500 mg/day

Hawthorn

Synonyms: *Crataegus laevigata; Crataegus monogyna; Crataegus oxyacantha; Crataegus pinnatifida*; English Hawthorn; Haw; Maybush; Whitehorn
Lactation: Contraindicated
Use: In herbal medicine, to treat cardiovascular abnormalities (arrhythmia, angina), increased cardiac output, increased contractility of heart muscle; used as a sedative
Mechanism of Action/Effect: Contains flavonoids, catechin, and epicatechin which may be cardioprotective and have vasodilatory properties; shown to dilate coronary vessels
Contraindications: Pregnancy

Drug Interactions: Antihypertensives (effect enhanced), ACE inhibitors, digoxin; effects with Viagra® are unknown

Adverse Reactions: Hypotension, bradycardia, hypertension, depression, fatigue, rash, nausea

Dosing: Daily dose of total flavonoids: 10 mg

Per Commission E: 160-900 mg native water-ethanol extract (ethanol 45% v/v or methanol 70% v/v, drug-extract ratio: 4-7:1, with defined flavonoid or procyanidin content), corresponding to 30-168.7 mg procyanidins, calculated as epicatechin, or 3.5-19.8 mg flavonoids, calculated as hyperoside in accordance with DAB 10 (German pharmacopoeia #10) in 2 or 3 individual doses; duration of administration: 6 weeks minimum

Horse Chestnut

Synonyms: *Aesculus hippocastanum*

Use: Oral and topical: Varicose veins, hemorrhoids, other venous insufficiencies; deep venous thrombosis, lower extremity edema

Mechanism of Action/Effect: Horse chestnut reportedly inhibits platelet aggregation and functions as an anti-inflammatory. It is also reported to support collagen structures. Horse chestnut's activity as an anti-inflammatory agent may also be related to quercetin's reported ability to inhibit cyclo-oxygenase and lipoxygenase, the enzymes which form inflammatory prostaglandins and leukotrienes. Quercetin is also an inhibitor of phosphodiesterase, which has been correlated to cardiotonic, hypotensive, spasmolytic, antiplatelet, and sedative actions.

Contraindications: May be contraindicated in individuals with active bleeding (eg, peptic ulcer, intracranial bleeding).

Warnings: Use with caution in individuals with a history of bleeding, hemostatic disorders, or drug-related hemostatic problems. Discontinue use prior to dental or surgical procedures (generally at least 14 days before). Use with caution in individuals with hepatic or renal impairment.

Drug Interactions: Warfarin, aspirin, aspirin-containing products, NSAIDs, or antiplatelet agents (eg, ticlopidine, clopidogrel, dipyridamole)

Adverse Reactions: May cause gastrointestinal upset

Dosing:

Oral: 300 mg 1-2 times/day, standardized to 50 mg escin per dose

Topical: Apply 2% escin gel 1-2 times/day to affected area

Kava

Synonyms: Awa; Kew; *Piper methysticum*; Tonga

Use: Treatment of nervous anxiety, stress, and restlessness (per Commission E); used for sleep inducement and to reduce anxiety

Restrictions: Do not use for more than 3 months without medical advice per Commission E

Mechanism of Action/Effect: Contains alpha-pyrones in root extracts; may possess central dopaminergic antagonistic properties

Contraindications: Per Commission E: Pregnancy, endogenous depression. Extended continuous intake can cause a temporary yellow discoloration of skin, hair, and nails. In this case, further application must be discontinued. In rare cases, allergic skin reactions occur. Also, accommodative disturbances (eg, enlargement of the pupils and disturbances of the oculomotor equilibrium) have been described.

Drug Interactions: Coma can occur from concomitant administration of kava and alprazolam; may potentiate alcohol or CNS depressants, barbiturates, psychopharmacological agents

Adverse Reactions: Euphoria, depression, somnolence, skin discoloration (prolonged use), muscle weakness, eye disturbances

Dosing: Per Commission E: Herb and preparations equivalent to 60-120 mg kavalactones

Melaleuca Oil

Use: Marketed as having fungicidal, bactericidal properties; used as a topical dermal agent for burns

Mechanism of Action/Effect: Consists of plant terpenes, pinenes, and cineole, derived from the *Melaleuca alternifolia* tree, the colorless or pale yellow oil can cause CNS depression; may be bacteriostatic

Adverse Reactions: Rarely causes allergic reactions or dermatitis

Dosing: Minimal toxic dose: Infant: <10 mL applied topically

HERBAL AND NUTRITIONAL PRODUCTS *(Continued)*

Melatonin

Lactation: Contraindicated
Use: Sleep disorders (eg, jet lag, insomnia, neurologic problems, shift work); aging; cancer; immune system support
Mechanism of Action/Effect: Melatonin is a hormone responsible for regulating the body's circadian rhythm and sleep patterns. Its release is prompted by darkness and inhibited by light. Secretion appears to peak during childhood, and declines gradually through adolescence and adulthood. Melatonin receptors have been found in blood cells, the brain, gut, and ovaries. This substance may also have a role in regulating cardiovascular and reproductive function through its antioxidant properties.
Contraindications: Immune disorders; pregnancy
Drug Interactions: Medications commonly used as sedatives or hypnotics, or those that induce sedation, drowsiness (eg, benzodiazepines, narcotics); CNS depressants (prescription, supplements such as 5-HTP); other herbs known to cause sedation include kava kava, valerian
Adverse Reactions: Reduced alertness, headache, irritability, increased fatigue, drowsiness, sedation
Dosing: Sleep disturbances: 0.3-5 mg/day

Red Yeast Rice

Synonyms: *Monascus purpureus*
Use: Hypercholesterolemic agent; may lower triglycerides and LDL cholesterol and raise HDL cholesterol
Mechanism of Action/Effect: Eight compounds with HMG-CoA reductase inhibitory activity have been identified, including lovastatin and its active hydroxy acid metabolite.
Contraindications: Based on pharmacological activity, use is contraindicated in pregnancy or lactation (or if trying to become pregnant). In addition, the use of red yeast rice is contraindicated in individuals with known hypersensitivity to rice or yeast. Keep out of reach of children, do not use if <20 years of age. Do not use in individuals with hepatic disease, a history of liver disease, or in those who may be at risk of liver disease. Do not use in individuals with serious infection, recent major surgery, other serious disease, or organ transplant individuals. Do not use in any individual who consumes more than 1-2 alcohol-containing drinks per day.
Warnings: Use with caution in individuals currently receiving other cholesterol-lowering medications. HMG-CoA reductase inhibitors have been associated with rare (less than 1% to 2% incidence) but serious adverse effects, including hepatic and skeletal muscle disorders (myopathy, rhabdomyolysis). The risk of these disorders may be increased by concomitant therapy with specific medications. Discontinue use at the first sign of hepatic dysfunction.
Drug Interactions: HMG-CoA reductase inhibitors, other cholesterol-lowering agents, anticoagulants, gemfibrozil, erythromycin, itraconazole, ketoconazole, cyclosporine, niacin, clofibrate, fenofibrate
Adverse Reactions: May cause gastrointestinal upset
Dosing: Oral: 1200 mg twice daily

SAMe

Synonyms: S-adenosylmethionine
Use: Depression
Mechanism of Action/Effect: Mechanism has not been defined; functions as a cofactor in many synthetic pathways
Contraindications: Active bleeding
Warnings: Use caution when combining SAMe with other antidepressants, tryptophan, or 5-HTP. SAMe is not effective in the treatment of depressive symptoms associated with bipolar disorder.
Drug Interactions: May potentiate activity and/or toxicities of MAO inhibitors, tricyclic antidepressants, or SSRIs; may potentiate the antidepressant effects of 5-HTP, tryptophan, and St John's wort
Adverse Reactions: Minor side effects, including dry mouth, nausea, and restlessness are occasionally reported.
Dosing: Oral: Dosage range: 400-1600 mg/day

Sassafras Oil

Synonyms: *Sassafras albidum*
Use: Banned by FDA in food since 1960; used as a mild counterirritant on the skin (ie, for lice or insect bites); should not be ingested

Mechanism of Action/Effect: Contains safrole (up to 80%) which inhibits liver microsomal enzymes; its metabolite may cause hepatic tumors
Adverse Reactions (primarily related to sassafras oil and safrole): Tachycardia, flushing, hypotension, sinus tachycardia, anxiety, hallucinations, vertigo, aphasia, contact dermatitis, vomiting, fatty changes of liver, hepatic necrosis, mydriasis, diaphoresis; little documentation of adverse effects due to ingestion of herbal tea
Absorption: Orally
Metabolism: Hepatic
Excretion: Renal primarily
Dosing: Sassafras tea can contain as much as 200 mg (3 mg/kg) of safrole.
Lethal: ~5 mL
Toxic: 0.66 mg/kg (based on rodent studies)
Patient Information: Considered unsafe by the FDA.

Saw Palmetto

Synonyms: Palmetto Scrub; *Sabal serrulata; Sabasilis serrulatae; Serenoa repens*
Lactation: Contraindicated
Use: Benign prostatic hyperplasia
Mechanism of Action/Effect: Liposterolic extract of the berries may inhibit the enzymes 5α-reductase, along with cyclo-oxygenase and 5-lipoxygenase, thus exhibiting antiandrogen and anti-inflammatory effects; does not reduce prostatic enlargement but may help increase urinary flow (not FDA approved)
Contraindications: Pregnancy
Adverse Reactions: Headache, gynecomastia, stomach problems (rare - per Commission E)
Absorption: Oral: Low
Dosing: Adults: Dried fruit: 0.5-1 g 3 times/day
Patient Information:

Schisandra

Synonyms: *Schizandra chinensis*
Use: Promoted as an adaptogen/health tonic, hepatic protection and detoxification, increased endurance, stamina, and work performance
Mechanism of Action/Effect: Stimulates hepatic glycogen synthesis, protein synthesis, and to increase microsomal enzyme activity; functions as an antioxidant
Contraindications: Contraindicated in pregnancy (uterine stimulation in animal studies)
Drug Interactions: Cytochrome P450 enzyme induction may alter the metabolism of many drugs (calcium channel blockers noted to be decreased)
Dosing: Oral: 100 mg twice daily

Senna

Synonyms: *C. angustifolia; Cassia acutifolia*; Senna Alexandria
Use: Catharsis
Mechanism of Action/Effect: Contains up to 3% anthraquinone glycosides which can cause colonic stimulation
Contraindications: Per Commission E: Intestinal obstruction, acute intestinal inflammation (eg, Crohn's disease), colitis ulcerosa, appendicitis, abdominal pain of unknown origin, children <12 years, and pregnancy
Drug Interactions: Per Commission E: Potentiation of cardiac glycosides (with long-term use) is possible due to loss in potassium; effect on antiarrhythmics is possible; potassium deficiency can be increased by simultaneous application of thiazide diuretics, corticosteroids, and licorice root.
Adverse Reactions: Palpitations, tetany, dizziness, finger clubbing (reversible), hypokalemia, vomiting (with fresh plant leaves or pods), diarrhea, abdominal cramping, nausea, melanosis coli (reversible), cachexia, red discoloration in alkaline urine (yellow-brown in acidic urine), hepatitis, oliguria, proteinuria, dyspnea. Per Commission E: Long-term use/abuse can cause electrolyte imbalance; in single incidents, cramp-like discomforts of GI tract requiring a reduction in dosage
Metabolism: Hydrolyzed by bacteria in the colon thus releasing active sennosides
Excretion: Urine and feces
Onset of Action: Oral: 6-8 hours; Suppository: 0.5-2 hours
Dosing:
Sennosides:
Children >6 years: 20 mg at bedtime
Adults: 20-40 mg with water at bedtime

HERBAL AND NUTRITIONAL PRODUCTS *(Continued)*

Senna granules: 2.5-5 mL (163-326 mg) at bedtime; maximum dose: 10 mL (652 mg)/day
Senna tablets:
Children >60 pounds: 1 tablet (187 mg) at bedtime; maximum daily dose: 2 tablets
Adults: 1-2 tablets (187-374 mg) at bedtime; maximum daily dose: 4 tablets (**Note:** Extra strength senna tablets contain 374 mg each.)
Senna syrup:
1 month to 1 year: 1.25-2.5 mL (55-109 mg) at bedtime, up to 5 mL/day
1-5 years: 2.5-5 mL (109-218 mg) at bedtime, up to 10 mL/day
5-15 years: 5-10 mL (218-436 mg) at bedtime, up to 20 mL/day
Adults: 10-15 mL (436-654 mg); maximum daily dose: 30 mL (1308 mg)
Senna suppositories:
Children >60 pounds: 1/2 suppository (326 mg)
Adults: 1 suppository (652 mg) at bedtime; can repeat in 2 hours
Tea: 1/2 to 2 teaspoons of leaves (0.5-4 g of the herb)

Soy Isoflavones

Synonyms: Isoflavones
Use: Decreased bone loss, hypercholesterolemia, menopausal symptoms
Mechanism of Action/Effect: Isoflavones contain plant-derived estrogenic compounds. However, the estrogenic potency has been estimated to be only 1/1000 to 1/100,000 that of estradiol. They have been claimed to inhibit bone reabsorption in postmenopausal women. In addition, isoflavones in soy have been reported to lower serum lipids, including LDL cholesterol and triglycerides, along with increases in HDL cholesterol.
Contraindications: History of estrogenic tumors (endometrial or breast cancer)
Warnings: May alter response to hormonal therapy; use with caution in individuals with history of thromboembolism or stroke
Drug Interactions: Soy isoflavones have a weak estrogenic effect. May interact with estrogen-containing medications, close monitoring is recommended.
Dosing: Oral: 500-1000 mg of soy extract daily

St John's Wort

Synonyms: Amber Touch-and-Feel; Goatweed; *Hypercium perforatum*; Klamath Weed; Rosin Rose
Use: Treatment of mild to moderate depression; traditionally for treatment of stress, anxiety, insomnia; topically for vitiligo; popular drug for AIDS patients due to possible antiretroviral activity; topically for wound healing. Per Commission E: Psychovegetative disorders, depressive moods, anxiety and/or nervous unrest; oily preparations for dyspeptic complaints; oily preparations externally for treatment of post-therapy of acute and contused injuries, myalgia, first degree burns
Mechanism of Action/Effect: Active ingredients are xanthones, flavonoids (hypericin) which can act as monoamine oxidase inhibitors, although *in vitro* activity is minimal; majority of activity appears to be related to GABA modulation; may be related to dopamine, serotonin, norepinephrine modulation also
Contraindications: Endogenous depression, pregnancy, children <2 years of age; concurrent use of indinavir or therapeutic immunosuppressants (cyclosporine)
Warnings: May be photosensitizing; caution with drugs metabolized by CYP 3A3/4; caution with tyramine-containing foods
Drug Interactions: Avoid amphetamines or other stimulants. Use with caution in patients taking MAO inhibitors, levodopa, and 5-hydroxytryptophan. Avoid concurrent use with SSRI or other antidepressants. Appears to induce hepatic cytochrome P-450 3A3/4 enzymes, potentially reducing effect of many medications.
Adverse Reactions: Sinus tachycardia, photosensitization is possible especially in fair-skinned persons (per Commission E), stomach pains, abdominal pain
Dosing: Based on hypericin extract content: Oral: 300 mg 3 times/day

Valerian

Synonyms: Radix; Red Valerian; *Valeriana edulis; Valeriana wallichi*
Use: Sleep-promoting agent and minor tranquilizer; used in anxiety, panic attacks, intestinal cramps, headache. Per Commission E: Restlessness, sleep disorders based on nervous conditions
Mechanism of Action/Effect: May affect neurotransmitter levels (serotonin, GABA, and norepinephrine); also has antispasmodic properties

Drug Interactions: Not synergistic with alcohol; potentiation of other CNS depressants is possible

Adverse Reactions: Cardiac disturbances (unspecified), lightheadedness, restlessness, fatigue, nausea, tremor, blurred vision

Dosing:

Sedative: 1-3 g (1-3 mL of tincture)
Sleep aid: 1-3 mL of tincture at bedtime
Dried root: 0.3-1 g

Vanadium

Synonyms:

Use: Type 1 and type 2 diabetes

Mechanism of Action/Effect: Vanadium is reported to be a cofactor in nicotinamide adenine dinucleotide phosphate (NADPH) oxidation reactions, lipoprotein lipase activity, amino acid transport, and hematopoiesis. May improve/augment glucose regulation.

Warning: May alter glucose regulation. Use with caution in individuals with diabetes or in those who may be predisposed to hypoglycemia. Effects of drugs with hypoglycemic activity may be potentiated (including insulin and oral hypoglycemics). The individual's blood sugar should be closely monitored, and the dosage of these agents, including insulin dosage, may require adjustment. This should be carefully coordinated among the individuals' healthcare providers.

Drug Interactions: Oral hypoglycemics or insulin

Adverse Reactions: No dietary toxicity or serious side effects have been reported, however industrial exposure has resulted in toxicity.

Dosing: Oral: RDI: 250 mcg 1-3 times/day

HERBS AND COMMON NATURAL AGENTS

The authors have chosen to include this list of natural products and proposed medical claims. However, due to limited scientific investigation to support these claims, this list is not intended to imply that these claims have been scientifically proven.

Proposed Medicinal Claims

Herb	Medicinal Claim
Agrimony	Digestive disorders
Alfalfa	Source of carotene (vitamin A); contains natural fluoride
Allspice	General health
Aloe	Healing agent
Anise seed	Prevent gas
Astragalus	Enhance energy reserves; immune system modulation; adaptogen
Barberry bark	Treat halitosis
Bayberry bark	Relieve and prevent varicose veins
Bay leaf	Relieves cramps
Bee pollen	Renewal of enzymes, hormones, vitamins, amino acids, and others
Bergamot herb	Calming effect
Bilberry leaf	Increases night vision; reduces eye fatigue; antioxidant; circulation
Birch bark	Treat urinary problems; used for rheumatism
Blackberry leaf	Treat diarrhea
Black cohosh	Relieves menstrual cramps; phytoestrogen
Blueberry leaf	Diarrhea
Blue Cohosh	Regulate menstrual flow
Blue flag	Treatment of skin diseases and constipation
Boldo leaf	Stimulates digestion; treatment of gallstones
Boneset	Treatment of colds and flu

HERBAL AND NUTRITIONAL PRODUCTS *(Continued)*

Proposed Medicinal Claims *(continued)*

Herb	Medicinal Claim
Bromelain	Digestive enzyme
Buchu leaf	Diuretic
Buckthorn bark	Expels worms; laxative
Burdock leaf and root	Treatment of severe skin problems; cases of arthritis
Butternut bark	Works well for constipation
Calendula flower	Mending and healing of cuts or wounds topically
Capsicum (Cayenne)	Normalizes blood pressure; circulation
Caraway seed	Aids digestion
Cascara sagrada bark	Remedies for chronic constipation
Catnip	Calming effect in children
Celery leaf and seed	Blood pressure; diuretic
Centaury	Stimulates the salivary gland
Chamomile flower	Excellent for a nervous stomach; relieves cramping associated with the menstrual cycle
Chickweed	Rich in vitamin C and minerals (calcium, magnesium, and potassium); diuretic; thyroid stimulant
Chicory root	Effective in disorders of the kidneys, liver, and urinary canal
Cinnamon bark	Prevents infection and indigestion; helps break down fats during digestion
Cleavers	Treatment of kidney and bladder disorders; useful in obstructions of the urinary organ
Cloves	General medicinal
Coriander seed	Stomach tonic
Cornsilk	Diuretic
Cranberry	Urinary tract health
Cubeb berry	Chronic bladder trouble; increases flow of urine
Damiana leaf	Sexual impotency
Dandelion leaf	Diuretic
Dandelion root	Detoxify poisons in the liver; beneficial in lowering blood pressure
Dill weed	Digestive health
Dong Quai root	Female troubles; menopause and PMS symptoms; anemia; blood pressure
Echinacea root	Treat strep throat, lymph glands; immune modulating
Eucalyptus leaf	Mucolytic
Elder	Antiviral
Elecampane root	Cough with mucus
Eyebright herb	Eyesight
Fennel seed	Remedies for gas and acid stomach
Fenugreek seed	Allergies, coughs, digestion, emphysema, headaches, migraines, intestinal inflammation, ulcers, lungs, mucous membranes, and sore throat
Feverfew herb	Migraines; helps reduce inflammation in arthritis joints
Garlic capsules	Lowers blood cholesterol; anti-infective
Gentian	Digestive health
Ginger root	Antiemetic

Proposed Medicinal Claims *(continued)*

Herb	Medicinal Claim
Ginkgo biloba	Improves blood circulation to the brain; asthma; vertigo; tinnitus; impotence
Ginseng root, Siberian	Resistance against stress; slows the aging process; adaptogen
Goldenseal	Treatment of bladder infections, cankers, mouth sores, mucous membranes, and ulcers
Gota kola	"Memory herb"; nerve tonic; wound healing
Gravelroot (Queen of the Meadow)	Remedy for stones in the kidney and bladder
Green barley	Antioxidant
Hawthorn	Antioxidant; cardiotonic
Henna	External use only
Hibiscus flower	Diuretic
Hops flower	Insomnia; used to decrease the desire for alcohol
Horehound	Acute or chronic sore throat and coughs
Horsetail (Shavegrass)	Rich in minerals, especially silica; used to develop strong fingernails and hair, good for split ends; diuretic
Ho shou wu	Rejuvenator
Hydrangea root	Backaches
Juniper berry	Diuretic
Kava kava root	Calm nervousness; anxiety; pain
Kelp	High contents of natural plant iodine, for proper function of the thyroid; high levels of natural calcium, potassium, and magnesium
Lavender oil	Wound healing; decrease scarring (topical)
Lecithin	Break up cholesterol; prevent arteriosclerosis
Licorice root	Expectorant; used in peptic ulceration; adrenal exhaustion
Malva flower	Soothes inflammation in the mouth and throat; helpful for earaches
Marjoram	Beneficial for a sour stomach or loss of appetite
Marshmallow leaf	Demulcent
Milk thistle herb	Liver detoxifier; antioxidant
Motherwort	Nervousness
Mugwort	Used for rheumatism and gout
Mullein leaf	High in iron, magnesium, and potassium; sinuses; relieves swollen joints; soothing bronchial tissue
Mustard seed	General medicinal
Myrrh gum	Removes bad breath; sinus problems
Nettle leaf	Remedy for dandruff; antihistiminic qualities
Nettle root	Used in benign prostatic hyperplasia (BPH)
Nutmeg	Gas
Oregano leaf	Settles the stomach after meals; helps treat colds
Oregon grape root	Gallbladder problems
Papaya leaf	Digestive stimulant; contains the enzyme papain
Paprika (sweet)	Stimulates the appetite and gastric secretions
Passion flower	Mild sedative
Pau d'arco	Protects immune system; antifungal
Peppermint leaf	Excellent for headaches; digestive stimulation
Pleurisy root	Mucolytic

HERBAL AND NUTRITIONAL PRODUCTS *(Continued)*

Proposed Medicinal Claims *(continued)*

Herb	Medicinal Claim
Poppy seed blue	Excellent in the making of breads and desserts
Prickly ash bark	Increases circulation
Psyllium seed	Lubricant to the intestinal tract
Red clover	Phytoestrogenic properties
Red raspberry leaf	Decreases menstrual bleeding
Rhubarb root	Powerful laxative
Rose hips	High content of vitamin C
Saw palmetto berry	Used in benign prostatic hyperplasia (BPH)
Scullcap	Nerve sedative
Seawrack (Bladderwrack)	Combat obesity; contains iodine
Senna leaf	Laxative
Shepherd's purse	Female reproductive health
Sheep sorrel	Diuretic
Slippery elm bark	Normalize bowel movement; beneficial for hemorrhoids and constipation
Solomon's seal root	Poultice for bruises
Spikenard	Skin ailments such as acne, pimples, blackheads, rashes, and general skin problems
Star anise	Promotes appetite and relieves flatulence
St John's wort	Mild to moderate depression
Summer savory leaf	Treats diarrhea, upset stomach, and sore throat
Thyme leaf	Ulcers (peptic)
Uva-ursi leaf	Diuretic; used in urinary tract health
Valerian root	Promotes sleep
Vervain	Remedy for fevers
White oak bark	Strong astringent
White willow bark	Used for minor aches and pains in the body; aspirin content
Wild alum root	Powerful astringent; used as rinse for sores in mouth and bleeding gums
Wild cherry	Cough suppressant
Wild Oregon grape root	Chronic skin disease
Wild yam root	Used in female reproductive health
Wintergreen leaf	Valuable for colic and gas in the bowels
Witch hazel bark and leaf	Hemorrhoids
Wormwood	Antiparasitic
Yarrow root	Fevers
Yellow dock root	Good in all skin problems
Yerba santa	Bronchial congestion
Yohimbe	Natural aphrodisiac
Yucca root	Reduces inflammation of the joints

Herb-Drug Interactions/Cautions

Herb	Drug Interaction / Caution
Acidophilus / bifidobacterium	Antibiotics (oral)
Activated charcoal	Vitamins or oral medications may be adsorbed
Alfalfa	Do not use with lupus due to amino acid L-canavanine; causes pancytopenia at high doses; warfarin (alfalfa contains a large amount of vitamin K)
Aloe vera	Caution in pregnancy, may cause uterine contractions; digoxin, diuretics (hypokalemia)
Ashwagandha	May cause sedation and other CNS effects
Asparagus root	Causes diuresis
Barberry	Normal metabolism of vitamin B may be altered with high doses
Birch	If taking a diuretic, drink plenty of fluids
Black cohosh	Estrogen-like component; pregnant and nursing women should probably avoid this herb; also women with estrogen-dependent cancer and women who are taking birth control pills or estrogen supplements after menopause; caution also in people taking sedatives or blood pressure medications
Black haw	Do not give to children <6 years of age (salicin content) with flu or chickenpox due to potential Reye's syndrome; do not take if allergic to aspirin
Black pepper (*Piper nigrum*)	Antiasthmatic drugs (decreases metabolism)
Black tea	May inhibit body's utilization of thiamine
Blessed thistle	Do not use with gastritis, ulcers, or hyperacidity since herb stimulates gastric juices
Blood root	Large doses can cause nausea, vomiting, CNS sedation, low BP, shock, coma, and death
Broom (*Cytisus scoparius*)	MAO inhibitors lead to sudden blood pressure changes
Bugleweed (*Lycopus virginicus*)	May interfere with nuclear imaging studies of the thyroid gland (thyroid uptake scan)
Cat's claw (*Uncaria tomentosa*)	Avoid in organ transplant patients or patients on ulcer medications, antiplatelet drugs, NSAIDs, anticoagulants, immunosuppressive therapy, intravenous immunoglobulin therapy
Chaste tree berry (*Vitex agnus-castus*)	Interferes with actions of oral contraceptives, HRT, and other endocrine therapies; may interfere with metabolism of dopamine-receptor antagonists
Chicory (*Cichorium intybus*)	Avoid with gallstones due to bile-stimulating properties
Chlorella (*Chlorella vulgaris*)	Contains significant amounts of vitamin K
Chromium picolinate	Picolinic acid causes notable changes in brain chemicals (serotonin, dopamine, norepinephrine); do not use if patient has behavioral disorders or diabetes
Cinnabar root (*Salviae multorrhizae*)	Warfarin (increases INR)
Deadly nightshade (*Atropa belladonna*)	Contains atropine
Dong quai	Warfarin (increases INR), estrogens, oral contraceptives, photosensitizing drugs, histamine replacement therapy, anticoagulants, antiplatelet drugs, antihypertensives
Echinacea	Caution with other immunosuppressive therapies; stimulates TNF and interferons
Ephedra	Avoid with blood pressure medications, antidepressants, and MAOIs
Evening primrose oil	May lower seizure threshold; do not combine with anticonvulsants or phenothiazines
Fennel	Do not use in women who have had breast cancer or who have been told not to take birth control pills

HERBAL AND NUTRITIONAL PRODUCTS *(Continued)*

Herb-Drug Interactions/Cautions *(continued)*

Herb	Drug Interaction / Caution
Fenugreek	Practice moderation in patients on diabetes drugs, MAO inhibitors, cardiovascular agents, hormonal medicines, or warfarin due to the many components of fenugreek
Feverfew	Antiplatelets, anticoagulants, NSAIDs
Forskolin, coleonol	This herb lowers blood pressure (vasodilator) and is a bronchodilator and increases the contractility of the heart, inhibits platelet aggregation, and increases gastric acid secretion
Foxglove	Digitalis-containing herb
Garlic	Blood sugar-lowering medications, warfarin, and aspirin at medicinal doses of garlic
Ginger	May inhibit platelet aggregation by inhibiting thromboxane synthetase at large doses; *in vitro* and animal studies indicate that ginger may interfere with diabetics; has anticoagulant effect, so avoid in medicinal amounts in patients on warfarin or heart medicines
Ginkgo biloba	Warfarin (ginkgo decreases blood clotting rate); NSAIDs, MAO inhibitors
Ginseng	Blood sugar-lowering medications (additive effects) and other stimulants
Ginseng (American, Korean)	Furosemide (decreases efficacy)
Ginseng (Siberian)	Digoxin (increases digoxin level)
Glucomannan	Diabetics (herb delays absorption of glucose from intestines, decreasing mean fasting sugar levels)
Goldenrod	Diuretics (additive properties)
Gymnema	Blood sugar-lowering medications (additive effects)
Hawthorn	Digoxin or other heart medications (herb dilates coronary vessels and other blood vessels, also inotropic)
Hibiscus	Chloroquine (reduced effectiveness of chloroquine)
Hops	Those with estrogen-dependent breast cancer should not take hops (contains estrogen-like chemicals); patients with depression (accentuate symptoms); alcohol or sedative (additive effects)
Horehound	May cause arrhythmias at high doses
Horseradish	In medicinal amounts with thyroid medications
Kava	CNS depressants (additive effects, eg, alcohol, barbiturates, etc); benzodiazepines
Kelp	Thyroid medications (additive effects or opposite effects by negative feedback); kelp contains a high amount of sodium
Labrador tea	Plant has narcotic properties, possible additive effects with other CNS depressants
Lemon balm	Do not use with Graves disease since it inhibits certain thyroid hormones
Licorice	Acts as a corticosteroid at high doses (about 1.5 lbs candy in 9 days) which can lead to hypertension, edema, hypernatremia, and hypokalemia (pseudoaldosteronism); do not use in persons with hypertension, glaucoma, diabetes, kidney or liver disease, or those on hormonal therapy; may interact with digitalis (due to hypokalemia)
Lobelia	Contains lobeline which has nicotinic activity; may mask withdrawal symptoms from nicotine; it can act as a polarizing neuromuscular blocker
Lovage	Is a diuretic
Ma huang	MAO inhibitors, digoxin, beta-blockers, methyldopa, caffeine, theophylline, decongestants (increases toxicity)

Herb-Drug Interactions/Cautions *(continued)*

Herb	Drug Interaction / Caution
Marshmallow	May delay absorption of other drugs taken at the same time; may interfere with treatments of lowering blood sugar
Meadowsweet	Contains salicylates
Melatonin	Acts as contraceptive at high doses; antidepressants (decreases efficacy)
Mistletoe	May interfere with medications for blood pressure, depression, and heart disease
L-phenylalanine	MAO inhibitors
Pleurisy root	Digoxin (plant contains cardiac glycosides); also contains estrogen-like compounds; may alter amine concentrations in the brain and interact with antidepressants
Prickly ash (Northern)	Contains coumarin-like compounds
Prickly ash (Southern)	Contains neuromuscular blockers
Psyllium	Digoxin (decreases absorption)
Quassia	High doses may complicate heart or blood-thinning treatments (quassia may be inotropic)
Red clover	May have estrogen-like actions; avoid when taking birth control pills, HRT, people with heart disease or at risk for blood clots, patients who suffer from estrogen-dependent cancer; do not take with warfarin
Red pepper	May increase liver metabolism of other medications and may interfere with high blood pressure medications or MAO inhibitors
Rhubarb, Chinese	Do not use with digoxin (enhanced effects)
St John's wort	Indinavir, cyclosporine, SSRIs or any antidepressants, tetracycline (increases sun sensitivity); digoxin (decreases digoxin concentration); may also interact with diltiazem, nicardipine, verapamil, etoposide, paclitaxel, vinblastine, vincristine, glucocorticoids, cyclosporine, dextromethorphan, ephedrine, lithium, meperidine, pseudoephedrine, selegiline, yohimbine, ACE inhibitors (serotonin syndrome, hypertension, possible exacerbation of allergic reaction)
Saw palmetto	Acts an antiandrogen; do not take with prostate medicines or HRT
Squill	Digoxin or persons with potassium deficiency; also not with quinidine, calcium, laxatives, saluretics, prednisone (long-term)
Tonka bean	Contains coumarin, interacts with warfarin
Vervain	Avoid large amounts of herb with blood pressure medications or HRT
Wild Oregon grape	High doses may alter metabolism of vitamin B
Wild yam	May interfere with hormone precursors
Wintergreen	Warfarin, increased bleeding
Sweet woodruff	Contains coumarin
Yarrow	Interferes with anticoagulants and blood pressure medications
Yohimbe	Do not consume tyramine-rich foods; do not take with nasal decongestants, PPA-containing diet aids, antidepressants, or mood-altering drugs

HERBAL AND NUTRITIONAL PRODUCTS *(Continued)*

Herbs Contraindicated During Lactation According to German Commission E

- Aloe (*Aloe vera*)
- Basil (*Ocimum basillcum*)
- Buckthorn bark and berry (*Rhamnus frangula, R. cathartica*)
- Cascara sagrada (*Rhamnus purshiana*)
- Coltsfoot leaf (*Tussilago farfara*)
- Combinations of senna, peppermint oil and caraway oil
- Kava kava root (*Piper methysticum*)
- Petasite root (*Pefasites* spp)
- Indian snakeroot (*Rauwolfia serpentina*)
- Rhubarb root (*Rheum palmatum*)
- Senna (*Cassia senna*)

Herbs Contraindicated During Pregnancy According to German Commission E

- Aloe (*Aloe vera*)
- Autumn crocus (*Colchicum autumnale*)
- Black cohosh root (*Cimicifuga racemosa*)
- Buckthorn bark and berry (*Rhamnus frangula, R. cathartica*)
- Cascara sagrada bark (*Rhamnus purshiana*)
- Chaste tree fruit (*Vitex agnus-castus*)
- Cinchona bark (*Cinchona* spp)
- Cinnamon bark (*Cinnamomum zeylanicum*)
- Coltsfoot leaf (*Tussliago farfara*)
- *Echinacea purpurea* herb (*Echinacea purpurea*)
- Fennel oil (*Foeniculum vulgare*)
- Combination of licorice, peppermint, and chamomile
- Combination of licorice, primrose, marshmallow, and anise
- Combination of senna, peppermint oil, and caraway oil
- Ginger root (*Zingiber officinale*)*
- Indian snakeroot (*Rauwolfia serpentina*)
- Juniper berry (*Juniperus comunis*)
- Kava kava root (*Piper methysticum*)
- Licorice root (*Glycyrrhiza glabra*)
- Marsh tea (*Ledum palustre*)
- Mayapple root (*Podophyllum peltatum*)
- Petasite root (*Petasites* spp)
- Rhubarb root (*Rheum palmatum*)
- Sage leaf (*Salvia officinalis*)
- Senna (*Cassia senna*)

*A subsequent review of the clinical literature could find no basis for the contraindication of ginger, a common spice, during pregnancy (Fulder and Tenne, 1996).

PHARMACOLOGIC INDEX

(Continued)

(Continued)

ANTITUBERCULAR AGENT *(Continued)*

ANTITUSSIVE

ANTITUSSIVE/DECONGESTANT

ANTITUSSIVE/DECONGESTANT/EXPECTORANT

ANTITUSSIVE/EXPECTORANT

ANTIVIRAL AGENT

ANTIVIRAL AGENT, OPHTHALMIC

AROMATASE INHIBITOR

BARBITURATE

BENZODIAZEPINE

BETA-ADRENERGIC BLOCKER, OPHTHALMIC

BETA BLOCKER

BETA BLOCKER, BETA$_1$ SELECTIVE

CATHARTIC

CAUTERIZING AGENT, TOPICAL

CENTRAL NERVOUS SYSTEM STIMULANT, AMPHETAMINE

CENTRAL NERVOUS SYSTEM STIMULANT, NONAMPHETAMINE

CEPHALOSPORIN (FIRST GENERATION)

CHELATING AGENT

CHOLINERGIC AGONIST

CHOLINESTERASE INHIBITOR

COLCHICINE

COLD PREPARATION

COLONY STIMULATING FACTOR

CONTRACEPTIVE

CONTRACEPTIVE, ORAL

CONTRACEPTIVE, PROGESTIN ONLY

CORTICOSTEROID, NASAL

CORTICOSTEROID, OPHTHALMIC

CORTICOSTEROID, ORAL

(Continued)

VASODILATOR *(Continued)*

VASOPEPTIDASE INHIBITOR

VASOPRESSIN ANALOG, SYNTHETIC

VITAMIN

VITAMIN A DERIVATIVE

VITAMIN D ANALOG

VITAMIN, FAT SOLUBLE

VITAMIN, TOPICAL

VITAMIN, WATER SOLUBLE

XANTHINE OXIDASE INHIBITOR

NOTES

NOTES

NOTES

NOTES

NOTES

NATURAL THERAPEUTICS POCKET GUIDE

by James B. LaValle, RPh, DHM, NMD, CCN; Daniel L. Krinsky, RPh, MS; Ernest B. Hawkins, RPh, MS; Ross Pelton, RPh, PhD, CCN; Nancy Ashbrook Willis, BA, JD

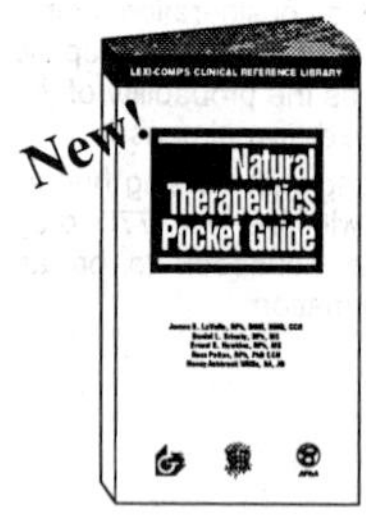

Provides condition-specific information on common uses of natural therapies.

Containing information on over 70 conditions, each including the following: review of condition, decision tree, list of commonly recommended herbals, nutritional supplements, homeopathic remedies, lifestyle modifications, and contraindications & warnings. Provides herbal/nutritional/nutraceutical monographs with over 10 fields including references, reported uses, dosage, pharmacology, toxicity, warnings & interactions, and cautions & contraindications.

Appendix: drug-nutrient depletion, herb-drug interactions, drug-nutrient interaction, herbal medicine use in pediatrics, unsafe herbs, and reference of top herbals.

DRUG INFORMATION HANDBOOK FOR CARDIOLOGY

by Bradley G. Phillips, PharmD; Virend K. Somers, MD, Dphil

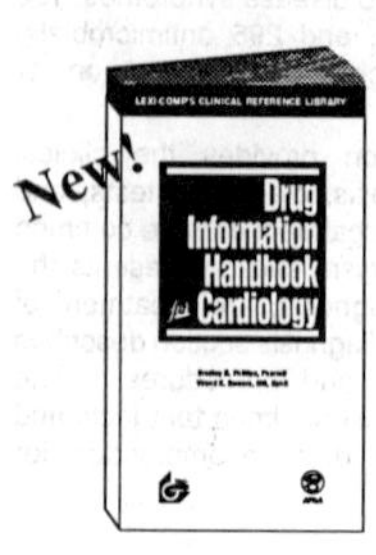

An ideal resource for physicians, pharmacists, nurses, residents, and students. This handbook was designed to provide the most current information on cardio-vascular agents and other ancillary medications.

- Each monograph includes information on Special Cardiovascular Considerations and I.V. to Oral Equivalency
- Alphabetically organized by brand and generic name
- Appendix contains information on Hypertension, Anticoagulation, Cytochrome P-450, Hyperlipidemia, Antiarrhythmia, and Comparative Drug Charts
- Special Topics/Issues include Emerging Risk Factors for Cardiovascular Disease, Treatment of Cardiovascular Disease in the Diabetic, Cardiovascular Stress Testing, and Experimental Cardiovascular Therapeutic Strategies in the New Millenium, and much more . . .

DRUG INFORMATION HANDBOOK FOR ONCOLOGY

by Dominic A. Solimando, Jr, MA; Linda R. Bressler, PharmD, BCOP; Polly E. Kintzel, PharmD, BCPS, BCOP; Mark C. Geraci, PharmD, BCOP

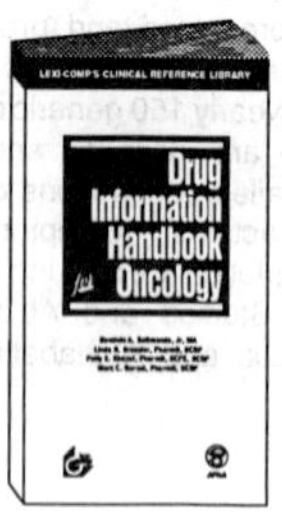

Presented in a concise and uniform format, this book contains the most comprehensive collection of oncology-related drug information available. Organized like a dictionary for ease of use, drugs can be found by looking up the *brand or generic name*!

This book contains 253 monographs, including over 1100 Antineoplastic Agents and Ancillary Medications.

It also contains up to 33 fields of information per monograph including Use, U.S. Investigational, Bone Marrow/Blood Cell Transplantation, Vesicant, Emetic Potential. A Special Topics Section, Appendix, and Therapeutic Category & Key Word Index are valuable features to this book, as well.

To order call toll free: 1-800-837-LEXI (5394)

DRUG INFORMATION HANDBOOK FOR ADVANCED PRACTICE NURSING

by Beatrice B. Turkoski, RN, PhD; Brenda R. Lance, RN, MSN; Mark F. Bonfiglio, PharmD

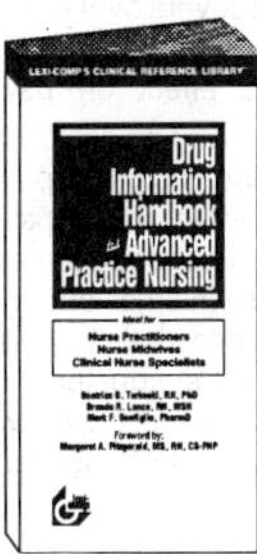

This handbook was designed specifically to meet the needs of Nurse Practitioners, Clinical Nurse Specialists, Nurse Midwives and graduate nursing students. The handbook is a unique resource for detailed, accurate information, which is vital to support the advanced practice nurse's role in patient drug therapy management.

A concise introductory section reviews topics related to Pharmacotherapeutics.

Over 4750 U.S., Canadian, and Mexican medications are covered in the 1055 monographs. Drug data is presented in an easy-to-use, alphabetically organized format covering up to 46 key points of information. Monographs are cross-referenced to an Appendix of over 230 pages of valuable comparison tables and additional information. Also included are two indices, Pharmacologic Category and Controlled Substance, which facilitate comparison between agents.

DRUG INFORMATION HANDBOOK FOR NURSING

by Beatrice B. Turkoski, RN, PhD; Brenda R. Lance, RN, MSN; Mark F. Bonfiglio, PharmD

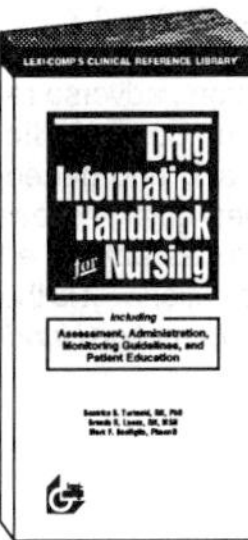

Registered Professional Nurses and upper-division nursing students involved with drug therapy will find this handbook provides quick access to drug data in a concise easy-to-use format.

Over 4750 U.S., Canadian, and Mexican medications are covered with up to 43 key points of information in each monograph. The handbook contains basic pharmacology concepts and nursing issues such as patient factors that influence drug therapy (ie, pregnancy, age, weight, etc) and general nursing issues (ie, assess-ment, administration, monitoring, and patient education). The Appendix contains over 220 pages of valuable information.

ANESTHESIOLOGY & CRITICAL CARE DRUG HANDBOOK

by Andrew J. Donnelly, PharmD; Francesca E. Cunningham, PharmD; and Verna L. Baughman, MD

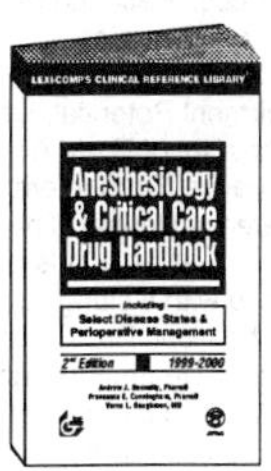

Contains over 512 generic medications with up to 25 fields of information presented in each monograph. It also contains the following Special Issues and Topics: Allergic Reaction, Anesthesia for Cardiac Patients in Noncardiac Surgery, Anesthesia for Obstetric Patients in Nonobstetric Surgery, Anesthesia for Patients With Liver Disease, Chronic Pain Management, Chronic Renal Failure, Conscious Sedation, Perioperative Management of Patients on Antiseizure Medication, Substance Abuse and Anesthesia.

The Appendix includes Abbreviations & Measurements, Anesthesiology Information, Assessment of Liver & Renal Function, Comparative Drug Charts, Infectious Disease-Prophylaxis & Treatment, Laboratory Values, Therapy Recommendation, Toxicology, *and much more . . .*

To order call toll free: 1-800-837-LEXI (5394)

DRUG INFORMATION HANDBOOK FOR PSYCHIATRY

(International edition available) by Matthew A. Fuller, PharmD; Martha Sajatovic, MD

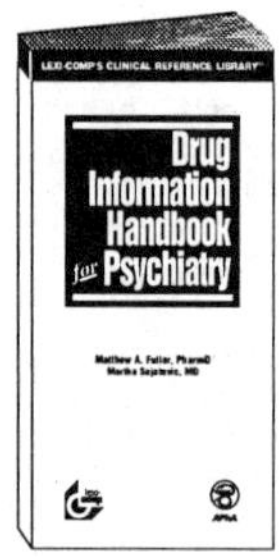

As a source for comprehensive and clinically relevant drug information for the mental health professional, this handbook is alphabetically arranged by generic and brand name for ease-of-use. It covers over 4,000 brand names and up to 32 key fields of information including effect on mental status and effect on psychiatric treatment.

A special topics/issues section includes psychiatric assessment, overview of selected major psychiatric disorders, clinical issues in the use of major classes of psychotropic medications, psychiatric emergencies, special populations, diagnostic and statistical manual of mental disorders (DSM-IV), and suggested readings. Also contains a valuable Appendix section, as well as, a Therapeutic Category Index and an Alphabetical Index.

PSYCHOTROPIC DRUG INFORMATION HANDBOOK

by Matthew A. Fuller, PharmD; Martha Sajatovic, MD

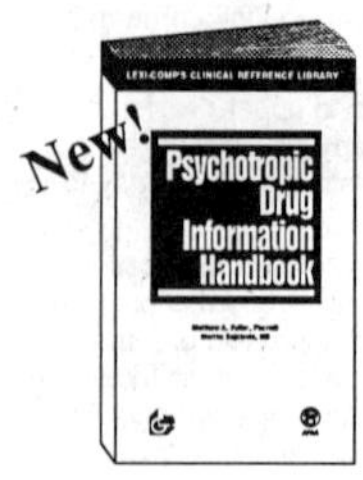

This portable, yet comprehensive guide to psychotropic drugs provides healthcare professionals with detailed information on use, warnings/precautions, drug interactions, pregnancy risk factors, adverse reactions, mechanism of action, and contraindications. Alphabetically organized by brand and generic name this concise handbook provides quick access to the information you need and includes patient education sheets on the psychotropic medications. It is the perfect pocket companion to the *Drug Information Handbook for Psychiatry.*

DRUG INFORMATION HANDBOOK FOR THE CRIMINAL JUSTICE PROFESSIONAL

by Marcelline Bums, PhD; Thomas E. Page, MA; and Jerrold B. Leikin, MD

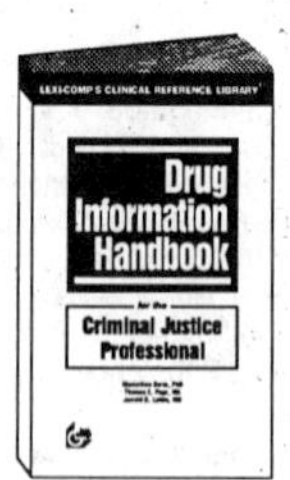

Compiled and designed for police officers, law enforcement officials, and legal professionals who are in need of a reference which relates to information on drugs, chemical substances, and other agents that have abuse and/or impairment potential. This handbook covers over 450 medications, agents, and substances. Each monograph is presented in a consistent format and contains up to 33 fields of information including Scientific Name, Commonly Found In, Abuse Potential, Impairment Potential, Use, When to Admit to Hospital, Mechanism of Toxic Action, Signs & Symptoms of Acute Overdose, Drug Interactions, Warnings/Precautions, and Reference Range. There are many diverse chapter inclusions as well as a glossary of medical terms for the layman along with a slang street drug listing. The Appendix contains Chemical, Bacteriologic, and Radiologic Agents - Effects and Treatment; Controlled Substances - Uses and Effects; Medical Examiner Data; Federal Trafficking Penalties, *and much more.*

To order call toll free: 1-800-837-LEXI (5394)

DRUG INFORMATION HANDBOOK FOR DENTISTRY

by Richard L. Wynn, BSPharm, PhD; Timothy F. Meiller, DDS, PhD; and Harold L. Crossley, DDS, PhD

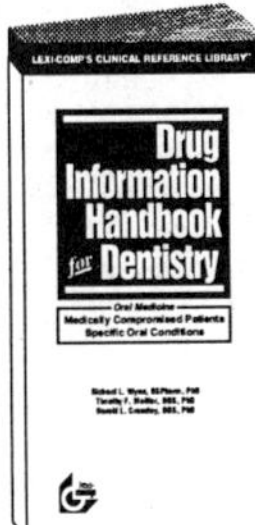

This handbook presents dental management and therapeutic considerations in medically compromised patients. Issues covered include oral manifestations of drugs, pertinent dental drug interactions, and dosing of drugs in dental treatment.

Selected oral medicine topics requiring therapeutic intervention include managing the patient with acute or chronic pain including TMD, managing the patient with oral bacterial or fungal infections, current therapeutics in periodontal patients, managing the patient receiving chemotherapy or radiation for the treatment of cancer, managing the anxious patient, managing dental office emergencies, and treatment of common oral lesions.

DENTAL OFFICE MEDICAL EMERGENCIES

by Timothy F. Meiller, DDS, PhD; Richard L. Wynn, BSPharm, PhD; Ann Marie McMullin, MD; Cynthia Biron, RDH, EMT, MA; Harold L. Crossley, DDS, PhD

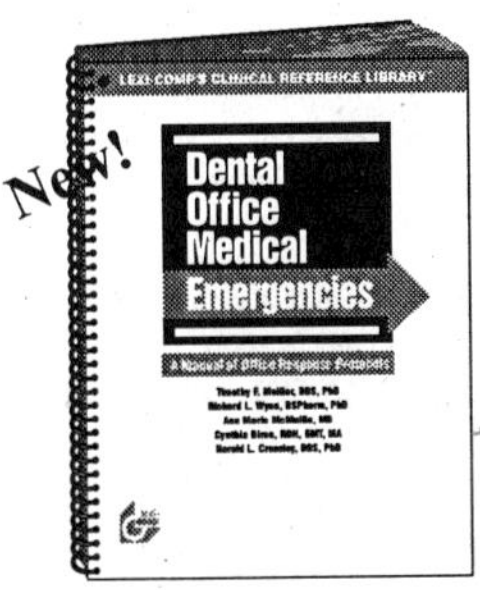

Designed specifically for general dentists during times of emergency. A tabbed paging system allows for quick access to specific crisis events. Created with urgency in mind, it is spiral bound and drilled with a hole for hanging purposes.

- Basic Action Plan for Stabilization
- Loss of Consciousness / Respiratory Distress / Chest Pain
- Allergic / Drug Reactions
- Altered Sensation / Changes in Affect
- Management of Acute Bleeding
- Office Preparedness / Procedures and Protocols

CLINICIAN'S ENDODONTIC HANDBOOK

by Thom C. Dumsha, MS, DDS; James L. Gutmann, DDS, FACD, FICD

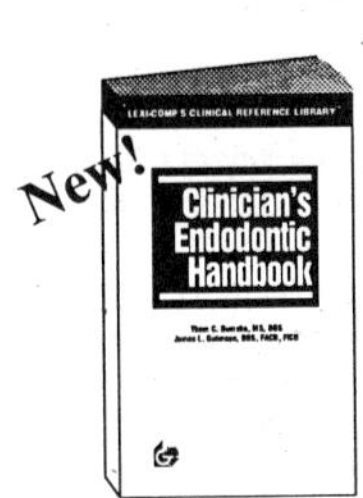

Designed for all general practice dentists.

- A quick reference addressing current endodontics
- Easy to use format and alphabetical index
- Latest techniques, procedures, and materials
- Root canal therapy: Why's and Why Nots
- A guide to diagnosis and treatment of endodontic emergencies
- Facts and rationale behind treating endodontically-involved teeth
- Straight-forward dental trauma management information
- Pulpal Histology, Access Openings, Bleaching, Resorption, Radiology, Restoration, and Periodontal / Endodontic Complications
- Frequently Asked Questions (FAQ) section and "Clinical Note" sections throughout.

To order call toll free: 1-800-837-LEXI (5394)